Physical Medicine and Rehabilitation

PRINCIPLES AND PRACTICE

Fourth Edition   *Volume 2*

Physical Medicine and Rehabilitation

PRINCIPLES AND PRACTICE

Fourth Edition   Volume 2

EDITOR-IN-CHIEF
Joel A. DeLisa, M.D., M.S.
PROFESSOR AND CHAIR
DEPARTMENT OF PHYSICAL MEDICINE AND REHABILITATION
UNIVERSITY OF MEDICINE AND DENTISTRY OF NEW JERSEY
NEW JERSEY MEDICAL SCHOOL
NEWARK, NJ
AND
PRESIDENT AND CEO
KESSLER MEDICAL REHABILITATION RESEARCH
AND EDUCATION CORPORATION
WEST ORANGE, NJ

EDITOR
Bruce M. Gans, M.D., M.S.
PROFESSOR
DEPARTMENT OF PHYSICAL MEDICINE AND REHABILITATION
UNIVERSITY OF MEDICINE AND DENTISTRY OF NEW JERSEY
NEW JERSEY MEDICAL SCHOOL
NEWARK, NJ
AND
CHIEF MEDICAL OFFICER
KESSLER INSTITUTE FOR REHABILITATION
WEST ORANGE, NJ

MANAGING EDITOR
Nicolas E. Walsh, M.D.
PROFESSOR AND CHAIRMAN
DEPARTMENT OF REHABILITATION MEDICINE
PROFESSOR
DEPARTMENT OF ANESTHESIOLOGY
UNIVERSITY OF TEXAS HEALTH SCIENCE CENTER AT SAN ANTONIO
AND
STAFF PHYSICIAN
PHYSICAL MEDICINE AND REHABILITATION SERVICE
SOUTH TEXAS VETERANS CARE HEALTH CARE SYSTEM
AUDIE L. MURPHY MEMORIAL VETERANS HOSPITAL
SAN ANTONIO, TEXAS

ASSOCIATE EDITORS
William L. Bockenek, M.D.   William S. Pease, M.D.
Walter R. Frontera, M.D., Ph.D.   Lawrence R. Robinson, M.D.
Steve R. Geiringer, M.D.   Jay Smith, M.D.
Lynn H. Gerber, M.D.   Todd P. Stitik, M.D.
Ross O. Zafonte, D.O.

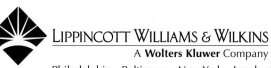
LIPPINCOTT WILLIAMS & WILKINS
A **Wolters Kluwer** Company
Philadelphia • Baltimore • New York • London
Buenos Aires • Hong Kong • Sydney • Tokyo

Acquisitions Editor: Robert Hurley
Developmental Editor: Jenny Kim
Supervising Editor: Tim Prairie
Production Editor: Print Matters, Inc.
Manufacturing Manager: Ben Rivera
Cover Designer: Christine Jenny
Compositor: Compset, Inc.
Printer: Quebecor World

© 2005 by LIPPINCOTT WILLIAMS & WILKINS
530 Walnut Street
Philadelphia, PA 19106 USA
LWW.com

Printed in the USA

Library of Congress Cataloging-in-Publication Data

Physical medicine and rehabilitation : principles and practice/
[edited by]
Joel A. DeLisa, Bruce M. Gans, Nicholas E. Walsh.—4th ed.
    p. ; cm.
    Re. ed. of: Rehabilitation medicine. 3rd ed. c1998.
    Includes bibliographical references and index.
    ISBN 0-7817-4130-0 (HC)
    1. Medical rehabilitation. 2. Medicine, Physical. I. DeLisa, Joel A.
II. Gans, Bruce M. III. Walsh, Nicholas E. IV. Rehabilitation medicine.
    [DNLM: 1. Physical Medicine—methods. 2. Rehabilitation.
WB 320 P5795 2004] RM930.R364 2004 617'.03—dc22
                                                          2004048722

Care has been taken to confirm the accuracy of the information presented and to describe generally accepted practices. However, the authors, editors, and publisher are not responsible for errors or omissions or for any consequences from application of the information in this book and make no warranty, expressed or implied, with respect to the currency, completeness, or accuracy of the contents of the publication. Application of this information in a particular situation remains the professional responsibility of the practitioner.

The authors, editors, and publisher have exerted every effort to ensure that drug selection and dosage set forth in this text are in accordance with current recommendations and practice at the time of publication. However, in view of ongoing research, changes in government regulations, and the constant flow of information relating to drug therapy and drug reactions, the reader is urged to check the package insert for each drug for any change in indications and dosage and for added warnings and precautions. This is particularly important when the recommended agent is a new or infrequently employed drug.

Some drugs and medical devices presented in this publication have Food and Drug Administration (FDA) clearance for limited use in restricted research settings. It is the responsibility of the health care provider to ascertain the FDA status of each drug or device planned for use in their clinical practice.

10 9 8 7 6 5 4 3 2 1

To our patients,
who challenge us to continually strive to improve their health,
function and quality of life

To our teachers,
who challenged us to develop a scientific approach to problem-solving
and instilled in us the need for continuous learning

To our students,
who challenge and stimulate us to keep at the cutting edge.
They are our hope for the future

To our families,
who provided the inspiration, support and patience necessary
to make this text a reality

To our colleagues,
who have gone before us, who are with us
and who will follow us

Contents

VOLUME 2. REHABILITATION MEDICINE

PART I
Principles of Evaluation and Management

PART II
Management Methods

PART III
Major Problems

PART IV
Specific Conditions

Contributing Authors

Geoffrey Abbott, MBBS, FAFRM (RACP)
Senior Lecturer
Rehabilitation Programme & Victorian
Rehabilitation Institute
Melbourne Health & University of
Melbourne
Melbourne, Victoria, Australia

Craig J. Alexander, Ph.D., MBA
Associate Professor
Miami Project to Cure Paralysis
Department of Neurological Surgery
Department of Rehabilitation Medicine
University of Miami School of Medicine
Miami, FL
and
Project Co Director, VA Rehabilitation
Research and Development
Center of Excellence in Functional
Recovery and SCI
Miami, FL

Annette Alves, M.A.
Performance Improvement Coordinator
Department of Psychiatry
St. Joseph's Regional Medical Center
Paterson, NJ

Karen L. Andrews, M.D.
Assistant Professor,
Department of Physical Medicine and
Rehabilitation
Mayo Clinic College of Medicine
Rochester, MN

Michael T. Andary, M.D., M.S.
Associate Professor
Physical Medicine and Rehabilitation
Michigan State University
E. Lansing, MI

Leigh Anderson, M.D.
Associate Professor and Vice Chair
Department of Physical Medicine and
Rehabilitation
University of Colorado Health Sciences
Center
Denver, CO
Chief of Staff
Veterans Affairs Medical Center,
Eastern Co H C System
Denver, CO

Michael Armento, M.D.
Clinical Assistant Professor
Department of Physcial Medicine and
Rehabilition
UMDNJ – New Jersey Medical School
Newark, NJ
and
Children's Specialized Hospital
Mountainside, NJ

John R. Bach, M.D.
Professor and Vice-Chair
Department of Physical Medicine and
Rehabilitation
UMDNJ – New Jersey Medical School
Newark, NJ

Richard D. Ball, M.D., Ph.D.
Physical Medicine & Rehabilitation
Traverse City, MI

Jeffrey R. Basford, M.D., Ph.D.
Professor and Consultant
Mayo Clinic College of Medicine
Department of Physical Medicine and
Rehabilitation
Rochester, MN

John Basmajian, M.D.
McMaster University
CheD.O.ke-McMaster Hospital
Division of Physical Medicine and
Rehabilitation
Hamilton, Canada

Alison J. Beck, Ph.D.
Assistant Professor
Department of Occupational Therapy
University of Texas Health Science Center
San Antonio, TX

Bruce E. Becker, M.D.
Clinical Professor
Department of Rehabilitation Medicine
University of Washington
Seattle, WA
and
St. Luke's Rehabilitation Institute
Spokane, WA

Kathleen Bell, M.D.
Associate Professor
Department of Rehabilitation Medicine
University of Washington
Seattle, WA

Keith A. Bengtson, M.D.
Assistant Professor
Department of Physical Medicine and
Rehabilitation
Director of Hand Rehabilitation
Mayo Clinic College of Medicine
Rochester, MN

Marla Bernbaum, M.D.
Associate Professor
Internal Medicine
Division of Endocrinology
St. Louis University Health Science Center
St. Louis, MO

Champa Bid, M.D.
Clinical Assistant Professor

Department of Physical Medicine and
Rehabilitation
UMDNJ – New Jersey Medical School
Newark, NJ

Karen J. Blankenship, M.A., R.N.
Faculty Online
School of Business
University of Phoenix
Phoenix, AZ
Director of Clinical Operations
Reeves Rehabilitation Center
University Health System
San Antonio, TX

William L. Bockenek, M.D.
Clinical Associate Professor
Physical Medicine and Rehabilitation
University of North Carolina—Chapel Hill
Chapel Hill, NC
And Director of Spinal Cord Injury
Charlotte Institute of Rehabilitation
Department of Physical Medicine and
Rehabilitation
Charlotte, NC

Cathy Bodine, Ph.D.
Assistant Professor
Department of Rehabilitation Medicine
University of Colorado School of Medicine
Denver, CO

Ross Bogey, D.O.
Assistant Professor
Department of Physical Medicine and
Rehabilitation
Feinberg School of Medicine Northwestern
University
Chicago, IL

Michael L. Boninger, M.D.
Assistant Professor and Research Director
Department of Physical Medicine and
Rehabilitation
University of Pittsburgh
Pittsburgh, PA
and
Research Scientist
Department of Veterans Affairs

Francis J. Bonner, Jr., M.D.
Clinical Professor of Medicine
Drexel University College of Medicine
Philadelphia, PA
And Medical Director
Rehabilitation Center at South Jersey
Vineland, NJ

Gordon Bosker, B.S.
Instructor
Department of Rehabilitation Medicine
University of Texas Health Science Center
San Antonio, TX

Brian L. Bowyer, M.D.
Associate Professional—Clinical
Department of Physical Medicine and
  Rehabilitation
The Ohio State University College of
  Medicine
Columbus, OH

Jay E. Bowen, D.O.
Assistant Professor
Physical Medicine and Rehabilitation
Department of Physical Medicine and
  Rehabilitation
UMDNJ – New Jersey Medical School
Newark, NJ
and
Kessler Insitute for Rehabilitation
West Orange, NJ

Victoria A. Brander, M.D.
Assistant Professor, Clinical
Physical Medicine and Rehabilitation
Feinberg School of Medicine Northwestern
  University
Consultant
Physical Medicine and Rehabilitation
Northwestern Memorial Hospital
McGaw Medical Center
Chicago, IL

Murray E. Brandstater, MBBS, Ph.D.
Professor and Chair
Department of Rehabilitation Medicine
Loma Linda University Affiliated
  Hospitals
Loma Linda, CA

Jeffrey S. Braullt, D.O.
Assistant Professor
Department of Physical Medicine and
  Rehabilitation
Mayo Clinic College of Medicine
Rochester, MN

Matthew A. Butters, M.D.
Assistant Professor
Department of Physical Medicine and
  Rehabilitation
Mayo Clinic College of Medicine
Rochester, MN
And Consultant
Department of Physical Medicine and
  Rehabilitation
Mayo Clinic Scottsdale
Scottsdale, AZ

Gregory T. Carter, M.D.
Clincial Associate Professor
Department of Rehabilitation Medicine
University of Washington School of
  Medicine
Seattle, WA
and
Co-Director
MDA/ALS Center
University of Washington Medical
  Center
Seattle, WA

John Chae, M.D.
Associate Professor
Department of Physical Medicine and
  Rehabilitation
and Biomedical Engineering
Case Western Reserve University School
  of Medicine
Cleveland, OH

Boquin Chen, M.D., Ph.D.
Clinical Assistant Professor
Department of Physical Medicine and
  Rehabilitation
UMDNJ – New Jersey Medical School
Newark, NJ

Charles H. Chesnut III, M.D.
Professor Radiology and Medicine
University of Washington School of
  Medicine
Seattle, WA
and
Director Osteoporosis Research Center
University of Washington School of
  Medicine
Seattle, WA

Andrea L. Cheville, M.D.
Assistant Professor
Department of Rehabilitation Medicine
University of Pennsylvania Health System
Philadelphia, PA

Nancy Chiaravalloti, Ph.D.
Assistant Professor
Department of Physical Medicine and
  Rehabilitation
UMDNJ – New Jersey Medical School
Newark, NJ
and
Associate Director, Neuroscience and
  Neuropsychology
Kessler Medical Rehabilitation Research
  and Education Corporation
West Orange, NJ

Mary L. Chipman, BSc,MA
Professor
Department of Public Health Science
Faculty of Medicine
University of Toronto
Toronto, Ontario
Canada

Charles H. Christiansen, Ed.D
Dean and George T. Bryan Distinguished
  Professor
School of Allied Health Sciences
University of Texas Medical Branch at
  Galveston
Galveston, TX

Alan W. Chu, M.D.
Assistant Professor
Department of Physical Medicine and
  Rehabilitation
University of Pittsburgh
Pittsburgh, PA

Gary S. Clark, MD, MMM, CPE
Professor and Chair
Department of Physical Medicine and
  Rehabilitation
Case Western Reserve University School of
  Medicine
MetroHealth Medical Center
Cleveland, OH

Rebecca R. Clearman, M.D.
Adjunct Assistant Professor
Department of Physical Medicine and
  Rehabilitation
College of Medicine
University of Texas Health Sciences
  Center
Houston, TX

Andrew J. Cole, M.D.
Clinical Associate Professor
Department of Rehabilitation Medicine
University of Washington
Seattle, WA

Jeffrey L. Cole, M.D.
Associate Professor of Physical and
  Rehabilitation
Director, Physiatric Interventional Pain
  Management
Physical Medicine and Rehabilitation
Nassau Medical Center
East Meadow, NY

Rory A. Cooper, Ph.D.
Distinguished Professor and Chair
Department of Rehabilitation Science and
  Technology
University of Pittsburgh
Pittsburgh, PA
and
Research Scientist
Department of Veterans Affairs
Pittsburgh, PA

Rosemarie Cooper, MPT, ATP
Clinical Instructor
Department of Rehabilitation Science and
  Technology
University of Pittsburgh
Pittsburgh, PA

Ann C. Cotter, M.D.
Clinical Assistant Professor
Department of Physical Medicine and
  Rehabilitation
UMDNJ – New Jersey Medical School
Newark, NJ
and
Medical Director
Atlantic Mind Body Center
Morristown, NJ

Graham H. Creasey, M.D.
Associate Professor
Physical Medicine and Rehabilitation
Case Western Reserve University School
  of Medicine
Cleveland, OH

Jimmy Y. Cui, M.D. Ph.D.
Clinical Assistant Professor
Department of Rehabilitation Medicine
University of Washington School of
  Medicine
Seattle, WA

Bess Dawson-Hughes, M.D.
Professor of Medicine
Endocrine Division
Tufts University
Director Bone Metabolism Laboratory
USDA Human Nutrition Research Center
  on Aging at Tufts University
Boston, MA

Gerben DeJong, Ph.D.
Professor
Department of Health
  Administration
College of Health Professions
University of Florida
Gainesville, FL

Joel A. DeLisa, M.D., M.S.
Professor and Chair

Department of Physical Medicine and
Rehabilitation
UMDNJ – New Jersey Medical School
Newark, NJ
and
President and CEO
Kessler Medical Rehabilitation Research
and Education Corporation
West Orange, NJ

Martin Diamond, M.D.
Clinical Associate Professor
Department of Physical Medicine and
Rehabilitation
UMDNJ – New Jersey Medical School
Newark, NJ
and
Children's Specialized Hospital
Mountainside, NJ

Anthony F. DiMarco, M.D.
Professor of Medicine
Case Western Reserve University School
of Medicine
Cleveland, OH

**Peter Disler, Ph.D. MBBCh, FRACP,
FAFRM (RACP)**
Professor and Director
Rehabilitation Programme & Victorian
Rehabilitation Institute
Melbourne Health & University of
Melbourne
Melbourne, Victoria, Australia

Eva Durand, M.D.
Private Practitioner
Valley Stream, New York

Daniel Dumitru, M.D., Ph.D.
Professor and Deputy Chair
Department of Rehabilitation
Medicine
Univeristy of Texas Health Science
Center
San Antonio, TX

Elizabeth A. Eastwood, Ph.D.
Associate Professor
Brooklyn College The City University of
New York
Health and Nutritional Sciences
Brooklyn, NY

Elie Elovic, M.D.
Associate Professor
Department of Physcial Medicine and
Rehabilitation
UMDNJ – New Jersey Medical School
Newark, NJ
and
Director of TBI Research Laboratories
Kessler Medical Rehabilitation Research
and Education Corporation
West Orange, NJ

Rolland P. Erickson, M.D.
Assistant Professor
Department of Physical Medicine and
Rehabilitation
Mayo Clinic College of Medicine
Rochester, MN
Consultant
Mayo Clinic Scottsdale
Department of Physical Medicine and
Rehabilitation
Scottsdale, AZ

Avital Fast, M.D.
Professor
Department of Rehabilitation Medicine
Montefiore Medical Center
Albert Einstein College of Medicine
Bronx, NY

Joseph H. Feinberg, M.D.
Assistant Professor
Department of Physical Medicine and
Rehabilitation
Presbyterian Hospital
Attending Physician
Hospital for Special Surgery
New York, NY

Gerald Felsenthal, M.D.
Clinical Professor
Department of Epidemiology and
Preventive Medicine
University of Maryland School of
Medicine
Chairman Emeritus
Department of Rehabilitation Medicine
Sinai Hospital of Baltimore
Baltimore, MD

Steven M. Fine, M.D., Ph.D.
Assistant Professor
Department of Internal Medicine,
Infectious Diseases Unit
University of Rochester Medical Center
Rochester, NY

Kathleen Fink, M.D.
Assistant Professor
Rehabilitation Medicine
Georgetown University
National Rehabilitation Hoospital
Washington, DC

Patrick M. Foye, M.D.
Assistant Professor
Department of Physical Medicine and
Rehabilitation
UMDNJ – New Jersey Medical School
Newark, NJ

Gerard E. Francisco, M.D.
Clinical Associate Professor
Department of Physical Medicine and
Rehabilitation
University of Texas
Associate Director for Research
Brain Injury and Stroke Prgram
The Institute for Rehabilitation and
Research
Houston, TX

Deborah J. Franklin, M.D.
Assistant Professor
Department of Rehabilitation Medicine
University of Pennsylvania Health
System
Philadelphia, PA

Michael Friedland, M.D.
Clinical Associate Professor of Medicine
University of North Carolina School of
Medicine
Chapel Hill, NC

Walter R. Frontera, M.D., Ph.D.
Earle P. and Ida S. Charlton Professor and
Chairman
Physical Medicine and Rehabilitation
Harvard Medical School

Chief of Service
Department of Physical Medicine and
Rehabilitation
Spaulding Rehabilitation Hospital
Harvard Medical School
Boston, MA

Gail L. Gamble, M.D.
Assistant Professor
Department of Physical Medicine and
Rehabilitation
Mayo Clinic College of Medicine
Rochester, MN

Bruce M. Gans, M.D.
Professor
Department of Physical Medicine and
Rehabilitation
UMDNJ – New Jersey Medical School
Newark, NJ
and
Chief Medical Officer
Kessler Institute for Rehabilitation
West Orange, NJ

Bryan K. Ganter, M.D.
Assistant Professor
Department of Physical Medicine and
Rehabilitation
Mayo Clinic College of Medicine
Rochester, MN
And Consultant
Department of Physical Medicine and
Rehabilitation
Mayo Clinic Scottsdale,
Scottsdale, AZ

Steve R. Geiringer, M.D
Professor
Physical Medicine and Rehabilitation
Wayne State University
Westland, MI

Lynn H. Gerber, M.D.
Clinical Professor
Internal Medicine
Georgetown University Medical
Center
Washington, DC
and
Chief
Rehabilitation Medicine Department
Warren G. Magnuson Clinical Center
National Institutes of Health
Bethesda, MD

Carol J. Gill, Ph.D.
Associate Professor
Disability and Human Development
University if Illinois at Chicago
Chicago, IL

Andrew Gitter, M.D.
Department of Rehabilitation
Medicine
University of Texas HSC at San
Antonio
San Antonio, TX

Peter Gloviczki, M.D.
Professor of Surgery
Chair, Division of Vascular Surgery
Mayo Clinic College of Medicine
Rochester, NY
and
Director, Gonda Vascular Center
Rochester, MN

Steve M. Gnatz, M.D. M.H.A.
Professor, Orthopaedic Surgery and
Rehabilitation
Medical Director, Rehabilitation Services
Loyola University Medical Center
Maywood, IL

Gary Goldberg, M.D.
Director of Traumatic Brain Injury
Program
Director Electrodiagnostic Medicine
Mercy Hospital
Pittsburgh, PA

Brian Greenwald, M.D.
Assistant Professor
Department of Rehabilitation Medicine
Mt. Sinai School of Medicine
New York, NY

Michael E. Groher, Ph.D.
Professor
Truesdail Center for Communicative
Disorders
University of Redlands
Redlands, CA

Janet Haas, M.D.
William Penn Foundation
Philadelphia, PA

Eugen M. Halar, M.D.
Professor Emeritus
Department of Rehabilitation Medicine
University of Washington School of
Medicine
Seattle, WA

Cassing Hammond, M.D.
Assistant Professor
Obstetrics and Gynecology
Northwestern University
Chicago, IL
and
Director
Obstetrics and Gynecology
Northwestern Memorial Hospital
Chicago, IL

Tessa Hart, PH.D.
Research Assistant Professor
Department of Rehabilitation Medicine
Jefferson Medical College, Thomas
Jefferson University
Institute Scientist
Moss Rehabilitation Research Institute
Philadelphia, PA

Marjorie Head, LPT
Faculty Associate
Department of Physical Medicine &
Rehabilitation
University of Texas Southwestern Medical
Center at Dallas
Dallas, TX

Phala M. Helm, M.D.
Professor
Department of Physical Medicine &
Rehabilitation
University of Texas Southwestern Medical
Center at Dallas
Dallas, TX

Stanley A. Herring, M.D.
Clinical Professor
Department of Rehabilitation Medicine

Puget Sound Sports and Spine Physicians
Seattle, WA

Jeanne E. Hicks, M.D., F.A.C.R.
Former Adjunct Associate Professor of
Rehabilitation Medicine
Department of Orthopedic Surgery
Georgetown University Medical Center
Washington DC
and
Former Deputy Chief
Department of Rehabilitation Medicine
Warren G Magnuson Clinical Center
National Institutes of Health
Bethesda, MD

Steven R. Hinderer, M.D., M.S., P.T.
Associate Professor
Department of Physical Medicine and
Rehabilitation
Wayne State University School of Medicine
Detroit, MI
and
Rehabilatation Insitute of Michigan
Detroit, MI

Kathleen A. Hinderer, Ph.D. M.P.T., P.T.
Ann Arbor, MI

Martin D. Hoffman, M.D.
Professor of Clinical Physical Medicine
and Rehabilatation
University of California–Davis School of
Medicine
Sacramento, CA
Chief
Physical Medicine and Rehabilitation
Service
VA Northern California Health Care
System
Mather, CA

Barbara Hopkins, MMScRD, LD
Director Dietetic Internship Program
Georgia State University
Atlanta, GA

Todd G. Holmes, M.D.
Clinical Assistant Professor
Department of Physical Medicine and
Rehabilitation
Michigan State University
East Lansing, MI
Private Practice
Eding Physical Medicine Consultants
St. Louis Park, MN

Debra Homa, M.A.
Institute of Psychology
Illinois Institute of Technology
Chicago, IL

Garrett S. Hyman, M.D.
Northwest Spine and Sports Physicians
Bellevue, WA

Galen O. Joe, M.D.
Staff Physiatrist
Rehabilitation Medicine Department
Warren G Magnuson Clinical Center
National Institutes of Health
Bethesda, MD

Mark V. Johnston, Ph.D.
Professor
Department of Physical Medicine and
Rehabilitation

UMDNJ – New Jersey Medical School
Newark, NJ
and
Director of Outcomes Research
Kessler Medical Rehabilitation Research
and Education Corporation
West Orange, NJ

David J. Jones, Ph.D.
Professor, Department of Anesthesiology
University of Texas Health Science
Center
San Antonio, TX

Vivek Kadyan, M.D.
Assistant Professor
Department of Physical Medicine and
Rehabilitation
The Ohio State University College of
Medicine
Columbus, OH

Teresa Kaldis, M.D.
Assistant Professor
Department of Physical Medicine and
Rehabilitation
Baylor College of Medicine
Houston, TX

Claire Z. Kalpakjian, Ph.D.
Project Manager
Physical Medicine and Rehabilitation
University of Michigan Health System
Ann Arbor, MI

Susan M. Kaschalk, M.S., P.A.-C
Pontiac, MI

Fary Khan, MBBS, FAFRM (RACP)
Lecturer
Rehabilitation Programme & Victorian
Rehabilitation Institute
Melbourne Health & University of
Melbourne
Melbourne, Victoria, Australia

Paul R. Kileny, Ph.D.
Professor and Director
Department of Otolaryngology and
Pediatrics
University of Michigan
Ann Arbor, MI
and
Director, Audiology and Electrophysics
Department of Otolaryngology
University of Michigan Health System
Ann Arbor, MI

Kevin L. Kilgore, Ph.D.
Assistant Professor of Biomedical
Engineering
Case School of Engineering
Cleveland, OH

David D. Kilmer, M.D.
Professor and Chair
University of California-Davis
Department of Physical Medicine and
Rehabilitation
Sacramento, CA

John C. King, M.D.
Professor
Department of Rehabilitation Medicine
University of Texas Health Center at San
Antonio
Director, Reeves Rehabilitation Center

University Hospital
San Anttonio, TX

Kristi L. Kirschner, M.D.
Associate Professor
Department of Physical Medicine and
Rehabilitation and of Medical
Humanities and Bioethics
Feinberg School of Medicine Northwestern
University
Chicago, IL
and
Director
Center for the Study of Disability Ethics
Rehabilitation Institute of Chicago
Chicago, IL

Steven Kirshblum, M.D.
Associate Professor
Department of Physical Medicine and
Rehabilitation
UMDNJ – New Jersey Medical School
Newark, NJ
and
Associate Medical Director and
Director of Spinal Cord Injury Services
Kessler Institute for Rehabilitation
West Orange, NJ

Mark D. Klaiman, M.D.
Consultant
Rehabilitation Medicine Department
Warren G Magnuson Clinical Center
National Institutes of Health
Bethesda, MD

Robert Klecz, M.D.
Clinical Assistant Professor
Department of Physical Medicine and
Rehabilitation
UMDNJ – New Jersey Medical School
Newark, NJ
and
Clinical Chief Orthopedic Rehabilitation
Kessler Insitute for Rehabilitation
East Orange, NJ

Eric L. Kolodin, D.P.M.
Assistant Attending
Department of Surgery, Section of Podiatry
Saint Barnabas Medical Center
Livingston, NJ

Sunil Kothari, M.D.
Assistant Professor
Department of Physical Medicine and
Rehabilitation
Baylor College of Medicine
Houston, TX

Karen Kowalske, M.D.
Associate Professor and Chairman
Department of Physical Medicine &
Rehabilitation
University of Texas Southwestern Medical
Center at Dallas
Dallas, TX

William J. Kraemer, Ph.D
Professor of Kinesiology
Physiology and Neurobiology
The University of Connecticut School of
Medicine
Storrs, CT

George Kraft, M.D.
Professor

Department of Rehabilitation Medicine
University of Washington School of
Medicine
Seattle, WA

Lisa S. Krivickas, M.D.
Assistant Professor
Harvard Medical School
Associate Chief
Physical Medicine and Rehabilitation
Director of EMG
Spaulding Rehabilitation Hospital
Boston, MA

David Kuo, M.D.
Clinical Assistant Professor
Department of Medicine
UMDNJ – New Jersey Medical School
Newark, NJ
and
Director of Outpatient Services
Morristown Memorial Hospital
Morristown NJ

Andrea Laborde, M.D.
Clinical Assistant Professor
Department of Physical Medicine and
Rehabilitation
University of Pennsylvania Health System
Philadelphia, PA
and
Director of Trauma Rehabilitation
University of Pennsylvania Health System
Philadelphia, PA

Indira Lanig, M.D.
Clinical Assistant Professor
Department of Physical Medicine and
Rehabilitation
University of Colorado Health Sciences
Center
Denver, CO

Stephen F. Levinson, M.D., Ph.D.
Associate Professor and Chair
Department of Physical Medicine and
Rehabilitation
University of Rochester Medical Center
Rochester, NY

Jan Lexell, M.D., Ph.D.
Associate Professor
Department of Rehabilition
Lund University Hospital
Medical Director of Department of
Rehabilition
and
Chief of Brain Injury Unit
Switzerland

Robert Lindsay, M.D.
Professor of Clinical Medicine
Columbia University
New York, NY
Chief, Internal Medicine
Helen Hayes Hospital
West Haverstran, NY

Todd A. Linsenmeyer, M.D.
Associate Professor
Department of Physical Medicine and
Rehabilitation and
Department of Surgery (Division of
Urology)
UMDNJ – New Jersey Medicine School
Newark, NJ
and

Director of Urology
Kessler Institute for Rehabilitation
West Orange, NJ

Jason S. Lipetz, M.D.
Assistant Professor
Rehabilitation Medicine
Albert Einstein College of Medicine
Bronx, NY
Director, Center for Spine Rehabilitation
North Shore—LIJ Health System
East Meadow, NY

David I. Lipetz, MSPT, OCS, Cert.MDT
Director of Rehabilitation
Westside Spine and Joint Rehabilitation
and
Adjunct Orthopedic Clinical Faculty
University of Southern California
Los Angeles, CA

Gerald A. Malanga, M.D.
Associate Professor
Department of Physical Medicine and
Rehabilitation
University of Medicine and Dentistry of
New Jersey
New Jersey Medical School
Newark, NJ
Director, Sports, Spine, and Orthopedic
Rehabilitation
Kessler Institute for Rehabilitation
West Orange, NJ

Nancy Mann, M.D.
Associate Professor
Department of Physical Medicine and
Rehabilitation
Wayne State University School of Medicine
Southfield, MI

Dennis Matthews, M.D.
Associate Professor and Chair
Department of Rehabilitation Medicine
University of Colorado School of Medicine
Denver, CO
and
Fischahs Chair Pediatric Rehabilitation
Medicine
Children's Hospital
University of Colorado Medical School
Denver, CO

B. Cairbre McCann, M.D.
Department of Rehabilitation Medicine
Maine Medical Center
Portland, OR

Mary Anne McDonald
General Counsel and Executive Vice
President
Henry H. Kessler Foundation
West Orange, NJ

Robert M. Miller, Ph.D., BCNCD
Lecturer, Speech and Hearing Sciences
University of Washington
Clinical Associate Professor
Rehabilitation Medicine and Otolaryngology
Head and Neck Surgery
University of Washington Medical Center,
Seattle, WA

Peter J. Moley, M.D.
Clinical Instructor of Physiatry
The Hospital for Special Surgery
New York, NY

Scott Millis, Ph.D.
Professor
Department of Physical Medicine and
Rehabilitation
UMDNJ – New Jersey Medical School
Newark, NJ
and
Director of Office of Clinical Trials
Kessler Medical Rehabilitation Research
and Education
Coporation
West Orange, NJ

Michael Munin, M.D.
Associate Professor
Department of Physical Medicine and
Rehabilitation
University of Pittsburgh
Pittsburgh, PA

Carol Mushett-Johnson, Med, CTRS, CSW
Department of Kinesiology and Health
Georgia State University
Atlanta, GA

Robert Nadler, C.P.O.
Hanger Prosthetics and Orthotics
Hamilton, NJ

Scott F. Nadler, D.O.
Professor and Director of Sports Medicine
Department of Physical Medicine and
Rehabilitation
UMDNJ – New Jersey Medical School
Newark, NJ

T. Russell Nelson, Ph.D.
Associate Clinical Professor
Department of Rehabilitation
University of Texas Health Science
Speech Pathologist
Audiology and Speech Pathology Service
South Texas Veterans Health Care System
San Antonio, TX

Stephen F. Noll, M.D.
Assistant Professor
Department of Physical Medicine and
Rehabilitation
Mayo Clinic College of Medicine
Rochester, MN
Medical Director, Rehabilitation
Department of Physical Medicine and
Rehabilitation
Mayo Clinic Scottsdale
Scottsdale, AZ

Kevin O'Connor, M.D.
Assistant Professor
Department of Physical Medicine and
Rehabilitation
Harvard Medical School
and
Medical Director, Spinal Cord Injury
Program
Spaulding Rehabilitation Hospital
Boston, MA

Zaliha Omar, MBBS, FAFRM (RACP)
Associate Professor and Director
Department of Rehabilitation
Faculty of Medicine University of Malaya
Kuala Lumpur, Malaysia

Liina Paasuke, M.A., C.R.C.
Rehabilitation Counselor
Physical Medicine and Rehabilitation

University of Michigan Health System
Ann Arbor, MI

Jeffrey B. Palmer, M.D.
Professor
Department of Physical Medicine and
Rehabilitation
The John Hopkins University School of
Medicine
Baltimore, MD

Karen E. Pape, M.D., F.R.C.P.C.
Medical Director
TASC Network, Inc.
Toronto, Ontario
Canada

Yong Park, M.D.
Philadelphia, PA

Shailesh Parikh, M.D.
Assistant Professor
Department of Physical Medicine and
Rehabilitation
UMDNJ – New Jersey Medical School
Newark, NJ
and
Kessler Institute for Rehabilitation
Saddle Brook, NJ

Scott Paul, M.D.
Rehabilitation Medicine Department
Warren G Magnuson Clinical Center
National Institutes of Health
Bethesda, MD

William S. Pease, M.D.
Ernest W. Johnson Professor and
Chairman
Department of Physical Medicine and
Rehabilitation
The Ohio State University College of
Medicine and Public Health
Medical Director, Dodd Hall Rehabilitation
Program
President, OSU Physical Medicine and
Rehabilitation. LLC
OSU Physicians, Inc.
The Ohio State University Hospital
Columbus, Ohio

Barbara Pippin, M.D.
Instructor
Department of Physical Medicine and
Rehabilitation
University of Pittsburgh,
Pittsburgh, PA

Ferne Pomerantz, M.D.
Medical Director
Department of Physical Medicine and
Rehabilitation
Westchester Medical Center
Valhalla, New York

Kristjan Ragnarsson, M.D.
Professor and Chair
Mount Sinai School of Medicine
Department of Rehabilitation
Medicine
New York, NY

Somayaji Ramamurthy, M.D.
Professor of Anesthesiology
University of Texas Health Science
Center
San Antonio, TX

James J. Rechtien, D.O., Ph.D.
Professor
Department of Physical Medicine and
Rehabilitation
Michigan State University School of
Medicine
East Lansing, MI

Thomas S. Rees, Ph.D.
Associate Professor
Department of Otolaryngology—Head
and Neck Surgery
and
Director of Audiology
University of Washington
Seattle, WA

Judith Panko Reis, M.A., M.S.
Director
Health Resources Center for Women with
Disabilities
Rehabilitation Institute of Chicago
Chicago, IL

Kenneth J. Richter, D.O.
Clinical Associate Professor
Department of Rehabilitation Medicine
Michigan State University
and
Wayne State University
Detroit, MI
and
Oakland Physiatry
Pontiac, MI

Joseph H. Ricker, Ph.D., ABPP
Associate Professor
And Director of Neuropsychology
Physical Medicine and Rehabilitation
University of Pittsburgh
Pittsburgh, PA

Keith M. Robinson, M.D.
Associate Professor
Department of Rehabilitation Medicine
University of Pennsylvania Health System
Philadelphia, PA

Lawerence R. Robinson, M.D.
Professor and Chair
Department of Rehabilitation Medicine
University of Washington School of
Medicine
Seattle, WA

James N. Rogers, M.D.
Professor of Anesthesiology
University of Texas Health Science Center
San Antonio, TX

Daniel E. Rohe, Ph.D.
Associate Professor of Psychology
Department of Psychiatry and Psychology
Mayo Clinic College of Medicine
Rochester, MN

Robert D. Rondinelli, M.D., Ph.D.
Medical Director
Younker Rehabilitation Center
Iowa Methodist Medical Center
Des Moines, IA

Thom W. Rooke, M.D., F.A.C.C.
Professor of Medicine
Head, Section of Vascular Medicine
Mayo Clinic College of Medicine
Rochester, MN

Mitchell Rosenthal, Ph.D.
Professor of Physical Medicine and
Rehabilitation
Department of Physical Medicine and
Rehabilitation
UMDNJ – New Jersey Medical School
Newark, NJ
and
Vice President for Research
Kessler Medical Rehabilitation Research
and Education Corporation
West Orange, NJ

Mya C. Schiess, M.D.
Associate Professor
Department of Neurology
University of Texas Health Science
Center
Houston, TX

Mark Schmeler, M.S., OTR/L, ATP
Clinical Instructor
Department of Rehabilitation Science and
Technology
University of Pittsburgh
Pittsburgh, PA

Carson D. Schneck, M.D., Ph.D.
Professor of Anatomy and Diagnostic
Imaging
Department of Anatomy and Cell Biology
Temple University School of Medicine
Philadelphia, PA

Lawerence S. Schoenfeld, M.D.
Professor
Department of Psychiatry
University of Texas Health Science Center
San Antonio, TX

Sarah Schuler, M.D.
Physical Medicine and Rehabilitation
Resident
JFK Johnson Rehabilitation Institute
UMDNJ – Robert Wood Johnson Medical
Edison, NJ

Subhashchandra K. Shah, MD
Mercy Hospital
Department of Rehabilitation Medicine
Chicago, IL

Andrew L. Sherman, M.D., M.S.
Assistant Professor of Clinical
Rehabilitation Medicine
Department of Rehabilitation Medicine
University of Miami School of Medicine
Miami, FL

Claudine Sherrill, Ed.D.
Professor
Adapted Physical Education
Texas Women University
Denton, TX

Lois M. Sheldahl, Ph.D.
Associate Professor, Medicine
Medical College of Wisconsin
VA Medical Center
Milwaukee, WI

Samuel C. Shiflett, Ph.D.
Director of Research
Continuum Center for Health and Healing
Beth Israel Medical Center
New York, NY
and

Assistant Professor
Family Medicine and Social Medicine
Albert Einstein College of Medicine
Bronx, NY

William H. Shull, M.D.
Department of Rehabilitation Medicine
University of Pennsylvania Health System
Philadelphia, PA

Hilary C. Siebens, M.D.
Professor of Physical Medicine and
Rehabilitation
Professor of Clinical Medicine
University of California Irvine College of
Medicine
Irvine, CA

Marca L. Sipski, M.D.
Professor and Interim Chair
Department of Rehabilitation Medicine
Miami Project to Cure Paralysis
University of Miami School of Medicine
Miami, FL
and
Project Director, VA Rehabilitation
Research and Development
Center of Excellence in Functional
Recovery and SCI
Miami, FL

Sue Ann Sisto, Ph.D.
Associate Professor
Department of Physical Medicine and
Rehabilitation
UMDNJ – New Jersey Medical School
Newark, NJ
and
Director of Human Performance and
Movement
Analysis Laboratory
Kessler Medical Rehabilitation Research
and Edcucation Corporation
West Orange, NJ

Jay Smith, M.D.
Associate Professor
Department of Physical Medicine and
Rehabilitation
Mayo Clinic College of Medicine
Rochester, MN

Steven A Steins, M.D. M.S.
Associate Professor
Department of Rehabilitation Medicine
and
Director of Fellowship Program
Spinal Cord Medicine University of
Washington
Attending Physician Spinal Cord Injury
Unit
VA Puget Sound Health Care System
Scattle, WA

Christopher J. Standaert, M.D.
Clinical Assistant Professor
Department of Rehabilitation Medicine
University of Washington School of
Medicine
Seattle, WA
and
Puget Sound Sports and Spine
Physicians
Seattle, WA

Margaret G. Stineman, M.D.
Associate Professor

Department of Physical Medicine and
Rehabilitation
University of Pennsylvania Health
System
Philadelphia, PA

Doreen Stiskal, PT, Ph.D.
Associate
Department of Physical Medicine and
Rehabilitation
UMDNJ – New Jersey Medical School
Newark, NJ
and
Assistant Chair
Graduation Programs in Health Sciences
School of Graduate Medical Education
Seton Hall University
West Orange, NJ

Todd P. Stitik, M.D.
Associate Professor
Department of Physical Medicine and
Rehabilitation
UMDNJ – New Jersey Medical School
Newark, NJ
and
Director, Occupational/Musculoskeletal
Medicine
Newark, NJ

James M. Stone, M.D.
Private Practice

David M. Strick, M.D.
Associate Professor of Physiology
and Instructor in P.T.
Mayo Clinic College of Medicine
Rochester, MN

S. David Stulberg, M.D.
Professor
Clinical Orthopaedic Surgery
Feinberg School of Medicine Northwestern
University
Chicago, IL

Jayson H. Takata, M.D.
Honolulu, Hawaii

Denise G. Tate, Ph.D. ABPP
Professor
Clinical Psychologist
Department of Physical Medicine and
Rehabilitation
University of Michigan
Ann Arbor, MI

Noc Thai, M.D., Ph.D.
Assistant Professor Department of Surgery
Division Transplant Surgery
University of Pittsburgh,
Pittsburgh, PA

Mark A. Thomas, M.D.
Associate Professor – Clinical
Rehabilitation Medicine
Department of Rehabilitation Medicine
Montefiore Medical Center
Albert Einstein College of Medicine
Bronx, NY

Ronald J. Triolo, Ph.D
Associate Professor
Department of Orthopedics
Case Western Reserve Univeristy School of
Medicine
Cleveland, OH

David S. Tulsky, Ph.D.
Associate Professor
Department of Physical Medicine and
 Rehabilitation
UMDNJ – New Jersey School of Medicine
Newark, NJ
and
Director of Northern New Jersey Spinal
 Cord Injury System
Kessler Medical Rehabilitation Research
 and Edcucation Corporation
West Orange, NJ

Margaret A. Turk, M.D.
Professor
Department of Physical Medicine and
 Rehabilitation
SUNY Health Science Center
Syracuse, NY

Thomas C. Turturro, M.S.
Assistant Professor
Department of Physical Therapy
University of Texas Health Science
 Center
San Antonio, TX

Heikki Uustal, M.D.
Clinical Assistant Professor
Department of Physical Medicine and
 Rehabilitation
UMDNJ – Robert Wood Johnson Medical
 School
Newark, NJ
and
JFK Johnson Rehabilitation Institute
Edison, NJ

Mary M. Vargo, M.D.
Assistant Professor
Department of Physical Medicine &
 Rehabilitation
Case Western Reserve Univeristy School of
 Medicine
Cleveland, OH

Thomas D. Vitale, D.P.M.
Instructor, Department of Surgery
New York College of Podiatric Medicine
New York, NY
Assistant Attending
Section of Podiatry
Saint Barnabas Medical Center
Livingston, NJ

Stanley F. Wainapel, M.D., M.P.H
Professor
Clinical Physical & Rehabilitation
 Medicine

Chief, Department of Physical Medicine &
 Rehabilitation
Montefiore Medical Center
Department of Rehabilitation Medicine
Bronx, NY

Nicolas E. Walsh, M.D.
Professor and Chairman
Department of Rehabilitation Medicine
Professor
Department of Anesthesiology
and
Staff Physician
Physical Medicine and Rehabilitation Service
South Texas Veterans Care Health Care
 System
Audie L. Murphy Memorial Veterans
 Hospital
San Antonio, TX

Robert J. Weber, M.D.
Professor and Chairman
Department of Physical Medicine and
 Rehabilitation
State University of New York Health
 Science
Center at Syracuse
Syracuse, NY

Stuart M. Weinstein, M.D.
Clinical Associate Professor
Department of Rehabilitation Medicine
University of Washington
Puget Sound Sports and Spine
 Physicians
Seattle, WA

Jodi S. Weiss, OTR
Randolph, NJ

John Whyte, M.D., Ph.D.
Professor
Department of Rehabilitation Medicine
Jefferson Medical College
Thomas Jefferson University
Director
Moss Rehabilitation Research Institute
Philadelphia, PA

J. Michael Wieting, D.O., M.Ed.
Associate Professor
Department of Physical Medicine and
 Rehabilitation
College of Osteopathic Medicine
Michigan State University
Medical Director
The Rehabilitation Center
Ingham Regional Medical Center
Lansing, MI

Deborah L. Wilkerson, M.A.
Director
Department of Research and Quality
 Improvement
CARF – The Rehabilitation Accreditation
 Commission
Tucson, AZ

Faren H. Williams, M.D., M.S., R.D.
Assistant Professor
Department of Physical Medicine and
 Rehabilitation
University of Pennsylviana Health
 System
and
Chief of Physical Medicine and
 Rehabilitation
Philadelphia Veterans Administration
Philadelphia, PA

Mark Young, M.D.
Assistant Professor
Department of Neurology
University of Maryland School of
 Medicine
Baltimore, MD

Kathryn M. Yorkston, Ph.D., BCNCD
Professor
Department of Rehabilitation Medicine
University of Washington School of
 Medicine
Seattle, WA

Ross O. Zafonte, D.O.
Professor and Chair
Department of Physical Medicine and
 Rehabilitation
University of Pittsburgh
Lillian Kaufman Building
Pittsburgh, PA

Eugenia F. Zimmerman, M.D.
Assistant Professor
Department of Physical Medicine and
 Rehabilitation
Michigan State University
Attending Physician
Rehabilitation Medicine
MSU—Clinical Center
East Lansing, MI

Teresa A. Zwolan, Ph.D.
Associate Professor
Department of Otolaryngology
Head and Neck Surgery
Director of Cochlear Implant Center
University of Michigan Medical Center
Ann Arbor, MI

Preface

Physical Medicine and Rehabilitation focuses on the restoration of function and reintegration into the community. These volumes are organized to assist the practitioner in these endeavors. This two-volume edition does not imply a division of physical medicine and rehabilitation medicine; this format was selected for ease of use by the practitioner and to accommodate the ever-increasing knowledge in the field of physical medicine and rehabilitation.

In response to the many advances in the field of physiatry, this textbook contains 88 chapters. Our goal was to provide comprehensive and multidisciplinary coverage of the depth and breadth of the field of physical medicine and rehabilitation, both in basic principles and in practical techniques of patient management. Each chapter was a collaborative effort by authors chosen for their expertise in the given topic area. This text reflects the efforts of over 223 contributing authors from all over the globe.

The editors express their appreciation to each of the authors who have contributed to this edition. Their hard work and dedication have made this an exciting and productive effort. As an essential resource for the training of medical rehabilitation professionals, this text will help ensure that the care they provide to people with disabilities is of the highest quality, encompassing improvement in their health, function and quality of life.

This fourth edition of *Physical Medicine and Rehabilitation* is dedicated to our colleagues of the past, present and future. Their passing is a loss of friendship, intellect and compassion to the field of physical medicine and rehabilitation. To ameliorate the void, we must challenge ourselves, and those around us, by our daily example, mentoring and care.

Joel A. DeLisa, M.D., M.S.
Bruce M. Gans, M.D.
Nicolas E. Walsh, M.D.
William L. Bockenek, M.D.
Walter R. Frontera, M.D.
Lynn H. Gerber, M.D.
Steve R. Geiringer, M.D.
William S. Pease, M.D.
Lawrence R. Robinson, M.D.
Jay Smith, M.D.
Todd P. Stitik, M.D.
Ross O. Zafonte, D.O.

Principles of Evaluation and Management

CHAPTER 43

Functional Evaluation and Management of Self-care and Other Activities of Daily Living

Charles H. Christiansen

INTRODUCTION

Enabling individuals to manage daily self-care is among the most important goals undertaken by the rehabilitation team. This is because such tasks relate directly to the business of living and their performance signifies a return to participation in the routines of daily life. Self-care tasks include dressing, eating, bathing, grooming, use of the toilet, and mobility within the home. These are basic tasks included within the general category of activities of daily living (ADL). Although able-bodied persons perform most self-care tasks routinely, such tasks can represent difficult challenges for persons with sensory, motor, and/or cognitive deficits.

Other important activities for living in the community are related to managing the everyday requirements of daily life. These extended ADLs go beyond basic self-care and have been labeled by Lawton as instrumental activities of daily living, or IADLs (1). These include food preparation, laundry, housekeeping, shopping, use of the telephone, use of transportation, use of medication, and financial management. Child care also is an important responsibility in the daily routine of many people.

Unfortunately, there is no consensus on the classification of human activity. As a result, many terms with similar definitions used for ADL categories are used in the medical, health, and rehabilitation literature. Table 43-1 lists some of these. In this chapter, basic ADLs (BADL), such as eating, dressing, grooming, hygiene, and mobility, are described as personal or self-care tasks. Essential tasks for maintaining the living environment and residing in the community are described as instrumental ADLs or extended activities of daily living (EADL) (see Table 43-1).

Self-care tasks may assume symbolic meaning for the individual in a rehabilitation program, because attending to eating, dressing, and toileting tasks are basic parts of the routine necessary for establishing a sense of identity (2) as well as for gaining acceptance in a social world (3). This is because appropriate dress, personal appearance, hygiene, and other expectations influence perceptions of the self and others (4).

In the developed nations, about 30% of a typical person's waking hours is spent performing self-maintenance activities, including basic self-care and household maintenance (5). For able-bodied persons, an average of more than 1 hour per day is spent in basic self-care activities (6,7). Research has shown that more than 70% of the variation in discharge decisions following stroke rehabilitation is determined by the ability to function independently in the performance of self-care tasks necessary for bathing, toileting, social interaction, dressing, and eating (8).

In the United States, recognition of the importance of functional independence is reflected in population survey data collected by governmental agencies, such as the National Center for Health Statistics (9). Moreover, an individual's functional ability is an important predictor of nursing home placement, with research showing a high correlation between the number of dependencies in activities of daily living and the risk of institutional placement (10).

TABLE 43-1.   Terminology of Functional Performance

Frequently Used Categories	Activities Typically Included in Category	Correspondence with ICF Descriptions of Categories and Activities
Self Care	bathing communication	Self Care: Caring for oneself, washing and drying oneself, caring for one's body and body parts, dressing, eating and drinking, and looking after one's health
Personal Care	dressing eating	Mobility: moving by changing body position or location or by transferring from one place to another, by carrying, moving or manipulating objects, by walking, running or climbing, and by using various forms of transportation.
Basic ADL (BADL)	grooming mobility toileting (sphincter control) transfers	Communication: general and specific features of communicating by language, signs and symbols, including receiving and producing messages, carrying on conversations, and using communication devices and techniques
Instrumental Activities of Daily Living (IADL)	childcare financial management food preparation	Domestic Life: Acquiring a place to live, food, clothing and other necessities, household cleaning and repairing, caring for personal and other household objects, and assisting others
Extended ADL (EADL)	housekeeping laundry medication use shopping telephone use transportation use	
Reintegration	Paid Work Volunteerism	Major Life Areas: Carrying out the tasks and actions required to engage in education, work and employment and to conduct economic transactions, including education, work and employment and economic life.
Community Participation	Leisure Recreation	Community, Social and Civic Life: The actions and tasks required to engage in organized social life outside the family, in community, social, and civic areas of life, such as participation in spirituality and religion, political life and citizenship, volunteerism, recreation and leisure.

Self-care and Activities of Daily Living in Context

Current international models of disability consider the multiple factors that influence daily life and the ability to perform necessary life tasks (11,12). These models recognize the importance of the physical and social setting in which an individual lives, and how these factors come together to support or limit task performance and participation as a member of society. Persons with whom an individual regularly spends time constitute that person's social nucleus, providing important support and social interaction and influencing activity choices and role requirements as well as the level of independence (13). This nucleus typically includes friends, acquaintances, and members of the individual's immediate and extended family.

It is within this social situation that the importance of self-care is most apparent, because meeting self-care needs is vital to success in meeting expectations within the social environment. Self-esteem, or the value accorded oneself, is determined by how well self-evaluation matches the values perceived as important in the social environment (14). Self-esteem is influenced by social acceptance and by one's success in achieving a desired social identity (15,16). Because the ability to perform self-care tasks contributes to both acceptance and identity, it can have a direct effect on self-esteem (17). In fact, social factors have been shown to explain life satisfaction and perceived well-being to a greater extent than functional limitations for those who must adjust to the consequences of aging (18), stroke (19), spinal cord injury (20), or arthritis (21).

Usually, self-care activities are taken for granted by the person and society unless difficulties are encountered. Limitations in self-care tasks and dependency on others for their completion serve to diminish an individual's self-concept and can lead to decreased morale and depression. A study of elderly patients found that a relationship existed between self-concept and functional independence and that people who were dependent in ADL scored lower in measures of self-concept (22).

Research has shown a clear relationship between self-concept, morale, and level of functional independence. For example, Chang and Mackenzie found that self-esteem was a consistent and significant predictor of functional ability at various intervals following stroke (23). Chemerinski and colleagues found that improvements in ADL performance were associated with remission of poststroke depression (24). These studies and others (25) indicate that an important goal of rehabilitation should be to help patients learn to take control of decisions about daily living, since this may contribute positively to their sense of efficacy, morale, and overall sense of well-being. More important, it may also increase life expectancy, since loss of hope and feelings of helplessness during early rehabilitation phases have been shown to be associated with shorter survival rates following stroke (26).

Within living settings, the presence of an individual with needs for care-giving affects the entire family or social group (27). When a member of the family can no longer perform expected activities, the daily routine may be upset, creating stress, diminished psychological well-being, and conflict (28, 29). Family members must adjust their expectations of the individual who is disabled as well as adjusting to changes in family routines and activities (30).

Because families are systems, they have lifecycles, with stages and time periods, each with characteristic issues. Important concerns related to self-care and care-giving needs must be considered in light of these stages, with recognition that needs change over time. The most significant change affecting care-giving is the number of family members who are available to provide support as a family life cycle matures.

Necessary adjustments made by families or caretakers confronted with rehabilitation challenges often include a reassignment of homemaking tasks or changes in priorities, and may impose additional financial or social burdens due to the need to hire outside assistance or rely on volunteers (31). Jones and Vetter found that the curtailment of the caretaker's social life as a result of the time needed to provide self-care assistance was more stressful than the actual tasks they performed (32). Their study and others (33,34) showed that levels of depression and anxiety, as well as somatic complaints, are more prevalent among caretakers and family members of disabled people living in the home environment than those typically found among members of the general population. Caregiver burden, a term given to the general strain, isolation, disappointment, and emotional demands of caring for a member of the household with a disability, seems to increase in proportion with ADL needs (35,36). A study of families involved in caring for survivors of stroke found that family adaptation after 1 year was related to family stresses and demands, family resources, and family perceptions. In particular, family functioning was poorer when the patient developed psychological morbidity, when the patient was less satisfied with the recovery, and when the health burden of the stroke was greater (37). In recognition of the increasing importance of the role of household caregivers, interventional strategies, including counseling, education and training, and social support, have been reported. A metaanalysis of 78 caregiver intervention studies was conducted by Sorenson and colleagues, indicating that such interventions are generally effective in improving well-being and reducing the "burden" of care (38).

During the rehabilitation process, the family can have a considerable influence on functional outcome (39,40). A stable and supportive family unit can be of great assistance, whereas families that are functioning poorly can impede rehabilitation. In some cases, poor outcomes can be traced to a lack of family involvement in the rehabilitation process. In other cases, too much support can encourage dependency (41). This indicates that the family should be involved in all aspects of rehabilitation, including evaluation and the setting of rehabilitation goals and treatment strategies before and after discharge.

A primary source of adjustment difficulties for people with physical disabilities comes from societal treatment of them as socially inferior. The common belief that strength, independence, and appearance are important aspects of self-worth is very damaging to people with disabilities. Interaction within a social group often depends on the ability to perform at the group's expected level; otherwise, the person will not be included as a significant group member (42).

Self-care tasks are not publicly valued in the same manner as gainful employment (43,44). Ironically, they assume importance principally when one's inability to perform them leads to perceived disadvantage or social stigma (45). Independence in ADL helps to refute the idea that a person with a disability may be a financial or social burden to society. It is important to realize that social participation and quality of life are the ultimate goals of patients, and this endpoint should influence goal setting for rehabilitation professionals. Physical health is an enabler of well-being, and the capacity to accomplish self-care represents the beginning set of tasks necessary for participation. As noted by Hogan and Orme, ambulation and self-care mastery alone are insufficient for attaining desired goals related to social participation (46). A recent research synthesis reported by Bays concluded that independence with activities of daily living, and social support were key variables in the quality of life experienced by survivors of stroke (47).

Self-care and Functional Performance

Traditionally, intervention for people who have difficulty performing self-care tasks begins with training in the hospital or acute rehabilitation environment. Typically, such intervention begins with instruction in procedures to regain dressing, grooming, hygiene, and eating skills and food preparation skills (45). In pursuit of these goals, rehabilitation sessions have been conducted within the patient's hospital room or in simulated ADL settings within occupational therapy clinics. Intervention strategies involve teaching the individual functional skills or the use of assistive technologies so that compensatory strategies can be performed at home after discharge.

Unfortunately, ADL training in a rehabilitation setting does not guarantee skill generalization to the discharge location (48). Patients may perform well in an occupational therapy clinic, but skills may not always transfer to the individual's bedside environment or, more important, his or her normal living setting (49). Environmental and psychosocial factors that directly influence task performance may be too varied between settings for the person receiving rehabilitation to generalize the learned skills (50). In addition, the individual may become dependent on the staff for self-care performance or lack the opportunity to perform new skills on a regular basis. Consequently, performance after discharge may reflect a lack of confidence or motivation.

Gill and colleagues argue that criteria emphasizing independence in basic ADL should also consider the degree of difficulty associated with performance. They found that persons experiencing difficulty with performance are significantly more likely to become dependent than those without difficulty (51).

Setting Rehabilitation Goals for the Discharge Environment

The growing costs of specialized rehabilitation care have led to a reduction in hospital lengths of stay and have resulted in more rapid discharge from special care facilities. More care is now provided in outpatient settings and in the home environment. This has advantages and disadvantages, since intervention in the home can be beneficial in achieving certain self-care skills and community reintegration (52,53), whereas functional gains may be attained more quickly in the rehabilitation setting (54), particularly in specialized units (55). The rehabilitation team can confront each problem with greater insight and sensitivity, and problems can be solved more rapidly than in more traditional therapy settings. The environment can be evaluated in terms of architectural, transportation, and communication barriers and how these support or limit the individual's daily living skills. In addition to expansion into the home and community, the use of high-technology assistive devices has greatly influenced the field of rehabilitation. These developments have the potential to help the patient gain environmental control for self-care and vocational and recreational pursuits. With the aid of computers and environmental control devices, some patients who previously required institutional care now can live in community settings (56,57).

Collaboratively Planning Self-care and ADL Goals

Current standards in rehabilitation encourage the involvement of the patient and members of the household in treatment planning. In the United States, a patient's bill of rights adopted by the American Hospital Association in the 1970s set the stage for a management approach toward self-care that fully informs and involves the individual receiving rehabilitation services (58). Subsequently, patient participation criteria have been included in accreditation standards (59,60) for hospitals and rehabilitation facilities. The President's Advisory Commission on Consumer Protection and Quality in the Health Care Industry recommended a Consumer Bill of Rights and Responsibilities that included strong provisions for patient participation in health-care decisions (61).

Despite the broad appeal of this philosophy, studies have shown that the goals of intervention are determined too frequently without significant input from the person receiving care and his or her social support system (62,63). A study of the extent to which occupational therapists practicing in adult physical rehabilitation settings met 23 patient and family involvement criteria showed that although involvement occurred, much potential for collaborative planning was unrealized (64). A study of housing decisions following discharge of persons recovering from stroke showed that in 86% of the cases, the affected family member was not included in the meetings of providers and family members where discharge-related decisions were made (65). Controlled studies have shown that active collaboration in rehabilitation goal setting increases client satisfaction with care (66).

When goals are set in collaboration with the individual receiving care, the motivation to learn and maintain a skill is better than if rehabilitation professionals or caregivers determine the goals. It also appears that agreement on goals may influence functional outcomes by establishing clearer and more realistic goals (67). Each self-care behavior should be evaluated to see if the individual is motivated to learn and maintain it. In a study by Chiou and Burnett (68), stroke patients' views of the importance of self-care skills were compared with the views of their occupational therapists and physical therapists. The results showed that the patients and therapists viewed the importance of specific self-care items differently. Moreover, a study comparing the rehabilitation goals and importance as viewed by adolescents and their parents showed a very low level of agreement (69). This suggests that rehabilitation goals and procedures should be individualized, that they should directly involve the clients themselves, and that assumptions about the importance of functional outcomes should be avoided.

The role of the rehabilitation team in self-care intervention is to set treatment goals collaboratively after determining the patient's preferences, resources, living situation, and limitations. One of the first options the professional and person receiving rehabilitation should explore concerning the performance of any self-care task is whether the task is necessary or desired. The individual may now choose not to perform some self-care tasks that were done before his or her illness. For example, a woman with hemiplegia who formerly rolled her hair on rollers on a daily basis may decide to have it cut in an easier-to-manage style rather than learn to use rollers with one hand. This type of decision should be based on individual preferences. Similarly, changes in societal styles and norms may also influence self-care goals, since greater diversity in clothing, hair style, and general appearance make it less likely that deviations from the norm will stand out.

In some instances, training procedures can be used to regain a desired skill. Following a cerebrovascular accident (CVA), for example, the therapist may be able to retrain the person to perform the task as it was performed before the CVA if there is sufficient return of voluntary movement. In some instances, the individual may no longer have the perceptual or physical capability to perform a task as before. However, he or she may be able to learn to accomplish the task using different movement patterns or with different body parts.

Environmental changes represent an additional array of intervention options that can be explored by the individual and his or her rehabilitation team as a means of gaining independence in self-care. In some instances simply rearranging the physical environment may allow the disabled person to perform tasks independently. For example, moving dishes to lower shelves so that the patient can reach them from a wheelchair would represent a modification of the environment requiring only simple rearrangement. Structural changes in the physical environment also may be necessary. These can include major changes such as the architectural modification of rooms to accommodate wheelchair movement or less extensive improvements such as replacing round doorknobs with lever handles for a person who has weak grasp, or installing bathroom rails and grab bars for persons with unsteady gait, or balance difficulties.

Bates (70) and others (71) have recommended that physical space also be considered from the standpoint of its *negotiability*, which suggests that in addition to being accessible, the environment must support its successful use with adaptive aids (if necessary) in a manner acceptable to the individual. For example, it does not matter that the doors to a food vending area at a workplace are wide enough for a wheelchair if persons with disability who can get there cannot use the machines themselves.

Assistive technology devices (ATDs) can be used to aid in the satisfactory performance of a desired task. These devices can range from simple, inexpensive articles, such as bathtub seats, to the use of expensive equipment such as computers for environmental control and communication. Many labor-saving devices are now widely available in catalogs and retail outlets catering to the general population. A line of fashionable apparel designed for easy dressing and maintenance is now available for persons with disability. The rehabilitation professional's role is to inform the patient of the existence and cost of these devices and to train the individual and caregiver in their use and maintenance.

Finally, assistance from other people for the partial or total completion of a desired task is another option available to the individual receiving care. Assistance may come from spouses, friends, or paid personal care attendants. The role of the professional in this case must be to instruct the individual and/or the care attendant on optimal approaches to working together for the completion of identified self-care tasks. Figure 43-1 provides a decision chart that describes the process of goal setting summarized in this section.

Collectively, the personal and environmental intervention options described in this section form the basis for collaborative decision making and treatment planning. It should be borne in mind that neither diagnosis alone nor the extent of impairment can serve as an adequate basis for planning self-care intervention. Together, the rehabilitation team and the individual receiving care must determine those approaches that represent the most realistic and achievable goals based on the abilities, values, and personal social circumstances of the recipient of care. Only in this way will optimal results be achieved after discharge.

ISSUES IN ADL EVALUATION

Granger (72) defines functional assessment as "a method for describing abilities and limitations and to measure an individual's use of the variety of skills included in performing tasks necessary to daily living, leisure activities, vocational pursuits, social interactions, and other required behaviors." Assessment must take place within a conceptual framework. A frequently cited model for this purpose is that of the World Health Organization's International Classification for Impairment, Disability and Handicap (ICIDH) (73). The ICIDH was revised in 2001 after a 7-year international revision effort, and is now

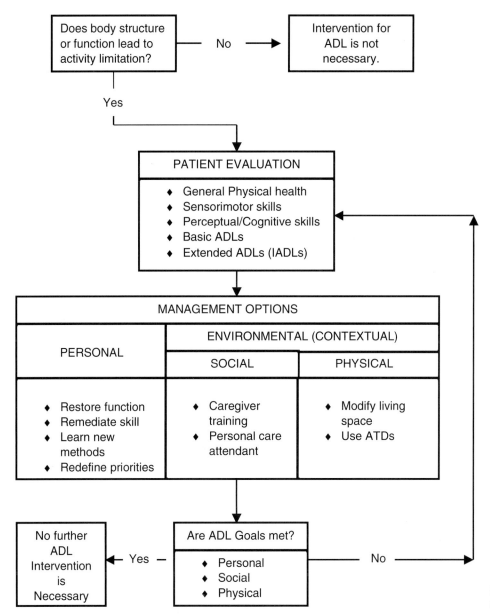

Figure 43-1. Decision-making process for self-care/ADL intervention.

called the International Classification of Functioning, Disability and Health, or ICF (74). This new classification structure broadens the overall scope of the taxonomy to include categories that conceptualize limitations to activities and participation as functional consequences that are influenced by environment, personal factors, and problems with body function or structure. The ICF also addresses concerns about terminology (such as use of the word *handicap*) and adopts terms and definitions that are global in application and reflect differences between developed and underdeveloped nations. The revised model for the ICF now has two parts, each with two components with defined domains and constructs as reflected in Table 43-2.

As a conceptual framework for considering self-care, the ICF provides a means for recognizing that self-care tasks take place within particular living environments and may be performed differently based on an individual's habits, culture, and social situation. This chapter attempts to recognize that these contexts should be reflected in the assessment process, the determination of patient goals, and the type and location of interventions chosen.

Assessment at any level has as its ultimate purpose the ability to make informed decisions. Scales and instruments designed to assess the ability of the individual to perform self-care tasks may assist in intervention or discharge planning by describing or documenting current abilities or monitoring changes in functional status. More global scales, which may include self-care components, are used to provide information on the effectiveness of rehabilitation programs, thus playing an important role in program evaluation.

Lawton has noted that formalized assessment of the patient's functioning yields a comprehensive picture of the strengths as well as the weaknesses of a patient and can provide objective evidence of clinical impressions (1). By providing a documented baseline of the individual's level of functioning, the formalized assessment facilitates communication with other members of the rehabilitation team.

Vash has suggested that because decisions made on the basis of assessment have the greatest ultimate impact on the individual receiving care, results of assessments should be shared with them (75). In this way, individuals receiving care enter into the decision-making process and become consultants.

TABLE 43-2.   International Classification of Functioning, Disability and Health, World Health Organization, 2001

	Part 1: Functioning and Disability		Part 2: Contextual Factors	
	Body Functions and Structures	Activities and Participation	Environmental Factors	Personal Factors
Domains	1. Body functions 2. Body structures	Life areas (tasks, actions)	External influences on functioning and disability	Internal influences on functioning and disability
Constructs	Change in body function (physiological) Change in body structures (anatomical)	Capacity Executing tasks in a standard environment Performance Executing tasks in the current environment	Facilitating or hindering impact of features of physical, social, and attitudinal world	Impact of attributes of the person

Adapted from World Health Organization. (2001). *International classification of functioning, disability and health.* World Health Organization. Available: www.who.int/icide/ICIDH-

Such involvement in decision making is viewed as an important collaborative dimension of the rehabilitation process.

Historical Development of Self-care Evaluation Tools

Assessment of the individual's ability to function independently has been conducted in medical rehabilitation for nearly 50 years. In an early review of the problems of measurement and evaluation in rehabilitation published in 1962, Kelman and Willner found that poorly conceptualized outcome criteria, lack of standardization, disagreement about methods, multidimensional scales, and the influence of the setting on performance were barriers to effective management (76).

Law and Letts reviewed several scales from the standpoint of clinical utility, scale construction, standardization, reliability, and validity (77). They concluded that the development of new scales should be curtailed, with greater effort devoted to the refinement and validation of existing scales. Other reviewers have reached similar conclusions (78–81). The challenges of functional assessment are summarized in the following sections.

Determining Capability Versus Characteristic Behavior

Current models of rehabilitation emphasize that function cannot be considered in isolation from its environmental context. This is made especially clear by the distinction between capability and actual behavior. Alexander and Fuhrer noted this distinction as it pertains to measures of functional ability (82). Measures of capability represent what the patient can do, whereas measures of actual behavior indicate what the patient does do.

Many self-care assessments in use during the past 30 years have been designed to measure what a patient is capable of doing within the traditional rehabilitation environment. An assessment of actual behavior, however, must take place in the daily living environment in which the person performs the tasks. This helps to explain why some studies have shown an apparent decline in patient function after discharge from the rehabilitation setting. Awareness of the distinction between capability and actual behavior and their relationship to the patient's environment has had an important impact on the development of new approaches to the assessment of self-care abilities.

As clients return home from hospitals, units, or residential facilities at an earlier stage, ease of administration becomes an issue for determination of client progress. Although one way of determining ability is through self-report or through reports by proxies living with the client, there is evidence that for certain categories, judgments of performance may not be sufficiently accurate to substitute for actual observation. A study of stroke survivors by Knapp and Hewison found that caregivers generally perceived stroke survivors as more functionally impaired than did the survivors themselves (83). A study by Kwakkel and others demonstrated that physical and occupational therapists consistently underestimated the degree of independence in ADL and level of recovery achieved by patients undergoing rehabilitation following stroke (84).

Contextual Factors in Self-care Evaluation

A complete assessment of self-care function should consider factors that include the patient's ability to manage devices that extend independence through environmental control; the family resources available to the patient in the environment to which he or she is to be discharged; the amount of time or energy required to perform tasks independently; and the degree of safety with which patients are able to perform tasks.

Developments in high technology for independent living have made it possible and important to assess people with severe disability in terms of their available movements and physical resources for controlling switches to activate environmental control units. Paradoxically, these devices are more likely to extend the patient's ability to perform instrumental ADL more proficiently than self-care tasks.

The inability to perform self-care tasks independently, of course, does not require discharge to institutional care if human resources are available in an alternative environment. Frequently, the client can, and does, rely extensively on the assistance of a partner, other family members, or friends, or personal care attendant to assist with self-care tasks. It can be argued that the presence of these resources, although commonly determined by the social worker in planning discharge, should be given early consideration in planning rehabilitation intervention.

Additional contextual considerations include the amount of time and energy required to perform the task independently versus the value of the task as perceived by the patient. It cannot be assumed, given competing requirements for time and energy, that all patients assign the independent performance of all self-care tasks the same degree of importance. Thus, the motivation to complete the task independently after discharge is likely to be a function of the alternatives available for task completion, the importance of the task to the patient, and the amount of time and energy required to perform the task independently in the face of competing demands.

Weingarden and Martin reported on a study of 10 postdischarge spinal cord–injured patients to determine if time was a factor in the decision to retain, modify, or completely delegate dressing activities (85). Although all 10 patients were capable of dressing independently at home, none did so routinely. The authors concluded that the person's concepts of appropriate time and energy expenditure are important considerations in postdischarge decisions on the use of functional skills. Another study by Pentland, Harvey, and Walker explored time use by 312 men with spinal cord injury living in the community. Their study showed that neither the level of the lesion, the level of functional independence, nor the setting predicted the amount of time spent in personal care, productivity, leisure, and sleep. Nor did the time spent in these activities predict outcomes such as life satisfaction, perceived health, or adjustment to disability (86).

The degree of safety with which a task is performed may be of obvious importance to the practitioner but may not be apparent to the patient or those caregivers in the environment who may be providing assistance with self-care tasks. It is therefore important that training in self-care assistance be provided as a part of the rehabilitation effort and that the ability of helpers to render this assistance in a safe and effective manner be assessed before the patient is discharged.

Defining Functional Outcomes

Many observers (87–89) have noted that increased emphasis on accountability and the need for determining the benefit–cost ratios of rehabilitation have revealed ambiguities and a lack of consensus regarding definitions of rehabilitation success. For example, gains in self-care ability, although important to the patient, may not be perceived as beneficial within a system that perceives employability as the sole criterion of success. This has created additional pressure for the development of evaluation tools that consider postdischarge function in the living setting.

Fortunately, the increased attention to these issues has resulted in increased research, which has encouraged the refinement or development and validation of several scales that assess self-care performance (90). Some of these scales possess characteristics suitable for program evaluation and research as well as clinical decision making. The need remains, however, for greater awareness of the problems associated with functional assessment, greater consensus on appropriate measurement items, and consistency in definitions and terminology. Although awareness of the importance of using instruments that possess necessary measurement characteristics has improved, a tendency to create ad hoc instrument modifications continues, making comparisons between studies more difficult.

Approaches to Obtaining Performance Data

Functional evaluation can be accomplished by direct and indirect means. Direct evaluation involves firsthand observation of skill performance. Indirect evaluation can occur by using client report (gathered through mailed surveys, face to face or with telephone interviews) or reported by proxies, such as members of the family or household. The validity of such indirect approaches is controversial (91). For example, McGinnis and colleagues compared therapists' ratings with patients' self-reports on the Barthel Index and found that the self-report scores were

significantly lower (92). Klein-Parris and colleagues found that interviews were more accurate when clients were high functioning and the items were less complex (93).

In addition to creating threats to reliability, indirect reporting of functional performance can create threats to validity. Kaufert notes that a number of factors make it difficult to establish the validity of functional ability indices (79). Specifically, he asserts that the impact of aids, adaptations, and helpers must be considered in measuring functional independence. Moreover, such factors as situational conditions, the patient's level of motivation, the professional perspective of the rater, and the role expectations of the patient can compromise efforts at establishing the validity of these scales.

Desirable Attributes of Self-care Scales

Recent reviews of functional status measures (94) have identified several criteria for evaluating the quality or suitability of scales. These criteria derive both from psychometric standards and from expert opinion, and include psychometric properties of validity, reliability, sensitivity to change, and methods for assessing scaling properties, such as Rasch analysis (95). Psychometric standards in the United States have been greatly influenced by The American Psychological Association and the American Educational Research Association (96). Within rehabilitation, the American Physical Therapy Association (APTA) published measurement standards (97) in 1991, and the American Congress of Rehabilitation Medicine developed Measurement Standards for Interdisciplinary Medical Rehabilitation in 1992 (98). These standards provide important guidelines for the appropriate use and interpretation of measures, including self-care scales. They also provide definitions of important terms relevant to test development, and refer to technical problems that should be avoided by developers and users. Table 43-3 summarizes important characteristics that can be used in evaluating, comparing, and selecting rehabilitation measures.

Resolving Measurement Problems in Functional Evaluation

A topic of considerable importance in the area of functional assessment is that of how numbers are assigned to performance observations and later interpreted. Most self-care scales use ordinal rankings to assign numbers to patient performance on selected items. Merbitz and colleagues have identified the limitations of such rankings, based on the characteristics of ordinal measurement scales (99). They point out that the properties of ordinal scales do not permit valid conclusions to be drawn on the summed or averaged scores obtained from them and that their misuse in this way is misleading and subject to invalid inferences. Further, because they are given equal weight in scoring, the implied assumption of most scales of functional ability is that the items being measured are equally important, either to the professional or to the individual being measured. This is clearly an invalid assumption.

Using techniques developed by George Rasch (100) and others (47), however, observations of functional ability (from items and persons) can be translated into linear measures. The logit unit of measurement produced by the Rasch model is the natural log of the odds of a correct response. This transformation allows the researcher to interpret the person and item information using the same units of measure. Once the scores for the persons and items have been transformed using Rasch scaling, other information about the persons and items can be obtained using a variety of statistical methods. These transformed scales possess the properties necessary for valid inferences (101). In

TABLE 43-3.   Desirable Criteria in Rehabilitation Measures of ADL Performance

Criterion	Explanation
Standardization	Scale has explicitly stated procedures for administration and scoring, performance data from a normal population, preferably of varying ages; information on the measurement properties of the scale (e.g., its computed reliability); and a statement of the necessary qualifications of the examiner. It is difficult to standardize scales that are useful both as measures of capability as well as measures of actual functioning, because of varying contextual factors.
Scalability	Scaling procedures serve to quantify a person's responses to a defined set of tasks so that they are distributed along a continuum of performance. For an assessment device to be considered a true scale, it must be established that the tasks performed will cumulatively yield a score or descriptor that represents increasing capability or independence.
Reliability	An acceptable scale should provide a reliable measure of the patient's level of performance. Reliability refers to a scale's accuracy and consistency in providing information, regardless of the time, setting, or person performing the assessment. Scales that have carefully defined methods and scoring criteria are likely to be more sensitive and consistent and present a more accurate picture of the patient than those that do not.
Validity	Validity is related to theoretical as well as methodological issues and depends on a number of factors. These include the extent to which the scores on the assessment are related to some external criterion, the degree to which the instrument contains items or tasks that represent the domain of interest, and the relationship of the instrument to other measures that collectively support various theoretical assumptions. A scale cannot be valid if it is not reliable.
Comprehensive	Self-care assessments are more useful if they determine performance levels for all basic ADL skills and are applicable to every diagnosis. Because patients have the universal need to perform or have performed for them basic self-care tasks, broad applicability is appropriate and facilitates comparison of research findings among differing patient groups. To the extent that extended ADLs can be assessed, a scale becomes more useful as a measure of independence everyday situations.
Performance Based	This characteristic eliminates measurement error due to selected observations or inaccurate memory. Although self-care abilities are increasingly being evaluated through interviews and surveys, this is most advisable only after discharge and if validation of such approaches has been demonstrated. Although performance-based scales should not emphasize speed, time can become an issue if the extent of time required makes it impractical.
Practical	The extent to which a scale is designed to facilitate decision-making and research is an important consideration in instrument selection. The number of items should be sufficient to permit reliability while requiring a reasonable length of time (i.e., 30 to 45 minutes) for administration. To the extent possible, items should not require equipment that would unduly limit locations where the scale could be administered. Scoring sheets should contain clear explanations of criteria and should be designed to permit accurate recording as well as coding for data processing. Terminology should be readily understandable, with abilities expressed using everyday language. The meaning of scores should clearly convey a patient's level of functional independence to professionals as well as to caregivers who will be living with the patient.

effect, these statistical transformations lead to scores, which are corrected for differences in items or raters. Such techniques are increasingly being applied to existing scales (102–104).

Patient Collaboration in Evaluation and Goal Setting

No discussion of functional evaluation is complete without a consideration of the values that may be reflected in the process. Although functional assessment is a judgmental process, it should not be unnecessarily value laden. In fact, the rehabilitation goal of independent functioning itself reflects a societal value not shared to the same extent by all cultures. There are profound differences in the cultural heritages and life experiences of individuals, and these differences bring differing sets of values about independence and self-care to the rehabilitation setting. Effective management of the patient requires an appreciation of these differences, and an appreciation that interdependence rather than independence is a condition typical of societal groups. It may therefore be important for the overall functional evaluation to include methods for determining premorbid activity patterns and leisure interests as well as values and attitudes toward assistance. Characteristic methods for performing basic and extended ADLs, as well as the characteristic aspects of the environment in which these have been performed, may be important information in planning successful intervention strategies for management of personal care and other activities of daily living necessary for life satisfaction and quality.

Selected Measures of Basic ADL (Self-care)

Although dozens of instruments designed to assess personal or self-care performance have been reported in the literature, con-

sensus has not been achieved for use of a single scale. Scales range from those that focus on personal or self-care ADL skills (basic ADLs) to those that focus on instrumental ADL or extended ADL skills. Still others are more global and include physical functioning and/or more extended ADL skills. These have been called *global scales.*

One such global scale is the Functional Independence Measure (FIM). The past decade has shown a marked growth in the use of the FIM developed in the United States by Granger and colleagues (72) in the 1980s and now translated into several languages. The FIM and its associated measurement systems have been adopted as a key part of decisions influencing public funding of rehabilitation services in the United States. The FIM has not been embraced universally, however, and the Barthel Index, developed by Mahoney and Barthel (105), with its modifications, continues to be used extensively throughout the world.

Besides the Barthel Index and the FIM, a handful of scales have demonstrated sufficient validity and frequency in the literature to warrant their review here. This review is not intended to be exhaustive, and it is acknowledged that there are other measures with self-care components that have been developed or are in use for specialized purposes that are not described here. To gain a complete picture of the client's level of function and community reintegration within the new WHO framework requires that items pertaining to household maintenance and community functioning also be considered. For this reason, the assessment of basic self-care items is often accompanied by additional items relating to household and community functioning.

The following paragraphs report the composition, measurement properties, and scoring of several scales. Brief summaries of selected studies describing their use with varying patient populations are also provided. Where available, evidence reporting reliability and validity is summarized. The scales to be reviewed in this section are the PULSES Profile (106), the Katz Index of Independence in ADL (107), the Barthel Index, and the FIM (108). These scales are reviewed here in the order of their development and appearance in the literature.

THE BARTHEL INDEX

In 1965, Mahoney and Barthel published a weighted scale for measuring basic ADL with chronically disabled patients (Table 43-4). Described as "a simple index of independence to score the ability of a patient with a neuromuscular or musculoskeletal disorder to care for himself," the Barthel Index included 10 items, including feeding, transfers, personal grooming and hygiene, bathing, toileting, walking, negotiating stairs, and controlling bowel and bladder. Items are scored differentially according to a weighted scoring system that assigns points based on independent or assisted performance. For example, a person who needs assistance in eating would receive five points, whereas independence in eating would be awarded 10 points. A patient with a maximum score of 100 points is defined as continent, able to eat and dress independently, walk at least a block, and climb and descend stairs. The authors were careful to note that a maximum score did not necessarily signify independence, since instrumental ADLs such as cooking, housekeeping, and socialization are not assessed.

The Barthel Index may be the most widely studied and used self-care scale globally. Several studies have shown that the scale has acceptable psychometric properties, including that it is sensitive to change over time, that it is a significant predictor of rehabilitation outcome, and that it relates significantly with other measures of patient status. Granger and colleagues (64) reported the stability (i.e., test–retest reliability) of the Barthel Index as 0.89, whereas interrater reliability coefficients were above 0.95. One study of interrater reliability between nursing staff and nonclinical research assistant showed that although overall agreement was within acceptable boundaries, two items out of 10 showed weakness for agreement (transfer and dressing) (109). Shortened versions of the Barthel Index (BI-3 and BI-5) have also been developed, and these have shown evidence of satisfactory psychometric characteristics and predictive validity acceptable for outcome use (110,111).

The initial Barthel Index score was found to be the most reliable predictor of final rehabilitation outcome in study of stroke patients conducted by Hertanu and colleagues (112). That study concluded that the Barthel Index was a more reliable predictor of rehabilitation outcome than estimates based on computed tomography showing the extent of the lesion after cerebrovascular accident. The Barthel Index also has been found to correlate significantly with type of discharge and shorter length of stay for patients with cerebrovascular accident (113,114) and independent living outcome for patients with spinal cord injury (115), as well as participation of young adults with disabilities (116). Scores on the Barthel Index and the PULSES Profile have been shown to correlate substantially (117).

A modified version of the Barthel Index, the Extended Barthel Index (EBI) (118), was developed to address perceived limitations of the FIM and existing Barthel Index by adding items for comprehension, expression, social interaction, problem solving, memory/learning/orientation, and vision/neglect. The Extended Barthel Index was administered to 342 neurologic patients in a study that showed the Extended Barthel Index to be a reliable, valid, and practical instrument that is sensitive to changes over time. Because of the manner in which the new items are administered, rater training is neces-

TABLE 43-4. Barthel Index Items and Scoring Weights

	With Help	Independent
1. Feeding (If food needs to be cut up = help)	5	10
2. Moving from wheelchair to bed and return (includes sitting up in bed)	5–10	15
3. Personal toilet (wash face, comb hair, shave, clean teeth)	0	5
4. Getting on and off toilet, (handling clothes, wipe, flush)	5	10
5. Bathing self	0	5
6. Walking on level surface (or, if unable to walk, propel wheelchair)	10 0[a]	15 5[a]
7. Ascend and descend stairs	5	10
8. Dressing (includes tying shoes, fastening fasteners)	5	10
9. Controlling bowels	5	10
10. Controlling bladder	5	10

[a]Score only if unable to walk.
A patient scoring 100 BI is cotinent, feeds himself, dresses himself, gets up out of bed and chairs, bathes himself, walks at least a block, and can ascend and descend stairs. This does not mean that he is able to live alone; he may not be able to cook, keep house, and meet the public, but he is able to get along without attendant care.
From Mahoney FI, Barthel DW. Functional evaluation: the Barthel index. *Maryland State Med* 1965;14:61–65.

sary. Time required to administer the Extended Barthel Index was described as significantly shorter than the time needed to administer the FIM.

THE KATZ INDEX OF INDEPENDENCE IN ACTIVITIES OF DAILY LIVING

The Katz Index of Independence in ADL was developed to study results of treatment and prognosis in the elderly and in those with chronic illness (119). Development of the index was originally based on observations of a large number of activities performed by a group of patients with fracture of the hip.

The index is based on an evaluation of the functional independence of patients in bathing, dressing, going to the toilet, transfers, continence, and feeding. Using three descriptors for rating independence in each of six subscales, the rater is able to derive an overall grade of independence with the aid of specific rating criteria. Depending on the determined level of independence, a patient is graded as A, B, C, D, E, F, G, or Other. According to the scale, a patient graded as A would be functioning independently in all six functions, whereas a patient graded as G would be dependent in all rated functions. Patients graded as Other are dependent in at least two functions but not classifiable as C, D, E, or F. Through observations over a defined period of time, the observer determines whether the patient is assisted or whether the patient functions on his or her own when performing the six activities. Assistance is classified as active personal assistance, directive assistance, or supervision.

In studies of the Katz Index involving more than 1,000 patients, the scale was found to result in an ordered pattern, so that a person able to perform a given activity independently also would be able to perform all activities done by those graded at lower levels (68). This hierarchical structure correctly classifies the functional ability of patients 86% of the time and reflects a desirable property of scalability (120).

The Katz Index of Independence in ADL has been used as a tool to accumulate information about recovery after cerebrovascular accident (121,122) and amputation from peripheral vascular disease (123,124), as a means of providing information about the need for care among patients with rheumatoid arthritis (68), and as an instrument to study information about the dynamics of disability in the aging process. Brorsson and Asberg used the scale in a study of internal medicine patients in a general hospital in Sweden (125). Their study found a high degree of interrater reliability as well as high coefficients of scalability.

Selected Measures of Instrumental ADL

Increasingly, as rehabilitation professionals give greater attention to the functional context of the patient, more consideration is being paid to instrumental ADLs, or the individual's ability to perform those tasks beyond basic self-care necessary to live in the community. Wade has suggested that these types of ADLs be described as Extended Activities of Daily Living (EADL) (90). Other terms in use for similar scale items are social ADL and advanced ADL (126). In this section, several scales that focus specifically on instrumental ADL (extended ADL) performance are reviewed, including the Assessment of Motor and Process Skills, the Nottingham Extended Activities of Daily Living Scale, and the Frenchay Activities Index (FAI).

ASSESSMENT OF MOTOR AND PROCESS SKILLS

The Assessment of Motor and Process Skills (AMPS) is an observational evaluation that is used to simultaneously examine both the ability to perform instrumental activities of daily living and the underlying motor and process capacities necessary for successful performance (127). The AMPS is an assessment system that requires a clinician to observe a person performing instrumental activities of daily living as he or she would normally perform them. The individual to be measured selects two or three familiar tasks from among more than 50 possibilities described in the AMPS manual. After the observation, the clinician rates the person's performance in two skill areas: instrumental ADL motor and instrumental ADL process. Table 43-5 lists the motor and process areas. Motor skills are defined as observable actions that are supported by underlying abilities, including postural control, mobility, coordination, and strength. The AMPS motor items represent an observable taxonomy of actions used to move the body and objects during actual performance. Process skills reflect the organization and execution of a series of actions over time in order to complete a specified task. Thus, process skills may be related to a person's underlying attentional, conceptual, organizational, and adaptive capabilities. Like the AMPS motor skill items, the AMPS process skill items represent a universal taxonomy of actions that can be observed during any task performance.

During each instrumental ADL task performed for the assessment, and for each of the 16 motor and 20 process skills (see Table 43-5), the person is rated on a four-point scale: 1 = deficit, 2 = ineffective, 3 = questionable, and 4 = competent. The raw ordinal scores are analyzed using the Rasch approach referred to as many-faceted Rasch analysis. This approach rests on a mathematical model of likelihood that the person will receive a given score on each of the motor and process skill items. The observed counts of the raw scores of instrumental ADL motor and process skill items constitute ordinal (ranked) data. These counts are converted by logistic transformation into additive, linear measures. Once the raw scores are computer analyzed, the derived person ability measures (motor and process) become estimates of the person's position on the two AMPS

TABLE 43-5. AMPS Motor and Process Skill Items by Group

Motor Skill Groups and Items	Process Skill Groups and Items
Posture	Using knowledge
Stabilizes	Chooses
Aligns	Uses
Positions	Handles
Mobility	Heeds
Walks	Inquires
Reaches	Notices
Bends	Temporal organization
Coordination	Initiates
Coordinates	Continues
Manipulates	Sequences
Flows	Terminates
Strength and effort	Space and objects
Moves	Searches
Transports	Gathers
Lifts	Organizes
Calibrates	Restores
Grips	Adaptation
Energy	Accommodates
Endures	Adjusts
Paces	Navigates
	Benefits
	Energy
	Paces
	Attends

Adapted from Fisher WP, Fisher AG. Applications of Rasch analysis to studies in occupational therapy. *Phys Med Rehab Clin North Am* 1993;4:493–516.

scales. That is, the AMPS motor and process scales represent continua of increasing instrumental ADL motor or process skill ability, and the person's estimated position on the AMPS motor and process scales, expressed in logits, represents his or her instrumental ADL motor and process skill ability (128).

The many-faceted Rasch analysis used in the AMPS allows simultaneous calibration of three aspects of performance: item easiness, task simplicity, and rater leniency. Each of these item characteristics is determined by using a probabilistic model. The ability measure produced by the Rasch analysis is the estimated person ability plotted on a linear scale and is defined by the skill item easiness and task simplicity but adjusted for the rater who scored the task performance (134,135).

Because the person ability measures on the AMPS are adjusted for task simplicity, a clinician can use the ability measure to predict whether a person possesses the motor and process skills necessary to perform tasks that are more difficult than those the person was observed performing. Also, since the AMPS includes 50 possible instrumental ADL tasks and each person is observed performing only two or three, the number of possible alternative task combinations is very large. Regardless of how many different tasks the individual performs, however, the ability measure will always be adjusted to account for the ease and simplicity of those particular tasks, so direct comparisons can be made among persons even though they performed completely different tasks.

Several investigations using the AMPS with persons who have psychiatric, orthopedic, neurologic (129), cognitive (130, 131), and developmental disabilities (132,133) have been reported. The ability of the AMPS to enable analysis of the separate contributions of motor and process variables has provided support for theoretical assumptions about the specific variables contributing to task limitations in various conditions. Validity studies have suggested that the AMPS can help predict home safety (134) and measure improvements following intervention for multiple sclerosis (135) and stroke (136). The AMPS has demonstrated consistency across different cultural groups (137,138). These investigations have established the reliability and validity of the AMPS. The AMPS is a new instrument and approaches the assessment of functional performance in a non-traditional manner, using many-faceted Rasch analysis with clients selecting the item to be performed from an inventory of possible instrumental ADL items. This approach has advantages, but it also has disadvantages. The logic of the Rasch approach is not familiar to many rehabilitation providers, and the mathematical modeling used to develop the scoring system is complex. For these reasons its routine clinical use outside of research may be less practical than other measures. However, the AMPS and other Rasch-based instruments are alternatives to traditional assessment approaches and represent an important new dimension in the evolution of functional assessment.

NOTTINGHAM EXTENDED ACTIVITIES OF DAILY LIVING INDEX

The Nottingham Extended Activities of Daily Living Index (NEADL) was developed by Nouri and Lincoln (139) in 1987 and is widely used throughout Europe and in other countries. This self-report scale has 21 items organized into four sections, which can serve as subscales. The sections include mobility, kitchen tasks, domestic tasks, and leisure activities. Scoring is along a four-item range of discrete categories, ranging from not done at all to done alone easily. Unfortunately, there are no guidelines for assigning scores. Because of the range of extended ADL tasks reported, the scale has intuitive appeal as an outcome measure of rehabilitation and social participation. Table 43-6 lists specific items included in the Nottingham EADL.

A growing literature on use of the scale is beginning to demonstrate that it is a suitable instrument for evaluating extended ADL function in the community. Although most reported studies involve subjects who have received rehabilitation following stroke (140–142), the measure has been used with other diagnostic groups such as those with pulmonary problems (143–146), elderly persons in the community (147,148), and patients with hip replacement (149). For this latter group, Harwood and Ebrahim compared the responsiveness of the Nottingham Extended ADL with two other measures. In that study, the NEADL was not viewed as sensitive to change in function as the SF-36 or the London Handicap Scale as a measure of activity and social participation for patients with hip replacement. Despite this the scales have shown evidence of acceptable scalability, concurrent validity, and construct validity. For example, Hsueh and colleague used the Nottingham Extended ADL in a study of stroke patients in Taiwan and found that with minor modification to two items, the Nottingham Extended ADL had satisfactory scalability and reproducibility and correlated with age and scores on the Barthel Index (150). The scale has also been useful as a measure of the effectiveness of rehabilitation strategies, such as ADL training (151).

FRENCHAY ACTIVITIES INDEX

The FAI was developed initially for use in clinical social work for stroke patients and has emerged as a frequently used measure of extended ADL (152,153). The index is designed as a mailed questionnaire to be completed by self-report. The FAI consists of 15 items divided into two sections or subscales. The first section pertains to activities performed within the 3 months preceding completion of the scale and includes standard mobility, household maintenance, and meal preparation items. The second section pertains to items performed in the 6 months before scale completion and reports on work, leisure, travel, and household/car maintenance. Items are scored on a four-point scale from 0 to 3 according to very-well-defined guidelines.

Turnbull and others studied 1,280 people to construct preliminary norms and to determine evidence of reliability and validity. They concluded that the FAI is reliable and shows good evidence of validity with an elderly population but would benefit from adding items relating to sport, physical ex-

TABLE 43-6. Nottingham Extended Activities of Daily Living Index				
Answers	Not at All	With Help	Alone with Difficulty	Alone Easily
Mobility Questions—Do you:				
Walk around outside?				
Climb stairs?				
Get in and out of the car?				
Walk over uneven ground?				
Cross roads?				
Travel on public transport?				
In the Kitchen—Do you:				
Manage to feed yourself?				
Manage to make yourself a hot drink?				
Take hot drinks from one room to another?				
Do the washing up?				
Make yourself a hot snack?				
Domestic Tasks—Do you:				
Manage your own money when you are out?				
Wash small items of clothing?				
Do your own shopping?				
Do a full clothes wash?				
Leisure Activities—Do you:				
Read newspapers or books?				
Use the telephone?				
Go out socially?				
Manage your own garden?				
Drive a car?				

ercise, and caring for children. This would make it a tool more useful for a broader segment of the population (154). Green and colleagues studied the test-retest reliability of the FAI and other scales of stroke outcome. They found that the FAI had only moderate reliability using kappa coefficients (mean differences for items 0.6 ± 7.1) and had higher random error when stroke survivors were measured twice within a 1-week interval (155).

Although most of the studies using the FAI have been related to outcomes following stroke (156–159), the index has also been used for other populations, including those with complex disabilities (160), patients with venous leg ulcers (161), and caregivers (162). The scale has also been translated for and used to study rehabilitation outcomes in Japan (163), China (164), Denmark (165), and Spain (166).

Carter and colleague compared the postal version of the FAI with an interviewer-administered version, using a population of stroke survivors discharged from the hospital. Kappa statistics for individual item agreement for the subjects tested ranged from .35 to 1.00. Overall, the correlation between total scores was .94. Piercy and associates estimated the interrater reliability of the FAI as .93 in a study of interview administered versions of the scale by two raters (167). A study by Schuling and others suggested that the reliability of the FAI could be improved by deleting two items and by creating two subscale scores, one for domestic and the other for outdoor activities (168). Studies using the FAI and measures of basic ADL (particularly the Barthel Index) have demonstrated that the scales measure different factors and may be useful in combination (164).

Combined ADL/IADL Measures

THE FUNCTIONAL INDEPENDENCE MEASURE

The FIM evolved from a Task Force of the American Congress of Rehabilitation Medicine and the American Academy of Physical Medicine and Rehabilitation, which met to develop a reliable and valid instrument that could be used to document the severity of disability as well as the outcomes of rehabilitation treatment as part of a uniform data system (169).

The FIM consists of 18 items organized under six categories, including self-care (e.g., eating, grooming, bathing, upper-body dressing, lower-body dressing, and toileting); sphincter control (i.e., bowel and bladder management); mobility (e.g., transfers for toilet, tub or shower, and bed, chair, wheelchair); locomotion (e.g., walking, wheelchair, and stairs); communication, including comprehension and expression; and social cognition (e.g., social interaction, problem solving, and memory). Using the FIM, patients are assessed on each item with a seven-point scale, ranging from complete independence (value = 7) to complete dependence (total assistance required = 1 (Fig. 43-2) (170).

The original components of the FIM were developed under a federal grant to the State University of New York at Buffalo. The FIM is now part of a system of data collection and outcome under proprietary license held through association with that university. The Uniform Data System for Medical Rehabilitation (UDSMR) holds the rights to the FIM instrument. In 1995, the Centers for Medicare and Medicaid Services (CMS) of the United States federal government (formerly known as HCFA) entered into an agreement with UDSMR to use the FIM system as the basis for the rehabilitation prospective payment system and to use the FIM instrument as part of a new patient assessment instrument known as The Inpatient Rehabilitation Facility–Patient Admission and Information Report (IRF–PAI). A

mastery test has been developed by UDSMR to encourage consistency among users of the FIM system (171).

Several studies have shown that the FIM is a reliable instrument. Ottenbacher and colleagues reported a metaanalysis of 11 reliability studies in 1996. Those 11 investigations included a total of 1,568 patients and produced 221 reliability coefficients. The analysis demonstrated a median interrater reliability for the total FIM of .95 and median test–retest and equivalence reliability values of .95 and .92, respectively. The median reliability values for the six FIM subscales ranged from .95 for Self-care to .78 for Social Cognition. For the individual FIM items, median reliability values varied from .90 for Toilet Transfer to .61 for Comprehension. The reliability of motor subscale items was generally higher than that for items in other subscales.

A large number of validity studies have been reported since the inception of the FIM that have demonstrated that the scale has concurrent (172–177), predictive (178–181), and construct validity (182–188). These results have also been demonstrated with foreign (translated) versions of the scale (189–192). Studies have also been conducted comparing various modes of test administration, including interviews, telephone reports, and direct observation (193). These suggest that the FIM retains acceptable reliability under different conditions of administration.

Some limitations regarding scalability and sensitivity in the FIM have been noted. A comprehensive analysis of the FIM reported in 1990 found that the burden of care for a person with a disability is a two-dimensional concept, reflecting both motor and cognitive dimensions. Consequently, the FIM was found to have acceptable scalability only when broken down into two parts that treat the 13 motor and five cognitive items as separate subscales. Hall and associates reported ceiling effects of the FIM at rehabilitation discharge, and particularly at 1 year after injury in a moderate to severely injured TBI population (194). Muecke and colleagues (195) studied the FIM as a predictor of rehabilitation outcome in lower-limb amputees. The FIM did not predict outcome of patients who were functioning lower (in bottom quartile) at admission, but it did predict rehabilitation success well in patients functioning at a higher level at admission.

To address the issue of sensitivity for use with brain injury survivors, an adjunct to the FIM, the Functional Assessment Measure (FAM) was developed by clinicians representing each of the disciplines in an inpatient rehabilitation program. Twelve items were developed in the areas of cognitive, behavioral, communication, and community functioning (196). These items are not designed to stand alone, but are intended to be added to the 18 items of the FIM. The total 30-item scale combination is referred to as the FIM+FAM and requires approximately 35 minutes to administer. In 1995 a users group in the United Kingdom developed a special version of the FAM, keeping the seven-level structure, but attempting to improve the objectivity of scoring for 10 items viewed as more subjective in scoring (197,198). According to Hall and Johnston the FAM appears to add sensitivity beyond the FIM only for post-acute rehabilitation functional assessment (199). Although the scale items have shown acceptable reliability (200), a 2-year study by Gurka and colleagues showed that the addition of the FAM items only modestly increased the ability to predict employability and community integration in survivors of brain injury (201).

Another adaptation of the FIM, the Self Reported Functional Measure, has been developed to quantify the ability of patients to care for themselves when they enter rehabilitation treatment and to chart their progress until they are discharged into the community or to another facility. Recent studies of the Self Re-

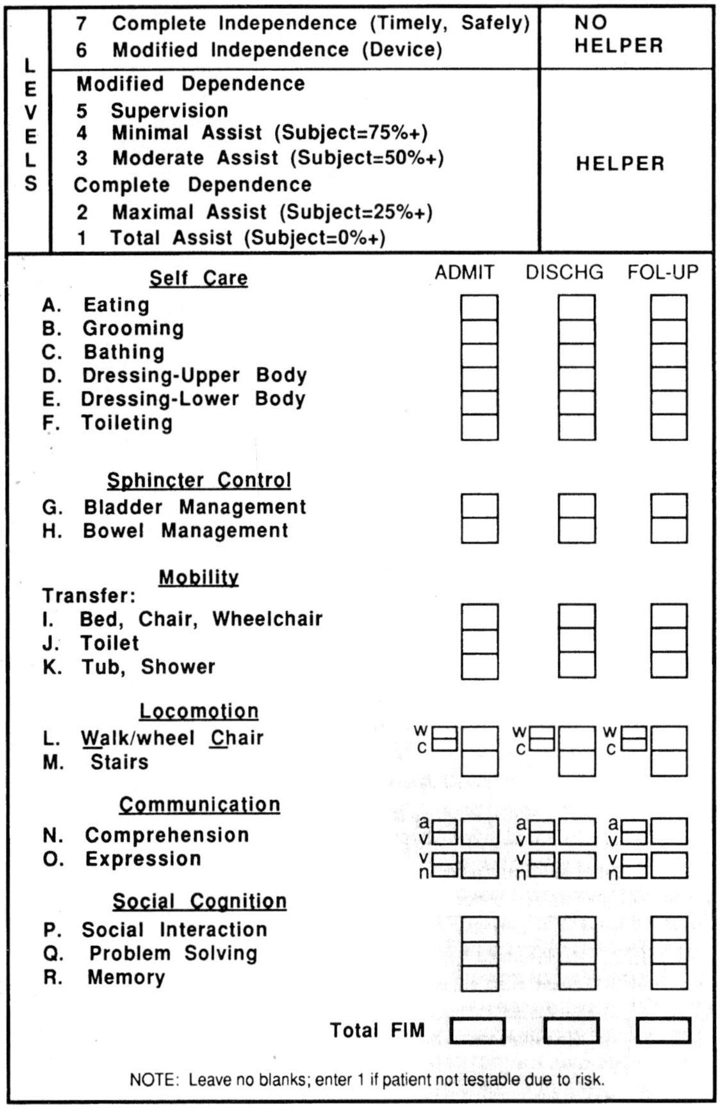

LEVELS		
	7 Complete Independence (Timely, Safely) 6 Modified Independence (Device)	NO HELPER
	Modified Dependence 5 Supervision 4 Minimal Assist (Subject=75%+) 3 Moderate Assist (Subject=50%+) Complete Dependence 2 Maximal Assist (Subject=25%+) 1 Total Assist (Subject=0%+)	HELPER

	ADMIT	DISCHG	FOL-UP
Self Care			
A. Eating			
B. Grooming			
C. Bathing			
D. Dressing-Upper Body			
E. Dressing-Lower Body			
F. Toileting			
Sphincter Control			
G. Bladder Management			
H. Bowel Management			
Mobility			
Transfer:			
I. Bed, Chair, Wheelchair			
J. Toilet			
K. Tub, Shower			
Locomotion			
L. Walk/wheel Chair	w c	w c	w c
M. Stairs			
Communication			
N. Comprehension	a v	a v	a v
O. Expression	v n	v n	v n
Social Cognition			
P. Social Interaction			
Q. Problem Solving			
R. Memory			
Total FIM			

NOTE: Leave no blanks; enter 1 if patient not testable due to risk.

Figure 43-2. Functional Independence Measure. (Copyright 1990 by the Research Foundation of the State University of New York. Reprinted with permission.)

ported Functional Measure show that the instrument predicts inpatient hospitalization but not outpatient health-care use (202) and that it can also predict caregiver hours (203).

THE PULSES PROFILE

The PULSES Profile, published by Moskowitz and McCann in 1957, has been described as the first major formalized functional assessment instrument to be widely used in American medical rehabilitation settings (204,205). The instrument evolved out of a perceived need for a more structured approach to functional assessment and represented an adaptation of a military classification system used by U.S. and Canadian armed forces in the 1940s to classify the overall physical status of military personnel. PULSES is an acronym formed of initials representing the subsections comprising the overall instrument, which is of the global variety. These subsections are designed to measure *P*hysical condition, performance using the *U*pper extremities, mobility as permitted by the *L*ower extremity function, communication and *S*ensory performance, bowel and bladder or *E*xcretory performance, and psychosocial *S*tatus. Within each section, numerical grades ranging from 1 (i.e., no abnormalities) to 4 (i.e., severe abnormalities limiting independence) are assigned based on the patient's functional ability as assessed by the examining professional.

The original PULSES Profile had notable weaknesses, including a lack of specifically defined criteria and an underlying assumption that impairment equates with disability. The profile was modified by Granger and associates in 1975 to include a scoring system and improved rating criteria (206). Studies since that time have demonstrated its usefulness in classifying the functional status of a wide variety of patient samples (207–210). Marshall and colleagues compared the PULSES Profile with the Functional Independence Measure in predicting the discharge of 197 patients from a stroke rehabilitation unit. The study showed that the PULSES Profile had an internal consistency of .74 and that it correlated highly with FIM admission and discharge scores (211). The PULSES Profile was able to accurately predict discharge from the unit. Research suggests that the PULSES Profile may be more useful in detecting change before discharge and is most effective in those situations in which substantial changes in functional status are likely to occur, such as in a patients with cerebrovascular accident or spinal cord injury (212).

CANADIAN OCCUPATIONAL PERFORMANCE MEASURE

The Canadian Occupational Performance Measure (COPM) is a criterion measure developed in consultation with the Department of National Health and Welfare and the Canadian Association of Occupational Therapy (213–215). The COPM incorporates roles and role expectations from within the client's living environment using a semistructured, individualized interview approach (139).

The COPM encompasses the areas of self-care, productivity, and leisure as the primary outcomes being measured but can also include an assessment of specific ability limitations in order to gain an understanding of why the client may be having difficulty in a particular functional area. The COPM was designed to help therapists establish functional performance goals based on client perceptions of need and to measure change objectively in defined problem areas.

The COPM measures the client's identified problem areas in daily functioning. In those instances where a client cannot identify problem areas (e.g., a young child, an individual with dementia) a caregiver may respond to the measure. The COPM considers the importance to the person, of the occupational performance areas as well as the client's satisfaction with present performance. The instrument takes into account client roles and role expectations and, in focusing on the client's own environments and priorities, ensures the relevance of identified areas in the assessment process.

The COPM can be used to measure a client outcome with different objectives for treatment, whether it is developmental, maintenance, restoration of function, or prevention of future disability. Because it is generic (not diagnosis specific) and can be used across different age groups, it has wide applicability. The instrument is administered in a five-step process using a semistructured interview conducted by the therapist together with the client and/or caregiver. The five steps in the process include problem identification/definition, initial assessment, occupational therapy intervention, reassessment, and calculation of change scores. The original version included a procedure whereby rated importance was used as a weighting factor in calculating performance and satisfaction scores. However, this has been eliminated in the second edition based on findings from pilot studies that indicated the equivalence of scores whether or not importance weights are included.

In administration of the measure, problems are identified and defined jointly with the client and appropriate caregivers. Once the problem areas are defined, the client is asked to rate the importance of each activity on a scale of 1 to 10. The client (or caregiver) is also required to rate his or her ability to perform the specified activities and his or her satisfaction with performance on the same scale of 1 to 10. These scores are then compared across time. There are two scores: one for performance and one for satisfaction. Administration time takes 30 to 40 minutes on average.

During initial development, the authors reported findings on an extensive pilot study of the COPM that involved administration in several countries, including New Zealand, Greece, and Great Britain (216). The scale has since been translated and used in several additional countries. Early findings indicated that the average change scores for performance and satisfaction were approximately 1.5 times the standard deviation of the scores, indicating sensitivity of the instrument to perceived changes in occupational performance by clients. The COPM is seen as a flexible instrument and appeals to clinicians who value the client-centered philosophy underlying its development (217). Some reports have indicated that patients occasionally experience difficulty with the process of self-rating of performance (218), and the suitability of the measure for use with patients demonstrating cognitive or affective difficulties has been questioned, although some studies have shown these concerns to be overstated (219).

Reliability studies have reported intraclass correlation coefficients of $r = 0.90$ and above for both performance and satisfaction scores (220). Trombly and colleagues studied the achievement of goals by adults with traumatic brain injury and found that client perceptions of progress as measured by the COPM were accompanied by improved scores on scales of independent living and social participation (221). A comparative study of rehabilitation settings for survivors of stroke using the COPM showed that participant satisfaction with goal achievement was independent of setting and consistent with the results of performance measured by instrumental ADL (IADL) and health outcome scales (222). A study by Simmons and colleagues found that the use of the COPM in combination with the FIM enhances accuracy in prediction of outcomes for rehabilitative services for persons in adult physical disabilities settings (223). These and several other studies have demonstrated that the COPM correlates well with other measures of ADL outcome, motivates active participation and adherence to rehabilitation regimens, and improves satisfaction with services for a variety of diagnostic groups and ages (224–231). The COPM appears to provide useful and important information regarding self-care performance from the standpoint of the recipient of care.

Self-care Evaluation of Children

Information presented to this point has been based on self-care and ADL assessment as it pertains to adults. It is worth noting, however, that self-care assessment of the pediatric patient requires a number of special considerations. These pertain to incorporating developmental milestones into the structure of the assessment, interacting with the child during the assessment process, and reporting information to parents. Two instruments have attained sufficient use to establish their value in the clinical setting as useful measures of functional performance in children. These are the WeeFIM and the Pediatric Evaluation of Disability Inventory. Specific information on these instruments is provided next.

FUNCTIONAL INDEPENDENCE MEASURE FOR CHILDREN (WEEFIM)

In 1987, the FIM was adapted to meet the need for a reliable and valid functional assessment tool that would be useful in measuring the severity of disability in children. The resulting Functional Independence Measure for Children (WeeFIM) (232) was designed to measure functional ability in a developmental context. Each of the 18 items is considered in relation to chronological age, developmental norms, and realistic expectations for children from 6 months to 7 years of age. Rather than replacing assessment tools that analyze individual component skills of ADL, the WeeFIM is meant to give clinicians an overall view of the child's actual daily performance in six areas, including self-care, mobility, locomotion, sphincter control, communication, and social cognition. The WeeFIM uses the same seven-point ordinal scale to assess level of function as its parent, the FIM.

Studies of the WeeFIM have shown a strong correlation between the scale scores and age, with the subscale scores involving gross and fine motor skill demonstrating the highest correlations (233). Data showed that tasks on the WeeFIM demonstrate a developmental sequence, with an observed positive relationship between the complexity of tasks and the age at which children achieve independence in their performance (234). Repeated evaluations of the scale and comparisons of personal and telephone interview ratings have demonstrated that the scale has good stability and equivalence reliability (235). In different studies and under varying conditions, the intraclass correlation coefficients for the six subscales have ranged from 0.73 to 0.99, and test–retest reliability has been estimated at 0.98 for children with disabilities and 0.99 for able-bodied children (235). Total score intraclass correlation coefficients values have consistently been greater than 0.95 (236). Comparisons of personal assessment and telephone interview ratings have found the scale to be consistent for items, subscales, and total test scores under those varying conditions of administration (235).

Comparisons of WeeFIM scores with other developmental tests, including the Vineland Adaptive Behaviors Scales and the Battelle Developmental Inventory Screening Test, found subscale correlations of 0.42 to 0.92 and total score correlations of 0.72 to 0.94 (236). Studies have shown that the WeeFIM demonstrates acceptable validity in tracking the developmental status of children without disability and across cultures (237–239) and those with genetic impairments (240), heart defects (241), cerebral palsy (242,243), spina bifida (244), Down's syndrome (245), and Rett syndrome. It is also useful in documenting progress and development following extreme preterm (246) and very-low-birth-weight delivery (247,248), primary brain tumors (249), and dorsal rhizotomy (250), in addition to rehabilitation following traumatic brain injury (251,252) and pediatric spinal injury (253).

PEDIATRIC EVALUATION OF DEVELOPMENT INVENTORY

The Pediatric Evaluation of Development Inventory (PEDI) is described as a comprehensive assessment that samples key functional capabilities and performance in children from the ages of 6 months to 7.5 years. The scale is designed to be used with children having a variety of disabling conditions and can be administered by professionals or by structured interview, or parental report. The PEDI addresses both capability and performance in the areas of self-care, mobility, and social function. Capability is determined by identifying the functional skills for which a child has demonstrated mastery, with scores reflected on the Functional Skills Scales. Two other subscales are provided. One is the Caregiver Assistance Scale, which measures the extent of help provided the child during typical daily situations, and the other is the Modifications Scale, a measure of environmental modifications and equipment used routinely in daily activities. The PEDI has 197 functional skill items and 20 items that measure caregiver assistance and environmental modifications. The scale was designed to detect functional deficit and developmental delay, to monitor progress, and to act as an outcomes measure (254). Table 43-7 lists item domains and complex activities included in the PEDI.

During development of the PEDI, content validity was determined through use of a multidisciplinary panel of experienced experts (255). Items were derived from a wide array of functional performance and development scales. Normative data were collected from 412 children and families from the northeastern United States with a sample stratified to represent national population demographics while retaining equal representation across the target age groups using 6-month intervals. A detailed manual with scale development data, administration instructions, and scoring has been developed. The scale also has published scoring forms and software.

Six domain scores are provided that enable a profile of relative strengths and weaknesses in both functional skills and caregiver assistance across the domains tested. No composite summary score is provided, with the rationale that this would obscure meaningful differences in functional performance within specific domains. Scaled scores can be computed to provide an indication of where a child's performance falls relative to the possible maximum. Item difficulty for the PEDI was determined through Rasch analysis, which was also used to estimate goodness of fit between individual subject profiles and the overall hierarchy, intended for each subscale. Since each scale is self-contained, it can be used individually or in combination with other scales. The average time for administration is 45 to 60 minutes.

The psychometric properties of the scale are reported in the administration manual. Reliability data (internal consistency) for the six scale scores were computed using Chronbach's alpha, with coefficients ranging from 0.95 to 0.99. Using the clinical samples, ICC values for interinterviewer reliability for the scales was estimated at 0.84 to 1.00. Values for independent respondents ranged from 0.74 to 0.96. Selected modifications in the PEDI were made based on these data. Initial scale data reflected an expected progression of functional skills according to age. Initial concurrent validity was established through comparison of scores on the PEDI with scores on the Battelle Developmental Inventory Screening Test and the Functional Independence Measure for Children (WeeFIM). These correlations were generally high for self-care and mobility but lower for social function. In early studies of the scale's ability to detect change, results were mixed, with one clinical sample of children with mild to moderate traumatic injuries demonstrating positive changes on the PEDI in all domains. Another clinical sample involving children with multiple significant disabilities showed positive change after 8 months only on the mobility scale. Some scores for this group decreased, indicating that the children were falling behind their peers in age-expected functional levels (254). Ludlow and Haley studied the influence of setting (context) on rating of mobility activities and found that parents in the home setting tend to use stricter criteria in their ratings than rehabilitation professionals in the school setting, although both can be trained to attain a satisfactory level of consistency (256).

Since its initial development and normative studies, several clinical studies using the PEDI have been reported. These have related to measuring the status of very-low-birth-weight children at age 5 and for various rehabilitation or surgical interventions with children in various diagnostic categories, including traumatic brain injury (257), spinal bifida (258), and osteogenesis imperfecta (259,260). In addition, several reports have been published where the PEDI has been used to measure outcomes following targeted medical and surgical interventions for cerebral palsy (261,262), including studies of posterior rhizotomy (263–265), the use of botulinum-A toxin injections (266,267), and surgical release (268). Ketelaar and colleagues studied the properties of 17 scales assessing the functional motor abilities of children with cerebral palsy and concluded that the PEDI was one of only two measures that demonstrated acceptable psychometric properties while having the capability to document changes in function over time (269).

Studies of children from outside the United States have been reported to ascertain the suitability of using the PEDI with other cultural groups. Custers and colleagues compared profiles of nondisabled Dutch children with normative profiles and found enough differences to recommend the cross-cultural validation of the PEDI before use in the Netherlands (270). Similar recommendations were made after a study of children in Puerto Rico (271). These studies led to recommended item modifications for use in those countries (271,272). In summary, the PEDI can be described as an instrument that is useful for measuring basic and extended functional ADL status and

TABLE 43-7.   Content of the Pediatric Evaluation of Disability Inventory

	Self-Care Domain	Mobility Domain	Social Function Domain
Function skills scales	Types of food textures Use of utensils Use of drinking containers Toothbrushing Hairbrushing Nose care Handwashing Washing body and face Pullover/front-opening garments Fasteners Pants Shoes/socks Toileting tasks Management of bladder Management of bowel	Toilet transfers Chair/wheelchair transfers Car transfers Bed mobility/transfers Tub transfers Method of indoor locomotion Distance/speed indoors Pulls/carries objects Method of outdoor locomotion Distance/speed outdoors Outdoor surfaces Upstairs Downstairs	Comprehension of word meanings Comprehension of sentence complexity Functional use of expressive communication Complexity of expressive communication Problem resolution Social interactive play Peer interactions Self-information Time orientation Household chores Self-protection Community function
Complex activities assessed with caregiver assistance and modifications scales	Eating Grooming Bathing Dressing upper body Dressing lower body Toileting Bladder management Bowel management	Chair/toilet transfers Car transfers Bed mobility/transfers Tub transfers Indoor locomotion Outdoor locomotion Stairs	Functional comprehension Functional expression Joint problem solving Peer play Safety

change in children with disabilities from age 6 months to 7.5 years.

MANAGEMENT OF BASIC SELF-CARE SKILLS

The functional evaluation process characterizes the strengths and weaknesses of each patient in relation to specific daily living skills. The practitioner or rehabilitation team uses this information to develop options for a plan of care that will assist or enable the patient to become more independent in selected activities. Figure 43-3 provides a hypothetical therapy plan of care for a patient with right hemisphere stroke. Research has shown that patients who collaborate in identifying goals and selecting treatment options become active and responsible participants in their own rehabilitation (229). Most rehabilitation options fall into one of four categories: remediation, compensation, disability prevention, or health promotion (273). These categories are consistent with what people do when they learn to cope with functional limitations, when they are acting without professional advice. A study of self-care and aging by Norburn and associates (274) identified three types of self-care coping strategies. These were related to the use of equipment or devices, specific changes in behavior, and modifications of the environment. The study also found that receiving assistance sometimes was used to supplement self-care coping strategies.

AN OVERVIEW OF INTERVENTION APPROACHES

The four major categories of ADL intervention described earlier are briefly described in the following sections.

Remediation

Remediation pertains to the resolution of functional or structural deficits or the acquisition of new skills in the area of skilled movement, cognition, or social function. Rehabilitation often involves an active learning process whereby patients must adapt to functional and environmental limitations as they affect the demands of everyday life. The initial acquisition of skills by those who are developmentally or congenitally disabled at birth is a markedly different learning process from the reacquisition of daily living skills by those who have been independent at such tasks before becoming disabled. When the goals of remediation are to develop skills in a person with a congenital condition, the training process is described as *habilitative*. When the goal is to achieve previous functional levels for a person with an acquired disability, the training process is described as *restorative*.

When able-bodied children learn self-care tasks initially, they do so over extended periods of time. Anthropologists note that there is a regular sequence of self-care independence that is supported by child development studies across cultures. Feeding, grooming, continence, transfers, undressing, dressing, and bathing usually occur in this order, with normal acquisition influenced by the appearance of readiness skills (275).

Even such limited information as this may be useful in habilitation training. Using a distributed practice schedule (i.e., teaching self-care activities only during those times they would normally be performed) is critical for the person unfamiliar with the concept of the task. Effectiveness in self-care training involves learning the appropriate times and natural sequences of daily activities. The patient who is relearning a task often retains an appreciation of when it is to be performed, but the patient being habilitated needs to learn not only the skills but also the context appropriate to each task (276). Thus, in habilitation training, the acquisition of self-care skills may occur over extended periods and involves the careful structuring of tasks, frequent monitoring to correct performance errors, and feedback.

Practice is an important aspect of all motor training. Mere repetition of activity is not therapeutic training. The therapist or other self-care trainer must provide task structuring, strategic prompts, and suggestions for improvement of performance. The patient or learner must learn to monitor and cor-

Evaluation Data	Problem List	ADL Goals	Intervention Strategies
HISTORY/NARRATIVE Client is male, 67 y.o, retired school administrator. Active premorbidly in volunteer work and outdoor hobbies.	**MEDICAL DIAGNOSES** Right CVA Depression	Client will demonstrate improved upper extremity endurance and strength so that with task modifications and assistive devices, he is able to dress independently in less than 30 minutes.	**REMEDIATION** Techniques to encourage use of affected extremity Improve strength, coordination
SENSORIMOTOR Proprioception intact Grade 3(Fair) muscle strength in Left wrist, elbow, and shoulder flexors and extensors No visual field cut 2 point discrimination absent on R digits	**PERFORMANCE LIMITATIONS** Unable to initiate or complete dressing or bathing tasks without verbal cues and physical assistance.	Client will shower independently using adaptive equipment and safe practices.	**COMPENSATION** Train in use of dressing skills Introduce dressing aids (stocking aid, zipper pull, velcro closures) Train family members
COGNITIVE Follows simple directions	**FUNCTIONAL LIMITATIONS**		
AFFECTIVE No interest in activities	Left Hemiparesis Apathy		**DISABILITY PREVENTION** Grab bars in tub/shower Non-slip surfaces

Figure 43-3. Self-care goals and intervention strategies.

rect performance errors. Over time, desirable behaviors must be systematically rewarded and undesirable behaviors ignored or extinguished.

Most often, operant conditioning is provided in which successive approximations toward each goal (e.g., feeding, bowel and bladder control, grooming, dressing, bathing) are rewarded. Four stages of learning are described by Snell, including acquisition, maintenance, fluency, and generalization. This incremental learning process, moving from initial instruction to mastery with graded assistance, is sometimes termed *scaffolding* (277).

Practice usually occurs only at the time or times each day that a task is appropriate (278). During the initial or acquisition stages of instruction, therapists can promote generalization and mastery by teaching under natural conditions, using real equipment rather than simulated tools, involving multiple teaching conditions (locations, instructors, materials), and selecting the instructional examples carefully, with attention to those that best sample the range of variation likely to be encountered in task performance. Learners are encouraged to do what they can to help–sometimes starting a task that the therapist will need to finish and sometimes completing a task that only the therapist can initiate (279).

For the patient with an acquired disability, relearning self-care independence is a distinctly different process than for the habilitation patient. First, there is a loss of self-esteem and sense of failure and frustration when one is unable to perform those tasks that often are taken for granted by the nondisabled. Initial learning usually is motivated by intrinsic rewards of increased competency at self-care tasks (280), as well as by the positive social reinforcement of parents and other caregivers. In learning a task, negative reinforcement (i.e., avoiding unpleasant experiences or consequences) such as avoiding embarrassment over having to ask for assistance for feeding or toileting may be far more effective than positive social reinforcement. The therapist who tries to use social praise to rein-

force practice of toileting skills will find that it is not effective. In fact, it probably will be viewed as demeaning to praise an adult in a situation reminiscent of a childhood experience.

Although many physically disabled adults with acquired deficits may not fit the above description, one category of patient clearly does not benefit from this approach. This category includes patients with closed head injury or cerebrovascular accident who also have significant cognitive or perceptual deficits. As Bjornby and Reinvang have pointed out, such conditions as apraxia may significantly influence the effects of self-care training and may in fact need to be remediated before or in conjunction with remediation of self-care dependency (281). For such patients and those for whom other approaches have failed to produce results, compensatory training should be considered.

Other remediation strategies focus on the restoration of biological, physiologic, or neurologic processes. For example, the practitioner may incorporate motor or sensory techniques to fully or partially develop or restore sufficient voluntary control or movement to enable task accomplishment. Techniques derived from theories of neuroscience, biomechanics, and motor control are included among remediative approaches. The objective is to recover sufficient perception, cognition, and voluntary movement to enable task performance in a safe and effective manner. It is noted, however, that studies have shown that body structure and function predict less than half of the variation in task performance. In particular, the literature on stroke rehabilitation shows that gains in organ/physiologic (impairment) skills are small and do not automatically result in improved functional performance (282,283). Trombly analyzed the results of several studies in which correlations between motor impairment and activities of daily living (ADL) were reported (284). Her findings indicate that the amount of variance in ADL accounted for by motor impairment was 31%. Most (approximately 69%) of the variance associated with ADL performance was derived from other factors unrelated to the physical impairment. Motivational and environmental factors explain most task performance variation (285).

In the restorative approach, training is frequently combined with compensatory strategies, such as the use of assistive technology devices, prostheses, or orthoses. For example, the individual with only one functional arm can continue to be independent in dressing by learning to select certain clothing and/or by substituting motions and using devices for dressing. When remediative approaches are inadequate or are too costly in terms of time, energy, or expense, compensatory or adaptive approaches are necessary.

Restoration of skills often involves a patient who may make considerable contributions to the therapy process based on his or her previous knowledge and understanding of how the task was performed. Such patients can monitor their own errors and often use appropriate strategies to minimize deficits. In this case the treatment session is used to develop a practice strategy and the patient practices self-care at each opportunity whether or not the therapist is present. Problems occurring between treatments are discussed, and possible solutions can be practiced during the next treatment session.

Compensatory Strategies

When habilitation or relearning fails or is inappropriate, compensatory options remain available. In compensatory intervention, the task to be performed can be adapted or eliminated, performed by a caregiver, or modified through changes to the environment.

One useful approach is to teach the individual to perform a task within his or her capabilities. A second strategy is to modify the environment to permit accomplishment of the task despite limitations in ability or skill. Systems or devices can be designed or acquired to enable performance, despite cognitive deficits, or diminished strength or sensation. Finally, an agent or caregiver can assist with task requirements or perform them entirely according to the requirements of the person receiving assistance.

COMPENSATORY TRAINING

Often a skill the patient would like to perform in a normal manner can be accomplished successfully some other way. The person with bilateral above-elbow amputations may not do well at feeding using prostheses but may develop superior toe prehension and use the feet rather than the hands to eat, write, and manipulate tools. Adaptive equipment may substitute for lost or impaired abilities that limit function. The use of such devices will be discussed in the next section.

Regardless of how compensatory training is approached, the philosophical principle that should guide intervention is that there are many approaches to accomplishing the same task. Innovative alterations in task performance may allow people to do something for themselves that under other circumstances they depend on others to perform. It is characteristic of compensatory training that the end result of a patient's activity, whether it is clean teeth or tied shoelaces, is most important, rather than the method used to perform the task.

ENVIRONMENTAL MODIFICATIONS

Both training and devices for aiding in independent self-care must be appropriate to the living space of the patient. Modifications of living spaces and the architectural barriers they often impose may greatly enhance meeting ADL goals. Necessary modifications may range from minimal, in the case of rearrangement of furniture, to extensive, when apartments or homes must be specially designed for the disabled. Intermediate to these extremes are the cases in which modifications or additions to existing space and equipment may be used to enhance function. A recent study by the National Center for Health Statistics reports that nearly one-quarter of adults more than 65 years of age require some type of assistive technology device or accessibility accommodation in the home, with this percentage steadily increasing as the age bracket increases (286). Tabbarah and colleagues examined the conditions that predict home modifications of community-dwelling seniors more than 70 years of age in the United States. They found that the experience of a hip fracture, fall, or joint replacement and greater limitations in ADL increased the likelihood of having some modifications. Unfortunately, disproportionately fewer home modifications are found among seniors from underrepresented cultural groups or from lower-income groups (287).

Although the ideal is to design facilities with sufficient flexibility to accommodate access and support the activities of a population of diverse abilities, many homes and public facilities currently in use create barriers to performance and participation. One compensatory strategy to support self-care needs is to recommend modifications in existing space. During the course of a home visit and with the aim of making environments accessible, usable, safe, and negotiable, the rehabilitation practitioner can suggest many simple accommodations that can facilitate the attainment of self-care goals.

It is useful to provide some examples of self-care modifications that support function when specific impairments are present. When upper-extremity range of motion is limited, pots, pans, cosmetics, canned goods, and other essential daily living items can be placed out on counters rather than kept in their traditional places, which often are difficult or impossible to reach. For the patient with a visual field deficit such as homonymous hemianopsia, moving the bed and furniture into the patient's intact visual field when viewed from the doorway may make it easier and safer to move around the room. Of course, the view and placement of objects relative to the bed also must be strategically considered for the same reasons.

The range of possibilities for modification of living space to meet the needs of disabled people is extensive. Examples of common modifications include widening doorways, adding ramps, converting dens or family rooms into a wheelchair-accessible bedroom, and modifying door handles and flooring to improve mobility.

Resources such as the American National Standards Institute's Specifications for Making Buildings and Facilities Accessible to and Usable by Physically Handicapped People give explicit guidelines for many common problems (288). Unfortunately, lack of information usually is not what prevents patients and caregivers from effecting changes in living space. Although cost is sometimes a barrier, one study showed that only 52% of recommended home modifications were made, with the primary reason for nonadherence being a lack of belief in the benefits of making changes (289). Some health-care providers have attacked these problems directly by developing partnerships between governmental and community agencies to fund programs designed to eliminate architectural barriers within the home.

USE OF ASSISTIVE TECHNOLOGY DEVICES

The use of assistive technology devices (ATDs) has as its special mission the application of technology to increase a person's performance capabilities by compensating for diminished function. Both low-technology and high-technology devices are available. High-technology systems are characterized by sophisticated electronic components. These include computers, robots, speech synthesizers, and environmental control systems. These electronic aids to daily living allow persons with very limited voluntary movement or degenerative neuromuscular conditions to operate a wide variety of household and workplace appliances without assistance. A recent study by Jutai and colleagues showed that electronic aids are perceived positively by patients using them and are expected to be useful by those who are not yet users but anticipate acquisition of the devices (290).

Low-technology items are simple mechanical aids, such as built-up handles for those with arthritis or shoelaces that can be tied with one hand. Such low-technology items are far more numerous than high-technology devices, yet they are less well known to many disabled people. The technology of remote control has become increasingly available in our society. For a person unable to reach a light switch, radio, television, thermostat, door lock, or curtain cord, an environmental control system can provide an important new degree of independence. Ultrasonic or infrared signals, sent from a command center, may allow a person with a disability to use a variety of electronically activated appliances.

Perhaps reflecting the growth in the specialty of rehabilitation engineering, the past several decades have seen an unprecedented increase in the numbers and kinds of devices available to assist persons with functional limitations (291). The increase in the number of assistive technology devices has been so significant that most rehabilitation practitioners cannot keep abreast of developments. Fortunately, in the United States, useful assistive technology databases are available to help identify suitable technologies. Two primary assistive technology databases currently exist, including REHABDATA, provided by the National Rehabilitation Information Center, and ABLEDATA, operated under contract with the National Institute of Disability and Rehabilitation Research. Each database is accessible through the Internet and describes commercially available rehabilitation products, providing equipment descriptions, information about manufacturers, and other comments.

Research provides insight into the most appropriate strategies for deploying devices and aids to living. For example, Verbrugge and colleagues studied device use and found that lower-extremity (mobility) technologies were most relied on for everyday tasks (292). Gitlin and colleagues (293) found that devices for older adults with mixed disabilities were seldom used, concluding that instruction within the home setting was frequently inadequate. Thompson reported that needs for assistive technology devices and needs for assistance with ADL change over time as people with disabilities become older. His study of individuals with spinal cord injury living in the community suggested the need for routine assessments to detect changes in functional status, and the provision of supportive services to alleviate or minimize the effect of these changes (294). Fuhrer has noted the need for maturation of outcomes research in assistive technology, calling for shared databases, the development of theory for assistive technology intervention, and the implementation of a multistakeholder approach for outcomes research (295). Loebl has proposed a decision model for using assistive technology that links task analysis with functional assessment (296).

To determine which systems or devices each person needs, a comprehensive team evaluation leads to a list of possible solutions for each identified problem, providing ample information for the patient to make the ultimate decision in the selection of equipment. In every instance, the goal of assessment is to find the simplest, least expensive device that best meets the needs for the ADL goal. Figures 43-4 through 43-7 provide examples

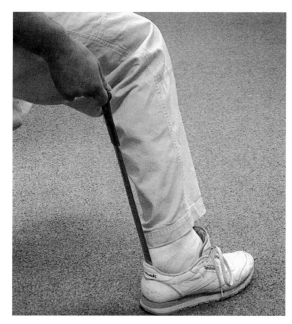

Figure 43-4. A long-handled shoe device can assist in dressing for persons with restricted range of motion.

of low-tech devices that are useful in different basic self-care tasks.

USE OF PERSONAL CARE ATTENDANTS

For many more people with severe disabilities, there is no combination of training, devices, or environmental modifications that will enable them to function independently in self-care. For such people to live independently outside an institution, they must depend on family members for support or personal care attendants (PCAs) to assist them. Part of the rehabilitation process for people who are going to require attendant care is that they learn to recruit, hire, supervise, and, if necessary, terminate personal care attendants.

Often the most difficult task for the patient is that of defining the tasks that require assistance, the degree of assistance that is desired, and the hours of the day when these tasks need to be performed. Because hours, pay, and working schedules (i.e., often attendants are needed 7 days per week) often are not

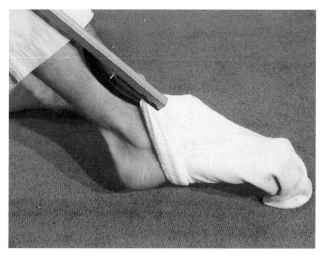

Figure 43-5. A reaching device with a claw end such as this stocking aid can be used to assist with dressing.

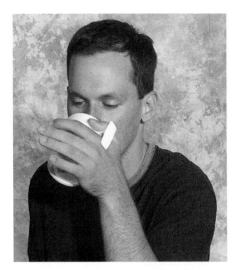

Figure 43-6. Specially designed cups can help compensate for weak palmar grasp.

competitive with other types of employment, turnover among attendants is high. The occupational therapist or other appropriately trained health-care professional often can assist the patient in writing the job description for a personal care attendant and in some cases may work with the patient to be an effective supervisor. Baum and Levesser note that selection and recruitment can be facilitated through the use of carefully defined tasks (297). The use of checklists with required tasks and procedures can serve as a specification for interviews, training, and performance appraisal (298).

An important and difficult aspect of working with a personal care attendants is to be able to define all the self-care and daily living activities that will require assistance. Many tasks, such as brushing one's teeth, dressing, and grooming, are performed on a daily basis. Other tasks, such as washing one's hair or having a bowel movement, may be performed less frequently but still quite regularly. Still other tasks, such as doing the laundry or changing the bed, are even less frequent but still are performed regularly. Finally, some tasks, such as mending torn clothing or washing windows, are infrequent and not performed regularly. This list must then be categorized into three

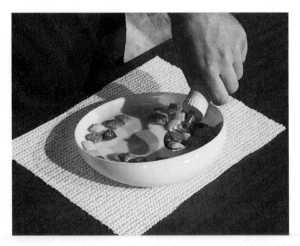

Figure 43-7. Eating devices such as a built-up spoon and plate with food guard can provide valuable mealtime assistance. A nonslip mat is also useful.

distinct classes of activities: those that the patient can perform alone, those that the patient can perform with some assistance, and those that must be performed by the personal care attendant. Research has shown that factors influencing success in the use of personal care attendants are mutual effort, skill, and commitment of the personal care attendants and employer with a disability (299).

Disability Prevention

Disability prevention pertains to those parts of a plan of care that promote safety or prevent health problems. These strategies seek to identify risk factors and implement preventive measures before an injury or adverse health event occurs. Disability prevention can take the form of training for the client and/or the caregiver, such as in teaching joint conservation techniques for patients with arthritis or in educating clients and caregivers with spinal cord injury on methods for preventing pressure sores or complications of bowel and bladder dysfunction. Monitoring for complications such as contractures, deep vein thrombosis (DVT), or recurrent stroke following cerebrovascular accident is also important.

Another approach to disability prevention involves exercise to promote fitness and counter the negative consequences of a sedentary lifestyle. Using a randomized controlled trial involving elders with osteoarthritis living in the community, Penninx and colleagues compared an aerobic exercise program, a resistance exercise program, and a control group (receiving attention only to control for socialization effects) for their effects on ADL disability assessed during an 18-month follow-up. The cumulative incidence of ADL-related disability was significantly reduced in the exercise groups in comparison to the control group (300).

Disability prevention also takes place through the use of environmental modifications oriented toward safety, such as attention to home hazards, lighting, and the installation of handrails and bathroom grab bars. Removal of throw rugs and other common obstacles for mobility or sensory limitations may make a nighttime trip to the bathroom considerably safer. Scales oriented toward the systematic assessment of living environments for safety and accessibility have been reported in the literature (301,302).

Another important area of safety and disability prevention concerns the prevention of falls. Fall prevention may include exercise programs to improve strength and postural control, improved medication management, careful attention to the selection and use of assistive technologies, and as indicated earlier, environmental modifications to improve safety. Rubenstein and colleagues have shown that a comprehensive fall prevention program can reduce falls and rehospitalization (303).

Health Promotion

A fourth intervention category involves strategies that promote health. Although some of the approaches in this category are similar to preventive strategies, because they may also serve to increase available resources of energy and time, they are considered to be health enhancing. One example of a strategy in this category is careful planning of the daily routines surrounding Basic and Extended Activities of Daily Living. Conserving available energy and time in the face of competing demands makes it appropriate for the client and caregiver to determine what tasks may be better assigned to caregivers even though the client is capable of performing them with or without assistance.

MAJOR SELF-CARE CONSIDERATIONS BY FUNCTIONAL LIMITATION

This section concerns special problems and issues related to ADL performance limitations associated with specific functional deficits. Perhaps the most important concept in rehabilitation aimed at daily living skills is that neither the type nor severity of the disability can be used exclusively to predict how independent a given patient will be. For example, Putzke and associates determined the predictors of ADL function among cardiac transplant candidates and found no correlation between certain expected physical variables and instrumental ADL capacity (304). Limited capacity for exertion, which is used by many occupational and physical therapists to recommend appropriate activities, was not a determinant of the activities those cardiac patients performed as part of their daily routine. The researchers concluded that patient perceptions and not cardiac symptoms accounted for the patterns of independence/dependence in household and social activities. Is it useful, then, to discuss self-care considerations by functional limitations? If the goal is to become aware of special problems or issues unique to a particular disability and not to predict outcomes, then the answer clearly is affirmative.

Some studies of physical function have provided useful theoretical associations between diseases and reports of difficulty with clusters of tasks within instrumental ADL routines. In a useful statistical analysis, Fried et al. studied 5,201 men and women age 65 and older in four U.S. communities (305). They analyzed difficulties associated with 17 tasks of daily life and found four clusters of activities where difficulty with one task was associated with reported difficulty for other tasks in that group. The groups included activities primarily dependent on mobility and exercise tolerance, complex activities heavily dependent on cognition and sensory input, selected basic self-care activities, and upper-extremity activities. These groups were then examined to see if they were associated with underlying impairments based on regression analysis using 15 chronic diseases and conditions. They found that physiologic and disease characteristics significantly correlated with difficulty in each of these four groups (Table 43-8). The implications of this study pertain to the appropriateness of outcome measures, which the authors suggest should be chosen with defined physiologic rationale. However, the study also provides a general indication of patterns of ADL/IADL consequences associated with the 15 conditions.

Several useful conclusions related to the performance of life tasks can be gleaned from this study. First, it is evident that problems with body structure and function seldom affect isolated tasks or task categories. Thus some health functional difficulties influence performance across all task categories. These could include depression, joint pain and stiffness, visual impairments, shortness of breath, and both generalized and hand grip weakness. Although these associations can help practitioners to anticipate certain activity and participation limitations associated with given diseases and their accompanying functional pathology, each case must be considered in the context of a particular patient's circumstances.

From the standpoint of rehabilitation intervention, these data suggest that some generalized strategies for improving endurance and strength can have the potential for broadly benefiting ADL/IADL performance on several tasks. In those cases where the underlying etiology of task difficulty cannot be addressed, such as with weakness and shortness of breath accompanying congestive heart disease, general compensatory strategies to address performance of self-care and instrumental ADL tasks will be necessary.

The following sections summarize recent studies related to interventions and outcomes for selected areas of task-related functional pathology. Practitioners are encouraged to consult

TABLE 43-8. ADL/IADL Task Groups Found to Be Statistically Associated with Underlying Medical Conditions[a]

Group	Mobility	Complex (Cognitive/Sensory)	Self-Care	Upper Extremity
Tasks	Walk 1/2 mile Climb 10 steps Transfer from bed to chair Walk in own home Heavy housework Lifting or carrying 10 pounds of groceries	Pay bills Meal preparation Shopping Light housework Telephone use	Using toilet Dressing Bathing Eating	Gripping Reaching
Pathology associated with task difficulty	Balance disorder Claudication Joint pain/stiffness Shortness of breath General weakness Hand grip weakness Depression Cognition/memory impairment Visual impairment	Cognition/memory impairment Claudication Joint pain/stiffness Hearing impairment Hand grip weakness Depression Shortness of breath Visual impairment General weakness	Joint pain/stiffness Hearing impairment Cognition/memory impairment General weakness Depression Hand grip weakness Visual impairment Shortness of breath	Joint pain/stiffness Shortness of breath Hand grip weakness General weakness Depression Visual impairment Balance disorder
Disease association (Difficulty with one or more tasks in group)	Congestive heart failure Cancer Arthritis Stroke Diabetes Emphysema Hypertension	Arthritis Stroke Diabetes Emphysema Hypertension	Myocardial infarction Arthritis Stroke Diabetes Emphysema Hypertension	Arthritis Stroke Diabetes Emphysema Hypertension

[a]Fried, LP et al, Physical Disability in Older Adults: A Physiological Approach. *Journal of Clinical Epidemiology*, 1994;47(7):747–760

the many intervention textbooks now available in the rehabilitation sciences for theoretical and applied (procedural) guidelines and details associated with implementing intervention strategies. Although many interventions have not yet been subjected to controlled study, it is important for practitioners to be aware of the literature in order to determine the available evidence underlying a particular intervention technique.

Cognitive and Perceptual Deficits

Diminished cognitive and perceptual function can be a consequence of senile dementia, traumatic brain injury, stroke, or developmental disability. The ability to attend; perceive and select relevant information in the environment; make logical decisions; plan and execute safe, goal-directed action; and remember events involves aspects of executive function, which may be compromised in cognitive dysfunction. Individuals with cognitive and/or perceptual loss must be approached and managed with greater care and attention than other patients.

The association between cognition (particularly executive function) and ADL/IADL performance is well documented. Studies of community-dwelling seniors (306), persons following hip fractures (307), patients with cerebral palsy (308), and stroke patients (309) are among those documenting this association.

Sometimes cognitive loss is associated with agitation, particularly following traumatic brain injury or in senile dementia. For example, Bogner and associates found that the presence of agitation predicted longer length of stay and decreased functional independence following traumatic brain injury (310).

In stroke, generalized cognitive deficits are most common in patient with frontal lobe insults. Cognitive deficits involving visuospatial abilities are associated with right hemisphere strokes and apraxia. Disorders of learned movement or motor planning are found with left hemisphere strokes. Unilateral neglect, or inattention to the side opposite the affected hemisphere, is also a difficult consequence of stroke and can occur in up to half of patients with right brain damage and less frequently in left hemisphere strokes. Unawareness of the stroke or its results can be found in patients with strokes in the nondominant hemisphere. This appears to be related to the severity of brain damage or the extent of cognitive impairment (311). Typically, these deficits interfere with regaining skills in ADLs. Patients with spatial constructional problems often have difficulty in eating, dressing, grooming, and walking. Those with unilateral neglect experience difficulty with reading and writing and numerical tasks, as well as in using a phone or driving. These results are consistent with other studies in which a clear relationship between apraxia and ADL skills was shown (312).

Several studies have found that perceptual motor abilities are significant predictors of self-care and ADL in patients with cerebrovascular accident (313–317). In a systematic review, Rubio and Van Dusen summarized the research on perceptual deficits and ADL-targeted intervention approaches following stroke (318). They acknowledged the convincing evidence associating perceptual difficulties with poorer ADL outcomes and noted that little attention has been paid to agnosia and that controlled studies comparing various intervention options are needed.

The literature documents many attempts to use perceptual training in addition to task-oriented (functional) training as a way of improving ADL outcomes in patients with perceptual problems such as unilateral neglect following cerebrovascular accident. Strategies for perceptual remediation include (a) visual scanning training with verbal cuing for visual anchoring,

(b) increased patient awareness of neglect to encourage use of compensatory mechanisms, (c) increased sensory stimulation to the affected side, and (d) activation of the affected extremity on the affected side of the body. Overall, although it has been shown that interventions targeted for perceptual skills can have short-term effects in improving perceptual skills (319–322), research has not demonstrated unequivocally that perceptual training in addition to traditional functional intervention improves outcomes in ADL over functional training alone (323). Patients with such limitations can and do make progress, albeit more slowly than similar patients without such deficits. At least one study has shown that training that includes specific compensation strategies along with traditional ADL strategies can improve overall performance in ADL skills for cerebrovascular accident patients with left hemisphere stroke (324). Unfortunately, there is a dearth of information on the long-term results of perceptual interventions (325).

Treatments for apraxia or motor planning and execution deficits have included such strategies as manual guided movement, the use of objects and situations that elicit automatic motor responses, and systematic stepwise training ("backward chaining"). Controlled studies of the long-term efficacy of these approaches for improving functional ADL skills have not been reported.

Depression

Numerous rehabilitation studies have shown that the presence of depression following stroke and other health events (such as hip fracture, postpolio syndrome, traumatic brain injury) can predict poorer functional outcomes and diminished well-being (47,326–330). Families and caregivers can be an important source of monitoring for depression, and mild depression often resolves or can be managed through behavioral interventions such as encouragement, attention, or active participation in suitable activities. More severe depression should be confirmed by accurate diagnosis. Symptoms may be effectively managed through medication (331). However, it appears for patients with cerebrovascular accident that the reduction in symptoms, particularly if started early, can result in improved levels of ADL function at discharge (332). One study, however, suggested that while treatment improves functional gains, the presence of depression among stroke survivors reduces the proportion of excellent outcomes in functional performance of ADL and mobility (333).

Craig and colleagues reported on a program of cognitive behavior therapy designed to reduce depression and improve self-esteem during rehabilitation following spinal cord injury. Their study improved anxiety, mood, and self-esteem of those receiving the intervention but did not result in outcomes that were significantly different from those of patients receiving traditional rehabilitation (334). Interestingly, studies of suicide following spinal cord injury show that frequencies are higher among those with marginal functional disability than in those with complete lesions (335).

Upper-Extremity Impairment

Upper-extremity impairment can be bilateral, as in spinal cord injury and arthritis, or unilateral, as may be the case following stroke, traumatic injury, amputation, peripheral nerve injury, or complex regional pain syndrome (CPRS/reflex sympathetic dystrophy). Bilateral upper-extremity amputation, loss of motion due to hemiparesis of nerve injury, and weakness are serious threats to self-care independence and may be helped with prosthetic and orthotic devices. Unilateral upper-extremity impairment most often is compensated for by use of the uninvolved extremity. When disability affects the preferred hand there will be a need to transfer skill to the other hand. This may or may not require coordination and dexterity training.

Persons with unilateral upper-extremity amputations will often be able to accomplish most of their activities of daily living with one arm. Thus, it is important to fit the unilateral upper-extremity amputation with prosthesis within 3 months of losing the arm in order to facilitate training for bilateral patterns of use. The prosthesis always functions as the nonpreferred extremity in stabilizing of objects (336). Functional electrical stimulation may also be effective in improving upper-extremity function for ADL (337).

Cosmesis may be a key factor for the patient in the selection of a prosthesis, which can be body powered, myoelectric, or hybrid. Bilateral upper-extremity amputations, particularly if above the elbow, are more challenging but can result in successful independence. The prosthetic training for a bilateral above-elbow amputee usually requires a carefully designed series of training sessions. Initial training of basic activities of daily living requires an extensive time, effort, and motivation on the part of the amputee. Often the basic tasks of writing, eating, brushing teeth, washing the face, and requiring assistance with dressing are the most realistic goals during rehabilitation following the prosthetic fitting. Later training can concentrate on additional activities in the daily routine (336). Motor control problems and spasticity related to cerebral palsy can also create ADL challenges. Some attempts to improve function using botulinum toxin have shown success, but more research is needed (338).

Lower-Extremity Impairment

Mobility and transfer limitations are the most significant self-care problems for lower-extremity impairments, including those with hip fractures, amputations, arthritis, and paraplegia. Often wheelchairs or other ambulation aids are needed for independent mobility. Bathroom safety equipment, dressing aids such as extended handle shoehorns, and raised seats often are useful items that may be used either temporarily or permanently. Rearrangement of living space to permit wheelchair access or access using other mobility aids often is necessary. Ramps, chairlifts, and additional railings may be needed if stairs are present. For the person dependent on a wheelchair, it also may be helpful to consider rearrangement of shelves, drawers, and closet space to permit frequently used items to be reached from the wheelchair. Narang and associates reported that more than half of the patients with lower-extremity amputations they studied were totally independent in all self-care, 40% required only additional aids to independence for self-care, and 5% were confined to wheelchairs or not totally independent (339). Haworth investigated the patterns of use of aids to independence in patients after total hip replacement and found that aids were used only as long as needed for bathroom safety, dressing, and toileting and that patients discarded them when they could manage independently (340).

Upper- and Lower-Extremity Impairment

Persons with tetraparesis or tetraplegia from traumatic spinal cord injury, cerebral palsy, muscular dystrophy, multiple sclerosis, or amyotrophic lateral sclerosis must rely on a wide range of options for self-care independence. In most cases there will be a need for attendant care, assistive devices, and modifi-

cations of living space. Such people often require high-technology devices, such as environmental controls, augmentative communications, and other microprocessor-based systems to be fully independent in their own homes (34). Promising developments are being shown in the technology associated with implanted neuroprostheses for restoring hand grasp in tetraplegia following spinal cord injury (341).

The disabling consequences of CRPS/Reflex Sympathetic Dystrophy frequently include intractable pain, sensory changes, edema, and movement disorder, which can include restricted or involuntary movement and atrophy of the upper or lower extremity. This syndrome can result in marked functional limitations affecting ADL performance, usually caused by pain rather than by restricted motion (342). Treatment often consists of medications or TENS to assist with pain control and compensatory training for alternative methods in accomplishing daily living tasks.

Hemiparesis

Perhaps the most important finding of studies related to ADL intervention for hemiparesis is that the side of the lesion may predict a pattern of problems but may not predict self-care outcomes. The cognitive and perceptual problems associated with different lesion sites and extent of damage were summarized earlier.

The differences between left- and right-side brain damage do not affect prognosis for self-care independence directly. Instead it appears that patients with left-sided brain damage are easier to train, receive more training, and progress more rapidly. Patients with right-sided damage tend to be more difficult to train, take longer to train, and tend to receive less training as a result. It remains possible that attitudes and skills of therapists and the economics of medical rehabilitation may be biased toward those with left-sided brain damage. Consequently, therapists and physicians need to be aware of the implications of their decisions about intensity and duration of training for patients with right- versus left-sided brain damage. It seems especially important to note that both groups show gains over time in self-care and that the hospital discharge prognosis for ADL independence is not necessarily the long-term self-care prognosis.

Historically, many therapeutic programs for stroke concentrated on the neurologic substrates of stroke, seeking to normalize muscle tone as a precursor to emphasis on functional training. More recent controlled studies have shown that motor learning strategies may represent a more effective approach in achieving improved outcomes in ADL (343).

An intervention approach known as constraint-induced (CI) movement therapy (also forced-use therapy) has received increasing attention. This approach uses a regimen involving intensive training of the affected extremity during which the unaffected arm is constrained in a sling for much of each day. The intent is to foster cortical reorganization to recruit other areas of the brain to assume motor planning and control functions. Some encouraging results, including improvements in ADL function, have been demonstrated in clinical studies, but the approach is still viewed as experimental (344–346).

Limitations in Joint Range of Motion

Problems of limited range of motion that result in difficulty reaching common ADL items are best addressed by rearrangement of living space. An occupational therapist or other health-care provider making a home visit can suggest safety equipment for the bathroom, removal of obstacles that could contribute to falls, and other adaptive devices that are needed. With respect to training, an emphasis on compensatory training regarding work simplification and energy conservation techniques is needed.

SUMMARY

Evaluation and management strategies for promoting independence in self-care represent, from the patient's standpoint, one of the most practical and important aspects of medical rehabilitation. As a rehabilitation goal, performance of basic and extended activities of daily living is now being viewed as an important outcome with profound implications for quality of life. In this chapter, emphasis has been given to the importance of patient/professional collaboration in setting goals and selecting methods for managing life tasks after discharge. These options include determining if the task is feasible, if retraining or new training is desirable, if the environment needs to be altered, if assistance needs to be provided through other people, or if assistive technology devices, including robotics and environmental control systems, may be useful.

In this collaborative process, the patient's preferences, experiences, and postdischarge living environment assume at least as much importance as the diagnosis or physical limitations. Moreover, such factors as costs of time and energy must enter into decisions about the value of various options for accomplishing daily living tasks. The active participation of the individual in determining a plan of care represents the desired outcome of rehabilitation. This goal is ultimately to enable the individual to participate in those activities that bring life satisfaction.

ACKNOWLEDGMENT

The work of Richard Schwartz, Karin Barnes and Kenneth Ottenbacher was instrumental to the development of earlier versions this chapter and is acknowledged with appreciation. I also thank Charles Hayden, Brian Berlin, Colin Adams, Jay J. Tanet, Margo Parr, and Judy Wolf for valuable assistance with the present chapter.

REFERENCES

1. Lawton MP. The functional assessment of elderly people. *J Am Geriatr Soc* 1971;14:465–81.
2. Christiansen CH. 1999 Eleanor Clarke Slagle Lecture: Defining lives: occupation as identity. An essay on competence, coherence and the creation of meaning. *Am J Occup Ther* 1999;53:547–558.
3. Christiansen C. The social importance of self-care intervention. In: Christiansen C, ed. *Ways of living: self care strategies for special needs*. Bethesda, MD: American Occupational Therapy Association, 2000:1–12.
4. Parsons T. Definitions of health and illness in the light of American values and social structure. In: Jaco EG, ed. *Patients, physicians and illness*. Glencoe, IL: Free Press, 1958:165–187.
5. Christiansen C. Three perspectives on balance in occupation. In: Zemke R, Clark F, eds. *Occupational science: the evolving discipline*. Philadelphia: FA Davis, 1996:431–451.
6. Gershuny J, Fisher K, Gauthier A, et al. A longitudinal, multinational collection of time–use data—the MTUS. In: J Gershuny, ed. *Changing times: work and leisure in postindustrial society*. Oxford: Oxford University Press, 2000: 270–288.
7. Eshun AB. Effective rehabilitation for older people. *Nurs Standard* 1999;13: 39–43.
8. Mauthe RW, Haaf DC, Hayn P, et al. Predicting discharge destination of stroke patients using a mathematical model based on six items from the Functional Independence Measure. *Arch Phys Med Rehabil* 1996;77:10–13.
9. Gabrel CS. Characteristics of elderly nursing home current residents and discharges: data from the 1997 National Nursing Home Survey. Advance data from vital and health statistics; No. 312. Hyattsville, MD: National Center for Health Statistics, 2000.
10. Wolinsky FD, Callahan CM, Fitzgerald FF, et al. The risk of nursing home placement and subsequent death among older adults. *Gerontology* 1992;47: S172–S182.
11. World Health Organization. International Classification of Functioning, Disability and Health. Geneva: WHO, 2001.
12. Christiansen CH, Baum CM, eds. *Occupational therapy: enabling function and well-being*, 3rd ed. Thorofare, NJ: Slack, Inc., 2003.
13. Tsouna-Hadjis E, Vemmos KN, Zakopoulos N, et al. First-stroke recovery process: the role of family social support. *Arch Phys Med Rehabil* 2000;81: 881–887.
14. Baumeister RF. Identity, self concept, and self esteem: the self lost and found. In: Hogan R, Johnson J, Briggs S, eds. *Handbook of personality psychology*. San Diego: Academic Press, 1997:681–711.
15. Hogan R. A socioanalytic theory of personality. *Nebr Symp Motiv* 1982;130: 55–89.
16. Murray SL, Griffin DW, Rose P, et al. Calibrating the sociometer: the relational contingencies of self-esteem. *J Pers Soc Psychol* 2003;85:63–84.
17. Backman K, Hentinen M. Factors associated with the self-care of home-dwelling elderly. *Scand J Caring Sci* 2001;15:195–202.
18. Bowling AP, Edelmann RJ. Loneliness, mobility, well-being and social support in a sample of over 85 year olds. *Pers Individ Dif* 1989;10:1189–1192.
19. Wyller TB, Holmen J, Laake P, et al. Correlates of subjective well-being in stroke patients. *Stroke* 1998;29:363–367.
20. Rintala D, Young ME, Hart, KA, et al. Social support and the well-being of persons with spinal cord injury living in the community. *Rehabil Psychol* 1992;37:155–163.
21. Affleck G, Pfeiffer CA. Social support and psychosocial adjustment to rheumatoid arthritis: quantitative and qualitative findings. *Arthritis Care Res* 1988;1:71–77.
22. Blair CE. Effect of self care ADLs on self esteem of intact nursing home residents. *Issues Ment Health Nurs* 1999;20:559–570.
23. Chang AM, Mackenzie AE. State self-esteem following stroke. *Stroke* 1998; 29:2325–2328.
24. Chemerinski E, Robinson RG, Kosier JT. Improved recovery in activities of daily living associated with remission of post stroke depression. *Stroke* 2001;32:113–117.
25. Smith GC, Kohn SJ, Savage-Stevens SE, et al. The effects of interpersonal and personal agency on perceived control and psychological well-being in adulthood. *Gerontologist* 2000;40:458–468.
26. Lewis SC, Dennis MS, O'Rourke SJ, et al. Negative attitudes among short-term stroke survivors predict worse long-term survival. *Stroke* 2001;32:1640–1645.
27. Berg-Weger M, Rubio DM, Tebb SS. Living with and caring for older family members: issues related to caregiver well-being. *J Gerontol Soc Work* 2000;33: 47–62.
28. Leathem J, Health E, Woolley C. Relatives' perceptions of role change, social support and stress after traumatic brain injury. *Brain Inj* 1996;10:27–38.
29. Forsberg-Wärleby G, Möller A, Blomstrand C. Spouses of first-ever stroke patients: psychological well-being in the first phase after stroke. *Stroke* 2001; 32:1646–1651.
30. Perlesz A, Kinsella G, Crowe S. Psychological distress and family satisfaction following traumatic brain injury: injured individuals and their primary, secondary, and tertiary carers. *J Head Trauma Rehabil* 2000;15:909–929.
31. Clark MS, Smith DS. Changes in family functioning for stroke rehabilitation patients and their families. *Int J Rehabil Res* 1999;2:171–179.
32. Jones DA, Vetter NJ. A survey of those who care for the elderly and home: their problems and their needs. *Soc Sci Med* 1984;19:511–514.
33. Evans RL, Bishop DS, Ousley RT. Providing care to persons with physical disability. Effect on family caregivers. *Am J Phys Med Rehabil* 1992;71:140–144.
34. Wilcox VL, Kasl SV, Berkman LF. Social support and disability in older people after hospitalization: a prospective study. *Health Psychol* 1994;13:170–179.
35. Elmstahl S, Malmberg B, Annerstedt L. Caregiver's burden of patients 3 years after stroke assessed by a novel caregiver burden scale. *Arch Phys Med Rehabil* 1996;77:177–182.
36. Blake H, Lincoln NB. Factors associated with strain in co-resident spouses of patients following stroke. *Clin Rehabil* 2000;14:307–314.
37. Clark MS. The double ABCX model of family crisis as a representation of family functioning after rehabilitation from stroke. *Psych Health Med* 1999;4:203–220.
38. Sorensen S, Pinquart M, Duberstein P. How effective are interventions with caregivers? An updated meta-analysis. *Gerontologist* 2002;42:356–372.
39. Dow-Richards C. Family involvement for optimal recovery. *Top Stroke Rehabil* 2000;7:44–49.
40. Bishop DS. Family and other psychosocial issues. *Top Stroke Rehabil* 1995;2: v–vii, 1–78.
41. Wilcox VL, Kasl SV, Berkman LF. Social support and physical disability in older people after hospitalization: a prospective study. *Health Psychol* 1994; 13:170–179.

42. Hogan R. A socioanalytic theory of personality. *Nebr Symp Motiv* 1982;30: 55–89.

43. Olkin R, Howson LJ. Attitudes toward and images of physical disability. *J SocBehav Pers* 1994;9:81–96.

44. Yuker HE. Variables that influence attitudes towardpeople with disabilities—conclusions from the data. *J Soc Behav Pers* 1994;9:3–22.

45. Goffman E. *Stigma: notes on the management of a spoiled identity.* Englewood Cliffs, NJ: Prentice-Hall, 1963.

46. Hogan K, Orme S. Measuring disability: a critical analysis of the Barthel Index: symposium on older people. *Br J Ther Rehabil* 2000;7:163–167.

47. Bays CL. Quality of life of stroke survivors: a research synthesis. *J Neurosci Nurs* 2001;33:310–316.

48. Haworth RJ, Hollings EM. Are hospital assessments of daily living activities valid? *Int Rehabil Med* 1979;1:59–62.

49. DiJoseph LM. Independence through activity: mind, body, and environment interaction in therapy. *Am J Occup Ther* 1982;36:740–744.

50. Iwarsson S, Isacsson A. On scaling methodology and environmental influences in disability assessments: the cumulative structure of personal and instrumental ADL among older adults in a Swedish rural district. *Can J Occup Ther* 1997;64:240–251.

51. Gill TM, Robison JT, Tinetti ME. Difficulty and dependence: two components of the disability continuum among community living older persons. *Ann Intern Med* 1998;128:96–101.

52. Willer B, Button J, Rempel R. Residential and home-based post-acute rehabilitation of individuals with traumatic brain injury: a case control study. *Arch Phys Med Rehabil* 1999;80:399–406.

53. Baskett JJ, Broad JB, Reekie G, et al. Shared responsibility for ongoing rehabilitation: a new approach to home-based therapy after stroke. *Clin Rehabil* 1999;13:23–33.

54. Neistadt ME, Marques K. An independent living skills training program. *Am J Occup Ther* 1984;38:671–676.

55. Drummond AER, Miller N, Colquohoun M, et al. The effects of a stroke unit on activities of daily living. *Clin Rehabil* 1996;10:12–22.

56. Lange ML, Smith RO. Technology and occupation: contemporary viewpoints. The future of electronic aids to daily living. *Am J Occup Ther* 2002; 56:107–109.

57. Trefler E. Assistive technology. In: Christiansen C, Baum C. eds. *Occupational therapy: enabling function and well-being.* Thorofare, NJ: Slack;1997:482–507.

58. Countryman KM, Gekas AB. *Development and implementation of a patient's bill of rights in hospitals.* Chicago: American Hospital Association, 1980.

59. Commission on Accreditation of Rehabilitation Facilities. *Standards manual for organizations serving people with disabilities.* Tucson, AZ: Commission on Accreditation of Rehabilitation Facilities, 1992.

60. *Accreditation Manual for Hospitals.* Chicago: Joint Commission on Accreditations of Hospitals, 1992.

61. Agency for Healthcare Research and Quality. *Quality first: better health care for all Americans.* Final Report of the President's Advisory Commission on Consumer Protection and Quality in the Health Care Industry. Silver Spring, MD: Agency for Healthcare Research and Quality, 1998.

62. Neistadt ME. Methods of assessing client's priorities: a survey of adult physical dysfunction settings. *Am J Occup Ther* 1995;49:428–436.

63. Wressle E, Oberg B, Henriksson C. The rehabilitation process for the geriatric stroke patient: an exploratory study of goal setting and interventions. *Disabil Rehabil* 1999;21:80–87.

64. Northen JG, Rust DM, Nelson CE, et al. Involvement of adult rehabilitation patients in setting occupational therapy goals. *Am J Occup Ther* 1995;49:214–220.

65. Unsworth C. Clients' perceptions of discharge housing decisions after stroke rehabilitation. *Am J Occup Ther* 1996;50:207–216.

66. Wressle E, Eeg-Ofsson AM, Marcusson J, et al. Improved client participation in the rehabilitation process using a client-centered goal formulation structure. *J Rehabil Med* 2002;34:5–11.

67. Schönherr MC, Groothoff JW, Mulder GA, et al. Prediction of functional outcome after spinal cord injury: a task for the rehabilitation team and the patient. *Spinal Cord* 2000;38:185–191.

68. Chiou IL, Burnett CN. Values of activities of daily living: a survey of stroke patients and their home therapists. *Phys Ther* 1985;65:901–906.

69. McGavin H. Planning rehabilitation: a comparison of issues for parents and adolescents. *Phys Occup Ther Pediatr* 1998;18:69–82.

70. Bates PS. Self care in context: enabling functional person–environment fit. In: Christiansen C, ed. *Ways of living: self care strategies for special needs,* 2nd ed. Bethesda, MD: American Occupational Therapy Association, 2000:361–382.

71. Norris-Baker C, Willems EP. Environmental negotiability as a direct measurement of behavior–environment relationships: some implications for theory and practice. In: Seidel AD, Danford S. eds. *Proceedings of the tenth annual conference of the environmental design research association.* Houston: Environmental Design Research Association, 1978:209–214.

72. Granger CV. A conceptual model for functional assessment. In: Granger CV, Gresham GE, eds. *Functional assessment in rehabilitation medicine.* Baltimore: Williams & Wilkins, 1984:14–25.

73. Wood PHN. Appreciating the consequences of disease: the international classification of impairments, disabilities and handicaps. *WHO Chron* 1980; 34:376–380.

74. *International classification of functioning, disability and health.* Geneva: World Health Organization, 2001.

75. Vash CL. Evaluation from the client's point of view. In: Halpern AS, Fuhrer MJ, eds. *Functional assessment in rehabilitation.* Baltimore: Paul H. Brookes, 1984:253–268.

76. Kelman HR, Willner A. Problems in measurement and evaluation of rehabilitation. *Arch Phys Med Rehabil* 1962;43:172–181.

77. Law M, Letts L. A critical review of scales of activities of daily living. *Am J Occup Ther* 1989;43:522–527.

78. Jette AM. Health status indicators: their utility in chronic-disease evaluation research. *J Chronic Dis* 1979;33:567–579.

79. Kaufert JM. Functional ability indices: measurement problems in assessing their validity. *Arch Phys Med Rehabil* 1983;64:260–267.

80. Keith RA. Functional assessment measures in medical rehabilitation: current status. *Arch Phys Med Rehabil* 1984;65:74–78.

81. Christiansen C. Continuing challenges in functional assessment. *Am J Occup Ther* 1994;48:333–335.

82. Alexander JL, Fuhrer MJ. Functional assessment of individuals with physical impairments. In: Halpern AS, Fuhrer MJ, eds. *Functional assessment in rehabilitation.* Baltimore: Paul H. Brookes, 1984:45–60.

83. Knapp P, Hewison J. Disagreement in patient and career assessment of functional abilities after stroke. *Stroke* 1999;30:934–938.

84. Kwakkei G, van Dijk GM, Wagenaar RC. Accuracy of physical and occupational therapists' early predictions of recovery after severe middle cerebral artery stroke. *Clin Rehabil* 2000;14:28–41.

85. Weingarden SL, Martin C. Independent dressing after spinal cord injury: a functional time evaluation. *Arch Phys Med Rehabil* 1989;70:518–519.

86. Pentland W, Harvey AS, Walker J. The relationships between time use and health and well-being in men with spinal cord injury. *J Occup Sci* 1998;5: 14–25.

87. Frey WD. Functional assessment in the 80s: a conceptual enigma, a technical challenge. In: Halpern AS, Fuhrer MJ, eds. *Functional assessment in rehabilitation.* Baltimore: Paul H. Brookes, 1984:11–44.

88. Keith RA. Functional assessment in program evaluation for rehabilitation medicine. In: Granger CV, Gresham GE, eds. *Functional assessment in rehabilitation medicine.* Baltimore: Williams & Wilkins, 1984.

89. Boschen KA, Gargaro J. Issues in the measurement of independent living. *Can J Rehabil* 1996;10:125–135.

90. Wade DT. *Measurement in neurological rehabilitation.* Oxford: Oxford University Press, 1992.

91. Guccione AA. Physical therapy diagnosis and the relationship between impairment and function. *Phys Ther* 1991;71:499–504.

92. McGinnis GE, Seward M, DeJong G, et al. Program evaluation of physical medicine and rehabilitation departments using self-report Barthel. *Arch Phys Med Rehabil* 1986;67:123–125.

93. Klein-Parris C, Clermont MT, O'Neill J. Effectiveness and efficiency of criterion testing versus interviewing for collecting functional assessment information. *Am J Occup Ther* 1986;40:486–491.

94. Cohen ME, Marino RJ. The tools of disability outcomes research: functional status measures. *Arch Phys Med Rehabil* 2000;81[Suppl 2]:S21–S29.

95. Andresen EM. Criteria for assessing the tools of disability outcomes research. *Arch Phys Med Rehabil* 2000;81[Suppl 2]:S15–S20.

96. American Psychological Association. *Standards for educational and psychological testing.* Washington, DC: American Psychological Association, 1985.

97. Anonymous. Task Force on Standards for Measurement in Physical Therapy. Standards for tests and measurements in physical therapy practice. *Phys Ther* 1991;71:589–622.

98. Johnston MV, Keith RA, Hinderer SR. Measurement standards for interdisciplinary medical rehabilitation. *Arch Phys Med Rehabil* 1992;73[Suppl]:S3–S23.

99. Merbitz C, Morris J, Grip JC. Ordinal scales and foundations of misinference. *Arch Phys Med Rehabil* 1989;70:308–312.

100. Rasch G. Probabilistic models for some intelligence and attainment tests. Copenhagen: Danmarks Paedogogistic Institut, 1960. Reprinted with foreword and afterword by Wright BD. Chicago: University of Chicago Press, 1980.

101. Wright B, Linacre JM. Observations are always ordinal: measurements, however, must be interval. *Arch Phys Med Rehabil* 1989;70:857–860.

102. Silverstein B, Kilgore K, Fisher W. *Implementing patient tracking systems and using functional assessment scales.* Wheaton, IL: Marianjoy Rehabilitation Center, 1989.

103. Heinemann AW, Linacre JM, Wright BD, et al. Prediction of rehabilitation outcomes with disability measures. *Arch Phys Med Rehabil* 1994;75:133–143.

104. Grimby G, Andran E, Daving Y, et al. Dependence and perceived difficulty in daily activities in community–living stroke survivors 2 years after stroke: a study of instrumental structures. *Stroke* 1998;29:1843–1849.

105. Mahoney FI, Barthel D. Functional evaluation: the Barthel Index. *Md State Med J* 1965;14:56–61.

106. Moskowitz E, Fuhn ER, Peters ME. Aged infirm residents in a custodial institution. *JAMA* 1959;169:2009–2012.

107. Katz S, Downs T, Cash H, et al. Progress in development of the index of ADL. *Gerontologist* 1970;10:20–30.

108. Granger CV, Hamilton BB, Sherwin FS. *Guide for use of the uniform data set for medical rehabilitation.* Buffalo, NY: Uniform Data System for Medical Rehabilitation, 1986.

109. Richards SH. Peters TJ. Coast J, et al. Inter-rater reliability of the Barthel ADL Index: how does a researcher compare to a nurse? *Clin Rehabil* 2000;14: 72–78.

110. Ellul J, Watkins C, Barer D. Estimating total Barthel scores from just three items: The European Stroke Database. *Age Ageing* 1998;27:115–122.

111. Hsueh IP, Lin JH, Jeng JS, et al. Comparison of the psychometric characteristics of the Functional Independence Measure, 5-item Barthel Index, and 10-item Barthel Index in patients with stroke. *J Neurol Neurosurg Psychiatry* 2002;73:188–190..

112. Hertanu JS, Demopoulos JT, Yang WC, et al. Stroke rehabilitation: correlation and prognostic value of computerized tomography and sequential functional assessments. *Arch Phys Med Rehabil* 1984;65:505–508.

113. Granger CV, Hamilton BB, Gresham GE, et al. The stroke rehabilitation outcome study: Part II: relative merits of the total Barthel Index score and a four-item subscore in predicting patient outcomes. *Arch Phys Med Rehabil* 1989;70:100–103.

114. Wylie CM, White BK. A measure of disability. *Arch Environ Health* 1964;8: 834–839.

115. DeJong G, Branch LG, Corcoran PJ. Independent living outcomes in spinal cord injury: multivariate analyses. *Arch Phys Med Rehabil* 1996;77:883–888.

116. Bent N, Jones A, Molloy I, et al. Factors determining participation in young adults with a physical disability: a pilot study. *Clin Rehabil* 2001;15:552–561

117. O'Toole DMK, Goldberg RT, Ryan B. Functional changes in vascular amputee patients: evaluation by Barthel Index, PULSES Profile and Escrow Scale. *Arch Phys Med Rehabil* 1985;66:508–511.

118. Prosiegel M, Boettger S, Give T, et al. The Extended Barthel Index: a new scale for the assessment of disability in neurological patients. *NeuroRehabil* 1996;1:7–13

119. Katz S, Ford AB, Moskowitz RW. Studies of illness in the aged: the Index of ADL: a standardized measure of biological and psychosocial function. *JAMA* 1963;185:914–919.

120. Guttman L. The basis for scalogram analysis. In: Stouffer SA, Guttman L, Suchman EA, et al., eds. *Measurement and prediction*. Princeton: Princeton University Press, 1950:60–90.

121. Anderson TP, Boureston N, Greenberg FR, et al. Predictive factors in stroke rehabilitation. *Arch Phys Med Rehabil* 1974;55:545–553.

122. Gibson CJ. Epidemiology and patterns of care of stroke patients. *Arch Phys Med Rehabil* 1974;55:398–403.

123. Hermodsson Y, Ekdahl C. Early planning of care and rehabilitation after amputation for vascular disease by means of Katz Index of Activities of Daily Living. *Scand J Caring Sci* 1999;13:234–239.

124. Assessing functional ability in patients with unilateral trans-tibial amputation for vascular disease. *Scand J Occup Ther* 1998;5:167–172.

125. Brorsson B, Asberg KH. Katz index of independence in ADL: reliability and validity in short-term care. *Scand J Rehabil Med* 1984;16:125–132.

126. Chong DK. Measurement of instrumental activities of daily living in stroke. *Stroke* 1995;26:1119–1122.

127. Fisher AG. *Assessment of motor and process skills,* 2nd ed. Fort Collins, CO: Three Star Press, 1997.

128. Fisher AG. The assessment of IADL motor skill: an application of the many-faceted Rasch analysis. *Am J Occup Ther* 1993;47:319–329.

129. Mercier L, Audet T, Herbert R, et al. Impact of motor, cognitive and perceptual disorders on ability to perform activities of daily living after stroke. *Stroke* 2001;32:2602–2608.

130. Nygard L, Bernspang B, Fisher AG, et al. Comparing motor and process ability of persons with suspected dementia in home and clinical settings. *Am J Occup Ther* 1994;48:689–696.

131. Darragh AR, Sample PL, Fisher AG. Environment effect on functional task performance in adults with acquired brain injuries: use of the assessment of motor and process skills. *Arch Phys Med Rehabil* 1998;79:418–423.

132. Fisher AG. The assessment of IADL motor skill: an application of the many-faceted Rasch analysis. *Am J Occup Ther* 1993;47:319–329.

133. Park S, Fisher AG, Velozo CA. Using the Assessment of Motor and Process Skills to compare occupational performance between clinic and home settings. *Am J Occup Ther* 1994;48:697–709.

134. McNulty MC, Fisher AG. Validity of using the Assessment of Motor and Process Skills to estimate overall home safety in persons with psychiatric conditions. *Am J Occup Ther* 2000;55:649–655.

135. Kinnman J, Andersson U, Wetterquist L, et al. Cooling suit for multiple sclerosis: functional improvement in daily living? *Scand J Rehabil Med* 2000; 32:22–24.

136. Tham K, Ginsburg E, Fisher AG, et al. Training to improve awareness of disabilities in clients with unilateral neglect. *Am J Occup Ther* 2001;55:46–54.

137. Fisher AG, Duran L. ADL performance of black Americans and white Americans on the assessment of motor and process skills. *Am J Occup Ther* 2000; 54:607–613.

138. Fisher AG, Liu Y, Velozo CA, et al. Cross-cultural assessment of process skills. *Am J Occup Ther* 1992;46:876–885.

139. Nouri FM, Lincoln NB. An extended activities of daily living scale for stroke patients. *Clin Rehabil* 1987;1:301–305.

140. Rodgers H, Soutter J, Kaiser W, et al. Early supported hospital discharge following acute stroke: pilot study results. *Clin Rehabil* 1997;11:280–287.

141. Walker MF, Gladman JRF, Lincoln NB, et al. Occupational therapy for stroke patients not admitted to hospital: a randomized controlled trial. *Lancet* 2000;354:278–280.

142. Lincoln NB, Gladman JR, Berman P, et al. Functional recovery of community stroke patients. *Disabil Rehabil* 2000;22:135–139.

143. Dyer CA, Singh SJ, Stockley RA, et al. The incremental shuttle walking test in elderly people with chronic airflow limitation. *Thorax* 2002;57:34–38.

144. Bestall JC, Paul EA, Garrod R, et al. Usefulness of the MRC dyspnea scale as a measure of disability in patients with chronic obstructive pulmonary disease. *Thorax* 1999;54:581–586.

145. Garrod R, Bestall JC, Paul EA, et al. Development and validation of a standardized measure of activity of daily living in patients with severe COPD: The London Chest Activity of Daily Living Scale (LCADL). *Respir Med* 2000; 94:589–596.

146. Yohannes AM, Roomi J, Winn S, et al. The Manchester Respiratory Activities of Daily Living questionnaire: development, reliability, validity and responsiveness to pulmonary rehabilitation. *J Am Geriatr Soc* 2000;48:1496–1500.

147. Burch S, Longbottom J, McKay M, et al. The Huntingdon Day Hospital Trial: secondary outcome measures. *Clin Rehabil* 2000;14:447–453.

148. Weatherall M. A randomized controlled trial of the Geriatric Depression Scale in an inpatient ward for older adults. *Clin Rehabil* 2000;14:186–199.

149. Harwood RH, Ebahim S. A comparison of the Nottingham Extended Activities of Daily Living Scale, London Handicap Scale and SF-36. *Disabil Rehabil* 2000;22:786–793.

150. Hsueh IP, Suang SL, Chen MH, et al. Evaluation of stroke patients with the extended activities of daily living scale in Taiwan. *Disabil Rehabil* 2000;22: 495–500.

151. Walker MF, Drummond AER, Lincoln NB. Evaluation of dressing practice for stroke patients after discharge from hospital: a crossover design study. *Clin Rehabil* 1996;10:22–31.

152. Buck D, Jacoby A, Massey A, Ford G. Evaluation of measures used to assess quality of life after stroke. *Stroke* 2000;31:2004–2010.

153. Holbrook M, Skilbeck CE. An activities index for use with stroke. *Age Ageing* 1983;12:166–170.

154. Turnbull JC, Kersten P, Habib M, et al. Validation of the Frenchay Activities Index in a general population aged 16 and over. *Arch Phys Med Rehabil* 2000;81:1034–1038.

155. Green J, Forster A, Young J. A test–retest reliability study of the Barthel Index, the Rivermead Mobility Index, the Nottingham Extended Activities of Daily Living Scale and the Frenchay Activities Index in stroke patients. *Disabil Rehabil* 2001;23:670–676.

156. Dennis M, Orourke S, Slattery J, et al. Evaluation of a stroke family care worker: results of a randomized controlled trial. *Br Med J* 1997;314:1071–1076.

157. Sveen U, Bautz-Holter E, Sodring KM, et al. Association between impairments, self care ability and social activities one year after stroke. *Disabil Rehabil* 1999;21:372–377.

158. Young J, Bogle S, Forster A. Determinants of social outcome measured by the Frenchay Activities Index at one year after stroke onset. *Cerebrovasc Dis* 2001;12:114–120.

159. Kwakkel G, Kollen BJ, Wagenaar RC. Long term effects of intensity of upper and lower limb training after stroke: a randomized trial. *J Neurol Neurosurg Psychiatry* 2002;72:473–479.

160. Haig AJ, Nagy A, Lebreck DB, et al. Outpatient planning for persons with physical disabilities: a randomized prospective trial of physiatrist alone versus a multidisciplinary team. *Arch Phys Med Rehabil* 1995;76:341–348.

161. Walters SJ, Morrell CJ, Dixon S. Measuring health-related quality of life in patients with venous leg ulcers. *Quality Life Res* 1999;8:327–336.

162. Mant J, Carter J, Wade DT, et al. Family support for stroke: a randomized controlled trial. *Lancet* 2000;356:808–813.

163. Hachisuka K, Saeki S, Tsutsui Y, et al. Gender related differences in scores of the Barthel Index and Frenchay Activities Index in randomly sampled elderly persons living at home in Japan. *J Clin Epidemiol* 1999;52:1089–1094.

164. Hsieh CL, Hsueh IP. A cross validation of the comprehensive assessment of activities of daily living after stroke. *Scand J Rehabil Med* 1999;31:83–88.

165. Pedersen PM, Jorgensen HS, Nakayama H, et al. Comprehensive assessment of activities of daily living in stroke. The Copenhagen Stroke Study. *Arch Phys Med Rehabil* 1997;78:161–165.

166. Carod-Artal FJ, Gonzalez-Gutierrez JL, Herrero JAE, et al. Functional recovery and instrumental activities of daily living: follow-up 1-year after treatment in a stroke unit. *Brain Inj* 2002;16:3207–3216.

167. Piercy W, Carter J, Mant J, et al. Inter-rater reliability of the Frenchay Activities Index in patients with stroke and their carers. *Clin Rehabil* 2000;14: 433–440.

168. Schuling J, Dehaan R, Limburg M, et al. The Frenchay Activities Index—assessment of functional status in stroke patients. *Stroke* 1993;24:1173–1177.

169. Hamilton BB, Granger CV, Sherwin FS, et al. A uniform national data system for medical rehabilitation. In: Fuhrer MJ, ed. *Rehabilitation outcomes: analysis and measurement.* Baltimore: Paul H. Brookes, 1987:137–147.

170. Hamilton BB, Granger CV. Disability outcomes following inpatient rehabilitation for stroke. *Phys Ther* 1994;74:494–503.

171. Granger C, Deutsch A, Linn R. Rasch analysis of the Functional Independence Measure FIM Mastery Test. *Arch Phys Med Rehabil* 1998;79:52–57.

172. Kidd D, Stewart G, Baldry J, et al. The Functional Independence Measure: a comparative validity and reliability study. *Disabil Rehabil* 1995;17:10–14.

173. Fisher WP Jr, Harvey RF, Taylor P, et al. Rehabits: a common language of functional assessment. *Arch Phys Med Rehabil* 1995;76:113–122.

174. Ottenbacher KJ, Mann WC, Granger CV, et al. Inter-rater agreement and stability of functional assessment in the community-based elderly. *Arch Phys Med Rehabil* 1994;75:1297–1301.

175. Segal ME, Schall RR. Determining functional health status and its relation to disability in stroke survivors. *Stroke* 1994;25:2391–2397.

176. Kaplan CP, Corrigan JD. The relationship between cognition and functional independence in adults with traumatic brain injury. *Arch Phys Med Rehabil* 1994;75:643–647.
177. Segal ME, Gillard M, Schall R. Telephone and in person proxy agreement between stroke patients and caregivers for the functional independence measure. *Am J Phys Med Rehabil* 1996;75:208–212.
178. Cowen CD, Meythaler JM, DeVivo MJ, et al. Influence of early variables in traumatic brain injury on functional independence measure scores and rehabilitation length of stay and charges. *Arch Phys Med Rehabil* 1995;76:797–803.
179. Granger CV, Divan N, Fiedler RC. Functional assessment scales: a study of persons after traumatic brain injury. *Am J Phys Med Rehabil* 1995;74:107–113.
180. Corrigan JD, Smith-Knapp K, Granger CV, et al. Validity of the functional independence measure for persons with traumatic brain injury. *Arch Phys Med Rehabil* 1997;78:828–834.
181. Muecke L, Shekar S, Dwyer D, et al. Functional screening of lower limb amputees: a role in predicting rehabilitation outcome? *Arch Phys Med Rehabil* 1992;73:851–858.
182. Segal ME, Schall RR. Determining functional health status and its relation to disability in stroke survivors. *Stroke* 1994;25:2391–2397.
183. Segal ME, Ditunno JF, Staas WE. Interinstitutional agreement of individual functional independence measure (FIM) items measured at two sites on one sample of SCI patients. *Paraplegia* 1993;31:622–631.
184. Heinemann AW, Linacre JM, Wright BD, et al. Relationships between impairment and physical disability as measured by the functional independence measure. *Arch Phys Med Rehabil* 1993;74:566–573.
185. Bunch WH, Dvonch VM. The "value" of functional independence measure scores. *Am J Phys Med Rehabil* 1994;73:40–43.
186. Granger CV, Cotter AC, Hamilton BB, et al. Functional assessment scales: a study of persons after stroke. *Arch Phys Med Rehabil* 1993;74:133–138.
187. Heinemann AW, Kirk P, Hastie BA, et al. Relationships between disability measures and nursing effort during medical rehabilitation for patients with traumatic brain injury and spinal cord injury. *Arch Phys Med Rehabil* 1997;78:143–149.
188. Heinemann AW, Hamilton BB, Betts HB, et al. *Rating scale analysis of functional assessment measures.* Chicago: Rehabilitation Institute of Chicago, 1991.
189. Weh L, Ramb JF. Functional Independence Measure as a predictor of expected rehabilitation outcome in patients with total endoprosthesis replacement and after apoplectic infarct. *Z Orthop Ihre Grenzgeb* 1992;130:333–338.
190. Tsuji T, Sonoda S, Domen K, et al. ADL structure for stroke patients in Japan based on the functional independence measure. *Am J Phys Med Rehabil* 1995;74:432–438.
191. Turkalj Z, Colja-Matic S, Vlah N, et al. Results of rehabilitation after ischemic cerebrovascular stroke. *Lijec Vjesn* 1995;117:268–271.
192. Smith PM, Ottenbacher KJ, Cranley M, et al. Predicting follow-up living setting in patients with stroke. *Arch Phys Med Rehabil* 2002;83:764–770.
193. Karamehmetoglu SS, Karacan I, Elbasi N, et al. The Functional Independence Measure in spinal cord injured patients: comparison of questioning with observational rating. *Spinal Cord* 1997;35:22–25.
194. Hall KM, Mann N, High WM, et al. Functional measures after traumatic brain injury: ceiling effects of FIM, FIM+FAM, DRS, and CIQ. *J Head Trauma Rehabil* 1996;11:27–39.
195. Muecke L, Shekar S, Dwyer D, et al. Functional screening of lower limb amputees: a role in predicting rehabilitation outcome? *Arch Phys Med Rehabil* 1992;73:851–858.
196. Hall KM. The Functional Assessment Measure (FAM). *J Rehabil Outcomes* 1997;1:63–65.
197. Alcott D, Dixon K, Swann R. The reliability of the scales of the Functional Assessment Measure (FAM): differences in abstractness between FAM scales. *Disabil Rehabil* 1997;19:355–358.
198. Hawley CA, Taylor R, Hellawell DJ, et al. FIM+FAM in head injury rehabilitation: a psychometric analysis. *J Neurol Neurosurg Psychiatry* 1999;67:749–754.
199. Hall KM, Johnston MV. Outcomes evaluation in TBI rehabilitation. Part II: Measurement tools for a nationwide data system. *Arch Phys Med Rehabil* 1994;75:SC10–SC18.
200. Donaghy S, Wass PJ. Interrater reliability of the Functional Assessment Measure in a brain injury rehabilitation program. *Arch Phys Med Rehabil* 1998;79:1231–1236.
201. Gurka JA, Felmingham KL, Baguley IJ, et al. Utility of the Functional Assessment Measure after discharge from inpatient rehabilitation. *J Head Trauma Rehabil* 1999;14:247–56.
202. Hoenig H, Hoff J, McIntyre L, et al. The self-reported functional measure: predictive validity for health utilization in multiple sclerosis and spinal cord injury. *Arch Phys Med Rehabil* 2001;82:613–618.
203. Samsa GP, Hoenig H, Branch LG. Relationship between self-reported disability and caregiver hours. *Am J Phys Med Rehabil* 2001;80:674–684.
204. Gresham GE, Labi MLC. Functional assessment instruments currently available for documenting outcomes in rehabilitation medicine. In: Granger CV, Gresham GE, eds. *Functional assessment in rehabilitation medicine.* Baltimore: Williams & Wilkins, 1984.
205. Moskowitz E, McCann CB. Classification of disability in the chronically ill and aging. *J Chronic Dis* 1957;5:342–346.
206. Granger CV, Albrecht GL, Hamilton BB. Outcome of comprehensive medical rehabilitation: measurement by PULSES Profile and the Barthel Index. *Arch Phys Med Rehabil* 1979;60:145–154.
207. Granger CV, Dewis LS, Peters NC, et al. Stroke rehabilitation: analysis of repeated Barthel Index measures. *Arch Phys Med Rehabil* 1979;60:14–17.
208. Kelly CR, Rose DL. Grading the rehabilitation effort. *J Kansas Med Soc* 1971;72:154–156.
209. Moskowitz E, Lightbody FEH, Freitag NS. Long term follow-up of the post stroke patient. *Arch Phys Med Rehabil* 1972;53:167–172.
210. Hopps SL, Pépin M, Arseneau I, et al. Disability related variables associated with loneliness among people with disabilities. *J Rehabil Med* 2001;67:42–48.
211. Marshall SC, Heisel B, Grinnell D. Validity of the PULSES profile compared with the Functional Independence Measure for measuring disability in a stroke rehabilitation setting. *Arch Phys Med Rehabil* 1999;80:760–765.
212. Mattison PG, Aitken RCB, Prescott RJ. Rehabilitation status in multiple handicap. *Arch Phys Med Rehabil* 1992;73:926–929.
213. Law M, Baptiste S, McColl MA, et al. The Canadian Occupational Performance Measure: an outcome measure for occupational therapy. *Can J Occup Ther* 1994;57:82–87.
214. Pollock N. Client-centered assessment. *Am J Occup Ther* 1993;47:298–301.
215. Pollock N, Baptiste S, Law M, et al. Occupational performance measures: a review of based on the guidelines for the client-centered practice of occupational therapy. *Can J Occup Ther* 1990;57:77–81.
216. Law M, Polotajko H, Pollock N, et al. Pilot testing of the Canadian Occupational Performance Measure: clinical and measurement issues. *Can J Occup Ther* 1994;61:191–197.
217. Toomey M, Nicholson D, Carswell A. The clinical utility of the Canadian Occupational Performance Measure. *Can J Occup Ther* 1995;62:242–249.
218. Bodiam C. The use of the Canadian Occupational Performance Measure for the assessment of outcome on a neurorehabilitation unit. *Br J Occup Ther* 1999;62:123–126.
219. Chesworth C, Duffy R, Hodnett J, et al. Measuring clinical effectiveness in mental health: is the Canadian Occupational Performance an appropriate measure. *Br J Occup Ther* 2002;65:30–34.
220. Sewell L, Singh SJ. The Canadian Occupational Performance Measure: is it a reliable measure in clients with chronic obstructive pulmonary disease? *Br J Occup Ther* 2001;64:305–310.
221. Trombly CA, Radomski MV, Davis ES. Achievement of self-identified goals by adults with traumatic brain injury: Phase I. *Am J Occup Ther* 1998;52:810–818.
222. Law M, Wishart L, Guyatt G. The use of a simulated environment (Easy Street) to retrain independent living skills in elderly persons: a randomized controlled trial. *J Gerontol Med Sci* 2000;55:M578–M584.
223. Simmons DC, Crepeau EB, White BP. The predictive power of narrative data in occupational therapy evaluation. *Am J Occup Ther* 2000;54:471–476.
224. Ripat J, Etcheverry E, Cooper J, et al. A comparison of the Canadian Occupational Performance Measure and the Health Assessment Questionnaire. *Can J Occup Ther* 2001;68:247–253.
225. Wressle E, Eeg-Olofsson A, Marcusson J, et al. Improved client participation in the rehabilitation process using a client-centered goal formulation structure. *J Rehabil Med* 2002;34:5–11.
226. Wressle E, Marcusson J, Henriksson C. Clinical utility of the Canadian Occupational Performance Measure—Swedish Version. *Can J Occup Ther* 2002;69:40–48.
227. Carpenter L, Baker GA, Tyldesley B. The use of the Canadian Occupational Performance Measure as an outcome of a pain management program. *Can J Occup Ther* 2001;68:16–22.
228. Gilbertson L, Langhorne P. Home-based occupational therapy: stroke patients' satisfaction with occupational performance and service provision. *Br J Occup Ther* 2000;63:464–468.
229. Boyer G, Hachey R, Mercier C. Perceptions of occupational performance and subjective quality of life in persons with severe mental illness. *Occup Ther Mental Health* 2000;15:1–15.
230. Cup EH, Scholte OP, Reimer WJ, Thijssen MC, et al. Reliability of the Canadian Occupational Performance Measure in stroke patients. *Clin Rehabil* 2003; 17:402–409.
231. Law M, Russell D, Pollock N, et al. A comparison of intensive neurodevelopmental therapy plus casting and a regular occupational therapy program for children with cerebral palsy. *Dev Med Child Neurol* 1997;39:664–670.
232. Uniform Data System. *Guide for the use of the pediatric functional independence measure.* Buffalo, NY: Research Foundation, State University of New York, 1990.
233. Ottenbacher KJ, Msall ME, Lyon N, et al. Measuring developmental and functional status in children with disabilities. *Dev Med Child Neurol* 1999;41:186–194.
234. Braun SL, Granger CV. A practical approach to functional assessment in pediatrics. *Occup Ther Practice* 1991;2:46–51.
235. Ottenbacher KJ, Taylor ET, Msall ME, et al. The stability and equivalence reliability of the functional independence measure for children (WeeFIM). *Dev Med Child Neurol* 1996;38:907–916
236. Ottenbacher KJ, Msall ME, Lyon NR, et al. Interrater agreement and stability of the functional independence measure for children (WeeFIM): use in children with developmental disabilities. *Arch Phys Med Rehabil* 1997;78:1309–1315.
237. Msall ME, Digaudio K, Duffy LC, et al. WeeFIM—normative sample of an instrument for tracking functional independence in children. *Clin Pediatr* 1994;33:431–438.
238. Liu MG, Toikawa H, Seki M, et al. Functional independence measure for children (WeeFIM): a preliminary study in nondisabled Japanese children. *Am J Phys Med Rehabil* 1998;77:36–44.

239. Wong V, Wong S, Chan K, et al. Functional independence measure (WeeFIM) for Chinese children: Hong Kong cohort. *Pediatrics* 2002;109:E36.

240. Msall ME, Tremont MR. Measuring functional status in children with genetic impairments. *Am J Med Genet* 1999;89:62–74.

241. Limperopoulos C, Majnemer A, Shevell ML, et al. Functional limitations in young children with congenital heart defects after cardiac surgery. *Am Acad Pediatr* 2001;108:1325–1331.

242. Azaula M, Msall ME, Buck G, et al. Measuring functional status and family support in older school-aged children with cerebral palsy: comparison of three instruments. *Arch Phys Med Rehabil* 2000;81:307–311.

243. Schneider JW, Gurucharri LM, Gutierrez AL, et al. Health related quality of life and functional outcome measures for children with cerebral palsy. *Dev Med Child Neurol* 2001;43:601–608.

244. Msall ME, Laforest S, Buck GM, et al. Use of the WeeFIM to facilitate functional independence in preadolescents with spina-bifida. *Pediatr Res* 1995; 37:A17.

245. Leonard S, Msall M, Bower C, et al. Functional status of school-aged children with Down syndrome. *J Pediatr Child Health* 2002;38:160–165.

246. Msall ME, Rogers BT, Buck GM, et al. Functional status of extremely preterm infants at kindergarten entry. *Dev Med Child Neurol* 1993;35:312–320.

247. Msall ME, Phelps DL, DiGaudio KM, et al. Severity of neonatal retinopathy of prematurity is predictive of neurodevelopmental functional outcome at age 5.5 years. *Pediatrics* 2000;106:998–1005.

248. Hogan DP, Park JM. Family factors and social support in the developmental outcomes of very low birth-weight children. *Clin Perinatol* 2000;27:433–438.

249. Philip PA, Ayyangar R, Vanderbilt J, et al. Rehabilitation outcome in children after treatment of primary brain tumor. *Arch Phys Med Rehabil* 1994;75: 36–39.

250. Loewen P, Steinbok P, Holsti L, et al. Upper extremity performance and self care skill changes in children with spastic cerebral palsy following selective posterior rhizotomy. *Pediatr Neurosurg* 1998;29:191–198.

251. DiScala C, Grant CC, Brooke MM, et al. Functional outcome in children with traumatic brain injury. Agreement between clinical judgment and the functional independence measure. *Am J Phys Med Rehabil* 1992;71:145–148.

252. Swaine BR, Pless IB, Friedman DS, et al. Effectiveness of a head injury program for children—a preliminary investigation. *Am J Phys Med Rehabil* 2001; 80:412–420.

252. Garcia RA, Gaebler-Spira D, Sisung C, et al. Functional improvement after pediatric spinal cord injury. *Am J Phys Med Rehabil* 2002;81:458–463.

254. Haley SM, Coster WJ, Ludlow LH, et al. *Pediatric evaluation of disability inventory–development, standardization and administration manual.* Boston: PEDI Research Group, 1992.

255. Haley SM, Coster WJ, Faas RM. A content validity study of the Pediatric Evaluation of Disability Inventory. *Pediatr Phys Ther* 1991;3:177–184.

256. Ludlow LH, Haley SM. Effect of context in rating of mobility activities in children with disabilities: an assessment using the pediatric evaluation of disability inventory. *Educ Psychol Measure* 1996;56:122–129.

257. Coster WJ, Haley S, Baryza MJ. Functional performance of young children after traumatic brain injury: a 6-month follow-up study. *Am J Occup Ther* 1994;48:211–218.

258. Tsai PY, Yang TF, Chan RC, et al. Functional investigation in children with spina bifida—measured by the Pediatric Evaluation of Disability Inventory (PEDI). *Childs Nerv Syst* 2002;18:48–53.

259. Engelbert RHH, Beemer FA, van der Graaf Y, et al. Osteogenesis imperfecta in childhood: impairment and disability—a follow-up study. *Arch Phys Med Rehabil* 1999;80:896–903.

260. Engelbert RHH, Gulmans VA, Uiterwaal CS, et al. Osteogenesis imperfecta in childhood: perceived competence in relation to impairment and disability. *Arch Phys Med Rehabil* 2001;82:943–948.

261. Msall ME, Rogers BT, Ripstein H, et al. Measurement of functional outcomes in children with cerebral palsy. *Ment Retard Dev Disabil Res Rev* 1997;3:194–203.

262. Ketelaar M, Vermeer A, Hart H, et al. Effects of a functional therapy program on motor abilities of children with cerebral palsy. *Phys Ther* 2001;81: 1534–1545.

263. Bloom KK, Nazar GB. Functional assessment following selective posterior rhizotomy in spastic cerebral palsy. *Childs Nerv Syst* 1994;10:84–86.

264. Nordmark E, Jarnlo GB, Hagglund G. Comparison of the gross motor function measure and paediatric evaluation of disability inventory in assessing motor function in children undergoing selective dorsal rhizotomy. *Dev Med Child Neurol* 2000;42:245–252.

265. Steinbok P. Outcomes after selective dorsal rhizotomy for spastic cerebral palsy. *Childs Nerv Syst* 2001;17:1–18.

270. Fehlings D, Rang M, Glazier J, et al. An evaluation of botulinum-A toxin injections to improve upper extremity function in children with hemiplegic cerebral palsy. *J Pediatr* 2000;137:331–337.

271. Fehlings D, Rang M, Glazier J, et al. Botulinum toxin type A injections in the spastic upper extremity of children with hemiplegia: child characteristics that predict a positive outcome. *Eur J Neurol* 2001;8:145–149.

268. McCarthy JJ, Finson R, Smith BT, et al. Cerebral palsy: results of surgical releases augmented with electrical stimulation. A case study. *Neuromodulation* 2002;5:113–119.

269. Ketelaar M, Vermeer A, Helders PJM. Functional motor abilities of children with cerebral palsy: a systematic literature review of assessment measures. *Clin Rehabil* 1998;12:369–380.

270. Custers JWH, Hoijtink H, van der Net J, et al. Cultural differences in functional status measurement: analyses of person fit according to the Rasch model. *Qual Life Res* 2000;9:571–578.

271. Gannotti ME, Handwerker WP, Groce NE, et al. Sociocultural influences on disability status in Puerto Rican children. *Phys Ther* 2001;81:1512–1523.

272. Custers JWH, Wassenberg-Severijnen JE, Van der Net J, et al. Dutch adaptation and content validity of the Pediatric Evaluation of Disability Inventory. *Disabil Rehabil* 2002;24:250–258.

273. Christiansen CH. Planning intervention for self care needs. In: Christiansen C, ed. *Ways of living: self care strategies for special needs.* Bethesda: American Occupational Therapy Association, 2000:46–55.

274. Norburn JE, Bernard SL, Konrad TR, et al. Self care and assistance from others in coping with functional status limitations among a national sample of older adults. *J Gerontol B Psychol Sci Soc Sci* 1995;50:S101–S109.

275. Schum TR, Kolb TM, McAuliffe TL. Sequential acquisition of toilet-training skills: a descriptive study of gender and age differences in normal children. *Pediatrics* 2002;109:E48.

276. Kayser JE, Billingsley FF, Neel RS. A comparison of in-context and traditional instructional approaches: total task, single trial versus backward chaining, multiple trials. *J Assoc Persons Severe Handicaps* 1986;11:28–38.

277. Snell MD, Vogtle LK. Methods for teaching self care skills. In: Christiansen C, ed. *Ways of living: self care strategies for special needs.* Bethesda, MD: American Occupational Therapy Association, 2000:58–81.

278. Snell ME. *Instruction of students with severe disabilities.* New York: Macmillan, 1993.

279. Cross KW. Role of practice in perceptual–motor learning. *Am J Phys Med Rehabil* 1967;46:487–510.

280. White RW. Motivation reconsidered: the concept of competence. *Psychol Rev* 1959;66:297–333.

281. Bjornby ER, Reinvang IR. Acquiring and maintaining self-care skills after stroke: the predictive value of apraxia. *Scand J Rehabil Med* 1985;17:75–80.

282. Wagenaar RC, Meijer OG. Effects of stroke rehabilitation: a critical review of the literature. *J Rehabil Sci* 1991;4:61–73.

283. Wagenaar RC, Meijer OG. Effects of stroke rehabilitation: a critical review of the literature. *J Rehabil Sci* 1991;4:97–109.

284. Trombly CA. Occupation: purposefulness and meaningfulness as therapeutic mechanisms. 1995 Eleanor Clarke Slagle Lecture. *Am J Occup Ther* 1995; 49:960–972.

285. Trombly CA. Anticipating the future: assessment of occupational function. *Am J Occup Ther* 1993;47:253–257.

286. LaPlante MP, Hendershot GE, Moss AJ. *Assistive technology devices and home accessibility features: prevalence, payment, need and trends.* Hyattsville, MD: National Center for Health Statistics, 1992;217:1–11.

287. Tabbarah M, Silverstein M, Seeman T. A health and demographic profile of non-institutionalized older Americans residing in environments with home modifications. *J Aging Health* 2000;12:204–228.

288. American National Standards Institute. *American National Standard specifications for making buildings and facilities accessible to and usable by physically handicapped people.* New York: American Standards Institute, 1986.

289. Cumming RG, Thomas M, Szonyi G, et al. Adherence to occupational therapist recommendations for home modifications for falls prevention. *Am J Occup Ther* 2001;55:641–648.

290. Jutai J, Rigby P, Ryan S, et al. Psychosocial impact of electronic aids to daily living. *Assist Technol* 2000;12:123–131.

291. Russell JN, Hendershot GE, LeClere F, et al. Trends and differential use of assistive technology devices: United States, 1994. Advance data from vital and health statistics, no. 292. Hyattsville, MD: National Center for Health Statistics, 1997.

292. Verbrugge LM, Rennert C, Madans JH. The great efficacy of personal and equipment assistance in reducing disability. *Am J Public Health* 1997;87:384–392.

293. Gitlin LN, Levine R, Geiger C. Adaptive device use by older adults with mixed disabilities. *Arch Phys Med Rehabil* 1993;74:149–152.

294. Thompson L. Functional changes in persons aging with spinal cord injury. *Assist Technol* 1999;11:123–129.

295. Fuhrer MJ. Assistive technology outcomes research: challenges met and yet unmet. *Am J Phys Med Rehabil* 2001;80:528–535.

296. Loebl D. A decision-making model for the provision of adaptive technology. *Am J Occup Ther* 1999;53:387–391.

297. Baum CM, Levesser P. Caregiver assistance: using family members and attendants. In: Christiansen C, ed. *Ways of living: self care strategies for special needs.* Bethesda, MD: American Occupational Therapy Association, 1994: 453–482.

298. Ulicny G, Jone, ML. Enhancing the attendant management skills of persons with disabilities. *Am Rehabil* 1985;2:18–20.

299. Opie ND, Miller ET. Attribution for successful relationships between severely disabled adults and personal care attendants. *Rehabil Nurs* 1989;14: 196–199.

300. Penninx BWJH, Messier SP, Rejeski WJ, et al. Physical exercise and the prevention of disability in activities of daily living in older persons with osteoarthritis. *Arch Intern Med* 2001;161:2309–2316.

301. Letts L, Marshall L. Evaluating the validity and consistency of the SAFER Tool. *Phys Occup Ther Geriatr* 1995;13:49–66.

302. Letts L, Scott S, Burtney J, et al. The reliability and validity of the safety assessment of function and the environment for rehabilitation (SAFER Tool). *Br J Occup Ther* 1998;61:127–132.

303. Rubenstein LZ, Robbins AS, Josephson KR, et al. The value of assessing falls in an elderly population: a randomized clinical trial. *Ann Intern Med* 1990: 131:308–316.

304. Putzke JD, Williams MA, Daniel FJ, et al. Activities of daily living among heart transplant candidates: neuropsychological and cardiac function predictors. *J Heart Lung Transplant* 2000;19:995–1006

305. Fried LP, Ettinger WH, Lind B, et al. Physical disability in older adults: a physiological approach. Cardiovascular Health Study Research Group. *J Clin Epidemiol* 1994;47:747–760.

306. Cahn-Weiner DA, Malloy PF, Boyle PA, et al. Prediction of functional status from neuropsychological tests in community-dwelling elderly individuals. *Clin Neuropsychol* 2000;14:198–195.

307. Heruti RJ, Lusky A, Barell V, et al. Cognitive status at admission: does it affect the rehabilitation outcome of elderly patients with hip fracture? *Arch Phys Med Rehabil* 1999;80:432–436.

308. Goldkamp O. Treatment effectiveness in cerebral palsy. *Arch Phys Med Rehabil* 1984;65:232–234.

309. Sveen U, Wsyller TB, Ljunggren AE, et al. Predictive validity of early cognitive assessment in stroke rehabilitation. *Scand J Occup Ther* 1996;3:20–27.

310. Bogner JA, Corrigan JD, Fugatge L, et al. Role of agitation in prediction of outcomes after traumatic brain injury. *Am J Phys Med Rehabil* 2001;80:636–644.

311. Levine DN. Unawareness of visual and sensorimotor deficits: hypothesis. *Brain Cogn* 1990;13:233–281.

312. Titus M, Gall N, Yerxa EJ, et al. Correlation of perceptual performance and activities of daily living. *Am J Occup Ther* 1991;45:410–418.

313. Bernsprang B, Asplund K, Erriksson S, et al. Motor and perceptual impairments in acute stroke patients: effects on self-care ability. *Stroke* 1987;18: 1081–1086.

314. Dudgeon BJ, DeLisa JA, Miller RM. Optokinetic nystagmus and upper extremity dressing independence after stroke. *Arch Phys Med Rehabil* 1985;66: 164–167.

315. Paolucci S, Antonucci G, Grasso MG, et al. The role of unilateral neglect in rehabilitation of right brain damaged ischemic stroke patients: a matched comparison. *Arch Phys Med Rehabil* 2001;82:743–749.

316. Katz N, Hartman-Maeir A, Ring H, et al. Functional disability and rehabilitation outcome in right hemisphere damaged patients with and without spatial neglect. *Arch Phys Med Rehabil* 1999;80:379–384.

317. Katz N, Hartman-Maeir A, Ring H, et al. Relationships of cognitive performance and daily function of clients following right hemisphere stroke: predictive and ecological validity of the LOTCA battery. *Occup Ther J Res* 2000;20:3–17.

318. Rubio KB, Van Deusen J. Relation of perceptual and body image dysfunction to activities of daily living of persons after stroke. *Am J Occup Ther* 1995; 49:551–559.

319. Schottke H. Rehabilitation of attention deficits after stroke: efficacy of a neuropsychological training program for attention deficits. *Verhaltenstherapie* 1997;7:21–33.

320. Gordon WA, Hibbard MR, Egelko S. Perceptual remediation in patients with right brain damage: a comprehensive program. *Arch Phys Med Rehabil* 1985; 66:353–359.

321. Edmonds JA, Webster J, Lincoln NB. A comparison of two approaches in the treatment of perceptual problems after stroke. *Clin Rehabil* 2000;14:230–243.

322. Beis JM, Andre JM, Baumgarten A, et al. Eye patching in unilateral spatial neglect: efficacy of two methods. *Arch Phys Med Rehabil* 1999;80:71–76.

323. Pedro-Cuesta J de, Widen-Holmqvist L, Bach-y-Rita P. Evaluation of stroke rehabilitation by randomized controlled studies: a review. *Acta Neurol Scand* 1992;86:433–439.

324. Donkervoort M, Dekker J, Stehmann-Saris FC, et al. Efficacy of strategy training in left hemisphere stroke patients with apraxia: a randomized clinical trial. *Neuropsychol Rehabil* 2001;11:549–566.

325. Cook EA, Luschen L, Sikes S. Case report-dressing training for an elderly woman with cognitive and perceptual impairments. *Am J Occup Ther* 1991; 45:652–654.

326. Bendsen BB, Bendsen EB, Lauitzen L, et al. Post stroke patients in rehabilitation. The relationship between biological impairment (CT scanning), physical disability and clinical depression. *Eur Psychiatry* 1997;12:399–404.

327. Berod AC, Klay M, Santos-Eggimann B, et al. Anxiety, depressive or cognitive disorders in rehabilitation patients: effect on length of stay. *Am J Phys Med Rehabil* 2000;79:266–273.

328. Corrigan JD, Bogner JA, Mysiw WJ, et al. Life satisfaction after traumatic brain injury. *J Head Trauma Rehabil* 2001;16:543–555.

329. Robinson-Smith G, Johnston MV, Allen J. Self-care self-efficacy, quality of life, and depression after stroke. *Arch Phys Med Rehabil* 2000;81:460–464.

330. Rosenthal M, Christensen BK, Ross TP. Depression following traumatic brain injury. *Arch Phys Med Rehabil* 1998;79:90–103.

331. Anderson G, Verstergaard K, Lauritzen L. Effective treatment of post stoke depression with the selective serotonin reuptade inhibitor citalopram. *Stroke* 1994;2:1099–1109.

332. van de Weg FB, Kuik DJ, Lankhorst GJ. Post-stroke depression and functional outcome: a cohort study investigating the influence of depression on functional recovery from stroke. *Clin Rehabil* 1999;13:268–272.

333. Paoulucci S, Antonucci G, Grasso MG, et al. Post stroke depression, antidepressant treatment and rehabilitation results: a case control study. *Cerebrovasc Dis* 2001;12:264–271.

334. Craig AR, Hancock K, Dickson H, et al. Long-term psychological outcomes in spinal cord injured persons: results of a controlled trial using cognitive behavior therapy. *Arch Phys Med Rehabil* 1997;78:33–38.

335. Hartkopp A, Bronnum-Hansen H, Seidenschnur A, et al. Suicide in a spinal cord injured population: its relation to functional status. *Arch Phys Med Rehabil* 1998;79:1356–1361.

336. Adkins D. Managing self care in adults with upper extremity amputations. In: Christiansen C, ed. *Ways of living: self care strategies for special needs.* Bethesda: American Occupational Therapy Association, 2000:221–230.

337. Davis SE, Mulcahey MJ, Smith BT, et al. Outcome of functional electrical stimulation in the rehabilitation of a child with C-5 tetraplegia. *J Spinal Cord Med* 1999;22:107–113.

338. Hurvitz EA, Conti GE, Flansburg EL, et al. Motor control testing of upper limb function after botulinum toxin injection: a case study. *Arch Phys Med Rehabil* 2000;81:1408–1415.

339. Narang IC, Mathur BP, Singh P, et al. Functional capabilities of lower limb amputees. *Prosthet Orthot Int* 1984;8:43–51.

340. Haworth RJ, Hollings EM. Are hospital assessments of daily living activities valid? *Int Rehabil Med* 1979;1:59–62.

341. Peckham PH, Keith MW, Kilgore KL, et al. Efficacy of an implanted neuroprosthesis for restoring hand grasp in tetraplegia: a multicenter study. *Arch Phys Med Rehabil* 2001;82:1380–1388.

342. Geertzen JHB, Dijkstra PU, van Sonderen ELP, et al. Relationship between impairments, disability and handicap in reflex sympathetic dystrophy patients: a long-term follow-up study. *Clin Rehabil* 1998;12:402–412.

343. Langhammer B, Stanghelle JK. Bobath or motor relearning program? A comparison of two different approaches of physiotherapy in stroke rehabilitation: a randomized controlled study. *Clin Rehabil* 2000;14:361–369.

344. Taub E, Uswatte G. A new approach to treatment and measurement in physical rehabilitation: constraint-induced (CI) movement therapy. In: Frank R, Elliott T, eds. *Handbook of rehabilitation psychology.* Washington, DC: American Psychological Association, 2000.

345. Dromerick AW, Edwards DF, Hahn M. Does the application of constraint induced movement therapy during acute rehabilitation reduce arm impairment after ischemic stroke? *Stroke* 2000;31:2984–2988.

346. Liepert J, Bauder H, Wolfgang HR, et al. Treatment induced cortical reorganization after stroke in humans. *Stroke* 2000;31:1210–1216.

CHAPTER 44

Psychological Aspects of Rehabilitation

Daniel E. Rohe

This chapter begins by reviewing the history and current status of rehabilitation psychology. This is followed by a description of the direct and indirect services typically provided by rehabilitation psychologists. Frequently encountered psychological measures are described, and their importance for rehabilitation planning is stressed. The final section examines theories of adjustment to disability.

REHABILITATION PSYCHOLOGY: HISTORY AND CURRENT STATUS

History

The field of rehabilitation psychology received initial impetus from veterans returning from the two world wars in the first half of this century. After World War II, the Veterans Administration focused on the psychological needs of the physically disabled, which led to acceptance of psychologists as providers of mental health services. During this same time period, Howard A. Rusk developed the first comprehensive rehabilitation center, which led, with the leadership of others, to the development of physical medicine and rehabilitation, as well as physical and occupational therapy. Thus, the birth and maturation of the disciplines comprising the rehabilitation team have overlapping histories (1,2).

As the number of psychologists working in rehabilitation settings grew, the need for a professional forum arose. In 1949, a special-interest group within the American Psychological Association (APA) was created and in 1958 was granted division status. The Division of Rehabilitation Psychology of the APA provides leadership in formulating federal legislation, and in various professional and lay organizations. The Rehabilitation Act of 1973 and the Education for All Handicapped Children Act of 1975 provided mandates for the participation of rehabilitation psychologists in services to the disabled (3). Rehabilitation psychologists promoted passage of the Americans with Disabilities Act of 1990 and its ongoing implementation (4).

Current Status

Rehabilitation psychologists have struggled with their identity since the field's inception. Shontz and Wright argued for the distinctiveness of rehabilitation psychology (5). More recently, Glueckauf argued that rehabilitation psychology is a subspe-

cialty within the larger domain of health psychology. In this model, rehabilitation psychology is grouped with the subspecialties of clinical neuropsychology, geropsychology, and pediatric psychology (6). To promote this model, an Interdivisional Healthcare Committee, with representatives from several divisions of the American Psychological Association, was formed to establish a common agenda (7).

The identity problem of rehabilitation psychologists arises from the fact that they typically have doctoral degrees in clinical or counseling psychology and enter the field through internship training. A general degree program initially molds their professional identity rather than training in rehabilitation theories, principles, literature, and research, training that is available in only a select number of doctoral programs. Depending on the quality of internship and postdoctoral training, some practitioners may lack training in theoretical models of rehabilitation. There has been ongoing debate within the field of rehabilitation psychology about the "best" training model. The key area of disagreement relates to timing of specialized training (predoctoral versus postdoctoral), with advocates for both points of view (8–12).

The training and practice of rehabilitation psychologists is changing for several reasons. First, the APA has developed a new model of education in which the graduate-level curriculum is generic, with specialization occurring through postdoctoral training. In 1995, the Division of Rehabilitation Psychology published guidelines for postdoctoral training in rehabilitation psychology (13). These guidelines define what constitutes comprehensive postdoctoral training of rehabilitation psychologists. Currently, there are 19 postdoctoral training programs in rehabilitation psychology in the United States. Second, the American Board of Rehabilitation Psychology (ABRP) was established in 1995, with the first diplomate in rehabilitation psychology awarded in 1996. The ABRP provided a comprehensive rationale for specialty definition and practice standards (14). Those awarded the diplomate have typically completed postdoctoral training and 5 years of clinical practice in rehabilitation psychology. The ABRP is part of the American Board of Professional Psychology (ABPP), an organization of psychologists that accredits subspecialties, much as the American Board of Medical Specialties does for medical specialties.

The goal of the Division of Rehabilitation Psychology is to expand knowledge and seek solutions to problems related to disability and the rehabilitation process. The mission of the organization states:

the Division of Rehabilitation Psychology will: 1) be APA's voice for the science and practice of psychology as it relates to changes in abilities and social roles arising from illness and disability; 2) be recognized by constituents internal and external to APA for the redefinition of "rehabilitation psychology" as an expanded spectrum of community and clinical services including prevention, rehabilitation, and postacute health care within the context of quality of life across the life-span; and 3) influence the health care marketplace such that rehabilitation psychology services are widely available and accessible, and that the quality of life perspective counterbalances both the economic and the medical/curative approaches [15].

The delivery of rehabilitation psychology services is adapting to the corporatization of health care and the reduction of expenditures in the Medicare and Medicaid programs (16–18). The impact of the Prospective Payment System (PPS) on rehabilitation psychologists is uncertain (19). Doctoral-trained rehabilitation psychologists can bill independently under Medicare Part B and hence are able to generate revenue in addition to the flat fee provided by the PPS. As a result, rehabilitation psychologists may assume expanded roles in patient evaluation and treatment planning. The shift to health maintenance and preferred provider organizations presents an evolving challenge, as payers are demanding psychological services that are brief, beneficial, and cost-effective. In response, rehabilitation psychologists are shifting their venues from hospitals to less expensive settings such as subacute and outpatient rehabilitation facilities, as well as to telehealth interventions (20).

The importance of aiding the process of adjustment to disability and preventing secondary conditions was acknowledged by the recent addition of six new current procedural technology (CPT) codes by the American Medical Association and their approval for reimbursement by the Medicare program. As of January 1, 2002, the new CPT codes for health and behavior assessment and intervention services apply to behavioral, social, and psychophysiologic procedures for the prevention, treatment, or management of physical health problems. These new "Health and Behavior Codes" recognize psychology's role as a health-care specialty and shift third-party reimbursement from a psychopathology model to a model focused on fostering individual adaptation and social accommodation. For example, CPT number 96152 pays for intervention services to modify the psychological, behavioral, cognitive, and social factors affecting health and well-being. Such services include using cognitive and behavioral interventions to initiate physician-prescribed diet and exercise programs. These new codes reimburse services such as patient adherence to medical treatment, symptom management, health-promoting behaviors, health-related risk-taking behaviors, and overall adjustment to physical illness. Federal reimbursement for these new codes will come from medical rather than from mental health funding, and hence will not draw from limited mental health dollars. The paradigm shift by the World Health Organization and the National Institutes on Disability and Rehabilitation Research from a biomedical to a social model of disability bodes well for the continued relevance of rehabilitation psychology services and research (21–25).

The direct and indirect services described in the following discussion reflect a traditional model of service delivery within an inpatient medical rehabilitation setting. As service delivery shifts to outpatient and community settings, adaptations in these services will evolve. Despite the consolidation of health-care payer and delivery systems, consumers continue to demand quality and value (26). The value of rehabilitation psychology services is acknowledged by the Commission on the Accreditation of Rehabilitation Facilities through their mandated provision for the availability of the rehabilitation psychologist as part of the rehabilitation team in both acute and subacute rehabilitation facilities. Rehabilitation psychology's focus on enhancing the quality of life for those with chronic illness and disability remains the central goal despite changes in health care.

DIRECT SERVICES

Nonstandardized Assessment: The Clinical Interview

The psychologist's first contact with a patient is pivotal in the development of a therapeutic relationship and may occur before transfer to a rehabilitation unit. The psychologist may visit the patient before the initial interview to explain his or her role. The patient's expectations of meeting with the psychologist are determined by previous exposure to mental health professionals; communications from other team members, including the physician; and preliminary explanations from the psychologist. The patient's willingness to interact meaningfully with the psychologist can be strongly influenced by the physician. At the introduction, the psychologist will state that comprehensive rehabilitation includes help with problematic thoughts and feelings associated with chronic illness or occasioned by the onset of disability. Frequently, patients are relieved to discover that contact with the psychologist is a routine part of comprehensive rehabilitation.

The initial interview may last an hour or more. Patients with cognitive impairment may be seen only long enough for a general determination of their information-processing capacity and emotional state. Further assessment will await improvement in their cognitive status or contact with an informed family member. The length of the initial interview with noncognitively impaired patients depends on the complexity of the medical or social issues. There are two major goals for the initial interview. First, a comprehensive history of the patient's social background is obtained. Table 44-1 lists frequently asked biographical questions. These data provide insight into previous learning experiences that may affect rehabilitation related attitudes and behaviors. Second, the psychologist attempts to understand the disability as the patient sees it. The foundation for a meaningful therapeutic relationship is laid in part by taking sufficient time to elicit the patient's perspective. The patient often faces a medical situation that he or she does not fully comprehend. Anxiety and fear often block the reception and communication of information between the patient and rehabilitation team members, especially physicians. The opportunity to have one's perspective, including cognitive and emotional aspects, aired in a supportive and clarifying manner is often therapeutic in itself.

The psychologist occupies an unusually difficult position. Although a team member, the psychologist has the professional responsibility of maintaining the confidentiality of the therapeutic relationship. The patient may confide information that is personally sensitive and inappropriate to share with other team members. If directly asked by other team members about such information, the psychologist may have to explain that the information is confidential. Usually the patient is told that any information considered sensitive by the psychologist or so indicated by the patient will not be communicated to others. General information of a less sensitive nature is provided in the form of an initial interview note. Subsequent therapeutic contacts are recorded in the hospital chart or summarized peri-

TABLE 44-1. Psychosocial Information Sought During Initial Interview

Data on Family of Origin
    Names, ages, occupations, marital status, and residence of parents and siblings
    Religious training
    Stability of family during early development
    History of major mental disorder in immediate and extended family, including a history of sexual abuse, chemical dependency, suicide, or psychiatric hospitalization
Relevant Patient Information
    Educational background and school achievement
    Occupation and vocational history
    Avocational activities
    History of adjustment to structured environments, such as school, work and military service
    Social adjustment, including any previous arrests, chemical dependency treatment, or psychiatric diagnosis
    Prior association with hospitals and health care
    Preinjury stresses at the time of injury
    Most difficult loss the patient has had to adjust to previously; success in that task
    Former associations with people having disabilities
Family Structure
    Names, ages, and quality of relationship with spouse and children
    Background of dating and sexual relationship with current spouse
    Marital adjustment
Understanding the Patient's Perspective
    The patient's understanding of the cause and probable course of the disability
    The patient's initial thoughts at the onset of the disability (if traumatic)
    The patient's most pressing immediate concern
    How well the patient thinks he or she is coping with the situation
    The patient's perception of how the disability will change lifestyle, including relationships, vocational future, and self-concept
    The patient's understanding of the behavioral expectations in the rehabilitation unit compared with those in the acute-care unit of the hospital
    The degree to which the patient's sense of self-esteem is related to physique or physical skills
    The patient's comfort in meeting with a psychologist
    Techniques the patient has used successfully to cope with stressful events
    Techniques the patient uses to get and maintain a sense of control over the environment

odically. The frequency of these contacts depends on the goals established during the initial interview, the current degree of psychological distress, the potential for behavioral decompensation, and staffing levels.

Standardized Assessment

Given the time-consuming and subjective nature of clinical interviews, rehabilitation psychologists use standardized tests to speed assessment and enhance interventions (27,28). This section describes several frequently used instruments. Standardized measures of personality, intellectual ability, and academic achievement are briefly discussed. The domains of neuropsychological and chemical use assessments are covered in more detail.

PERSONALITY

A personality test conventionally refers to a measure of personal characteristics, such as emotional status, interpersonal relations, motivation, interests, and attitudes. Personality in-

ventory development has generally relied on one or more methods, including content validation, empirical criterion keying, factor analysis, and personality theory. Personality measurement has generated controversy over two issues. The first concerns the stability of personality traits across situations as opposed to the situational specificity of behavior (29). The second issue involves the degree to which a given personality characteristic reflects a merely transitory state rather than a stable underlying trait. Anastasi provided a thorough overview of these issues and of other psychological measurement concepts, including norms, item analysis, reliability, and validity (30). Elliott and Umlauf caution that the insensitive use of personality measures with individuals who have medical symptoms or limited physical abilities can produce misleading results (31). The most frequently used personality inventory designed to measure psychopathology is the Minnesota Multiphasic Personality Inventory-2 (MMPI-2). Two personality measures of nonpathologic, or "normal," personality relevant to rehabilitation are the Revised NEO Personality Inventory (NEO-PI-R) and the Strong Interest Inventory (SII). Space limitations preclude discussion of the measurement of mood in persons with physical disability. Eliott and Frank reviewed the literature on depression and spinal cord injury (32). Rohe discussed the differentiation of grief from depression after onset of disability (33).

Minnesota Multiphasic Personality Inventory-2

The MMPI-2 is the revised version of the MMPI, the most widely used and thoroughly researched objective measure of personality (34–38). The MMPI-2 is composed of statements describing thoughts, feelings, ideas, attitudes, physical and emotional symptoms, and previous life experiences. In general, the material included on the MMPI-2 is usually covered in a clinical interview. However, factors of privacy, clinician time savings, and the clinical relevance of the items have ensured its acceptance in health-care settings.

The MMPI-2 was originally designed to yield information about personality factors related to the major psychiatric syndromes. The 567 true–false questions are grouped into 10 clinical scales (Table 44-2) that continue to reflect important aspects of personality despite their obsolete psychiatric titles. The items composing each scale were determined statistically. An item was included only if a carefully diagnosed group of patients (e.g., those hospitalized for depression) answered that question in a manner statistically different from that of other carefully diagnosed groups of patients (e.g., schizophrenics) and from the normal standardization sample. The MMPI-2 standardization sample consisted of 2,600 persons from seven states chosen to reflect several national census parameters, including minority group status. This system of item selection (i.e., empirical criterion keying) fostered the inclusion of subtle items, items that make the MMPI-2 less easily faked when compared with other personality measures.

The 10 clinical scales are interpreted with the aid of four validity scales (see Table 44-2). These scales provide information on the client's response style, such as literacy, cooperation, malingering, comprehension, and defensiveness. The empirical nature of the inventory has permitted construction of special scales. For example, there are scales to help predict rehabilitation motivation, headache proneness, and tendencies toward the development of alcoholism. Additionally, there are extensive MMPI norms on persons with specific diagnoses such as multiple sclerosis and spinal cord injury (39). Norms are reported as standard scores with a mean of 50 and a standard deviation of 10. A score of 65 or greater is the point at which the

TABLE 44-2. Brief Description of the Minnesota Multiple Personality Inventory–2: Validity and Clinical Scales

Scale		Number of Items	Elevated Scores Suggest
Number	**Name**		
Q	Cannot say	567	A large number of items have not been answered, a possible indication that the patient is resentful or is uncomfortable with ambiguity
L	L scale	15	An effort to create the impression of being a person with high moral, social, and ethical values
F	F scale	60	The questionnaire has been invalidated by some factor, including lack of comprehension, poor reading ability, mental confusion, a deliberate desire to fake psychiatric difficulty, random marking of responses, or scoring errors
K	K scale	30	A self-view of being well adjusted, capable, and confident, which, at higher scale elevations, is likely to represent a denial of the true state of affairs
1	Hypochondriasis	32	Undue concern with bodily states and preoccupation with possible symptoms of physical illness
2	Depression	57	Depression, sadness, pessimism, guilt, passivity, and tendency to give up hope easily
3	Hysteria	60	Psychological immaturity, self-centeredness, superficial relationships, and frequent use of denial in everyday life, and a tendency to develop physical symptoms under stress
4	Psychopathic deviate	50	Assertiveness and nonconformity at moderate elevations; angry rebelliousness and noncompliance with social mores at extreme levels
5	Masculinity–femininity	56	The degree of identification with roles and interests traditionally assigned to the sex opposite that of the respondent
6	Paranoia	40	Interpersonal oversensitivity and irritability about motives or behavior of others, and at extreme elevations, suspicious thinking similar to that of people with paranoid personality traits
7	Psychasthenia	48	General feelings of anxiety, with excessive rumination about personal inadequacies
8	Schizophrenia	78	Feelings of detachment from the social realm, extending to frank mental confusion and interpersonal aversiveness
9	Hypomania	46	Talkativeness, distractibility, physical restlessness, and, at times, impatience, irritability, or rapid mood swings
0	Social introversion	69	Social introversion and a lack of desire to be with others

normal and the pathologic groups are most reliably discriminated. However, depending on the scores obtained on the validity scales, this "cut-score" may be adjusted by the trained interpreter.

The MMPI-2 requires an eighth-grade reading level and is intended for adults 18 years of age and older. A version of the MMPI, entitled the MMPI-A, is preferred for use with adolescents (40). The MMPI-2 requires between 1 and 2 hours for completion. Although many computerized scoring services are available, this does not obviate the need for interpretation by an experienced psychologist. A variety of factors—including race, socioeconomic status, unique family circumstances, ethnic background, and physical disability—may distort the MMPI-2 profile (41).

An important goal in the development of the MMPI-2 was to preserve sufficient item continuity with the original MMPI to allow for the generalizability of the voluminous MMPI research literature to the MMPI-2. Unfortunately, Humphrey and Dahlstrom reported that profiles generated by the MMPI and the MMPI-2 on the same subjects are too frequently at variance to be able to consider the two instruments interchangeable (42). Hence, it would be an error to assume that the MMPI clinical research literature can be uncritically generalized to the MMPI-2 for all patients. Moreover, many of the original criticisms of the MMPI remain problematic for the MMPI-2 (43).

NEO Personality Inventory Revised

The NEO Personality Inventory Revised (NEO-PI-R) reflects the culmination of decades of personality research that concludes that personality traits can be summarized in terms of the so-called five-factor model (44,45). The NEO-PI-R was designed to measure the five major dimensions, or domains, thought to be central to normal adult personality. These dimensions are enti-

tled Neuroticism (N), Extraversion (E), Openness (O), Agreeableness (A), and Conscientiousness (C). Each domain scale has six facet scales resulting in a total of 35 scales on the inventory. Neuroticism refers to a general tendency to experience negative affect, self-consciousness, poor coping, irrational ideas, feelings of vulnerability, and difficulties controlling cravings and urges. Extroversion relates to interpersonal warmth, gregariousness, assertiveness, activity, excitement-seeking, and the tendency to experience positive emotions. Openness pertains to depth of imagination, aesthetic sensitivity, intensity of feelings, preference for variety, intellectual curiosity, and independence of judgment. Agreeableness includes the characteristics of trust, straightforwardness, altruism, methods of handling interpersonal conflict, humbleness, and sympathy for others. Finally, conscientiousness encompasses the characteristics of competence, organization, reliability, achievement striving, self-discipline, and deliberation before acting.

NEO-PI-R item construction was based on rational-theoretical methods. Item selection was determined by internal consistency and factor analytic data. The scale's 240 items are rated on a five-point continuum from "strongly disagree" to "strongly agree." The inventory is designed for adults, 17 years of age and older. The inventory requires a sixth-grade reading level and about 45 minutes for completion. There are separate adolescent norms for those less than 21 years old. The NEO-PI-R has a self-report (Form S) and an observer rating form (Form R). This dual-form feature is unique among personality measures and is especially relevant to rehabilitation research. Also noteworthy, the NEO-PI-R items do not contain references to physical abilities or sensations that might distort a physically disabled subject's responses.

The NEO-PI-R is a reliable and valid measure. Validity has been established through numerous studies that correlate the

NEO-PI-R with other measures of personality. All these correlations have been in accord with theory and expectation (46). There are two limitations to the NEO-PI-R. The NEO-PI-R assumes an honest respondent; no subtle items or validity scales are provided. In addition, it remains unclear to what degree the subject's current mood (state) may impact the response to test items that describe long-standing personality characteristics (trait).

The NEO-PI-R has been used in a limited number of rehabilitation studies. Rohe and Krause administered the initial version of the NEO-PI-R to males with traumatic spinal cord injury (SCI) 16 years after injury (47). The subjects scored lower on the scales of conscientiousness, assertiveness, and activity; they scored higher on the scales of excitement seeking and fantasy when compared with the adult male normative sample. Scales reflective of negative affect were not elevated. The subjects' reduced conscientiousness and nonelevated neuroticism scale scores have negative implications for adherence to rehabilitation regimens but positive implications for long-term coping abilities. A subsequent study on the same sample correlated personality and self-reported life adjustment. Krause and Rohe discovered that elevated scores on the depression scale were associated with poorer outcomes, whereas elevated scores on the scales dealing with warmth, positive emotions, actions, and values were associated with superior outcomes. The authors suggested that personality assessment may be an invaluable aid in predicting long-term outcomes and can help delineate those individuals most vulnerable to negative outcomes, perhaps indicating a need for more careful follow-up and supportive services for this subgroup (48). In a seminal study using the NEO-PI-R, the authors assessed whether SCI is associated with personality change by comparing the personality test scores of identical twins, one of whom sustained an SCI. The authors found no significant differences between the NEO-PI-R scores of the twins with SCI and their non-SCI twins (49).

The Strong Interest Inventory

The Strong Interest Inventory (SII) is traditionally considered a measure of vocational interests; however, research has supported its use as a valid non-pathology-oriented measure of personality (50). First published in 1927, the SII is one of the most thoroughly researched, highly respected, and frequently used psychological tests. The SII asks the respondent to indicate liking, indifference, or dislike for occupations, school subjects, activities, leisure activities, and types of people. Two subsections ask for preferences between two occupational activities and between pairs of work dimensions. Finally, one section asks the respondent to rate their possession of 13 personal characteristics. The test contains 317 items, requires 35 to 40 minutes to complete, and is written at an eighth- to ninth-grade reading level (51).

The General Occupational Themes, one of the three types of scales on the SII, are based on trait theory as derived by John Holland (52). Holland drew on factor-analytic studies of personality and interests to produce a typology of six basic personality types. These types are titled Realistic, Investigative, Artistic, Social, Enterprising, and Conventional. Rohe and Athelstan administered the SII to a national sample of persons with spinal cord injury (SCI) (53). Contrary to previous research, they found unique personality characteristics associated with persons having SCI of traumatic onset. These characteristics included an interest in activities requiring physical interaction with things, such as machinery, and a disinterest in activities that require intense or complex interaction with either data or people. Malec used the Eysenck Personality Inventory with people having SCI of traumatic onset and discovered a pattern of personality characteristics congruent with that found in Rohe and Athelstan's study (54).

Rohe's review of the literature suggested that when a disability is of traumatic onset and secondary to the individual's behavior, earlier statements in the literature about the lack of relationship between disability and personality characteristics appear to be inaccurate (55). He noted the previous literature either used pathology-oriented measures (e.g., MMPI) or studied individuals whose disability was not the result of trauma associated with their behavior. An additional study sought to determine if those personality characteristics associated with people having SCI would change after years of living with the disability. The data indicated that personality characteristics remained constant over an average of 10 years (56). Rohe and Krause conducted a follow-up study to the aforementioned personality stability study. They found that males with traumatic SCI displayed marked consistency in personality characteristics over an 11-year follow-up period (57).

The MMPI-2, NEO-PI-R and SII represent three measures of personality relevant to clinical rehabilitation settings. These measures can help answer diagnostic and management questions. For example, the MMPI-2 has been used successfully to diagnose the presence of psychopathology expressed in the form of physical disability—the so-called conversion disorder. Additionally, a patient's unwillingness to comply with requested medical interventions or the structure imposed by the hospital environment may be discerned with the use of personality measures. Knowledge of such personality characteristics can help prevent ill-advised interventions and can create a treatment environment designed to maximize patient compliance.

INTELLECTUAL ABILITY

Intellectual ability tests provide a summary score that serves as a global index of a person's general problem-solving ability, frequently referred to as an IQ, or intellectual quotient score. This summary score is validated against a broad criterion, such as scholastic achievement or occupational success. Although such tests are constructed of a number of subtests that sample facets of intellectual functioning, they are usually weighted toward tasks requiring verbal ability. The most frequently encountered measure of intellectual ability is the Wechsler Adult Intelligence Scale, III (WAIS-III) (58).

Wechsler Adult Intelligence Scale, III

The Wechsler Adult Intelligence Scale, III (WAIS-III) is the second revision of the Wechsler Adult Intelligence Scale originally published in 1955 and revised in 1981 (Wechsler Adult Intelligence Scale—Revised, WAIS-R). The WAIS-III was standardized on a normative sample of 2,450 "normal adults" from ages 16 to 89, divided into 13 age groups. They were chosen to be representative of the U.S. population as determined by the 1995 census update. The sample was stratified by gender, educational level, ethnicity, and region of the country. On the WAIS-III, items from earlier versions of the test that had become obsolete because of societal changes or bias against ethnic groups were altered or eliminated and the artwork was updated. Other improvements include extending the range of possible scores both downward and upward (Full Scale IQ range = 45 to 155), decreased reliance on timed tests, and addition of a new subtest that requires conceptual reasoning using abstract symbols (matrix reasoning). The WAIS-III must be administered by a trained examiner and requires 75 to 90 minutes for completion.

The WAIS-III consists of 14 subtests, one of which is optional. Table 44-3 lists, in their order of administration, these

TABLE 44-3. The 14 Subtests of the Wechsler Adult Intelligence Scale–III

Test Number	Test Title	Number of Items	Task	Measures
Verbal Scale				
2	Vocabulary	35	Define the meaning of words presented both orally and visually	Verbal and general mental ability
4	Similarities	14	Explain the way in which two things are alike	Verbal concept formation
6	Arithmetic	14	Solve arithmetic problems presented in a story format without using pencil or paper	Concentration and freedom from distractibility
8	Digit span		Listen to and orally repeat increasingly long lists of numbers, with separate lists presented in forward and reverse directions	Ability to attend; immediate auditory recall
9	Information	29	Answer oral questions about diverse information acquired through living in the United States	Retention of long-term general knowledge
11	Comprehension	16	Explain what should be done under certain circumstances and why certain social conventions are followed; interpret proverbs	Common sense, abstract reasoning, and social judgment
13	Letter-number sequencing[a]	7	Order sequentially a series of numbers and letters initially presented in a specified, random order	Working memory and attention
Performance Scale				
1	Picture completion	20	Determine which part is missing from a picture of an object or scene	Visual recognition, remote memory, and general information
3	Digit symbol-coding		In a timed code substitution task, pair nine symbols with nine digits	Concentration and psychomotor speed
5	Block design	9	Reproduce a two-dimensional design on a card by using 1-inch block whose sides are red, white, or red and white	Visuospatial organizing ability
7	Matrix reasoning	26	Continuous and discrete pattern completion, classification, reasoning by analogy, serial reasoning	Visual information processing and abstract reasoning skills
10	Picture arrangement	10	Arrange sets of cards containing cartoonlike drawings so that they tell a story	Social judgment, sequential thinking, foresight and planning
12	Symbol search[a]	60	Visually scan a target group and a search group of symbols, then indicate whether the target symbols appear in the search group	Visual scanning and divided visual attention
14	Object assembly[b]	4	Properly arrange four cut-up cardboard figures of familiar objects	Visual concept formation and visual

[a]Supplementary subtest.
[b]Optional subtest.

subtests and what they measure. On the WAIS-III, six subtests are used in the computation of the verbal IQ, and five subtests determine the performance IQ. In general, the WAIS-III has deemphasized speed of responding by reducing the number of items with time bonus points, eliminating the picture arrangement subtest and replacing the timed object-assembly subtest with the nontimed matrix reasoning subtest. Object assembly remains available when time and motoric response capabilities are not an issue. All WAIS-III subtest scores are corrected for age and standardized with a mean of 10 and a standard deviation of 3. The full-scale IQ is calculated by averaging scores obtained from the verbal and performance IQs.

The WAIS-III incorporates earlier research of Cohen, who discovered that three underlying factors accounted for most of the WAIS-R test variance (59). The Cohen factors are now codified as three of the four WAIS-III "index scores." The names of the index scores and the subtests used to compute them are *verbal comprehension* (vocabulary, similarities, information), *perceptual organization* (picture completion, block design, matrix reasoning), *working memory* (arithmetic, digit span, letter-number sequencing), and *processing speed* (digit symbol-coding, symbol search). As with the traditional IQ scores, index scores have a mean of 100 and a standard deviation of 15. They are sometimes reported in lieu of the traditional IQ scores. The subtests

of digit symbol coding and symbol search were added to the WAIS-III to measure the proposed fourth factor, *speed of information processing,* as suggested by Malec and colleagues (60). The test exceeds all standards of reliability and validity. Reviewers have been uniformly impressed with the quality of the resulting instrument (61,62).

Given the emotional significance of IQ scores, psychologists usually convert both IQ scores and discussions about them into either percentiles or classifications (Table 44-4). When the physician is confronted with questions about test results from patients, the use of either percentiles or classifications is recommended. Measures of intellectual ability help the physiatrist set appropriate expectations about the rate and complexity of learning legitimately expected from the patient. They also serve as the cornerstone for determining the presence of organic brain dysfunction and provide guidance for postdismissal vocational planning.

ACADEMIC ACHIEVEMENT

A frequently overlooked but nonetheless important factor within rehabilitation settings is academic achievement. Reading and mathematics achievement are of particular concern not only during inpatient rehabilitation but also for longer-range educational and vocational planning. The patient's reading

TABLE 44-4.   IQ Scores, Percentile Ranges, and Classifications for the Wechsler Adult Intelligence Scale–III

IQ Score	Percentile Range	Classification
130 and above	98 or greater	Very superior
120–129	91 to 97	Superior
110–119	74 to 89	High average
90–109	25 to 73	Average
80–89	9 to 23	Low average
70–79	2 to 8	Borderline
69 and below	<2	Extremely low

level is a potential limiting factor in tasks ranging from filling out hospital menus to incorporating ideas presented in patient education materials. The average reading level in the United States is roughly that of the sixth grade, the level required to read a newspaper. Patient education materials, however, often reflect the reading levels of the professionals who devise them. As the patients' reading level falls below the national average, progressively greater reliance on oral instruction and audiovisual materials becomes necessary. Patients are often expected to use mathematics when recording fluid intake and taking correct dosages of medications. Two frequently used measures of reading and mathematical achievement are the Wide Range Achievement Test-3 and the Woodcock-Johnson Psycho-Educational Battery-III.

Wide Range Achievement Test-3

The Wide Range Achievement Test-3 (WRAT-3) is the current edition of the Wide Range Achievement Test (63). The test provides assessment of three types of academic achievement: reading, spelling, and arithmetic. The test is for individuals from 5 through 75 years of age. There are alternate forms, entitled "Tan" and "Blue." The reading subtest requires the subject to recognize and name letters and correctly pronounce individual words, ranging from *see* to *synecdoche*. Critics highlight that the reading test is not a measure of reading comprehension but rather a rough gauge of an individual's potential reading level. They stress that when the goal of assessment is accurate measurement of reading achievement, other tests should be employed. The spelling test requires correct spelling of words presented by the examiner in the context of a sentence. Finally, the mathematics test ranges in difficulty from simple counting to performing advanced algebra and has a time limit of 15 minutes. The entire test can be completed in roughly 30 minutes, and results are presented in the form of standard scores, percentiles, and grade equivalents. The WRAT-3 is reliable, and the national stratified sample of 5,000 individuals is a significant improvement over the previous version of the test.

Woodcock–Johnson Psycho-Educational Battery-III

The Woodcock–Johnson Psycho-Educational Battery-III (WJ-III) contains 42 subtests subdivided into two parts: cognitive ability (20 subtests) and academic achievement (22 subtests). The WJ-III replaces the Woodcock–Johnson-Revised, which received critical acclaim for ease of administration, reliability, validity, and normative sampling procedures. Improvements in the current version include expanding the number of subtests; co-norming the cognitive ability and the academic achievement tests on a large nationally representative sample of 8,818 subjects from 100 geographically diverse U.S. communities; providing age norms from 2 to more than 90 years; and decreasing testing time through focusing testing at the subject's

ability level. Efforts were made to minimize the use of manipulatives and eliminate items that might be culturally insensitive to individuals with disabilities. Both improvements are helpful when assessing those with disabilities (64).

The academic achievement subtests are grouped into five broad curricular areas: reading, oral language, mathematics, writing, and academic knowledge. The achievement tests are further organized into groupings that aid interpretation. Reading achievement is determined by averaging three subtests requiring about 15 minutes to complete. These three subtests assess letter–word identification, reading fluency, and passage comprehension. Thus, the resulting score reflects diverse aspects of reading, including reading decoding, reading speed, and reading comprehension. Achievement scores are reported in age- and grade-normed percentiles, and reading ranges from easy to difficult. Mathematics achievement is based on three subtests consisting of calculation, math fluency, and applied problems that require about 20 minutes to complete. The three remaining achievement clusters are of less relevance to inpatient rehabilitation but may be useful in postdismissal planning. The WJ-III is an exceedingly well-constructed test that will become the standard to which other tests of ability and achievement will be compared. The cognitive test portions of the WJ-III can serve as an alternative to the WAIS-III when a broad-based, well-constructed measure of intellectual ability is desired (65,66).

NEUROPSYCHOLOGICAL ASSESSMENT

Individuals with cognitive dysfunction represent one of the largest groups receiving rehabilitation services. For many, the deficits are transient. For some, cognitive deficits are permanent and not only will complicate the learning of independent living skills, but also will determine future living arrangements, social interactions, and vocational prospects. In both situations, the rehabilitation psychologist is frequently asked to clarify the nature and type of cognitive deficits. This section describes three helpful screening tests of cognitive status entitled the Short Test of Mental Status, the Galveston Orientation and Amnesia Test, and the Repeatable Battery for the Assessment of Neuropsychological Status (RBANS). Next, two approaches to neuropsychological assessment—the quantitative approach, as exemplified by the Halstead–Reitan Neuropsychological Battery, and the qualitative approach, as exemplified by the Boston Process Approach—are described.

Screening Measures of Cognitive Status

The physician frequently encounters patients of doubtful potential for a rehabilitation program. A question that often arises is whether the patient shows evidence of organic brain dysfunction. Mental status scales can be divided into three groups: lengthy scales with multiple content, abbreviated scales with one or two items per cognitive area, and short scales of 10 or fewer items. Lengthy scales often require 1 hour to administer and may not provide enough information to warrant the time required. Short scales tend to focus on orientation questions, ignoring the diversity of cognitive abilities. Kokmen and colleagues devised the Short Test of Mental Status to address the preceding limitations (67).

The Short Test of Mental Status

The Short Test of Mental Status has diverse content, is easily learned, and only requires 5 minutes to administer. Content includes orientation, attention, learning, calculation, abstraction, information, construction, and delayed recall. The test was normed by comparing 93 consecutive neurologic outpatients without dementia to 87 outpatients with dementia. The maximum possible score is 38. A cut-off score of 29 or less resulted in a sensitivity of 92% and a specificity of 91% for the diagnosis of dementia. When this test was compared with standardized tests of cognitive function, a high degree of correlation was demonstrated (68).

Although the Short Test of Mental Status is useful for answering the question of whether to refer for neuropsychological assessment, the physician must decide when to refer for testing. This is particularly true for individuals with a closed head injury or slowly resolving coma. The Glasgow Coma Scale is useful for assessment of wakefulness during the acute stage of head injury but is not designed to guide the timing of psychological assessment (69).

The Galveston Orientation and Amnesia Test

The Galveston Orientation and Amnesia Test (GOAT) was developed by Levin and colleagues and measures amnesia and disorientation after head injury (70). The scale consists of 10 questions that focus on temporal orientation, recall of biographical data, and memory of recent events. The patient can obtain a maximum of 100 points; the final score is computed by subtraction of the number of error points. The GOAT was standardized on a group of 50 young adults (median age 23) who had recovered from mild closed head injury, usually consisting of a momentary loss of consciousness. Scores below those received by all members of the control group (<65) are designated impaired; scores between 66 and 75 are designated borderline; and those above 75 are considered normal. The greatest scoring difficulty occurs where points are assigned for the patient's accuracy in recalling events before trauma. More recently, Bode and colleagues rescored the items as dichotomies and identified three strata of posttraumatic amnesia (PTA). Equal-interval measures of PTA were created, and a self-scoring key was developed to assess PTA more efficiently (71). Posttraumatic amnesia is defined as the time during which the GOAT score is 75 or less. Validity data were generated by a comparison of the length of the posttraumatic amnesia with the variables of initial neurologic impairment and scores on the Glasgow Outcome Scale. In both cases, the GOAT score readily discriminated according to the severity of head injury. Scaling recovery of cognitive function in the noncomatose patient permits meaningful discussion with the family and rehabilitation team members. Most important, attempts at more involved neuropsychological assessment usually prove nonproductive until the patient consistently obtains scores of 70 or greater. Once a score of 70 is achieved, neuropsychological test data usually are reliable for further rehabilitation and postdismissal planning.

The Repeatable Battery for the Assessment of Neuropsychological Status

The Repeatable Battery for the Assessment of Neuropsychological Status (RBANS) is a recently developed, brief battery that fills an important niche between brief screening measures of cognitive status and comprehensive neuropsychological assessment. The RBANS is an individually administered instrument designed to measure attention, language, visuospatial–constructional abilities, and immediate and delayed memory (72). The test requires about 30 minutes to complete. The RBANS is intended for use with adults between 20 and 89 years. Norms are based on a stratified, nationally representative sample of 540 healthy adults. The RBANS subtests are subdivided into five cognitive domains: immediate memory, visuospatial reasoning, language, attention, and delayed recall. A total scale score is also generated. The 12 subtests are entitled *list learning*, *story memory*, *figure copy*, *line orientation*, *picture naming*, *semantic fluency*, *digit span*, *coding*, *list recall*, *list recognition*, *story recall*, and *figural recall*. An alternate form is available. The test is a collection of item types from other well-known tests that are used to assess memory and cognitive function. Although there are some limitations to the depth of the test manual and associated data, the RBANS has acceptable reliability and validity coefficients (73). The RBANS is useful for a broad-based but intermediate level of screening for cognitive deficits in acute-care settings and for tracking improvements or declines in cognitive function over time.

Goals of Neuropsychological Assessment

The field of neuropsychological assessment has come full circle since 1935, when Ward Halstead established his laboratory (74). Halstead observed the behavior of individuals with brain damage and then developed psychological tests to measure the characteristics that he observed. Thus, the initial goal of assessment was a better understanding of brain–behavior relationships, particularly in individuals with brain impairments. Halstead's assessment methods quickly proved their worth when used by experienced clinicians, by reliably and validly diagnosing brain damage and localizing malfunctioning regions of the brain. Their use as a neurodiagnostic instrument gained prominence and is now routine. Their diagnostic validity has been shown to be equal to that of neurodiagnostic techniques in use before the introduction of computed tomography and magnetic resonance imaging (75). As brain imaging technology has improved, however, the importance of neuropsychological assessment has returned to the original goal of describing brain–behavior relationships.

The field of neuropsychological assessment is increasingly focusing on the development of new methods for assessing rehabilitation potential, functional competence, and valid cognitive remediation procedures for patients with brain damage (76–80). For example, Sherer and colleagues demonstrated how early brief cognitive assessment combined with severity of head injury indicators can more reliably predict long-term employment outcome (81). Unfortunately, most neuropsychological tests were designed with diagnosis, not prediction or remediation, as their major goal. The tests were not constructed to determine which combinations of cognitive abilities are minimally necessary for survival in complex environments. Heaton and Pendleton, in an early comprehensive review of the neuropsychological literature, lamented that prediction of everyday functioning is a largely ignored topic of research in a field still dominated by diagnostic issues (82). Optimal prediction about the satisfactory matching of persons with environments will require new approaches to the measurement of environments and careful attention to the ecological validity of neuropsychological tests (83,84).

Halstead–Reitan Neuropsychological Battery

The Halstead–Reitan Neuropsychological Battery (HRNB) consists of three batteries (i.e., child, intermediate, and adult) (85). The adult version consists of Halstead's original five tests of seven variables selected for their ability to distinguish adults who have frontal lobe dysfunction. Halstead's first graduate student, Ralph Reitan, established his own laboratory and added measures of aphasia, sensory-perceptual integrity, grip strength, and sequential visual scanning, collectively entitled "Allied Procedures." In addition to the HRNB, a complete battery usually includes the WAIS-III and a measure of personality (e.g., the MMPI-2). The results of the HRNB can be presented as the Halstead Impairment Index, which is not a meaningful indicator of brain damage by itself but must be understood in the context of other test data that have been analyzed using inferential methods. Reitan described these inferential methods as follows:

Level of performance. The individual's score is compared with that of a criterion group and the normality of the score is determined. Statements describing the amount or degree of a specific attribute are provided.

Pattern of performance. Variations of scores within and between tests can be analyzed for specific strengths and weaknesses.

Specific behavioral deficits or pathognomonic signs. Behaviors occurring only with brain damage (e.g., anomia, hemianopsia, and hemiplegia) can be detected.

Comparison of performance of the right and left sides of the body. Measures of motor, sensory, and sensory-perceptual functions from one side of the body are compared with those of the opposite side. Significant discrepancies may reflect brain dysfunction and can help rule out competing explanations of poor performance on more complex neuropsychological tests.

In rehabilitation, as opposed to general medicine, the issue of diagnosing the presence of brain damage is of reduced importance. Brain damage is frequently the criterion for entry into a rehabilitation unit. Rehabilitation team members are more concerned with the degree to which the patient will be able to understand and profit from rehabilitation services or function in their home environments. As noted in the introduction to this section, a lengthy test battery may not be physically possible because of recent onset of impairment or because of shortened lengths of stay in acute rehabilitation. In these cases, the rehabilitation psychologist may administer select portions of the standard HRNB or use tests that place fewer demands on the patient such as the RBANS. A comprehensive battery of neuropsychological tests may be administered on an outpatient basis to more fully assess cognitive function and provide guidance on such issues as supervision, return to driving, and ability to return to work.

The HRNB is not without its limitations. For example, Halstead's original cutting scores were based on the performance of young patients, with age-graded norms becoming available recently (86). Patients with minimal education may spuriously score in the impaired range. Finally, the battery's ability to consistently localize lesions and discriminate psychiatric from organically impaired patients remains problematic (87).

The Boston Process Approach to Neuropsychological Assessment

The Boston Process Approach to Neuropsychological Assessment (BPA) is the designation given to neuropsychological assessment that focuses on the manner in which the patient produced his or her response rather than concentrating solely on test norms and patterns of scores. The three goals of the BPA are to (a) understand the qualitative nature of the behavior being assessed, (b) reconcile descriptive richness with the reliability and validity of quantitative tests, and (c) relate the behavior assessed to neuropsychological theory (88).

The BPA emphasizes developmental psychology's distinction between "process and achievement" to understand cognition in individuals with brain damage. Systematic observation of the problem-solving strategies used by patients during standardized testing is the hallmark of this approach. This method allows both a quantitative assessment and a dynamic description of the information-processing style of each patient.

The BPA uses a core set of tests with supplementary tests to clarify problem areas and confirm clinical hypotheses. The core set consists of frequently used tests that assess functions in six cognitive domains, including intellectual and conceptual, memory, language, visuoperceptual, academic achievement, self-control, and motor control (88). The BPA is concerned with the extent the patient gives priority to processing low-level detail or "featural" information versus higher-level "configural" or "contextual" information. Patients with impairments in contextual processing often have difficulties organizing their behavior (89).

Both the quantitative and qualitative approaches to neuropsychological assessment have proponents. The process approach is perhaps more compatible with the rehabilitation emphasis on practical and functional improvements. Given its focus on qualitative observation, the process approach provides potential insights regarding the most effective cognitive rehabilitation methods to use for remediation of cognitive deficits. Lezak noted that the use of fixed neuropsychological test batteries is waning in favor of a flexible choice of tests (87). Increasingly, the norm is for neuropsychologists to flexibly borrow from both the quantitative and qualitative traditions to design briefer batteries that are appropriate to a particular assessment question and setting (90). Moreover, the current trend toward reduced lengths of initial rehabilitation often precludes administration of a comprehensive neuropsychological test battery. A common alternative is to perform a brief assessment of cognitive function before discharge from inpatient rehabilitation, followed by comprehensive assessment weeks to months after discharge. This brief initial assessment provides a "benchmarking" of current levels of cognition and can provide guidance about the amount of supervision needed for the patient. A recent report by the American Academy of Neurology confirmed the efficacy of neuropsychological assessment (91).

CHEMICAL USE ASSESSMENT

Background

In the mid-1980s, Rohe and DePompolo highlighted the failure of rehabilitation professionals to assess and intervene in the domain of chemical health among those with disabilities. In 2002, Basford, Rohe, and Depompolo found significant improvements in chemical health screening for those with disabilities but a continued failure to provide staff training on the issue of chemical health assessment and intervention (92). Throughout this section, alcohol and drug abuse are considered jointly. The focus of discussion, however, is on alcohol, the more frequently abused substance.

The importance of alcohol screening is related to both the drug's impact on bodily functions and the associated behavioral aberrations occasioned by its excessive use. Eckardt and colleagues reviewed the detrimental effect of alcohol on most organs, especially the liver, pancreas, and heart (93,94). Alcohol ingestion may potentiate the action of prescribed medications, most notably central nervous system (CNS) depressants. This potentiation is of particular importance for rehabilitation patients. For example, medications that control blood clot formation and reduce spasticity are frequently used with rehabilitation patients. Alcohol may decrease blood-clotting activity and act in an additive manner with muscle relaxants such as diazepam (Valium) and baclofen (Lioresal). In addition, altered consciousness may result in less vigilance in health-compromising situations. If alcohol is ingested in the form of beer, the large fluid volume could seriously compromise a bladder-retraining program (95).

The cognitive and behavioral aberrations associated with drug intoxication often result in the onset of a disability. Rohe and DePompolo noted that vehicular crashes and falls, especially while the individual is under the influence of alcohol, account for a large proportion of admissions to rehabilitation units (96). Retrospective chart reviews of persons with CNS trauma often show alcohol present at the time of injury. Heinemann and associates found that 39% of their spinal cord–injured patients admitted to being intoxicated at the time of injury (97). Corrigan's review of the literature found that as many as two-thirds of head-injured patients have a history of substance abuse that preceded their injury. These studies revealed alcohol intoxication present in one-third to one-half of hospitalizations (98). Heinnemann, Schmidt, and Semik found that drinking patterns before and after spinal cord injury are strongly related (99). In a study of long-term spinal cord–injured patients, problems resulting from substance abuse were reported by more than one-half of the patients sampled (100). Rivara and colleagues found that 47% of general trauma patients had a positive blood alcohol level and that 36% were intoxicated (101). The preceding data suggest that individuals admitted to rehabilitation units with traumatic CNS injuries are not a random sample of the drinking public. Assessment and intervention with this population represents an opportunity at reducing future medical, social, and personal costs. Corrigan argues that rehabilitation professionals, under scrutiny from third-party payers, cannot afford to have a significant proportion of their patients display poor long-term outcomes secondary to failure to address substance abuse (98).

The screening of chemical health for all rehabilitation patients must become a standard of care. For this to occur, the administrators of rehabilitation facilities will have to require that drug screening be standard policy and that rehabilitation professionals, especially physiatrists, have necessary screening skills. Although one recent survey of rehabilitation unit administrators indicated that chemical health screening has become common, as recently as 1996 Schmidt and Gavin found that only 4% of persons receiving initial traumatic brain injury rehabilitation were screened for substance abuse (92,102). Thus, the data on administrators' perception of the adequacy of chemical health screening occurring in their facilities versus actual practice appear inconsistent. Unfortunately, staff training on this issue remains sorely lacking, with only 23% of rehabilitation unit administrators reporting that staff were provided education (92). Obtaining accessible substance abuse treatment for those with physical disabilities remains difficult (103). Perhaps the most overlooked chemical health issue is screening and intervention for nicotine dependence in those with disabilities. Basford, Rohe, and DePompolo point out that rates of smoking may be higher in those with disabilities when compared with the general population, and the health consequences in terms of lung function and wound healing may be particularly devastating to this population (92).

Screening for Chemical Dependency

Individual attitudes about alcohol use are diverse, are strongly held, and determine the perception of another person's use. Unless one first examines personally held attitudes and values about alcohol use, perceptions of another's use may be biased. A training program developed by the Center for Substance Abuse Prevention stresses the importance of attitudes in prevention programs (104). The two most frequent problems encountered during screening are viewing alcohol as a moral problem and judging the deviance of the patient's drinking through comparison with the interviewer's personal pattern of use. Weinberg stated that the most important aspects of interviewing about alcohol use are (a) getting a detailed history; (b) demonstrating nonjudgmental acceptance; (c) asking direct, specific, and factual questions; (d) maintaining persistence; (e) never discussing alibis; and (f) titrating hostility (105).

The most promising approach to helping people change their alcohol use is "motivational interviewing," which is based on Prochaska's stages of change model (106,107). Two measures useful in assessing alcohol use are the Cage Questionnaire and the Alcohol Use Disorders Identification Test (AUDIT).

The Cage Questionnaire. The CAGE Questionnaire was originally developed on 130 randomly selected medical and surgical inpatients at North Carolina Memorial Hospital. The goal was to find the least number of questions that would reliably identify those suffering from alcoholism. The four CAGE questions are

1. Have you ever felt you ought to cut down on your drinking?
2. Have people annoyed you by criticizing your drinking?
3. Have you ever felt bad or guilty about your drinking?
4. Have you ever had a drink first thing in the morning to steady your nerves or to get rid of a hangover (i.e., an eye opener)?

Ewing summarized the scale's development and data on four normative samples (108). One positive response to any of the questions raises the suspicion that alcohol dependence is present. Two positive responses identified 97% of his alcoholic sample correctly, and only 4% of his nonalcoholic sample incorrectly. Three or more responses are clearly symptomatic of alcohol dependence. The CAGE has sensitivity of from 60% to 95% and specificity ranging from 40% to 95% (109).

The Alcohol Use Disorders Identification Test. The Alcohol Use Disorders Identification Test (AUDIT) is a measure designed to aid in the process of accurate and reliable assessment of alcohol use. The AUDIT was developed by the World Health Organization to detect alcohol problems in primary medical care settings. The AUDIT consists of 10 questions: three on alcohol consumption, four on alcohol-related problems, and three on alcohol dependence symptoms. The AUDIT requires 2 minutes to administer and 1 minute to score, with a recommended cutoff score of 8. Sensitivities are typically above 90%, with specificities in the 80% to 90% range (110).

Summary. The field of rehabilitation has yet to fulfill its responsibility in the screening and treatment of chemical abuse and dependency, especially nicotine dependence. Research data suggest that patients with traumatic CNS injuries have a high probability of chemical abuse. Physiatrists have a responsibility for learning the skills needed for systematic screening of their patients. This intervention, early in the rehabilitation process, is a crucial aspect of prevention of future medical complications.

Psychotherapeutic Interventions

INDIVIDUAL PSYCHOTHERAPY

Psychotherapy is a generic term denoting psychological interventions that ameliorate emotional and behavioral difficulties. Psychotherapy can be defined as an interpersonal process whose goal is modification of problematic affect, behavior, or cognition (111). Of the more than 130 varieties of psychotherapy, research has yet to demonstrate that any specific variety shows clear superiority. Instead, effectiveness seems related to a therapist's degree of training in, and enthusiasm for, the theory and methods espoused by the particular therapy. Data suggest that psychotherapy does produce measurable change in patients. This change, however, can be negative as well as positive. The important principle of "above all, do no harm" is as important in psychotherapy as it is in medicine. Inadequately trained therapists are thus a source of concern in a field lacking firm boundaries.

The three basic assumptions underlying psychotherapy are as follows:

1. The person seeking services desires change.
2. The dysfunctional affect, behavior, or cognition is understood and amenable to change.
3. The process is a collaborative endeavor that assumes active client participation.

Psychotherapeutic intervention is thus contraindicated in patients on whom it must be forced or in those with significant communication or learning impediments. Additionally, if the difficulties are due to factors solely in the patient's environment (e.g., long hospitalization, unpleasant medical interventions, prejudice, nonunderstanding staff), the focus of the psychotherapist's intervention may shift from the patient to the environment (112).

The qualities of effective therapists have been studied and delineated. Therapeutic effectiveness initially depends on good assessment skills. Knowing when and how to intervene and, conversely, when to do nothing is fundamental to the process. Effective therapists are able to instill trust, confidence, and hope in their clients. Regardless of the type of therapy practiced, effective therapists have been shown to communicate the specific attitudinal qualities of genuineness, unconditional positive regard, and empathy. As opposed to mere friendship, the therapist provides an atmosphere of acceptance, respect, understanding, warmth, and help in conjunction with deliberate efforts to avoid criticizing, judging, or reacting emotionally with the patient. The creation of this atmosphere results in a framework unmatched by any other human relationship, one conducive to therapeutic change.

Most patients in rehabilitation units are faced with discovering and coping with permanent physical, cognitive, and social losses. This discovery is frequently accompanied by anger, anxiety, dysphoria, grief, and fear. Clinical experience suggests that the patient population can be divided into thirds according to the severity of their reactions. One-third of the patients copes extremely well through use of previously established skills and the support of significant others. Another one-third has greater difficulties, but through limited psychotherapeutic intervention is able to successfully manage the crisis. The final one-third has significant difficulties in coping. These patients frequently have histories of difficulties in adjustment, such as chemical abuse, major mental disorder, and inability to tolerate structured living environments. This group is of paramount concern to the rehabilitation psychologist and consumes disproportionate amounts of professional time.

Because of the pressing practical problems faced by rehabilitation inpatients and the increasingly short periods of hospitalization, rehabilitation psychologists tend to use time-limited forms of therapy, also known as brief therapy. Brief therapy is a general term denoting therapies with a small number of sessions (i.e., six to 10) and limited, focused, and readily attainable goals. These goals often include amelioration of the most disabling symptoms, reestablishment of previous levels of functioning, and development of enhanced coping skills. The sessions are focused on concrete content and the "here and now." Rehabilitation psychologists frequently apply techniques termed *cognitive–behavioral*. This concept is described by Turk and associates (113).

There are several common elements of cognitive–behavioral therapy. Interventions are active, time-limited, and fairly structured, with the underlying assumption that affect and behavior are largely determined by the way in which the individual construes the world. Therapy is designed to help the patient identify, reality-test, and correct maladaptive, distorted conceptualizations and dysfunctional beliefs. The patient is assisted in recognizing the connections among cognition, affect, and behavior, together with their joint consequences, and is encouraged to become aware and monitor the role that negative thoughts and images play in the maintenance of maladaptive behavior.

BEHAVIORAL MANAGEMENT AND OPERANT CONDITIONING TECHNIQUES

In contrast to other areas of medicine, in rehabilitation medicine there is a strong and systematic interaction between the medical and the behavioral sciences. Although the physiatrist would not be expected to devise or implement a detailed behavioral modification program, knowledge of the laws of behavior is essential when problems are conceptualized.

This section discusses the three types of learning:

1. Observational learning
2. Classic or respondent conditioning
3. Operant conditioning or behavior modification

Because of their relevance to rehabilitation, the principles underlying behavior modification are discussed in detail. Included are the topics of token economies, behavioral contracting, and misconceptions about behavior modification. The following material is drawn from the writings of Martin and Pear (114), Reynolds (115), Kazdin (116), and Brockway and Fordyce (117).

Three Types of Learning

Observational Learning. Observational learning, also known as modeling, occurs when a person observes a model's behavior but makes no overt response and receives no direct consequences. The behavior is learned through watching a model without actually performing the behavior. In modeling, a critical distinction is made between learning and performance. The only requirement for learning by modeling is observation of the model. Performance of the learned response, however, depends on the response consequences or incentives connected with the response. Thus, although rehabilitation professionals can effectively use observational learning when instructing patients about desired responses, the principles of behavior modification operate to determine if the observed behavior is actually performed. The likelihood of spontaneously emulating a model depends on a variety of factors, including whether the model is rewarded after the behavior; the similarity of the model to the observer; and the prestige, status, and expertise of the model.

Classic Conditioning. Classic, or respondent, conditioning is the process of repeatedly pairing a neutral stimulus with stimuli that automatically elicit respondent behavior. Some examples of respondents are salivation in response to food in the mouth, muscle flexion in response to pain, and accelerated heart rate in response to loud, unexpected noise. Thus, respondents are responses associated with the organism's glands, reflexes, and smooth muscle. Respondent conditioning does not involve the learning of new behavior but rather involves the capacity of a previously neutral stimulus to elicit a respondent. Respondent behavior is innate, part of the inherited structure of the organism. In respondent conditioning, stimuli that precede the behavior elicit the response. The resulting behavior is stereotyped and rather invariant across species, whereas in operant conditioning, behavior is emitted without any apparent prior stimulus.

The principles of respondent conditioning are used in the treatment of phobias and compulsions. For example, the relatively well-known therapeutic procedure of systematic desensitization involves pairing subjective states of deep muscle relaxation with graded approximations of the stimuli identified as eliciting the pathologic anxiety or fear response. Respondent conditioning techniques have been applied to enuresis, excessive eating, smoking, drinking, and deviant sexual behavior.

Operant Conditioning. Operant conditioning is a process by which the frequency of a bit of behavior is modified by the consequences of the behavior. Such behaviors are termed *operants* because they are emitted responses that operate on the environment. Operants are behaviors involving the striated muscles. Most behaviors occurring in everyday life, including those in rehabilitation units, are operants. When an operant is followed by a positive consequence (i.e., reinforcer), its frequency increases. Behavior that results in the termination of an aversive stimulus (e.g., turning off an alarm clock) is "negatively reinforced." When an operant is followed by a negative consequence (i.e., punisher), its frequency decreases. Operants no longer followed by reinforcers decrease in frequency and eventually disappear, a process known as extinction. An additional method of decreasing an undesirable behavior is to reinforce an alternative behavior, one that is incompatible with undesirable behavior. In simple terms, rehabilitation is the process of reinforcing disability-appropriate behaviors and extinguishing or punishing disability-inappropriate behaviors.

Environmental events that regularly precede and accompany operants are said to "set the occasion" on which the operant has been reinforced. These environmental stimuli, also known as discriminative stimuli, signal the availability of reinforcement should the previously reinforced behavior occur. Examples of such stimuli are a doorbell ringing, a traffic light turning green, and an "open" sign on the front door of a business. Discriminative stimuli are important, because their presence increases the likelihood that a previously reinforced behavior will be emitted.

The speed, amount, and schedule of reinforcement are major determinants of the effectiveness of reinforcement. If possible, the reinforcer should be delivered immediately after the response to maximize the effect of reinforcement. The greater the amount of the reinforcer, the more frequent the response. Schedules of reinforcement have a major impact on the rate of emission of a behavior. When one is increasing a low-frequency behavior, it is best to reinforce each occurrence of the behavior. Once the behavior is established, the frequency can be maintained with less frequent (i.e., intermittent) reinforcement. Table 44-5 lists the steps for setting up a behavioral modification program.

Types of Reinforcers

There are three types of reinforcers. *Primary* or *unconditioned reinforcers* are present at birth. They include food, water, sexual stimulation, rest after activity and activity after rest, a band of temperatures, air, and cessation of aversive stimuli. *Conditioned reinforcers* are stimuli that have been repeatedly paired with primary reinforcers. They are idiosyncratic and are based on the learning history of the person. *Generalized reinforcers* are stimuli that have been paired with two or more conditioned re-

---

TABLE 44-5. Steps in Setting Up a Behavior Modification Program

1. Define the behavior to be increased or decreased.
2. Define units of that behavior that can be readily measured.
3. Record the rate of occurrence of the behavior (i.e., movement cycle or time).
4. Identify potentially effective and readily controlled reinforcers.
5. Determine a schedule of reinforcement.
6. Implement and modify the program on the basis of outcome obtained.

---

inforcers. The prime example of a generalized reinforcer is money; however, verbal responses such as "thank you," "correct," and "great" also are in this category. In addition to the three types of reinforcers, there is an important principle, the Premack principle, which states that any high-frequency behavior can be used to reinforce a low-frequency behavior. For example, a high-frequency behavior such as watching television can be made contingent on performing a low-frequency behavior such as stretching exercises.

Token Economies

A token economy refers to a reinforcement system based on tokens. The tokens, frequently poker chips, function as generalized reinforcers and can be exchanged at agreed-on rates for back-up reinforcers, such as food, activities, and privileges. The behaviors to be changed (i.e., target behaviors) are specified along with the number of tokens earned for their performance. The stipulations of the economy are usually written in the form of a contract. a "reinforcement menu," that indicates exchange rates and back-up reinforcers and is displayed in a prominent place. Token economies have been used extensively in special education and psychiatric settings. They can be useful with troublesome rehabilitation patients for such behaviors as arriving at therapy sessions late, lack of compliance with fluid schedules, and failure to perform activities of daily living. As with behavioral contracts, ethical considerations and the success of the program mandate full involvement of the patient in the initial design of the program.

Behavioral Contracts

Behavioral contracts, also known as contingency contracts, are written agreements between people who desire a change in behavior. The contract precisely indicates the relationship between behaviors and their consequences. The contract serves four important functions. First, it ensures that the rehabilitation team and the patient agree on goals and procedures. Second, because the goals are specified behaviorally, evidence is readily available regarding fulfillment of the contract. Third, the patient has a clear picture of what behaviors are expected if he or she is to remain in the rehabilitation program. Fourth, the signing of a document functions as a powerful indicator of commitment and helps ensure compliance with the agreement.

Common Misconceptions About Behavior Modifications

Behavior modification arouses concerns usually because of a misunderstanding of its underlying principles. Kazdin presented a succinct overview of common objections, two of which are iterated here (116). A frequent objection is that use of tangible reinforcers is the same as bribery. Bribery can be differentiated from reinforcement, because bribery is used to increase behavior that is considered illegal or immoral and usually involves delivery of the payoff before performance of the behavior, not, as in behavior modification, after. Bribery and reinforcement share the similarity of being ways of influencing behavior, but that is where the similarity ends.

A second objection is that behavior modification is "coercive." Although behavior modification is inherently controlling and designed to alter behavior, multiple safeguards prevent its misapplication. These safeguards include involving the patient when contingencies are negotiated, constructing programs that rely on positive reinforcement rather than negative reinforcement or punishment, and making response requirements for reinforcement lenient at the beginning of the program (118). The use of behavioral modification in rehabilitation units requires careful training of staff. A limiting factor in many inpatient rehabilitation units is the lack of stability in team membership, especially where nursing personnel change frequently.

SOCIAL SKILLS TRAINING

Changes in Social Interaction After Disability

Although only a limited number of the recently disabled may profit from psychotherapy, most can benefit from social skills training. Research on the social psychology of disability is plentiful and underscores the social disadvantages encountered by the disabled, especially the recently disabled (119–131). Richardson summarized the literature and found consistently negative public attitudes toward the disabled (126). He noted that when first encountering a disabled person, the nondisabled experience heightened emotional arousal, anxiety, and feelings of ambivalence. These learned but somewhat involuntary reactions usually result in distorted social interactions.

Often the nondisabled focus solely on the disability and ignore personal characteristics normally used to evaluate people and establish relationships. The disabled also suffer from the societal norm to be kind to the disabled, which results in a lack of honest feedback and concomitant decreased accuracy in social perception by the disabled person (132). Consequently, the physically disabled often learn to discount praise and pay close attention to criticism. The factors mentioned earlier suggest that social interactions between the disabled and the nondisabled are complex, ambiguous, and unpredictable. Interventions that ameliorate difficulties with social interaction might help reduce emotional distress, speed the slow process of community reintegration, and reduce the risk of future medical problems (133).

Social Skills: Types and Methods of Assessment

Social skills is an inexact term used to describe a wide range of behavior thought necessary for effective social functioning. Dunn and Herman listed three types of social skills: general, general disability-related, and specific disability-related (Table 44-6) (134). Patients with onset of disability before adolescence may require intensive remedial help with the development of general social skills. Patients with onset of disability after adolescence enter the social arena with various competencies in general social skills. However, those with onset after adolescence experience social situations for which they have no previous socialization experiences, hence the importance for training to handle these situations. General social skills can be assessed through a variety of means, including paper and pencil tests, behavioral assessment, and observational techniques.

A social skill frequently identified as a problem is assertiveness; hence, it is used here to illustrate three assessment methods. A paper-and-pencil measure of assertiveness is the Gam-

---

TABLE 44-6.   General, General Disability, and Disability-Specific Social Skills

General Social Skills
  Listening
  Positive and negative assertion
  Self-disclosure
  Receiving compliments
  Confrontation
  Touching
  Conversation
  Maximizing physical attractiveness
  Meeting new people
  Use of humor
  Heterosocial skills
General Disability-Related Social Skills
  Acknowledgment of the disability
  Asking for help
  Acknowledgment of unstated attitudes (making the implicit explicit)
  Refusing undesired help
  Managing unwelcome social advances
  Dealing with staring
  Handling unwanted questions
Disability-Specific Social Skills
  Facilitating communication
  Overcoming early deficits in socialization
  Managing bowel and bladder problems
  Handling reactions to deformity and disfigurement
  Disclosing nonvisible disabilities
  Dealing with reactions to prostheses

From Dunn ME. Social skills and rehabilitation. In: Caplan B, ed. *Rehabilitation psychology desk reference*. Rockville, MD: Aspen Publishers, 1987:345–381, by permission of the publisher.

---

brill Assertion Inventory (GAI) (135). The GAI presents 40 situations described by a short phrase—for example, "turn off a talkative friend." The subject then rates his or her degree of discomfort for each situation on a five-point scale ranging from "none" to "very much." Next, the subject rates his or her response probability for each situation on a five-point scale ranging from "always do it" to "never do it." Normative data allow comparisons with the general population and with those having assertiveness difficulties. A measure of assertiveness more relevant to disability is the Spinal Cord Injury Assertion Questionnaire (136). The format of this questionnaire is similar to that of the GAI, but social situations that are potential problems for wheelchair users are described.

Behavioral measures help clarify the frequently found discrepancy between what people say they do and what they actually do. Behavioral measures offer direct and quantifiable data on both verbal and nonverbal aspects of social interactions. Such measures might include checklists or rating scales that permit counting responses, measuring length of time spent interacting, and so on. For example, studies using behavioral measures have shown that disabled people receive offers of help from strangers less frequently than do the nondisabled. However, if help is offered to the disabled, it tends to be overly solicitous (137,138). Hastorf and associates found that strangers were more willing to work on a cooperative project if the disabled partner assertively acknowledged the handicap at the beginning of the interaction (132). Finally, behavioral measures have been used during evaluation of the efficacy of assertion training with disabled people (139–142).

Observational techniques can be used by the person, significant others, or staff members. Generally, this type of assessment is less objective than that provided by behavioral measures. Nonetheless, reduced precision is counterbalanced by the opportunity to observe qualitative aspects of the social skill in a natural setting. Several research projects (e.g., Longitudinal Functional Assessment System and Rehabilitation Indicators Project) use observational techniques in the form of diaries, self-reports, and environmental surveys. Thorough descriptions of methods of assessing social skills can be found in a variety of publications (139,143,144). The reader is encouraged to consult relevant social skills training manuals for intervention techniques (145,146). Social skills training programs for wheelchair users are described by Dunn and Herman (134). Brotherton and colleagues describe a program for the traumatic brain injured (147).

INDIRECT SERVICES

The rehabilitation psychologist's overall aim is to enhance the quality of rehabilitation outcomes for patients. Indirect services such as maximizing team interaction skills, staff development, administration, and research provide avenues for enhancing patient outcomes that are as important as those of direct patient services.

The rehabilitation team is a unique structure in the delivery of health-care resources (148). Nowhere else are so many professionals with diverse backgrounds of training expected to communicate in a clear, timely, and comprehensive manner. This communication may become tenuous because of different professional terminologies, overlap in roles, and the pressures of productivity in a competitive health-care environment (149). The psychologist can enhance patient outcomes by facilitating cohesion of the rehabilitation team (150). This task can be accomplished through a variety of methods, including chairing committees to improve interdisciplinary cooperation and leading staff meetings to clarify overlap in professional roles. The rehabilitation psychologist's knowledge of normal and abnormal behavior is frequently called on for staff in-service training. Although some in-service topics focus on patient variables, such as practical management suggestions and brain–behavior relationships, other topics include personal concerns of the staff such as job stress and communication skills. The psychologist's strengths in interpersonal communication frequently prompt their selection for administrative positions.

Rehabilitation psychologists trained at the doctoral level are typically the only team members with specific expertise in research design and statistical methods. As such, they frequently consult with other team members interested in conducting research. They often coordinate research or direct research committees. The research expertise of psychologists is reflected in their presence on editorial boards of numerous rehabilitation-related publications. They are also found in local, state, and national organizations whose function is to promote quality rehabilitation or social justice for the physically disabled.

PSYCHOLOGICAL ADJUSTMENT TO DISABILITY

This section is divided into two parts. The first part reviews theories of adjustment to disability. The second part describes three models of adjustment to disability. The stage model emphasizes internal cognitions; the behavioral model emphasizes external events; and the coping skills model emphasizes both internal cognition and external events in the adjustment to disability.

Overview of Theories of Adjustment to Disability

Theories of adjustment to disability can be grouped along an internal to external continuum (151). On one end are theories that emphasize internal cognitive events, termed *mentalistic theories,* and on the other end are theories that emphasize events external to the individual, termed *social theories* or *behavioral theories.* The middle of the continuum contains integrative theories that attempt to meld the internal with the external determinants.

Before formal theorizing about adjustment to disability, most people thought that the primary source of suffering connected with disability was the disability itself. Hence, removal or amelioration of the disability would presumably reduce distress. However, experience demonstrated that after removal of a disability, some people remained incapacitated. The search for understanding the adjustment process shifted to the then contemporary principles of dynamic psychology and focused on internal events such as motivation. Patients' difficulties in adjusting to disability were conceptualized in psychodynamic terms, and their incapacitation was transformed into a mental health problem.

As time progressed, dynamic psychology models, especially the classic psychoanalytic model with its emphasis on psychopathology, provided insufficient explanatory power. Professionals came to recognize that physical and social barriers, barriers external to the patient, produce the major source of adjustment problems. Emphasis on sociologic concepts such as "sick role" (152) and "illness behavior" (153) ensued. These sociologic theories added to the understanding of adjustment to disability on a societal level (154). When an individual's adjustment to disability behavior is the focus, however, learning theory's emphasis on the sensitivity of behavior to its consequences provides significant explanatory power. The behavioral model of adjustment to disability is described more fully in a later section.

Theories that attempt to simultaneously take into account the internal events of the person and the external demands of the environment are called *integrative field theories* (151,155). Integrative field theories grew out of Lewin's concept of life space (156). These theories state that behavior is a joint function of the person and his environment [$B = f(P,E)$]. Meyerson, Trieschmann, and Wright applied Lewin's basic formulation to problems encountered by the physically disabled (124,157,158). For example, Trieschmann expanded Lewin's model and described the "educational model of rehabilitation" in which behavior is the function of personal, organic, and environmental variables, designated by the formula $B = f(P \times O \times E)$. Her acknowledgment of organic variables highlights the concept that behavior is fundamentally dependent on and limited by the physical capacities of the person.

Models of Adjustment to Disability

STAGE MODEL

Stage theory states that people undergoing a life crisis follow a predictable, orderly path of emotional response. Shontz is the major contributor to the application of stage theory to adjustment to disability (159). Stage theory appears both explicitly and implicitly in a wide variety of rehabilitation-related literature, including that on cancer, hemodialysis (160,161), spinal cord injury (162–165), and amputation (166). Additional writers who make implicit or explicit reference to a stage model of adjustment to disability are Dembo and associates, Siller, and Gunther (121,127,167). Unfortunately, these studies are merely descriptive and are based on interview data or anecdotal reports.

Most stage theories propose a series of three to five steps beginning with shock and ending with some form of adaptation. Three commonly held assumptions appear to underlie stage theory formulations applied to the disabled. First, people respond to the onset of disability in specific and predictable ways. Second, they go through a series of stages over time. Finally, they eventually accept or resolve their emotional crises. The following discussion draws on the work of Silver and Wortman (168–170) and Trieschmann (157). Much of the stage theory literature is derived from the study of bereavement. Although there are important differences between the death of a significant other and loss (death) of a body part or function, it is reasonable to assume that the process of coping with death and coping with disability are psychologically similar if not equivalent.

ARE THERE UNIVERSAL RESPONSES TO DISABILITY ONSET?
Both Gunther (167) and Shontz (159) indicated that once the crisis of disability is realized, virtually all people experience shock. Unfortunately, most studies report retrospective accounts of initial feelings and behavior. In one such study, Parkes interviewed widows and amputees after their losses (166). Initial feelings of shock and numbness were reported by only 50% of the sample. Tyhurst observed disaster victims and described three types of reactions (171). One group reacted with classic signs of shock, another group appeared cool and collected during the acute situation, and a third group responded with reactions of paralyzing anxiety and hysterical crying. Shock was far from a universal reaction. Silver and Wortman's 1980 literature review concluded that there is little evidence supporting the belief that people react in specific and predictable ways to undesirable life events (168). Although some patterns are evident, individual variation is inevitably present. Their updated (2001) literature review found no research that would compel them to revise their earlier conclusion. This author's clinical experience supports this conclusion. The initial reaction to onset of disability is diverse. Moreover, the more accurate the first thought after the onset of disability (termed by this author the *sign-on cognition*) and the more honest the self-acknowledgment, the better the initial and longer-term adjustment appears to be. Further research on the concept of sign-on cognition may prove useful in understanding the process of adjustment to disability.

DO EMOTIONAL RESPONSES FOLLOW A PATTERN AFTER INJURY?
The belief that people follow a predictable pattern of emotional response after the onset of a disability is widely held. References to stage models of emotional response occur in the professional literature of nurses (172,173), social workers (174), clergy (175), health-care professionals (176), and psychologists (127,159,167).

Silver and Wortman were unable to discover any studies specifically testing stage theory by measurement of affective states over time (168,170). Four related studies, all conducted on patients with spinal cord injury, failed to support state theory. Dunn studied seven psychological variables during three time periods of inpatient rehabilitation (157). He found no pattern of change in mood over time; variability was the norm. McDaniel and Sexton assessed psychological status over four points in time from ratings by rehabilitation team members (174). Ratings of negative mood states remained relatively constant over the length of the study and were independent of staff ratings of the patient's degree of acceptance of loss. Dinardo, in a cross-sectional study, found that the degree of depression experienced by his subjects was independent of the

time that had elapsed since their injury (177). Finally, Lawson, in a longitudinal study, used a variety of methods to assess the presence of depression (178). He found no period of at least a week when any of his patients scored consistently in the depressive range on any of the measures. His results suggest that patients with spinal cord injury do not experience a stage of depression during initial rehabilitation.

Although there is considerable popular and professional literature attesting to the veracity of stages of adjustment to disability, the empirical data do not support such a contention. Silver and Wortman summarized the available data by stating, "Perhaps the most striking feature of available research, considered as a whole, is the variability in the nature and sequence of people's emotional reactions and coping mechanisms as they attempt to resolve their crises" (168). Their follow-up review of the literature highlighted that there are deep-seated assumptions about how people "should" react to loss. These assumptions include that (a) individuals suffering a loss are supposed to go through a period of intense distress; (b) failure to experience intense distress is suggestive of a problem; (c) successful adjustment requires that the individual "work through" his or her feelings; (d) continued attachment to the deceased (in the case of disability, attachment to previous levels of body function) is viewed as pathologic; and (e) within a year or two people will recover from their loss and return to earlier levels of functioning (170). They note that individuals who do not comply with these assumptions may incur negative reactions from their peers and subsequently shift their behavior to be in accord with others' expectations.

IS A FINAL STAGE OF RESOLUTION REACHED?
Do people who have suffered a major undesirable life event eventually reach a final stage of resolution or acceptance of their disability? The findings across studies suggest that a large minority of people continue to suffer years after a traumatic life event. The unquestioned expectation of resolution or acceptance appears unwarranted for such traumatic life events as severe burns, spinal cord injury, cancer, death of a spouse, and rape (168,179). For example, Shadish and associates studied a cross-sectional sample of patients with spinal cord injury (180). They found that those who had been disabled for as long as 38 years continued to think about and miss physically impossible activities.

Wortman, Silver, and Kessler discuss a theoretical framework that suggests that the impact of a major undesirable life event is determined by whether the event can be incorporated into an individual's view of the world (181). The term *world-view* denotes the system of beliefs, assumptions, or expectations related to oneself, others, and the world that provides a sense of coherence and meaning (182). Losses that are sudden, uncontrollable, and random may readily shatter people's assumptions about the world. Thus, the extent to which an individual's world-view is violated will determine the intensity of the disequilibrium and distress that they experience. The degree to which they can reconcile the event with their preexisting world-view or create a new world-view that adequately accounts for the event will determine their long-term adjustment. Hence, disability of sudden onset would have a greater impact on world-view than disability caused by chronic illness.

Given the lack of support for three common assumptions underlying stage theory, one must consider alternative explanations of why such beliefs permeate clinical folklore and descriptive writing in the area. As suggested earlier, stage theory may represent a codification of strongly but implicitly held culturally determined expectations about reaction to loss. Two additional reasons come to mind. First, professionals working with the recently disabled often encounter unpredictable and emotionally charged situations. One way to help neutralize fears occasioned by such situations is to label the patient as being in a particular stage. This may help transform potentially threatening and seemingly unpredictable behavior into meaningful and predictable categories. A negative outcome of such conceptualizing may be the documented tendency for rehabilitation personnel to overdiagnose psychopathologic conditions in patients (183). This interpretation of behavior may also result in the staff inappropriately distancing themselves from the patient by negating the necessity for careful listening. A second reason may be the enticing belief that all patients eventually resolve the negative effect occasioned by their disability and achieve a final stage of adjustment or resolution. Such a belief has intrinsic appeal to health-care professionals who strive to maximize functional abilities and enhance quality of life.

Behavioral Model

The behavioral model of disability adjustment emphasizes the importance of external factors in determining a person's adjustment. In this model there is reduced interest in the patient's cognitions and a primary focus on observable behaviors. The most frequently cited proponent of this model is Fordyce, and much of what follows is culled from his writings (117,184). Additional applications of the behavioral model to rehabilitation problems can be found in the works of Ince (185), and Berni and Fordyce (186). In the behavioral model of adjustment to disability, the newly disabled face four tasks. The patient must remain in the rehabilitation environment, eliminate disability-incongruent behaviors, acquire disability-congruent behaviors, and maintain the output of disability-congruent behaviors.

The onset of physical disability and entry into the rehabilitation environment represent punishment. In learning theory, punishment is defined as the loss of access to positive reinforcers or the response-contingent onset of aversive stimuli. Thus, the newly disabled find themselves initially operating under a pattern of punishment. Two types of behavior follow the onset of aversive stimuli. The first is escape or avoidance, and the second is aggression. Escape or avoidance behavior is frequently seen in the rehabilitation setting in the form of daydreaming, verbal disclaimers of disability, unauthorized forays off the medical unit, and refusal to participate in scheduled treatments. Aggressive behaviors may consist of either rebellious behavior or verbal and sometimes physical attack. If avoidant or aggressive behaviors are not understood and dealt with therapeutically, rehabilitation may end prematurely.

The intervention strategy for these problems involves the discovery and, if possible, reduction of aversive aspects of the rehabilitation environment. This is accompanied by reinforcement of approximations to active participation in the rehabilitation program. Selecting and systematically graphing a mutually agreed indicator of rehabilitation progress can help the patient focus on tangible improvements. Patient reactions of hostility are common and should be tolerated within limits. These reactions should never be dealt with through counter-hostility, which only increases the probability that the environment, including the treatment staff, will become conditioned aversive stimuli. Systematically ignoring unwanted behavior and establishing therapeutic rapport enhance the probability that the patient will remain in the rehabilitation environment.

The reduction of disability-inappropriate behaviors and the acquisition of disability-congruent behaviors are synonymous with the concept of "adjustment to disability." Disability-inappropriate behaviors are decreased by withdrawal of reinforcers

after their occurrence, a process known as extinction. Paradoxically, the laws of behavior demonstrate that withdrawal of reinforcers initially results in a temporary increase in the rate of behavior. This is true for both verbal and performance behaviors.

The patient's verbal behavior is likely to change more slowly than performance behavior. Statements indicating a belief in the eventual return of physical function may require years to extinguish. The staff should neither reinforce nor punish unrealistic verbalizations. Rather, a verbal response suggesting the need to maintain hope tempered with a focus on the present is least likely to offend the patient. These statements of patients are more frequent at the onset of rehabilitation and may reflect the beginning of extinction. Detailed explanations of anticipated recovery of functional abilities help decrease unrealistic patient or family verbalizations and keep everyone focused on achievable functional goals. This is especially important for family members, who may erroneously believe that the proper way to help the disabled family member cope is through agreeing with unrealistic fantasies about eventual recovery of function.

Difficulties in the acquisition of disability-congruent behaviors are usually considered to be problems in motivation. Learning theory rejects this formulation because it relies on an inference about the internal state of the person. Usually, this label is applied to people who have failed to reach expected levels of performance set by the rehabilitation staff. In learning theory, the problem is that of adjusting contingencies to increase the rate of desired behavior or reduce the rate of behaviors competing with the desired behavior. Unfortunately, most disability-congruent behaviors are initially of low frequency, strength, and value. The steps in changing this situation include establishing reinforcing relationships with the treatment staff, enhancing long-term reinforcers for disability-congruent behaviors, and introducing contingency management interventions that promote the acquisition of disability-congruent behaviors.

Maintaining the output of disability-appropriate behaviors is the final and most important step in adjustment to disability. Rehabilitation is unsuccessful if the behaviors learned in the rehabilitation unit cannot be transferred to the patient's home environment (187). Although the patient may demonstrate the ability to perform a task, the probability of its occurrence depends on contingencies operating in the home environment. Disability-congruent behaviors, such as propelling a wheelchair, maintaining a fluid schedule, and using gait aids are unlikely to be reinforcing in themselves.

Two strategies for improving generalization are bringing disability-congruent behaviors under the control of reinforcers occurring naturally in the environment and reprogramming the patient's home environment to deliver appropriate reinforcement contingently. The first strategy is promoted through interventions designed to reengage the patient in meaningful vocational and avocational activities after dismissal. Therefore, vocational counseling and therapeutic recreation are important as part of inpatient rehabilitation. Gradual and systematic rehearsal of newly learned skills in the home environment during weekend visits is an additional method encouraging generalization. The second strategy is promoted through such interventions as home modifications, assigning a family member to monitor and reinforce home therapy programs, and contracting with the patient for continued compliance. Unfortunately, powerful contingencies may be operating to prevent generalization. For example, the patient may receive reinforcers in the form of increased attention or financial rewards from litigation, a condition also known as secondary gain. Inability to control sources of secondary gain may prevent generalization of disability-congruent behaviors to the home environment. Family interventions are critical to prevent these problems.

Coping Skills Model

The coping skills model (188), which emphasizes both cognitive and behavioral factors, is based on the crisis theory originally formulated by Lindemann (189). Crisis theory asserts that people require a sense of social and psychological equilibrium. After a traumatic event, a state of crisis and disorganization occurs. At the time of the crisis, a person's characteristic patterns of behavior are ineffectual in establishing equilibrium. This state of disequilibrium is always temporary, and a new balance is achieved within days to weeks. Veninga and Snyder provide two practical guides for negotiating the dilemma of a crisis (190,191). The coping skills model comprises seven major adaptive tasks and seven major coping skills. The coping skills are elaborated in the following discussion.

DENYING OR MINIMIZING THE SERIOUSNESS OF A CRISIS

This coping skill may be directed at the illness or at its significance and helps to reduce negative emotions to manageable levels. This reduction enhances the mental clarity needed for effective action in emergency situations. The likelihood of implementing a greater range of coping responses is also increased.

SEEKING RELEVANT INFORMATION

Often, misunderstanding of medical diagnoses and procedures causes emotional distress. Understanding often reduces anxiety and provides a sense of control. Gathering information gives the patient and family a concrete task and the accompanying feeling of purposefulness. One longitudinal study of people with chronic illness showed that information-seeking has salubrious effects on adjustment (192).

REQUESTING REASSURANCE AND EMOTIONAL SUPPORT

The literature shows that perceived social support, adjustment during a crisis, and improved health outcomes are interrelated (193–195). Component parts of social support include perceiving that one is cared for, being encouraged to openly express beliefs and feelings, and being provided material aid. Social support may enhance coping by reducing counterproductive emotional states, building self-esteem, and increasing receptivity to new information. Cobb suggested that social support enhances health outcome either directly through neuroendocrine pathways or indirectly through increased patient compliance (196). He cited evidence showing that patients who receive social support are more likely to stay in treatment and follow their physicians' recommendations. Turner found a reliable association between social support and psychological well-being, especially during stressful circumstances (197).

LEARNING SPECIFIC ILLNESS-RELATED PROCEDURES

Learning specific illness-related procedures is a skill that reaffirms personal competence and enhances self-esteem, which is often undermined by physical disability. Bulman and Wortman asked social workers and nurses on a rehabilitation unit to define good and poor coping in patients with spinal cord injury (198). Both groups agreed that good coping included the willingness to learn physical skills that would minimize disability. Conversely, the definition of poor coping included an unwillingness to improve the condition or attend physical therapy.

SETTING CONCRETE LIMITED GOALS

Limited goal setting breaks a large task into small and more readily mastered components. As each component is mastered, self-reinforcement accrues and sets the stage for further learning. Limited goal-setting decreases feelings of being overwhelmed and enhances the opportunity to achieve something considered meaningful.

REHEARSING ALTERNATIVE OUTCOMES

Activities such as mental rehearsal, anticipation, discussions with significant others, and incorporation of medical information are involved in this skill. Here the patient considers possible outcomes and determines the most fruitful manner of handling each. Recalling previous periods of stress and how these were successfully managed is an example of this coping skill. The patient engages in behaviors that alleviate feelings of anxiety, tension, fear, and uncertainty. A cognitive road map is delineated to provide guidance on how any of a variety of possible future stressors will be minimized.

FINDING A GENERAL PURPOSE OR PATTERN OF MEANING IN THE COURSE OF EVENTS

Physical disability is a crisis that can destroy a person's belief that the world is a predictable, meaningful, and understandable place. There appears to be a compelling psychological need to believe that the world is just (199) and to make sense out of a crisis experience. The previously discussed concept of world-view, with its focus on coherence and meaning, is relevant in this context. Some theorists claim that the search for meaning is a basic human motivation (200). Bulman and Wortman studied 29 subjects with spinal cord injury and concluded that the "ability to perceive an orderly relationship between one's behaviors and one's outcomes is important for effective coping" (198). Krause, in a 15-year prospective study of persons with spinal cord injury, found that survival was directly related to higher activity levels and being employed (201).

SUMMARY

This chapter reviewed the history and current status of rehabilitation psychology, followed by an overview of services offered by the rehabilitation psychologist and theories of adjustment to disability. Although the rehabilitation psychologist provides a wide variety of direct and indirect services, certain skills are particularly relevant to rehabilitation, including psychological assessment, behavior modification, and research. Rehabilitation environments represent settings in which people under physical and emotional distress are asked to learn. Many of these people not only are emotionally upset but may have brain injuries that further impair learning efficiency. Standardized measurement of personality, intellectual ability, academic achievement, neuropsychological integrity, and chemical health provide a reliable base on which to set rehabilitation goals.

Rehabilitation is concerned with the functional performance of a person. Rehabilitation team members provide diverse interventions to ensure that the person can physically perform specific activities. Whether this person will actually do so is determined by contingencies in the rehabilitation unit and home environment. The rehabilitation psychologist's behavioral modification skills permit the careful assessment and harnessing of these contingencies in the service of the patient.

Progress in any scientific field depends on quality research. Such research is of particular concern for rehabilitation because outcomes are determined by a complex set of physical and social variables. Doctoral-level psychologists are typically the only rehabilitation team members with training in research. Traditionally, this training stresses asking practical research questions relevant to clinical problems.

Theories of adjustment to disability can be grouped along a continuum stressing internal cognitive events on the one end and external social and behavioral events on the other. Stage theory is a widely held but largely unsubstantiated model that stresses internal events. Alternative models worth considering include the behavioral model and the coping skills model.

REFERENCES

1. Eisenberg MG, Jansen MA. Rehabilitation psychology: state of the art. *Ann Rev Rehabil* 1983;3:1–31.
2. Fraser RT. An introduction to rehabilitation psychology. In: Golden CJ, ed. *Current topics in rehabilitation psychology.* Orlando, FL: Grune & Stratton, 1984:1–15.
3. DeLeon PH, Forsythe P, VandenBos GR. Federal recognition of psychology in rehabilitation programs. *Rehabil Psychol* 1986;31:47–56.
4. Bruyere SME. Special issue on the implications of the Americans with Disabilities Act of 1990 for psychologists. *Rehabil Psychol* 1993;38:71–148.
5. Shontz FC, Wright BA. The distinctiveness of rehabilitation psychology. *Prof Psychol* 1980;11:919–924.
6. Glueckauf RL. Doctoral education in rehabilitation and health care psychology: principles and strategies for unifying subspecialty training. In: Frank RG, Elliott TR, eds. *Handbook of rehabilitation psychology.* Washington, DC: American Psychological Association, 2000:615–627.
7. Glueckauf RL. Interdivisional Healthcare Committee: speaking with one voice on cross-cutting issues in health care psychology. *J Clin Psychol Med Settings* 1999;6:171–181.
8. Kaplan SP. Full circle to Boulder: a commentary on rehabilitation psychology training. *Rehabil Psychol* 2001;46:203–208.
9. Pape DA, Tarvydas VM. Responsible and responsive rehabilitation consultation on the ADA: the importance of training for psychologists. *Rehabil Psychol* 1993;38:117–131.
10. Thomas KR, Chan F. On becoming a rehabilitation psychologist: many roads lead to Rome. *Rehabil Psychol* 2000;45:65–73.
11. Wegener ST, Hagglund KJ, Elliott TR. On psychological identity and training: Boulder is better for rehabilitation psychology. *Rehabil Psychol* 1998;43 Spr 1998:17–29.
12. Wegener ST, Elliott TR, Hagglund KJ. On psychological identity and training: a reply to Thomas and Chan (2000). *Rehabil Psychol* 2000;45:74–80.
13. Patterson DR, Hanson SL. Joint Division 22 and ACRM guidelines for postdoctoral training in rehabilitation psychology. *Rehabil Psychol* 1995;40:299–310.
14. Cox RH. Fellows Address: Excellence in rehabilitation psychology—the ABPP diplomate in rehabilitation psychology. *Rehabil Psychol* 1998;43.348–352.
15. Caplan B. Statement of vision and mission: APA division 22. *Rehabil Psychol News* 1996;23:14.
16. Chan L, Ciol M. Medicare's payment system: its effect on discharges to skilled nursing facilities from rehabilitation hospitals. *Arch Phys Med Rehabil* 2000;81:715–719.
17. Frank RG, Elliott TR. *Handbook of rehabilitation psychology.* Washington, DC: American Psychological Association, 2000.
18. Klapow JC, Pruitt SD, Epping-Jordan JE. Rehabilitation psychology in primary care: preparing for a changing health care environment. *Rehabil Psychol* 1997;42:325–335.
19. Hagglund KJ, Kewman DG, Ashkanazi GS. Medicare and prospective payment systems. In: Frank RG, Elliott TR, eds. *Handbook of rehabilitation psychology.* Washington, DC: American Psychological Association, 2000:603–614.
20. Liss HJ, Glueckauf RL, Ecklund-Johnson EP. Research on telehealth and chronic medical conditions: critical review, key issues, and future directions. *Rehabil Psychol* 2002;47:8–30.
21. National Institute on Disability and Rehabilitation Research Long Range Plan, 64: *Federal Register* 234, December 7, 1999.
22. Dijkers MP, Whiteneck G, El-Jaroudi R. Measures of social outcomes in disability research. *Arch Phys Med Rehabil* 2000;81[Suppl 2]:S63–S80.
23. Halbertsma J, Heerkens YF, Hirs WM, et al. Towards a new ICIDH. International Classification of Impairments, Disabilities and Handicaps. *Disabil Rehabil* 2000;22:144–156.
24. Post MWM, de Witte LP, Schrijvers AJP. Quality of life and the ICIDH: towards an integrated conceptual model for rehabilitation outcomes research. *Clin Rehabil* 1999;13:5–15.
25. World HO. *ICIDH–2: International classification of functioning and disability.* Geneva: World Health Organization, 2000.
26. Banja JD, DeJong G. The rehabilitation marketplace: economics, values, and proposals for reform. *Arch Phys Med Rehabil* 2000;81:233–240.
27. Cushman LA, Scherer MJ, eds. *Psychological assessment in medical rehabilitation.* Washington, DC: American Psychological Association, 1995.
28. Plake BS, Impara JC, eds. *The fourteenth mental measurements yearbook.* Lincoln, NE: The Buros Institute of Mental Measurements, 2001.
29. Epstein S, O'Brien EJ. The person–situation debate in historical and current perspective. *Psychol Bull* 1985;98:513–537.
30. Anastasi A, Urbina S. *Psychological testing,* 7th ed. Upper Saddle River, NJ: Prentice Hall, 1997.
31. Elliott TR, Umlauf RL. Measurement of personality and psychopathology following acquired physical disability. In: Cushman LA, Scherer MJ eds. *Psychological assessment in medical rehabilitation: measurement and instrumentation in psychology.* Washington, DC: American Psychological Association, 1995:325–358.
32. Elliott TR, Frank RG. Depression following spinal cord injury. *Arch Phys Med Rehabil* 1996;77:816–823.
33. Rohe DE. Loss, grief and depression in persons with laryngectomy. In: Keith RL, Darley FL, eds. *Laryngectomy rehabilitation.* 3rd ed. Austin: Pro-Ed Publications, 1993:487–514.
34. Butcher JN. *MMPI-2: Minnesota Multiphasic Personality Inventory-2: manual for administration, scoring, and interpretation,* rev. ed. Minneapolis: University of Minnesota Press, 2001.
35. Graham JR. *MMPI-2: assessing personality and psychopathology,* 3rd ed. New York: Oxford University Press, 2000.
36. Greene RL. *The MMPI-2: An interpretive manual,* 2nd ed. Needham Heights, MA: Allyn & Bacon, 2000:vii, 696.
37. Friedman AF. *Psychological assessment with the MMPI-2.* Mahwah, NJ: L. Erlbaum Associates, 2001.
38. Nichols DS. *Essentials of MMPI-2 assessment.* New York: John Wiley, 2001.
39. Levitt EE, Gotts EE. *The clinical application of MMPI special scales,* 2nd ed. Hillsdale, NJ: Lawrence Erlbaum Associates, 1995.
40. Butcher JN. *MMPI-A: Minnesota Multiphasic Personality Inventory—Adolescent: manual for administration, scoring, and interpretation.* Minneapolis: University of Minnesota Press; distributed by National Computer Systems, Inc., 1992.
41. Rodevich MA, Wanlass RL. The moderating effect of spinal cord injury on MMPI-2 profiles: a clinically derived T score correction procedure. *Rehabil Psychol* 1995;40:181–190.
42. Humphrey DH, Dahlstrom W. The impact of changing from the MMPI to the MMPI-2 on profile configurations. *J Pers Assess* 1995;64:428–439.
43. Helmes E, Reddon JR. A perspective on developments in assessing psychopathology: a critical review of the MMPI and MMPI-2. *Psychol Bull* 1993;113:453–471.
44. Digman JM. Personality structure: emergence of the five-factor model. *Ann Rev Psychol* 1990;41:417–440.
45. Goldberg LR. The structure of phenotypic personality traits. *Am Psychol* 1993;48:26–34.
46. Costa PT, McCrae RR. *NEO-PI-R professional manual.* Odessa, FL: Psychological Assessment Resources, 1992.
47. Rohe DE, Krause JS. The five-factor model of personality: findings in males with spinal cord injury. *Assessment* 1999;6:203–213.
48. Krause JS, Rohe DE. Personality and life adjustment after spinal cord injury: an exploratory study. *Rehabil Psychol* 1998;43:118–130.
49. Hollick C, Radnitz CL, Silverman J, et al. Does spinal cord injury affect personality? A study of monozygotic twins. *Rehabil Psychol* 2001;46:58–67.
50. Costa PT, McCrae RR, Holland JL. Personality and vocational interests in an adult sample. *J Appl Psychol* 1984;69:390–400.
51. Harmon LW, Hanson JC, Borgen FH, et al. *Strong Interest Inventory: applications and technical guide.* Palo Alto: Consulting Psychologists Press, 1994.
52. Holland JL. *Making vocational choices: a theory of vocational personalities and work environments,* 3rd ed. Odessa, FL: Psychological Assessment Resources, 1997.
53. Rohe DE, Athelstan GT. Vocational interests of persons with spinal cord injury. *J Couns Psychol* 1982;29:283–291.
54. Malec J. Personality factors associated with severe traumatic disability. *Rehabil Psychol* 1985;30:165–172.
55. Rohe DE. Personality and spinal cord injury. *Top Spinal Cord Inj* 1996;2:1–10.
56. Rohe DE, Athelstan GT. Change in vocational interests after spinal cord injury. *Rehabil Psychol* 1985;30:131–143.
57. Rohe DE, Krause J. Stability of interests after severe physical disability: An 11-year longitudinal study. *J Vocational Behav* 1998;52:45–58.
58. Wechsler D. *Wechsler Adult Intelligence Scale,* 3rd ed. San Antonio: The Psychological Corporation, 1997.
59. Cohen J. The factorial structure of the WAIS between early adulthood and old age. *J Consult Psychol* 1957;21:283–290.
60. Malec JF, Ivnik RJ, Smith GE, et al. Mayo's older Americans normative studies: utility of corrections for age and education for the WAIS-R. *Clin Neuropsychol* 1992;6[Suppl]:31–47.
61. Hess AK. Review of the Wechsler Adult Intelligence Scale, 3rd ed. In: Conoley JC, Impara JC, eds. *The twelfth mental measurements yearbook.* Lincoln: The University of Nebraska–Lincoln, 1995:1332–1336.
62. Rogers BG. Review of the Wechsler Adult Intelligence Scale, 3rd ed. In: Conoley JC, Impara JC, eds. *The twelfth mental measurements yearbook.* Lincoln: The University of Nebraska–Lincoln, 1995:1336–1340.
63. Wilkinson JS. *Wide-range achievement test administration manual.* Wilmington, DE: Wide Range, Inc., 1993.
64. McGrew KS, Woodcock RW. *Technical manual. Woodcock–Johnson III.* Itasca, IL: Riverside Publishing, 2001.

65. Mather N. *Woodcock–Johnson III tests of cognitive abilities: examiner's manual.* Itasca, IL: Riverside Publishing, 2001.

66. Mather N, Jaffe L. *Woodcock–Johnson III: reports, recommendations, and strategies.* New York: Wiley, 2002.

67. Kokmen E, Naessens JM, Offord KP. A short test of mental status: description and preliminary results. *Mayo Clin Proc* 1987;62:281–288.

68. Kokmen E, Smith GE, Petersen RC, et al. The Short Test of Mental Status: correlations with standardized psychometric testing. *Arch Neurol* 1991;48: 725–728.

69. Teasdale G, Jennett B. Assessment of coma and impaired consciousness. A practical scale. *Lancet* 1974;2:81–84.

70. Levin HS, O'Donnell VM, Grossman RG. The Galveston Orientation and Amnesia Test. A practical scale to assess cognition after head injury. *J Nerv Ment Dis* 1979;167:675–684.

71. Bode RK, Heinemann AW, Semik P. Measurement properties of the Galveston Orientation and Amnesia Test (GOAT) and improvement patterns during inpatient rehabilitation. *J Head Trauma Rehabil* 2000;15:637–655.

72. Randolph C. *Repeatable Battery for the Assessment of Neuropsychological Status manual.* San Antonio: The Psychological Corporation, 1998.

73. Freeman SJ. Review of the repeatable battery for the assessment of neuropsychological status. In: Conoley JC, Impara JC, eds. *The twelfth mental measurements yearbook.* Lincoln: University of Nebraska–Lincoln, 1995:1008–1009.

74. Boll TJ. The Halstead–Reitan Neuropsychological Battery. In: Filskov SB, Boll TJ, eds. *Handbook of clinical neuropsychology.* New York: John Wiley & Sons, 1981:577–607.

75. Filskov SB, Goldstein SG. Diagnostic validity of the Halstead–Reitan Neuropsychological Battery. *J Consult Clin Psychol* 1974;42:382–388.

76. Conway T, Crosson B. Neuropsychological assessment. In: Frank RG, Elliott TR, eds. *Handbook of rehabilitation psychology.* Washington, DC: American Psychological Association, 2000:327–343.

77. Cicerone KD, Dahlberg C, Kalmar K, et al. Evidence-based cognitive rehabilitation: recommendations for clinical practice. *Arch Phys Med Rehabil* 2000; 81:1596–1615.

78. Dunn EJ, Searight HR, Grisso T, et al. The relation of the Halstead–Reitan Neuropsychological Battery to functional daily living skills in geriatric patients. *Arch Clin Neuropsychol* 1990;5:103–117.

79. Heinrichs R. Current and emergent applications of neuropsychological assessment: problems of validity and utility. *Prof Psychol Res Pract* 1990;21: 171–176.

80. Wilson BA, McLellan DL. *Rehabilitation studies handbook.* New York: Cambridge University Press, 1997.

81. Sherer M, Sander AM, Nick TG, et al. Early cognitive status and productivity outcome after traumatic brain injury: findings from the TBI model systems. *Arch Phys Med Rehabil* 2002;83:183–192.

82. Heaton RK, Pendleton MG. Use of neuropsychological tests to predict adult patients' everyday functioning. *J Consult Clin Psychol* 1981;49:807–821.

83. Wicker AW. Nature and assessment of behavior settings: recent contributions from the ecological perspective. In: McReynolds P, ed. *Advances in psychological assessment.* San Francisco: Jossey-Bass Publishers, 1981.

84. Sbordone RJ. The ecological validity of neuropsychological testing. In: Horton AM, Wedding D, Webster J, eds. *The neuropsychology handbook,* vol. 1. *Foundations and assessment.* New York: Springer, 1997:365–392.

85. Reitan RM, Wolfson D. *The Halstead–Reitan neuropsychological test battery: theory and clinical interpretation.* Tucson, AZ: Neuropsychology Press, 1993.

86. Heaton RK, Grant I, Matthews CG. *Comprehensive norms for an expanded Halstead–Reitan battery.* Odessa, FL: Psychological Assessment Resources, 1991.

87. Lezak MD. *Neuropsychological assessment,* 3rd ed. New York: Oxford University Press, 1995:1026.

88. Milberg WP, Hebben N, Kaplan E. The Boston approach to neuropsychological assessment. In: Grant I, Adams KM, eds. *Neuropsychological assessment of neuropsychiatric disorders.* New York: Oxford University Press, 1986:65–86.

89. Kaplan E, Fein D, Morris R, et al. *WAIS-R as a neuropsychological instrument.* San Antonio: The Psychological Corporation, 1991.

90. Bauer RM. The flexible battery approach to neuropsychological assessment. In: Vanderploeg RD, ed. *Clinician's guide to neuropsychological assessment.* Hillsdale, NJ: Erlbaum, 1994:259–290.

91. Anonymous. Assessment: neuropsychological testing of adults. Considerations for neurologists. Report of the Therapeutics and Technology Assessment Subcommittee of the American Academy of Neurology. *Neurology* 1996;47:592–599.

92. Basford JR, Rohe DE, Barnes CP, et al. Substance abuse attitudes and policies in US rehabilitation training programs: a comparison of 1985 and 2000. *Arch Phys Med Rehabil* 2002;83:517–522.

93. Eckardt MJ, Harford TC, Kaelber CT, et al. Health hazards associated with alcohol consumption. *JAMA* 1981;246:648–666.

94. Eckardt MJ, File SE, Gessa GL, et al. Effects of moderate alcohol consumption on the central nervous system. *Alcohol Clin Exp Res* 1998;22:998–1040.

95. Cameron JS, Halla-Poe D. *Alcohol and spinal cord injury.* Minneapolis: Brad Thompson Publishing Company, 1985.

96. Rohe DE, DePompolo RW. Substance abuse policies in rehabilitation medicine departments. *Arch Phys Med Rehabil* 1985;66:701–703.

97. Heinemann AW, Mamott BD, Schnoll S. Substance use by persons with recent spinal cord injuries. *Rehabil Psychol* 1990;35:217–228.

98. Corrigan JD. Substance abuse as a mediating factor in outcome from traumatic brain injury. *Arch Phys Med Rehabil* 1995;76:302–309.

99. Heinemann AW, Schmidt MF, Semik P. Drinking patterns, drinking expectancies, and coping after spinal cord injury. *Rehabil Couns Bull* 1994;38: 134–153.

100. Heinemann AW, Doll MD, Armstrong KJ, et al. Substance use and receipt of treatment by persons with long-term spinal cord injuries. *Arch Phys Med Rehabil* 1991;72:482–487.

101. Rivara FP, Jurkovich GJ, Gurney JG, et al. The magnitude of acute and chronic alcohol abuse in trauma patients. *Arch Surg* 1993;128:907–912; discussion 912–913.

102. Schmidt MF, Heinemann AW, Semik P. The efficacy of inservice training on substance abuse and spinal cord injury issues. *Top Spinal Cord Inj* 1996;2: 11–20.

103. Cherry L. *Summary report. Alcohol, drugs and disability II: Second national policy and leadership development symposium.* San Mateo, CA: Institute on Alcohol, Drugs and Disability, 1994.

104. Center for Substance Abuse Prevention. *Rehabilitation specialists prevention training system.* Rockville, MD: Center for Substance Abuse Prevention, United States Department of Health and Human Services, 1994.

105. Weinberg JR. Interview techniques for diagnosing alcoholism. *Am Fam Physician* 1974;9:107–115.

106. Miller WR, Rollnick S. *Motivational interviewing: preparing people for change,* 2nd ed. New York: Guilford Press, 2002.

107. Prochaska JO, DiClemente CC, Norcross JC. In search of how people change: applications to addictive behaviors. *Am Psychol* 1992;47:1102–1114.

108. Ewing JA. Detecting alcoholism. The CAGE questionnaire. *JAMA* 1984;252: 1905–1907.

109. Cooney NL, Zweben A, Fleming MF. Screening for alcohol problems and at-risk drinking in health-care settings. In: Hester RK, Miller WR, eds. *Handbook of alcoholism treatment approaches: effective alternatives,* 2nd ed. Needham Heights, MA: Allyn & Bacon, Inc, 1995:45–60.

110. Allen JP, Litten RZ, Fertig JB, et al. A review of research on the Alcohol Use Disorders Identification Test (AUDIT). *Alcohol Clin Exp Res* 1997;21:613–619.

111. Bergin AE, Garfield SL. *Handbook of psychotherapy and behavior change,* 4th ed. New York: John Wiley & Sons, 1994.

112. Olkin R. *What psychotherapists should know about disability.* New York: Guilford Press, 1999.

113. Turk DC, Meichenbaum D, Genest M. *Pain and behavioral medicine: a cognitive–behavioral perspective.* New York: Guilford Press, 1983.

114. Martin G, Pear J. *Behavior modification: what it is and how to do it,* 7th ed. Upper Saddle River, NJ: Prentice Hall, 2002.

115. Reynolds GS. *A primer of operant conditioning,* rev. ed. Glenview, IL: Scott Foresman, 1975.

116. Kazdin AE. *Behavior modification in applied settings,* 6th ed. Belmont, CA: Wadsworth/Thomson Learning, 2001.

117. Brockway JA, Fordyce WE. Psychological assessment and management. In: Kottke FJ, Lehmann JF, eds. *Krusen's handbook of physical medicine and rehabilitation,* 4th ed. Philadelphia: WB Saunders, 1990:153–170.

118. Malec JF, Lemsky C. Behavioral assessment in medical rehabilitation: traditional and consensual approaches. In: Cushman LA, Scherer MJ, eds. *Psychological assessment in medical rehabilitation measurement and instrumentation in psychology.* Washington, DC: American Psychological Association, 1995:199–236.

119. Asch A. The experience of disability: a challenge for psychology. *Am Psychol* 1984;39:529–536.

120. Davis F. Deviance disavowal: the management of strained interaction by the visibly handicapped. *Soc Prob* 1961;9:120–132.

121. Dembo T, Leviton GL, Wright BA. Adjustment to misfortune: a problem of social–psychological rehabilitation. *Rehabil Psychol* 1975;22:1–100.

122. Goffman E. *Stigma: notes on the management of spoiled identity.* New York: J. Aronson, 1974.

123. Hanks M, Poplin DE. The sociology of physical disability: a review of the literature and some conceptual perspectives. In: Nagler M, ed. *Perspectives on disability. Text and readings on disability.* Palo Alto, CA: Health Markets Research, 1990:179–189.

124. Meyerson L. The social psychology of the physical disability: 1948 and 1988. *J Soc Issues* 1988;44:173–188.

125. Nagler M. *Perspectives on disability: text and readings on disability.* Palo Alto, CA: Health Markets Research, 1990.

126. Richardson SA. Attitudes and behavior toward the physically handicapped. *Birth Defects: Original Article Series* 1976;12:15–34.

127. Siller J. Psychological situation of the disabled with spinal cord injuries. *Rehabil Lit* 1969;30:290–296.

128. Tajfel H. Social psychology of intergroup relations. *Ann Rev Psychol* 1982; 33:1–39.

129. Yuker HE. *Attitudes toward persons with disabilities.* New York: Springer Publishing, 1988.

130. Dunn DS. Social psychological issues in disability. In: Frank RG, Elliott, TR eds. *Handbook of rehabilitation psychology.* Washington, DC: American Psychological Association, 2000:565–584.

131. Harper DC. Presidential address: Social psychology of difference: stigma, spread, and stereotypes in childhood. *Rehabil Psychol* 1999;44:131–144.

132. Hastorf AH, Northcraft GB, Picciotto SR. Helping the handicapped: how realistic is the performance feedback received by the physically handicapped? *Pers Soc Psychol Bull* 1979;5:373–376.

133. Cogswell BF. Self-socialization: readjustment of paraplegics in the community. *J Rehabil* 1968;34:11–13, 35.

134. Dunn M, Herman SH. Social skills and rehabilitation. In: Caplan B, ed. *Rehabilitation psychology desk reference*. Rockville, MD: Aspen Publishers, 1987: 345–364.

135. Gambrill ED, Richey CA. An assertion inventory for use in assessment and research. *Behav Ther* 1975;6:550–561.

136. Dunn M. Social discomfort in the patient with spinal cord injury. *Arch Phys Med Rehabil* 1977;58:257–260.

137. Piliavin IM, Piliavin JA, Rodin J. Costs, diffusion, and the stigmatized victim. *J Pers Soc Psychol* 1975;32:429–438.

138. Soble SL, Strickland LH. Physical stigma, interaction, and compliance. *Bull Psychon Soc* 1974;4:130–132.

139. Dunn M, Van Horn E, Herman SH. Social skills and spinal cord injury: a comparison of three training procedures. *Behav Ther* 1981;12:153–164.

140. Ginsburg ML. *Assertion with the wheelchair-bound: measurement and training.* Storrs, CT: U Connecticut, 1979.

141. Mischel MH. Assertion training with handicapped persons. *J Couns Psychol* 1978;25:238–241.

142. Morgan B, Leung P. Effects of assertion training on acceptance of disability by physically disabled university students. *J Couns Psychol* 1980;27:209–212.

143. Curran JP, Monti PM. *Social skills training: a practical handbook for assessment and treatment.* New York: Guilford Press, 1982.

144. Hersen M, Bellack AS. *Handbook of comparative interventions for adult disorders*, 2nd ed. New York: Wiley, 1999.

145. Bellack AS, Hersen M. *Comprehensive clinical psychology.* New York: Pergamon, 1998.

146. Wilkinson J, Canter S. *Social skills training manual: assessment, programme design, and management of training.* New York: John Wiley & Sons, 1982.

147. Brotherton FA, Thomas LL, Wisotzek IE, et al. Social skills training in the rehabilitation of patients with traumatic closed head injury. *Arch Phys Med Rehabil* 1988;69:827–832.

148. Keith RA. The comprehensive treatment team in rehabilitation. *Arch Phys Med Rehabil* 1991;72:269–274.

149. Rothberg JS. The rehabilitation team: future direction. *Arch Phys Med Rehabil* 1981;62:407–410.

150. Diller L. Fostering the interdisciplinary team, fostering research in a society in transition. *Arch Phys Med Rehabil* 1990;71:275–278.

151. Shontz FC. Psychological adjustment to physical disability: trends in theories. *Arch Phys Med Rehabil* 1978;59:251–254.

152. Parsons T. Illness and the role of the physician: a sociological perspective. *Am J Orthopsychiatry* 1951;21:452–460.

153. Mechanic D. The concept of illness behavior. *J Chronic Dis* 1962;15:189–194.

154. Kutner B. The social psychology of disability. In: Neff WS, ed. *Rehabilitation psychology.* Washington, DC: American Psychological Association, 1971:143–167.

155. Livneh H. Psychosocial adaptation to chronic illness and disability: a conceptual framework. *Rehabil Couns Bull* 2001;44:151–160.

156. Lewin K, Heider F, Heider GM. *Principles of topological psychology.* New York: McGraw-Hill, 1936.

157. Trieschmann RB. *Spinal cord injuries: psychological, social and vocational rehabilitation*, 2nd ed. New York: Demos Publications, 1988.

158. Wright BA. *Physical disability: a psychosocial approach*, 2nd ed. New York: Demos Publications, 1983.

159. Shontz FC. *The psychological aspects of physical illness and disability.* New York: Macmillan, 1975.

160. Beard BH. Fear of death and fear of life: the dilemma in chronic renal failure, hemodialysis, and kidney transplantation. *Arch General Psychiatry* 1969;21: 373–380.

161. Reichsman F, Levy NB. Problems in adaptation to maintenance hemodialysis. A four-year study of 25 patients. *Arch Internal Medicine* 1972;130:859–865.

162. Bray GP. Rehabilitation of spinal cord injured: a family approach. *J Appl Rehabil Couns* 1978;9:70–78.

163. Cohn N. Understanding the process of adjustment to disability. *J Rehabil* 1961;27:16–18.

164. Weller DJ, Miller PM. Emotional reactions of patient, family, and staff in acute-care period of spinal cord injury: II. *Soc Work Health Care* 1977;7–17.

165. Weller DJ, Miller PM. Emotional reactions of patient, family, and staff in acute-care period of spinal cord injury: I. *Soc Work Health Care* 1977;369–377.

166. Parkes CM. Components of the reaction to loss of a limb, spouse or home. *J Psychosom Res* 1972;16:343–349.

167. Guenther MS. Emotional aspects. In: Ruge D, ed. *Spinal cord injuries.* Springfield, IL: Charles C Thomas, 1979:93–108.

168. Silver RC, Wortman CB. Coping with undesirable life events. In: Garber J, Seligman MEP, eds. *Human helplessness: theory and applications.* New York: Academic Press, 1980:279–340.

169. Wortman CB, Silver RC. The myths of coping with loss. *J Consult Clin Psychol* 1989;57:349–357.

170. Wortman CB, Silver RC. The myths of coping with loss revisited. In: Stroebe MS, Hansson RO. eds. *Handbook of bereavement research: consequences, coping, and care*, Washington, DC: American Psychological Association, 2001:405–429.

171. Tyhurst JS. Individual reactions to community disaster; the natural history of psychiatric phenomena. *Am J Psychiatry* 1951;107:764–769.

172. Engel GL. Grief and grieving. *Am J Nurs* 1964;64:93–98.

173. Zahourek R, Jensen JS. Grieving and the loss of the newborn. *Am J Nurs* 1973;73:836–839.

174. McDaniel JW, Sexton AW. Psychoendocrine studies of lesions. *J Abnorm Psychol* 1970;76:117–122.

175. Nighswonger CA. Ministry to the dying as a learning encounter. *J Thanatol* 1971;1:101–108.

176. Bernstein L, Bernstein RS, Dana RH. *Interviewing: a guide for health professionals*, 4th ed. Norwalk, CT: Appleton-Century-Crofts, 1985.

177. Dinardo QE. Psychological adjustment to spinal cord injury. *Dissert Abstr Int* 1972;32:4206–4207.

178. Lawson NC. Depression after spinal cord injury: a multimeasure longitudinal study. *Dissert Abstr Int* 1976;37:1439.

179. Davis CG, Wortman CB, Lehman DR, et al. Searching for meaning in loss: are clinical assumptions correct. *Death Studies* 2000;24:497–540.

180. Shadish WR, Hickman D, Arrick M. Psychological problems of spinal cord injury patients: emotional distress as a function of time and locus of control. *J Consult Clin Psychol* 1981;49:297.

181. Wortman CB, Silver RC, Kessler RC. The meaning of loss and adjustment to bereavement. In: Stroebe MS, Stroebe W, Hansson RO, eds. *Handbook of bereavement: theory, research, and intervention.* New York, Cambridge University Press, 1993:349–366.

182. Janoff-Bulman R. *Shattered assumptions: towards a new psychology of trauma.* New York: Free Press, 1992.

183. Gans JS. Depression diagnosis in a rehabilitation hospital. *Arch Phys Med Rehabil* 1981;62:386–389.

184. Fordyce WE. *Behavioral methods for chronic pain and illness.* St Louis: CV Mosby, 1976.

185. Ince LP. *Behavioral psychology in rehabilitation medicine: clinical applications.* Baltimore: Williams & Wilkins Co, 1980.

186. Berni R, Fordyce WE. *Behavior modification and the nursing process*, 2nd ed. St Louis: CV Mosby, 1977.

187. Davidoff G, Schultz JS, Lieb T, et al. Rehospitalization after initial rehabilitation for acute spinal cord injury: incidence and risk factors. *Arch Phys Med Rehabil* 1990;71:121–124.

188. Moos RH, Tsu VD, Schaefer JA. *Coping with physical illness.* New York: Plenum Medical Book Co, 1977.

189. Lindemann E. Symptomatology and management of acute grief. *Am J Psychiatry* 1944;101:141–148.

190. Veninga RL. *A gift of hope: how we survive our tragedies.* Boston: Little, Brown, 1985.

191. Snyder CR. *Coping: the psychology of what works.* New York: Oxford, 1999.

192. Felton BJ, Revenson TA. Coping with chronic illness: a study of illness controllability and the influence of coping strategies on psychological adjustment. *J Consult Clin Psychol* 1984;52:343–353.

193. Cutrona C, Russell D, Rose J. Social support and adaptation to stress by the elderly. *Psychol Aging* 1986;1:47–54.

194. Gottlieb BH. Social support as a focus for integrative research in psychology. *Am Psychol* 1983;38:278–287.

195. Schaefer C, Coyne JC, Lazarus RS. The health-related functions of social support. *J Behav Med* 1981;4:381–406.

196. Cobb S. Social support as a moderator of life stress. *Psychosom Med* 1976;38:300–314.

197. Turner RJ. Social support as a contingency in psychological well-being. *J Health Soc Behav* 1981;22:357–367.

198. Bulman RJ, Wortman CB. Attributions of blame and coping in the "real world": severe accident victims react to their lot. *J Personal Soc Psychol* 1977;35:351–363.

199. Lerner MJ. *The belief in a just world: a fundamental delusion.* New York: Plenum Press, 1980.

200. Frankl VE. *Man's search for meaning; an introduction to logotherapy.* Boston: Beacon Press, 1963.

201. Krause JS. Survival following spinal cord injury: a fifteen-year prospective study. *Rehabil Psychol* 1991;36:89–98.

CHAPTER 45

Speech, Language, Swallowing, and Auditory Rehabilitation

Robert M. Miller, Michael E. Groher, Kathryn M. Yorkston, Thomas S. Rees, and Jeffrey B. Palmer

Speech and language are dynamic, multidimensional behaviors that are continuously influenced by physiologic, psychological, and environmental factors. Speech uses anatomic structures and physiologic reflexes that are common to both respiration and swallowing. Language is intimately related to cognition and the integration of sensory modalities, most commonly the auditory sense. Because of the complexity of human communication, a number of specialists are involved in studying and treating components of these communication behaviors and the disease states that impair their function.

An introduction to the processes of human communication, a description of disorders that are recognized at each level of the process, and a rationale for the evaluation and rehabilitation procedures that are used for each condition are presented in this chapter. Because of the complexity of these behaviors, the discussion is limited to the major areas of acquired dysfunction found in an adult population. The major divisions include normal processes for human speech and language, motor speech disorders, laryngectomy rehabilitation, language and intellectual disorders, swallowing evaluation and management, and auditory evaluation and the management of hearing loss.

NORMAL PROCESSES

The process of human speech is accomplished through the systems of cerebration, ventilation, phonation, and articulation. Neural organization by the brain programs and sequences the physical processes. The resonating cavities of the pharynx, mouth, and nose influence the acoustic product.

Respiration

Two forms of respiration are recognized: chemical and mechanical. Chemical respiration is concerned with the exchange of oxygen and carbon dioxide to and from the blood, whereas mechanical respiration (or ventilation) is concerned with the tidal movement of air in and out of the lungs. The expiration of air through the vocal mechanism, the larynx, is the energy source for audible speech. Inhalation is an active process that is accomplished by the contraction of the diaphragm, which in-

creases the vertical dimension of the thorax. The decrease in air pressure within the thoracic cavity causes air to flow into the lungs. Other notable muscles of inhalation are the clavicle elevators, serratus muscles, and certain muscles of the neck and back that elevate the ribs.

Exhalation is more passive than inhalation. Tissue elasticity and gravity contribute to this act as the diaphragm returns to its relaxed position. The abdominal and intercostal muscles can provide force to exhalation or help to control exhalation for speech.

Phonation

Energized air passes from the lungs into the subglottic region, where the vocal folds are capable of modifying the air stream. Complete glottic closure can result in a Valsalva effect, whereas close approximation increases subglottic pressure and creates a mucosal wave cycle that results in audible sound energy or voice production. Raising the level of subglottic pressure increases vocal intensity. Higher pitch is achieved primarily by increasing the length and tension of the vocal folds and by elevating the larynx. A normal voice is therefore the product of a controlled exhalation of air, steady maintenance of subglottic air pressures, and delicately balanced vocal folds capable of producing regular mucosal wave patterns.

Resonation

The raw vocal tone is modified and amplified by resonance within the pharyngeal, oral, and nasal cavities, which are referred to collectively as the vocal tract. The shape of the vocal tract is altered by (a) changing the tension of the pharyngeal walls; (b) raising or depressing the larynx; (c) modifying the position of the jaw, tongue, and lips; and (d) occluding or lowering the soft palate. The innumerable configurations of the shape of the vocal tract provide the human voice with a tremendous range of variation in quality.

Articulation

The physical event that lends meaning to the resonating voice is articulation. The coordinated action of the tongue, lips, jaw, and soft palate regulates the air stream and produces the meaningful sounds of speech called phonemes. These structures may shape the vocal tract to produce vowels or voiced consonants, or they may relax, compress, or momentarily stop the air stream to produce unvoiced consonants.

Cerebration

Thought transformed into symbols and communicated by speech, writing, or gestural sign is considered language. A broad area of associational cortex in the left hemisphere of the brain is responsible for converting thoughts into symbols, and then into words or language. The words are organized into a meaningful arrangement using rules of grammar and are eventually transmitted either through the physical efforts previously described for speech or through gesture or writing. The brain, or more specifically the left frontal cortex, is responsible for organizing and patterning the muscle actions of respiration, phonation, and articulation to produce recognizable speech.

COMMUNICATION PATHOLOGY

A pathologic condition that affects any one of the organs involved in the process of speech or language influences the final product in total. At times the pathologic condition is limited to a single speech or language organ, and the speech dysfunction can be detected in only one component of the process such as an isolated voice or articulation impairment. More commonly, however, the pathologic condition of a single organ influences other elements of the communication process in ways that are predictable when one considers the integrated nature of speech and language. For example, severe obstructive pulmonary disease does not just impair the respiratory support for speech but results in alterations in vocal pitch, vocal intensity and phrasing or prosody, as the speaker compensates for an impaired ability to sustain airflow. Certain disease states, involving organs that are not directly involved in speech or language, can affect the final vocal product in a secondary manner. Some endocrine disorders, such as hypothyroidism, can influence voice quality as an isolated component of speech and can lead to language confusion and impaired memory. Because of the complexity and interactive nature of the speech and language processes, whenever one evaluates or treats a patient with a communication disorder, some considerations must be given to overall human physiology, as well as to the dynamics of speech and language systems.

Dysarthria

DEFINITIONS AND DIFFERENTIAL DIAGNOSIS

The dysarthrias are a group of motor speech disorders characterized by slow, weak, imprecise, or uncoordinated movements of speech musculature. Rather than a single neurologic disorder, the dysarthrias vary along a number of different dimensions. The neuroanatomic site of a lesion can be either the central or peripheral nervous system, or both, including the cerebrum, cerebellum, brainstem, and cranial nerves. One or a combination of pathophysiologic processes may be involved, including spasticity, flaccidity, ataxia, tremor, bradykinesis, rigidity, and chorea (1). A number of diagnoses may be associated with dysarthria, including cerebral palsy, parkinsonism, multiple sclerosis, amyotrophic lateral sclerosis, brainstem stroke, cortical stroke, and traumatic brain injury. All or several speech subsystems may be involved to varying degrees, including the respiratory, phonatory, velopharyngeal, and oral articulatory components.

As a first step, differential diagnosis involves distinguishing the dysarthrias from other neurogenic communication disorders. The dysarthrias are distinct from aphasia in that language function (i.e., word retrieval, comprehension of both verbal and written language) is preserved in dysarthria but impaired in aphasia. Although both apraxia and dysarthria are considered motor speech disorders, they can be distinguished on the basis of several clinical features. In apraxia, automatic (i.e., nonspeech) movements are intact, whereas in most dysarthrias they are not. Highly consistent articulatory errors are characteristic of dysarthria, whereas inconsistent errors are a hallmark of apraxia. Finally, in most dysarthrias, all speech subsystems, including respiration and phonation, are involved; in apraxia, respiratory or phonatory involvement is rare. It should be recognized that patients can have elements of both dysarthria and apraxia, particularly those with bilateral brain damage.

Differential diagnosis among the dysarthrias is an area that has received more systematic attention than any other aspect of the disorder. Table 45-1 summarizes information related to the various dysarthrias (2). In studies carried out at the Mayo Clinic, the perceptual features of the speech of seven groups of dysarthric patients were examined (3,4). These groups contained patients who were unequivocally diagnosed as having one of the following conditions: pseudobulbar palsy, bulbar palsy, amyotrophic lateral sclerosis, cerebellar lesions, parkinsonism, dystonia, and choreoathetosis. Speech samples were rated along 38 dimensions that described dimensions of pitch characteristics, loudness, vocal quality, respiration, prosody, articulation, and general impression. Results of these studies indicated that each of the seven neurologic disorders could be characterized by a unique set of clusters of deviant speech dimensions and that no two disorders had the same set of clusters. Thus, differential diagnosis among the dysarthrias can be made, in part, on the basis that one type of dysarthria sounds different from the others. However, single features such as imprecise consonants or nasal emission may not be sufficient to distinguish one type of dysarthria from another. Instead, differential diagnosis is made on the basis of clusters of features reflecting underlying pathophysiology and the findings on examination of the musculature. The following are perceptual descriptions of the unique features of selected types of dysarthria (5).

Pseudobulbar Palsy
Speech is slow and labored, and the articulation is rather consistently imprecise, especially on more complicated groups of consonant sounds. Pitch is low and monotonous. Voice quality is harsh, and often strained or strangled.

Bulbar Palsy
Hypernasality is associated with nasal emission of air during speech. Inhalation often is audible and exhalation breathy. Air wastage is manifest by short phrases. Articulation often is imprecise because consonants are weak due to failure of sufficient intraoral breath pressure owing to velopharyngeal incompetence. There may be immobility of tongue and lips due to impairment of the hypoglossal and facial nerves, which prevents normal production of vowels and consonants.

Amyotrophic Lateral Sclerosis
The progressive nature of amyotrophic lateral sclerosis (ALS) with combined spastic and flaccid dysarthria in this disorder causes continuous deterioration of speech. In an early stage of

TABLE 45-1.   Summary of the Etiologies, Neuropathologies, and Neuromuscular Deficits Characteristic of the Common Dysarthrias

Type	Example	Location of Neuropathology	Neuromuscular Deficit
Flaccid	Bulbar palsy	Lower motor neuron	Muscular weekness; hypotonia
Spastic	Pseudobulbar palsy	Upper motor neuron	Reduced range, force, speed; hypertonia
Ataxic	Cerebellar ataxia	Cerebellum (or tracts)	Hypotonia; reduced speed; inaccurate range, timing, direction
Hypokinetic	Parkinsonism	Extrapyramidal system	Markedly reduced range; variable speed of repetitive movements; movement arrest rigidity
Hyperkinetic			
Quick	Chorea Myoclonus Gilles de la Tourette syndrome	Extrapyramidal system	Quick, unsustained, random, involuntary movements
Slow	Athetosis Dyskinesias Dystonia	Extrapyramidal system	Sustained, distorted movements and postures; slowness; variable hypertonus
Tremors	Organic voice tremor	Extrapyramidal system	Involuntary, rhythmic, purposeless, oscillatory movements
Mixed	Amyotrophic lateral sclerosis Multiple sclerosis Wilson's disease	Multiple motor systems	Muscular weakness, limited range and speed

Adapted from Rosenbek JC, LaPointe LL. The dysarthrias: description, diagnosis and treatment. In: Johns DF, ed. *Clinical management of neurogenic communication disorders.* Austin TX: ProEd, 1985: 97–152.

disease, either spastic or flaccid speech and nonspeech signs can predominate; while in an advanced stage, both sets of features described previously are present. Slow rate, low pitch, hoarse and strained–strangled quality, highly defective articulation, marked hypernasality, and nasal emission combine to make the speaker struggle to produce short, barely intelligible phrases.

Parkinsonism

In this hypokinetic dysarthria vocal emphasis, peaks and valleys of pitch, and variations of loudness are flattened, resulting in monotony. Short rushes of speech are separated by illogically placed pauses, with the rate being variable and often accelerated. Consonant articulation in contextual speech and syllable repetition is blurred as muscles fail to go through their complete excursion. Difficulty initiating articulation is shown by repetition of initial sounds and inappropriate silences. The voice often is breathy, and loudness is reduced, at times to inaudibility.

Dystonia

Involuntary body and facial movements cause unpredictable voice stoppages, disintegration of articulation, excessive variations of loudness, and distortion of vowels. Perhaps in anticipation of these interruptions normal prosody is altered by slowing of rate, reduction in variations of pitch and loudness, prolongation of interword intervals, and interposition of inappropriate silences.

Choreoathetosis

The involuntary movements alter the normal breathing cycle and result in sudden exhalatory gusts of breath, bursts of loudness, elevations of pitch, and disintegration of articulation. The overall loudness level may be increased. Anticipated breakdowns are managed by varying the rate, introducing and prolonging pauses, and equalizing stress on all syllables and words.

ASSESSMENT

The World Health Organization model of chronic disease has been applied to the area of dysarthria (6,7). *Impairment* refers to "any loss or abnormality of psychological, physiological, or anatomical structure or function." *Activity limitation*, on the other hand, refers to "any restriction or lack (resulting from impairment) of the ability to perform any activity in the manner or within the range considered normal for the human being."

In a dysarthric speaker, the impairment would include the movement deficits seen in the respiratory, phonatory, velopharyngeal, and oral articulatory subsystems. As a consequence of these motor speech impairments, activity limitations may occur because of the patient's reduced intelligibility, altered speech rate, and loss of naturalness. In the assessment of a dysarthric speaker, both the impairment and the activity limitation must be considered (8).

Assessing the Impairment

During the assessment of the impairment, focus is placed on the speech production process. The clinician seeks to understand how the weakness, slowness, discoordination, or abnormal tone of the speech musculature has influenced points or places along the speech mechanism, including respiratory, phonatory, velopharyngeal, or oral articulatory subsystems (9). A number of perceptual or instrumental tools are available for measuring speech performance (10,11). The perceptual tools are those that rely on the trained eyes and ears of the clinician, whereas instrumental approaches to assessment include devices that provide information about the acoustic, aerodynamic movement, or myoelectric aspects of speech.

Before we proceed with a more detailed description of the assessment of the various speech subsystems, a word of caution is warranted. Viewing speech as a series of isolated points or components would seriously oversimplify a complex process. In dysarthria, the impairment almost never is restricted to a single dimension. Rather, impairments of varying levels of severity may occur at numerous points, all of which are interdependent. For example, consider the function of the muscles and structures of respiration as a pump to provide breath support for speech. The adequacy of respiratory support may be influenced by the efficiency of other organs that affect the flow of air. For example, inadequate laryngeal, velopharyngeal, or oral articulatory control interacts with poor respiratory support to create a cumulative negative effect on the voice.

Assessment of the respiratory subsystem begins with perceptual measures, including ratings of the number of words produced per breath, the loudness of samples of connected speech, or visual observations of the presence of clavicular breathing. Instrumental approaches to the measurement of respiratory function may include acoustic measures of vocal intensity and utterance durations. Respiratory performance may also be assessed by estimating the subglottic air pressure generated by the speaker (12,13). Respiratory inductive plethysmography, commercially available as the Respitrace, is an instrument capable of obtaining information about the movements of the rib cage and abdomen during breathing and speech.

Assessment of the phonatory or laryngeal subsystem typically begins with perceptual ratings of pitch characteristics (e.g., pitch level, pitch breaks, monopitch, and voice tremor), loudness (e.g., monoloudness, excess loudness, variation of volume), and voice quality (e.g., harsh voice, hoarseness, wet voice, breathiness, strained–strangled voice). Vocal fundamental frequency and intensity can be measured acoustically in the clinical setting (14,15). Measures of laryngeal resistance to airflow can also be obtained (16).

Assessment of the velopharyngeal mechanism can be made with perceptual judgments of hypernasality or the occurrence of nasal air emission. Nasalization also can be measured acoustically. Precise inferences can be made about the timing of velopharyngeal closure by obtaining simultaneous pneumatic measures of air pressure and air flow during selected speech samples (17,18). Movement of the velopharyngeal mechanism can be observed through cineradiographic techniques.

Assessment of oral articulation can be made by the rating of consonant and vowel precision. Although movements can be recorded using cineradiographic technique and myoelectric activity with electromyographic recordings, these techniques are not used in routine clinical practice.

Assessing the Functional Limitation

The overall speech disability observed in dysarthric speakers may be characterized by abnormalities in speech intelligibility, rate, and naturalness. Of these measures of disability, intelligibility has received the most attention in the clinical literature for a number of reasons. First, measures of speech intelligibility, when accompanied by measures of speaking rate, provide a useful index of the severity of the impairment in the disorder. Second, reduced speech intelligibility and speaking rate is a nearly universal characteristic of dysarthria, regardless of the underlying neuromotor impairment (19). Finally, intelligibility appears to be closely related to other aspects of the impairment, including measures of information conveyed (20), movement rates, sounds produced recognizably, and judgments of speech disability (21,22).

Despite the importance of intelligibility, care must be taken in clinically measuring this aspect of dysarthria (23). Research literature contains numerous examples of how intelligibility scores can be changed, depending on the speakers' task, the transmission system, and conditions imposed on listeners (19,24). Standard tools are available for measuring sentence and single-word intelligibility and speaking rate using reading or imitation tasks (19). These measures are used clinically as an index of severity of the disability to monitor change over time,

and as a measure of the effectiveness of specific intervention techniques such as rate control or palatal lift fitting.

TREATMENT CONSIDERATIONS

Decisions about the management of dysarthric speakers are twofold. The first level involves the most general decisions about goals of treatment, and the second involves the selection of specific treatment approaches to achieve those goals. General goals of treatment vary with the severity of the disability and with the natural course of the disorder (8).

For severely involved speakers, whose intelligibility is so poor that they are unable to communicate verbally in some or all situations, the general goal of treatment involves establishing a functional means of communication using augmentative approaches. The term *communication augmentation* refers to any device designed to augment, supplement, or replace verbal communication for someone who is not an independent verbal communicator. Systems range from communication boards and books to computer-based speech synthesis systems (25–27). The selection of an appropriate augmentation system necessitates a thorough evaluation of the person's communication needs. These needs may vary considerably; some people need a system for survival communication, whereas others manage basic communication well but need assistance in educational or vocational communication. Physical and cognitive capabilities, including cognition, language, memory, physical control, vision, and hearing, are assessed concurrent with the evaluation of communication needs. Because of the person's limited response abilities, these tests must be carefully selected or modified for the individual. Once the individual's capabilities have been ascertained, system components can be selected, and an appropriate system developed.

For those moderately involved speakers who are able to use speech as their primary means of communication but who are not completely intelligible, the goal of treatment involves improving intelligibility. The term *compensated intelligibility* aptly describes the goal of this phase of intervention (1). Achieving compensated intelligibility may take a variety of forms, depending on the speaker and the nature of the underlying impairment. For some severely dysarthric people, use of an alphabet supplementation system, in which they point to the first letter of each word as they say the word, assists in the transition to intelligible speech (26). For other dysarthric people, treatment involves an attempt to decrease the impairment by exercises that will improve performance on selected aspects of speech production. For example, exercises may involve developing more adequate respiratory support for speech (28), whereas for others, treatment may include training to establish an appropriate speech rate (29). Management may involve orthotically managing a severely impaired velopharyngeal mechanism through the use of a palatal lift (30,31), which is a dental retainer with a shelf attached to elevate the soft palate to the height necessary to reduce hypernasality and nasal air emission. An appropriately fitted palatal lift will allow certain dysarthric speakers to better produce speech sounds that require the buildup of oral air pressure, such as for the consonants /p/, /t/, and /d/. In other cases, maximizing intelligibility involves improving prosody, including teaching dysarthric speakers to emphasize speech sounds in the final position of words, to control the number of words per breath, and to stress important words in a sentence.

For the mildly involved dysarthric speaker whose speech is characterized as intelligible but less efficient and less natural than normal, treatment planning must first determine whether there is a handicap. For some speakers, these mild reductions in speech efficiency pose no problems. For other mildly involved speakers, however, treatment is warranted. The general goals of treatment for dysarthric people with mild disabilities include maximizing communication efficiency while maintaining intelligibility and maximizing speech naturalness. Maximizing naturalness is accomplished by teaching appropriate phrasing, stressing patterning, and intonation (32).

Treatment approaches for patients with progressive disorders such as parkinsonism, multiple sclerosis, and amyotrophic lateral sclerosis are different from those used with the dysarthric speaker who is recovering from a single event (33). Initially, the patients are encouraged to maximize the functional communication level by paying specific attention to the clarity and precision of their speech. At some point, the patients will need to modify their speaking patterns by controlling rate and consonant emphasis, and by reducing the number of words per breath. Some patients with progressive dysarthria make the adjustments in their speech pattern without specific treatment; others may need to practice these modifications with a speech pathologist or trained family member until the changes become habitual. In severe cases, a communication augmentation system may be considered. These augmentation systems usually are chosen or designed to accommodate the life-style of the patient while serving his or her anticipated communication needs over the longest period of time.

Laryngectomee Rehabilitation

Cancer of the larynx may be treated by a single treatment modality or a combination of modalities, including surgery, irradiation, and chemotherapy. Generally, the surgical options include the following: tumors that are limited to the region above the glottis may be treated by supraglottic laryngectomy; lesions lateralized to one side may be treated with hemilaryngectomy; and tumors that involve the glottic area with one mobile arytenoid may be dealt with by a subtotal laryngectomy. In each of these organ-conserving operations, the patient's laryngeal tumor is removed, yet voice is maintained. Postoperative rehabilitation for subtotal laryngectomy usually centers more on training compensations for swallowing than voice restoration.

Total laryngectomy remains a common procedure for the treatment of advanced laryngeal cancer. In addition to the obvious need for speech rehabilitation, these patients require education for care of their tracheostoma and adjustment to tracheostomal breathing. The patient must adjust to the relatively dry air entering the lungs without benefit of mucosal humidification from the nose, mouth, and pharynx. Humidifiers and moist stomal covers often are required to prevent crusting and the formation of dry mucus plugs, especially in the first few postoperative months. Shower bibs, neck wear, and stoma filters may assist the patient in adjusting to neck breathing and the changes in appearance.

SPEECH OPTIONS
Several options for speaking are available to postlaryngectomy patients. External prosthetic devices, specifically electrolarynxes and pneumatic external reeds, offer most patients an opportunity to speak within days of surgery. A tracheal–esophageal puncture (TEP) with insertion of a small one-way-valved prosthesis enables some laryngectomees to produce an esophageal vibratory voice. A third option, which is effective for a small percentage of patients, is to learn esophageal speech.

Electrolarynx
Commercially available electrolarynxes are designed to introduce air vibrations either directly into the oral cavity through a

catheter or indirectly through the neck tissues. In each case, the tones resonate within the oral and pharyngeal cavities and are modified by articulation into audible, intelligible words. Often an intraoral electrolarynx can be used 2 or 3 days after surgery, providing the patient with a means of communication. Speech therapy that is begun early can prevent the problem of trismus, which is common when head and neck surgical patients do not use their jaw muscles in speech or mastication for 2 weeks after surgery. Intraoral devices can also be used long term for patients with necks that are unsuitable for indirect transmission of vibration, usually because of pain, edema, or scar tissue. Experience suggests that good speech is slower to develop using an intraoral device than with a neck device. Therefore, care must be taken to help the patient avoid early frustration associated with not being understood immediately. Although most electrolarynxes designed for neck placement can be easily converted for intraoral use, they are primarily intended to transmit the vibration through the submandibular or neck tissue into the oral and pharyngeal cavities. Patients usually can begin to use a hand-held neck instrument when they are allowed to take nutrition by mouth. In patients with a suitable neck, intelligible speech can be achieved after only one or two practice sessions with a hand-held neck vibrator.

Pneumatic Reeds
Another type of external voice prosthesis is the pneumatic reed. This device is placed over the tracheostoma to allow exhaled air to pass across a reed to produce a tone that is carried into the mouth, much like an intraoral electrolarynx. Although these devices are inexpensive and capable of producing a pleasant quality of voice, they are cumbersome and conspicuous to use and have not gained wide popularity.

Tracheal–Esophageal Puncture
Tracheal–esophageal puncture procedures have been used since 1980 as a relatively simple means of voice restoration (34). The TEP can be performed either as a primary procedure at laryngectomy (35) or at almost any time during the postoperative period. A small, one-way-valved voice prosthesis is inserted through the TEP to allow the patient to shunt pulmonary air into the esophagus without having esophageal contents enter the TEP. Air passing through the prosthesis and up the esophagus vibrates the pharyngoesophageal segment to produce an esophageal voice. The prosthesis is not the source of sound vibrations, but the speech outcome does depend on the size and the design of the prosthesis chosen for the patient. Prostheses may be chosen that require weekly cleaning and replacement or indwelling devices that remain in place for 5 to 8 months (36). Early speech success following TEP and voice prosthesis fitting has been reported in almost 90% of cases (37,38). Long-term success is reported at between 93% for patients given primary TEP and 83% for those given secondary procedures (39). Success largely depends on patient selection, and in some cases, success can be enhanced by surgical techniques that can prevent pharyngoesophageal segment spasm (40), such as pharyngeal plexus neurectomy or cricopharyngeal myotomy. Other factors to consider in patient selection are motivation, intellect, dexterity, eyesight, stoma size and sensitivity, hand hygiene, surgical risk, and cost.

Esophageal Speech
Esophageal speech is accomplished by training the patient to move air from the oral and pharyngeal cavities into the esophagus by injection or suction methods, to hold the air in this esophageal reservoir, and then to release it in a controlled manner through the pharynx and esophagus. This method of voice

production uses the same anatomic vibratory site as the TEP technique but is accomplished without the necessity of occluding the tracheostoma. Because the volume of air maintained in the esophagus is much less than the pulmonary capacity used by the TEP speaker, the reservoir must be replenished constantly. Accomplished esophageal speakers can speak clearly and effortlessly; however, many laryngectomy patients are unable to learn this technique. Failure to learn esophageal speech may represent insufficient or excessive pharyngoesophageal segment tone, scarring, nerve damage, or learning difficulties.

LANGUAGE DISTURBANCE

An understanding of the mechanisms responsible for the processing and formulation of language is critical to good rehabilitation practice. Success in rehabilitation depends on a patient learning a new skill. Learning this new skill depends on how well the clinician and patient communicate. The success of this interaction is crucial to the speed, efficiency, and retention of newly learned behavioral patterns. Loss or disruption of input and output communication modalities can impede the learning process unless compensations are made. The necessary compensations are achieved with an understanding of how to assess the patient's language strengths and weaknesses, and how these modalities compare with nonlanguage learning modalities. A description of the learning strengths and limitations of patients with those language disorders frequently associated with cortical and subcortical disease, both focal and diffuse, is presented in this section.

Aphasia

Aphasia is a disorder of both the expression and reception of language secondary to cortical or subcortical disease, usually in the left hemisphere. It interferes with the ability to manipulate the meaning (i.e., semantics) or order (i.e., syntax) of words and gestures. There are three important points to emphasize in this definition, as follows:

1. The term *aphasia* implies impairment in both receptive and expressive language modalities. Expression may be more severely involved than reception, and reception can appear grossly intact. If the testing instrument is sensitive to subtle change in language behavior, pathology can be identified in the more intact modality.
2. Aphasia is consistent only with focal disease, usually of the left hemisphere. Aphasic symptoms may be part of a diffuse pathologic condition. However, these patients evidence more than disruptions in their ability to manipulate linguistic symbols, such as disorientation. Prognosis and recovery for this group is markedly different from those who evidence aphasia alone.
3. Although it is well known that aphasic disturbances are usually a consequence of cortical disease, the identification and classification of more atypical aphasic syndromes are also associated with subcortical infarction and hemorrhage (41).

Language Characteristics

Comprehension impairment of spoken language includes deficits of auditory perception and auditory retention. Auditory misperceptions are characterized by a tendency to confuse words that are similar in either meaning or sound. These confusions create a distorted message resulting in errors of com-prehension. Most aphasics will experience more errors in comprehension as the length of the auditory input increases. In general, the speed of auditory input, combined with increased length, leads to errors in auditory retention. In addition, increased sentence length often presupposes a more difficult syntax and vocabulary, combining to make comprehension more liable to error. It has been demonstrated that some aphasics retain more information from the beginning of an utterance, whereas others retain information from the end (42). Evaluation of this aspect of the patient's auditory capacity is especially important if rehabilitation is to succeed. Comprehension of reading material also is impaired. The severity of this impairment often is greater than that of the linguistic deficits in other modalities.

Expressively, patients might evidence anomia, agrammatism, paragrammatism, or paraphasia, or they may produce jargon, stereotypic, or echolalic language patterns. Although most aphasics display an overall reduction in word classes available for production, they show particular deficits in the retrieval of nouns (i.e., anomia). Because nouns carry a large part of the meaning during an intended message, the language of the anomic patient is described as "empty" because sentences often lack a subject or referent. In their attempts to retrieve words, aphasics make "paraphasic" language errors. When the substitution for the intended word is from the same word class, such as *chair* for *table*, it is a semantic paraphasia. The substitution of like sounds or syllables, such as *flair* for *chair* is classified as a phonemic paraphasia. A final class of paraphasic error is the neologism. Neologisms are attempts at the target that bear no phonemic or semantic relationship to that target, such as: "I want to brush my ploker." Patients who find word retrieval difficult may also circumlocute, or talk around the intended noun, such as saying, "I wear it on my wrist" instead of *watch*.

Agrammatism is a form of expressive deficit characterized by reliance on nouns and verbs (i.e., content words) to the exclusion of articles, verb auxiliaries, pronouns, and prepositions (i.e., function words). Agrammatic productions often are described as *telegraphic*. Paragrammatic language is characterized by the misuse, rather than the omission, of grammatical elements

Patients whose expressive output is largely incomprehensible, even though the utterance is well articulated and verbose, may display a form of expressive deficit called jargon. Concentrations of neologisms are called neologistic jargon and may be associated with stereotypes such as "blam, blam, blam" substituted for all attempts at verbalization. A preponderance of unrelated semantic paraphasias is semantic jargon. Finally, some patients evidence echolalia, typified by the patient echoing back the same utterance he or she has just heard.

Expressive writing output also is impaired in typical aphasia, as is the ability to use gestures as a substitute form of expression (43). Table 45-2 provides a summary of the terminology used to describe expressive language deficits in aphasia.

Classification of Aphasic Syndromes

Historically, there have been many attempts to place pathologic language symptoms into homogeneous groups, permitting reference to specific aphasic subtypes. The Boston classification system standardizes terminology beginning with a broad classification of disorders into those in which expressive skills are predominantly fluent and those in which they are predominantly nonfluent (44). Although such a distinction might be useful clinically, it often can be difficult to make this classification, as in the case of a conduction aphasic (a fluent

TABLE 45-2.   Summary of the Terminology Used to Describe Expressive Disorders of Aphasia

Term	Definition
Agrammatism	The absence of recognized grammatical elements during speech attempts
Anomia	Difficulty producing nouns
Circumlocution	Attempts at word retrieval end in descriptions or associations related to the word
Echolalia	An accurate repetition of a preceding utterance when repetition is not required
Empty speech	A fluent utterance that lacks substantive parts of language, such as nouns and verbs
Jargon	Mostly incomprehensible, but well-articulated language
Neologistic jargon	Mostly incomprehensible, some words are partially recognizable, others are contrived or "new"
Paragrammatism	Misuse of grammatical elements, usually during fluent utterances
Phonemic paraphasia	*Flair* for *chair*, also called *literal paraphasia*
Press for speech	Excessively lengthy, often incomprehensible, well-articulated language
Semantic jargon	A combination of unrelated semantic and phonemic paraphasia, together with recognizable words
Semantic paraphasia	*Table* for *chair*, also called *nominal paraphasia*
Stereotypes	Nonsensical repetition of similar syllables for all communicative attempts, such as *dee dee dee*
Telegraphic speech	Language similar to a telegram, mostly nouns and verbs

TABLE 45-3.   Summary of the Boston Classification System of Aphasia

Type	Language Characteristics
Nonfluent	
Broca	Telegraphic, agrammatic expression often associated with apraxia; good comprehension except on more abstract tasks
Transcortical motor	Limited language output; fair naming; intact repetition; fair comprehension
Global	Severe expressive and receptive reduction in language
Mixed transcortical	Severe reduction in expression and reception; repetition intact
Fluent	
Anomia	Word-finding difficulty without other serious linguistic deficits
Conduction	Phonemic paraphasic errors; good comprehension; fluency in bursts; deficits in repetition of low-probability phrases
Wernicke	Phonemic and semantic paraphasias; poor comprehension
Transcortical sensory	Fluent neologistic language; poor comprehension; intact repetition

aphasia) who may have long pauses and expressive struggle (nonfluency) during speech. The eight major types of aphasia in the Boston system include the more common forms of Broca's aphasia, Wernicke's aphasia, anomia, conduction aphasia, and global aphasia, as well as the less frequent transcortical types (Table 45-3). Each of these aphasic syndromes is correlated with a specific localized cortical lesion, some with subcortical extension.

Improvements in brain imaging have made it possible to correlate disturbances in language with lesions in the corpus striatum and thalamus. The data are still incomplete, but most of the syndromes described differ from those associated with confirmed cortical disease. Although some characteristics of speech show patterns that are consistent with each of the sites, not every investigator describes the same speech and language deficits from identical lesions.

Preliminary evidence suggests that the speech and language disorders are confined to left hemispheric subcortical structures (45). There is a suggestion that an infarct or a hemorrhage at the same site may produce different effects. Lesion size also is important, of course. Lesions involving the putamen and caudate with anterosuperior extension into the internal capsule reportedly have produced more dysarthria with reduced vocal volume and labored speech (46,47). Grammar and comprehension were unaffected. Paraphasia and poor comprehension were associated most with a posterior extension of the lesion. A combination of anterior and posterior capsular lesions resulted in global aphasia. Patients with anterior capsular lesions have been found to have articulation disturbances consistent with buccofacial apraxia plus disturbances of comprehension (48).

Linguistic deficits secondary to thalamic hemorrhage also have been reported (49,50). A great deal of variation is observed in language performance, with some patients having almost normal language performance and others demonstrating marked paraphasia and periods of fluctuating unconsciousness (50). These fluctuations may be related more to the role of the thalamus in arousal and selective attention as prerequisites to communication than to its role in actual deficits of language (49). Although most studies confirm the notion that the symptoms associated with subcortical disease may be transitory, patients seen in our clinic who evidence attentional and arousal deficits beyond the acute stage of illness have not been able to learn compensations for their communication failures in spite of nearly normal comprehension skills.

Differentiation from Other Disorders

Aphasia, particularly in the acute stages, may be difficult to differentiate from other disorders that compromise communication. Accurate differentiation is necessary because each communication disorder requires separate treatment and management approaches. It should be noted that aphasia may occur in conjunction with other syndromes. Table 45-4 provides a comparison of linguistic and nonlinguistic behaviors among disorders that commonly interfere with communication.

AGNOSIA

Agnosia is the inability to interpret or recognize information when the end organ is intact. For example, a patient with auditory agnosia would have normal audiometric hearing thresholds but cannot interpret speech signals at the cortical level. Hence, auditory comprehension will be severely compromised. Patients with agnosia can be differentiated from those with aphasia because they will be impaired in only one modality. For example, the patient with auditory agnosia who has severe comprehension deficits can read the same words through the intact visual modality.

TABLE 45-4.   Aphasia Differentiated from Other Cortical and Subcortical Speech and Language Disorders

Characteristic	Agnosia	Aphasia	Apraxia	Confusion	Dementia	Dysarthria	Subcortical Aphasia
Auditory comprehension	±	±	+	±	±	±	±
Auditory memory	+	±	+	−	−	+	±
Visual memory	+	+	+	−	−	+	±
Naming	+	±	+	±	−	+	±
Reading/writing	±	−	+	−	−	+	±
Generalized cognitive deficits	+	+	+	−	−	+	±
Inappropriate behaviors	+	+	+	−	−	+	±
Disturbance of attention	+	+	+	−	−	+	−
Learn well	+	+	+	±	−	+	±
Disorder confined to one input/output modality	−	+	−	+	±	+	+
Regular errors of speech output	+	+	+	+	+	−	±
Irregular errors of speech output	+	+	−	+	+	+	±

In acute stages: +, usually unimpaired; -, usually impaired; ±, patient dependent.

APRAXIA

In its pure form, apraxia of speech (AOS) is the motor counterpart of agnosia. AOS occurs in the absence of significant weakness and incoordination of muscles, with automatic and reflexive movements undisturbed. Lesions in the premotor cortex are a frequent finding (51). AOS is characterized by labored and dysprosodic productions, resulting in errors of omission, substitution, and repetition. There is debate as to whether AOS is a pure motor or linguistic (i.e., phonemic) disturbance (43,52,53). Patients have difficulty programming the positioning of the speech musculature and sequencing the movements necessary for speech. It is seen by some as a distinct condition that often coexists and complicates aphasia, whereas others regard the characteristics as part of the nonfluent Broca's aphasia. AOS carries a negative prognosis for recovery when there is a moderate to severe aphasia in tandem. When it occurs without the concomitant language disturbance, therapy can focus on retraining the patient's ability to program sound patterns, to shift from one sound to another, and to use preserved melodic and rhythmic patterns to facilitate speech.

DEMENTIA

Dementia is a syndrome of progressive cognitive deterioration that adversely affects the ability to communicate (54). Although specific expressive and receptive language disturbances can present as part of an underlying disease process, the aphasic patient does not show evidence of cognitive deficits in such areas as orientation, judgment, self-care, and visual-perceptual skills. The distinction between those patients with language deficits secondary to aphasia and those with diffuse disease is particularly relevant in rehabilitation because the prognosis for retraining specific skills and developing independence is more favorable for the patient with aphasia alone.

CONFUSION

Confused language is characterized by reduced recognition, reduced understanding of and responsiveness to the environment, faulty memory, unclear thinking, and disorientation (54). It often is associated with head trauma. In contrast to the language disorders of dementia, the prognosis for recovery after traumatic injury is more favorable and the course is not progressive.

Tests for Aphasia

Tests for aphasia measure the patient's receptive and expressive language capacities by sampling different types of language skills through systematically controlled channels. For example, an examination of reception via the visual input system might begin with a concrete task such as copying or matching, and then proceed to more difficult tasks such as reading sentences for comprehension. Tests of expression might range from simple repetition, to naming, to providing definitions. Most test batteries currently in use provide a representative sample from which inferences can be made about performance in similar linguistic situations. Although most tests of aphasia do sample linguistic competencies, they are not equipped to measure either the least severe or the most severe disorders. Therefore, the examination will have to be supplemented by other specialized formal and informal measures in selected cases.

THE MINNESOTA TEST FOR DIFFERENTIAL DIAGNOSIS OF APHASIA

The Minnesota Test for Differential Diagnosis of Aphasia is the most comprehensive test battery, taking an average of 3 hours to administer (55). The test has 47 subtests and is particularly useful for recognizing and classifying deficits of auditory comprehension. Means and standard deviations are available for each subtest, and patients can be rated from 0 to 6 in each major area of performance (e.g., comprehension, reading, expression, and writing). Because of the length of the test, it must be given in multiple sessions. Scoring is cumbersome, and subtest instructions for the examiner are not always clear. Patients can be classified into groups by aphasia type, which is the basis of a prognosis for recovery.

THE BOSTON DIAGNOSTIC APHASIA EXAMINATION

The Boston Diagnostic Aphasia Examination (BDAE) provides the examiner with 27 subtests and an additional group of non-language-based subtests as part of a battery to evaluate parietal lobe dysfunction (44). It is particularly valuable as a classification tool because it assesses deficiencies in language consistent with the Boston schema of aphasia classification. The examiner rates the patient's conversational speech and auditory comprehension on a seven-point scale. This scale is used for patient classification and is related to a lesion site. Test scores are summarized by modality and are presented as percentiles compared with a large sample of patients.

THE WESTERN APHASIA BATTERY

The Western Aphasia Battery is a modification and expansion of the BDAE (56). Subtest scores provide the information used in classification. Auditory and expressive modality scores yield an aphasia quotient (AQ) that is calculated taking spontaneous recovery into account. An AQ score below 93 (8) is consistent with aphasia. The patient is assigned a performance quotient (PQ) on the basis of tests of reading, writing, drawing, calculation, block design, and portions of the Raven's Progressive Matrices. A summary of cognitive function combines the PQ and AQ scores. This summary score is useful in assessing patients with cognitive deficits after traumatic injury.

THE PORCH INDEX OF COMMUNICATIVE ABILITY

The Porch Index of Communicative Ability contains 18 subtests and uses 10 common objects to elicit patient responses (57). Examiners must be trained a minimum of 40 hours and then meet reliability criteria before using the test. The uniqueness of this battery is its 16-point scoring scale. Every response on each subtest is scored from 1 to 16, based on the completeness, accuracy, promptness, responsiveness, and efficiency of the patient's response. Percentile scores by modality can be compared with a database of patients with bilateral or left hemisphere damage. Modality or overall test scores can be used to predict recovery. The test is particularly useful in planning programmed treatment and research. It is not particularly sensitive to patients with mild or severe linguistic deficits because it assesses a narrow range of verbal functions.

THE TOKEN TEST

The Token Test is designed to detect subtle auditory comprehension disorders and often is administered to patients who reach ceiling levels on standardized aphasia batteries (58). The patient is given 20 tokens with two shapes, two sizes, and five colors, and then is asked through nonredundant language to manipulate them. The five sections, comprised of 62 total items, increase in difficulty by length and linguistic complexity. Normative data do not come with the test but are available from the literature (59,60). Test interpretation can be difficult because patients can make errors owing to pure linguistic auditory comprehension problems or auditory memory deficits. A more standardized version, The Revised Token Test, also is available (61). A version in which the examiner moves the tokens and the patient describes what he or she has seen is the Reporter's Test (62).

THE READING COMPREHENSION BATTERY

The Reading Comprehension Battery comprises 10 subtests that are used to assess reading skills in greater detail than most standardized aphasia batteries (63). Subtests include comprehension of morphosyntactic structure, functional reading, synonym recognition, and sentence and paragraph comprehension. This popular test is useful to specify the degree of reading impairment for patients at all levels of severity.

Approaches to Treatment

Aphasia treatment should be patient dependent and maximize communication in actual interactive situations. Aphasics, even those with similar types of lesions, represent a heterogeneous group. Because of this heterogeneity, outcomes of treatment are often unpredictable. In addition to building on the patient's communicative strengths, remediation should be directed toward helping the patient, family, and friends accept and adapt to the person's liabilities.

Traditionally, the focus of aphasia remediation has been on the stimulation–facilitation approach, in which the patient and clinician interact within a stimulus–response framework on tasks that are thought to be related to communication (64,65). Although this approach may be most beneficial for the more severely impaired, its relevance in helping the patient solve everyday communicative needs remains questionable. The notion that the clinician's role should be guided toward helping the patient adjust to his or her own particular environment presupposes that family, friends, and employers will receive as much remediation as the patient, and that they will learn how to enhance the patient's communicative competencies. To accomplish this, the speech pathologist must analyze the patient's communicative strengths and weaknesses and then objectify and teach the pragmatics of communication to the language-impaired person and to his or her significant others.

In general, patients who evidence diffuse cortical signs in addition to their linguistic deficits, those with unilateral multilobe disease secondary to hemorrhage, and those with a severe reduction of test scores after the first month will not be candidates for direct daily speech and language remediation. Reassessment of these patients with either standardized or informal testing instruments is used to identify any emerging communicative strengths so that they can be further enhanced with treatment. This reassessment should continue monthly for 6 months after the onset, and then in 2-month intervals for up to 1 year. Treatment with globally involved patients should focus on their ability to learn a new task in a prescribed amount of time. Such tasks usually do not require a great deal of complex processing, such as matching picture to object, object to object, or word to object. Data should be kept on the patient's accuracy and processing time as measures of change. Learning success provides prognostic information for further daily remediation in using direct approaches to treatment.

Training in communicative interaction must focus on the following:

- Appropriate rates of auditory presentation and the importance of pause times
- Differences between concrete and abstract language
- Use of redundancy to improve comprehension
- Ways to carry the load of a conversation while still involving the patient
- Utilization of contextual cues to comprehend what the patient may be communicating
- Ways to verify messages from the patient
- Ways to combine gesture and oral language to facilitate communication
- Allowing the appropriate amount of time for a patient to formulate a response before restimulation (i.e., questioning or repeating)

The training modules should be divided into four parts: direct work with the patient and clinician, demonstrations of pragmatics with the family, patient–family interactions critiqued by the clinician, and environmental control training.

Environmental controls are similar to environmental language stimulation described by Lubinski (66). The patient's environment should be evaluated to determine how it might be manipulated to enhance communicative skills and compensate for deficits. These manipulations should focus on ways to con-

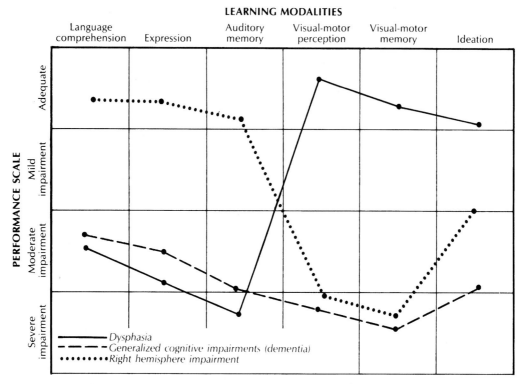

Figure 45-1. Comparison of learning strengths and weaknesses of patients with right and left hemisphere pathology and dementia. (From DeLisa JA, Miller RM, Melnick RR, et al. Stroke rehabilitation. Part I. Cognitive deficits and prediction of outcome. *Am Fam Physician* 1982;26:208, with permission.)

trol for distractions, to provide favorable seating and lighting when possible, to control the number of speakers, to suggest the time of day when the patient's performance is best, to control daily situations so that the patient has a need to communicate, and to provide adequate reinforcement for communication. Other environmental controls that enhance communication because they allow for linguistic predictability include the design of a daily regimented schedule and keeping items in the environment such as chairs, utensils, and food items in familiar places. These controls can maximize communicative effectiveness. However, patients who react favorably to such controls should also have them removed at prescribed times, forcing them to practice using their language in reaction to less predictable situations. These encounters, if positive, can lead to significant improvement in communication.

Communication Impairment After Right Hemisphere Damage

It is well known that the right hemisphere plays a major role in initiating planned action, making judgments based on visual perception, and remembering information that must be visually coded. In some patients, neglect or denial of the situation makes these deficits more pronounced and harder to manage. It is easy to overlook these deficits because of the patient's stronger communication skills. Typically, the verbal performance is so strong that the reasons for the poor visual motor skills might be questioned (Fig. 45-1). Evidence suggests that even though the patient with right hemisphere damage may suffer more from visual than from linguistic deficits, there is also affective and extraverbal communication impairment.

The right hemisphere's role in affective aspects of communication is continuing to be explored. Affective aspects, such as the lack of facial expression while speaking, failure to maintain eye contact, failure to use gesture, and lack of vocal inflection, all have been described in the patient with right hemisphere damage (67). Loss of inflectional patterns that signal anger or frustration is not surprising, given the role the right hemisphere plays in decoding and recalling melodies. The clinician must be alert to the possibility of such a pathologic process because loss of these affective cues often is mistaken for the functional states of rudeness or unconcern for another's feelings.

Additional problems with extraverbal aspects of communication also help to explain the "difficult-to-get-along-with" personality of the patient with right hemisphere damage. Extraverbal skills include behaviors such as appreciation of humor and figurative language, and the use of pragmatics such as the ability to maintain a conversational topic and turn-taking during conversation. These patients have difficulty in organizing information, and they fail to make use of contextual cues. Failure to recognize these cues results in many conversational irrelevancies, as well as poor monitoring of rate and amount of expressive language when they stray from, or completely lose, the thread of the conversation. Failure to recognize humor and metaphoric language structures may be misunderstood by family members as a noncaring, depressed personality. Problems in interpreting incoming visual and auditory information, long known to be a right hemisphere function, make it difficult for these patients to get the point of discourse, leading to the further frustration of friends and family.

ASSESSMENT

Before the clinical management of right hemisphere dysfunction (68), no formal assessment tool was available for the systematic evaluation of the communication skills of the patient with right hemisphere damage. This test offers a scoring system for the use of pragmatics, nonverbal skills such as eye contact and facial gestures, interpretation of metaphoric language,

should include environmental controls, capitalization on the preserved procedural memory, and family education. Environmental structure provides orientation and reinforces memory that, in turn, will improve the accuracy of linguistic attempts. Interactions with the patient should be structured to reduce demands beyond the limits of the cognitive system as established by psychometric evaluation. Frequent measures of linguistic function are part of the treatment and are necessary so that family and friends can be informed about how much to expect from the patient both receptively and expressively. This knowledge will reduce frustration for the patient and family. Some patients retain skills longer than others do, and knowledge of the best input and expected output modalities is useful in management. Because dementia often results in diminution of all linguistic modalities, performance may be strengthened through the use of multiple channels such as the combination of gestural, written, and verbal language. This multimodality strategy is a process that should be taught to family members.

Recent evidence suggests that combining exercise activities with cognitive stimulation tasks may facilitate the communicative process (86). This may be related either to increased blood flow to the brain during periods of aerobic exercise or to stress management. Therapy to enhance communicative skills applied during rest periods from aerobic exercise also may be of importance for patients with dementia (87). Although the evidence that certain medications facilitate memory in patients with dementia remains controversial, no data are available to support the use of facilitative drugs to enhance language.

SWALLOWING IMPAIRMENT

Swallowing is an essential life function that begins *in utero*. It is necessary to survival both because it is the source of hydration and alimentation, and because it has a crucial role in maintaining airway integrity by clearing residue from the oral cavity and pharyngeal tract. Abnormal swallowing (dysphagia) may lead to dehydration, starvation, aspiration pneumonia, or airway obstruction. Dysphagia is frequently associated with cerebrovascular disease, traumatic brain injury, head and neck cancer, and other conditions common in rehabilitation patients. In many cases, swallowing impairments are amenable to rehabilitation treatment.

Physiology of Swallowing

Swallowing is coordinated with other patterned behaviors, including respiration and mastication; and each is controlled by a central pattern generator in the brainstem. For convenience, swallowing is typically divided into three phases based on the anatomic location of the bolus. These phases may overlap in their timing and coordination.

ORAL PHASE

The oral phase begins with the oral preparation of the bolus, which precedes the swallow per se. The manner in which the bolus is prepared for swallowing varies, depending on the consistency of the material. Liquids may be held either between the tongue and palate or in the lingual sulcus, but generally they pass through the oral cavity in a continuous process. Soft foods may be held immediately between the tongue and anterior hard palate or lateralized for mastication before resuming a midline position for swallowing.

The preparation for solid food entails several distinct but overlapping processes (88). Ingestion is passage of food through the lips and into the mouth by biting or manual placement. This is followed immediately by stage I transport, in which food is propelled from the anterior to the middle or posterior oral cavity. If food particles are still too large or coarse for swallowing, they remain in the mouth. During mastication, food is softened, and food particles are reduced in size by chewing (incising, crushing, and grinding) and mixing with saliva. Food in the mouth stimulates mechanoreceptors for the fifth cranial nerve located in the periodontal membrane and palate. Stimulation of these receptors activates the central pattern generator for mastication, producing sequential contraction and relaxation of the elevator and depressor muscles of the mandible and resulting in cyclic opening and closing of the mouth. This cyclic grinding motion of the jaws is coordinated with rotation of the tongue, which pushes the food between the upper and lower teeth. Saliva is excreted from the salivary glands, helping to break down the food and stimulate the taste buds. The physical consistency of the food is monitored continuously by oral mechanoreceptors.

Once a small portion of the food is fully prepared (triturated), a cycle of stage II transport is initiated. The tongue pushes upward and forward in the mouth, contacting the anterior portion of the hard palate. The area of tongue–palate contact expands backward, propelling the small portion of the triturated food through the faucial arches and into the oropharynx. This small portion of food may remain in the oropharynx while chewing continues for several more jaw cycles, and additional small portions of triturated food may be propelled into the oropharynx. When a large enough bolus has been prepared, a swallow is initiated. The pharyngeal phase of swallowing follows immediately.

PHARYNGEAL PHASE

When appropriate sensory input reaches the medullary central pattern generator for swallowing, a complex motor sequence is elicited to propel a bolus through the pharynx, around the larynx, through the pharyngoesophageal (PE) sphincter, and into the esophagus. The events of the pharyngeal phase occur almost simultaneously, having a duration of about 1 second. Respiration ceases, and the palatopharyngeal isthmus closes to seal off the nasopharynx. The tongue pushes back into the pharynx like a plunger, pushing the bolus downward. The epiglottis inverts, deflecting the bolus around the larynx and away from the airway. The larynx closes via contraction of the vocal folds and sealing of the laryngeal vestibule. The PE sphincter opens, allowing the bolus to pass into the esophagus. Opening of the PE sphincter is a complex process: the cricopharyngeus muscle relaxes, allowing the sphincter to open; the submandibular muscles pull the hyoid bone, the larynx, and the attached anterior wall of the pharynx upward and forward (away from the posterior pharyngeal wall); and the pressure of the descending bolus helps push the PE sphincter open (89). The pharyngeal constrictors contract sequentially with a peristaltic wave from top to bottom, clearing the pharynx of residue.

ESOPHAGEAL PHASE

The pharyngeal constricting wave that cleared the bolus into the esophagus continues throughout the esophagus as a primary peristaltic wave that propels the bolus through the gastroesophageal sphincter (GES) and into the stomach. Esophageal clearance is assisted by gravity but also requires relaxation of the GES. Reflux of stomach contents is prevented by tonic contraction of the GES and reflex esophageal swallowing that is triggered by esophageal distension (secondary peristalsis).

Evaluation of Swallowing

When dysphagia is recognized, or a complaint about swallowing is registered, a special evaluation is required (90,91). Such an evaluation should consist of a complete medical history, a detailed description of the complaint, and a physical examination of the peripheral deglutitory motor and sensory system, including trial swallows under observation. Diagnostic studies, including videofluorography, manometry, electromyography, and fiberoptic endoscopy, are indicated in selected cases.

HISTORY

Data should be compiled from a review of the patient's general health history. Special attention should be paid to the neurologic history, which might suggest contributing factors such as stroke, head trauma, parkinsonism, or multiple sclerosis, each of which may cause dysphagia. All prior operations should be noted, especially those involving the head and neck. All current prescription and nonprescription medications should be listed. Those that have side effects of sedation, muscle weakness, drying of mucous membranes, disorientation, or dyskinesia may contribute to dysphagia. Anticholinergic and psychoactive medications are specially noted.

Psychosocial factors may have a significant impact on swallowing, especially for elderly individuals. An individual living alone may be unable to obtain supervision during meals. For a nursing home resident, prescribing a special diet may be unrealistic. Swallowing must also be considered in the context of feeding. Feeding dependency is an enormous problem for the elderly. Problems with feeding may be difficult to differentiate from impairments of swallowing per se (92).

DESCRIPTION OF THE COMPLAINT

In many instances the subjective complaint gives the examiner clues to the cause of the swallowing problem. Critical data include a sensation of food sticking in the throat or chest, difficulty initiating swallowing, occurrence of coughing or choking spells associated with eating, drooling or difficulty clearing oral secretions, weight loss, change in diet or eating habits, episodes of aspiration pneumonia, and symptoms referable to gastroesophageal reflux. Difficulties swallowing solids and liquids should be contrasted and compared.

With liquids, patients may complain of coughing or choking during drinking. These symptoms are suggestive of aspiration (misdirection of food through the larynx and into the trachea) and are common in patients with neurogenic swallowing impairment. A complaint of food sticking in the throat or chest is common with solid food and raises the possibility of foodway obstruction. It may have many causes, however, including bulbar palsy, pharyngoesophageal diverticula, tumor, stricture, or esophageal dysmotility. The sensation of food sticking in the chest (thoracic dysphagia) is usually associated with disease of the esophagus or GES. Pharyngeal dysphagia, however, has poor localizing value and may be caused by dysfunction of the pharynx, PE sphincter, esophagus, or GES. Nasal regurgitation is associated with weakness or incompetence of the palatopharyngeal mechanism. Oral malodor may suggest a pharyngoesophageal diverticulum, but may also be associated with mastication problems, poor oral hygiene, pharyngeal retention of food, tumor, or infection. Pain on swallowing (odynophagia) is a worrisome symptom, often associated with cancer of the esophagus. Heartburn, acid or sour regurgitation, and regurgitation of digested food suggest gastroesophageal reflux disease (GERD). Reflux of stomach contents due to GERD, especially at night, can lead to severe aspiration pneumonia. Instances of aspiration pneumonia should be recorded as a measure of sever-

ity. Because the shared anatomic and neuromuscular systems are used for both speech and swallowing, any speech or voice changes should be carefully noted and described. Weight loss or changes in eating habits often reflect an underlying problem with swallowing.

CLINICAL EXAMINATION

A general physical examination is essential to look for evidence of cardiopulmonary, gastrointestinal, or neurologic disease that may impair swallowing. This exam includes an assessment of mental status, as well as the patient's ability to cooperate. A screening of language functions (e.g., following spoken commands, expressing thoughts), memory, and visual–motor–perceptual function is helpful (93). Cranial nerves should be assessed carefully. The respiratory system is examined for signs of obstruction or restriction such as tachypnea, stridor, use of accessory muscles, paradoxic motion of the chest wall, or labored breathing. Speech is examined for evidence of dysarthria or dysphonia.

The head and neck are inspected and palpated for structural lesions. The hyoid bone and laryngeal cartilages are palpated carefully and gently mobilized. Facial sensation is checked bilaterally. The muscles of the face, mouth, and neck are examined beginning with the muscles of facial expression, carefully comparing movement of the two sides of the face for signs of asymmetric weakness. The masseter and temporalis can be palpated as the patient bites and chews. Movements of the lower jaw are assessed in three directions of movement.

The examination proceeds to inspection of the intraoral mucosa. Careful attention should be paid to the presence of lesions, oral debris, abnormal movement, and dryness. Palpation with gloved hand on the floor of the mouth, gum lines, tonsillar fossa, and tongue serves to help rule out neoplastic growth. Atrophy, weakness, and fasciculations of the tongue should be noted. Tongue strength can be assessed by placing fingers against the outer cheek and resisting the patient's tongue as it is pushed into the inner cheek. The palate is inspected for symmetry at rest and during phonation. Each side of the palate is stimulated to elicit gag reflexes, observing whether the soft palate and pharyngeal walls contract briskly and symmetrically. However, gag reflexes may be difficult to elicit in some normal individuals. The presence of primitive reflexes associated with chewing and swallowing (such as the sucking, biting, or snout reflexes) should be noted. These pathologic reflexes are often found in patients with damage to both hemispheres or frontal lobes, and may indicate impairments of oral motor control.

The comprehensive examination includes observing the patient eating and drinking (91). Trial swallows are an essential portion of the examination, but they do carry a small risk of aspiration. It is advisable initially to use a substance that is relatively safe if aspirated and to ensure that the patient is able to cough to protect the airway. (A sip of water is relatively innocuous.) The examiner observes for the promptness of the swallow and palpates the anterior neck to assess the adequacy of laryngeal elevation. Behaviors that should be noted include drooling, slow rate of eating, residual food in the mouth after swallowing, frequent throat clearing, change in voice quality, and posturing of the head and neck with swallowing. A spoonful of crushed ice may elicit chewing because of its texture and temperature. The examiner can observe the chewing action and feel for the laryngeal elevation to indicate that a swallow has occurred. Once it has been determined that the patient adequately elevates the larynx and that there is an adequate protective cough, other substances with varying textures and consistencies can be tried. Soft solid foods will also elicit chewing and allow the examiner to feel for laryngeal elevation. The mouth is always reinspected for retention after swallowing.

The purposes of the history and physical examination are to assess components of the swallowing mechanism, to characterize the nature and severity of the swallowing deficit, to assess the patient's ability to perform compensatory maneuvers, and to determine whether further diagnostic studies are necessary. The physical examination is neither sensitive nor specific for identifying aspiration and cannot prove or disprove that a patient aspirates (94).

DIAGNOSTIC STUDIES

The videofluorographic swallowing study (VFSS) is the *sine qua non* of diagnostic tests for dysphagia. The rehabilitation approach to videofluorography is to have the patient eat various radio-opacified foods, using appropriate modifications, toward the goal of establishing a safe and efficient method of eating. An empirical approach is used to identify variables associated with safe and unsafe swallowing such as physical consistency of food, posture of the patient (especially position of the head and neck), and the means for presenting the food. These variables are altered systematically during the VFSS, and the effects on swallowing are observed (95–97).

Indications for a VFSS include frequent choking episodes, difficulty managing secretions, wet-hoarse voice quality, respiratory complications, and unexplained weight loss. Relative contraindications include inability to cooperate with the examination and severe respiratory dysfunction. Although static x-ray films may be valuable to detect morphologic changes in the pharynx or esophagus, they are not useful in studying the dynamics of swallowing. A complete examination should be conducted beginning with a small amount of liquid barium. Both lateral and anteroposterior views should be obtained with the patient in an upright posture. The oral and pharyngeal stages of swallowing should be studied with the camera focused superiorly on the hard palate and inferiorly on the cervical esophagus. Many clinicians recommend using a variety of textures (e.g., thin and thick liquid barium, puree, and cookie). Because simultaneous disorders of the pharynx and esophagus are frequent, the examination should include a study of the esophagus whenever possible. The esophagus and GE junction are best visualized with the patient in a prone position.

A protocol for fiberoptic endoscopic examination of swallowing (FEES) has been described by Langmore and colleagues (98) as a means to detect aspiration in patients for whom radiographic studies are difficult. A FEES carries the added benefit of directly visualizing the pharynx and larynx, to inspect for mucosal lesions or motion impairment of the vocal folds. Esophagoscopy is essential for detecting a variety of esophageal and GES disorders and provides the opportunity for diagnostic biopsy. Electrodiagnostic studies may be helpful for detecting motor unit dysfunction of the larynx, pharynx, and oral musculature but cannot substitute for VFSS (99).

Management of Swallowing Impairment

Once the patient's swallowing has been described, the impairment identified, and the compensatory strengths recognized, a recommendation is made to feed the patient by mouth or to manage nutrition by an alternative route such as feeding tube. When oral feeding is recommended, a plan is needed that will maintain optimum calorie and fluid intake while minimizing the patient's risk for aspiration. Each plan must be individualized and based on what is known about the normal physiology of swallowing, the specific physiologic abnormality, the cause of the disorder, and the prognosis for recovery (100). Table 45-5 lists some of the therapeutic and compensatory techniques that can be employed for patients with oral–pharyngeal forms of dysphagia.

MECHANICAL DISORDERS

Disruptions in the transmission of food and beverage from the anterior oral cavity into the pharynx and esophagus caused by structural abnormalities such as mucosal inflammation, trauma, tumor, or surgical alteration (in the mouth, pharynx, or larynx) may be described as mechanical disturbances of swallowing (101).

One type of mechanical disorder is found in the patient with partial or total glossectomy. If pharyngeal sensation and motor function are preserved, a special feeding spoon with a plunger to propel food into the posterior oral cavity can be used. A cohesive bolus of soft food can be pushed toward the back of the tongue. Liquids can be placed directly into the posterior oral cavity or oropharynx by using a syringe and length of tubing that will reach the faucial pillars.

Complications to swallowing for many surgical head and neck cancer patients are caused by radiation therapy. Xerostomia, or dry mouth, results from destruction of the salivary glands and other moisture-producing cells in the mucous lining. Artificial saliva may be used just before meals to provide moisture. Lemon-glycerin swabs, used to clean out oral debris, can be helpful for some patients, although others complain

---

TABLE 45-5. Some Therapeutic and Compensatory Techniques for Managing Patients with Dysphagia

Technique	Desired Effect
Flex neck	Reduce aspiration
Turn head to one side	Direct bolus to the ipsilateral side (away from side of weakness)
Hold breath before swallowing	Seal larynx, reduce aspiration
Thicken liquids (avoid thin)	Reduce aspiration, improve bolus control
Thin liquids (avoid thick)	Reduce pharyngeal retention
Slow rate of eating	Improve oral bolus control, avoid overloading pharynx
Mendelsohn maneuver	Prolong pharyngoesophageal sphincter opening, improve pharyngeal clearance
Glottic adduction exercises	Improve airway protection, reduce aspiration
Use glossectomy spoon	Bypass anterior mouth, place food directly into posterior oral cavity
Stimulate soft palate with cold	Increase sensitivity for eliciting swallow
Feeding gastrostomy	Bypass oral cavity and pharynx

they increase dryness. The diet of these patients should emphasize foods lubricated with sauces, gravies, and butter. Mucosal pain associated with irradiation can be managed in part by the use of topical anesthetics; however, patients with impaired pharyngeal swallowing will have a greater aspiration risk because of the reduction of sensation.

Patients who have undergone a supraglottic laryngectomy are at risk for aspiration because of the loss of the epiglottis and altered sensation. Aspiration can be minimized by training the patient to inhale and hold breath before swallowing, to swallow, to cough gently while exhaling, and then to reswallow. This procedure ensures that the patient has an adequate amount of air in the lungs to cough out debris that has penetrated the unprotected laryngeal region. Logemann and colleagues have described a "super" supraglottic swallow maneuver in which patients are instructed to hold their breath tighter and to bear down with this (Valsalva). Improved airway closure and decreased aspiration have been reported in irradiated patients with this technique (102).

DISORDERS OF THE MOTOR UNIT
Diseases that affect the lower motor neuron, neuromuscular junction, or muscle may result in weakness or paralysis of the swallowing musculature. These include brainstem stroke or tumor (particularly lateral medullary syndrome), motor neuron disease, myasthenia gravis, botulism, and inflammatory muscle disease. If the condition is progressive, and examination indicates that oral intake is reasonably safe, management centers on minimizing aspiration risks and preventing the secondary complications of dehydration and malnutrition (91, 103). The posture should be adjusted to keep the patient upright with the neck flexed and chin down toward the chest. This posture typically helps to reduce aspiration. In lateral medullary syndrome, there is unilateral weakness of pharyngeal constrictor muscles. Turning the head toward the side of pharyngeal weakness directs the bolus to the stronger side, and improves pharyngeal clearance (104). Some can be trained either in the breath-holding technique described for the patient with supraglottic laryngectomy or to prolong laryngeal elevation while swallowing repeatedly, the Mendelsohn maneuver (105). Care providers should be taught assistive coughing techniques but also should be instructed to recognize that the patient must be allowed every opportunity to clear material independently with an unassisted cough. The diet should be adjusted to provide foods that hold together as cohesive boluses. Dry and sticky foods should be avoided.

In those patients with potentially improving conditions, the same principles of management apply; however, exercise may hasten recovery of some motor functions. Vocal cord adduction may be strengthened by performing Valsalva maneuvers for exercise. The use of surface EMG biofeedback has also been demonstrated to be beneficial in retraining swallowing for patients who have suffered from brainstem strokes (106,107).

Some patients with specific muscle weakness can be assisted in swallowing and airway protection by surgical intervention. For example, laryngeal surgical procedures can be used to improve glottic function in some patients with vocal cord paralysis. Cricopharyngeal myotomy, a surgical procedure to slit the cricopharyngeal muscle and facilitate its opening during the swallow, may be beneficial to patients with demonstrated impairment of sphincter opening (89). In the event of persistent aspiration, surgical closure of the glottis with tracheostomy can be considered. Some techniques are potentially reversible should the patient recover function, whereas others, including total laryngectomy, are permanent

(108). After laryngectomy, an alternative form of communication becomes the primary consideration.

SUPRANUCLEAR IMPAIRMENTS
Supranuclear or pseudobulbar swallowing impairments result from neurologic lesions above the level of the somatic motor nuclei in the brainstem. These include hemispheric stroke, brain tumor, and parkinsonism. In supranuclear impairments, there may be cognitive, sensory, and upper motor neuron dysfunction. The active swallowing muscles may be spastic or poorly coordinated, with diminished speed and delayed initiation of motion. Unlike patients with paralysis of swallowing, the patients with pseudobulbar impairment generally retain reflexes associated with airway protection, such as the gag and cough. The voluntary initiation of swallowing and coughing may be impaired, but each can be elicited by sensory stimulation.

Cognitive deficits can mimic or exacerbate supranuclear swallowing difficulties. Perceptual–motor impairments, judgment deficits, and language disorders are common in these patients and may complicate the feeding process (93). Behavioral manifestations include failing to chew and swallow, owing to impaired awareness or distractibility; taking excessively large bites or eating quickly, owing to impaired judgment or motor planning, and causing oral and pharyngeal overload; retaining food in the mouth between bites and ignoring food on the one side of the tray because of sensory neglect; and failing to appreciate the importance of eating, which may be attributed mistakenly to depression or lack of motivation in patients with various forms of attention deficits.

Management of the patient with cognitive deficits is similar in many respects to the principles described for the patient with paralysis of swallowing (103). Placing patients in an upright posture with the neck flexed, providing foods that maintain a cohesive bolus, and ensuring that patients are in an optimal state of nutrition and hydration are very important considerations. Maintenance of good oral hygiene is a necessity. Additional attention should be paid to selecting foods that stimulate receptors associated with swallowing. Temperature, texture, volume, and taste may all help to elicit a swallow. Foods should be pleasant in appearance and aroma. Items that are sticky, dry, or tough to chew or that fall apart in the mouth should be avoided.

Each patient with supranuclear swallowing difficulty must be evaluated individually to determine the nature and extent of cognitive impairment. The dysphagia treatment plan must be adapted to compensate for intellectual deficits. For example, the patient with distractibility or language deficits may require an environment for eating that is free of distracting conversation. Patients with motor planning deficits may need verbal cues to begin eating and to maintain the process. Patients with impaired perception, judgment, or neglect require close, quiet supervision and monitoring. Most patients with supranuclear swallowing problems function best in a quiet setting with simple verbal instructions.

AUDITORY REHABILITATION

Hearing loss is the most common type of acquired sensory impairment, and affects about 28 million persons in the United States. With increasing life expectancy as well as increasing noise exposure, the number of Americans who will suffer the effects of hearing loss will become even greater. Unfortunately, hearing loss is a disorder that is frequently unrecognized, frequently misunderstood, and all too often neglected, both by those who are affected and by health-care providers.

The rehabilitation professional may often have patients presenting with hearing loss in association with other physical and cognitive problems. Hearing loss can occur following head injury, having been caused by longitudinal temporal bone fractures, transverse temporal bone fractures, or labyrinthine concussion. Older rehabilitation patients may have preexisting hearing impairments as a result of presbycusis, hereditary factors, or past occupational noise exposure. Hearing loss is the third most prevalent major chronic disability in those more than 65 years of age. The prevalence of hearing loss increases substantially with age. Although only slightly more than 1% of people under the age of 17 have hearing loss, the prevalence rises to 12% for those between the ages of 45 and 64, to 24% for those between the ages of 65 and 74, and up to 39% for those more than 75 years of age.

The ear is a complex organ, capable of transforming airborne sound waves into mechanical energy, transferring this mechanical energy into electrochemical signals and then to neural impulses that are processed as auditory information. The external ear collects sound waves and funnels them through the 2.5- to 3-cm-long external ear canal to the tympanic membrane. The tympanic membrane, approximately 9 mm in diameter, changes the airborne sound waves into mechanical vibrations, which are transmitted to the ossicular chain (malleus, incus, and stapes). The stapes, the smallest bone in the body, rests in the oval window of the cochlea (inner ear). The transduction of mechanical energy to electrochemical neural potentials takes place in the cochlea. Vibratory displacements of the oval window send fluid waves through the cochlea. There are approximately 16,000 sensory hair cells in the cochlea. Serving these hair cells are approximately 31,000 sensory nerve fibers. The hair cells are stimulated by the fluid wave within the cochlea, and nerve impulses are then transmitted via the 8th cranial nerve to the auditory centers of the brain.

Psychosocial Implications of Hearing Loss

The psychosocial impact of hearing loss is poorly understood and poorly appreciated. Indeed, even people who live with a hearing-impaired person rarely fully grasp the all-pervasive effects of hearing impairment on daily living. The many ways in which we depend on our hearing are simply not recognized until hearing loss is experienced directly or unless a very close acquaintance has impaired hearing. Few aspects of daily living are not impacted by hearing loss in some way. Hearing loss impairs communication, subtly at first, and increasingly so as the magnitude of the hearing loss increases.

Misunderstanding, mistrust, and lack of sympathy for the hearing impaired seems to be built into our cultural heritage. These attitudes are certainly quite different from our perceptions and treatment of blindness. Often the symptoms of hearing loss (e.g., not answering when spoken to, answering inappropriately, or requiring repetition) encourage other people to talk to and treat the hearing impaired as if their cognitive abilities were also diminished.

The two most commonly reported consequences of hearing loss are depression and social isolation. In addition, adverse effects on general well-being and on physical, cognitive, emotional, behavioral, and social functions have been reported. Social and emotional handicaps are present even in those with only mild to moderate hearing loss. Not being able to hear may create frustration, anger, and suspiciousness that others are talking about the hearing-impaired person. Over time, social

relationships may deteriorate, leaving the individual in isolation and with diminished quality of life.

A major goal of medical practice is to help patients maintain function. The capacity for independent living requires maintenance of functional health. Functional health refers not only to physical health, but also emotional, cognitive, and social health. Physicians are in an excellent position to identify treatable conditions that may compromise their patients' functional performance. Unfortunately, many caregivers tend to view hearing loss as a benign problem that does not threaten functional health.

Assessment of Auditory Function

OTOLOGIC EVALUATION

The management of the person with hearing loss should begin with a complete otologic evaluation. A thorough otologic history should be obtained, including questions about the time of onset, whether the loss was sudden or gradual, and whether associated symptoms are present, such as tinnitus, vertigo, discharge, aural fullness, or pain. In addition, questioning should review family history of hearing loss, as well as loud noise exposure, head trauma, and ototoxic drug use. The otologic examination should include otoscopic evaluation and pneumootoscopy to assess tympanic membrane mobility. Some practitioners may use tympanometry, a measurement of the compliance of the tympanic membrane and middle ear system. The standard audiologic evaluation is then administered, and any special audiologic tests are recommended. The use of associated neurologic, laboratory, and radiologic studies also may be helpful. Only after the assessment has been completed and a diagnosis has been established should rehabilitation of the hearing loss be initiated.

BASIC HEARING EVALUATION

The clinical assessment of hearing loss includes the completion of an audiogram (Figure 45–2). The frequency scale along the abscissa is measured in Hertz (Hz) for the octave frequencies of 250 Hz through 8,000 Hz. The most critical frequencies for speech reception and understanding are 500, 1,000, 2,000, and 3,000 Hz.

The intensity scale on the ordinate of the audiogram is measured in decibels (dB), ranging from a very faint level of -10 dB hearing level (HL) up to a very loud level of 110 dB HL. Sensitivity thresholds are obtained for each frequency for each ear separately using earphones. This air conduction (AC) testing measures the responsiveness of the entire auditory system, from the ear canal through the middle ear to the cochlea and the associated neural pathways to the brain. Any loss by air conduction may be due to a disorder anywhere in the entire auditory system. The use of bone conduction (BC) audiometry defines the general anatomic location of the hearing disorder, since sound transmission by bone conduction bypasses the outer and middle ear. An oscillator is placed behind the ear to be tested and sensitivity thresholds are obtained for the frequencies 250 Hz through 4,000 Hz.

In addition to pure tone threshold measurements, the basic audiologic evaluation includes the measurement of threshold sensitivity for speech and the assessment of word-recognition abilities. The speech reception threshold (SRT) test serves primarily as a reliability check on the pure tone threshold levels. Familiar two-syllable words are presented to each ear separately through earphones, and the intensity level at which 50% of the words are correctly repeated is defined as the SRT. The

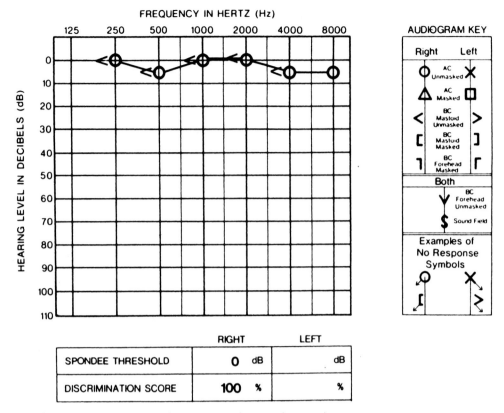

Figure 45-2. Audiogram of a normal ear.

SRT should agree within ±10 dB of the pure tone average (PTA) threshold levels at 500, 1,000, and 2,000 Hz.

A hearing impairment may be reflected not only in a sensitivity loss but also in the reduced ability to understand speech, even when speech is sufficiently loud. The assessment of word recognition (speech discrimination) analyzes the patient's ability to understand speech at comfortably loud levels; it is not a threshold or sensitivity test. Standardized lists of 25 to 50 single-syllable words are presented to each ear separately at comfortably loud intensity levels. These words are repeated back by the patient, and the percentage of correct responses is the word recognition score. Scores of 90% to 100% correctly recognized are considered normal.

AUDIOMETRIC TEST INTERPRETATION

Location of Auditory Impairment

The general anatomic location of a hearing impairment can be determined by comparing the air conduction and bone conduction thresholds. A *conductive* hearing loss is present when air conduction results demonstrate a hearing loss but bone conduction results are within the normal range (Fig. 45-3). The difference between the air and bone conduction thresholds reflects the amount of conductive involvement and is called the *air–bone gap*. A conductive hearing loss could be caused by any obstruction in the sound-conducting mechanism of the ear, from the external auditory canal through the middle ear. The specific etiology and site of the hearing loss cannot be predicted solely on the basis of audiometric results. Although otoscopic evidence of a cerumen impaction, tympanic membrane perforation, or serous otitis media could account for a conductive hearing loss, there are also conductive pathologies that present with normal otoscopic examinations, such as otosclero-

sis or ossicular discontinuity. Patients with pure conductive hearing loss demonstrate normal speech discrimination scores, since the sensorineural system is intact. Speech needs only to be presented at louder levels than normal to compensate for the conductive deficit.

When a hearing loss is present by air conduction and similarly by bone conduction, the impairment is called a *sensorineural* loss (Fig. 45-4). The hearing disorder could be located in the cochlea, the associated neural pathways, or both. The specific etiology of the sensorineural hearing loss cannot be determined by the audiometric results alone. Speech discrimination test results often provide important diagnostic and rehabilitative signs in sensorineural hearing loss. In general, cochlear involvement demonstrates speech discrimination scores compatible with the degree of hearing loss. The greater the hearing loss in cochlear disorders, the poorer the speech discrimination. On the other hand, neural auditory disorders often yield speech discrimination scores disproportionately poorer than would be expected from the pure-tone thresholds. That is, a 40-dB HL sensorineural hearing loss with a 72% speech discrimination score would be consistent with cochlear involvement, whereas a similar amount of hearing loss with only a 10% speech discrimination score would suggest the possibility of eighth-cranial nerve involvement. From a rehabilitative standpoint, the higher the speech discrimination score, the better the prognosis for hearing aid success, as there is less distortion in the auditory system.

A loss in hearing sensitivity for bone conduction with a greater loss for air conduction represents a *mixed* hearing loss (Fig. 45-5). A sensorineural hearing loss is present, as reflected by the reduced bone conduction levels, and conductive loss also is present, as reflected by the air–bone gaps. Speech discrimination performance reflects the amount and etiology of

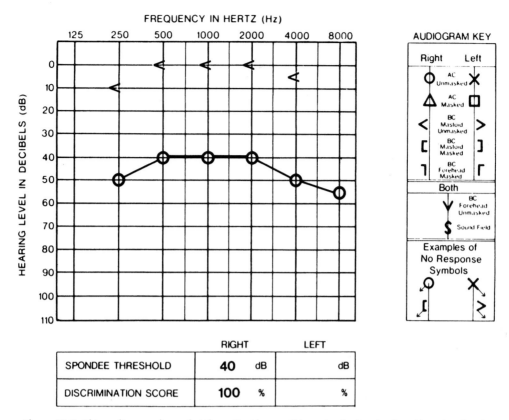

Figure 45-3. This audiogram shows that the patient has a mild conductive hearing loss. Note that the air conduction thresholds reveal a hearing impairment of 40 dB, but the bone conduction responses are within the normal range. Therefore, an air–bone gap of 35 dB is present. Speech discrimination is normal because no sensorineural involvement is present.

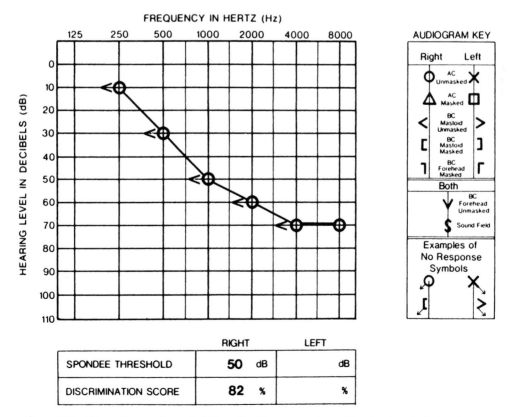

Figure 45-4. This audiogram shows that the patient has a sensorineural hearing loss: both the air conduction and the bone conduction thresholds are similarly depressed. Speech discrimination at a comfortable level is relatively good in this illustration (82%) but is reduced from normal performance.

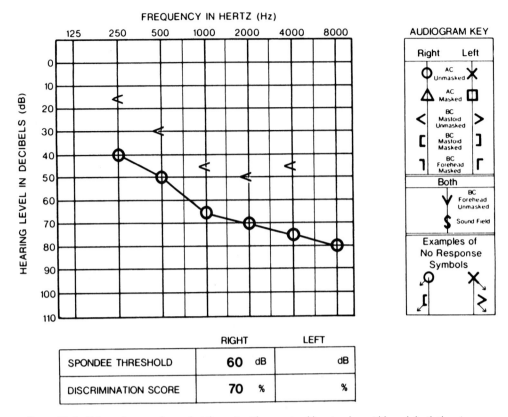

Figure 45-5. This audiogram shows that the patient has a mixed hearing loss. Although both the air conduction and the bone conduction thresholds are reduced, a greater impairment is evident for air conduction. Speech discrimination is reduced (70%), reflecting the sensorineural component of the loss.

the sensorineural involvement. Correction of the conductive component by medical or surgical treatment should result in a sensorineural loss alone, as reflected by the bone conduction levels.

Degree of Hearing Loss

The results obtained from the air conduction evaluation provide quantitative information as to the amount of hearing loss. Classification systems have been devised in an effort to relate the amount of air conduction hearing loss to the expected degree of handicap imposed by a hearing loss. Such systems typically use the pure tone average (PTA) to estimate various hearing loss categories and the expected effects of the loss on understanding of speech. Table 45-6 gives an example of such a classification system.

The most widely accepted formula for calculating hearing handicap is that proposed in 1979 by the American Academy of Otolaryngology and subsequently accepted by the American Medical Association in 1984 (Table 45-7). This formula averages the most important frequencies for speech understanding, 500, 1,000, 2,000 and 3,000 Hz recorded bilaterally. Impairment is defined at a 25-dB HL. The HL of the better ear is weighted in the average to be five times more important than the poorer ear. Any type of audiometric classification system must be interpreted with caution because most are based on pure-tone air conduction thresholds alone and do not incorporate the effects of speech discrimination difficulties, etiologic factors, or hearing loss configuration. In addition, those with similar amounts of pure-tone hearing loss may be affected in very different ways, depending on their life-styles, hearing demands, and other psychosocial factors.

EXTENDED HEARING EVALUATION

Additional audiologic tests are sometimes needed in hearing assessment to rule out exaggerated hearing loss or to define the site of the hearing loss in the auditory system. Tympanometry is an objective test procedure that measures the middle ear pressure, the ear canal volume, and the mobility of the tympanic membrane/middle ear system. Electrophysiologic measurements, such as Brainstem Auditory Evoked Potentials (BAEPs), can help in determining the general degree of hearing loss, although not providing discrete frequency sensitivity thresholds. Electrocochleography (ECoG) also is available for measuring the electrophysiologic activity originating within the cochlea and can supplement information provided by BAEP audiometry.

Transient and distortion product otoacoustic emissions (OAEs) have been widely used during the 1990s. The outer hair cells of a healthy ear emit faint sounds (echoes) when moderate-level clicks or tones are presented to the ear. Robust OAEs are usually obtained in ears with thresholds less than or equal to 30 dB HL. Individuals who offer voluntary thresholds in excess of 30 dB HL and have normal OAEs are most likely displaying exaggeration of hearing loss. Although OAEs do not quantify the exact amount of hearing loss, they do serve to provide the clinician with a means of validating or invalidating the voluntary audiometric results. The use of OAEs and BAEPs are also of assistance in the evaluation of those populations that are difficult to test, such as neonates and those with mental retardation.

The evaluation of asymmetric sensorineural hearing loss or clinical suspicion of eighth nerve or central auditory involvement requires special audiologic procedures to define the site

TABLE 45-6. Classification System for Hearing Loss

Pure Tone Average	Classification	Effects on Speech Understanding
0–25 dB HL	Normal	No significant difficulty
25–40 dB HL	Mild	Difficulty with soft speech
40–55 dB HL	Moderate	Difficulty with normal speech
55–70 dB Hl	Moderately-Severe	Difficulty with loud speech
70–90 dB HL	Severe	Can only understand shouted or amplified speech
90–110 dB HL	Profound	Usually cannot understand even amplified speech

of auditory impairment. The evaluation of the integrity of the stapedius (acoustic) reflex by immittance measurement is a helpful test in differentiating between cochlear and auditory nerve involvement. BAEPs are also used to help differentiate cochlear involvement from eighth-nerve involvement.

Management of Hearing Impairment

MEDICAL-SURGICAL REHABILITATION

Medical or surgical treatment of hearing loss most often is available for people with impairments of the conductive auditory system. When hearing loss originates in the external auditory canal, it usually is related to a mechanical obstruction in the form of cerumen or foreign body. Cerumen impaction is the most common cause of conductive hearing loss, and removal of the obstruction will improve or restore hearing. Infections of the lining of the external canal, otitis externa, can be treated with topical antibiotics. Hearing impairment originating in the middle ear system may be treated with otologic surgery. Surgical procedures such as myringoplasty (i.e., repair of tympanic membrane perforation), tympanoplasty (i.e., ossicular reconstruction), stapedectomy for otosclerosis, and myringotomy with placement of ventilating tubes for middle ear effusion often can correct the conductive hearing loss.

Otologic surgery sometimes is required for treatment of life-threatening disease and not for hearing improvement. Pathologic conditions such as cholesteatoma, glomus tumor, or chronic middle ear disease necessitate surgery. In addition, otoneurosurgery is necessary for sensorineural impairment caused by eighth-nerve tumors (vestibular schwanomas). Al-

though hearing preservation is possible in some patients, the primary goal is the removal of the neoplasm.

Otologic treatment of congenital or hereditary sensorineural hearing loss, noise-induced hearing loss, presbycusis, and most other types of sensorineural impairment is not possible at this time. Perhaps the greatest advance in the surgical rehabilitation of sensorineural impairments is now available with the development of the cochlear implant for severe to profound hearing loss.

HEARING AID AMPLIFICATION

Although hearing loss due to conductive deficits such as otosclerosis, otitis media, and eardrum perforations can be most often successfully treated with medical or surgical intervention, the most common site of hearing loss is dysfunction in the cochlea or associated neural structures. Of all patients with cochlear hearing loss, fewer than 5% can be helped medically. Hearing aids are the principal resource for improving communication and reducing hearing handicaps in persons with sensorineural hearing loss. Unfortunately, only 10% of people who might benefit from an aid actually own one, which indicates a substantial underservice (109).

Significant improvements in hearing aid design have made possible greater flexibility in selecting and fitting hearing aids for the typical hearing loss patterns. The past decade has witnessed an increase of technological innovations that has made possible a wide assortment of hearing aids, both in physical size and in technological sophistication. Current hearing aid styles include devices that fit behind the ear, in the ear, in the canal and most recently, completely in the canal. Since many

TABLE 45-7. Sample Audiogram and Calculation of Impairment (AAO-79 method)

Hertz (Hz)	500	1,000	2,000	3,000	4,000	6,000	8,000
Right ear (dB)	25	35	35	45	50	60	45
Left ear (dB)	25	35	40	50	60	70	50

1. Unilateral impairment:
   (Average dB at 500, 1,000, 2,000, 3,000 Hz) − 25 dB (low fence) × 1.5% = Percentage of unilateral impairment

   Right ear = ((25 + 35 + 35 + 45 divided by 4) − 25) × 1.5% = 15%
   Left ear = ((25 + 35 + 40 + 50 divided by 4) − 25) × 1.5% = 18.8%

2. Bilateral impairment:
   [(Percentage of unilateral impairment in better ear × 5) + (Percentage of unilateral impairment in poorer ear)] divided by 6 = Percentage of bilateral impairment

   [(15 × 5) + (18.8%)] divided by 6 = 15.6%

people unfortunately associate hearing loss with the "stigma" of aging, the introduction of the smaller devices, which fit entirely in the ear canal, has had obvious cosmetic appeal. However, people with dexterity problems or vision impairments are often unable to insert and adjust the smaller aids properly, and they are better served with larger hearing aids. The audiologist reviews such issues with the hearing-impaired individual during the prefitting session.

Technological advances in hearing aids now offer the patient a wide variety of amplification options. Hearing aids no longer merely provide linear amplification but may include compression circuitry to reduce the amplification for loud sounds, automatic loudness adjusting circuits that automatically decrease amplification of continuous background sounds, and hearing aids without volume controls that automatically increase the loudness of soft sounds while decreasing loud level inputs. There are also hearing aids that offer several programs for use at the listener's discretion, since a single amplification paradigm may not be optimal for all listening situations. One may choose a wide frequency amplification for quiet environments, another program that eliminates low frequencies for noisier situations, or a program specifically suited for telephone use. These hearing aids are digitally programmed by a computer through the use of a microchip within the hearing aid itself. Individual programming of the hearing aid enables the audiologist to make significant modifications to an individual's needs. Such multimemory hearing aids typically include a user-operated remote control to facilitate program changes or volume changes. Some hearing aids have multiple microphones, one for use to improve directionality in background noise situations and another for use in other environments where a broad range of acoustic input is desired. The most recent introduction in hearing aid technology is the fully digital hearing aids, which have the processing power of a desktop personal computer and can be fit into the small canal-sized instruments. These aids have many features not available in analog hearing aids and will undoubtedly provide greater improvements in hearing and speech understanding for the hearing-impaired in future years. These new, innovative hearing aid systems require a higher level of training and sophistication on the part of the user and the audiologist. In addition, these new amplification systems are considerably more expensive than conventional hearing aids. The specific hearing needs, lifestyle, and adaptability of the hearing aid wearer must be taken into account during the prefitting process.

Hearing Aid Candidacy

It is a disservice to the patient to discourage a hearing aid trial because of the outdated notion that a hearing aid does not help "nerve deafness." Hearing aids were not very helpful for sensorineural deficits many years ago, but this is not the case today, thanks to the substantial improvements in hearing aid technology. Also, some physicians merely tell their patients that they can probably "get by" without a hearing aid and should wait until the hearing loss progresses. Discouraging a hearing aid trial for an individual with communicative difficulties and a potentially remediable hearing loss serves only to invite isolation and frustration. Unless assurance and support are provided, hearing-impaired patients may unfortunately postpone and avoid the use of amplification.

Once a hearing loss has been identified and medical or surgical treatment is not indicated, referral to a certified clinical audiologist should be made. The clinical audiologist is a university-trained professional in the nonmedical management of hearing loss, whether with hearing aid amplification, rehabilitation therapies, assistive listening devices, or a combination of rehabilitative approaches. Although some hearing aid dealers are relatively skilled in the evaluation of hearing aids, others possess only minimal training and are more oriented to sales. Many states, in fact, require that a hearing aid dealer meet only the minimum requirement of being 18 years old and passing a state licensing examination; there are typically no educational requirements. The clinical audiologist, on the other hand, holds at least a master's degree in the evaluation and rehabilitation of hearing loss. The audiologist is uniquely qualified to provide a full range of auditory assessment and rehabilitative services to those who are hard of hearing.

After the initial interview and evaluation, an audiologist will recommend the type of hearing aid or aids, specify the acoustical requirements of the aids, and provide training in the use of amplification. The potential advantages and limitations of hearing aids are reviewed, and follow-up is provided during the initial trial as well as during the postpurchase period. It is usual to provide patients with a free or low-cost 30-day hearing aid trial period before purchasing the aid(s). This trial period provides patients with the opportunity to wear the aid(s) in their own home and social environment to determine their satisfaction.

There are no accepted rules or criteria as to who should be considered a hearing aid candidate. Hearing loss greater than 40 dB HL certainly warrants consideration for the fitting of amplification; however, there are those with even moderate to severe hearing impairment who reject such advice. Anyone who has hearing difficulties that handicap daily social or professional activities should be considered a prospective hearing aid candidate. This recommendation for possible hearing aid use should be accompanied by a very positive and uplifting approach by the practitioner. Psychological attitudes such as denial of a hearing loss, putting the blame of hearing difficulties on others (e.g., people just don't speak clearly), and fear that a hearing loss reflects aging result in some people being poor hearing aid candidates and rejecting hearing aids. The most important criteria for successful hearing aid use relate to the person's self-perceived hearing difficulties, acceptance of the hearing loss, and motivation to use amplification. Critical to successful hearing aid usage are factors unrelated to the audiologic assessment, such as lack of motivation, negative attitudes, family pressure, denial of hearing difficulties, and other psychosocial factors.

Assistive Listening Devices

Although substantial improvements have been achieved in hearing aid design and application, few of the hearing-impaired can ever come close to achieving "normal" auditory function with the use of a hearing aid alone. Assistive listening devices (ALDs) comprise a growing number of situation-specific amplification systems designed for use in difficult listening environments. ALDs commonly use a microphone placed close to the desired sound source (e.g., a television, theater stage, or speaker's lectern), and sound is directly transmitted to the listener. Transmission methods include infrared, FM radio, or direct audio input. Such transmission of sound directly to the listener improves the signal-to-noise ratio. That is, the desired sounds are enhanced while competing extraneous noises are decreased, thus improving understanding. These ALDs in many churches, theaters, and classrooms enable hearing-impaired persons to avoid the isolation imposed by the inability to hear a sermon, play, or public address.

Amplified telephones, low-frequency doorbells, amplified ringers, and closed-captioned TV decoders are just a few examples of the number of devices currently available for the hearing impaired for everyday use. Pressure-release alarms are available with low-frequency alarms for those persons with high-frequency hearing losses who cannot hear the higher-pitch alarms. Flashing alarm clocks, alarm bed vibrators, and flashing smoke detectors provide alerting for severely hearing-impaired individuals.

Although the "treatment" of sensorineural hearing impairments with hearing aid amplification, assistive listening devices, and aural rehabilitation therapy does not "cure" the impairment or restore hearing and communicative efficiency to normal, such approaches represent the best treatments available at this time. They will improve the ability of most people to communicate effectively and reduce the handicapping consequences of hearing loss.

Speech Reading and Auditory Training

Speech reading (lip reading) is the use of visual cues in the recognition of speech and incorporates the interpretation of facial expressions, body movements, and gestures. Everyone uses speech reading to some extent, although usually we are not conscious of the importance of visual input in helping us to recognize what is being said. Many hearing-impaired people, particularly those with gradually progressive hearing loss, develop this skill through necessity.

The use of speech reading alone cannot be the sole rehabilitative approach in providing the hearing-impaired patient with complete understanding of speech. Although a considerable amount of the speech signal can be perceived visually, only about one-third of English speech sounds are clearly visible. Certain sounds (e.g., *f* and *th*) are relatively easy to see on the lips, whereas others, such as *k* and *g*, are not visible, and some (e.g., *p* and *b*) are indistinguishable from one another.

Speech reading usually is taught in conjunction with a program of auditory training. Auditory training teaches the patient to make the most effective use of the minimal auditory cues imposed by the hearing loss. The combination of visual input and auditory input is superior to either one alone in understanding speech. Aural rehabilitation strategies also try to teach the hearing-impaired person to become a more assertive listener. Those who quietly accept not hearing and not understanding merely invite continued social isolation. The hearing-impaired listener needs to inform others of his or her impairment and advise them as to the most effective means of communication. Self-help groups are available, most notably the Self Help for Hard of Hearing People organization, which offers local groups as well as an active national organization and journals.

COCHLEAR IMPLANT

The cochlear implant is an auditory prosthesis designed to provide hearing for those with bilateral severe to profound sensorineural hearing loss by electrically stimulating residual eighth-nerve neurons in the cochlea (See Chapter 87). Cochlear implants have been FDA approved for two decades and are regarded as safe and effective. More than 20,000 people have received cochlear implants, including more than 8,000 children.

Prospective implant candidates require an extensive audiologic evaluation to document that powerful hearing aids would not be of help. The 2- to 3-hour implant operation involves placing an electrode array into the cochlea and connecting it to an internal coil, which is placed under the skin behind the ear and is aligned with an external coil placed behind the ear. After the healing period, the patient is fitted with a microphone and stimulator/signal processor unit. The microphone, usually worn at ear level, transmits the sound to a signal processor unit that resembles a body-type or ear-level hearing aid. The processor converts the sound to electrical signals that are transmitted to the external coil, through the skin to the internal coil and to the electrodes in the cochlea. Current flows between the active electrodes and a ground electrode placed in the Eustachian tube, stimulating remaining nerve fibers and producing a sensation of sound.

The cochlear implant, unlike a hearing aid, does not change the electrical impulses back into amplified sounds. Rather, sound is changed into electrical impulses that are delivered directly to the cochlea. Most implant users are able to detect speech at comfortable listening levels and can learn to recognize environmental sounds. Cochlear implants aid in communication by improving the person's ability to understand speech. The cochlear implant procedure costs between $30,000 and $50,000 and is often covered by medical insurance.

REFERENCES

1. Duffy JR. *Motor speech disorders: substrates, differential diagnosis and management.* St. Louis: CV Mosby, 1995.
2. Rosenbek JC, LaPoint LL. The dysarthrias: description, diagnosis and treatment. In: Johns DF, ed. *Clinical management of neurogenic communication disorders.* Austin, TX: ProEd, 1985:97–152.
3. Darley FL, Aronson AE, Brown JE. Differential diagnostic patterns of dysarthria. *J Speech Hear Res* 1969; 12:246–269.
4. Darley FL, Aronson AE, Brown JE. Clusters of deviant speech dimensions in the dysarthrias. *J Speech Hear Res* 1969; 12:462–496.
5. Darley FL, Aronson AE, Brown JE. Motor speech signs in neurologic disease. *Med Clin North Am* 1968; 52:835–844.
6. Yorkston KM, Strand EA, Kennedy MRT. Comprehensibility of dysarthric speech: implications for assessment and treatment planning. *Am J Speech-Lang Pathol* 1996; 5:55–66.
7. *International Classification of Function, Disability and Health.* World Health Organization. From World Wide Web: http://www3.who.int/icf/icftemplate.cfm.
8. Yorkston KM, Beukelman DR, Strand EA, Bell KR. *Management of motor speech disorders in children and adults.* Austin, TX: Pro-Ed, 1999.
9. Netsell R. Speech physiology. In: Minifie FD, Hixon TJ, Williams F, eds. *Normal aspects of speech, hearing, and language.* Englewood Cliffs, NJ: Prentice-Hall, 1973.
10. Gerratt BR, Till JA, Rosenbek JC, Wertz RT, Boysen AE. Use and perceived value of perceptual and instrumental measures in dysarthria management. In: Moore CA, Yorkston KM, Beukelman DR, eds. *Dysarthria and apraxia of speech: perspectives on management.* Baltimore: Paul H. Brookes, 1991:77–94.
11. Murdoch BE, Ward EC, Theodoros DG. Dysarthria: clinical features, neuroanatomical framework and assessment. In: Papathanasiou I, ed. *Acquired neurogenic communication disorders: a clinical perspective.* London: Whurr Publishers, 2000:103–148.
12. Hixon TJ, Hoit J. Physical examination of rib cage wall by the speech-language pathologist. *Am J Speech-Language Pathology.* 2000;9:179–196.
13. Netsell R, Hixon TJ. A noninvasive method of clinically estimating subglottal air pressure. *J Speech Hear Disord* 1978;43:326–350.
14. Keller E, Vigneuz P, Lafamboise M. Acoustic analysis of neurologically impaired speech. *Br J Disord Commun* 1991;26:75–94.
15. Ramig LA, Scherer RC, Tize IR, et al. Acoustic analysis of voices of patients with neurologic disease: rationale and preliminary data. *Ann Otol Rhinol Laryngol* 1988;97:164–172.
16. Smitheran J, Hixon TJ. A clinical method for estimating laryngeal airway resistance during vowel production. *J Speech Hear Disord* 1981;46:138–146.
17. Barlow SM. High-speed data acquisition for clinical speech physiology. In: Yorkston KM, Beukelman DR, eds. *Recent advances in dysarthria.* Boston: College-Hill Press, 1989:39–52.
18. Hardy JC, Netsell R, Schweiger JW, et al. Management of velopharyngeal dysfunction in cerebral palsy. *J Speech Hear Disord* 1969;34:123–137.
19. Yorkston KM, Beukelman DR, Tice R. *Sentence intelligibility test.* Lincoln, NE: Tice Technology Services, Inc., 1996.
20. Beukelman DR, Yorkston KM. The relationship between information transfer and speech intelligibility of dysarthric speakers. *J Commun Disord* 1979;12:189–196.
21. Platt LJ, Andrews G, Young M, et al. The measurement of speech impairment of adults with cerebral palsy. *Fol Phoniatr* 1978;30:30–58.

22. Platt LJ, Andrews G, Young M, et al. Dysarthria of adult cerebral palsy: intelligibility and articulatory impairment. *J Speech Hear Res* 1980;23:28–40.

23. Yorkston KM, Dowden PA, Beukelman DR. Intelligibility as a tool in the clinical management of dysarthric speakers. In: Kent RD, ed. *Intelligibility in speech disorders: theory, measurement and management.* Amsterdam: John Benjamins, 1992:265–286.

24. Yorkston KM, Beukelman DR, Traynor CD. Articulatory adequacy in dysarthric speakers: a comparison of judging formats. *J Communication Disord* 1988;21:351–361.

25. Beukelman DR, Yorkston KM, Reichle J. *Augmentative and alternative communication for adults with acquired neurologic disabilities.* Baltimore: Paul H. Brookes Publishing, 2000.

26. Yorkston KM, Beukelman DR. Motor speech disorders. In: Beukelman DR, Yorkston KM, eds. *Communication disorders following traumatic brain injury: management of cognitive, language, and motor impairment.* Austin, TX: ProEd, 1991:251–316.

27. Beukelman DR, Mirenda P. *Augmentative and alternative communication: management of severe communication disorders in children and adults,* 2nd ed. Baltimore: Paul H. Brookes, 1998.

28. Netsell R, Daniel B. Dysarthria in adults: physiologic approach to rehabilitation. *Arch Phys Med Rehabil* 1979;60:502–508.

29. Yorkston KM, Hammen VL, Beukelman DR, et al. The effect of rate control on the intelligibility and naturalness of dysarthric speech. *J Speech Hear Disord* 1990;55:550–561.

30. Gonzalez J, Aronson A. Palatal lift prosthesis for treatment of anatomic and neurologic palatopharyngeal insufficiency. *Cleft Palate J* 1970;7:91–104.

31. Yorkston KM, Honsinger MJ, Beukelman DR, et al. The effects of palatal lift fitting on the perceived articulatory adequacy of dysarthric speakers. In: Yorkston KM, Beukelman DR, eds. *Recent advances in clinical dysarthria.* Austin, TX: ProEd, 1989:85–98.

32. Bellaire K, Yorkston KM, Beukelman DR. Modification of breath patterning to increase naturalness of a mildly dysarthric speaker. *J Commun Disord* 1986;19:271–280.

33. Yorkston KM, Miller RM, Strand EA. *Management of speech and swallowing disorders in degenerative disease,* 2nd ed. Austin, TX: Pro-Ed, In press.

34. Singer MI, Blom ED. An endoscopic technique for restoration of voice after laryngectomy. *Ann Otol Rhinol Laryngol* 1980;89:529–533.

35. Hamaker RC, Singer MI, Blom ED, et al. Primary voice restoration at laryngectomy. *Arch Otolaryngol* 1985;111:182–186.

36. Hilgers FJM, Balm AJM. Long-term results of vocal rehabilitation after total laryngectomy with the low-resistance, indwelling Provox voice prosthesis system. *Clin Otolaryngol* 1993;18:517–523.

37. Singer MI, Blom ED, Hamaker RC. Further experience with voice restoration after total laryngectomy. *Ann Otol Rhinol Laryngol* 1981;90:498–502.

38. Wetmore SJ, Johns ME, Baker SR. The Singer–Blom voice restoration procedure. *Arch Otolaryngol* 1981;107:674–676.

39. Kao WW, Rose MM, Kimmel CA, et al. The outcome and techniques of primary and secondary tracheoesophageal puncture. *Arch Otolaryngol Head Neck Surg* 1994;120:301–307.

40. Singer MI, Blom ED, Hamaker RC. Pharyngeal plexus neurectomy for alaryngeal speech rehabilitation. *Laryngoscope* 1986;96:50–54.

41. Robin DA, Schienberg S. Subcortical lesions and aphasia. *J Speech Hear Disord* 1990;55:90–100.

42. Brookshire RH. Recognition of auditory sequences by aphasic, right hemisphere damaged and non-brain damaged subjects. *J Commun Disord* 1975;8:51–59.

43. Duffy RJ, Duffy JR, Pearson KL. Pantomime recognition in aphasics. *J Speech Hear Res* 1975;18:115–132.

44. Goodglass H, Kaplan E. *The assessment of aphasia and related disorders.* Philadelphia: Lea & Febiger, 1983.

45. Wallesch G, Kornhuber H, Brunner R, et al. Lesions of the basal ganglia, thalamus, and deep white matter: differential effects on language functions. *Brain Lang* 1983;20:286–304.

46. Naeser MA. CT scan lesion size and lesion locus in cortical and subcortical aphasias. In: Kertesz A, ed. *Localization in neuropsychology.* New York: Academic Press, 1983;63–120.

47. Naeser MA, Alexander MP, Helm-Estrabrooks N, et al. Aphasia with predominantly subcortical lesion sites: description of 3 capsular/putaminal aphasia syndromes. *Arch Neurol* 1982;39:2–14.

48. Damasio A, Damasio H, Rizzo M, et al. Aphasia with non-hemorrhagic lesions in the basal ganglia and internal capsule. *Arch Neurol* 1982;39:15–20.

49. Alexander MP, LoVerme SR. Aphasia after left hemisphere intracerebral hemorrhage. *Neurology* 1980;30:1193–1202.

50. Mohr JP, Watters WC, Duncan GW. Thalamic hemorrhage and aphasia. *Brain Lang* 1975;2:3–17.

51. Darley FL. *Aphasia.* Philadelphia: WB Saunders, 1982.

52. Buckingham HW. Explanation in apraxia with consequences for the concept of apraxia of speech. *Brain Lang* 1979;8:202–226.

53. Martin AD. Some objections to the term apraxia of speech. *J Speech Hear Disord* 1974;39:53–64.

54. Bayles KA, Kaszniak AW. *Communication and cognition in normal aging and dementia.* Austin, TX: ProEd, 1987.

55. Schuell H. *The Minnesota test for the differential diagnosis of aphasia.* Minneapolis: University of Minnesota Press, 1965.

56. Kertesz A. *The Western aphasia battery.* New York: Grune & Stratton, 1982.

57. Porch BE. *The Porch index of communicative ability.* Palo Alto, CA: Consulting Psychology Press, 1967.

58. DeRenzi E, Vignolo LA. The token test: a sensitive test to detect receptive disturbances in aphasia. *Brain* 1962;85:665–678.

59. Noll JD, Randolph SR. Auditory semantic, syntactic, and retention errors made by aphasic subjects on the token test. *J Commun Disord* 1978;11:543–553.

60. Swisher LP, Sarno MT. Token test scores of three matched patient groups: left brain damaged with aphasia; right brain damaged without aphasia; non-brain damaged. *Cortex* 1969;5:264–273.

61. McNeil MR, Prescott TE. *Revised token test.* Baltimore: University Park Press, 1978.

62. DeRenzi E, Ferrai C. The reporter's test: a sensitive test to detect expressive disturbances in aphasics. *Cortex* 1978;14:279–293.

63. LaPoint LL, Horner J. *Reading comprehension battery.* Tigard, OR: CC Publications, 1979.

64. Albert ML, Helm-Estabrooks N. Diagnosis and treatment of aphasia. Part I. *JAMA* 1988;259:1043–1047.

65. Albert ML, Helm-Estabrooks N. Diagnosis and treatment of aphasia. Part II. *JAMA* 1988;259:1205–1210.

66. Lubinski R. Environmental language intervention. In: Chapey R, ed. *Language intervention strategies in adult aphasia.* Baltimore: Williams & Wilkins, 1981:223–245.

67. Simmons N. Interaction between communication and neurologic disorders. In: Darby JK, ed. *Speech and language evaluation in neurology: adult disorders.* Orlando, FL: Grune & Stratton, 1985:3–28.

68. Burns MS, Halper AS, Mogil SI. *Clinical management of right hemisphere dysfunction.* Rockville, MD: Aspen Systems Corporation, 1985.

69. West JF, Leader BJ, Costagliola C. *Screening battery assessing cognition in patients with right cerebrovascular accidents.* Paper presented at New York State Speech and Hearing Association meeting, 1982.

70. Beukelman DR, Yorkston KM, eds. *Communication disorders following traumatic brain injury: management of cognitive, language, and motor impairments.* Austin, TX: Pro-Ed, 1991.

71. Groher M. Language and memory disorders following closed head trauma. *J Speech Hear Disord* 1977;20:212–220.

72. Hagen C, Malkmus D, Burditt G. *Intervention strategies for language disorders secondary to head trauma.* Paper presented at short course, American Speech and Hearing Association convention, Atlanta, 1979.

73. Hagen C, Malkmus D, Durham E. Levels of cognitive functioning. In: *Rehabilitation of the head injured adult.* Downey, CA: Professional Staff Association, 1979.

74. Coelho CA, Liles BZ, Duffy RJ. Analysis of conversational discourse in head-injured adults. *J Head Trauma Rehabil* 1991;6:92–99.

75. Little AJ, Templer DI, Persel CS, et al. Feasibility of the neuropsychological spectrum in prediction of outcome following head injury. *J Clin Psychol* 1996;52:455.

76. Helm-Estabrooks N, Hotz G. *The brief test of head injury.* Chicago: Riverside, 1991.

77. Adamovich B, Henderson J. *Scales of cognitive ability for traumatic brain injury.* Chicago: Paradigm Publishing, 1991.

78. Groher M. Communication disorders in adults. In: Rosenthal M, Griffith ER, Bond MR, Miller JD, eds. *Rehabilitation of the adult and child with traumatic brain injury.* Philadelphia: FA Davis, 1990.148–162.

79. Wertz RT. Neuropathologies of speech and language: an introduction to patient management. In: Johns DF, ed. *Clinical management of neurogenic communication disorders.* Boston: Little, Brown, 1991:1–96.

80. Bayles K. Language function in senile dementia. *Brain Lang* 1982;16:265–280.

81. Bayles KA, Salmon DP, Tomoeda CK, et al. Semantic and letter category naming in Alzheimer's patients: a predictable difference. *Dev Neuropsychol* 1989;5:335–347.

82. Brun A. Frontal lobe degeneration of non-Alzheimer type 1 neuropathology. *Arch Gerontol Geriatr* 1987;6:193.

83. Obler L. *Language in age and dementia. Short course abstract.* Washington, DC: American Speech, Language, and Hearing Association, 1985.

84. Mattis S. *The dementia rating scale.* Odessa, FL: Psychological Assessment Resources, Inc., 1988.

85. Bayles KA, Tomoeda C. *Arizona battery for communication disorders of dementia.* Tucson, AZ: Canyonland, 1991.

86. Palleschi L, Vetta F, deGennaro E, et al. Effects of aerobic training on the cognitive performance of elderly patients with senile dementia of the Alzheimer type. *Arch Gerontol Geriatr* 1996;5:47.

87. Arkin S. Volunteers in partnership: an Alzheimer's disease rehabilitation program delivered by students. *Am J Alz Dis* 1996;11:12.

88. Palmer JB, Rubin NJ, Lara G, et al. Coordination of mastication and swallowing. *Dysphagia* 1992;7:187–200.

89. Goyal RK. Disorders of the cricopharyngeus muscle. *Otolaryngol Clin North Am* 1984;17:115–130.

90. Miller RM. Evaluation of swallowing disorders. In: Groher M, ed. *Dysphagia: diagnosis and management.* Boston: Butterworths, 1984:85–110.

91. Palmer JB, DuChane AS. Rehabilitation of swallowing disorders in the elderly. In: Felsenthal G, Garrison SJ, Steinberg FU, eds. *Rehabilitation of the aging and older patient.* Baltimore: Williams & Wilkins, 1994:275–287.

92. Siebens H, Trupe E, Siebens A, et al. Correlates and consequences of eating dependency in institutionalized elderly. *J Am Geriatr Soc* 1986;34:192–198.

93. Martin BJW, Corlew MM. The incidence of communications disorders in dysphagic patients. *J Speech Hear Disord* 1990;55:28–32.
94. Horner J, Massey EW. Silent aspiration following stroke. *Neurology* 1988;38: 317–319.
95. Palmer JB, DuChane AS, Donner MW. The role of radiology in the rehabilitation of swallowing. In: Jones B, Donner MW, eds. *Normal and abnormal swallowing: imaging in diagnosis and therapy.* New York: Springer-Verlag, 1991;215–225.
96. Palmer JB, Kuhlemeier KV, Tippett DC, et al. A protocol for the videofluorographic swallowing study. *Dysphagia* 1993;8:209–214.
97. Logemann JA. *Manual for the videofluorographic study of swallowing.* Boston: College-Hill, 1986.
98. Langmore SE, Schatz K, Olsen N. Fiberoptic endoscopic examination of swallowing safety: a new procedure. *Dysphagia* 1988;2:216–219.
99. Palmer JB, Holloway AM, Tanaka E. Detecting lower motor neuron dysfunction of the pharynx and larynx with electromyography. *Arch Phys Med Rehabil* 1991;72:237–242.
100. Miller RM, Groher M. General treatment of swallowing disorders. In: Groher M, ed. *Dysphagia: diagnosis and management.* Boston: Butterworths, 1984: 113–132.
101. Fleming SM. Treatment of mechanical swallowing disorders. In: Groher M, ed. *Dysphagia: diagnosis and management.* Boston: Butterworths, 1984:157–172.
102. Logemann JA, Pauloski BR, Rademaker AW, et al. Super-supraglottic swallow in irradiated head and neck cancer patients. *Head and Neck* 1997;19: 535–540.
103. Palmer JB, DuChane AS. Rehabilitation of swallowing disorders due to stroke. *Phys Med Rehabil Clin North Am* 1991;2:529–546.
104. Logemann JA, Kahrilas PJ, Kobara M, et al. The benefit of head rotation on pharyngoesophageal dysphagia. *Arch Phys Med Rehabil* 1989;70:767–771.
105. Ding R, Larson CR, Logemann JA, et al. Surface electromyographic and electroglottographic studies in normal subjects under two swallow conditions: normal and during the Mendelsohn maneuver. *Dysphagia* 2002;17:1–12.
106. Crary MA. A direct intervention program for chronic neurogenic dysphagia secondary to brainstem stroke. *Dysphagia* 1995;10:6–18.
107. Huckabee M, Cannito MP. Outcomes of swallowing rehabilitation in chronic brainstem dysphagia: a retrospective evaluation. *Dysphagia* 1999;14:93–109.
108. Lindemann RC. Diverting the paralyzed larynx: a reversible procedure for intractable aspiration. *Laryngoscope* 1975;85:157–180.
109. Gates GA, Rees TS. Hear ye! Hear ye! Successful auditory aging. *West J Med* 1997;167:247–252.

CHAPTER 46

Rehabilitation Team Function and Prescriptions, Referrals, and Order Writing

John C. King, T. Russell Nelson, Karen J. Blankenship, Thomas C. Turturro, and Alison J. Beck

Comprehensive rehabilitation patients require the services of multiple health-care providers who possess unique skills, training, and expertise that is employed for the full restoration of these patients' function and their optimal reintegration into all aspects of life. The competent physiatrist must be able to communicate in an optimal fashion to all these providers to meet the many needs of the patient. Prescriptions, referrals, and orders are basic tools by which the physiatrist may communicate the desired involvement of other rehabilitation or medical specialties in assessment, treatment planning, treatment delivery, provision of equipment, and fitting of adaptive devices. Medical specialties that are commonly involved with the rehabilitation patient include neurosurgery, neurology, geriatrics, primary care (including family practice, internal medicine, and pediatrics), psychiatry, urology, and orthopedics. Many other medical and surgical specialties are consulted as needed. Assessment, treatment planning, and therapy are often provided by rehabilitation clinicians specializing in occupational therapy, physical therapy, kinesiotherapy, prosthetics and orthotics, psychology and neuropsychology, recreational therapy, speech and language pathology, rehabilitation nursing, social work, dietary science, case management, and others (Fig. 46-1, Table 46-1) (1,2). Which professions are involved with a particular patient and the extent of those involvements are largely determined by the nature of the patient's deficits and the structure of the setting in which rehabilitation is being conducted. As indicated by an initial comprehensive physiatric assessment, the physiatrist requests the participation of other rehabilitation specialists for their assistance in determining the appropriate rehabilitation services and level of care, as well as for comprehensive rehabilitation planning, conduct, and monitoring of treatment, discharge planning, and patient and family education.

The health-care team is a group of health-care professionals from different disciplines who share common values and objectives (3). Halstead performed a literature review, covering the years 1950 to 1975, on team care in chronic illness and concluded that a coordinated team care approach appears to be more effective than fragmented care for patients with long-

term illness (3). More recently, the efficacy and efficiency of team care has continued to be lauded (1,4–9).

Writing physical medicine and rehabilitation (PM&R) therapy referrals, equipment prescriptions, and coordinating care requires the skills of a well-rounded clinician who is adept in both therapist and patient interactions to form an effective health-care team individualized to the needs of that particular patient. Deficits in knowledge base or team and patient interaction skills lead to suboptimal treatment plans and care. The well-trained rehabilitation medicine specialist is able to develop comprehensive PM&R treatment plans of substantial detail when warranted. The degree of documentation and specification required depends on the mode of team interaction and treatment adopted by the professionals involved. Effective participation in treatment planning nevertheless requires the ability both to generate and to support the rationale behind multiple interventions. These interventions must be appreciated in terms of their impact on function as well as on each patient's pathophysiologic processes.

Treatment plans are generated from goals that arise from the problem list developed during evaluation. The evaluation (see Chapters 1, 2, 5, and 43) results in a set of identified problems that can be classified in various ways, but typically are organized as medical, rehabilitation, and social problems. A set of goals or desired treatment outcomes is generated, along with an initial estimate of the duration of therapy necessary to accomplish each. Such goals form the heart of a comprehensive treatment plan. This plan is a tool that patients, families, therapists, and other treating professionals examine for prognosis and expectations. It forms the basis from which all team members may suggest additions, deletions, or modifications. The treatment plan is not a static document but remains dynamic as goals are accomplished, new goals are identified and added, or some goals, which become irrelevant or unachievable, are eliminated.

Treatment strategies are developed to accomplish the identified goals. The specific strategies can be physician directed, therapist directed, or, ideally, mutually derived by the patient and team through the interdisciplinary process. The rehabilita-

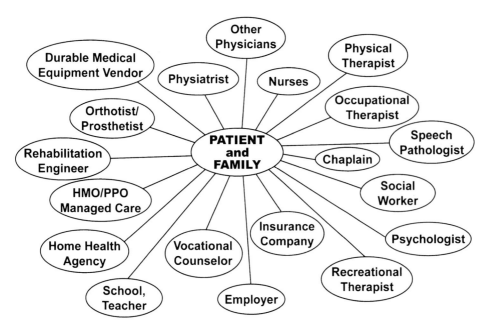

Figure 46-1. Multiple caregivers that may be required in comprehensive rehabilitation.

tion medicine specialist should be knowledgeable about all pertinent therapies and their potential benefits plus risks to optimally apply the specific interventions desired from each therapy specialty that will help to accomplish the desired patient goals. The availability, benefits, and risks of adaptive equipment and their use to facilitate independence in activities of daily living (ADL); improve mobility, communication, and leisure activities; or decrease pain must be well understood to be prescribed and proscribed appropriately. A knowledge of expected effects and potential side effects, as well as a pathophysiologic and pharmacologic knowledge base, allows therapeutic interventions to be made with the least possible morbidity. This occurs when treatment is supervised by a physiatrist who can offer appropriate precautions and monitoring of referrals and prescriptions. The comprehensive treatment plan is initiated by referrals, prescriptions, and direct physician interventions. Factors that influence the form and details of the written therapy referral or equipment prescription include team communication needs, styles of interaction, and need for ongoing quality control.

Health-care teams may be classified into one of four groups: the traditional medical model, the multidisciplinary model, the interdisciplinary model, and the transdisciplinary models. These will be more fully discussed later, along with pertinent regulatory issues, within the context of the communication styles and needs of these differing team interactions.

TEAM DYNAMICS

The focus of the comprehensive rehabilitation team is the well-being, quality of life, and functional reintegration of the patient into all aspects of life. An effective team is efficient in reaching its goals and creates an exciting and stimulating work environment for its members. Douglas McGregor developed one of the first descriptions of an effective team, noting that it must have the 11 characteristics outlined in Table 46-2 (6). When a team exhibits McGregor's characteristics, it has a built-in feedback mechanism through which it constantly monitors itself and maintains its effectiveness. When a team is not functioning well, effective function can be developed or restored through the process of team building (6). Team building requires com-

mitments of time and energy, but the rewards of improved patient outcomes and satisfaction of the team members are worth the effort (6,10,11).

A newly formed team, or a team with several new members, faces several major tasks if the team is to function effectively (6,11). The members must build a working relationship and establish a facilitative climate. This is particularly challenging in training atmospheres, since new members are frequently being added or removed for new rotations, and new trainees must learn and adapt to the culture of the permanent team in which negotiated roles have already been established. New teams must work out methods for setting goals, solving problems, making decisions, ensuring follow-through on task assignments, developing collaboration of effort, establishing lines of open communication, and ensuring an appropriate support system that will let team members feel accepted yet allow open discussion and disagreement. In a newly formed team it is advisable to designate meetings in which members can share personal expectations and develop working policies.

CONFLICT AND DISAGREEMENT

Conflict is a normal, necessary, and not necessarily destructive part of team development (7,10). The potential for conflict is high in health services organizations (12). How it is handled will determine its effect on team objectives and the group process. A good rehabilitation team creates an atmosphere in which members can agree to disagree without making personal accusations or faulting each others' personalities. In this atmosphere, conflict can be used as a vehicle for growth and innovation.

The interactionist perspective is one current view toward conflict. According to this view, a certain level of conflict is healthy and leads to a group that is viable, self-critical, and innovative. A group can have too little conflict. Without conflict, it may be viewed as harmonious, cooperative, and tranquil, but the team may become apathetic, noninnovative, and nonresponsive to needs for change, and may show low productivity. Team members may leave the apathetic team because they are bored. If this occurs, then it becomes the responsibility of team leaders to stir up enough conflict or tension to promote creativ-

TABLE 46-1. Facts About Some Rehabilitation Team Members

Discipline	Organization	Journal	Certification Required
Occupational therapist	American Occupational Therapy Association 4720 Montgomery Lane P.O. Box 31220 Bethesda, MD 20824-1220 Tel: (301) 652-2682 Fax: (301) 652-7711	*American Journal of Occupational Therapy* (monthly) *OT Practice* (monthly)	Yes
Physical therapist	American Physical Therapy Association 1111 North Fairfax Street Alexandria, VA 22314 Tel: 1-800-999-APTA Fax: (703) 706-3169	*Physical Therapy Journal* (monthly)	Yes
Prosthetist/ orthotist	American Orthotic and Prosthetic Association 330 John Carlyle Street Suite 200 Alexandria, VA 22314 Tel: (800) 229-7530 Fax: (877) 734-9384	*The Journal of Prosthetics and Orthotics* (quarterly) *The Almanac* (annually)	Yes
Rehabilitation nurse	Association of Rehabilitation Nurses 4700 West Lake Avenue Glenview, IL 60025 Tel: (800) 229-7530 Fax: (877) 734-9384	*Rehabilitation Nursing* (bimonthly)	Yes
Speech pathologist	Amerian Speech Language Hearing Association 10801 Rockville Pike Rockville, MD 20852 Tel: (301) 897-5700 Fax: (301) 571-0457	*Journal of Speech and Hearing Research* (bimonthly) *American Journal of Audiology* (3 issues per year)	Yes
Social worker	National Association of Social Workers 750 First Street NE Suite 700 Washington, DC 20002 Tel: (202) 408-8600 Fax: (202) 336-8310	*Social Worker* (quarterly) *Health and Social Work* (quarterly) *Social Work Research* (quarterly) *Social Work Abstracts* (quarterly)	Yes
Vocational counselor	American Counseling Association 5999 Stevenson Avenue Alexandria, VA 22304 Tel: (703) 823-9800 Fax: (703) 823-0252	*Journal of Counseling and Development* (4 issues per year) *Counseling Today* (monthly newspaper)	Yes
Child life specialist	Child Life Council 11820 Parklawn Drive Suite 202 Rockville, MD 20852-2529 Tel: (800) 252-4515 Fax: (301) 881-7092	*The Bulletin* (quarterly, for members only)	Certification not required but strongly recommended
Kinesiotherapist (corrective therapist)	American Kinesiotherapy Association P.O. Box 1390 Hines, IL 60141-1390 Tel: (800) 296-2582	*Clinical Kinesiotherapy* (quarterly)	Certification not required but strongly recommended
Horticultural therapist	American Horticulture Therapy Association 909 York Street Denver, CO 80206-3799 Tel: (800) 634-1603 or (303) 370-8087 Fax: (303) 331-5766	*Journal of Therapeutic Horticulture* (annually)	Yes
Music therapist	American Music Therapy Association 8455 Colesville Road Suite 1000 Silver Spring, MD 20910 Tel: (301) 589-3300 Fax: (301) 589-5175	*Journal of Music Therapy* (quarterly) *Music Therapy Perspectives* (two issues yearly)	Yes
Recreation therapist	National Therapeutic Recreation Society 22377 Belmont Ridge Road Ashburn, VA 20148-4501 Tel: (703) 858-0784 Fax: (703) 858-0794 American Therapeutic Recreation Association 1414 Prince Street Suite 204 Alexandria, VA 22314 Tel: (703) 683-9420 Fax: (703) 683-9431	*Therapeutic Recreation Journal* (quarterly) *Annual of Therapeutic Recreation*	Yes
Dance therapist	American Dance Therapy Association 2000 Century Plaza Suite 108 10632 Little Patuxent Parkway Columbia, MD 21044 Tel: (410) 997-4040 Fax: (410) 997-4048	*American Journal of Dance Therapy* (semi-annually)	Yes

---

TABLE 46-2.   McGregor's Characteristics of an Effective Work Team

1. The atmosphere tends to be informal, comfortable, and relaxed. There are no obvious tensions. It is a working atmosphere in which people are involved and interested. There are no signs of boredom.
2. There is a lot of discussion in which virtually everyone participates, but it remains pertinent to the task of the group. If the discussion gets off the subject, someone will bring it back in short order.
3. The task or the objective of the group is well understood and accepted by the members. There will have been free discussion of the objective at some point, until it was formulated in such a way that the members of the group could commit themselves to it.
4. The members listen to each other! The discussion does not have the quality of jumping from one idea to another unrelated one. Every idea is given a hearing. People do not appear to be afraid of being foolish by putting forth a creative thought even if it seems fairly extreme.
5. There is some disagreement. The group is comfortable with this and shows no signs of having to avoid conflict or to keep everything on a plane of sweetness and light. Disagreements are not suppressed or overridden by premature group action. The reasons are carefully examined, and the group seeks to resolve them rather than to dominate the dissenter. On the other hand, there is no "tyranny of the minority." Members who disagree do not appear to be trying to dominate the group or to express hostility. Their disagreement is an expression of a genuine difference of opinion, and they expect a hearing so that a solution may be found. Sometimes there are basic disagreements that cannot be resolved. The group finds it possible to live with them, accepting them but not permitting them to block its efforts. Under some conditions, action will be deferred to permit further study of an issue between the members. On other occasions, when the disagreement cannot be resolved and action is necessary, it will be taken but with open caution and recognition that the action may be subject to later reconsideration.
6. Most decisions are reached by a consensus, in which it is clear that everybody is in general agreement and willing to go along. However, there is little tendency for members who oppose the action to keep their opposition private and thus let an apparent consensus mask real disagreement. Formal voting is at a minimum; the group does not accept a simple majority as a proper basis for action.
7. Criticism is frequent, frank and relatively comfortable. There is little evidence of personal attack, either openly or in a hidden fashion. The criticism has a constructive flavor in that it is oriented toward removing an obstacle that faces the group and prevents it from getting the job done.
8. Team members are free in expressing their feelings as well as their ideas both on the problem and on the group's operation. There is little pussyfooting, there are few hidden agendas. Everybody appears to know quite well how everybody else feels about any matter under discussion.
9. When action is taken, clear assignments are made and accepted.
10. The chairman of the group does not dominate it, nor does the group defer unduly to him or her. In fact as one observes the activity, it is clear that the leadership shifts from time to time, depending on the circumstances. Different members, because of their knowledge or experience, are in a position at various times to act as resources for the group. The members use them in this fashion and they occupy leadership roles while they are thus being used. There is little evidence of a power struggle as the group operates. The issue is not who controls but how to get the job done.
11. The group is self-conscious about its own operations. Frequently, it will stop to examine how well it is doing or what may be interfering with its operation. The problem may be a matter of procedure, or it may be a member whose behavior is interfering with the accomplishment of the group's objectives. Whatever it is, it gets open discussion until a solution is found.

Adapted from McGregor D. *The human side of enterprise.* New York: McGraw-Hill, 1960:232–235.

---

ity, innovation, and productivity among the team members. The manager who creates conflict must use great skill to see that the conflict does not accelerate to the point where it becomes disruptive, divisive, or chaotic. If conflict is not controlled, then communication suffers, cooperation ceases, and the quality of patient care decreases (7). When conflict repeatedly occurs with no resolution, action must be taken to restore the team's effectiveness. An appropriate setting for conflict resolution is a team-building session.

TEAM BUILDING AND DEVELOPMENT

A group of professionals brought together for the purpose of helping a particular patient or set of patients will not automatically form the most efficient and effective force to accomplish that purpose. Understanding the factors that lead to the development of a team in which members are synergistic in their care of patients is of paramount importance to the physiatrist. To make interdisciplinary rehabilitation teams effective, Rothberg believes the following functions must be performed (13):

- Show/teach team members how to work together and provide sufficient practice time in teamwork.
- Ensure that all members learn, understand, and respect the knowledge and skills of others.
- Develop clear definitions of the roles and behaviors expected of team participants and lessen ambiguities regarding expectations of others.

- Encourage use of the full potential of each member.
- Direct attention to initiation and maintenance of communication and to the breaking down of barriers to interdisciplinary communications.
- Attend to the maintenance of the teams in the same way that other organizations engage in activities that strengthen their cohesion and offer satisfaction to their personnel.
- Acknowledge that leadership should shift as necessary in terms of the patients' needs.
- Ensure that the person in the leadership role respects the other members, as evidenced by consultation, active listening, and their inclusion in planning.
- Develop an internal system for demonstrating the accountability of each team member to the group, as well as to the institution in which the team practices.
- Develop a process to acknowledge conflict as it arises and to address it in a manner that strengthens the group and its members.

Table 46-3 lists individual characteristics that help one integrate into an interdisciplinary health-care team. A professional who is unwilling to accept such roles cannot participate in a significant way in the interdisciplinary health-care process.

New Team Development

Initiating an effective team is a particular challenge. No matter what type of team is being developed, whether formal or informal, multidisciplinary, interdisciplinary, or transdisciplinary

TABLE 46-3. Personal Characteristics of Successful Interdisciplinary Team Participants

1. Accept differences and perspectives of others
2. Function interdependently
3. Negotiate role with other team members
4. Form new values, attitudes, and perceptions
5. Tolerate constant review and challenge of ideas
6. Take risks
7. Possess personal identity and integrity
8. Accept team philosophy of care

Adapted from Given B, Simmons S. The interdisciplinary health-care team: fact of fiction? *Nurs Forum* 1977;16:165–183, with permission.

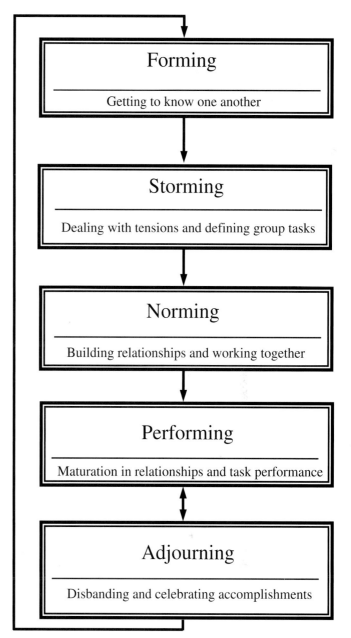

Figure 46-2. Phases of new team development. (Modified from Schermerhorn JR, Flint JG, Osborn RN. *Organizational behavior,* 7th ed. Philadelphia: John Wiley & Sons, 2000:178–181.)

(as defined later), or a business group or committee, five basic stages of group development are encountered (Fig. 46-2). These are (a) forming, (b) storming, (c) norming, (d) performing, and (e) adjourning (14).

- During the *forming* stage, initial entry and identification with the group are the primary concerns. Group members are interested in what the group can offer them and what they can offer the group. During this stage individuals are usually on their best behavior and may temporarily overlook conflicts for the good of the group.
- *Storming* is the most difficult stage and is characterized by high emotional tension. The level of trust becomes low during this phase. Team members tend to pressure the rest of the group to accept their preferences. Status and control in the group may become an issue during this phase. Cliques and coalitions may form here, and "hostility and infighting" (14) are common. During this phase members begin to understand each other's interpersonal styles and learn to interact within those parameters (15). Team members also attempt to find ways to work toward the team's goals while they seek concurrently to meet their individual needs.
- The *norming* phase is a transition to more comfortable and stable interaction, and is referred to as *initial integration.* Balance begins to emerge during this phase, and the team begins to function more as a unit. This initial balance is not completely stable and can give way at any time, but balance and focus are usually reestablished fairly quickly. The new-found harmony usually comes as a great relief after the storming and may become the primary objective of the team for a period of time. Trust improves; however, the group has not yet matured, and the balance between group needs versus individual needs is precarious.
- *Performing,* also referred to as complete integration, is characterized by maturity and a high level of functional efficiency. Complex tasks and disagreements no longer suspend or preoccupy the group. They are quickly resolved, often creatively, and the group moves on toward goal accomplishment. Trust is a key component of the successful team and becomes very high during this phase.
- The *adjourning* phase occurs when the team disbands. The ability to do this and reconvene in the future as needed is the true test of a team's integration, maturity, and ultimate success.

The physiatrist, as team leader, must appreciate that these phases of team development are normal, realizing that to some extent they are inevitable, are acceptable, and represent progress toward the desired goals of an effective and efficient team (14). Leading the team through these tumultuous times takes calm, steady leadership, and the leader must have the ability to remind the members of the group of these normal phases as they pass through them, with the goal of something better resulting eventually. The team must be reminded that complete integration is the goal, but this may not necessarily occur without these other, less effective and efficient phases of negotiation processes first. The leadership qualities defined by Lundberg should be cultivated by rehabilitation team leaders approaching this task (Table 46-4) (16). During the storming and early norming phases extra care needs to be taken to avoid the appearance of selling out for personal gain during this time of naturally high distrust. Emphasizing the value and importance of each member will help to establish trust and facilitate progress through these tumultuous phases of team development.

Established Team Complacency

Another factor that may be detrimental to the team's effectiveness is complacency among established teams (2,6,7). Whereas

---

TABLE 46-4. Some Qualities of a Leader

- Knows where he or she is going
- Knows how to get there
- Has courage and persistence
- Can be believed
- Can be trusted not to "sell out" a cause for personal advantage
- Makes the mission seem important, exciting, and possible to accomplish
- Makes each person's role in the mission seem important
- Makes each member feel capable of performing his or her role

Modified from Lundborg LB, *The art of being an executive*. Reprinted with the permission of The Free Press, a Division of Macmillan, Inc. © 1981 by Barbara W. Lundborg.

---

much transitional energy is present on initial team development and negotiation of roles, a mature team may lose its edge by accepting routine patterns of behaviors even when change is indicated. A complacent team may be recognized by one or more of the following characteristics: the same members seem to be doing the same things the same way year after year despite advances in the field; products prescribed are predictable; new members transfer out of the team because of the lack of challenge; there is a fear of, or resistance to, risk taking; and the rewards go to team members with average performance. These characteristics are especially detrimental to the rehabilitation team because external conditions that define the team's direction and individual patient's needs are always changing.

Despite similar diagnoses, each patient presents a unique picture; thus, treatment goals and procedures should always vary in some customized way. Treatment techniques should change in response to new research finding, and creativity and problem solving should be important to the operation of a rehabilitation team. Steiner has identified the following characteristics of a creative team: unusual types of people, open channels of communication, interaction with outside sources, openness to new ideas, freedom (i.e., not run as a "tight ship"), an atmosphere in which members have fun, rewards go to people with ideas, and risk taking occurs (2,6).

Barriers to Communication

Communication networks associated with rehabilitation are complex, and there are many potential barriers to effective communication (2). Understanding flows of communication and strategies to overcome communication barriers can improve internal communication within the rehabilitation team and health-care organization and thus improve patient care. Communicating well in a rapidly changing health-care market, especially external communication with stakeholders outside the rehabilitation facility, can benefit the health-care organization in ways that ensure the health, or even survival, of the organization. For example, the rehabilitation organization that communicates well may benefit in terms of being selected as the first-choice provider of rehabilitation services, obtaining contracts at favorable reimbursement levels, or helping to establish favorable regulatory policies (17). Communication skills enhancement is also important for marketing to external stakeholders, as emphasized by the Rehabilitation Accreditation Commission (CARF) (18).

An important issue in facilitating rehabilitation team communication is the identification and resolution of barriers to communication. Given and Simmons have identified communication barriers that can interfere with the achievement of treatment goals (11):

- Autonomy
- Individual members' personal characteristics that may contribute to personality conflicts
- Role ambiguity
- Incongruent expectations
- Differing perceptions of authority
- Power and status differentials
- Varying educational preparation of the patient care team members
- Hidden agendas

These barriers stem from interpersonal, interprofessional, and practice issues, and these are not intrinsic defects of the team concept (11).

A special barrier to effective communication on rehabilitation teams is the presence of many professional disciplines in rehabilitation, particularly the differing perspectives of professionals with a physical background (e.g., physiatrists and physical therapists) and a psychosocial background (e.g., psychologists and social workers) (19). This adds strength to the holistic assessment and consideration of all aspects of the individual patient's life needs but can permit a frustrating set of varying backgrounds, priorities, and initial perspectives that may not be well understood by other team members of a differing discipline. A portion of this barrier can be varying definitions and understanding of rehabilitation-related terminology by different members of the rehabilitation team. A recent study provided objective evidence that members of rehabilitation teams have "a disturbing lack of common understanding for some basic rehabilitation terminology" and that "only about half of the personnel providing rehabilitation services are currently sensitive to this issue" (20). The authors suggested several courses of action for this problem: alert rehabilitation professionals that it exists, adopt a standardized rehabilitation glossary for the team, avoid the use of vague terms, define terms operationally, and express descriptions of patients and their progress objectively using standardized functional assessment instruments (20). The use of a communication instrument to help keep the information comprehensible, relevant, and compact can help improve discussion between professionals with different backgrounds (19).

Lack of effective communication can be detrimental to the rehabilitation process, as well as uncomfortable for team members. Time must be designated to maintain an effective team process and to help overcome any existing communication barriers. When a team is functioning suboptimally because of conflict, complacency, or poor communication, the problem can be resolved through the team-building process (6).

Dyer cites three prerequisites for conflict negotiation:

1. All parties must agree to come together and work on the problems.
2. Members must agree that there are problems that need to be solved and that solving them is everyone's responsibility.
3. Members accept the position that the end result is that the team will communicate better, thus enhancing the rehabilitation process (6).

Once these prerequisites have been met, the team identifies the conflicts or barriers in need of resolution. It is important that concrete suggestions be made for the resolution of these problems and that the team agree on the solutions. This creates a problem-solving session rather than a detrimental process in which the members attempt to determine fault or place blame.

Once solutions are agreed on, each member has the responsibility to follow through according to his or her role.

An outside consultant may be extremely helpful, since some signs of poor team function are more easily discerned by an outsider (6). Other symptoms are more easily observed by team members, but an outside consultant can help interpret and resolve these symptoms. The consultant can guide the team away from interpretations of problems that are not likely to lead to resolution, such as erroneously labeling incomplete or inadequate conflict resolution as personality conflict, or placing blame rather than finding effective solutions (6). Consultants can guide the team toward constructive ways to resolve problems such as appreciating the expectation theory, which simply states that negative reactions can be predicted whenever the behavior of one person violates the expectations of another (15). A vicious cycle of escalating conflict can result when the negative reaction itself violates the expectations of the first person. However, because this theory focuses on behavior rather than personality, it allows a greater possibility for conflict resolution. If the parties involved, or even one of the parties, can identify the behaviors that violate expectations, then behaviors can be changed or agreements can be reached. Team members can then reward each other's behaviors rather than negatively reinforce them (6,15). Appreciating our differences and anticipating how others desire to be treated, including how they prefer to communicate, has been called the Platinum Rule (15). A consultant can help the team learn to sustain healthy communication by developing its own internal mechanisms for problem identification and diagnosis, planning remediation, implementing changes, and evaluating its own results in a healthy feedback loop. The beneficiaries of healthy communication on the rehabilitation team are both the patients and the team members.

It is especially important that health-care teams and organizations be able to manage a particular type of conflict—the conflict that arises when something goes wrong. Even in the best-managed organization, things will go wrong. In a health-care organization, the result of mistakes can be injury, pain, suffering, or even death. In such cases the rehabilitation team and the organization also experience distress. There are always ripple effects that can affect multiple stakeholders inside and outside the organization. Excellent communication skills in this situation can contain the damage and may help to redress the consequences, the most difficult step. Healthy communication can help to build trust and even strengthen future relationships with affected stakeholders, and demonstrate a proactive approach toward helping to prevent recurrences of similar mishaps (2,17).

REHABILITATION TEAM COMMUNICATION METHODOLOGY

Comprehensive medical rehabilitation requires the interactions of multiple caregivers to provide the breadth of services needed by people with physical and cognitive impairments (3,4,21,22). Patient needs range from acute and chronic medical problems to physical impairments, their complex interactions, and the impact each has on the patient's psychological, vocational, and social integration. The primary goal of interactions between care providers is communication of the patient's needs and coordination of his or her efforts in a synergistic manner (23). Physician-initiated prescriptions, referrals, or orders are written communications that are intended to provide for patient needs by initiating the services to be provided by multiple caregivers. The form such written communications

take depends in part on the style of interaction adopted by involved professionals. Redundant, noncoordinated, or incomplete care can occur when a patient's desires and needs are addressed from multiple vantage points without effective communication and coordination among the different caregiving professionals. Despite the widespread perception that a coordinated team effort enhances the effectiveness of such complex patient care, definitive studies are not available to prove this point. The results of the available studies have varied outcomes related to different measured variables (4,5,7).

Accrediting agencies such as the Rehabilitation Accreditation Commission (CARF) and, more recently, the Joint Commission on the Accreditation of Healthcare Organizations (JCAHO), as well as federal regulations in certain instances, require "interdisciplinary teams" (5,9,24,25), yet many styles of interaction exist that are influenced in part by the practice environment (26). Four general styles of interaction between physicians and other professional caregivers will be discussed: the traditional *medical model* without a formal team; the *multidisciplinary team*, which some call the traditional medical model of team interaction; the *interdisciplinary* model; and the *transdisciplinary* model. Each model's advantages and disadvantages are outlined, and its impact on prescriptions, orders, referrals, and treatment plan writing is discussed. These four models of interaction are described in pure form, though features of each are often combined to take the greatest advantage of the benefits each model's features may offer for a particular practice setting. Effective team dynamics and communication discussed earlier are always important, but they are especially necessary for successful implementation of the interdisciplinary and transdisciplinary models.

STYLES OF INTERACTIONS

Medical Model

Traditional medical care results in a model in which a physician attends to the patient's needs. If services of another discipline are desired, that professional is consulted and given either specific or general requests for assistance to meet the needs of the patient as perceived by the attending physician. The quality of the service rendered by the consultant, and thus future consultations, depends on meeting those needs, as perceived by the attending physician. The consultant identifying additional needs would usually discuss them with the attending physician before proceeding with the additional treatment, in recognition of the fact that the attending physician may have additional information and insight not available to the consultant. This traditional system results in a clear chain of responsibility that continues to be well respected and that is reinforced medicolegally. This traditional autocratic model of leadership, in which the physician assumes an authoritarian role and other team members obey, is not effective in the rehabilitation setting (10). Multiple consultations may result in many professionals doing multiple tasks. Coordination of these efforts by the attending physician or among the involved professionals can often be difficult or incomplete, resulting in less efficient and sometimes redundant patient care. This is one of the major disadvantages to the medical model of patient care (21,23,27).

Rehabilitation professionals have recently favored the concept of "client-centered therapy." This is not meant to trivialize the patient's needs as physicians may suppose, but rather to emphasize the patient as the director and arbiter of the interventions according to the patient's own desires (28). The term *client* is used in the place of *patient* in order to indicate that the role is an active one. The client, his or her caregivers, and the service providers enter into a collaborative relationship with the assumption that the client is the most knowledgeable about his own functional needs. The professionals advise and educate, and assist in creating an optimal environment for the client to achieve independence in those areas that the client has identified as being important. Some advantages of this approach include empowerment and decreased dependency for the client, and a truly individualized treatment program, since each patient identifies the issues that he or she wishes to master. However, client-centered care is challenging to provide within the structure of current health-care systems, which emphasize professional assessment and medical necessity over patient desires in establishing allowed treatment interventions. It also assumes a fluid interaction that can be problematic within the bounds of the medical model in which a particular attending defined problem was the cause for the initial referral and for which authorization for treatment was received.

Medical ethics in recent decades has prioritized patient autonomy over attending beneficence (paternalistic actions deemed by the practitioner to be in the patient's best interest), which is also consistent with patient-centered care (2,29,30). The medical model, as compared with more team interactive models in which the patient is part of the team, is not particularly well suited for patient-directed care because of the additional effort required of the physician in this system. This is because all therapies and consultant plans are coordinated by the attending, and not by the patient. For patient autonomy to have priority, the full weight of patient education, advice regarding all possible interventions and their respective risks and potential benefits, and recommendations is borne by the attending physician. This has become more difficult in an era of time-limiting managed care. Indeed, much of the decision making over what is best for the patient's health care is defined by what the patient's health insurance is willing to cover, and is frequently removed from both patient and attending preferences by the coverage certification mechanisms of managed-care systems. These decisions are based more on economic considerations than on considerations of optimal health benefit.

Multidisciplinary Team Model

The multidisciplinary team model provides a means for multiple professionals who require frequent interactions to meet and coordinate efforts on a consistent basis. The multidisciplinary model is analogous to the classic pyramid-shaped model of management, which features vertical communication between supervisor and subordinates. It typically remains an attending-physician-controlled team in which most interactions are between consultants and the primary attending. Discussion between consulting professionals is held to a minimum or, when necessary, directed by the attending physician. This emphasis on vertical communication (Fig. 46-3) evolved from the medical model attending physician's role and relationship with consultants (26).

Team conferences can be conducted efficiently with such clear lines of authority and control, but lateral communication may suffer (27,31) (see Fig. 46-3). This tendency to impede the free, horizontal flow of communication between the team members is recognized as an obstacle to the optimal use of each participant's specific expertise and problem-solving skills. This may negate the possible group synergism that can create a product greater than the sum of its parts; or, in clinical terms, a care plan better than any one participant could have developed alone (26,32). The interdisciplinary team model does attempt to improve this communication and enhance group synergism, thus fostering a sense of mutual authority and responsibility (22,31, 32).

Interdisciplinary Team Model

Interdisciplinary teams benefit from lateral communication flow that occurs as easily as vertical communication in the multidisciplinary team. Because the interdisciplinary model is designed to facilitate such lateral communication, it is theoretically better suited for rehabilitation teams (34–36). The expected norm is group decision making and group responsibility for developing optimal care planning (31). The problem orientation and ease of flow of lateral communication in the interdisciplinary team processes are similar in function to the project orientation and communication patterns of matrix organization (33,34). The patient is considered part of this planning group and has a central role in the team's considerations (Fig. 46-1) (23,37,38). With the emphasis on mutual communication and responsibility, the patient care-coordinating conferences may be led by any team member (Fig. 46-4) (27,39). One objective of this model is to allow a freer exchange of ideas and thereby benefit from the group synergy concept (23,40). The interdisciplinary model has been described as a compromise between the benefits of specialization and the need for continuity and comprehensiveness of care (13). Its disadvantages can include considerably less time-effectiveness in completing patient care conferences. In theory, this inefficiency is offset by improved communication and better problem solving. Such teams also require considerable training in the team process,

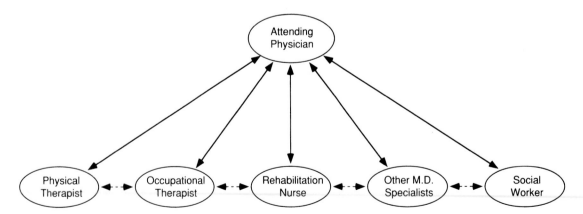

Figure 46-3. Multidisciplinary team conference structure. Vertical communication *(solid lines)* may serve to limit horizontal communication *(dotted lines)* between team care providers.

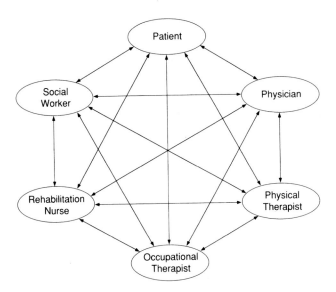

Figure 46-4. In an interdisciplinary team, communication and decision-making mutualism are encouraged. One team member usually acts as the patient care coordinator, but lack of role dominance allows any team member to be eligible for this role.

their own professional expertise. A future corps of rehabilitation generalists as the main therapy providers has been predicted and advocated by some (47,48). Whether such informally shared professional knowledge and cotreatment lead to competent therapists in each other's fields is doubtful. The issues of technically competent care, professional society opposition, state licensure, and qualifications may limit the development of truly transdisciplinary rehabilitation on a widespread scale. To further differentiate transdisciplinary from interdisciplinary or multidisciplinary team approaches, attributes from the literature have been defined by Walker and Avant (49). They define five premises that need to be met before the transdisciplinary approach is possible. They are role extension, role enrichment, role expansion, role release, and role support (42).

Role extension is a process whereby one's own discipline-specific knowledge is continually increasing (50). "Feeling secure in one's role and knowing that individual contributions are facilitating positive patient outcomes are essential components in creating an environment where each discipline is comfortable collaborating with the other" (51). Role extension involves understanding one's own discipline well and understanding how it compares to the aspects of other disciplines that can benefit the patient. Further, "having the security in

generally not received during the years of formal training in the individual disciplines (31). Team communication, development, and conflict resolution have been discussed earlier. This non-patient-care training is expensive and does not ensure success (22,31,41). The commitments and personality traits found in the members of a successful interdisciplinary team are similar to those that engender good referral patterns between physicians (Table 46-3 and Table 46-5) (27,41). The physician may be uncomfortable with the team decision-making process because the physician is the one who must usually assume the greatest medicolegal responsibility for the team's actions and plans. There may be difficulty in having the physician complete the appropriate prescription for such team-generated plans, especially if the plans seem to be different from what the physician recalled or desired. Such conflicts are ideally resolved in team meetings, but delays in completion of the paperwork can jeopardize the optimal patient care.

Transdisciplinary Team Model

Transdisciplinary teams, a more recent development, encourage not only communication but cross-treatment between disciplines. This atypical strategy has developed with the central focus on improving patient care through a team approach in which responsibilities are shared as in the interdisciplinary team, but also where the normal boundaries of the various health-care professions are blurred (42,43,44,45,46). These teams have mostly developed out of educational models (21, 26,43,44) and have been justified on the basis of economic market forces, and in part by shortages in adequate numbers of therapy professionals (22,47,48). Cross-training, or multiskilling, of available teachers and aides is reported to be very helpful in providing the needed educational services. Such programs, when self-rated against no integration of the disciplines, are rated very favorably (43,45,46). The transdisciplinary team has also found favor with traumatic brain injury teams (26,46). Consistency of information exchange, with the patient intrinsic to cotreatment, is cited as an advantage (43,44,46). Furthermore, the exchange of information between disciplines is highly valued, with therapists or teachers noting expansion of

---

TABLE 46-5.   Personal Practices that Engender Referrals from Other Physicians

1. Never say anything bad about another physician, especially in front of a patient.
2. Send a typed note to the referring physician every time you see the patient as an outpatient.
3. Tell the referring physician in person or by phone of major changes in a patient's condition or treatment plan.
4. Never discharge another physician's patient from a hospital without informing that physician.
5. Do not provide care to referred patients that is in the area of expertise of the referring physicians, unless they have asked you to do so.
6. Regardless of your opinion on providing free care, do not refuse to see a patient who cannot pay or who has poor insurance if referred by a physician who also sends you many paying patients.
7. Do not communicate with the referring physician directly in hospital chart notes, particularly about an item of disagreement. Remember that the chart is a legal document. A lawyer may ask you to read your chart notes in court.
8. Get to know your referring physicians and their individual ways of handling patients. Avoid violating personal habits and biases.
9. Never send a patient who has been referred to you to another specialist unless the referring physician concurs.
10. Never leave a referring physician uninformed about the disposition of his or her patient. Physicians usually stop sending you patients if they know they will never see them again.
11. Answer consultations promptly.
12. Keep up your competence. Your referring physicians expect you to be on the cutting edge of your field.
13. Give the referring physician some suggestions or leads if you cannot definitively help him or her with a referred patient.
14. Let physicians' calls come through to you, but take a number and call back other persons.
15. Use a tickler file to keep up with patient needs.
16. Have a method for handling angry patients. Let them get all their emotion out—do not interrupt. Lower your voice and talk slowly. Never argue with their feelings, only with the facts of the case.

From Braddom RL. Practice issues in the hospital-based rehabilitation unit. In: Melvin JL, Odderson IR, eds. Clinical rehabilitation and physiatric practice. *Phys Med Rehabil Clin North Am* 1996; 7:31–41, with permission.

one's own role leads to the resolution of role, turf, and status issues" (52).

Role enrichment is gaining awareness and knowledge of the other disciplines present on the team (50). Although health-care personnel recognize and appreciate the various other professionals, the level of role enrichment to which this defining attribute refers is only achieved through a high degree of collaboration. Team members are encouraged to communicate, collectively plan and implement assessments, discuss results, and develop integrated treatment goals during team meetings (53).

Through team meetings, role expansion is expressed. Each team member from a particular discipline educates the others regarding his or her own expertise (52). Knowledge is shared as team members teach each other to make specific judgments and decisions about interventions that transcend the boundaries of traditional roles (52).

The fourth critical characteristic, role release, is frequently lauded in the literature. Incorporating the skills acquired from other disciplines can help in problematic settings and enhance an individual's skill set, but such actions tend to blur the traditional discipline boundaries (54). A simple example would be that of a speech-language pathologist (SLP) helping a patient to sit more comfortably for speech therapy by applying proper body mechanics principles learned from a physical therapy colleague. This health-care provider assumed responsibility for a needed task by applying techniques learned from another discipline.

Role support, the fifth defining attribute, would be best captured if the physical therapist should walk by at just the moment the SLP was helping the patient to a more comfortable position and gave the SLP feedback on how he or she was instructing the patient about body mechanics. Support of others and feedback about the implementation of a particular skill are the hallmarks of role support (50).

One application of transdisciplinary team approach is the "arena" or group assessment, in which the patient and all therapists gather at one setting. One primary team facilitator conducts the initial assessment, with all the other disciplines observing, adding, or questioning as needed. This approach limits the number of times the patient is required to answer the same question or demonstrate the same activity or skill, and is considered the best for detecting difficulties because of its thoroughness by several specialties observing the same patient at the same time but from differing perspectives (55).

Though collegiality is enhanced by the transdisciplinary approach, the blurring of roles is discouraged by many specialties and regulatory agencies. The question is whether adequate competence can be developed by the informal training of transdisciplinary teams as compared with the years of formal training during which individual specialists have acquired their competence. Billing rules and regulations can also offer practical problems for appropriate billing for transdisciplinary treatments sessions.

Which Team Approach to Use

Research is lacking on which of the previous models is most effective. The usefulness of such studies almost certainly will depend on which parameters are examined (i.e., team and patient satisfaction versus outcome). It may be that different models are more effective in different practice environments. The medical care, multidisciplinary team, interdisciplinary team, and transdisciplinary team models can be found in various settings in rehabilitation. The medical care model often is used in a freestanding office practice or in inpatient consultations in an acute-care hospital. This becomes especially true when referrals are made to therapists who are geographically distant or with whom frequent interaction may be difficult. Standing hospital programs that often include nonphysiatric physicians, such as cardiac rehabilitation, pulmonary rehabilitation, geriatrics, prosthetics clinic, myelomeningocele clinic, and the like, may use the multidisciplinary model with one physician in charge. Interdisciplinary teams generally consist of a stable population of health caregivers that often can be found in association with specialized units in a comprehensive rehabilitation hospital, unit, or service. Transdisciplinary teams are more common when a stable population of professionals is to provide long-term care for a patient, and cognitive-educational needs are more prominent than intense physical needs.

These models of interaction are meant to enhance communication and thereby coordination of care. The practicing physiatrist may prefer one style over the others but often finds it necessary to communicate with patients and multiple care providers in all these models, or some combination, depending on practice setting. Specificity of orders and the methods in which treatment plans are developed will vary with the treatment and communication models that are adopted.

Regulatory Organizations

The two primary regulatory organizations for rehabilitation programs are the Joint Commission for Accreditation of Health Care Organizations (JCAHO) and the Rehabilitation Accreditation Commission (CARF). Both JCAHO and CARF have standards addressing the rehabilitation treatment team and its composition as it relates to the individual needs of the person served. Both use the term *interdisciplinary team*, but they generalize the application of this term in ways that suggest that multidisciplinary teams as defined here would also qualify. CARF uses specific language about the interdisciplinary team and its role and composition. Specifically, CARF indicates in the standard for comprehensive integrated inpatient rehabilitation programs, CIIRP2.9, that the interdisciplinary team includes the following (18):

1. An occupational therapist
2. A physical therapist
3. A psychologist
4. A rehabilitation nurse
5. A rehabilitation physician
6. A social worker
7. A speech-language pathologist
8. A therapeutic recreational specialist

The intent statement for this standard indicates that this dynamic, changing team always includes the person served, the rehabilitation physician, and the rehabilitation nurse. Other team members are determined by the assessment and individual planning processes (18).

JCAHO, although less specific, implies the importance of the interdisciplinary team approach. Standard TX.6.1 indicates that, "An interdisciplinary team implements and coordinates planned treatment and services" (24). Standard TX.6.3 and its intent statement indicate that a "collaborative interdisciplinary approach" helps to achieve optimal outcomes. This plan is developed by the interdisciplinary team based on the needs of, and in conjunction with, the person served.

These regulatory standards do not address the various types of team formats specifically, but they do address the need for the person served to have a team approach and they define the various disciplines that are likely to be needed for the assessment, planning, and implementation of a comprehensive treat-

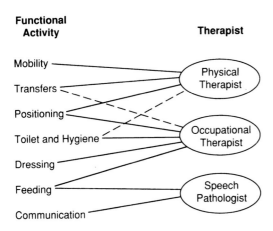

Figure 46-5. The appropriate therapy specialties must be chosen for the patient's specific deficiencies. Examples from physical therapy, occupational therapy, and speech pathology are shown. Team coordination is required to prevent duplication of services and avoid gaps in services needed.

ment plan for rehabilitation. This developed plan should be goal oriented and should produce positive, measurable outcomes for the person served (18,24).

Managing a Team Meeting

Although the rehabilitation health-care team makes effective use of the combined expertise of all participants, this increased communication comes with a cost, and that is time (2). Because much of the communication occurs during scheduled weekly staffings, or patient care conferences, these meetings must be run in an efficient and effective manner. A good team meeting is productive, stimulating, and goal oriented, and it involves creativity and problem solving through facilitated interdisciplinary interaction. The team leader, frequently the physiatrist, has the responsibility of facilitating the meeting, including maintaining the team's investment, productivity, and efficiency, while not inhibiting effective problem-solving contributions by all participants.

The structure of a team meeting can facilitate an effective team process. The simplest and most popular structure for team meetings is for a member from each discipline to give a progress report for each patient with opportunity for comment by other disciplines, especially when problems arise. This structure can work well because each member tends to focus on the problems particular to his or her discipline. Where cross interactions occur (Fig. 46-5) the observations of other disciplines can be added during the discussion of progress in the common area or task.

Another approach is the problem-oriented agenda, where the problem list for each patient is reviewed in sequence. As each problem on the agenda is discussed, any team member may address his or her role in managing that particular problem. This format tends to promote team ownership to solve

problems and to promote the synergistic interdisciplinary approach. It may be easier to keep the meeting goal-oriented because the problem list inherently defines the objectives for the meeting. However, this model requires more skill on the part of the team leader to keep the meetings efficient. For unusually complex problems, it may be prudent to delegate a subgroup to explore resources and possible solutions outside the larger group, and then have the subgroup report on their solutions, to be discussed by all, at the following large group meeting.

Regardless of model used, it is the team leader's responsibility to keep the group focused and on task. This involves facilitating discussion, ensuring that ideas are understood, negotiating compromises, and clarifying responsibilities as well as minimizing non-problem-solving discussions (56). The documentation for the meeting should include an action summary of the agreed responsibilities with assignments and deadlines (Fig. 46-6).

Another important factor to facilitate communication within a team meeting is the physical setting. A specific meeting time must be designated, and team members must be committed to respecting this time. The meeting room's size, lighting, and temperature may help or hinder effective group process. Seating should allow face-to-face communication among all members. This criterion typically is met by sitting around a table or in a circle. Adequate physical space and time can help minimize some easily discernible barriers to effective communication (2).

MULTIPLICITY OF CARE PROVIDERS

Comprehensive rehabilitation of people with physical and cognitive impairments can be an enormously complex task. The treatment goals are not disorder-specific but rather are patient individualized. The patient's psychological, religious, vocational, social, and personal needs, desires, and priorities are used to establish and prioritize rehabilitation goals. As an integrated member of the treatment team, the patient is expected to make a transition from the passive observer role common during the acute treatment phase of an injury or debilitating disease to an active participatory role. This shift in roles requires some patient orientation and education about the team process of evaluating and establishing goals. Patient autonomy should be supported and encouraged. Not only are the patient's medical needs addressed, but the psychological, social, religious, and vocational impacts of her disabling disorder require attention. Planning and facilitating all desired interventions can be accomplished best by each of the disciplines evaluating patient issues from their unique point of expertise. This knowledge from each professional must then be shared and formulated into a cohesive team plan of treatment.

Professional health-care givers in the many disciplines common to rehabilitation (see Fig. 46-1, Table 46-1) spend many years acquiring specific skills necessary to effectively assess patient problems that fall within their professional expertise. This often includes the use of test instruments standardized for specific disorders. They learn to formulate and communicate their

Decision	Who is to do it	Date of completion	Date to report progress
Train to do safe independent car transfers with a sliding board	Jan Hoover, PT. Patient's mother is to bring her car in for use in the training sessions	May 23	May 27 (next scheduled team meeting)

Figure 46-6. Example of an action summary.

discipline-specific treatment plans and goals; educate patients, family, and other professionals; apply discipline-specific individualized interventions; and monitor patient progress. From their unique vantage points, they often uncover problems or issues not apparent to others. Although physiatrists have the most wide-based training among physician specialties in the issues involved in physical impairments, disabilities, and handicaps, their perspective generally will not be as specific in any one area as that of a therapist who focuses exclusively in that treatment area. Because the interventions required are more than any one provider can reasonably give, the expertise of many professionals is used to divide up needs according to areas of treatment or intervention expertise. To avoid fracturing or neglecting needs and goals that cross disciplines, team communication is used to formulate comprehensive treatment plans (22). The specific capabilities and general roles of the various health-care providers commonly found on the rehabilitation team (see Fig. 46-1 and Table 46-1) must be learned, well understood, and appreciated by the competent physiatrist for optimal application of these disciplines' capabilities toward enhancing the function of any particular patient.

Through the medical model, the patient often first encounters a physiatrist, a specialist in PM&R, by referral from another physician. With rehabilitation as the first goal, the physiatrist also will address associated medical problems unique to disabling disorders such as dysfunctional spasticity or optimal pharmacologic bladder management in the spinal-cord-injured patient. The physiatrist often initiates the referrals to the necessary rehabilitation professionals. In the inpatient comprehensive rehabilitation setting, the physiatrist may be the sole physician involved.

A physiatrist is knowledgeable in the medical care issues of physically debilitating diseases and trauma, and has the broadest knowledge of the expertise available from each of the other team professionals (see Fig. 46-1). Identifying the areas of patient need addressed by each of these professionals will ensure that appropriate resources are used (examples are shown in Fig. 46-5). The physician who specializes in medical rehabilitation must be aware of the techniques and therapeutic interventions available from each discipline that could have positive impacts on the care of patients as well as the interventions that are specifically contraindicated.

The appropriately consulted professionals, the patient, and the family form the rehabilitation team. The multitude of potential needs (medical, physical, psychological, vocational, educational, social, or spiritual) require multiple health-care professionals to whom referrals, orders, or prescriptions may be sent. The combined input of the team members should form the basis for a coordinated, comprehensive treatment plan, including methods, goals, and estimates of length of time for completion of each. The treatment plan is dynamic and will require frequent modifications, updates, and revisions as the patient progresses.

THERAPY REFERRALS AND ORDER WRITING

Therapy referrals and order writing are based on the initial evaluation (see Chapters 1 and 2). This may or may not include team evaluation input or consensus toward the treatment plan. In the medical model and multidisciplinary team model, orders and treatment plans usually are developed initially by the physiatrist, although they may be modified later as input is received from consultants. In the interdisciplinary team model, a period of evaluation by appropriate disciplines occurs before group development and consensus on the comprehensive

treatment plan. Depending on frequency of team meetings, this may introduce a delay before coordinated team interventions begin. In the transdisciplinary model, group evaluations are the rule, frequently allowing team treatment plans to be developed during the same evaluation and treatment session. Although time efficient, the transdisciplinary team may have less time available for deliberation or complex problem solving, since the concurrent patient treatment is occurring.

Once the problems and treatment goals have been delineated, the process of referrals and order writing can proceed. Often this can be facilitated by organizing problems into functional areas of concern. One organizational scheme is to list problems that are primarily medical in nature first, followed by functional limitations or rehabilitation problems, and then associated social–environmental problems. This allows orders to be broken down into medical, therapeutic, and psychosocial issues, although overlap of problems between these categories is common. Problem-based management of medical issues is now commonplace and integrates well into this scheme.

Interactions with the other professionals providing rehabilitation of complex problems requires the physiatrist to possess both a diverse professional knowledge and a highly developed communication skill. The resources available should be applied optimally to obtain the best results for the patient. Through correct identification of the suitable providers, appropriate referrals or orders communicate in as complete a fashion as possible without limiting creative problem solving or the reciprocal feedback that helps take full advantage of the available expertise. The format of these orders and referrals depends on the practice setting and the model of communication customary in that setting.

Medical Model Referrals and Orders

In the outpatient setting, the practice may involve a well-integrated cohesive team, but more often the rehabilitation medicine specialist is a sole practitioner using community-wide resources. The former type is discussed later under the appropriate team model section. The latter outpatient practice is similar to inpatient physiatric consultations in an acute-care hospital where individual therapy departments may exist without organized teams. In such settings, referrals and orders need to be more specific because frequent verbal feedback and clarification are not as readily available. Recording notes in the hospital chart helps with inpatient coordination and communication, but the chart is less available in the outpatient setting. Written prescriptions help avoid ambiguity and ensure that the patient is being treated as desired (see the section entitled "Written Protocols, Prescriptions, Orders, and Referrals").

Although treatment recommendations ideally are based on clear physiologic rationales and clinically proven efficacy, such a literature base often is lacking or incomplete. Practitioners tend to be strongly influenced by their own successes and failures, applying lessons learned from past patients to future patients. If the physiatrist does not know which approach to treatment a consulted discipline is taking, then it is unlikely any specific learning will occur from that interaction to benefit the rehabilitation physician's future management of similar patients. Thus, knowing the particular interventions to be used will help enhance the clinical acumen of the referring physiatrist. Indeed, knowledge of how to prescribe in as much detail as is necessary is one measure the American Board of Physical Medicine and Rehabilitation examiners use to determine certification.

Another unique advantage the physiatrist holds is the understanding of how therapeutic interventions affect the pathophysiologic process of disease states. This knowledge may serve as a safety check for his or her patients. The physical medicine aspect of physiatry demands that the physics, biophysics, physiology, and pathophysiology of all prescribed physical modalities be well appreciated. This allows rational prescription of intensity, application methods, sites, duration, frequency, and precautions as warranted for such treatments. The physiatrist must both prescribe appropriate interventions and proscribe inappropriate interventions. It is from such patient safety concerns that legal requirements for physician prescriptions were mandated. Without specific understanding of and concurrence in the treatment strategies used, this safety net of supervision is lost.

The major disadvantage in an extremely precise prescription format is that it may be taken as a signal by the consultant not to think, question, or be creative in addressing the patient's problems but, rather, merely to perform the services as a technician. This perception may occur even though an order to evaluate the patient has been included, which often is legally required by state rules, whether prescribed or not. To minimize this potential negative impact on professional creativity and problem-solving expertise, requests for feedback should be specifically included. It often is helpful to request phone consultation with therapists after their evaluation but before they begin treatment to explore additional options or to convey significant yet sensitive information. If a phone consultation is requested, priority must be given to receiving such calls. Otherwise, this form of feedback and collaboration will not be reinforced enough to be maintained. Phone consultations may allow a better treatment approach to be pursued through modifications of orders by phone while providing the attending rehabilitation physician with the knowledge to adequately coordinate the specific interventions being applied. This will also help provide the order specifics often necessary for reimbursement of therapist-provided services.

Occasionally, team members are found who are unwilling to follow specific treatment orders and who proceed on a treatment plan based on their impression of what is in the patient's best interests, without consulting the prescribing physician. This violates the trust placed in the consultant and the rules by which one should engender referrals between health-care providers (see Table 46-5) (57). Such practices also expose the therapist and patient to medically unsupervised care. If this situation cannot be corrected, the patient, for his or her safety and optimal care, should be redirected to more cooperative and collegial therapy professionals. General orders requesting "evaluate and treat," sometimes because of lack of better knowledge, tend to promote such cross-purpose practices. Although this takes advantage of the therapist's creativity and expertise, it may restrict the physician's ability to supervise or coordinate patient care and may reduce the advantage of multiple professionals' synergism. Habitual poor physician support has, in part, encouraged some therapy groups to seek independent practices (also called direct access), available in 30 of the 50 United States, wherein no medical supervision is required (58). The relationship between a physiatrist and consulted professionals should be collegial and mutually supportive because a domineering, rigid posture serves only to dampen creativity and problem solving among professionals and thus may diminish the quality of patient care (45). Managed care may restrict access to only certain providers. This adds weight to the value of being able to generate rapport, collegiality, and a sense of teamwork with many different rehabilitation professionals in many different settings.

A physiatrist may evaluate patients in the outpatient setting, in which no other professional consultations are required.

TABLE 46-6. Patient Education Resources
Channing Bete Company 1 Community Place South Deerfield, MA 01373-7328 Phone 1-800-628-7733 Krames Staywell 780 Township Line Road Yardley, PA 19067 Phone 1-800-333-3032 The source book of patient education materials for physical medicine and rehabilitation, an extremely complete resource for patient education materials for people with any disability, can be obtained by telephoning Dr. Sandra J. Koch, at (903) 596-3587.

In this situation, instructions to the patient about medications, side effects, therapeutic exercise home programs, or simple modalities (e.g., heating pads, ice packs, home traction) are the important communications. Informational brochures and pictographic flyers frequently are available from national advocacy groups (Table 46-6) or can be devised to help reinforce patient comprehension and therefore compliance with the prescribed home program. Without the benefit of a therapist who interacts frequently with the patient and reports problems regularly, more frequent reevaluations may be necessary to ensure both compliance and progress. Increasingly, case management nurses are involved and may serve as valuable coordination resources and advocates for the patient with third-party payers.

When formal therapy is ordered, treatment referrals should specify any patient education or instruction desired. This includes requesting home programs and follow-up to verify compliance as necessary. Home health-care services often terminate treatment because of funding constraints before all goals have been accomplished. Using therapy time before such terminations to provide patient and family training in home programs may significantly extend gains.

Multidisciplinary Team Referrals and Orders

In the multidisciplinary team setting, the physiatrist may be a team member, a consultant, or more often one who acts as the primary attending physician. In such a group, the same specificity of orders often is required to initiate therapy but is modified more readily after input from team members at regularly scheduled patient care conferences. Priorities of goals and treatments also are more easily discussed verbally than in the written form. This allows some of the subtleties of comprehensive management to be more effectively conveyed and coordinated. Some degree of coordination between consultants also occurs at multidisciplinary conferences, but the flow of problem-solving creativity is not as free as that at interdisciplinary team conferences. Format usually consists of consultants giving their reports (i.e., initial evaluations or progress since last conference) and recommendations. Other members ideally monitor the input, but the primary consultant determines the solution to any perceived problems and organizes all the input into a modified problem list and treatment plan. Many treatment modifications are made by verbal orders, with feedback guaranteed by regular meetings. In this setting, it is not necessary to include the time until next physician follow-up or desired frequency and mechanism of follow-up therapy reports on the original orders.

Interdisciplinary Team Referrals and Orders

The format of initial orders to consultants who comprise an interdisciplinary team often is based on requesting a general evaluation, with specific evaluation instruments and the comprehensive treatment plans to be discussed and mutually derived. Occasionally, to avoid delays in initiating therapy, broad categories of intervention also are requested (e.g., "ADL training"). The specifics, however, should be discussed and integrated by the team into a comprehensive individualized patient treatment plan. The shortcomings of a setting with no dynamic, creative problem-solving interactions may persist when the patient's treatment plan is not specified and discussed but consists only of general orders for initial evaluations and general treatment, or treatment ordered according to a protocol (e.g., "quadriplegic protocol"). Such a generalized order format implies little attention to the patient's specific and unique needs. It may be countered that therapists adapt the program to this patient's unique needs, but each team member's professionalism still functions in isolation, which defeats the advantage of the interdisciplinary team process. Although the mutualism of the interdisciplinary team implies no dominant specialty, it does not exclude any member from the responsibility to be interdependent with the creative input from other members in establishing his or her own specific treatment interventions. This means the physician should consider input from the physical therapist and therapeutic recreation specialist as well as from a consulting psychiatrist before starting antidepressant medications. Territory is both relinquished by all and embraced by all, although, in the end, specific needs and interventions are assigned by the group to those individual team members who have the greatest expertise in that area.

Because the comprehensive treatment plan is not developed solely by the admitting physician, and specific interventions are decided by mutual consensus among all team members, the actual specifics of treatment can be difficult to grasp in the training environment for the PM&R resident physician. This is especially true if the medicolegally required orders remain generalized or if the specific treatment plans are signed much later by the attending physician without the resident necessarily being in the loop. This may occur because only the attending signature is required to meet hospital and third-party payer rules. Much of resident training is funded by inpatient rehabilitation hospitals or units in which the interdisciplinary team process is most often used. It is necessary not only that generalized order formats be appreciated but that the specifics of therapy interventions and efficacy be prescribed for other, less-integrated settings. If the specifics are not discussed in team meetings, then the full benefit of the interdisciplinary team process is not being realized. Many times, multidisciplinary teams with good mutual interactive skills will be labeled interdisciplinary, but each professional maintains full control of his or her specialty's area, with little cross-disciplinary discussion of methods and approaches. Such teams remain multidisciplinary despite labels to the contrary. In this setting, general orders may become accepted but may be counterproductive to the educational process of the physician, the medical supervision of the patient, and the collective group synergism that can enhance creative problem solving. Becoming interdisciplinary is threatening, challenging, and time-consuming, but satisfying in increasing collegial relationships and in deriving optimal treatment plans. Marginally competent professionals become exposed, but the team process can partially compensate for such member weaknesses (5). Professional expertise is challenged by the team, and many are not comfortable in such a vulnerable position (see Table 46-3).

Transdisciplinary Team Referrals and Orders

All members are involved collaboratively in treatments in the transdisciplinary team approach. Collective hands-on treatment is an excellent method for learning, especially when the information shared among the treating professionals is pertinent and applicable to the moment of care needs. Having another professional depend on your input as you are cotreating is both rewarding and self-affirming. The importance of each member's beliefs can be emphasized and appreciated in a very practical hands-on experience. The team member does not have to wonder whether a communication about a belief's importance was received adequately when it becomes essential to the treatment approach integrated between professionals during a cotreatment. Many reports on the transdisciplinary approach emphasize the high ratings such approaches receive by the treating disciplines (43,44,46). Collaboration and coordination of effort certainly are optimized because the disciplines have the opportunity to communicate throughout both the evaluation and the treatment of patients. There may not be a need for a formal team meeting apart from ongoing patient care, except as necessary to provide regulatory or third-party payer required documentation. If all the disciplines in comprehensive rehabilitation could be integrated sufficiently that each felt comfortable treating any patient's problem, regardless of usual discipline specificity, then a rehabilitation therapy generalist could be envisioned (47). Such a corps of professionals would certainly appreciate problems from a broader perspective and, in an era of shortage, allow for a certain ease of cross-coverage. The greatest impediment to such a development is the necessity by certification laws and ethical considerations of providing skilled, competent professional care (5,22). Billing also can be an ethical dilemma. Should a single patient treated for 1 hour by three cotreating professionals be billed for 1 hour of therapy or 3? Should the therapy time be billed on the schedule of the best-paying specialty present or equally divided among the therapy disciplines treating? It remains an open question as to whether cotreatment results in each participating professional becoming more globally competent or merely exposes the patient to less than fully professional care in those areas in which the cotreating caregiver lacks certified expertise and competence.

The advantage of dynamic, fluid, and constantly changing treatment plans that adapt to the patient's changing status can be a disadvantage when such plans must be developed on the spot. This allows little time for deliberation or consideration of alternatives because treatment must be given promptly. Written plans may not keep up with the current flow of treatment, causing difficulties when a patient must make the transition to other care providers. Indeed, written treatment plans often are generated as a retrospective report of the patient's past treatments and progress.

If the physician team member is a part of the treatment team, then any concerns about medical safety and medical treatment coordination can be addressed as treatment progresses. This, however, is unusual, with the rehabilitation physician often referring patients to such teams in which the physician will not act as a cotherapist. In such a setting, the more generalized order format may not allow adequate communication of the physician's concerns and treatment goals, especially because formal team conferences may not be frequent. Because the treating professionals may be addressing areas outside their specific expertise, the comprehensiveness with which all specific therapy issues are addressed may be of concern. In such a setting, it may be to the patient's advantage for the physician to write more specific and detailed orders to ensure that the breadth of patient issues identified by the physician will be addressed. Some mechanism to allow flexibility in approaches while maintaining direction toward the desired goals is important. Thus, treatment orders or referrals are written in a very goal-directed way, giving guidelines for treatment methods or intervention models. A mechanism for feedback on the approaches taken also is important to enhance the prescribing physician's supervision and learning experience. Without such interaction, prolonged ineffectiveness or perhaps even contraindicated approaches may result without the benefit of a physiatrist's professional expertise. Because of the possible professional "dilution" in the transdisciplinary approach, even closer re-evaluation of care by the prescribing professional may be indicated.

WRITTEN PROTOCOLS, PRESCRIPTIONS, ORDERS, AND REFERRALS

Communication

The purpose of physician-generated protocols, prescriptions, orders and referrals is to communicate patient needs ade-

quately and to request services from another professional. In the case of medications, this applies to the prescription sent to the pharmacist. In rehabilitation, it applies to the services requested from the various professionals described earlier. The rehabilitation medicine specialist must use his or her expertise first to decide what the patient's needs are. The physiatrist's broad knowledge of the capabilities of various rehabilitation professionals allows selection of the appropriate consulting professionals (see Figs. 46-1 and 46-5). Each professional is then sent a referral or orders, depending on the setting. The content depends on the team process in effect in that setting. Referrals in the medical model or multidisciplinary team model should include all elements listed in the first part of Table 46-7 to provide adequate communication (22). The referral should include a mechanism for feedback and possibly an invitation for pretreatment discussion as to the most efficacious plan of treatment. If such an approach is taken, priority must be given to responding to therapist-initiated phone consultations, similar to the courtesy that should be offered to referring physicians (see Table 46-5) (57). Referrals to interdisciplinary team members often are requests for evaluation, with the specifics of treatment to be discussed and agreed on at the next team confer-

---

TABLE 46-7. Seven Requirements for Therapy Referrals

Required of *All* Referrals
1. Discipline of therapist to whom referral is directed: may include referral to a specific team
2. Diagnosis for which treatment is being requested
3. Request for evaluation
4. Goals of treatment with expected duration
5. Intensity, frequency, and initial duration of treatment desired: may be modified after consultation with therapy professional according to patient's rate of progress
6. Precautions: include other diagnoses or problems that could impede or contraindicate certain interventions, and necessary patient monitoring during therapy with recommended limitations to maintain patient's safety
7. Mechanism for feedback, date, and signature: date when physician is to reevaluate patient, request for phone consultation or progress reports, or implied team staffing if referred to an established team

Specifics *Possibly* Needed in Therapy Referrals
1. a. If a specific therapist is desired may be listed as "*Discipline*/Attention: *Therapist's Name*"
   b. If to a specific team, may include each therapy discipline desired or left to be defined, implying referrals will be generated to all disciplines for an initial evaluation; specific therapy orders would then be determined at team conference
2. a. Onset of diagnosis or associated problem
   b. Include both physical problem and relevant medical diagnosis and onset
   c. May include multiple relevant problems and respective underlying diagnoses
   d. Associated psychosocial problems that may affect goals or outcome
3. a. Specify desired testing and reporting mechanisms
   b. Specify intervals between any retesting or reevaluation desired.
4. a. Detailed short- or long-term goals usually based on problems listed above, or
   b. Detailed component tasks to be accomplished and sequence desired
   c. Estimated length of time expected to accomplish each of the above goals
5. a. Location of therapy desired (e.g., bedside, department or gym, inpatient, outpatient)
   b. Desired duration of each treatment session
   c. Specific therapeutic modalities desired, with intensity, duration, frequency, and timing with other therapeutic interventions described (see Chapters 17 through 29)

   d. Endpoints or decision points and criteria for increasing or decreasing therapy in general, or a specific intervention's frequency
   e. Specific education for patient and mechanism to evaluate effectiveness of this teaching
   f. Home program training desired, including timing or criteria for such transition
   g. Nature of home program to be taught: frequency, duration, and intensity of modalities, therapeutic exercise, or other interventions
   h. Handout materials specifically desired
   i. Anticipated or desired home equipment training or trials
   j. Duration until therapist follow-up, if any desired, to reverify or enhance compliances with home program and maintenance of gains
6. a. Specifics of monitoring desired: type, frequency, timing during therapeutic interventions, and criteria to discontinue or specifically modify intervention
   b. Criteria for immediate physician notification
   c. Specific precautions to ensure therapist safety (e.g., infectious, patient behavior, or violence risks)
   d. Specific modality precautions given the patient's diagnoses
   e. Complete list of patient problems or complete diagnosis list
   f. May include physician's evaluation report
7. a. Next physician follow-up date
   b. Anticipated physician follow-up frequency
   c. Possibly desired phone consultation before initiating therapy
   d. Desired frequency of follow-up reports and mechanism (written or phone)
   e. Details desired in follow-up reports
   f. Third-party reporting required or desired
   g. Criteria to discontinue or duration to continue therapy should physician follow-up not be obtained
   h. Date or week desired first to discuss this patient at team conference
   i. Frequency of team conferencing desired, especially if different from team's norm
   j. Desired emergency health system to be activated should patient decompensate
   k. Provision of phone, address, and paging numbers to contact the referring physician; mechanism for emergency contact provided

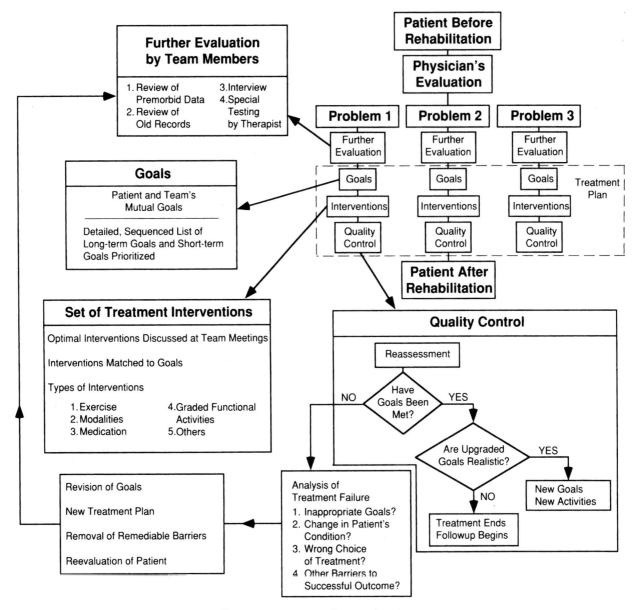

Figure 46-7. Treatment-planning algorithm.

ence, at which time a written treatment plan and orders will be developed. Referrals that are to be addressed by a transdisciplinary team can be performed in a way similar to the interdisciplinary team, if a postevaluation conference can be planned; otherwise, they are best left in the detailed format of the medical model. Protocols may be established by the collective consensus of a treatment team, especially for commonly seen disorders that require little variation in approach. These should be agreed on by all treating professionals before their implementation and often require significant development time. A protocol must not become an excuse not to think or customize the treatment approach according to the patient's unique needs and circumstances. All formats for orders should provide a mechanism for feedback, and the treating team should discuss any changes in treatment required as the patient progresses.

Therapy Quality Control

Without appropriate follow-up, the efficacy of any intervention cannot be evaluated or documented. Referrals for therapy, as well as any prescribed equipment or medication, require follow-up. Often what was desired and presumed to be well communicated by written prescription or referral by the physician is not what occurred with the patient and the therapist. Feedback enhances the accuracy of conveying the correct messages and should be encouraged (32). Receiving feedback helps the rehabilitation physician obtain a broader and more complete perspective on the patient's required needs and provides information necessary to evaluate progress. A certain degree of feedback is built into the multidisciplinary and interdisciplinary models as well as the transdisciplinary model if the physician is a cotherapist. Otherwise, mechanisms to ensure feedback are essential to good written referrals and orders. Quality control requires not only feedback and follow-up but appropriate corrective actions (Fig. 46-7).

In the medical model, the attending physician alone bears the responsibility for ensuring feedback, providing appropriate follow-up, and initiating additional contacts as problems arise. The physician's judgment determines whether outcomes are adequate and whether treatment is brought to closure.

TABLE 46-8. Examples of Detailed Prescriptions for Durable Medical Equipment (DME) and Therapy Generated from Problem List, Leading to Goals, Which Lead to Specific Interventions

This level of specificity may not be required when working with a known therapist with whom treatment protocols have been previously discussed; however, the required 7 elements from Table 46-7 should be included. This is for both patient safety and billing needs as well as to optimize care.

Problems ↓	Peroneal palsy, likely recovery within 6 months	Left shoulder adhesive capsulitis
Goals ↓	Eliminate toe catching with ambulation	Improve shoulder external rotation and then abduction, while avoiding impingement, to functional and, if possible, normal range.
Interventions	DME prescription: Please fit with off-the-shelf polypropylene ankle-foot orthosis set at 90°, and provide single cane adjusted to patient. Diagnosis: Foot drop secondary to peroneal palsy; needed for more than 6 months; medically necessary to provide safe gait. Date: _____	DME prescription: Please issue yellow, red, and green theraband exercise elastic cords. Diagnosis: Deficient rotator cuff on left; medically needed over 6 months for proper shoulder function Date: _____
	Therapy referral: Date: _____ P.T. X 1 visit Dx: Peroneal palsy with footdrop. Goals: Improved gait safety and efficiency, and eliminate toe catching during gait; prevent heel cord contracture. Precautions: Mildly decreased sensation on foot dorsum, gait instability, chronic intermittent hepatitis B, fluid precautions, and train in the use of AFO. Please evaluate and train in the use of AFO; including donning, doffing and skin checks. Teach home program for gastroc. stretching. Also, train in proper gait, including stairs and rough terrain, with cane to be used until patient becomes comfortable with balance. I will follow up pt. at 2 weeks; please send report. Thank you.	Therapy referral: Date: _____ P.T. 3 times per week for 4 weeks. Dx: Left shoulder adhesive capsulitis Goals: Improve external rotation by 20° and shoulder abduction by 30° in 4 weeks. Precautions: Patient S/P rotator cuff repair 2 weeks ago with weak rotator cuff muscles and increased impingement risk; pulleys are contraindicated. Please evaluate and manually stretch left shoulder, including scapular mobilization, avoiding shoulder impingement, while applying ultrasound to anterior, then posterior joint to start at 1.5 watts/cm² and adjust to highest level comfortable for 10 minutes at each site. Teach home program for self-stretching of external rotation only (abduction) and rotator cuff muscle strengthening with progressive therabands will be added later. Pt. will be reevaluated in 4 weeks. Please send progress report, including shoulder active and passive range of motion measurements every 2 weeks. Please call 123-4567 for any questions. Thank you.

Table 46-8 shows examples of referrals and orders that arise from this model.

In the multidisciplinary team, the members give input as to whether goals are being achieved and, if not, why. Problems with progress also can be discussed in team conferences, with solutions derived between the consultants and the primary team-leading physician. Identification of problems and necessary corrective actions becomes a more joint effort as the consultants collectively discuss a single patient's care.

In the interdisciplinary team, a sense of mutual responsibility demands rapid identification and problem solving by the team for any problem perceived by a member. Solutions are achieved by interactive discussions, brainstorming, and finally mutual consensus over the optimum course to be taken. Problem identification and corrective actions are a team process. It is this process that forms the strength of the interdisciplinary team and occupies the greatest time in patient care team conferences.

In the transdisciplinary team, problems are agreed on so rapidly during treatment that larger-scale or longer-term problems may be ignored or not formally considered. If such a problem currently is affecting treatment, it should be solved by mutual discussion and problem solving. Feedback, discussion, and problem solving occur so fluidly and rapidly that the physician member may be left out until after a solution has been decided and enacted. This diminishes the value of the physician's expertise to the team and can create conflicts should the physician subsequently believe alternative approaches are indicated. Even if by mutual consent the treating therapist and patient concur, the patient may come to doubt the treatment team's or physician's expertise. More likely, the physician's opinion will be viewed as obtrusive, given the relative paucity of time he or she has been involved in the patient's team care. Thus, corrective action can be a disjointed process in the transdisciplinary model unless the physician is an integral cotherapist.

Diagnosis-related groups (DRGs), implemented in 1983 to cap Medicare expense growth, created incentives for improved efficiency in terms of hospital costs. This prompted the development of care paths in an attempt to optimize hospital resource utilization. Now the Centers for Medicare and Medicaid Services (CMS), which supplanted the Health Care Finance Administration, has implemented a prospective payment system (PPS) for rehabilitation based on the functional independence measure (FIM) with Case Mix Groups (CMGs) defining reimbursement, similar to the DRG system for acute care (48,59; and see Website at cms.hhs.gov). Besides increasing the efficiency of cost containment, managed care desires to document maintenance of quality. The ability to measure quality requires some degree of uniformity of approach across institutions for comparisons. Care paths, or protocols for patient treatment, help establish a greater degree of uniformity of patient care. Care paths are ideally targeted for populations for whom 75% are expected to follow a typical course. More customization is typically required in rehabilitation than for other medical care. Care paths are most easily developed for postsurgical patients in whom few complications are expected, such as elective orthopedic cases. In the acute-care setting, 20% to 60% shorter lengths of stay have been obtained by implementing such protocols. Few studies have been done in rehabilitation settings, but one study showed no impact on cost or length of stay when a care path was used versus the usual interdisciplinary team approach. The high level of coordinated care that already exists in comprehensive rehabilitation settings may explain this result (60).

Managed care continues to dominate many markets, as was predicted (61). Competition for these contracts and the quality improvement management techniques fostered by the JCAHO and CARF promote the development and implementation of care paths even in rehabilitation, where their value has yet to be firmly established (9,24,60). Care paths or treatment protocols have many labels, including critical paths, practice guidelines or parameters, clinical guidelines, clinical pathways, care maps, flow charts, anticipated recovery plans, or case management (60,62). Care paths for inpatient comprehensive rehabilitation units will become more common as managed care increases. The development of such paths always needs to be customized to each particular setting, ideally by an interdisciplinary team. It is hoped that such protocols will improve efficiency without sacrificing the individualization of care required by most complex rehabilitation inpatients.

EQUIPMENT PRESCRIPTIONS

Prescriptions can involve not only needed therapies but also necessary adaptive equipment. The use of adaptive equipment or tools is an important component of the rehabilitation of people with disabilities (63,64). Frequently, appropriate equipment may represent the difference between being functionally independent and requiring the assistance of a caregiver to perform necessary tasks for self-care and activities of daily living (ADL). The ultimate goal in rehabilitation is for the patient to achieve the highest level of independence possible. This requires the effective integration of adaptive equipment into the patient's individualized treatment as necessary (65).

The importance of adaptive equipment and devices is illustrated by the diversity of items available to enhance mobility or perform ADL (66). Adaptive devices and equipment are categorized according to the functional skills they are devised to facilitate. These include ADL (e.g., dressing sticks, sock-aides, rocker knife, reachers, etc.), mobility (e.g., gait aids, positioning and transfer equipment, wheelchairs, etc.), communication (e.g. picture boards, Passy-Muir valves, Electrolarynx, computer augmentation, etc.), environmental management (e.g., adaptations, environmental controls, etc.), and leisure and recreation (e.g., adaptive sports and leisure equipment, specialized prostheses, etc.).

Concomitant with the availability of an increasing array of adaptive aids is the inconsistent evaluation of the efficacy of these devices (67). Both information regarding development and research as well as printed information resources are variable in quality and content.

Changes in a patient's functional status through the rehabilitative process introduce another aspect of consideration in adaptive equipment use and length of need. Improved function through time could mean decreased need for adaptive equipment. However, patients with progressive neurologic conditions may require more sophisticated assistive technology if they are to be as functional as they wish to be. The goal would be the attainment of the highest level of independence with the least adaptive equipment. All these factors are part of the process for the selection of adaptive equipment.

Devices and equipment can be very costly. Costs can be minimized by using rentals or 30-day trial usage when utility is uncertain. When items are more unique and customized, costs increase, whereas more commonly used devices can be mass-

produced and become more economical. Some costs may be decreasing because some adaptive devices are being increasingly used by a normative aging population to facilitate their self-care and functional performance (e.g., a reacher rather than standing on a step stool to reach items in the closet or pantry, a long-handled shoe horn that makes it unnecessary to bend over when putting on shoes, etc.).

Frequently, commercial devices must be adapted to the patient to provide for appropriate, individualized fit. Training also is required for the patient to achieve proper and optimum use of the equipment. In addition, the items of adaptive equipment on the market do not remain static; there are ongoing additions to the available repertoire. These changes can represent refinements on current items, new adaptations, or equipment using new technology.

Types of Adaptive Equipment and Devices

SELF-CARE AND ACTIVITIES OF DAILY LIVING EQUIPMENT

Equipment that aids in self-care and facilitates the activities of daily living constitutes a category that encompasses a wide variety of items. These adaptive devices generally contribute to the patient's independence in performing these activities, with the ADL dysfunction dictating the type of adaptive equipment needed. For example, a stroke patient may be able to perform only one-handed activities, owing to upper-extremity hemiparesis. Therefore to facilitate eating, a plate guard and adaptive eating utensils such as a rocker knife may be appropriate. The use of the equipment should serve the two purposes of providing the patient with independence in eating a meal and releasing the caretaker from the supervisory or assistive task during the eating process. Other examples for this patient might include a suction-based hand brush to assist in hygiene and a dressing stick to help in performing dressing activities independently with one hand. (See Chapter 77 for additional details.)

The diagnosis, prognosis, and residual function of the patient indicate the types and extent of equipment (68,69). A general rule of thumb is that the more restricted the patient is in performing ADL, the more adaptive the equipment must be and the more extensive will be the collaboration among occupational therapists, physical therapists, and speech-language pathologists to provide adequately for the patient. Rehabilitation engineers also can be helpful members, particularly when the custom adaptations are extensive or complex. Common vendor sources are listed in Table 46-9; data bases, in Table 46-10; and consumer sources, in Table 46-11. Many consumer advocacy groups and their patient information resource materials can now be accessed through Internet searches. Table 46-11 lists some of the more germane Internet addresses.

Mobility

There are several types of mobility equipment. There are many items that help to facilitate ambulation. Canes and walkers are frequently used, with each offering a method of facilitating ambulation as well as enhancing ambulation safety. Prostheses or orthoses also are designed to assist in ambulation and mobility. (See Chapters 60, 63, and 64 for additional details.)

Positioning adaptations and seating systems can range from the very simple to the intricate. Proper positioning provides the preliminary and necessary basis of posture for the teaching and development of other life skills. Good body support and head control are essential for many activities. Positioning can be simple, such as the placement of a wedge or bolster. It also can involve elaborate seating configurations that require training for proper measurements and construction. The mainte-

TABLE 46-9. Major Sources of ADL Devices
AliMed 297 High Street Dedham, MA 02026 (800) 225-2610
Concepts ADL, Inc. 10804 Mark Twain Road West Frankfort, IL 62896 (800) 626-3153
Independent Living Aids, Inc. P.O. Box 9022 Hicksville, NY 11802 (800) 537-2118
Don Johnston Incorporated 26799 West Commerce Drive Volo, IL 60073 (800) 999-4660
Graham-Field Health Products, Inc. 2935 Northeast Parkway Atlanta, GA 30360 (800) 347-5678
Maddak, Inc. 661 Route 23 South Wayne, NJ 07470 (800) 443-4926
North Coast Medical, Inc. 18305 Sutter Boulevard Morgan Hill, CA 95037-2845 (800) 821-9319
Sammons Preston Roylan, Inc. P.O. Box 5071 Bolingbrook, IL 60440-5071 (800) 323-5547
ADL, activities of daily living

TABLE 46-10. Databases and Resources for Rehabilitation
ABLEDATA Listings of assistive technology products and devices for people with disabilities and seniors. The database includes architectural elements, communication, computers, controls, education management, home management, orthotics, personal care, prosthetics, recreation, seating, sensory disabilities, therapeutic aids, transportation, vocational management, walking, and wheeled mobility. Sponsored by the National Institute on Disability and Rehabilitation Research, U.S. Department of Labor. ABLEDATA 8630 Fenton Street Suite 930 Silver Springs, MD 20910 (800) 227-0216 *http://www.abledata.com*
Accent on Living Information on rehabilitation aids and devices, disability service organizations, and publications; buyers' guide biannually. Accent on Information P.O. Box 700 Bloomington, IL 61702 (800) 787-8444 *http://www.blvd.com/accent*
CTG (Closing the Gap) Solutions Focuses on computer services and applications for the disabled. Closing the Gap P.O. Box 68 Henderson, MN 56044 (507) 248-3294 *http://www.closingthegap.com*
National Health Information Center This health information referral service was established by the Office of Disease Prevention and Health Promotion (ODPHP) within the Public Health Service. The objectives are to identify health information resources, channel requests for information to these resources, and to develop publications in print and electronic form on health-related topics of interest to health professionals, health-related media, and the public. National Health Information Center P.O. Box 1133 Washington, DC 20013-1133 (800) 336-4797 *http://nhic-nt.health.org(NHIC)*
National Rehabilitation Information Center (NARIC) This is a library and information center on disability and rehabilitation funded by the National Institute on Disability and Rehabilitation Research (NIDDR). The collection includes commercially published books, journal articles, and audiovisuals, as well as federally funded research projects. Documents cover all aspects of disability and rehabilitation, including physical disabilities, independent living, employment, mental retardation, medical rehabilitation, assistive technology, psychiatric disabilities, special education, and law and public policy. REHABDATA is the bibliographic database that contains citations and abstracts of the materials in the collection. REHABDATA 8455 Colesville Road Suite 935 Silver Spring, MD 20910-3319 (800) 346-2742(V/TT) *http://www.naric.com/naric*

nance of skin integrity is another aspect of seating and positioning equipment that must be considered. As with adaptive devices, the more involved the seating requirements are, the more important it is to have representatives from occupational therapy and physical therapy with the physiatrist to formulate the seating requirements. (See Chapter 58 for additional information.)

Transfer equipment to facilitate a patient's movement from one place to another will depend on the amount of assistance required by the patient for the transfer. A transfer board is the simplest item of equipment for transfer. This is used to facilitate safe movement of the patient from a wheelchair to a bed, a chair, or an automobile. The less able the patient is to assist in the transfer process, the more elaborate or complex is the equipment needed. Transfer equipment can be manually or electronically operated and may require little or no exertion by the person being transferred or the person assisting in the transfer.

Wheelchairs are another category of mobility equipment and may be manually or electronically operated. (Wheelchairs are discussed further in Chapter 59.) The selection of the type of mobility aid will depend on the person's residual motor power to facilitate the process. Car and van adaptations, as well as community mobility in general, are discussed in Chapter 60.

Communication

Augmentative and alternative communication systems are a major area of equipment provision. These devices are becom-

ing increasingly more involved and more readily available. They range from low-tech communication boards and pointing devices through complex computer-based communication systems. The physiatrist should collaborate with a speech-language pathologist and an occupational therapist in selection of the optimal augmentative communication system for the pa-

TABLE 46-11.   Sources for Direct Consumer Adaptive Aids
Adapt-Ability, Inc.   9355 Dielman Industrial Drive   St. Louis, MO 63132   (314) 432-1101
Bruce Medical Supply   411 Waverly Oaks Road   P.O. Box 9166   Waltham, MA 02454-9166   (800) 225-8446
Enrichments Catalog   c/o Sammons Preston Roylan, Inc.   P.O. Box 5071   Bolingbrook, IL 60440   (800) 323-5547
Independent Living Aids, Inc.   P.O. Box 9022   Hicksville, NY 11802   (800) 537-2118
North Coast Medical, Inc.   18305 Sutter Blvd.   Morgan Hill, CA 95307-2845   (800) 821-9319

tient. The speech-language pathologist would recommend the most appropriate device for communication. For the motorically challenged patient, the occupational therapist would recommend the most appropriate switch- and control-operated devices for the patient. The provision of adapted computer inputs is now an important area of consideration in the lives of people of all ages (70). (See Chapter 45 for additional information.)

Environmental Management

Various adaptive devices are available to provide assistance in the home (71). Most of the devices are engineered for use in the kitchen. These can include one-handed cutting boards, one handed sandwich holders, stove overhead mirrors for wheelchair-mobile people to see the top of the stove, and other items. Adaptations also are available for washer and dryer operation. Numerous devices are available for the bathroom to assist in independence and safety. Environmental controls for home management are another example of assistive devices. Electronic Aids to Daily Living (EADLs), formerly known as environmental control units, can consist of a few simple devices (e.g., for turning on and off a light or television) or more elaborate systems that manage many of the electric functions in a home. These can be introduced in the rehabilitation unit environment (hospital-based EADLs) (70). (See Chapter 60 for additional details.)

Adaptations can also be made in the work environment to facilitate use by those requiring accommodations. Frequently this is done on an individualized basis. If necessary, site visits are made to determine the needs for either adaptations or equipment. Considerations such as space needed for a wheelchair to turn or to pass through a door, and alterations of table position or height to a comfortable work level are examples of work adaptations.

Leisure and Recreation

People may want to pursue old hobbies or develop new leisure and recreational activities. Because of dysfunction, adaptations

of equipment required for an activity may be indicated. Just as with other previously described devices, coordination would be indicated for equipment provision. The therapeutic recreation specialist may assist in the identification of the leisure or recreational activity that a patient wants to pursue. The occupational therapist or orthotist may assist in the provision and fitting of the appropriate adaptation or splint needed to perform tasks involved in the activity of interest. (See Chapter 24 for additional information.)

Resources

Commercial vendors sell equipment and many adaptive devices (72). Most items can be used as purchased; others will need adaptations that customize the devices for the person. At other times, equipment will have to be individually designed and constructed to meet patient needs. These special items are done on an individual basis by bioengineering or orthotics with professional input from occupational or physical therapy, or others.

There is wide variation in the cost of equipment, the requirements for documentation for procurement of equipment, and the availability of equipment for patient evaluation trials for efficacy. Some items, such as wheelchairs and EADLS, can be very costly to procure. Ideally, there would be a range of items within each category (e.g., ADL, mobility, communication) available to use for patient assessment or training, but often this is not economically feasible. Vendors sometimes can provide equipment for patient assessment and use. Equipment pools are another resource where equipment no longer needed by people or equipment shared among several facilities in an area can be used to assist in the evaluative and training process.

Prescriptions for Devices

Any device, be it a simple plate guard for eating or the most elaborately configured electric wheelchair, typically requires a physician prescription for insurance coverage, including Medicare. Even without insurance coverage, a physician's prescription often allows medically necessary devices to be purchased free of sales tax in many states. Those items that are considered durable medical equipment (DME) require specific information for prescription coverage. Not all items are DME. To avoid confusion and minimize patient expense, it is useful to provide a comprehensive equipment prescription for all medically necessary devices.

The patient's name and diagnosis are included in the information part of the prescription. Then the initial part of the prescription is the name of the item, the stock number or other identifiers, and, when appropriate, the source of the item. All parts, sizes, adaptations, colors, and so on, are included, as applicable. The justification and rationale for the item are included, as well as the estimated duration of use. A permanent need is documented as "greater than 12 months" for Medicare prescriptions. When expensive devices are being requested, it usually is necessary to receive approval from the third-party payer before ordering such equipment.

DME Quality Control

Regardless of what adaptive equipment or device is ordered for a patient, there is a responsibility to ensure that the patient receives training in its use. Also, some items, such as wheelchairs, require fitting. Both the physician and therapist requesting the equipment are responsible for ensuring that the equipment fits the patient and that the equipment received is operational for its intended purpose. This is especially true in managed-care settings, in which negotiated DME contracts may exist and determine what equipment is available. Timely follow-up is indicated for reassessment of the patient's use of the equipment and to ensure that the items serve the purpose for which they were initially ordered.

PRESCRIPTION, REFERRALS AND ORDER-WRITING SUMMARY

The ability to comprehensively define the rehabilitation needs of the patient and to request specific, individualized, and appropriate therapeutic interventions distinguishes the physiatrist from all other medical specialties. To successfully identify and accomplish the goals of rehabilitation, the physical medicine and rehabilitation physician works closely with the allied health rehabilitation disciplines and other medical specialties. Referrals, orders, and equipment prescriptions are basic mechanisms by which the physiatrist requests the participation of the other professions in assessment, planning, and delivery of patient care. The necessary elements and specificity of detail included in the referrals or orders are largely determined by the mode of professional interaction and style of communication developed among the members of the rehabilitation team. A cohesive team with well-developed mechanisms for clear communication among its members can result in an approach to rehabilitation that exceeds the sum of its parts. Nevertheless, the rehabilitation medicine physician must be knowledgeable about the treatment strategies used and their potential interactions with the patient's medical problems. Providing appropriate therapy precautions is a particular responsibility of physiatrists. Effectively written referrals, orders, and equipment prescriptions will fully communicate patient needs, desired interventions, appropriate precautions, and expectations, and provide adequate mechanisms for feedback and quality control.

ACKNOWLEDGMENT

Significant contributions were taken and modified from Chapter 1 by Joel A. DeLisa, Donald M. Currie, and Gordon M. Martin of the 3rd edition of this text as referenced, which also included substantial historical perspective not included here. The prior contributions, now revised, of coauthors to Chapter 13 of the 3rd edition of this text, Mary E. Heye and Mary Nelle Titus, are also acknowledged and appreciated.

REFERENCES

1. Greshan GE, Duncan PW, Stason WB, et al. *Post-stroke rehabilitation, clinical practice guideline, no. 16.* Rockville, MD: U.S. Department of Health and Human Services, Public Health Service, Agency for Health Care Policy and Research, AHCPR Publication No. 95–0662, May 1995.
2. DeLisa JA, Currie DM, Martin GM. Rehabilitation medicine: past, present, and future. In: DeLisa JA, Gans BM, eds. *Rehabilitation medicine: principles and practice,* 3rd ed. Philadelphia: Lippincott-Raven, 1998.
3. Halstead LS. Team care in chronic illness: critical review of literature of past 25 years. *Arch Phys Med Rehabil* 1976;57:507–511.
4. Keith RA. The comprehensive treatment team in rehabilitation. *Arch Phys Med Rehabil* 1991;72:269–274.
5. Portilo RB. Ethical issues in teamwork: the content of rehabilitation. *Arch Phys Med Rehabil* 1988;69:318–322.
6. Dyer WG. *Team building: issues and alternatives.* Reading, MA: Addison-Wesley, 1977.
7. Robbins SP. *Organizational behavior: concepts, controversies, and applications,* 4th ed. Englewood Cliffs, NJ: Prentice Hall, 1989.
8. Cochrane: *Database of systematic reviews. BMJ,* Tavistock Square, London, BMA House, 1995.
9. Teasell RW, Grant A. Failure to adhere to rehabilitation principles—painful lessons learned. *Am J Phys Med Rehabil* 1999;78:166–168.
10. Sharf BF (in consultation with Flaherty JA). *The physician's guide to better communication.* Glenview, IL: Scott, Foresman & Co, 1984:82–91.
11. Given B, Simmons S. Interdisciplinary health care team: fact or fiction? *Nurs Forum* 1977;15:165–184.
12. Longest BB. *Management practices for the health professional,* 4th ed. Norwalk, CT: Appleton & Lange, 1990:168–170.
13. Rothberg JS. The rehabilitation team: future direction. *Arch Phys Med Rehabil* 1981;62:407–410.
14. Schermerhorn JR, Flint JG, Osborn RN. *Organizational behavior,* 7th ed. New York: John Wiley & Sons, 2000:178–181.
15. Alessandra T, O'Connor M, Van Dyke J. *People smart.* La Jolla, CA: Keynote Publishing Co., 1995.
16. Lundberg LB. What is leadership? *J Nurse Admin* 1982;12:32–33.
17. Longest BB. *Health professionals in management.* Stamford, CT: Appleton & Lange, 1996:277–305.
18. CARF, *2002 medical rehabilitation standards manual: 2.CIIRP.* Tucson: The Rehabilitation Accreditation Commission, 2002.
19. Jelles F, van Bennekom CAM, Lankhorst GJ. The interdisciplinary team conference in rehabilitation medicine: a commentary. *Am J Phys Med Rehabil* 1995; 74:464–465.
20. Wanlass RL, Reutter SL, Kline AE. Communication among rehabilitation staff: "mild," "moderate," or "severe" deficits? *Arch Phys Med Rehabil* 1992;73: 477–481.
21. Nevlud GN. The team approach: current trends and issues in rehabilitation. *Texas J Audiol Speech Pathol* 1990;16:21–23.
22. Spencer WA. Changes in methods and relationships necessary within rehabilitation. *Arch Phys Med Rehabil* 1969;50:566–580.
23. Schulz IL, Texidor MS. The interdisciplinary approach: an exercise in futility or a song of praise? *Med Psychother* 1991;4:1–8.
24. JCAHO, *2002 hospital accreditation standards manual.* Oakbrook Terrace, IL: Joint Commission on Accreditation of Healthcare Organizations, 2002.
25. Melvin JL. Status report on interdisciplinary medical rehabilitation. *Arch Phys Med Rehabil* 1989;70:273–276.
26. Deutsch PM, Fralish KB. *Innovations in head injury rehabilitation.* New York: Matthew Bender, 1989.
27. Rothberg JS. The rehabilitation team: future directions. *Arch Phys Med Rehabil* 1981;62:407–410.
28. McColl MA, Gerein N, Valentine F. Meeting the challenges of disability: models for enabling function and well-being. In: Christiansen C, Baum C, eds. *Occupational therapy: enabling function and well-being,* 2nd ed. Thorofare, NJ: SLACK, Inc., 1997:511–513.
29. Laine C, Davidof F. Patient-centered medicine, a professional evolution. *JAMA* 1996;275:152–156.
30. Haas JF. Ethical considerations of goal setting for patient care in rehabilitation medicine. *Am J Phys Med Rehabil* 1995;74:S16–S20.
31. Given B, Simmons S. The interdisciplinary health-care team: fact or fiction? *Nurs Forum* 1977;16:165–183.
32. Walton RE, Dutton JM. The management of interdepartmental conflict: a model and review. *Admin Sci Q* 1969;14:73–84.
33. Gaston EH. Developing a motivating organizational climate for effective team functioning. *Hosp Commun Psychiatry* 1980;31:407–417.
34. Longest BB. *Management practices for the health professional,* 4th ed. Norwalk, CT: Appleton & Lange, 1990.
35. Longest BB. *Health professionals in management.* Stamford, CT: Appleton & Lange, 1996:166–168.
36. Melvin JL. Interdisciplinary and multidisciplinary activities and the ACRM. *Arch Phys Med Rehabil* 1980;61:379–380.
37. Anderson TP. An alternative frame of reference for rehabilitation: the helping process versus the medical model. *Arch Phys Med Rehabil* 1975;56:101–104.
38. Becker MC, Abrams KS, Onder J. Goal setting: a joint patient–staff method. *Arch Phys Med Rehabil* 1974;55:87–89.
39. Halstead LS, Rintala DH, Kanellos M, et al. The innovative rehabilitation team: an experiment in team building. *Arch Phys Med Rehabil* 1986;67:357–361.
40. Tollison CD. Preface. In: Tollison CD, ed. *Handbook of chronic pain management.* Baltimore: Williams & Wilkins, 1989:ix–x.
41. Mazur H, Beeston JJ, Yerxa EJ. Clinical interdisciplinary health team care: an educational experiment. *J Med Educ* 1979;54:703–713.
42. Reilly Carolyn. Transdisciplinary approach: an atypical strategy for improving outcomes in rehabilitative and long-term acute care settings. *Rehabil Nurs* 2001;26:216–220.
43. Lyon S, Lyon G. Team functioning and staff development: a role release approach to providing educational services for severely handicapped students. *J Assoc Severe Handicap* 1980;5:250–263.
44. Gast DL, Wolery M. Severe developmental disabilities. In: Berdine WH, Edward AE, eds. *An introduction to special education,* 2nd ed. Boston: Little, Brown, 1985:469–729.
45. Darling LA, Ogg HL. Basic requirements for initiating an interdisciplinary process. *Phys Ther* 1984;64:1684–1686.
46. Hoffman LP. Transdisciplinary team model: an alternative for speech-language pathologists. *Texas J Audiol Speech Pathol* 1990;16:3–6.
47. Melvin JL. Rehabilitation in the year 2000. *Am J Phys Med Rehabil* 1988;67: 197–201.
48. Tresolini CP, Bailit HL, Conway-Welch C, et al. *Health professions education and managed care: challenges and necessary responses.* San Francisco: Pew Health Professions Commission, 1995.
49. Walker LO, Avant KC. *Strategies for theory construction in nursing,* 3rd ed. Norwalk, CT: Appleton & Lange, 1995.

50. Woodruff G, McGonigel M. The transdisciplinary model. In: Jordan J, Gallagher J, Huttinger P,et al., eds. *Early childhood special education: birth to three.* Reston, VA: Council for Exceptional Children, 1988.

51. Akhavain P, Amaral D, Murphy M, et al. Collaborative practice: a nursing perspective of the psychiatric interdisciplinary treatment team. *Holistic Nurs Pract* 1999;13:1–11.

52. Lamorey S, Ryan S. From contention to implementation: a comparison of team practices and recommended practices across service delivery models. *Infant–Toddler Interv* 1998;8:309–331, 335.

53. Rosen C, Miller AC, Cate IMP, et al. Team approaches to treating children with disabilities: a comparison. *Arch Phys Med Rehabil* 1998;79:430–434.

54. Lyon S, Lyon G. Team functioning and staff development: a role release approach to providing integrated educational services for severely handicapped students. *J Assoc Severely Handicapped* 1980;5:250–263.

55. Smith DL. Tele-assessment: a model for developmental assessment of high-risk infants using a televideo network. *Infant Young Child* 1997;9:58–61.

56. Melvin JL. Interdisciplinary and multi-disciplinary activities and the ACRM. *Arch Phys Med Rehabil* 1980;61:379–380.

57. Braddom RL. Practice issues in the hospital-based rehabilitation unit. In: Melvin JL, Odderson IR, eds. Clinical rehabilitation and physiatric practice. *Phys Med Rehabil Clin North Am* 1996;7:31–41.

58. Colachis SC. New directions in health care. *Arch Phys Med Rehabil* 1984;65: 291–294.

59. *IRF–PAI training manual.* Buffalo, NY: UB Foundation Activities, Inc., 2002.

60. Odderson IR. Pathways to quality care at lower cost. In: Melvin JL, Odderson IR, eds. Clinical rehabilitation and physiatric practice. *Phys Med Rehabil Clin North Am* 1996;7:147–165.

61. Odderson IR, Melvin JL. Overview of the spectrum of rehabilitation services. In: Melvin JL, Odderson IR, eds. Clinical rehabilitation and physiatric practice. *Phys Med Rehabil Clin North Am* 1996;7:1–4.

62. Lumsdon K, Hagland M. Mapping care. *Hosp Health Netw* 1993;20:3440.

63. Hall M. Unlocking information technology. *Am J Occup Ther* 1987;41:722–725.

64. Vanderheiden GC. Service delivery mechanisms in rehabilitation technology. *Am J Occup Ther* 1987;41:703–710.

65. Loeble D. A decision-making model for the provision of adaptive technology. *Am J Occup Ther* 1999;53:387–391.

66. Enders A, ed. *Technology for independent living sourcebook.* Washington, DC: Association for the Advancement of Rehabilitation Technology, 1984.

67. American Occupational Therapy Association. *Technology review '89: perspectives on occupational therapy practice.* Rockville, MD: The Association, 1989.

68. Hopkins H, Smith H, eds. *Willard and Spackman's occupational therapy,* 7th ed. Philadelphia: JB Lippincott, 1989:498–513.

69. Trombly C, Radowski MV, eds. *Occupational therapy for physical dysfunction,* 5th ed. Baltimore: Williams & Wilkins, 2001:632–663.

70. Cook AM, Hussey SM. *Assistive technologies: principles and practice,* 2nd ed., St. Louis: CV Mosby, 2002:382–398.

71. Dickey R, Shealey SH. Using technology to control the environment. *Am J Occup Ther* 1987;41:717–721.

72. American Occupational Therapy Association. *Technology review '90: perspectives on occupational therapy practice.* Rockville, MD: The Association, 1990.

CHAPTER 47

Vocational Rehabilitation, Independent Living, and Consumerism

Denise G. Tate, Claire Z. Kalpakjian, Liina Paasuke, and Debra Homa

From their inception, vocational rehabilitation (VR) programs have been designed to promote employment opportunities for people with disabilities. Being a productive member of society through the activity of holding a job has been a major goal of rehabilitation in the United States. Our society's values suggest that our self-identity is closely related to our work and our ability to financially support ourselves independently. Historically, VR services have emphasized the provision of services for people with disabilities who have vocational potential. It was not until 1978 that VR services were also provided for those without clear vocational goals. Title VII, Comprehensive Services for Independent Living (IL), an amendment to the Rehabilitation Act of 1973 (PL 93–112), authorizes services for people with severe disabilities, those who require multiple services over an extended period of time, and those whose disability prevents them from working or participating in other major life activities.

This chapter provides the reader with an overview of both the VR and IL programs. The authors review the legislative history and purpose of VR and IL services, and discuss some contrasts between these two service paradigms. In doing so, program service settings and staff are described as well as the processes and services that are utilized to reach individual goals. A brief review of key research findings is offered to assist readers in better understanding the current state of knowledge and implications for practice. Based on these findings, conclusions are offered.

PURPOSE AND CHARACTERISTICS OF VR AND IL SERVICES

The primary purpose of VR has been to assist and enable people with disabilities to increase their productivity, usually through competitive employment (e.g., paid work). VR counselors work with individuals who have a wide range of disabilities. These include physical disabilities, such as spinal cord injury, stroke, arthritis, multiple sclerosis, congenital or orthopedic difficulties, chronic pain, or amputations; cognitive disabilities, such as traumatic brain injury, organic brain syndromes, developmental and learning disabilities; and emotional disorders, including substance abuse problems (1).

The VR process is focused on the individual seeking assistance with the aim of identifying a feasible employment goal and outlining the services needed to achieve employment. This process generally involves (a) individual assessment and planning, which may include interviewing, paper-and-pencil tests, and performance evaluation in real or simulated work situations; (b) service provision, which may include counseling, education, skill training, medical restoration, and procurement of adaptive equipment; and (c) job placement, which may include trial work placements, job development, marketing, and placement in permanent employment. Services provided by public agencies under the Department of Education and private agencies include vocational assessment, work hardening and reconditioning, work capacity evaluation, job site analysis, job accommodations, job-seeking skills, vocational training, job placement, follow-up services, and employer development.

The service provision plan is formalized with an Individual Plan for Employment (IPE), which is jointly developed by the individual and counselor. Once job placement has been achieved, follow-up services are continued for a minimum of 90 days to provide support and consultation to the new employee, and to his or her employer. This helps to ensure that the employment situation is working out satisfactorily for all parties.

In contrast, independent living services are most often provided by a national network of Centers for Independent Living (CILs) across the country. There are currently more than 400 CILs in the United States (2). An IL program can be defined as a community-based program with substantial consumer involvement that provides direct or indirect services (through referral) for people with severe disabilities. These services are intended to increase self-determination and promote independence. Services typically provided include housing, attendant care, reading or interpreting, and information about other necessary goods and services. They may also include transportation, peer counseling, advocacy or political action, training in IL skills, equipment maintenance and repair, and social and recreational services (3). VR programs may provide these services, but on a limited basis as a secondary or supplementary means of achieving the primary vocational objective.

Although the VR and the IL paradigms share a client-centered approach, they differ in their respective emphases. The VR process can be described as deductive in nature. Client characteristics, the nature and extent of the handicap, socioeconomic factors, and other factors are carefully assessed. This information is then reviewed by the counselor and consumer to develop an employment plan. The IL process is equally client centered, but inductive in nature and focuses on achieving independence while the status of the individual continues to be recognized as dependent. The type of intervention is dictated by the type of problem (e.g., housing, transportation, or health). Multiple goals are targeted, and any increase in self-determination and personal participation in the targeted goal areas represents movement away from dependency (4).

Evaluation is an important part of the VR process. It is essential to understanding the effect of the disability on the client. Services are planned on the basis of the findings from the evaluation, and the final goal of VR results from those services. IL services, on the other hand, acknowledge the effect of disability on the client but do not require a thorough analysis of the client, or the disability, as a prerequisite to the provision of services. The success of IL programs depends on the people and resources in the community for direction and support. Consumer involvement is key, ensuring that programs do not lose touch with individual needs and that they maintain their practical and down-to-earth characteristics.

Consumer sovereignty and empowerment have always been hallmarks of the IL movement. The Rehabilitation Act Amendments of 1998 also formalized consumer choice in the vocational rehabilitation process and planning. *Consumer sovereignty*, sometimes referred to as *consumer involvement*, asserts that people with disabilities are the best judges of their own interests and should ultimately determine what services are provided to them. This current rise of consumerism directly challenges the traditional service delivery system. There has been a gradual deemphasis on professional decision making with respect to case planning. Accordingly, service provision plans are now drawn up jointly by the individual with the disability along with his or her counselor. Because of the increased awareness created by advocacy skills training at CILs, many people with disabilities are better informed about their benefits and the regulations of the agencies with which they must deal (5).

LEGISLATIVE HISTORY

Two world wars and federal legislation since the early twentieth century have had a significant impact on VR programs and the IL movement. For a summary of legislative highlights, see Table 47-1.

The VR program was formally inaugurated in the United States in 1918 with passage of the Soldiers' Rehabilitation Act. The Federal Board for Vocational Education, established in 1917 by the Smith–Hughes Act (PL 65–178), was authorized to create VR programs for veterans with disabilities, and the U.S. Department of Labor was charged with locating jobs for these veterans. In part, because of the immensity of this task and the priority given to returning servicemen, civilian rehabilitation did not begin until 1920, with passage of the Smith–Fess Act (PL 66–236), also known as the Civilian Rehabilitation Act. From the beginning, civilian rehabilitation was set up as a grant-in-aid program to encourage participation of the states. This was in contrast to the veterans' rehabilitation program, which was run solely by the federal government.

There was little preexisting knowledge about the VR process, and this knowledge was eventually gained through much trial and error. One of the important principles that emerged early on was that VR is an individualized process, as each person with a disability presents a somewhat different set of issues

and characteristics. Consequently, a casework approach was adopted to address each person's needs. For example, issues of training, education, transportation, functional limitations, vocational interests and aptitudes, family, public stereotypes, work attitude, and job market factors were seen to impact differentially on each individual's ability to obtain suitable employment. This was in sharp contrast to the Worker's Compensation system, which was much more narrowly focused on obtaining a fair monetary settlement for an injured worker. This conceptual and fundamental difference has been largely responsible for the lack of coordination between these two large disability programs.

Over the years, there have been opponents to the provision of VR services by the federal government. Some believed the program to be too socialistic, outside the purview of the federal government, and unconstitutional. The 1920 bill had to be reauthorized every few years and consequently was frequently in danger of being discontinued. However, during the Depression years, a number of new economic security programs were instituted under the direction of President Franklin Roosevelt. The ground-breaking Social Security Act of 1935 included unemployment compensation, old age insurance, aid to dependent children, maternal and child health services, and other important programs. Lobbyists of the National Rehabilitation Association were successful in attaching an amendment to this legislation that permanently authorized annual VR grants to participating states. By 1939, $3.5 million was being given annually to the states for VR service provision, and the program eventually developed solid support among the majority of federal legislators. Like the veterans' rehabilitation program, federal oversight of civilian rehabilitation had become the responsibility of the Federal Board for Vocational Education. Although there were several administrative shifts during the first 20 years, rehabilitation remained under the auspices of vocational education. The Randolph–Sheppard Act of 1936 and Wagner–O'Day Act of 1938 expanded opportunities for individuals with visual impairment to operate vending stands on federal property and required the federal government to purchase certain products from workshops for the blind.

World War II was a catalyst for major changes to both the veterans' and civilian rehabilitation systems. The Servicemen's Readjustment Act (PL 73–346) of 1944, known as the GI Bill of Rights, guaranteed up to 4 years of tuition and a stipend for living expenses for returning veterans, whether disabled or not. Between 1943 and 1953, more than 600,000 World War II veterans obtained VR services, and another 8 million took advantage of the GI Bill. Civilian rehabilitation also was significantly expanded with the Vocational Rehabilitation Act Amendments of 1943 (Barden–LaFollette; PL 78–113). Eligibility for VR services was broadened to include people with emotional disturbances and developmental disabilities. In addition, medical services and income maintenance for trainees were authorized for the first time. Services helped 44,000 civilians with disabilities to find employment in 1949 at an average cost of $150. At that same time, it was estimated that more than 1.5 million citizens were considered vocationally disabled (5).

The Vocational Rehabilitation Act Amendment of 1954 (PL 83–565) laid the groundwork for a tremendous expansion of the rehabilitation programs. Important facets of this legislation included authorization for the use of federal funds to build and expand rehabilitation facilities, authorization of training grants to institutions for the education of new rehabilitation professionals, and extensive funding for research and demonstration projects to improve and disseminate knowledge of rehabilitation treatment. This legislation promoted the professionalization of VR and ultimately led to its legitimacy as an academic

TABLE 47-1. Legislative Highlights of VR and IL Programs

1917	Smith-Hughes Act: Established Federal Board for Vocational Education.
1918	Soldier's Rehabilitation Act: Created vocational rehabilitation programs for disabled veterans.
1920	Smith-Fess (Civilian Rehabilitation Act): Established civilian rehabilitation programs.
1935	Social Security Act: Vocational rehabilitation became permanent federal program.
1936	Randolph-Sheppard Act: Allowed blind individuals to operate vending stands on federal property.
1938	Wagner-O'Day Act: Required federal government to purchase products from workshops for the blind.
1943	Vocational Rehabilitation Act Amendments: Eligibility expanded to include people with emotional disturbance and developmental disabilities; medical services and income maintenance for trainees.
1944	The Serviceman's Readjustment Act: Tuition and stipends for returning WWII veterans.
1954	Vocational Rehabilitation Act Amendment: Authorized federal funds to build and expand rehabilitation facilities; training grants to educational institutions for rehabilitation professionals.
1965	Vocational Rehabilitation Act Amendment: Expanded federal–state funding ratio; included "behavior disorder" as new category (but dropped in Rehabilitation Act of 1973).
1973	Rehabilitation Act, Title V: Creation of Individualized Written Rehabilitation Plan (now IPE) and consumer grievance procedures. Title V guaranteed nondiscrimination against people with disabilities.
1974	Rehabilitation Act Amendments: Gave broader definition of "handicapped" emphasizing limitations in major life activities, not only employment.
1978	Title VII of the Rehabilitation Act Amendments—Comprehensive Services for Independent Living: Authorized grants to organizations receiving federal funds to provide IL services to those with little potential for employment.
1986	Rehabilitation Act Amendments: Authorized supported employment services to individuals who could not be placed in competitive employment; increased use of rehabilitation engineering services.
1990	Americans with Disabilities Act: Prohibited discrimination against people with disabilities in employment, public services, public transportation, public accommodation and telecommunications.
1992	Rehabilitation Act Amendments: Emphasized consumer involvement in development of rehabilitation plans; mandated state rehabilitation agencies establish Rehabilitation Advisory Councils.
1996	Telecommunications Act: Mandated that telecommunication services and equipment be designed and fabricated to be accessible to people with disabilities.
1998	Assistive Technology Act: Provided states funding to develop and expand consumer-responsive technology programs for people with disabilities.
1998	Workforce Investment Act and Rehabilitation Act Amendments: "One-stop" shopping for employment services; emphasized consumer role in service selection and access to information.
1999	Ticket to Work and Work Incentive Improvement Act: Provides SSI and SSDI beneficiaries a "ticket" to purchase VR services from employment network of their choosing.
2001	New Freedom Initiative and Executive Order 13217: Nationwide effort to eliminate barriers to community participation of people with disabilities; six federal agencies directed to review their policies in accordance with new emphasis on community access.

discipline (6). However, this increasing professionalism led to the alienation of many people who became part of the disability rights movement of the 1970s and 1980s. Federal expenditures for VR increased from $23 million in 1954 to $125 million in 1964.

The Vocational Rehabilitation Act Amendments of 1965 expanded federal–state funding ratio to 75% to 25% and provided for extended evaluation for individuals with severe disabilities to determine if VR services would be beneficial. The amendments also extended eligibility to include "behavior disorders," which made it possible for those with substance abuse problems, public offenders, and those who were socially disadvantaged to obtain VR services. However, this category was subsequently dropped in the Rehabilitation Act of 1973, as these individuals required a significant amount of already limited resources, reducing what was available to the more traditional clientele (7). In 1967, VR was charged with applying its methods to assist people who were disadvantaged by reason of educational attainment, ethnic or cultural factors, criminal history, or impoverishment (5), but this was discontinued under the Nixon administration of the early 1970s.

Between 1959 and 1971, there were several attempts in the U.S. Congress to pass legislation authorizing comprehensive rehabilitation services for those with severe disabilities without vocational potential. In 1959, a bill (HR 361) was introduced that contained the term *independent living services* for the first time. In 1961, other bills were introduced calling for the state VR agencies and other organizations to provide IL services; however, they failed to pass. In 1972, a new bill (HR 8395) was written and passed to replace existing VR legislation by including comprehensive rehabilitation services and IL provisions. This legislation was vetoed by President Nixon, who believed that IL would dilute the resources of the VR program. The bill was resubmitted in 1973 and once again vetoed, as the president's advisors felt that the rehabilitation of people without vocational potential was too expensive. In 1973, a compromise was reached and the Rehabilitation Act was made into law. Although the IL provisions were eliminated, the bill emphasized the delivery of VR services to individuals with severe disabilities.

The Rehabilitation Act of 1973 had a major impact on VR programs. Additional important features of the Act were the creation of the Individual Written Rehabilitation Plans (now called the Individual Plan for Employment, or IPE) and consumer grievance procedures. These two innovative measures emphasized for the first time the notion of consumer empowerment with simultaneous changes in language from "client" to "consumer" (8,9). Perhaps the most significant feature of the 1973 Act was the inclusion of a civil rights clause (Section 504) that guaranteed nondiscrimination against people with disabilities in any federally assisted program or activity. The law was interpreted to mean that employers or institutions receiving federal funds were required to make "reasonable accommodations" for otherwise qualified people with disabilities. This provision in the legislation represented cost implications for educational institutions and public transportation systems in the years to follow. For employers this meant job restructuring, workplace modifications, provision of specialized training, or ongoing support. Other sections of the 1973 Rehabilitation Act provided for affirmative action programs for the employment of the "handicapped," barrier-free work areas, and creation of the Architectural and Transportation Barrier Board.

In 1974, the Rehabilitation Act of 1973 was amended to include a broader definition of the term *handicapped individual.* The new definition emphasized limitations in major life activities rather than only vocational objectives. In 1978, several amendments were made to the Rehabilitation Act of 1973, the most important of which was Title VII, entitled "Comprehensive Services for Independent Living." Its purpose was to authorize grants to states to provide services for individuals with significant disabilities who had little potential for employment but who could benefit from services that would enable them to live and function independently. A major limitation of the Rehabilitation Act was that nondiscrimination against people with disabilities was restricted to the federal sector or to organizations receiving federal funds. Furthermore, "despite annual expenditures of $200 to $300 billion on direct subsidies and supports for people with disabilities, more than 70 percent of those who were capable of working and desired to work were still unemployed" (10). The Rehabilitation Act Amendments of 1986 authorized state VR agencies to provide supported employment services to individuals with significant disabilities who could not be placed in competitive employment. As such, long-term placement in workshops was deemphasized. This amendment also increased the use of rehabilitation engineering (7).

The Americans with Disabilities Act (ADA; PL 101–336) was passed in 1990 with extensive bipartisan support after 2 years of intensive lobbying by disability rights groups. This bill was to people with disabilities what the Civil Rights Act of 1964 (PL 88–392) was to African-Americans (11). The ADA prohibits discrimination against people with disabilities in employment, public services, public transportation, places of public accommodation (e.g., hotels and restaurants), and telecommunications. Businesses with more than 15 employees are required to make reasonable accommodations for qualified candidates with disabilities unless such accommodations would impose "undue hardship." Such accommodations might include improving worksite accessibility, equipment modification, work schedule modification, or provision of interpreters. The ADA also spells out regulations for making public accommodations accessible with a distinction between existing facilities and newly created facilities, the latter having more stringent requirements. Accessibility to public transportation was hotly contested because of the potential expense. In the end, it was decided that modification of the transportation system would be phased in over a period of years. Because the bill is so broad and far-reaching, its application to specific circumstances requires some measure of interpretation. In fact, debate on this bill has continued, with some members of Congress still calling for repeal. Nevertheless, the ADA was a historic, landmark piece of legislation that guarantees civil rights for people with disabilities.

The Rehabilitation Act Amendments of 1992 emphasized consumer involvement in the policies and procedures of state VR agencies. This included consumer participation in the development of IPEs. In addition, Rehabilitation Advisory Councils were created and were required to be comprised primarily of people with disabilities (7).

In 1998, President Clinton signed the Workforce Investment Act (WIA; PL 105–220), which included the Rehabilitation Act Amendments. The WIA reformed federal job training programs, creating a new, comprehensive workforce investment system. Its intention was to be a consumer-focused program to help individuals access the tools needed to manage their careers and meet the needs of U.S. businesses to find skilled workers. The WIA is based on a "one-stop" concept of locating job training, education, and employment services available at a single location. As of 2002, the WIA was still in the process of implementation with consumer empowerment facilitated through Individual Training Accounts (ITAs) that allow individuals to "purchase" services they determine best meet their needs (12).

The Rehabilitation Act Amendments of 1998 comprise a major portion of the WIA. Perhaps most important to issues of empowerment and involvement of individuals with disabilities is a change in the language of the Amendments, emphasizing the consumer's role in rehabilitation planning and exercising informed choice through information and support services. Additional changes in language included "significant disability" in place of "most severe disability," and renaming the Individualized Written Rehabilitation Plan as the Individual Plan for Employment. The 1998 amendments require federal agencies to provide, use, and maintain electronic and information technology that gives comparable access to people with disabilities (13).

In 1999, the Ticket to Work and Work Incentive Improvement Act (TWWIIA; PL 106–170) was passed, providing SSI and SSDI beneficiaries with a "ticket" for VR services from an employment network of their choice. By definition, an employment network is any agency or state/political subdivision or private entity that provides or arranges for delivery of services. For example, CILs, state VR agencies, educational institutions, and employment agencies are examples of potential employment networks. The TWWIIA also provided for the removal of work disincentives that many people with disabilities face, namely, the loss of medical coverage. Starting in October 2000, Medicare and Medicaid coverage was expanded to more people with disabilities who were employed. Effective January 1, 2002, the TWWIIA prohibited the use of work activity as a basis of medical review of an individual entitled to insurance benefits, moving away from the either-or thinking that characterized the historical approach to people with disabilities and employment. Earning guidelines also were made more flexible and took into account the cost of living. The TWWIIA was phased in nationally, between 2002 and 2003 (14).

On February 1, 2001, President Bush announced the New Freedom Initiative as part of a nationwide effort to eliminate barriers in the community for people with disabilities. Its primary goals are to (a) increase access to assistive technologies and universally designed technologies, (b) expand educational opportunities, (c) promote homeownership, (d) integrate Americans with disabilities into the workforce, (e) expand transportation, and (f) promote full access to community life. As part of the New Freedom Initiative, President Bush issued Executive Order 13217, entitled "Community-Based Alternatives for Individuals with Disabilities" on June 18, 2001. This order directed six federal agencies, including the departments of Justice, Health and Human Services, Education, Labor, and Housing and Urban Development, as well as the Social Security Administration to evaluate their policies in accordance with this new emphasis on community access for people with disabilities. On March 25, 2002, the department of Health and Human Services presented President Bush with reports from all participating agencies, entitled "Delivering on the Promise: Compilation of Individual Federal Agency Reports of Actions to Eliminate Barriers and Promote Community Integration" (15).

With the passage of the ADA and the New Freedom of Initiative greater emphasis has been placed on making the environment accessible, including the work environment, through the use of adaptive technologies for people with disabilities. This combined legislative effort is expected to positively influence VR and IL practice, thus resulting in more opportunities for employment and a better quality of life for people with disabilities.

Consumerism, Accessibility, and Assistive Technology

Architectural barriers have long been a problem for people with disabilities in accessing work, education, and otherwise actively participating in their communities. The concept of "universal design" refers to the design of products that can be used by all people, as much as possible, without the need for individual adaptation or specialized design. Assistive technology (AT) also has made an important contribution to the independence of people with disabilities, not only through the technology itself, but also through consumer involvement in decisions related to the use of AT. Sherer contends that the broadening of rehabilitation's involvement to the larger community has meant a shift in philosophy from normalization to empowerment, and that AT makes a meaningful contribution to this expansion of rehabilitation's purview (16). Universal design and AT can be thought of along a continuum, with universal design allowing access into the mainstream and AT meeting specific needs of the individual, with some overlap in products that can be either universal in design or AT (17).

AT was officially defined in the 1998 Assistive Technology Act as "any item, piece of equipment or product system, whether acquired commercially off the shelf, modified or customized, that is used to increase, maintain, or improve functional capabilities of individuals with disabilities" (16). AT can range from "low-tech" devices such as walkers or canes to "high-tech" devices such as speech synthesizers or stair-climbing wheelchairs. The 1986 and 1990 amendments to the Individuals with Disabilities Education Act (IDEA) mandated the inclusion of AT devices and services in education, although in practice, fear of excessive costs has limited the inclusion of AT in education plans and programs (18). In 1990, the ADA greatly increased public awareness of physical barriers and mandated uniform national standards for accessibility. Guidelines for accessible design were issues by the Architectural and Transportation Barriers Compliance Board in 1991, which were modified and adopted by the U.S. Department of Justice and became enforceable ADA Standards for Accessible Design (19).

Under a 1990 Rehabilitation Services Administration directive, state VR agencies were expected to include considerations of AT in IPEs and to make available rehabilitation engineering support and services (18). The Telecommunications Act of 1996 (PL 104–104) mandates that telecommunications services and equipment be "designed, developed and fabricated to be accessible to and usable by individuals with disabilities, if readily achievable" (20). The Technology-Related Assistance Act of 1988 (PL 100–407), amended and renamed the Assistive Technology Act of 1998, provides the states with funding to develop, expand, and coordinate statewide, consumer-responsive technology programs. The Act also places a special emphasis on identifying the individual's needs for accommodation throughout the rehabilitation process (21).

Recognition of AT's capacity to allow people with disabilities to have greater control over their lives; greater participation in home, school, work, and community; enhanced interaction with people without disabilities; and a greater array of opportunities were essential to the AT Act's passage (18). The Act's language clearly recognizes the involvement of consumers themselves in "decisions related to the provision of AT devices and AT services." The use of "consumer-responsive" is also an important contribution, referring to "respect for individual dignity, personal responsibility, self-determination, pursuit of meaningful careers, based on informed choice" (21).

THE CONSUMER MOVEMENT IN REHABILITATION

With the emergence of the consumer (in contrast to patients or clients) movement in the early 1970s and its emphasis on self-help and self-direction, the stage was set for the emergence of the IL and Disability Rights movements. Pioneered by Ed Roberts and other individuals with severe disabilities during the early 1970s, the philosophy of IL asserted that individuals with severe disabilities were capable of managing and directing their own lives. Furthermore, the services and supports that people with disabilities need are best delivered by individuals who themselves have disabilities and whose knowledge about both disability and services is derived from firsthand experience.

Empowerment of Consumers

Federal disability legislation increasingly reflects a growing understanding that all people with disabilities need and have the right to make decisions about their own lives (22). Since 1973, political action has been based on a foundation of assumed consumer–counselor partnerships:

- The 1978 Rehabilitation Act Amendments provided that those individuals with disabilities be guaranteed more substantial involvement in the policies governing their rehabilitation.
- The 1986 Rehabilitation Act Amendments added support for individual consumer rights and revised the IPE format to include consumers' statements of their own rehabilitation goals.
- The 1990 Americans with Disabilities Act furthered self-determination by consumers by ensuring rights in the areas of employment, transportation, public services, and public accommodations.
- The 1992 Amendments to the Rehabilitation Act further supported this movement toward self-determination.

Consumer empowerment has become the manifestation of today's rehabilitation policy and practice. Since its beginning, the independent living movement has placed a very high value on consumer control and direction, not only of the services needed by its individual constituents, but also of the institutions and organizations that house its activities and administer its resources. Thus, the 1992 Amendments to the Rehabilitation Act required that a majority of CIL staff, management, and directors be individuals with disabilities.

Increasingly, CILs distinguish themselves from traditional rehabilitation providers by their emphasis on teaching individuals with disabilities how to procure and direct services to meet their own needs, as they define the needs. This is in contrast to medically oriented rehabilitation programs, which rely on the diagnosis of a doctor or evaluation by a therapist to determine the need. Nowhere has consumer empowerment been more strongly embraced by CILs than in the area of advocacy. With the increasing emphasis placed on advocacy by the Rehabilitation Services Agency (federal), many CILs have shifted from active involvement in the process of removing barriers for their individuals to teaching individuals with disabilities how to overcome obstacles, remove barriers, and advocate for change on their own. In addition, a sea of change in attitudes is reflected in legislation such as the ADA, 1998 Rehabilitation Act Amendments, and TWWIIA, which in both spirit and letter promote empowerment of people with disabilities through expansion of choices of services, involvement in rehabilitation planning, and something as simple as a change in language.

Consumer-Related Services and Centers for Independent Living

The specific features of individual IL programs are determined by the individual needs of the consumers served, availability of existing community resources, physical and social make-up of the community, and goals of the program itself. IL support services can be provided by a variety of community-based programs such as self-help and information referral centers, service providers, transitional programs, and residential programs. Between 1977 and 2002, the number of IL programs in the United States grew from 52 to more than 400.

With the 1992 Amendments to the Rehabilitation Act, many CILs are currently placing greater emphasis on systems advocacy and consumer empowerment. Systems advocacy aimed at improving the working conditions of people with disabilities may be focused at the local, state, regional, or national level, depending on the nature of the underlying issue being addressed. Both VR counselors and IL specialists agree that their role is to educate consumers about systems advocacy and the benefits of including people with disabilities in policy-making roles that regulate services available to them.

SERVICE NETWORKS AND STAFF

VR and IL services fostering consumer-driven choices and services are provided by a network of agencies and organizations that are often connected by common goals and principles, as well as funding mechanisms. The following section describes these networks in greater detail.

VR Networks and Services

Either state VR agencies or private, for-profit rehabilitation firms, both of which are described later, have typically provided VR services. However, as noted earlier, the TWWIIA has opened up possibilities for various agencies to provide VR services and receive compensation. In addition, more and more CILs are providing VR services, many in coordination with state VR agencies.

STATE VOCATIONAL REHABILITATION AGENCIES

Although many CILs require that those providing services have firsthand experience with disability, VR counselors hired by state agencies or private rehabilitation firms are formally trained to provide employment counseling for people with disabilities. Typically, the counselor has a master's degree in rehabilitation counseling, guidance and counseling, or social work. A rehabilitation counselor may be certified through the Commission on Rehabilitation Counselor Certification (CRCC) or licensed through their state. Although licensure or certification is not a standard requirement, state agencies typically require it.

VR services are offered in various settings, with state agencies comprising the largest of these. State agencies work with multiple community partners, both to increase awareness of services to individuals and to implement services. These partners can include school systems, CILs, community mental health agencies, hospitals and health-care clinics, substance abuse centers, local support groups, other state and county employment programs, and a host of social service agencies. State or private rehabilitation providers may also contract with community, private, or not-for-profit organizations, which may provide vocational evaluation, sheltered or transitional employment, job coaching, or other specialized job placement services.

PRIVATE REHABILITATION

In the late 1970s and 1980s there was a tremendous growth in the number of private, for-profit rehabilitation firms. Similarly, graduates of rehabilitation counselor training programs were increasingly taking jobs in the private sector rather than with the state and federal VR system. This was due in part to a lack of growth in the established VR system. Another important factor was the increasing attention that insurance companies were paying to controlling costs in an ever-growing medical care reimbursement system. Payers found that, in many cases, contracting VR services relatively early in the return-to-work process could minimize disability payments to injured or ill members. Private rehabilitation firms tend to be smaller, less bureaucratic, and more efficient in their approach to return to work than their state VR counterparts. Their services typically focus more intensely on vocational guidance and placement and they can be less holistic in their approach to the individual. Counselors working in the private sector require basic business skills, knowledge of the insurance industry, an understanding of the worker's compensation system, expertise in legal and medical case management, and the ability to provide vocational expert testimony (23). Many rehabilitation counselors in the private sector are self-employed or co-owners of small firms (24). Private rehabilitation counselors often contract with insurance carriers to provide VR services to those who qualify for these services through workers compensation, auto no-fault, or long-term disability policies; and their services are provided within the insurers' parameters. Consequently, private rehabilitation firms are usually very responsive to the payer's goals and objectives. Because worker's compensation laws are governed by each state, rather than federal law, provision of VR services will vary among different states.

VR SERVICES

Although services vary according to individual needs, the VR process is essentially comprised of evaluation, job-seeking skills training, job analysis, job placement, and job follow-up. (See Fig. 47–1 for an overview of possible VR pathways.)

Cultivating relationships with local employers for employment of people with disabilities also is an important component of the VR process. The following are the various services offered by VR agencies. Whether an agency is public or private will determine the extent to which particular services are emphasized. For example, public agencies (e.g., state VR) will focus more attention on assessment than will a private agency, which will focus heavily on job placement.

The Individual Plan for Employment

The Individual Plan for Employment (IPE), mandated by the Rehabilitation Act of 1973 and required by state VR agencies, must document (a) long-term vocational goal and intermediate objectives; (b) services to be provided; (c) financial responsibilities for the services to be provided; (d) counselor and consumer responsibilities; (e) criteria and procedures for evaluating progress; and (f) an annual review for as long as the case is

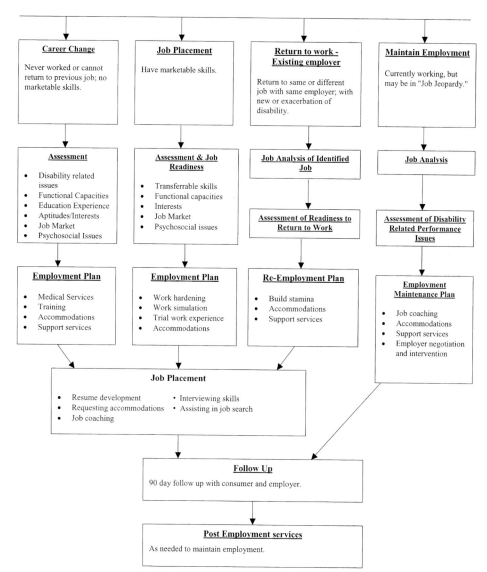

Figure 47-1. Vocational rehabilitation services—possible pathways.

open. Objectives in the plan might include provision of a service such as medical evaluation or treatment, training (e.g., college, on-the-job training, vocational schools), job placement, and specialized adaptive equipment or transportation.

There are several considerations in writing an effective IPE. The barriers to employment and the steps needed to overcome them must be identified in the evaluation process. The evaluation can often be a learning experience for the consumer, who may need help in understanding what the barriers are as well as their own vocational assets and limitations. The counselor also is responsible for understanding the consumer's unmet needs, aspirations, and potentials. The development of a schedule of when and how services will be provided permits periodic evaluation of the program's progress, enabling adjustments to be made as necessary. If the consumer and counselor disagree about the IPE, an ombudsman may mediate the dispute. Provision of this service is required by federal statute and is intended as a safeguard for consumer rights.

Vocational Assessment

Vocational rehabilitation begins with assessment of the consumer's vocational interests, abilities, and vocational potential. By providing information about an individual's strengths and weaknesses and identifying needed services, the vocational assessment helps the consumer and VR counselor set goals and establish a rehabilitation plan. Assessment may also be used to determine eligibility for services and potential to benefit from vocational rehabilitation. Vocational assessment can help the counselor and consumer answer the following questions:

1. Can you return to your former occupation?
2. Would you be able to return to your previous occupation with job accommodations and AT?
3. Which of your skills may be transferable to another occupation?
4. What training or other services would help you become successfully employed?

Assessment is a multidisciplinary process that initially involves gathering data from a variety of sources, such as work and educational history, as well as medical records. For individuals who have received physical rehabilitation services, these records may include a medical examination and reports from the rehabilitation team, such as occupational and physical therapy. The VR counselor may also refer the consumer for additional assessment services, such as a psychological evaluation or a vocational evaluation. The psychological evaluation can provide helpful information regarding the individual's learning abilities, coping skills, and personality characteristics, whereas the vocational evaluation describes important work-related behaviors, capabilities, and interests.

Although the terms *vocational evaluation* and *vocational assessment* are often used interchangeably, *vocational assessment* is a general term that includes many different forms of evaluation. *Vocational evaluation* is defined specifically as a comprehensive assessment that utilizes a variety of tools, including paper-and-pencil tests, structured interviews, and real or simulated work (25). With its focus on work-related abilities, a vocational evaluation may use work samples, situational assessments, and on-the-job evaluations. The work sample approach to measurement has been used most often in vocational evaluation, often through commercial work sample systems (e.g., VALPAR or Singer) designed to simulate specific jobs or a cluster of jobs; a vocational evaluation may also incorporate actual work samples from industry.

Using a variety of evaluation procedures can help verify other assessment data and thereby contribute to more accurate findings and recommendations (25). Cross-validating assessment data may be especially important for persons with disabilities, as concerns have been raised about the validity of paper-and-pencil tests for this population, particularly for individuals with severe disabilities (26). In addition, vocational evaluation may incorporate AT during the assessment process—for example, by modifying work samples or other test instruments, and by making recommendations that include consideration of specific AT devices that would maximize the consumer's vocational potential (27). For example, the vocational evaluator may recommend speech-recognition software to enable a consumer with limited hand function to perform a job requiring computer access.

Evaluation of an individual's functional skills is an important part of the assessment process and can be applied to various domains, such as independent living skills, interpersonal communication, sensory awareness, emotional stability, learning ability, and stamina. Many functional skills can be observed as part of a situational assessment or on-the-job evaluation, as well as through more formal methods, such as work samples and inventories. Sophisticated systems designed to measure a wide range of physical capacities such as lifting strength are also available, including the ERGOS Work Simulator and the BTE Simulator. These systems are more likely to be used as part of a Functional Capacities Evaluation (FCE) conducted at a work-hardening center, rather than during a vocational evaluation.

Employment Readiness

Several key dimensions are assessed to determine job readiness. Medical stability is an important concern, as many conditions fluctuate over time (e.g., multiple sclerosis), interfering with maintaining employment. Stamina and endurance are also important when considering both job demands and work schedules (i.e., part-time vs. full-time). Psychosocial factors such as the individual's support systems are critical to employment success, as is the availability of adequate attendant care. Transportation is another critical element in job success, as public transportation can be inaccessible and is often unreliable.

The individual's psychological readiness to go to work also must be addressed. This includes motivation, self-confidence, interpersonal flexibility, coping resources, and realistic expectations about work. Motivation to work is not simply a personal characteristic, but also a function of a person–environment interaction (28). People have needs beyond the financial, such as satisfying interpersonal contact, achieving a sense of belonging, being productive, and enjoying creative expression, all of which can greatly contribute to motivation for work.

Job Placement Strategies

Once the individual is ready to seek employment, he or she must develop or refine the employment skills that will be required for success in the job search, which will largely be determined by past experience. For example, the individual who acquired a disability later in life and who has a long work history will likely need to refine job-seeking skills that include addressing disability issues with potential employers. The individual with virtually no work history will require far more extensive job-seeking-skills training, which typically includes identifying and following up on job leads, resume writing, application completion, and interviewing skills.

Job placement activities can be viewed along a continuum, ranging from self-placement to the counselor assuming all placement responsibility. The skills and personality traits of the job seeker, the nature of the disability, local market conditions, and even luck influence the extent of counselor involvement. The IPE will target the consumer's job goal, specify acceptable geographic and environmental criteria, consider the types of job accommodations needed, and specify follow-up and support services required. A primary role of the VR counselor is to assist the consumer in developing job-seeking skills using such tools as coaching, role playing, or video taping. In addition to job seeking skills, he or she must also know how to respond to questions about disability, either on an application or in an interview. Knowledge of legal protections, such as those stipulated by the ADA, is critical for the individual with a disability who is seeking employment.

Job Analysis

Job analysis can be critical to the ultimate success of job placement efforts. By analyzing a particular job in a certain environment, suitable accommodation recommendations can be made. The job must be analyzed for factors in the work environment, job tasks, and productivity. An analysis of environmental factors may consider parking at the worksite, restrooms, cafeteria, and building accessibility. The physical requirements of the job must be assessed, such as lifting, grasping, standing, walking, sitting, talking, hearing, writing, and reading. For people with cognitive or affective limitations, other critical factors might include the work atmosphere (e.g., busy or relaxed) and cognitive demands (e.g., memory, reasoning, problem solving). Because of the need for being knowledgeable about state and national standards for accessibility, occupational safety and health standards, business practices and organizational structure, and roles of labor and management, along with employer needs in order to best represent the consumer, job analysis is one of the more demanding tasks of the VR counselor (23).

Job Accommodations

Requesting a job accommodation is another skill that should be developed. Although the individual is expected to know what accommodations are required, the VR counselor can often act as a consultant to the employer and can help to negotiate these. As stipulated by the ADA, the employer is required to make reasonable accommodations; however, this term is not clearly defined in current legislation. Some employers view this as prohibitively expensive, although the majority of accommodations cost less than $500 (29). In fact, job accommodations can reduce worker's compensation and other costs. Some accommodations may be as simple as a rearrangement of equipment. For example, for individuals using wheelchairs, a height-adjustable desk, a voice-activated speakerphone, or moving office supplies to accessible drawers are low-cost and simple accommodations. Other examples of accommodations include job restructuring (e.g., trading off essential job tasks), flexible schedules, large print, allowing use of personal care attendants or service animals, and large-button phones.

Job Follow-up Services

Follow-up services for both consumer and employer help to ensure a successful outcome and are an important step in the job placement process. Intervention may be needed to help solve problems the consumer may be having that affect work performance or work relationships (30). Accommodations may require further adjustments after the individual actually begins the job. Finally, it is important that an employee who cannot function successfully be removed from the job, as the primary goal of VR is a successful outcome for both the individual and the employer.

Employer Development

Many employers still object to hiring individuals with disabilities on grounds of increased cost and risk in insurance rates, environmental modifications, safety, job performance, and job stability. Thus, a primary goal of the VR counselor continues to be to dispel these misconceptions of both employers and workers with disabilities (30). Toward this end, it is essential for rehabilitation professionals to be visible and active in business organizations and to continue to build credibility within the community. Services that can be marketed include recruitment and referral of qualified applicants, consultant services (e.g., ADA compliance, job accommodation, and disability awareness training programs), employee assistance programming, and support and follow-up services.

IL SERVICES

The IL process of assisting individuals to adapt themselves and their environment to the reality of disability is often more fluid and multifocused than is the VR process, which focuses its attention on employment. Living independently with a severe disability in a physical and social world that is often less than accommodating presents a lifetime of challenges. Attention to individual needs also is critical, as people with disabilities do not stop along the developmental trajectory because of the onset of disability. For example, the same individual who may appear totally unhampered by his or her disability in one area of life, or during one stage of development, may at another time or under different circumstances be completely overwhelmed by any one of the myriad challenges presented by a severe disability.

The IL process begins when an individual with a disability realizes that an obstacle exists because of a limitation, preventing realization of a desired goal. For some individuals, this realization may come with the acquisition of a disability, whereas for others it may come after years of institutionalization. In other cases, the IL process may begin when an individual who has lived independently with a severe disability encounters new circumstances, such as a change in employment, housing, physical capacity, or relational status.

For an individual with a developmental disability who may have lived all his or her life in an institution and now wants to live in his or her own apartment, the IL assessment will need to be comprehensive. It will typically include such areas as personal hygiene, medication management, problem-solving and decision-making skills, social skills, housekeeping, shopping, meal preparation, money management, telephone skills, and emergency procedures. In contrast, for a middle-aged individual returning home after a spinal cord injury, the initial assessment may focus on the ability to perform a standard list of ADLs, the need for social services, emotional concerns, the impact of disability on personal relationships, and the needs for home modification and personal assistance. In either case, the goal of the IL assessment is to identify the individual's goal and provide the IL counselor with the information necessary to assist that individual in developing a plan to achieve his or her goal.

As consumers are assisted in growing and adapting to disability, the IL program provides concurrent services directed at changing the environment by removing barriers to the realization of personal goals and by remediating discriminatory practices (31). The IL programs can also offer housing assistance, attendant care training and referral, reader and interpreter referral, financial benefits counseling, and community awareness and barrier removal programs. Other services may include family counseling, vocational counseling, legal service counseling, health-care or nutrition education, equipment maintenance and repair, and social and recreational programs.

Attendant care is one of the services most closely associated with the IL movement. The attendant care concept touches nearly all the themes considered important to the IL movement, as it assumes that the person with a disability is well informed about his or her own medical care needs and has the necessary skill and ability to direct and monitor his or her own personal care (32). The Medicaid program has become one of the main sources of funding for consumer-directed attendant care services. The CILs are responsible for educating consumers about their rights and benefits under Medicaid and about how to recruit and train their own attendants. The IL program's focus on the cognitive and emotional aspects of independence uses the peer role model; that is, a person with a severe disability living independently who can provide motivation and counseling about dealing with the realities of living with a disability. Specific areas in which peer counselors can provide help can include management of personal care attendant services, equipment purchase, exploration of community resources, dealing with grief and anxiety, and self-advocacy (33).

EMPLOYMENT OUTCOMES: A REVIEW OF FINDINGS

An overview of rehabilitation studies on employment, VR, and IL outcomes among people with physical disabilities suggests a number of factors that may assist VR counselors and IL specialists in identifying those who have a great need for their services. This type of research can be helpful in informing rehabilitation professionals about personal and environmental conditions that facilitate or limit employment after disability. Based on these findings, specialized programs can be put into practice to assist individuals at risk or who can benefit most from these programs.

Several studies have reported certain demographic and injury-severity and disability characteristics as factors related to vocational outcomes (34–37). In most cases, those returning to work are more likely to be white, younger, and more educated, and to have been employed before the onset of disability (38–40). Age at the time of disability, premorbid employment status, work status, and psychological distress were also found to be significant predictors of successful employment for a group of people with traumatic brain injury (36).

While results are inconclusive about the association of level of disability to employment, several authors have commented on functional independence as a predictor of positive VR and IL outcomes. Tomassen et al. found that functional independence measured by the Barthel index predicted employment after spinal cord injury (SCI) (41). Anderson and Vogel have found that education, community mobility, functional independence, and decreased medical complications were significantly associated with employment, community integration, and IL (34). However, Goldberg and Freed report that level of injury in a sample of SCI patients was associated with motivation to work but not with employment status (42).

Motivation to work appears to predict employment status across several disability groups (38–40). Internal locus of control is frequently discussed as an important predictor of job search and employment success (43). McShane and Karp reported that strong motivation, greater social support, and ability to drive one's car were directly predictive of paid employment (44). Similarly, the vocational satisfaction of people with limb loss was improved by better workplace modifications, depending on the level of functional capabilities of the person and job demands (45). Such worksite improvements can be achieved by VR and IL programs working closely with potential employers and at an early stage of the rehabilitation process.

While return to work has been held as the gold standard of benefits achieved by VR programs, little has been said about the effect of IL programs on broader life outcomes such as community reintegration, adjustment, and improved quality of life. Findings reviewed so far suggest that both types of programs can contribute significantly to restoring productivity to a person with a disability, as well as enhance self-dignity and provide a greater measure of personal control. These results can guide VR counselors and IL specialists in designing better approaches and programs targeting individuals at risk; using appropriate methods to determine their functional, personal, and cognitive needs; working with prospective employers; and emphasizing the use of technologies to facilitate employment and access to work environments.

CONCLUSIONS

Although philosophically at different ends of the continuum, the VR and IL processes are becoming increasingly similar as both stress the importance of the environment and of AT in rehabilitation. These programs also complement each other in many ways. The VR programs are goal oriented and provide people with disabilities with resources and training needed to find employment or to further education, which can lead to vocational opportunities. In contrast to VR, IL programs promote a greater sense of inner control, self-reliance, and personal achievement. They offer options and encourage self-sufficiency and self-determination in the conduct of daily routines, establishment of social identity, and life choices. IL promotes independence, which in turn can facilitate vocational options.

The role and nature of professional involvement comprise another difference between the two models of service. IL specialists are seen as agents of change and facilitators to help people with disabilities become as independent as possible. Their success in the rehabilitation process is based on their ability to enable consumers to achieve their own goals. Once these personal decisions have been made, the availability of training and other resources external to the individual as offered by traditional VR programs become more meaningful to people with disabilities. The VR emphasis on restoring the individual's

functional independence is complemented by the IL focus on assisting people with disabilities to maintain independent life styles, and to improve their community environment.

The emphasis on outcomes selected from both programs accentuates differences between the VR and IL approach as well. VR programs emphasize competitive, paid employment as a successful outcome. The IL services focus on broader and more comprehensive outcomes that tend to be less quantifiable and concrete. The IL outcomes relate to improvement in one's overall quality of life and self-dignity. These more individualized outcomes are often more difficult to document as identifiable and immediate benefits to payers of rehabilitation services.

As noted in this chapter, technology is also an important issue for both VR and IL programs. Through technology, independence in the basic ADL necessary to getting an education or gaining employment is possible. Technology can help to compensate for functional loss and increase physical and psychological independence. Assistive technology projects more recently being offered in conjunction with VR programs are vital to promote independence in the workplace and beyond. Similarly, according to the IL philosophy, technology is key to the removal of barriers facing people with disabilities in the areas of transportation, housing self-care, and mobility.

In summary, the delicate balance between competency and autonomy fostered by the VR and IL model of services need not be viewed as exclusive of each other. Although most people with disabilities are able to maintain the capacity to make decisions concerning their needs and life-styles, they may need time to be educated and empowered about new roles and options in learning to cope with disability.

REFERENCES

1. Tate D, Heinrich R, Paasuke L, et al. Vocational rehabilitation, independent living and consumerism. In: DeLisa J, Gans B, eds. *Rehabilitation medicine: principles and practice*, 3rd ed. Philadelphia: Lippincott-Raven, 1998:1151–1162.
2. National Council on Independent Living. Available at http://www.ncil.org. Accessed July 24, 2002.
3. Frieden L. Understanding alternative program models. In: Crewe N, Zola I, eds. *Independent living for physically disabled people*. San Francisco: Jossey-Bass, 1983:62–72.
4. DeJong G. Defining and implementing the independent living concept. In: Crewe N, Zola I, eds. *Independent living for physically disabled people*. San Francisco: Jossey-Bass, 1983:4–27.
5. Wright B. *Total rehabilitation*. Boston: Little, Brown, 1980.
6. Berkowitz E. *Disabled policy: America's programs for the handicapped*. Cambridge: Cambridge University Press, 1987.
7. Rasch J. World Wide Web review guide for the CRC examination. Available at http://luna.cas.usf.edu/~rasch/areas.html. Accessed July 31, 2002.
8. Nosek M. A response to Kenneth R. Thomas commentary: some observations on the use of the word consumer. *J Rehabil* 1993;59:9–10.
9. Thomas K. Commentary: some observations on the use of the word consumer. *J Rehabil* 1993;59:6–8.
10. Anderson D. The ADA: our next step toward liberty and justice for all. *Mich Mun Rev* 1994;67:240–243.
11. Treanor R. *We overcame: the story of civil rights for disabled people*. Falls Church, VA: Regal Direct Publishing, 1993.
12. U.S. Department of Labor Employment and Training Administration. Workforce Investment Act of 1998. Available at http://www.usdoj.gov/crt/508/508law.html. Accessed April 30, 2004.
13. Michigan Department of Career Development. Highlights of the 1998 Amendments to the Rehabilitation Act. Available at http://www.michigan.gov/mdcd. Accessed April 30, 2004.
14. Social Security Administration. Social Security Legislative Bulletin. Available at http://www.ssa.gov/legislation/legis_bulletin_120399.html. Accessed April 30, 2004.
15. U.S. Department of Health and Human Services. The new freedom initiative. Available at http://www.hhs.gov/newfreedom/init.html.Accessed April 30, 2004.
16. Sherer M. Introduction. In: Sherer M, ed. *Assistive technology: matching device and consumer for successful rehabilitation*. Washington, DC: American Psychological Association; 2002:3–13.

17. The Center for Universal Design, North Carolina State University. The principles of universal design. Available at http://www.design.ncsu.edu/cud/univ_design/princ_overview.htm. Accessed April 30, 2004.
18. Gradel K. Funding and public policy. In: Olson D, DeRuyter F, eds. *Clinician's guide to assistive technology*. St. Louis: Mosby, 2002:75–88.
19. The Center for Universal Design, North Carolina State University. History and background. Available at http://www.design.ncsu.edu/cud/univ_design/udhistory.htm. Accessed April 30, 2004.
20. Federal Communications Commission. Telecommunications Act of 1996. Available at http://www.fcc.gov/telecom.html. Accessed July 29, 2002.
21. Maryland Technology Assistance Program. Assistive Technology Act of 1998. Available at http://www.mdtap.org/tt/1998.09/1b-art.html. Accessed July 18, 2002.
22. Empowerment counseling: consumer-counselor relationships in the rehabilitation process. *Rehabil Brief* 1994;16.
23. Lynch R, Martin T. Rehabilitation counseling in the private sector: a training needs story. *J Rehabil* 1982;48:51–73.
24. Matkin R. Rehabilitation services offered in the private sector: a pilot investigation. *J Rehabl* 1982;48:31–33.
25. Smith F, Lombard R, Neubert D, et al. Position paper of the interdisciplinary council on vocational evaluation and assessment. Available at http://www.vecap.org/council.html. Accessed April 30, 2004.
26. Power P. *Guide to vocational assessment*. 3rd ed. Austin, TX: Pro-Ed; 2000.
27. Vocational Evaluation and Work Adjustment Association. VEWAA Position Paper on the Role of Assistive Technology in Assessment and Vocational Evaluation. Available at http://www.vecap.org/atrole.html. Accessed April 30, 2004.
28. Keilhofner G. Functional assessment: toward a dialectic view of person–environment relations. *Am J Occup Ther* 1993;47:248–251.
29. Job Accommodation Network. Available at http://www.jan.wvu.edu. Accessed July 19, 2002.
30. Davis D, Paasuke L. Vocational evaluation and rehabilitation. In: DeLisa J, ed. *Rehabilitation medicine: principles and practice*, 3rd ed. Philadelphia: JB Lippincott, 1988:83–94.
31. Nosek M, Zhu Y, Howland C. The evolution of independent living programs. *Rehabil Couns Bull* 1992;35:174–189.
32. DeJong G, Wenker T. Attendant care. In: Crewe N, Zola I, eds. *Independent living for physically disabled people*. San Francisco: Jossey-Bass, 1983:151–170.
33. Saxton M. Peer counseling. In: Crewe N, Zola I, eds. *Independent living for physically disabled people*. San Francisco: Jossey-Bass, 1983:171–186.
34. Anderson C, Vogel L. Employment outcomes of adults who sustained spinal cord injuries as children or adolescents. *Arch Phys Med Rehabil* 2002;83:791–801.
35. Hess D, Ripley D, McKinley W, et al. Predictors for return to work after spinal cord injury: a 3-year multicenter analysis. *Arch Phys Med Rehabil* 2000;81:359–363.
36. Felmingham K, Baguley I, Crooks J. A comparison of acute and post discharge predictors of employment 2 years after traumatic brain injury. *Arch Phys Med Rehabil* 2001;82:435–439.
37. Keyser-Marcus L, Bricout J, Wehman P, et al. Acute predictors of return to employment after traumatic brain injury: a longitudinal follow-up. *Arch Phys Med Rehabil* 2002;83:635–641.
38. DeVivo M, Rutt R, Stover S, et al. Employment after spinal cord injury. *Arch Phys Med Rehabil* 1987;68:494–498.
39. Goldberg R, Freed M. Vocational development, interests, values, adjustment and rehabilitation outlook of spinal cord patients: Four year follow-up. *Arch Phys Med Rehabil* 1976;57:532.
40. Goldberg R, Bigwood A. Vocational adjustment after laryngectomy. *Arch Phys Med Rehabil* 1975;56:521–524.
41. Tomassen P, Post M, van Asbeck F. Return to work after spinal cord injury. *Spinal Cord* 2000;38:51–55.
42. Goldberg R, Freed M. Vocational development of spinal cord injury patients: an 8-year follow-up. *Arch Phys Med Rehabil* 1982;63:207–210.
43. Crisp R. Locus of control as a predictor of adjustment to spinal cord injury. *Austr Dis Rev* 1984;1:53–57.
44. McShane S, Karp J. Employment following spinal cord injury: a covariance structure analysis. *Rehabil Psychol* 1993;38:2–41.
45. Schoppen T, Boonstra A, Groothoff J, et al. Job satisfaction and health experience of people with a lower-limb amputation in comparison with health colleagues. *Arch Phys Med Rehabil* 2002;83:628–634.

CHAPTER 48

Ethical Issues in Rehabilitation Medicine

Janet F. Haas

A 59-year-old man suffered a left hemispheric cerebrovascular accident. Two weeks later, he was admitted to a rehabilitation unit for treatment of deficits resulting from expressive language impairment and right-sided weakness. He did not agree with the self-care, mobility, and speech goals proposed by the rehabilitation team. Instead, he was anxious to return to his home and work. His wife of 30 years was apprehensive about caring for him at his current level of disability and urged the team to continue therapy.

Patients, family members, and practitioners often disagree about the goals, processes, or utility of rehabilitation therapy. Healthcare practitioners face difficult dilemmas as they attempt to set a course that all can promote. In this patient's case, pracitioners were torn between honoring the patient's desire to be discharged and respecting the concerns and wishes of his wife. They did not want to treat a patient who failed to provide informed consent. On the other hand, the practitioners realized that the patient's wife was not prepared to care for him at home. They knew that training would improve his functional abilities and enhance his eventual return home.

Rehabilitation practitioners confront moral quandaries often during the course of practice. A single moral principle—such as that of autonomy or beneficence—may not outweigh all others, yet choices must be made. Practitioners must attempt to reconcile and assign priority to conflicting moral obligations (1). Decisions of a moral nature are distinguishable from those of the law, technology, religion, and politics. They focus on what is proper rather than on what is possible or legally permissible. Considerations of etiquette, cost, and convenience play an insignificant role in moral decision-making.

The terms *moral* and *ethical* are closely related; Cicero apparently used the Latin word *moralis* to translate the Greek *ethikos* (2). Both terms stress manners, customs, and character. Contemporary usage reflects a divergence of meaning, however. *Ethics* refers to theoretical and contemplative descriptions of values. *Morality* describes conduct—that is, whether behaviors are right or wrong.

HISTORICAL DEVELOPMENT

Religious Influences

In the fifth century B.C., Hippocrates described scientific, technological, and ethical facets of medical care (3). The Hippo-

cratic oath developed from the traditions of a religious sect known as the Pythagoreans. The oath pertained to a small group of physicians who lived on the Isle of Cos. It required them to vow secrecy and loyalty to their teachers, to refuse to give deadly drugs to their patients, and to strive to attain virtues of purity and holiness. Physicians were compelled to help patients and forbidden from harming them. They alone were qualified to determine how to benefit sick patients.

Religious traditions influenced the development of medical ethics through the Middle Ages, when monks dominated medical practice, and beyond (4). Since that time, Catholics have integrated principles of medical decision making into their moral theology (3). Protestants have examined specific ethical topics in detail and have incorporated concepts of medical ethics into a larger, systematic theology (3). Orthodox Jews historically have linked Talmudic and rabbinical teachings to the practice of medicine, emphasizing values of preservation and sanctity of life (3).

Secular Influences

During the Age of Enlightenment, the influence of religion on morality in medicine was eclipsed by secular theories of reason and philosophy. Discussion and controversy flourished as scholars studied and debated varied viewpoints. A number of works were published and disseminated (3).

Codes of medical practice developed in time; the first followed an epidemic of typhoid in 1789. Chaos erupted in an English hospital when staff members were required to assume additional, unfamiliar tasks. As tension heightened and some staff members resigned, a retired physician named Thomas Percival sought to restore calm. He designed a code of professional conduct later published in a book titled *Medical Ethics* (3). The virtues of physicians, "tenderness with steadiness and condescension with authority," were expected to "inspire the minds of their patients with gratitude, respect, and confidence" (5). Percival's very words were included in the first professional code of ethics, published in 1847 by the American Medical Association. Physicians were instructed to address the needs of individual patients rather than those of the larger society (3).

Recent Developments

The nature of medicine has changed dramatically in the past 40 years. Technological advances have established a scientific basis for medical treatment. Many diseases can now be cured.

Developments in the biological sciences and health-care fields have given rise to complex and profound moral dilemmas. The study of ethical problems, a central focus of contemporary medicine, transcends discrete professional boundaries.

Daniel Callahan describes five factors that underlie the development of ethical issues in medicine (6). First, technologies such as renal dialysis, organ transplantation, genetic engineering, and embryonal transplantation have expanded our ability to intervene in nature. A strong social commitment to health care coupled with a compelling tendency to apply available technology has made it difficult to restrict technology's use.

Second, medical resources are costly. When medicine could do little to help people, care tended to be cheap. But now that improved neonatal, emergency, and acute care medicine saves many lives, the chronicity and cost of disease have skyrocketed. Americans spent $1.4 trillion on health care in 2001, accounting for 14.1% of the gross national product. Spending over the previous year increased at an unprecedented level, 0.8%. During the years 1992 through 2000, health care spending had ranged from 13.1% to 13.4% of the gross national product (7).

Callahan cites an expanded role of the public as a third factor prompting recognition of ethical issues (6). The solitary and secretive aura of Hippocratic medicine has been supplanted by an environment that is more receptive to public input. More than 80% of Americans die in hospitals. Taxpayers support medical research and fund health-care entitlement programs. Research on human subjects is regulated by federally mandated Institutional Review Boards. Legal issues are increasingly salient in medicine (8).

The language of rights is another evolving concept. Support for individualism in American society and our increasing respect for rights of racial minorities, women, and disabled persons have catalyzed discussion about patients' rights. Medical personnel who respect self-determination and personal dignity acknowledge that patients have a right to make their own decisions (3).

Finally, Callahan cites increasing concern about quality of life. Certainly, many lives are now preserved and extended. We may wonder, however, what kind of life some people will be able to lead (9). At times, the cure clearly is worse than the disease, with its burdens outweighing its benefits (10).

Dramatic change has occurred in the health-care insurance industry in recent years. Mechanisms of reimbursement for health care have shifted as systems of managed care, many operating on a for-profit basis, have spread rapidly. Expectations, relationships, and roles of payers, providers, and consumers have been profoundly altered.

What About Rehabilitation?

Until the recent past, little formal attention was directed to the ethical aspects of rehabilitative care. A number of explanations exist (11). Still a relatively young field, rehabilitation medicine has concentrated on acquiring recognition and acceptance by the medical community (12). Its chronic care dilemmas may seem to lack the drama of life-and-death decisions. Patients often are treated over an extended period of time by a broad range of professionals, none of whom clearly possess responsibility for addressing ethical issues. Educational and training programs have not always sought to promote student awareness of ethical issues.

As moral problems have been identified in fields of chronic care, however, descriptions of ethical dilemmas inherent to rehabilitative practice have appeared in the literature as well (11,13–29). Questions have been raised about duties of profes-

sionals, dynamics of professional–patient relationships, roles and expectations of family members, and goals of care. A discussion of fundamental ethical principles furnishes a conceptual framework to study these issues.

Ethical Principles: Beneficence, Autonomy, and Justice

The term *beneficence* connotes kindness, charity, and the doing of good; it refers to a moral obligation to help other people, refrain from harming them, and attempt to balance benefits with harms. In the health-care setting, beneficence entails an obligation to promote the health and well-being of patients and to prevent disease, injury, pain, and suffering (2).

However, the issue of beneficence becomes complicated when patients' values conflict with traditional medical values of healing and care. There can be a difference of opinion among patients, family members, and professionals about what should be considered the best interests of patients or about what constitutes a good quality of life. Balancing many different interests within a moral framework can pose difficulties. Beauchamp and McCullough wrote that "beneficence includes the obligation to balance benefits against harms, benefits against alternative benefits, and harms against alternative harms" (4). It may not be possible to objectify so many conditions, much less to determine whose perspective should serve as the standard.

The principle of autonomy is grounded in the notion of respect for the values and beliefs of other people. Humans are entitled to privacy and to make decisions about their lives. They are seen to possess a right to self-determination that ensures freedom to make personal choices and to resist the intervention of others. The principle of autonomy gives rise to the principle of respect for other people. Within the context of health care, autonomy underlies the medical doctrine of informed consent. There is an obligation to give patients accurate information about their diagnoses and treatment alternatives, as well as to seek their permission before instituting treatment. Decisions are respected, even if they appear to be unwise (2,4).

Many authors describe tension between the principles of beneficence, which requires acting in a patient's best interests, and autonomy, which entails respecting patient choices (4–30). Balancing the two principles is a perpetual struggle for health-care givers who deem some patient decisions harmful. When patients refuse to accept information, they may be seen to be acting autonomously or, conversely, they may in fact be shirking autonomy. To Englehardt, "the moral obligation to respect persons will often constrain physicians to acquiesce in patients' choices—choices that most likely will lead to the loss of important goods" (30). In fact, health-care givers may be tempted to act paternalistically to restrict patient freedom to make autonomous choices if these are seen to compromise the patient's best interests.

The principle of justice concerns questions of what is due to whom and how to distribute the burdens and benefits of living in a society. An egalitarian model obliges society to provide all its members with a fair share of health-care resources and to treat people equitably. Scarcity of resources or competition for them can create conflict (2). It may be that people should share social goods equally or that an unequal distribution of goods should benefit those who are favored least.

American society has yet to define the basic medical services required by all people. For example, despite the fact that measles and sexually transmitted diseases are public health hazards, some people receive neither prevention nor treatment efforts. Others, however, can obtain organ transplants or extensive cosmetic surgery. Emergency treatments generally are available, but aftercare and rehabilitation to improve the lives saved often are not funded adequately. Entitlement programs in some states pay for procedures not funded in others. Millions of Americans, many of whom work, do not qualify for publicly funded insurance programs yet cannot afford to buy private health-care insurance. Insurance plans, which are often linked to employment, provide widely differing levels of benefit coverage.

Our emphasis on individual desires and dignity has transcended our concern with society's needs. Daniel Callahan ponders what kind of medicine is needed by a good society, one that has other needs such as education, housing, welfare, and culture (9). Determining how much health care to afford spurs us to reflect on how we want to live meaningfully within our larger society. Fundamental questions are challenging to frame and to answer; it is not surprising, then, that we have yet to develop and implement a sound health-care delivery system based on a just social policy.

CLINICAL PRACTICE ISSUES

Acute care physicians attempt to reverse the course of pathologic processes, relieve symptoms, save lives, and discharge medically stable patients. Unlike acute care medicine, rehabilitation does not center on a sick patient whom treatment is expected to cure. Rather, rehabilitation practitioners treat dysfunctions that are chronic, often irreversible, and rarely curable. Residual disability may well persist throughout a person's life.

Medical rehabilitative care addresses impairment caused by pathologic processes that include disease, accident, and congenital abnormality. Disabled persons experience restricted ability to perform activities in a normal manner. When unable to execute activities important to role fulfillment, a person is said to be handicapped (31). Rehabilitation therapy attempts to ameliorate handicap by restoring skills and capabilities through functional retraining and environmental adaptation. Many professionals—including but not limited to physicians, nurses, psychologists, social workers, and educators, as well as physical, speech, occupational, recreational, and vocational therapists—contribute to this effort. They must address and also reach beyond pathologic condition and physiologic function to learn about the unique familial, social, vocational, psychological, and financial characteristics of patients. An unanticipated stairway, an unavailable family member, or limited skin-pressure tolerance may compromise an otherwise successful discharge plan.

Relationships integral to rehabilitation are more complicated than those of a traditional medical dyad of doctor and patient; in fact, a team of professionals and family members concerns itself with each patient's treatment. The many relationships involved can be portrayed by a triangle with points bearing patient; family, which often includes at least several people; and health-care team, with representatives of several disciplines. Individuals at each point of the triangle share concerns with the others but have unique considerations as well. Competing rights and obligations of patients, family members, and practitioners can trigger conflict. Blurred responsibilities and loyalties can cause confusion.

Two studies, building on the seminal description of ethical issues in rehabilitation medicine published in the Hastings Center Report in 1987, have identified ethical issues of most concern to rehabilitation clinicians (17,32,33). Practicing clinicians completed questionnaires in which they were asked to

TABLE 48-1. Clinical Practice and Policy Issues Inherent to Rehabilitation Care

Clinical Practice Issues	Policy Issues
1. Selection of patients	1. Allocation of resources
2. Goal setting for patients	2. Insurance and rehabilitation
3. Patient–practitioner relationships	3. Professional responsibility
4. Professional and team issues	
5. Duties and rights of family members	
6. Quality of life and termination of treatment	

describe ethical conflicts encountered in daily practice. A broad range of clinicians described four primary issues: reimbursement and allocation of scarce resources; setting rehabilitation goals; compromised decision-making capacity in patients; and concerns about confidentiality (32). When asked to scrutinize a pregenerated list of topics, the practitioners prioritized clinical issues involving the treatment team (such as conflicts about legitimate goals of rehabilitation) above their concerns about allocation of scarce resources. Nonetheless, they expressed considerable angst about attempting to balance their obligations to payers with their roles as patient advocates. Ensuring justice in treatment decisions and releasing patients without adequate discharge plans were of substantial concern as well.

In another study, experienced registered nurses, many of whom currently held management positions, reported that they were most seriously troubled about fair allocation of resources, including both overtreatment and substandard treatment of patients. Achieving an optimal balance for each patient of doing good and avoiding harm, while simultaneously respecting patient autonomy, concerned many of the nurses (33). Ethical issues identified in these surveys and additional clinical and policy dilemmas inherent to rehabilitation care (Table 48-1) are described in the remainder of this chapter.

Selection of Patients

Provision of medical care in the United States is based only in part on demonstrated need; in 2000, more than 38 million Americans lacked health insurance for the entire year (34). Even for patients who are insured by a single plan such as Medicare, studies have shown that factors such as race and income affect the care given (35). Persons whose lives have been saved by acute care interventions may not be entitled to reimbursement for rehabilitative care; supply and payment for rehabilitation has fallen far short of demand historically.

To distribute available resources wisely, rehabilitation practitioners screen potential patients before selecting those to treat. They recognize that not all patients will benefit from therapy; some have impairments that cannot be rehabilitated, others are too ill to participate in therapy, and still others have relatively insignificant deficits of functional skills (36). To assess prospective patients, practitioners consult with referring and other treating professionals, review information derived from hospital records, and may examine patients or interview family members.

MEDICAL AND NONMEDICAL FACTORS
Providers consider a variety of specific factors when determining whether to initiate therapy (16). Medical diagnosis and

prognosis are paramount. For example, people with spinal cord injury, amputation, or stroke may be viewed as more likely to achieve functional gains than patients with progressive disorders. Impairments in cognitive or sensory capacity must not preclude effective therapy. Factors such as secondary diseases, medical complications, and requirements for respirators or other specialized equipment must be manageable in a rehabilitation environment.

A patient's ability to learn and retain information is considered crucial to successful rehabilitation, which often requires patients to solve problems by applying new approaches to meet their functional needs. Patient age and predicted course of recovery also influence decisions to initiate care. Despite severe dysfunction, those patients who are expected to make significant progress are usually viewed as good candidates.

Practitioners also explore nonmedical parameters when considering patient admission. They direct particular attention to whether family members are available geographically and emotionally to help patients; strong social support correlates with positive patient outcomes (37). Ability to pay is also a powerful determinant of access to services, because comprehensive coverage permits optimal rehabilitation, and gains made during treatment are more likely to be retained in a setting with adequate financial resources to secure further services and equipment.

Features of the rehabilitation unit also influence selection of patients. Some units specialize in treating specific impairments or in addressing priorities set by regional or national treatment centers. Facilities that emphasize training patients for work require prospective patients to demonstrate vocational potential. Fluctuating bed availability or staffing patterns may affect selection; surplus program capacity at a given time may prompt admission of patients who would otherwise be rejected (16).

VALUES

Practitioners are guided in the selection process by a patient's potential to benefit, ability to pay, and the burden of care that is likely to be placed on staff. The absence of formal, publicly disclosed admission criteria confers significant flexibility on decision makers, but also a potential for injustice resulting from bias or subjectivity. Practitioners who have not received training with respect to moral problems are likely to make judgments that reflect their personal experience, beliefs, and values (16). Their judgments may be influenced by society's desire to save money while caring for its disabled members (17).

Dilemmas abound. Who should be selected: a patient with considerable need but a relatively poor prognosis, or one with lesser disability and the promise of a better outcome? A young person who will use his or her training during a long life span, or an older person who has contributed to society over many years? Should patients who bear responsibility for their disability or who have been noncompliant with past treatment be given a chance?

Our current approach to selection seems to favor those already well off, consistent with Engelhardt's description of "lotteries." The "natural lottery" describes one's talents and abilities, diseases and illnesses; the "social lottery" refers to educational and work status, finances and insurance, and social desirability (38). "Winners" are prepared to manage a complex medical system that can help them cope with disease, but "losers" lack sophisticated resources and may be uninformed about available services. Patients who are already disadvantaged by socioeconomic factors may thus experience restricted access to rehabilitation, but absent an explanation for their rejection, they are unable to challenge selection decisions effectively.

RECOMMENDATIONS

An enormous potential for injustice exists in a system that fails to provide clear criteria or standards for those making difficult selection determinations. Although screening is necessary to assure that patients are medically stable and have remediable functional disabilities, shortcomings of the screening process must be addressed. We should document the factors and processes used to select candidates for treatment, carefully and transparently explain our reasons for rejecting patients, and commit to reevaluating patients in the future. Otherwise, a single decision made relatively early in the course of disease may preclude rehabilitative care. Staff discussions could help practitioners develop consensus about more objective selection guidelines; formulating those guidelines in writing, accompanied with a mechanism for patient appeals, could provide valuable checks and balances to the selection process.

Goal-Setting for Individual Patients

After reviewing a patient's history and physical examination, staff members seek information from the patient and family about personal goals and requirements of the postdischarge environment in order to develop a treatment plan. During the course of treatment, goals are reviewed and adjusted periodically to ensure that they are appropriate and realistic.

Several authors have addressed goal-setting during patient care (22,24,25,39–41). Trieschman asserts the importance of consulting patients and family members to cast and refine goals, and refraining from imposing goals on patients who may reject them in the long run anyway. She cautions caregivers against assuming that skills mastered in the rehabilitation setting will transfer readily to a home environment (42). Becker and associates emphasize the importance of promoting family and staff interaction, and of sharing written goals with the full team in order to identify discrepancies (39).

PROBLEMS OF CURRENT PRACTICE

Although rehabilitation practitioners encourage most patients to take an active role in designing their treatment program, patients may have difficulty setting goals initially. They may feel vulnerable as a result of pain, weakness, fatigue, depression, or anxiety, and may not have come to terms with new or exacerbated disability (43). They may know little about what they will achieve from rehabilitation and may find the rehabilitation unit unfamiliar and unsettling. Behaviors that seemed desirable on the acute care ward—cooperation, passivity, acceptance of frightening or painful interventions—no longer apply. Instead, patients are encouraged to socialize with strangers who may have visible, and perhaps distressing, bodily scars and dysfunctions. Deprived of most daytime visitors, feeling stranded, insecure, and scared, patients are nonetheless expected to assume responsibility for their actions and to participate in treatment. Yet they may lack knowledge about the demands of their new situation; they have yet to return home to live with disability and have been isolated from the real-life experiences that could illuminate their postdischarge needs (25).

VALUES

Different people interpret data about probabilities and outcomes differently. A person's approach to information about risks and benefits, pain, cost, health, and disability is influenced by his or her personal values. Thus, patients, family members, health-care teams, and insurers may advocate for discrepant or even mutually exclusive goals. Patients are likely to want to make decisions that are meaningful to them personally; they also know best how exhausted or disheartened they feel. At the same time, they may feel indebted to family members who seek different goals. Their relatives may believe that, as caretakers, their opinions should take priority. Practitioners, respecting professional experience with disability perhaps more than the wishes of inexperienced laymen, may be inclined to usurp decision-making power rather than to accept choices that will expend time, money, or effort unnecessarily.

RECOMMENDATIONS

The principle of autonomy holds self-determination as paramount regardless of whether patients make ill-advised choices. We know that people often lose autonomy just by becoming patients and knowing less about medicine than do their caregivers. But technical expertise does not imply moral authority. Professionals should refrain from imposing their values on patients; people generally know best what is possible for themselves. Ultimately, when free to do as they wish, patients may refuse tasks that require extensive time, patience, or concentration and discard equipment that is ugly, cumbersome, or unreliable. They may ignore home exercise programs or allow themselves to be taken care of by others. Finances, transportation, or social networks may be insufficient to support the progress they made in the rehabilitation setting (25).

The process of setting goals may unveil tension in patient–provider relationships (25–27). Practitioners should understand their position in regard to patients who have experienced profound, often sudden, loss of physical abilities, and always be cognizant of the power of their recommendations. They should educate patients about costs, risks, and effectiveness of treatment, and discuss with them the medical and functional ramifications of alternative approaches. They should keep in mind that statistical prediction based on objective data is more accurate than clinical predictions, even those based on personal experience (44). On the other hand, it has been argued that an effective and proper role of physicians in medical decision making may entail more guidance on the part of professionals than a model in which the physician is strictly a provider of information to an autonomous patient. But in order to give appropriated recommendations, it is surely necessary for physicians to understand their patient's values and preferences. They must also be aware that persistent beneficence, however well meaning, may compromise a patient's best interests, and that patients should be able to overturn their recommendations.

Clinicians should signal the values, ethical norms, and institutional priorities that underlie their recommendations. Tauber emphasizes that sustained, deliberate efforts to explicate values held by all interested parties and to delineate major value conflicts are essential to resolving the moral issues that impact care of disabled persons (45). Over time and with experience, as patients become accustomed to disability and to their evolving capabilities and challenges, their preferences should be respected. Specific issues of patient competence will be addressed below.

Patient–Practitioner Relationships

Relationships between rehabilitation patients and health-care providers are likely to be of long duration, unlike some acute care relationships (15). The nature of the moral rules and principles that determine exchange of information and provision of services bears exploration.

CONTRACTUAL MODEL

As patients have been accorded greater rights, a new and more egalitarian relationship has replaced the paternalistic connection between patients and providers (17). This arrangement, known as a contractual model, requires practitioners to tell patients the truth, to present options in an accurate and balanced manner, and to avoid deceiving patients. The duty to act beneficiently toward patients is constrained by respect for their autonomy. Physicians supply the medical care that autonomous people, making informed decisions, desire and permit. Respect for confidentiality and privacy are central to developing trusting and egalitarian relationships between patients and physicians.

Caplan describes a number of factors that compromise the relevance of the contractual model to rehabilitation (15). The model presumes a relationship between two parties, a physician and a patient. In rehabilitation, patients work with many health-care providers, only some of whom are physicians, and family members often assume an integral role in treatment as well. Circumstances under which informed consent should be obtained are not always clear. A general consent for rehabilitation treatment and specific permission for invasive procedures are usually obtained, but informed consent is often not requested for many procedures that are performed during a patient's treatment. Perhaps patients should consent to all interventions and should renew their general consent periodically over the weeks, months, or even years during which treatment continues.

The competence of patients during the earliest phases of rehabilitative treatment may be questioned (17,22,26,27). People who have experienced sudden, severe impairment need time to adjust to the reality of disability. Many experience anguish as a result of altered function. They may fear the future and feel unprepared to make decisions for themselves. Even those who retain decision-making capacity may know little about disability and how it may affect their choices. Similarly, family members may not understand a patient's remaining capacities, nor know about decisions that will be faced in the future.

COMPETENCY AND RECOMMENDATIONS

Caplan believes that rehabilitation professionals are justified in overriding autonomous wishes of patients who have not had sufficient opportunity to adapt to impairment and to appreciate future possibilities (15). He argues that early in therapy, practitioners are warranted in using persuasion and other means designed to restore patient identity, capacity to cope, and autonomy in the long run. His conceptualization of an educational model of rehabilitative care underscores earning the patient's understanding and cooperation rather than giving orders, and respecting the complex and evolving nature of relationships between patients and providers. The model emphasizes the importance of instructing patients about disability and encouraging their participation in rehabilitation. It tolerates a greater level of beneficence on the part of providers than is usually accepted in contemporary medicine.

If an educational model for relationships were to be adopted in rehabilitation, periodic assessment of patients' capacities to make autonomous choices would be needed. An independent committee could appraise the evolution of patient autonomy during treatment, for practitioners would need to be mindful that paternalism is appropriate only in a limited sense, and only in the service of restoring autonomous control to patients (17). Patients would be consulted incrementally about the nature of their treatments, and after having an opportunity to adjust to the consequences of impairment, they would resume decision making.

Assessments of patient competency, particularly in persons with neuropsychological dysfunction, focus on specific, contextual competencies rather than global competency. Information should be presented in ways consistent with patient processing skills. Patients are judged competent if they recognize that a decision is needed, understand the pros and cons of proposed options and likely consequences, and can communicate their decisions effectively (44,46). When patients and caregivers disagree, the extent to which disagreements are value laden must be discerned. Identifying relevant values helps elucidate the potential risks and harms of treatment and nontreatment, and underscores the importance of identifying methods to evaluate outcomes. Only in such a manner are clinicians likely to avoid compromising patient autonomy (44,47).

Professional and Team Issues

Rehabilitation treatment is delivered by a multidisciplinary group of professionals who work as a team to address patients' functional deficits and psychosocial and vocational needs. Professionals believe that teams provide a coordinated and comprehensive approach not offered by individual caregivers working independently. Teams can render services efficiently as a result of their experience, economies of scale, and organization of functions (19,22).

MORAL PROBLEMS OF TEAMS

Patients and family members may be relatively unaccustomed to health-care teams whose locus of authority is often unclear. They may tell "secrets" to a provider who is instructed not to tell team members. If the information is important to the patient's rehabilitation, practitioners may be conflicted about whether to honor confidentiality or to act in the patient's apparent best interests. Team members may gather discrepant information from patients and relatives that is difficult to reconcile without alienating some family members.

Members of a rehabilitation team should recognize the vulnerability of patients to subtle pressure. Patients who are exhausted, frightened, or confused may be intimidated by professionals. Purtilo suggests that when outnumbered by the team, patients may feel compelled to follow recommendations with which they do not agree (19).

CONFLICTS AND LOYALTIES

Practitioners serve as teachers or guides to enhance individual patient function and assist adjustment to disability. Team members must address the needs of many patients simultaneously in an efficacious and cost-effective manner. Activities of patients, including smoking, eating, dressing, watching television, and other pursuits, are often governed by institutional policies. When those policies clash with the desires of particular patients, the team must balance the interests of individuals with those of the collective (17).

Controversy about authority and responsibility can arise among team members who recommend discrepant goals for patients or who disagree about how to set priorities among goals. Team members may work with patients in dissimilar or conflicting ways (48). They may disagree about the arrangement of patients' schedules or about the amount of time patients should spend with each professional. Dissension may be difficult to resolve within a team that functions in an egalitarian manner. Team members who share long and difficult hours of work may develop a sense of mutual loyalty that deters questioning another's competency.

RECOMMENDATIONS

Purtilo suggests that a "common moral language" is needed to frame ethical decisions and that teams would benefit from exercises to help them clarify values (19). Training about team dy-

namics and conflict resolution is important, as is the use of sound administrative mechanisms that support timely identification and resolution of conflicts (17,32). Team members must be accountable to the team for their actions and should be willing to raise questions about professional behaviors that appear to compromise patient interests. Recognizing that the team itself may inadvertently intimidate patients, its members must strive to be accessible and to listen carefully to the wishes of patients and families. Team members must treat patients respectfully, even those who are noncompliant or difficult to manage.

Professionals should explain to patients and their relatives the manner in which team members share responsibility and designate authority (17). Similarly, they should clarify lines of communication to alleviate patient uncertainties and anxieties, and should discuss with the family their expectations regarding the nature and extent of family input into decision-making. Practitioners should protect patient privacy and confidentiality to the extent possible, but must emphasize to patients and relatives the need to share relevant information among those concerned with a patient's care. If confidential information must be divulged, patients and their families should be informed. Team members should seek to resolve promptly the inevitable conflicts among patients, family members, and teams to assure effectiveness of patient care. They should be mindful that, on occasion, a rational and supportive decision-making process can be advanced with input from professionals who are not directly involved in a particular patient's care (47). Ethics committees can also be called on to offer a neutral forum for discussion.

Duties and Rights of Family Members

Family members often play an extremely important role in the care of disabled people. The presence of interested and committed family may actually determine whether a patient is admitted for rehabilitation. During treatment, family members meet with the team to discuss goal-setting and postdischarge arrangements.

OBLIGATIONS

There is an expectation on the part of society that family members will assist one another when needs arise. Family or family-like relationships are considered unique in extensiveness and interdependence (17). Family members often undertake special caretaking duties with the understanding that they can provide special emotional support and affection as well as the physical care that patients require (14).

The need for family caretaking has increased over time (49). Outpatient or home settings are less expensive than inpatient facilities and are preferred by many patients. Early discharge often enhances patient autonomy and enables patients to test their skills and the feasibility of their goals in a real-life setting. Thus, some rehabilitative care has shifted to home settings.

A randomized controlled trial of stroke patients with moderately severe disability compared routine hospital rehabilitation with early discharge with continuity of rehabilitation care at home. Patients in the latter group showed better recovery of activities of daily living, ambulation, motor capacity, manual dexterity, socialization, and satisfaction. These patients required half as many hospital resources as the hospitalized group and experienced no difficulties in the use of home help or negative impact on family caregivers (50).

Callahan has noted that many families discover that providing care to their disabled members is mutually satisfying and rewarding (14). Caretakers develop skills and resources that enable them to adapt effectively to new demands. They may take pride in their ability to identify patient needs and to give care in a kind and sensitive way. They may be exceptionally responsive to the patient's situation and offer the care most compatible with it.

Other families experience difficulties, however. Unresolved problems between patients and caregivers may interfere with satisfactory relationships. The demands of caring for a disabled person may exceed the capacities of family members. Strain may result from limited financial resources or inadequate physical facilities. Family members may feel angry, sad, or depressed about the patient's condition. They may question whether they are equipped to deal with a disabled person who has an uncertain prognosis or who faces years of severe disability. Plunged into an unexpected and involuntary situation, they may find their own happiness and welfare threatened.

LIMITS OF DUTY

There is no simple formula to determine how much family members ought to give to patients or what the limits of duty may be. Some people may gladly dedicate the remainder of their days to care for a patient; others may view this as unjustified self-sacrifice (14). Commitments are complicated by the fact that families today are smaller and more dispersed than in the past; several people may not be available to share caregiving tasks. Women may feel a special responsibility to become caretakers, but many work outside the home and have limited availability to perform traditional caretaking roles. Some families are not in a position to provide adequate care despite wishing to do so, whereas others have inadequate financial or emotional resources to do so.

Health-care providers rarely have sufficient knowledge about the lives and relationships of patients and family members to know best how to advise them. It may be difficult to identify the nature of trust and intimacy within specific relationships in a family. Practitioners realize that although patients' needs and vulnerabilities may best be addressed by family caregivers who provide a nurturing and regenerative environment, family members may be unwilling to relinquish plans, hopes, or dreams of their own (14).

RECOMMENDATIONS

Practitioners may be uncertain about how much persuasion is justified as they attempt to convince potential caregivers to commit themselves to patients. When patient needs are minor and family members are likely to sacrifice little, serving the patient's best interests may well entail encouraging relatives to fulfill obligations. When disability is severe and great sacrifice will be required, however, strong persuasion does not appear justified. Callahan points out that our society neither rewards nor honors people who transcend their own needs to care for others; such people are more likely to meet with social isolation than with commendation. They are not treated as heroes, nor should they be expected to act as such (14).

As a society, we have yet to develop mechanisms to reimburse the financial and psychological services that could minimize the burden on caregivers. We need to furnish family members with tools to sustain them, such as daycare centers, respite care, counseling and self-help groups, and adequate physical facilities (49). Only then can society expect any but the most extraordinary people to embrace an opportunity to care for a seriously disabled relative.

Quality of Life and Termination of Treatment

Many factors contribute to decisions to terminate treatment in the rehabilitation setting (17). During rehabilitation care, pa-

tients are expected to make steady and measurable progress toward attaining their goals. When progress slows significantly or patients appear to have reached a plateau in degree of improvement, members of the treatment team may doubt whether continuation of therapy is justifiable. Questions about the efficacy of treatment are typically raised first by professionals, often without consulting patients and relatives—who themselves may well desire to continue working toward goals that professionals deem insignificant or unrealistic. On the other hand, clinicians may be concerned that patients who are about to be discharged have received insufficient treatment (33).

WHOSE VALUES?

Moral values of team members influence termination decisions. Practitioners must assess somewhat nebulous concepts such as "benefit," "productivity," "functional improvement," and "integration into society" as they delineate meaningful and reasonable end points of treatment (39–41,51). Their subjective judgments about the ability of patients to cope with impairment outside the rehabilitation setting affect their appraisals. Their perceptions about acceptable levels of function do likewise, yet their personal values may differ significantly from those of patients (17). The potential for overtreatment likewise concerns professionals; families often request services and equipment that are not clinically indicated.

Our society lacks a commonly accepted way to relate ambiguous concepts of health, function, and quality of life to cherished personal values such as autonomy and independence. Medical practitioners surely do not have the final word on quality of life, nor are their theoretical views—particularly if unexamined—more important than those of others.

Many articles have described subjective quality of life as viewed by persons with disability and demonstrated that adversity does not necessarily cause a person to appraise his quality of life negatively (52). Rather, an individual who adapts to disability may be wholly satisfied with the meaningfulness of his or her life (53). If there is a shortfall between one's aspirations and his accomplishments, however, quality of life suffers to the extent that one has attached significance to his goals (54). Practitioners who make sound decisions to terminate treatment understand patients' values and subjective assessments of a satisfying life.

The progress of some rehabilitation patients may be examined sooner than that of others. Certain patients—those who may be considered noncompliant, uncooperative, or poorly motivated—may be so difficult to manage that the team discusses discharge relatively early in the course of treatment. Many patients have limited insurance coverage. Treating professionals may feel pressure to use scarce resources for new patients, and thus decide to wean care from longer-term patients. A patient's home setting and anticipated level of assistance affect the timing of the decision to curtail care as well.

In recent years, it has become increasingly common for patients to be transferred to rehabilitation before they are able to participate fully in training. Yet they may not be eligible for readmission were they to be discharged until further recovered; practitioners may thus be reluctant to terminate treatment. At other times, onset of medical complications requires transfer to acute care, regardless of patient progress in rehabilitation. Whether to later readmit such a patient for further treatment can be another source of disagreement among professionals and patients.

RECOMMENDATIONS

Even wise and morally sensitive caregivers find it challenging to allocate care among patients. Sometimes rehabilitation teams fail to explain the criteria influencing decisions to end treatment; at other times, nonprofessionals may not appreciate the significance of the many factors assessed. Surely patients and their relatives have a right to learn about the parameters that are used to measure patient progress and the standards that determine whether treatment will be continued. Practitioners have a duty to document information about patient progress so that more objective data underlie the decision to stop care. Patients and relatives should be informed about team discussions concerning termination of care, and their opinions should be sought and honored to the extent possible (17).

POLICY ISSUES

Allocation of Resources

The number of patients who can benefit from rehabilitation grows steadily. Babies who would have died from complications of prematurity or congenital abnormality only a few years ago now survive, but often with significant residual disability. Many injured and sick people overcome life-threatening conditions. Americans live considerably longer than did previous generations; by 2040, 23% of the population is expected to be older than 65 years (55). Not surprisingly, then, chronic disease is becoming increasingly prevalent as a result of population growth, extended life span, and successful acute care interventions. At some point, many persons with chronic disease will require rehabilitation services to enhance their functional skills at work, school, or in the home (49).

COSTS OF HEALTH CARE

The costs of health care skyrocketed in the 1980s and early 1990s and once again are rising rapidly. In 1998, health expenditures were 15% of the gross national product, by far the highest in the world, and nearly double that of the nearest competitor (56). Costs are increasing well above inflation; for example, in a single year, from 1989 to 1990, the cost of health-care premiums increased by more than 17% (57). Even middle-income Americans worry that they could be excluded from necessary health-care services because of inability to pay (58,59).

Yet our national appetite for health-care services increases. Our willingness to provide medical care for patients who will experience marginal benefit serves to increase costs, as does use of hospital-based services and a preoccupation with expensive technology. Fee-for-service reimbursement plans and the practice of defensive medicine are incentives for physicians to render more services (55). People who in the past would have died of trauma to the spinal cord or brain may receive early care worth several hundred thousand dollars; additional costs are incurred from replacing lost wages with income and social supports. Increasing numbers of patients augment demand for acute care and rehabilitation resources. Yet higher costs of care and tighter economic times have forced Americans to choose among health-care services. An unwillingness to afford health care for all Americans who want it has created a system that curtails access to care.

LIMITED ACCESS

A strong national economy led in 1999 to the first decline in the number of uninsured patients in more than a decade. The decrease of 1.8 million that year was followed in 2000 by an additional decrease of 600,000 uninsured persons, primarily attributed to an increase in numbers of children who secured coverage through Medicaid and the State Children's Health In-

surance Program. Nonetheless, in 2000, more than 38 million Americans younger than age 65 were completely uninsured throughout the entire year, and many more had inadequate coverage (59,60). According to the Census Bureau's March 2000 Current Population Survey, more than a third of the poor and a quarter of the near-poor (families with incomes between 100% and 199% of the poverty level) lacked health coverage. Categorical restrictions and income eligibility ceilings in the Medicaid program excluded from coverage many working people with low incomes (61). The presence of a full-time worker does not assure coverage; in fact, 72% of uninsured persons live in families with at least one full-time worker. Impoverished adults are more likely than children to be uninsured (43% compared with 26%, respectively), despite the fact that 71% have at least a high school education and more than a third have had some college education.

Racial and ethnic minorities, 32% of the nonelderly population, make up half of the uninsured; a large majority of the uninsured, 81%, are native or naturalized citizens (59,60). Urban and rural people who are poor receive relatively little medical care. Geographic maldistribution of health-care resources restricts access to care when insufficient numbers of physicians practice in inner city and rural areas. Innovations such as diagnosis-related groups, health maintenance organizations, and preferred provider organizations have reduced health care for underinsured people by precluding practices used in the past to shift costs to insured patients (55). People who lack medical services are known to have worse health than those who receive services, even if factors such as increased stress and poor hygiene are controlled (62). Less healthy people, despite being more likely to qualify for public coverage, are more likely than their healthier counterparts to be uninsured.

Churchill states that despite considering the idea morally repugnant, Americans do ration health care according to ability to pay (55). Physicians have little public accountability regarding whom they treat. Even desperately needed care is typically provided only sporadically to those without financial resources. Many uninsured people forego basic preventive care and therapeutic services such as eyeglasses, hearing aids, and routine dental care. Patient interest groups compete with one another at the federal and state levels to capture and retain limited amounts of funding.

Interventions designed to extend life are often emphasized over those that enhance its quality. The heroism and drama of rescue medicine prevails over more mundane preventive medicine. The United States lacks a coherent and comprehensive approach to address the needs of people of all ages, income levels, and medical needs. Our fragmented system of private health insurance and publicly funded entitlement programs fails many. We struggle to place the needs of one individual within a context of others and to identify and weigh priorities when making allocation decisions (9).

PRINCIPLE OF JUSTICE

A system of medical care should be considered morally acceptable only if it serves principles of equity and justice. A just society does not allocate health care to favor those who are insured, wealthy, and white; rationing is not simply unfortunate, it is unfair. We can respect a community that offers mutual and reciprocal assistance to its members and one that honors its social obligations to care for those who are sick. After all, no one is immune to unexpected disease or calamity. Misfortune can in fact serve to link us to one another (55).

But what services should be offered in a society that cannot afford everything? Principles of utility emphasize services that provide the greatest good for the greatest number of people (2). Principles of justice imply that services should be based on need, a concept that may be subjective and readily confused with highly individualistic desires, hopes, and preferences (9).

When health care is apportioned, as it must be in an era of limited resources, we should avoid discriminating among individuals. Limits should derive from generic guidelines applied to people with common conditions. Private, personal appeals for specialized services should be discouraged (55). Quality, rather than simply length of life, should be stressed. Americans should be assured universal access to basic and primary care services, but access to additional care should depend on its effectiveness and the efficiency with which it can be provided. Costly care of marginal benefit should be discouraged.

We do not actually know how to define an optimal level of medical care, although it is clear that enhanced supplies of medical services lead to greater use, often with little evidence of improved patient outcomes. In a recent study, patients in Minneapolis, Miami, Portland, and Orange County, California were evaluated in their last 6 months of life. The Medicare program pays twice as much per person annually in Miami than in Minneapolis, and the typical lifetime spending for a 65-year-old in Miami is more than $50,000 higher than for a 65-year-old in Minneapolis. Patients in Miami visited medical specialists more than six times as often as those in Minneapolis, spent twice as much time in the hospital, and were admitted to intensive care units more than twice as often. Yet, neither their life expectancy nor their quality of life was improved by their much greater level of treatment (63).

Another study examined the distribution of newborn intensive care specialists and the death rate among newborns; a tripling of numbers of specialists did not improve infant mortality (64). Only when supplies of care dwindle below adequate levels do outcomes deteriorate. Thus, some health-care planners are concluding that maldistribution of medical services can be harmful in two ways: by compromising persons who have inadequate access to care and by encouraging wasteful spending on patients who receive excessive services.

Descriptions of health characteristics such as "quality," "efficiency," and "benefit" are elusive (65). Specialties such as rehabilitation must demonstrate how their treatments promote health, contribute to useful functioning, and prevent illness and deterioration. Services that are demonstrably important and effective are most likely to be considered worthy of continued funding.

Insurance and Rehabilitation

Despite enjoying the most advanced medical technology in the world, Americans worry that this care may one day be beyond their economic reach. In 1993, cognizant of concern about health-care security, President Clinton assembled a task force to draft a health reform act that would guarantee universal, affordable health care (66). Although legislation failed, the intense focus on the health-care industry catalyzed widespread changes within it as employers and the government turned to the marketplace (56).

Managed care is based on the concept of utilitarianism and predicated on an assumption that payers are more qualified to oversee treatment than are either users or providers. Seeking to enhance access to comprehensive, coordinated care delivered in a cost-effective manner, managed care has markedly altered medical practice and transformed relationships among patients, payers, and providers, who are now supervised by payers. It has led to major discordances in the care that patients desire, providers wish to give, and payers are willing to reim-

burse (29). Managed-care plans have reduced hospitalization rates and lengths of stay dramatically, and have restricted access to specialists, expensive tests, and complicated treatments. Many do not cover significant rehabilitation services. Nonetheless, health maintenance organizations are failing to contain costs (60).

Administrators of managed-care plans have been slow to measure quality of outcome after treatment. Rather than being assessed on the basis of patient outcomes, plans compete to attract customers on the basis of price and the results of internal surveys of consumer satisfaction. Information about quality of care has been difficult to access; it is still an open question whether the health status of enrollees has improved (56,67).

In the past, professionals were expected simply to provide services, but today they must also delineate probable outcomes of therapy. It is necessary not only to align expectations of patients, families, providers, and payers in regard to outcome, but for payers and providers to negotiate about the finances required to implement treatment programs. Knowledge about likely patient outcomes plays an essential role in the struggle to balance ethically appropriate services with fiscally responsible expenditures.

Professionals who act as "gatekeepers" to managed-care services experience tension between containing medical costs and advocating for additional resources to benefit individual patients. They often feel that they have lost the ability to guide the care of their patients. More than 75% of physicians surveyed believe that personal financial incentives to restrain testing, treatment, and referrals are not ethical; 87% disagree with payers who discourage physicians from describing restraints in coverage to patients. A similar percentage thinks that professional loyalty to patients has diminished during the last decade. More than half believe that their own patients' trust in them has declined in the past 5 years (68).

Physicians are reluctant to reconceive their traditional role of loyalty to their patients in order to balance the care of each patient with stewardship of collective health-care resources. Caplan agrees that gatekeeping at the bedside is not an ethical solution to the problem of limited resources, but instead serves to undermine patient ability to trust caregivers. Coverage decisions should rest on broad guidelines determined publicly with input from providers, patients, and families (69). National standards are needed to delineate minimal services that must be offered by treatment plans. Appeals processes for patients who find their treatment alternatives unreasonably limited are also important (70).

The many and varied needs of a particularly vulnerable population of patients may be difficult to meet within the resource constraints of managed-care organizations. Ethical questions at the confluence of managed care and the rehabilitation of severely disabled individuals concern use of research and outcome information, roles and responsibilities of practitioners, respect for individualism, patient privacy, informed consent, and the moral character of a responsible rehabilitation institution (28).

Managed care has had a significant impact on the integrity of the practice of informed consent. Gag rules may prohibit physicians from informing patients about potentially beneficial services and the financial incentives and constraints that pertain to professionals who practice within the plan (68). Yet in order to make informed decisions, patients must receive and understand all relevant information (70). A bias to limit treatment inherent to managed-care systems may especially compromise rehabilitation and other lesser-known medical fields.

Despite the promise of various reforms—health maintenance organizations, diagnostic-related groups, managed care within Medicaid and Medicare, heath-care rationing in Oregon, high-risk insurance pools, and for-profit facilities—health-care costs are once again rising rapidly. No program appears to have made a significant dent in controlling costs or capping our ever-swelling medical bureaucracy, or in significantly decreasing the number of uninsured Americans. Bureaucracy now accounts for nearly 30% of health-care expenditures (60).

Moral values that underscore respect for individual rights and freedoms have had a powerful influence on contemporary health care. Values that foster individualism discourage mutual obligations to one another, including to disabled persons who may not be deemed capable of contributing fully to society. A just health-care system should seek to remedy the characteristics of disease and disability that lead to social disadvantage, but managed-care plans often compromise the quality and duration of treatment for chronic impairment (71).

Rehabilitation institutions should seek to benefit vulnerable patients with disability as well as the broader community. The principle of utilitarianism should not necessarily be applied to already marginalized patients. A virtuous institution conveys morally sound values as it assures skillful care of patients and responsiveness to families within a fiscally responsible environment (72).

Professional Responsibilities

RESEARCH

Rehabilitation professionals claim that treatment helps patients improve the quality of their lives as well as the efficacy of their skills (73). Therapy is thought to diminish the burden of disability on patients and their relatives. But many rehabilitation interventions have been based on empirical rather than scientifically collected information. Prospective, controlled epidemiologic studies have been largely unavailable; even retrospective studies of sizable patient populations are few in number. In fact, methods to document outcomes of therapy have been developed only relatively recently (74). Practitioners must emphasize and respond to the need for further research to validate current practices. Sound research protocols, using the gold standard of double blind/placebo treatments to the extent possible, are needed to assure that clinical practice is guided by factual knowledge (12). Patients should be informed when treatments have been recommended for their theoretical potential rather than for demonstrated efficacy.

Many treatments are expensive, time-consuming, and labor intensive. The importance of validating even well-established interventions should not be underestimated. For example, not unlike rehabilitation, surgical procedures often become incorporated into standard clinical practice despite a lack of rigorous evaluation through randomized, placebo-controlled experiments. In a controlled trial to assess the efficacy of arthroscopic surgery to relieve pain in patients with osteoarthritis of the knee, investigators found no difference in improvement of knee pain after treatment than after placebo operation (75). Patients' subjective symptoms improved with each type of treatment and nontreatment, but neither arthroscopic lavage nor débridement improved comfort or self-reported functional outcome more than sham surgery. Nonetheless, 3.25 billion dollars is spent annually on arthroscopy for osteoarthritis of the knee (76).

Some may wonder whether it is justifiable to withhold from control and placebo groups a treatment that is thought generally to be effective. But failing to test efficacy in clinical trials may result in unnecessary morbidity as well as needless expense. Many procedures in rehabilitation, similar to orthopedic

procedures, may appear to be clinically effective, but have not been subjected to scientific study. Particularly when the primary outcome of a procedure is to improve a subjective symptom, use of a placebo in clinical trials is necessary to test efficacy of the targeted treatment.

Critics of the use of placebo in more invasive approaches, such as sham surgery, believe that the potential value of knowledge to be gained from a well-controlled clinical trial does not justify risks to the patient. Yet it has been argued that, for procedures with limited risks that do not substantially exceed other well-accepted research interventions (such as muscle biopsy, bronchoscopy, or testing of experimental drugs), this risk may well be justified in order to understand clinically important information (77). The placebo effect is known to powerfully benefit patients psychologically and emotionally, and has been shown to confer measurable physiologic effects, such as improved patient ability to control hypertension and elevated blood sugar, the discomfort of arthritis, pain, and panic. It has also been shown to alter levels of neurotransmitters, such as dopamine, in the brain (77,78). Even patients who know that they are taking placebo often demonstrate improvement, which may be due simply to the expectation of lessened symptoms or the patient's increased access to medical attention.

Yet another reason exists to prove the efficacy of treatments and new processes (79). Controlled clinical trials and outcome-related research make the strongest case for demonstrating the effectiveness of rehabilitation treatments. In a competitive funding environment, factual evidence helps those who wish to secure additional public funding for rehabilitation (12). Rehabilitation practitioners continually seek to increase the prominence of their field in the eyes of those who fund scientific studies. There is more money available now for scientific evaluation of rehabilitation processes than at any time in the past (17). However, Fuhrer cites three factors that inhibit public support of rehabilitation research:

- Insufficient appreciation of the potential of disabled people for self-sufficiency and economic productivity
- Skepticism on the part of those who fund research about studies directed to palliative efforts rather than to cures for underlying impairments
- Belief that research will produce technology that is excessively sophisticated and expensive

Fuhrer advises practitioners to seek to increase federal funding of research by creating greater awareness of past research successes and demonstrating the monetary benefit of treating disabled people (80).

Clearly such investigation is moral only if informed consent is secured. The medical literature often refers to the importance of using the local institutional review board and adhering to federal and state laws that are intended to ensure patient safety and offer a reasonable balance between risks and benefits. Stineman and Musick describe challenges of obtaining truly informed consent for research studies that involve rehabilitation patients who have significant cognitive, physical, sensory, or developmental disabilities (81). They stress the vulnerability of disabled persons to undue influence as a result of their social isolation, dependency for physical care, or potentially unrealistic therapeutic optimism. The authors distinguish between a patient's global competency and specific decision-making capacity, and cite concern about patient and provider overreliance on proxy decision makers. They also advise that persons should neither be systematically selected nor excluded from studies on the basis of disability.

The prevalence of expensive technologies has made research increasingly important. Rapidly evolving technologies underscore the need to develop criteria for selecting those that will be embraced. At the same time, we must learn to harness sophisticated technologies without allowing technology to become an end in itself. We must decide for whom to provide customized environmental control systems, complicated physical therapy, and sophisticated vocational training, and we must determine how to respond to the ever-expanding demands of people who want unlimited services and equipment.

PROFESSIONAL DUTIES

Rehabilitation professionals have a duty to maintain personal and professional standards of competence in their field. Discipline-specific codes of ethics define appropriate behaviors expected of professionals in a variety of clinical fields. Of increasing concern, however, are relationships among healthcare providers and commercial interests, such as pharmaceutical, assistive device, and medical equipment companies. Weber et al. describe the risk of professionals becoming inadvertently but inappropriately influenced by relationships with biomedical companies that provide not only gifts, free samples, and loans of equipment, but also influence provider opinions by sponsoring educational and informational programs for professionals (82). Commercial sponsorship of research introduces a serious potential for bias in academic research. Ownership of substantial equity in a company, or the availability of stock options and patents with unlimited potential for profit, signify meaningful financial interests that can bias professionals. Professional codes of ethics, including instruments that specify ethics of business conduct, must be enforced to protect the interests of patients and the integrity of professionals in connection with commercial interests (82–85).

Professional interfaces can also raise issues of concern that require attention (17). For example, practitioners need appropriate safeguards in order that they might question the conduct of co-workers or colleagues in other institutions when necessary. Individual clinicians must be supported in situations in which they wish to oppose team norms or expectations. They must feel empowered to decline roles that may be required by the team but that have not been part of their professional training and experience.

Principles of justice confer a duty on practitioners to serve all patients, even those with serious infections. Persons who entered the medical profession did so of their own accord with the knowledge that exposure to contagious disease is an inherent condition of practice. Professionals thus have a duty to treat patients when there is a limited risk of incurring infection themselves, as is likely in a rehabilitation setting (84). Universal precautions should be followed when working with patients who have human immunodeficiency virus (HIV) infection or acquired immunodeficiency syndrome (AIDS). For patients who are approaching death, rehabilitative treatment will be too strenuous or yield minor benefit, but for the many patients who will live for years after diagnosis, rehabilitation care is likely to be of significant benefit (23).

PREVENTION EFFORTS

Some rehabilitation patients became disabled as a result of accident or unwise choices of lifestyle; altered behavior patterns might have avoided disability altogether. For example, alcohol use leads to accidents of all kinds. Excessive speed commonly precedes traffic accidents. Road injuries are more serious when seat belts or car seats are not used. Absence of helmets worsens head injuries of motorcyclists and bicyclists. Firearms produce severe and disabling accidental injuries.

The knowledge that so many of their patients have sustained disability that was preventable should mobilize rehabilitation practitioners to advocate measures such as gun control, stiff penalties against drunk driving, moderate speed limits, and reasonable laws with respect to individual rights and responsibilities. Regardless of their own choices of lifestyle, it would seem that practitioners have an obligation to influence public policies in order to prevent needless disability; no one can portray more vividly the devastating ramifications of impairments such as spinal cord injury or severe brain injury. Practitioners must work to ensure that laws such as the 1990 Americans with Disabilities Act are enforced properly.

PEDAGOGIC ISSUES

In recent years, a number of medical institutions and professional societies have made significant efforts to include ethics topics in their educational programs. Until recently, very few professional training programs in rehabilitation medicine, nursing, allied health, or social work offered courses on this topic, nor were faculty members encouraged to choose ethics as a focus of their teaching and research. Relatively few articles and case materials that apply specifically to rehabilitation have been published (17).

If ethics is to be considered as important to the education of rehabilitation students as it is to students of other disciplines, faculty members will need resources and time to familiarize themselves with ethics; effective teaching requires competent and committed professionals. Some professions (e.g., nursing) and specialties (e.g., family practice, internal medicine) have introduced an ethics requirement into their certification process. Rehabilitation accrediting agencies could likewise emphasize formal teaching of ethics (17). As the number of knowledgeable instructors increases, rehabilitation practitioners might add formal certification requirements in ethics for students in specialty training programs.

Continuing education in rehabilitation should also emphasize the study of ethics. Some rehabilitation institutions have initiated "ethics grand rounds" to discuss topics in ethics, and others have developed ethics committees similar to those in acute care hospitals to explore educational issues through discussion and workshops. Working closely with these committees enables rehabilitation professionals to increase their understanding of ethical problems. A Scholars Program at the Rehabilitation Institute of Chicago and the University of Illinois trains selected clinicians on traditional medical ethics, disability studies, and practical clinical topics part-time over the course of a year. Completion of this professional training program leads to a certificate in disability ethics. Associated efforts include monthly interdisciplinary disability ethics seminars, quarterly grand rounds, and in-house ethics newsletters (32, 86). Expansion of such efforts will increase the ethical literacy of professionals.

Journal editors could encourage examination of clinical case studies and more scholarly writing about policy aspects of rehabilitation. Organizers of medical ethics conferences could sponsor or solicit symposia and panel discussions on interesting ethical topics of rehabilitation. Rehabilitation professionals should work closely with community groups and organizations to enhance discussion about ethical aspects of care. Educating advocacy groups, institutional trustees, staff, patients, and family members about the ethical challenges that confront patients and practitioners is invaluable (17).

CONCLUSION

Rehabilitation practitioners will continue to confront important moral challenges in the coming years. Certainly they must strive to ensure excellent patient care that is based on sound scientific research. They must also assure that patients are treated with compassion and respect in an era dominated by intense financial competition and rapid technological innovation. Close attention should be directed to the personal qualities, manners, sensibilities, and everyday practice procedures of practitioners. The extent to which they tolerate differences and the manner in which they listen to and understand their patients are more important than ever in a rapidly evolving, complex, and somewhat intimidating health-care environment. Providing reassurance and comfort in conjunction with competent care has never been more important.

Health-care practitioners also have a duty to recognize and address problems and inequities of our current medical system. Our competitive, market-based structure has prompted development not only of managed-care systems and for-profit facilities, but an ever-increasing array of commercial opportunities, including the option for practitioners to invest in laboratories, imaging centers, physical therapy clinics, and hospitals. Treatment offered by some "joint ventures" costs more than that delivered at similar facilities not owned by doctors. A study of doctor-owned physical therapy facilities in Florida reported a lower quality of care, fewer licensed therapists, and shorter patient treatment sessions than in facilities not owned by doctors (87).

As rehabilitation practitioners examine the quality and availability of medical resources, they must respond to society's failure to provide millions of Americans with basic medical resources. For-profit facilities, including some rehabilitation facilities, have a negligible commitment to medically indigent people, who are considered highly unprofitable. Access to all medical care for poor people or those who live in rural areas is limited (86). Many insurers preferentially select persons with good health histories while turning away others with chronic diseases who are expected to require costly treatment. Sometimes commercial insurers cancel individual policies.

Rehabilitation clinicians should identify conflicts of interest in their practices and set high and exacting standards for professional conduct. Practitioners have a responsibility to ponder the role of medical rehabilitation in an era of limited resources. Conscious of the fact that some medical needs will remain unmet in a society that has other important needs, they must identify and limit care of marginal benefit or excessive cost. They must inform and educate Americans about important medical needs and help society in its attempt to balance needs of individuals with those of the larger society.

REFERENCES

1. Ross WD. *The right and the good.* Oxford: Oxford University Press, 1930.
2. Beauchamp TL, Childress JF. *Principles of biomedical ethics.* New York: Oxford University Press, 1989.
3. Veatch RM. *A theory of medical ethics.* New York: Basic Books, 1981.
4. Beauchamp TL, Mcullough LB. *Medical ethics: the moral responsibilities of physicians.* Englewood Cliffs, NJ: Prentice Hall, 1984.
5. Percival T. *Percival's medical ethics.* [Originally published 1803.] Reprint, Leake CD, ed. Baltimore: Williams & Wilkins, 1927.
6. Callahan D. Personal communication (Telephone Conversation, January 21, 1998).
7. Pear R. Spending on health care increased sharply in 2001. *New York Times* 2003 Jan 8:13. .
8. Relman AS, Kassirer JP, Angell M, et al. Legal issues in medicine—a new series. *N Engl J Med* 1991;325:354– 355.
9. Callahan D. *What kind of life: the limits of medical progress.* New York: Simon & Schuster, 1990.
10. Dutton DB. *Worse than the disease: pitfalls of medical progress.* Cambridge: Cambridge University Press, 1988.
11. Haas JF. Ethics in rehabilitation medicine. *Arch Phys Med Rehabil* 1986;67: 270–271.
12. deLateur BJ. Fostering research in the physiatrist's future. *Arch Phys Med Rehabil* 1990;71:1–2.
13. Brody BA. Justice in allocation of public resources to disabled citizens. *Arch Phys Med Rehabil* 1988;69:333–336.
14. Callahan D. Families as care givers: the limits of morality. *Arch Phys Med Rehabil* 1988;69:323–328.
15. Caplan AL. Informed consent and provider-patient relationships in rehabilitation medicine. *Arch Phys Med Rehabil* 1988;69:312–317.
16. Haas JF. Admission to rehabilitation centers: selection of patients. *Arch Phys Med Rehabil* 1988;69:329–332.
17. Caplan AL, Callahan D, Haas J. Ethical and policy issues in rehabilitation medicine. *Hastings Cent Rep* 1987;17(suppl):1–20.
18. Jennings B, Callahan D, Caplan AL. Ethical challenges of chronic illness. *Hastings Cent Rep* 1988; 18(special suppl):1–16.
19. Purtilo RB. Ethical issues in teamwork: the context of rehabilitation. *Arch Phys Med Rehabil* 1988;69:318–322.
20. Haas JF, MacKenzie CA. The role of ethics in rehabilitation medicine. *Am J Phys Med Rehabil* 1993;72:48–51.
21. Callahan D. Allocating health care resources: the vexing case of rehabilitation. *Am J Phys Med Rehabil* 1993;72:101–105.
22. Meier RH III, Purtilo RB. Ethical issues and the patient-provider relationship. *Am J Phys Med Rehabil* 1994;72:365–366.
23. Strax TE. Ethical issues of treating patients with AIDS in a rehabilitation setting. *Am J Phys Med Rehabil* 1994; 73:293–295.
24. Purtilo RB, Meier RH III. Team challenges: regulatory constraints and patient empowerment. *Am J Phys Med Rehabil* 1993;72:327–330.
25. Haas J. Ethical considerations of goal setting for patient care in rehabilitation medicine. *Am J Phys Med Rehabil* 1993;72:228–232.
26. Venesy BA. A clinician's guide to decision making capacity and ethically sound medical decisions. *Am J Phys Med Rehabil* 1994;73:219–226.
27. Jennings B. Healing the self: the moral meaning of relationships in rehabilitation. *Am J Phys Med Rehabil* 1993;72:401–404.
28. Haas JF. Ethical issues in physical medicine and rehabilitation: conclusion to a series. *Am J Phys Med Rehabil* 1995;74(suppl):54–58.
29. Haas JF, Mattson Prince J. Ethics and managed care in rehabilitation medicine. *J Head Trauma Rehabil* 1997;12:vii–xiii.
30. Englehardt HT Jr. *The foundations of medical ethics.* New York: Oxford University Press, 1986.
31. Acton N. The world's response to disability: evolution of a philosophy. *Arch Phys Med Rehabil* 1982;63:145–149.
32. Kirschner KL, Stocking C, Wagner LB, et al. Ethical issues identified by rehabilitation clinicians. *Arch Phys Med Rehabil* 2001;82(suppl 2):S2–S8.
33. Redman BK, Fry ST. Ethical conflicts reported by certified registered rehabilitation nurses. *Rehab Nurs* 1998;23:179–184.
34. Ubel PA. "What should I do, doc?" *Arch Intern Med* 2002;162:977–980.
35. Gornick M, Eggers P, Reilly TW, et al. Effects of race on mortality and use of services among Medicare beneficiaries. *N Engl J Med* 1996;335:791–799.
36. Kottke FJ, Lehman JF, Stillwell GK. Preface. In: Kottke FJ, Stillwell GK, Lehman JF, eds. *Krusen's handbook of physical medicine and rehabilitation,* 3rd ed. Philadelphia: WB Saunders, 1982:xi–xix.
37. De Vellis RF, Sauter SVH. Recognizing the challenges of prevention in rehabilitation. *Arch Phys Med Rehabil* 1985;66:52–54.
38. Englehardt HT Jr, Rie MA. Intensive care units, scarce resources, and conflicting principles of justice. *JAMA* 1986;255:1159–1164.
39. Becker MC, Abrams KS, Onder J. Goal setting: joint patient-staff method. *Arch Phys Med Rehabil* 1974;55:87–89.
40. Kottke FJ. Future focus of rehabilitation medicine. *Arch Phys Med Rehabil* 1980;61:1–6.
41. Wallace SG, Anderson AD. Imprisonment of patients in the course of rehabilitation. *Arch Phys Med Rehabil* 1978;59:424–429.
42. Trieschmann RB. Coping with a disability: a sliding scale of goals. *Arch Phys Med Rehabil* 1974;55:556–560.
43. Anderson TP. Educational frame of reference: an additional model for rehabilitation medicine. *Arch Phys Med Rehabil* 1978;59:203–206.
44. Macciocchi SN, Stringer A. Assessing risk and harm: the convergence of ethical and empirical considerations. *Arch Phys Med Rehabil* 2001;82(suppl 2): S15–S19.
45. Tauber AI. Putting ethics into the medical record. *Ann Intern Med* 2002; 36:559–563.
46. Callahan CD, Hagglund KJ. Comparing neuropsychological and psychiatric evaluation of competency in rehabilitation: a case example. *Arch Phys Med Rehabil* 1995;76:909–912.
47. Malec JF. Ethical conflict resolution based on ethics of relationships for brain injury rehabilitation. *Brain Injury* 1996;10:781–795.
48. Booth J, Davidson I, Winstanley J, Waters K. Observing washing and dressing of stroke patients: nursing intervention compared with occupational therapists. What is the difference? *J Adv Nurs* 2001;33:98–105.
49. Lubin IM. *Chronic illness: impact and interventions.* Boston: Jones & Bartlett, 1990;200–217.
50. Holmqvist LW, von Koch L, de Pedro-Cuesta J. Use of healthcare, impact on family caregivers and patient satisfaction of rehabilitation at home after stroke in southwest Stockholm. *Scand J Rehabil Med* 2000;32:173–179.
51. Rusk HA. Rehabilitation medicine: knowledge in search of understanding. *Arch Phys Med Rehabil* 1978;59:156–160.
52. Diener E. Subjective well-being. *Psychol Bull* 1984;95:542–575.
53. van Dijk AJ. Quality of life assessment: its integration in rehabilitation care through a model of daily living. *Scand J Rehabil Med* 2000;32:104–110.

54. Montgomery H, Persson L-O. Importance and attainment of life values among disabled and non-disabled people. *Scand J Rehabil Med* 1998;30:61–63.

55. Churchill LR. *Rationing health care in America: perceptionsand principles of justice.* Notre Dame, IN: University of Notre Dame Press, 1987.

56. Dalen JE. Health care in America. *Arch Intern Med* 2000;160:2573–2576.

57. Freudenheim M. Health care: a growing burden. *New York Times* 1991 Jan 29: D1.

58. Wine M, Pear R. President finds he has gained even if he lost on health care. *New York Times* 1996 Jul 30: 1.

59. The Kaiser Commission on Medicaid and the Uninsured. Washington, DC: February 2002.

60. Woolhandler S, Himmelstein DU. National health insurance. *Arch Intern Med* 2002;162:973–975.

61. Davis K, Rowland D. Uninsured and underserved: inequities in health care in the US. *Milbank Mem Fund Q* 1983:61:149–152.

62. Bayer R, Caplan A, Daniels N, eds. *In search of equity: health needs and the health care system.* New York: Plenum, 1983.

63. Kolata G. Research suggests more health care may not be better. *New York Times* 2002 Jul 21: 1.

64. Goodman DC, Elliott SF, Little G, et al. The relation between the availability of neonatal intensive care and neonatal mortality. *N Engl J Med* 2002;346: 1538–1543.

65. Blumenthal D. Quality of care—what is it? *N Engl J Med* 1996;335:891–893.

66. Haas JF. Recent changes in health care insurance. *J Head Trauma Rehabil* 1997; 12:1–9.

67. Prince JM, Haas JF. A vision for the future: an interview with Gerben De-Jong, Ph.D. *J Head Trauma Rehabil* 1997;12:71–86.

68. Sulmasy DP, Bloche MG, Mitchell JM, et al. Physicians' ethical beliefs about cost-control arrangements. *Arch Intern Med* 2000;160:649–656.

69. Caplan AL. The ethics of gatekeeping in rehabilitation medicine. *J Head Trauma Rehabil* 1997;12:29–36.

70. Dougherty C. Managed care and (un)informed consent. *J Head Trauma Rehabil* 1997;12:21–28.

71. Banja J. Values, function and managed care: an ethical analysis. *J Head Trauma Rehabil* 1997;12:60–70.

72. Thobaben J. The moral character of rehabilitation institutions. *J Head Trauma Rehabil* 1997;12:10–20.

73. Rusk HA. *World to care for.* New York: Random House, 1972.

74. Granger CV, Hamilton BB, Forer S. Development of a uniform national data system for medical rehabilitation. *Arch Phys Med Rehabil* 1985;66: 538.

75. Moseley JB, O'Malley K, Petersen NJ, et al. A controlled trial of arthroscopic surgery for osteoarthritis of the knee. *N Engl J Med* 2002;347:81–88.

76. Horng S, Miller FG. Is placebo surgery unethical? N *Engl J Med* 2002;347: 137–139.

77. Burling S. Maybe it's all in your head. *Philadelphia Inquirer* 2002 Jul 15: F1.

78. Interview on Placebo: Paul Volpe and Walter Brown. Philadelphia, WHYY 90.9 FM radio, July 22, 2002.

79. Why is physiatric research important? *Am J Phys Med Rehabil* 1991;70(suppl):23.

80. Fuhrer MJ. Issues in the federal funding of rehabilitation research. *Arch Phys Med Rehabil* 1985;66:661–668.

81. Stineman MG, Musick DW. Protection of human subjects with disability: guidelines for research. *Arch Phys Med Rehabil* 2001;82(suppl):S9–S14.

82. Weber LJ, Wayland MT, Holton B. Health care professionals and industry: reducing conflicts of interest and established best practices. *Arch Phys Med Rehabil* 2001;82(suppl):S20–S24.

83. Angell M. Is academic medicine for sale? *N Engl J Med* 2000;342:1516–1518.

84. Daniels N. Duty to treat or right to refuse? *Hastings Cent Rep* 1991;21:36–46.

85. Drazen JM, Curfman GD. Financial associations of authors. *N Engl J Med* 2002;346;1901–1902.

86. Kirschner K. Personal communication (Telephone Conversation, December 10, 2001).

87. Pear R. Study says fees are often higher when doctor has stake in clinic. *New York Times* 1991 Aug 9:1.

CHAPTER 49

The International Classification of Functioning, Disability, and Health: ICF Empowering Rehabilitation through an Operational Bio-Psycho-Social Model

Margaret G. Stineman, Donald J. Lollar, and T. Bedirhan Üstün

INTRODUCTION

This chapter introduces and describes the International Classification of Functioning, Disability and Health: ICF (hereafter referred to as the ICF) (1). It begins with basic relevant principles defining body structures and functions, activity and participation, and contextual factors. Historical background is reviewed, placing development of the ICF in contexts with the International Classification of Diseases (ICD) (2), other models of disablement, and the national and international human rights movement. Principles of relevance to medical and rehabilitation practices are presented through the introduction of concepts such as "empowerment medicine" and the analyses of "personal ecology." The practical application of ICF codes is illustrated through a clinical example, with formulation of a clinical problem list. The chapter concludes by discussing the utility and challenges of implementing the ICF in the United States and internationally.

BASIC PRINCIPLES AND DESCRIPTION OF THE ICF

The ICF, now accepted by 191 countries, is fast becoming the world standard for describing health and disabilities. It defines health and some health-related components of well-being in two parts. Part 1 classifies functioning and disability. Part 2 expresses environmental and personal contextual factors. Functioning and disability in Part 1 are described from the perspectives of the body, the individual, and society, formulated in two components: (a) body functions and structures, and (b) activities and participation. The new terms are intended to extend the scope of classification, enabling the description of positive functioning as well as negative experience associated with disability. *Functioning* is a broad term intended to encompass all body functions, activities, and participation. Similarly, *disability* is used as an umbrella term that encompasses impairments, activity limitations, and participation restrictions. *Activity limitations* replaces the former "disabilities," and *participation restrictions* replaces the more negative term "handicaps," used in the precursor International Classification of Impairment, Disabilities and Handicaps (ICIDH) (3).

The contextual factors, Part 2 of the ICF, are expressed as having to do with background of the individual's life and the surrounding environment. Contexts are believed to interact with the individual's health condition, forming facilitators and barriers. Facilitators enhance function, whereas barriers increase limitations and restrictions. Contextual factors are grouped into (a) personal factors and (b) environmental factors. Personal factors include background contexts, such as the individual's particular attitudes, experiences, gender, age, race, and vocation. A classification of personal factors is not listed in the ICF, mainly because these are difficult to standardize internationally, and also there may exist special international schemes, such as those for education, labor, and occupations. Environmental factors are divided into those that are physical, such as features of the home setting, and those that are societal, such as politics and social attitudes. Body functions and structures are classified according to main physiological systems. Activities and participation are classified according to meaningful sets of related life areas, and these domains are expressed as capacity or performance. Each of the domains of ICF parts is detailed through a series of chapters and categories at different levels. The full detailed version can be aggregated into a short version when summary information is required. Various qualifiers are used to express severity (extent or magnitude), capacity or performance, and facilitators or barriers.

Body Functions and Structures ("Body Level")

The body functions and structures sections are organized as a series of eight chapters describing broad areas of the human body. Body function and structure codes are designed to be used in parallel, as shown in Table 49-1. For example, "mental

ICF Chapter	Body Functions	Body Structures
	TABLE 49-1. The Parallel Lists of Body Function and Structure	
1	Mental functions	Structures of the nervous system
2	Sensory functions and pain	The eye, ear, and related structures
3	Voice and speech functions	Structures involved in voice and speech
4	Functions of the cardiovascular, hematologic, immunologic, and respiratory systems	Structures of the cardiovascular, immunologic, and respiratory systems
5	Functions of the digestive, metabolic, and endocrine systems	Structures related to the digestive, metabolic, and endocrine systems
6	Genitourinary and reproductive functions	Structures related to the genitourinary and reproductive systems
7	Neuromusculoskeletal and movement-related functions	Structures related to movement
8	Functions of the skin and related structures	Skin and related structures

ICF, the International Classification of Functioning, Disability and Health.

functions" corresponds to the structural correlate "structures of the nervous system," which in turn can be linked to specific diagnoses (ICD-10 codes) (2). Body functions are "physiological functions of body systems (including psychological functions.)" (p. 40). Body structures are "anatomical parts of the body, such as organs, limbs and their components" (p. 105). Impairments are "problems in body function or structure as a significant deviation or loss" (p. 47). Severity of impairment is described based on a generic qualifier, which indicates the extent or magnitude of impairment. The qualifiers include ranges of percentages for use in those cases in which assessment instruments or other standards are available to quantify impairment. Impairments can be temporary, permanent, progressive, regressive, static, intermittent, or continuous.

Each chapter is subdivided into more detailed categories that form the actual classification. A series of "b" codes express the classification taxonomy in the body function scheme in great detail. For example, mental functions (Chapter 1) include global mental functions (b110 b139), among other categories. Consciousness function forms the first subdivision. Consciousness function is further subdivided into b1100 "state of consciousness"; b1101 "continuity of consciousness"; b1102 "quality of consciousness"; b1108 "consciousness functions, other specified"; and b1109 "consciousness functions, unspecified."

The parallel body structure classification system operates the same way through a series of "s" codes that describe the area of the body involved. For example, Chapter 1, structures of the

nervous system, describes areas of the brain that could explain the mental impairments detailed above. Biological foundations guided the classification of impairments of structure and attempt to be in congruence with knowledge about tissues, cells, and molecules. Rather than expressing pathology, impairments are manifestations of pathology. Combining information from Table 49-2 with the example codes above, it becomes immediately apparent that a patient with a moderately impaired state of consciousness would be assigned a code of b1100.2. If severe damage to the structure of the brainstem was documented, the companion impaired structure code would be s1105.3.

Activity and Participation (Person and Society Levels)

Activity is "the execution of a task or action by an individual." Participation is "involvement in a life situation" (p. 123). Activity limitations are "difficulties an individual may have in executing activities." Participation restrictions are problems an individual may experience with involvement in life situations. The activity and participation components are expressed in a single list of domains characterized as "d" codes (Table 49-3). They cover a broad range of life areas (from basic learning and watching to composite tasks such as participation in civic life). Each domain (d) can specify activities (a) or participation (p). In the current scheme, for which there is international consensus and the World Health Organization (WHO) will use for reporting purposes, activity is measured as capacity and partici-

TABLE 49-2. The Generic ICF Qualifiers

Qualifier	Definition	Extent of Magnitude of Impairment
xxx.0 No impairment	None, absent, negligible	0–4%
xxx.1 Mild impairment	Slight, low	5–24%
xxx.2 Moderate impairment	Medium, fair	25–49%
xxx.3 Severe impairment	High, extreme	50–95%
xxx.4 Complete impairment	Total	96–100%
xxx.8 Not specified		
xxx.9 Not applicable		

ICF, the International Classification of Functioning, Disability and Health.

TABLE 49-3. Activities and Participation

	Domains
d1	Learning and applying knowledge
d2	General tasks and demands
d3	Communication
d4	Mobility
d5	Self-care
d6	Domestic life
d7	Interpersonal interactions and relationships
d8	Major life areas
d9	Community, social, and civic life

TABLE 49-4.   Capacity and Performance Qualifiers

Qualifier	Definition	Extent of Magnitude of Difficulty
xxx.0 No difficulty	None, absent, negligible	0–4%
xxx.1 Mild difficulty	Slight, low	5–24%
xxx.2 Moderate difficulty	Medium, fair	25–49%
xxx.3 Severe difficulty	High, extreme	50–95%
xxx.4 Complete difficulty	Total	96–100%
xxx.8 Not specified		
xxx.9 Not applicable		

TABLE 49-5.   Environmental Factors

Chapter	Factors
1	Products and technology
2	Natural environment and human-made changes to environment
3	Support and relationships
4	Attitudes
5	Services, systems, and policies

pation as performance, both expressed in terms of two qualifiers. However there are three other alternatives for coding the d list, as explained in Annex 2 (1).

The capacity qualifier is most relevant to day-to-day measurement in a standardized environment, such as the physical and occupational therapy setting, because capacity expresses what an individual can do when elements of the environment are defined. Once the patient returns to his or her own home environment, performance is measured in the current environment. Codes on the environmental factors are particularly useful here to describe the features of the current environment. Because of the differing environments associated with individuals' lives, it would be extremely difficult to measure capacity. Presumably a change in environmental contexts, holding the health condition constant, can lead to changes in activity limitation (1) That is why the capacity qualifier must be measured in a uniform or standard environment intended to be the same for all people and countries facilitating international comparisons. The gap between performance and capacity suggests how that standard environment will improve performance.

Limitations or restrictions are evaluated against the norm of a person without similar disease, disorder, or injury. Activities are broadly interpreted as the "person level" or the individual perspective. Participation takes the societal perspective. The single ICF list of activities and participation can be used in four ways. The user can choose to (a) designate some domains as activities and others as participation without overlap, (b) allow some overlap across the domains, (c) designate all detailed domains as activities but the broader category headings as participation, or (d) use all domains as both activities and participation. Further information is given on the ICF coding guidelines and on the WHO Web site, http://www.who.int/classification/icf.

Activity and participation include nine chapters involving broad areas of function, ranging from learning and applying knowledge through community, social, and civic life. The chapters on communication, mobility, self-care, and other life areas

contain the functions that are among those most often applied in setting goals during rehabilitation. Each chapter is further divided into blocks and then categories/domains. For example, mobility (Chapter 4) includes changing and maintaining body position as one of its blocks designated d410-d429. Lying down (d4100), squatting (d4101), and kneeling (d4102) are examples of categories or domains included in that block. Table 49-3 shows the activity and participation chapters. Table 49-4 shows how those domains are described relative to severity of limitations in performance or capacity.

Contextual Factors

The environmental factors are organized into five chapters, as expressed from the perspective of the person being described. The five chapters are listed in Table 49-5. These are qualified, as shown in Table 49-6, based on whether a factor is a facilitator or a barrier. Environmental factors have a complex effect on the lives of people with health conditions and disabilities, and integration between the health condition and environmental factors is poorly understood. Because this area of classification is less well understood in physiatry, those chapters are described below.

The first chapter is products and technology (including food, drugs, and technical aids) in an individual's immediate environment used by people with disability in preventing, compensating, monitoring, or relieving activity limitation or participation restriction.

The second chapter is about animate and inanimate elements of the local physical world that surround or will surround the person. The clinician may need to consider land forms, local populations, plants, animals, climate, light, sound, air quality, and other elements that could have particular bearing on the patient's activities and participation.

The third chapter is support and relationships, including the individuals who provide physical support, emotional support, or assistance. This includes family, friends, peers, working ani-

TABLE 49-6.   Qualifiers for Measuring Environmental Contexts

Factor			
Barrier	Facilitator	Presence	Quantity
xxx.0 No	xxx+0 No	None, absent, negligible	0–4%
xxx.1 Mild	xxx+1 Mild	Slight, low,	5–24%
xxx.2 Moderate	xxx+2 Moderate	Medium, fair	25–49%
xxx.3 Severe	xxx+3 Substantial	High, extreme	50–95%
xxx.4 Complete	xxx+4 Complete	Total	96–100%
xxx.8 Not specified	xxx+8 Not specified		
xxx.9 Not applicable			

TABLE 49-7. The Relationship of Common Functional Status Measures to the ICF

Instrument	Measures	Describes
Physical Performance Test (15,16)	Balance, coordination, endurance, speed etc.	Body function
	Eating, lifting a book, putting on and taking off a jacket, etc.	Activity
Barthel Index (17,18)	Feeding, transfers, grooming, bowel and bladder, walking, etc.	Activity
FIM™ Instrument (19,20)	Items included in the domains of self-care, sphincter management, mobility, and cognitive	Activity has components of body function, urination and defecation, mental functions, and voice and speech functions
Rehabilitation Institute of Chicago Functional Assessment Scale (RIC-FAS) (21)	Extends the FIM to include measures of community integration	Activity participation
Mini Mental State (22)	Orientation, memory, attention, ability to name, verbal commands, follow written commands, write a sentence, and copy a figure	Requires body function primarily involving mental functions, voice and verbal, and vision. Also has components of activity such as copying.
Timed "Up and Go" Test (23)	Measures the time it takes to stand up from a chair, walk 3 meters, turn around, walk back to chair, and sit down	Activity
Berg Balance Scale (24–26)	Tests balance by progression from sitting to bilateral to tandem and single leg stance	Body function

ICF, the International Classification of Functioning, Disability and Health.

mals, those in positions of authority, those in subordinate positions, and health professionals.

The fourth chapter is about attitudes, customs, ideologies, values, and norms. These attitudes are addressed relative to how they influence individual behaviors, interpersonal relationships, stigma, stereotyping, positive practices, or prejudice as arising from specific people in the patient's circle of acquaintances.

Services, systems, and policies are represented in the fifth chapter. This includes structured programs, systems, and poli-

cies that operate in various sectors of society. Examples of particular relevance to people with disability include architectural policies with regard to the design and construction of buildings, systems of communication, transportation services, legal policies, media systems that govern the provision and content of information provided to the general public, and economic or social security policies.

The expansive nature of the ICF becomes clear when comparing its classification contents with existing measures. There is a plethora of functional status measures available to rehabilitation practice and research. Table 49-7 illustrates a few of the most common instruments and their relationship to the ICF framework. Some might be cross-walked to the ICF. Table 49-8 shows a suggested crosswalk between Functional Independence Measure (FIM™) instrument performance levels and ICF qualifiers. Existing instruments and measures classify patients primarily by Part 1 components. Few measures express Part 2.

TABLE 49-8. Proposed FIM Performance Level to ICF Performance Qualifiers

FIM Performance Levels	Equivalent ICF Qualifier[a]
1 Total assistance Subject = 0% + effort	Complete difficulty 0%–4% + capacity (96%–100% performance problem) —or—
2 Maximal assistance Subject = 25% effort	Severe difficulty 5%–50% capacity (50%–95% performance problem)
3 Moderate assistance Subject = 50% + effort	Moderate difficulty 51%–75% capacity (25%–49% performance problem)
4 Minimal assistance Subject = 75% + effort	Mild difficulty 76%–95% capacity (5%–24% performance problem) —or—
5 Supervision 6 Modified independence —or—	No difficulty 96%–100% capacity (0%–4% performance problem)
7 Complete Independence	

ICF, the International Classification of Functioning, Disability and Health.
[a]The ICF is rescaled to reflect performance so that the percentage values can be compared with the FIM performance levels. The actual ICF qualifier ranges appear in parentheses. The two scales are not absolutely equivalent.
From FIM™ instrument. Copyright ©1996. Uniform Data System for Medical Rehabilitation (UDSMR), a division of UB Foundation Activities, Inc. (UBFA). FIM is a trademark belonging to UBFA.

HISTORICAL BACKGROUND

The ICF was developed for use with the ICD, which is the basis for clinical encounter information throughout the world and at the heart of describing medical practice. WHO, which also spearheaded development of the ICF, became the conservator of the ICD in 1946, after the ICD had been in use almost 100 years. The development of the ICF, to some extent, parallels development of the ICD, although there are some differences because of the dissimilarities in the biomedical approach of the ICD and more social orientation of the ICF.

In 1853 the first International Statistical Congress convened and encouraged that the causes of death be classified in a uniform way (4). Two separate lists were presented at the next Congress meeting, based on different principles. The first principle, proposed by William Farr, listed causes of death that were due to disease by anatomic site, developmental diseases, and deaths as a result of violence. The second principle, proposed by Marc D'Epsine, classified deaths by the nature of disease, such as gouty, herpetic, or hematic. After 35 years of controversy, the concept of classification by anatomic site survived and was incorporated into the evolving classification of causes of death led by the French statistician, Jaques Bertillon. That original classification system was based on distinguishing general diseases from those localized to a specific organ or anatomic site. In 1898 the American Public Health Association recommended adoption of the Bertillon Classification in Canada, Mexico, and the United States. They further recommended revision every decade. In 1948, WHO developed a list of causes of morbidity that was integrated with causes of death, leading to the ICD, which has been updated through many versions over the years and is now in its tenth version (2).

There are two primary reasons for placing the ICF in context with development of the ICD. First, the classification of function is a natural extension of the emphasis on health outcomes: death first, disease or morbidity second, and, now, "disability" third (5). As the field of public health statistics has evolved, it has become apparent that diagnostic categories do not adequately describe the breadth of experience needed to address concrete issues, such as service provision, much less broader well-being concerns, such as quality of life (6). Second, as this evolution has occurred, it is reasonable to include the role of the environment in health outcomes.

In 1979, at the time of the ninth revision to form ICD-9, it was recognized that diagnostic codes did not adequately cover the breadth of experience related to chronic illness, injuries, and developmental conditions. The ICIDH, introduced in 1980, grew out of this concern (3). The ICIDH, from the beginning, provided an extraordinary conceptual approach, suggesting that the experience of what is generally called "disability" is a multidimensional experience that occurs on several planes—at the body level, the personal activity level, and the societal level. It included definitions across these different planes. Although the ICIDH included a coding scheme, it had weaknesses, which compromised its acceptance in the medical, public health, and disability advocacy communities. In spite of these problems, the ICIDH was revised in 1993 and translated into 13 languages, and 25,000 copies of the manual were distributed.

The ICF in Context with Other Disablement Models and Existing Measures

Zola (7), who founded the Society for Disability Studies in the 1980s, emphasized that health states do not result from pathology and impairment alone, but rather from interactions between impairments and the social, political, economic, and physical environments. Minaire (8), in the early 1990s, criticized the ICIDH as placing too much emphasis on individual experience and too little on the role of the environment. Minaire saw disablement as a process, which unfolds with time depending on life situations, which take place at different moments of the life process. Thus, life is a combination of micro-situations (eating, driving, opening and closing doors . . .), all of which occur in a particular environment. Occupational therapists view environment as influencing volition, the need for certain skills, and the demands for performance. These factors affect the individual's engagement (9), a concept closely aligned with the ICF concept of participation.

In the model championed by Nagi (10), the disability construct relates to the performance of socially defined roles and tasks, which can be encumbered by environmental barriers. The National Center for Medical Rehabilitation Research (NCMRR) defines societal limitation as structural or attitudinal, barriers in social policy, which limit fulfillment of roles or deny access to services and opportunities that are associated with full participation in society (11). The Institute of Medicine concluded in its report that "disability is not inherent in the individual, but is rather a product of the interaction of the individual with the environment" (12). The concept of health environmental integration (HEI) (13) views functioning and disability as a four-way interaction among patients' mental and physical health states and the physical and societal environments, yielding a specific quantity (14). Maximal functioning (expanded HEI) occurs when the individual's physical and mental states are in balance, and the person is able to fully integrate into the environment. Disability results (restricted HEI) when mental and physical injury or illness inhibits environmental integration. Potential for activity and participation in a given environment, as defined by the ICF, is analogous to the HEI quantity.

Although the dimensions of the various models are similar—body, person, and society—the terminology across these conceptual frameworks is not interchangeable. For example, functional limitation, as defined by the NCMRR and Nagi models, shares certain elements with impairment and activity limitation, as characterized by the ICF. Although the proliferation of these models is confusing in many respects, they are noteworthy because of the consistent emphasis on the importance of environmental effects.

Most instruments currently in use to measure function in rehabilitation fail to incorporate the environment. Many can only be classified roughly within the Part 1 domains of the ICF framework (see Table 49-7) (15–26). It might also be possible in some cases to form a crosswalk to the ICF severity qualifiers as illustrated (see Table 49-8) for the FIM™. After review of the various disability frameworks and instruments for measuring them, it becomes clear that the ICF is the only one that includes both a conceptual model and a classification coding scheme, making it applicable to clinical practice.

The ICF from the Perspective of Disability Advocacy and Human Rights

The ICF incorporates a human rights perspective in recognition of importance of the worldwide disability rights movements. The advocacy or independent living movement (27–29) in the United States was established in the 1970s largely to protest paternalistic ways in which society at large and physicians in general viewed people with disabilities. Advocates objected to concepts of defined abnormality and dependency, which they believed legitimized their being marginalized from mainstream society. They further resented the position of being forced to accept orders from physicians and other experts with little explanation. Some people with disabilities, fearing stigma resulting from diagnostic classification, were reluctant to establish formal relationships with providers in the health-care industry. Rejecting the medical model, advocates proposed a social model of disablement. Disability is seen largely as a societal, cultural, and environmental problem arising from the architectural and attitudinal barriers that permeate society at large. This model formed the underpinnings of the independent living movement (30). Supported by a nationwide network of independent living centers, the movement focuses on community integration, barrier removal, the availability of personal assistants to facilitate independence, and the procurement of human rights. It triumphed in passage of the Americans with Disability Act (ADA) (31), the federal antidiscrimination statute designed to remove barriers that prevent people with disabilities from enjoying the same rights to employment, access to federal building or programs, and liberty as everyone else.

During United Nations (UN) Decade of Disabled Persons (1983–1992) the "Standard Rules on the Equalization of Opportunities for Persons with Disabilities" (32) were put forth.

Many international human rights mandates formed the political and moral foundations of the standard rules. The intention was to "offer an instrument for policy making and action to persons with disabilities and their organizations" to ensure that "girls, boys, women and men with disabilities . . . may exercise the same rights and obligations as others" (p. 8). People with disabilities are seen as partners in the process of equalization of opportunities.

The ICF is intended to be a force championing the Standard Rules and is accepted as the principal classification for disability among the UN's social classifications. Thus, the ICF provides an instrument for testing and measuring progress toward implementation and the benefits of international and national human rights legislation, including the ADA. The overarching emphasis of the human rights approach is on establishing an inclusive community, so that society at large takes responsibility for overcoming those prejudicial attitudes and physical barriers that limit the participation of people with disabilities. The term *inclusive community* focuses on and is intended to treat all citizens equally regardless of disability. The underlying human rights perspective permeates the ICF and, if implemented, could change the way rehabilitation is practiced worldwide.

RELEVANCE TO MEDICAL AND REHABILITATION PRACTICE

Shifting the Paradigm from "Restoration" to "Empowerment"

By addressing components of health and human rights, the ICF scheme has moved away from the "consequences of disease" classification approach taken by the ICIDH (3). It takes a neutral stand, emphasizing function rather than pathology. As relevant to people regardless of disability status, the ICF removes the stigma of difference associated with pathology. Through the addition of environmental contexts, the ICF will engender expansion of the restorative rehabilitation paradigm to include empowerment. The expanded rehabilitation objective is to both maximize physical and mental abilities, and to equalize opportunities for community inclusion (33,34). The process seeks to guarantee the rights of all people with disabilities to live within our communities, to enjoy maximal health and well-being, and to fully participate in educational, social, cultural, religious, economic, and political activities. With this broadened approach, it becomes even more in society's interest to support rehabilitation. When persons with disabilities gain the same rights, opportunities, and duties as others, they become empowered to become productive members of society. The concept of charity is replaced with the concepts of equalization of opportunities and human rights (34).

This broadened focus in support of the alignment of the persons served with the environment (1,13,35) incorporates principles of independent living into the process of rehabilitation. Although the precise mechanisms of combining such principles remain contentious (36), it has, in part, been addressed by community-based rehabilitation. Community-based rehabilitation is a "radical approach" that reflects the structure and functions of the indigenous culture (37) and springs from the grassroots of the community, with branches to rehabilitation institutions (38). This constitutes a dramatic paradigm shift for physiatry. With blending of the "medical" and "social" models, "empowerment medicine" emerges.

Empowerment medicine (13,39,40) gives power or authority to the patient through knowledge in efforts to place him or her in the best position to take control of the direction of his or her own life. Effective rehabilitation helps the patient regain the control of his or her life often lost during the acute phase of disabling illness. Evidence-based practices are applied to reduce impairment and enhance function in contexts with the often-idiosyncratic needs, responses, and desires of the individual. As the individual evolves toward empowerment, potential for activity and opportunities for participation can be visualized as the integrating and overlapping functions of four spheres: the body, the mind, the physical world, and the social environment represented by the HEI quantity (14). Empowerment is sought by seeking full integration of the mind with the body, to the extent allowed by one's health state. It further includes finding ways to alter or integrate with the environment in a manner that maximizes functional performance and the capacity to participate in life situations fully. With disabling health conditions, mental and physical balance is disrupted, and the full integration between the person and environment is lost. Environmental factors can have as great a causal role in the production of activity limitation and participation restriction as health conditions. HEI can be increased by interventions targeted to the person (the reduction of mental or physical impairment) or to the environment (enhancement of facilitators of function).

The introductions of ICF "e" codes to the routine of rehabilitation practices encourages the emergence of a new form of assessment that might be referred to as "personal ecology." Personal ecology is the study of how life contexts influence functioning, restrict activity, and produce participation restriction. Those contexts are built structures, personal and societal attitudes, caregivers, personal goals, and motivations. An environmental intervention expands personal space for living through combinations of technology (assistive devices) and the enhancement of environmental facilitators. Appropriate selection and prescription of a wheelchair is a prime example of a clinical decision needing the assessment of personal ecology. Information from the history and physical examination—including the patient's weight and size, seating needs, and required method of propulsion—is required to optimize the "person-machine interface." Information about personal ecology, including terrain, the use of the type of transportation available, and cosmesis, optimizes the "machine-environment interface" and thus is ultimately required to maximize quality of the linkage between the person and physical world.

Simultaneous with improving access to the physical world, the wheelchair is also stigma laden. Patient empowerment can go a long way in reducing perceptions of stigma associated with disability equipment. By encouraging the patient to be a full partner in selection of technology, he or she gains a sense of ownership and empowerment.

ICF Coding Example

The ICF classification is intended to provide a unified and standard language for describing health-related states (1). As part of the family of international classifications developed by the WHO, when combined with other classifications, it becomes possible to include a wide range of information about diagnoses, functioning, disabilities, and the reasons for contact with various components of the health-care system. For example, the WHO's ICD-10 (4) provides an etiologic framework describing the underlying diseases, disorders, injuries, etc., that link to the ICF impairment categories expressing body function "b" or structure "s." Functioning and disability associated with those health conditions are described by the ICF activity and participation "d" codes. Social and environmental factors are expressed by "e" codes. The numeric "s," "b," "d," and "e" codes can each be followed by a qualifier (following a decimal point) that expresses severity for the "s," "b," and "d" codes, and the strength of the barrier or facilitator for "e" codes.

TABLE 49-9.   Case Example: ICF Problem List

Body Functions

b1140.2	Orientation to time, moderate impairment (oriented to person, place, not time; thinks it is Thanksgiving in April)
b134.2	Sleep functions, moderate impairment (some difficulty falling asleep at night)
b1304.1	Impulse control, mild impairment (mildly impaired impulse control)
b1440.2	Short-term memory, moderate impairment (moderate-deficit short-term memory)
b320.1	Articulation functions, mild impairment (mild receptive and expressive aphasia)
b4101.2	Heart rhythm, moderate impairment (Cardiovascular: irregular rhythm)
b6202.3	Urinary continence, severe impairment (loss of bladder control)
b7302.2	Power of muscles of one side of the body, moderate impairment (moderately increased tone right side of the body with dense hemiparesis)
b735.2	Muscle tone functions, moderate impairment (light touch is markedly diminished on the inside of her right cheek and on the right side of her body)
b740.2	Muscle endurance functions, moderate impairment (no hand grasp or finger motion, able to reach arm forward, but not above shoulder)

Body Structures[a]

s11000.27	Frontal lobe, moderate impairment (a lesion of the left temporal lobes of her central nervous system)
s11002.27	Parietal lobe, moderate impairment (a lesion of the parietal lobes of her central nervous system)

Activities and Participation [a]

d330.88	Speaking, no specified performance problem, no specified capacity limitation (difficulty communicating)
d4200.34	Transferring oneself, severe performance problem, complete capacity limitation (transfers bed to chair, totally dependent)
d4500.34	Walking, severe performance problem, complete capacity limitation (walks 5 feet, maximum assistance of two people)
d550.12	Eating, mild performance problem, moderate capacity limitation (eating, minimum assistance)
d540.23	Dressing, moderate performance problem, severe capacity limitation (dressing, moderate assistance, dressing upper body, moderate assistance)
d7600.0_	Parent child relationships, no performance problem (she has a positive and supportive relationship with her one daughter who lives about 15 minutes away)
d7500.0_	Informal relationships with friends, no performance problem
d7501.0_	Informal relationships with neighbors, no performance problem (there are a number of close friends and neighbors who are devoted to her and will be able to stop in and help during the day, should she be discharged home)

Environmental Factors

e155.3	Design, construction and building products and technology of buildings for private use, severe barrier (Mrs. Whyte's house has five steps to enter, no bathroom on the first floor, and the doorways into the kitchen and bathroom are too narrow for wheelchair or walker passage)
e165.+3	Assets, substantial facilitator (there are sufficient personal economic resources for a companion to be hired, and the daughter has agreed to oversee the process)
e310.+3	Immediate family, substantial facilitator (she has a positive and supportive relationship with her one daughter . . . this daughter works full-time but can spend several hours doing errands for her on Saturdays)
e320.+3	Friends, substantial facilitator (there are a number of close friends and neighbors who are devoted to her and will be able to stop in and help during the day, should she be discharged home)

ICF, the International Classification of Functioning, Disability and Health.
[a]The first qualifier is performance, and the second qualifier is capacity without assistance. Generally, the capacity qualifier describes the individual's true ability as not enhanced by an assistance device or personal assistance. The performance qualifier relates to the individual's current environment, including assistive device, personal assistance, or directly observable barriers. The nature of those facilitators or barriers is then described by the environmental factors classification.

The multilayered coding structure of the ICF enables expression of both global information appropriate to broad population-level analyses and specific details necessary to guide clinical practices. Although ICF coding is complex, it is clear that as electronic reporting of patient information is more fully implemented, the capacity for handheld devices and other application instruments (e.g., ICF Checklist, ICF Core Sets) (41) to easily prompt medical personnel toward appropriate and useful data collection will increase. The hypothetical case study below is used to show how something as complex as a clinical problem list can be formulated using ICF codes (Table 49-9). The qualifier following the decimal point indicates severity when sufficient information was offered.

A CASE STUDY

History

Mrs. Whyte is a 62-year-old woman (a hypothetical patient) who presented to the emergency department 6 days before admission to rehabilitation with sudden onset right-sided hemi-

paresis, loss of bladder control, and difficulty communicating. She was stabilized on the neurology service and found on magnetic resonance imaging to have an ischemic lesion of the left temporal and parietal lobes of her brain.

Review of Systems
The patient has marked frequency of urination and incontinence, some difficulty falling asleep at night.

Social and Family History
Mrs. Whyte lives alone.

Personal Ecology
Mrs. Whyte has a positive and supportive relationship with her one daughter, who lives about 15 minutes away. Her daughter sees her mother as a hard worker and wants the best for her care. This daughter works full-time but can spend several hours doing errands for her on Saturdays. There are sufficient personal economic resources for a companion to be hired, and the daughter has agreed to oversee the process. The patient

worked as a bookkeeper before admission, and she was an avid crossword puzzler. There are a number of close friends and neighbors who are devoted to her and will be able to stop in and help during the day, should she be discharged home. Mrs. Whyte's house has five steps to enter, no bathroom on the first floor, and the doorways into the kitchen and bathroom upstairs are too narrow for wheelchair or walker passage.

Functional Status

Eating, minimum assistance; dressing, moderate assistance; dressing upper body, moderate assistance; transfers bed to chair, totally dependent; walks 5 feet, maximum assistance of two people.

Physical Examination

Oriented to person, place, not time (thinks it is Thanksgiving in April), high energy level, mildly impaired impulse control, moderate deficit short-term memory with mild receptive and expressive aphasia.

Cardiovascular

Irregular rhythm.

Neurologic

Moderately increased tone right side of the body with dense hemiparesis, no hand grasp or finger motion, able to reach arm forward, but not above shoulder. Light touch is markedly diminished on the inside of her right cheek and on the right side of her body.

Utility and Critique of the ICF

In the United States, likely the major potential strength—and, at the same time, the major challenge—to implementation is the ICF aim to "establish a common language for describing health and health-related states in order to improve communication. . . ." (p. 5). Discipline-specific language and professional enculturation are often at the core of our communication, yielding unique terminology to describe a particular discipline's perspective on a person's functioning, along with the professional role. Some may be reluctant to learn a new or second language, yet being able to communicate beyond one's discipline using ICF terminology can substantially increase efficiency and quality of communication. This first basic premise, uniformity of concepts and terminology, should provide a major motivation for finding ways to use this framework. Having a clear, concise summary of this information can enhance both medical and rehabilitation decision making. Moreover, widespread implementation of the ICF could permit comparison of disability case mix, outcome, and disability management strategies over time across rehabilitation disciplines, long-term care services, acute medical and surgical settings, and across states and countries. In addition, this common language could improve communication between health-care professionals and disparate users, including researchers, architects, policy makers, city planners, transportation planners, people with disabilities, insurance agencies, educational institutions, and the public at large. The contributions of all these disciplines to the well-being of people with disability will be magnified if coordination, communication, and collaboration is enhanced (42).

There are many aspects of ICF that are clearly congruent across various groups within the broadly defined "disability community," including advocates, service providers, researchers, and policy makers. There are two overarching conceptual themes that find substantial agreement around the world and across sectors. The first of these is the notion that the experi-

ence of disability is a universal phenomenon. In addition to more than 50 million people in the United States reporting a limitation in basic activities, there are substantially more family members affected by those with disabling conditions (43). Across the life span, everyone will experience some degree of functional limitation, and in this sense, disability is part of the universal human condition (44,45).

The second concept is the importance of environmental factors to the disabling experience. This operationalization of the role of environmental factors paves the way for clinicians, researchers, and policy makers to frame environmental interventions in cooperation with the disability community. These conceptual strengths provide the foundation and the energy to begin addressing some thorny issues surrounding the clinical utility of the current ICF. As indicated earlier, the ICD explicitly showed its growth over time. There is little doubt that the ICF will continue to grow in use and will change as knowledge is gained through its implementation. The following issues need attention.

The basic problem of ICF application is the operationalization of the rubrics of the classification as dimensions and domains. To operationalize is to create, for each entity, a logical definition that allows for clinical assessment or quantitative measurement. If we have standard definitions, then we can easily establish population norms for any function. Although certain biological functions, such as seeing and hearing, are traditionally measured with standard tools such as eye charts or audiometry, such precise measurement is more difficult in areas such as self-care, usual activities, or societal participation. Not only are these more complex constructs but also there is a larger degree of interaction with contextual factors, including environmental ones.

Additionally, there has always been a controversy between the boundaries among the three levels—body, person, and society. At times it is difficult to distinguish differences between body functions and personal activity, such as specific body movements that combine to allow an activity, for example, hand strength and flexibility combined with eating. Is the therapeutic intervention at the body function/impairment level or at the activity limitation level? Similarly, body functions of "seeing" and "hearing" are difficult to distinguish from the activity/participation components labeled "watching" and "listening." Related to this conceptual issue is the explicit combination of activities and participation into a single component list, even though the definitions of each suggest difference. Basically each human activity is a composite function of smaller subfunctions, and distinctions between certain planes should be defined either by some scientific method or arbitrarily by consensus. Current options are listed in the Annex 3 of the ICF, and future use will enable revisions of the ICF to have a better empirical database of preferred options. For classification purposes, the distinction between capacity and performance has been the internationally accepted solution in the current version of the ICF and will be used by the WHO for international reporting purposes. The distinction between capacity and performance attempts to define the differences between individuals' current functioning in a nonobstructing environment (capacity) and their functioning in their usual environment (performance). The coding rules also suggest using the environmental factor codes for identifying the features of a standard environment and current environment in order to identify the barriers and facilitators. In addition, the notion of accomplishing personal or societal functions with and without assistance is included as additional qualifiers. Without fully developing the strengths and weaknesses of the inclusion of these notions, it is clear that the classification gets complicated very quickly—beyond the capacity of practitioners to efficiently record information. This matrix of information, including the component (body, person/society) delineated by capacity and performance and further delineated by the presence or absence of assistance, would be difficult for a researcher with a reasonably lengthy time period. It is all but impossible for a fast-paced clinical practitioner. For the ICF to gain credibility in service provision, the bits of information to be recorded will need to be substantially reduced. Which components and qualifiers are chosen will depend on the use made of the information. Even with electronic data, reporting will require brief, clean coding elements. For this purpose, WHO has developed the ICF Checklist (41) and ICF core sets, and is also developing further clinical applications.

Medicare compiles information about medical conditions and procedures through what is referred to as the "patient encounter form." The National Committee on Vital and Health Statistics (46) recently completed a report suggesting that additional information on functioning be considered for addition to that standard form. The committee specifically recommended that the ICF be considered as the framework for collecting functional status. If this direction is to be considered, the recording burden will need to be minimized. Toward this end, attention should be given by all medical specialties and health professionals to deciding the most useful functional information. A starting point for rehabilitation might be to code person-level activity limitations and their severity as measured during the clinical encounter, without and with assistance. This information provides a bridge between the ICD and clinical (current procedure terminology) codes currently being collected on the patient encounter form.

Although the concept of capacity, as expressed through functioning in a standard universal environment, is theoretically useful for international comparisons of function, the gap between performance and capacity as measured against current and standard environments is not a complete measure of the extent to which environmental alterations can improve performance for all individuals with activity limitations. Certain environmental elements represent a barrier for people with one type of disability while representing facilitators for people with other types of disabilities. Witness the curb cuts at street crosswalks that eliminate clues delineating sidewalk and street for mobility-trained people who are blind yet are required to ease wheelchair mobility.

If this all seems just too much information to manage, it is a sign that the ICF developers have worked to include all relevant dimensions for classifying and coding functioning and disability. While the classification is in its neonatal period, there will continue to be serious issues to be resolved and difficult questions to be answered. It is clear to many of us, however, that developing more standard and relevant data about the experience of individuals with disabilities is crucial for improving the health and well-being of the growing disabled population. The ICF moves us toward that goal. The ultimate usefulness of the ICF must be determined based on evidence through implementation in practice and research settings.

Implications to Policy Determination Worldwide

ICF has provided a standardized operational tool for the measurement of health and disability. It has created a new paradigm viewing health and disability as related multidimensional constructs. Rather than restricting health and disability within narrow biomedical or social models, the ICF has identified all major dimensions in an integrated bio-psycho-social model. Such a model strongly advocates the integration of the environment in which the disability experience takes place.

Assessment of health and disability in the full spectrum of various human functions spanning from simple sensory functions to full participation in the community activities is the major advance in the ICF. Unlike the former disability models, ICF does not restrict disability to a minority model that belongs to a small subset of the society with certain bodily impairments. ICF takes a "universal model" that expands the functioning into the total human experience and tries to capture the full spectrum of life (44,45).

At the population level this would give a more comprehensive picture of the need for rehabilitation services. Firstly, the need could be defined as a threshold in a given population distribution, and then we can calculate the met need and unmet need. This will provide a useful planning tool as to how best to redirect future rehabilitation resources and activities.

At the clinical level, the ICF provides a common framework to measure the health outcomes from various interventions, including rehabilitation (47). Given the expanding nature of rehabilitation, from bodily functions to daily activities and community-based interventions, ICF provides the necessary assessment framework to measure and manage the effectiveness of such (42,48).

Using these evaluations, we can then assess the efficiency of rehabilitation activities in a more rational way and plan better for the allocation of resources. Having a road map that shows how far and well we have traveled will help to improve rehabilitation activities. ICF is a great tool as a yardstick that measures how well we are doing for evidence-based medicine, rehabilitation management, and policy making. In this way we can identify priorities in a better way by measurement of needs and resources.

The use of ICF at population and clinical levels will make the importance of disability and rehabilitation more visible and consequently place them in the center of the international public health debate. From an international perspective, this might be the most important contribution of ICF for empowering rehabilitation.

SUMMARY

The ICF was developed by WHO to provide a common framework for describing and measuring health and disability. ICF complements the ICD-10, and together they constitute the WHO Family of International Classifications. The ICF includes standard codes that describe how diseases, injuries, and disorders impair body function and structure, limit activities, and restrict participation. These codes can provide a rich base of information useful in rehabilitation settings for patient assessment and tracking, for justifying service provision, and for research. The ICF also includes specific codes that express the environmental contributors to disability, realizing that personal functioning can be substantially undermined or facilitated by characteristics of the environment at both the personal and societal levels. This later set of codes is important to physiatry. It allows focus on the generalization of skills learned in standard rehabilitation clinic environments to the community setting. It will facilitate description of those environments that are most associated with successful community integration. Knowledge of how to create facilitating environments may represent the next frontier in rehabilitation science.

REFERENCES

1. World Health Organization. *International classification of functioning, disability and health:ICF.* Geneva: WHO, 2001.

2. World Health Organization. *International statistical classification of diseases and related health problems*, 10th re, vols. 1–3. Geneva: WHO, 1992–1994.
3. World Health Organization. *International classification of impairments, disabilities, and handicaps*. Geneva: WHO, 1980.
4. World Health Organization. Introduction. *Manual of the international classification of diseases, injuries and causes of death (ICD)*. Geneva: WHO, 1977.
5. Üstün TB, Chatterji S, Rehm J. Limitations of diagnostic paradigm: it doesn't explain "need" [Letter]. *Arch Gen Psychiatry* 1998;55(12):1145–1146.
6. Üstün TB. A new paradigm: assessment of functioning and WHO's ICIDH. *SAMJ* 1996;86(12):1575.
7. Zola IK. Toward the necessary universalizing of a disability policy. *Milbank Q* 1989;67(Suppl 2, Pt. 2):401–428.
8. Minaire P. Disease, illness and health: theoretical models of the disablement process. *Bull World Health Organn* 1992;70(3):373–379.
9. Barris R. Environmental interactions: an extension of the model of occupation. *JAm Occ Ther* 1982:36(10);637–644.
10. Nagi S. Disability concepts revisited: implications for prevention. In: Pope AM, Tarlov AR (eds). *Disability in America: toward a national agenda for prevention*. Washington, DC: National Academy Press, 1991.
11. National Institutes of Health. *Research plan for the National Center for Medical Rehabilitation Research*. Washington, DC: U.S. DHHS, 1993.
12. Brandt EN, Pope AM, eds. *Enabling America: assessing the role of rehabilitation science and engineering*. Washington, DC: National Academy Press, 1997.
13. Stineman MG. Medical humanism and empowerment medicine. *Disability Studies Quarterly* 2000; 20(1):11–16.
14. Stineman MG. Defining the population, treatments, and outcomes of interest: reconciling the rules of biology with meaningfulness. *Am J Rehabil Med* 2001;80:147–159.
15. Reuben D, Siu A, Kimpau S. The predictive validity of self-report and performance-based measures of function and health. *J Geronotol* 1992;47:M106–M110.
16. Reuben D, Siu A. An objective measure of physical function of elderly outpatients: the Physical Performance Test. *J Am Geriatr Soc* 1990;38:1105–1112.
17. Collins C, Wade D, Davies S, et al. The Barthel ADL Index: a reliability study. *Int Disabil Studies* 1988;10:61–63.
18. Mahoney F, Barthel D. Functional evaluation: the Barthel Index. *MD State Med J* 1965;14:61–65.
19. Granger CV, Hamilton BB, Keith RA, et al. Advances in functional assessment for medical rehabilitation. *Top Geriatr Rehabil* 1986;57:103–108.
20. Uniform Data System for Medical Rehabilitation. *Guide for the uniform data set for medical rehabilitation (including the FIM^SM instrument), version 5.0*. Buffalo, NY: State University of New York at Buffalo, 1996.
21. Cichowski KC. The Rehabilitation Institute of Chicago Functional Assessment Scale. *J Rehabil Outcomes Measurement* 1997;1:66–71.
22. Folstein MF, Folstein SE, McHugh PR. Mini-mental state: a particular method for grading the cognitive state of patients for a clinician. *J Psychiatr Res* 1975;12:189–198.
23. Podsiadlo D, Richardson S. The timed "up & go": a test of basic functional mobility for frail elderly persons. *J Am Geriatr Soc* 1991;39:142–148.
24. Berg KO, Wood-Dauphinee SL, Williams JI. The Balance Scale: reliability assessment for elderly residents and patients with an acute stroke. *Scand J Rehabil Med* 1995;27:27–36.
25. Berg KO, Wood-Dauphinee S,L Williams JI, et al. Measuring balance in the elderly: preliminary development of an instrument. *Physiotherapy Canada* 1989;41:304–311.
26. Berg KO, Wood-Dauphinee SL, Williams JI, et al. Measuring balance in the elderly: validation of an instrument. *Can J Public Health* 1992;83:S7–S11.

27. Beatty PW, Richmond GW, Tepper S, et al. Personal assistance for people with physical disabilities: consumer-direction and satisfaction with services. *Arch Phys Med Rehabil* 1998;79(6):675–677.
28. DeJong G. Health care reform and disability: affirming our commitment to community. *Arch Phys Med Rehabil* 1993;74:1017–1024.
29. DeJong G. Independent living: from social movement to analytic paradigm. *Arch Phys Med Rehabil* 1979;60(10):435–446.
30. DeJong G, Wenker T. Attendant care as a prototype independent living service. *Arch Phys Med Rehabil* 1979;60(10):477–482.
31. Americans with Disabilities Act of 1990. Public Law 101–336, July 26, 1990 104 STAT.327.
32. United Nations. *The standard rules on the equalization of opportunities for persons with disabilities*. Adopted by the United Nations General Assembly at its 48th session on 20 December 1993 (Resolution 48/96). New York: United Nations Department of Public Information, 1994.
33. *Community-based rehabilitation for and with people with disabilities*. 2000 Joint Position Paper. Geneva: ILO, UNESCO, UNICEF, WHO, draft 2000–11–04.
34. Disability and Rehabilitation Team. *Proposed strategy paper 1999–2000*. Geneva: Disability/Injury Prevention and Rehabilitation Department, Social Change and Mental Health Cluster, World Health Organization, 1998.
35. Seibens H. Applying the Domain Management Model in treating patients with chronic disease. *J Qual Impr* 2001;27(6):302–314.
36. Lysack C, Kaufert J. Some perspectives on the disabled consumers' movement and community based rehabilitation in developing countries. *Action-aid Disability News* 1996;7(1):5–9.
37. Agar A. The importance of sustainability in the design of culturally appropriate programmes of early intervention. *International Disability Studies* 1990; 12(2):89–92.
38. Maison Halls G, O'Toole B. Community based participation: rehabilitation rooted in community action. In: Finkenflugel H, ed. *Primary health care publications 7*. Amsterdam: VU University Press, 1993:89–94.
39. Hahn H. An agenda for citizens with disabilities: pursuing identity and empowerment. *J Voc Rehabil* 1997;9:31–33.
40. Nosek MA. Women with disabilities and the delivery of empowerment medicine. *Arch Phys Med Rehabil* 1997;78:S1–S2.
41. Stucki G, Cieza A, Ewert T, et al. Application of the International Classification of Functioning, Disability and Health: ICF in clinical practice. *Disabil Rehabil* 2002;24:281–282.
42. McNeil JM. Americans with disabilities: 1994–95. *Current Population Reports Series P70–61*. Washington, DC: Department of Commerce, Economics and Statistics Administration, Bureau of the Census, 1997.
43. Üstün TB, Rehm J, Chatterji S, et al., and the WHO/NIH Joint Project CAR Study Group. Multiple-informant ranking of the disabling effects of different health conditions in 14 countries. *Lancet* 1999;354 (9173):111–115.
44. Bickenbach JE, Chatterji S, Badley EM, et al. Models of disablement, universalism and the international classification of impairments, disabilities and handicaps. *Soc Sci Med* 1999;48(9):1173–1187.
45. Üstün TB, Bickenbach JE, Badley E, et al. A reply to David Pfeiffer: "The ICIDH and the Need for its Revision." *Disability and Society* 1998; 13(5):829–831.
46. National Committee on Vital and Health Statistics. *Classifying and reporting functional status*. Washington, DC: Department of Health and Human Services/Center for Disease Control/National Center for Health Statistics, 2001.
47. Üstün TB, Chatterji S. Measuring functioning and disability: a common framework. *Internat J Methods in Psych Res* 1998;7(2):79–83.
48. Üstün TB, Chatterji S, Bickenbach JE, et al., eds. *Disability and culture: universalism and diversity*. Göttingen, Germany: Hogrefe and Huber Publishers, 2001.

CHAPTER 50

Research in Physical Medicine and Rehabilitation

Joel A. DeLisa, Scott R. Millis, and Bruce M. Gans

For any field of medicine, research is an essential foundation for its growth, refinement, and improvement. Research is also critical for acceptance of the teachings and beliefs of that field. For physiatry to flourish as a clinical and academic discipline, it must develop a stronger research base (1–4). Much of the research recently published in the core journals of physical medicine and rehabilitation has been observational, rather than based on prospective randomized clinical trials. Over the past 2 years, only 15% of the articles in the *Archives of Physical Medicine and Rehabilitation* are clinical trials of any sort, with the vast majority of these being longitudinal observational work. The demand for evidence-based medical practice is fueling the need for randomized clinical trials in all specialties. Proof of efficacy and efficiency of interventions are high priority and are effectively addressed through clinical research. Innovations in care are also an essential component of applied research. Studies in rehabilitation engineering seeking to demonstrate that modern technology (i.e., new designs for orthoses, prostheses, adaptive devices, and wheelchairs) can facilitate functional gains are unique to this field. In addition to the invention of new and improved devices, the need for clinical investigation of their effectiveness is also evident.

Clinical research in physical medicine and rehabilitation is the unique type of scientific investigation that is meaningful to the field, and it is the focus of this chapter. It includes studies intended to provide knowledge that contributes to our understanding of the prevention, diagnosis, treatment, rehabilitation, or cure of human disease. It also includes health services research and may seek to relate to research on organs, tissues, cells, subcellular elements, proteins, and genes derived from humans (5).

An ideal research program should improve the quality of patient care by integrating research findings into ongoing clinical activities and engaging interested clinical staff in research activities. An experienced clinician with an analytic, inquiring mind can help to formulate clinical questions that do not have a scientific answer (6). Integrating research and clinical programs can be achieved by (a) educating staff in new treatment approaches and technology. (b) allowing staff to participate in the development and testing of new treatment methods. (c) heightening awareness among staff regarding critical issues in the objective evaluation and treatment of rehabilitation patients, and (d) fostering an intellectually stimulating and pro-

fessionally rewarding environment that attracts and retains staff of high professional caliber with excellent clinical skills (6).

Basic science research forms a foundation for rehabilitation treatment advances as in all other fields of medicine. Nevertheless, clinical science can and should influence the basic science agenda as well. Based on their clinical experience, clinicians can help to formulate basic science questions about the biological or psychological aspects of disability and human performance. They can help focus basic scientists as they apply their scientific findings to the clinical realities. The field of rehabilitation requires a collaborative effort between basic and clinical scientists. For example, understanding how functions mediated by the motor cortex appear to "shift" following amputation or spinal cord injury can guide the development of new treatment methods for persons with these impairments.(6)

THE RESEARCH PROCESS

The foundation of any research study is the formulation of an answerable research question (6) (Table 50-1). The genesis of a problem may stem from clinical observation, the literature, previous or ongoing research, or from colleagues. How the question is asked will determine which data should be collected, the method of research design, what statistical analyses should be performed, and the conclusions that are reached. The problem should be original, as well as clinically relevant and pertinent. The conduct of the study must be consistent with research ethics—e.g., the data should be credible, and the rights, integrity, and confidentiality of subjects must be protected. The research question should be distinctive, but supported by a critical review of the literature. In short, the research project meets the FINER criteria: the study is feasible, interesting, novel, ethical, and relevant (7) (see Table 50-1).

Hypothesis

Once the research problem or question is articulated, the next step in the scientific method is to formulate the hypotheses to be proven or disproved. The key to this phase of the process is to keep the question clearly defined and focused. It is probably better to ask what may seem to be a simple question that can be

TABLE 50-1.   Basic Research Skills

- Defining a research question and formulating testable hypotheses
- Critical review of the scientific literature in a selected area
- Specifying subjects and sampling techniques
- Precision and accuracy of measurements
- Development and use of questionnaires
- Using secondary data
- Cohort study design
- Cross-sectional and case-control design
- Evaluation of diagnostic tests
- Observational studies and inferences of causality
- Experimental sample size
- Ethical issues
- Project management
- Use of descriptive statistics
- Use of analytic statistics
- Use of statistical consultants
- Organizing a pilot study: pretest, quality control
- Technical skills in equipment, procedures, and questionnaires
- Scientific writing
- Oral presentation
- Grant preparation
- Computer use: word processing, database, statistics
- Library reference search

From Findley TW, DeLisa JA. Research in physical medicine and rehabilitation: XI. Research training: setting the stage for lifelong learning. *Am J Phys Med Rehabil* 1991;70(1):S107–S113.

successfully answered rather than a broad one with many parts.

The hypothesis can be viewed as the research question reexpressed in operational language. An explicit research hypothesis forces the investigator to state what is measured and what is proposed to be found; e.g., "There will be a significant increase in health-related quality of life, as measured by the SF-36, in the therapy-intervention group compared with the placebo group (an average increase of 15 points)." This degree of specificity assists the investigator and reviewers to determine whether a study is worthwhile.

Study Sample

In addition to hypothesis, investigators need to define their study sample. This is typically accomplished by clearly specifying inclusion and exclusion criteria (e.g., injury or illness severity of patients to be recruited, age range, comorbidities and medications that will preclude participation in study, and stage of illness). Before initiating the study, it behooves the investigator to determine how difficult it will be to recruit participants. Estimates of treatment impact are necessary for sample size calculations (as discussed in the following section). An explicit hypothesis may alert the investigator that a particular focus of a study may require a huge sample. Knowing this before initiating the study helps the investigator to salvage the research proposal; the research focus can be changed, or more sensitive outcome measures can be chosen.

Research Design

Next, the proper experimental design has to be determined. Different medical research problems require different types of studies. An appropriate study design will generate results that should be reproducible.

Research designs can be broadly classified into two categories: observational designs and experimental designs. There are three common types of observational designs: (a) cohort study, in which a group of persons is observed for a set of variables and followed over time; (b) cross-sectional study, in which a group is examined on a set of variables at a single time point; and (c) case-control study, in which a group of persons of with a disorder ("cases") are compared with a group of persons without the disorder ("controls").

The experimental design is best exemplified by randomized clinical trials, in which persons are randomly assigned to a treatment group or control group (e.g., placebo or standard treatment group). Ideally, both research participant and investigator are blinded to group assignment. At times, it is not feasible to assign research participants randomly to groups. In those cases, a different type of experimental design known as "quasiexperimental" may be used (8).

The above focuses on group designs in which many participants are studied. Another experimental design, known as a single-subject or within-subject design, is a technique in which a single participant is repeatedly measured. At its core, the single-subject design has a baseline phase and intervention phase (9). The simplest single-subject design has single baseline and intervention phases. Multiple baseline designs can be used when the withdrawal of an intervention is associated with a return to baseline status. In this case, inference of a causal connection between an intervention and status change is stronger when change is observed repeatedly during the multiple intervention phases. Findings from single-subject designs have limited generalizability, but may be quite useful when studying low-prevalence disorders or when an investigator is refining theory and technique in preparation for a larger group study.

Sample Bias

Conclusions drawn from biased sampling can be as harmful to the scientific literature as poorly designed clinical trials. The steps described thus far are designed to reduce error or bias. One can never totally eliminate error from a study, but steps can be taken to minimize it. For example, increasing a study's sample size will decrease error. Error can also be reduced by increasing the precision and accuracy of how measurements are made in a study: standardizing tests, training persons making the measurements, improving the tests, automating the measurement process, and repeating measurements (7).

Additional threats include selection bias, performance bias, exclusion bias, and detection bias (10). Selection bias occurs when there are systematic differences between groups. In clinical trials, randomization generally minimizes selection bias, but selection bias can be more of a problem in case-control studies. Performance bias becomes an issue when groups are treated differently apart from the study intervention. For example, performance bias may occur when the active medication group is given more attention and monitoring than the placebo group. Exclusion bias occurs when participants systematically drop out of a study; e.g., the study medication has a high frequency of noxious side effects. In detection bias, the groups' outcomes are assessed differently; e.g., the active treatment group undergoes additional diagnostic testing at the end of the trial.

Study Outcomes

Along with subject selection criteria, the investigator will need to identify the specific predictor and outcome variables to be used in the study. For example, in a proposed study of depression associated with traumatic brain injury, it is insufficient to simply state that "depression will be examined" in the research protocol. It is necessary to specify the instruments that will be used to measure depression, e.g., Beck Depression Inventory or Center for Epidemiologic Studies–Depression Mood Scale.

If a construct or outcome cannot be validly measured, there is little reason to undertake a study. Carefully developing the research hypothesis before data collection increases the likelihood that the investigator has considered measurement options.

A clearly stated research hypothesis can assist investigators and reviewers in assessing the relative costs, risks, and benefits of both observational and experimental studies. Although cost-benefit analyses are obviously important in randomized clinical trials, similar analyses are needed even in retrospective archival data analyses. For example, studies based on archival data are often hampered by unrepresentative samples.

ISSUES IN STATISTICAL ANALYSIS IN MEDICAL REHABILITATION RESEARCH

There are many excellent and comprehensive textbooks in biostatistics that are readily accessible to nonstatisticians. Rather than cataloging a variety of statistical techniques in this chapter, the reader is referred to these references for a full treatment of the content (11–14). The focus here is to highlight and discuss a number of issues in statistical analysis that are particularly relevant in medical rehabilitation research: (a) the overreliance on null hypothesis testing and P values in particular, (b) determining optimal sample sizes, (c) dealing with small samples, (d) handling missing data, (e) measuring change, (f) adopting a systematic multivariable modeling approach, (g) the overuse of parametric statistical procedures, and (h) new developments in item response theory. These topics were chosen because they have posed particularly vexing challenges to rehabilitation research in the past. Fortunately, advances in statistical science have provided new analytic approaches and techniques for dealing with the challenges.

P Values

One summer afternoon in Cambridge, England, in the late 1920s, a group of university professors, their wives, and some guests were sitting around an outdoor table for afternoon tea. "One of the women was insisting that tea tasted different depending on whether the tea was poured into the milk or whether the milk was poured into the tea. The scientific minds among the men scoffed at this as sheer nonsense. What could be the difference? A thin, short man, with thick glasses and a Vandyke beard beginning to turn gray, pounced on the problem. 'Let us test the proposition,' he said excitedly." (15)

The man was Sir Ronald Fisher, the British statistician. The woman was Muriel Bristol of the Wedgwood family. He gave Mrs. Bristol eight cups of tea in random order in which four had the tea added first and in the other four cups, milk was added first. She correctly identified six of the eight cups. Did Mrs. Bristol prove her claim?

This experiment demonstrates aspects of null hypothesis significance testing and the use of P values that are pervasive in biomedical research. The P value is the probability of the observed data given that the null hypothesis is true. That is, the probability of observing a difference of 10 points of the SF-36 between two groups, given that there really is no difference between the groups. By convention, $P < 0.05$ has been used to define a rare event. Hence, if P is less than 0.05, we typically reject the null hypothesis and conclude that the group differences did

not occur by chance. The null hypothesis in this experiment was that Mrs. Bristol could not distinguish between the tea-first or milk-first conditions. She had a 50% chance of being correct even if she could not tell the difference between the conditions. Fisher needed to figure out all of the possible outcomes in this experiment and compute the probability for each outcome. If the probability of Mrs. Bristol's outcome were less than 0.05, we would say that this outcome was not due to chance. We would reject the null hypothesis. It suggests "there is not nothing" (16).

But is this meaningful? To know that there is "not nothing" does not seem to tell us very much. Yet, null hypothesis significance testing and the calculation of P values tend to be carried out reflexively without investigators being aware of the major limitations to this approach. Many researchers continue to confuse statistical significance with clinical significance or practical significance. P values alone cannot provide information on the magnitude of an intervention or an association (17). For example, a negligible difference between placebo and an intervention can be statistically significant if the sample size is large enough. Conversely, a small sample and a nonsignificant P value can mask a clinically meaningful effect. It is worth stressing that the nonsignificant P value does not mean that there is no difference but, rather, *no statistical evidence* was found that there is a difference. This distinction is more than semantic word play because, as Mathews and Altman (18) point out, "A P value is a composite which depends not only on the size of an effect but also on how precisely the effect has been estimated (its standard error). So differences in P values can arise because of differences in effect sizes or differences in standard errors or a combination of the two" (p. 808). There is inherently less precision in estimating effect with small samples because there is less information.

Confidence Intervals

The null hypothesis significance testing is still useful in determining whether there is an effect or association (19). However, null hypothesis significance testing needs to be supplemented with additional statistical information. At the minimum, this should include the point estimate and associated confidence intervals (CIs). The CI is a measure of the precision of the study findings (18). A technical interpretation of the 95% CI is that if the same study were done 100 times with different samples of patients, 95% of these intervals would contain the true population values (e.g., group difference, mean, proportion). The wider the CI is, the less precise the estimate will be.

CIs are particularly useful in interpreting nonsignificant results. Sung et al. (20) compared octreotide infusion to sclerotherapy for the treatment of acute variceal hemorrhage in a group of 100 patients. There were no significant differences in controlled bleeding rates (octreotide = 84% and sclerotherapy = 90%, $P = 0.55$). The authors concluded that both treatments were equally effective. On the surface, it does seem that a 6% difference (i.e., the point estimate) is not a big difference. However, the 95% CI for the treatment difference of 6% is -7.7% to 19.7%. This CI is wide and suggests that there could be quite large differences in the treatments despite the nonsignificant P value. Similarly, in a randomized trial of cognitive rehabilitation for traumatic brain injury, Salazar et al. (21) found that there was no significant difference between patients who received an in-hospital cognitive program versus those receiving the limited home program with regard to fitness for duty (73% vs. 66%, $P = 0.43$). Yet, the 95% CI (-10% to 24%) suggests that one cannot necessarily conclude that the treatments are equivalent.

We recommend that investigators routinely report the point estimate (e.g., difference in means, difference in proportions, etc.) and its associated 95% CI. Moreover, in clinical trials, we recommend that researchers state what they consider to be the minimum difference or effect needed to conclude that an intervention is clinically important. When an intervention's entire 95% CI falls below this specified minimum difference, there is evidence to suggest that the outcome is not clinically significant (22). When the entire CI lies above the minimum difference, there is a clinically important difference. When the CI straddles the minimum difference, the evidence is inconclusive.

Sample Size Calculations

Before embarking on any study, it is helpful to make some initial estimate of the number of participants needed for enrollment. For example, if too few participants are enrolled in a clinical trial, one may fail to detect a clinically meaningful treatment effect. Conversely, enrolling too many subjects is wasteful and potentially exposes participants to unnecessary medical risks. Yet, sample-size calculation, also known as power analysis, is shrouded in mystery to most investigators. Indeed, the statistical complexities should not be minimized; however, researchers should be familiar with the rudiments of power analysis. Bare-bones knowledge saves time and resources: (a) studies requiring unachievable large samples may be identified early in the planning process, (b) necessary data are gathered early to help the investigator communicate more effectively with the statistician to complete the formal power analysis, and (c) gathering the data for a power analysis helps the researcher to determine whether a study is worthwhile.

A good introduction to power analysis is to become familiar with a basic formula for sample-size determination. This example will focus on a formula for two groups in which the outcome variable is continuous. Suppose the hypothesis is that the treatment will reduce hospital stay. A parallel groups design will be used with patients randomly assigned to a control group or to a treatment group. The dependent variable is the number of days. In order to obtain a rough estimate for the number of subjects needed for this study, the following data are required: (a) an estimate of the number of days patients in the control group will be hospitalized; (b) the number of days patients in the treatment group will be hospitalized; and (c) an estimate of group variation, i.e., the standard deviation in days. The following sample size formula is adapted from Van Belle (23):

$$n = \frac{16}{d^2}, where$$

$$d = \frac{\mu_{control} - \mu_{treatment}}{sd}$$

Although the data needed for this formula may be based on previous studies, it is crucial that the investigator critically evaluate the plausibility of the estimates. For example, is it likely that the treatment will reduce length of stay by 30 days? On the other hand, is it a clinically meaningful change and worth the cost of the intervention if treatment reduces length of stay by 1 day? This particular formula determines the sample size for alpha = 0.05 with a power of 0.80. It is hypothesized that the intervention will reduce length of stay by 5 days. The average length of stay without treatment is estimated to be 20 days, with a standard deviation of 4.5 days. Given these parameter estimates, this formula estimates that we will need about 13 patients per group for a total of 26 patients.

Rehabilitation investigators often use multiple regression models in which there may be several predictor variables. If the model contains too many predictor variables, there is a high risk of spurious associations between the predictor and outcome variables. How many is too many? Generally, it is desirable to have 10 to 20 subjects per predictor variable (24). Harrell provides additional guidelines for sample sizes for logistic regression and survival analysis (24).

Small Samples

Even when a power analysis indicates that more participants are required, small samples may be unavoidable. The investigator may wish to study a disorder that has a low prevalence rate, or resource constraints may limit the investigation to a small pilot study. Use of conventional statistical procedures can be a problem under these circumstances. Conventional statistical procedures available in commercial software packages are based on large sample (asymptotic) statistical theory. For example, when comparing the means of two groups on a single variable with a t-test, the result is a P value. If the groups are compared on age and the difference between the groups is 15 years, the P value is the probability of observing a group difference of 15 years or greater, given that there was no difference in the mean age between the groups. Typically, if P is less than 0.05, it is concluded that this is a rare occurrence that is unlikely to have occurred by chance. The hypothesis of no age difference between the groups is rejected. This P value is based on statistical distributions and theory that hold when large sizes are sufficiently large. However, when samples are small, data are sparsely distributed, or data have skewed distributions, the P values may not be accurate. An example of sparsely distributed data is a two-by-two contingency table in which the expected cell count is less than five. An unbalanced data set is illustrated in the case in which only 5% of the sample has the disorder or condition of interest.

Statistical procedures known as "exact tests" are designed to handle small or unbalanced data sets. Software to implement exact tests includes StatXact 5 (25), LogXact 4.1 (26), and SAS 8.2 (27). A wide variety of exact procedures are available, including logistic regression and Poisson regression. An example of an application of exact tests is taken from Mehta and Patel (25), in which they report the results from a chemotherapy pilot study (Table 50-2). Five chemotherapy regimens were used, and tumor regression was measured on a three-point ordinal scale. Small pilot studies can be precursors to larger randomized trials but this example nicely illustrates one of the common problems encountered in pilot studies: i.e., small and unbalanced data. In this case, almost half of the cells are empty. The standard asymptotic procedure found no statistically significant difference in chemotherapy regimens, $P = 0.07$. How-

TABLE 50-2. Chemotherapy Pilot Data			
Treatment	No Response	Partial Response	Complete Response
CTX	2	0	0
CCNU	1	1	0
MTX	3	0	0
CTX + CCNU	2	2	0
CTX + CCNU + MTX	1	1	4

CTX, cyclophosphamide; CCNU, lomustone; MTX, methotrexate.

From Mehta CR, Patel NR. *StatXact 5 manual.* Cambridge, MA: Cytel Software Corporation; 2001.

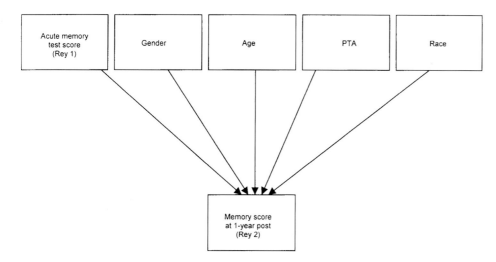

Figure 50-1. Model to predict memory test performance at one-year postinjury.

ever, the exact test yielded a *P* value of 0.039. In this case, the investigator would conclude there is sufficient evidence to suggest that there are treatment differences. Reliance on standard methods of analysis would have missed the differential responses to treatments.

Missing Data

Medical rehabilitation by nature is concerned with multiple variables and factors. For example, several variables are typically required when describing rehabilitation outcome following an intervention. A single binary variable (e.g., cured versus not cured) will rarely be meaningful in a rehabilitation context. Yet, collecting data from patients on several variables can be problematic. Whether a study is a randomized clinical trial or retrospective chart review, it is inevitable that there will be some patients with missing data for some variables. The causes are many. Research participants drop out of studies, and investigators are unable to locate them. Data collectors forget to collect information for selected items in the protocol. Participants may be too ill or impaired to complete some medical or psychological tests. Case report forms are lost, or computer data files become corrupt. Over time, a protocol may be changed, and variables are dropped. Hospitalized research participants may be discharged before all data are collected.

Millis (28) presented methods for handling missing data commonly encountered in medical rehabilitation research. Using data from the Traumatic Brain Injury Model Systems, his goal was to predict performance on a memory test at 1 year postinjury, based on the patient's score on the same memory test during acute rehabilitation. Other variables considered were the patient's sex, age at time of injury, length of posttraumatic amnesia, and race (Fig. 50-1). Memory and new learning capacity are often compromised following brain injury. Models that accurately predict memory outcome can be useful in treatment planning and family counseling. The study had data for 532 patients, but only 69 patients had complete data for all variables (Fig. 50-2). In addition, some of the variables had a substantial proportion of missing data (Fig. 50-3). For example, more than 60% of the sample had missing data on the memory test at 1 year postinjury (Rey2). The variable Rey2 is the total number of words recalled on the five acquisition trials of the Rey Auditory Verbal Learning Test. The most common and simple approach to handling missing data is to analyze only those cases having complete data for all variables. In fact, this is typically the default option used in standard statistical software. This approach is known as listwise deletion or complete case

analysis. However, there are several problems with complete case analysis. The sample size may shrink to a handful of cases when even a few variables have some degree of missing data. In this example, Millis would have analyzed data from only 13% of his sample. There is also a consequent loss of statistical power to detect group differences or to determine which variables are reliable predictors of outcome. In addition, results and parameter estimates may be severely biased because the complete case subsample fails to represent the entire sample. People drop out of studies for a variety of reasons. Unfortunately, their missing data are rarely missing completely at random.

However, it is often a reasonable assumption that the data are missing at random. Missing at random means that participants with incomplete data may differ from participants with complete data, but the pattern of missing data is predictable from other variables in the data set (29). For example, some, but not all, patients with severe traumatic brain injury in inpatient acute rehabilitation are able to complete neuropsychological tests. The inability to complete the tests is often related to injury severity. In other words, the missing neuropsychological test data may be able to be explained by injury severity variables, e.g., length of posttraumatic amnesia, time-to-follow commands, or initial Glasgow Coma Scale score. If data are missing at random, there are some recently developed statistical techniques available to handle missing data: (a) full information maximum likelihood and (b) multiple imputation. Full information maximum likelihood finds the set of parameter values that would have most likely given us our observed data (30). Full information maximum likelihood is particularly useful for handling missing data in multiple linear regression models. It can be implemented in several statistical software packages, e.g., LISREL 8 (31) or AMOS 4.0 (32).

A second method, multiple imputation, can handle missing data in both linear and nonlinear models (e.g., Cox proportional hazards model or ordered logistic regression model). There are three steps in the multiple imputation process. First, multiple imputation typically creates 5 to 10 data sets in which raw data are generated that can be used to "fill in" the missing data. Next, the complete data sets are analyzed with standard statistical procedures. Finally, the results from the analyses of the complete data sets are combined to produce parameter estimates (29). There are a wide variety of statistical software options for performing multiple imputation: SAS 8.2 (PROC MI and PROC MIANALYZE) (27), SOLAS 3 (33), and the Missing Data Library for S-Plus 6.1 (34).

Before the development of full information maximum likelihood and multiple imputation methods to handle missing

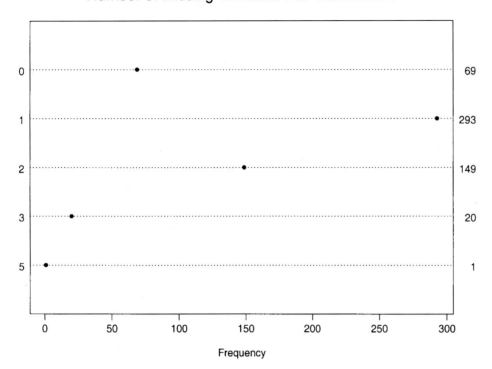

Figure 50-2. Number of missing variables per observation.

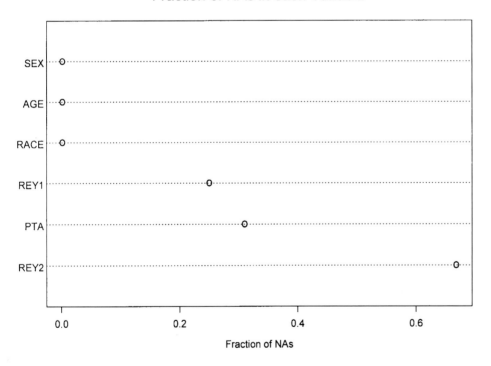

Rey 1 – Rey Auditory Verbal Learning Test Score at inpatient rehabilitation

PTA – Post-Traumatic Amnesia

Rey 2 – Rey Auditory Verbal Learning Test Score at 1 year post injury

Figure 50-3. Fraction of missing values for each variable. [From Millis SR. Dealing with missing data. *Outcome Oriented* 2001 (Winter);1–3.]

TABLE 50-3. Regression Coefficients (and Standard Errors) for Different Missing Data Methods

	Listwise Deletion	Pairwise Deletion	Mean Substitution	Maximum Likelihood	Multiple Imputation
Memory test	.66[a]	.66[a]	.08[a]	.72[a]	.78[a]
	(.10)	(.08)	(.03)	(.06)	(.08)
Sex	−1.01	−.78	−1.00	−2.73	−3.37
	(2.42)	(2.42)	(.78)	(1.82)	(1.86)
Age	−.16[a]	−.09	−.08[a]	−.12[a]	−.13
	(.08)	(.08)	(.02)	(.06)	(.07)
PTA	.03	.06[a]	.01	.03	.04
	(.04)	(.03)	(.01)	(.03)	(.03)
Race	−2.07	1.50	1.52[a]	1.58	1.11
	(2.24)	(2.13)	(.68)	(1.61)	(2.97)

PTA, posttraumatic amnesia.
[a]($p < .05$).

data, some investigators used mean substitution or pairwise deletion. Neither method can be recommended. In mean substitution, a variable's mean value is calculated from the available cases and is then used as the imputed value for the missing cases. Mean substitution produces biased results because it artificially reduces variance (29). The method of pairwise deletion is sometimes used with missing data in regression or factor analysis because a covariance matrix can be calculated with cases having data for pairs of variables. This method also produces biased results.

Table 50-3 contains the estimated regression coefficients (i.e., unstandardized beta weights) and their standard errors for the model to predict memory test performance (see Fig. 50-1). All methods identified the memory test given during acute rehabilitation as a significant predictor of memory performance at year 1. However, the size of the coefficient varied widely across methods, from 0.08 (mean substitution) to 0.78 (multiple imputation). The size of the standard errors was also quite variable. Equally notable were which variables were found to be significant predictors of memory performance at 1 year postinjury. Pairwise deletion found length of posttraumatic amnesia to be a significant predictor, whereas mean substitution identified race as significant. In contrast, the other methods of handling missing data did not find posttraumatic amnesia or race as significant. The maximum likelihood and multiple imputation methods had the greatest concordance in terms of size of regression coefficients and standard errors. Which method is correct? Simulation studies have clearly determined that listwise deletion, pairwise deletion, and mean substitution methods produce biased estimates unless data are missing completely at random, which is not likely to have been the case with the data set. Hence, maximum likelihood and multiple imputation probably provide the best estimates under the circumstances. This example shows how some methods of handling missing data cannot only be inefficient but also may inaccurately identify variables as significant predictors, which, in fact, are not.

Measuring Change

In clinical trials, it is a common practice in the parallel groups design to measure participants before the intervention or placebo control condition and at the end of the trial. If the treatment is effective, we expect to detect a difference between the intervention and control groups. It would seem that the analysis of this change should be simple. Yet, the investigator faces a bewildering choice of statistical methods to analyze change: (a) analysis of variance (ANOVA) on the post-

test scores alone, (b) ANOVA on difference (gain) scores, (c) ANOVA on percentage change scores, (d) analysis of covariance (ANCOVA), (e) blocking by initial scores (stratification), (f) repeated measures analysis of variance (RMAOV), and (g) generalized estimating equations (GEE), in which the pretest and posttest scores are treated as a bivariate vector in a restricted moment model.

Investigators often choose the RMAOV approach to analyze pretest–posttest data. This is not the optimal strategy. First, investigators often interpret the wrong component of the model, i.e., the treatment factor. RMAOV assumes that all measurements are made after a treatment (35). This cannot possibly occur in the pretest–posttest design because the intervention by design occurs between the pretest and posttest. Thus, the treatment affects only the posttest, and this causes the F test for the treatment effect to be biased. Second, the treatment-by-trials interaction in the RMAOV produces an unbiased estimate of the treatment effect. This is the proper component for analysis of change in the pretest–posttest design. However, in this particular design, the treatment-by-trials interaction is equivalent to the analysis of difference scores (35). Moreover, differences scores do not control for pretest imbalance because of regression to the mean (11,13). As a consequence, the treatment effect will be overestimated if the pretest scores were lower in the group receiving the intervention (36).

In most pretest–posttest designs, ANCOVA should be considered for use first for data analysis. ANCOVA takes regression to the mean into account and tends to be the most powerful and efficient approach in the analysis of pretest–posttest data (36–38). If the assumptions of parametric ANCOVA are violated, then nonparametric, rank-transformed ANCOVA should be used. Alternatively, use of GEE might be considered, particularly when sample sizes are 50 or greater (38).

There is, however, an inherent weakness in designs that collect data at only two time points that no statistical procedure can overcome (39). One can only detect a linear trajectory with two time points. However, response to treatment or recovery from a disorder may not be linear. Future studies in rehabilitation medicine should consider using multiple-time-point designs to assess response to treatment or for describing change or growth over time. There have been significant advances over the past 5 years in the statistical analysis of multiple-time-point data. Different names have been used to describe essentially the same analytic approach, e.g., random effects models, mixed models, and hierarchical linear models. Mixed models can be analyzed with a wide range of statistical software, including, but not limited to, SAS (PROC MIXED and PROC NLMIXED),

S-Plus, LISREL, AMOS, Mplus, and EQS. In addition to considering multiple-point designs, multivariable models hold great promise in the assessment change in clinical trials.

Multivariable Modeling Approach

Many of the statistical issues discussed thus far (e.g., P values, sample size, missing data, detecting change, and selecting variables) come together when the hypotheses are operationalized. Many of the phenomena of interest in rehabilitation research are complex. For this reason, multivariable models are required. Development of adequate multivariable models necessarily involves consideration of sample size, missing data, and variable selection. In addition, multivariable models are often desirable for use in randomized clinical trials. It is common in randomized clinical trials to use null hypothesis testing to evaluate treatment effectiveness. However, finding a "statistically significant difference" between treatment and control groups may not take full advantage of the data. We are often interested in estimating the absolute effects of a treatment. In this case, it is necessary to develop a multivariable model of the response variable (24). Most patients enrolled in rehabilitation studies do not have the same risk factors. Multivariable models can account for this circumstance. As Harrell (24) notes, "This approach recognizes that low-risk patients must have less absolute benefit of treatment (lower change in outcome probability) than high-risk patients, a fact that has been ignored in many clinical trials" (p. 4). Even if randomization results in balanced baseline characteristics in our samples, the estimate of the treatment effect will be incorrect when there is even moderate heterogeneity among participants unless a multivariable model is used to estimate adjusted effects (24).

In his textbook on regression modeling, Harrell (24) presents a comprehensive approach to multivariable modeling. Below are guidelines from Harrell and other sources that have broad applications in rehabilitation research:

1. Allow the research hypotheses, theory, and past research findings to guide variable selection. Critically evaluate whether each variable should be included in the model. "More" is not necessarily better when building models. Parsimony should be a guiding principle.
2. Select variables that have wide score distributions. Variables having limited range will have limited variance and an attenuated capacity to detect differences or to predict. Histograms or other graphic methods can be useful in detecting a variable's range, as well as other aspects of its shape and distribution. Figure 50-4 contains an array of histograms of the continuous variables used by Millis (28) in the prediction of memory performance following traumatic brain injury. For example, posttraumatic amnesia appears to have a relatively restricted range, whereas the memory tests (Rey1 and Rey2) have more variability. In certain cases, transformations can improve model fit.
3. Consider eliminating variables that have or will likely have high levels of missing data.
4. Do not use stepwise regression to select variables. Stepwise techniques produce biased standard errors and inflated R^2 values. Harrell (24) found that ". . . variables selected for the final model represented noise 20% to 74% of the time and that final model usually contained less than half of the actual number of authentic predictors" (p. 58). Menard (40) also notes that ". . . there appears to be general agreement that computer-controlled stepwise procedures to select variables is inappropriate for theory testing because it capitalizes on random variations in the data, and produces results that tend to be idiosyncratic and difficult to replicate

in any sample other than the sample in which they were originally obtained" (p. 63).
5. Examine your data for missing data. Consider using full information maximum likelihood or multiple imputation strategies when the proportion of missing data exceeds 0.15.
6. Fit the model on the entire data set.
7. Linear regression has a number of assumptions about model errors (e.g., constant variance, normal distribution, uncorrelated error terms, no correlation between errors and predictor variables). Violations of these assumptions can have serious consequences. For example, nonconstant variance (heteroscedasticity) will tend to inflate standard errors and cause the statistical tests to be inaccurate (40). Analysis of the model's residuals can assist the researcher in detecting violation. Examination of residual plots and numerical analysis of the residuals should be the next step once the model has been fit. There are several types of residuals from which to choose; the Studentized residual is a good choice. Values of less than -2 or greater than $+2$ deserve some attention (40,41)
8. In addition to residual analysis, one should check for overly influential observations in the model. A useful set of diagnostic indicators include the hat-value (leverage values), Cook's D, DFFITS, DFBETAS, and COVRATIO (41). Unusual or influential data should initially alert the investigator to check for data-entry errors. If the data are correct, the researcher needs to determine whether the unusual observation can be understood in the context of the study. At times, transformation of the variable is warranted. Robust regression is another alternative. Rarely should the observation be simply discarded. Table 50-4 contains cutoff score guidelines for selected regression diagnostics as suggested by Fox (41).
9. Use the variance inflation factor to screen for multicolinearity among the predictor variables. If the square root of the variance inflation factor is equal to or greater than 2, multicolinearity may be a problem. Fox (41) discusses methods for addressing this problem.
10. Leave insignificant predictor variables in the model. Taking out the insignificant predictors and then refitting the models with only the significant predictors produces a biased model.

Additional Issues

There is a reflexive tendency among many data analysts to use standard parametric statistical procedures not only for small samples but also in all situations, even when there are gross violations of basic parametric statistical assumptions, e.g., variances

---

TABLE 50-4.   Cutoff Scores for Selection Regression Diagnostic Indexes

- Hat-values: exceeding twice the average $(k + 1) / n$, where k is the number of predictors and n is the sample size

- DFBETAS: $2/\sqrt{n}$

- DFFITS: $2/\sqrt{(k + 1)/(n - k - 1)}$

- Cook's D: $4/(n - k - 1)$

- COVRATIO: $3(k + 1)/n$

From Fox J. *Applied regression analysis, linear models, and related methods.* Thousand Oaks, CA: Sage, 1997.

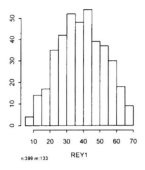
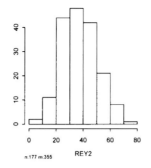
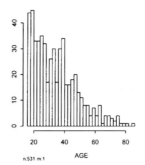

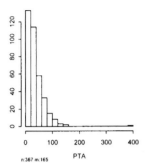

Rey 1 – Rey Auditory Verbal Testing Score at inpatient rehabilitation

PTA – Post-Traumatic Amnesia

Rey 2 – Rey Auditory Verbal Learning Test Score at 1 year post-injury

Figure 50-4. Histograms of continuous variables. [From Millis SR. Dealing with missing data. *Outcome Oriented* 2001 (Winter); 1–3.]

among groups that are wildly heterogeneous and parent distributions of variables that are nonnormal. As has been noted, erroneous conclusions may be drawn. Fortunately, there are several nonparametric and robust statistical methods now available that can be used to deal with messy data. Wilcox (42) provides an excellent discussion with applications of current methods.

Many of the phenomena that are measured in rehabilitation are complex. Hence, instrument development is formidable. Item response theory is an important tool for test item selection and score interpretation. One type of item response theory method that has been popular in rehabilitation research has been Rasch analysis. Rasch analysis focuses on a single parameter: item difficulty. It should be noted, however, that there are alternative approaches to item response theory; the two-parameter and three-parameter logistic models, for example, may be more suitable for developing tests for complex phenomena (43). As with parametric methods for general data analysis, there has been an unfortunate overreliance on simple Rasch models in rehabilitation research. Investigators need to be aware of alternative methods.

RESEARCH ETHICS

In this section it would be useful to make reference to issues of protection of human subjects (how we have come from the Nuremberg to Helsinki to Belmont Report), and the watchdog of this is the Institutional Review Board (IRB), whose role is established through 45CFR46. The physician's duty is to promote and safeguard the health of the people (44). Simply, biomedical researchers' duty is to improve diagnostic, therapeutic, rehabil-itative, and prophylactic procedures and add to our understanding of the etiology, pathogenesis, and treatment of disease while protecting human subjects involved in research. To provide guidance to physicians and others in medical research involving human subjects, the World Medical Association developed the Declaration of Helsinki (44). Investigators are strongly encouraged to read this document and adhere to its four basic principles. The ethical issues associated with clinical research involve four moral principles. These are beneficence and nonmaleficence, concern for other's welfare, justice, and trust (Table 50-5).

Federal law requires approval of any research project involving human subjects by an IRB. It is the IRB's responsibility to review the research proposal and consent forms and to weigh the potential benefits and risks to participants. IRBs now have formal educational requirements for investigators in biomedical research. All investigators are strongly advised to follow the rules, regulations, and educational requirements of their institutional IRB. Special caution and additional requirements apply to research that affects the welfare of animals. Experimental devices and drugs, additionally, may require approval from the Food and Drug Administration.

Conflict of Interest

Conflict of interest in a research study exists when a participant in the study or peer evaluation process has financial or other types of interest that could bias the results. Financial relations with industry through employment, consultation, honorarium, expert testimony, and stock options are usually considered to be the most important conflicts of interest. However, conflicts

TABLE 50-5.   Moral Principles Applied to Conduct of Research

1. Beneficence and Nonmaleficence
   • Maximize potential benefits and minimize possible harms
   • Difficult to balance; necessitates autonomous, informed consent from participants
2. Concern for Other's Welfare
3. Justice
   • Concern about power imbalances related to special, potentially vulnerable populations, e.g., sex, ethnic minority, and socioeconomic status
   • Researchers are concerned about and work to mitigate the causes of human suffering. When undertaking research, they strive to advance human welfare, science, and practice.
4. Trust
   • Explicit agreement about what participants will experience and its consequences, and the researcher's obligations in conducting the research
   • Giving adequate opportunity, at multiple points, to ask questions and to receive simple answers as to the nature or experiments and what is expected

TABLE 50-6.   Intellectual Property
• *Patents:* Grant by the government to exclude others from using or selling his/her claimed invention, e.g., device • *Copyright:* Protection of original ideas from presentation by others, e.g., book • *Trademarks:* Protection of an emblem, symbol, or object that distinguishes an idea, service, or product, e.g., logo

can also stem from personal relationships, academic competition, etc. It is important for investigators to disclose any potential conflict of interest at the beginning of a research study so that a determination may be made as to whether the conflict is tolerable, once disclosed.

Grant Ownership

Usually, a grant to support research is awarded to the institution, not the actual investigator. The investigator who is the lead on the project is charged with the responsibility for directing the expenditure of the grant funds by the institution to achieve the research objectives that have been funded. If a principal investigator leaves an institution, the grant is not automatically transferable. Approval by both the granting agency and the institution are generally required for transfer of the work and assets associated with the studies. These are delicate issues that require tactful resolution.

Data Ownership

The grantee university or research institution holds legal title to the original primary research data acquired as part of a grant-supported research project, unless the institution explicitly relinquishes legal rights to data ownership (45). Investigators need to maintain data files for 3 and in some cases 5 years after completion of their research studies.

Scientific Integrity

It is the investigator's responsibility to conduct all research activities in accordance with the rules and regulations promulgated by federal and state agencies, as well as the host institution. In rehabilitation research, relevant organizations are the Department of Health and Human Services, National Institutes of Health (NIH), and NIDRR. NIH defines scientific fraud as the fabrication, falsification, plagiarism, or other practices that seriously deviate from those that are commonly accepted within the community for proposing, conducting, or reporting research. Serious deviation includes theft, vandalism, and violation of intellectual property. It does not include honest errors or honest differences in interpretations or judgments of data.

Authorship

Unless the results of research are presented and published, they will not benefit other investigators or clinicians. Establishing authorship becomes an important issue when multiple individuals have participated in a study (as is common in clinical investigations). All persons designated as authors should have participated sufficiently in the work to take public responsibility and accountability for the intellectual content. Authorship credit should be based only on substantial contributions to conception and design or analysis and interpretation of data; drafting the manuscript or revising it critically for important intellectual content; and on final approval of the version to be published (46,47).

Personnel who anticipate authorship of a paper are advised to discuss this with the senior investigator in advance to avoid disappointment. Individual project members may feel they have had a major role in the project, although their contribution may not warrant authorship according to international standards. Senior investigators and first authors are similarly advised to discuss authorship with other participants early in the research project.

Intellectual Property

Universities and other research organizations support the preparation and publication of copyrightable works resulting from the teaching, research, scholarly, and artistic endeavors of the faculty, staff, and students as part of their roles at the institution. They respect, acknowledge, and promote the intellectual property of its members, and they strive to maintain a balance knowing the interests of the creators, the funding agency, and themselves in copyrightable material and income resulting from such works. Each institution has a royalties and revenue distribution arrangement, as well as a policy with respect to the intellectual property, which usually deals with patients, copyright, trademark, and data ownership. Investigators are advised to familiarize themselves with the local policy. These are defined in Table 50-6.

RESEACH FUNDING SOURCES

It is very difficult to sustain even a minimal research program without external funding. In 1991, Davidoff and co-workers showed that the lack of research funding from other sources may reflect the lack of initiative and enthusiasm in many physical medicine and rehabilitation departments to develop methods for funding research programs outside their own financial base (48). It is essential that researchers learn how to write grants and that they view this as a core responsibility.

The largest sponsor of health research in the United States is the federal government. Close behind are health-oriented corporations, but they are devoted largely to product application development, be it pharmaceutical or device. Philanthropic contributions by private corporations represent only about 5%

TABLE 50-7. Budgets of Rehabilitation Research Granting Agencies (in Millions USD) and Rates of Growth (by Percentage)

Year	NIH	NICHD	NCMRR	NIDRR
2001	20,300 (14.2%)	976 (13.9%)	46 (22%)	100
2000	17,800 (13.7%)	857 (14.1%)	38 (41%)	86
1999	15,600 (14.7%)	71 (11.7%)	27 (25%)	81
1998	13,600 (7%)	672 (6.5%)	21 (−5%)	76
1997	12,800 (6.9%)	6.31 (6.5%)	19 (25%)	70
1996	11,900 (5.8%)	594 (4.5%)	19 (25%)	70
1995	11,300 (3.3%)	570 (2.8%)	15 (8%)	70
1994	10,900 (5.9%)	559 (5.1%)	14 (40%)	68
1993	10,300 (2.6%)	528 (5.8%)	10 (50%)	67

NIH, National Institutes of Health; NICHD, National Institute of Child Health and Human Development; NCMRR, National Center for Medical Rehabilitation Research; NIDRR, National Institute on Disability and Rehabilitation Research.

of the total U.S. investment in health research, and they generally are in somewhat restricted fields of interest. However, it is advantageous to know the priorities of the foundations in your state and region, as well as those of the larger foundations, such as Robert Wood Johnson, Pew, and Macy.

Within the federal government, the major funding agencies that fund rehabilitation research are the NIDRR (www.ed.gov/offices/OSERS/NIDRR/), an agency of the U.S. Department of Education; NIH (www.nih.gov/), an agency with the Department of Health and Human Services (HHS), the Centers for Disease Control and Prevention (CDC) (www.cdc.gov); the Agency for Healthcare Research and Quality (www.ahrq.gov) within the U.S. Public Health Service, also under HHS; and the Office of Research and Development within the Department of Veterans Affairs.

The two largest programs are NIDRR and NIH. NIDRR was founded in 1978 and for many years was the main source of rehabilitation research funding. The mission of NIDRR is to generate, disseminate, and promote the use of new knowledge that will substantially improve the capacities of people with disabilities to perform work and other activities in the community (49). NIDRR funds model research and demonstration programs in spinal cord injury, traumatic brain injury, and burns. It also funds rehabilitation research and training centers, rehabilitation engineering research centers, field-initiated research grants, innovative grants, and specific calls for proposals, as well as research training grants and fellowships.

Within the NIH, the National Center for Medical Rehabilitation Research (NCMRR) (www.nichd.nih.gov/about/ncmrr/ncmrr.htm) was created by statute in 1990 by P.L. 101–613. NCMRR is part of the National Institute of Child Health and Human Development (NICHD), and its director reports to the director of the NICHD, who in turn, reports directly to the director of NIH. The mission of NCMRR is to enhance the quality of life for people with disabilities through the support of research that will restore, replace, enhance, or prevent deterioration of function (49).

Table 50-7 depicts the NCMRR budget from the inception of the agency through fiscal year 2001. Most NIH awards are the regular or investigator-initiated research award (RO-1), which supports research on a single topic over a 1- to 5-year period. The topics range from acquisition of new knowledge to evaluation of the effectiveness of clinical therapies. Training grants are available to develop the skills to conduct research on rehabilitation-related topics. NCMRR offers two additional programs that further physician research skills: the clinical investigator award (KO8) and the physician scientist award (K11).

Most funding sources welcome questions from prospective applicants about their mission and focus of funding. Most institutions engaged in research operate an office for grants and contracts, which may offer invaluable assistance to investigators seeking grant support. It is also helpful to know the grant review process of the funding agency in advance of submitting a grant.

CONCLUSION

The conduct of rehabilitation research is complex and demanding. It requires talented and creative individual investigators who can dedicate time to asking meaningful questions in a supportive research environment. The methods of conducting this research are available, and funding can usually be secured for well-conceptualized important studies. There are, however, no shortcuts or work-arounds to the hard work that is required to conduct this research. Despite its difficulty, the future of the field depends on these efforts.

REFERENCES

1. DeLisa JA. Compounding the challenge for PM&R in the 1990s. *Arch Phys Med Rehabil* 1985;66:792–793.
2. Grabois M, Fuhrer MJ. Physiatrists' view on research. *Am J Phys Med Rehabil* 1988;67:171–174.
3. Fowler WM Jr. Viability of physical medicine and rehabilitation in the 1980s. *Arch Phys Med Rehabil* 1982;63:1–5.
4. Stolov WC. Rehabilitation research: habit analysis and recommendations. *Arch Phys Med Rehabil* 1983;64:1–5.
5. Kelley WN. Careers in clinical research: obstacles and opportunities: a postscript. *Pediatr Res* 1996;39:903–905.
6. Findley TW, DeLisa JA. Research in physical medicine and rehabilitation: XI. Research training: setting the stage for lifelong learning. *Am J Phys Med Rehabil* 1991;70(1):S107 S113.
7. Hully SB, Cummings SR, Browner WS, et al. *Designing clinical research,* 2nd ed. Philadelphia: Lippincott, Williams & Wilkins, 2001.
8. Campbell DT, Stanley JC. *Experimental and quasi-experimental designs for research.* Boston: Houghton Mifflin, 1963.
9. Helewa A, Walker JM. *Critical evaluation of research in physical rehabilitation.* Philadelphia: W. B. Saunders, 2000.
10. Greenhalgh T. *How to read a paper.* London: BMJ Publishing Group, 1997.
11. Altman AG. *Practical statistics for medical research.* Boca Raton, FL: Chapman and Hall/CRC, 1999.
12. Armitage P, Berry G, Matthews JNS. *Statistical methods in medical research,* 4th ed. Oxford: Blackwell Science, 2002.
13. Bland M. *An introduction to medical statistics,* 3rd ed. New York: Oxford University Press, 2000.
14. Riffenburgh RH. *Statistics in medicine.* San Diego: Academic Press, 1999.
15. Salsburg D. *The lady tasting tea.* New York: W. H. Freeman & Co., 2001.
16. Dawes RM. Probabilistic versus causal thinking. In: Cicchetti D, Grove WM, eds. *Thinking clearly about psychology.* Minneapolis: University of Minnesota Press, 199:235–264.

17. Borenstein M. The case for confidence intervals in controlled clinical trials. *Control Clin Trials* 1994;15:411–428.

18. Matthews JNS, Altman DG. Statistics notes: Interaction 2: Compare effects sizes not p value. *BMJ* 1996;313:808.

19. Frick RW. The appropriate use of null hypothesis testing. *Psychol Methods* 1996;1:379–390.

20. Sung JJ, Chung SC, Lai CW, et al. Octreotide infusion or emergency sclerotherapy for variceal hemorrhage. *Lancet* 1993;342:637–641.

21. Salazar AM, Warden DL, Schwab K, et al. Cognitive rehabilitation for traumatic brain injury. *JAMA* 2000;283:3075–3081.

22. Braitman LE. Confidence intervals assess both clinical significance and statistical significance. *Ann Intern Med* 1991;114:515–516.

23. Van Belle G. *Statistical rules of thumb*. New York: Wiley, 2002.

24. Harrell FE Jr. *Regression modeling strategies*. New York: Springer; 2001.

25. Mehta CR, Patel NR. *StatXact 5 manual*. Cambridge, MA: Cytel Software Corporation, 2001.

26. Mehta C, Patel N. *LogXact 4.1 manual*. Cambridge, MA: Cytel Software Corporation, 1999.

27. SAS Institute. *SAS/STAT software*: reference (version 8.2). Cary, NC: SAS Institute, 2001.

28. Millis SR. Dealing with missing data. Outcome Oriented 2001 (Winter):1–3.

29. Allison PD. *Missing data*. Thousand Oaks, CA: Sage, 2001.

30. Wothke W. Longitudinal and multi-group modeling with missing data. In: Little TD, Schnabel KU, Baumert J, eds. *Modeling longitudinal and multiple group data*. Mahwah, NJ: Lawrence Erlbaum Associates, 1998.

31. Joreskog K, Sorbom D. *LISREL 8: User's reference guide*. Chicago: Scientific Software International, 1996.

32. Arbuckle JL, Wothke W. *Amos 4.0 user's guide*. Chicago: Smallwaters Corporation, 1999.

33. Statistical Solutions. *Solas for missing data analysis 3*. Saugus, MA: Statistical Solutions, 2001.

34. Insightful. S-Plus 6.1. Seattle: Insightful Corporation, 2002.

35. Bonate PL. *Analysis of pretest–posttest designs*. Boca Raton, FL: Chapman & Hall/CRC, 2000.

36. Vickers AJ, Altman DG. Analyzing controlled trials with baseline and follow up measurements. *BMJ* 2001;323:1123–1124.

37. Frison L, Pocock SJ. Repeated measures in clinical trials: analysis using mean summary statistics and its implications for design. *Stat Med* 1992;11:1685–1704.

38. Yang L, Tsiatis AA. Efficiency study of estimators for a treatment effect in a pretest–posttest trial. *American Statistician* 2001;55:314–321.

39. Raudenbush SW, Bryk AS. *Hierarchical linear models*, 2nd ed. Thousand Oaks, CA: Sage, 2002.

40. Menard S. *Applied logistic regression analysis*, 2nd ed. Thousand Oaks, CA: Sage, 2002.

41. Fox J. *Applied regression analysis, linear models, and related methods*. Thousand Oaks, CA: Sage, 1997.

42. Wilcox RR. *Fundamentals of modern statistical methods*. New York: Springer;, 2001.

43. Embretson SE, Hershberger SL. *The new rules of measurement*. Mahwah, NJ: Lawrence Erlbaum Associates, 1999.

44. World Medical Association Declaration of Helsinki: Ethical principles for medical research involving human subjects. *JAMA* 2000;284:3043–3045.

45. Fishbein EA. Ownership of research data. *Acad Med* 1991;66(3):129–133.

46. International Commission of Medical Journal Editors. Uniform requirements for manuscripts submitted to biomedical journals: writing and editing for biomedical publications. Available at http://www.icmje.org. Accessed April 26, 2004.

47. Rennie D, Yank V, Emanuel L. When authorship fails: A proposal to make contributors accountable. *JAMA* 1997;278:579–585.

48. Davidoff GN, Ditunno JF, Findley TO, et al. Elements of academic productivity: a comparison of PM&R units versus other clinical science units. *Arch Phys Med Rehabil* 1991;72:874–876.

49. Gray DB, Groves WH, Cole TM. Federal funding of medical rehabilitation research: the National Center for Medical Rehabilitation Research. *Phys Med Rehabil State Art Rev* 1993;70(2):381–392.

CHAPTER 51

Administration and Management in Physical Medicine and Rehabilitation

Steve M. Gnatz

The need for physician leadership in rehabilitation hospitals and facilities has never been greater than it is today. The competing interests of financial constraints and patient care needs create an environment that may be difficult for nonphysician administrators to navigate. Physiatrists are particularly well suited to work in the area of administration and management because of our experience with teams and teamwork. Many physiatrists become acquainted with administrative duties through medical direction of a rehabilitation unit or hospital, but there are many other aspects of administration and management that will be covered in this chapter. In particular, the roles of chief of staff and vice president of medical affairs are ones that extend beyond the boundaries of rehabilitation medicine. These roles may offer new experiences for the clinician/administrator and an enhanced career path. Given the benefits of an administrative career, why would physicians choose not to assume these duties? Despite the attractiveness of an administrative career, some physicians find that the responsibilities can be difficult to master. Different skills are required than those we are familiar with from clinical medicine. For example, the art of negotiation is neither taught nor used very much in clinical medicine, yet good negotiation skills are required to be a successful administrator. Another key skill is the ability to tolerate ambiguity. In clinical medicine, the patient lives or dies, the lab value is normal or abnormal, etc. These clear distinctions tend to be less so in rehabilitation medicine, in which gray areas are more common. For example, the patient's functional outcome has no absolute end point, and many factors influence attainment of the final goal. Nonetheless, the physician who has difficulty tolerating the often-ambiguous nature of medical administration will not travel far on this career path. Often there is no clear right or wrong, no clear pathway to success or failure in medical administration. Often decisions that are made based on the best data available at the time are only seen to be incorrect in retrospect. This is both the challenge and the curse of medical administration. I hope that using the skills outlined in this chapter will assist the clinician/administrator to navigate the stormy waters of medical administration and achieve the rewards and satisfaction that this area holds.

ADMINISTRATION AND MANAGEMENT VERSUS LEADERSHIP

The day-to-day operations of a hospital or medical rehabilitation entity require management skills appropriate to the task at hand. Budgets must be adhered to, schedules made, customer-service issues resolved. These operational management issues, although critically linked to the success or failure of any facility, should be distinguished from leadership. Managers do things right, but leaders do the right things (1).

Physicians often like to expound on what *should be* done but may have limited ability to see the steps necessary to operationalize the changes. This tends to lead to a state of perpetual dissatisfaction between medical groups and medical facilities. True leadership is the ability to visualize the organization of the future and facilitate the changes across the organization that result in attaining that goal.

There is no more powerful engine driving an organization toward excellence and long-range success than an attractive, worthwhile and achievable vision of the future, widely shared.
Burt Nanus (2)

A leader's role is to develop that attractive, worthwhile, and achievable vision of the future and to garner individual buy-in by stakeholders in the organization.

LEADERSHIP STYLES

How a leader helps achieve the goal of excellence and long range success of the organization is somewhat dependent on his or her personality and leadership style. It may be instructive to learn about your own personality type through the use of one or more of the many systems that have been designed for this purpose. Probably the most commonly used system is the Myers-Briggs Type Indicator (www.capt.org) personality inventory, which assesses personality traits along introversion-extroversion, sensing-intuition, thinking-feeling, and judging-perceiving axes. Awareness of these personality traits can aid the leader in understanding the ways that they interact with others and lead to strategies for personal development and growth.

Good leaders pull, they don't push (3). Although it is true that some authority is required to be an effective leader, power and authority alone will not be sufficient to lead an organization into the future. Autocratic leaders can be very effective in the short term because their authoritative style is efficient. However, the long-term result for organizations led by such autocrats is less than ideal. At best, the organization may develop a culture in which creativity and innovation are stifled, and there is risk that a culture of fear can develop in which the people who work in the organization can become paralyzed and unable to think and act independently. The ability to share a vision of the future and then empower people within the organization to create the tactics and steps to achieve that vision makes for an effective leader.

> Keys to success in leadership
> *Know your mission*
> *Articulate and spread your vision*
> *Stick to your values*
> *Be flexible*
> *Look for "win-win" solutions*
> *Don't re-invent the wheel*
> *Delegate authority, let people under you take chances,*
>   *make mistakes and grow*

In the Deming model of total quality, more than 90% of defects in quality relate more to processes than to people (4). Although this model was developed for the manufacturing industry, this seems equally true in health care. Effective leadership realizes this principle and works on improving the processes using input from the stakeholders within and outside the organization.

MISSION, VISION, VALUES, AND THE STRATEGIC PLANNING PROCESS

Organizations only live in their statements, whether they be written down or spoken. Statements of mission or purpose play a significant role in the effective leadership of any organization. They should be developed with input from all of the stakeholders. Often this is done as the first step of the strategic planning process.

Mission statements target customers and markets, indicate the principle services offered by the organization, specify the geographic area within which the organization intends to concentrate, identify the organization's philosophy, include confirmation of the organization's preferred self-image, and specify the organization's desired public image. Most organizations have some sort of mission or purpose statement already in place; however, it is important to review this statement from time to time to assure that it continues to reflect the current status of the organization.

A vision statement reflects what the organization aspires to be and the expectations of the stakeholders when the mission is being accomplished. It is affected by the history of the organization and its internal capacity. The external and internal environment of the organization also affects it. It is the hope for the future that we want to create as an organization. Like the mission statement, the vision statement is usually developed through the strategic planning process with input from stakeholders and needs to be updated from time to time.

Value statements reflect our guiding principles. For example, "We believe that rehabilitation is effective, both cost-effective and in quality of life" or "We believe in treating our patients with compassion, excellence, and respect" or "We believe in teamwork, innovation, and integrity." These types of statements usually will not change within an organization over time, but they should be reviewed periodically to assure that they reflect the true values of the organization.

Once the mission, vision, and values have been developed or reviewed, the strategic planning process can proceed as shown in Figure 51-1.

In the planning process, the mission, vision, and values are reviewed and confirmed or modified to meet the needs of the organization in its current environment. Once that is accomplished, there are several methods for developing a strategic plan. Probably the most commonly used strategic planning technique is the situational analysis or SWOT (strengths, weakness, opportunities, and threats), which incorporates a group technique of analyzing these elements both within and external to the organization. The SWOT technique can then be used to develop tactics and strategies particularly related to how the organization will develop the opportunities that are identified or handle the threats. Another useful technique for strategic planning is the use of scenario analysis. In this technique, the group is led through different scenarios that may range from the likely to the nearly absurd. For example, "What if the medical school decided that the department of physical medicine and rehabilitation should be a division of orthopedics?" or "What if we lost our largest referral source?" Using these types of questions, the group can formulate plans based on the scenarios presented and develop tactics to deal with each. This technique is usually used by more mature organizations that are already familiar with the SWOT analysis.

Once the strategic objectives and tactics are outlined, the group can prioritize, assign time frames, and establish responsible parties for each of the tactics. It is important at this stage to relate the tactics to key performance areas of the organization. For example, the tactics might have financial implications, relate to the functional outcomes for patients participating in clinical programs, or be related to customer satisfaction measures—all key performance areas for many organizations. If there are budgetary ramifications of the tactics, these should be discussed and agreed on by the leadership, because it is unlikely that a tactic that requires budgetary support will be accomplished in the absence of allocation of resources.

Unfortunately, at this point in the strategic planning process, many organizations stop, print out the strategic plan in a large tome, and put it on a shelf to collect dust until the next strategic planning retreat. A critical step in the success of this process is the feedback loop that is shown in Figure 51-1, wherein the organization monitors the progress of the tactics and strategic objectives and subsequently modifies its behavior, adapting to the conditions that occur moving forward. The link between the strategic plan and the budget is critical here because financial goals are routinely monitored by organizations. Also, this feedback loop gives the strategic planning process the essence of continuous quality improvement. As processes are identified that require redesign with specific objectives in mind and these changes are effected, the feedback loop of strategic planning becomes a continuous quality improvement initiative, lifting the organizational quality with every revolution of the strategic planning cycle.

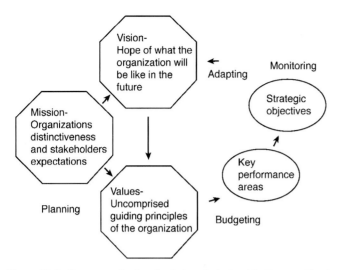

Figure 51-1. From organizational mission strategic objectives and back.

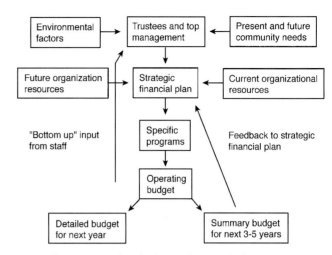

Figure 51-2. Where budgeting fits in to the big picture.

FINANCIAL DECISION MAKING

Physician leaders are often involved in financial decision making, whether as a leader of their practice group or in a hospital administrative role. Because financial training in most medical schools is lacking (although recently more attention has been paid to this area by curriculum committees), physicians either learn these skills on the job or through formalized programs. Given the risk associated with error in this area, formalized training is recommended if one is considering an administrative career. Several resources are available to physicians, including executive programs offered by many business schools in health administration or business administration leading to an MHA or MBA degree. Also, courses offered by the American College of Physician Executives (www.acpe.org) lead to a Master of medical management (MMM) degree. A significant amount of information on practice management in physical medicine and rehabilitation is available through the American Academy of Physical Medicine and Rehabilitation (www.aapmr.org).

Tools for Financial Decision Making

The most recognizable financial decision-making tool in most organizations is the budget. The budget compares expected revenue streams with expected operational expenses and is used to make predictions about the financial workings of the organization over a period of time (usually the fiscal year). One of the most important aspects to recognize about budgets is that they are always wrong. The extent to which the budget reflects what actually happens financially to the organization during the upcoming year reflects the art and science of the leaders making up the budget. Most budgets are built to predict the profit margin or, for not-for-profit organizations, the revenues in excess of expenses.

> *No margin, no mission*
>
> Attributed to the Sisters of Charity

Because without revenues in excess of expenses (or profit margin) no organization can exist for long, effective budgeting is required for all organizations. There are, however, some important considerations when building and analyzing budgets. If one is overly conservative, the organization will not be able

to take advantage of new opportunities. That is, in order to grow and expand, the organization must invest sufficient resources to programs and services that may not return revenue immediately. However, if one is too optimistic about revenue associated with fixed expenses, the organization will have cash flow issues at best and at worst will sustain a financial loss that will either require tapping of reserves or lead to insolvency. If the organization does not have good information about what resources are needed to get the job done, and what organizational capacities it has, then the budgeting process will be inaccurate, leading to error. Figure 51-2 shows how the budget process fits in with the strategic planning process for organizations.

Other Financial Tools Available

PRO FORMA OR BUSINESS PLAN

Unfortunately, in most hospitals and medical practices, the use of a pro forma or formal business plan is underutilized as a financial planning technique. Many health-care organizations initiate and maintain clinical programs based on intuition and the will of strong clinical champions (often physicians) rather than a well-thought-out business plan. Certainly without physicians who have a strong clinical interest in an area, there is little hope of a successful program. However, one of the main reasons for excess capacity in health care in America today is the wanton disregard for whether there is a business case that can be made for a program to be developed. A pro forma statement is a projection of how a financial statement would appear if the project were developed as planned. It is a prediction of the financial aspects of a program to be developed. A well-thought-out business plan incorporating such a pro forma statement, although not a guarantee of success, will at least assure an organization that it has been sufficiently diligent in determining if there is a chance that the program will meet its financial and operational goals.

FINANCIAL STATEMENTS

Most organizations use financial statements such as statements of income and expense (also know as profit and loss statements or statements of position), cash flow statements, or balance sheets to display financial information for their stakeholders and for the purposes of required reporting to federal agencies, such as the Securities and Exchange Commission or the Inter-

TABLE 51-1.   Examples of Ratios Used in Health Care

$$\text{Net operating margin} = \frac{\text{Net income or revenues in excess of expenses}}{\text{Net operating revenue}}$$

$$\text{Average collection period} = \frac{\text{Net accounts receivable}}{\text{Average daily gross or net patient revenue}}$$

$$\text{Collection rate} = \frac{\text{Net collections}}{\text{Gross charges}}$$

$$\text{Clinic space utilization} = \frac{\text{Number of patient office visits}}{\text{Number of clinic rooms available}}$$

$$\text{Net collections per RVU} = \frac{\text{Net collections}}{\text{Physician relative value units produced}}$$
By physician

nal Revenue Service (IRS). The detailed analysis of these financial tools is beyond the scope of this chapter, and the reader is referred to the suggested reading list for resources available. Also, training in the interpretation of financial statements is a typical part of the business school curriculum for those who take the path of formal training.

RATIOS

Useful tools in the armamentarium of an administrator are ratio measures to assist with decision making. Some common ratios are shown in Table 51-1, however, there are essentially an unlimited number of ratios that can be invented to answer questions of financial performance within an organization. Because these ratios yield a simple number, they can be benchmarked against either the organization's historical performance or external benchmarks (if available).

Ratios lend themselves well to performance "dashboards." These are relatively simple, often 1-page reports with graphs that track key operational indicators for monitoring of organizational performance on a regular basis. Most administrators have favorite ratios and other indicators that they have reported to them in this fashion so that they can get an at-a-glance look at key performance indicators and spot trouble areas that may be developing.

MARKET ANALYSIS

When evaluating new or existing programs and making predictions about financial performance, market analysis is an essential tool. A great deal of information is required to be made publicly available by hospitals. For example, the Health Plan Employer Data and Information Set indicators provide information about discharge DRGs from the acute care hospitals that rehabilitation facilities can use to predict the market for inpatient rehabilitation patients. Knowing the demographics of the potential patient population in an area may help an administrator predict if demand for a new program is likely to allow it to succeed. A qualified market analyst will use publicly available information from databases and privately obtained information to answer focused questions from administration regarding the market into which the organization is planning to move. Analysis of competitors and their competencies may assist in differentiating the organization from those competitors in the eyes of the public. This type of analysis may lead to marketing strategies as well, but the primary focus is on assuring

to the best of our ability that a business plan has viability in the marketplace.

Financing for Rehabilitation

PHYSICIAN PROFESSIONAL FEE PAYMENT SCHEMES

Administrative physicians must become facile with several health-care financing realms. Physicians are most often reimbursed for their professional services on a discounted fee-for-service (FFS) basis today, but may occasionally practice in a capitated environment. In a traditional undiscounted FFS environment, the more services are provided, the more remuneration is paid at full rates. Hence, historically, the payers have concentrated on controlling utilization. This could be accomplished through denial of care as medically unnecessary, requiring authorization before procedures, etc. This system of payment is often referred to as the good old days of physician compensation. Under the system of discounted FFS payment, the concept is the same as FFS, but physicians have offered payers discounts based on the promise or hope of capturing a larger market share. In the case of Medicare, the physician agrees to accept the Medicare fee schedule, almost always at a discount compared with the usual, customary, and reasonable fees of most physician practices. A discounted FFS system may encourage "milling" (i.e., the practice of increasing volume by not providing the same amount of patient contact per encounter) or "up-coding" (i.e., billing a higher charge code than the actual work of the visit would normally allow). The response from payers has been to attempt to control utilization and to discover and prosecute fraudulent physician billing practices.

In a capitated payment system, the physician or medical group assumes financial risk for a defined patient population. In this payment scheme, the payer agrees to pay in advance for medical services for their enrollees, called "covered lives." The physician or medical group agrees to provide all of the medical services required to maintain the health of the enrolled population. This is the model of the health maintenance organization. Under a capitated system of payment, the fewer physician services are provided, the more revenue is retained by the physician or group. This system avoids the perverse incentive of FFS, wherein unnecessary service provision brings higher revenues, but may create an even less desirable environment in which health-care services are not provided to patients when necessary. In a capitated environment, the payers focus on controlling quality and patient outcomes because they have paid for the services up front.

Physician administrators should be particularly aware of the incentives generated by the payment schemes under which the members of their physician practice are working. It is not uncommon for there to be a variety of the payment schemes noted above at play simultaneously in a group practice. This can lead to confusion among the medical staff. The time-honored advice to the physicians is to practice medicine in the most cost-effective and ethically correct manner, and let the financial chips fall where they may.

INPATIENT REHABILITATION FACILITY PAYMENT

One of the biggest changes to ever affect the rehabilitation hospital industry is the introduction of the Inpatient Rehabilitation Facility Prospective Payment System (IRF PPS) for inpatient rehabilitation facilities by Medicare. The Balanced Budget Amendment of 1997 set in motion a plan to bring inpatient rehabilitation facilities under a system of prospective payment.

After a series of delays, the IRF-PPS started taking effect for fiscal reporting periods as of January 1, 2002.

> *Between the 1980's and today, the paradigm in rehabilitation has shifted from attempting to produce the highest quality outcome for the patient to attempting to produce the highest quality outcome for the patient **with the resources allowed.***
>
> Attributed to Barry S. Smith, MD

Nearly 20 years ago, the Diagnosis Related Group form of prospective payment revolutionized acute medical/surgical hospital financing (as well as patient care). The resultant declines in acute hospital lengths of stay and innumerable other changes in medical practice in the United States are due, in great measure, to this change in the payment system. As noted previously, in any prospective payment system, the focus shifts from control of utilization to control of quality and outcome. Inpatient rehabilitation has mature and reliable outcome measurement systems that have been refined over many years. In fact, Medicare incorporated elements of the Functional Independence Measure (FIM®) into its assessment and payment tool, the Inpatient Rehabilitation Facility Patient Assessment Instrument.

The IRF-PPS system distinguishes patients within 21 rehabilitation impairment categories based on their diagnosis and subdivides these rehabilitation impairment categories into case mix groups based on severity and other criteria. Because the payment is determined prospectively, based on the assessment at the time of admission, there is a known amount of resources available to provide all of the care required to reach the desired outcome. However, this is the average amount of resources that will be needed to rehabilitate the patient; some will require more, others less. By understanding the costs associated with the rehabilitation care within the hospital, the physician administrator can assist with the refinement of patient care protocols and pathways to help assure the highest level of outcome at the lowest cost.

COMPLIANCE WITH LAWS AND REGULATIONS

This section of the chapter is meant as a general introduction to the topic of some of the more common legal and legislative aspects that the administrative physician may encounter. It is not meant as legal advice or counsel. If you believe that you or your organization have concerns in the areas listed below, it is recommended that you engage an attorney familiar with this area of the law.

Although not officially designated as a regulated industry, health care certainly labors under a huge, and seemingly ever-increasing, number of governmental and nongovernmental rules and regulations. These regulations may be confusing for health-care providers and challenges to achieve compliance. Further, they may occasionally be applied retroactively to health-care organizations by the federal government. Nonetheless, administrators have a duty to provide a good faith effort to comply with the wide array of different laws, rules, and regulations. In this chapter, an attempt will be made to list the general categories and essential principles of many of the current regulations. It is without a doubt that before this text is published, regulatory changes will be enacted that will make some of the information obsolete. The reader is therefore cautioned to constantly scan for new information in this important area.

Despite the commitment of time and resources to compliance activities, there is a distinct advantage to remaining aware of and attempting to comply with laws and regulations. The federal sentencing guidelines recognize such a good faith effort in assigning penalties for being out of compliance. Such punitive measures as treble damages and incarceration are usually reserved for individuals and organizations that demonstrate willful noncompliance or no attempt at an effective compliance program.

Federal Regulation

PARTICIPATION IN MEDICARE
As one of the largest payers purchasing health-care services, the Center for Medicare and Medicaid Services (CMS) promulgates a large number of rules and regulations regarding how providers act. In order to be a participating provider under Medicare, both physicians and hospitals must abide by the Medicare conditions of participation. These regulations are publicly available on the CMS Web site at (www.cms.hhs.gov). Many of these regulations are echoed by other health-care accrediting bodies, such as the Joint Commission on Accreditation of Health Care Organizations (JCAHO), but there are some specific rules as well. CMS has become more aggressive in using its right to remove (either temporarily or permanently) providers who do not abide by the conditions of participation. Most providers cannot financially sustain prolonged exclusion from this important payer.

MEDICARE TEACHING PHYSICIAN RULES
Primarily affecting academic medical centers (AMC), the Medicare teaching physician rules have evolved over the past 20 years or so. Essentially these rules changed the face of attending-resident practices over that time period. Before these rules being promulgated, residents often were supervised by attending physicians without separate and independent documentation on the part of the attending physician. Because the CMS position is that no documentation equals no billable service provided, this led to large fines and reimbursements to Medicare by several AMCs over the past 10 years. These regulations evolved slowly and were often enacted retrospectively, however, so it was very difficult for AMCs to comply. Nonetheless, most, if not all, AMCs have enacted changes in resident and attending interaction that produce specific documentation of resident and attending work under clearer guidelines from CMS.

FRAUD AND ABUSE
Private practitioners and academic physicians alike have become ensnared in fraud and abuse charges. Legally, many of these cases are tried under the federal False Claims Act, which makes it illegal for anyone to fraudulently bill the federal government. Most of these cases stem from insufficient physician documentation for services billed to Medicare recipients. The government has become quite aggressive in enlisting seniors to "whistle-blow" on physicians and other providers who they believe have overbilled or otherwise abused the Medicare program. The practice of up-coding or billing a higher level of service than that substantiated by the documentation has led to many settlements against providers. This risk has led some practitioners to practice an equally illegal (but not usually enforced) act of down-coding, or billing a lower level service than the documentation would allow. Obviously, down-coding has significant negative financial ramifications for a physician practice. Clearly, educational efforts aimed at the medical staff to follow the rules and "right-code" are a priority for every hospital and medical practice in America today.

TABLE 51-2.   Under the Current Interpretation of the Stark Law

A doctor owns an interest in a Physical Therapy (PT) service, and therefore he or she may not directly refer to that company and bill the Medicare program . . .
He or she admits patients to a Skilled Nursing Facility (SNF) in which he/she has a financial interest (OK to do) . . .
Even if that SNF contracts with unrelated PT company (doctor does not own) but he/she orders the PT . . .
If the service is arranged by the SNF, it may be illegal if the SNF bills Medicare Part A for the PT because then the doctor would potentially benefit from ordering the PT as a part of the profit on the SNF.

STARK SELF-REFERRAL LEGISLATION

The Omnibus Budget Reconciliation Act of 1989 (Stark I) and the Omnibus Budget Reconciliation Act of 1993 (Stark II) made physician self-referral to clinical laboratories, physical therapy, durable medical equipment suppliers, and certain other entities illegal except for certain safe harbors. A significant safe harbor applies to integrated practice groups that employ physicians and have the business entities mentioned above. Further "clarification" of the Stark Law is currently pending. It is safe to say that this is an area in which great confusion abounds. Most, if not all, independent physicians divested themselves of any ventures that were outside the safe harbors years ago, but the potential of family members or relatives who are in health care may still pose a threat. See the example in Table 51-2.

Confusing? You bet. Would it be possible that a physician could be out of compliance with the Stark Law and not even know? Absolutely. Does that ignorance protect the physician? Not likely.

ANTIKICKBACK LEGISLATION

The Antikickback Act of 1986 forbids the payment of any remuneration for referrals of patients. This applies to either in-cash or in-kind payments. It applies to all contractual arrangements with the federal government, including Medicare. Discounts to specific groups of patients (so-called professional courtesy), waiving of copayments, and other inducements may be considered illegal under this act as well.

ANTITRUST

Antitrust law prohibits conspiracies to dominate markets and other impermissible activities to gain competitive advantage over others in the process. Antitrust law prohibits health-care providers and organizations from sharing information that would confer a significant competitive advantage in the marketplace. Examples of this would be sharing physician or hospital charges with other entities for the purposes of price fixing. Sharing of physician salary information or administrative stipend levels, once again with the goal of price fixing or gaining a competitive advantage in the market, is illegal. Survey data on physician salaries or other financial information is allowable when not used for the purpose of price fixing. It may be of interest to note that the insurance industry is considered a regulated industry and therefore immune from antitrust law. Our payers are free to share information about physician and hospital charges and to fix prices without the risk of antitrust exposure.

HEALTH INFORMATION PORTABILITY AND ACCOUNTABILITY ACT

With regulations only partially promulgated at the time of this writing, Health Information Portability and Accountability Act (HIPAA) legislation promises to bring many measures that will require monitoring for compliance. The HIPAA law is aimed at ensuring security and privacy of personally identifiable health information, and requiring the transmission of health transactions electronically and uniformly (with standard code sets required).

The security measures relate to the way medical records are stored and transmitted. A significant potential side benefit of HIPAA to providers is the requirement that all payers accept electronic transfer of information in a standardized format. The privacy measures are more difficult compliance issues however. These provisions, although not fully resolved at the time of this writing, provide penalties for disclosure of personally identifiable health information by health-care organizations. Additionally, patients are granted specific rights by the act to direct certain use and disclosure of their personally identifiable health information. Health-care providers must abide by these restrictions or face penalties. The use of personally identifiable health information for research or marketing purposes may be limited. The patient has the statutory right under HIPAA to review and amend any information in his or her medical record. Despite the administrative burdens on health-care providers, HIPAA carries with it the promise of more secure and private health information for all citizens.

State-Level Regulation

Individual states have enacted substantial health-care laws over the years related to the regulation of medical practice and health-care facilities. State law governs medical licensure and requirements for the practice of medicine within the state. Additionally, because it has an interest in the welfare of its citizens, the state takes an active role in the monitoring of physician and hospital misadventures. The state department of public health usually promulgates hospital regulations, which may specify everything from the temperature of the food to the handling of medical waste to the nursing staffing levels. Discipline of physicians is the purview of the board of professional regulation (or its equivalent) within the state. Because states administer the Medicaid program, regulation and oversight of this program for indigent and low-income patients is highly variable. Some states have extensive case review and utilization programs for Medicaid, whereas others are less active.

Local-Level Regulation

Generally, health care is not extensively regulated at the local level, with a few exceptions. There may be county-level restrictions of land use and zoning regulations related to health-care enterprises. Also, one should note that for the purposes of malpractice law, the local medical community standard of care is the benchmark by which physicians are judged, although national and regional standards are frequently considered, especially with the increasing use of telemedicine.

Other Regulatory Entities

THE JOINT COMMISSION ON ACCREDITATION OF HEALTH CARE ORGANIZATIONS

In an attempt to be self-regulating, many nongovernmental organizations have developed in medicine to promulgate voluntary standards that health-care organizations may comply with if they wish to be accredited. JCAHO (www.jcaho.org) was formed in 1951 through an alliance of many professional organizations in health care, including the American Medical Association, American Hospital Association, and others. Over the years, JCAHO has developed and refined its standards continuously to challenge health-care organizations to assure high-quality care. Hospitals voluntarily submit to be surveyed by JCAHO on a schedule that allows for a maximum of 3-year accreditation. The standards cover a wide range of hospital and medical staff operations, including physician credentialing. JCAHO standards often are the same as the Medicare conditions of participation. In fact, JCAHO has been granted deemed status, which allows JCAHO accreditation to be accepted as equivalent to certification by CMS itself.

THE COMMISSION ON ACCREDITATION OF REHABILITATION FACILITIES

Founded in 1966, the Commission on Accreditation of Rehabilitation Facilities (CARF; www.carf.org) promulgates standards specific to rehabilitation facilities and programs. CARF offers many voluntary accreditation programs, including comprehensive integrated inpatient rehabilitation, brain injury, and spinal cord injury. CARF surveyors are practicing providers in the field, so they tend to be more consultative than JCAHO surveyors, with a better knowledge of rehabilitation. CARF accreditation is voluntary and, with a few exceptions, does not confer any preferred status with payers. However, with quality providers being sought by all payers, CARF accreditation signifies that the organization holds itself up to the highest standards in the field.

ADMINISTRATIVE ROLES FOR PHYSICIANS

The Role of Medical Director

Often one of the first administrative roles that physicians in physical medicine and rehabilitation may be exposed to is that of medical director of a rehabilitation program, unit, or facility. There are approximately 1,000 rehabilitation units within acute care hospitals and 200 freestanding rehabilitation hospitals in the United States (5) currently, and each is required to have a medical director according to the Medicare conditions of participation, JCAHO, and CARF. Generally, medical directors are paid a stipend to compensate for the time spent in administrative duties. Under Stark regulations, such a stipend must represent a fair market value for the time allocated. Physicians who take on an administrative role such as a medical director should be aware of the potential Stark and Antikickback Act implications of negotiating a better than fair market value stipend based on supply and demand. The usual duties of a medical director are listed in Table 51-3.

Depending on the size of the medical staff, the medical director may have a role in physician credentialing and privileging; however, in larger organizations, this function usually falls to the medical staff president or the vice president for medical affairs (VPMA).

Medical directors usually have a role in working with the medical staff on resource utilization. The challenge of the medical director is to manage the process so that on average, fewer resources are consumed than the reimbursement that will be provided while high-quality patient care is rendered.

Medical directors generally have a limited role in the other financial aspects of the hospital and must effect change

TABLE 51-3.   Usual Duties of a Medical Director
1. Working with the facility to assure overall quality of the programs and services offered
2. Resolving Customer Service issues
3. Developing and maintaining admission, continued stay, and discharge criteria
4. Interface between the Medical Staff and administration
5. Awareness of and compliance with laws, rules, and regulations as they relate to the facility
6. Working with the medical staff to increase cost effectiveness through application of evidence based medicine
7. Collaborating on the development and improvement of clinical pathways or protocols
8. Development of new programs
9. Recruitment and retention of physicians to the medical staff
10. Lots and lots of committee work

through interaction with the chief executive officer (CEO) and chief operating officer. This can be frustrating for medical directors if resources are not allocated to initiatives that they believe are required for compliance or medical quality reasons. Nonetheless, in most organizations, a balance can be struck between the financial constraints and medical quality needs. This is the art of the medical director.

As an individual clinician, you affect one patient at a time; as a medical director, your efforts affect everyone who receives services from the organization. A job well done in this important medical administration area can be very fulfilling.

Medical Staff President

Often an elected position, the president of the medical staff performs certain administrative functions in the context of the medical staff. Most medical staff bylaws require an organized medical staff that is self-regulating in many respects. Medical staff rules and regulations require monitoring and enforcement. Hospital personnel usually support a medical staff office. Given the often-transient nature of the medical staff leadership based on their elected status, the staff may provide continuity of policy and procedures related to medical staff issues. The main functions of the medical staff office within the hospital are physician credentialing, hospital privileging, and medical peer review.

Physician credentialing has developed over many years as a mechanism for the hospital and society to be assured that physicians practicing within a hospital have the appropriate and legitimate qualifications to do so. An effective physician credentialing program is required by CMS, JCAHO, and CARF. Physician credentialing is required to use primary source verification. That is, the hospital must verify with the original source of the credential (medical license, school diploma, etc.) that it is true and accurate. Obviously, in the interest of patient safety, applicants to the medical staff who falsify any of these documents must not be granted privileges within the hospital. Because some credentials are time limited (licenses, DEA registration, certain board certificates, etc.), keeping the physician credentialing files up to date is a perpetual job. Also, physicians are generally required to renew membership on the medical staff on a regular basis (usually every 2 years), and at that time they are required to be reevaluated by the credentials committee of the hospital. The president of the medical staff often chairs this committee.

Hospital medical staff privileges govern the practice of any physician granted medical staff membership. They may specify the types of patients that may be admitted or the procedures that the physician is able to perform within the hospital. The granting of hospital medical staff privileges is fairly simple within medical staffs associated with rehabilitation hospitals and units compared with the complexity of acute care hospitals. Nonetheless, the responsibility of the medical staff to decide the privileges that may be exercised by any physician practicing at the facility is under the purview of the credentials committee and the medical staff president. Contentious issues between specialties wishing to protect their turf are less common, but not unheard of, in rehabilitation facilities. The hospital medical staff has a duty to grant privileges based on the needs of the patient population. The potential that decisions in this area could be construed as restraint of trade by a medical staff applicant must be carefully avoided by clearly basing such decisions on patient-care needs, not business or turf considerations. Careful attention should be paid to the capacities and competencies of the hospital personnel (especially nursing) when granting medical staff privileges. Granting physicians medical staff privileges for a procedure for which the facility does not have the infrastructure necessary to support is not a formula for success. Additional considerations for the credentials committee when granting medical staff privileges include determining if proper equipment and supplies are available and will be stocked, as well as how the outcomes will be monitored.

The medical staff has an obligation to review its own medical quality through the process of peer review. Organized peer review holds a special legal standing in that it is not "discoverable" for the purpose of malpractice litigation. That is, because of this special legal status, medical staffs may review the medical quality of their fellow medical staff members without the fear that such activity could be used against that member in a malpractice suit. The special legal standing of peer review does not apply to criminal cases, however. Nonetheless, hospital medical staffs should take advantage of this special status to have a robust and effective internal peer review process. Recently, JCAHO has promulgated a standard that calls for the medical staff to determine under what circumstances external peer review would be required. In response, medical staffs have developed criteria under which such an external peer review would be triggered.

The president of the medical staff may chair required medical staff meetings and the medical staff executive committee. At such meetings, information regarding the medical practice within the hospital will be shared and decisions made regarding policy and procedures that affect the medical staff. Often the medical staff bylaws will specify the minimum required reports that are to be presented to the medical staff as a whole. These may include such reports as patient outcomes, financial parameters, and infection rates.

Vice President for Medical Affairs or Medical Services

In larger health-care systems, an administrative role has developed that may incorporate a wide range of duties. The VPMA generally answers to the president of the corporate entity that leads a health-care system or integrated network. Such a system often includes a network of hospitals, outpatient facilities, and physicians. In some cases, the VPMA acts as the CEO for a group of employed physicians within the network. The VPMA generally has budgetary authority over the medical services that he/she manages. As a member of the senior leadership team, the VPMA takes an active role in strategic planning and budgeting for the health-care network. The role of the VPMA may include physician recruitment and retention across the entire network of facilities. Working with or overseeing the physician practice manager, the VPMA may be responsible to the system CEO for the fiscal bottom line of the employed physician practice. Involvement in the front-end office practice as well as the back-end billing and collections system for the physician practice may be a part of the responsibilities of the VPMA. As the most senior medical administrator in the system, the VPMA may evaluate and develop all of the other medical personnel within the system. Working with the marketing department to promote the physician practice and development of new programs are often duties of the VPMA as well. Given the extensive administrative duties of the VPMA, they are often compensated more like other senior executives within the organization than clinicians within the practice. Most either have a very limited clinical practice or have moved completely into medical administration. Similar to the role of medical director, however, decisions made by the VPMA affect most, if not all, of the patients who contact the system, and therefore a job well done in this administrative area can have far-reaching impact. The VPMA sets the tone for the whole health-care system.

Private Practice Administrative Roles

Medicine has a long history as a cottage industry in which legions of solo practitioners hung out their shingle and became individual small businesses. Recent history has demonstrated considerable consolidation. Nonetheless, the American Medical Association estimates that almost one-half of physicians in the United States are in solo (that is, individual) private practice. There are several possible reasons for the increased popularity of group practice over solo practice over the last several years. First and foremost is the economic pressure that the solo practitioner has come under as a result of increasing overhead. The Medical Group Management Association calculates that between 1989 and 1999, operating costs as a percentage of revenue increased from 54.3% to 58.2% (6). Group practices offer some advantages with regard to economies of scale. That is, a solo practitioner must often hire staff (e.g., front office staff or a medical records clerk) to fulfill roles that could only be cost-effective if they supported additional physicians. Also, with increased regulatory pressures and compliance requirements, solo practices do not have ability to spread responsibilities among the members that group practices have. The solo practitioner must be clinician, practice manager, customer service representative, compliance officer, and human resources director, among other roles. Under HIPAA, they might now also be the required privacy officer and information security officer for the practice. On the positive side, the solo practitioner has complete authority and control of their practice. Any decisions that they make will only affect themselves and their staff. In both solo and group practices, all of the required business functions are the ultimate responsibility of the owner(s). A budgeting process must be developed to track revenue and expenses. The required financial reporting (to the IRS, etc) must be performed. Decisions will need to be made about hiring, firing, and benefits for staff. The private practice administrative physician will be involved in decisions regarding whether to lease or buy space and equipment. They may outsource functions for which they do not have internal competencies, such as billing and collections or legal advice. As physician groups grow and develop, there may be a hierarchy that develops with the original partner or partners hiring new physicians under arrangements that may or may not include ownership rights. Legal contracts are the preferable way to structure these relationships. Also, as groups grow, there is an opportunity for the members to diversify in their roles. One partner may take on the role of human resources director, for example, taking responsibility for the payroll, benefits, routine employee evaluations, hiring and firing of staff, etc.

Academic Administrative Roles

DEPARTMENT CHAIRPERSON
Physicians in academic health-care settings have specific administrative roles available. Medical schools and hospitals are usually organized by departments. There are approximately 80 departments of physical medicine and rehabilitation in the United States with a residency training program in physical medicine and rehabilitation (7). Each one of these departments has an administrative structure generally headed by a department chairperson. Department chairs generally have budgetary discretion over the department. In many institutions, the department chair sets the policies and procedures for the department. This is somewhat dependent on how centralized or decentralized the organization is, but in most, the department chair has final authority over matters within the department. The department chair develops the budget and is responsible for delivering a black bottom line with excess revenues over expenses—not always an easy task in the current academic environment. With decreasing state and private support to graduate medical education and increased dependence on shrinking clinical net revenue, department chairs have to be creative and innovative to survive. Department chairs play a major role in the development and evaluation of faculty. They chair department meetings of their faculty. They may have a role in graduate medical education or delegate this duty to a residency program director. Nonetheless, chairs usually have final authority over all of the clinical, educational, and research activities within an academic department. Clearly, the future of medical education in physical medicine and rehabilitation (and thereby the future of our field itself) rests on the shoulders of the 80 or so department chairs. This challenging administrative role can be very fulfilling, but requires excellent negotiation and fiscal skills to be successful.

RESIDENCY PROGRAM DIRECTOR
Many department chairs and medical directors started their administrative careers in the role of residency program director. The residency program director is responsible for assuring that the graduate education program meets the requirements of the residency review committee (RRC) of the Accreditation Council on Graduate Medical Education (ACGME). The ACGME has promulgated rules and regulations specific to the specialty of physical medicine and rehabilitation that govern the postgraduate training requirements and experiences that lead to eligibility for the residents to sit for their board exams given by the American Board of Physical Medicine and Rehabilitation. In order for residency programs to maintain accreditation by the ACGME, they must undergo survey by the RRC on a regular basis with the time frame governed by the extent to which the residency program complies with these standards and other factors. The residency program director has authority over these educational issues delegated to him or her by the department chair. Often the residency program director chairs a departmental graduate medical education committee. The di-

rector generally has some discretionary budget allocated from the department for resident materials, such as books, and outside speakers, such as visiting professors and the like. The residency program director is the first-line arbitrator in any issues brought forward by the residents, with the department chair generally having ultimate authority in such matters.

CONFLICTS AND CONTROVERSIES

In this final section, some real-life scenarios and conundrums will be presented.

The administrative physician is neither fish nor foul. That is, he or she will be seen as an administrator in the eyes of physicians and as a physician in the eyes of the administrators. The administrative physician always straddles this proverbial fence and can never please everyone completely.

I don't know the key to success—but the key to failure is trying to please everybody.
—Bill Cosby

Accordingly, the administrative physician is often placed in a position where compromise may result in both sides feeling as though they have lost. The administrative physician is always on the lookout for a win-win solution, and these often come through looking at the problem creatively or using an innovative solution that neither the administration nor the medical staff has considered. Technological solutions, if feasible, often have the advantage of solving problems in innovative ways that allow the organization to "work smarter, not harder." For example, an organization was struggling with the requirement to assess the outcome for procedures performed within the hospital but had no way to track such procedures. Their solution was to require that the physicians log procedures in a book that was kept in the procedure room. Because the physicians did not buy in to this process, the book was routinely not filled out, leading to incomplete capture of the procedures performed. The medical director was called in to the CEO's office and asked to bring the physicians into line on this requirement. The medical director thought through the problem and recognized that each procedure required that a special procedure tray was ordered and delivered to the procedure room from central supply. These trays were already tracked in the hospital information system, along with the name of the physician requesting them. By obtaining a report of the trays ordered, the medical director could deliver a list of all of the procedures to the CEO without having to attempt to enforce an (onerous in their mind) bookkeeping requirement on the physicians.

In health-care systems that own hospitals and employ physicians, conflicting interests may arise. This is often the case in AMCs, where both the hospitals and physician practices are under the same corporate umbrella. The hospital in this scenario may be the stronger partner with regard to revenue generated and net income produced. Administration may not fully appreciate or value the physician practice choosing to allocate resources preferentially to the hospital. Information systems may not be equal between the practice group and the hospital. When the physician practice group admits patients to many facilities within the network, conflicts between the physicians and the hospital may develop based on a perceived lack of loyalty by the physicians to the hospitals. This may occur either between hospitals within the system or between the hospitals in the system and the competing facilities. Physicians may sometimes tend to value patient preference and geographic

TABLE 51-4.   Framework for Ethical Decision Making
Identify the significant facts of the case:
What are the relevant facts of the case?
What individuals/groups have an important stake in the outcome?
Identify the values at risk:
Name the values at stake.
Include ethical values (e.g. justice, autonomy) as well as organizational values.
Determine the major value conflict:
What is the "ethical" issue at hand?
Is there a conflict of values and/or are there competing values?
Is the choice between the lesser of two "bad" choices or the "greater" of two good choices?
How does the decision affect people? The organization?
Identify possible courses of action/decisions/alternatives:
Which alternative promotes the most good/does the least harm?
Which alternative respects the rights and dignity of all stakeholders?
If someone is "left out", how is that person's situation addressed?
Which alternative promotes the common good and the responsible stewardship of resources?
Choose one course of action:
Which of the alternatives identified is the "right thing to do"? Why is this choice better than the others?
Support the decision by identifying the values that support it.
Support the decision by identifying the probable consequences of it.
Act, then reflect on the outcomes of the decision:
Be clear on what needs to happen to carry out the decision.
Plan a time/meeting to reflect on how the decision turned out for all concerned.
If you had to confront this issue again, what would you do differently?

Adapted from David Thomasma, PhD, Loyola University Medical Center

convenience factors over allegiances to hospitals within their own system.

Additionally, what is good for the physician practice may not be good for the hospital, and vice versa. For example, in contracting for managed-care business, integrated health-care delivery systems may make choices that adversely affect one or the other entity for the good of the order. Usually, in my experience, these decisions benefit the hospital at the expense of the medical practice. If the system does not correct these inequities internally through a proper funds-flow analysis, the inequities may lead to dissatisfaction of physicians in the practice plan. A specific example of this is the decision for a health-care system to apply to CMS for what are designated as hospital-based (also called provider-based) clinics. Under this designation, Medicare reimburses the integrated health-care system at a slightly higher rate overall, based on the higher costs associated with physician practice in this location. However, although the hospital collects a new revenue stream from hospital-based clinics, physician reimbursement is reduced. The net effect is slightly higher reimbursement for the system as a whole, but the physician practice will see revenue decline for those physicians practicing in the hospital-based clinics. Most physicians are keenly aware of financial indicators such as their personal collection rate. Often their pay is related to productivity, which may be calculated on their collections from clinical activities. A health-care system that does not make ac-

commodation for this inequity through analysis of the funds flow and subsidization back to the practice group may find that the outcome of this change is not as positive as anticipated.

It should be noted that although integrated health-care systems are immune from Stark law considerations regarding self-referral, they may be unable to directly compensate physicians based on their referrals into system hospitals based on anti-kickback legislation. Because the employed physicians in an integrated health-care system are stakeholders in the organization, they may benefit from the overall financial well-being of the system (if there is any), once again being clear that such incentives are not tied to the referral of individual patients.

The administrative physician may need to make decisions in a time frame that is not consistent with determining all of the facts relevant to the case at hand. Incomplete information, inaccurate information, individuals who have personal agendas, and other obstacles to perfect decision making are often factors in administrative medicine. It may be helpful to practice using a framework for ethical decision making as shown in Table 51-4.

Budgets in health care are tighter than ever before. Physicians and administrators alike are being asked to do more with less. Payers continue to exert pressure leading to failing revenues and increasing costs. Governmental regulations are continually increasing and always arrive in the form of unfunded mandates. Only by working together as physicians and administrators can we succeed in our endeavor to provide high-quality patient care in a cost-effective manner.

REFERENCES

1. Bennis W, Nanus B. *Leaders.* New York: 1985.
2. Duncan WJ, Ginter PM, Swayne LE. *Strategic management of health care organizations,* 2nd ed. Cambridge, MA: Blackwell, 1995:173.
3. Covey SR. *Principle-centered leadership.* New York: Simon and Schuster, 1992.
4. Deming WE. *Out of the crisis.* Cambridge, MA: Massachusetts Institute of Technology, 1986.
5. *AMRPA Magazine* 2002; 5(10):38.
6. *American Medical News,* January 7, 2002.
7. Association of Academic Physiatry. *Directory of physical medicine and rehabilitation residency training programs.*

SUGGESTED READINGS

American Academy of Physical Medicine and Rehabilitation. *Guide to practice marketing.* Chicago: American Academy of Physical Medicine and Rehabilitation, 1998.

Conrad DA, Hoare GA, eds. *Strategic alignment: managing integrated health systems.* Ann Arbor, MI: AUPHA Press/Health Administration Press, 1994.

Duncan WJ, Ginter PM, Swayne LE. *Strategic management of health care organizations,* 2nd ed. Cambridge, MA: Blackwell, 1995.

Furrow BR, Johnson SH, Jost TS, Schwartz RL. *Health law: cases, materials and problems,* 2nd ed. St. Paul, MN: West Publishing Co., 1991.

Johnson S. *Who moved my cheese?* New York: GP Putnam's Sons, 1998.

Joint Commission Resources. *How the medical staff can help achieve Joint Commission accreditation,* 4th ed. Oak Brook, IL: Joint Commission on Accreditation of Heath Care Organizations, 2000.

Maloney FP. Administration and management in physical medicine and rehabilitation. In: DeLisa JA, Gans BM, eds. *Rehabilitation medicine: principles and practice,* 3rd ed. Philadelphia: Lippincott-Raven, 1998.

Neumann BR, Suver JD. *Financial management: concepts and applications for health care providers,* 3rd ed. Dubuque, IA: Kendall Hunt Publishing Co., 1995.

Shortell SM, Kaluzny AD. *Health care management: organization design and behavior,* 3rd ed. Albany, NY: DelMar Publishing, 1994.

Silver JK. *The business of medicine.* Philadelphia: Hanley and Belfus, 1998.

Stanley K, ed. *The physiatrist's guide to practice management.* Chicago: American Academy of Physical Medicine and Rehabilition, 1997.

CHAPTER 52

International Aspects of Rehabilitation

Peter Disler, Fary Khan, Zaliha Omar, and Geoffrey Abbott

The aim of rehabilitation is to help people with "impairments" achieve the "activities" and "participation" that they desire, and have the capacity to attain. This dictum is based on the World Health Organization International Classification (ICF) (1), which stresses that the outcome may be influenced just as strongly by "personal factors" and the physical, social, and cultural "environment"as by the nature or extent of the impairment. As the latter may be unique to the country in which rehabilitation is practiced, and to the disparate groups of people resident there, rehabilitation varies more internationally than any other field of medical practice: hence this chapter. We believe that this topic is relevant to all rehabilitation professionals, not only those interested in sociological research or working in countries other than their own. International travel is now commonplace, and most of us include people from other countries in our practices, who are often further challenged by living in a society to which they are unaccustomed and by a language which is not their own.

This is a large topic; many aspects impinge on rehabilitation practice, and we can consider only some that seem most relevant. In this respect, it may be important to dispel any concern that the reader has about the bias toward Australia in the authorship of this chapter. We live in a mobile world, and the primary authors have worked in South Africa, the United Kingdom, the United States, Canada, New Zealand, Pakistan, Israel, and the Association of Southeast Asian Nations (ASEAN) countries, as well as both the remote and urban parts of Australia. Our travels have taken us to many parts of the globe, and where our experience was lacking, we have been assisted generously by colleagues, all of whom are acknowledged in the chapter.

"Culture defines the experience of living with a disability within a society" (2), and this determines both societal and personal attitudes; social stigma may prevent access to the resources available, and also determine whether people seek, or accept, help. For example, witchcraft may be blamed for disability in some parts of the world, whereas in other areas, religious doctrine may influence others to accept disablement as "God's will" or fate; either may dissuade people with disabilities from seeking advice from rehabilitation professionals. At a less philosophical level, some Pacific islanders attribute congenital impairments to tension between the parents or their promiscuous behavior, and the family may be unwilling to reveal a child who exposes them to such criticism (3). Such factors must be understood by the treating rehabilitation professionals and incorporated into their therapeutic programs.

Particular groups of people with disability may be more vulnerable to societal prejudice than others: Literature abounds with the sorry fate of lepers. Moreover, an Indian study showed that people with psychiatric and drug-related disability experience far more discrimination than those with physical disability (4), and such a "hierarchy" is probably common to many countries. Furthermore, the world seems to suffer from perpetual "troubled times;" hence, the close dependence of people with disabilities on environmental resources means that local changes have devastating effects. Political and economic instability, and war, will have even more of an adverse effect on people with disabilities than their able-bodied peers.

OVERVIEW

In the first instance, we will briefly consider the history of international liaison in rehabilitation and how rehabilitation professionals have met to exchange ideas. We will then look at the new International Classification of Functioning, Disability and Health (ICF) (1) in more detail, as this will provide a template for the interchange of such ideas and may be the key to understanding this topic better in the future.

We will then illustrate some aspects of international similarities and differences in clinical practice through case scenarios. This is potentially a limitless topic, and we have room to describe only a few small segments of the world. We hope that we offend no one in being selective; we know there are many more models of rehabilitation, some of which are undoubtedly more or less successful than those we have chosen. We sought to provide principles, not an exhaustive travelogue, and have illustrated these through examples familiar to the authors and other colleagues. We have also not attempted to encompass the full spectrum of impairments and have repeated some such as stroke, which respects neither class, nationality, nor creed; causes a large range of impairments; and demands a wide variety of rehabilitation professionals. In doing so, we have also undoubtedly neglected other vitally important areas, such as impairments more common in children, and the important rehabilitation domain of chronic pain; we are in no way implying that these are less important, and we hope that the reader will be able to extrapolate from this text to other impairments.

Finally, we will also look specifically at community-based rehabilitation, as this model, which has been the dominant pattern of practice in many parts of the "third world" for years, is now capturing the attention of the "first world." This will emphasize how much we can all learn from others in the world; education is never a unidirectional process. We are not trying to provide an exhaustive analysis of community-based rehabilitation, and we will again focus on stroke, partly for the reasons given above, and because we wanted to look at an area that has a strong evidence base. Paradoxically, much of this research evidence will come from the first world; that is the unfortunate reality of research and publications. The need for research in other environments is clear, and again, we trust that the principles can be applied across the spectrum.

HISTORY OF INTERNATIONAL LIAISON IN REHABILITATION MEDICINE

The world has a general shortage of rehabilitation professionals, and many will spend their professional lives working in relative isolation. International liaison thus becomes a critical force in peer communication, which is so important to productive professional life. Many people in many spheres have worked hard to promote such interchange. We will not attempt an exhaustive history of this, but will focus on three bodies that seem to exemplify the principles.

The first of these is the International Federation of Physical Medicine and Rehabilitation (IFPMR). When founded in 1950, its title reflected physical medicine only, but this was amended in 1972 to add rehabilitation. It set out to link existing national and regional societies and organize regular international congresses. The first meeting took place in London in 1952, followed every 4 years by a meeting in different parts of the world, including Denmark, France, the United States, Canada, Spain, Brazil, Sweden, Israel, East Germany, and Australia. The themes of the meetings were ambitious and included "Scientific Research," "Humanitarian, Social, and Economic Factors," and the more philosophical "Under the Sign of Rehabilitation" and "Rehabilitation: The Bridge between Medical Science and Society.'

Links with the World Health Organization were cemented by the recognition of the Federation in 1964 as an affiliated nongovernmental organization, and in 1974, a landmark *White Book on Education and Training* was produced, this being one of the first attempts to develop international standards for rehabilitation training.

As membership of the IFPMR was restricted to national societies of rehabilitation medicine, it unfortunately only represented countries in which the field was relatively well recognized. Isolated rehabilitation physicians, who perhaps had the greatest need, were thus excluded from membership. This deficit was addressed in 1968 by the foundation of the International Rehabilitation Medicine Association, which had 670 members from 62 countries by 1970. Again, it was somewhat restrictive, as membership was limited to medical doctors, and exclusion of other rehabilitation health professionals remained a cause of disagreement throughout its lifespan. Regular conferences were held in many parts of the world, including Italy, Mexico, Switzerland, Puerto Rico, the United States, Japan, and the Philippines. International contributions included a major role in the preparation of World Health Organization International Classification of Impairments, Disabilities and Handicaps taxonomy in 1980, the founding of an international rehabilitation journal (*International Rehabilitation Medicine*), and an important program for the International exchange of experts in rehabilitation medicine.

Although the two societies had different charters, duplication of effort was inevitable. A decision was thus made in the early 1990s to join forces through a new combined organization, the International Society of Physical and Rehabilitation Medicine. The last International Rehabilitation Medicine Association conference was in 1997, and that of the International Federation of Physical Medicine and Rehabilitation in 1999; in 2001. the first International Society of Physical and Rehabilitation Medicine meeting took place in Amsterdam.

The rehabilitation world thus now has a corporate entity that invites membership from both rehabilitation societies and individuals, the latter being open to both physicians and other health professionals. The International Society of Physical and Rehabilitation Medicine also encourages regional conferences that address "local" issues (e.g., regular Mediterranean and ASEAN meetings), and a strong World Health Organization liaison continues (e.g., in the International Classification of Functioning, Disability and Health project). In the future, rehabilitation professionals must continue to play an active role in international rehabilitation policy, and organizations such as those described above are critical to this. We live in a world that hovers between international conflict and cooperation; rehabilitation may have a specific role in leading the way forward.

THE INTERNATIONAL CLASSIFICATION OF FUNCTIONING, DISABILITY, AND HEALTH

One of the challenges facing people who are interested in comparative international models of rehabilitation is the many different ways in which concepts and terms are described. A uniform language and taxonomy is thus an essential prerequisite for international exchange of ideas, research, and experience.

An attempt to provide such a tool has recently resulted in the International Classification of Functioning, Disability, and Health (ICF) (Table 52-1), developed by the World Health Organization through a worldwide consensus process and endorsed by the World Health Assembly. This grew out of the former International Classification of Impairments, Disabilities and Handicaps (ICIDH) (5) and was initially called ICIDH-2. However, the well-known ICIDH definitions reflect *deficits* only, whereas the new paradigm recognizes that any of the domains may have either positive or negative influences, and thus has the capacity to record a far wider range of health-related information and better describe the departure from "health" that is perceived as "disability." It is intended for use in multiple sectors. including education and policy, and in the clinical context should be useful for needs assessment, rehabilitation goal-setting, and outcome evaluation.

However, we still face the challenge of making this practical and transportable. Previous attempts have been made to develop a uniform rehabilitation outcome measure, one example being the Pro-ESOR project (6), which has attempted to standardize the use, and comparison of the Functional Independence Measure (FIM™) (7) in patients with stroke in six countries (United Kingdom, France, Belgium, Slovenia, Israel, and Italy). The FIM™ was chosen because it has been well standardized, and training through a detailed manual is a prerequisite for its use. Despite this, however, Rasch analysis has shown that several of the FIM™ items are interpreted and applied differently in these selected countries (8), and one can only speculate as to the differences that might emerge if the countries had been even more culturally disparate than these.

The comprehensiveness and broad base of the International Classification of Functioning, Disability, and Health may help to overcome this; however, this also makes it unwieldy, and in the clinical (or clinical research) context, brevity is critical. An international collaborative project is currently under way with

TABLE 52-1. The International Classification of Functioning, Disability, and Health

	Part 1: Functioning and Disability		Part 2: Contextual Factors	
Components	Body functions and structures	Activities and participation	Environmental factors	Personal factors
Domains	Body functions and structures	Life areas	External influences on functioning and disability	Internal influences on functioning and disability
Constructs	Change in body functions or structure	Executing tasks in a standard environment (capacity) or the current environment (performance)	Facilitating or hindering the impact of the physical, social, and attitudinal world	Impact of attributes of the person
Positive aspect	Functional and structural integrity Functioning	Activities participation	Facilitators	Not yet developed (2003)
Negative aspect	Impairment Disability	Limitation of activities Restriction of participation	Barriers and hindrances	Not yet developed (2003)

From World Health Organization: *International classification of functioning, disability, and health.* Geneva: WHO, 2001.

the stated aim of making the International Classification of Functioning, Disability, and Health clinically useful. The first step is to link specific diseases or conditions (classified by the ICD-10) to the "core-set" of domains most likely to be relevant to the person who is disabled by the condition (e.g., low back pain is extremely likely to constrain bending and lifting, and most unlikely to affect speech). Empirically selected core-sets will be field tested to ensure that they are robust and practical for everyday clinical use. We look forward to a tool that allows rehabilitation professionals to understand how others practice; the potential advantages of this are clear.

INTERNATIONAL MODELS OF REHABILITATION PRACTICE AND TRAINING

This section will look at international differences and similarities in rehabilitation practice, as well as training programs for medical rehabilitation specialists. Although the latter will focus on physicians, there is no doubt that the same principles apply to all other rehabilitation professionals, all of whom are in as short (or even shorter) supply as doctors in this field.

Physicians in Rehabilitation Practice in Various Parts of the World

Much of the data discussed below was initially presented at an international symposium in Washington in 1999, hosted by the American Board of Physical Medicine and Rehabilitation, and published in an abbreviated form as a series of articles thereafter (9–15).

NUMBER OF PHYSICIANS PRACTICING IN REHABILITATION MEDICINE

An international survey of physicians practicing in the field was undertaken in 1999 (9). Respondents from 45 countries reported 25,404 physicians practicing the specialty of physical medicine and rehabilitation; their regional distribution is shown in the Table 51-2.

Within these regions, the individual countries with the biggest numbers of specialists were the United States with 6,000; Japan with 3,000; and Germany, Spain, France, and Italy, each with 1,000–2,000. Therefore, physical medicine and rehabilitation physicians are found in many countries, but the distribu-

tion is patchy, and some areas such as Africa and Central America have very few.

COMPONENTS OF REHABILITATION MEDICINE PRACTICE

In the United States, physical medicine and rehabilitation practitioners spend about 40% of their clinical time dealing with inpatients, during which 76% of American physiatrists acknowledged participating in the care of patients with stroke, 59% in the care of patients with traumatic brain injury, and 57% in the care of patients with spinal cord injury. About 40% of their clinical time is spent dealing with outpatients, during which nearly 80% of American physicians participated in pain management and 51% in sports medicine. In addition, 16% of clinical practice time is spent doing diagnostic electromyography.

In the rest of the world, the mean time spent with inpatients is similar (35%), but there is a wide range in different countries (5% to 85%). Electromyography is less commonly part of practice (only 7%), but the overall distribution of work is relatively similar.

In the USA, subspecialization is common; 76% of physical medicine and rehabilitation specialists restrict their practice to neurologic rehabilitation; this happens less often elsewhere in the world.

Training in Rehabilitation

Of the 45 countries that were surveyed by Brandstater, 43 offer clinical training in the specialty of physical medicine and rehabilitation, with 4,217 doctors in training. The number of years required for training after graduation from medical school

TABLE 52-2. Number of Physicians Practicing in Rehabilitation Medicine

Region	Countries (*n*)	Physicians (*n*)
Europe	23	11,574
North America	2	6,500
Asia/Pacific	11	5,084
Middle East/Africa	6	1,049
Central/South America	3	1,197
Totals	45	25,404

varies from 3 to 6, some countries requiring completion of a period of training in internal medicine before clinical training in physical medicine and rehabilitation can begin, and many countries demanding time be spent in the specialities of rheumatology, orthopedics, and neurology. All countries who responded prescribe training in inpatient rehabilitation (usually 12 to 24 months), with rotations in stroke and spinal cord injury rehabilitation units; a considerable number have some formal requirement in geriatrics, and 29 of the 43 require a pediatric rehabilitation experience. Musculoskeletal medicine is required in 40 of 43 countries, and 28 require experience with pain management. Twenty-three countries require electromyography training.

In most countries, speciality training is formalized, and some have established national training standards. Of the 45 countries surveyed, 41 provide certification in the specialty of physical medicine and rehabilitation, either independently or in collaboration with other countries. The number of physical medicine and rehabilitation candidates taking annual national certification examinations varies from very few to more than 400, the median being 13; many countries therefore have small training programs. Thirty countries set a written examination, mainly comprising multiple-choice questions; 31 have oral examinations; and 2 only have an oral examination. In 37 countries, formal training in physical medicine and rehabilitation that was completed in other countries is recognized and may satisfy prerequisites for admission to the certification examination.

Although a relatively wide range of practice and training patterns appears to exist internationally, there are perhaps more similarities than differences. It is reassuring that physical medicine and rehabilitation has gained a degree of international acceptance, but unfortunately no data are available that compare the types of patients who need the service and to answer the important questions that arise: Is physical medicine and rehabilitation practice internationally based on the "western" model? Does this meet the needs of patients in other countries as well as it does in the United States? Are the training programs successful, and do they produce the kind of professionals that are needed? Good research is clearly needed in this field and in allied fields such as nursing, physiotherapy, and occupational therapy.

Rehabilitation Case Scenarios from Various Parts of the World

The following case histories describe the rehabilitation of patients in disparate parts of the world. These countries were mainly chosen because they reflect the experience and contacts of the chapter authors; all are real patients, although none is called by his/her real name. Credit is given when the details were supplied by someone other than the authors.

AUSTRALIA: METROPOLITAN: THE "FIRST WORLD"
A 44-year-old single parent of two teenage sons who was working as a florist was admitted to the Stroke Care Unit of a tertiary hospital with a history of headache, nausea, dizziness, ataxia, and impaired balance. She underwent magnetic resonance imaging and magnetic resonance angiography 1 hour after admission, which revealed a 2-cm cerebellar hemorrhage secondary to an arteriovenous malformation. Angiographic embolization of the arteriovenous malformation was undertaken, but unfortunately, during the procedure, she developed an upper brainstem infarct, leading to dense hemiparesis, impaired lateral gaze, complex cranial nerve deficits, urinary and

fecal incontinence, dysarthria, and dysphagia [the latter demanding percutaneous endoscopic gastronomy (PEG) feeding]. She was assessed on the combined neurology/rehabilitation ward rounds. Given the level of care, intensity of rehabilitation required, and lack of support at home, inpatient rehabilitation was considered necessary. When she was medically stable, on the sixth day after the stroke, she was transferred to a freestanding rehabilitation hospital, where she improved steadily. Four weeks after admission, she was continent, tolerated a soft diet and free fluids, and had intelligible, slurred speech. She was mobile in an electric wheelchair, but required assistance with transfers.

Discussions with her, her former partner, and children revealed that all wished her to go home, but none could provide "hands-on" help during daylight hours. By 8 weeks after admission, however, she could transfer independently and could go home; government funding was obtained for the employment of a personal care attendant 2 hours daily, a district nurse came in three times weekly to assist with showering, and she received interdisciplinary domiciliary rehabilitation three times per week. After a further 4 weeks, she achieved independence with car transfers and was able to continue a rehabilitation program in a community rehabilitation center, which she attended twice weekly for a further 2 months.

Points That This Scenario Demonstrates
- The passage of this woman after stroke through the spectrum of acute and rehabilitation care, from inpatient to domiciliary to community-based rehabilitation, provided free of charge by the government
- A modern "Western" rehabilitation approach, comparable with others in many parts of the United States, Europe, and the United Kingdom

AUSTRALIA: RURAL: THE "THIRD WORLD"
A 20-year-old Aboriginal man, who lives with his family in a small village in Arnhem Land in the "Top End" of Australia, was diagnosed at 14 years with Machado-Joseph disease (spinocerebellar ataxia type 3), a progressively disabling disorder, found in a number of people living in this region. Locomotor ataxia and spasticity limited his walking to a few steps only, aggravated by involuntary eye movements and diplopia. He thus spent most of the day in his wheelchair and developed grade 1 pressure ulcers on both buttocks. He became increasingly housebound and depressed, and had intermittent bladder and bowel incontinence, and recurrent urinary tract infections. He reported dysphagia and a recurrent productive cough. The original diagnosis was made by specialist medical staff at the regional hospital, in Darwin, 100 km (60 miles) from where he lives. He refused to come to Darwin for rehabilitation, partly because of the travel expense, and because Aboriginal people have strong traditional links within the family, local community, and land, and are reluctant to be treated away from family and the local community. An attempt was therefore made to offer him rehabilitation in his home. Problems identified included a sandy, poorly wheelchair-accessible local terrain and an overcrowded home with poor internal access (he shared a bedroom with two siblings). Management of his skin and urinary incontinence was complicated by the heat, humidity, and poor sanitation in the house, and despite a large residual volume, he was unwilling to catheterize intermittently. Rehabilitation professionals from Darwin trained his mother and sister as primary caregivers, as cultural prejudices limited the personal care role to women; other community members were trained to provide respite. The local

church minister counseled the man and his family, and management was monitored by the community nurse. With time, the patient's skin healed, and he agreed to intermittent catheterization. His mood improved, and he communicated better with those around him.

The general health of indigenous Australians is poorer than that of other Australians, and the life expectancy about 20 years less; drug and alcohol abuse is common. This type of situation is common to many rural people, and not unique to Australia. There is often little alternative to compromise "first world" rehabilitation principles—e.g., we know that intermittent catheterization will improve his health, but it will fail unless he is persuaded of the advantages thereof; this may take a good deal of input over a long period. Some of his needs have been met by training those around him; such training programs demand diversion of money from central high-tech services. Rehabilitation programs must be culturally appropriate if they are to have any chance of success, and the support of local community and religious leaders is essential.

Points That This Scenario Demonstrates

- How difficult it is to provide high-quality rehabilitation in a rural area, even if it is relatively close to an academic regional hospital where sophisticated diagnoses can be made
- The effect of the physical environment on activities and participation
- How close family members can be trained to provide high-quality care
- How cultural and economic issues impact rehabilitation

CHINA

A 36-year-old journalist, working at a county television station, was injured in a train accident, sustaining traumatic brain injury and multiple internal injuries. After initial surgical treatment, he remained unconscious and appeared to have "brain death." From the Western medicine perspective, there appeared to be no hope of improvement, but as his family insisted on trying traditional Chinese medicine, he was transferred to a provincial hospital. On admission (30 days after the accident), he was unconscious but medically stable, with no pressure ulcers or joint contracture (reflecting good initial medical care). The rehabilitation program combined a "Western" approach with Chinese herbs, acupuncture, and Chinese massage, all of which have been used traditionally for more than 2,000 years. This included daily calculus bovis (which stimulates the brain to "wake up" from coma) and body and scalp acupuncture, twice daily for 20 to 30 minutes. The acupuncture points were carefully selected according to traditional Chinese medicine meridians and were modulated regularly as his condition improved. One hour of Chinese massage was also given twice daily, and this comprised passive movement of upper and lower extremities, applied to prevent joint stiffness and muscle atrophy while he was restricted to bed.

After 46 days of this approach, he opened his eyes, and after another 14 days, he spoke a few words. After another 2 months, he could sit independently, and after 6 months, he could stand and walk for a few steps with the assistance of careers.

Points That This Scenario Demonstrates

- Even though he is still severely disabled, his progress attests to the value of combining traditional medicine with Western medicine in developing countries

- Local "medicine" techniques are not only effective, but also economical
- Cultural issues impact rehabilitation

THE PACIFIC ISLANDS: FIJI

A 25-year-old Fijian villager, married with one child, had recently commenced employment in the Beche-de-mer (sea slug) export industry. After limited training with SCUBA apparatus, he worked at 40 meters for almost 2 hours. When the surface air compressor failed, he ascended rapidly to the boat, and within 5 minutes he developed low back pain, numbness, and weakness in both legs. It took 3 hours to return to shore by boat, followed by bumpy half-hour ride in the back of a jeep to the settlement where divers and their families from the outer islands are accommodated. At that stage, he was unable to move or feel his legs and had not passed urine. He was then driven a further hour by jeep to the capital city, Suva. A doctor diagnosed paraplegia at T-10 caused by spinal decompression illness (16). He was catheterized and rehydrated intravenously, and transferred to the Fiji Recompression Chamber Facility, which he reached 16 hours after symptoms first developed. No improvement occurred with this treatment, and he was transferred to the National Rehabilitation Medicine Hospital, where a 6-cm sacral pressure area was noted, as were superficial burns on both his feet (attributed to a hot-water bottle placed there during the journey). After 3 months of rehabilitation, he had achieved wheelchair and activities of daily living independence, and was independently doing urinary catheterization. He returned to his home to the other side of Fiji, 120 km away. The family lives in rented accommodations, and cannot afford home modifications; poor access makes it impossible for him to leave the home independently or use the bathroom without help. His wife has found it difficult to comprehend his medical problems, even through an interpreter. Although Fiji has a network of Western-style medical facilities, traditional beliefs drive a parallel health-care system. Fijians often have far more faith in the latter (17,18), and he is regularly visited by faith healers, who pray for him and provide herbal medication.

Points That This Scenario Demonstrates

- Poorly regulated work practices may lead to injury and disability in workers; migrant workers have particular problems in this regard
- The nexus between traditional belief and belief in Western health care models

THE MIDDLE EAST: PAKISTAN AND AFGHANISTAN

A 13-year-old Afghan girl lost her leg below the knee after stepping on a land mine while trying to escape into Pakistan. Her family tied a tourniquet of string around her leg and carried her for 2 days across the border, where first aid (including antitetanus toxoid and antibiotics) was provided by a UN relief mission. She was taken to a crowded refugee camp, where she underwent transtibial amputation (in a tent), but after 3 days, the stump became infected. Antisepsis and antibiotics were limited, and she developed gangrene, treated with transfemoral amputation. Little analgesia was available. She was nursed on the floor by her mother and was given the bulk of the family's food rations.

Funding in Pakistan for people with disability is limited, and refugees with disabilities are a particularly vulnerable group. This young girl may have to be content with a "peg leg" or crutches, as she will find it hard to access the resources and expertise to provide a more appropriate, cosmetically preferable prosthesis. This will make it difficult, and perhaps painful, to walk on the rough terrain.

In addition, she will face great social hardship, as her impairment is visible, and her family may keep her out of sight of others; she has had no education, and although she is of marriageable age, she will find it difficult to find a husband. Financially her support is thus likely to come from her family or traditional *Zakat* funding (a tax on Muslim earners to support those who are less fortunate), although some programs have been set up to teach women "cottage industry" skills, which may result in a degree of economic self-sufficiency.

Points That This Scenario Demonstrates
- The plight of disabled refugees, particularly if young
- The problems faced by amputees when rehabilitation facilities are poor

THE ASIA PACIFIC RIM: MALAYSIA
A 42-year-old college lecturer was referred to the rehabilitation service at the University of Malaya Medical Centre, Kuala Lumpur, 5 days after onset of brainstem stroke. Initial referral was delayed as the family consulted a traditional healer because the local emergency department was so busy. Transfer by air from his hometown of Kota Kinabalu took 2 hours, and he was accompanied by a doctor and four family members. On arrival, he was drowsy, could not speak, was quadriplegic, and was incontinent of urine and feces. A multidisciplinary stroke rehabilitation program commenced, and a PEG tube was inserted for feeding. He required antihypertensive medication and developed depression sufficient to require treatment with citalopram.

He was discharged home after 12 weeks, by which stage he was alert and able to follow commands, but could communicate only via eye movements. Sitting tolerance was 5 hours in a reclining wheelchair, and he could stand with a tilt table for 1 hour. Two personal caregivers were trained by the hospital staff to manage all aspects of his personal care, including PEG feeds, urinary catheterization, skin and respiratory care, and bowel management. The family were counseled regarding the limited chance of functional improvement.

Follow-up and maintenance of his gains was challenging. Initially, a nurse from Kuala Lumpur stayed in his home for a week, and this reassured the patient and family; she also made contact with health professionals in the town. The next 18 months were difficult, as his local doctor had little experience with severe brain damage, so the family frequently contacted the rehabilitation team in Kuala Lumpur, even for relatively trivial matters. It was also hard to maintain a supply of good caregivers; training of replacement caregivers had to be undertaken several times, and this predisposed the patient to complications. The caregivers were often contradicted by elderly family members who prescribed traditional treatment, and they had to be taught to work together; e.g., a traditional masseur successfully maintained joint mobility.

PEG feeding solutions and technical aids (e.g., a suction pump for respiratory toilet) were difficult to obtain in his local area and could not be repaired locally. Most of the costs were borne by the family, including the major expense of transporting him to Kuala Lumpur, caregivers, catheters, PEG tubes, and incontinence pads. However, the government paid for medications, therapy, and medical care, as his wife is a public servant.

His wife faced particular problems, as she was only 36 years old and had married at 17. They have four children, the youngest being only 3 years. Before the stroke, she was at the height of her own professional career, but committed herself to putting her husband's needs first, as long as he lived. She got some support from her extended family, however, she particularly wanted to discuss sexual matters, which were taboo with her family and peers. She could not obtain help from a skilled psychologist.

Points That This Scenario Demonstrates
- The complexities of rehabilitative care of a profoundly disabled patient in a developing country bound by traditional beliefs and values, but which has developed a center of excellence in one area
- The needs and problems of the spouse are critical, but often neglected

COSTA RICA
A 53-year-old divorced man from a small town was referred by his local doctor to the medical rehabilitation facility in San Jose, 100 km from his home, with a diagnosis of "right hemiplegia due to stroke." The acute event had occurred 8 months earlier; he had received little therapy, and little improvement had occurred. In San Jose, he was found to have weakness of all four limbs, fasciculation, and difficulty swallowing, and a diagnosis of motor neuron disease was made (amyotrophic lateral sclerosis variety) clinically and with electromyographic confirmation.

The fact that he needed help in his activities of daily living made the possibility of his returning to home difficult. His half-sister agreed to take him into her home, and she was trained to help him with his personal care; both he and she were counseled as to the likely prognosis and future. As he had not previously had a formal job, he had not contributed actively to the social security system, and so could not obtain state disability benefits or other financial support. He was, however, provided with a wheelchair, and his sister received government assistance to modify her residence, which was a two-room tin house on a steep riverside hill. His urine and feces were emptied directly into the river via a tin slide.

Points That This Scenario Demonstrates
- General medical care is provided throughout Costa Rica, but rehabilitation services are less widely distributed.
- Rehabilitation is rarely part of medical school training, and incorrect diagnoses may be made.
- Resources are limited with respect to funding technical aids for disabled people, personal care, community-based rehabilitation services, or other financial benefits.
- Rehabilitation professionals often have to deal with social issues that prevent integration of people with disabilities into society and allow them to live with dignity.

Community-Based Rehabilitation

Community-based rehabilitation was defined in 1994 in a joint International Labor Organization, United Nations Educational, Scientific and Cultural Organization, and World Health Organization Position Paper (19) as a strategy "for the rehabilitation, equalization of opportunities and social integration of all children and adults with disabilities. Community-based rehabilitation is implemented through the combined efforts of disabled people themselves, their families and communities, and the appropriate health, education, vocational and social services." As such, it has been advocated internationally for more than 20 years as the core strategy for improvement of the quality of life of persons with disabilities. Although traditionally tailored for developing countries, first-world countries are currently facing a demand for community-based rehabilitation too. As a case can be made for community-based rehabilitation being the approach that will bring rehabilitation to less well–served countries, it seemed appropriate to briefly discuss this topic in this chapter.

The 1997 statement of the Economic and Social Commission for Asia and the Pacific, "Understanding CBR" (20), concluded that community-based rehabilitation programs have the following essential criteria:

- Persons with disabilities must be included at all stages and have distinct decision-making roles.
- As the primary objective of community-based rehabilitation is the improvement of the quality of life of persons with disabilities, programs must focus on eliminating stigma and increasing the recognition of disabled persons as resourceful members of family and society, making the environment and existing service delivery systems accessible to persons with disabilities, and supporting persons with *all* types of disabilities according to their specific needs.

Recent research in Ghana, Guyana, and Nepal has shown that from the perspective of persons with disabilities, community-based rehabilitation has been effective in reaching some of these objectives (21). Based on interviews with a sample of persons with disabilities or their parents, community-based rehabilitation was felt to have affected positively on self-esteem, empowerment, influence, self-reliance, and social inclusion. However, the expectation that the community would provide the necessary resources, once awareness was raised, was not regularly fulfilled. The study outlined a number of recommendations suggesting how community-based rehabilitation programs could be improved in the areas of awareness-raising, medical care, rehabilitation, education, and income generation.

The authors also suggested that the title "community-based rehabilitation (CBR)" no longer reflects the nature of such programs, because they target many levels of society, not only the community level, and address all issues affecting the quality of life of persons with disabilities, not only rehabilitation. Notwithstanding the definitions given above, the corollary is that there is no uniform international concept of community-based rehabilitation, the paradigm varying markedly within countries and in different parts of the world (22).

A facet of community-based rehabilitation, which has excited a good deal of discussion, is the provision of rehabilitation in the home, or home-based rehabilitation. This has many protagonists, who have argued that rehabilitation must be practiced in the environment in which people live, for which hospitals are a questionable surrogate, and that home-based rehabilitation means less isolation of "patients," particularly if they are not fluent in the language of the hospital or have dietary or religious idiosyncrasies. It also frees the family from long, expensive journeys to hospital and permits the continuation of child, parent, and grandparent relationships. There are also cogent counterarguments; e.g., where there are only few rehabilitation staff, they can make the greatest impact where the patient concentration is highest, in large hospitals, and rehabilitation in the home means taking travel time out of limited therapy time. "Hotel costs" may also be more than balanced by travel cost, and for the family, hours lost in travel may be more than equaled by hours of demanding personal care, sometimes after a long day at work, often followed by disturbed sleep.

However, in this era of evidence-based medicine, some aspects of home-based rehabilitation have been subjected to high-quality research scrutiny. Home-based stroke rehabilitation, for example, has been the subject of several systematic reviews (23–25); although these have largely focused on the first world, and the need for high-quality research in other environments is clear, they do provide a base for analytic argument. In essence, although (not surprisingly) home-based stroke rehabilitation substantially reduces the length of hospital stay, no difference has been found in either patient outcomes or resource utilization. Given that some studies quoted showed trends toward higher levels of patient satisfaction in the home-based rehabilitation group, this is perhaps an argument for home-based rehabilitation.

What is certain is that community rehabilitation needs far more skillful case management than conventional hospital care. Pulling together all the threads of rehabilitation is challenging in the closed hospital environment and far more difficult in the open community, where voluntary organizations and family members are far more likely to play a role. Appointment of individual case managers to supervise and monitor care plans may be the difference between success and failure.

CONCLUDING REMARKS

We have attempted in this chapter to explore some of the ways in which rehabilitation differs in various parts of the world. What we have written may be criticized in many ways; as authors, what concerns us most is the fact that what we have described is changing as we write and is likely to change even more in the future. Indeed we hope so; rehabilitation is a dynamic speciality that is based on iterative learning and that must be as responsive to change as we expect our patients to be. However, we must avoid "reinventing the wheel" when there are others who have done the same, or done it better, elsewhere in the world. International comparisons may provide the key to the constructive advances that we all seek.

ACKNOWLEDGMENTS

Information regarding the patient in "Australia: Rural: The 'Third World'"was kindly provided by Dr. Howard Flavell, Royal Darwin Hospital, Darwin, Northern Territory, Australia. Information regarding the patient in "China"was kindly provided by Professor Dengkun of Tongji Hospital, Wuhan, China, and Professor Tiebin Yan, Sun Yat-sun University, Guangzhou, China. Information regarding the patient in "The Pacific Islands: Fiji" was kindly provided by Dr Jagdish Maharaj, Suva Hospital, Fiji. And the "Costa Rica" case scenario was prepared by Dr Christine Ares-Rivet, San Jose, Costa Rica.

REFERENCES

1. World Health Organization. *International classification of functioning, disability and health.* Geneva: WHO, 2001.
2. Armstrong MJ. Culture and disability studies: an anthropological perspective. *Rehabilitation Education* 1996;10:247–304.
3. Parsons CD. *Healing practices in the South Pacific.* Honolulu: University of Hawaii Press, 1985.
4. Pal HR. Issues related to disability in India: a focus group. *National Medical Journal of India* 2000;13:237–241.
5. World Health Organization. *International classification of impairments, disabilities and handicaps.* Geneva: WHO, 1980.
6. Tesio L. Standardising outcome measurement in PM&R across Europe. Proceedings 13th European Congress of Physical and Rehabilitation Medicine. 2002: 140–141.

7. *Guide for the uniform data set for medical rehabilitation (including the FIM(TM) instrument), version 5.1.* Buffalo, NY: State University of New York at Buffalo, 1997.

8. Tennant A. The Rasch model and standardising outcome in rehabilitation: the PRO-ESOR project. Proceedings 13th European Congress of Physical and Rehabilitation Medicine. 2002: 142–143.

9. Brandstater M. International survey of training and certification in physical medicine and rehabilitation. *Arch Phys Med Rehabil* 2000;81:1234–1235.

10. DeLisa J. Certifying and measuring competency in the United States. *Arch Phys Med Rehabil* 2000;81:1236–1237.

11. Disler PB. Certifying and measuring competency in Australia and New Zealand. *Arch Phys Med Rehabil* 2000;81:1245–1247.

12. Ring H. Certification and measuring competency in Israel. *Arch Phys Med Rehabil* 2000;81:1250–1252.

13. Chino N. Certification and measuring competency in Japan, South Korea, and the Philippines. *Arch Phys Med Rehabil* 2000;81: 248–1249.

14. Ward AB. Training and certifying in the United Kingdom and Europe. *Arch Phys Med Rehabil* 2000;81:1242–1244.

15. Anton H. Certification and measuring competency in physical medicine and rehabilitation in Canada. *Arch Phys Med Rehabil* 2000;81:1253–1254.

16. Maharaj JC. Epidemiology of spinal cord paralysis in Fiji. *Spinal Cord* 1996; 34:549–559.

17. Braun KL. Cultural themes in health, illness and rehabilitation for native Hawaiians: observations of rehabilitation staff and physicians. *Topics in Geriatric Rehabilitation* 1987;12:19–37.

18. Fitzgerald MH. Rehabilitation services for the Pacific. *West J Med* 1993;159: 50–55.

19. International Labour Organization, United Nations Educational, Scientific and Cultural Organization, and World Health Organization. *Community-based rehabilitation for and with people with disabilities: joint position paper.* Geneva: ILO, UNESCO, and WHO, 1994.

20. United Nations Economic and Social Commission for Asia and the Pacific. *Understanding CBR.* Bangkok: United Nations Economic and Social Commission for Asia and the Pacific, 1997.

21. Nilsson A, Nilsson L. *Community-based rehabilitation as we have experienced it: voices of persons with disabilities.* Geneva: World Health Organization, 2002.

22. Wade DT. Community Rehabilitation. *Clin Rehabil* 2001;15:575.

23. Rodgers H. *Rehabilitation—hospital or home? An overview.* Royal College of Physicians of the United Kingdom, 2000.

24. Geddes J, Chamberlain MA. Home-based rehabilitation for people with stroke: a comparative study of six community services providing co-ordinated, multidisciplinary treatment. *Clin Rehabil* 2001;15:589–599.

25. Early Supported Discharge Trialists. Services for reducing duration of hospital care for acute stroke patients (Cochrane Review). In: The Cochrane Library, Issue 2, 2002. Oxford: Update Software, 2002.

CHAPTER 53

Principles and Applications of Measurement Methods

Steven R. Hinderer and Kathleen A. Hinderer

Objective measurement provides a scientific basis for communication between professionals, documentation of treatment efficacy, and scientific credibility within the medical community. Federal, state, private third-party payer, and consumer organizations increasingly are requiring objective evidence of improvement as an outcome of treatment. Empirical clinical observation is no longer an acceptable method without objective data to support clinical decision making. The lack of reliability of clinicians' unaided measurement capabilities is documented in the literature (1–7), further supporting the importance of objective measures. In addition, comparison of alternative evaluation or treatment methods, when more than one possible choice is available, requires appropriate use of measurement principles (8–11).

Clinicians and clinical researchers use measurements to assess characteristics, functions, or behaviors thought to be present or absent in specific groups of people. The application of objective measures uses structured observations to compare performances or characteristics across individuals (i.e., to discriminate), or within individuals over time (i.e., to evaluate), or for prognostication based on current status (i.e., to predict) (12,13). It is important to understand the principles of measurement and the characteristics of good measures to be an effective user of the tools. Standards for implementation of tests and measures have been established within physical therapy (14, 15), psychology (16), and medical rehabilitation (17) to address quality improvement and ethical issues for the use of clinical measures.

The purpose of this chapter is to discuss the basic principles of tests and measurements and to provide the reader with an understanding of the rationale for assessing and selecting measures that will provide the information required to interpret test results properly. A critical starting point is to define what is to be measured, for what purpose, and at what cost. Standardized measurements meeting these criteria should then be assessed for reliability and validity pertinent to answering the question or questions posed by the user. Measurements that are shown not to be valid or reliable provide misleading information that is ultimately useless (18).

The initial section of this chapter discusses the psychometric parameters used to evaluate tests and measures. Principles of evaluation, testing, and interpretation are detailed in the second section. The third section provides guidelines for objective measurement when a standardized test is not available to measure the behavior, function, or characteristic of interest.

The complexity and diversity of the tests and measures used in rehabilitation medicine clinical practice and research preclude itemized description in a single chapter. Appendix A, which appears at the end of this chapter, provides sources of available objective tests and measures and serves as a resource for the reader to seek further information on measures in their domain or domains of interest. Reviewing the references provided in Appendix A in conjunction with the principles provided in this chapter will enable the reader to become a more sophisticated user of objective measurement tools. Although there are several good measures listed in Appendix A, there is much developmental work that needs to be completed for many of these tests. A measurement is not objective unless adequate levels of reliability have been demonstrated (18). Therefore, it is imperative that the user be able to recognize the limitations of these tests to avoid inadvertent misuse or misinterpretation of test results.

PSYCHOMETRIC PARAMETERS USED TO EVALUATE TESTS AND MEASURES

The methods developed primarily in the psychology literature to evaluate objective measures generally are applicable to the standardized tests and instruments used in rehabilitation medicine. The topics discussed in this section are the foundation for all useful measures. Measurement tools must have defined levels of measurements for the trait or traits to be assessed and a purpose for obtaining the measurements. Additionally, tests and measures need to be practical, reliable, and valid.

Levels of Measurement

Tests and measures come in multiple forms because of the variety of parameters measured in clinical practice and research.

Despite the seemingly overwhelming number of measures, there are classified levels of measurement that determine how test results should be analyzed and interpreted (19). The four basic levels of measurement data are nominal, ordinal, interval, and ratio. Nominal and ordinal scales are used to classify discrete measures because the scores produced fall into discrete categories. Interval and ratio scales are used to classify continuous measures because the scores produced can fall anywhere along a continuum within the range of possible scores.

A nominal scale is used to classify data that do not have a rank order. The purpose of a nominal scale is to categorize people or objects into different groups based on a specific variable. An example of nominal data is diagnosis.

Ordinal data are operationally defined to assign individuals to categories that are mutually exclusive and discrete. The categories have a logical hierarchy, but it cannot be assumed that the intervals are equal between each category, even if the scale appears to have equal increments. Ordinal scales are the most commonly used level of measurement in clinical practice. Examples of ordinal scales are the manual muscle test scale (20–24) and functional outcome measures (e.g., Functional Independence Measure) (25).

Interval data, unlike nominal and ordinal scales, are continuous. An interval scale has sequential units with numerically equal distances between them. Interval data often are generated from quantitative instrumentation as opposed to clinical observation. An example of an interval measurement is range-of-motion scores reported in degrees.

A ratio scale is an interval scale on which the zero point represents a total absence of the quantity being measured. An example is force scores obtained from a quantitative muscle strength testing device.

Interval and ratio scales are more sophisticated and complex than nominal and ordinal scales. The latter are more common because they are easier to create. However, analysis of nominal and ordinal scales requires special consideration to avoid misinference from test results (26,27). The major controversies surrounding the use of these scales are the problems of unidimensionality and whether scores of items and subtests can be summed to provide an overall score. Continuous scales have a higher sensitivity of measurement and allow more rigorous statistical analyses to be performed.

Purpose of Testing

After the level of the measure has been selected, the purpose of testing must be examined. Tests generally serve one of two purposes: screening or in-depth assessment of specific traits, behaviors, or functions.

SCREENING TESTS

Screening tests have three possible applications:

1. To discriminate between "suspect" and "normal" patients
2. To identify people needing further assessment
3. To assess a number of broad categories superficially

One example of a screening test is the Test of Orientation for Rehabilitation Patients, administered to individuals who are confused or disoriented secondary to traumatic brain injury, cerebrovascular accident, seizure disorder, brain tumor, or other neurologic events (28–31). This test screens for orientation to person and personal situation, place, time, schedule, and temporal continuity. Another well-developed screening test is the Miller Assessment for Preschoolers (MAP) (32). This test screens preschoolers for problems in the following areas: sensory and motor, speech and language, cognition, behaviors, and visual-motor integration.

The advantages of screening tests are that they are brief and sample a broad range of behaviors, traits, or characteristics. They are limited, however, because of an increased frequency of false-positive results that is due to the small sample of behaviors obtained. Screening tests should be used cautiously for diagnosis, placement, or treatment planning. They are used most effectively to indicate the need for more extensive testing and treatment of specific problem areas identified by the screening assessment.

ASSESSMENT TESTS

Assessment tests have four possible applications:

1. To evaluate specific behaviors in greater depth
2. To provide information for planning interventions
3. To determine placement into specialized programs
4. To provide measurements to monitor progress

An example of an assessment measure is the Boston Diagnostic Aphasia Examination (33). The advantages of assessment measures are that they have a lower frequency of false-positive results; they assess a representative set of behaviors; they can be used for diagnosis, placement, or treatment planning; and they provide information regarding the functional level of the individual tested. The limitations are that an extended amount of time is needed for testing, and they generally require specially trained personnel to administer, score, and interpret the results.

Criterion-Referenced versus Norm-Referenced Tests

Proper interpretation of test results requires comparison with a set of standards or expectations for performance. There are two basic types of standardized measures: criterion-referenced and norm-referenced tests.

CRITERION-REFERENCED TESTS

Criterion-referenced tests are those for which the test score is interpreted in terms of performance on the test relative to the continuum of possible scores attainable (18). The focus is on what the person can do or what he or she knows rather than how he or she compares with others (34). Individual performance is compared with a fixed expected standard rather than a reference group. Scores are interpreted based on absolute criteria, for example, the total number of items successfully completed. Criterion-referenced tests are useful to discriminate between successive performances of one person. They are conducted to measure a specific set of behavioral objectives. The Tufts Assessment of Motor Performance (which has undergone further validation work and has been renamed the Michigan Modified Performance Assessment) is an example of a criterion-referenced test (35–39). This assessment battery measures a broad range of physical skills in the areas of mobility, activities of daily living, and physical aspects of communication.

NORM-REFERENCED TESTS

Norm-referenced tests use a representative sample of people who are measured relative to a variable of interest. Norm referencing permits comparison of a single person's measurement with those scores expected for the rest of the population. The normal values reported should be obtained from, and reported for, clearly described populations. The normal population should be the same as those for whom the test was designed to detect abnormalities (34). Reports of norm-referenced test results should use scoring procedures that reflect the person's position relative to the normal distribution (e.g., percentiles, standard scores). Measures of central tendency (e.g., mean, median, mode) and variability (e.g., standard deviation, standard error of the mean) also should be reported to provide information on the range of normal scores, assisting with determination of the clinical relevance of test results. An example of a norm-referenced test is the Peabody Developmental Motor Scale (40). This developmental test assesses fine and gross motor domains. Test items are classified into the following categories: grasp, hand use, eye-hand coordination, manual dexterity, reflexes, balance, nonlocomotor, locomotor, and receipt and propulsion of objects.

Practicality

A test or instrument should ideally be practical, easy to use, insensitive to outside influences, inexpensive, and designed to allow efficient administration (41). For example, it is not efficient to begin testing in a supine position, switch to a prone position, then return to supine. Test administration should be organized to complete all testing in one position before switching to another. Instructions for administering the test should be clear and concise, and scoring criteria should be clearly defined. If equipment is required, it must be durable and of good quality. Qualifications of the tester and additional training required to become proficient in test administration should be specified. The time to administer the test should be indicated in the test manual. The duration of the test and level of difficulty need to be appropriate relative to the attention span and perceived capabilities of the patient being tested. Finally, the test manual should provide summary statistics and detailed guidelines for appropriate use and interpretation of test scores based on the method of test development.

Reliability and Agreement

A general definition of reliability is the extent to which a measurement provides consistent information (i.e., is free from random error). Granger and associates (42) provide the analogy "it may be thought of as the extent to which the data contain relevant information with a high signal-to-noise ratio vs. irrelevant static confusion." In contrast, agreement is defined as the extent to which identical measurements are made. Reliability and agreement are distinctly different concepts and are estimated using different statistical techniques (43). Unfortunately, these concepts and their respective statistics often are treated synonymously in the literature.

The level of reliability is not necessarily congruent with the degree of agreement. It is possible for ratings to cluster consistently toward the same end of the scale, resulting in high-reliability coefficients, and yet these judgments may or may not be equivalent. High reliability does not indicate whether the raters absolutely agree. It can occur concurrently with low agreement when each rater scores patients differently, but the relative differences in the scores are consistent for all patients rated. Conversely, low reliability does not necessarily indicate that raters disagree. Low-reliability coefficients can occur with high agreement when the range of scores assigned by the raters is restricted or when the variability of the ratings is small (i.e., in a homogeneous population). In instances in which the scores are fairly homogeneous, reliability coefficients lack the power to detect relationships and are often depressed, even though agreement between ratings may be relatively high. The reader is referred to Tinsley and Weiss for examples of these concepts (44). Both reliability and agreement must be established on the target population or populations to which the measure will be applied, using typical examiners. There are five types of reliability and agreement:

1. Interrater
2. Test-retest
3. Intertrial
4. Alternate form
5. Population specific

Each type will be discussed below, along with indications for calculating reliability versus agreement and their respective statistics.

INTERRATER RELIABILITY AND AGREEMENT

Interrater or interobserver agreement is the extent to which independent examiners agree exactly on a patient's performance. In contrast, interrater reliability is defined as the degree to which the ratings of different observers are proportional when expressed as deviations from their means; that is, the relationship of one rated person to other rated people is the same, although the absolute numbers used to express the relationship may vary from rater to rater (44). The independence of the examiners in the training they receive and the observations they make is critical in determining interrater agreement and reliability. When examiners have trained together or confer when performing a test, the interrater reliability or agreement coefficient calculated from their observations may be artificially inflated.

An interrater agreement or reliability coefficient provides an estimate of how much measurement error can be expected in scores obtained by two or more examiners who have independently rated the same person. Determining interrater agreement or reliability is particularly important for test scores that largely depend on the examiner's skill or judgment. An acceptable level of interrater reliability or agreement is essential for comparison of test results obtained from different clinical centers. Interrater agreement or reliability is a basic criterion for a measure to be called objective. If multiple examiners consistently obtain the same absolute or relative scores, then it is much more likely that the score is a function of the measure, rather than of the collective subjective bias of the examiners (18).

Pure interrater agreement and reliability are determined by having one examiner administer the test while the other examiner or examiners observe and independently score the person's performance at the same point in time. When assessing some parameters, when the skill of the examiner administering the test plays a vital role (e.g., sensory testing, range of motion testing) or when direct observation of each examiner is required (e.g., strength), it is impossible to assess pure interrater agreement and reliability. In these instances, each examiner must test the individual independently. Consequently, these interrater measures are confounded by factors of time and variation in patient performance.

TEST-RETEST RELIABILITY AND AGREEMENT

Test-retest agreement is defined as the extent to which a patient receives identical scores during two different test sessions when rated by the same examiner. In contrast, test-retest reliability assesses the degree of consistency in how a person's score is rank ordered relative to other people tested by the same examiner during different test sessions. Test-retest reliability is the most basic and essential form of reliability. It provides an estimate of the variation in patient performance on a different test day, when retested by the same examiner. Some of the error in a test-retest situation also may be attributed to variations in the examiner's performance. It is important to determine the magnitude of day-to-day fluctuations in performance so that true changes in the parameters of interest can be determined. Variability of the test or how it is administered should not be the source of observed changes over time. Additionally, with quantitative measuring instruments, the examiner must be knowledgeable in the method of and frequency required for instrument calibration.

The suggested test-retest interval is 1 to 3 days for most physical measures and 7 days for maximal effort tests in which muscle fatigue is involved (45). The test-retest interval should not exceed the expected time for change to occur naturally. The purpose of an adequate but relatively short interval is to minimize the effects of memory, practice, and maturation or deterioration on test performance (46).

INTERTRIAL RELIABILITY AND AGREEMENT

Intertrial agreement provides an estimate of the stability of repeated scores obtained by one examiner within a test session. Intertrial reliability assesses the consistency of one examiner rank-ordering repeated trials obtained from patients using the same measurement tool and standardized method for testing and scoring results within a test session. Intertrial agreement and reliability also are influenced by individual performance factors such as fatigue, motor learning, motivation, and consistency of effort. Intertrial agreement and reliability should not be confused with test-retest agreement and reliability. The latter involves test sessions usually separated by days or weeks as opposed to seconds or minutes for intertrial agreement and reliability. A higher level of association is expected for results obtained from trials within a test session than those from different sessions.

ALTERNATE FORM RELIABILITY AND AGREEMENT

Alternate form agreement refers to the consistency of scores obtained from two forms of the same test. Equivalent or parallel forms are different test versions intended to measure the same traits at a comparable level of difficulty. Alternate form reliability refers to whether the parallel forms of a test rank order people's scores consistently relative to each other. A high level of alternate form agreement or reliability may be required if a person must be tested more than once and a learning or practice effect is expected. This is particularly important when one form of the test will be used as a pretest and a second as a posttest.

POPULATION-SPECIFIC RELIABILITY AND AGREEMENT

Population-specific agreement and reliability assess the degree of absolute and relative reproducibility, respectively, that a test has for a specific group being measured (e.g., Ashworth scale scores for rating severity of spasticity from spinal cord injury). A variation of this type of agreement and reliability refers to the population of examiners administering the test (18).

INTERPRETATION OF RELIABILITY AND AGREEMENT STATISTICS

Because measures of reliability and agreement are concerned with the degree of consistency or concordance between two or more independently derived sets of scores, they can be expressed in terms of correlation coefficients (34). The reliability coefficient is usually expressed as a value between 0 and 1, with higher values indicating higher reliability. Agreement statistics can range from −1 to +1, with +1 indicating perfect agreement, 0 indicating chance agreement, and negative values indicating less than chance agreement. The coefficient of choice varies, depending on the data type analyzed. The reader is referred to Bartko and Carpenter (47), Hartmann (48), Hollenbeck (49), Liebetrau (50), and Tinsley and Weiss (44) for discussions of how to select appropriate statistical measures of reliability and agreement. Table 53-1 provides information on appropriate statistical procedures for calculating interrater and test-retest reliability and agreement for discrete and continu-

TABLE 53-1.   Interrater Reliability, Test-Retest Reliability, and Agreement Analysis: Appropriate Statistics and Minimum Acceptable Levels

Data Type	Reliability Analysis		Agreement Analysis	
	Appropriate Statistic	Level	Appropriate Stastic	Level
Discrete				
Nominal	ICC or κ_W	>0.75	κ	>0.60
Ordinal	ICC	>0.75	κ_W	>0.60
Continuous				
Interval	ICC	>0.75	χ^2 and T	$P < 0.05$
Ratio	ICC	>0.75	χ^2 and T	$P < 0.05$

References: ICC: discrete (47,55), ordinal (47), continuous (44,47), minimal acceptable level (56); Cohen's κ—κ (44,47,57,58), κ_W (47,59,60), κ_W equivalence with ICC for reliability analysis of minimal data (61–64), minimal acceptable level (65); Lawlis and Lu's χ^2 and T; statistical and minimal level (43,44). ICC, intraclass correlation; κ, kappa; κ_W, weighted kappa; T, T index.

ous data types. No definitive standards for minimum acceptable levels of the different types of reliability and agreement statistics have been established; however, guidelines for minimum levels are provided in Table 53-1. The acceptable level varies, depending on the magnitude of the decision being made, the population variance, the sources of error variance, and the measurement technique (e.g., instrumentation versus behavioral assessments). If the population variance is relatively homogeneous, lower estimates of reliability are acceptable. In contrast, if the population variance is heterogeneous, higher estimates of reliability are expected. Critical values of correlation coefficients, based on the desired level of significance and the number of subjects, are provided in tables in measurement textbooks (51,52). It is important to note that a correlation coefficient that is statistically significant does not necessarily indicate that adequate reliability or agreement has been established, because the significance level only provides an indication that the coefficient is significantly different from zero (see Table 53-1).

Agreement and reliability both are important for evaluating patient ratings. As discussed earlier, these are distinctly different concepts and require separate statistical analysis. Several factors must be considered to determine the relative importance of each. Decisions that carry greater weight or impact for the people being assessed may require more exact agreement. If the primary need is to assess the relative consistency between raters, and exact agreement is less critical, then a reliability measure alone is a satisfactory index. In contrast, whenever the major interest is either the absolute value of the score, or the meaning of the scores as defined by the points on the scale (e.g., criterion-referenced tests), agreement should be reported in addition to the reliability (44). Scores generated from instrumentation are expected to have a higher level of reliability or agreement than scores obtained from behavioral observations.

A test score actually consists of two different components: the true score and the error score (34,53). A person's true score is a hypothetical construct, indicating a test score that is unaffected by chance factors. The error score refers to unwanted variation in the test score (54). All continuous scale measurements have a component of error, and no test is completely reliable. Consequently, reliability is a matter of degree. Any reliability coefficient may be interpreted directly in terms of percentage of score variance attributable to different sources (18). A reliability coefficient of 0.85 signifies that 85% of the variance in test scores depends on true variance in the trait measured and 15% depends on error variance.

SPECIFIC RELIABILITY AND AGREEMENT STATISTICS

There are several statistical measures for estimating interrater agreement and reliability. Four statistics commonly used to determine agreement are the frequency ratio, point-by-point agreement ratio, kappa (κ) coefficients, and Lawlis and Lu's χ^2 and T-index statistics. For reliability calculations, the most frequently used correlation statistics are the Pearson product-moment (Pearson r) and intraclass correlation coefficients (ICC). When determining reliability for dichotomous or ordinal data, specific ICC formulas have been developed. These nonparametric ICC statistics have been shown to be the equivalent of the weighted kappa (κ_w) (55–58). Consequently, the κ_w also can be used as an index of reliability for discrete data, and the values obtained can be directly compared with equivalent forms of ICCs (56). The method of choice for reliability and agreement analyses partially depends on the assessment strategy used (44,47,50,59). In addition to agreement and reliability statistics, standard errors of measurement (SEM) provide a clinically relevant index of reliability expressed in test score units. Each statistic is described below.

Frequency Ratio

This agreement statistic is indicated for frequency count data (46). A frequency ratio of the two examiners' scores is calculated by dividing the smaller total by the larger total and multiplying by 100. This statistic is appealing because of its computational and interpretive simplicity. There are a variety of limitations, however. It only reflects agreement of the total number of behaviors scored by each observer; there is no way to determine whether there is agreement for individual responses using a frequency ratio. The value of this statistic may be inflated if the observed behavior occurs at high rates (59). There is no meaningful lower bound of acceptability (48).

Point-by-Point Agreement Ratio

This statistic is used to determine if there is agreement on each occurrence of the observed behavior. It is appropriate when there are discrete opportunities for the behavior to occur or for distinct response categories (46,60,61). To calculate this ratio, the number of agreements is totaled by determining the concurrence between observers regarding the presence or absence of observable responses during a given trial, recording interval, or for a particular behavior category. Disagreements are defined as instances in which one observer records a response and the other observer does not. The point-by-point agreement percentage is calculated by dividing the number of agreements by the number of agreements plus disagreements, and multiplying by 100 (61). Agreement generally is considered to be acceptable at a level of 0.80 or above (61).

The extent to which observers are found to agree is partially a function of the frequency of occurrence of the target behavior and of whether occurrence and/or nonoccurrence agreements are counted (60). When the rate of the target behavior is either very high or very low, high levels of interobserver agreement are likely for occurrences or nonoccurrences, respectively. Consequently, if the frequency of either occurrences or nonoccurrences is high, a certain level of agreement is expected simply owing to chance. In such cases, it is often recommended that agreements be included in the calculation only if at least one observer recorded the occurrence of the target behavior. In this case, intervals during which none of the observers records a response are excluded from the analysis. It is important to identify clearly what constitutes an agreement when reporting point-by-point percentage agreement ratios because the level of reliability is affected by this definition.

Kappa Coefficient

The κ coefficient provides an estimate of agreement between observers, corrected for chance agreement. This statistic is preferred for discrete categorical (nominal and ordinal) data because, unlike the two statistics discussed above, it corrects for chance agreements. In addition, percentage agreement ratios often are inflated when there is an unequal distribution of scores between rating categories. This often is the case in rehabilitation medicine, in which the frequency of normal characteristics is much higher than abnormal characteristics (62,63). In contrast, κ coefficients provide accurate estimates of agreement, even when scores are unequally distributed between rating categories (63).

Kappa coefficients are used to summarize observer agreement and accuracy, determine rater consistency, and evaluate scaled consistency among raters (59). Three conditions must be met to use κ:

1. The patients or research subjects must be independent.
2. The raters must independently score the patients or research subjects.
3. The rating categories must be mutually exclusive and exhaustive (62, 63).

The general form of κ is a coefficient of agreement for nominal scales in which all disagreements are treated equally (44,47, 50,64–67). The κ_w statistic was developed for ordinal data (47,50,68,69), in which some disagreements have greater gravity than others (e.g., the manual muscle testing scale, in which the difference between a score of 2 and 5 is of more concern than the difference between a score of 4 and 5). Refer to the references cited above for formulas used to calculate κ and κ_w.

Several other variations of κ have been developed for specific applications. The kappa statistic κ_v provides an overall measure of agreement, as well as separate indices for each subject and rating category (70). This form of κ can be applied in situations in which subjects are not all rated by the same set of examiners. The variation of κ described by Fleiss et al. is useful when there are more than two ratings per patient (57); a computer program is available to calculate this statistic (62). When multiple examiners rate patients and a measure of overall conjoint agreement is desired, the kappa statistic κ_m is indicated (71). Standard κ statistics treat all raters or units symmetrically (57). When one or more of the ratings is considered to be a standard (e.g., scores from an experienced rater), alternate analysis procedures should be used (71–73).

Lawlis and Lu χ^2 and T Index

These measures of agreement are recommended for continuous data (44). They permit the option of defining seriousness of disagreements among raters. A statistically significant χ^2 indicates that the observed agreement is greater than that expected owing to chance. The T index is used to determine whether agreement is low, moderate, or high. The reader is referred to Tinsley and Weiss (44) for a discussion of the indications for, calculation of, and interpretation of these statistics.

Pearson Product-Moment Correlation Coefficient

Historically, the Pearson r has been used commonly as an index of reliability. It has limited application, however, because it is a parametric statistic intended for use with continuous bivariate data. The generally accepted minimum level of this coefficient is 0.80; however, levels above 0.90 often are considered more desirable (34,51). The Pearson r provides only an index of the strength of the relationship between scores and is insensitive to consistent differences between scores. Consequently, a linear regression equation must be reported in addition to the Pearson r to indicate the nature of the relationship between the scores (18). Because the Pearson r is limited to the analysis of bivariate data, it is preferable to use an ICC to assess reliability because ICC can be used for either bivariate or multivariate data. The Pearson r and ICC will yield the same result for bivariate data (74).

Intraclass Correlation Coefficients

ICCs provide an index of variability resulting from comparing rating score error with other sources of true score variability (42,52,75). As indicated above, it is the coefficient of choice for reliability analyses. The ICC is based on the variance components from an analysis of variance (ANOVA), which includes not only the between-subject variance, as does the Pearson r, but also other situation-specific variance components, such as alternate test forms, maturation of subjects between ratings, and other sources of true mean differences in the obtained ratings (76). The individual sources of error can be analyzed to determine their percentage contribution to the overall error variance using generalizability analysis (53,54). For further information regarding the use of generalizability theory to distinguish between sources of error, the reader is referred to Brennan (77) and Cronbach and associates (78).

There are six different ICC formulas (54). The correct ICC formula is selected based on three factors:

1. The use of a one-way versus two-way ANOVA
2. The importance of differences between examiners' mean ratings
3. The analysis of an individual rating versus the mean of several ratings (44,54)

Selection of the proper formula is critical and is based on the reliability study design (54,76,79). It is important to report which type of ICC is used to compute reliability because the calculations are not equivalent. Variations of the ICC formulas also exist for calculating ICCs using dichotomous (80) and ordinal (44) nonparametric data. The marginal distributions do not have to be equal, as was originally proposed for nonparametric ICCs (56). These nonparametric ICC formulas have been demonstrated to be equivalent to weighted κ coefficients, provided that the mean difference between raters is included as a component of variability and the rating categories can be ordered (56).

Standard Error of Measurement

It has been suggested that measurement error estimates are the most desirable index of reliability (18,34,75). The SEM is an estimate, in test score units, of the random variation of a person's performance across repeated measures. The SEM is an expression of the margin of error between a person's observed score and his or her true ability (46). The SEM is an important indicator of the sensitivity of the test to detect changes in a person's performance over time.

The formula for the SEM is

$$SD \sqrt{1 - r_{rr}}$$

where SD is the standard deviation of the test scores and r_{rr} is the reliability coefficient for the test scores (34,45,75). Correlating scores from two forms of a test is one of several ways to estimate the reliability coefficient (75) and often is used in psychology when parallel forms of a test are available. In rehabilitation medicine, however, equivalent forms of a test often are not available. The test-retest reliability coefficient

therefore is the coefficient of choice for calculating the SEM in most rehabilitation applications because the primary interest is in the variation of subject performance. The SEM is a relatively conservative statistic, requiring larger data samples (approximately 300 to 400 observations) in order to not overestimate the error (15).

It is best to report a test score as a range rather than as an absolute score. The SEM is used to calculate the range of scores (i.e., confidence interval) for a given person; that is, the person's true performance ability is expected to fall within the range of scores defined by the confidence interval. A person's score must fall outside of this range to indicate with confidence that a true change in performance has occurred. Based on a normal distribution, a 95% confidence interval would be approximately equal to the mean ±2 SEM. A 95% confidence interval is considered best to use when looking for change over time. This rigorous level of confidence minimizes the likelihood of a type I error (i.e., there is only a 5% chance that differences between scores obtained from a given person during different test sessions will not fall within the 95% confidence interval upper and lower values). Consequently, there is less than a 5% chance that differences between scores exceeding the upper end of the confidence interval are due to measurement error (i.e., they have a 95% chance of representing a true change in performance).

FACTORS AFFECTING RELIABILITY

There are four sources of measurement error for interrater reliability (18,45):

1. Lack of agreement among scorers
2. Lack of consistent performance by the individual tested
3. Failure of the instrument to measure consistently
4. Failure of the examiner to follow the standardized procedures to administer the test

Threats to test-retest reliability similarly are caused by four factors:

1. The instrument
2. The examiner
3. The patient
4. The testing protocol

Sources and prevention of examiner error will be discussed in the section on principles of evaluation, testing, and interpretation.

There are several factors conducive to good reliability of a measure (45). These factors are the power to discriminate among ability groups; sufficient time allotted so that each patient can show his or her best performance without being penalized for an unrepresentative poor trial; test organization to optimize examinee performance; and test administration and scoring instructions that are clear and precise. Additionally, the testing environment should support good performance, and the examiner must be competent in administering the test. For tests designed to be appropriate for a wide age range, reliability should be examined for each age level rather than for the group as a whole (53).

In summary, reliability and agreement are essential components to any objective measurement. Measurements lacking test-retest reliability contain sufficient error as to be useless because the data obtained do not reflect the variable measured (18). Reliability is an important component of validity, but good reliability or agreement does not guarantee that a measure is valid. A reliable measurement is consistent, but not necessarily correct. However, a measurement that is unreliable cannot be valid.

Validity

Validity is defined as the accuracy with which a test measures that which it is intended to measure. Application of the concept of validity refers to the appropriateness, meaningfulness, and usefulness of a test for a particular situation (18). Validity is initially investigated while a test or instrument is being developed and confirmed through subsequent use. Four basic aspects of validity will be discussed: content, construct, criterion-related, and face validity.

CONTENT VALIDITY

Content validity is the systematic examination of the test content to determine if it covers a representative sample of the behavior domain to be measured. It should be reported in the test manual as descriptive information on the skills covered by the test, number of items in each category, and rationale for item selection. Content validity generally is evidenced by the opinion of experts that the domain sampled is adequate. There are two primary methods that the developer of a test can use for obtaining professional opinions about the content validity of an instrument (81). The first is to provide a panel of experts with the items from the test and request a determination of what the battery of items is measuring. The second method requires providing not only the test items but also a list of test objectives so that experts can determine the relationship between the two. For statistical analysis of content validity, the reader is referred to Thorn and Deitz (82).

CONSTRUCT VALIDITY

Construct validity refers to the extent to which a test measures the theoretical construct underlying the test. Construct validity should be obtained whenever a test purports to measure an abstract trait or theoretical characteristics about the nature of human behavior such as intelligence, self-concept, anxiety, school or work readiness, or perceptual organization. The following five areas must be considered with regard to construct validity in test instruments (34, 81).

Age Differentiation

Any developmental changes in children or changes in performance due to aging must be addressed as part of the test development.

Factor Analysis

Factor analysis is a statistical procedure that can be performed on data obtained from testing. The purpose of factor analysis is to simplify the description of behavior by reducing an initial multiplicity of variables to a few common underlying factors or traits that may or may not be pertinent to the construct or constructs that the test was originally designed to measure. The reader is referred to Cronbach (75), Wilson et al. (83), Wright and Masters (84), and Wright and Stone (85) for in-depth discussions of factor analysis. The more recent development of confirmatory factor analysis (86,87) overcomes the relative arbitrariness of traditional factor analysis methods. Confirmatory factor analysis differs from traditional factor analysis in that the investigator specifies, before analysis, the measures that are determined by each factor and which factors are correlated. The specified relationships are then statistically tested for goodness of fit of the proposed model compared with the actual data collected. Confirmatory factor analysis is therefore a more direct assessment of construct validity than is traditional factor analysis. Rasch modeling (88) is a further expansion on confirmatory factor analysis methods for the purpose of establishing construct validity of a measurement tool. Rasch models start with a carefully thought-out and systemati-

cally implemented analogy used to facilitate the construction of the concepts of the measurement tool in concrete terms, then use a developmental pathway analogy to develop the Rasch concepts of unidimensionality, fit, difficulty/ability estimation and error, locations for item difficulties, and locations for person abilities.

Internal Consistency

In assessing the attributes of a test, it is helpful to examine the relationship of subscales and individual items to the total score. This is especially important when the test instrument has many components. If a subtest or item has a very low correlation with the total score, the test developer must question the subtest's validity in relation to the total score. This technique is most useful for providing confirmation of the validity of a homogeneous test. A test that measures several constructs would not be expected to have a high degree of internal consistency. For dichotomous data, the Kuder-Richardson statistic is used to calculate internal consistency (34). Cronbach's coefficient alpha (α) is recommended when the measure has more than two levels of response (34). The minimum acceptable level of α generally is set at 0.70 (89).

Convergent and Divergent Validity

Construct validity is evidenced further by high correlations with other tests that purport to measure the same constructs (i.e., convergent validity) and low correlations with measures that are designed to measure different attributes (i.e., divergent validity). It is desirable to obtain moderate levels of convergent validity, indicating that the two measures are not measuring identical constructs. If the new test correlates too highly with another test, it is questionable whether the new test is necessary because either test would suffice to answer the same questions. Moderately high but significant correlations indicate good convergent validity, but with each test still having unique components. Good divergent validity is demonstrated by low and insignificant correlations between two tests that measure theoretically unrelated parameters, such as an activities of daily living assessment and a test of expressive language ability.

Discriminant Validity

If two groups known to have different characteristics can be identified and assessed by the test, and if a significant difference between the performance of the two groups is found, then incisive evidence of discriminant validity is present.

CRITERION-RELATED VALIDITY

Criterion-related validity includes two subclasses of validity: concurrent validity and predictive validity (34,46). The commonality between these subclasses of validity is that they refer to multiple measurement of the same construct. In other words, the measure in question is compared with other variables or measures that are considered to be accurate measures of the characteristics or behaviors being tested. The purpose is to use the second measure as a criterion to validate the first measure.

Criterion-related validity can be assessed statistically, providing clear guidelines as to whether a measure is valid. Frequently, the paired measurements from the tests under comparison have different values. The nature of the relationship is less important than the strength of the relationship (18). Ottenbacher and Tomchek (90) showed that the limits of agreement technique provided the most accurate measurement error when comparing test results versus other statistics frequently used for such comparisons.

Concurrent Validity

Concurrent validity deals with whether an inference is justifiable at the present time. This is typically done by comparing results of one measure against some criterion (e.g., another measure or related phenomenon). If the correlation is high, the measure is said to have good concurrent validity. Concurrent validity is relevant to tests used for diagnosis of existing status, rather than predicting future outcome.

Predictive Validity

Predictive validity involves a measure's ability to predict or forecast some future criterion. Examples include performance on another measure in the future, prognostic reaction to an intervention program, or performance in some task of daily living. Predictive validity is difficult to establish and often requires collection of data over an extended period of time after the test has been developed. Hence, very few measures used in rehabilitation medicine have established predictive validity. A specific subset of predictive validity that is important to rehabilitation medicine practice is ecological validity. This concept involves the ability to identify impairments, functional limitations, and performance deficits within the context of the person's own environment. Measures with good concurrent validity sometimes are presumed to have good predictive validity, but this may not be a correct assumption. Unless predictive validity information exists for a test, extreme caution should be exercised in interpreting test results as predictors of future behavior or function.

FACE VALIDITY

Face validity is not considered to be an essential component of the validity of a test or measure. It reflects only whether a test appears to measure what it is supposed to, based on the personal opinions of those either taking or giving the test (91). A test with high face validity has a greater likelihood of being more rigorously and carefully administered by the examiner, and the person being tested is more likely to give his or her best effort. Although it is not essential, in most instances, face validity is still an important component of test development and selection. Exceptions include personality and interest tests when the purpose of testing is concealed to prevent patient responses from being biased.

Summary

The information discussed in this section provides the basis for critically assessing available tests and measures. The scale of the test or instrument should be sufficiently sophisticated to discriminate adequately between different levels of the behavior or function being tested. The purposes for testing must be identified, and the test chosen should have been developed for this purpose. The measure selected should be practical from the standpoint of time, efficiency, budget, equipment, and the population being tested. Above all, the measure must have acceptable reliability, agreement, and validity for the specific application it is selected. Reliability, agreement, and validity are important for both clinical and research applications. The power of statistical tests depends on adequate levels of reliability, agreement, and validity of the dependent measures (92). Consequently, it is essential that adequate levels of reliability, agreement, and validity be assessed and reported for dependent measures used in research studies.

For additional information on the test development process, the reader is referred to Miller (93). For information on the principles of tests and measurements, the reader is referred to Anastasi and Urbina (34), Baumgartner and Jackson (45), Cronbach (75), Safrit (51), Rothstein (18), Rothstein and Echternach (15), and Verducci (52).

Identification of the most appropriate test for a given application, based on the psychometric criteria discussed above, does not guarantee that the desired information will be obtained. Principles of evaluation, testing, and interpretation must be followed to optimize objective data acquisition.

PRINCIPLES OF EVALUATION, TESTING, AND INTERPRETATION

Systematic testing using standardized techniques is essential to quantify a patient's status objectively. Standardized testing is defined as using specified test administration and scoring procedures, under the same environmental conditions, with consistent directions (34,46). Standardized testing is essential to permit comparison of test results for a given person over time and to compare test scores between patients (91). In addition, consistent testing techniques facilitate interdisciplinary interpretation of clinical findings among rehabilitation professionals and minimize duplication of evaluation procedures.

Examiner Qualifications

Assessments using objective instrumentation or standardized tests must be conducted by examiners who have appropriate training and qualifications (14,16,17,34,91,94). The necessary training and expertise varies with the type of instrument or test used. The characteristics common to most rehabilitation medicine applications will be discussed. Examiners must be thoroughly familiar with standardized test administration, scoring, and interpretation procedures. Training guidelines specified in the published test manual must be strictly adhered to. A skilled examiner is aware of factors that might affect test performance and takes the necessary steps to ensure that the effects of these factors are minimized. Interrater reliability needs to be attained at acceptable levels with examiners who are experienced in administering the test to ensure consistency of test administration and scoring.

Examiners also must be knowledgeable about the instruments and standardized tests available to assess parameters of interest. They need to be familiar with relevant research literature, test reviews, and the technical merits of the appropriate tests and measures (14,16,17,34). From this information, examiners should be able to discern the advantages, disadvantages, and limitations of using a particular test or device. Based on the purpose of testing and characteristics of the person being assessed, examiners need to be able to select and justify the most appropriate assessment method from the available options.

When interpreting test results, examiners must be sensitive to factors that may have affected test performance (34). Conclusions and recommendations should be based on a synthesis of the person's scores, the expected measurement error, any factors that might have influenced test performance, the characteristics of the given person compared with those of the normative population, and the purpose of testing versus the recommended applications of the test or instrument. Written documentation of test results and interpretation should include comments on any potential influence of the above factors.

Examiner Training

Proper training of examiners is critical to attaining an acceptable level of interrater reliability for test administration and scoring (91). Examiners should be trained to minimize later decrements in performance (59). Training methods should be documented carefully so that they can be replicated by future examiners.

TRAINING PROCEDURES

As part of their training, examiners should read the test manual and instructions carefully. Operational definitions and rating criteria need to be memorized verbatim (95). A written examination should be administered to document the examiners' assimilation of test administration and scoring procedures (59). This information should be periodically reviewed to produce close adherence to the standardized protocol. It is helpful for examiners to view a videotape of an experienced examiner conducting the test. If test administration and scoring techniques need to be adjusted for the varying abilities of the target population (e.g., children of different age levels), the experienced examiner should be observed testing a representative sample from the target population to demonstrate the various testing, scoring, and interpretation procedures.

Videotapes also are useful to clarify scoring procedures and establish consistency of scoring between and within raters (66, 91). Once scoring procedures have been reviewed adequately, interrater reliability can be established by having trainees view several patients on videotape, then compare their scores with those from an experienced examiner. Scoring discrepancies should be discussed, and trainees should continue to score videotaped segments until 100% agreement is established with an experienced examiner (95). Intrarater consistency of scoring also can be established by having an individual examiner score the same videotape on multiple occasions. Sufficient time should elapse between multiple viewings so examiners do not recall previous ratings.

For assessments that involve multiple trials (e.g., strength assessments), intertrial reliability can be calculated to provide a measure of the examiner's consistency of administering multiple trials within a given test session. As was mentioned previously, intertrial reliability also is influenced by factors such as fatigue, motor learning, motivation, and the stability of performance over a short period of time. Multiple trials administered during a given session generally are highly correlated; thus, intertrial reliability coefficients are expected to be very high. Although this measure provides feedback on consistency in administering multiple trials, it should not be considered a substitute for establishing other types of reliability during the training phase.

ESTABLISHING PROCEDURAL RELIABILITY

Procedural reliability is defined as the reliability with which standardized testing and scoring procedures are applied. As part of training, examiners should be observed administering and scoring the test on a variety of people with characteristics similar to those of the target population (91). Procedural reliability should be established by having an experienced examiner observe trainees to determine if the test is being administered and scored according to the standardized protocol. Establishing procedural reliability greatly increases the likelihood that the observed changes in performance reflect true changes in status and not alterations in examiner testing or scoring methods. Unfortunately, this type of reliability often is neglected. According to Billingsley and associates (96), failure to assess procedural reliability poses a threat to both the internal and external validity of assessments.

Procedural reliability is assessed by having an independent observer check off whether each component of an assessment is completed according to the standardized protocol while

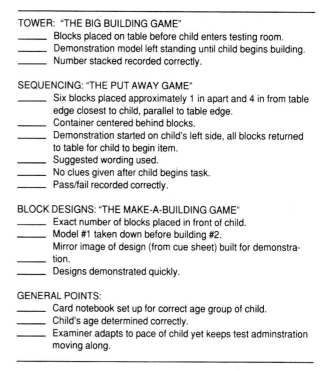

Figure 53-1. Procedural reliability checklist for selected items on the Miller Assessment for Preschoolers. (Reprinted with permission from Gyurke J, Prifitera A. Standardizing an assessment. *Phys Occup Ther Pediatr* 1989;9:71.)

viewing a live or videotaped assessment. Specific antecedent conditions, commands, timing of execution, and positioning are monitored, and any deviations are noted. Procedural reliability is calculated as a percentage of correct behaviors (96). Checklists should include all essential components of the standardized protocol. An example of a procedural reliability checklist for selected items on the MAP is provided in Figure 53-1 (91). In this example, the checklist varies for each item administered. Another example of procedural reliability is referenced for strength testing using a myometer (97). In this case, the protocol was standardized across muscle groups, including the command sequence, tactile input, myometer placement, start and end positions, and contraction duration.

Deviation from the standardized protocol can be minimized by conducting periodic procedural reliability checks (96). Procedural reliability should be assessed on an ongoing basis at random intervals in clinical or research settings, in addition to the training period. Assessments should be conducted at least once per phase during a research study. Examiners should be informed that procedural reliability checks will occur randomly, and ideally should be unaware of when specific assessments are conducted to avoid examiner reactivity. A minimum acceptable level of procedural reliability should be established for clinical or research use (generally, 90% to 100%). During the training phase, a 100% level should be attained. Feedback on procedural reliability assessments should be provided to examiners. If an examiner's score decreases below the acceptable level, pertinent sections of the standardized protocol should be reviewed.

ESTABLISHING INTERRATER RELIABILITY AND AGREEMENT

Once an examiner has demonstrated consistency in scoring by viewing videotaped assessments and reliability in test administration through procedural reliability checks, then interrater reliability and agreement should be established with an experienced examiner (59,91). Both examiners should independently rate people with characteristics similar to the target population. Reliability and agreement assessments should be conducted under conditions similar to those of the actual data collection procedures (60). As with procedural reliability, interrater assessments should be conducted periodically in both clinical and research settings. It is essential to establish interrater reliability and agreement at least once per phase in a research study to determine the potential influence of examiner rating differences on the data recorded (59,60). When calculating interrater agreement when the experienced examiner's scores are considered to be a standard, specific statistical procedures are indicated (71–73).

For assessments where the person's performance can be observed directly (e.g., developmental or activities of daily living assessments), it is preferable to establish interrater reliability and agreement with the examiner in training administering the test while the experienced examiner simultaneously observes and independently scores the person, so that pure interrater reliability and agreement can be assessed. When measuring parameters such as range of motion, sensation, or strength, it is imperative that both examiners independently conduct the tests because the measurement error depends to a large extent on the examiner's skill and body mechanics in administering the test. In addition, direct observation of these parameters by each examiner is required. In these instances, interrater reliability and agreement are confounded by factors of time and variation in patient performance, as discussed above in the section on interrater reliability and agreement.

If examiners are aware that interrater reliability and agreement is being assessed, the situation is potentially reactive (60). Reactivity refers to the possibility that behavior may change if the examiners realize they are being monitored. Examiners demonstrate higher levels of reliability and agreement when they are aware that they are being observed. It is difficult, however, to conduct reliability and agreement assessments without examiner awareness; consequently, during a research study, it might be best to lead examiners to believe that all of their observations are being monitored throughout the investigation (60). It is important to note that levels of reliability and agreement attained when examiners are aware that they are being monitored are potentially inflated compared with examiner performance in a typical clinic setting where monitoring occurs infrequently.

DETECTING EXAMINER ERRORS

When training examiners in the use of rating scales, interrater reliability and agreement data should be examined to determine if there are any consistent trends indicative of examiner rating errors. These data should be obtained from testing patients who represent a broad-range sample of pertinent characteristics of the population, so that a relatively normal score distribution is expected. In many circumstances, a representative group of patients can be observed efficiently on videotape by multiple examiners. The distribution of examiners' scores across patients is then compared for error trends (52). If only one examiner is using a given rating scale, so that multiple examiners' scores cannot be compared for rating errors, rating errors still can be detected by examining the distribution of one examiner's ratings across multiple patients. Rasch analysis is another useful method for detecting examiner errors on specific items or as an overall trend. Rating errors can be classified into five categories:

1. Error of central tendency
2. Error of standards

3. Halo effect error
4. Logical error
5. Examiner drift error

An indication of an error of central tendency is when one rater's scores are clustered around the center of the scale and the other rater's scores are spread more evenly over the entire scale. Errors of standards occur when one rater awards either all low or all high scores, indicating that his standards are set either too high (i.e., error of severity) or too low (i.e., error of leniency), respectively. Leniency errors are the most common type of rating error (52). Halo effect errors can be detected if several experienced examiners rate a number of people under identical conditions and the score distributions are examined. There should be little variability between well-trained examiners' scores. If one examiner's scores fall outside of this limited range of variability, a halo rating error may have occurred as a result of preset examiner impressions or expectations. A logical error occurs when multiple traits are rated and an examiner awards similar ratings to traits that are not necessarily related.

A fifth type of rating error is examiner drift. Examiner drift refers to the tendency of examiners to alter the manner in which they apply rating criteria over time (60). Examiner drift is not easily detected. Interrater agreement may remain high even though examiners are deviating from the standardized rating criteria (59,60). This occurs when examiners who work together discuss rating criteria to clarify rating definitions. They may inadvertently alter the criteria, diminishing rating accuracy, and yet high levels of interrater agreement are maintained. If examiners alter rating criteria over time, data obtained from serial examinations may not be comparable. Examiner drift can be detected by assessing interrater agreement between examiners who have not worked together, or by comparing ratings from examiners who have been conducting assessments for an extended period of time with scores obtained from a newly trained examiner (60). Presumably, recently trained examiners adhere more closely to the original criteria than examiners who have had the opportunity to drift. Comparing videotaped samples of patient performance from selected evaluation sessions with actual examiner ratings obtained over time is another method of detecting examiner drift.

REDUCING EXAMINER ERRORS

Examiner ratings can be improved in several ways (52,59,60). Operational definitions of the behavior or trait must be clearly stated, and examiners must understand the rating criteria. If examiners periodically review rating criteria, receive feedback on their adherence to the test protocol through procedural reliability checks, and are informed of the accuracy of their observations through interrater agreement checks, examiner drift can be minimized. Examiners should be aware of common rating errors and how these errors may influence their scoring. Adequate time needs to be provided to observe and rate behaviors. If the observation period is too brief for the number of behaviors or people to be observed, rating accuracy is adversely affected. The reliability of ratings also can be improved by averaging ratings from multiple observers because the effects of individual rater biases tend to be balanced. Averaging multiple scores obtained from one rater is not advantageous for reducing rating error, however, because a given rater's errors tend to be relatively constant.

The complexity of observations negatively affects interrater reliability and agreement because observers may have difficulty discriminating between rating criteria (60). With more complex observations, examiners need to attain higher levels of agreement for each behavior during the training phase.

These high levels of interrater agreement need to be achieved under the exact conditions that will be used for data collection (60). If multiple behaviors are observed on several patients, it is best to rate all patients on one behavior before rating the next behavior. This practice facilitates more consistent application of operational definitions and rating criteria for the individual behavior. It also tends to reduce the incidence of logical errors.

Another method for improving scoring is to make raters aware of examiner idiosyncrasies or expectations that can affect ratings. According to Verducci (52), there are five patient-rater characteristics that may affect scoring:

1. If an examiner knows the person being evaluated, ratings can be either positively or negatively influenced. The longer the prior relationship has existed, the more likely the ratings will be influenced.
2. The rater tends to rate more leniently if the rater is required to disclose ratings directly to the person, or if the person confronts the examiner about the ratings.
3. Examiner gender also can influence ratings. In general, male examiners tend to rate more leniently than female examiners.
4. There is a tendency to rate members of one's sex higher than those of the opposite sex.
5. Knowledge of previous ratings may bias examiners to rate similarly. Consequently, examiners should remain blind to previous scores until current ratings have been assigned.

Other potential sources of rater bias are the examiner's expectations about the patient's outcome and feedback received regarding ratings (59,60). If examiners expect improvement, their ratings are more likely to show improvement. This is especially true when examiners are reinforced for patient improvement. In a research setting, examiner bias can be minimized if the observers remain blind to the purposes and hypotheses of the study. In a clinical setting, the baseline, intervention, and follow-up sessions often can be videotaped. Blind, independent observers can then rate the behaviors when shown the videotaped sessions in a random order.

Test Administration Strategies

Consistency in test administration is essential to permit comparison of test results from one session to another or between people. Multiple factors that might influence performance must be held constant during testing. These factors include test materials and instrumentation, the testing environment, test procedures and scoring, state of the person being assessed, observers present in the room, and time of day. Examiners must be aware of the potential influence of these factors and document any conditions that might affect test performance. Examiners ideally should remain blind to previous test results until after conducting the evaluation to avoid potential bias.

If more than one method is acceptable for testing, it is important to document which protocol is used so that the same method can be used during future evaluations. If it is necessary to alter the method of measurement as a result of a change in status or the development of an improved measurement technique, measurements should be taken using both the new and old methods so there is overlap of at least one evaluation. This overlap permits comparison with previous and future test results so that trends over time can be monitored.

Multiple trials should be administered when assessing traits, such as muscle strength, which require consistent efforts on the part of the patient. An average score of multiple trials is more stable over time than a single effort (97). A measure of central tendency and the range of scores both should be reported.

Standardized test positions always should be used unless a medical condition prevents proper positioning (e.g., joint contractures). In this event, the patient should be positioned as closely as possible to the standardized position, and the altered position should be documented. It is important to make sure that patients are posturally secure and comfortable during the evaluation. For patients with neurologic involvement, the head should be positioned in neutral to avoid subtle influences of tonic neck reflexes. An exception occurs when testing is conducted in the prone position. In this case, the head should be turned consistently toward the side being tested.

A key to obtaining reliable and valid test results is providing clear directions and demonstrations to the patient. Standardized instructions always must be provided verbatim and may not be modified or repeated unless specifically permitted in the test manual. Verbal directions often are enhanced by tactile, kinesthetic, and visual cues, if permitted. If confusion about the task is detected, this should be documented. If the examiner believes that a given patient could complete a task successfully with further instructions that are not specified in the standardized protocol, this item can be readministered at the end of the test session. The person's test score should be based solely on performance exhibited when given standardized instructions. Test performance with augmented instructions can be documented in the clinical note but should not be considered when scoring.

When conducting tests that do not have standardized instructions (e.g., strength testing), it is important to use short, simple, consistent commands. If repetitive or sustained efforts are required, the examiner's voice volume needs to be consistent and adequate to heighten the arousal state and motivate patients to give their best effort.

Verbal reinforcement and feedback regarding performance can influence performance levels (98). Consequently, it must be provided consistently, according to the procedures specified in the test manual. For tests in which reinforcement and feedback intervals are not specified and are permitted as needed, the frequency and type of feedback provided should be documented.

Test Scoring, Reporting, and Interpretation of Scores

Examiners should be thoroughly familiar with scoring criteria so that scores can be assigned accurately and efficiently during evaluation sessions. It is not appropriate for examiners to look up scoring criteria during or after the evaluation. Uncertainty about the criteria prolongs the evaluation and leads to scoring errors. It is helpful to include abbreviated scoring criteria on the test form to assist the examiner during the evaluation. Test forms should be well organized and clearly written to facilitate efficient and accurate recording of test results. If multiple types of equipment and test positions are required, it is useful if the equipment and position are identified on the score sheet using situation codes for each item. Such a coding system expedites test administration by assisting the examiner in grouping test items with similar positioning and equipment requirements. Examples of well-organized test forms that use situation codes are the Bayley Scales of Infant Development (99), the MAP (32), and the revised version of the Peabody Developmental Motor Scales test forms (40).

If the scoring criteria for a test are not well defined, it may be necessary for examiners within a given center or referral region to clarify the criteria. This was the case for many items on the Peabody Developmental Motor Scales. Interrater reliability levels of highly trained examiners were low for several items, so therapists at the Child Development and Mental Retardation Center in Seattle, Washington, clarified the scoring criteria to improve reliability. Examiners in the surrounding referral area were educated about the clarified criteria by means of in-services and videotapes to ensure that all examining centers in the area would be using identical criteria (40). If scoring criteria are augmented to improve reliability, it is imperative to document that the test was administered with altered criteria. Future results are comparable only if administered using identical scoring criteria. Additionally, if scores are compared with normative data, it is important to document that the test scores obtained may not be directly comparable because altered scoring criteria were used.

Raw scores obtained from testing are meaningless in the absence of additional interpretive data. To compare meaningfully a person's current test results to previous scores, the SEM of the test must be known. To determine how a person's performance compares with that of other people, normative data must come from a representative standardized sample of people with similar characteristics. In the latter case, the raw score must be converted into a derived or relative score to permit direct comparison with the normative group's performance. These concepts are discussed in detail below.

Raw scores may be compared with previous scores obtained from a given person to monitor changes in status. However, the SEM of the test must be known to determine if a change in a score is clinically significant. A change in a test score exceeding the SEM is indicative of a meaningful change in test performance. As was discussed earlier, in the section on reliability and agreement, it is best to report test scores as a range, based on confidence intervals, rather than as an absolute score. This is because a person's score is expected to vary as a result of random fluctuations in performance. It is only when a score changes beyond the range of random fluctuation that we can

be confident that a true change in performance has occurred. This true score range usually is based on the 95% confidence interval. This rigorous level of confidence minimizes the likelihood of a type I error (i.e., believing a change occurred when actually there was no change) and is considered the confidence level of choice when looking for improvement in performance, resulting from a specific treatment regimen or improved physical status. A lower level of confidence (e.g., 75%, 50%) may be desirable when monitoring the status of people who are at risk for loss of function over time. For these people, it is important to minimize the likelihood of a type II error (i.e., believing no change occurred when actually there was a change). In such cases, if a person's score falls outside a true score range that is based on a lower level of confidence, it may indicate the need to conduct further diagnostic tests or to monitor the person more closely over time.

If normative data are available for a given test, a person's score can be compared directly to the normative group performance by converting the score into a derived or relative score. Normative scores provide relative rather than absolute information (100). Normative data should not be considered as performance standards but rather as a reflection of how the normative group performed. Derived scores are expressed either as a developmental level or as a relative position within a specified group. Derived scores are calculated by transforming the raw score to another unit of measurement that enables comparison with normative values. Most norm-referenced tests provide conversion tables of derived scores that have been calculated for the raw scores so that hand calculations are not required. However, it is important for examiners to understand the derivation, interrelationship, and interpretation of derived scores. Specific calculation of these scores is beyond the scope of this chapter. For computational details and the practical application of these statistical techniques, the reader is referred to

TABLE 53-2. Descriptive and Standard Scores Commonly Reported in Rehabilitation Medicine

Summary Statistic	Definition and Interpretation
Descriptive Score	
Raw Scores	Expressed as number of correct items, time to complete a task, number of errors, or some other objective measure of performance
Percentage Scores	Raw scores expressed as percent correct
Percentile Scores	Expressed in terms of the percentage of people in the normative group who scored lower than the client's score (e.g., a client scoring in the 75th percentile on a norm-referenced test has performed better than 75% of the people in the normative group). Often stratified for age, gender, or other pertinent modifying varieties
Age-equivalent Score	Average score for a given age group
Grade-equivalent Score	Average score for a given grade level
Developmental Age	The basal age score, plus credit for all items earned at higher age levels (up to the ceiling level of the test). Also called motor age for tests of motor development. The basal age level is defined as the highest age at and below which all test items are passed.
Scaled Score	The client's total score, summed across all sections of the test. Used for comparison to previous and future scores.
Standard Scores	
Z Score	The client's raw score minus the mean score of normative group, divided by the standard deviation of the normative group. The mean of a z score is 0 with a standard deviation of 1. Scores may be plus or minus. Reported to two significant digits.
T Score	Z-score times 10 plus 50. The mean of a T score is 50 with a standard deviation of 10.
Stanine	Standard scores which range from 1 to 9. A stanine of 5 indicates average performance and the standard deviation is 2. Often used to minimize the likelihood of overinterpreting small differences between individual scores.
DMQ	The ratio of the client's actual score on the test (expressed as developmental age) and the client's chronologic age, DMQ = DA/CA. The DMQ equals the z score times 15, plus 100. The mean DMQ is 100, with a standard deviation of 15.
Deviation IQ	A standard score deviation of the ratio between the client's actual score on the test, expressed as a mental age and the client's chronological age. The mean deviation IQ is 100, with a standard deviation of 15, based on the Wechsler deviation IQ distribution.

CA, chronological age; DA, developmental age; DMQ, developmental motor quotient; IQ, intelligence quotient; MA, motor age.

textbooks on psychological or educational statistics and measurement theory (91,93,100).

Selection of the particular type of score to report depends on the purpose of testing, the sophistication of the people reading the reports, and the types of interpretations to be made from the results (100). Table 53-2 summarizes various descriptive and standard scores that are commonly used. Figure 53-2 shows the relationship of these scores to the normal distribution and the interrelationship of these scores. Calculation of standard scores (e.g., z scores, T scores, stanines, developmental motor quotients, deviation IQ) is appropriate only with interval or ratio data. They express where a person's performance is with regard to the mean of the normative group, in terms of the variability of the distribution. These standard scores are advantageous because they have uniform meaning from test to test. Consequently, a person's performance can be compared between different tests.

Written Evaluation

Thorough documentation of testing procedures and results is essential in both clinical and research settings to permit comparison of test results between and within individuals. The tests administered should be identified clearly. Any deviations from the standardized procedures, such as altered test positions or modified instructions, should be documented (14). If multiple procedural options are available for a given test item (e.g., measuring for a flexion contracture at the hip), the specific method used should be specified in the report. The patient's behavior, level of cooperation, alertness, attention, and motivation during the evaluation should be documented. Any potential effect of these factors on test performance should be stated. Other factors that might have influenced the validity of

test results also should be noted (e.g., environmental factors, illness, length of test session, activity level before the test session). It should be indicated whether optimal performance was elicited. If a person's performance is compared with normative data, the degree of similarity of the person's characteristics to those of the normative group should be stated. It is imperative to distinguish between facts and inferences in the written report.

The use of a standard written evaluation format facilitates communication between and within disciplines. In addition, computerized databases provide standardized formats useful for both clinical and research purposes. Serial examinations of a given person can be reviewed easily, and a patient's status can be compared directly with that of other people with similar characteristics. Clinical and research applications of computer data bases for documentation in rehabilitation medicine are discussed by Shurtleff (101) and Lehmann and associates (102).

OBJECTIVE MEASUREMENT WHEN A STANDARDIZED TEST IS NOT AVAILABLE

Rationale for Systematically Observing and Recording Behavior

Standardized tests and objective instrumentation are not always available to measure the parameters of clinical and research interest. Consequently, rehabilitation professionals often resort to documentation of subjective impressions (e.g., "head control is improved," "wheelchair transfers are more independent and efficient"). However, functional status and behaviors can be documented objectively by observing behavior using standardized techniques that have been demonstrated to be re-

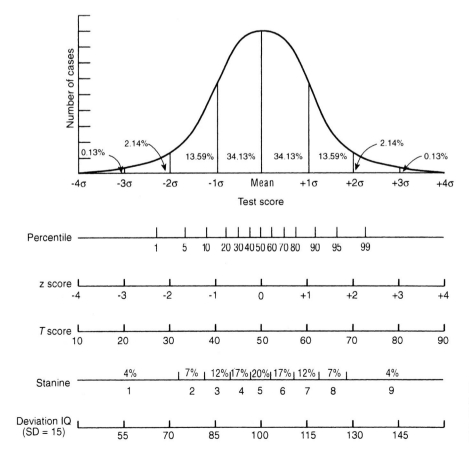

Figure 53-2. Relationships among standard scores, percentile ranks, and the normal distribution. (Adapted with permission from Anastasi A. *Psychological testing,* 6th ed. New York: Macmillan, 1988:97.)

liable. Systematically observing and recording behavior provides objective documentation of behavior frequency and duration, identifies the timing and conditions for occurrence of a particular behavior, and identifies small changes in behavior. Several of the procedures for objective documentation described below are based on the principles of single-case research designs. These research designs have been suggested to be the most appropriate method of documentation of treatment-induced clinical change in rehabilitation populations, owing to the wide variability in clinical presentation, even within a given diagnostic category (94,103). In addition, such designs have been recommended to evaluate and compare the effects of two different treatments on individual patients (104). Selected single-case research concepts that specifically pertain to objective documentation for either clinical or research purposes are presented in this chapter. The reader is referred to Hayes and colleagues (105), Barlow and Hersen (59), Bloom and colleagues (46), Kazdin (60), and Ottenbacher (94) for more thorough discussions of documentation using single-case research standardized testing techniques.

Procedures for Objective Observation and Recording of Behavior

STEP 1: IDENTIFY THE TARGET BEHAVIOR TO BE MONITORED

The target behavior must be identified by specifying the parameters of interest and their associated conditions. The prerequisite conditions required must be defined, such as verbal directions, visual or verbal cues, or physical assistance provided. In addition, environmental conditions must be described because different responses may be observed in the therapy, inpatient ward, or home setting. The duration, frequency, and timing of the observation period also must be specified. Ideally, these conditions should be constant from one observation period to the next for comparison purposes.

STEP 2: OPERATIONALLY DEFINE THE TARGET BEHAVIOR

An operational definition is stated in terms of the observable characteristics of the behavior that is being monitored. The definition must describe an observable or measurable action, activity, or movement that reflects the behavior of interest. The beginning and ending of the behavior must be clearly identified. Objective, distinct, and clearly stated terminology should be used (59,94). The definition should be elaborated to point out how the response differs from other responses. Examples of borderline or difficult responses, along with a rationale for inclusion and exclusion, should be provided. An example of an operational definition used to determine success or failure in drawing a circle is provided in Figure 53-3.

STEP 3: IDENTIFY THE MEASUREMENT STRATEGY

There are five methods of sampling behavior: event recording, rate recording, time sampling, duration recording, and discrete categorization (46,59,94). Each of these methods will be described below, along with indications and contraindications for their use.

Event Recording

The number of occurrences of the behavior is tallied in a given period of time, or per given velocity in the case of mobility activities. Indications for event recording include when the target response is discrete, with a definite beginning and end, or when the target response duration is constant. The target behavior frequency should be low to moderate, and the behavior duration should be short to moderate. It is best to augment the

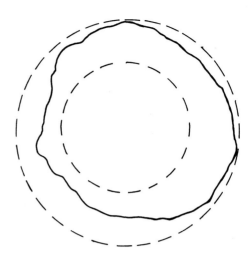

Figure 53-3. The operational definition of a circle (*dashed lines*, circle path template; *solid line*, patient's drawing of a circle). The patient is instructed to draw a circle inside the two dashed lines. An adequate circle is one in which the two ends meet, and the line of the circle stays within the circle path template. It can touch the edges of the template but cannot extend beyond the edges.

number of occurrences with real-time information to permit sequential, temporal, and reliability and agreement analyses. Contraindications for using event recording techniques include behaviors that have a high incidence of occurrence because of the increased probability of error in counting the high-frequency behavior and behaviors that have an extended duration or that occur infrequently (59,94) (e.g., wheelchair transfers). Duration recording should be used in the latter case. The following is an example of event recording:

A man with hemiplegia successfully fastened 5 of 10 shirt buttons during a 10-minute period of time using his involved hand to hold his shirt and his uninvolved hand to manipulate the buttons. The number of successes, number of trials, and duration of the observation period were recorded.

Rate Recording

The number of occurrences of the behavior is divided by the duration of the observation period (e.g., the number of occurrences per minute). This method is indicated when the observation period varies from session to session. Rate recording is advantageous because it reflects changes in either the duration or frequency of response and is sensitive for detecting changes or trends because there is no theoretical upper limit. The following is an example of rate recording.

A child with Down syndrome exhibits five occurrences of undesirable tongue thrusting during a 10-minute observation period the first day and eight times during a 20-minute observation period the second day. The observations were made from videotapes recorded immediately after the child's oral motor therapy program. An independent observer, who was blind to the child's intervention program, performed the frequency counts. The rate of responding was 0.5 behaviors per minute (five per 10 minutes) for the first day and 0.4 behaviors per minute (eight per 20 minutes) for the second day.

Time Sampling

This method involves recording the state of a behavior at specific moments or intervals in time. It also has been described in the literature as scan sampling, instantaneous time sampling, discontinuous probe time sampling, and interval sampling. Time sampling is analogous to taking a snapshot and then examining it to see if a particular behavior is occurring. This method often is used in industrial settings to determine exposure to risk factors or compliance with injury prevention techniques.

To monitor behavior using this method, the behavior of interest is observed for a short block of time (e.g., a 5-second observation period) at specified recording intervals (e.g., 5-minute intervals) during a particular activity (e.g., a 30-minute meal period). The recording interval is signaled to the observer by means of a timer, audiotape cue, or a tone generator. The target behavior is scored as either occurring or not occurring during the observation period of each recording period. Fixed (i.e., preset) or random intervals can be used, but it is important to avoid a situation in which the signal coincides with any regular cycle of behavior. The sampling should occur at various times throughout the day and in different settings to obtain a representative picture of the behavior frequency. The recording interval length depends on the behavior duration and frequency, as well as on the observer's ability to record and attend to the person. The more frequent the behavior, the shorter the interval. For low to medium response rates, 10-second intervals are recommended. For high response rates, shorter intervals should be used (106). An advantage of this type of recording is that several patients can be observed simultaneously by one rater in a group setting (e.g., during meal times or recreational events) by staggering the recording intervals for each patient.

Variations of time sampling include observing the behavior during a single block of time that is divided into short intervals (i.e., interval recording) or during brief intervals that are spread out over an entire day (i.e., time sampling); combining time sampling and event recording, when the number of responses occurring during a given interval are recorded; and combining time sampling and duration recording, when the duration of the response during a given interval is recorded. The following are examples of time sampling.

To document a patient's ability to maintain his head in an upright position, the nursing staff observed him for 15 seconds at 5-minute intervals during one 30-minute meal period, during one 30-minute self-care/dressing period, and during one 30-minute recreation period.

To estimate compliance of 12 industrial workers with suggestions provided in a back school program, the time individual workers spent in appropriate versus inappropriate postures was recorded for 5 minutes each hour during an 8-hour shift.

Duration Recording

Either the duration of the response or the length of the latency period is recorded. The duration is reported as the total time if the observation period is constant, or as the percentage of time that a behavior occurred during observation periods of varying length. Indications for this method include continuous target responses, behaviors with high or even response rates, and behaviors with varying durations, such as a wheelchair transfer, for which a frequency count would be less meaningful. The behavior duration is timed with a stopwatch, electromechanical event recorder, or electronic keyboard. Variations of duration recording include timing the response latency (i.e., the time that elapses between a cue and a response); measuring the time required to complete a particular task; or monitoring the time spent performing a particular activity. The following are examples of duration recording:

- The amount of time that it takes an adult with a spinal cord injury to dress in the morning
- The length of time that a child is able to stand independently with and without orthotics before losing his or her balance.

Discrete Categorization

With this method of behavior measurement, several different behaviors of interest are listed and checked off as being performed or not performed. This method is useful in determining whether certain behaviors have occurred. It is indicated when behavioral responses can be classified into discrete categories (e.g., correct/incorrect, performed/not performed). An example of this method is a checklist of the different steps for performing a wheelchair transfer, such as positioning the wheelchair, locking the brakes, removing feet from footrests, and so forth. The observer checks off whether each of these steps was performed during a given transfer.

STEP 4: ESTABLISH INTERRATER RELIABILITY

There are four reasons for assessing interrater (i.e., interobserver) reliability and agreement.

1. To establish how consistently two observers can measure a given behavior.
2. To minimize individual observer bias by establishing interrater reliability and then retraining observers if the level of reliability is unacceptable.
3. To reduce the chances of an examiner altering or "drifting" from the standard method of rating by implementing periodic interrater reliability or agreement checks to ensure that observers are consistent over time.
4. To examine the adequacy of operational definitions, rating criteria, and scoring procedures. Items that have poor agreement should be revised.

Before the onset of data collection, two people should independently observe and score pilot subjects who have characteristics that are similar to those of the clinical or study population. Behaviors of interest are rated according to predetermined operational definitions. Interrater reliability and agreement are then calculated using an appropriate statistic (see section on reliability and agreement). The minimum acceptable level of agreement depends on the type of statistic calculated (see Table 53-1).

If interrater reliability or agreement is below the target level, improvement may occur by discussing operational definitions of the behaviors. If problems with reliability or agreement continue, it may be necessary to redefine behaviors, improve observation and recording conditions, reduce the number of behaviors being recorded, provide additional training, and, if necessary, further standardize the data collection environment (64,84). Interrater reliability or agreement should be reestablished once remedial steps have been taken. As stated previously, periodic checks of interrater reliability or agreement should be conducted in the clinic and at least once during each phase of a research study (64,65). Reliability and agreement data should be plotted along with clinical or research data to show the level of consistency in measurements.

STEP 5: REPORT SCORES AND GRAPH DATA

Baseline, intervention, and follow-up data should be plotted on a graph or chart to provide a pictorial presentation of the results. Graphing strategies include using standard graph paper or a standard behavior chart (i.e., six-cycle graph paper). Advantages of the latter are that it permits systematic, standardized recording using a semilog scale that allows estimation of linear trends. Extremely high and low rates can be recorded on the chart. Behavior rates that range from once per 24 hours to 1,000 per minute can be accommodated; therefore, data are not lost as a result of floor or ceiling effects. In addition, continuous recording of data for up to 20 weeks is permitted. For further information on graphing strategies, the reader is referred to

White and Haring (107) and Carr and Williams (108) for use of the standard behavior chart in clinical settings.

The time period of data collection is plotted on the horizontal axis (e.g., hours, days, weeks) and changes in the target behavior on the vertical axis. Appropriate scaling should be used to accommodate the highest expected response frequency and the longest anticipated documentation period duration. The measurement interval on both axes should be large enough to permit visual detection of any changes in behavior. Interrater reliability data from each phase should be plotted on the same graph, along with the study results, as discussed previously.

Considerations When Reporting Scores

The percentage of correct scores often is reported because of the ease of calculation and interpretation. However, usefulness of this summary statistic is limited because it does not provide information on the number of times a patient has performed correctly (94). Consequently, it can be misleading if the total number of opportunities varies from day to day. For example, three successes of six trials on day 1 versus three successes out of four trials on day 2 would yield percentages of 50% and 75%, respectively. Based on percentage scores, it would appear that the patient's performance was improved, and yet the absolute number of successes has not changed. Additionally, if an odd number of trials is administered on some days and an even number of trials on other days, performance changes may occur based on percentage scores simply because it is not possible to receive half-credit for a trial on days when an odd number of trials are given (e.g., five successes out of 10 trials versus three successes out of five trials).

SUMMARY

Rehabilitation practitioners and researchers in rehabilitation medicine increasingly are using objective tests and measurements as a scientific basis for communication, to establish credibility with other professionals, and to document treatment effectiveness. The increased use of such measures has resulted in greater responsibility of the user for appropriate implementation and interpretation of tests and measures. Rehabilitation professionals must be familiar with the principles of objective measurement to use the tools properly.

The initial section of this chapter described the psychometric parameters used to evaluate the state of development and quality of available objective measures. The four basic levels of measurement—nominal, ordinal, interval, and ratio scales—were defined. The purposes for testing were discussed, including screening tests, in-depth assessment tests, and criterion-referenced tests. Several issues of practicality for selection and use of tests also were identified. The various forms of reliability, agreement, and validity described are of great importance for using the various measurements effectively. A test that does not provide reproducible results, or does not measure what it is purported to measure, is of no value and is potentially harmful by giving a false implication of meaningfulness. Consequently, caution in the use and interpretation of test results must be exercised when information on reliability or validity of a measure is not available or if their values are below accepted levels.

The second section of this chapter discussed the principles of evaluation, testing, and interpretation that help to ensure that adequate reliability and validity are obtained from test administration. The issues of standardization, interrater reliability, and procedural reliability are of particular importance. Care must be taken during test administration to control for the potential rater errors of central tendency, standards, halo effect, logical errors, and examiner drift.

For many applications in rehabilitation medicine practice and research, standardized measures have not yet been developed. Methods derived from single-subject research paradigms provide guidelines for objective measurement when a standardized test is not available. These guidelines, which are discussed in the third section of this chapter, include identifying the behavior to be monitored; operationally defining the behavior; identifying the measurement strategy (e.g., event recording, rate recording, time sampling); establishing interrater reliability; and properly reporting scores and graphing the data.

Specific tests and objective measurement instruments are not discussed because of the number and broad spectrum of measures used by rehabilitation professionals. Rather, a detailed table of references (see Appendix A) describing measures is provided, categorizing measures by the domains assessed.

The principles discussed in this chapter provide the framework for the readers critically to assess the measures available for their specific application needs. Such critical analysis will further emphasize the need for ongoing development and improvement of objective measures at the disposal of rehabilitation professionals.

REFERENCES

1. Frese E, Brown M, Norton BJ. Clinical reliability of manual muscle testing: middle trapezius and gluteus medius muscles. *Phys Ther* 1987;67:1072–1076.
2. Harris SR, Smith LH, Krukowski L. Goniometric reliability for a child with spastic quadriplegia. *J Pediatr Orthop* 1985;5:348–351.
3. Hinderer KA, Hinderer SR. Muscle strength development and assessment in children and adolescents. In: Harms-Ringdahl K, ed. *Muscle strength series: international perspectives in physical therapy: muscle strength.* Edinburgh: Churchill-Livingstone, 1993.
4. Hinderer SR, Nanna M, Dijkers MP. The reliability and correlations of clinical and research measures of spasticity [Abstract]. *J Spinal Cord Med* 1996;19:138.
5. Iddings DM, Smith LK, Spencer WA. Muscle testing, part 2: reliability in clinical use. *Phys Ther Rev* 1961;41:249–256.
6. Lilienfeld AM, Jacobs M, Willis M. A study of the reproducibility of muscle testing and certain other aspects of muscle scoring. *Phys Ther Rev* 1954;34: 279–289.
7. Sackett DL. *Clinical epidemiology: a basic science for clinical medicine.* Boston: Little, Brown, 1991.
8. Bartlett MD, Wolf LS, Shurtleff DB, Staheli LT. Hip flexion contractures: a comparison of measurement methods. *Arch Phys Med Rehabil* 1985;66:620–625.
9. Hinderer KA, Gutierrez T. Myometry measurements of children using isometric and eccentric methods of muscle testing [Abstract]. *Phys Ther* 1988; 68:817.
10. Hinderer KA, Hinderer SR. Stabilized vs. unstabilized myometry strength test positions: a reliability comparison [Abstract]. *Arch Phys Med Rehabil* 1990;71:771–772.
11. Hinderer KA, Hinderer SR, Deitz JL. *Reliability of manual muscle testing using the hand-held dynamometer and the myometer: a comparison study.* Paper presented at: American Physical Therapy Association Midwinter Sections Meeting; February 11, 1988; Washington, DC,.
12. Gowland C, King G, King S, et al. *Review of selected measures in neurodevelopmental rehabilitation: a rational approach for selecting clinical measures.* Research report no. 91–2. Hamilton, Ontario: McMaster University, Neurodevelopmental Clinical Research Unit, 1991.
13. Kirshner B, Guyatt G. A methodological framework for assessing health indices. *J Chronic Dis* 1985;38:27–36.
14. American Physical Therapy Association. Standards for tests and measurements in physical therapy practice. *Phys Ther* 1991;71:589–622.
15. Rothstein JM, Echternach JL. *Primer on measurement: an introductory guide to measurement issues.* Alexandria, VA: American Physical Therapy Association, 1993.
16. American Educational Association, American Psychological Association, National Council on Measurement in Education. *Standards for educational and psychological testing.* Washington, DC: American Psychological Association, 1985.
17. Johnston MV, Keith RA, Hinderer SR. Measurement standards for interdisciplinary medical rehabilitation. *Arch Phys Med Rehabil* 1992;73[suppl 12S]:S3–S23.
18. Rothstein JM. Measurement and clinical practice: theory and application. In: Rothstein JM, ed. *Measurement in physical therapy:clinics in physical therapy,* vol. 7. New York: Churchill-Livingstone, 1985:1–46.

19. Krebs DE. Measurement theory. *Phys Ther* 1987;67:1834–1839.
20. Hislop HJ, Montgomery J. *Daniels and Worthingham's muscle testing: techniques of manual examination,* 7th ed. Philadelphia: WB Saunders, 2002.
21. Janda V. *Muscle function testing.* Boston: Butterworths, 1983.
22. Cutter NC, Kevorkian CG. *Handbook of Manual Muscle Testing.* New York: McGraw-Hill, 1999.
23. Clarkson HM. *Musculoskeletal assessment,* 2nd ed. Philadelphia: Lippincott Williams & Wilkins, 2000.
24. Kendall FP, McCreary EK, Geise PG. *Muscles, testing and function,* 4th ed. Baltimore: Williams & Wilkins, 1993.
25. Granger CV, Gresham GE, eds. *Functional assessment in rehabilitation medicine.* Baltimore: Williams & Wilkins, 1984.
26. Merbitz C, Morris J, Grip JC. Ordinal scales and foundations of misinference. *Arch Phys Med Rehabil* 1989;70:308–312.
27. Wright BD, Linacre JM. Observations are always ordinal; measurements, however, must be interval. *Arch Phys Med Rehabil* 1989;70:857–860.
28. Deitz JC, Beeman C, Thorn DW. *Test of orientation for rehabilitation patients (TORP).* Tucson, AZ: Therapy Skill Builders, 1993.
29. Deitz JC, Tovar VS, Beeman C, et al. The test of orientation for rehabilitation patients: test-retest reliability. *Occup Ther J Res* 1992;12:172–185.
30. Deitz JC, Tovar VS, Thorn DW, Beeman C. The test of orientation for rehabilitation patients: interrater reliability. *Am J Occup Ther* 1990;44:784–790.
31. Thorn DW, Deitz JC. A content validity study of the Test of Orientation for Rehabilitation Patients. *Occup Ther J Res* 1990;10:27–40.
32. Miller LJ. *Miller assessment for preschoolers,* 2nd ed. San Antonio, TX: Psychological Corporation, 1999.
33. Peterson HA, Marquardt TP. *Appraisal and diagnosis of speech and language disorders,* 3rd ed. Englewood Cliffs, NJ: Prentice-Hall, 1994.
34. Anastasi A, Urbina S. *Psychological testing,* 7th ed. Upper Saddle, NJ: Prentice-Hall, 1997.
35. Gans BM, Haley SM, Hallenborg SC, et al. Description and inter-observer reliability of the Tufts Assessment of Motor Performance. *Am J Phys Med Rehabil* 1988;67:202–210.
36. Haley SM, Ludlow LH, Gans BM, et al. Tufts Assessment of Motor Performance: an empirical approach to identifying motor performance categories. *Am J Phys Med Rehabil* 1991;72:359–366.
37. Ludlow LH, Haley SM. Polytomous Rasch models for behavioral assessment: the Tufts Assessment of Motor Performance. In: Wilson M, ed. *Objective measurement: theory into practice,* vol. 1. Norwood, NJ: Ablex Publishing, 1992:121–137.
38. Haley SM, Ludlow LH. Applicability of the hierarchical scales of the Tufts Assessment of Motor Performance for school-aged children and adults with disabilities. *Phys Ther* 1992;72:191–206.
39. Ludlow LH, Haley SM, Gans BM. A hierarchical model of functional performance in rehabilitation medicine: the Tufts Assessment of Motor Performance. *Evaluation Health Prof* 1992;15:59–74.
40. Hinderer KA, Richardson PK, Atwater SW. Clinical implications of the Peabody Developmental Motor Scales: a constructive review. *Phys Occup Ther Pediatr* 1989;9:81–106.
41. Chaffin DB, Anderson GBJ, Martin BJ. *Occupational biomechanics,* 3rd ed. New York: Wiley-Interscience, 1999.
42. Granger CV, Kelly-Hayes M, Johnston M, et al. Quality and outcome measures for medical rehabilitation. In: Braddom RL, ed. *Physical medicine and rehabilitation,* 2nd ed. Philadelphia: WB Saunders, 2000.
43. Lawlis GF, Lu E. Judgment of counseling process: reliability, agreement, and error. *Phys Occup Ther Pediatr* 1989;9:81–106.
44. Tinsley HE, Weiss DJ. Interrater reliability and agreement of subjective judgments. *J Counsel Psychol* 1975;22:358–376.
45. Baumgartner TA, Jackson AS. *Measurement for evaluation in physical education and exercise science,* 7th ed. Boston: McGraw-Hill, 2003.
46. Bloom M, Fischer J, Orme JG. *Evaluating practice: guidelines for the accountable professional,* 4th ed. Boston: Allyn and Bacon, 2003.
47. Bartko JJ, Carpenter WT. On the methods and theory of reliability. *J Nerv Ment Dis* 1976;163:307–317.
48. Hartmann DP. Considerations in the choice of interobserver reliability estimates. *J Appl Behav Anal* 1977;10:103–116.
49. Hollenbeck AR. Problems of reliability in observational research. In: Sackett GP, ed. *Observing behavior: data collection and analysis methods,* vol. 2. Baltimore: University Park Press, 1978:79–98.
50. Liebetrau AM. *Measures of association. Sage University paper series on quantitative applications in the social sciences.* Series no. 07–032. Newbury Park, CA: Sage, 1983.
51. Safrit MJ. *Introduction to measurement in physical education and exercise science,* 2nd ed. St. Louis: Times Mirror/Mosby College Publishing, 1990.
52. Verducci FM. *Measurement concepts in physical education.* St. Louis: CV Mosby, 1980.
53. Deitz JC. Reliability. *Phys Occup Ther Pediatr* 1989;9:125–147.
54. Shrout PE, Fleiss JL. Intraclass correlations: uses in assessing rater reliability. *Psychol Bull* 1979;86:420–428.
55. Fleiss JL. Measuring agreement between two judges on the presence or absence of a trait. *Biometrics* 1975;31:651–659.
56. Fleiss JL, Cohen J. The equivalence of weighted kappa and the intraclass correlation coefficient as measures of reliability. *Educ Psychol Measure* 1973;33:613–619.
57. Fleiss JL, Harvey B, Park MC. The measurement of interrater agreement. In: Fleiss JL, ed. *Statistical methods for rates and proportions,* 3rd ed. Chichester: Wiley, 2002.
58. Krippendorff K. Bivariate agreement coefficients for reliability of data. In: Borgatta EF, ed. *Sociological methodology.* San Francisco: Jossey-Bass, 1970: 139–150.
59. Barlow DH, Hersen M. *Single case experimental designs:strategies for studying behavior change,* 2nd ed. New York: Pergamon, 1984.
60. Kazdin AE. *Single-case research designs.* New York: Oxford University Press, 1982.
61. Harris FC, Lahey BB. A method for combining occurrence and nonoccurrence interobserver agreement scores. *J Appl Behav Anal* 1978;11:523–527.
62. Haley SM, Osberg JS. Kappa coefficient calculation using multiple ratings per subject: a special communication. *Phys Ther* 1989;69:90–94.
63. Plewis I, Bax M. The uses and abuses of reliability measures in developmental medicine. *Dev Med Child Neurol* 1982;24:388–390.
64. Cicchetti DV, Aivano SL, Vitale J. Computer programs for assessing rater agreement and rater bias for qualitative data. *Educ Psychol Measure* 1977;37: 195–201.
65. Cohen J. A coefficient of agreement for nominal scales. *Educ Psychol Measure* 1960;20:37–46.
66. Landis JR, Koch GG. The measurement of observer agreement for categorical data. *Biometrics* 1977;33:159–174.
67. Hubert L. Kappa revisited. *Psychol Bull* 1977;84:289–297.
68. Cicchetti DV, Lee C, Fontana AF, Dowds BN. A computer program for assessing specific category rater agreement and rater bias for qualitative data. *Educ Psychol Measure* 1978;38:805–813.
69. Cohen J. Weighted kappa: nominal scale agreement with provision for scaled disagreement or partial credit. *Psychol Bull* 1968;70:213–220.
70. Fleiss JL. Measuring nominal scale agreement among many raters. *Psychol Bull* 1971;76:378–382.
71. Light RJ. Measures of response agreement for qualitative data: some generalizations and alternatives. *Psychol Bull* 1971;76:365–377.
72. Wackerly DD, McClave JT, Rao PV. Measuring nominal scale agreement between a judge and a known standard. *Psychometrika* 1978;43:213–223.
73. Williams GW. Comparing the joint agreement of several raters with another rater. *Biometrics* 1976;32:619–627.
74. Fleiss JL. *The design and analysis of clinical experiments.* New York: John Wiley & Sons, 1986:1–32.
75. Cronbach LJ. *Essentials of psychological testing,* 5th ed. New York: Harper & Row, 1990.
76. Krebs DE. Computer communication. *Phys Ther* 1984;64:1581–1589.
77. Brennan RL. *Elements of generalizability theory.* Iowa City, IA: ACT Publications, 1983.
78. Cronbach LJ, Gleser GC, Nanda H, Rajaratnam N. *The dependability of behavioral measurements.* New York: Wiley, 1972.
79. Lahey MA, Downey RG, Saal FE. Intraclass correlations: there's more there than meets the eye. *Psychol Bull* 1983;93:586–595.
80. Fleiss JL. Estimating the accuracy of dichotomous judgments. *Psychometrika* 1965;30:469–479.
81. Dunn WW. Validity. *Phys Occup Ther Pediatr* 1989;9:149–168.
82. Thorn DW, Deitz JC. Examining content validity through the use of content experts. *Occup Ther J Res* 1989;9:334–346.
83. Wilson M, Engelhard G, Draney K, eds. *Objective measurement: theory into practice.* Norwood, NJ: Ablex, 1992.
84. Wright BD, Masters GN. *Rating scale analysis.* Chicago: Mesa Press, 1982.
85. Wright BD, Stone MH. *Best test design: Rasch measurement.* Chicago: Mesa Press, 1979.
86. Francis DJ. An introduction to structural equation models. *J Clin Exp Neuropsychol* 1988;10:623–639.
87. Long JS. Confirmatory factor analysis. *Sage University paper series on quantitative application in the social sciences.* Series no. 07–033. Newbury Park, CA: Sage Publications, 1983.
88. Bond TG, Fox CM. *Applying the Rasch model: fundamental measurement in the human sciences.* Mahwah, NJ: Lawrence Erlbaum Associates, 2001.
89. Law M. Measurement in occupational therapy: scientific criteria for evaluation. *Can J Occup Ther* 1987;54:133–138.
90. Ottenbacher KJ, Tomchek SD. Measurement variation in method comparison studies: an empirical examination. *Arch Phys Med Rehabil* 1994;75:505–512.
91. Gyurke J, Prifitera A. Standardizing an assessment. *Phys Occup Ther Pediatr* 1989;9:63–90.
92. Cleary TA, Linn RL, Walster GW. Effect of reliability and validity on power of statistical tests. In: Borgatta EF, ed. *Sociological methodology.* San Francisco: Jossey-Bass, 1970:130–138.
93. Miller LJ, ed. Developing norm-referenced standardized tests. *Phys Occup Ther Pediatr* 1989;9:1–205.
94. Ottenbacher KJ. *Evaluating clinical change: strategies for occupational and physical therapists.* Baltimore: Williams & Wilkins, 1986.
95. Paul GL, Lentz RJ. *Psychosocial treatment of chronic mental patients: milieu versus social-learning programs.* Cambridge, MA: Harvard University Press, 1977.
96. Billingsley F, White OR, Munson R. Procedural reliability: a rationale and an example. *Behav Assess* 1980;2:229–241.
97. Hinderer KA. Reliability of the myometer in muscle testing children and adolescents with myelodysplasia. Unpublished master's thesis, University of Washington, Seattle, WA, 1988.
98. Schmidt RA. Feedback and knowledge of results. In: Schmidt RA. Lee TD, eds. *Motor control and learning,* 3rd ed. Champaign, IL: Human Kinetics Publishers, 1999.

99. Bayley N. *The Bayley scales of infant development,* 2nd ed. New York: Psychological Corporation, 1993.

100. Cermak S. Norms and scores. *Phys Occup Ther Pediatr* 1989;9:91–123.

101. Shurtleff DB. Computer data bases for pediatric disability: clinical and research applications. *Phys Med Rehabil Clin N Am* 1991;2:665–687.

102. Lehmann JF, Warren CG, Smith W, Larson J. Computerized data management as an aid to clinical decision making in rehabilitation medicine. *Arch Phys Med Rehabil* 1984;65:260–262.

103. Martin JE, Epstein L. Evaluating treatment of effectiveness in cerebral palsy. *Phys Ther* 1976;56:285–294.

104. Guyatt G, Sackett D, Taylor W, et al. Determining optimal therapy. *N Engl J Med* 1986;314:889–892.

105. Hayes SC, Barlow DH, Nelson-Gray RO. *The scientist practitioner: research and accountability in the age of managed care,* 2nd ed. Boston: Allyn & Bacon, 1999.

106. Repp AC, Roberts DM, Slack DJ, et al. A comparison of frequency, interval, and time-sample methods of data collection. *J Appl Behav Anal* 1976;9:501–508.

107. White OR, Haring NG. *Exceptional teaching: a multimedia training package.* Columbus, OH: Charles E Merrill, 1976.

108. Carr BS, Williams M. Analysis of therapeutic techniques through the use of the Standard Behavior Chart. *Phys Ther* 1982;62:177–183.

109. Hughes CJ, Weimar WH, Sheth PN, Brubaker CE. Biomechanics of wheelchair propulsion as a function of seat position and user-to-chair interface. *Arch Phys Med Rehabil* 1992;73:263–269.

110. Fife SE, Roxborough LA, Armstrong RW, et al. Development of a clinical measure of postural control for assessment of adaptive seating in children with neuromotor disabilities. *Phys Ther* 1991;71:981–993.

111. McClenaghan BA, Thombs L, Milner M. Effects of seat-surface inclination on postural stability and function of the upper extremities of children with cerebral palsy. *Dev Med Child Neurol* 1992;34:40–48.

112. Myhr U, von Wendt L. Improvement of functional sitting position for children with cerebral palsy. *Dev Med Child Neurol* 1991;33:246–256.

113. Deitz JC, Jaffe KM, Wolf LS, et al. Pediatric power wheelchairs: evaluation of function in the home and school environments. *Assist Technol* 1991;3:24–31.

114. Bader DL, ed. *Pressure sores: clinical practice and scientific approach.* London: Macmillan, 1990.

115. Webster JG, ed. *Prevention of pressure sores.* Bristol, England: Adam Hilger Publishers, 1991.

116. Harris GF. A method for the display of balance platform center of pressure data. *J Biomech* 1982;15:741–745.

117. Shumway-Cook A, Horak FB. Assessing the influence of sensory interaction on balance. *Phys Ther* 1986;66:1548–1554.

118. Nashner LM. Adapting reflexes controlling the human posture. *Exp Brain Res* 1976;26:59–72.

119. Winter DA. *Biomechanics and motor control of human movement,* 2nd ed. New York: Wiley, 1990.

120. Schmidt RA. Methodology for studying motor behavior. In: Schmidt RA, Lee TD, eds. *Motor control and learning,* 3rd ed. Champaign, IL: Human Kinetics Publishers, 1999.

121. Bernstein N, Wilberg RB, Woltring HJ. The techniques of the study of movement. In: Whiting HTA, ed. *Human motor actions: Bernstein reassessed.* Amsterdam: Elsevier, 1984:1–73.

122. University of Pittsburgh. *Health instruments file database.* Pittsburgh, PA: University of Pittsburgh, 1992.

123. Educational Testing Service. *Medical/health science bibliographies.* Princeton, NJ: Educational Testing Service, 1992.

124. Medical Device Register, Inc. *Medical device register: United States and Canada.* Montvale, NJ: Medical Economics Co., 1996–2001.

125. Institute for Scientific Information, Inc. *Science citation index.* Philadelphia: Institute for Scientific Information, Inc., 1945–present.

126. Siu AL, Reuben DB, Moore AA. Comprehensive geriatrics assessment. In: Hazard WR, ed. *Principles of geriatric medicine and gerontology,* 4th ed. New York: McGraw-Hill, 1999.

127. Dumitru D. *Electrodiagnostic medicine,* 2nd ed. Philadelphia: Hanley & Belfus, 2002.

128. Delisa JA, Lee HJ, Baran EM, et al. *Manual of nerve conduction velocity and clinical neurophysiology,* 3rd ed. New York: Raven, 1994.

129. Bruett BS, Overs RP. A critical review of 12 ADL scales. *Phys Ther* 1969;49:857–862.

130. Law M, Letts L. A critical review of scales of activities of daily living. *Am J Occup Ther* 1989;43:522–528.

131. Halpern AS, Fuhrer MJ, eds. *Functional assessment in rehabilitation.* Baltimore: Paul H Brookes, 1984.

132. Barer D, Nouri F. Measurement of activities of daily living. *Clin Rehabil* 1989;3:179–187.

133. Jebsen RH, Taylor N, Trieschmann RB, Trotter MH. Measurement of time in a standardized test of patient mobility. *Arch Phys Med Rehabil* 1970;51:170–175.

134. Shores M. Footprint analysis in gait documentation. *Phys Ther* 1980;60:1163–1167.

135. Lerner-Frankiel MB, Vargas S, Brown M, et al. Functional community ambulation: what are your criteria? *Clin Manage* 1986;6:12–15.

136. Perry J. *Gait analysis: normal and pathological function.* Thorofare, NJ: Slack, 1992.

137. Eastlack ME, Arvidson J, Synder-Mackler L, et al. Interrater reliability of videotaped observational gait-analysis assessments. *Phys Ther* 1991;71:465–472.

138. Krebs DE, Edelstein JE, Fishman S. Reliability of observational kinematic gait analysis. *Phys Ther* 1985;65:1027–1033.

139. Rose SA, Ounpuu S, DeLuca PA. Strategies for the assessment of pediatric gait in the clinical setting. *Phys Ther* 1991;71:961–980.

140. Winter DA. *The biomechanics and motor control of human gait,* 2nd ed. Waterloo, Ontario: University of Waterloo Press, 1991.

141. Rondinelli RD, Katz RT, eds. *Impairment rating and disability evaluation.* Philadelphia: WB Saunders, 2000.

142. Lister MJ, Currier DP. Clinical measurement. *Phys Ther* 1987;67:1829–1897.

143. Rothstein JM, ed. *Measurement in physical therapy.* New York: Churchill-Livingstone, 1985.

144. Johnston MV, Findley TW, DeLuca J, Katz RT. Research in physical medicine and rehabilitation. XII: measurement tools with application to brain injury. *Am J Phys Med Rehabil* 1991;70[Suppl]:114–130.

145. McDowell I, Newell C. *Measuring health: a guide to rating scales and questionnaires,* 2nd ed. New York: Oxford University Press, 1996.

146. Spilker B, ed. *Quality of life assessments in clinical trials.* New York: Raven, 1990.

147. Salek S, ed. *Compendium of quality of life instruments.* New York: John Wiley & Sons, 1998.

148. Tulsky DS, Rosenthal M, eds. Quality of life measurement: applications in health and rehabilitation populations, part I. *Arch Phys Med Rehabil* 2002;83[Suppl]:S1–S54.

149. Blake BS, Impara JC. *The fourteenth mental measurements yearbook.* Lincoln, NE: University of Nebraska, Buros Institute of Mental Measurements, 2001.

150. Amundsen LR, ed. *Muscle strength testing: instrumented and noninstrumented systems.* New York: Churchill-Livingstone, 1990.

151. Kellor M, Kondrasuk R, Iversen I, et al. *Technical manual: hand strength and dexterity tests.* Minneapolis, MN: Sister Kenny Institute, 1977.

152. Bohannon RW, Smith RB. Interrater reliability of a modified Ashworth scale of muscle spasticity. *Phys Ther* 1987;67:206.

153. Lee KC, Carson L, Kinnin E. The Ashworth scale: a reliable and reproducible method of measuring spasticity. *J Neurol Rehabil* 1989;3:205.

154. Meythaler JM, Guin-Refroe S, Grabb P. Long-term continuous infused intrathecal baclofen for spastic-dystonic hypertonia in traumatic brain injury: 1-year experience. *Arch Phys Med Rehabil* 1999;80:13.

155. Frollo I, Kneppo P, Krizik M, Rosik V. Microprocessor-based instrument for Achilles tendon reflex measurements. *Med Biol Eng Comput* 1981;19:695–700.

156. Lehmann JF, Price R, de Lateur BJ, et al. Spasticity: quantitative measurements as a basis for assessing effectiveness of therapeutic intervention. *Arch Phys Med Rehabil* 1989;70:6–15.

157. Katz RT, Rymer WZ. Spastic hypertonia: mechanisms and measurement. *Arch Phys Med Rehabil* 1989;70:144–155.

158. Rodgers SH. *Ergonomic design for people at work,* vols. 1 and 2. Rochester, NY: Eastman Kodak, 1983, 1986.

159. Asher IE. *An annotated index of occupational therapy evaluation tools.* Rockville, MD: American Occupational Therapy Association, Inc., 1989.

160. Wittmeyer M, Barrett JE. *Housing accessibility checklist.* Seattle: University of Washington, Health Sciences Learning Resources Center, 1980.

161. Hemphill BJ, ed. *Mental health assessment in occupational therapy.* Thorofare, NJ: Black Publishers, 1988.

162. Crepeau EB, Cohn ES, Willard AS, Scheil BAB. *Willard and Spackman's occupational therapy,* 10th ed. Baltimore: Lippincott, 2003.

163. Haley SM, Coster WJ, Ludlow LH. Pediatric functional outcome measures. *Phys Med Rehabil Clin N Am* 1991;2:689–723.

164. Gledhill N. Discussion: assessment of fitness. In: Bouchard C, Shephard RJ, Stephens T, et al., eds. *Exercise, fitness, and health.* Champaign, IL: Human Kinetics Books, 1990:121–126.

165. Skinner JS, Baldini FD, Gardner AW. Assessment of fitness. In: Bouchard C, Shephard RJ, Stephens T, et al, eds. *Exercise, fitness, and health.* Champaign, IL: Human Kinetics Books, 1990:109–119.

166. Edwards RHT. Human muscle function and fatigue. In: *Ciba Foundation symposium 82 on human muscle fatigue: physiological mechanisms.* London: Pitman Medical, 1981:1–18.

167. Hashimoto K, Kogi K, Grandjean E. *Methodology in human fatigue assessment.* London: Taylor & Francis, 1971.

168. Minor MAD, Minor SD. Patient evaluation methods for the health professional. Reston, VA: Reston, 1985.

169. Comrey AL, Backer TE, Glaser EM. *A sourcebook for mental health measures.* Los Angeles: Human Interaction Research Institute, 1973.

170. Lezak MD. *Neuropsychological assessment,* 3rd ed. New York: Oxford University Press, 1995.

171. Bellack AS, Hersen M. *Behavioral assessment: a practical handbook,* 4th ed. Boston: Allyn and Bacon, 1998.

172. Nicol AC. Measurement of joint motion. *Clin Rehabil* 1989;3:1–9.

173. Norkin CC, White DJ. *Measurement of joint motion: a guide to goniometry,* 2nd ed. Philadelphia: FA Davis, 1995.

174. Batti MC, Bigos SJ, Fisher LD, et al. The role of spinal flexibility in back pain complaints within industry. *Spine* 1990;15:768–773.

175. Burton, AK. Regional lumbar sagittal mobility: measurement by flexicurves. *Clin Biomech* 1986;1:20–26.

176. Domjan L, Nemes T, Balint GP, et al. A simple method for measuring lateral flexion of the dorsolumbar spine. *J Rheumatol* 1990;17:663–665.

177. Hart DL, Rose SJ. Reliability of a noninvasive method for measuring the lumbar curve. *J Orthop Sports Phys Ther* 1986;8:180–184.

178. Lovell FW, Rothstein JM, Personius WJ. Reliability of clinical measurements of lumbar lordosis taken with a flexible rule. *Phys Ther* 1989;69:96–105.

179. Mellin GP. Physical therapy for chronic low back pain: correlations between spinal mobility and treatment outcome. *Scand J Rehabil Med* 1985;17:163–166.
180. Mellin GP. Accuracy of measuring lateral flexion of the spine with a tape. *Clin Biomech* 1986;1:85–89.
181. Merrit JL, McLean TJ, Erickson RP, Ojford KP. Measurement of trunk flexibility in normal subjects: reproducibility of three clinical methods. *Mayo Clin Proc* 1986;61:192–197.
182. Rose MJ. The statistical analysis of the intra-observer repeatability of four clinical measurement techniques. *Physiotherapy* 1991;77:89–91.
183. Frattali CM, ed. *Measuring outcomes in speech-language pathology.* New York: Thieme, 1998.
184. Johnson AF, Jacobsen BH, eds. *Medical speech-language pathology: a practitioner's guide.* New York: Thieme, 1998.

APPENDIX A: MEASUREMENT SCALES AND TEST METHODS USED IN PHYSICAL MEDICINE AND REHABILITATION: CRITIQUES AND REFERENCES

Adaptive Equipment Assessments for Positioning and Function

- Biomechanics of wheelchair propulsion as a function of seat position and user-to-chair interface (109). Describes an experimental protocol for determining three-dimensional wheelchair propulsion kinematics with varied hand placements (push-levers versus hand rims) and seat positions
- Development of a clinical measure of postural control for assessment of adaptive seating in children with neuromotor disabilities (110). Reviews the literature on seating assessment, including measures that require complex instrumentation and clinical evaluation scales. Describes the development of a clinical evaluation scale, the Seated Postural Control Measure (SPCM) for use with children requiring adaptive seating systems. The SPCM consists of postural alignment and functional movement items, scored on a four-point scale. A modified version of the Level of Sitting Ability Scale (LSAS) also is described. The LSAS is used to rate sitting ability based on the amount of support required to maintain sitting and the degree of sitting stability. Interrater and test-retest reliability data are reported for both scales.
- Effects of seat-surface inclination on postural stability and function of the upper extremities of children with cerebral palsy (111). Describes methods of evaluating optimal seating surface inclination through postural, center of pressure, and upper-extremity function data. Postural data were obtained by means of videotape analysis. Center of pressure data were acquired using a force platform. Upper-extremity performance was assessed through six motor control tasks.
- Improvement of functional sitting position for children with cerebral palsy (112). Describes a method of determining the most optimal functional sitting position by using videotapes and photographs. The Sitting Assessment Scale was used to rate head control, trunk control, foot control, arm function, and hand function. Interrater reliability of this scale is reported.
- Pediatric power wheelchairs: evaluation of function in the home and school environments (113). Describes a standardized functional task assessment for use in evaluating indoor function in a wheelchair, both at home and at school. The tasks assessed are classified into three categories: positioning, reaching, and driving.
- Pressure sores: clinical practice and scientific approach (114). Describes pressure distribution measurements, movement studies during sleep, and remote monitoring mechanical force measurements, wound-healing measurements, tissue-distortion measurements, and compressive loading regimens of wheelchair sitting behavior
- Prevention of pressure sores: engineering and clinical aspects (115). Describes skin blood flow measurement, seat cushion evaluation techniques, pressure measurement using bladder pressure sensors and conventional pressure sensors, interface pressure distribution visualization, and sheer measurement techniques.

Balance Measurement Techniques

- Method for the display of balance platform center of pressure data (116). Describes the measurement of center of pressure.
- Assessing the influence of sensory interaction on balance (117). Describes procedures for assessing balance under six conditions in the typical clinic setting. Three visual conditions (i.e., normal, blindfolded, visual-conflict dome) are tested with two surface inputs (i.e., normal, standing on foam). Suggestions of quantifying postural sway under each condition are provided.
- Adapting reflexes controlling the human posture (118). Describes a method of assessing balance using a displacement platform and a visual surround, which is used to assess the influence of various sensory conditions on balance.

Biomechanics and Motor Control Assessment Techniques

- Biomechanics and motor control of human movement (119). Describes measurement of kinematic data (e.g., by using goniometers, accelerometers, and imaging techniques); anthropometric data (e.g., density, mass, center of mass, moment of inertia, joint centers of rotation, muscle anthropometry); kinetic data (e.g., joint reaction forces, bone-on-bone forces, force transducers, force plate data, muscle force estimates); mechanical work, energy, and power measurements; muscle mechanics; and electromyography.
- Methodology for studying motor behavior (120). Describes methods of measuring movement kinematics, electromyography, movement errors, tracking, balance, coordination, reaction time, movement time, and motor skills.
- Techniques of the study of movement (121). Describes methods of studying movements, including cinematography, stroboscopic photography, cyclography, stereoscopic recording, determining masses and centers of gravity, electrogoniometry, ultrasound, optoelectronics, accelerometry, photogrammetry, rigid-body kinematics, derivative estimation, state-space modeling, force plates, body segment description, kinetic modeling, and data processing. Includes descriptions of historical techniques and compares these with contemporary methods.

Computerized Assessment Data Bases and Techniques

- Computer databases for pediatric disability: clinical and research applications (101). Reviews computer-based medical records and evaluation systems for individuals with disabilities. These systems have applications for clinical and research settings.
- Computerized data management as an aid to clinical decision making in rehabilitation (102). Describes a computerized database that has been developed for clinical decision making in rehabilitation. Multidisciplinary patient performance data can be stored and accessed by all team members.

Computerized Medical Instrument Databases and Citation Indexes

- Health instruments file database (122). A computerized database that contains information on instruments (e.g., questionnaires, interview protocols, observation checklists, index measure, rating scales, projective techniques, tests) in health, health-related, and behavioral sciences. Designed to identify measures needed for research studies, clinical assessments, and program evaluation. The database contains information on selected measurement instruments, instruments constructed for a particular study, and modifications of existing instruments.

- Medical/health science bibliographies (123). A computerized database of annotated test bibliographies. The database includes tests of personality, sensory-motor function, vocation/occupation, behavior, developmental scales, family interaction, environmental influences, manual dexterity, learning, social skills, and social perception and judgment.
- Medical device register: United States and Canada (124). Cross-references lists of medical instruments and devices.
- Science citation index (125). References that have cited specific instruments are indexed according to the specific name of the instrument.

Elderly Assessment Instruments

- Assessing the elderly (126). Reviews selected instruments for measuring physical health, physical functioning, activities of daily living, cognitive functioning, affective functioning, general mental health, social interactions and resources, person-environment compatability, and multidimensional measure.

Electrodiagnostic Assessment Techniques

- Electrodiagnostic evaluation of the peripheral nervous system (127). Describes electrodiagnostic procedures, including sensory nerve conduction studies, motor nerve conduction studies, single-fiber electromyography, needle electrode examination, and findings for specific diagnostic categories.
- Manual of nerve conduction velocity and somatosensory evoked potentials (128). Describes techniques and normal value ranges for nerve conduction studies and somatosensory evoked potentials.

Functional Assessment Instruments

- A critical review of 12 activities of daily living (129). Discusses parameters measured, type of scoring, scaling of scores, and the advantages and disadvantages of each scale.
- A critical review of scales of activities of daily living (130). Reviews scales of basic self-care according to standard criteria. The evaluation criteria include purpose, clinical utility, test construction, standardization, reliability, and validity. Specific recommendations are made regarding which activities of daily living scales are most suitable for describing, predicting, or evaluating activities of daily living function.
- Functional assessment in rehabilitation (131). Reviews functional assessments for people with physical disabilities, mental retardation, and psychiatric impairments, functional communication assessments, quantitative muscle function testing, upper-extremity functional capabilities, job-related social competence, learning potential for people with mental retardation, environmental influences on behavior, rehabilitation indicators, self-observation and report techniques, and vocational rehabilitation assessments.
- Functional assessment in rehabilitation medicine (25). Reviews functional assessment instruments used in outcome measurement, rehabilitation nursing, and in assessing the elderly, the arthritic patient, and people with mental retardation. Also reviews functional measurement of verbal impairments, assessments of support systems for the elderly, assessment of family functioning, and functional assessments used in primary care.
- Measurement of activities of daily living (132). Reviews the characteristics of several commonly used standardized activities of daily living assessments. The characteristics reviewed include number of test items, target population, parameters assessed, method of administration, and reliability.
- Measurement of time in a standardized test of patient mobility (133). Describes a standardized assessment for evaluating the efficiency of bed mobility, wheelchair activities, transfer activities, and ambulation. Normative values are provided for 20- to 69-year-old people.

Gait Assessment Techniques

- Footprint analysis in gait documentation (134). Provides instructions for obtaining footprint data in the typical clinic setting. Instructions for measuring velocity, cadence, foot progression angle, base of support, stride length, and step length are provided. Observations of toe drag and symmetry of pressure also are suggested.
- Functional community ambulation: what are your criteria (135). Criteria are provided for evaluating functional community ambulation. Distances required for independent community ambulation at the post office, bank, doctor's office, supermarket, department store, drugstore, and to cross intersections are provided. Typical curb heights and crosswalk times also are presented.
- Gait analysis: normal and pathological function (136). Discusses observational gait analysis, oxygen consumption measures, ground reaction force measurements, dynamic electromyography, and gait assessment using motion analysis systems. Normal and pathologic gait patterns are described. Applications of assessment techniques to specific patient populations are discussed.
- Interrater reliability of videotaped observational gait analysis assessments (137). Interrater reliability of 54 therapists observing videotapes of patients exhibiting abnormal gait was determined. The parameters assessed included knee flexion, genu valgum, cadence, step length, stride length, stance time, and step width. The therapists received no special training in preparation for this study, beyond their physical therapy education. The results indicate that observational gait analysis, in the absence of common rater training, has low to moderate interrater reliability.
- Reliability of observational kinematic gait analysis (138). Methods of observational analysis are discussed. Descriptions are provided of the procedures used to develop a reliable observational gait analysis format and the protocol used to train raters. Interrater and test-retest reliability data were obtained by having raters observe gait videotapes. The results indicate that observational kinematic gait analysis is a convenient but only moderately reliable technique.
- Strategies for the assessment of pediatric gait in the clinical setting (139). Describes observational and video gait analysis, measurement of time-distance parameters, electromyography, kinematics, kinetics, and energy expenditure. The pros and cons of each method are discussed, and instrumentation required is described. The use of gait analysis measurements for surgical and orthotic decision making also is presented.
- Biomechanics and motor control of human gait (140). Discusses gait terminology, temporal and stride measures, kinematics, kinetics, electromyography. Selected normal values are provided.

- Impairment rating and disability evaluation (141). Section two of this text provides assessment tools for rating musculoskeletal impairment and work disability; functional capacity evaluation; psychological, social, and behavioral assessment tools; and physician assessment of work capacity.

Multifactorial Rehabilitation Assessment References

- Clinical measurements (142). Reviews measures of isokinetic strength, clinical measures, functional disability, sensorimotor performance, range of motion, developmental parameters, infant movement, postural control and cardiopulmonary function.
- Measurement in physical therapy (143). Reviews measures of strength testing (e.g., manual muscle testing, instrumented muscle performance measures), joint motion, functional assessment, gait assessment, children with central nervous system dysfunction, pulmonary function testing, cardiovascular function, nerve conduction velocity, and electromyographic testing.
- Measurement tools with application to brain injury (144). Reviews measures of coma and global function, disability measures, communicative function, cognitive function, degree of handicap, general outcome measures, environmental measures, preinjury history, and sensory impairments.
- Measuring health: a guide to rating scales and questionnaires (145). Reviews measures of functional disability and handicap, activities of daily living, psychological well-being, social health, quality of life and life satisfaction, pain measurements, and general health measurements.
- Quality of life assessments in clinical trials (146). Reviews economic scales and tests, quality of life assessments, social interaction tests and scales, psychological tests and scales, and functional disability scales. Applications of these scales in rehabilitation and for specific patient populations are discussed.
- Compendium of quality of life instruments (147). Contains more than 150 questionnaires and translations covering a wide range of disorders. It is divided into four parts to ensure easy access to the required instruments: (a) general section containing nondisease specific quality of life measures; (b) disease- or disorder-specific questionnaires; (c) section devoted to caregivers, children, elderly, and women; and (d) economic specific quality of life indices.
- Quality of life measurement: applications in health and rehabilitation populations, part I (148). Special journal edition sponsored by the American Congress of Rehabilitation Medicine addressing an agenda for future QOL test development, SF-36, and other health-related QOL measures to assess persons with disabilities, measuring QOL in chronic illness, QOL issues in individuals with spinal cord injury, activity-related QOL in rehabilitation and traumatic brain injury, measuring health outcomes in stroke survivors, QOL outcomes perspective, and abstracts covering QOL issues.
- Fourteenth-Mental Measurements Yearbook (149, www.unl.edu/buros). Reviews standardized tests in the areas of achievement, aptitude, development, education, intelligence, neuropsychology, personality, sensory-motor, speech and hearing, and vocation. Bibliographies of references for specific tests, related to the construction, validity, or use of the tests in various settings, also are included. The tests are indexed by periodical, author, publisher, tests or book title, and tests classification. Reviews, descriptions, and references associated with older tests are contained in previous editions of the Yearbook.

Muscle Strength Assessment Techniques

- Manual muscle strength assessment methods (20–24). Describes standard tests positions and grading criteria for manual assessment of strength.
- Muscle strength development and assessment in children and adolescents (3). Reviews the literature pertaining to the reliability and validity of strength testing using manual muscle testing and objective techniques. Describes principles of strength testing with both traditional manual methods and objective myometry techniques. Suggestions for testing infants, children, and adolescents are provided.
- Muscle strength testing: instrument and noninstrumented systems (150). Discusses strength assessment techniques, including skeletal muscle strength testing with instrumented and noninstrumented systems, isometric testing with fixed-load cells, dynamic strength testing, trunk strength testing, and grip and pinch strength measurements.
- Technical manual: hand strength and dexterity tests (151). Describes tests of grip strength, pinch strength, and finger-hand coordination, and provides normative values.

Muscle Tone Assessment Techniques

- Clinical measures of spasticity: are they reliable? (4). Intertrial, interrater, and test-retest reliability results of clinical measures of spasticity, including clonus and tendon tap reflexes obtained on a group of people with traumatic spinal cord injuries are reported.
- Modified Ashworth Scale (152–154). Describes reliability testing results for the Modified Ashworth Scale in stroke, multiple sclerosis, and traumatic brain injury subjects .
- Microprocessor-based instrument for Achilles tendon reflex measurements (155). Describes quantification of reflex responses by means of tendon tapping with measured forces.
- Spasticity: quantitative measurements as a basis for assessing effectiveness of therapeutic intervention (156). Detailed description of a method for measuring mechanical output from spastic reflex muscle response to sinusoidal ankle motion at varying frequencies of oscillation and confirming spastic muscle response with surface electromyographic monitoring.
- Spastic hypertonia: mechanisms and measurement (157). Describes a device with a servo-controlled motor that applies ramp and hold movements to the elbow. Surface electromyographic activity of the biceps, brachioradialis, and lateral triceps muscles are measured in response to the stretch stimulus.

Occupational Biomechanics, Ergonomics, and Work Capacity Evaluation Techniques

- Ergonomic design for people at work (158). Volume 1 discusses design issues for the workplace, equipment, hand tools, and the environment. Volume 2 describes evaluation of job demands, lifting, manual materials handling by means of surveys, timed activity analysis, biomechanical analysis, energy expenditure measurements, and motion analysis techniques.
- Occupational biomechanics (41). Reviews measurement of anthropometry, joint motion, muscle strength, motion analysis, postural analysis, force platform data, work capacity, vibration exposure, manual materials handling, hand tool analysis, preemployment screening, job analysis, and ergonomic assessments in clerical and industrial settings. Man-

ual work evaluation techniques also are discussed, including motion time measurement methods, physical demands analysis, manual lifting analysis, job static strength analysis, and job postural analysis.

Occupational Therapy Evaluation Techniques

- An annotated index of occupational therapy evaluation tools (159). Reviews the purposes, advantages, and limitations of standardized and nonstandardized tests of activities of daily living, adaptive skills, cognitive skills, developmental skills, oral function, person-environment interactions, play skills, psychosocial skills, roles and habits, sensory integration, visual-perceptual skills, and vocational skills.
- Housing accessibility checklist (160). Specific criteria are described for determining housing accessibility. Recommended minimum standards are provided for parking areas, walks and ramps, curbs, stairs, doorways, elevators, and interior rooms.
- Mental health assessment in occupational therapy (161). Reviews selected assessments of human function pertaining to mental health, including checklists, interest inventories, assessment of older adults, prevocational assessments, work tolerance screening, research analysis of evaluation tools used to assess mental health patients, and the Milwaukee Daily Living Skills and Kohlman Evaluation of Living Skills assessment scales.
- Willard and Spackman's occupational therapy (162). Reviews tests of manual dexterity, motor function, developmental, sensory integration, intelligence, and psychological tests.

Quality of Life Assessments

PEDIATRIC ASSESSMENT INSTRUMENTS
- Pediatric functional outcome measures (163). Reviews the technical and clinical merits of selected functional outcome measures used in pediatric rehabilitation practice. Review of selected measures in neurodevelopmental rehabilitation. Reviews measures of gross and fine motor function, activities of daily living, general cognitive abilities, speech and language, and child and parent adjustment.

PHYSICAL FUNCTION ASSESSMENT TECHNIQUES
- Assessment of fitness (164,165). Discusses methods of objective assessment and interpretation of test results for objective evaluation of flexibility, body composition (e.g., body density, anthropometry, total body water, muscle mass estimation), muscle strength and endurance, anaerobic abilities, aerobic abilities, leisure time and occupational activity, and physiologic fitness (e.g., blood pressure, blood lipids and lipoproteins, glucose intolerance). References for specific tests are provided.
- Human muscle function and fatigue (166). Describes the mechanism of muscle fatigue, distinguishing between central and peripheral factors. Describes tests of contractile function and electromyographic changes with fatigue.
- Introduction to measurement in physical education and exercise science (51). Reviews measures of physical fitness, including body composition (e.g., hydrostatic weighing, skinfold thickness), aerobic fitness tests, performance-based measures, muscle strength and endurance, balance, flexibility, posture, and motor ability.
- Measurement for evaluation in physical education and exercise sciences (45). Reviews measures of physical abilities (e.g., muscle strength, power, endurance, flexibility, balance,

kinesthetic perception), youth fitness, aerobic fitness, body composition (e.g., hydrostatic weighing, skinfold thickness), and skill achievement.
- Methodology in human fatigue assessment (167). Describes methods of assessing fatigue, including psychological ratings, the blink method, urinary metabolite measurements, assessment of fatigue at work, direct estimation of circulatory fatigue using bicycle ergometry, determination of muscular work performed with different muscle groups, increasing workloads under different environmental conditions, mental fatigue and stress, and fatigue assessments of specific worker populations.
- Patient evaluation methods for the health professional (168). Describes standardized techniques for measuring limb girth, limb length, limb volume, joint range of motion, muscle length, activities of daily living, motor control, and neurologic parameters.

PSYCHOSOCIAL ASSESSMENT INSTRUMENTS
- A sourcebook for mental health measures (169). Contains 1,100 abstracts of mental health-related psychological measures that describe questionnaires, scales, inventories, tests, and other types of measuring devices. The emphasis is on instruments that have been developed for research or clinical purposes and are less well known than commercially published tests. Abstracts are grouped into 45 categories. These categories include alcoholism, cognitive tests, counseling and guidance, crime and juvenile delinquency, differential psychological diagnosis, drugs, educational adjustment, environments, family interaction, generations differences, geriatrics, marriage and divorce, mental health attitudes, mental retardation, mental status and level of psychological functioning, occupational adjustment, parent behavior and viewpoints, personal history and demographic data, personality, physical handicap, racial attitudes, psychiatric rehabilitation, service delivery, sex, social issues, student and teacher attitudes, suicide and death, therapeutic outcomes, therapeutic processes, and vocational tests. A description of each instrument is provided, along with the source. In addition, the sourcebook references several other sources of mental health measures.
- Evaluating practice: guidelines for the accountable professional (46). Reviews a group of nine instruments that measure generalized contentment, self-esteem, marital satisfaction, sexual satisfaction, parental attitudes, child's attitudes, family relations, and peer relations. Also provides references and briefly discusses reviews of various psychological measures, including mental health measures, psychotherapy change measures, behavioral assessment questionnaires, behavior checklists, psychological assessment, social attitudes, social functioning, adult assessment, rapid assessment instruments for practice, and rating scales which are useful to evaluate patient performance using an interview or observation format.
- Neuropsychological assessment (170). Reviews measures of intellectual abilities, verbal functions, perceptual functions, constructional functions, memory functions, conceptual function, executive functions, motor performance, orientation, attention, tests for brain injury, observational methods, rating scales, and inventories, and tests of personal adjustment and functional disorders.
- Psychological testing (34). Reviews intelligence and developmental tests for the general population and special populations, educational achievement and competency tests, creativity and reasoning tests, projective testing techniques, environmental attitudes tests, vocational aptitude tests, oc-

cupational cognitive screening, psychomotor tests, aptitude tests, personality tests, behavioral assessments, measures of interests, values, and personal orientation, and tests for learning disabilities and neuropsychological dysfunctions.
- Self-report inventories in behavioral assessment (171). Reviews instruments that measure fears, anxiety, assertiveness, social skills, and depression.

RANGE-OF-MOTION AND MUSCLE EXTENSIBILITY ASSESSMENT TECHNIQUES
- Measurement of joint motion (23,172). Reviews static and dynamic methods of measuring joint motion.
- Measurement of joint motion: a guide to goniometry (173). Describes standardized procedures for measuring range of motion of the extremities, spine, and temporomandibular joint. Photos show each test position. Normative values are provided for ranges of motion of each joint.
- Measurement of trunk motion and flexibility (174–182). This series of references describe measurement techniques and reliability of trunk lateral flexion (176,179,180,182), forward flexion (174,181), and extension (175,177,178,182).

SPEECH ASSESSMENT TECHNIQUES
- Appraisal and diagnosis of speech and language disorders (33). Reviews measures of articulation, speech-sound discrimination, language, developmental skills, motor skills, nonverbal intelligence, speech production, structural disorders, fluency, and neurologic disorders.

- Measuring outcomes in speech-language pathology (183). Comprehensive text covering multiple content domains, including definitions, dimensions, perspectives, and requirements of measurement; measuring modality-specific behaviors, functional abilities, and quality of life; measuring consumer satisfaction; collecting, analyzing, and reporting financial outcomes; treatment efficacy research; program evaluation; quality improvement; outcomes measurement in culturally and linguistically diverse populations; outcomes measurement in aphasia; outcomes measurement in cognitive communication disorders (traumatic brain injury, right hemisphere brain damage, dementia); efficacy outcomes and cost-effectiveness in dysphagia; outcomes in motor speech disorders; outcomes measurement in voice disorders; outcomes measurement in fluency disorders; outcomes measurement in child language and phonologic disorders; outcomes measurement in specific settings (schools, health-care facilities, universities, private practice).
- Medical speech-language pathology: a practitioner's guide (184). Clinically oriented text with practical measurement methods for selected issues such as measures of swallowing useful in defining the efficacy of treatment during radiographic study of oropharyngeal swallow; neurocommunicative monitoring tools; indicators of malnutrition; ASHA Functional Assessment of Communication Skills; electrodiagnostic testing for neuromuscular disorders; language and communication assessment measures to use with dementia patients.

CHAPTER 54

Systematically Assessing and Improving the Quality and Outcomes of Medical Rehabilitation Programs

Mark V. Johnston, Elizabeth Eastwood, Deborah L. Wilkerson, Leigh Anderson, and Annette Alves

It was once commonly said that the quality of health care could not be defined but could be recognized when seen. While this view is still occasionally heard, the characteristics of quality health care have become increasingly well defined and scientifically based. Quality health care involves the standardized implementation of effective treatments with favorable risk/benefit ratios. Treatment interventions should be delivered in a skilled manner sensitive to the patient's rights, needs, and lifestyle. Scientific evidence of treatment effectiveness is required, usually evidence from controlled trials. Health care quality is understood to be complex and individualized, and both authority structures and multidisciplinary teams are typically involved in its delivery.

A large number of outcome scales are now available in both rehabilitation and health care in general. Although identification and implementation of practical validated measures of key processes and outcomes often remain a challenge, debate has moved from issues of measurement to evaluation of strategies designed to improve patient outcomes by improving the actual delivery of evidence-based care process. There is much to learn from rehabilitation's long experience with program evaluation (PE) and from older quality assurance (QA) strategies, but new and more promising models of outcomes-oriented QA and quality improvement (QI) are now available from areas of health care related to medical rehabilitation.

The broad thesis of this chapter is that multiple strategies and systems are useful for assuring and improving the quality and effectiveness of medical rehabilitation in practice. The most effective strategy for improving care and outcomes will depend on varying local circumstances. Process-focused and outcomes-focused strategies are both needed. Key processes, for which there is evidence and good reason to believe they are effective, need to be implemented and monitored, and relevant outcomes measured. QI efforts draw from all of the knowledge in this thick textbook—and more. The chapter is designed to be a guide and reference work for physicians, administrators, QI specialists, and other professionals concerned with quality and patient outcomes in medical rehabilitation.

MOTIVATIONS AND BACKGROUND

Demands for accountability, improved quality, and delivery of expected outcomes have grown throughout health care as a whole and in rehabilitation in particular. As the Institute of Medicine's *Crossing the Quality Chasm* states: "The frustration levels of both clinicians and patients have probably never been higher. Health care today harms too frequently and routinely fails to deliver its potential benefits" (1, p. 1).

The health care industry in the United States is a tangled, fragmented web rather than a system. This nonsystem often duplicates efforts, wasting resources, while at the same time leaving great gaps in coverage and failing to employ the strongest skills of all health care professionals. In rehabilitation, the growth of managed care and prospective payment has pressured rehabilitation facilities to reorganize and shorten length of stay (LOS) to lower costs. Effects of cutbacks on rehabilitation quality have been little studied, but it is known that rehospitalization rates after discharge from inpatient rehabilitation have increased (2).

Numerous studies have documented systematic problems in the quality of medical care. Errors in medical care have received particular attention in recent years. While reports that massive numbers of patients have their lives needlessly shortened by medical errors appear to be exaggerated (3,4), avoidable morbidity and even mortality have clearly been documented (5). Adverse reactions to drugs or other drug errors may occur in about 10% of hospitalized patients; these errors increase morbidity and even mortality and extend hospital stays by 1.7 to 2.2 days (6). Tens of millions of Americans continue to experience chronic illness and disability (7,8), but there are no data on avoidable disablement due to inadequate or poor quality rehabilitation programs.

The primary motivation for quality and outcomes improvement systems in rehabilitation, however, is not avoidance of outright bad care and patient injury. Medical rehabilitation facilities are caring environments, and the great majority of rehabilitation patients clearly improve in function (9). The motivation is public accountability and the ability to demonstrate efficacy in improvement of the function and quality of life of persons with disabilities. Accountability systems for rehabilitation are best developed by rehabilitation professionals because we are the ones who are best able to improve the quality and effectiveness of rehabilitation services. Detailed quality control regulations of payers and government, though not without merit or necessity, have been known to be highly problematic (10). The position, influence, and even perhaps the very survival of rehabilitation as a specialty may hinge on its ability to develop and implement quality and outcomes management systems based on evidence and data.

PARTICULAR CONSIDERATIONS IN MEDICAL REHABILITATION

The goals of medical rehabilitation are broad and encompass both physiological dysfunctions and functional and quality of life objectives (11–16). Medical rehabilitation typically treats patients with chronic impairments which cannot be totally "cured," although recovery can be enhanced and complications, prevented. Improving the person's functioning and participation in everyday life in the community after discharge have long been enunciated as major goals of rehabilitation (11,12,13,16). Priority clinical objectives are individually tailored (17,18). Individual responses to care and individual priorities are typically sought. QI and PE system in rehabilitation, however, have traditionally been linked to group outcomes, providing little information on quality of patient management and even confusing priority clinical issues. Rehabilitation goals are measurable, or potentially so, but the complexity and individualization involved present a challenge in practice.

Clinical Treatment Objectives

The clinical care process involves assessing (diagnosis and fact finding), planning (and deciding), treating, checking (measuring the result), and then assessing again whether to alter, continue, or discontinue the treatment, leading to another treatment process or ultimately to patient discharge (Fig. 54-1). Clinical practice involves all of these steps, including some check of the success of any preceding diagnostic-planning-treatment sequence. In this sense, clinical outcomes measurement is intrinsic and essential to clinical practice. The relevant clinical measures may be indicators of short-term responsiveness to treatment, such as a serum level, an oral response from the patient, or slightly increased strength or normalization of gait. Efforts to improve the quality and outcomes of rehabilitation address all elements of this basic cycle.

Improving the rehabilitation process requires that long-term outcome goals be addressed as well as short-term treatment objectives (14,15,19). Rehabilitation *outcome goals* are defined at a broader, less specific, but still highly meaningful level of improvements in the person's life at the level of activities or community participation (also known as handicap) and quality of life (14–17). Outcome goals are measured after termination of services, when patient function has stabilized to some degree. Implementations of this model have measured rehabilitation outcomes in terms of productive activity (e.g., paid work, schooling, housework, or other uses of time considered normal for such a person) or independent living (e.g., noninstitutional living arrangement and total support requirements) (14–17, 20,21). Attainment of outcome goals provides information on the local system of rehabilitation programming as a whole, and is employed in PE systems and individual case management systems that involve major responsibility for persons with disability over the long term.

In contrast, *treatment objectives* are shorter-term and have a close scientific, logical relationship to the particular interventions provided to the person (19). Shorter-term and intermediate measures are valuable in identifying recovery associated with rehabilitation, distinguishing them from events due to exogenous factors (22,23). Other experts in quality and clinical outcomes research also affirm the need to measure *intermediate-outcomes* to connect long-term outcomes to clinical care (24). We emphasize the need for clinicians to define and measure treatment objectives in rehabilitation case management or outcomes management.

Dual Accreditation

Medical rehabilitation is both medical and rehabilitative. It is a pragmatic combination of medical interventions designed to reduce impairments, therapies involving practice and learning, and equipment provision. Reflecting this duality, accreditation of medical rehabilitation facilities involves both the Joint Commission on Accreditation of Healthcare Organizations (JCAHO) and the Commission on Accreditation of Rehabilitation Facilities (CARF).

The JCAHO is of course the primary agency for accreditation of health care facilities in the United States. JCAHO accreditation is usually essential for hospital licensure and reimbursement in the United States. JCAHO standards address numerous aspects of organizational structure and care processes, discussed in greater detail later in this chapter.

Continuous efforts to maintain and improve quality are to be made. QI should be embedded throughout the organization, with responsibility centered at leadership.

Recognizing the limitations of an exclusive emphasis on structure and processes, JCAHO initiated an "Agenda for Change" in 1987. The process has led to increased emphasis on indicators of the routine quality and effectiveness of care and outcomes as well as continuous efforts to improve quality. This effort—ORYX—culminated in standards related to formal

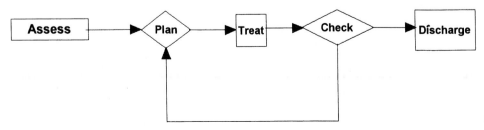

Figure 54-1. The clinical care process.

monitoring systems in the 1990s, encompassing sets of both process and outcome indicators. JCAHO has supported the development of objective indicators of clinical events and mostly short-term outcomes (examples of which are provided later in the chapter) and has recently developed a standard requiring functional assessment for all patients admitted to the hospital.

Medical rehabilitation facilities voluntarily apply for accreditation by CARF to attest to their commitment to maximize the rehabilitation of disabled persons. It has long been recognized that rehabilitation of persons with disability requires more than medical interventions, in the narrow sense of the term. Generalization of learning and attaining a significant impact on real-world outcomes is integral to quality rehabilitation. CARF standards are pragmatic, detailed, and optimized for rehabilitation. CARF has long emphasized function and attainment of outcomes after discharge (11). CARF has long specified characteristics of rehabilitation organizations believed to indicate quality, effective care. CARF has long required that rehabilitation programs eventually establish outcomes monitoring systems. Requirements for "program evaluation," the older term, were modified in the mid-1990s, replaced by "outcomes measurement and management" (11). CARF standards identify the domains or general indicators that programs should use in their own information systems, but the actual values reported by the data system are not usually integral to the accreditation standards or the survey process.

The focus for accreditation by both CARF and JCAHO is on a program's conformance with standards during a site survey. Standards primarily reflect the structure and process aspects of programs or services—that is, the ways services should be organized and how activities should be conducted in the provision of services. CARF has historically been oriented toward outcomes via PE and requires performance monitoring that includes some sort of outcomes assessment (usually Functional Independence Measures, or FIMs), but with ORYX, JCAHO now requires definite outcomes measurement as well. In sum, accreditation—like QI in general—requires attention to structure, processes, inputs, and outcomes.

Dual CARF-JCAHO accreditation has been an expense. During the late 1990s, the two accrediting bodies began work on a collaborative process to streamline rehabilitation accreditation and minimize duplication of effort. Whatever happens to accreditation in the future, medical rehabilitation will need to continue to deal with both medical problems and broad issues of patients' function and quality-of-life.

Approaching Performance Improvement

The complex of ideas and experience designated as *continuous quality improvement* (CQI) (25–28) and *total quality management* (TQM) have had great influence on QI throughout health care (29,30). It is now widely accepted that quality is a property of the total, complex, adaptive "system," not just isolated parts (1). Measures of processes and outcomes may be employed, but such measures are not to be relied upon in isolation from knowledge of wider considerations (26,27). The insights of TQM and CQI are found throughout this chapter.

Although TQM and CQI are process-oriented, their philosophic basis transcends a pure process approach (26,29,30). Outcomes measurement is an important tool, and systematic outcome measurement is essential in health care, where the results produced are not as obvious as the products of manufacturing. CQI assumes a scoreboard of process or outcome measures (25–27,30). Accreditation agencies require process or outcomes measurement. As in the rest of health care, systematic QA and QI in medical rehabilitation require the implemen-

tation of processes which use scientific methods by developing a plan, gathering data on both system and patient problems, acting to improve processes, checking results, and reassessing on a regular basis. Both short-term and longer-term outcomes should be regularly addressed.

TERMS AND CONCEPTS

This section will explain basic terms and concepts that underlie both quality and outcomes monitoring and improvement systems.

Basic Quality of Care Concepts

The general features of quality of care are definable. Quality is always positive, connoting activities that benefit the person served in the short- or long-term. The Institute of Medicine has defined quality as the "degree to which health services for individuals and populations increase the likelihood of desired health outcomes and are consistent with current professional knowledge" (31,32). In other words, quality involves achieving desired health outcomes to a degree that is consistent with current knowledge of diagnosis and effective treatment. A first approximation to measurement of quality in rehabilitation involves measurement of the degree to which the objectives of care are met for appropriate groups of patients.

Quality care involves the following components (10,18):

1. *Choosing appropriate care.* That is, care that optimally addresses the patient's impairments and activity limitations. Diagnosis, planning, and clinical judgment are involved in the attempt to match treatments to patient conditions and to balance likely benefits against possible risks. The treatments chosen should be established as effective for the condition or problem addressed.
2. *Implementing it well.* Needed care should be available (access), provided at the most beneficial time (timeliness), in the correct manner (technical correctness), minimizing safety risks. The skills and sustained efforts of individual professionals and the coordination of the clinical team are involved.

In addition, quality care also requires treating patients with dignity and sensitivity to their individual needs, expectations, and circumstances. In rehabilitation, patient involvement is particularly important because engaging the patients' motivations is essential to the success of activity therapies. Communication, concern, empathy, honesty, sensitivity, and responsiveness to individuals are important (33). Patients not only want to be informed about what is going on but also want to be involved in selection of treatment goals. The disability rights movement insists on empowerment of persons with disabilities, and rehabilitation accreditation requires patient involvement in decisions about care and placement (11).

Quality medical rehabilitation should engender sustained improvement in the function, health, and quality of life of patients beyond any improvements that would have occurred with nonprofessional care. Although duration of life is relevant, functional improvement and quality of life are the main issues in medical rehabilitation. In rehabilitation of patients with complex problems and differing personal circumstances, quality of care surely involves a degree of tailoring of the rehabilitative plan to the individual. The durability of outcomes—whether valued functional gains are sustained—is a major and recurring issue in judging the success of rehabilitation, motivating requirements for patient follow-up.

Quality health care is based on provision of effective care. Specification of optimally effective care is difficult in a field as complex and broad as rehabilitation, but the evidence basis for rehabilitation is growing and increasingly defined. Explication, implementation, and improvement of guidelines for care are basic to efforts to assure and improve the routine core quality of care.

Accreditation organizations judge conformance of programs with *standards*. Standards are usually defined in terms of the structure and process of programs. Standards may specify necessary services, staffing, or administrative organization. They may identify the domains or indicators that programs should use in their performance information systems, but the actual values reported in the data are not usually integral to the accreditation standards. For example, a CARF *standard* might require a program to use measures of function in evaluating rehabilitation outcomes but would not specify the exact measure or vendor. Standards relevant to outcomes and patient gains are under development at both CARF and JCAHO.

We retain the term *quality assurance* (QA). The term has fallen out of vogue, perhaps because it at one time led to reliance on external policing of clinicians, peer review alone, and other limited techniques. QA means activities to assure that implicit or explicit standards of care are met. Such activities are still needed. Assuring provision of sensitive, effective care is a particularly critical issue given cutbacks in rehabilitation imposed by managed care and by payment systems that provide an incentive to provide less care.

PERFORMANCE INDICATORS

The term "performance indicator" has come into widespread use to designate key outcomes and processes that need to be measured and reported to judge the effectiveness and efficiency of service delivery. The choice, implementation, and use of performance indicators are central concerns to performance monitoring and improvement. Performance indicators are used in QI and reported to stakeholders such as consumers, payers, governing boards, accreditation organizations, and the public. Both CARF and JCAHO use the term.

To improve quality systematically, objective comparison data are needed as a basis for evaluation. The necessity for data and preestablished standards of quality and outcome is asserted by JCAHO, CARF, and government agencies, although the nature of what is to be measured varies.

OUTCOMES

The classic outcomes-oriented method of connecting outcomes to processes involves routine assessment of diagnostic and therapeutic outcomes; related process variables are assessed if outcomes do not meet accepted standards (34). In process-oriented approaches, proximal or short-term clinical results of interventions are assessed.

The term *"outcome"* is commonly used in different ways: *life outcomes*—in the sense of role restoration and quality of life generally; *health-related quality of life*—those aspects of life or experience or function that are logically related to physical health or recognized mental disorders; and the *outcomes of care*, or *rehabilitation outcomes*. The latter terms imply a connection to preceding treatments as well as impact on patient functioning or well-being. Although rehabilitation improves aspects of the quality of patients' lives, it would not be honest to suggest that medical rehabilitation can routinely produce or assume responsibility for massive, global improvements in patients' lives. Although we are concerned with the person's quality of life as a whole (large circle in Fig. 54-2), medical rehabilitation is primarily directed at health-related quality of life (smaller oval).

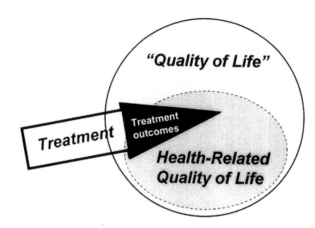

Figure 54-2. Quality of life, health, and rehabilitation outcomes.

Medical rehabilitation professionals are primarily and directly responsible for those aspects of patients' lives that they can affect, namely *treatment outcomes* (the small triangle in Fig. 54-2).

At a substantive level, JCAHO has defined rehabilitation outcomes as "restoration, improvement or maintenance of the patient's optimal level of functioning, self-care, self-responsibility, independence and quality of life" (23, Tx. 6.5). The term *rehabilitation outcomes* also connotes connection to rehabilitative treatments. Hence, an *outcome of rehabilitation* is an aspect of function or life due to rehabilitative treatments. Such outcomes are not directly measured but are inferred or estimated after adjustment for case severity and factors influencing likely responsiveness.

BENCHMARKING

Benchmarking is basic to both quality and outcomes monitoring. A *benchmark* is a target value of a performance indicator. JCAHO requires that facilities compare their processes and outcomes with those known to be attainable elsewhere (35). CARF also writes of benchmarks . CQI assumes a scoreboard of process or outcome measures (25–27,30). Severity or risk adjustment is usually needed to develop benchmarks that enable us to evaluate outcomes and processes as well.

TREATMENT EFFECTIVENESS

Knowledge of treatment effectiveness ties together processes and outcomes. *Effectiveness* may be defined as the sustained improvement in patient function produced by rehabilitative care beyond those improvements that occur with the natural healing and adjustment that occurs even with less intensive, non-specialized care. Effectiveness is assumed by use of the term "rehabilitation outcomes" and is the core attribute of quality professional medical rehabilitation. Effectiveness encompasses appropriateness of care, the technical competence with which procedures are carried out, risks, and unintended as well as intended consequences.

Validated Indicators of Causal Processes

Both QI and outcomes monitoring systems should be based on established knowledge regarding effective treatment. *Clinical practice guidelines* or practice parameters are needed if this knowledge is to be explicit. Generally, health care guidelines encompass recommendations for patient diagnosis and evaluation, followed by treatment recommendations, and monitoring of patient responsiveness. Input, process, and outcome measures are, then, needed to judge whether appropriate, effective care is provided. Guidelines are most valuable if based on controlled research. Inference of effectiveness requires controlled research and at least a simple theory of what constitutes effective treatment (36).

Surrogate Indicators of Effectiveness

In practice, PE and outcomes management in rehabilitation have commonly been based on implicit beliefs and practical but flawed surrogate estimates of effectiveness. In PE, the term "effectiveness" is usually used to mean how successful a program is in accomplishing its goals or average functional gain by patients. Rates of functional improvement distinguish rehabilitation hospitals from chronic disease programs and nursing facilities (37).

Some QI publications have defined effectiveness as "the degree to which the care is provided in the correct manner, given the current state of the art" (23,38). Effectiveness is then adherence to normatively based standards and methods of care. This is a good pragmatic definition. Studies in acute hospitals, for instance, have clearly demonstrated that better adherence to the best practices would clearly improve patient outcomes (18,39–41).

EFFICIENCY AND VALUE

Improving the quality of care would be easy if money were free. Resources, however, are always limited. As economic constraints have increased, assuring the provision of high-quality care has become an increasingly challenging issue.

Efficiency means delivering appropriate, effective care within cost constraints. *Straightcost* considerations must be distinguished from *cost-effectiveness*, which involves evaluating costs of treatment against gains in patient outcomes. Measures of service use (e.g., LOS, treatments units) are often useful surrogates for detailed computations of cost. In a managed care environment, we especially need to know whether the imposed limitations have compromised patient outcomes. In a prospective payment environment, if one spends too much effort on one patient, there will be fewer resources available for others. Data systems are needed to guide us in determining where the optimum lies.

Rehabilitative care not only needs to be provided efficiently: it must be of *value* to its customers, including most of all patients but also including payers (42). Patients, payers, and society commonly demand a robust improvement in the patient's functioning or quality of life that endures in everyday life after discharge. While this can happen, the improvements associated with rehabilitative interventions are frequently limited in magnitude and type. Honest projection and communication of the likely results and value of interventions is challenging in rehabilitation but important to provision of quality care.

Levels of Health and Functioning

Health and functioning are rich concepts that involve a number of levels which need to be understood, given the central importance of these to systematic performance improvement. Chapter 49 in this book explains components of health outcomes as defined by the newer *International Classification of Functioning, Disability, and Health* (43). In brief, distinctions between functioning at the biological level, the level of the individual per se, and of the individual in actual society and environment (previously designated as impairment—disability—handicap) (44) are replaced by *impairment, activity,* and *participation.* Measures of *pathology*—dysfunction at the cellular or biochemical level—and *disease* are also needed in QI and outcomes management in medical settings. The term *functional limitation* is also valuable

to denote very specific limitations or activity restriction of the person, as measured in a controlled or clinical environment (8,12), in contrast to indicators of broader activities in daily life.

Impairments are of focal importance in *medical* rehabilitation treatments. Performance monitoring systems in medical rehabilitation must at least group patients by their primary etiology or impairment group, and ideally, severity adjustment is in terms of the primary diagnosis or impairment [e.g., severity and level of paralysis in spinal cord injury (SCI)] (45). If an impairment is used as an outcome measure, there should be evidence—not merely an assumption—that the impairment is significantly related to functional outcomes or quality of life. Numerous medical and nursing conditions treated in medical rehabilitation—infection control, reduction of decubitus ulcers, control of blood pressure, prevention and treatment of deep vein thrombosis, diabetes management, pain relief—meet this criterion. In many circumstances in rehabilitation, however, a pathology or impairment can be treated and reduced without alteration of the primary disease or the functional status of the patient (46). Range of motion and even spasticity reduction, for instance, are poorly correlated with functional outcomes (47), probably because they are not the primary barriers to improved function for many patients with these impairments. Discriminating more worthwhile from less worthwhile but still technically effective interventions is a challenge for rehabilitation physicians and case managers.

While medical rehabilitation deals with all these levels, it has long focused on improving basic activity capabilities of its patients [e.g., reducing assistance requirements in activities of daily living (ADLs)]. There are many reasonably reliable and valid scales of physical functioning that can be used for performance monitoring in rehabilitation, the most popular being the Functional Independence Measure (FIM). Its limitations have been in the areas of speech, language, and cognition, but progress is being made in measurement of cognitively based problems in daily life (48). Activities and disabilities are determined not only by impairments but also by the extent of compensating functional strengths. Disability and activity can have a loose connection to community participation or life satisfaction (45,49).

Health Status Measures

Medical rehabilitation outcome measures may be considered to be a subcategory of health status and quality of life measures in general. Books summarizing different scales of health-related quality of life are now available (45,50–54). These books are filled with scales that should be of use in rehabilitation outcomes assessment, though their sensitivity and logical applicability to medical rehabilitation requires verification. Perhaps the most commonly used measures of general health are the Sickness Impact Profile (55) (SIP) and the Medical Outcomes Study Short-Form 36 (SF-36) (56). Some of the subscales within these instruments appear to be too broad or are otherwise not directed at problems treated in medical rehabilitation, but many dimensions—such as pain relief, general feelings of health and well-being, and physical function—are relevant. In general *quality of life (QOL)* measures are relevant to rehabilitation outcomes assessment. Subjective or affective quality of life is so important that it deserves assessment, even though it is not part of the World Health Organization (WHO) scheme, although without qualification. *Subjective well-being* and *life satisfaction* have been increasingly studied for use as ultimate rehabilitation outcomes measures (57). Subjective well-being is statistically associated with health and function, community participation, and a loving and satisfying social life, but the inconsistency of these associations demonstrates that subjective well-being cannot be reduced to indicators of objective health and circumstance (49,57): the person's own expectations or implicit standards regarding his or her own life are critical. Chapter 55 discusses QOL assessment in greater detail. At this point, indices of patient well-being are sufficiently well validated to be used in research but have not yet been validated for use as routine indicators of the performance of individual rehabilitation programs.

Criteria for Choice of Measures

Criteria for choice of measures for performance monitoring and improvement projects include: (a) psychometric or biometric soundness (reliability and validity or accuracy) (58); (b) sensitivity to patient gain; and (c) a basis in validated treatment theory and evidence-based guidelines, that is, relatedness to the documented effects of provision of proven, high-quality interventions (22,36). The last of these has grown to be so important that it is treated in a separate section below. In practice, ease of administration and expense are critical considerations. This section considers principles that apply to measurement of inputs, processes, and outcomes.

VALIDITY AND RELIABILITY

Evidence of reliability and validity is needed to choose and interpret scales or ratings employed in performance monitoring. The Measurement Standards for Interdisciplinary Medical Rehabilitation are available to guide clinicians, quality professionals, and researchers in choice of scales in rehabilitation (59). Scales employed in performance monitoring should meet recognized standards of reliability and validity (59). In brief, we need to know the *reliability*—that is, the stability, agreement, and reproducibility of measures used for QI or outcomes monitoring. Without this information, results are more subject to error and charges of subjectivity. Error-prone indices of the appropriateness of medical care have been shown to overstate the frequency of inappropriate care (60).

Validity is a concept associated with use. Validity is always *validity for* some defined purpose or construct. Validity may be seen as the sum of the correct inferences that one can make from a measure in defined circumstances. *Accuracy* is the relevant criterion to evaluate the validity of a measure when an extremely accurate, objective "gold standard" is available. Knowledge of sensitivity and specificity are of course basic to interpretation of categorical tests (59).

To add up items to provide a meaningful summary number, one should know the degree to which the items are internally consistent, additive, and unidimensional (58,61,62). The FIM, for instance, consists of at least two dimensions: motor ADLs and cognitive-psychosocial function (63).

Limited range of item difficulty has also been a problem with some scales employed in rehabilitation, since rehabilitation deals with an enormous range of human performance—from coma or total paralysis through return to community living and paid employment. Many existing scales are sensitive to the typical range of improvement seen in medical rehabilitation hospitals (12,13,48,64) but still have ceiling or floor problems, that is, they may be insensitive to very real improvements that occur in some patients who remain at a "total assist" level in ADLs or in individuals who are independent in ADLs but need speed, endurance, or higher level skills to sustain a productive lifestyle in the community (65).

To employ parametric analysis techniques (e.g., reporting means, *t*-tests, or Pearson correlations), the scales employed should have equal-interval characteristics. Measures developed using Rasch analysis have probabilistic equal-interval properties (58,61,62,66). The technique is applicable to items with much wider ranges of difficulty than previous techniques, lessening floor and ceiling problems (58,62). The method also has the advantage of identifying "misfitting" persons, that is, individuals whose pattern of functioning is so atypical that the conventional method of assessing and interpreting their outcomes is likely to be misleading. Different methods of scoring functional scales may be needed for different diagnostic groups. Walking, for instance, is relatively easy for a person with brain injury but is near impossible for a person with complete paraplegia; its significance as a marker of progress is radically different between the diagnostic groups. Chapter 53 presents additional criteria for choice of measures.

SENSITIVITY TO CHANGE AND EVIDENCE BASES

A minimum simple criterion for choice of indicators for quality and outcomes monitoring is demonstrated change in association with treatment. Older works in medical rehabilitation interpreted improvement per se as indicating provision of effective treatment. While improved function is generally good, causation cannot be reliably inferred from improvement alone. Causation is inferred from a pattern of improvement highly associated with treatment but not associated with case severity or other exogenous (i.e., nontreatment) factors (67). Previous controlled research is necessary to establish the efficacy of treatments and to identify attainable outcomes. The emerging standard is that performance indicators chosen should be sensitive to provision of efficacious treatment. Indicators of such outcomes are not only scientifically sound but also actionable.

SEVERITY ADJUSTMENT AND STATISTICAL CONSIDERATIONS

The need for *severity adjustment* or *risk adjustment* of performance data can hardly be overemphasized. QI and outcomes monitoring systems that are unadjusted or poorly adjusted for disease severity, functional limitations, and other factors that affect likely outcomes are likely to provide misleading reports. While all factors cannot be controlled statistically, outstanding confounding factors can be measured, and their effect, projected. A risk factor for a particular functional or health outcome is a characteristic of patients or of their environment that influences the likelihood of occurrence of a (usually negative, dichotomous) health outcome.

Knowledge of statistical principles is needed to interpret performance monitoring data. Rehabilitation outcomes are generally stochastic, not deterministic. Sample size is always a consideration: a single bad outcome may well be a fluke; a pattern of outcomes below severity-adjusted norms indicates a possible process problem needing further investigation.

Change in function is a prototypical goal in medical rehabilitation, and its computation involves statistical considerations. While simple change scores (discharge minus admission values) are often used, the resulting difference scores are subject to regression artifacts because of error of measurement and the stochastic nature of the change itself: residualizing outcome scores by their probabilistic relationship to pre-test scores is often more justified statistically (68). The statistical analysis of change scores is a complex issue which depends on one's theory or model of recovery curves or stages (69).

Causal Knowledge and Guidelines

Inference of quality or effective treatment in rehabilitation depends on our total knowledge of medical therapies as well as healing and adaptive processes. Rehabilitation involves provision of an array of medical and nursing interventions as well as therapies that work through the activity of the person, such as physical therapy (PT), occupational therapy (OT), and speech/language pathology (SLP). A well-validated theoretical basis is needed to make results credible and to enable results to be generalized to practice (19). Clinical practice guidelines can be written that encompass such a multidisciplinary array, and hence can form the basis for connecting such interventions to relevant outcomes.

Quality and outcomes evaluation systems are commonly thought to be looser than scientific research. Indeed, uncontrolled data systems do not usually provide unambiguous evidence of causation or intervention effectiveness or cost-effectiveness. Rather, performance monitoring systems need to be based on validated, or at least accepted, knowledge regarding effective treatment. Although elaborate controlled trials are necessary to establish the efficacy of different approaches to treatment, the implementation of such treatments can usually be monitored in practice with a less elaborate set of measures.

Performance monitoring and QI require a basis in causal knowledge. Evidence-based clinical guidelines are therefore needed for QI in rehabilitation, as in other fields of health care. While complexity will defeat attempts to define appropriate clinical interventions for every patient, the process of developing workable guidelines that define key features of rehabilitative processes, along with indicators of relevant outcomes, has begun, and guidelines have already been created for the more common, better-defined patient problems and groups seen in rehabilitation, as will be discussed below.

PROGRAM EVALUATION AND OUTCOMES MANAGEMENT

This section discusses systems of measurement, monitoring, and interpretation focused on the outcomes attained by patients after care. We will begin by discussing the older term—"program evaluation" (PE) and its associated schema. Over several decades, PE models in rehabilitation have become well developed, and knowledge of the strengths and limitations of these models provides a basis for more recent approaches. We will then describe more recent, but less defined, "outcomes management" concepts.

Program Evaluation

Program evaluation (PE) refers to a variety of information-gathering activities designed to aid in program development or functioning (i.e., formative evaluation) or to decide whether a program as a whole is worthwhile (i.e., summative evaluation). Many approaches to PE have been employed over the last three decades (70). "Performance monitoring" is a more current term which includes both PE and monitoring of key processes. Accountability to the public and internal management have overarching purposes regardless of rubric. These systems have multiple uses, including marketing, profitability, program planning and development, research, prognosis, utilization review, and improved clinical planning and treatment.

CARF AND THE DEVELOPMENT OF PROGRAM EVALUATION
Beginning in the 1970s, leaders in rehabilitation realized that the field needed to demonstrate its benefits to the public. Providing a forum for this realization, CARF assumed leadership and developed standards that required established rehabilitation facilities to develop PE systems that measure outcomes. In the mid-to-late 1970s and 1980s, workable prototype PE de-

signs and guides (71) were developed and implemented in numerous rehabilitation facilities.

PE has been be defined as "a systematic procedure for determining the effectiveness and efficiency with which results are achieved by persons served following services" (11). These results are collected on a "regular or continuous basis" for all patients or for a systematic sample of patients (11,72). PE and outcomes management involve setting goals and expectancies. If goals are not attained, action should be taken to determine why. In its usual form, PE does not provide answers to specific problem areas but merely identifies that a problem or strength exists. Answers are identified through more in-depth investigations involving further analyses of data, chart review, examination of QI measures (i.e., monitors), and discussions with the knowledgeable staff (25,73–76). PE systems are to be used to help make clinical management decisions and improve program operations.

Many programs, realizing the need for objective comparative data, have joined mass data systems. Since 1998 CARF standards have incorporated standards asking that organizations do some kind of comparison of their own results to those of internal or external benchmarks by whatever method these can be gathered (e.g., pooled data systems), the organization's own larger network, or the published literature.

CARF has long emphasized meaningful outcomes in the real world after discharge. The goal is to maximize patient functioning and QOL in the community after discharge. Medical outcomes are emphasized when these may affect functional or general health outcomes. CARF standards ask that rehabilitation programs assess patient outcomes in terms of the WHO's International Classification of Function, Disability, and Health (ICF) (43), emphasizing as well durability of outcomes, characteristics of the person's environment, and satisfaction with services (77). (See Chapter 49 for a more complete discussion of the ICF.)

Experience with PE systems resulted in a shift of emphasis away from choice of measures and formal design of the PE system. Use of PE information, regardless of details of system design, became the key point as early as the 1980s. Between 1995 and 1998 CARF standards changed to use the terms "outcomes measurement and management" rather "program evaluation" in order to emphasize the need for more operationally oriented approaches. CARF's concern about outcomes has remained, and much of the substance of data collection and emphasis on use of information has not changed. The need to demonstrate the effectiveness and value of care provided remains. Through PE, medical rehabilitation has two decades of experience with the uses and limitation of outcomes measurement, as much and perhaps more experience than any other sector of the medical care industry.

THE STANDARD REHABILITATION PROGRAM EVALUATION MODEL
In the 1970s and 1980s, medical rehabilitation programs developed their own tradition in PE (72). These PE systems were designed to provide an overview of program outcomes. In effect, they were designed to assure outcomes to the public, that is, to be summative evaluation systems. In operation, however, these systems functioned as formative evaluation systems (74). Information on outcomes is given primarily to program staff, who constitute the main audience for reports. Improved program management was, in fact, a primary expectation, leading to the relabeling as "outcomes management."

Standard PE systems in rehabilitation have three components: design, goals and objectives, and reports. The standard model sketched here is based on the work of Robert Walker, a chief CARF consultant in the 1970s. While this basic model is still widely used, updating has occurred as part of CARF's strategic outcomes initiative to incorporate notions of outcomes management. CARF offers training, guidance, and materials on outcomes management. Anyone developing, implementing, or using a PE or QI system in rehabilitation should consult the CARF standards manual or the CARF office or Web site (www.carf.org) for references to the most recent information (11).

Major components of a PE system are summarized below.

Program Purpose and Description

The PE design is based on a mission statement describing who the organization serves, what services it provides, and what goals it expects to accomplish. Goals should be anchored in the concerns of the persons served and other stakeholders—groups or entities with an interest in the success of the program. The programs that constitute the organization are then described (e.g., stroke program, brain injury, spinal injury, pain program, general inpatient rehabilitation, transitional living center). Key influencers are listed to ground the statement in reality. These are external agencies that constrain and direct the rehabilitation program, such as the rehabilitation market and clients, referral sources, patients, staff, Medicare, third-party payers, and key government agencies.

Each program within an organization and the population it serves are to be described in terms that should be well known.

1. General program objectives. These are anticipated results to the primary clients. (Here the term "objectives" is used for what we call more general "goals.")
2. Admission criteria, or definition of the population served in the program. Both inclusionary [e.g., cerebrovascular accident (CVA)] and exclusionary (e.g., free from communicable disease, over 18, noncomatose, dependent in ADLs and ambulation, medically stable for 3 hours per day of therapy, likely to survive at least 6 months) criteria are defined.
3. Persons served, described with regard to diagnosis, functional issues and problems to be addressed, and relevant demographics.
4. Services provided or readily available to the patient, such as routine physiatry, PT, OT, SLP, psychology, social services, and rehabilitation nursing.

General Program Objectives

CARF standards require the measurement of program performance in the domains of effectiveness (results or outcomes for persons served), efficiency (relationship between outcomes and resources used), and satisfaction (experience of the persons served and other stakeholders (11). These three domains for PE have been in the CARF standards for at least three decades. Data elements to assess these domains are measured at admission, discharge, and follow-up, depending on the appropriate time for each data element. Outcomes are assessed after discharge. Follow-up data collection usually takes place 3 months after discharge but other periods can also be justified.

Also needed are progress objectives or intermediate outcomes in terms of patient improvement in the clinical setting toward outcomes such as improved independence in mobility, self-care, communication, or medical self-management. These are similar to (but less specific than) our concept of treatment objectives.

Efficiency objectives are also needed. Resources consumed such as staff time, LOS, number of treatment sessions, and dollars should be monitored and related to the results achieved. For example, the functional gain for a given LOS can be monitored to ensure that outcome is not sacrificed with resource restriction.

Program Evaluation and Outcomes Monitoring Measures

The Functional Independence Measure (FIM) is the most commonly used functional outcomes measure in medical rehabilitation. It became the basis for the prospective payment system for medical rehabilitation hospitals in the United States beginning January 1, 2002. The FIM is an 18-item scale that rates each item along a scale ranging from 1 (i.e., total assist) to 7 (i.e., completely independent). The FIM consists of two overall factors (i.e., motor function and cognition), and recent reports indicate acceptable-to-good reliability (66).

Typical constituents of a rehabilitation inpatient hospital PE system are shown in Figure 54-3. The sparseness of measures (italicized) in the process box and the larger set of admission (i.e., input) and outcomes (i.e., discharge and follow-up) measures show the emphasis of conventional PE systems. Scales of independence in ADLs like the FIM constitute the primary input (e.g., admission, baseline) and output (e.g., discharge, follow-up) measures. Cost and LOS are classified here as process or input measures because they indicate the degree of effort or *resource use* devoted to benefiting the patient. PE systems also address quality of routine nursing care, hotel services, and patient satisfaction (29,78).

Supplementary Measures

PE systems usually have measures used for general descriptive or comparative purposes (Fig. 54-3). Demographic variables (e.g., age, gender, race) are often considered to be input or independent variables. They are listed here as supplemental measures because they may not be very good measures of case severity. However, these variables may help segment the population into homogeneous groups for analysis of other differences (e.g., access to care, service type). Data and reasons for death are essential supplementary measures in PE and quality monitoring. Inpatient medical rehabilitation programs frequently deal with aged, infirm, and chronically ill patients. Although the main purpose of medical rehabilitation is not to decrease mortality, research has shown that medical rehabilitation programs can substantially increase survival (79).

DEFINING A PE SYSTEM IN REHABILITATION

For several decades, rehabilitation programs employed a certain specific model of PE. This model is only one of several alternatives; textbooks provide lessons in the variety of approaches and issues encountered in PE more generally (70,80). We describe this standard or classic model because examples of it became well defined and tested over many years of use and because development and lessons from PE form a basis for current performance monitoring systems. The standard PE model in rehabilitation involved the following:

- Program objectives, such as improved function in self-care, mobility, and continence; communication; target LOS; and patient satisfaction.
- Appropriate indicators and the operational measures, such as percent who improve in bladder management as measured by the FIM.
- Specification of who the measure applies to. In the conventional PE model, program objectives are applied to all patients in the program. Newer approaches (and CARF standards after 1998) require analysis of outcomes in meaningful groupings of patients, recognizing that the nature of relevant outcomes and degree of improvement vary across groups.
- Specification of how measures are implemented and when they are applied. Most programs measure function at admission and discharge. Assessment of function 1 to 6 months after discharge gives a more valuable picture of patient outcomes. Follow-up of outcomes has become common and is

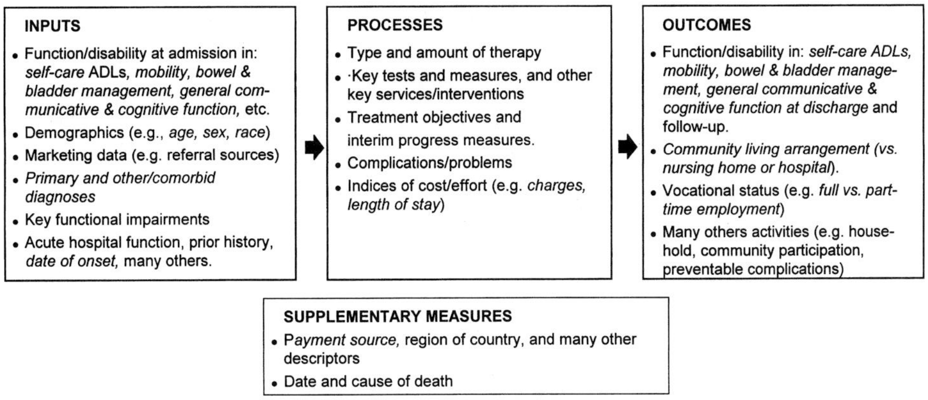

INPUTS	PROCESSES	OUTCOMES
• Function/disability at admission in: *self-care ADLs, mobility, bowel & bladder management, general communicative & cognitive function*, etc. • Demographics (e.g., *age, sex, race*) • Marketing data (e.g. referral sources) • *Primary and other/comorbid diagnoses* • Key functional impairments • Acute hospital function, prior history, *date of onset,* many others.	• Type and amount of therapy • ·Key tests and measures, and other key services/interventions • Treatment objectives and interim progress measures. • Complications/problems • Indices of cost/effort (e.g. *charges, length of stay*)	• Function/disability in: *self-care ADLs, mobility, bowel & bladder management, general communicative & cognitive function at discharge* and follow-up. • *Community living arrangement (vs. nursing home or hospital).* • Vocational status (e.g. *full vs. part-time employment*) • Many others activities (e.g. household, community participation, preventable complications)

SUPPLEMENTARY MEASURES
• *Payment source,* region of country, and many other descriptors
• Date and cause of death

Figure 54-3. Basic conventional framework for evaluation of rehabilitation programs. Items from the Inpatient Rehabilitation Facility-Patient Assessment Instrument (IRF-PAI) are shown in italics.

required by CARF standards. The person who does the measurement should also be specified.

• Establishment of expectancies—specific statements of the expected level or range for objective performance indicators. The classic PE model involves specifying a range of performance expectancies: minimal, optimal, and the maximal thought to be attainable under ideal circumstances. Outcomes were not to fall below the minimum. If they did, action was to be taken (71,72). Expectancies are commonly based on a combination of internal trends and targets, and where known, regional or national norms for the population of interest.

• Consideration of the relative importance of objectives. In the traditional PE model, program success was to be summarized in a single number. Actual objectives attained were multiplied by weights and expectancies chosen so that optimal attainment of outcome was signified by 100. The weighting system is no longer required by CARF, although concept of weighting outcomes may still be in use in some circumstances.

A drawback of this system was that when performance expectancies were not met, a common response was simply to change the expectancy. Even though accreditation standards allowed completely local measures and standards, the flimsiness of completely local, subjective expectancies has been recognized. Recognizing this, rehabilitation programs have voluntarily created regional and national outcomes data systems, beginning with the "Hospital Utilization Project" (HUP) in the 1970s and more recently the Uniform Data System, eRehabData, and other firms. The use of normative benchmarks is highly valuable to performance monitoring but provides a challenge when the available benchmark data do not correspond exactly to the program's objectives or population. Recognition of the need for severity adjustment based on shared data with other programs has grown. In sum, the evaluation, and especially the action component of the classic PE model, was weak, but the process has taught rehabilitation much about realistic outcome expectations.

OUTCOME MONITORING MODELS FOR DIFFERENT POPULATIONS

Patient populations need to be divided into major groups, usually by etiology or impairment group and functional severity. This is so important that we elaborate on methods of comparison and severity adjustment (e.g., "Function-Related Groups" or FRGs) below. Uncontrolled comparisons across facilities are rarely interpretable.

Reports to subscribers to shared data systems typically describe average functional outcomes or gain, percentages of patients discharged to home, and "efficiency" in terms of functional gain per day of stay or $1,000 charged. Follow-up data

services also can provide the subscribing program with indicators such as percent of patients who maintain functional status from discharge to follow-up, percent satisfied with various aspects of the program, percent who have been re-hospitalized since discharge, among others.

The most widely used set of rehabilitation performance indicators at present is found in the Inpatient Rehabilitation Facility-Patient Assessment Instrument (IRF-PAI) data set. This data set contains information on impairment group, functional independence at admission and discharge (FIM), and demographic information, and LOS. It is a general purpose dataset whose primary purpose is to categorize patients so that they can be grouped by estimate expense for the prospective payment system (PPS). For purposes of PE or clinical performance monitoring, however, the information system needs to be tailored to diagnostic and functional groups. References are available on how to tailor a PE system for:

• general inpatient medical rehabilitation, including stroke (12,64,81)
• SCI (12,64,82)
• traumatic brain injury (TBI) (14,15,17,45)
• chronic pain management programs (83)
• outpatient rehabilitation clinics (71)
• postacute community reentry (17,20,64) and vocational programs (17,64)
• other conditions requiring rehabilitation (64,84).

Materials on PE are being updated to reflect "outcomes management." Readers should contact CARF to obtain its most recent offerings.

Because inpatient rehabilitation programs must contend with numerous mixed-diagnosis cases, comorbidities, and rare diagnoses, mixed-diagnosis evaluation systems are a necessity if outcomes (and processes) are to be monitored for all patients. Functional improvement is a meaningful if imperfect way of quantifying the benefits in mixed-diagnosis groups. Mixed-diagnosis systems that focus on functional and handicap-level outcomes appear to be relatively successful for later stages of rehabilitation, including transitional living, community integration, vocational rehabilitation, and long-term nursing home care. Both function and diagnosis are critical in evaluation of processes and outcomes of inpatient, outpatient, and at-home medical rehabilitation programs.

ADDITIONAL DESIGN POINTS

Here are some additional points for design of outcomes monitoring systems:

• Cases that stay only a few days are not comparable to full-stay cases and need to be looked at as a separate group. Long-stay outliers also need to be examined.

- Outcomes monitoring systems center on episodes of illness rather than on administratively convenient units such as a stay in rehabilitation. Readmissions need to be collapsed or analyzed separately. Efficiency cannot be achieved by cycling difficult cases back and forth between facilities.
- Some rehabilitation programs distinguish between cases admitted for different reasons. Some patients, for instance, are admitted largely for care of certain medical-nursing problems that rehabilitation hospitals are particularly adept at treating (e.g., decubitus ulcers, urinary tract infections, weaning a patient from a ventilator). Incorporating measures relevant to the reasons for admission and for rehabilitative treatment enhances the meaningfulness of outcomes monitoring reports.

Outcomes Measurement

This section treats issues distinctive of measurement of *outcomes* for rehabilitation PE.

GENERALITY OF MEASURES

PE goals have been designed to credit the program with the larger benefits it produces, such as general independence from assistance (72). These goals are more general than treatment or case management objectives. Measures of long-term outcomes in the community are valuable for marketing and are ultimately needed for policy and accountability (73,74). Data on how a program has reduced the frequency with which patients are institutionalized in nursing homes and hospitals after discharge, for instance, are meaningful and even influential with boards of directors, government officials, insurers, families, and referral sources. While reports of such benefits are useful in communication of the benefits of rehabilitation to the public, more proximal outcome measures are usually more closely related to interventions and hence are more likely to be related to action to improve clinical processes.

TIMING OF OUTCOMES MEASUREMENT

Outcomes for persons served are best measured following discharge (72). Measurement at discharge is less expensive but may be less informative, as clinical staff are already aware of patient function at discharge. Information on durability of outcomes is valuable. Patterns of under-preparation, or of long stays by patients otherwise ready for discharge, should be actionable. Whatever time is chosen, data need to be obtained from all persons served or from a representative sampling (11).

There is no perfect time for follow-up, as there are contrasting advantages to both short-term and long-term follow-up. Three months has been the most common period for follow-up of rehabilitation outcomes, but periods of 1 to 6 months after discharge are also found. Rehabilitation involves enhancing healing and adaptation processes, so recovery processes should ideally be measured repeatedly over time.

PERFORMANCE VERSUS ABILITY

Primary outcomes should be measured in terms of actual patient performance rather than capability or other terms (64,72,84). This has long been the standard and usual practice, because actual performance is usually a more reliable and objective measure than judged ability and because frequently used skills tend to provide greater benefit than rarely used ones. Exceptions exist when dealing with performance capabilities that are important though infrequently needed (e.g., safety skills).

FOLLOW-UP METHODS

Longer-term outcomes are usually assessed by telephone calls or clinic visits. PE systems in rehabilitation have long employed telephone follow-up. A great deal of research has shown that telephone follow-up using structured questionnaires of demonstrated reliability and validity (59) provides a good balance of reliability, low rate of missing data, and modest-to-moderate costs. The number of self-report scales for assessing health and function with basic knowledge of reliability and validity is now large (12,13,48,50–55). In-clinic follow-up methods are required to objectively assess medical problems. Missing data, however, can be a problem if patients do not return for their follow-up visit in the clinic. Tele-rehabilitation technologies may improve our capacity to provide objective patient assessment following inpatient discharge.

Benchmarking Functional Outcomes

The availability of benchmarks or standards of comparison is, as introduced at the beginning of this chapter, basic to systematic QA and QI. While they may be obtained from many sources, including the published literature, contemporary benchmarks are most commonly obtained from shared data systems which pool data from a number of facilities. The typical outcomes benchmark in rehabilitation has been average functional outcome or gain for major diagnostic groups. Accurate adjustment for case mix and severity is essential for meaningful comparison of raw quality and outcome indicators across patient groups and programs.

SEVERITY ADJUSTMENT FOR FUNCTIONAL OUTCOMES

To compare a program's outcome or improvement scores to a benchmark, one should examine major factors that drive these scores. There are a number of factors that generically affect functional outcomes across many diagnostic groups in rehabilitation (12,37,62,85):

1. Functional severity at admission. Improvement may not be equally likely or meaningful across all levels of an admission measure. Some studies have reported curvilinear relationships, that is, greater improvement among patients admitted at intermediate levels of severity (37,85).
2. Chronicity (i.e., onset-admission interval). After the acute phase of many severe injuries, there is a period of relatively rapid recovery, followed by increasingly slow improvement and eventual asymptote, at least on a group basis. Control for natural history recovery curves is needed.
3. Length of stay (LOS). Improvement in rehabilitation tends to be correlated with LOS.
4. Differences in comorbidities, and severity of illness or injury (45). Differences in improvement across facilities may be due to differences in medical-nursing severity or case mix. Diagnostic complexity and comorbid conditions adversely affect outcomes and increase LOS in rehabilitation (86). Further development of indices and models of such factors is needed to identify patients with high medical-nursing needs and to establish clinically useful performance benchmarks for them.

Longitudinal research has identified relatively powerful outcome predictors within diagnostic groups. General severity of disease or impairment is typically a major predictor [e.g., severity of spinal paralysis and American Spinal Cord Injury Association (ASIS) motor scores in SCI (45), Glasgow Coma Scale and duration of unconsciousness or posttraumatic amnesia for TBI (48), severity of paralysis as measured by Fugl-Meyer

Motor Scores in stroke (87)]. Premorbid factors can be powerful predictors of long-term community outcomes after rehabilitation, even more powerful than severity of injury (e.g., 88). A great deal of research has been done on predictors of outcome following rehabilitation, and this research is applicable to quality-outcomes improvement.

There are several methods of case mix or severity adjustment for medical rehabilitation (89). As methods of risk or severity adjustment, all these are approximate and typically predict a minority of the variance of LOS or functional gain. Rankings of acute hospital outcomes are sensitive to the method of adjustment employed (90). One would expect similar results for rankings of rehabilitation hospitals by functional gain.

FUNCTION-RELATED GROUPS AND CASE MIX GROUPS

Function-Related Groups (FRGs based on the FIM) were developed to adjust inpatient medical rehabilitation caseload for case mix factors affecting LOS (91). Relabeled Case Mix Groups (CMGs), they are now used as a basis for Medicare prospective payment for patients admitted to inpatient rehabilitation programs in the United States. CMGs group patients based primarily upon admissions FIM and impairment group. Average LOS can be projected. FIM-FRGs predict about 31% of the variance of LOS in rehabilitation, which is similar to the performance of Diagnosis-Related Groups (DRGs) for acute hospital LOS. FRGs and CMGs are more detailed than previous PE systems that reported by broad etiologies. Strokes, for instance, were grouped into multiple diagnostic-functional subgroups (92). FRGs classify rehabilitation patients into groups which are more clinically homogeneous and interpretable than groupings by primary diagnosis alone. FIM-FRGs have been used to investigate the "efficiency" of rehabilitation, that is, the relationship of functional gain to cost or LOS (93).

The main use of FRGs/CMGs is as case-mix adjusters to identify groups whose costs are higher or lower than expected. They are used to identify patients concurrently whose LOS exceeds the average for the FRG. They are, however, potentially applicable to analysis of efficiency and QI in rehabilitation, defining patient groups whose gains in function are unexpectedly low given LOS (92,93). In contrast, European groups are developing "Rehabilitee Management Categories" and classifications of therapeutic services. These resemble FRGs in some ways, but TQM and quality standards (guidelines) are an explicit aim (94).

FUNCTIONAL GAIN AS AN INDICATOR OF QUALITY

It was once thought that functional gain—or at any rate, severity-adjusted gain in function—would provide a robust indicator of the quality of rehabilitation programs. While greater gain in function is undoubtedly desirable and better outcome is the sine qua non of quality, research connecting functional gain of actual ongoing rehabilitation programs to indicators of care processes or program characteristics is scarce. Recent, relatively large studies have failed to find an appreciable correlation between staffing intensity and other characteristics of inpatient rehabilitation programs and severity-adjusted functional gain (85). Functional outcomes and LOS, however, are relatively predictable, and managed care clearly constrained LOS in rehabilitation hospitals. "Relationships between rehabilitation practices and functional gains by patients do not appear to be either simple or overt" (85). With continued research, one may expect that reliable connections will be identified between characteristics of certain kinds of rehabilitation programming and certain severity-adjusted outcomes for selected patient groups. Knowledge of such connections is essential to QA and QI.

MEASUREMENT AND STATISTICS: SUMMARY

Medical rehabilitation has reached agreement on basic typical domains for inpatient programs (e.g., mobility and self-care ADLs in the FIM), but measures of other critical domains still have to be developed or agreed-upon (e.g., measures of treatment objectives clearly linked to therapies prescribed, extended or instrumental ADLs, ecologically valid measures of communicative and cognitive outcomes, family and environmental factors (45,48,50,59). Methods of statistical control for severity of disease, comorbid conditions, and of environmental factors that affect outcomes have been inadequately developed.

Outcomes Management

The term "outcomes management" has become increasingly popular. The term is loosely associated with outcomes measurement, PE, case management, and managed care (84). Paul Ellwood provided the original conceptualization of outcomes management as "a technology of patient experience designed to help patients, payers, and providers make rational medical care-related choices based on better insight into the effect of these choices on the patient's life" (95). Outcomes management is based on the increasingly scientific basis of medical care, including the increasing ability to predict outcomes and on advances in measurement of health and function at the level of patient experience rather than at the level of mortality or disease rates. Professional analyses of huge, population-based databases were to provide estimates of the effectiveness and efficiency of medical services in practice. Rather general outcomes measures were to be used, so implications would be primarily at the aggregate level—for systems of intervention or programs rather than for management of individual patients.

The term "outcomes management" has also been used to refer to systems that manage individual patients. We define a *clinical outcomes management system* as a system that involves routine monitoring of the treatment objectives for individual patients and indicators of patient responsiveness to treatments. Clinical outcomes management, as defined here, differs from traditional PE in that standard goals are not routinely applied mechanically across a group but are modified to fit the individual. Treatment objectives and outcomes need to be risk-adjusted, necessitating a computerized system. Objective measures are possible for important, high-frequency objectives and outcomes.

CARF's *Standards Manual* treats information and outcomes management in very general terms:

> Information is gathered and analyzed to measure and manage outcomes. The information gathered is relevant to the core values and mission of the organization and to the needs of all stakeholders. Analyzed information is used to improve performance in a variety of areas. It is the responsibility of the organization to share relevant information with stakeholders at a frequency that meets their needs. The information shared with stakeholders accurately reflects the performance of the organization and considers the requests and input of stakeholders. (11, p. 50)

CARF has fostered a process of discussion toward indicators for rehabilitation outcomes management (96), but reflecting uncertainty in the field, has not specified details (11).

Outcomes management in medical rehabilitation involves four techniques:

1. The use of treatment guidelines (or standards) to help clinical professionals to evaluate patients and choose appropriate treatments.

2. Routine and systematic measurement of both indicators of disease and of patients' functioning, health, and well-being, and of changes in these related to the likely effects of treatments.
3. Combining data on inputs (severity), processes, and outcomes into large databases to permit scientific analyses.
4. Analysis and dissemination of results in a form useful to different stakeholders.

The term "outcomes management" has sometimes been used to imply regulation of outcomes to an unrealistic degree. While quality rehabilitation enhances a patient's likely recovery and adaptation, an exact level of outcomes cannot generally be manufactured.

Although U.S. health care as a whole is far from operationalizing Ellwood's grand vision for outcomes management, elements of it are being implemented on a piecemeal basis as integrated health organizations create their own clinical databases and smaller organizations voluntarily join health outcomes databases. Rehabilitation, with its long experience with outcomes-oriented PE systems, should be ready to operationalize outcomes management.

CARF Performance Indicators

CARF has historically been oriented toward outcomes, but CARF standards increasingly use the term "performance indicator." CARF has worked to develop performance indicators for medical and other rehabilitation programs, at least since its Quality and Accountability Initiative in 1996 (96). This work has evolved on the basis of concerns of major stakeholders to the rehabilitation process, including not only providers but also payers, researchers, and persons receiving rehabilitation services. Core questions have been addressed: What does a stakeholder want to know about a program's performance in order to assess its quality and choose among programs? How should these concerns be quantified? Key concerns and draft indicators have been identified for further indicator development.

Many of the proposed indicators are outcomes-oriented (96). Outcome concerns include: percentage of clients reporting improvement after service provision; durability of outcomes; functional gain; increased productivity, participation, and activities; reduced impairment and disability; satisfaction with processes of care; satisfaction with results of care; QOL after care; efficiency concerns; reduced downstream costs; and value (outcome relative to cost). Examples of possible outcome indicators include:

- for "durability of outcomes"—percent of persons in a program who maintain or increase level of motor function from discharge to follow-up; or percent of persons who have not been rehospitalized for the same impairment within 6 months of discharge.
- for "satisfaction with results of care"—percent of persons with mobility impairments who respond "satisfied" or "very satisfied" to the question "How satisfied are you with the amount you are able to move around outside following your rehabilitation?"

Structure and process indicators are also proposed:

- Structure concerns—types and numbers of persons served, staff credentials and education, legal status of organization, accreditation status.
- Process concerns—cost and resource use, communication effectiveness, involvement of persons served in rehab decisions, collaboration of providers with payers.

Specific performance indicators and dataset are not yet required by 2002–2003 CARF standards, and CARF does not endorse or specify any particular measure, tool, or vendor for outcomes management or PE. The information systems of many existing rehabilitation programs provide possible indicators of the concerns identified. Indicators and measures need to be specified in such a way that stakeholders can know they are looking at comparable information from different programs (96).

CARF's indicators are a good beginning and serve as a guide for the kinds of indicators needed, although they are not yet fully developed or implemented. More knowledge of their validity in practice—that is, demonstrations that they can be used as tools to improve performance—is needed.

Critique of PE and Outcomes Management

The standard PE model has a number of strengths. It provides an overview of primary patient outcomes, progress, and cost. If used with a shared national or regional data system, standard PE systems provide an index or benchmark of the effectiveness of the program in improving patient function and placing patients in community settings. Efficiency, or at least an operational utilization review system, is demonstrated if the facility shows a direct correlation between cost or LOS and improvement (37,71), and if improvement/day rates are similar to those in other rehabilitation facilities for similar diagnostic-functional groups. PE data have numerous administrative and clinical uses (84). PE systems have begun to tell us whether rehabilitation programs attain an outcome for their patients.

Dissatisfaction with the traditional PE model has grown over time. The main problem has been that PE systems have not provided staff with the specific information they need to improve program operations or outcomes within budgetary constraints. The tie between functional improvement, typically reported in PE, and the real effectiveness of treatment has remained weak. The necessary construct validation work to develop ties between set measures and inferences of effective rehabilitative interventions has not been done. Controlled studies are needed to validate the theoretical and causal basis for such inferences.

When "expectancies" for outcome gain in PE systems are not met, the usual response has been to change the expectancy rather than take action to improve the system of care. While such changes in expectations are undoubtedly self-serving and convenient, they are not unreasonable. Admission of more severe patients is probably the most common reason for declines in outcomes, though reductions in resources and the subsequent elimination of large components of the rehabilitation team process (e.g., social work, vocational rehabilitation) may also be suspected. Since these patients probably also needed care, action implications have been unclear. These problems remain regardless of whether the approach is labeled "PE", "outcomes management", or "performance monitoring. "Regardless of rubric, the basic concerns remain the same: whether the program is effective—that is, whether participants benefit—and how effectiveness can be improved.

There has been a contradiction between the design of most outcomes monitoring systems in medical rehabilitation and the audience they have had. Conventional PE systems are designed to give an overview of program outcomes. They provide data that, if pooled and analyzed at a nationwide level, could be valuable for identifying systems and strategies of care that best help persons with disabilities. The basic measure set constitutes a useful summative evaluation system for many patient groups. The audience for most PE systems, however, has been internal clinical staff, who already know roughly what is happening to their patients and need more detailed measures and insightful analyses to help them give better care within realistic constraints. PE and outcomes monitoring systems in medical rehabilitation are often not used because they are designed for public accountability, yet the public and even researchers often do not have access to the data. Solutions to this problem will involve continuing access to data by researchers to enable the needed in-depth analyses and the development of methods of connecting processes to intermediate- and long-term outcomes. These strategies, involving indicators of implementation of treatment guidelines and "second-stage screens" (24), are discussed later in this chapter.

QUALITY ASSESSMENT AND IMPROVEMENT

To ensure quality in medical care, it should meet standards that are in some sense predefined (35,97,98). Although efforts to systematically ensure quality in medical care go back to the first quarter of the 20th century, pressure for accountability has increased in recent decades, driven by explosive growth of costs, and by higher expectations of medical care (97). The federal government and the JCAHO have been major institutional forces behind hospital-care quality assessment and improvement in general. In rehabilitation, CARF has played an important role in defining and improving quality (11). This section will begin by discussing TQM and CQI techniques and their application to medical rehabilitation. Discussion of professional QI terminology and then JCAHO accreditation will follow.

TQM and CQI in Healthcare

An important insight of TQM and CQI (26,27), based on experience, is this: Quality and effectiveness primarily depend on the routine system. The root causes of problems are more commonly at the level of the system or of sequences of care processes than at the level of individuals or even single departments. The causes of error or undesirable variation in the sequence of activities must be identified and rooted out. The aim is to improve systems, not to blame individuals. Improved protocols for activities and processes need to be developed and implemented as a key element of QI (29,99). Global organizational commitment is the dominant requirement (26,29,30). The philosophy has moved health care toward improving routine processes.

In practice TQM and CQI emphasizes knowledge of effective processes and involvement of the staff directly involved in the process. They involve fact finding, emphasize prevention of problems, and use measures of processes or of shorter- or longer-term results, depending on the problem. In Deming's terms, "profound knowledge"—detailed, expert, first-hand understanding—of what is really happening in the organization and of the complex processes involved in producing a product are required to improve quality; knowledge of "general variation" (i.e., statistics and scientific measures) alone is insufficient (26,27,100). The emphasis is on understanding of the total system and involvement of everyone to diagnose, to plan, and to fix problems or improve systems. Both the specific problem and systems in which it is embedded need attention. CQI emphasizes review of systems and sequences rather than discrete inspections (25). One must acquire deep and broad knowledge about the system, not just identify errors or outliers as in traditional QA. When variation outside normally observed limits occurs, knowledge of the system is needed to infer the cause and mend problematic processes.

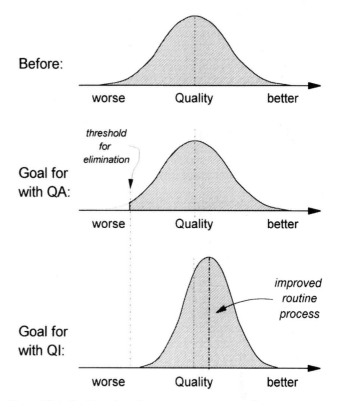

Figure 54-4. Traditional quality assurance versus quality improvement.

To improve medical care, knowledge of diagnosis and treatment alternatives as well as an evidence basis is required. *Clinical practice guidelines* are, if well-developed and based on evidence, invaluable tools for QA and QI; so valuable that we treat them separately in the following sections below. Guidelines need to be integrated with and adapted to actual team processes to assure and improve the quality and effectiveness of care.

The superior effectiveness of improving routine processes, compared to simply trying to eliminate the worse problems or the worst performers, is graphically displayed in Figure 54-4. This conventional display assumes that measured quality or results are distributed normally. An approach aimed at eliminating unacceptably poor care would, if successful, eliminate poor care for only a small fraction of patients (the small left tail of the distribution). An approach aimed as improving the process of care and eliminating inappropriate variations in the process (bottom of Fig. 54-4) would improve results for most patients. As a by-product, the fraction of results or care which is clearly below the old threshold is also greatly diminished.

As with CQI in other industries, the majority of problems, especially remediable ones, in medical settings are most likely problems with systems or procedures rather than the incompetence of individuals. Many works give examples of systems problems (e.g., in nursing care or the hospital pharmacy) (1,25,101). In contrast, the claims history of individual physicians, for instance, only weakly predicts future claims proneness, so use of such data to target individual physicians is scientifically problematic (102). Malpractice claims data have been used to identify problem-prone clinical processes and to suggest improvements to reduce the likelihood of negligence (41).

Another insight is that QA systems that *depend* on mass inspection of discrepancies in outcomes are often ineffective or inefficient (25,29). If QA simply counts errors and points them out to staff, QA can be perceived as an unpleasant policing activity, and the substantial effort to detect outcome anomalies may not be paralleled by efforts to improve production or treatment processes. The problem is not that outcome measures are wrong, but in how they are used: data should function as scoreboards for team efforts to improve their own processes (27). Multiple statistical approaches are needed, including process and outcome measures to both identify defects and verify improvements. CQI integrates knowledge, processes, at least short-term outcomes, and action to improve them.

The literature now reports many examples of successful system improvement in health care organizations, especially hospitals. Limited quantitative evidence of effectiveness exists (103), but CQI and TQM are difficult to test as they transcend any particular setting or method. TQM has often been implemented by managers and applied to administrative organization so that clinicians have difficulty seeing its use to improve clinical processes. CQI/TQM teams led by clinical professionals may have a different experience.

Experience has shown that approaches to quality and outcomes improvement from manufacturing or provision of hotel services need major modifications to be applied to health care. Patients are not uniform material input to a manufacturing process, and customer satisfaction is not the only, or even the primary, relevant outcome in health care. The response of patients to treatments is hardly as predictable as the response of physical material to manufacturing processes. Rather than being assumed or predicted on the basis of processes, patient responses to treatment must be tested in controlled research and monitored in practice. Comorbid conditions and idiosyncratic patient characteristics and needs alter ordinary patterns of treatment and response. "Context" has fundamental effects on activity therapies in rehabilitation (104). The principle of reducing variance in processes is relevant to parts of rehabilitation, but quality rehabilitation also involves the tailoring of treatments to the priority needs of the individual.

Professional QI Terminology

A few basic terms assist in professional assessment and improvement (97,105). *Norms* are measures of actual clinical practice. Examples are average LOS, average improvement in FIM scores, and average hours of physical therapy (PT). Norms are most clinically useful when they are specific to a patient diagnosis or otherwise graded to patient characteristics. *Benchmarks* apply to processes as well as outcomes. Rehabilitation professionals need to have benchmarks against which to compare their staffing, education, costs, initial evaluation, intervention types and intensities, patient satisfaction, and short-term outcomes as well as long term ones. Norms and benchmarks have greater authority when they are based on large samples or when they tell us what is done and achievable by the "best" or at least better programs.

Criteria are statements that define appropriate or correct clinical care (97,106). Criteria are typically developed on the basis of professional experience and scientific literature. Some distinguish between a criterion and a *standard* (107), using the former as the more general dimension and the latter as the specific numeric cut-point. We will not rigidly distinguish the two, because a general dimension separate from a quantitative decision point is of little use (97). For instance, the statement that "stroke patients will have a blood level of Coumadin in the therapeutic range" is useless without specification of what the range is (e.g., prothrombin time of 1.2 to 1.5 × control). An-

other example of a criterion or standard is the assertion that inpatients in medical rehabilitation should receive 3 hours per day of PT, OT, and SLP treatment combined. Criteria and standards may describe structure, process, or outcome, and in practice involve all three.

Sentinel Events

In practice, action to maintain quality of care frequently depends on *sentinel events* (108)—single occurrences that are highly problematic or socially unacceptable. Litigation following patient injury, staff quitting over unacceptable quality or ethical issues, and cockroaches on the walls are not definitive evidence of global quality problems, but they should motivate a review to determine whether there are remediable problems. Sentinel events require a response. The point of systematic QI is to go beyond concern for negative outliers alone. Maintaining quality care requires conservative, proactive processes to avoid embarrassment or worse.

An *indicator condition* is a frequent, treatable clinical situation (97,100). In JCAHO terms, an *indicator* is a specific instrument to measure an aspect of care to guide the assessment of performance (109). Clinical indicators point to clinical processes or procedures that need further analysis to determine if improvements can be made. Improved clinical procedures should lead to improved outcomes.

A *threshold* indicates a preestablished point in an *indicator* that should trigger more in-depth investigation to determine whether a problem or opportunity to improve care exists (97). Action should follow to actually improve the system of care. As an example, a threshold of 5% might be set for rehabilitation patients discharged back to acute care and 15% to a nursing home. In the past, thresholds have been either rather arbitrary or set by expert judgment; some have suggested statistical criteria (97,110,111). The JCAHO has had difficulty in setting and implementing thresholds. Benchmarks based on both regional and local experience are needed to set thresholds.

There are situations where a 0% or 100% threshold is needed (112). For sentinel events, such as death or suicide within rehabilitation or within 7 days of discharge, a threshold of 0% would be justifiable: every case needs to be individually reviewed. In general, however, a threshold of 100% success or 0% problems is unrealistic. Setting thresholds at less-than-perfect levels avoids disproportionate use of time to evaluate a few discrepant cases that will probably be found to be clinically justified (97,113). QI in rehabilitation usually requires discrimination and amelioration of frequently occurring or significant problems, not undiscriminating compulsiveness.

The term "monitor" has been commonly used to describe any routinely collected measure on a group of patients. Staff engaged in activities to improve or oversee care *monitor* aspects of these processes or their outcomes. Because formal indicators have yet to be validated, QI efforts for rehabilitation must be undertaken with the use of ad hoc monitors. Specific JCAHO indicators are discussed below.

Statistical Issues

Statistical control principles are as relevant to quality monitoring as outcomes monitoring. Sample size needs to be specified to set a threshold in QI. A 20% rate of apparent error with 5 patients is very different from the same rate with 50 patients. Patient groups for which indicators are applied must be well defined. Interpretation of process and intermediate outcomes data is greatly facilitated by severity adjustment, just as with monitoring of long-term outcomes.

JCAHO Approaches and Standards

JCAHO standards have evolved over the years, and there are lessons in this evolution. Structural and process indicators of quality were first propounded. Care had to be provided by licensed practitioners with certain staffing patterns and authority relationships. Extensive record keeping, facility, and equipment standards were prescribed. Although certain structural indicators have been retained today, emphasis has shifted. The aim now is to improve the actual provision of high-quality, effective care, not just to assure the capacity to do so.

In past decades (1950s through 1970s), great reliance was placed on peer review, methodologies for which became increasingly elaborate and focused. Although peer review methods remain useful in certain circumstances, the method came to face increasing criticism. There was little evidence that it improved the actual process or effectiveness of care provided, although it did improve medical records. Current health data systems also face the challenge of proving that they improve care and outcomes rather than record keeping.

Ideas of objective indicators or monitoring, introduced into JCAHO standards during the 1980s, are now increasingly operationalized in terms of systems of standardized severity-adjusted, objective performance indicators (97), arbitrarily labeled ORYX. Only implicit standards and thresholds exist for many conditions in rehabilitation, but the movement is clearly and strongly toward objective ones.

In the past (before 1992), standards were organized around departments and services, distinguished processes and outcomes, and defined specific leadership responsibilities. Influenced by TQM and CQI, the departmental focus was deemphasized, and the chapter on "Improving Organizational Performance" treats both quality and outcomes issues. "Quality assessment and improvement" was replaced by "quality assurance" in the 1992 Accreditation Manual for Hospitals (AMH). JCAHO now emphasizes continuous improvement of organizational performance, the identification of processes that most significantly impact care effectiveness or patient outcomes, their improvement, and integration of systems and processes across departments and functions.

CURRENT STANDARDS

JCAHO standards today emphasize care processes as well as structure. Objective indicators of care processes and linked indicators of care effectiveness (outcomes) are increasingly required. Current JCAHO standards relate to care and assessment of patients, patient education, consistency across the continuum of care, environment of care, management of human resources (staff competency assessment and training), management of information, infection control, patient rights and organizational ethics, leadership, governance, nursing care, medical care, and improving organizational performance (35). The JCAHO evaluates quality of care in terms of:

- *what* is done—the degree to which care is *appropriate* and *efficacious* for the patient, and *how well* it is done—the degree to which care is *available* in a *timely* manner, is *safe and effective*, is *respectful and caring*, and is *continuous* with other care.

Continuous efforts to maintain and improve quality are to be made. Performance improvement should be embedded throughout the organization.

The chapter "Improving Organizational Performance" expresses much of the philosophy of CQI and TQM, without losing sight of the ultimate purpose of improving patient outcomes. The JCAHO requires that "the leaders establish a

planned, systematic, organization-wide approach to process design and performance measurement, analysis and improvement" (35, p. 1). The performance improvement plan is to be based on the organization's mission, vision, and values. The plan is to reduce variation in processes and outcomes, to increase patient satisfaction, decrease or control the cost per patient, and increase the effectiveness of information management. Performance improvement efforts should be prioritized according to: (a) expected impact on performance; (b) high-risk, high-volume, or problem-prone processes; (c) relationship of potential improvement to JCAHO dimensions; and (d) organizational resources.

There are several methods that health care organizations can use to implement performance improvement consistent with JCAHO. These methods include a 10-step method outlined by JCAHO in the past and the Deming cycle or the Plan-Do-Check-Act (PDCA) methodology (114). The Focus PDCA method specifies (F) finding a process to improve, (O) organizing a team, (C) clarifying the current knowledge, and (U) uncovering root cause of variation, before (S) starting the PDCA cycle. These methods include the following (35):

- *Plan.* Planning is a multidisciplinary, includes input from relevant stakeholders, and includes an understanding of the current process and outcomes.
- *Implement.* Implementation involves developing potential solutions, benchmarking best practices, and pilot testing new processes.
- *Check.* New processes and processes that involve risks must be monitored and measured. To measure performance, a hospital collects data on: processes; outcomes; a comprehensive set of performance measures (indicators); high-risk, high-volume, and problem-prone processes; and other sensors of performance.
- *Assessment.* Assessment is defined as transforming data into information by analyzing it (35). Benchmark data, trends over time, and adherence to regulatory requirements are all useful in determining whether a process improvement has been successful. Appropriate statistical quality control techniques are to be used.
- *Improve.* Once improvements have been realized, process changes need to be standardized and gains maintained.

Regardless of how many detailed steps are counted, measurement of processes and results is to be embedded into the total, continuous process of action to maintain and improve quality.

JCAHO has defined general elements of inpatient rehabilitation (e.g., a requirement for assessment of "functional rehabilitation status") (standard tx.6, 35). Detailed standards and indicators for inpatient or outpatient medical rehabilitation programs have not been established at the time of this writing, but standards and indicators for related areas of health care may be informative [e.g., standards manuals for home medical equipment, respiratory therapy and rehabilitation technology (115), ORYX indicators for home care (116)].

DATA COLLECTION RECOMMENDATIONS AND STANDARDS

JCAHO considers measurement and data collection to be the foundation for performance improvement activities (35). The organization's leadership is responsible for establishing an information system to monitor quality-related events. JCAHO requires that organizations (35):

1. collect data to monitor performance
2. aggregate and analyze their data on an ongoing basis

3. compare performance over time with other sources of information.

Arbitrary thresholds and standards particular to a program are not enough. Benchmark values may come from an external multifacility database, the published research literature, and other sources.

To maximize the impact of limited resources, QI and data collection efforts should focus on high-volume, high-risk, and problem-prone processes. Additional foci include:

- patient outcomes (e.g., functional improvement in rehabilitation)
- targeted areas of study (e.g., a new or redesigned process)
- comprehensive performance measures
- client needs, expectations, and feedback (e.g., patient satisfaction)
- infection control measures (e.g., urinary tract infection rates)
- safety of the environment (e.g., hazard surveillance monitoring)
- quality control and risk management indicators (e.g., medication incidents, patient falls).

Indicator sets to operationalize the domains are in varying stages of development, discussed below.

JCAHO has developed more stringent patient safety standards in recent years. Prevention of errors is a major focus. Effective in 2002, health care organizations were mandated to perform at least two Failure Mode and Effect Analyses (FMEA) annually (35). An FMEA analysis is similar to a root cause analysis, but is proactive rather than reactive. For example, rather than reacting to a sentinel event, an FMEA analysis is performed before a negative outcome occurs. The organization first identifies a high-risk process (e.g., maintaining security of medication carts) or population (e.g., admitting and monitoring ventilator-dependent patients). "Sentinel Event Alerts," published by JCAHO, may be used to identify patients or processes at high risk. The next potential "failure modes" or hazards are identified, and the process is redesigned to minimize potential risk.

PERFORMANCE INDICATORS

JCAHO has devoted considerable attention to developing and identifying appropriate performance measurement sets or systems. Difficulties have been encountered, and development continues after more than a decade of work. Priority was given to high-volume, high-risk, or problematic clinical practices. Most performance indicators developed thus far are short-term clinical indicators for acute medical conditions rather than long-term outcomes, structure, or processes measures. Indicators developed have been subsumed into what is now called the ORYX initiative (described below). Health care organizations are required to send data to an approved data organization on a continuing basis.

JCAHO's *National Library of Healthcare Indicators* describes over 200 measures of clinical conditions, functional health status, or satisfaction in a standard format (109). Key hospital-wide processes—infection control and prevention of medication errors—have been a special focus. The Agency for Health Care Research and Quality now operates the National Quality Measures Clearinghouse (http://www.qualitymeasures.ahrq.gov/) and distributes a database (CONQUEST 2.0) that describes numerous sets of performance indicators for many important clinical conditions and settings (117). In these listings, single measures are becoming the exception: sets of measures—specifying very specific patient groups or subgroupings of patients,

processes, and outcome indicators—are required to evaluate quality.

According to JCAHO, three types of performance indicators are acceptable: (a) "clinical indicators," (b) health status scales, and (c) patient perceptions of care and service. Clinical indicators evaluate processes or proximal outcomes of care and must be condition-specific, procedure-specific, or address important functions of patient care (e.g., medication use, infection control). Health status scales may address health in general or in relation to specific patient conditions. Patient perceptions and reports are also accepted, including patient satisfaction with services, effectiveness of pain management, adequacy of information and education provided, and perceived changes in health.

Core Measures

JCAHO has been developing a standardized set of consensus and evidence-based "core measures" or indicators to be compared across health care organizations. An initial set of core indicators was developed and tested for certain conditions commonly seen in acute care hospitals, including acute myocardial infarction, heart failure, community-acquired pneumonia, pregnancy, and related conditions. It is anticipated that core measures will be developed for rehabilitation facilities in the future.

ORYX

Performance indicators accepted by JCAHO are given their ORYX seal of approval. There are now over 200 performance measurement systems with over 8,000 indicators, and the number increases regularly (http://www.jcaho.com/pms/oryx/index.htm). Qualified performance measurement systems have transmitted their data to the JCAHO since 1999. Health care organizations are required to select a number of measures (currently, 6) and to report their data to JCAHO on a quarterly basis. Since 2000, JCAHO surveyors have been provided with organization-specific presurvey reports, with ORYX data, to use during the accreditation survey. More standardized, evidence-based "core measures" are being developed to enable more rigorous comparisons. The long project of development and validation of indicators, still underway, should ultimately enable accreditation decisions to be based more directly on the actual performance of the health care organizations.

INDICATORS FOR REHABILITATION

JCAHO standards describe rehabilitation outcomes in general terms as involving "improvement ... of ... functioning, self-care, self-responsibility, independence and quality of life" (35, standard tx.6.5, p. tx.7). Actual rehabilitation-specific indicators, however, are still under development. Many of the indicators discussed above, such as satisfaction with care, infection control, and medication monitoring are also appropriate to medical rehabilitation (118,119). Quality indicators for nursing practice are becoming increasingly well defined, with available benchmarks (120).

The Functional Independence Measure (FIM) is currently an accepted health status measure for rehabilitation. Rehabilitation facilities currently submit FIM data as indicators (e.g., change in FIM score from admission to discharge). FIM scores at discharge, LOS, and number of days from onset to admission might also be submitted. The rate of unplanned program interruptions, acute hospital discharges, and discharges to nursing homes might also be employed as problem indicators, as they have been employed for decades in rehabilitation PE.

Comprehensive rehabilitation is required, at minimum, to meet the most frequently encountered physical and psychosocial needs of the patient. The services of physical rehabilitation encompass rehabilitation medicine, rehabilitation nursing, PT, OT, SLP, psychology, and social work or case management. Older JCAHO publications have discussed quality monitoring, goals, and evaluation for specific physical rehabilitation service departments (121). Possible "monitors" for physical rehabilitation services have included: increase in self-care ADLs, mobility, reduction in pain, patient satisfaction with services overall and with specific aspects of services (e.g., satisfaction with fit and functioning of prosthetic and orthotic services); cognitive and emotional adaptation of the patient and family to disability; improvement in communication skills; health maintenance; and reduction or prevention of preventable complications commonly seen in the impairment group. Such goals and indicators resemble the objectives and goals in PE systems in medical rehabilitation. A difference is that PE goals were typically for the entire program or a broad diagnostic group rather than for a clinically well-defined group of patients. Interdisciplinary team objectives are preferable to departmental goals where such a team is routinely critical to achievement of outcomes for the patient. In comprehensive rehabilitation, the attainment of functional goals for the patient typically involves such a team.

Guidelines and Evidence-Based Practice

The movement to develop clinical practice guidelines and the closely associated movement toward evidence-based medicine (EBM) or evidence-based clinical practice has continued to grow. *Clinical practice guidelines*—also called *care protocols or practice parameters*—are standardized, explicit descriptions of how patients should be evaluated and treated in different circumstances. EBM attempts to provide clinical professionals, patients, and policy makers with the information they need to make decisions based on the best evidence available. Both EBM and guidelines involve synthesis of the best available clinical (efficacy) evidence to inform decisions about patient care. Guidelines aim to define standard clinical practice for commonly seen and well-understood patient problems. The main purpose of guidelines is to improve clinical practice. Because they explicitly define standards of care, guidelines development is intrinsic to performance monitoring and improvement.

Guidelines should include enough detail to specify ordinarily appropriate decisions and processes. They typically involve a sequence of initial measures, alternative clinical processes, at least some decision rules, and subsequent assessment of patient responsiveness or clinical outcome. Well-developed guidelines are designed to be more clearly applicable to clinical practice than review articles, and should be based on evidence of assured, standard quality (122). Guidelines should be sufficiently developed so that they are useful for clinical education.

Clinical paths are similar to guidelines but tend to be less detailed. *Critical paths* also are typically simpler and oriented toward administrative issues, such as controlling LOS. A critical path, for instance, might specify that a swallowing evaluation for stroke patients and a PT evaluation occur no later than the second day after admission. A clinical guideline or path would go further, describing the nature of the evaluation, the differing interventions needed depending on differing patient characteristics, and how patient responses (clinical outcomes) are to be measured and evaluated.

Bases for Guidelines

High-quality guidelines are developed using increasingly standardized, formal methods of synthesizing information from expert judgment as well as from research studies (123). The combination of systematic evidence review and expert consensus can result in an authoritative and reliable guideline which can give clinicians greater confidence in making treatment decisions (124). Randomized clinical trials (RCTs) are the most widely accepted standard for evaluation of treatments. When strong evidence of treatment effectiveness is synthesized into guidelines, clinical applicability is clear.

In early stages of the guideline movement, it was felt that quality would be improved by reducing variation in care provided (99). While variation in practice remains an important consideration, evidence basis is even more important. Guidelines without adequate scientific basis may merely codify custom and inhibit innovation. In the absence of evidence, one does not know whether the average represents optimal care.

Direct evidence for the effectiveness of many types of rehabilitative care is limited, but relevant RCTs and a larger number of less highly controlled studies do exist, with the strength of evidence varying across diagnostic groups and interventions (19,125). Synthesizing evidence of the effectiveness of rehabilitation is not a simple chore, as rehabilitation employs and adapts interventions from allied fields, making the total amount of relevant knowledge large. Interventions based on learning and physical conditioning surely "work," as do many environmental modifications, prostheses, orthoses, nursing interventions, and pharmaceutical interventions from general medical care (19). Reviews (e.g., by the Cochrane Collaboration http://www.cochrane.org), metaanalyses, and textbooks provide a useful basis for defining quality of care and understanding outcomes. Well-developed clinical practice guidelines make such evidence more clinically usable and authoritative (18,99, 119).

GUIDELINES FOR COMMON CONDITIONS

Initially led by the Institute of Medicine and the Agency for Health Care Policy and Research (now the Agency for Health Care Quality and Research), work to develop clinical practice guidelines and similar clinical paths and practice parameters has spread throughout the health care industry (99). Thousands of clinical practice guidelines have been developed. An outstanding current source for these is the National Guidelines Clearinghouse (http://www.guideline.gov/). At the time of this writing the site lists 102 guidelines relevant to medical rehabilitation (excluding psychiatric and substance use rehabilitation, purely preventive guidelines, non-reconstructive plastic surgery and dental problems, and developmental learning disorders). Some of the more relevant guidelines listed here include those for:

- poststroke rehabilitation (126)
- several pain syndromes, including low back problems
- medical complications following SCI, including depression, autonomic dysreflexia, and prevention of thromboembolism
- brain injuries (an authoritative National Institutes of Health review, but so general it should hardly be called a guideline)
- cardiac rehabilitation (127)
- treatment of lower-limb osteoarthritis, with rehabilitative implications [as with other guidelines, they vary in quality and use (128)]
- deep vein thrombosis
- treatment of depression in primary care
- treatment of pressure ulcers (129) and their prediction and prevention (130)
- acute and chronic management of urinary incontinence (131)
- fall prevention
- exercise and strength training

- several other neurological and neuromusculoskeletal conditions.

Other sources also provide information on guidelines, critical paths, and related forms for medical rehabilitation (132,133).

The strengths and limitations of guidelines in medical rehabilitation can be better understood by discussion of guidelines on which implementation research has been done.

LESSONS FROM STROKE GUIDELINES

Developing and implementing guidelines in stroke rehabilitation is particularly difficult, given the multiplicity of presenting problems and consequent complexity of needed treatment. This very complexity, however, is typical of patient management in rehabilitation. Stroke is also the most frequently seen diagnostic group in inpatient rehabilitation hospitals in the United States. For these reasons, stroke guidelines may be of particular interest.

Implementation of astute clinical pathways under a skilled physiatrist has been shown to reduce LOS while reducing complications in acute stroke care, but rehabilitation is another matter, being even more complex (134). One randomized trial has compared an explicit clinical pathway with traditional team rehabilitation of stroke (135). The pathway resulted in no advantage in either cost or patient gains; it even decreased patient satisfaction. An explanation was that stroke rehabilitation is highly developed and routinized, though complex, and the path merely codified existing practice. The simple pathway seemed time-consuming to the team and sometimes also seemed insensitive to priorities. In a clinical trial results depend as much on the control group as on the experimental group. In stroke rehabilitation, interdisciplinary teams, addressing issues of feasible functional gain and outstanding remediable medical problems, are well established, and it would appear to be difficult to write guidelines that improve functional gain, complication rates, patient satisfaction, and LOS attained by existing experienced, coordinated rehabilitation teams. Guidelines for such care will need to be complex, and provisions need to be made for variations in clinical priorities depending on patient needs.

The Agency for Health Care Policy and Research's guideline for stroke rehabilitation (126) attempted to explicate the complex practice of stroke rehabilitation. The limited evidence basis for many practices was a problem; most recommendations were based on expert opinion. Nonetheless, there is evidence of their validity. Closer adherence to stroke rehabilitation guidelines is associated with greater functional recovery (136) and patient satisfaction (137) in a Veterans' Administration study. The placement algorithm, however, which attempts to specify which patients should receive rehabilitation, and if so, where and what type, is of variable reliability (138).

IMPLEMENTATION AND IMPACT OF GUIDELINES ON PRACTICE

Research on the impact of guidelines on clinical practice and outcomes is emerging. Initial hopes that guidelines would greatly improve the quality of medical care, improving health outcomes and constraining the growth of medical care expenditures as a whole, have been dashed. Many guidelines appear to have been little used after publication. Adherence to evidence-based guidelines is often suboptimal.

Researchers have documented 30% reduction in adverse events from antibiotics, a 27% decline in mortality, and decreased costs when using computer programs that help physi-

cians choose antibiotic treatment (139). A detailed treatment protocol for mechanical ventilation can reduce unwarranted variations from good practice and substantially improve survival (140). Randomized trials have shown that, when combined with feedback on performance and education by respected peers, practice guidelines can improve medical care processes and outcomes (124). Experience with implementation of well-developed guidelines shows that knowledge and acceptance can be high. Guideline implementation has repeatedly been associated with small-to-moderate improvements in care processes (141,142), though effects on health outcomes have been less studied and are less clear. Guidelines designed to explicate only basic care requirements may define only what virtually everyone is already doing.

Clinical guidelines and paths can assist in the coordination of multidisciplinary teams by defining procedures more clearly (143). Key clinical process and expected results can be tracked in a checklist to be addressed by members of the team. Successful clinical paths should enable teams to provide quality of care more reliably and efficiently, with discussion focusing on a minority of exceptions from the usual path rather than the normal process. For new team members, the path should be educational. Requirements for documentation can potentially be reduced without loss of meaning.

Well-designed computer decision-support systems have similarly demonstrated improvements in clinical practices (144). Using a touch-screen, for instance, patients or staff can complete a questionnaire, and responses can be processed against evidence-based guidelines at the time of the clinical encounter. Care suggestions, targeted to the patient's history, comorbid conditions, and current symptoms, can be provided. Reminder and suggestion systems have only begun to be developed, but both patients and health care practitioners have been satisfied with some of them (145).

Research on guidelines for depression deserves further mention, not only because persons with disability exhibit depressive symptomatology more frequently than the general population, but also because research on their implementation is instructive. A substantial body of research has elucidated effective methods of recognizing depression and improving its treatment in ordinary care settings; reductions in frequency of depression have clearly been demonstrated (146). Implementation research has shown that clinical information and education is necessary but insufficient. To achieve levels of treatment and outcome recommended by the guideline, patients too must be educated and encouraged. "Quality improvement efforts that focus resources on improving systems of care and the active participation of patients offer the best evidence of improved patient outcomes" (147). Knowledge of organizational tactics and factors enhances the likelihood of successful implementation of guidelines (148).

A final important practical factor is that costs are frequently not considered in development of guidelines. Cost, however, is a huge factor in health policy and in provision of actual rehabilitative care. Implementation of cost-conscious guidelines has been reported to save substantial sums in certain circumstances (134,149). However, methods of ethically incorporating costs into guidelines are not yet well developed or widely accepted (150). The cost-effectiveness of alternative approaches to assuring and improving the quality of care, including EBM, TQM, and patient partnerships, needs to be examined (151). Even with all these shortcomings, we can expect the development and use of clinical guidelines to increase in the future.

Multifaceted approaches to guideline implementation, involving provision of written information, talks with local consensus discussions, and individualized contact by colleagues (academic detailing) appear to be most effective in dissemination (141). Guidelines and attempts to implement them should be pilot tested and built into normal, ongoing channels for improving care. Obstacles to implementation vary across organizations, so a preliminary diagnosis of the organization itself is logically needed to identify barriers and optimal implementation strategies—a topic on which more research is needed.

CRITIQUE

Evidence-based guidelines are now widely accepted by clinical professionals and policy makers as essential bases for clinical practice. Expert, best-practice guidelines can improve clinical performance and serve as a tool for clinicians and a source of information for patients. Evidence-based guidelines are a necessary and potentially powerful tool for accountability and QI, as well as to achieve effective and efficient care, though limitations are becoming clearer (152,153).

Guidelines can be rigid, based on the assumption that one single method of care is best when several approaches may be effective. Proliferation of forms and applicability to varying local circumstances remain concerns. Patient acceptance has not been considered in development of some guidelines, and though patient involvement may be recommended, specifics of how this is to occur are often not given. Guidelines need to be tested to evaluate their use in practice and whether they actually improve clinical processes and patient outcomes. They will also need recurrent revision.

While the feasibility of guidelines in rehabilitation—at least for certain better-understood problems—has been established, most existing guidelines focus on medical/nursing pathologies rather than on producing functional gains, the core goal of medical rehabilitation. Most conditions and clinical practices in rehabilitation are not covered by guidelines or by direct efficacy research. Rehabilitation is so complex that one might expect that only sophisticated, flexible, multifaceted guidelines would actually improve practice.

Peer review is needed to determine whether deviations from guidelines are justifiable. In general, peer review and other external quality mechanisms are necessary and established techniques for QA and QI and their continued development is warranted (154).

Guidelines vary in their quality. Some are well based on evidence, while others are based largely on expert opinion. The few guidelines that have been produced for rehabilitation involve substantial expert opinion (e.g., for stroke rehabilitation) or target highly specific conditions (e.g., deep vein thrombosis prophylaxis). Criteria now exist for appraisal of the quality of clinical practice guidelines (155,156). Guidelines need to be developed to the point that they are useful for professional and patient education and should be sufficiently detailed and clear that one can objectively evaluate the degree to which patients have received the needed care and experience the expected health benefits.

INFORMATION SYSTEMS FOR PERFORMANCE MONITORING

Due to inherent complexity, risks, and lack of national standards, "health care delivery has been relatively untouched by the revolution in information technology that has been transforming nearly every other aspect of society" (1, p. 15). The mass of information on personal health collected in encounters with health care professionals is a great potential resource for improved quality of care, but that information is dispersed in poorly organized, sometimes illegible paper records at a variety of sites, inhibiting access to the information needed to monitor and manage patients with chronic illnesses.

Systematic improvement of care quality and outcomes involves attention to information flow, the medical record, and the clinical data system. A sophisticated system for reporting and analysis is required to extract useful meaning from the mass of data collected and to convey information to clinicians in a useful, timely way.

Data System Structure: Inputs, Processes, and Outcomes

Performance monitoring systems involve measures of three types—inputs, processes, and outcomes. Figure 54-5 shows two schemata for outcomes-oriented monitoring systems. In traditional PE systems in medical rehabilitation, the emphasis has been on outcomes, and the process box is sparse. There is no explicit theory or guideline to determine what aspects of intervention should be measured, so that rehabilitative processes are treated virtually as a black box (at the top of the figure). The approach has been useful to characterize patient gains associated with comprehensive medical rehabilitation programs, where processes are so multiple and complex their complete explication would appear to be an intractable task. Many current data systems in medical rehabilitation are like this, including data systems for the prospective payment system (PPS) based in the Inpatient Rehabilitation Facility-Patient Assessment Instrument (IRF-PAI). A minimal ability to analyze the effect of general factors such as intensity of treatment, primary impairment, payer, and demographic factors for somewhat similar patient groups (e.g., FRGs or CMGs) may be provided. However, the limitations of this model have been increasingly recognized (19,22,36,111,157). When needed processes are not stipulated and measured in the data system, it is extremely difficult to identify what might be done to improve the appropriateness or outcomes of care.

More sophisticated data systems—tied to the actual process of rehabilitation planning and treatment provision—have been attempted in rehabilitation (14,15,158). As displayed at the bottom of Figure 54-5, treatment objectives and progress are represented by arrows. While some functional and medical measures may be constant across all patients, others vary to permit needed individualization. Treatment objectives are chosen to fit the priority needs of the individual (14,15). Ongoing patient reassessment is part of quality rehabilitation (35, JCAHO Standard 6.2), so a more adequate rehabilitation data system incorporates change in patient functioning and treatment objectives. Whether medical and functional goals have been attained (and possible reasons if not) is determined in patient follow-up. Requirements for attainment of a productive, independent lifestyle are evaluated. Given the importance of discharge planning to quality rehabilitation (35, JCAHO standard tx.6.1.1), environmental, family, and other requirements for discharge to a maximally independent living arrangement need to be evaluated.

The provision of rehabilitation services should be guided by an interdisciplinary plan (35, JCAHO standard tx.6.3). When the objectives in a performance monitoring system are based on actual rehabilitation plans for individuals, it is a true *clinical outcomes management data system*. With such a system, the team can be provided with specific and potentially valuable feed-

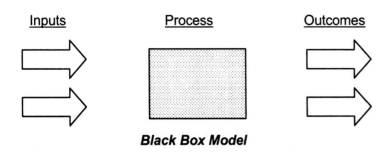

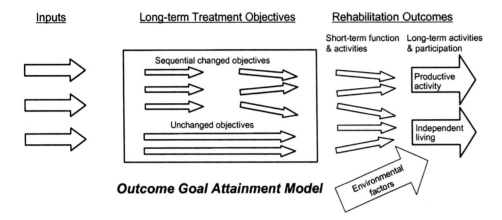

Figure 54-5. Simplified schemata for rehabilitation program evaluation and outcomes management.

back on their ability to choose objectives, implement effective interventions, and attain outcomes for individuals served.

Information System Design and Integration

A fully automated medical record is not needed to achieve QI (1). Automated order entry systems can reduce errors in prescription and delivery of medications (159). Reminder systems have recurrently been shown to improve compliance with clinical practice guidelines (160). Although current examples are few and limited to specific structured problems, computer-assisted diagnosis and management promise to improve quality in the future (1,161).

Much data in current medical records are entered in free form, nearly illegible notes. If entered into computers, new natural language search engines, such as those used on Web portals, make retrieval of information from free-text notes possible. Even so, natural language recording yields results of limited reliability, given individual variations in style and completeness of recording.

Information systems, whether on computer or paper, can present clinicians with standardized, relevant considerations and information to assist them in their diagnosis and treatment decisions and in monitoring response to treatment. Common evaluative and intervention processes can be presented in a format (e.g., reminders or a flow sheet) that reminds clinicians of standard best practices and simultaneously facilitates recording of whether these are done. Additional screens or pages can facilitate standardized measurement of patient responsiveness. The importance, appropriateness, simplicity, and *transparency* (understandability) of items presented to clinicians are critical to a usable clinical data system. While structured input is needed for systematic QI and outcomes monitoring, free text

notes are still required to record individual variations and for the numerous clinical situations for which validated, structured guidelines do not exist.

The idea of integrating information systems is hardly new, but it is still common for health care organizations to have multiple, poorly integrated recording systems. Clinical data may be recorded in paper medical records, professional files, or in pharmacy and other departmental computers. Billing records may be in an entirely separate system. The integration of clinical, financial, case management, QI, and outcomes data systems increases the potential use of these systems (14,78).

Reporting and Uses

Computerization assists QI by increasing the amount of data available but does not in itself provide more information, in the sense of relevant or useful information. With the spread of automation, the information available to clinicians and managers is expanding rapidly. This mass of information can enhance decision making, but it can also confuse the process. The bottleneck in many facilities is not in collection of data but in organizing it and analyzing it to draw out its meaning. One could argue that the performance monitoring literature has concentrated too much on measurement and too little on how to use the data. Routine performance reports give rise to hypotheses about problems in the program or why outcomes are or are not attained. Targeted, special in-depth analyses are needed to discover *reasons* why performance is better or worse than expected. The information system must facilitate professional statistical investigation and interpretation.

Information systems are justified not by single use but by their multiplicity of uses. Following sections will discuss clinical and then management uses.

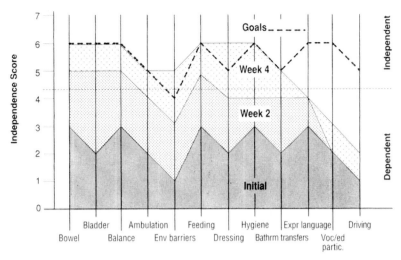

Figure 54-6. Status and goal profile of a possible discharge candidate (From Silverstein B, Kilgore KM, Fisher WP. Implementing patient tracking systems and using functional assessment scales. Vol 1. In: Harvey RF, ed. Center for Rehabilitation Outcome Analysis. Monograph series on issues and methods in outcome analysis. Wheaton, IL: Marianjoy Rehabilitation Center, 1989, with permission.)

CLINICAL REPORTING AND USES

Reports of functional gains by patients have been used in rehabilitation for decades, not only to evaluate the rehabilitation program as a whole and to assist in QI but also to organize communication and set goals in the rehabilitation team conference (162). Patient functioning and improvement are key indicators in utilization review and assessment of readiness for discharge in rehabilitation (12,162). Data on functional history and gains have also been used to assist case managers by predicting outcomes.

Rehabilitation information systems can produce informative, graphic displays of individual patient progress used in team conference, case management, and reports to referral sources or payers. Figure 54-6 presents an example of such a report (64,162). Functional tasks are ordered by difficulty: the easiest, first-to-recover activities are presented to the left with more difficult activities to the right. The case displayed is a possible discharge candidate. Team discussion of the patient's functioning, lifestyle preferences, special needs, and family support is needed for quality rehabilitative management and a safe, high-quality community placement.

As noted previously, clinical reminder and decision-support systems are being developed that will surely affect medical rehabilitation. To be most useful, information should be available when and where it is needed to accomplish the current tasks. Astute design of reports and reminders is essential (163).

Interpreting Clinical Outcomes Data

Well-designed routine reports tell us whether desired, attainable results are in fact routinely attained and whether interventions are being applied to patients who are most likely to benefit from them. Performance monitoring systems, however, infrequently provide unequivocal evidence of quality or outcomes by themselves. Rather, data patterns strengthen some ideas about program quality and effectiveness, and weaken other ideas.

There are several common, avoidable traps in interpretation of clinical outcomes data. First is the common tendency to assume a massive effect of treatments. Rehabilitative interventions will tend to lessen complications and augment healing and adjustment, but quick cures are not ordinarily expected. A second common error is assuming that improvement is due entirely to rehabilitation. Improvement can be due also to natural healing and family and environmental processes that can occur

at home. Conversely, failure to improve may not reflect provision of inadequate treatment. Reports need to incorporate sophisticated severity adjustment to identify patients with anomalously poor outcomes. Even then, detailed clinical data are needed to judge whether failure to improve is associated with provision of substandard care (17).

CASE MANAGEMENT DATA BASES AND THEIR USES

Difficulties in use of traditional routine clinical monitoring data systems are not entirely due to technical deficiencies, although these exist. When there is a concrete motive (e.g., a financial motive), clinical data systems are used. Managed care organizations, for instance, have developed their own databases to track the appropriateness of medical care, including medical rehabilitation. These databases concentrate on financial factors but increasingly include detailed clinical data. If the case management agency does not like the care or outcomes of patients sent to a rehabilitation provider, it does not send new cases to that provider. Only a minority of expensive cases are managed with the use of such databases, but for this minority the external party's data system is essentially the operational outcomes management database. These case management systems are typically proprietary, but their adequacy and impact on patient care and outcomes are of public interest.

MANAGEMENT REPORTING AND USES

Management reports are the routine product of performance monitoring systems. Patient progress, indicators of clinical outcomes and processes, goal attainment rates, efficiency, caseload, service intensity or frequency, and trends are reported periodically. Reports may go to the governing board and staff as well as clinicians and managers. Both frontline staff and key decision makers should receive findings and use them. Performance reports should engage staff at all the levels of the organization involved in actually implementing possible improvements based on the findings. Data on patient progress or outcomes may also be formatted for release to purchasers of services and the public (11,73,74).

Managing Length of Stay and Cost-Effectiveness

QI efforts need to be practical. By relating data on program quality and outcomes to costs, quality can be managed and improved within practical constraints.

Management of LOS and readiness for discharge is critical in rehabilitation facilities in the United States and is a major use of clinical information systems. Additional uses include marketing (164), refined profitability analyses, planning, accreditation, and estimation of patient acuity for determination of staffing requirements (14,15,17,75,76,78). LOS, however, is not an indicator of quality. Shortening LOS in rehabilitation has been accompanied by an increase in the frequency of rehospitalization after discharge (2). Discharges of hip fracture patients from acute hospitals with active clinical issues (e.g., temperature, blood pressure, other vital signs) or with new impairments have been associated with increased rates of rehospitalization and mortality, and patients who develop new impairments have worse functional mobility (165). Information systems need to present information on patient readiness for discharge.

Improvement per day or per dollar has often been labeled as "efficiency" or cost-effectiveness. Though not entirely illogical, the label is questionable, as patient improvement and costs are driven by many factors exogenous to treatment effectiveness, including natural healing, referral sources, comorbid conditions, base reimbursement rates, cost-charge ratios, the adequacy of postdischarge support systems, and family support. Ratios of gain-to-cost are a heuristic or first-stage screen, meaningful only if further analysis is done.

Interpretation of cost-effectiveness data requires understanding of basic relationships. More severe cases tend to receive and require longer care (37,63). While outcomes per se often have little relation to effort or even an inverse one, improvement in medical rehabilitation hospitals is and should be probabilistically related to LOS (37,62). Strategies for cost-benefit and cost-effectiveness analysis in rehabilitation are presented in other works (166).

Regardless of the details of the data system, oral or written narrative interpretations are usually essential for data to be meaningful and useful.

STRATEGIES FOR USE OF QUALITY AND OUTCOMES DATA

Both process-focused and outcomes-focused monitoring systems have limitations—and complementary strengths. Quality monitoring systems may focus on clinical processes which are already performed when needed, so that incremental improvements are of little value. They may also focus on processes that are not actual clinical priorities or that have little demonstrated relationship to long-term function or QOL. Systems focusing on such processes may not be worth the effort or may distract attention from interventions that hold promise to provide greater long-term benefit to patients. Outcomes monitoring systems have their own limitations, the principal one being the difficulty of connecting the outcome to specific antecedent processes. The use of any data system depends on motivations and how the system is built into clinical, administrative, public reporting, and accountability operations.

Outcomes-Focused Quality Improvement

Given the lack of evidence for a single best way to deliver rehabilitative care, it makes sense to monitor functional outcomes, giving programs leeway in how they produce these outcomes. Shaughnessey and colleagues have shown that outcomes-based QI (OBQI) can substantially improve patient outcomes (167). In a study of over 300,000 patients receiving services from home health agencies, OBQI reduced rehospitalization for targeted conditions in OBQI agencies by 22% to 26% over 3- to 4-year demonstration projects, compared to a 1% reduction in matched non-OBQI agencies. "The risk-adjusted rates of improvement in OBQI target outcome measures of health status

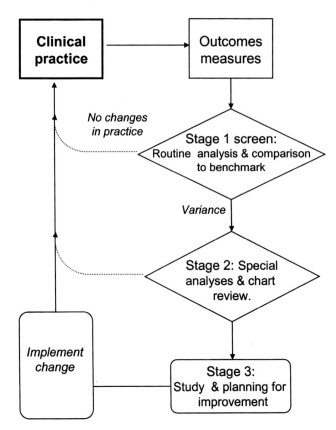

Figure 54-7. The outcomes-focused quality improvement cycle.

averaged 5% to 7% per year in both demonstration trials and were significantly greater ($P < .5$) than analogous improvement rates for nontarget comparison outcomes, which averaged about 1% per year." There is no reason why outcomes-focused approaches should not work for other forms of rehabilitation as well. Outcomes-focused approaches, however, have frequently been misunderstood.

In general, *when a program or patient group has higher or lower outcomes than projected, this by itself does not constitute evidence for high or low quality or effectiveness of care* (85). Although FRGs can be modified to predict up to 63% of the variance of discharge FIM scores, current severity-adjustment methods typically predict only a minority of the variance of patient *gains*, so that much is left unexplained (85,168). Outcomes after rehabilitation are due to many factors beyond the control of even high-quality care. As a consequence, a discrepancy between expected and actual outcomes is validly usable (only) *as a first-stage screen*—an indicator of a possible problem or opportunity to improve operations (Fig. 54-7). The discrepancy indicates that further investigation is needed.

Second stage screens or investigations are required to determine whether there are deviations in care processes, or whether outcome deviations reflect unmeasured patient or environmental factors. Many studies show that appropriate use of outcomes data to improve clinical processes "virtually always requires detailed clinical data" (119, p. 868). Peer review of charts may be employed to determine reasons for deviations but are expensive. Chart review may focus on patients whose outcomes are particularly discrepant, but ad hoc methods may fail to detect remediable problems

A defined system of in-depth analyses of detailed clinical data, based on well-developed guidelines, is needed to confirm whether a discrepancy in outcomes is associated with process deficiencies or other factors. The difficult process of determining reasons for suboptimal outcomes should not be left to harried local QI committees or part-time PE staff without well-developed tools to guide their efforts. Objective review criteria that connect outcomes to process deviations are feasible and have begun to be developed for home health services (140) and stroke rehabilitation (136,137). Perhaps the greatest technical problem with current approaches to QI in rehabilitation is that the evidence-based guidelines and methods of operationalizing them in second-stage analyses have not been developed and validated.

When a problem or opportunity for improvement in care processes is identified, the quality task force should direct effort toward solving the problem. In this *third stage*, detailed practical planning should occur, followed by implementation and change in care processes. Continued monitoring will reveal the impact on patient outcomes.

In principle, performance improvement efforts can and should have the capacity to focus on several points in the causal chain connecting clinical processes to intermediate and long-term outcomes. QI analyses, for instance, can identify patients who experience variances in care processes and determine if their severity-adjusted outcomes are in fact below expectation. If so, action is indicated. Evidence-based clinical guidelines and methods of operationalizing them are needed to improve performance, whether the initial examination focuses on processes or outcomes.

OTHER APPROACHES TO PERFORMANCE IMPROVEMENT

Professional Education and Development

Education of professional and other staff is an essential component of QA and QI. The quality of care provided in practice is surely dependent primarily on professionals' pride, ownership, and self-regulation. In appropriate learning environments, clinical professionals will strive toward improved competence and improved practice. These assumptions underlie current professional licensure, testing, and continuing medical education (CME).

Classic CME approaches involving courses, provision of written educational materials, and conferences have empirically demonstrated only limited effectiveness in improving clinician performance (153,169). A variety of improved educational methods with greater interactivity and realism may prove to be more effective than classic CME. Educational outreach and personally tailored approaches are promising; small group learning and physician peer-review are also useful (153). Methods involving more realistic, behavioral learning and testing, such as objective-structured clinical examinations, are promising (170) but have not yet proven their superiority to traditional methods. Bottom-up approaches, involving clinical education and formation of groups of clinicians dedicated to improving clinical practice and accountability, have repeatedly been shown to improve clinical practice (153).

A variety of new and revised educational techniques will be needed to provide the skills required to enhance the quality of health care. Enhanced skills will be needed to: synthesize, apply, and communicate evidence and guidelines; properly use decision support systems; understand the course of illnesses and patients' experience; measure the quality of care in terms of both process and outcomes; design and improve interdisciplinary care processes; and communicate with patients both as full partners in decision making and to enhance compliance

with guidelines (1). Traditional emphases on disease processes need to be expanded.

Professional groups can sometimes develop a culture of hiding errors and maximizing income rather than of true quality and cost-effectiveness. Systems of QI based on professional culture need to be linked to systems that ensure public accountability.

Patient-Centered Approaches

Patient- or "customer-"centered approaches have been increasingly advocated to improve the quality of health care delivery, both in the United States and Europe. We will primarily consider the monitoring of patient satisfaction, a clearly practical matter, and then comment on broader issues of patient involvement or empowerment. Although details may vary, assessment of quality from a patient's perspective is clearly an essential and valuable component of performance monitoring in health care.

PATIENT SATISFACTION

The monitoring of patient satisfaction has deservedly become a ubiquitous, standard part of performance monitoring in health care. Patient satisfaction is both a process and an outcome issue.

There are persuasive practical reasons for organizations to have a strong emphasis on patient satisfaction. Patient satisfaction is quite measurable at a modest cost (171). A facility's reputation is largely based on satisfied clients. Marketing is enhanced by high customer satisfaction, both by word-of-mouth and presentation of satisfaction information. Patient perceptions of quality have been found to be robustly correlated with hospital profitability (172). Increased patient satisfaction has been associated with decreased risk of malpractice suits (173).

Measuring patient satisfaction helps both clinicians and administrators understand patients' experiences with care. Patient satisfaction assessment can identify problematic processes. Dissatisfaction rates are much higher in facilities that misrepresent the services they offer (18,171,174). Satisfied patients tend to be more compliant to treatment recommendations (175).

Well-validated, reliable questionnaires, with available normative data, are available for assessment of patient satisfaction, and should be used. Multipoint rating scales have become standard (e.g., ratings from "very poor" to "very good" or "excellent"). Valid satisfaction questionnaires avoid bias, giving customers freedom to complain if they feel like it. The point is to get information rather than to manipulate a vote of approval. Mail provides more anonymous results than phone calls, and at lower cost, but low-response rates can be a problem. Patient satisfaction questionnaires have been published for general medical settings (176) and for inpatient (177) and outpatient (178) rehabilitation programs (27). Many large group health organizations have adopted standard formats for assessment of patient satisfaction based on Ware's research (179). Third-party firms provide standard satisfaction monitoring systems, including reports of comparative data across settings. Reports are needed for different types of patients and should target different actionable areas of care.

Patient satisfaction measures have limitations and need to be presented to staff in a positive light. Care issues are often viewed positively. Patients tend to express high satisfaction with medical rehabilitation services. "The most consistent finding is that the characteristics of providers or organizations that result in more 'personal' care are associated with higher levels of satisfaction" in medical settings (171), while patient satisfaction is poorly or inconsistently related to technical effectiveness and professional standards. Satisfaction measures often elicit comments about food, temperature, billing hassles, and other hotel and personal services. Billing and cost issues typically receive ratings that are distinct from care issues and should be summed and reported separately from care issues. Administrative journals provide advice on how to interpret and use patient satisfaction data (180).

PATIENT INVOLVEMENT AND EMPOWERMENT

Increased patient involvement or empowerment has been propounded as a way to improve the quality of rehabilitation programs. CARF accreditation particularly emphasizes and even requires patient involvement (11), and JCAHO standards now also state that the rehabilitation plan is "developed by qualified professionals, in conjunction with the patients and/or his or her family, social network or support system" (35, tx.6.3). Patient autonomy is a basic ethical value, and involving "consumers" is seen as essential to enabling them to receive the individualized care they desire. Patients' valuation of outcomes may differ from those of professionals, and individual patients have differing functional needs. "Consumers" of rehabilitative services may choose cognitive and communicative abilities over physical abilities (181), although conventional outcome measures weight them equally or even give greater weight to physical outcomes. The significance of the same disability can vary among patients (17,18,182). Patients have different desired lifestyles. Improved ability to prepare meals or to climb stairs, for instance, may be critical to one person but irrelevant to another.

Differing methods of empowering or involving patients have been employed, including satisfaction surveys, complaint procedures, communication training for professionals, surveys of patient needs, and enhanced provision of educational information. All these methods make sense. One of the few studies on the topic has reported encouraging results of a system involving a patient care notebook in a rehabilitation setting (183). Patient, family, and team are all involved in the notebook, which also educates the patient in self-care and is used as a resource when the patient goes home.

Many studies have been done on physician-patient communication, and reviews show that various indicators of sensitive caring communication and patient-centeredness lead to greater patient satisfaction and even to better compliance with prescribed treatment (184). While most patients want to receive information on their condition and treatment alternatives, many do not want to make key decisions regarding necessary treatment; seriously ill patients in particular may not want to take responsibility for management of their disease (185).

After decades of simplistic advocacy of patient involvement and professional suspicion of patient opinions, new conceptualizations of patient-centered care have been propounded. "Dialog-centered care", based on a clearer definition of the rights and responsibilities in communicative process between clinicians and patients, is among the most promising of these (153). Research is needed to clarify methods and circumstances for appropriately involving patients in such a way that satisfaction and outcomes are improved.

CLINICAL PRACTICE IMPROVEMENT (CPI)

Systematic "clinical practice improvement" (CPI) has led to insights and improved care processes in a number of areas of medical care (186,187). Developed by Dr. Susan Horn, CPI is a data driven "bottom-up" approach involving collection of both extensive process and outcomes data. It typically begins with clinician's ideas and experience, rather than a review of the evidence. Clinicians who choose different practices from those in the protocol are given the opportunity to present their reasoning to the team so that the protocol can be modified or consensus can be reached. The goal of the CPI process is to enable clinicians to improve severity-adjusted outcomes within cost limits or to maintain relevant outcomes while decreasing costs.

CPI involves collection of great quantities of data on care processes, outcomes, and patient characteristics, including indicators of severity. All three types of data—patient characteristics, steps in the process of care, and relevant outcomes—must be measured, or one cannot tell whether outcomes are associated with care processes or to differences in case severity.

Compared to randomized clinical trials, CPI has less internal validity, but greater external validity, that is, greater generalization to practice. Sophisticated multivariate statistics are used to control for factors that confound process-outcome relationships for selected subsets of patients. Process variations are lessened through ongoing feedback from statistical analyses, discussion, and consensus.

Proponents of CPI argue that clinical practice guidelines are often based on a consensus of experts, and what scientific evidence is available is often limited or based on selected patient groups and programs that vary from those seen in practice. In such circumstances, CPI is particularly justifiable scientifically. By taking a comprehensive view of the care process, CPI studies have identified actionable factors that have been associated with improved outcomes. Repeatedly, too, these factors had been excluded from previous RCTs and written guidelines. The CPI literature provides examples of how a team comprised of CPI researchers and experienced clinicians can implement data collection systems and use them in a way that leads toward improvements in the quality and effectiveness of care. Research applying CPI to stroke rehabilitation is currently ongoing.

PUBLIC ISSUES

Trends in health care as a whole suffuse rehabilitation, which is a relatively small part of the total health care "system." Payment policies impel the organization of rehabilitation, and current payment policies are complex and contradictory and may provide no incentive (or even disincentives) for improving the quality and even the efficiency of care (1). Rehabilitation may face a "market" that disempowers its "customers"—persons with disability (188).

Changes in the Health Care Industry

Cost control mechanisms, including various managed care mechanisms, risk-sharing arrangements, and Medicare's prospective payment system—have heightened concern about the quality of rehabilitative care. Although reports on the quality of care have not always shown that managed care arrangements provide worse care to persons with disabilities and chronic conditions, these firms have incentives to do so, as these patients cost much more to care for than average (42). Under-capitated payment arrangements and disabled and chronically ill individuals are money losers, so the incentive is not to enroll such individuals, to treat them as cost-effectively as possible, and hope that limited services will induce them to sign up for alternatives. Severely disabled individuals lose their private insurance and shift to Medicaid or Medicare. The disabled individuals affected may be poor and limited in mobility, and some cannot communicate articulately. As a consequence of all these factors, organizations may decline to participate in studies of rehabilitation quality and outcomes. In sum, rehabilitation is vulnerable to adverse pressure in the changing

TABLE 54-1.   Rehabilitation Impairment Categories (RICs)

01	Stroke (Stroke)
02	Traumatic brain injury (TBI)
03	Nontraumatic brain injury (NTBI)
04	Traumatic spinal cord injury (TSCI)
05	Nontraumatic spinal cord injury (NTSCI)
06	Neurological (Neuro)
07	Fracture of lower extremity (FracLE)
08	Replacement of lower extremity joint (Rep1LE)
09	Other orthopedic (Ortho)
10	Amputation, lower extremity (AMPLE)
11	Amputation, other (AMPNLE)
12	Osteoarthritis (OsteoA)
13	Rheumatoid, other arthritis (RheumA)
14	Cardiac (Cardiac)
15	Pulmonary (Pulmonary)
16	Pain Syndrome (Pain)
17	Major multiple trauma, no brain injury or spinal cord injury (MMT NBSCI)
18	Major multiple trauma, with brain or spinal cord injury (MMT BSCI)
19	Guillain-Barré (GB)
20	Miscellaneous (Misc)
21	Burns (Burns)

From *Federal Register,* August 7, 2001:41342–41344.

health care system in the United States, and quality of rehabilitative care is or should be a public issue as well as a professional one.

PROSPECTIVE PAYMENT

Function-Related Groups (FRGs)—patient groups defined by Functional Independence Measures (FIMs) at admission, primary impairment group, and age with similar lengths of stay or costs—were developed by Stineman as a basis for prospective payment for medical rehabilitation hospitals (89,91). The system, as extended by Carter at the Rand Corporation, was finally adapted by the federal government. Implementation began on January 1, 2002, with blended prospective payment system (PPS) and TEFRA (Tax Equity and Fiscal Responsibility Act) payment, with the phase-in to be completed by October 1, 2003.

Payment is based on data in the "Inpatient Rehabilitation Facility-Patient Assessment Instrument" or IRF-PAI, a modified version of the FIM-Uniform Data System (UDS) dataset. The IRF-PAI provides the data necessary to classify patients into the "Case Mix Groups" (CMGs) on which payment is based. Table 54-1 displays the 21 primary Rehabilitation Impairment Categories (RICs) on which CMGs are based. RICs are further subdivided. As an example, stroke is further divided into five diagnostic subcategories and 21 CMGs.

The PPS provides an incentive for rehabilitation hospitals in the United States to further reduce LOS. Will PPS accentuate the already-documented trend toward increased rehospitalization rates (2) after inpatient rehabilitation? Effects of the PPS on quality will need to be monitored. The CMS has expressed its intention to develop quality indicators for rehabilitation (e.g., functional independence including discharge to the community, incidence of worsening pressure ulcers as measured by the Pressure Ulcer Scale for Healing scale, and prevention of falls) (189). Although this list is limited, it provides a starting point for the development of quality indicators for medical rehabilitation.

PUBLIC REPORTING OF PERFORMANCE

Fears regarding simplistic misinterpretation of quality and outcomes data are still with us, leading to restrictions on access impairing the use of the data. The data in rehabilitation clinical information systems, like that in other medical information systems, have been private, the property of the facility. Consumers and the public, however, are major stakeholders to the rehabilitation process, and they have a valid claim to disidentified performance information (that is, information that does not identify any individual patient). Medicare now releases severity-adjusted data on quality of care in nursing homes (see http://www.medicare.gov/). The Center for Medicare and Medicare Services may be expected to release similar reports on functional gain and outcomes in rehabilitation.

Payers and large health care institutions have developed methods of profiling the cost and case mix of physicians and facilities. Little, however, has been published regarding the reliability or validity of these systems. Because nonspecialist physicians may encounter only a small number of patients with a specific disease, the profile could easily be unreliable, and individual physicians could game the system by avoiding just a few severe, high-cost, or poorly adherent patients (190).

HEALTH PLAN REPORT CARDS: NATIONAL COMMITTEE ON QUALITY ASSURANCE'S HEALTH PLAN EMPLOYER DATA AND INFORMATION SET

The National Committee on Quality Assurance (NCQA) was formed to address the issue of QA of health care in managed health care plans. Without objective measures and credible data, competition between such plans is possible only on the basis of cost. The NCQA accredits health plans, and its Health Plan Employer Data and Information Set (HEDIS) was developed to provide needed data on sponsored care processes, professional resources, and outcomes (see http://www.ncqa.org/Programs/HEDIS/).

Although still limited, the number of HEDIS quality indicators has increased over time. The current (2004) version of HEDIS has expanded to include 59 quality indicators sets, including 22 indicators of effectiveness, 8 on access/availability, 3 on satisfaction, 2 on plan stability, 18 on intensity of care utilization, and 6 structural descriptors (http://www.ncqa.org/Programs/HEDIS/index.htm). A few outcome indicators or surveys are specified (e.g., the Medicare Health Outcome Survey), but most are process indicators. Although quality indicators are specified for a half dozen chronic conditions (e.g., diabetes, cholesterol management after acute cardiovascular events), HEDIS currently has no items on the neurological, traumatic, or orthopedic conditions most commonly seen in inpatient rehabilitation hospitals.

HEDIS data are compiled into a national database, and report cards are issued on health plans. Whether HEDIS is measuring the most important factors is controversial. HEDIS quality indicator sets, however, continue to evolve, expand, and improve. Case studies attest to the use of the database in organizational QI efforts (http://www.qualityprofiles.org/). A broader issue is that accreditation and much reporting is voluntary. Health management organizations (HMOs) with lower quality-of-care scores have tended to stop disclosing their quality data (191). Gaming of quality data invalidates, or at least biases, quality-of-care reports, undermining accountability and decision making. In sum the quality of managed care organizations remains a pressing issue for health care professionals and patients.

INCOMPATIBLE DOCUMENTATION REQUIREMENTS

Incompatibility between requirements of various payers, regulatory agencies, and clinical needs is more than a technical issue. The multiplicity of differing and even conflicting documentation requirements and standards for coverage from different payers is part and parcel of the extreme levels of administrative waste that afflict health care in the United States (192). Standard documentation requirements, measures, and accepted clinical guidelines would reduce this waste while facilitating the use of performance benchmarks. Progress will involve communication to reach agreement on standards within the professional rehabilitation community and with major stakeholders.

Incorporating Wider Considerations into Performance Monitoring

The monitoring of the quality of the specific services provided can beg the question of whether a different type of service might provide superior benefits to patients and whether the person served has major unmet service needs. Although monitoring of current care processes is appropriate, performance improvement systems have greater potential use if they consider all interventions known to be effective for patients' problems, regardless of whether they are currently offered by the program. Studies of quality in acute care hospitals have reported that errors of omission (e.g., a physician not detecting a major diagnostic problem) were more common than errors of commission (not providing the correct treatment for the diagnosis) (40). Errors of omission of needed rehabilitative treatments may be frequent as well, especially given today's cost and LOS constraints. The results of inpatient rehabilitation, for example, may be compromised if quality follow-up care is not provided. A wider consideration of patient needs might lead to QI efforts that address patient referral, adding or changing service mix, and education of payers regarding service needs. Patients, their families, and disability advocates can be influential allies in such education.

FOLLOW-UP AND SYSTEMS ISSUES

The problems of patients undergoing rehabilitation are usually long-enduring, and patient needs and outcomes often cannot be reliably projected on the basis of short-term clinical responses. Follow-up and follow-along of patients has traditionally been considered to be important to quality rehabilitation and has long been incorporated into rehabilitation accreditation (11). Practical difficulties of follow-up include its expense, funding restrictions on continuing outpatient care, a lack of payment for educational or evaluative follow-up, and the fact that continuing outpatient care may involve a different provider than inpatient care. Nonetheless, rehabilitation programs can be improved by ongoing knowledge of whether new, unexpected problems or complications arise after discharge, and if so, to whom and why. Monitoring of long-term outcomes is also needed to assess whether changes in health care designed to control costs have compromised the health or functioning of patients undergoing rehabilitation.

COST AND VALUE

Awareness of the critical importance of cost has spread throughout health care, including rehabilitation. Even in the midst of pressures, however, it would be naïve to believe that cost alone is the only issue: the issue is the balance of cost to benefits, or in more general terms, value (42).

Interventions which are likely to produce small improvements in functioning of patients with severe chronic conditions are commonly available, but are these improvements and hence, the interventions—worth the money? Systematic research is needed to provide evidence regarding the value of various rehabilitative interventions, bearing in mind that this value may vary depending on context. CARF accreditation regulations have touched on the issue. They have addressed the need for rehabilitation programs to formulate feasible objectives, involving the patient in this process, and to communicate appropriate information regarding associated results to stakeholders (72,77). The agreement provides prima facie evidence that attaining the objective is probably of some worth to individuals involved, but it is difficult to summarize the value of attainment of such diverse individualized results to payers and policy makers. In any case, honest communication regarding patient benefits associated with rehabilitation, including objective data on goal attainment and evidence regarding treatment effectiveness, to major stakeholders remains essential to promoting a reputation for quality care and for nurturing the resources needed to maintain that quality.

Rehabilitation managers today are charged to develop systems that place each individual in a care setting that optimizes both outcomes and cost containment. The ability to predict outcome and to tier rehabilitative care to the level needed for the individual's improvement is becoming a necessity. To assure that each patient is provided the most effective rehabilitative care, objective indicators need to be developed that specify the level, type, and dosages of rehabilitation that should be provided.

SUMMARY AND CONCLUSIONS

The Institute of Medicine (IOM) has documented the "quality chasm" between care realistically possible and that actually provided (1). To cross the quality chasm, the IOM has proposed six objectives for the 21st century health care system: health care should be safe, effective, patient-centered, timely, efficient, and equitable. The current nonsystem of care for persons with disabilities in the United States does not meet these objectives, and care in other countries is limited as well. Persons with disability frequently are unable to obtain needed items and services from their health insurance plans and "experience more problems than others with follow-up care, availability of specialists, getting to doctors, and obtaining help during off hours" (188). Few would contest the assertion that there is a chasm between the quality of rehabilitation possible and that commonly provided to patients with disabling conditions.

Strategies for Performance Improvement

Health care quality monitoring and use of QA data has changed greatly since QA programs were originally established. The focus has shifted from identifying poor care toward identification of feasible improvements that will benefit the majority of patients with frequently encountered problems and the implementation of these improvements. Quality of care is now understood to be complex and multifaceted, and no aspect of the total system of care can be excluded from consideration if quality is truly to be improved.

More than a decade after their initial vogue, TQM and CQI remain theoretically attractive approaches (151). The emphasis on quality care, not as performance of a defined action or even sequence of defined steps but as processes organized around patient problems remains persuasive, as does the emphasis on improving systems, improving cultures, and developing smooth transitions between systems. Rehabilitation will do well to learn from CQI and TQM efforts in health care more generally, including acute medical care, psychiatric care, geriatric medicine, home health care, and long-term care (98,140, 193,194). Cooperation within specially trained multidisciplinary QI teams leads to improved quality in medical care (195). Multidisciplinary team approaches are also particularly valuable approaches to operational QI in rehabilitation.

At the same time, limitations of TQM/CQI have become evident. As Grol points out, "the current TQM approaches should be better adapted to the realities of health care. Links to other approaches (e.g., professional development and external assessment should be established. Physicians should be actively involved and occupy leadership roles, and the quality improvement activities should be related to their needs and to patient-related problems more directly" (153, p. 2583).

Multiple approaches are needed to assure and improve the quality and effectiveness of rehabilitative care. Processes and short-term and long-term outcomes all need to be measured either continuously or in occasional focused studies to identify opportunities for performance improvement and to keep score. Professionals—and patients—will need education, improved access to health information, and appropriate incentives. Involvement and accountability are required at all levels of the rehabilitative process. The emerging problem is that of identifying the QI strategy or tool most needed at any particular site.

The development, implementation, and monitoring of practice guidelines are critical to systematic efforts to assure and improve the quality of rehabilitative care. Without well-developed, evidence-based guidelines, there is no standard by which quality of care can be evaluated and neither process nor outcomes monitoring has definite action implications. The development of practice guidelines in rehabilitation is difficult in rehabilitation, given its breadth and complexity and limited funding for the extensive needed studies. Much work remains to be done to determine the most valuable rehabilitative care processes and to incorporate the needed tailoring of treatment objectives to patient priorities. Evidence-based guidelines will not be possible for all rehabilitation problems, but even when evidence is limited (e.g., stroke rehabilitation) it is possible to develop guidelines based on the best-validated of existing theories and whatever direct evidence exists. These guidelines can then be tested to determine their validity, that is, if closer adherence to the guideline in fact is associated with better severity-adjusted outcomes. No current system of performance monitoring can presently determine the "best practice" of rehabilitation, but guidelines are being improved and will increasingly provide standards for care.

Building Bridges

Improving the quality of medical care in general requires "building bridges among professional pride, payer profit, and patient satisfaction" (153). In rehabilitation, too, multifaceted approaches are needed that engage major stakeholders in the rehabilitation process. Changing health care to support the more uniform provision of quality rehabilitation will require the building of alliances among professionals, persons with disability, and others at risk in current fragmented systems.

Medical rehabilitation has a long history of concern for persons with disabilities. Public education and advocacy for policies to provide needed care naturally include rehabilitation as well as long-term care and social and environmental policies designed to alleviate disabling conditions. Education of payers, referral sources, and the public promotes the motivation and partnerships necessary for provision of quality rehabilitative care. Patients and family also need to be educated and engaged as allies. Professional educational communications should not only promote notions of the general value of rehabilitation but also state what specifically constitutes quality, effective rehabilitation. Evidence-based guidelines, studies, and relevant local

data, in a form readable by nonexperts, facilitate such communication. Data on local quality and outcomes can also facilitate such communications. For instance, data on late or inappropriate admission or referrals or other barriers to provision of required rehabilitative services may persuade referral sources or payers to ameliorate the barriers.

In summary, advances in systematic QI and outcomes management are critical to improve rehabilitative care and to justify it to the medical community, payers, and patients. Formal QI and outcomes monitoring systems aim to improve the effectiveness of care, to reduce errors, and to improve function and QOL by providing comparative data and decision-support information. These systems enable patients, family, referral sources, and payers to make better choices regarding level and type of rehabilitation needed. Medical rehabilitation has developed systems for monitoring patient gains in basic functional activities, but more work is needed to develop full-featured performance improvement systems that monitor key aspects of care quality and that demonstrably improve that care and associated patient outcomes. Evidence-based guidelines especially need to be developed to establish standards for multifaceted rehabilitative care. Efforts to improve the quality and outcomes of medical rehabilitation now have available a toolkit with a variety of methods. A major challenge in practice is communication to stakeholders to build support for high-quality rehabilitation. Defining the parameters of quality care and associated patient outcomes is the responsibility of all rehabilitation professionals and will be essential to preserving and enhancing the field.

REFERENCES

1. Institute of Medicine, Committee on Quality of HealthCare in America, William C. Richardson, Chair. *Crossing the quality chasm.* Washington, DC: National Academy Press, 2001.
2. Ottenbacher KJ, Smith PM, Illig SB, et al. Length of stay and hospital readmission for persons with disabilities. *Am J Public Health* 2000;90(12):1920–1923.
3. Leape LL. Error in medicine. *JAMA* 1994;272:1851–1857.
4. Hayward RA, Hofer TP. Estimating hospital deaths due to medical errors: preventability is in the eye of the reviewer. *JAMA* 2001;;286(4):415–420
5. Institute of Medicine, Kohn LT, Corrigan JM, Donaldson MS, et al., eds. *To err is human: building a safer health system.* Washington, DC: National Academy Press, 2000.
6. Lindquist R, Gersema LM. Understanding and preventing adverse drug events. *AACN Clin Issues* 1998, 9(1):119–128.
7. DeJong G, Batavia AI, Griss R. America's neglected health minority: working-age persons with disabilities. *Milbank Q* 1988;67:311–351.
8. Institute of Medicine. *Disability in America.* Washington, DC: National Academy of Sciences, 1991.
9. Iwanenko W, Fiedler RC, Granger CV. Uniform data system for medical rehabilitation: report of first admissions to subacute rehabilitation for 1995, 1996 and 1997. *Am J Phys Med Rehabil* 1999;78:384–388.
10. Blumenthal D. Quality of health care: Part 1: Quality of care—what is it? *N Engl J Med* 1996;335(12):891–894.
11. Commission on Accreditation of Rehabilitation Facilities. *Medical rehabilitation standards manual.* Tucson: CARF, 2002.
12. Granger CV, Gresham G, eds. *Functional assessment in rehabilitation medicine.* Baltimore: Williams & Wilkins, 1984.
13. Keith RA. Functional assessment measures in medical rehabilitation: current status. *Arch Phys Med Rehabil* 1984;65:74–78.
14. Haffey WJ, Johnston MV. An information system to assess the effectiveness of brain injury rehabilitation. In: Wood R, Eames P, eds. *Models of brain injury rehabilitation.* London: Chapman Hall, 1989:205–233.
15. Haffey WJ, Johnston MV. A functional assessment system for real world rehabilitation outcomes. In: Tupper D, Cicerone K, eds. *The neuropsychology of everyday life.* Boston: Martinus Nijhoff, 1989:99–124.
16. DeJong G, Hughes J. Independent living: methodology for measuring long-term outcomes. *Arch Phys Med Rehabil* 1982;63:68–73.
17. Haffey WJ, Lewis FD. Programming for occupational outcomes following traumatic brain injury. *Rehabil Psychology* 1989;34:147–158.
18. Brook RH. Quality of care: do we care? *Ann Intern Med* 1991;115:486–490.
19. Johnston MV, Stineman M, Velozo CA. Foundations from the past and directions for the future. In Fuhrer M, ed. *Assessing medical rehabilitation practices: the promise of outcomes research.* Baltimore: Paul H. Brookes, 1997:1–41.

20. Johnston MV, Lewis FD. The outcomes of community re-entry programs for brain injury survivors. Part 1: independent living and productive activities. *Brain Inj* 1991;5:141–154.

21. Johnston MV. The outcome of community re-entry programs for brain injury survivors. Part 2: further investigations. *Brain Inj* 1991;5:155–168.

22. Glueckauf RL. Program evaluation guidelines for the rehabilitation professional. *Adv Clin Rehabil* 1990;3:250–266.

23. Joint Commission on Accreditation of Healthcare Organizations. Characteristics of clinical indicators. *Qual Rev Bull* 1989;15:330–339.

24. Shaughnessy PW, Crisler KS, Schlenker RE, et al. Measuring and assuring the quality of home health care. *Health Care Financing Review* 1994;16(1): 35–67.

25. Kritchevsky SB, Simmons BP. Continuous quality improvement. *JAMA* 1991;266(13):1817–1823.

26. Deming WE. *Out of the crisis*. Cambridge, MA: Massachusetts Institute of Technology Center for Advanced Engineering Study, 1986.

27. Lubeck RC, Davis PK. W.E. Deming's 14 points for quality: can they be applied to rehabilitation? *J Rehabil Admin* 1991;15:216–222.

28. Thompson R. Some practical applications of Deming's fourteen points. *J Qual Assur* 1990;12:22–23.

29. Casalou RF. Total quality management in health care. *Hosp Health Services Admin* 1991;36(1):134–176.

30. Juran J. *Quality control handbook*, 4th ed. New York: McGraw-Hill, 1988.

31. Lohr KN, Donaldson MS, Harris-Wehling J. Medicare: a strategy for quality assurance. Quality of care in a changing health care environment. *Qual Rev Bull* 1992;18:120–126.

32. Lohr KN, ed. *Medicare: a strategy for quality assurance*. Washington, DC: National Academy Press, 1990.

33. Donabedian A, Palmer RH. Considerations in defining quality of health care. In: Palmer RH, Donabedian A, Povar GJ, eds. *Striving for quality in health care*. Ann Arbor, MI: Health Administration Press, 1991:1–53.

34. Williamson JW. Evaluation quality of patient care: a strategy relating outcome and process assessment. *JAMA* 1971;218(4):564–569.

35. Joint Commission on the Accreditation of Healthcare Organizations: The 2002 Automated Comprehensive Accreditation Manual for Hospitals [CD-ROM]. Oakbrook Terrace, IL: JCAHO, , 2002.

36. Lipsey M. Theory as method: small theories of treatments. In: Sechrest L, Perrin E, Bunker J, eds. Research methodology: strengthening causal interpretations of nonexperimental data Rockville, MD: DHHS, PHS, AHCPR; 1990:33–52; PHS 90–3454.,.

37. Carey RG, Seibert JH, Posavac EJ. Who makes the most progress in inpatient rehabilitation? An analysis of functional gain. *Arch Phys Med Rehabil* 1988; 69:337–343.

38. Joint Commission on Accreditation of Hospitals. *Primer on clinical indicator development and application*. Chicago: JCAHO, 1990.

39. Donabedian A. Explorations in quality assessment and monitoring. In: *Methods and findings of quality assessment and monitoring*. Vol 3. Ann Arbor, MI: Health Administration Press, 1985.

40. Brennan TA, Leape LL, Laird NM, et al. Incidence of adverse events and negligence in hospitalized patients. Results of the Harvard Medical Practice Study I. *N Engl J Med* 1991;324:370–376.

41. Kravitz RL, Rolph JE, McGuigan K. Malpractice claims data as a quality improvement tool. I. Epidemiology of error in four specialties. *JAMA* 1991; 266:2087–2092.

42. DeJong G, Sutton JP. Rehab 2000: the evolution of medical rehabilitation in American health care. In: Landrum-Kitchell P, Schmidt ND, McLean A Jr, eds. *Outcome-oriented rehabilitation*. Gaithersburg MD: Aspen, 1995:3–42.

43. World Health Organization. International Classification of Functioning, Disability and Health. Geneva: WHO, 2001. Available at: http://www3.who.int/icf/icftemplate.cfm. Accessed February 25, 2004..

44. World Health Organization. *International Classification of Impairments, Disabilities, and Handicaps*. Geneva: WHO, 1980.

45. Whiteneck GG, Charlifue SW, Gerhart KA, et al. Quantifying handicap: a new measure of long-term rehabilitation outcomes. *Arch Phys Med Rehabil* 1992;73: 519–526.

46. Whyte J. Towards a methodology for rehabilitation research. *Am J Phys Med Rehabil* 1994;73(6):428–435.

47. Hinderer SR, Gupta S. Functional outcome measures to assess interventions for spasticity. *Arch Phys Med Rehabil* 1996;77(10):1083–1089.

48. Johnston MV, Hall K, Carnevale G, et al. Functional assessment and outcome evaluation in TBI rehabilitation. In: Horn LJ, Zasler ND, eds. *Medical rehabilitation of traumatic brain injury*. Philadelphia: Hanley and Belfus, 1996: 197–226.

49. Johnston M, Nissim EN, Wood K, et al. Objective and subjective handicap following spinal cord injury: interrelationships and predictors. *Spinal Cord Med* 2002;25:11–22.

50. Wade DT. *Measurement in neurological rehabilitation*. New York: Oxford University Press, 1992.

51. McDowell I, Newell C. *Measuring health: a guide to rating scales and questionnaires*, 2nd ed. New York: Oxford, 1996.

52. Dittmar SS, Gresham GE. *Functional assessment and outcome measures for the rehabilitation health professional*. Gaithersburg, MD: Aspen Publishers, Inc., 1997.

53. Bowling A. *Measuring health: a review of quality of life measurement scales*, 2nd ed. Buckingham, UK: Open U Press, 1997.

54. Bowling A. *Measuring disease: a review of disease-specific quality of life measurement scales*, 2nd ed. Buckingham, UK: Open University Press, 2001.

55. Bergner M, Bobbit RA, Carter WB, et al. The Sickness Impact Profile: development and final revision of a health status measure. *Med Care* 1981;19: 787–805.

56. Stewart AL, Ware JE Jr, eds. *Measuring functioning and well-being*. Durham NC: Duke University Press, 1992.

57. Fuhrer MJ. Subjective well-being: implications for medical rehabilitation outcomes and models of disablement. *Am J Phys Med Rehabil* 1994;73(5):358–364.

58. Allen MJ, Yen WM. *Introduction to measurement theory*. Monterey, CA: Brooks/Cole, 1979.

59. Johnston MV, Keith RA, Hinderer S. Measurement standards for interdisciplinary medical rehabilitation. *Arch Phys Med Rehabil* 1992;73[Suppl 12-Sj]:S6–S23.

60. Phelps CE. The methodologic foundations of the appropriateness of medical care. *N Engl J Med* 1996;329(17):1241–1245.

61. Silverstein B, Kilgore KM, Fisher WP, et al. Applying psychometric criteria to functional assessment in medical rehabilitation: I. Exploring unidimensionality. *Arch Phys Med Rehabil* 1991;72:631–637.

62. Silverstein B, Kilgore KM, Fisher WP. Implementing patient tracking systems and using functional assessment scales. Vol 1. In: Harvey RF, ed. Center for Rehabilitation Outcome Analysis monograph series on issues and methods in outcome analysis. Wheaton, IL: Marianjoy Rehabilitation Center, 1989.

63. Linacre JM, Heinemann AW, Wright BD, et al. The structure and stability of the Functional Independence Measure. *Arch Phys Med Rehabil* 1994;75(2): 127–132.

64. Fuhrer MJ, ed. *Rehabilitation outcomes: analysis and measurement*. Baltimore: Paul Brookes, 1987.

65. Hall KM, Mann N, High WM Jr, et al. Functional measures after traumatic brain injury: ceiling effects of FIM, FIM + FAM, DRS, and CIQ. *J Head Trauma Rehab* 1966;11(5):27–39.

66. Heinemann AW, Linacre JM, Wright BD, et al. Relationships between impairment and physical disability as measured by the Functional Independence Measure. *Arch Phys Med Rehabil* 1993;4(6):566–573.

67. Johnston MV, Ottenbacher K, Reichardt K. Strong quasi-experimental designs for research on the effectiveness of rehabilitation. *Am J Phys Med Rehabil* 1995;74(5);383–392.

68. Cohen J, Cohen P. *Applied multiple regression/correlation analysis for the behavioral sciences*, 2nd ed. Hillsdale, NJ: Lawrence Erlbaum, 1983.

69. Collins LM, Johnston MV. Analysis of stage-sequential change in rehabilitation research. *Am J Phys Med Rehabil* 1995;74:163–170.

70. Posavac EJ, Carey RG. *Program evaluation: methods and case studies*, 4th ed. Englewood Cliffs, NJ: Prentice Hall, 1992.

71. Commission on Accreditation of Rehabilitation Facilities. *Program evaluation in outpatient medical rehabilitation programs*. Tucson: CARF, 1980.

72. Commission on Accreditation of Rehabilitation Facilities. *Program evaluation in inpatient medical rehabilitation programs*. Tucson: CARF, 1988.

73. Commission on Accreditation of Rehabilitation Facilities. *Program evaluation: a guide to utilization*. Tucson: CARF, 1989.

74. Commission on Accreditation of Rehabilitation Facilities. *Program evaluation: utilization and assessment principles*. Tucson: CARF, 1989.

75. Forer SK. Outcome analysis for program service management. In: Fuhrer MJ, ed. *Rehabilitation outcomes: analysis and measurement*. Baltimore: Paul Brookes, 1987.115 136.

76. Forer SK, Magnuson RI. Feedback reporting. In: Granger C, Gresham G, eds. *Functional assessment in rehabilitation medicine*. Baltimore: Williams & Wilkins, 1984:171–193.

77. Commission on Accreditation of Rehabilitation Facilities. *Standards manual for medical rehabilitation, July 2002–June 2003*. Tucson: CARF, 2002.

78. Gray CS, Swope MG. Integrated program evaluation and quality assurance processes. In: England B, Glass RM, Patterson CH, eds. *Quality rehabilitation: results-oriented patient care*. Chicago: American Hospital Publishing, 1989: 53–59.

79. Rubenstein LZ, Josephson KR, Wieland GD, et al. Effectiveness of a geriatric evaluation unit: a randomized clinical trial. *N Engl J Med* 1984;311:1664–1670.

80. Glueckauf RL. Use and misuse of assessment in rehabilitation: getting back to the basics. In: Glueckauf RL, Secrest LB, Bond GR, et al., eds. *Improving assessment in rehabilitation and health*. Newbury Park, CA: Sage Publications, 1993:135–155.

81. Gonnella C. Program evaluation. In: Fletcher GF, Banja JD, Jann BB, et al., eds. *Rehabilitation medicine: contemporary clinical perspectives*. Philadelphia: Lea & Febinger, 1992:243–268.

82. Commission on Accreditation of Rehabilitation Facilities. *Program evaluation in spinal cord injury programs*. Tucson: CARF, 1987.

83. Commission on Accreditation of Rehabilitation Facilities. *Program evaluation in chronic pain management programs*. Tucson: CARF, 1987.

84. Forer S. *Outcomes management and program evaluation made easy: a toolkit for occupational therapy practitioners*. Bethesda, MD: American Occupational Therapy Association, 1996.

85. Johnston MV, Wood K, Fiedler R. Characteristics of effective and efficient medical rehabilitation programs. *Arch Phys Med Rehabil* 2002;83, 2003;84(3), 410–418.

86. Stineman MG, Ross RN, Williams SV, et al. A functional diagnostic complexity index for rehabilitation medicine: measuring the influence of many diagnoses on functional independence and resource use. *Arch Phys Med Rehabil* 2000;81(5):549–557.

87. Chae J, Johnston M, Kim H, et al. Admission motor impairment as a predictor of physical disability after stroke rehabilitation. *Am J Phys Med Rehabil* 1995;74:218–223.

88. Novack TA, Bush BA, Meythaler JM, et al. Outcome after traumatic brain injury: pathway analysis of contributions from premorbid, injury severity, and recovery variables. *Arch Phys Med Rehabil* 2001;82(3):300–305.

89. Stineman MG. Case-mix measurement in medical rehabilitation. *Arch Phys Med Rehabil* 1995;76(12):1163–1170.

90. Iezzoni LI, Ash AS, Shwartz M, et al. Predicting who dies depends on how severity is measured: implications for evaluating patient outcomes. *Ann Intern Med* 1995;123(10):763–770.

91. Stineman MG, Escarce JJ, Goin JE, et al. A case-mix classification system for medical rehabilitation. *Med Care* 1994;32(4):366–379.

92. Stineman MG, Granger CV. Outcome, efficiency, and time-trend pattern analyses for stroke rehabilitation. *Am J Phys Med Rehabil* 1998;77(3):193–201.

93. Stineman MG, Goin JE, Hamilton BB, et al. Efficiency pattern analysis for medical rehabilitation. *Am J Med Qual* 1995;10(4):190–198.

94. Spyra K, Muller-Fahrnow W. Rehabilitee management categories (RMKs)—a new approach to case group formation in medical rehabilitation. *Rehabilitation (Stuttgart)* 1998;37[Suppl 1]:S47–S56.

95. Ellwood P. Outcomes management: a technology of patient experience. *N Engl J Med* 1988;318:1549–1556.

96. Wilkerson D, Shen D, Duhaime M. Version 1.1: Performance Indicators for Rehabilitation Programs. Tucson: Commission on Accreditation of Rehabilitation Facilities, 1998. Available at: http://www.carf.org. Accessed February 25, 2004.

97. Fauman MA. Quality assurance monitoring in psychiatry. *Am J Psychiatry* 1989;146:1121–1129.

98. Brook RH, McGlynn EA, Cleary PD. Quality of health care: Part 2: measuring quality of care. *N Engl J Med* 1996;335(13):966–970.

99. Committee to Advise the Public Health Service on Clinical Practice Guidelines, Field MJ, Lohr KN, eds. *Clinical practice guidelines*. Washington, DC: National Academy Press, 1990.

100. Marder R. Relationship of clinical indicators and practice guidelines. *Qual Rev Bull* 1990;16:60–61.

101. Kleefield S, Churchill W, Laffel G. Quality improvement in a hospital pharmacy department. *Qual Rev Bull* 1991;17:138–143.

102. Kravitz RL, Rolph JE, McGuigan K. Malpractice claims data as a quality improvement tool. II. Is targeting effective? *JAMA* 1991;266:2093–2097.

103. Shortell S, Bennet C, Byck G. Assessing the impact of continuous quality improvement on clinical practice: what it will take to accelerate progress. *Milbank Q* 1998;76:593–624.

104. Haley SM, Costner WJ, Binda-Sundberg K. Measuring physical disablement: the contextual challenge. *Physical Ther* 1994;74(5):443–451.

105. Batalden P. Building knowledge for quality improvement in healthcare: an introductory glossary. *J Qual Assur* 1991;13:8–12.

106. Donabedian A. *Explorations in quality assessment and monitoring*. Vol 2. Ann Arbor, MI: Health Administration Press, 1982.

107. Donabedian A. Criteria and standards for quality assessment and monitoring. *Qual Rev Bull* 1986;12:99–108.

108. Rutstein DD, Berenberg W, Chalmers TC, et al. Measuring the quality of medical care: a clinical method. *N Engl J Med* 1976;194;582–588.

109. Joint Commission on Accreditation of Healthcare Organizations. *National Library of Healthcare Indicators*. Oakbrook Terrace, IL: JCAHO, 2001.

110. Bush D. Quality management through statistics. J Qual Assur 1991;13(Sept/Oct):40–48.

111. McAuliffe WE. Measuring the quality of medical care: process versus outcome. *Milbank Mem Fund Q* 1979;57:118–152.

112. Andrews S. QA vs. QI: the changing role of quality in health care. *J Qual Assur* 1991;13(Jan/Feb):14–15.

113. Marx L, Haskin J. Nursing QA: step VI—determining thresholds for evaluation. *J Qual Assur* 1991;10:5, 15.

114. Gaucher EJ, Coffey RJ. *Total quality in healthcare: from theory to practice*. San Francisco: Jossey-Bass Health Series, 1993.

115. Joint Commission on Accreditation of Healthcare Organizations. *2003 standards for home medical equipment, respiratory therapy, and rehabilitation technology*. Chicago: JCAHO, 2002.

116. Joint Commission on Accreditation of Healthcare Organizations. *2003 comprehensive accreditation manual for home care*. Chicago: JCAHO, 2002.

117. Agency for Health Care Policy and Research. CONQUEST 2.0: A computerized needs-oriented quality measurement evaluation system. Rockville MD: US Department of Health and Human Services, Public Health Service, AHRQ Clearinghouse; 1999; AHCPR publication no 99-DPO1.

118. Mayhall CG. *Hospital epidemiology and infection control*. Philadelphia: Williams & Wilkins, 1966.

119. Association of Practitioners in Infection Control (APIC). *Infection control and applied epidemiology: principles and practice*. St. Louis: Mosby, 1966.

120. Kobs AE. Getting started on benchmarking. *Outcomes Manage Nurs Pract* 1998;2(1):45–48.

121. Gray CS, Upton BM, Berman S. *Monitoring and evaluation: physical rehabilitation services*. Chicago: Joint Commission on Accreditation of Healthcare Organizations, 1988.

122. Lutters M, Vogt N. What's the basis for treating infections your way? Quality assessment of review articles on the treatment of urinary and respiratory tract infections in older people. *J Am Geriatr Soc* 2000;48(11):1454–1461.

123. Leape L. Practice guidelines and standards: an overview. *Qual Rev Bull* 1990;16:42–49.

124. Chassin MR. Quality of health care. Part 3: improving the quality of care. *N Engl J Med* 1996;335(14):1060–1063.

125. Birch and Davis Associates, National Rehabilitation Hospital Research Center. The state-of-the-science in medical rehabilitation. Vol. II. Report submitted to Office of the Civilian Health and Medical Program for the Uniformed Services, Department of Defense. Falls Church VA: Birch and Davis Associates, 1996.

126. Post-stroke Rehabilitation Guideline Panel. Post-stroke rehabilitation. Clinical Practice Guideline Number 16.. Rockville MD: US Department of Health and Human Services, Public Health Service, Agency for Health Care Policy and Research; 1995; AHCPR publication no 95–0662.

127. Wenger NK, Froelicher ES, et al. (Guideline Panel). Cardiac rehabilitation. Clinical Guideline Number 17.. Rockville MD: US Department of Health and Human Services, Public Health Service, Agency for Health Care Policy and Research; 1996; AHCPR publication no 96–0672.

128. Pencharz JN, Grigoriadis E, Jansz GF, et al. A critical appraisal of clinical practice guidelines for the treatment of lower-limb osteoarthritis. *Arthritis Res* 2002;4(1):36–44.

129. Bergstrom N, Bennett MA, Carlson CE, et al (Guideline Panel). Treatment of pressure ulcers. Clinical Practice Guideline Number 15. Rockville, MD: US Department of Health and Human Services, Public Health Service, Agency for Health Care Policy and Research; 1994; AHCPR publication no 95–0652.

130. Bergstrom N, Allman RM, Carlson CE, et al. (Guideline Panel). Pressure ulcers in adults: prediction and prevention. Clinical Practice Guideline Number 3. Rockville MD: US Department of Health and Human Services, Public Health Service, Agency for Health Care Policy and Research; 1992; AHCPR publication no 92–0047.

131. Fantl JA, Newman DK (chairs), et al. (Guideline Update Panel). Urinary incontinence in adults: acute and chronic management. Clinical Practice Guideline Number 2, 1996 Update. Rockville, MD: US Department of Health and Human Services, Public Health Service, Agency for Health Care Policy and Research; 1996; AHCPR publication no 96–0682.

132. Aspen Reference Group. *Medical rehabilitation services: forms, checklists, & guidelines*. Frederick, MD: Aspen, 1995.

133. Schunk C, Reed K, eds. *Clinical practice guidelines: examination and intervention for rehabilitation*. Gaithersburg, MD: Aspen Publishers, 2000.

134. Odderson IR. Pathways to quality care at lower cost. In: Melvin JL, Odderson IR, eds. *Clinical rehabilitation and physiatric practice. PM&R Clin North Am* 1996;7(1):147–166.

135. Falconer JA, Roth EJ, Sutin JA, et al. The critical path method in stroke rehabilitation: lessons from an experiment in cost containment and outcome improvement. *Qual Rev Bull* 1993;19(1):8–16.

136. Duncan PW, Horner RD, Reker DM, et al. Adherence to postacute rehabilitation guidelines is associated with functional recovery in stroke. *Stroke* 2002;33(1):167–177.

137. Reker DM, Duncan PW, Horner RD, et al. Postacute stroke guideline compliance is associated with greater patient satisfaction. *Arch Phys Med Rehabil* 2002;83(6):750–756.

138. Johnston MV, Wood K, Stason WB, et al. The Reliability of the AHCPR's Clinical Practice Guideline for Rehabilitative Placement of Post-Stroke Patients. *Arch Phys Med Rehabil*, 2000;81:539–548.

139. Pestotnik SL, Classen DC, Evans RS, et al. Implementing antibiotic practice guidelines through computer-assisted decision support: clinical outcomes and financial outcomes. *Ann Intern Med* 1966;124:884–890.

140. James BC. Implementing practice guidelines through clinical quality improvement. *Frontiers Health Serv Manage* 1993;10(1):3–37.

141. Grol R. Successes and failures in the implementation of evidence-based guidelines for clinical practice. *Med Care* 2001;39[8 Suppl 2]:II46–54.

142. Grimshaw JM, Russel IT. Effects of guidelines on medical practice: a systematic review of rigorous evaluations. *Lancet* 1993;342:1317–1322.

143. Angstman G. Getting physician and organization buy-in. In: Kaegi L, ed. Practice guidelines: from paper to practice to point of care. *Jt Comm J Qual Improv* 1996;22(8):551–555.

144. Hunt DL, Haynes RB, Hann SE, et al. Effects of computer-based clinical decision support systems on physician performance and patient outcomes: a systematic review. *JAMA* 1998;280:1339–1346.

145. Hunt DL, Haynes RB, Hayward RS, et al. Patient-specific evidence-based care recommendations for diabetes mellitus: development and initial clinic experience with a computerized decision support system. *Int J Med Inf* 1998;51(2–3):127–135.

146. Von Korff M, Katon W, Unutzer J, et al. Improving depression care: barriers, solutions, and research needs. *J Fam Pract* 2001;50(6):E1.

147. Callahan CM. Quality improvement research on late life depression in primary care. *Med Care* 2001;39(8):772–784.

148. Randall G. Taylor DW. Clinical practice guidelines: the need for improved implementation strategies. *Healthcare Manage Forum* 2000;13(1):36–42.

149. O'Brien JA Jr, Jacobs LM, Pierce D. Clinical practice guidelines and the cost of care. A growing alliance. *Int J Technol Assess Health Care* 2000;16(4):1077–1079.

150. Eccles M. Mason J. How to develop cost-conscious guidelines. *Health Technol Assess* 2001;5(16):1–69.

151. Grol R. Between evidence-based practice and total quality management: the implementation of cost-effective care. *Int J Qual Health Care* 2000;12(4):297–304.

152. Woolf SH, Grol R, Hutchinson A, et al. Clinical guidelines: potential benefits, limitations, and harms of guidelines. *BMJ* 1999;31:527–530.

153. Grol R. Improving the quality of medical care: building bridges among professional pride, payer profit, and patient satisfaction. *JAMA* 2001;286(20):2578–2585.

154. Shaw CD. External quality mechanisms for health care: summary of the ExPeRT project on visitatie, accreditation, EFQM and ISO assessment in European Union countries. External Peer Review Techniques. European Foundation for Quality Management. International Organization for Standardization. *Int J Qual Health Care* 2000;12(3):169–175.

155. The AGREE Collaboration. Writing Group: Cluzeau FA, Burgers JS, Brouwers M, et al. Development and validation of an international appraisal instrument for assessing the quality of clinical practice guidelines: the AGREE project. *Qual Safety Health Care* 2003;12(1):18–23. Instrument available at: http://www.agreecollaboration.org. Accessed February 25, 2004.

156. Graham ID, Calder LA, Hebert PC,. et al. A comparison of clinical practice guideline appraisal instruments. *Int J Technol Assess Health Care* 2000;16(4): 1024–1038.

157. Wilkerson DL, Johnston MV. Outcomes research and clinical program monitoring systems: current capability and future directions. In: Fuhrer M, ed. *Medical rehabilitation outcomes research.* Baltimore: Paul H. Brookes, 1997:275–305.

158. Johnston MV, Wilkerson DL. Program evaluation and quality improvement systems in brain injury rehabilitation. *J Head Trauma Rehabil* 1993;7(4);68–82.

159. Bates DW, Teich JM, Lee J et al. The impact of computerized physician order entry on medication error prevention. *J Am Med Inform Assoc* 1999;6(4): 313–321.

160. Balas EA, Weingarten S, Garb CT et al. Improving preventive care by prompting physicians. *Arch Int Med* 200;160(3);301–308.

161. Durieux P, Nizard R, Ravaud P, et al. A clinical decision support system for prevention of venous thromboembolism. *JAMA* 2000;283(21):2816–2821.

162. Harvey RF, Jellinek HM. Patient profiles: utilization in functional performance assessment. *Arch Phys Med Rehabil* 1983;64:268=271.

163. Tierney WM. Improving clinical decisions and outcomes with information: a review. *Int J Med Informatics* 2001;62(1):1–9.

164. Widmer TG, Matthews CB, Gray LW, et al. Marketing program quality. In: England B, Glass RM, Patterson CA, eds. *Quality rehabilitation: results-oriented patient care.* Chicago: American Hospital Publishing, 1989: 69–101.

165. Halm EA, Magaziner J, Hannan EL, et al. Frequency and impact of active clinical issues and new impairments on hospital discharge in patients with hip fracture. *Arch Intern Med* 2003;;163(1):108–113.

166. Johnston MV. Cost-benefit methodologies in rehabilitation. In: Fuhrer M, ed. *Rehabilitation outcomes: analysis and measurement.* Baltimore: Paul Brookes, 1987:99–114.

167. Shaughnessy PW, Hittle DF, Crisler KS, et al. Improving patient outcomes of home health care: findings from two demonstration trials of outcome based quality improvement. *J Am Geriatr Soc* 2002;50(8):1354–1365.

168. Stineman MG, Goin JE, Granger CV, et al. Discharge motor FIM-function related groups. *Arch Phys Med Rehabil* 1997;78(9):980–985.

169. David D, O'Brien MA, Freemantle N, et al. Do conferences, workshops, rounds and other traditional continuing education activities change physician behavior or health outcomes? *JAMA* 1999;282:8867–8874.

170. Jain SS, DeLisa JA, Nadler S, et al. One program's experience of OSCE vs. written board certification results: a pilot study. *Am J Phys Med Rehabil* 2000;79(5):462–467.

171. Cleary PD, McNeil BJ. Patient satisfaction as an indicator of quality care. *Inquiry* 1988;25:25–36.

172. Nelson E, Rust R, Zahorik A, et al. Do patient perceptions of quality relate to hospital financial performance? *J Health Care Marketing* 1992;12(4):6–13.

173. Press I. The predisposition to file claims: the patient's perspective. In: G Troyer, Salam SL, eds. *Handbook of health care risk management.* Rockville, MD: Aspen, 1986.

174. Linn LS, DiMatteo MR, Chang BL, et al. Consumer values and subsequent satisfaction ratings of physician behavior. *Med Care* 1984;22(9):804–812.

175. Donabedian A. Patient satisfaction: an indicator of nursing care quality? *Nurs Manage* 1987;7:31–35.

176. Ware JE. Research methodology: how to survey patient satisfaction. *Drug Intell Clin Pharm* 1981;15:892–899.

177. Courts NF. A patient satisfaction survey for a rehabilitation unit. *Rehabil Nursing* 1988;13:79–81.

178. Davis D, Hobbs G. Measuring outpatient satisfaction with rehabilitation services. *Qual Rev Bull* 1989;15:192–197.

179. Ware JE Jr, Hays RD. Methods for measuring patient satisfaction with specific medical encounters. *Med Care* 1988;26(4):393–402.

180. Mylod DE. How satisfied are your patients? Surveys can help you benchmark quality. *Advance for Directors in Rehabilitation* 1998;8(6):17–20.

181. Stineman MG, Maislin G, Nosek M, et al. Comparing consumer and clinician values for alternative functional states: application of a new feature trade-off consensus building tool. *Arch Phys Med Rehabil* 1998;79(12):1522–1529.

182. McNeil BJ, Pauker SG, Sox HC Jr, et al. On the elicitation of preferences for alternative therapies. *N Engl J Med* 1982;306:1259–1262.

183. Siebens H, Weston H, Parry D, et al. The patient care notebook: quality improvement on a rehabilitation unit. *J Qual Improve* 2001;27(10):555–567.

184. Steward MA. Effective physician-patient communication and health outcomes: a review. *CMAJ* 1995;152:1423–1433.

185. Guadagnoli E, Ward P. Patient participation in decision making. *Soc Sci Med* 1998;47: 329–399.

186. Horn SD (ed). *Clinical practice improvement methodology: implementation and evaluation.* New York: Faulkner and Gray, 1997.

187. Horn SD. Clinical practice improvement: a data driven methodology for improving patient care. *J Clin Outcomes Management* 1999;6(3):20–32.

188. Iezzoni LI. The canary in the mine. *Arch Phys Med Rehabil* 2002;83(10):1476–1478.

189. US Department of Health and Human Services, Center for Medicare and Medicaid Services. Federal Register, 42 CFR Parts 412 and 413. *Federal Register,* August 7, 2001:41315–41364.

190. Hofer TP, Hayward RA, Greenfield S, et al. The unreliability of individual physician "report cards" for assessing the costs and quality of care of a chronic disease. *JAMA* 1999;281(22):2098–2105.

191. McCormick D, Himmelstein DU, Woolhandler S, et al. Relationship between low quality-of-care scores and HMOs' subsequent public disclosure of quality-of-care scores. *JAMA* 2002;288(12):1484–1490.

192. Himmelstein D, Woolhandler S. Cost without benefit: administrative waste in U.S. health care. *N Engl J Med* 1986;314(7): 441–445.

193. Kane RL. Improving the quality of long-term care. *JAMA* 1995;273(17): 1376–1380.

194. Wilson L, Goldschmidt P. *Quality management in health care.* New York: McGraw-Hill, 1995.

195. Clemmer TP, Spuhler VJ, Berwick DM, et al. Cooperation: the foundation of improvement. *Ann Intern Med* 1998;128:1004–1009.

CHAPTER 55

Measuring Quality of Life in Rehabilitation Medicine

David S. Tulsky and Nancy D. Chiaravalloti

Thanks to significant advances in technology and medicine throughout the last century, individuals are living longer following a catastrophic accident or serious illness. This produces a need for more sensitive and varied outcomes measures. No longer is it appropriate to rate medical success by the length of time that someone lives postinjury. Functional ability and independence have become significant outcome criteria in rehabilitation medicine. The measurement of an individual's functional ability, however, tells only one part of the story.

Quality of life (QOL) has emerged as an important endpoint in clinical trials research. It is crucial to evaluate the impact and value of any new treatment intervention. In the medical field, this end point emerges as a variable that is equal in importance to, or perhaps even more important than, increased survival time. In the rehabilitation field, this variable is broader than analyses of functional ability. As more and more medical advances occur, more refined measurement tools need to be developed for evaluating how the individual responds to their disability, its associated limitations, and its secondary conditions. The purpose of this chapter is to provide background into the science of QOL measurement and review current methods in key disability groups.

BACKGROUND

Although health-care professionals desire to improve the health and functioning of their patients, when pressed to offer a definition of *quality of life*, few could operationally define the term. Moreover, fewer still would be able to measure it reliably and validly. In fact, QOL is a term that many people use but few people really understand. Often, QOL definitions are interchanged with terms like *psychological well-being* or *happiness*.

Before the 1960s or 1970s, QOL was thought to be synonymous with material wealth, and it was measured in quantifiable units, such as the size of house one owned, the type of car one drove, the amount of income one received, and other material and economic indices. Campbell, Converse, and Rogers (1) cited a quotation by Herbert Hoover who promised Americans a "car in every garage and a chicken in every pot" as his way of improving QOL. Such a definition emphasizes materialistic possessions, and this conceptualization was common throughout much of the twentieth century. As Cella and Tulsky (2) have

pointed out, financial statistics, such as economic growth in gross national product or income per capita, were common methods of measuring QOL.

In the 1960s, more emphasis was placed on the construct of QOL, and its measurement started moving toward more social aspects of an individual's life. Lyndon B. Johnson developed the "Great Society" plan during his presidency, which emphasized improvement in the quality of the daily lives of Americans. He hoped that his policies would improve individual happiness and that there would be objective measures that could reflect the success of his policy through an increase in QOL. Thus, the indicators of QOL shifted from simple measurement of tangible goods to those that reflected an improved lifestyle. There became an increased emphasis on measures of social quality. However, constructs such as "psychological well-being" and a more global "quality of life" had not been systematically studied and measurement tools had not yet been developed.

It was shortly after this time that sociologists and social psychologists like Agnus Campbell and Norman Bradburn initiated research on psychosocial measures of QOL. Bradburn (3) first advanced the term *psychological well-being* and conducted one of the most thorough psychological studies of happiness and well-being of the era. Bradburn believed that psychological well-being could be measured from looking at the discrepancy between positive and negative affect. Within the sociology literature, the term *quality of life* was introduced in research in 1976 by Agnus Campbell and his colleagues (1), who set out " . . . to document and provide understanding of certain experiences which might be said to describe the quality of people's lives" (p. 13). The team placed great emphasis on subjective experiences rather than conditions of life and advanced the idea that the way people evaluate their experiences and conditions is a crucial component of QOL.

Several researchers have pointed out that this shift in the 1960s away from materialistic things to the measurement of more personal, subjective perceptions and response to life situations was a crucial development for the medical field (2,4,5). These events marked a transition in conceptualization that involved the individual and his/her reaction to the environment. By the late 1970s and early 1980s, the term *quality of life* was beginning to be applied to the health field. This application was most noticeable in the development of new means of assessing an individual's QOL, including the Nottingham Health Profile (6), the Sickness Impact Profile (7), the McMaster Health Index Questionnaire (8), the Duke Health Profile (9), and the RAND health measures (10,11). The latter set of indices were developed for some of the earliest studies in health care, including the Health Insurance Study and the follow-up Medical Outcomes Study, which were designed, in part, to study variations in patients' outcomes in competing systems of care (12).

In the rehabilitation field, Alexander and Willems (4) felt that "continuous functioning" and "reciprocal interactions between persons and their environments" were important components of the concept of QOL in individuals with spinal cord injury (SCI). Marcus Fuhrer (13) claimed that the term *subjective quality of life* is a synonym of *subjective well-being* and refers to "individuals' global judgments of their life experience along a continuum that ranges from positive to negative" (p. 359). This has not always been done in rehabilitation medicine, as several studies have focused on observer-rated measures of functional ability.

So, just what is this term that everyone seems to write about, and why is important to rehabilitation medicine? Cella and Tulsky (2) have offered three reasons why health professionals may be interested in measuring QOL. They cite its use (a) as a clinical tool to augment the evaluation of rehabilitation needs, (b) as an endpoint in evaluating clinical trials, and (c) as a predictor of an individual's response to future treatment. For instance, Cella (14) pointed out the importance of using QOL variables in oncology clinical trials as he describes the importance of the shift from solely measuring outcome by survival to applying indices of QOL by pointing out that increased "time without quality is of questionable value" (p. 57). Such sentiments began being expressed in the literature on cancer patients approximately 15 to 20 years ago (15–20). Fuhrer (21) acknowledged that subjective QOL or subjective well-being should be utilized as an outcome variable to evaluate medical rehabilitation interventions. He goes on to point out that the improvement of QOL is at the crux of the aims of the field of rehabilitation medicine. Dijkers (5) also made that point, writing that ". . . the field of rehabilitation medicine is in the forefront of concern for life's quality" (p. 153). Bach (22) illustrated how an evaluation of QOL is extremely important in making critical end-of-life decisions and advanced directives. Clearly, QOL is currently a vital concern in the field of rehabilitation medicine. The remainder of this chapter will look at the current conception of QOL measurement and review the status of how this measurement is done with select patient groups.

THE CONSTRUCT OF QUALITY OF LIFE: DEFINITION

One of the first formal definitions of health-related QOL was published as the initial principle in the World Health Organization's (WHO) Constitution, which was adopted in 1946 and published in six different languages (23). The WHO designated health (and QOL) as " . . . a state of complete physical, mental, and social well-being and not merely the absence of disease or infirmity" (p. 2). Today, most descriptions of QOL refer to it as a multidimensional construct involving the physical, emotional, functional, and social domains (2,11,24–29). Individuals, healthy or ill, with or without disability, view their life in whole and seek to have adequate well-being in a wide variety of areas, including the physical, functional, emotional, social, and spiritual domains. The conceptualization of QOL as a mul-

tidimensional construct allows us to view the impact of a disability or illness on the person as a whole (and not simply the specific function or system that is affected). Valid and adequate measurement of each of these domains is therefore necessary.

When referring to the potential impact of illness or injury on QOL, it is often referred to as Health Related QOL (HRQOL). HRQOL is by definition subjective in nature, and any preferred conceptualization of the construct states that QOL measures should be obtained directly from patient ratings and not from outside observers (e.g., physicians, nurses, family members) (25,30,31). Researchers tend to agree that the patient's subjective experience is an essential element in measuring this construct, which only the patients themselves can provide. These researchers pointed to findings that observer ratings of QOL do not correlate with patient-reported measures; soon, these health-care researchers incorporated into their definitions the view that individual perception, expectations, and subjective importance were paramount to adequate assessment of this construct. For instance, Calman (26,32,33) suggested that in health settings, QOL could be measured by the gap or disparity between an individual's expectations and achievements. Cella and Cherin (31) wrote that, for cancer patients, "quality of life refers to patients' appraisal of, and satisfaction with, their current level of functioning as compared to what they perceive to be possible or ideal" (p. 70). As Cella and Nowinski (27) point out, "there is seldom a good substitute for asking the patient, and for asking about a broad spectrum of functioning and well-being, such as symptoms, physical functioning, mood, cognition, family functioning, and social activity)" (p. S11).

GENERIC VERSUS TARGETED MEASUREMENT

QOL measures can be broken down into generic scales, disease-specific scales, and scale batteries (34,35). A key question that has confronted outcomes researchers is whether "disease-specific" or "population-specific" measures should be used versus generic measures. Both forms of questionnaires have been important and can serve different purposes.

Generic measures are more general in nature and thus have broad applicability across many populations and illnesses. The items on these measures tend to measure basic human values and are universally relevant to a wide variety of individuals, even those without medical problems (36) (Table 55-1). A benefit of using a generic scale is the possibility for cross-population comparisons. That is, QOL can be examined across populations, and individuals with a multitude of illnesses and disabilities can be measured on the same metric. This would allow a comparison of the impact of different illnesses or injuries on QOL between populations. Additionally, Cella and Nowinski (27) point out that these generic QOL measures can be tied to population norms when the scores of healthy individuals have set the standard upon which group scores from specific medical and rehabilitation populations are "benchmarked." Furthermore, Ware (36) discussed the benefit of such comparison studies, describing that these scales will become the common denominator, allowing us to identify the sensitivity of the illness or disability to treatment and examine the impact of differences in severity and treatment within or between diagnostic groups. At the same time, generic scales, while widely applicable to multiple populations, are not always sufficient to address the specific problems of certain medical populations (37). When using such instruments, many of the specific details are lost. This issue will be illuminated further in a later section.

TABLE 55-1.   Generic Quality of Life Measures That Have Been Used in Rehabilitation Populations

Scale	Citation
The SF-36 (from the Medical Outcomes Study)	Ware, J.E. Jr., Snow, K.K., Kosinski, M., Gandek, B. SF-36 Health Survey: manual and interpretation guide. Boston: The Health Institute, New England Medical Center; 1993.
Satisfaction with Life Scale	Diener, E., Emmons, R., Larson, R., Griffin, S. The Satisfaction with Life Scale. J Pers Assess 1985;49:71–5
Sickness Impact Profile	Bergner, M., Bobbitt, R.A., Pollard, W.E. Sickness Impact Profile: Validation of a health status measure. Med Care 14:57–61, 1976
	Bergner, M., Bobbitt, R.A., Carter, W.B., Gilson, B.S. The Sickness Impact Profile: Development and final revision of a health status measure. Med Care 19:787–806, 1981
Quality of Life Index	Ferrans, C.E., Powers, B. Psychometric assessment of the Quality of Life Index. Research in Nursing and Health. 1992;15:19–38.
Psychosocial Adjustment to Life	Derogatis, L.R., Lopez, M.: PAIS & PAIS-SR: Administration, scoring and procedures manual—I. Baltimore: Clinical Psychometric Research, 1983.
	Derogatis, L.R., Derogatis, M.F. The Psychosocial adjustment to illness scale (PAIS & PAIS-SR). Administration, Scoring, & Procedures Manual-II. Towson, M.D. Clinical Psychometric Research; 1983.
Nottingham Health Profile	Hunt, S.M., McEwen, J., McKenna, S.P. Measuring health status: a new tool for clinicians and epidemiologists. J R Coll Gen Pract 1985;35:185–8
McMaster Health Index Questionnaire (MHIQ)	Chambers, L.W., Macdonald, L.A., Tugwell, P., Buchanan, W.W., Kraag, G. The McMaster Health Index Questionnaire as a measure of quality of life for patients with rheumatoid disease. J Rheumatol 9:780–784, 1982

To address this limitation in generic measures, "disease-specific" or "targeted" measures have been developed specifically to measure distinct issues and problems that patients experience in a defined population. These problems or issues tend to be very focused and often are irrelevant when extracted to other populations. Cella and Nowinski (27) described that using these measures are ". . . akin to using a telephoto lens. They leave out some of the overall picture, but are more precise" (p. S11). Disease specific QOL scales have been developed for rheumatoid disorders (38), stroke (39), cancer (16), and cardiovascular diseases (40). Moreover, targeted measures have been developed for subgroups of certain illnesses or disability groups. For instance, David Cella and his colleagues have developed targeted instruments for various types of cancer (e.g., lung, breast, colorectal, etc.), with each set of items focusing on the specific condition (e.g., see 28, 41, 42 for examples of these targeted subscales). Although these scales are limited in the sense that they do not allow QOL comparisons across diseases, they are focused enough to provide sufficient, meaningful information about the specific patient population for which they were developed (37) and may be more sensitive for detection of small, yet important, changes (34).

In trying to determining which type of instrument is "better," most health-care researchers will argue that generic and disease-specific instruments should be used in a complementary fashion (27,36). Generic measures tend to enhance the sensitivity and allow greater comparison across groups, whereas the targeted measures tend to enhance the specificity of the measurement, allowing greater understanding of the specific functioning for the condition being assessed. Ware (36) writes that "the greatest progress in understanding outcomes for cancer patients is going to occur, not by substituting one measure or assessment strategy for another, but by mastering them in concert" (p. 776). This is true of any medical population.

Perhaps it is because of this goal of integrating these two forms of measurement that modular systems like the Functional Assessment of Chronic Illness Therapy system and the European Organization for Research and Treatment of Cancer Quality of Life Questionnaire systems were developed (27,43, 44fo). In these systems, a core generic instrument is used to assess the common QOL dimensions that are relevant to all patients and subjects (regardless of disability or illness). Supplementing the core questionnaire are subscales composed of items that are specific to the diagnostic group being studied.

QUALITY OF LIFE IN REHABILITATION MEDICINE

Much like early researchers in oncology focused on survival and increased life span, researchers in the field of rehabilitation medicine focused primarily on improving functional ability. After all, following a traumatic injury, serious illness, or other medical condition, key clinical questions exist in regard to classifying and improving the patients' ability to return to their prior level of functioning and, especially, function independently. Such questions are at the core of rehabilitation medicine, and classification systems like the WHO's *International Classification of Impairment, Disability, and Handicap* (ICIDH-2) (45) and Nagi's scheme of disablement (46,47) served important functions in the field by offering methods to describe and conceptualize an individual's disability. Similarly, a measure like the Uniform Data System's *Functional Independence Measure* (FIM™) (48,49) became a core outcome instrument in the field as it could be used to document increased functioning following a rehabilitation intervention.

This traditional outcome variable, functional ability, is only part of a broader range of outcome variables that are important to the field of rehabilitation medicine. Recent publications, such as the supplement edition of *Archives of Physical Medicine and Rehabilitation* (December 2000) suggested a need for new disability outcome measures that would broaden the measurement of outcomes in rehabilitation populations (50–52).

QOL is one such outcome variable, and indeed, there have been numerous studies of QOL that have been conducted within many rehabilitation populations. Despite the proliferation of research in this topic area, there is a dearth of studies that have developed new targeted scales for use in rehabilitation populations; nor are there many studies that even adapted generic instruments for rehabilitation populations. This is despite the fact that much of the research demonstrates the importance of tailoring the assessment tool to meet the needs of the specific patient population in question. A major challenge in evaluating the impact of an injury or illness on QOL is the fact that there is no gold standard for evaluating QOL, and the results of some studies may in fact be a by-product of the measures utilized (53). The following sections discuss QOL measurement in common disease etiologies seen in a medical rehabilitation setting, including traumatic brain injury (TBI), stroke, SCI, and multiple sclerosis (MS). (See Table 55-2 for a synopsis of instruments targeted to a specific population).

QUALITY OF LIFE IN SPECIFIC POPULATIONS

Quality of Life in Traumatic Brain Injury

It is estimated that in the United States alone 1.5 million to 2 million individuals per year experience TBI (54). Recent years have shown tremendous increases in the number of people surviving TBI, but 70,000 to 90,000 people incurring TBI sustain a substantial, long-term loss of functioning (54). These staggering statistics lead to questions regarding the quality of an individual's life following TBI. Despite this widespread impact of TBI, research on QOL following TBI remains limited. Not surprisingly, severity of TBI is not the lone contributor to QOL following TBI. The evidence indicates that social expectations and needs fulfillment affect QOL more than the severity of TBI (55). Johnston and Miklos (55) suggest that we first need to under-

stand the personal experience of the individual, only after which we can begin to understand the impact of TBI.

Although research examining QOL following TBI has been limited, numerous scales have been utilized to evaluate QOL in this population. Most scales used in TBI however, have been developed as global QOL assessment tools and therefore fail to contain questions specific to the experience of TBI. Strictly subjective QOL scales used within a TBI population include the Life Satisfaction Index-A (56), the Perceived Wellness Survey (57), and the Satisfaction with Life Scale (58). More commonly applied to TBI samples are scales with both subjective and objective components, including the Bigelow Quality of Life Questionnaire (59), the Brain Injury Community Rehabilitation Outcome—39 (60), the European Head Injury Evaluation (61), the Ferrans and Powers Quality of Life Index for Cancer (62), Flanagan's Quality of Life Scale (63), the Mayo-Portland Adaptability Inventory (64), the Neurobehavioral Functioning Inventory (61), the Psychosocial Adjustment to Illness Scale—Self Report (65), the Quality of Life Interview (66), the Quality of Life Questionnaire (67), the Quality of Life Rating Scale (68), the Reintegration to Normal Living Index (69), the Self-Rated Quality of Life Scale (70), the SF-36 (Ware et al., 1993), and the Wisconsin HSS Quality of Life Inventory (71).

Recent years have shown an interest in individually weighted measures of QOL, which allow the patient to weight items according to their importance to them. Such measures applied to the study of QOL following TBI include the Ferrans and Powers Quality of Life Index for Cancer (72), the Quality of Life Interview (66), the Reintegration to Normal Living Index

TABLE 55-2.   Targeted Quality of Life Measures by Population

	Scale	Citation
TBI	No targeted measures that have been published to date	
SCI	No targeted measures that have been published to date	
Stroke	Border of Stroke Scale (BOSS)	Doyle, P.J. Measuring health outcomes in stroke survivors. Arch Phys Med Rehabil. 2002;83:S39–43.
	Stroke specific—Quality of Life	Williams, L.S., Weinberger, M., Harris, L.E., Clark, D.O., Biller, J. Development of a stroke-specific quality of life scale. Stroke. 1999;30:1362–9.
	Quality of Life Index—Stroke Version	Ferrans, C.E., Powers, M.J. Psychometric assessment of the Quality of Life Index. Res Nurs Health 1992;15:29–38.
		Ferrans, C.E., Powers, M.J. Quality of Life Index: development and psychometric properties. Adv Nurs Sci 1985;1:15–24.
	Stroke adapted sickness impact profile	Van Straten, A., De Haan, R.J., Limburg, M., Schuling, J., Bossuyt, P.M., Van Den Bos, G.A. A stroke-adapted 30-item version of the sickness impact profile to assess quality of life (SA-SIP30). Stroke. 1997;28:2155–61.
	Stroke impact scale	Duncan, P.W., Wallace, D., Lai, S.M., Johnson, D., Embretson, S., Laster, L.J. The stroke impact scale version 2.0 evaluation of reliability, validity, and sensitivity to change. Stroke. 1999;30:2131–40.
MS	Multiple sclerosis quality of life index	The Consortium of Multiple Sclerosis Centers Health Services Research Subcommittee; MSQLI: Multiple Sclerosis Quality of Life Inventory: A User's Manual. New York: The National Multiple Sclerosis Society; 1997.
	Functional assessment of multiple sclerosis	Cella, D.F., Dineen, K., Arnason, B., et al. Validation of the functional assessment of multiple sclerosis quality of life instrument. Neurology. 1996;47:129–39.
	Quality of life multiple sclerosis version	Ferrans, C., Powers, M. Quality of life index: Development and psychometric properties. Advances in Nursing Science. 1985;8:15–24.
	Leeds multiple sclerosis quality of life scale	Ford, H.L., Gerry, E., Tennant, A., Whalley, D., Haigh, R., Johnson, M.H. Developing a disease-specific quality of life measure for people with multiple sclerosis. Clin Rehabil. 2001;15:247–58.
	Hamburg quality of life scale in multiple sclerosis	Gold, S.M., Heesen, C., Schulz, H., et al. Disease specific quality of life instruments in multiple sclerosis: validation of the Hamburg Quality of Life Questionnaire in Multiple Sclerosis (HAQUAMS). Mult Scler. 2001;7:119–30.

(69), and the Self-Rated Quality of Life Scale (70). The Personal Evaluation of Community Integration is a survey instrument that asks the person about his/her activities first, and then asks the person to evaluate feelings of satisfaction/dissatisfaction with them. The weighting approach to QOL measurement appears to be particularly promising to the evaluation of QOL following TBI (73). This is due to the fact that all people do not engage in the same activities, and all activities do not hold equal importance for different individuals. The loss of such an activity therefore has differential impact on individuals, and QOL will be affected uniquely for each person.

Often, in TBI research, the construct of QOL is not well defined, and studies have confounded the measurement of functional ability, assessment of the degree to which basic human needs are met, and traditional QOL measurement. Although the instruments purported to evaluate needs [e.g., Bigelow Quality of Life Questionnaire(59)] have been shown to be quite predictive of global QOL [as measured by various instruments, including Flanagan's QOL questionnaire (63), the Wisconsin HSS Quality of Life Inventory (71), and the SF-36 (74)] the construct of QOL is often blurred and not operationally defined. Similarly, well-known scales have been developed to assess health and functioning following TBI and have been mistakenly thought to measure the construct of QOL. Such measures include the Functional Independence Measure (FIM™) (75,76), the Sickness Impact Profile (77), the Functional Status Examination (78), and the Craig Handicap and Reporting Technique (CHART: 79,80). Although the inclusion of these measures in rehabilitation studies is essential to measure outcome, it is important to note that these measures do not assess overall QOL following TBI. Rather, they are designed to assess functional abilities and limitations. This is only one subcomponent of overall QOL.

Although QOL following TBI is traditionally assessed with generic measures not specifically designed for the TBI population, numerous characteristics have been identified as distinctive of individuals sustaining TBI. The experience of TBI goes beyond what is directly observable in that some report a loss of "normality" (81). Two ends of a continuum likely ensue. Either the person is treated as if nothing has changed, with performance expectations identical to that which was expected before the injury, or the person becomes stigmatized. These conditions are equally frustrating for the individual and often affect their overall QOL.

Research has indicated QOL following TBI to be generally poor (82,83), with emotional symptomatology prevailing. Specifically, major depression has been reported in 25% to 50% of individuals sustaining TBI (84), and dysthymia has been reported to occur in 15% to 30% of the population, sustaining for years after the injury (85). In fact, a lack of depressive feelings was shown to have a profound impact on the perception of a high QOL in TBI (83). Anxiety, apathy, and emotional distress have also been reported in this population (84), as well as posttraumatic stress disorder (85), all of which can impact QOL. Interestingly, QOL does not appear to improve over time in this population; rather, it may worsen (86,87).

QOL has been shown to correlate with a number of factors, including physical and social independence (83,88), employment activities (76,89–91), social/emotional support (83,89–91), social integration (92), and perceived mental and physical health (89). Blaming oneself for the injury is also associated with decreased QOL (88). Interestingly, severity of TBI shows a weak inverse relationship with QOL. Specifically, Fordyce and colleagues(86) reported that survivors of mild to moderate TBI show lower QOL than survivors of severe TBI, whereas Findler and colleagues (93) noted that individuals with mild TBI reported more health problems on the SF-36 than individuals with moderate to severe TBI. Other researchers have noted similar relationships, with those individuals sustaining mild TBI reporting more distress and lower QOL than those individuals with moderate-severe TBI (66,94). Hanks and colleagues (95) also noted greater adjustment difficulties for those with moderate TBI than those with mild and severe TBI. Dawson and colleagues (96) examined the ability of duration of posttraumatic amnesia, duration of loss of consciousness, and the Glasgow Coma Scale to predict QOL at 4 years postinjury, noting duration of PTA (days to recall three words) to be the only significant variable in predicting QOL 4 years after injury.

Some TBI patients present challenges to the assessment of QOL, such those with aphasia. Aphasia is a relative inability to either speak, comprehend language (either spoken or written), or both (97). If one cannot communicate in general, communications regarding QOL would clearly be impacted. As stated previously, the thoughts of the patient himself are essential to the accurate evaluation of QOL. This unique subgroup of TBI patients with aphasia is therefore largely overlooked in the TBI QOL literature.

Quality of Life in Stroke

Given the fact that the survival rate following stroke has been increasing over the past few decades (98) and 85% of individuals who sustain a stroke now survive (99), the QOL of stroke survivors has become a major public health concern. There is a substantial body of literature indicating that the experience of a stroke has considerable impact on an individual's QOL. Viitanen and colleagues (100) noted that 61% of their sample of individuals sustaining stroke had experienced a decrement in their QOL, mainly focusing on global, sexual, and leisure satisfaction. Many factors have been identified as associated with QOL following stroke, including depression (101–105), cognitive deficits (104,106,107), physical limitations (37,101–103,108), social factors (34, 103,108–110), and functional abilities (103,105, 111). In addition, Robinson-Smith and colleagues (111) noted the perceived ability to perform self-care tasks and levels of functional independence at discharge from inpatient rehabilitation to be related to QOL ratings 6 months after stroke. Although motor impairment is a major factor in QOL ratings (100), both qualitative (112) and quantitative (113) means of QOL assessment indicate that recovery extends beyond the regaining of physical symptoms. In fact, Hackett et al. (113) noted that individuals who survived to 6 years after a stroke demonstrated adequate QOL even though as many as 50% had not completely recovered from the stroke physically.

Numerous investigators have studied QOL after stroke using generic QOL measures. Some of these measures include the COOP Charts (114), the McMaster Health Index Questionnaire (115), the Nottingham Health Profile (6,116), the Sickness Impact Profile (7), the Medical Outcomes Study Short-Form Health Survey (117), the Karnofsky Performance Status Scale (118) the Quality of Life Index (119), the EuroQol (120), and the Quality of Life Well-being Scale (121). The Barthel Index is one of the most commonly used outcome measures in the stroke population. However, the Barthel Index has been noted to show some limitations, including ceiling and floor effects in stroke populations (122–125). The SF-36 is another generic QOL index that has gained wide usage within the stroke population, used in numerous stroke studies (122,125–128). Although the SF-36 is a well-constructed and widely applied QOL instrument, it does have significant limitations within the stroke population (122,127,128) and has thus been recommended for use only as a core QOL measure following stroke (129). As is evident, many generic QOL measures have been accused of failing to capture many clinically meaningful changes experienced as a result of stroke, such as changes in communication abilities or cognition (130).

The Burden of Stroke Scale (BOSS) is a comprehensive patient-report measure of functioning following stroke. It measures specific components of health frequently impacted by stroke that may be the target of clinical intervention, rather than broader aspects of QOL. In this respect, the BOSS is not the typical QOL measure. Rather, it quantifies the contribution of perceived limitations in one's physical, cognitive, and psychological world to the perceived burden resulting from stroke (130). The Stroke Specific Health Related Quality of Life Measure is also a relatively new QOL measure developed specifically for the assessment of QOL following stroke that shows good reliability, validity, and responsiveness in a stroke population (131). Williams et al. (132) noted such disease-specific QOL scores to be more sensitive to meaningful changes poststroke than the more generic QOL measures, namely the SF-36. The Frenchay Activities Index is a stroke-specific QOL measure (39) that has shown adequate reliability and validity, although it only assesses three of the important areas in QOL measurement (domestic chores, outdoor activities, and leisure/work) (133). Buck and colleagues (133) noted the Niemi Quality of Life Scale (107), the Ferrans and Powers Quality of Life Index—Stroke Version (QLI) (103), and the Stroke Adapted–Sickness Impact Profile–30 (SA-SIP30)(134)) each to have adequate reliability and validity within the stroke population, with the Niemi and the QLI assessing four relevant domains of life functioning and the SA-SIP30 measuring eight domains. Van Straten and colleagues (134) examined the SA-SIP30 for its clinical utility in stroke research, noting the SA-SIP30 scores to primarily represent aspects of physical functioning as opposed to health-related QOL. However, the authors also noted the SA-SIP30 to provide more clinical information than the more frequently used disability measures, concurring with previous findings that the SA-SIP30 is a feasible and sound measure for assessing QOL following stroke (134). Buck et al. (133) reported the Viitanen Life Satisfaction Interview (100), the Stroke Rehabilitation Outcome Study (135), and the Ahlsio Quality of Life Interview (101) to demonstrate adequate validity, but insufficient reliability. The Stroke Impact Scale (124) is an additional measure of QOL developed fairly recently specifically for the stroke population.

Many different factors have been shown to correlate with QOL poststroke. Kauhanen et al. (136) found that, overall, stroke significantly affects one's QOL, impairing the physical and psychosocial domains. Interestingly, depression was the most important reason for decreased QOL in this study. Jonkman et al. (137) also noted a significant relationship between QOL following stroke and depression, with QOL scores improving from 3 months to 1 year after stroke, but remaining abnormal at 1 year poststroke. Other studies have also noted a significant relationship between depression and QOL ratings (105).

Although different types of strokes have been demonstrated to result in vastly different outcomes in terms of mortality and morbidity, few studies have examined their differential effect on QOL. In a study examining QOL 6 months after stroke, de Haan and colleagues (138) found substantial limitations in most life areas, most notable in household management and recreation. Interestingly, except for communication abilities, there was little relationship between lesion laterality and QOL 6 months after the stroke. In addition, there were no significant differences in QOL between those patients with hemorrhagic

stroke and those with ischemic stroke, but relatively better QOL is noted in those who sustained lacunar infarcts and infratentorial stroke (138). However, age may be an important factor in this study; patients with lacunar infarcts were significantly younger, experienced less severe strokes, and had fewer poststroke handicaps compared with patients with supratentorial infarctions and hemorrhages. With findings such as this in mind, Hamedani and colleagues (139) began to validate an instrument specifically for the measurement of QOL following hemorrhagic stroke, the HSQuale. The HSQuale was found to be a reliable instrument for assessing QOL following hemorrhagic stroke. Subarachnoid hemorrhage survivors were found to show higher scores on the HSQuale than other stroke groups. In addition, 39% of the subarachnoid hemorrhage group was noted to show an improvement in overall QOL following the stroke as compared with their premorbid status, with occupational outcomes being very important to overall QOL in this younger sample of stroke patients (139).

The quality-adjusted life year is a common metric for the assessment of health-related QOL and length of life (140). With this metric, each year of life following a stroke is adjusted for the individual's perceived QOL during that year (141). This measure has been used frequently to evaluate the cost-effectiveness of interventions (141,142). In their review of the QOL literature in stroke, Tengs et al. (142) found that QOL weights for a major stroke ranged from −0.02 (worse than death) to 0.71; for a moderate stroke, QOL weightings ranged from 0.12 to 0.81; and for a minor stroke, QOL weightings ranged from 0.45 to 0.92. Interestingly, some studies presented weightings for a major stroke that were higher than weightings for a moderate stroke seen by other investigators. This indicates that QOL is not always more severely affected by a major stroke than by a moderate stroke. These authors noted a significant amount of variation in QOL weights following stroke, as well as various degrees of vigor in methods used to assess QOL after stroke (142).

As with TBI, stroke presents some interesting challenges to researchers and clinicians interested in measuring QOL. Most notably, survivors who are unable to communicate are consequently unable to provide QOL ratings (143). For such individuals, other means of QOL assessments have been found useful, including proxy ratings (144) and QOL inferences from performance-based evaluations (145). However, as mentioned previously, the use of proxy ratings may undermine the accuracy of the data collected given that the patient's perspective is thought to be paramount to the valid assessment of QOL.

Quality of Life in Spinal Cord Injury

With improvements in health care, life expectancy following SCI has also increased significantly in recent years. However, many individuals sustaining SCI are left with permanent limitations in motor functioning and the perception of sensation. This leads to concern regarding the quality of an individual's life following SCI.

A number of studies have noted that individuals with SCI report lower subjective well-being than nondisabled individuals (5,83,146,147). However, QOL ratings following SCI are not poor (53) and have even been determined to be good by some authors (148). Krause (149) found that SCI participants were less satisfied with economic satisfaction than they were with more general satisfaction, and were least satisfied with areas of life outside of their control.

A number of factors have been shown to be related to life satisfaction following SCI, including physical functioning (83), the experience of pain (150), health problems (151), social functioning (5,152–155), leisure satisfaction (156), ability to drive a car (155), coping effectiveness (157), sexual functioning (153), degree of dependency (151), occupational status and functioning (150,153,154,158,159), marital status (83,152,158,160,161), psychological functioning (83,151,152), number of rehospitalizations (153), social support (154,162), self-blame for the injury (88), and perceived loss of independence or perceived control (83,154). Access to the community has also been identified as an important predictor of QOL following SCI (153), however, this is one factor that has been shown to improve over time (163). In addition, research comparing individuals with SCI living in the community with those living in a nursing home has found that individuals living in a nursing home show lower QOL, even when controlling for factors such as age, education, race, marital status, and impairment level (164). A significant relationship has also been noted between physical fitness and QOL following SCI, with physical deconditioning significantly decreasing QOL (165). Duggan and Dijkers (166) carried out a qualitative study of QOL following SCI. They noted that financial security, material assets, meaningful social roles, and a longer time since injury were important prerequisites for higher QOL. Importantly, Craig and colleagues (167) noted cognitive behavioral therapy during inpatient rehabilitation to improve some aspects of long-term adjustment following SCI.

Data regarding the relationship between time since injury and QOL is conflicting, with some studies reporting a significant relationship (146,163,168) and others failing to find a relationship between the two (152,169,170). Tate et al. (168) noted the level of psychological distress to be significantly higher 1 year following SCI than at rehabilitation admission and discharge. Significant predictors of psychological distress at 1 year included distress at admission, neurologic completeness of SCI, type of rehabilitation insurance payor, occupational status before SCI, and participation in an independent living program. Krause (149) noted positive changes in adjustment over a 15-year period in a sample of 135 SCI participants, with long-term adjustment following SCI determined to be at least stable, but potentially improving significantly over time. Interestingly, there is evidence that the criteria an individual uses to measure QOL following SCI changes over time, with unattainable goals becoming less important and attainable goals becoming more desirable (53). Weitzenkamp and colleagues (171), in fact, found that the criteria used by an SCI sample to evaluate QOL changed over time. Differences were noted between the criteria used by the SCI sample and the criteria used by a sample of healthy controls, with priority values in the SCI group being related to what the individual has actually achieved.

Much of the SCI literature attempts to divide SCI participants into subgroups to evaluate the impact of injury level (tetraplegia versus paraplegia) and completeness of injury (complete versus incomplete) on QOL. Most studies have found no significant difference in QOL ratings between groups of SCI patients with tetraplegia versus paraplegia (83,146,147, 155,172), groups of patients requiring ventilator assistance versus those not requiring ventilator assistance (173), or groups of patients with complete versus incomplete injuries (152). In addition, cause of injury (e.g., traffic accident) has been shown to be unrelated to postinjury QOL (147,174). Kannisto and colleagues (175) divided SCI participants into three groups: (a) those who sustained pediatric SCI, (b) newly injured patients at the beginning of acute rehabilitation, and (c) patients with chronic SCI. The health-related QOL scores of the pediatric SCI group (assessed by a generic 15 dimensional self-administered instrument) was significantly higher than the other two groups.

Clayton and Chubon (176) also noted lower ratings of QOL to be associated with greater severity of disability.

Current measures of QOL are significantly limited in their use with an SCI population because they were not developed particularly for this population with their specific challenges in mind (53). They therefore tend to have items with limited relevance and lack the sensitivity to detect changes in QOL following SCI. Of particular concern is the impact of response shift on the documented changes in QOL following SCI (53). That is, if an individual is using a different criteria to measure QOL years after their SCI than initially following their SCI, current measurement tools are not adequate to capture these changes.

Numerous measures have been used to examine QOL following SCI. The Health Status Questionnaire (SF-12, SF-36) has been used frequently within an SCI population. However, a major limitation of the SF-36 within an SCI population is the appropriateness of the physical functioning items. Specifically, several of the items on the physical functioning scale are not sensitive to the paralysis associated with SCI, and slight modifications to item wording have consequently been published (177).[177] Other measures used to assess QOL following SCI have included an adapted version of the Older Americans Research and Services Questionnaire (178), the Index of Psychological Well-Being (179), the Life Satisfaction Index (180), the Life Satisfaction Index—A (151,154), the Satisfaction with Life Scale (153), the Quality of Life Index (157), the Life Situation Questionnaire (181), the Life Situation Survey (176), the Diener Satisfaction with Life Scale (182), and the Quality of Life and Individual Needs Questionnaire (183). Andresen et al. (52) evaluated the performance of five health-related QOL questionnaires with an SCI sample. Findings indicated good construct validity for the physical health measures of the Behavioral Risk Factor Surveillance System, the Quality of Well-Being Scale, the Instrumental Activities of Daily Living Scale, and the SF-36, with greater impairment noted in quadriplegia than paraplegia. A simple, subjective globally rated questionnaire has also been used with SCI patients (184). As with the stroke population, Quality of Life Adjusted Years have also been applied to SCI (165).

Quality of Life in Multiple Sclerosis

MS can have a considerable impact on an individual's QOL, largely as a result of common manifestations of the disease (185). Specifically, common symptoms often include motor and sensory impairment, bowel and bladder difficulty, vision problems, alterations in sexual functioning, fatigue, and cognitive deficits (186). In addition to the wide range of affected realms of functioning, MS typically has a young age of onset: between the ages of 20 and 40. Given the fact that MS often surfaces during the third and fourth decades of life, and younger adults tend to expect a higher level of functioning than older adults, MS symptoms may have a disproportionate impact on QOL.

In diseases such as MS, in which death is an unlikely consequence, the goal of health care is often to maximize a patient's health-related QOL (187). Disability in MS is often measured by Kurtze's Expanded Disability Status Scale (188), which focuses mainly on motor limitations. Other disease manifestations, such as visual impairment, cognitive impairment, or urinary incontinence, also exert a significant impact on the quality of one's life, yet are not reflected in the scale (187). A valid and reliable means of assessing all aspects of QOL in MS is therefore necessary, especially given that QOL is a main goal of clinical intervention. Multiple measures have been constructed for this purpose, some of which have been recently applied to an MS population. For example, Hermann and colleagues (189) used the RAND SF-36 to examine differences in QOL between individuals with MS, epilepsy, and diabetes. Results indicated that the MS group showed significantly lower health-related QOL than both the epilepsy and diabetes groups on physical functioning, role-limitation—physical, energy, and social functioning. It was therefore concluded that MS specifically influences specific health-related QOL issues not attributable to simply having a chronic medical condition or neurologic illness. Similar findings were noted by the Canadian Burden of Illness Study Group (190), in which the SF-36 was administered to 198 MS patients. The authors concluded that the QOL in MS patients is dramatically reduced compared with both a normal population and other chronic medical illnesses, even at very mild disease stages. Nortvedt and colleagues (191) also noted significantly lower scores on the SF-36, the SF-12, and the RAND-36 physical summary scales, as well as the mental summary scale of the RAND-36 in MS patients. However, they concluded these measures to be difficult to interpret in this population, noting that they tend to underestimate mental health problems in MS. The Canadian Study Group (190) also noted that MS disease progression resulted only in a lowering of physical functioning scale of the SF-36.

Gulick (192) used the Life Situations Survey (LSS) as a measure of QOL in an MS and a SCI sample. Results indicated the SCI and MS samples to demonstrate similar scores on the LSS. However, both groups had scores that were significantly lower than a healthy control group, indicating lowered QOL for these samples. In attempting to identify significant contributors to this decreased QOL, Gulick (192) identified living with a spouse and employment as the most important of six demographic variables in affecting QOL. Employment was thought to be important not only for income, but also due to the increased structure in daily life, the health insurance, and the opportunity for social interaction. Among activities of daily living functions, recreation/socializing was demonstrated to be important to one's QOL, consistent with findings in other populations including SCI (176,193) and cancer (194). Other factors found to have a relationship with QOL in MS include pain (192), cognitive functioning (195), and depression (196).

In addition to the identification of the presence of health-related QOL difficulties in MS, researchers have also identified lower QOL scores in the presence of more severe and more progressed MS, with a longer disease duration (185). That is, these authors noted that patients with MS have lower health-related QOL scores than a healthy reference group, regardless of the subtype of MS; this is true on both the SF-36 and the Disability and Impact Profile. In addition, the progression and severity of MS and time since diagnosis have been shown to exert a negative impact on QOL.

Although many studies have used the SF-36 with an MS population (190,197,198), other measures of QOL have been developed and applied to MS and should be considered when assessing QOL in MS. For example, the Farmer QOL Index has been used to study QOL in an MS population (199). The Quality of Life Index (QLI)—MS Version (62) was originally developed to measure the QOL of healthy individuals and subsequently adapted to assess QOL in persons with MS (200). The Leeds Multiple Sclerosis Quality of Life Scale is a brief disease-specific measure of QOL, with only eight items (201,202). The Hamburg Quality of Life Questionnaire in Multiple Sclerosis has been determined to be a reliable, valid, appropriate measure for assessing QOL in MS, distinguishing between patient groups differing in disease severity, cognitive impairment, and emotional symptomatology (203). The Functional Assessment of Multiple Sclerosis (FAMS) was also specifically developed for use with the MS population and has been shown to have adequate reliability and validity within this population. The FAMS is a 59-item questionnaire organized into six subscales: mobility, symptoms, emotional well-being, general contentment, thinking/fatigue, and family/social (204).

The Multiple Sclerosis Quality of Life Inventory (MSQLI) was developed recently by the Consortium of Multiple Sclerosis Centers Health Services Research Subcommittee (205) to respond to a need in the field to develop and test QOL measures in the MS population. A major emphasis was the development of a measure that would be specific to MS while also allowing a comparison with other patient populations. Given this goal, the MSQLI is a compilation of both generic and MS-specific measures. The SF-36 was included as a generic measure, whereas, for example, measures of bladder dysfunction and fatigue were included because these are common difficulties in MS. The MSQLI is actually a combination of a set of 10 scales. The authors recommend that the MSQLI be administered in its entirety, but each of the scales can be used in isolation. These scales are the SF-36, the Modified Fatigue Impact Scale, the MOS Pain Effects Scale, the Sexual Satisfaction Scale, the Bladder Control Scale, the Bowel Control Scale, the Impact of Visual Impairment Scale, the Perceived Deficits Questionnaire, the Mental Health Inventory, and the MOS Modified Social Support Inventory (206).

Despite the evidence of lower health-related QOL with disease progression, there is evidence indicating that health-related QOL can improve with treatment in an MS population. Specifically, Jonsson and colleagues (207) examined QOL with the Disability and Impact Profile before and after treatment with a cognitive retraining program. Significant improvement in ratings of disability and mood were noted following treatment, as well as less of an impact of difficulty with stair climbing and work. The authors interpreted these findings to indicate an overall improvement in QOL following treatment.

In summary, recent developments in medicine and technology have improved survival following traumatic injury and lessened the impact of neurologic disease progression of physical symptoms. However, many individuals are left with long-term deficits in physical, cognitive, social, and emotional functioning that have been shown to negatively impact one's QOL. It is important to recognize that each rehabilitation population presents with unique challenges to the assessment of QOL given that the life challenges associated with each population are different and the factors affecting QOL are consequently different. Such challenges make the development of QOL instruments tailored to individual populations necessary, and future research should focus on the development and validation of such measures.

THE FUTURE OF THE MEASUREMENT OF QUALITY OF LIFE IN REHABILITATION MEDICINE

A consistent theme running through the rehabilitation medicine literature is that existing generic scales of health-related QOL [e.g., SF-36 (208–210)] and life satisfaction [Satisfaction with Life Scale (58,211)], have been used in several studies across rehabilitation populations. Sometimes there were minor adaptations that had been made to these existing generic scales. However, it is unclear as to how appropriate these "measures of generic HRQOL" have been in populations of people with disabilities, as they have not been thoroughly tested (52,212–214). Unfortunately, with few exceptions, there has been little effort put forth to develop specific scales that are targeted toward individual disability groups.

Tulsky and Rosenthal (214) pointed out that QOL scales should tap a wide range of functioning, and if key elements are omitted from the measurement tool, the scale may suffer from "construct underrepresentation," which is a threat to the validity of the scale. So, when examining QOL in rehabilitation populations, it is important to identify which factors are most important to the specific population at hand. Rehabilitation researchers and clinicians alike should be aware that although health researchers are most often interested in factors that are affected by health care and illness (185), such as emotional symptoms, marital functioning, or mobility, other important issues for individuals with disabilities (e.g., such as housing or finances) may be overlooked, or if examined, they may be considered less important than other factors. It is therefore incumbent on the clinician to identify issues that may be important for a particular patient that may not be commonly examined, such as housing. Measure selection should then flow from the identification of these factors.

Additionally, QOL is differentially affected by disabilities, varying with the disability itself, as well as its impact or importance for a patient. This observation leads to the thought that the disability itself, as well as the impact of that disability on different activities, requires measurement. This realization has led researchers and clinicians to embrace newer, more creative means of assessing QOL. For example, a parallel approach to assessment is often used in which not only the disability is measured, but also its impact (35). The Disability and Impact Profile is used for this purpose (187). Designed as a parallel assessment, the Disability and Impact Profile ranks the degree of disability experienced by an individual, as well as the importance of the activity to the individual. In this way, scores are weighted according to their importance to the patients (187). The Personal Evaluation of Community Integration is another survey instrument that asks the person about his/her activities first, and then asks the person to evaluate feelings of satisfaction/dissatisfaction with them. The weighting approach to QOL measurement appears to be particularly promising (73), observing differences between rehabilitation populations in terms of the effects of the illness or injury as well as differences between individuals in terms of the aspects of life that are important to them.

In summary, in order to improve our capacity to accurately and validly evaluate QOL in different rehabilitation populations, a number of obstacles must be overcome. First, the development and refinement of QOL assessment tools appropriate to the individual patient populations is needed. The attainment of such tools will likely incorporate both disease-specific and generic QOL questionnaires in hopes of maximizing sensitivity and specificity in QOL measurement. Second, QOL measures should meet the professional consensus standards of obtaining subjective self-reported QOL and measuring multiple domains of well-being and functioning. Third, state-of-the-art assessment tools will also require creativity in terms of their capacity to circumvent identified obstacles. For example, Tate et al. (53) and Weitzenkamp and colleagues (171) discuss evidence that the criteria an individual uses to measure QOL following SCI changes over time. Ratings of QOL are thus improved. However, these improvements in QOL ratings are not due to QOL improving per se, but rather the individual's expectations of himself change over time. QOL measures need a means by which such changes can be accounted for in assessing changes in QOL. Finally, future QOL research should focus on the needs of specific patient populations. For example, stroke and TBI often result in aphasia. This inability to communicate precludes one's ability to truly assess QOL from the patient's perspective. Effective means for dealing with such an obstacle must be developed to avoid overlooking an important rehabilitation population.

QOL research has moved to the forefront of rehabilitation medicine over the past few decades. As a result, significant progress has been achieved in terms of learning about the QOL of diverse rehabilitation populations, developing and refining measurement tools for examining QOL effectively, and identifying factors within each population that are associated with increased or decreased QOL. However, as outlined above, many tasks lie ahead. Advances in medicine and technology will likely continue, facilitating the physical recovery of a larger proportion of individuals sustaining injury and adjusting to illness. This advancement will result in an even greater focus on the assessment and improvement of QOL following rehabilitation.

REFERENCES

1. Campbell A, Converse PE, Rogers WL. *The quality of American life*. New York: Sage, 1976.
2. Cella DF, Tulsky DS. Quality of life in cancer: definition, purpose, and method of measurement. *Cancer Invest* 1993;11:327–336.
3. Bradburn NM. *The structure of psychological well-being*. Chicago: Aldine; 1969.
4. Alexander JL, Willems EP. Quality of life: some measurement requirements. *Arch Phys Med Rehabil* 1981;62:261–265.
5. Dijkers M. Quality of life after spinal cord injury: a meta analysis of the effects of disablement components. *Spinal Cord* 1997;35:829–840.
6. Hunt SM, McKenna SP, McEwen J, et al. The Nottingham Health Profile: subjective health status and medical consultations. *Soc Sci Med [A]* 1981;15:221–229.
7. Bergner M, Bobbitt RA, Carter WB, et al. The Sickness Impact Profile: development and final revision of a health status measure. *Med Care* 1981;19:787–805.
8. Chambers LW, Macdonald LA, Tugwell P, et al. The McMaster Health Index Questionnaire as a measure of quality of life for patients with rheumatoid disease. *J Rheumatol* 1982;9:780–784.
9. Parkerson GR, Gehlbach SH, Wagner EH, et al. The Duke–UNC Health Profile: an adult health status instrument for primary care. *Med Care* 1981;19:806–828.
10. Ware JE, Johnston SA, Brook R, et al. *Conceptualization and measurement of health for adults in the health insurance study*, vol. 3. *Mental Health*. Rand Corp.; 1979:162.
11. Stewart AL, Sherbourne CD, Hays RD, et al. Summary and discussion of MOS measures. In: Stewart A., Ware JE, eds. *Measuring functioning and well being: the medical outcomes study approach*. Durham: Duke University Press, 1992:345–371.
12. Stewart AL, Greenfield S, Hays RD, et al. Functional status and well-being of patients with chronic conditions: results from the Medical Outcomes Study. *JAMA* 1989;262:907–913.
13. Fuhrer MJ. Subjective well-being: implications for medical rehabilitation outcomes and models of disablement. *Am J Phys Med Rehabil* 1994;73:358–364.
14. Cella DF. Quality-of-life measurement in oncology. In: Baum A, Anderson S, eds. *Psychosocial interventions for cancer*. American Psychological Association, 2001.
15. Brinkley D. Quality of life in cancer trials. *BMJ* 1985:291;685.
16. De Haes J, Van Knippenberg F. The quality of life of cancer patients: a review of the literature. *Soc Sci Med* 1985;20:809–817.
17. Donovan K, Sanson-Fisher RW, Redman S. Measuring quality of life in cancer patients. *J Clini Oncol* 1989;7:959–968.
18. Duncan W. Caring or curing: conflicts of choice. *Journal of Research in Social Medicine* 1985;78:526–535.
19. Greer DS, Mor V. An overview of National Hospice Study findings. *J Chronic Dis* 1986;39:5–7.
20. Peck A, Boland J. Emotional reactions to radiation treatment. *Cancer* 40:180–184.
21. Fuhrer MJ. Postscript and commentary. In: Fuhrer MJ, ed. *Assessing medical rehabilitation practices: the promise of outcomes research*. Baltimore: Paul H. Brooks Publishing Company; 1997:443–451.
22. Bach JR. Threats to "Informed" advance directives for the severely physically challenged? *Archives of Physical Medicine and Rehabilitation* 2003:84[Suppl]:523.
23. World Health Organization. *Constitution of the World Health Organization*. Geneva: Basic Documents, 1947.
24. Aaronson NK. Quantitative issues in health-related quality of life assessment. *Health Policy* 1988;10:217–230.
25. Aaronson NK, Meyerowitz BE, Bard M, et al. Quality of life research in oncology: past achievements and future priorities. *Cancer* 1991;67[Suppl]:844–850.

26. Calman KC. Definitions and dimensions of quality of life. In: Aaronson NK, Beckman, J, eds. *The quality of life in cancer patients.* New York: Raven Press, 1987.

27. Cella D, Nowinski CJ. Measuring quality of life in chronic illness: the functional assessment of chronic illness therapy measurement system. *Arch Phys Med Rehabil* 2002;83:S10–S17.

28. Cella DF, Bonomi AE, Lloyd SR, et al. Reliability and validity of the functional assessment of cancer therapy—lung (FACT-L) quality of life instrument. *Lung Cancer* 1995;12:199–220.

29. Wellisch D. Work, social, recreation, family and physical status. *Cancer* 1984; 53:2290–2298.

30. Aaronson NK. Methodologic issues in assessing the quality of life of cancer patients. *Cancer* 1991;67 [Suppl]:844–850.

31. Cella EA, Cherin DF. Quality of life during and after cancer treatment. *Compr Ther* 1988;14:69–75.

32. Calman KC. Quality of life in cancer patients. *Current Concepts in Oncology* 1984;6:2–3.

33. Calman KC. Quality of life in cancer patients–: an hypothesis. *J Med Ethics* 1984;10:124–127.

34. Wyller TB, Holmen J, Laake P, et al. Correlates of subjective well-being in stroke patients. *Stroke* 1998;29:363–367.

35. Guyatt GH, Eagle DJ, Sackett B, et al. Measuring quality of life in the frail elderly. *J Clin Epidemiol* 1993;46:1433–1444.

36. Ware JE. Conceptualizing and measuring generic health outcomes. *Cancer* 1991;67[Suppl]:779.

37. DeHaan R, Aaronson N, Van Limburg M, et. al. Measuring quality of life in stroke. *Stroke* 1993;24:320–327.

38. Liang MH, Fossel AH, Larson MG. Comparisons of five health status instruments for orthopedic evaluation. *Med Care* 1990;28:632–642.

39. Holbrook M, Skilbeck CE. An activities index for use with stroke patients. *Age Ageing* 1983;12:166–170.

40. Wenger NK, Furberg CD. Cardiovascular disorders. In: Spilker B, ed. *Quality of life assessment in clinical trials.* New York: Raven Press, 1990:335–345.

41. Brady MJ, Cella DF, Mo F, et al. Reliability and validity of the functional assessment of cancer therapy breast quality of life instrument. *J Clin Oncol* 1997;15:974–986.

42. Ward W, Hahn E, Mo F, et al. Reliability and validity of the functional assessment of cancer therapy–colorectal (FACT-C) quality of life instrument. *Quality of Life Research* 1999;8:181–195.

43. Cella DF, Tulsky DS, Gray G, et al. The Functional Assessment of Cancer Therapy scale: development and validation of the general measure. *J Clin Oncol* 1993;11:570–579.

44. Aaronson NK, Ahmedzai S, Bergman B, et al. The European Organization for Research and Treatment of Cancer QLQ-C30: a quality-of-life instrument for use in international clinical trials in oncology. *J Natl Cancer Inst* 1993;85:365–376.

45. Gray DB, Hendershot GE. The ICIDH-2: developments for a new era of outcomes research. *Arch Phys Med Rehabil* 2000;81:S10–S14.

46. Nagi SZ. Some conceptual issues in disability and rehabilitation. In: Sussman MB, ed. *Sociology and rehabilitation.* Washington, D.C.: American Sociology Society, 1965.

47. Enabling America: assessing the role of rehabilitation, science and engineering. In: Branch N, Pope AM, eds.Washington, D.C.: Institute of Medicine/ National Academy Press, 1997:5–10.

48. *Guide for uniform data set for medical rehabilitation (adult FIM).* Buffalo, NY: State University of New York at Buffalo, 1993.

49. Cohen ME, Marino RJ. The tools of disability outcomes research functional status measures. *Arch Phys Med Rehabil* 2000;81:S21–S29.

50. Andresen EM, Lollar DJ, Meyers AR. Disability outcomes research: why this supplement, on this topic, at this time? *Arch Phys Med Rehabil* 2000; vol 81(12 Suppl 2)S1–S4.

51. Meyers AR, Andresen EM. Enabling our instruments: accommodation, universal design, and access to participation in research. *Arch Phys Med Rehabil* 2000;81:S5–S9.

52. Andresen EM, Fouts BS, Romeis JC, et al. Performance of health-related quality-of-life instruments in a spinal cord injured population. *Arch Phys Med Rehabil* 1999;80:877–884.

53. Tate DG, Kalpakjian CZ, Forchheimer MB. Quality of life issues in individuals with spinal cord injury. *Arch Phys Med Rehabil* 2002;83:S18–25.

54. NIH Consensus Development Panel on Rehabilitation of Persons with Traumatic Brain Injury. Rehabilitation of persons with traumatic brain injury. *JAMA* 1999;282:974–983.

55. Johnston MV, Miklos CS. Activity-related quality of life in rehabilitation and traumatic brain injury. *Arch Phys Med Rehabil* 2002;83:S26–38.

56. Neugarten BL, Havighurst RS, Tobin SS. The measurement of life satisfaction. *Journal of Gerontology* 1961;16:134–143.

57. Bezner JR, Hunter DL. Wellness perception in persons with traumatic brain injury and its relation to functional independence. *Arch Phys Med Rehabil* 2001;82:787–792.

58. Pavot W, Diener E. Review of the satisfaction with life scale. *Psychol Assess* 1993;5:164–172.

59. Bigelow D, Gareau M, Young D. A quality of life interview. *Psychol Rehabil J* 1992;14:94–98.

60. Powell JH, Beckers K, Greenwood RJ. Measuring progress and outcome in community rehabilitation after brain injury with a new assessment instrument—the BICRO-39 scales. Brain Injury Community Rehabilitation Outcome. *Arch Phys Med Rehabil* 1998;79:1213–1225.

61. Johnston MV, Hall K, Carnevale G, et al. Functional assessment and outcome evaluation in traumatic brain injury rehabilitation. In: Horn LJ., Zasler ND, eds. *Medical rehabilitation of traumatic brain injury.* Philadelphia: Hanley & Belfus, Inc., 1996:197–226.

62. Ferrans C, Powers M. Quality of life index: development and psychometric properties. *Advances in Nursing Science* 1985;8:15–24.

63. Flanagan JC. Measurement of quality of life: current state of the art. *Arch Phys Med Rehabil* 1982;63:56–59.

64. Malec JF, Moessner AM, Kragness M, et al. Refining a measure of brain injury sequelae to predict postacute rehabilitation outcome: rating scale analysis of the Mayo-Portland Adaptability Inventory. *J Head Trauma Rehabil* 2000;15:670–682.

65. Derogatis LR, Derogatis MF. The psychosocial adjustment to illness scale (PAIS & PAIS-SR). *Administration, Scoring, & Procedures Manual-II.* Towson, MD: Clinical Psychometric Research, 1983.

66. Brown M, Vandergoot D. Quality of life for individuals with traumatic brain injury: comparison with others living in the community. *J Head Trauma Rehabil* 1998;13:1–23.

67. Evans DR, Cope MA. *Quality of Life Questionnaire manual.* New York: Multi-Health Systems, 1989.

68. Walker DE, Blankenship V, Ditty JA, et al. Prediction of recovery for closed-head-injured adults: an evaluation of the MMPI, the Adaptive Behavior Scale, and a "Quality of Life" Rating Scale. *J Clin Psychol* 1987;43: 699–707.

69. Wood-Dauphinee SL, Opzoomer MA, Williams JI, et al. Assessment of global function: the Reintegration to Normal Living Index. *Arch Phys Med Rehabil* 1988;69:583–590.

70. Hadorn DC, Sorensen J, Holte J. Large-scale health outcomes evaluation: how should quality of life be measured? Part II. Questionnaire validation in a cohort of patients with advanced cancer. *J Clin Epidemiol* 1995;48:619–629.

71. Collins R, Lanham RA Jr, Sigford BJ. Reliability and validity of the Wisconsin HSS Quality of Life inventory in traumatic brain injury. *J Head Trauma Rehabil* 2000;15:1139–1148.

72. Ferrans CE, Powers B. Psychometric assessment of the Quality of Life Index. *Research in Nursing and Health* 1992;15:19–38.

73. Gorbatenko-Roth KG, Levin IP, Altmaier EM, et al. Accuracy of health-related quality of life assessment: what is the benefit of incorporating patients' preferences for domain functioning? *Health Psychol* 2001;20:136–140.

74. Ware JE, Snow KK, Kosinski M, et. al. *SF-36 health survey manual and interpretation guide.* Boston, MA: The Health Institute, New England Medical Center, 1993.

75. Granger CV, Hays KM, Johnston MV, et al. Quality and outcome measures. In Braddom RL., Buschbacher R, eds. *Physical medicine and rehabilitation,* 2nd ed. Philadelphia: Saunders, 2000:151–164.

76. Corrigan JD, Bogner JA, Mysiw WJ, et al. Life satisfaction after traumatic brain injury. *J Head Trauma Rehabil* 2001;16:543–555.

77. McLean A Jr, Dikmen SS, Temkin NR. Psychosocial recovery after head injury. *Arch Phys Med Rehabil* 1993;74:1041–1046.

78. Dikmen S, Machamer J, Miller B, et al. Functional status examination: a new instrument for assessing outcome in traumatic brain injury. *J Neurotrauma* 2001;18:127–140.

79. Corrigan JD, Smith-Knapp K, Granger CV. Outcomes in the first 5 years after traumatic brain injury. *Arch Phys Med Rehabil* 1998;79:298–305.

80. Boake C, High WM. Functional outcome from traumatic brain injury: unidimensional or multidimensional? *Am J Phys Med Rehabil* 1996;75:105–113.

81. Prigatano GP. The problem of lost normality after brain injury. *J Head Trauma Rehabil* 1995;10:87–95.

82. Heinemann AW, Sokol K, Garvin L, et al. Measuring unmet needs and services among persons with traumatic brain injury. *Arch Phys Med Rehabil* 2002;83:1052–1059.

83. Kreuter M, Sullivan M, Dahllof AG, et al. Partner relationships, functioning, mood and global quality of life in persons with spinal cord injury and traumatic brain injury. *Spinal Cord* 1998;36:252–261.

84. Hibbard MR, Uysal S, Kepler K, et al. Axis I psychopathology in individuals with traumatic brain injury. *J Head Trauma Rehabil* 1998;13:24–39.

85. Hoofien D, Gilboa A, Vakil E, et al. Traumatic brain injury (TBI) 10–20 years later: a comprehensive outcome study of psychiatric symptomatology, cognitive abilities and psychosocial functioning. *Brain Inj* 2001;15: 189–209.

86. Fordyce DJ, Roueche JR, Prigatano GP. Enhanced emotional reactions in chronic head trauma patients. *J Neurol Neurosurg Psychiatry* 1983;46:620–624.

87. Koskinen S. Quality of life 10 years after a very severe traumatic brain injury (TBI): the perspective of the injured and the closest relative. *Brain Inj* 1998; 12:631–648.

88. Warren L, Wrigley JM, Yoels WC, et al. Factors associated with life satisfaction among a sample of persons with neurotrauma. *J Rehabil Res Dev* 1996;33:404–408.

89. Steadman-Pare D, Colantonio A, Ratcliff G, et al. Factors associated with perceived quality of life many years after traumatic brain injury. *J Head Trauma Rehabil* 2001;16:330–342.

90. O'Neill J, Hibbard MR, Brown M, et al. The effect of employment on quality of life and community integration after traumatic brain injury. *J Head Trauma Rehabil* 1998;13:68–79.

91. Webb CR, Wrigley M, Yoels W, et al. Explaining quality of life for persons with traumatic brain injuries 2 years after injury. *Arch Phys Med Rehabil* 1995;76:1113–1119.

92. Burleigh SA, Farber RS, Gillard M. Community integration and life satisfaction after traumatic brain injury: long-term findings. *Am J Occup Ther* 1998; 52:45–52.

93. Findler M, Cantor J, Haddad L, et al. The reliability and validity of the SF-36 health survey questionnaire for use with individuals with traumatic brain injury. *Brain Inj* 2001;15:715–723.

94. Brown M, Gordon WA, Haddad L. Models for predicting subjective quality of life in individuals with traumatic brain injury. *Brain Inj* 2000;14:5–19.

95. Hanks RA, Temkin N, Machamer J, et al. Emotional and behavioral adjustment after traumatic brain injury. *Arch Phys Med Rehabil* 1999;80:991–997.

96. Dawson DR, Levine B, Schwartz M, et al. Quality of life following traumatic brain injury: a prospective study. *Brain Cogn* 2000;44:35–49.

97. Ayd FJ. *Lexicon of psychiatry, neurology, and the neurosciences.* Baltimore: Williams & Wilkins, 1995.

98. National Heart, Lung and Blood Institute, National Institutes of Health (2000). *Morbidity and mortality: 2000 chart book on cardiovascular, lung and blood disease.* http://www.nhlbi.nih.gov/resources/docs/00chtbk.pdf (10 Aug 2000).

99. National Stroke Association. *Recovery and rehabilitation.* http://www.stroke.org/recov_rehab.cfm (10 Aug 2000).

100. Viitanen M, Fugl-Meyer KS, Bernspang B, et al. Life satisfaction in long-term survivors after stroke. *Scand J Rehabil Med* 1988;20:17–24.

101. Ahlsio B, Britton M, Murray V, et al. Disablement and quality of life after stroke. *Stroke* 1984;15:886–890.

102. Clarke PJ, Black SE, Badley EM, et al. Handicap in stroke survivors. *Disabil Rehabil* 1999;21:116–123.

103. King RB. Quality of life after stroke. *Stroke* 1996;27:1467–1472.

104. Sisson RA. Cognitive status as a predictor of right hemisphere stroke outcomes. *J Neurosci Nurs* 1995;27:152–156.

105. Carod-Artal J, Egido JA, Gonzalez JL, et al. Quality of life among stroke survivors evaluated 1 year after stroke: experience of a stroke unit. *Stroke* 2000; 31:2995–3000.

106. Kwa VI, Limburg M, de Haan RJ. The role of cognitive impairment in the quality of life after ischaemic stroke. *J Neurol* 1996;243:599–604.

107. Niemi ML, Laaksonen R, Kotila M, et al. Quality of life 4 years after stroke. *Stroke* 1988;19:1101–1107.

108. Johansson BB, Jadback G, Norrving B, et al. Evaluation of long-term functional status in first-ever stroke patients in a defined population. *Scand J Rehabil Med Suppl* 1992;26:105–114.

109. Tate DG, Dijkers M, Johnson-Greene L. Outcome measures in quality of life. *Top Stroke Rehabil* 1996;2:1–17. 110.

110. Shimoda K, Robinson RG. The relationship between social impairment and recovery from stroke. *Psychiatry* 1998;61:101–111.

111. Robinson-Smith G, Johnston MV, Allen J. Self-care self-efficacy, quality of life, and depression after stroke. *Arch Phys Med Rehabil* 2000;81:460–464.

112. Pilkington FB. A qualitative study of life after stroke. *J Neurosci Nurs* 1999; 31:336–347.

113. Hackett ML, Duncan JR, Anderson CS, et al. Health-related quality of life among long-term survivors of stroke: results from the Auckland Stroke Study, 1991–1992. *Stroke* 2000;31:440–447.

114. Nelson E, Wasson J, Kirk J, et al. Assessment of function in routine clinical practice: description of the COOP chart method and preliminary findings. *J Chronic Dis* 1987;40[Suppl 1]:55S–69S.

115. Sackett DL, Chambers LW, MacPherson AS, et al. The development and application of indices of health: general methods and a summary of results. *Am J Public Health* 1977;67:423–428.

116. Ebrahim S, Barer D, Nouri F. Use of the Nottingham Health Profile with patients after a stroke. *J Epidemiol Community Health* 1986;40:166–169.

117. Stewart AL, Hays RD, Ware JE Jr. The MOS short-form general health survey: reliability and validity in a patient population. *Med Care* 1988;26:724–735.

118. Schag CC, Heinrich RL, Ganz PA. Karnofsky performance status revisited: reliability, validity, and guidelines. *J Clin Oncol* 1984;2:187–193.

119. Spitzer WO, Dobson AJ, Hall J, et al. Measuring the quality of life of cancer patients: a concise QL-index for use by physicians. *J Chronic Dis* 1981;34: 585–597.

120. The EuroQol Group. EuroQol—a new facility for the measurement of health-related quality of life. *Health Policy* 1990;16:199–208.

121. Anderson JP, Kaplan RM, Berry CC, et al. Interday reliability of function assessment for a health status measure: the Quality of Well-Being scale. *Med Care* 1989;27:1076–1083.

122. Duncan PW, Samsa GP, Weinberger M, et al. Health status of individuals with mild stroke. *Stroke* 1997;28:740–745.

123. Kelly-Hayes M, Robertson JT, Broderick JP, et al. The American Heart Association Stroke Outcome Classification. *Stroke* 1998;29:1274–1280.

124. Duncan PW, Wallace D, Lai SM, et al. The stroke impact scale version 2.0: evaluation of reliability, validity, and sensitivity to change. *Stroke* 1999; 30:2131–2140.

125. Kappelle LJ, Adams HP Jr, Heffner ML, et al. Prognosis of young adults with ischemic stroke: a long-term follow-up study assessing recurrent vascular events and functional outcome in the Iowa Registry of Stroke in Young Adults. *Stroke* 1994;25:1360–1365.

126. Hop JW, Rinkel GJ, Algra A, et al. Quality of life in patients and partners after aneurysmal subarachnoid hemorrhage. *Stroke* 1998;29:798–804.

127. Anderson C, Laubscher S, Burns R. Validation of the Short Form 36 (SF-36) health survey questionnaire among stroke patients. *Stroke* 1996;27:1812–1816.

128. Dorman P, Slattery J, Farrell B, et al. Qualitative comparison of the reliability of health status assessments with the EuroQol and SF-36 questionnaires after stroke. United Kingdom Collaborators in the International Stroke Trial. *Stroke* 1998;29:63–68.

129. Ware JE. The SF-36. In: B. Spilker, ed. *Quality of life and pharmacoeconomics in clinical trials,* 2nd ed. Philadelphia: Lippincott-Raven, 1996:337–345.

130. Doyle PJ. Measuring health outcomes in stroke survivors. *Arch Phys Med Rehabil* 2002;83:S39–S43.

131. Williams LS, Weinberger M, Harris LE, et al. Development of a stroke-specific quality of life scale. *Stroke* 1999;30:1362–1369.

132. Williams LS, Weinberger M, Harris LE, et al. Measuring quality of life in a way that is meaningful to stroke patients. *Neurology* 1999;53:1839–1843.

133. Buck D, Jacoby A, Massey A, Ford G. Evaluation of measures used to assess quality of life after stroke. *Stroke* 2000;31:2004–2010.

134. van Straten A, de Haan RJ, Limburg M, et al. A stroke-adapted 30-item version of the Sickness Impact Profile to assess quality of life (SA-SIP30). *Stroke* 1997;28:2155–2161.

135. Granger CV, Hamilton BB, Gresham GE. The stroke rehabilitation outcome study—Part I: general description. *Arch Phys Med Rehabil* 1988;69:506–509.

136. Kauhanen ML, Korpelainen JT, Hiltunen P, et al. Domains and determinants of quality of life after stroke caused by brain infarction. *Arch Phys Med Rehabil* 2000;81:1541–1546.

137. Jonkman EJ, de Weerd AW, Vrijens NL. Quality of life after a first ischemic stroke: long-term developments and correlations with changes in neurological deficit, mood and cognitive impairment. *Acta Neurol Scand* 1998;98:169–175.

138. de Haan RJ, Limburg M, Van der Meulen JH, et al. Quality of life after stroke: impact of stroke type and lesion location. *Stroke* 1995;26:402–408.

139. Hamedani AG, Wells CK, Brass LM, et al. A quality-of-life instrument for young hemorrhagic stroke patients. *Stroke* 2001;32:687–695.

140. Gold MR, Siegel JE, Russell LB, et al. *Cost-effectiveness in health, and medicine.* New York: Oxford University Press, 1996.

141. Turner S. Quality-adjusted life years: cost-effective medical decision-making. *J Cardiovasc Manag* 1997;8:34–39.

142. Tengs TO, Yu M, Luistro E. Health-related quality of life after stroke: a comprehensive review. *Stroke* 2001;32:964–972.

143. LaPointe LL. Quality of life with aphasia. *Semin Speech Lang* 1999;20:5–16; quiz 16–17.

144. Sneeuw KC, Aaronson NK, de Haan RJ, et al. Assessing quality of life after stroke: the value and limitations of proxy ratings. *Stroke* 1997;28:1541–1549.

145. McEwen S, Mayo N, Wood-Dauphinee S. Inferring quality of life from performance-based assessments. *Disabil Rehabil* 2000;22:456–463.

146. Westgren N, Levi R. Quality of life and traumatic spinal cord injury. *Arch Phys Med Rehabil* 1998;79:1433–1439.

147. Post MW, Van Dijk AJ, Van Asbeck FW, et al. Life satisfaction of persons with spinal cord injury compared to a population group. *Scand J Rehabil Med* 1998;30:23–30.

148. Whiteneck GG. Outcome evaluation and spinal cord injury. *NeuroRehabil* 1992;2:31–41.

149. Krause JS. Longitudinal changes in adjustment after spinal cord injury: a 15-year study. *Arch Phys Med Rehabil* 1992;73:564–568.

150. Lundqvist C, Siosteen A, Blomstrand C, et al. Spinal cord injuries: clinical, functional, and emotional status. *Spine* 1991;16:78–83.

151. Krause JS, Dawis RV. Prediction of life satisfaction after spinal cord injury. *Rehabilitation Psychology* 1992;37:49–60.

152. Post MW, de Witte LP, van Asbeck FW, et al. Predictors of health status and life satisfaction in spinal cord injury. *Arch Phys Med Rehabil* 1998;79:395–401.

153. Dijkers MP. Correlates of life satisfaction among persons with spinal cord injury. *Arch Phys Med Rehabil* 1999;80:867–876.

154. Fuhrer MJ, Rintala DH, Hart KA, et al. Relationship of life satisfaction to impairment, disability, and handicap among persons with spinal cord injury living in the community. *Arch Phys Med Rehabil* 1992;73:552–557.

155. Siosteen A, Lundqvist C, Blomstrand C, et al. The quality of life of three functional spinal cord injury subgroups in a Swedish community. *Paraplegia* 1990;28:476–488.

156. Coyle CP, Lesnik-Emas S, Kinney WB. Predicting life satisfaction among adults with spinal cord injuries. *Rehabilitation Psychology* 1994;39:95.

157. Nieves CC, Charter RA, Aspinall MJ. Relationship between effective coping and perceived quality of life in spinal cord injured patients. *Rehabil Nurs* 1991;16:129–132.

158. McColl MA, Stirling P, Walker J, et al. Expectations of independence and life satisfaction among aging spinal cord injured adults. *Disabil Rehabil* 1999;21: 231–240.

159. Krause JS, Anson CA. Adjustment after spinal cord injury: relationship to participation in employment or educational activities. *Rehabilitation Counseling Bulletin* 1997;40:203.

160. Putzke J, Elliott T, Richards J. Marital status and adjustment 1 year post spinal cord injury. *Journal of Clinical Psychology Medical Settings* 2001;8:101–107.

161. Holicky R, Charlifue S. Aging with spinal cord injury: the impact of spousal support. *Disabil Rehabil* 1999;21:250–257.

162. Rintala DH, Young ME, Hart KA, et al. Social support and the well-being of persons with spinal cord injury living in the community. *Rehabilitation Psychology* 1992;37:155.

163. Richards JS, Bombardier CH, Tate D, et al. Access to the environment and life satisfaction after spinal cord injury. *Arch Phys Med Rehabil* 1999;80:1501–1506.

164. Putzke JD, Richards JS. Nursing home residence: quality of life among individuals with spinal cord injury. *Am J Phys Med Rehabil* 2001;80:404–409.

165. Noreau L, Shephard RJ. Spinal cord injury, exercise and quality of life. *Sports Med* 1995;20:226–250.

166. Duggan CH, Dijkers M. Quality of life after spinal cord injury: a qualitative study. *Rehabilitation Psychology* 2001;46:3–27.

167. Craig A, Hancock K, Dickson H. Improving the long-term adjustment of spinal cord injured persons. *Spinal Cord* 1999;37:345–350.

168. Tate DG, Maynard F, Forchheimer M. Predictors of psychologic distress one year after spinal cord injury. *Am J Phys Med Rehabil* 1993;72:272.

169. Crewe N, Krause J. An eleven-year follow-up of adjustment to spinal cord injury. *Rehabilitation Psychology* 1990;35:205–210.

170. Kennedy P, Rogers B. Reported quality of life of people with spinal cord injuries: a longitudinal analysis of the first 6 months post-discharge. *Spinal Cord* 2000;38:498–503.

171. Weitzenkamp D, Gerhart K, Charlifue S, et al. Ranking the criteria for assessing quality of life after disability: evidence for priority shifting among long-term spinal cord injury survivors. *B J Health Psych* 2000;5:57–69.

172. Manns PJ, Chad KE. Determining the relation between quality of life, handicap, fitness, and physical activity for persons with spinal cord injury. *Arch Phys Med Rehabil* 1999;80:1566–1571.

173. Hall KM, Knudsen ST, Wright J, et al. Follow-up study of individuals with high tetraplegia (C1-C4) 14 to 24 years postinjury. *Arch Phys Med Rehabil* 1999;80:1507–1513.

174. Putzke JD, Richards JS, DeVivo MJ. Quality of life after spinal cord injury caused by gunshot. *Arch Phys Med Rehabil* 2001;82:949–954.

175. Kannisto M, Merikanto J, Alaranta H, et al. Comparison of health-related quality of life in three subgroups of spinal cord injury patients. *Spinal Cord* 1998;36:193–199.

176. Clayton KS, Chubon RA. Factors associated with the quality of life of long-term spinal cord injured persons. *Arch Phys Med Rehabil* 1994;75:633–638.

177. Tate D, Forchheimer M, Karunas R. Relationship of health status and functional independence to neurological impairment in spinal cord injury. *Arch Phys Med Rehabil* 1998;79:1322.

178. Duke University. *OARS multidimensional functional assessment questionnaire.* Durham, NC.: Duke University Center for the Study of Aging and Human Development, 1978.

179. Berkman PL. Measurement of mental health in a general population survey. *Am J Epidemiol* 1971;94:105–111.

180. Wood V, Wylie ML, Sheafor B. An analysis of a short self-report measure of life satisfaction: correlation with rater judgments. *J Gerontol* 1969;24:465–469.

181. Krause JS. Life satisfaction after spinal cord injury: a descriptive study. *Rehabilitation Psychology* 1992;37:60.

182. Diener E. Assessing subjective well-being: program and opportunities. *Soc Indicators Res* 1994;31:103–157.

183. Flanagan JC. A research approach to improving our quality of life. *Am Psychol* 1978;2:138–147.

184. Whiteneck GG. Long-term outlook for persons with high quadriplegia. In: Whiteneck GG, Adler C, Carter RF, et. al., eds.. *The management of high quadriplegia*. New York: Demos Publications, 1989.

185. Pfennings L, Cohen L, Ader H, et al. Exploring differences between subgroups of multiple sclerosis patients in health-related quality of life. *J Neurol* 1999;246:587–591.

186. Kurtze JF, Beebe GW, Nagler B, et al. Studies on the natural history of multiple sclerosis. *Acta Neurol Scand* 1972;48:19–46.

187. Lankhorst GJ, Jelles F, Smits RC, et al. Quality of life in multiple sclerosis: the disability and impact profile (DIP). *J Neurol* 1996;243:469–474.

188. Kurtze JF. Rating neurological impairments in multiple sclerosis: an expanded disability status scale (EDSS). *Neurology* 1983;33:1444–1452.

189. Hermann BP, Vickrey B, Hays RD, et al. A comparison of health-related quality of life in patients with epilepsy, diabetes and multiple sclerosis. *Epilepsy Res* 1996;25:113–118.

190. The Canadian Burden of Illness Study Group. Burden of illness of multiple sclerosis: Part II: Quality of life. *Can J Neurol Sci* 1998;25:31–38.

191. Nortvedt MW, Riise T, Myhr KM, et al. Performance of the SF-36, SF-12, and RAND-36 summary scales in a multiple sclerosis population. *Med Care* 2000;38:1022–1028.

192. Gulick EE. Correlates of quality of life among persons with multiple sclerosis. *Nurs Res* 1997;46:305.

193. Crisp R. The long-term adjustment of 60 persons with spinal cord injury. *Australian Psychologist* 1992;27:43–47.

194. Kreitler S, Chaitchik S, Rapoport Y, et al. Life satisfaction and health in cancer patients, orthopedic patients and healthy individuals. *Soc Sci Med* 1993;36:547–556.

195. Cutajar R, Ferriani E, Scandellari C, et al. Cognitive function and quality of life in multiple sclerosis patients. *J Neurovirol* 2000;6[Suppl 2]:S186–190.

196. Wang JL, Reimer MA, Metz LM, et al. Major depression and quality of life in individuals with multiple sclerosis. *Int J Psychiatry Med* 2000;30:309–317.

197. Vickrey BG, Hays RD, Genovese BJ, et al. Comparison of a generic to disease-targeted health-related quality-of-life measures for multiple sclerosis. *J Clin Epidemiol* 1997;50:557–569.

198. Nortvedt MW, Riise T, Myhr KM, et al. Quality of life in multiple sclerosis: measuring the disease effects more broadly. *Neurology* 1999;53:1098–1103.

199. Rudick RA, Miller D, Clough JD, et al. Quality of life in multiple sclerosis: comparison with inflammatory bowel disease and rheumatoid arthritis. *Arch Neurol* 1992;49:1237–1242.

200. Stuifbergen AK. Health-promoting behaviors and quality of life among individuals with multiple sclerosis. *Sch Inq Nurs Pract* 1995;9:31–50; 51–55.

201. Ford HL, Gerry E, Tennant A, et al. Developing a disease-specific quality of life measure for people with multiple sclerosis. *Clin Rehabil* 2001;15:247–258.

202. Ford HL, Gerry E, Johnson MH, et al. Health status and quality of life of people with multiple sclerosis. *Disabil Rehabil* 2001;23:516–521.

203. Gold SM, Heesen C, Schulz H, et al. Disease specific quality of life instruments in multiple sclerosis: validation of the Hamburg Quality of Life Questionnaire in Multiple Sclerosis (HAQUAMS). *Mult Scler* 2001;7:119–130.

204. Cella DF, Dineen K, Arnason B, et al. Validation of the functional assessment of multiple sclerosis quality of life instrument. *Neurology* 1996;47:129–139.

205. The Consortium of Multiple Sclerosis Centers Health Services Research Subcommittee. *MSQLI: Multiple Sclerosis Quality of Life Inventory: a user's manual.* New York: The National Multiple Sclerosis Society, 1997.

206. Fischer JS, LaRocca NG, Miller DM, et al. Recent developments in the assessment of quality of life in multiple sclerosis (MS). *Mult Scler* 1999;5:251–259.

207. Jonsson A, Dock J, Ravnborg MH. Quality of life as a measure of rehabilitation outcome in patients with multiple sclerosis. *Acta Neurol Scand* 1996;93:229–235.

208. Hays RD, Sherbourne CD. The MOS 36-item health survey 1.0. *Health Econ* 1993;2:217–227.

209. Ware JE, Sherbourne CD. The MOS 36-item short-form health survey: (SF-36) I. Conceptual framework and item selection. *Med Care* 1992;30:473–483.

210. Ware JE, Snow KK, Kosinski M, et al. *SF-36 health survey: manual and interpretation guide.* Boston: The Health Institute, New England Medical Center, 1993.

211. Diener E, Emmons R, Larson R, et al. The satisfaction with life scale. *J Pers Assess* 1985;49:71–75.

212. Andresen EM, Meyers AR. Health related quality of life outcome measures. *Arch Phys Med Rehabil* 2000;81:S30–S45.

213. Hays RD, Hahn H, Marshall G. Use of the SF-36 and other health-related quality of life measures to assess persons with disabilities. *Arch Phys Med Rehabil* 2002;83:S4–S9.

214. Tulsky DS, Rosenthal M. Quality of life measurement in rehabilitation medicine: building an agenda for the future. *Arch Phys Med Rehabil* 2002;83:S1–S3.

PART II

Management Methods

CHAPTER 56

Pharmacotherapy of Disability

Todd P. Stitik, Robert Klecz, and Brian Greenwald

This chapter is intended to provide the physiatrist with clinically useful material about many medications that are used in both adult inpatient and outpatient physiatric practice. While it is not the chapter's intent to serve as an all-inclusive detailed source of information on every aspect of all the medications prescribed by physiatrists, it provides a good blend of basic information about mechanism of action, relevant pharmacokinetics, dosing, potential side effects, and drug interactions to facilitate basic and evidence-based clinical studies. It is a major objective of the chapter to illustrate common physiatric uses and potential positive or negative impact on a patient's rehabilitation course. As was true of the chapter in the previous edition of this book, much of the information is in tabular form so that it is "user friendly" for the busy clinician who needs to quickly look up information and expeditiously apply it. Although the tables list most of the medications from the various categories, all of them could not be included. Table 56-1 provides a list of the abbreviations used throughout the chapter.

The chapter is structured so that sections have been arranged according to medication class whereas others have been more logically grouped based upon disease entities. Some of this chapter's information overlaps with chapters pertaining to disease-specific entities and with Chapter 15, "Pharmacology of Pain Management." This is an inevitable consequence of a comprehensive textbook but does give the reader the advantage of more than one perspective on medication use. In contrast, discussion about other medications has been left for specific chapters devoted to certain disease entities. As is true of the last edition, a separate section on pharmacotherapy of traumatic brain injury is presented.

Although certain biases based on the authors' experiences are presented, this does not necessarily endorse one medication over another. This chapter primarily addresses medication for adults and does not discuss vitamins, supplements, or homeopathic medications (see Chapter 19).

ANALGESICS

The treatment of patients with pain is a major focus of many outpatient physiatric practices and is becoming even more important as the Joint Commission on Accreditation of Healthcare Organizations (JCAHO) has mandated pain as the fifth vital sign and Congress has declared, as of January 1, 2001, that this is the Decade of Pain Control and Research. Physiatrists, therefore, should have familiarity with analgesics. In this chapter, analgesic medications are grouped into classes and discussed in alphabetical order.

Overview of Pharmacologic Pain Management by the Physiatrist

Analgesics, particularly opioids are being prescribed with greater frequency. New analgesic medication options have become available over the last several years, including additional medications within previously available medication classes and a new class of oral antiinflammatory medications.

Although pain can be classified as nociceptive or neuropathic, patients often present with mixed pain syndromes (1). Currently, optimal medication choice for neuropathic pain is unclear, even though a better understanding of the pathophysiology of neuropathic pain suggests that nonopioid agents, such as antidepressants and anticonvulsants, should be more efficacious than opioids or nonsteroidal antiinflammatory drugs (NSAIDs). Although clinical studies have not consistently demonstrated this, the many confounding factors involved in neuropathic pain states make study interpretation difficult (2).

TABLE 56-1.   Abbreviation Key

μ μg	mu microgram	LSD	lysergic acid diethylamide
ACE	angiotensin converting enzyme	MAOI(s)	monoamine oxidase inhibitor(s)
Ach	acetylcholine	mg(s)	milligram(s)
ADP	adenosine 5′ diphosphate	MI(s)	myocardial infarction(s)
AED	anti-epileptic drug	mL(s)	milliliter(s)
AF	atrial fibrillation	MT	multiple trauma
AF/flut	atrial fibrillation/flutter	Na+	sodium
APAP	acetaminophen	NE	norepinephrine
aPTT	activated partial thromboplastin time	NMDA	N-methyl-D-aspartate
ASA	aspirin	NNT	number needed to treat
AV node	atrioventricular node	NO-NSAIDs	nitric oxide NSAIDs
bid	twice per day	NSAID(s)	nonsteroidal antiinflammatory drug(s)
BNZs	benzodiazepine(s)	OA	osteoarthritis
BP	blood pressure	OTC	over-the-counter
BUN	blood urea nitrogen	po	by mouth
C_{max}	maximum concentration	pr	by rectum
Ca2+	calcium	PCP	phencyclidine
CaCB(s)	calcium channel blocker(s)	PE	pulmonary embolus
cAMP	3′,5′-cyclic adenosine monophosphate	prn	as needed
CBC	complete blood count	PSVT	paroxysmal supraventricular tachycardia
CHF	congestive heart failure	PT	prothrombin time
CNS	central nervous system	PVC	premature ventricular contraction
COPD	chronic obstructive pulmonary disease	q	every
COX-2	cyclooxygenase-2	qd	once per day
CVA(s)	cerebrovascular accident(s)	qid	four times per day
DA	dopamine	qod	every other day
DP	dipyridamole	RVR	rapid ventricular rate
DVT	deep venous thrombosis	s.c.	subcutaneous
ECG	electrocardiogram	SCI	spinal cord injury
ER	extended-release	SL	sublingual
FDA	Food and Drug Administration	SP	substance P
GERD	gastroesophageal reflux disease	SR	sustained release
GI	gastrointestinal	SSRI(s)	selective serotonin reuptake inhibitor(s)
H/S	at bedtime	SVT	supraventricular tachycardia
H2	histamine 2 receptor	$t_{1/2}$	half-life
HDL	high-density lipoprotein	TBI	traumatic brain injury
HIV	human immunodeficiency virus	TCA	tricyclic antidepressant
HTN	hypertension	TD	transdermal
i.m.	intramuscular	THA	total hip arthroplasty
INR	international normalized ratio	tid	three times per day
IR	immediate release	TKA	total knee arthroplasty
i.v.	intravenous	UFH	unfractionated heparin
JCAHO	Joint Commission on Accreditation of Healthcare Organizations	V tach	ventricular tachycardia
LDL	Low-density lipoprotein	VLDL	very low-density lipoprotein
LFTs	liver function tests	WBCs	white blood cells
LMWH	low-molecular-weight heparin	VF	ventricular fibrillation

ANALGESIC MEDICATIONS

Acetaminophen (Tylenol)

RELEVANCE TO PHYSIATRY

Although acetaminophen (APAP) is unsatisfactory as a single agent in patients requiring a powerful analgesic, it can be an effective primary or adjuvant medication for pain of mild to moderate intensity. In particular, it is considered to be the initial medication of choice for patients with osteoarthritis (OA) of the knee or hip who present without obvious signs of inflammation (see Chapter 32) (3). APAP also offers a viable alternative for some patients who experience gastrointestinal (GI) side effects with NSAIDs or cyclooxygenase II (COX-II) inhibitors or who are at particular risk for renal toxicity associated with these agents. In addition, it is often used in combination with both opioid and nonopioid medications so as to decrease potential side effects (and thereby lessen interference with a rehabilitation program) by lowering the dose requirement of these other medications. It

is often used in the pediatric rehabilitation setting due to the lack of an association with Reye's syndrome, in contrast to aspirin (ASA).

In addition to its use in nociceptive and neuropathic pain states, APAP has other advantages. For headache, it can be used as a single agent or can be used as a combination agent along with various narcotic analgesics, as well as with butalbital and caffeine (i.e., Fioricet or Esgic). In the inpatient setting, APAP is the primary agent used to treat fever

APAP does not possess antiinflammatory effects, therefore it cannot be substituted for antiinflammatory agents when treating conditions such as rheumatoid arthritis.

Due to the potential for chronic APAP overdosage leading to hepatoxicity, patients must be counseled to stay within the dosage limitations when they are placed on scheduled doses of APAP. Patients might not realize that over-the-counter (OTC) headache or cold/flu remedies often contain APAP and this can lead to inadvertent APAP overdosage if they are also placed on APAP either in the form of Tylenol or in combination analgesic medications.

MECHANISM OF ACTION AND PHARMACOKINETICS

Although APAP, like the NSAIDs and (COX-II) inhibitors, inhibits the COX isoenzymes and thereby diminishes prostaglandin synthesis, it is unclear why APAP fails to exert peripheral antiinflammatory effects. Since it does have analgesic and antipyretic effects however, one theory is that APAP preferentially inhibits central nervous system (CNS) prostaglandins without affecting prostaglandin levels at peripheral sites of inflammation (4).

APAP is rapidly and almost completely absorbed from the upper GI tract. Part of it is bound by plasma proteins, and the unbound portion exerts the therapeutic effects. The liver then metabolizes it and the kidneys excrete it.

PREPARATIONS AND DOSING

The brand name Tylenol is frequently used interchangeably with the generic term APAP. There are three major oral dosing regimens of Tylenol as shown in Table 56-2 which lists the dosing regimens that would provide a maximum dose of 4 g per 24 hours for those patients with normal hepatic function. For those with abnormal liver function, specific dosing information should be consulted prior to prescribing. It is also available in liquid and suppository preparations.

RELEVANT SIDE EFFECTS AND DRUG INTERACTIONS

APAP has an extremely favorable side-effect profile when used within recommended dosage limitations (5). In those with normal hepatic function the maximum daily recommended dose is 4 g per day. When used chronically in excess of this, or at more than approximately 2 g per day in patients who consume excessive amounts of alcohol (defined as more than 3 alcoholic drinks per day) or when taken as a single dose in excess of approximately 15 g, an intermediary substance of metabolism (N-acetyl-benzoquinoneimine) can have a detrimental effect upon hepatocytes to the point of fatal hepatic necrosis (6). APAP overdosage in children less than 6 years of age is rarely associated with hepatotoxicity. Fatalities in children due to confusing doses of infant Tylenol drops with children's Tylenol liquid have been reported.

An association between chronic use of APAP and end-stage renal disease remains controversial. Aside from cases of overdosage, acute nephrotoxic effects of APAP have not been reported other than in alcoholics (7). Thus, the National Kidney Foundation recommends APAP as the drug of choice for analgesia in those with renal dysfunction (8).

APAP has a very favorable medication interaction profile. One potentially important exception however is the fact that large APAP doses can potentiate the effect of warfarin by prolonging its half-life (9). Although this is believed to only be clinically significant in patients with a relatively high international normalized ratio (INR), monitoring of the INR should be performed in patients who are chronically taking APAP and are on warfarin (10).

Antidepressants

RELEVANCE TO PHYSIATRY

Physiatrists have gained some familiarity with these agents, as depression is a common consequence of illnesses and injuries, particularly if they are associated with functional loss. Antidepressants are also used off-label to treat chronic nonmalignant pain syndromes and neuropathic pain (11–13). Some studies attribute their analgesic effect to resolution of the associated depression often seen in chronic pain (14). There is evidence, however, that antidepressants help chronic pain even if there

TABLE 56-2. Acetaminophen Preparations and Dosing		
Tylenol Formulation	Acetaminophen Content	Dose (Maximum No. of Units)
Tylenol	325 mg	2 po q4h
Extra-strength Tylenol (ES-Tylenol)	500 mg	1 q3h or 2 q6h
Tylenol Arthritis	650 mg	2 q8h

are no symptoms of depression (15). Others feel that antidepressants help with chronic pain by improving sleep patterns. However, improvements in pain have been noted in the absence of effects on sleep. (15) This chapter will address their use as analgesics as the treatment of depression is covered elsewhere (see Chapter 44).

The tricyclic antidepressant (TCA), amitriptyline is the prototypical antidepressant agent used for neuropathic pain. Other TCAs that have been used for this purpose include nortriptyline and desipramine. There is some evidence that desipramine is as effective as amitriptyline and has fewer side effects (e.g., drowsiness) (16,17). Another TCA, doxepin has shown efficacy as a topical analgesic (3.3%) in chronic neuropathic pain (18).

A relatively newer class of antidepressants, the selective serotonin reuptake inhibitors (SSRIs), is hypothesized to affect brain stem pain-modulating systems. Case reports involving the successful use of the first SSRI, fluoxetine, in fibromyalgia prompted at least one randomized controlled trial that yielded somewhat inconclusive results (19,20). An ensuing controlled trial concluded that the combination of fluoxetine at 20 mg per day along with amitriptyline at 25 mg per day may offer more benefit than either alone (21). In painful diabetic neuropathy, fluoxetine was found to only relieve pain in patients who were also depressed (17). There have been several studies on paroxetine at doses of 40 mg per day and at least one each on citalopram and sertraline (22–24). One major systematic review of SSRI effectiveness in chronic pain concluded that SSRIs are effective for mixed chronic pain, but it is unclear whether they are beneficial for tension headaches, migraine headaches, diabetic neuropathy, and fibromyalgia (25). Overall, proof of SSRI analgesic efficacy is not as convincing as for TCAs. Another SSRI, fluvoxamine, has also been examined as an analgesic but has received less attention compared to other SSRIs. One randomized controlled trial (n = 53) of patients with depression and chronic pain compared it to fluoxetine and concluded that fluvoxamine led to an improvement in neuropathic pain independent of its effect on depression whereas fluoxetine's analgesia depended on its antidepressant effect (26). Another randomized controlled trial found it to be beneficial in chronic tension-type headache (27).

Other antidepressants that have been studied as analgesics include several that do not fall into any one particular chemical class, including trazodone, venlafaxine, and bupropion. Each of these has received somewhat less attention than TCAs and SSRIs but deserve further comment. Additional antidepressants in this category include mirtazapine and nefazodone. At the time of this writing, there is only one case report in the peer-reviewed literature on mirtazapine and one basic science study on nefazodone in the setting of pain (28,29).

Trazodone is chemically unrelated to other antidepressants. It is rarely used for depression, but is more commonly used as a hypnotic. Although there is some literature on it as an analgesic, a review of 59 randomized placebo-controlled trials of antidepressants as analgesics concluded that trazodone is not effective (30,31).

Interest is growing in venlafaxine, one of the newer generation antidepressants, for neuropathic pain (32–35). Preliminary indications are that it may outperform SSRIs in neuropathic pain states, although the available evidence comes primarily from uncontrolled open trials and case reports, including two in diabetic neuropathy and radiculopathy (36–41).

After an uncontrolled pilot study suggested that bupropion may be an effective and tolerated treatment for neuropathic pain, a subsequent placebo-controlled crossover trial confirmed that bupropion SR (sustained release, 150 to 300 mg qd) was effective and well tolerated in neuropathic pain (42).

MECHANISM OF ACTION AND PHARMACOKINETICS

TCAs increase aminergic transmission by inhibiting norepinephrine and serotonin reuptake at presynaptic nerve-ending terminals. As a result, they elevate pain thresholds in depressed and nondepressed patients. Analgesic doses are usually lower than those for primary depression. These agents are rapidly absorbed and metabolized, and then renally excreted. Nortriptyline is a demethylated active metabolite of amitriptyline.

SSRIs selectively inhibit serotonin reuptake with less of an effect on norepinephrine reuptake. This mechanism offers the advantage of a superior side-effect profile. Paroxetine and sertraline are the most frequently used agents in this class and both have a chemical structure that is unique among the SSRIs as well as other antidepressants. As a whole, this class is well absorbed orally and then undergoes hepatic metabolism followed by renal excretion.

Bupropion's exact mechanism of action is not known. It is hepatically metabolized and excreted in the urine.

Trazodone possibly acts via serotonin reuptake inhibition and mixed serotonin agonist-antagonist effects. It has variable clearance that may lead to accumulation in some patients.

Venlafaxine is a norepinephrine inhibitor via α_2-adrenergic receptor blockade, a serotonin reuptake inhibitor, and it binds to opioid receptors. Overall, its combined mechanism of action is somewhat similar to tramadol.

PREPARATIONS AND DOSING

Table 56-3 lists dosage, side effects, and miscellaneous information about the most commonly used antidepressants for neuropathic and chronic pain.

Elderly and otherwise medically fragile patients should probably be started on nortriptyline rather than amitriptyline given nortriptyline superior side-effect profile. Orthostatic hypotension and significant morning sedation are relatively common initial TCA side effects in this patient population and can potentially interfere with rehabilitation efforts.

RELEVANT SIDE EFFECTS AND DRUG INTERACTIONS

Antidepressants in general are associated with a high incidence of sexual dysfunction that is often underreported in product literature (43). Those antidepressants that inhibit serotonin reuptake (e.g., SSRIs, Desyrel, Effexor) can cause "serotonin syndrome," a hyperexcitable state of nervousness and insomnia.

TCA side effects are mainly anticholinergic and include dry mouth, blurred vision, tachycardia, constipation, and urinary retention. Their main antihistaminergic side effects are sedation (thus explaining why they are often prescribed as a single bedtime dose), and weight gain related to an increased appetite for carbohydrates. TCAs also exert some quinidinelike cardiac effects including atrioventricular conduction-time prolongation. Leukopenia is less commonly seen. Nortriptyline is better tolerated than amitriptyline.

Since SSRIs have a relatively specific effect on serotonin reuptake without a significant effect on norepinephrine reuptake, their side-effect profile is generally superior to TCAs, especially with respect to cardiovascular issues, and they are

---

TABLE 56-3.   Antidepressants Used in the Treatment of Neuropathic Pain[a]

[Class] Generic (Trade) Name	Dose (mg) Neuropathic Pain (Depression)	Miscellaneous
[TCAs]		
Amitriptyline (Elavil, Vanatrip)	10–100 @ H/S (150–300/d); begin @ 12.5–25 qH/S, and titrated as tolerated	Dry mouth and sedation very common Demethylated to nortriptyline
Nortriptyline (Aventyl, Pamelor)	10–30 @ H/S (50–150/d)	First metabolite of amitriptyline; less side effects but not as potent
[SSRIs]		
Citalopram (Celexa)	20–40 qd (20–60 qd)	Relatively short half-life
Fluoxetine (Prozac) (Prozac Weekly)	20 qd (20–80 qd or 90 qw of "Prozac Weekly")	Very popular when first released; blamed in the press as a contributing factor to several high-profile murders
Fluvoxamine (Luvox)	100 qd (50–150 bid)	Least studied of the SSRIs for pain
Paroxetine (Paxil)	20–50 qd (20–50 qd)	Most selective of the SSRIs
Sertraline (Zoloft)	50–150 qd (50–200 qd)	Tablets and oral concentrate; serotonin syndrome (hyperserotonergic state) with tramadol co-administration; also used for obsessive-compulsive disorder (OCD) and posttraumatic stress disorder (PTSD)
[Other antidepressants]		
Bupropion SR (Wellbutrin SR)	150–300 qd (100–400 qd)	SR formulation have a better side effect profile vs. IR preparation, esp. for sexual dysfunction and seizures; also used for smoking cessation (Zyban)
Trazodone (Desyrel)	50–150 @ H/S (200–300 bid)	Priapism that can be severe; less anticholinergic side effects vs. TCAs
Venlafaxine (Effexor)	18.75–75 qd divided bid or tid (37.5–75 divided bid or tid)	An extended release form (Effexor XR) is used for depression but not studied yet for pain

[a] Note: Only those generally considered used for neuropathic pain are shown in the table.

much safer in cases of overdose. Recently, an SSRI antidepressant discontinuation syndrome has been described as dizziness, light-headedness, insomnia, fatigue, anxiety/agitation, nausea, headache, and sensory disturbance (44). It may last up to three weeks but lessens by restarting the agent or starting another one with a similar profile.

Bupropion has caused seizures and interference with cardiac conduction (ventricular arrhythmias and third-degree heart block). Idiosyncratic reactions including Stevens-Johnson syndrome and rhabdomyolysis have also been reported. The sustained release (SR) bupropion is generally better tolerated than the immediate release (IR) form.

Trazodone also possesses some anticholinergic effects but these are less than for the TCAs. Sedation is its most common side effect, thus its use as a hypnotic. Due to α-adrenergic blocking properties, it has caused penile and very rarely clitoral priapism that in some cases required surgical intervention or resulted in permanent erectile dysfunction (45).

TCAs, SSRIs and bupropion should not be used in patients taking monoamine oxidase inhibitors (MAOIs) and should be instituted cautiously in patients who have been off of MAOIs for at least 2 weeks. Concomitant use of TCAs or SSRIs and MAOIs can cause hyperpyretic crises, seizures, and death. TCAs should also be used cautiously in patients taking other anticholinergic medications, neuroleptics, or CNS depressants.

It is not known whether interactions occur between trazodone and MAOIs. Trazodone can increase serum digoxin and phenytoin levels, and can cause either an increase or a decrease in prothrombin times in patients on warfarin.

Venlafaxine's most common side effects are from increased serotonin levels (irritability, insomnia, and sexual dysfunction) but also include hypertension (HTN), constipation, and nausea.

Corticosteroids

RELEVANCE TO PHYSIATRY

Antiinflammatory effects of corticosteroids are usually more important to the physiatrist than mineralocorticoid or androgenic/estrogenic effects. Corticosteroids are being used increasingly by physiatrists for injection procedures, including fluoroscopic-guided spinal injection procedures and peripheral joint injection procedures for patients with OA. They are used orally in short tapering courses (e.g., Medrol dose pack) for radiculopathy and other localized musculoskeletal conditions, and are used chronically for systemic inflammatory diseases. In addition to their oral and injectable forms, corticosteroids can be delivered transdermally by iontophoresis or phonophoresis.

MECHANISM OF ACTION AND PHARMACOKINETICS

Corticosteroids bind to receptors within a target cell's nucleus and cause an alteration in protein synthesis. These altered proteins then exert various mineralocorticoid, androgenic/estrogenic, and glucocorticoids effects. Corticosteroids are classified into one of these three categories depending upon their predominant effect. At physiologic but not pharmacologic doses, the glucocorticoid class of corticosteroids exerts antiinflammatory and immunosuppressive effects via several mechanisms: Inhibition of prostaglandin and leukotriene synthesis, probably by preventing arachidonic acid release from phospholipids (in contrast, NSAIDs and COX-II inhibitors act at a later step in prostaglandin synthesis via inhibition of COX isoenzymes); inhibition of chemotactic factor release leading to a diminished attraction of white blood cells (WBCs) to sites of inflammation; decrease in circulating lymphocytes and monocytes; reduction

of vascular permeability by acting as vasoconstrictors or by inhibiting vasodilator release (e.g., histamines and kinins); and stabilization of lysosomal membranes (occurs only at higher steroid doses).

Oral glucocorticoids are hepatically metabolized and renally excreted at a rate proportional to the particular agent's water solubility. Hence, longer-acting glucocorticoids are less water soluble.

PREPARATIONS AND DOSING

The two most commonly used oral steroid preparations in many physiatric practices are prednisone and the Medrol dose pack. One dose pack provides an initial 24 mg of Medrol (equivalent to 30 mg of prednisone) and tapers to 0 mg over 7 days. It is convenient both for the prescribing physician and the patient as the instructions are printed on the package. This eliminates the need to count out a certain number of pills each day and probably increases compliance. Potential drawbacks are its expense compared to generic prednisone and the fact that a dose pack provides a peak equivalent prednisone dose of only 30 mg. Some physicians overcome this somewhat low dose by prescribing a "double Medrol dose pack" (two packs taken simultaneously).

At the time of this writing there is a shortage of several injectable corticosteroids. Injectable triamcinolone diacetate and triamcinolone hexacetonide are in short supply due to manufacturing difficulties and raw material shortage. The resultant increased demand for other injectable corticosteroids has led to a short supply of methylprednisolone acetate suspension, betamethasone acetate, betamethasone sodium phosphate, and triamcinolone acetonide.

Corticosteroid selection can be made on the basis of equivalent cortisone doses, relative antiinflammatory potency, relative mineralocorticoid potency, and duration of action (46,47) (Table 56-4). For comparison, physiologic steroid doses are equivalent to 30 mg per day of hydrocortisone (7.5 mg day of prednisone), whereas stress doses are equivalent to 300 mg per day of hydrocortisone (75 mg/day of prednisone). Dosing guidelines have also been developed (48) (Tables 56-4 and 56-5).

RELEVANT SIDE EFFECTS AND DRUG INTERACTIONS

Although not a true side effect, a potential problem is that corticosteroids often just mask disease-associated inflammation rather than affecting a cure. Thus, there is a tendency for patients to feel better from the antiinflammatory effects of corticosteroids and ignore the underlying disorder. An example is a patient who has received a subacromial steroid injection and soon resumes repetitive overhead activities that initially led to impingement. Most of the true side effects occur after prolonged administration and many of these are basically manifestations of Cushing's syndrome as shown in Table 56-6.

Steroid myopathy and avascular necrosis are two interesting catabolic side effects that are directly pertinent to physiatry. Physiatrists who routinely perform electrodiagnostic studies are likely familiar with the request to "rule out steroid myopathy." Femoral or humeral head avascular necrosis is a rare idiosyncratic event that can occur after a short course of prednisone.

Skin depigmentation and subcutaneous atrophy are dermatological complications that can occur with corticosteroid injections but can be minimized by adding local anesthetic or normal saline vehicle into the injectate, and by flushing the needle of residual corticosteroid with saline or local anesthetic injection through it before removal from the skin. Skin changes from chronic oral corticosteroids can lead to pressure ulcers and easy bruising.

TABLE 56-4. Corticosteroid Preparations

Corticosteroid Generic (Trade) Name	Route	Equivalent Oral Dose (mg)	Relative Potencies: Antiinflammatory (Mineralocorticoid)	Relative Duration
Betamethasone (Celestone)	po/i.m.	0.6–0.75	20–30 (0)	Long
Cortisone (Cortone)	po	25	0.8 (2)	Short
Dexamethasone (Decadron)	po/i.m./i.v.	0.75	20–30 (0)	Long
Hydrocortisone (Cortef, Solu-Cortef)	po/i.m./i.v.	20	1 (2)	Short
Methylprednisolone (Medrol, Medrol Dosepack, SoluMedrol)	po/i.m./i.v.	4	5 (0)	Intermediate
Prednisolone (Hydeltra)	po/i.m./i.v.	5	4 (1)	Intermediate
Prednisone (Deltasone, Orasone)	po	5	4 (1)	Intermediate
Triamcinolone (Aristocort, Kenacort, Kenalog)	po/i.m.	4	5 (0)	Intermediate

Acceleration of corticosteroid metabolism occurs with medications that induce hepatic microsomal enzymes, especially phenobarbital, phenytoin, carbamazepine, and rifampin. In contrast, corticosteroid potency is increased by NSAIDs and exogenous estrogens (47). Clinicians should consider discontinuing NSAIDs or switching to a COX-II inhibitor if concomitant corticosteroid use is needed as corticosteroids are risk factors for NSAID-induced GI bleeding.

Membrane-Stabilizing Medications: Antiarrhythmics

RELEVANCE TO PHYSIATRY

There are three circumstances under which a physiatrist might prescribe antiarrhythmics. First, some patients in the inpatient rehabilitation setting are taking antiarrhythmics for existing cardiac conditions. Second, type I antiarrhythmics (i.e., mexiletine, tocainide, lidocaine, and phenytoin) are used off-label as agents for neuropathic pain. Third, mexiletine and tocainide are occasionally used off-label for myotonia-associated pain from certain neuromuscular disorders. Intravenous (i.v.) lidocaine as an analgesic agent will not be discussed in detail in this chapter as it is generally only used in highly specialized pain management clinics as a predictive test for mexiletine treatment (49). In brief, those who report good pain relief with i.v. lidocaine (2 to 5 mg/kg i.v. over 30 minutes) in a nonpainful limb with earlier termination if either significant pain relief or

intolerable side effects are reported, are more likely to benefit from undergoing a titrating trial of mexiletine. In contrast, an i.v. lidocaine infusion should not be used as a definitive diagnostic test for neuropathic pain since false-negatives occur frequently (50).

The literature pertaining to oral antiarrhythmics for neuropathic pain is somewhat limited to mexiletine. (51) Earlier case reports and prospective studies suggested that mexiletine is efficacious and safe in various neuropathic pain states including pain from peripheral nerve damage, diabetic neuropathy, alcoholic neuropathy, phantom limb pain, multiple sclerosis complicated by painful dysesthesias, and thalamic pain syndrome (52–61).

In contrast to the aforementioned favorable studies, some have found that mexiletine lacks efficacy in other disorders such as central pain, spinal cord injury (SCI) with spinal dysesthetic pain, trigeminal neuralgia, and human immunodeficiency virus (HIV)-related peripheral neuropathic pain. (62–64). In addition, a double-blinded placebo-controlled study concluded that it was ineffective in the treatment of allodynia associated with various neuropathic pain conditions (65). This study, however, failed to achieve adequate mexiletine plasma levels. A subsequent human study on experimentally induced pain also concluded that mexiletine had minimal effects and that it was severely limited by side effects (66).

The literature on tocainide for neuropathic pain unrelated to neuromuscular conditions essentially only includes trigeminal neuralgia (67). In contrast, there have been case reports on the

TABLE 56-5. Corticosteroid Dosing Guidelines

- Use these only after less toxic therapy has been ineffective or is not an alternative
- Use the smallest corticosteroid amount that can control symptoms
- Administer the corticosteroid locally rather than systemically whenever possible
- Short-term use: Dosing qd (preferably in the a.m.) is more convenient and causes less adrenal suppression than qid dosing @ ¼ the total dose
- Chronic use: Dosing qod is less likely to suppress adrenal function
- Do not use the term "steroids" because of this word's negative connotations. Although the terms *cortisone* or *prednisone* may also have negative connotations, explain that osteoporosis and truncal obesity only occur with chronic use
- Forewarn patients that oral steroids typically cause a metallic taste
- Adrenal suppression is likely for dose, potency, and duration as follows:
  Doses ≥100 mg hydrocortisone (25 mg prednisone) daily × 3 d
  Doses ≥30 mg hydrocortisone (7.5 mg prednisone) daily × 30 d
- Wean patients off over weeks or months if taking steroids for more than several weeks
- If unsure that patient has become adrenally suppressed, refer to endocrinologist for metyrapone or insulin-tolerance testing. Recovery of adrenal function is variable
- For corticosteroid injections:
  Can decrease chance of corticosteroid arthropathy with limit of: 3/year; 20/lifetime
  Never inject directly into a tendon and avoid weight-bearing peritendinous injections (e.g., Achilles, patellar, posterior tibial) or risk tendon rupture

TABLE 56-6.   Corticosteroid Side Effects

Organ System	Side Effect
Central nervous system	Behavior and mood alteration
Cardiovascular	Fluid retention; hypertension
Endocrine/metabolism	Adrenal atrophy; amenorrhea; appetite increase; glucose tolerance impairment; hypernatremia and hypokalemia; weight gain leading to "moon facies"
Gastrointestinal	Aggravation of peptic ulcer disease
Musculoskeletal	Avascular necrosis; bone demineralization; steroid myopathy
Skin	Acne, depigmentation, and subcutaneous atrophy with injection, fatty deposition leading to "buffalo hump", hirsutism, skin thinning

successful treatment of myotonic pain in paramyotonia congenita and Thomsen-Becker myotonia (68). There is also a case report of its beneficial effect on fecal incontinence in patients with myotonic muscular dystrophy (69). Although both mexiletine and tocainide are considered to be potent antimyotonic agents, one paper argued against tocainide for the treatment of myotonia because of potential hematologic toxicity, including aplastic anemia (70). Another study found significant improvement of disabling cramps and muscle spasms in nine patients with motor neuron diseases, tetany, and myotonic disorders who were treated with tocainide (71). The only side effect was light-headedness and fatigue in one patient who had intraventricular conduction-time prolongation. A two-patient case series found that cramping and difficulty in muscle relaxation after voluntary contraction were improved after tocainide (72).

MECHANISM OF ACTION AND PHARMACOKINETICS

As is true of other type I antiarrhythmics (e.g., lidocaine, mexiletine, and tocainide), amides act by blocking Na+ channels in nerve and muscle cell membranes. This reduces abnormal ectopic impulse generation by dysfunctional peripheral nerves. Although structurally similar to lidocaine these agents are orally active due to low first pass metabolism.

PREPARATIONS AND DOSING

Mexiletine is available in 150, 200, and 250 mg caplets. Neuropathic pain doses are lower (150 to 300 mg tid) than those used for arrhythmias (200 to 400 mg tid). So as to minimize the most common side effect (nausea), it can be begun at 150 mg per day and titrated weekly.

Tocainide is available in 400 and 600 mg tablets. Although rarely used as an antiarrhythmic, it is dosed at 400 to 800 mg tid. Insufficient information is available on tocainamide as a neuropathic pain agent to reliably comment on dosages in this setting.

RELEVANT SIDE EFFECTS AND DRUG INTERACTIONS

Mexiletine's potential side effects are only acute and are GI, neurologic, and cardiovascular (CV). One mexiletine study of experimentally induced pain found that the higher doses used for analgesia caused side effects at an average daily dose of 993 mg (600 to 1,350 mg range), whereas another study found negligible side effects at doses up to 900 mg per day (56,63). GI side effects include nausea, anorexia, and gastric irritation in up to 40%. Neurologic side effects occur in up to 10% and are similar to those of other class I antiarrhythmics, including dizziness,

visual disturbances, tremor, altered coordination, and anxiety in those with a previous anxiety disorder. In patients with normal cardiac conduction, it has minimal effects on cardiac impulse generation and propagation, whereas in patients with abnormal cardiac conduction, the most common side effect is exacerbation of the cardiac condition. It is contraindicated in second- or third-degree heart block in those without a pacemaker. An electrocardiogram (ECG) is recommended prior to starting mexiletine.

Mexiletine's hepatic metabolism is induced by phenytoin and rifampin whereas mexiletine may increase theophylline plasma levels. Since mexiletine reduces caffeine clearance by 50%, it can potentially interact with caffeine-containing agents such as Norgesic.

Tocainide's side-effect profile is similar to mexiletine's except for potential hematologic toxicity (e.g., aplastic anemia). Drug interactions are minimal.

Membrane-Stabilizing Medications: Anticonvulsants

RELEVANCE TO PHYSIATRY

When anticonvulsants are used for neuropathic pain, they are more logically referred to as membrane-stabilizing medications. Their use as antineuralgic drugs perhaps derived from clinical observations that pain thresholds of epileptic patients seemed to be higher than those of healthy subjects (73). This was attributed to the fact that most anticonvulsants are also analgesic. Similarities in the pathophysiology in some epilepsy and neuropathic pain models may explain their dual role (74). Supportive evidence of anticonvulsant efficacy in neuropathic pain continues to evolve and anticonvulsants (e.g., gabapentin) have marked a new era in neuropathic pain. There are several different agents, each with its own properties. Although all have antihyperalgesic and antinociceptive actions in animal neuropathic pain models, their efficacy (except for gabapentin, carbamazepine, and to a lesser extent lamotrigine) in human neuropathic pain has not yet been fully determined in clinical trials. Neuropathic pain relief has been shown for lamotrigine in two controlled clinical trials, although another randomized trial showed no effect (74). The agents will be discussed individually as there are significant differences among them, however sedation and cerebellar dysfunction (nystagmus, tremor, and incoordination) seem to be common to all (Table 56-7).

The exact analgesic mechanism of action is not completely known for several of these medications. Further understanding should help with rational initial medication selection and medication changes in cases of poor efficacy or side effects (Table 56-8).

GABAPENTIN (NEURONTIN)

Relevance to Physiatry

Gabapentin is a first-line treatment for neuropathic pain now approved for post-herpetic neuralgia. There is evidence, including a limited number of placebo controlled trials, supporting its efficacy (particularly in painful diabetic neuropathy and postherpetic neuralgia) (75–79). It has also been investigated for spasticity reduction in SCI patients (80). Its very favorable side-effect profile and minimal medication interactions make it perhaps the most commonly used first-line agent for neuropathic pain.

Mechanism of Action and Pharmacokinetics

See Tables 56-7 and 56-8.

TABLE 56-7. Anticonvulsant Efficacy and Pharmacokinetics in Neuropathic Pain

Efficacy	Medication	Specific Neuropathic Pain Uses	Pharmacokinetics
Efficacious			
	Gabapentin (Neurontin)	Especially diabetic neuropathy and postherpetic neuralgia (FDA-approved)	Not protein bound or metabolized; renal excretion
	Carbamazepine (Tegretol)	Trigeminal neuralgia (FDA-approved), glossopharyngeal neuralgia, diabetic neuropathy, and postherpetic neuralgia	Highly plasma protein- bound, variable $t_{1/2}$ as it induces its own metabolism
Probable			
	Lamotrigine (Lamictal)	Some efficacy in trigeminal neuralgia; peripheral neuropathy post-stroke syndromes	Good oral absorption; hepatic conjugation; renal excretion
Unclear			
	Clonazepam (Klonopin)	Some efficacy in trigeminal neuralgia	Good absorption; highly plasma protein-bound and hepatically metabolized
	Oxcarbazepine (Trileptal)	Efficacy in trigeminal neuralgia and possibly in other neuropathic pain conditions	Hepatically metabolized to its active metabolite; renal excretion
	Phenobarbital (Solfoton)	No clinical studies in humans in peer-reviewed literature	Moderate protein binding; hepatic metabolism; pH-dependent renal excretion
	Phenytoin (Dilantin)	Conflicting results in trigeminal neuralgia and diabetic neuropathy	Metabolism saturable at high plasma levels, thus large concentration increases from additional small doses
	Tiagabine (Gabitril)	One successful trial in painful sensory neuropathy	Highly protein-bound; at least 2 metabolic pathways
	Topiramate (Topamax)	Some evidence in refractory intercostal neuralgia and trigeminal neuralgia but not in central pain	Rapidly absorbed orally and subsequently renally eliminated unchanged
	Valproate (valproic acid)	Efficacy in neuropathic cancer pain but not paraplegia central pain	Highly protein-bound; no consensus about monitoring free vs. bound drug levels
	Zonisamide (Zonegran)	Studies in neuropathic pain are lacking	Renally excreted intact and as a glucuronide metabolite

Gabapentin's exact mechanism is unknown. Since it is structurally related to gamma-aminobutyric acid (GABA), the major CNS excitatory neurotransmitter, gabapentin was originally developed as an anticonvulsant that was thought to inhibit GABA receptors. However, it does not interact with GABA receptors, is not metabolically converted into GABA or a GABA agonist, and it does not inhibit GABA uptake or GABA degradation. It apparently does not bind to other common receptors including benzodiazepine, glutamate, glycine, β-adrenergic, cholinergic, muscarinic, nicotinic, histaminic, serotonergic, dopaminergic, calcium (Ca2+) channels, or sodium (Na+) channels. Its action at the N-methyl-D-aspartate (NMDA) receptor is also controversial as study results are conflicting. One hypothesis is that it acts by altering the concentration or metabolism of the brain's amino acids (41). There is evidence that it may raise the interneuron pool excitability threshold of polysynaptic reflexes (81).

TABLE 56-8. Proposed Mechanism of Action of Anticonvulsants in Neuropathic Pain

Proposed Mechanism	Medications
Na+ channel blocker	Carbamazepine; lamotrigine; oxcarbazepine; phenytoin; valproate; zonisamide
Ca++ channel blocker	Gabapentin; oxcarbazepine; zonisamide
GABA receptor activity	Barbiturates; benzodiazepines
GABA metabolism	Gabapentin; tiagabine; valproate
Glutamate receptor activity	Carbamazepine; lamotrigine; topiramate
Glutamate metabolism	Gabapentin

Preparations and Dosing

The usual dosage range reported for neuropathic pain is 900 to 2,400 mg divided tid. When starting gabapentin, it is recommended that a 300 mg dose be given at bedtime on day one, then bid dosing on day two, and tid dosing thereafter. It is felt that this regimen will help patients accommodate to potential CNS side effects. A 3,600 mg per day maximal dose has been well tolerated in a small number of patients for a relatively short duration.

Relevant Side Effects and Drug Interactions

Gabapentin's main side effects relate to CNS depression, and include somnolence, dizziness, ataxia, and fatigue. Nystagmus has also been reported. Side effects are generally transient with resolution in 2 weeks. There have been only rare reports of adverse events which required its discontinuation. These have included rash, leukopenia, increased blood urea nitrogen (BUN), thrombocytopenia, and various nonlethal ECG abnormalities. Given the rarity of these events, routine laboratory monitoring and monitoring of gabapentin levels is not indicated.

There are no known drug interactions except with cimetidine, which slightly decreases renal gabapentin excretion to a degree that is not felt to be clinically significant, and Maalox which reduces gabapentin's bioavailability by 20%. The lack of drug-drug interactions is expected since gabapentin is not highly protein bound, not appreciably metabolized, does not induce hepatic enzymes, and does not undergo tubular secretion by the pathway blocked by probenecid.

CARBAMAZEPINE (TEGRETOL)

Relevance to Physiatry

Carbamazepine was the first anticonvulsant to be studied in neuropathic pain clinical trials. Results from these trials support its use in trigeminal neuralgia (FDA-approved), glossopharyngeal neuralgia, painful diabetic neuropathy, and postherpetic neuralgia. It has not been as extensively studied for other neuropathic conditions. Traditional teaching is that it is especially useful for neuropathic pain of a sudden and lancinating quality as often occurs due to postamputation neuroma. Its relative lack of CNS side effects compared to other anticonvulsants offers an obvious advantage with respect to functional activities. Unfortunately, serious potential toxicity with the need for lab monitoring as well as baseline and periodic eye examinations, and numerous medication interactions are disadvantages.

Mechanism of Action and Pharmacokinetics (41)
See Tables 56-7 and 56-8.

Preparations and Dosing
Carbamazepine is available in tablets, chewable tablets, and suspensions. Although specific neuropathic pain dosing recommendations are not available, it has been used for trigeminal neuralgia at 100 mg bid and increased based on pain resolution or side effects to a maximum of 400 mg tid. Given potential hematologic toxicity, its dose should be reduced to the minimum effective one. An extended release form, Tegretol-XR can be given bid using the same total daily dose as the nonextended release form.

Relevant Side Effects and Drug Interactions
Very serious toxicity can occur including bone marrow suppression (most commonly leukopenia and thrombocytopenia but also rarely including aplastic anemia and agranulocytosis), hepatotoxicity, skin reactions (including Stevens-Johnson syndrome and toxic epidermal necrolysis) and, to a lesser degree, renal dysfunction. A pretreatment complete blood count (CBC), liver function tests (LFTs), BUN, and urinalysis, and possibly a pretreatment reticulocyte count and serum iron level, are recommended. Although exact guidelines have not been developed, periodic CBC and liver function testing should also be done and, if toxicity is found, consideration for discontinuation should be given.

Due to the significant hepatic enzyme induction by carbamazepine, it has the potential to both affect and be affected by many medications (Table 56-9). It should not be given to those hypersensitive to TCAs as it is structurally related or be used within 2 weeks of an MAOI.

LAMOTRIGINE (LAMICTAL, LAMICTAL CD)

Relevance to Physiatry
Although lamotrigine is indicated as adjunctive therapy in adults with partial seizures and generalized seizures of Lennox-Gastaut syndrome in children and adults, its most common physiatric application is neuropathic pain (81,82). It is not currently considered to be a first-line agent due in part to the lack of clear evidence supporting its use for this purpose and its potentially severe side-effect profile, including fatal allergic-mediated skin reactions.

There is some evidence that lamotrigine is effective in neuropathic pain from trigeminal neuralgia, painful HIV peripheral neuropathy, and poststroke syndromes (83–85). Additional proof includes anecdotal evidence, two randomized controlled trials and a small trigeminal neuralgia trial (86). In contrast, another randomized trial showed no benefit (87).

Mechanism of Action and Pharmacokinetics
See Tables 56-7 and 56-8.

Preparations and Dosing
Lamotrigine is available in both tablets and chewable tablets (Lamictal CD) of various strengths. Specific dosing regimens have not been established for neuropathic pain. It was used in one study at doses as high as 200 mg bid (88). It is therefore recommended that seizure management guidelines be followed, as the risk of potentially life-threatening rash may be increased by exceeding recommended initial doses or recommended dose escalation rates.

Relevant Side Effects and Drug Interactions
Most side effect information is from its anticonvulsant use. Serious rashes (including Stevens-Johnson syndrome) have been reported at an incidence of approximately 1% in children (age <16 years) and 0.3% in adults. In worldwide postmarketing experience, rare cases of toxic epidermal necrolysis and rash-related death have been reported, but their numbers are too few to permit a precise rate estimate. Other than age, there are as yet no known factors that predict the risk of occurrence or rash severity. Although benign rashes also occur, it is not possible to reliably predict which rashes will become serious. Thus, it should be discontinued at the first sign of rash. Besides rash, the most common (≥5%) adverse effects are CNS- and GI-related.

CLONAZEPAM (KLONOPIN)

Relevance to Physiatry (48,89)
Although controlled trials are lacking, two main physiatric applications are neuropathic pain (especially in patients with trigeminal neuralgia who are either intolerant to or have failed carbamazepine, baclofen, or phenytoin), and movement disorders such as sleep-related nocturnal myoclonus, restless legs

---

TABLE 56-9. Potential Drug-Drug Interactions with Carbamazepine

Interaction	Decreased serum level	Increased serum level
Medications whose serum levels are affected by carbamazepine	Acetaminophen, alprazolam, clonazepam, clozapine, dicumarol, doxycycline, ethosuximide, haloperidol, lamotrigine, methsuximide, oral and other hormonal contraceptives, phensuximide, phenytoin, theophylline, tiagabine, topiramate, valproate, warfarin	Clomipramine, phenytoin, primidone
Medications that affect serum carbamazepine levels	Cisplatin, doxorubicin, felbamate, phenobarbital, phenytoin, primidone, rifampin, theophylline	Calcium channel blockers, cimetidine, clarithromycin, erythromycin, danazol, fluoxetine, isoniazid, itraconazole, ketoconazole, loratadine, macrolides, niacinamide, nicotinamide, propoxyphene, terfenadine, troleandomycin, valproate

syndrome, tardive dyskinesia, and opioid-related myoclonic jerks.

Mechanism of Action and Pharmacokinetics
See Tables 56-7 and 56-8.

Preparations and Dosing
Because its name can be confused with other medications, 0.5 mg, 1 mg, and 2 mg tablets have a specially designed K-shaped perforation so that the pill is easily recognized. For movement disorders, clonazepam is begun at 0.5 mg at bedtime or tid and increased up to 2 mg tid. For trigeminal neuralgia, 0.5 to 1.0 mg is recommended (90).

Relevant Side Effects and Drug Interactions
Early in the treatment course, ataxia and personality changes can occur but may partially subside with long-term use. As is true for other benzodiazepines, long-term use can lead to psychological addiction and physical tolerance. Withdrawal symptoms include a flulike syndrome, and abrupt discontinuation of chronic high doses can cause convulsions. Caution should be exercised when it is given with other CNS depressants.

OXCARBAZEPINE (TRILEPTAL)

Relevance to Physiatry
Oxcarbazepine was developed via structural variation of carbamazepine. It has been used in the treatment of epilepsy since 1990. There is convincing evidence of efficacy in newly diagnosed and refractory trigeminal neuralgia. In addition, there are encouraging initial results in other neuropathic pain states and in bipolar disorders (91).

Mechanism of Action and Pharmacokinetics
See Tables 56-7 and 56-8.

Preparations and Dosing
It is available as 150 mg, 300 mg and 600 mg scored tablets and as a 60 mg/mL suspension. Trigeminal neuralgia dosing has ranged from 600 to 1,800 mg per day.

Relevant Side Effects and Drug Interactions
The most commonly observed adverse events are CNS- and GI-related. Between 20% to 25% of patients discontinue it due to a side effect. Although it is a carbamazepine analogue, serious hematologic toxicity has not been associated with it. Strong cytochrome P450 enzyme system inducers, including carbamazepine, phenobarbital, and phenytoin decrease mean plasma oxcarbazepine concentrations by 40%. Antiepileptic drug (AED) co-administration, however, is most likely in the setting of epilepsy and not neuropathic pain. Two other situations that are more relevant to the physiatrist are the co-administration of felodipine with calcium channel blockers (CaCBs) or oral contraceptives. Since Ca2+ channel blockade is believed to be part of its mechanism, it has been studied in the setting of CaCB co-administration. Specifically, verapamil decreased oxcarbazepine concentration by 20% and oxcarbazepine decreased felodipine concentration by 30%. They may render contraceptives ineffective.

PHENOBARBITAL (LUMINAL, SOLFOTON)
There is limited neuropathic pain animal model evidence for phenobarbital (92). As is true of barbiturates, human neuropathic pain studies are lacking and significant sedation occurs with its use. It thus has a very limited role in neuropathic pain management.

PHENYTOIN (DILANTIN)

Relevance to Physiatry
Besides its well-known anticonvulsant use, phenytoin is also used off-label in much lower doses as a neuropathic pain agent. Phenytoin was the first anticonvulsant to be used as an antinociceptive agent and was found to be successful in trigeminal neuralgia and diabetic neuropathy via controlled clinical trials conducted more than 20 years ago. More recent clinical trials however have shown conflicting evidence for its efficacy (86). In addition to its unclear efficacy, there is a significant potential for medication interactions due to its high degree of protein binding and extensive hepatic metabolism. Although cerebellar ataxia can interfere with rehabilitation, it usually only occurs at seizure management doses.

Mechanism of Action and Pharmacokinetics
See Tables 56-7 and 56-8.

Preparations and Dosing
Phenytoin is available in extended-release capsules, tablets, Infatabs, an injectable solution, and oral suspension. Neuropathic pain doses are often less than those used for seizures. Due to saturation of its metabolism at higher doses, it is important to monitor serum levels since further dose increases cause greater than expected drug levels.

Relevant Side Effects and Drug Interactions
Side effects can be classified into three different categories: toxic (i.e., dose-related) effects, true side effects, and idiosyncratic reactions:

- *Toxic effects* generally occur with 20 to 40 µg/mL plasma levels and include sedation, ataxia, and nystagmus. There is marked individual variation with respect to toxic phenytoin plasma levels. At high doses over time, painful sensory peripheral neuropathy can occur.
- *True side effects* from long-term use include osteomalacia and hypocalcemia from vitamin D metabolism interference, megaloblastic anemia from low serum folate levels, hirsutism, and gingival hyperplasia due to interference with fibroblastic activity.
- *Idiosyncratic reactions* include blood dyscrasias and a rare clinical picture that resembles malignant lymphoma.

Drug interactions relate to serum protein binding and hepatic metabolism (Table 56-10).

TIAGABINE (GABITRIL)

Relevance to Physiatry
Tiagabine became available a few years ago. Although it demonstrated antihyperalgesic and antinociceptive activity in animal neuropathic pain models, its efficacy in human neuropathic pain has not been determined in clinical trials (74,93). At the time of this writing, there was only one published small clinical trial in painful sensory neuropathy that concluded it may be beneficial (94).

Mechanism of Action and Pharmacokinetics (95)
See Tables 56-7 and 56-8.

Preparations and Dosing
Tiagabine is available in multiple strength tablets (2 mg, 4 mg, 12 mg, 16 mg, and 20 mg). Its neuropathic pain dose has not been fully established. The one published clinical trial to date involved 4 to 16 mg dose ranges. When used as an anticonvul-

TABLE 56-10. Potential Phenytoin Drug Interactions

Can interfere with phenytoin absorption	Antacids (calcium-containing), Moban brand of molindone HCl
Can raise phenytoin levels	Alcohol (acute intake), amiodarone, chloramphenicol, chlordiazepoxide, diazepam, dicumarol, disulfiram, estrogens, halothane, H2 antagonists, isoniazid, methylphenidate, phenothiazines, phenylbutazone, salicylates, succinimide, sulfonamides, tolbutamide, trazodone
Can decrease phenytoin levels	Alcohol (chronic abuse), carbamazepine, reserpine, sucralfate
Can raise or decrease phenytoin levels (or its level can be raised or decreased by phenytoin)	Phenobarbital, sodium valproate, valproic acid
Efficacy is impaired by phenytoin	Corticosteroids, coumarin anticoagulants, digitoxin, doxycycline, estrogens, furosemide, oral contraceptives, quinidine, rifampin, theophylline, vitamin D

sant however, it should be initiated at 4 mg q day. The total daily dose of tiagabine may be increased by 4 mg at the beginning of week 2. Thereafter, the total daily dose may be increased by 4 to 8 mg at weekly intervals until clinical response is achieved or up to 32 mg per day is given. The total daily dose should be given in divided doses (bid-qid). Doses greater than 32 mg per day have been tolerated in a small number of adolescents for a relatively short duration.

Relevant Side Effects and Drug Interactions

The most common adverse events in placebo-controlled epilepsy trials associated with tiagabine use in combination with other anticonvulsants were CNS- and GI-related. Approximately 20% of those who received tiagabine in clinical epilepsy trials discontinued it due to an adverse event. Since it is a nonenzyme-inducing anticonvulsant, it offers the advantage of not affecting the metabolism of other medications that induce hepatic enzymes.

TOPIRAMATE (TOPAMAX)

Relevance to Physiatry

Like the other anticonvulsants, topiramate is FDA-approved for seizure management but is also used off-label for neuropathic pain and is used for myoclonic jerks (96). One small study found pain relief in refractory intercostal neuralgia but it has not been helpful for central neuropathic pain (97,98). Other possible indications with less direct physiatric relevance are tinnitus, cluster headaches, and trigeminal neuralgia (99).

Mechanism of Action and Pharmacokinetics

See Tables 56-7 and 56-8.

Preparations and Dosing

It is available in tablet, capsule and sprinkle capsule forms of various strengths. The recommended total daily dose as adjunctive therapy for seizure prophylaxis is 400 mg per day divided bid. In neuropathic pain it has been used at 200 to 400 mg per day dose ranges.

Relevant Side Effects and Drug Interactions

Topiramate causes two general CNS-related side effects: psychomotor slowing (concentration difficulty, and speech or language problems, especially word-finding difficulties) and somnolence/fatigue. Although these are more common at seizure prophylaxis doses, somnolence does not appear to be dose-related and psychomotor slowing is only marginally dose-related. Kidney stone formation occurs from weak carbonic an-

hydrase inhibition leading to reduced urinary citrate excretion and urinary pH increase. Concomitant carbonic anhydrase inhibitor use should be avoided as renal stone formation risk may increase. Due to hepatic enzyme induction, alterations in topiramate and other anticonvulsant concentrations can occur.

VALPROATE (VALPROIC ACID) (DEPAKENE)

Relevance to Physiatry

Valproate has been used as a third-line agent for epilepsy and headaches. Valproate is more recently being studied for cancer-related neuropathic pain (100–102). Previously it was the subject of a small randomized clinical trial in paraplegic central pain and was not effective (103). It has yielded variable results in experimentally induced central pain (104).

Mechanism of Action and Pharmacokinetics (105)

See Tables 56-7 and 56-8.

Side Effects and Drug Interactions

Pancreatic complications range from asymptomatic hyperamylasemia to fatal acute pancreatitis. Interference with ammonia metabolism may play an important role in valproate-induced toxic encephalopathy (106).

ZONISAMIDE (ZONEGRAN)

Relevance to Physiatry

Although developed and FDA-approved as an anticonvulsant, neuropathic pain is a relatively recent potential physiatric indication. At the time of this writing, there are no published peer-reviewed clinical trials on the use of this agent for neuropathic pain.

Mechanism of Action and Pharmacokinetics (107,108)

See Tables 56-7 and 56-8.

Preparations and Dosing

Zonisamide 100 mg capsules are given every day for the first 2 weeks, after which the dose may be increased to 200 mg per day for at least 2 weeks. It can be increased to 300 mg per day and 400 mg per day, with the dose stable for at least 2 weeks to achieve steady-state at each level. Evidence from controlled trials as an anticonvulsant suggests that 100 to 600 mg per day doses are effective, but there is no suggestion of increasing efficacy above 400 mg per day.

Relevant Side Effects and Drug Interactions

Zonisamide is contraindicated in sulfonamide allergy. Rare cases of aplastic anemia and agranulocytosis have been reported. It can also cause adverse psychiatric CNS events (depression and psychosis), psychomotor slowing (concentration difficulties and speech/language problems, especially word-finding difficulties) and somnolence and fatigue. Concomitant phenytoin or carbamazepine use increases zonisamide clearance.

LOCAL ANESTHETICS

Relevance to Physiatry

In the outpatient physiatric setting, local anesthetics are frequently used prior to a variety of procedures and are used diagnostically during nerve blocks. More recently, a lidocaine-impregnated patch (Lidoderm) has been FDA-approved for postherpetic neuralgia pain but is also being used for other neuropathic and musculoskeletal pain conditions (109–111).

The short-acting local anesthetic lidocaine is the most commonly used agent for percutaneous infiltration anesthesia as well as for diagnostic blocks and injections. Long-acting local anesthetics such as bupivacaine are used for procedures in which at least several hours of analgesia are desired. A classic example is the shoulder impingement test in which the physiatrist may inject a long-acting local anesthetic along with a corticosteroid preparation into the subacromial bursa of a patient who has had a good response to lidocaine. Local anesthetics are also generally added to corticosteroids for intraarticular injections so that the joint can be more fully bathed and so that the patient can feel some immediate pain relief for both psychological reasons and for providing treatment feedback to the physician (47). Lidocaine (0.5% or 2%) is often a component of proliferant solutions used in prolotherapy.

Mechanism of Action and Pharmacokinetics

Local anesthetics are classified as esters (e.g., procaine) or amides (e.g., bupivacaine and lidocaine) based upon their chemical structure. Both classes interfere with nerve conduction by an incompletely understood mechanism. At the cellular level, they compete with $Ca2+$ for receptor binding that controls $Na+$ flux across the cell membrane. When this occurs, action potential depolarization rate slows as does nerve impulse propagation. Overall, they affect small, unmyelinated fibers prior to larger, myelinated fibers. Thus, the general order of loss of function following neural blockade is: pain, temperature, touch, proprioception, skeletal muscle tone.

Ester class local anesthetics are quickly hydrolyzed by plasma pseudocholinesterase enzymes, whereas amides are hepatically metabolized. Serum levels peak at approximately 5 to 25 minutes depending upon the administration route and the rate of renal excretion. To enhance the duration, epinephrine can be added to the anesthetic solution.

Preparations and Dosing

Two of the most commonly used local anesthetics in physiatric practice are reviewed in Table 56-11. Although additional concentrations are also available and are employed for various procedures, the ones that are most relevant to percutaneous infiltration anesthesia are listed. The maximum doses for percutaneous infiltration shown in Table 56-11 are guidelines and the doses should ideally be individualized for each patient based upon several factors including the patient size and physical status as well as the usual rate of systemic absorption from a particular injection site. In general, the lowest concentration and smallest dose that will achieve a given effect should be employed. When doses larger than those shown in the table are to be used, preparations containing epinephrine should be employed. The reader is referred to other sources for dosing guidelines for other specific procedures. Preservative-free local anesthetic solutions should be used for epidurals since the safety of preservative in epidural and subarachnoid spaces is unknown (47).

BUPIVACAINE (MARCAINE, SENSORCAINE)

For reasons discussed previously, bupivacaine is especially used within corticosteroid-containing solutions for procedures where a prior lidocaine test injection has provided good pain relief. When bupivacaine is used for intraarticular injections, some recommend that it be restricted to non-weightbearing joints so that the patient does not inadvertently traumatize the joint while it is has been rendered relatively insensate by this long-acting anesthetic.

LIDOCAINE (XYLOCAINE)

Given its more favorable side-effect profile, lidocaine has replaced procaine (Novocain) in both medicine and dentistry as the short-acting local anesthetic of choice. A burning sensation that is evident upon intradermal or subcutaneous injection is due to the acidity of the solution which helps to increase the lidocaine's shelf-life and is especially true of solutions that contain epinephrine as this lowers the pH even more. This can be largely eliminated via buffering lidocaine solutions with 7.5% sodium bicarbonate added directly in a 9:1 ratio of lidocaine-to-sodium bicarbonate (e.g., 2 mL sodium bicarbonate added to 20 mL of 1% lidocaine) (112,113). The resultant multidose buffered solution vial should probably be discarded within 24

TABLE 56-11. Commonly Used Local Anesthetics

Generic (Trade) Name	Applicable Preparations & Concentrations	Onset of Action (Duration)	Usual Dosage (mL): Bursal Injection (A); (IP); (Ish); (SA); (T) [a]	Usual Dosage (mL): Joint Injection Small (Large)	Dosage: Percutaneous Infiltration (Maximum Amount)
Bupivacaine (Marcaine, Sensorcaine)	0.25% or 0.5%	5 min (2–4 h)	(A) 2½–4½; (IP) 4–4½ (Ish) 2½–4; (SA) 4–6; (T) 4½–9	1–2 mL (2–4 mL)	Up to 70mL
Lidocaine (Xylocaine)	0.5% or 1%	½–1 min (½ h)	(A) 2½–4½; (IP) 4–4½; (Ish) 2½–4; (SA) 4–6; (T) 4½–9	1–2 (2–4 mL)	Up to 60 mL

[a](A), anserine bursa; (IP), iliopectineal bursa; (Ish), ischial bursa; (SA), subacromial bursa; (T), trochanteric bursa.

hours to decrease risk of contamination. Since sodium bicarbonate can produce a cloudy solution when added to lidocaine, distinguishing a contaminated solution from a noncontaminated one by simple inspection is not possible.

A 2% lidocaine concentration is also available and is especially useful for procedures in which the total injection volume should be minimized. Examples include digital nerve blocks due to the possibility of developing a compartment syndrome and subsequent digital ischemia, and small joints such as the acromioclavicular joint since rebound pain can occur.

Relevant Side Effects and Drug Interactions

Although local anesthetics predominantly affect the circumscribed area into which they have been administered, they are also absorbed systemically and can therefore cause CV and CNS side effects. CNS toxicity occurs prior to CV toxicity and may manifest either as excitation in the form of a seizure or as a central respiratory depressant at even higher medication levels. At nontoxic concentrations, local anesthetics act as antiarrhythmics whereas at toxic levels, they are pro-arrhythmic and negative inotropes. The local anesthetic toxicity syndrome consists of salivation, tremor, convulsions, coma, hypertension, and tachycardia, followed by hypotension.

True allergic reactions to amide local anesthetics, such as lidocaine and bupivacaine, are quite rare. In contrast, allergic reactions are more common with ester class local anesthetics (e.g., procaine). There is no cross-sensitivity among these two classes.

Certain precautions should be observed when injecting local anesthetics in order to avoid inadvertent toxic serum levels. For example, aspiration should be performed in order to prevent inadvertent intravascular injection. Some feel, however, that the needle must be rotated in two planes before it can be concluded that the needle tip is not within a blood vessel, and that needles smaller than 25-gauge are not reliable when aspirating for blood (47). If blood is found, the needle should then be repositioned and aspiration done again. Another precaution is to dose-adjust by taking into account the procedure being performed since this in part dictates potential lidocaine serum levels. For example, high serum concentrations occur after intercostal nerve blocks as the intercostal regions are highly vascularized, whereas the lowest concentrations occur after subcutaneous administration. The epidural region is another highly vascular region from which dangerously high serum concentrations can occur. In general, the smallest dose that can produce effective anesthesia should be used when injecting local anesthetics into these regions. Lumbar and caudal epidural steroid injections are procedures that in particular have the potential to produce significant toxicity due to inadvertent intrathecal administration. Another factor involved in the potential for local anesthetic toxicity is patient age and general health. For example, children, the elderly, and debilitated and acutely ill patients have a greater potential for toxicity. In addition, since amide local anesthetics are hepatically metabolized, they should be used cautiously in hepatic dysfunction or reduced hepatic blood flow such as that which occurs in patients taking β-blockers or with congestive heart failure (CHF) (47).

In an effort to prolong the local anesthetic effect and to help prevent potential systemic side effects, epinephrine is sometimes added at a concentration that varies from 2 to 10 μg/mL (i.e., 1:500,000 to 1:100,000). However, when epinephrine is also present, additional side effects (e.g., anxiety, tachycardia, and hypertension) may occur. Epinephrine solutions also contain sodium metabisulfite, a chemical that can cause allergic reactions including anaphylaxis. Although the incidence of sulfite sensitivity in the general population is unknown, it is probably relatively low. Epinephrine is also capable of causing tissue ischemia when injected into body regions that are supplied by end arteries (e.g., digits) or have a compromised blood supply. An increased incidence of injection pain and wound infection potentially can also occur when epinephrine is present (47).

When local anesthetics are used in patients already taking CNS depressants, the risk of CNS side effects increases (47). Local anesthetics can potentially enhance the action of neuromuscular blocking agents. Local anesthetic solutions containing epinephrine should not be given to patients taking MAOIs or TCAs due to the potential for severe hypertension. In contrast, epinephrine's vasoconstrictor effects can be diminished or reversed by phenothiazines or by butyrophenones such as haloperidol.

NONINJECTABLE LOCAL ANESTHETICS

In addition to the injectable local anesthetics, a local anesthetic cream and a transdermal lidocaine preparation are also available. Both have applicability to a physiatric practice. Although EMLA is the most commonly used topical local anesthetic cream, several new topical anesthetic agents have been released recently and claim to have an increased efficacy and a faster onset of action (114).

EMLA Cream (Eutectic Mixture of Local Anesthetics)

EMLA cream is composed of 2.5% prilocaine (Citanest) and 2.5% lidocaine. This topical compound can be used to anesthetize the skin prior to a needle stick procedure. At least four European studies have compared EMLA cream applied for at least one hour with placebo cream, ethyl chloride, subcutaneous lidocaine, and intradermal lidocaine prior to i.v. cannulation. EMLA was more efficacious than placebo cream and ethyl chloride, comparable to subcutaneous lidocaine and less effective than intradermal lidocaine, yet preferable to lidocaine infiltration. EMLA was also as efficacious as lidocaine via iontophoresis prior to venipuncture in children (115).

Lidocaine Patch 5% (Lidoderm Patch)

The lidocaine patch is FDA-approved for postherpetic neuralgia pain but is also being used in other pain states. Two small, prospective, uncontrolled clinical studies reported clinically significant pain relief in reflex sympathetic dystrophy (RSD)/complex regional pain syndrome, stump neuroma pain, intercostal neuralgia, postthoracotomy pain, and meralgia paresthetica (109,116). Past response to EMLA might not predict response to the lidocaine patch since vehicle preparation within EMLA is crucial to efficacy (117,118).

MECHANISM OF ACTION AND PHARMACOKINETICS
The lidocaine patch potentially has a dual mechanism including blockade of local nerve fiber abnormal Na+ channels that have developed on damaged nociceptors and sensory nerve fibers. It can also act as a barrier against skin rubbing which can provoke allodynia in some. Although it is unclear if lidocaine is metabolized in the skin, it is hepatically metabolized to several active and inactive metabolites. There is a negligible concentration of one minor metabolite that is carcinogenic in rats.

DOSAGE AND PREPARATIONS

The lidocaine patch is a soft, stretchy 10 × 14 cm adhesive containing 700 mg of 5% lidocaine (50 mg/g adhesive). Up to 3 patches for a 12-hour duration (so as to lessen skin irritation) within 24 hours can be applied over intact skin. Patches may be cut into smaller sizes to fit the dimensions of painful skin regions. Smaller areas are recommended for debilitated patients, or for those with impaired function. Clothing may be worn over the application area.

RELEVANT SIDE EFFECTS AND DRUG INTERACTIONS

Potential side effects include local skin irritation and systemic toxicity. In clinical studies it has been associated with few adverse events, the most frequent being mild skin redness or irritation at the application site which occurred with a similar incidence for lidocaine and vehicle patch. These local reactions do not necessarily indicate allergy to lidocaine or another patch component. It should be used cautiously in patients on class I antiarrhythmics (e.g., tocainide and mexiletine) since the toxic effects are potentially synergistic. The concentration released from the lidocaine patch is not high enough to cause complete analgesic block and hence protective sensation loss (119). No serious adverse events have been observed in more than 120,000 patch-hours and patients have used the patch in clinical trials for periods of up to 8.7 years without adverse events that lead to patch discontinuation (120,121).

MUSCLE RELAXANTS

Relevance to Physiatry (122)

Muscle relaxants are often reserved for short-term use in painful musculoskeletal conditions where muscle "tightness" is believed to be playing a role as a pain generator. Unlike antispas-

ticity agents, muscle relaxants are not indicated for true skeletal muscle spasticity. The various medications that comprise the muscle relaxant category diminish muscle excitability and thus decrease pain associated with increased muscle tension. They are not believed to directly relax tense skeletal muscle. Since sedation usually occurs, shorter-acting agents can be prescribed for bedtime use only. Unlike true antispasticity agents, they do not significantly impair strength.

Perhaps the most common muscle relaxant emergency room and primary care physicians prescribe is cyclobenzaprine (Flexeril). It is structurally very similar to TCAs. Patients often mistake "muscle relaxants" with NSAIDs or other analgesics when asked about past medications.

A metaanalysis of cyclobenzaprine for back pain found that cyclobenzaprine's analgesic effect is modest and comes at the price of significant adverse effects—especially sedation. Analgesia is greatest in the first 4 days of treatment, suggesting that shorter courses may be better. Studies comparing the relative value of APAP, NSAIDs, and cyclobenzaprine individually and in combination for back pain are needed (123).

Mechanism of Action and Pharmacokinetics

Muscle relaxants are part of different medication groups, with different mechanisms and pharmacokinetics (Table 56-12). A common denominator however is that they interrupt the following pathway: Nociceptive input from skeletal muscles after injury or during inflammatory conditions travels along IA afferent nerve fibers to the spinal cord. This results in α-motor neuron stimulation which causes skeletal muscle contraction and leads to metabolite accumulation, particularly lactate. Lactate and other metabolites further stimulate α-motor neurons. Alpha-motor neuron impulse transmission causes muscle fiber contraction (122).

TABLE 56-12. Muscle Relaxants

[Class] Generic (Trade) Name	Structural Analog	Dose (mg)	Other Properties & Side Effects
[Single agents]			Sedation often occurs from muscle relaxants
Carisoprodol(Soma) (Rela)	Meprobamate (Equanil) Miltown)	350 po tid–qid	? mechanism but centrally acting; sedation; first dose idiosyncratic reactions; contraindicated in acute intermittent porphyria; addictive
Cyclobenzaprine (Flexeril)	Tricyclic antidepressants	10–20 po tid	? mechanism but centrally acting; widely used; plasma levels vary widely; sedation and other anticholinergic side effects
Diazepam (Valium)	Benzodiazepines	2–10 po bid–qid 5–10 i.v./i.m. q3–4h	Enhances GABA effect by binding to benzodiazepine receptors; also used as an antispasticity agent
Metaxalone (Skelaxin)	None	800 po tid–qid	? mechanism but centrally acting; drowsiness or CNS paradoxical excitation; hematologic toxicity, esp. hemolytic anemia or leukopenia; avoid if hepatic dysfunction
Methocarbamol (Robaxin)	Mephenesin (first muscle relaxant)	1,500 qid load × 48–72 h, then 1,000–1,500 po/i.m./i.v. qid	? mechanism but centrally acting; i.m. form inconvenient since should inject into each buttock rather than entire dose into one; lowers seizure threshold
Orphenadrine (Norflex)	Antihistamines	100 po bid 60 i.v./i.m. bid	? mechanism but centrally acting; sedation; reports of anaphylaxis in some asthmatics with i.m./i.v. dosing
[Muscle relaxant/ analgesic]			
Norgesic Norgesic forte		1–2 tabs po tid–qid	Norgesic [Norgesic forte] contents (mg): orphenadrine 50 [100]/ASA 385 [385]/caffeine 30 [30]; addition of ASA and caffeine is based upon a presumed synergistic effect with the muscle relaxant and decreased sedation
Soma compound		1–2 tabs po qid	Contents (mg): carisoprodol 200/ASA 325; addictive
Soma compound with codeine		1–2 tabs po qid	Contents (mg): carisoprodol 200/ASA 325/codeine 16; potentially quite sedative; highly addictive
Robaxisal		2 tabs po qid	Contents (mg): methocarbamol 400/ ASA325

Preparations, Dosing, Relevant Side Effects, and Drug Interactions

See Table 56-12.

N-METHYL-D-ASPARTATE-RECEPTOR ANTAGONISTS

Relevance to Physiatry

CNS excitation and inhibition is in part a balance between the excitatory amino acids glutamate and aspartate, and the inhibitory substance, GABA. Nerve or soft-tissue injury causes activation of the NMDA receptor for glutamate. Blocking the NMDA receptor in the brain and spinal cord prevents generation of central acute and chronic pain sensations from peripheral nociceptive stimuli and thus can potentially influence pain perception. NMDA receptor antagonists (i.e., NMDA glutamatergic antagonists) represent a new analgesic class. In addition to studies that report analgesia from NMDA antagonists, others have shown synergistic co-analgesia from combined use of NMDA antagonists and opioids, while opioid tolerance was prevented by reversing the rightward shift of the opioid-response curve (124).

Agents from this class include ketamine, dextromethorphan, and amantadine, as well as two opioids (methadone and dextropropoxyphene) that also possess NMDA blocking properties. Individual agents are discussed below. Other NMDA-receptor antagonists have phencyclidine site affinity, but are significantly limited by side effects.

Oral NMDA-receptor antagonists seem to alleviate NMDA-related neuropathic pain, including lumbosacral radiculopathy, trigeminal neuralgia, postherpetic neuralgia, cancer, and RSD (125–131). NMDA-receptor antagonists administered by nonoral routes have been investigated. Four patients with postherpetic neuralgia pain that was refractory to NSAIDs and antidepressants reported pain reduction after epidural ketamine (5 mg to 20 mg) (132). There is also a case report on i.v. ketamine in RSD (133).

Multiple NMDA-receptor antagonist clinical trials have been discontinued due to psychomimetic adverse effects as well as ataxia and incoordination (134). Since this is especially true of agents that completely block NMDA receptors, this has led to the development of moderate affinity channel blockers (e.g., glycine(B) and NR2B selective antagonists) that show a better profile in animal models since they block peripheral NMDA receptors without crossing the blood–brain barrier (135). These "therapeutically" safe NMDA-receptor antagonists have also diminished or prevented opioid tolerance, suggesting use with opioids in chronic pain.

Other potential applications include oral or epidural preemptive analgesia prior to surgery (136–139). They have also been co-administered with opioids to improve postoperative pain relief. Although this has been shown with ketamine, dextromethorphan studies have yielded variable results (140,141).

KETAMINE (KETALAR)

Ketamine hydrochloride has been most commonly used as a general anesthetic for children, persons of poor health, and in veterinary medicine. In 1999 it was classified as schedule III since it is used illicitly (referred to as "special K", "cat valium", "K", "Ket", "KitKat", "blind squid", "super acid", "vitamin K") with diversion occurring primarily from veterinary clinics. The dissociative anesthetic state (separation of perception from sensation) it produces after it is snorted, placed in alcoholic drinks, injected intramuscularly, or smoked with marijuana, reportedly is similar to the altered consciousness due to phencyclidine (PCP) with the lysergic acid diethylamide (LSD)-like visual effects. Users tout it as preferable to PCP or LSD because its overt hallucinatory effects are short-acting, lasting an hour or less. However, ketamine can adversely affect the senses, judgment, and coordination for up to 24 hours. Ketamine abuse is reportedly increasing, particularly among teenagers attending rave parties (142).

It is currently approved as a general anesthetic (i.v. or i.m. administration) and a preoperative sedative (po or pr administration) without an official pain indication. There are no specific recommended doses for analgesic use, although one trigeminal neuralgia study used 0.4 mg/kg i.m. doses (126). Its side-effect profile has been best established for its use as an anesthetic.

DEXTROMETHORPHAN

A review of dextromethorphan's (DM) role in pain control found that DM attenuated acute pain at doses of 30 to 90 mg divided q 4 to q 6 hours (5–10 mg/mL), without major side effects, and reduced analgesic requirements in 73% of postoperative DM-treated patients (141). However, secondary pain model studies in healthy volunteers and in those in chronic pain found suboptimal analgesia. In polyneuropathy pain, the number needed to treat (NNT) from placebo-controlled trials was 1.9 versus 2.5 for anticonvulsant Na+ channel blockers, 2.6 for TCAs, 3.4 for tramadol, 4.1 for gabapentin, and 6.7 for SSRIs. Its oral availability is an advantage.

AMANTADINE

Amantadine is widely used in Parkinson's disease and traumatic brain injury (TBI). Although literature on its use in pain is scant, case reports have been favorable (124,143,144).

NONSTEROIDAL ANTIINFLAMMATORY DRUGS

Relevance to Physiatry

At higher doses, NSAIDs are antiinflammatory in addition to being analgesic. Both of these effects are generally achieved without causing sedation, and thereby interfering with rehabilitation. Although there are numerous NSAIDs, they share a common mechanism of action and basic side-effect profile. Most agents however, have at least one somewhat unique characteristic. Since superior efficacy of a given NSAID has not been demonstrated and COX-II inhibitors are occasionally unavailable due to cost or insurance denial, physiatrists should become familiar with at least one agent from each of the major NSAID classes in order to switch medication classes in case of side effects or lack of efficacy of a particular agent.

Mechanism of Action and Pharmacokinetics

Like ASA, the prototypical oral antiinflammatory agent, NSAIDs exert their primary effects by inhibiting the synthesis of prostaglandins and other related compounds such as thromboxanes and leukotrienes. The four primary properties of NSAIDs are analgesia (mild to moderate pain), antiinflammatory effects, antipyresis and reversible antiplatelet effects. Antiinflammatory effects contribute to analgesia as inflammatory mediators sensitize nociceptors.

Oral NSAIDs are absorbed in the upper GI tract, a large percentage is then plasma protein bound and the unbound drug exerts its effects. Hepatic metabolism and renal excretion then occur. Both short-acting and long-acting NSAIDs (half-life of 30 to 50 hours at steady-state) exist. Although the significance of drug accumulation in long-acting agents in terms of toxicity is unclear, its potential occurrence is of concern and has been studied in detail for two of the long-acting agents, oxaprozin (Daypro) and piroxicam (Feldene) (145).

Preparations and Dosing

Table 56-13 shows a chemical structure classification scheme. Additional information about each of the NSAID classes is as follows:

- *Salicylates:* These include ASA and three nonacetylated salicylates. Compared to other NSAIDs, nonacetylated salicylates are less potent but have a favorable side-effect profile, especially for the GI tract and platelet inhibition. Within this medication category, however, it is not clear that any one particular agent offers a particular advantage over the other two.
- *Propionic acids:* This is perhaps the most popular NSAID class due to widespread prescription of and the OTC availability of ibuprofen and naproxen.

TABLE 56-13.   Nonsteroidal Antiinflammatory Drugs (NSAIDs)

[Class] Generic (Trade) Name	Dose (Oral in mg)	Other Properties & Side Effects
[Salicylates: acetylated] Aspirin	325–650 q4–6h	Used: esp. for antipyretic and cardioprotective effects Other formulations available:
(Ecotrin)		800 mg controlled release (prescription)
(Empirin)		975 mg enteric-coated (prescription) suppositories: 100, 200, 300,
(Bayer)		600 mg combined with narcotics and muscle relaxants
(Entrophen)		Side effects: allergy esp. if triad of nasal polyps, hay fever, asthma; GI toxicity but enteric-coated and buffered forms exist; tinnitus; Reye syndrome in children
[Salicylates: non-acetylated] Diflunisal (Dolobid)	500–1,000 load → 250–500 q8–12h	Relatively weak antiinflammatory effect; lacks antipyretic activity
Salicylate (Disalcid) (Salflex)	3,000/d divided q8–12h	Relatively weak antiinflammatory effect; no platelet inhibition
Salicylate combination (Trilisate)	1,500 bid	Relatively weak antiinflammatory effect; ? no ASA-allergic reactions; liquid preparation available (500 mg/5 mL)
[Propionic acids] Flurbiprofen (Ansaid)	200–300/d divided bid–qid	Available in ophthalmic solution (Ocufen); TD form available
Ibuprofen (Motrin)	600–800 tid–qid	Inexpensive and widely used; frequent dosing; [OTC]: Advil, Motrin IB; Nuprin, Rufen; TD form available
Ketoprofen (Orudis)	50–75 tid	Accumulates if poor renal function
(Oruvail) (Orafen)	200 qd	[OTC]: Orudis-KT; Actron; TD form available
Naproxen (Naprosyn)	250–500 bid	High incidence GI side effects; advantage of enteric-coated form ?,
(EC-Naprosyn)	375–500 bid	although expensive; [OTC]: Aleve;
Naproxen-Na (Naprelan)	750–1,000 qd	Naprelan has Intestinal Protective Drug Absorption System (IPDAS);
(Anaprox)	275–550 bid	immediate- and sustained-release components
Oxaprozin (Daypro)	600 bid; 1,200 qd	qd or bid dosing
[Acetic acids] Diclofenac (Cataflam)	50 bid–tid	LFT monitoring if prolonged use; side effects in up to 20%;
(Voltaren)	50 bid–tid	Arthrotec = diclofenac (50 or 75 mg) + misoprostol (200 µg)
(Voltaren-XR)	100 qd	
Etodolac (Lodine)	200–400 bid–tid	Gastric-sparing properties?
(Lodine XL)	400–1,200 qd	
Indomethacin (Indocin)	25–50 tid	Most potent and toxic NSAID; pr preparation (Indotec); drug of choice
(Indocin-SR)	75 qd	in ankylosing spondylitis; indicated in other highly inflammatory conditions (e.g., acute gouty arthritis); prevents heterotopic ossification s/p total hip replacement (THR) and used for myositis ossificans; dose-related CNS/ hematologic side effects in up to 25–50%; GI toxicity
Ketorolac (Toradol)	10 qid (po) 15–60 (i.m.) Lower doses if age >65 or renal dysfunction	FDA-approved only for 5 consecutive days; GI bleeding at higher doses; rapid analgesia with i.m. form—decrease dose for age ≥65, renal dysfunction, weight <110; i.v. preparation also available
Nabumetone (Relafen)	500–1,000 bid	qd or bid dosing; nonacidic prodrug that undergoes hepatic biotransformation into active metabolite; preliminary studies suggest that unlike other NSAIDs, no evidence of enterohepatic recirculation of active metabolite—this may be an advantage
Sulindac (Clinoril)	150–200 bid	Prodrug; possibly renal-sparing because urinary excretion, primarily as biologically inactive forms, may be more GI toxic
Tolmetin (Tolectin)	200–600 tid–qid	Frequent dosing; frequent GI toxicity
[Fenemates] Meclofenamate (Meclomen)	50–100 tid–qid	Frequent dosing; diarrhea common
Mefenamic acid (Ponstel)	500 × 1, then 250 qid	Frequent dosing; used for dysmenorrheic pain
[Oxicams] Piroxicam (Feldene)	20 qd or 10 bid	qd dosing; accumulation in older adults possibly due to enterohepatic recirculation; dermatologic side effects and cases of serum sickness; pr form (Fexicam)

- *Acetic acids*: This class is the most potent and hence the most potentially toxic NSAID group. It includes two NSAIDs which can be administered via i.m. and pr routes, (i.e., ketorolac and indomethacin) and includes the two prodrug NSAIDs (i.e., sulindac and nabumetone).
- *Fenemates*: Meclofenamate can cause significant GI toxicity whereas mefenamic acid has been marked for dysmenorrheic pain.
- *Oxicams*: Piroxicam has true once-daily dosing but has also been associated with severe dermatologic reactions, such as exfoliative dermatitis and pemphigus vulgaris.

Relevant Side Effects and Drug Interactions

GI side effects are the most frequently observed form of NSAID-related toxicity and most commonly occur in older patients and in those with a prior history of peptic ulcer disease. Due to widespread use and the relatively high incidence of GI side effects, NSAID-induced GI pathology is the most prevalent adverse drug reaction in the United States (146). It is unclear if any traditional NSAID offers the advantage of less GI side effects compared to the others. Indomethacin and ketorolac (used for more than 5 consecutive days) have high GI side-effect rates.

GI side effects occur from a direct mucosal irritant effect and via the systemic effect of prostaglandin inhibition, since prostaglandins normally protect the lining of the GI tract by stimulating the production of a gastric mucosal barrier. The direct irritant effect differs among NSAID preparations and only occurs with the oral route of administration, whereas the systemic effect will occur regardless as to how the medication is administered and regardless if the drug is a prodrug or if it is enteric-coated. There is laboratory evidence that differences in the systemic effects of NSAIDs on prostaglandin metabolism exist (3). The metabolic breakdown of different NSAIDs might also in part dictate the medication's GI side-effect profile. In particular, NSAIDs such as indomethacin, diclofenac, naproxen, piroxicam, and sulindac that undergo extensive biliary excretion of active metabolites, and hence prolonged intestinal mucosal contact, might predispose to increased GI toxicity (3). Strategies can be used to decrease the chance of this: NSAIDs can be taken with meals so that absorption is delayed and food is present to directly protect the mucosa from the stomach's acid environment. Some NSAIDs are enteric-coated so that duodenal rather than gastric absorption occurs. In cases of prior significant GI toxicity due to NSAIDs or in patients with a prior history of peptic ulcer disease, other prophylactic medications including antacids, H2 blockers, misoprostol, proton pump inhibitors, or sucralfate can be given concomitantly (Table 56-14). Of these, only Cytotec is FDA-approved for gastric ulcer prevention, and should be taken for the duration of NSAID therapy. In controlled studies of 3 months' duration, it had no effect, compared to placebo, on NSAID-associated GI pain or discomfort (147) (Table 56-14). A COX-II inhibitor can be prescribed instead.

It would be useful to identify patients at particular risk for NSAID-induced GI side effects, especially since the majority of NSAID-induced ulcers are asymptomatic and bleeding is often the initial symptom. Unfortunately, periodic fecal occult blood testing is not helpful in screening for NSAID-induced ulcers due to a high false-positive rate (3). There is epidemiologic support in patients with OA for a few risk factors. (32)

Since nitric oxide is a crucial mediator of GI mucosal defense, another protective strategy is the coupling of a nitric oxide-releasing moiety to NSAIDs (148). These nitric oxide NSAIDs (NO-NSAIDs) have been shown in experimental, and preliminary clinical studies to reduce upper GI bleeding risk, but are not yet clinically available (148).

Less common GI side effects involve the esophagus, the nonduodenal portion of small bowel, the colon, and the liver. Esophageal side effects include esophagitis and benign esophageal strictures. As in the duodenum, the remainder of the small bowel can develop ulcers, erosions, and weblike strictures. The colon can also ulcerate or erode, and irritable bowel disease can be unmasked. This NSAID enteropathy is not believed to occur via an acid mechanism and is therefore not likely to be prevented by antacids, H2 blockers, or proton pump inhibitors. Hepatotoxicity is rare except in those with preexisting liver disease. Clinically significant hepatic enzyme elevations occur with some agents, particularly diclofenac and it is therefore suggested that LFTs, specifically alanine aminotransferase (ALT, previously referred to as serum glutamic-oxaloacetic transaminase, or SGPT) be monitored when this NSAID is being taken. Unfortunately, the optimal times for measuring these levels have yet to be determined.

Renal side effects can especially occur in those with preexisting kidney disease or in those with comorbid medical conditions such as CHF and hypovolemia that impair renal blood flow. Acute renal failure, nephrotic syndrome, and interstitial nephritis are examples of NSAID-induced renal toxicity. It has been suggested but not proven that sulindac is somewhat renal-sparing compared to other NSAIDs (147).

True NSAID allergic reactions occur in 1% and range from simple skin rashes and rhinitis to anaphylaxis. NSAIDs should not be used in patients allergic to ASA.

CYCLOOXYGENASE-II INHIBITORS

Relevance to Physiatry

COX-II inhibitors have direct applicability to day-to-day clinical physiatric practice. They represent a better alternative to NSAIDs for those who would benefit from oral antiinflammatory agents but are at high risk for GI side effects (149). Their

TABLE 56-14.   Agents Used in NSAID-Induced Upper GI Toxicity Prophylaxis/Treatment

Medication	Dose Range	Gastric Ulcer (NSAID-Induced)	Duodenal Ulcer (NSAID-Induced)
Antacids	Standard	Not preventative	Not preventative
H2 Blockers	Standard	Not preventative	Preventative
	High dose	Preventative?	Preventative
Misoprostol (Cytotec)	Standard (200 μm qid)	Preventative (FDA-approved)	Not preventative
	Low (200 μg bid–tid)	Preventative?	Not preventative
Proton pump inhibitors	Standard	Not preventative	Preventative?
Sucralfate (Carafate)	Standard (1 g qid)	Not preventative	Healing (if stop NSAIDs)

exact role is still being defined as postmarketing experience accumulates and studies are published. At the time of this writing, three oral coxibs [celecoxib (Celebrex), rofecoxib (Vioxx), and valdecoxib (Bextra)] have been FDA-approved. Valdecoxib's prodrug, an i.m./i.v. injectable coxib (parecoxib or Dynastat) is also close to FDA-approval, as is etoricoxib (Arcoxia), the most COX-II selective coxib.

Mechanism of Action and Pharmacokinetics

COX-II inhibitors reduce prostaglandin synthesis via COX-II inhibition, without inhibition of cyclooxygenase-I (COX-I) at therapeutic concentrations.

The COX-I isoenzyme is constitutively expressed and COX-I–derived prostaglandins function to protect the GI mucosa while thromboxanes derived from the COX-I isoenzyme increase platelet aggregation. COX-II isoenzyme prostaglandins mediate inflammation, pain, and fever, and are constitutively expressed in the brain and kidney. The degree of relative COX-II/COX-I inhibition varies according to the agent, with rofecoxib being the most, followed by valdecoxib, and celecoxib being the least COX-II selective. Although the coxibs differ with respect to these *in vitro* COX-II/COX-I inhibition ratios, the clinical significance of this is unclear. At usual therapeutic doses, food has no significant effect on either peak plasma concentration or absorption, thus coxibs can be taken without regard to meals. Conversely, higher celecoxib doses (≥400 mg bid) should be given with food to improve absorption.

Preparations and Dosing

COX-II inhibitors are currently only approved for oral administration for the indications as shown in Table 56-15. At the time of this writing, the first parenteral COX-II inhibitor is close to being released and approved for acute pain. In patients with moderate hepatic impairment, doses should be decreased by approximately 50% for all three coxibs.

Relevant Side Effects and Drug Interactions

COX-II inhibitors cause less gastropathy than traditional NSAIDs as shown by several major studies, most notably the VIGOR (Vioxx Gastrointestinal Outcomes Research) and the CLASS Trial (Celebrex Long-term Arthritis Safety Study) (150, 151).

Potential renal toxicity is the same for coxibs and traditional NSAIDs and includes fluid retention leading to edema, renal hypertension, interstitial nephritis, and papillary necrosis (152). The lack of renal sparing is due to the constitutive expression of the COX-II isoenzyme in the kidney (153,154). As is true for traditional NSAIDs, coxibs should not be used in patients with renal insufficiency or in those at risk for renal failure. Coxibs are not associated with decreased platelet aggregation and hence prolongation in bleeding time (155). They can therefore be used concomitantly with antiplatelet medications. They can also be used in patients who will be undergoing lumbar epidural steroid injections and other fluoroscopic-guided spinal injection procedures where the risk of inadvertent bleeding makes the use of medications with an antiplatelet effect somewhat dangerous. In contrast, patients should be taken off of NSAIDs for at least 5 days on average to allow thromboxane synthesis to return to a functional level.

Mean INR increases of approximately 10% have been seen in patients receiving warfarin and COX-II inhibitors (147). There have been infrequent postmarketing reports of INR increases associated with bleeding events, predominantly in the elderly for both celecoxib and rofecoxib (147,155). Therefore, standard monitoring of INR should be performed in those receiving warfarin or similar agents, when treatment with a COX-II inhibitor is initiated or changed, particularly for the first few days.

Celecoxib is contraindicated in patients allergic to sulfonamide (about 3% of the general population) (156). Whereas rofecoxib does not contain a sulfonamide group, valdecoxib does but for unclear reasons does not invoke an antigenic response in patients allergic to sulfonamide allergic.

With respect to contraindications, none of the COX-II inhibitors should be given to patients with a history of ASA or NSAID allergy, or to patients with advanced renal or hepatic dysfunction. COX-II inhibitors should be used with caution and introduced at the lowest recommended doses in those with HTN or CHF, given their potential to cause renal prostaglandin-mediated fluid retention. Potential blood pressure (BP) increases in hypertensive patients are similar for NSAIDs and COX-II inhibitors (157).

The issue of increased thromboembolic events in patients receiving coxibs has been controversial (158). At the time of this writing, there is insufficient data to justify the conclusion that coxibs are thrombogenic. It is instead believed that these events were due to the lack of antiplatelet effect from coxibs and that this manifested as myocardial infarctions (MIs) and cerebrovascular accidents (CVAs) in patients with subclinical CV pathology (159,160). As coxibs are clearly not substitutes for cardioprotective ASA, all patients with appropriate CV risk factors who are receiving COX-II inhibitors should also be placed on cardioprotective ASA. Since NSAIDs have a mild reversible antiplatelet effect they should probably not be used concomitantly with cardioprotective ASA due to the possibility of a less predictable bleeding time prolongation. For example, treatment with daily ibuprofen undermines the cardioprotec-

Indication	Celecoxib (Celebrex): Capsules (mg) 100; 200	Rofecoxib (Vioxx): Tablets (mg): 12.5; 25; 50 Oral Suspension: 12.5 or 25 mg/5 mL	Valdecoxib (Bextra): Tablets (mg): 10
Acute pain	(Day 1): 400 mg × 1, then 200 mg × 1 prn; then 200 mg bid prn thereafter	50 mg qd prn (50 mg doses for >5 d has not been studied	Not FDA-approved
Osteoarthritis	200 mg qd or 100 mg bid	12.5–25 mg qd	10 mg qd
Familial adenomatous polyposis	200 mg bid	N/A	N/A
Primary dysmenorrhea	50 mg qd prn	50 mg qd prn/5 d	20 mg bid
Rheumatoid arthritis	100–200 mg bid	N/A	10 mg qd

TABLE 56-15.   Currently Available Coxibs and Recommended Doses for Approved Indications

TABLE 56-16. A Sample of COX-2 Inhibitor-Medication Interactions

COX-2 Inhibitor	Medications That Alter COX-2 Inhibitor Concentration	Medications Whose Concentration Is Altered by COX-2 Inhibitor
Celecoxib	Fluconazole (increases)	Lithium (increases)
Rofecoxib	Rifampin (decreases)	Methotrexate (increases)
Valdecoxib	Fluconazole (increases)	Dextromethorphan (increases)
	Ketoconazole (increases)	Lithium (decreases)

tive effect of ASA (161). Traditional NSAIDs are also not substitutes for cardioprotective ASA. Hence, patients with CV risk factors who are receiving NSAIDs should be switched to cardioprotective ASA and a COX-II inhibitor.

There are some similarities and differences between potential drug interactions for the COX-II inhibitors (Table 56-16). The differences relate to disparities in hepatic metabolism. Specifically, celecoxib is metabolized via the cytochrome P450, rofecoxib via cytosolic enzyme reduction, and valdecoxib by both cytochrome P450 isoenzymes and non-P450 dependent pathways. When COX-II inhibitor therapy is desired, these potential medication interactions can be considered in guiding COX-II inhibitor selection. All COX-II inhibitors may diminish the antihypertensive effect of angiotensin-converting enzyme (ACE) inhibitors. It is unclear how clinically significant this is. For example, in those with mild to moderate hypertension, use of rofecoxib 25 mg q day with the ACE inhibitor benazepril (10 to 40 mg for 4 weeks), was associated with an average increase in mean arterial pressure of about 3 mm Hg (147). Clinical studies and postmarketing observations show that NSAIDs and COX-II inhibitors can reduce the natriuretic effect of furosemide and thiazides in some patients. This response is due to renal prostaglandin synthesis inhibition.

Future Developments

In the near future, another class of oral antiinflammatory agents, the prostaglandin receptor blockers may become clinically available. These may offer certain advantages over COX-II inhibitors.

OTHER ADJUVANT ANALGESICS

Tizanidine (Zanaflex)

RELEVANCE TO PHYSIATRY
Tizanidine was developed as an antispasticity agent but has also been studied for headache and neuropathic pain conditions including trigeminal neuralgia and phantom pain syndrome (162–166). Although there are no published controlled trials to date, tizanidine may play a role in refractory neuropathic pain, unrelated to spasticity. As is true of clonidine, another centrally acting α_2-adrenergic agonist, tizanidine has been investigated for managing narcotic withdrawal symptoms (167). Some older studies have also examined it for painful muscular "spasm" and acute low back pain (168–170). Other uses not as directly applicable to physiatry include its use along with long-acting NSAIDs for detoxification of rebound headache and chronic tension headache (171–173).

MECHANISM OF ACTION AND PHARMACOKINETICS
Tizanidine is a centrally acting α_2-adrenergic agonist which presumably reduces spasticity by increasing presynaptic motor neuron inhibition. After oral administration, 95% of the dose undergoes first-pass hepatic metabolism and peak plasma levels occur in 1.5 hours. Since food increases maximum concentration (C_{max}) by approximately one third and shortens time to peak concentration by 40 minutes, it should not be given around mealtimes as this can cause increased sedation (174).

PREPARATIONS AND DOSING
Tizanidine is available in 2 and 4 mg tablets. Dosing for spasticity is accomplished by gradually increasing the amount over 1 month until a maximum of 24 mg divided tid is reached, the desired therapeutic effect is achieved, or dose-limiting side effects occur. Although the total daily dose should not exceed 36 mg, experience beyond 24 mg is limited. Myofascial or neuropathic pain dosing regimens are unclear.

SIDE EFFECTS AND MEDICATION INTERACTIONS
The most clinically significant side effect is potential hepatotoxicity. In controlled clinical studies, 5% had serum transaminase elevations to greater than three times the upper limit of normal (or two times if baseline levels were elevated). Although most resolved rapidly upon medication withdrawal with no reported sequelae, some developed nausea, vomiting, anorexia, and jaundice. In postmarketing experience, there have been three deaths due to liver failure. In one case, tizanidine was clearly the cause. In the two other cases, patients were also taking other potentially hepatotoxic medications. Aminotransferase-level monitoring is recommended during the first 6 months (i.e., baseline, 1, 3, and 6 months) and then periodically. It should be used only with extreme caution in those with impaired hepatic function.

The most frequent side effects include dry mouth, CNS depression (i.e., somnolence/sedation), asthenia (weakness, fatigue, or tiredness), and dizziness or hypotension associated with its α_2-adrenergic antagonism. In controlled clinical trials, 48% reported sedation. Only 10% rated sedation as severe, compared to less than 1% of patients receiving placebo.

Despite extensive first-pass metabolism, reports of medication interactions are essentially limited to oral contraceptives. Analyses have shown a 50% lower tizanidine clearance in women on oral contraceptives compared to controls. It is thought not to be associated with muscle weakness to the same extent as other antispasticity agents (175).

OPIOID ANALGESICS

Relevance to Physiatry

Narcotic analgesics are often referred to as opioid or opiate analgesics as some are opium-derived. They are indicated for moderate to severe pain, especially that which is of a nociceptive quality (i.e., dull and constant) rather than of a neuropathic quality (i.e., sharp, burning, and intermittent). The perception of opioid analgesics as being relatively ineffective in neuropathic pain is changing (40,176,177). It is still unclear as to which patient subgroups with neuropathic pain are most likely to respond to them. Evolving concepts in opioid analgesic use include the recognition that oxycodone appears to be in part a κ-opioid-receptor agonist and may offer enhanced analgesia when combined with morphine. Also, opioid rotation might help to avoid tolerance to therapeutic effects with the need to increase dose and incur side effects (178–180).

Pertinent physiatric uses besides pain management include control of diarrhea and cough, particularly in those with a nonproductive cough that is interfering with sleep and thus reha-

bilitation. Potential side effects can have a detrimental effect upon a patient's ability to participate in a rehabilitation program. The absence of end-organ toxicity with pure opioid analgesics except for Demerol is a major advantage for those requiring chronic opioid therapy.

Mechanism of Action and Pharmacokinetics

Endorphins, enkephalins, and dynorphins are the three endogenous opioid families and the three primary opioid-receptor types are named mu (μ), kappa (κ), and delta (δ). Each of these receptors has a different CNS distribution and can cause

TABLE 56-17.   Narcotic Analgesics

[Narcotic Class] *Subclass* Generic (Trade) Name	Usual Dosage Range (mg) (Time = h)	Relative Potency po (i.m.) [Other]
[AGONIST]		
Codeine	15–60 po q4–6h; 15–60 i.m. q4–6h	200 (120)
Fentanyl-transdermal (Duragesic patch)	1 patch q72h	Refer to PDR for table of equivalent doses
Hydromorphone (Dilaudid)	2–4 mg po q4–6h; 3 mg pr q6–8h	1.5
	0.5–2 mg i.m./s.c. or slow i.v. q4–6h	
(Dilaudid-5)	5 mg/5 mL liquid po q6h	
Meperidine (Demerol)	1–1.8 mg/kg po/i.m./s.c. q3–4h; max 150 mg	300 (75)
	slow i.v. q3–4h	
Morphine sulfate		60
• sustained release tabs (MS Contin; Oramorph SR)	30 q8–12h	
• sustained release caps (Kadian)	20 q12–24h	
• oral solution (Roxanol)	various concentrations: 10–30 q4h	
• immediate release (MS IR)	10–30 q4h	
Oxycodone		30
• immediate release tabs (OxyIR; Roxicodone)	5 q6h	
• immediate release tabs (Percolone)	10–30 q4h	
• oral concentrate solution (OxyFAST)	5 mg q6h of a 20mg/mL solution	
• sustained release (OxyContin)	10–40 q12h	
Propoxyphene		130
(Darvon Pulvules)	65 q4h	
(Darvon-N)	100 q6h	
[PARTIAL AGONISTS]		
Buprenorphine (Buprenex)	Parenteral only	N/A
[MIXED AGONIST-ANTAGONISTS]		
Butorphanol tartrate nasal spray (Stadol NS)	1 mg (1 spray per nostril) q3–4h	N/A
Pentazocine		N/A
(Talwin)	1 tab po q3–4	
(Talwin NX) {pentazocine: 50 mg /Naloxone: 0.5 mg}	1–2 tabs po q3–4	
[ANALGESIC COMBINATIONS]		
Narcotic/acetaminophen		
Propoxyphene/acetaminophen (Darvocet) {N-50 = 50/325; N-100 = 100/650}	1–2 tabs po q4h	N/A
Hydrocodone/acetaminophen (Lortab) {2.5/500, 5/500, 7.5/500}	1–2 tabs po q4–6h	N/A
Anexsia (hydrocodone/acetaminophen) {5/500, 7.5/650, 10/660}	1 tab po q4–6h	
Hydrocodone/acetaminophen (Lorcet) {5/500}	1 tab po q6h	N/A
Oxycodone/acetaminophen (Percocet){5/325}	1 tab po q6h	N/A
Pentazocine/acetaminophen (Talacen) {25/650}	1 caplet po q4h (max 624 h)	
APAP/codeine (Tylenol with codeine) {Tylenol #2, #3, #4 = 300/15; 300/30; 300/60}	1–2 tabs po q4–6h	
Oxycodone/acetaminophen (Tylox) {5/500}	1 po q6h	
Hydrocodone/acetaminophen (Vicodin) {5/500}	1–2 tabs po q4–6h	N/A
Vicodin-ES {7.5/750}	1 tab po q4–6h	N/A
Narcotic/aspirin		
Propoxyphene/ASA/caffeine (Darvon compound-65 Pulvules) {65/389/32.4}	1 tab po q4h	N/A
Oxycodone/aspirin (Percodan){5/325}	1 tab po q6h	N/A
ASA/Codeine (Empirin with Codeine #3){325/30}		N/A
Empirin with Codeine # 4 (ASA/Codeine) {325/60}		
Pentazocine/ASA (Talwin compound) {12.5/325}	2 caplets po q6–8h	N/A

slightly different physiologic responses upon activation. Although the biochemical alterations that follow opioid-receptor binding are not completely clear, the basic analgesic mechanism is inhibition of pain impulse transmission to higher centers and alteration of pain perception. Opioid receptors have been recently identified in peripheral nerves and joints where they are thought to regulate pain perception associated with inflammation (40). Intraarticular morphine is being studied in knee OA (181,182).

There are two important opioid-receptor binding characteristics: affinity (how tightly it binds) and intrinsic activity (amount of receptor stimulation). Based on these two properties, narcotic analgesics are classified as full agonists (bind and stimulate a receptor), partial agonists (bind but less intrinsic activity), mixed agonists/antagonists (bind and activate some receptors but not others), or antagonists (bind but devoid of activity). Unlike the other three categories, agonists have no analgesic ceiling.

Opioid analgesics have several different administration routes including oral, intramuscular, intravenous, subcutaneous, intranasal, and transdermal. Most metabolism is hepatic but some also occurs in the kidney, lung, and CNS. Renal excretion then occurs.

Preparations and Dosing

There are several important principles of narcotic analgesic administration. One is that short-acting preparations should be used initially in order to titrate the dose prior to starting a long-acting agent. Short-acting agents generally peak in 30 to 60 minutes and last for 4 hours. In contrast, sustained-release oral compounds peak within 2 to 3 hours and last for 12 hours, whereas sustained-release transdermal fentanyl peaks within 24 to 72 hours and lasts up to 72 hours. Long-acting agents are obviously more convenient for patients and their sustained effect help to prevent serum medication concentrations peaks and troughs that are inherent with short-acting medications. By maintaining analgesic efficacy through the night, long-acting agents also help prevent pain-related nocturnal awakening. Allowing patients an otherwise uninterrupted night's sleep should help with rehabilitation.

Around-the-clock rather than as needed (prn) dosing is another narcotic analgesic principle. It offers the advantage of more constant blood levels, thus better tolerance to side effects since these tend to occur with blood level peaks. Regularly scheduled dosing also helps to limit breakthrough pain due to serum medication troughs. The anticipation of regularly scheduled doses may reduce pain behavior reinforcement based on prn dosing regimens.

Narcotic preparations of particular importance to the physiatrist along with their usual dosage ranges and relative potencies are shown in Table 56-17. Due to significant first-pass metabolism with oral dosing, required oral doses are larger than the parenteral ones. Several of the more commonly used agents are discussed in some detail below. Although the most commonly used dosage ranges are shown, doses should be titrated as high as necessary to relieve pain as long as they are tolerated well. Partial agonists and mixed agonists-antagonists are shown in Table 56-17, although their use is quite limited. Dosing software for personal digital assistants (PDAs) that assists with converting opioid analgesics is available.

Finally, the issue of incomplete cross-tolerance among opioids deserves further comment. Specifically, switching to an alternate opioid in the setting of poor pain relief or intolerable side effects may prove to be of benefit due to this phenomenon.

INDIVIDUAL AGENTS

Agonists (Weak)

CODEINE PREPARATIONS
Codeine is used as an antitussive as well as a mild to moderately potent analgesic. After oral, i.m., or s.c. administration, codeine is partly demethylated to morphine, the active metabolite and partly converted to the inactive metabolite norcodeine. Codeine is not analgesic in some patients who are unable to convert codeine to morphine. These metabolites are then hepatically conjugated and most are renally excreted. Adverse effects are typical of other narcotics but with an increased frequency of CNS side effects. In addition, some codeine-containing preparations such as various forms of APAP with codeine contain sodium metabisulfite, a potentially allergenic preservative in susceptible patients. Thus codeine per se commonly becomes mistakenly identified as the allergen by the patient or treating physician. A new formulation, sustained-release codeine (Codeine Contin) is available outside the United States (183).

PROPOXYPHENE (DARVON, DARVON PULVULES, DOLENE)
This narcotic analgesic is structurally related to methadone but was originally considered to be a nonopioid. After it was found to be associated with tolerance, dependence, and addiction, it was reclassified as an opioid. It has an analgesic efficacy of approximately one half to two thirds that of oral codeine, and is therefore used to manage mild to moderate pain. It undergoes extensive first-pass metabolism with conversion to a metabolite (norpropoxyphene) that is associated with CNS toxicity similar to normeperidine (from meperidine), and may accumulate with repeated dosing. It produces local anesthetic and antiarrhythmic depressant effects similar to those of lidocaine and quinidine which are clinically significant if overdosed. When it accumulates, either from chronic administration or acute overdose, norpropoxyphene can lead to arrhythmias, cardiogenic shock, mental status changes, seizures, coma, and death. Propoxyphene therapy has also been associated with abnormal LFTs and, more rarely, with instances of reversible jaundice (including cholestatic jaundice), and therefore should be used cautiously in patients with preexisting hepatotoxicity. By strict definition this drug should have no ceiling but because of the metabolite norpropoxyphene, doses should not exceed 390 mg per day. In excessive doses, either alone or in combination with other CNS depressants, it can cause death. Consensus committees have concluded that it should not be used in geriatric patients (184).

Agonists (Strong)

FENTANYL-TRANSDERMAL (DURAGESIC)
Fentanyl is a potent, short-acting opioid agonist that is used for pain control when administered in the form of a transdermal patch with an average duration of 72 hours or transmucosally for breakthrough pain from a lozenge (Actiq or Oralet). The success of the patch can be attributed to fentanyl's low molecular weight and its highly lipophilic nature, which enables it to be readily absorbed through the skin and subsequently distributed throughout the body. The fentanyl patch is generally used in patients with chronic pain syndromes who require regular doses of narcotic analgesics. Due to its potential for significant hypoventilation in narcotic-naïve patients, it should not be used for acute pain syndromes. In addition to pain, it is used as

a preprocedural anxiolytic and sedative and as a supplement to anesthesia.

When initiating opioid therapy with the fentanyl patch, the lowest available dose (25 µg per hour) should be selected. If further dose titration is needed, the other available patch strengths include the 50 µg per hour (5.0 mg), 75 µg per hour (7.5 mg), and 100 µg per hour (10 mg) formulations. Patches of different strengths can also be simultaneously applied to achieve a variety of fentanyl doses. For patients who are already on opioids, the dose should be expressed in terms of the equianalgesic morphine dose and this should then be converted to the equivalent fentanyl patch dose as can be determined using a standard table. At the start of treatment, depot accumulation of fentanyl within skin tissue results in a significant delay (17 to 48 hours) before maximum plasma concentration is achieved. There is wide variability between patients in fentanyl absorption from the patch (185). In addition, the physiatrist should become familiar with other details of fentanyl patch use including dosage titrations, the concomitant use of other analgesics, and weaning patients off of the patch. An advantage of transdermal fentanyl over oral opioid analgesics is less constipation associated with its use as suggested by open studies (186–189).

Two notes of caution include the potential for diversion and accidental overdose related to increases in body temperature. Various methods of diversion of fentanyl from the patch have been reported. Specifically, there have been reports of patches being removed from patients, even dead ones, and then used for illicit purposes (190). Since approximately 20% on average of the medication remains in a patch that has been removed after 3 days of application, this underscores the importance of proper patch disposal and the need for strict policies and guidelines in patient care settings regarding their disposal (191). In addition, there is a published case report of fentanyl intoxication caused by heating and inhaling the contents from a fentanyl patch (192). The fentanyl patch can also serve as a drug reservoir by withdrawing the liquid medication from the patch by using a tuberculin syringe. There have also been anecdotal reports of diversion via freezing the patches using dry ice followed by oral ingestion of a portion of the patch that has been subsequently cut up. Patients should be cautioned that use of the patch during febrile episodes or other conditions involving extreme increases in body temperature (as can occur when a person is in a sauna or hot tub) should probably be avoided (193,194). As is true of transdermal medications in general, most cutaneous reactions are limited to localized dermatitis; however, systemic effects may occur. Others details of patch application and use can be explained to the patient with the help of a pictorial guide from the manufacturer. Some patients, particularly the elderly with thinning skin, may have difficulty tolerating the patch (195).

HYDROMORPHONE (DILAUDID)

This semisynthetic opioid is derived from morphine and has a pharmacokinetic profile similar to it. Due to its high solubility it can be prepared from a powder in high concentration and therefore is particularly useful for pain relief in opioid-tolerant patients who require larger than usual opioid doses. Because of its lack of any identified metabolites, it is sometimes recommended for patients with renal failure. Literature on the use of hydromorphone is not as extensive as for morphine but studies available suggest that there is little difference between their analgesic efficacy, adverse effect profile, and patient preference (196). A new SR formulation is in clinical trials and preliminary evidence suggests that once a day dosing (rather than q 4 hour

dosing required with conventional hydromorphone) provides effective analgesia (197).

MEPERIDINE (DEMEROL)

Although traditionally prescribed by surgeons to parenterally treat postoperative pain, meperidine is of limited use to the physiatrist for two major reasons. First, it has a short duration of action that necessitates frequent dosing with the inherent peaks and troughs in serum concentrations. Second, meperidine is metabolized to normeperidine, a toxic metabolite which lowers the seizure threshold and causes other manifestations of CNS excitation such as anxiety, tremors, and myoclonus. Normeperidine has about half the analgesic potency of meperidine but a much longer half-life and accumulates with prolonged use (more than several days), particularly in patients with compromised renal function. In fact, normeperidine accumulates just as much with oral doses as with i.v. doses, even though oral doses have only about 25% of the analgesic effect. Unfortunately, naloxone not only fails to reverse these effects, but may worsen them. Overall, there is a sentiment to replace meperidine with other more efficacious and less toxic opioids (198).

METHADONE

Methadone along with dextropropoxyphene is unique among the opioids because of weak, noncompetitive antagonistic binding to NMDA receptors in addition binding to traditional opioid µ-receptors. NMDA-receptor antagonism is believed to explain its efficacy in the treatment of neuropathic pain as the NMDA nonopioid receptor is a likely component of neuropathic pain (199,200). Many opioid conversion charts have traditionally underestimated the potency of methadone, leading to safety concerns due to confusion about dosage. To add to the confusion, it has been proposed but not proven that the equianalgesic dose of hydromorphone or morphine to methadone will be different in patients with neuropathic pain than in patients with nonneuropathic pain (201). A greater understanding of dosing and pharmacokinetics has led to methadone becoming increasingly used as a second-line agent in treating cancer pain unresponsive to conventional opioids (202). There is also specific literature on its use as a neuropathic pain agent in other conditions. Examples include a case series in phantom limb pain and a case report in neuropathic burn pain (199,203). Advantages include its lack of active metabolites, high lipid solubility, excellent absorption after oral and rectal delivery, and extremely low cost (204). Disadvantages include its slightly unpredictable long half-life and social stigma associated with it due to its use as part of maintenance programs for opiate addicts.

OXYCODONE PREPARATIONS

Oxycodone is a morphine derivative that is available as a generic short-acting form, in a short-acting immediate release form (Oxyir), a long-acting form (OxyContin) as well as in several combination analgesic products. Pure oxycodone products offer the advantage of not being limited by the potential for toxicity associated with increasing doses of ASA or APAP.

OxyContin has been the subject of some controversy related to illicit use of the medication (i.e., diversion) (205). This in fact has led to a black box warning and suspended distribution of 160 mg OxyContin tabs at the time of this writing. Despite this, it is still a valuable medication with a prompt onset yet prolonged effect despite bid dosing. Its prolonged analgesic effect can eliminate the problem of nocturnal wakening due to pain exacerbations. In addition, since narcotic side effects in general are most often associated with high peak serum drug levels, drugs with steady plasma levels in theory should be better tolerated since more constant blood levels are maintained. The apparent dichotomy of prompt yet sustained analgesia can be explained on the basis of its AcroContin delivery system. With this system some oxycodone is released relatively quickly after ingestion of OxyContin and continues to be released in a steady fashion over time until the next dose. The relatively short half-life of the oxycodone allows for OxyContin to reach steady-state in a relatively short time period, thereby allowing assessment of analgesia and side effects within a day or two, rather than after a week or two as with opioids that have long half-lives. Other advantages of this medication include its absorption which is independent of pH, thereby allowing the patient to take the medication without regard to meal time. This is a potential advantage over opioids with a greater pH dependency such as MS Contin which has a higher dissolution rate in an acidic medium. After absorption, it undergoes minimal first-pass metabolism, thus its high bioavailability and absence of active metabolites make it relatively independent of hepatic function, especially compared to opioids with low bioavailability (high first-pass effect) and active metabolites (e.g., morphine).

The short-acting immediate release form, OxyIR, can be used as premedication prior to therapy sessions. It can also be used to treat breakthrough pain, generally at one-fourth to one-third the 12-hour dose of OxyContin. When used in this manner, if more than two rescue doses are needed in any 24-hour period, consideration should be given to increasing the OxyContin dose. Efficacy and adverse events are believed to be similar for both OxyIR and OxyContin (206,207).

PARTIAL AGONISTS

Partial agonists bind to opioid receptors and activate them to a lesser degree than agonists do. At the time of this writing, there are no currently available oral partial agonists. The prototype from this class, buprenorphine is available for parenteral administration only. Outside of the U.S., it is available via the sublingual route and a transdermal delivery system recently has been reported with good efficacy in patients with chronic moderate to severe pain (208). Its slow dissociation from the μ-receptor has several implications besides its long duration of action. For example, there are fewer withdrawal signs and symptoms and hence less abuse potential relative to other agonists. It therefore may eventually play a role in the management of opioid addiction. In addition, it is not reversed well by naloxone. As it binds mostly to μ- receptors, it has minimal effects upon GI motility and sphincter tone.

MIXED AGONISTS-ANTAGONISTS

Mixed agonists-antagonists act at opioid receptors in both an agonistic and antagonistic fashion. For example, the prototype agent, pentazocine (Talwin) is an antagonist at μ- receptors but an agonist at κ- and δ-opioid receptors. This class of medications does not offer any advantage over opioid agonists other than a diminished risk of respiratory depression due to a ceiling effect. This advantage is of diminishing benefit compared to traditional opioids as tolerance to this side effect occurs with time for narcotic agonists. There are several disadvantages to the mixed agonist-antagonist class, including the presence of a therapeutic ceiling effect and the potential for precipitation of a

withdrawal syndrome. Pentazocine is approximately equivalent to codeine on a milligram per milligram basis in analgesic effect. Several different pentazocine combinations are available as shown in Table 56-17. It is unclear how this medication or pentazocine-containing medications are best used in pain management. Pentazocine is also subject to illicit use as a pentazocine and methylphenidate (Ritalin) combination (known by various street terms including "crackers", "one and ones", "poor man's heroin", "ritz and T's", "T's and rits", "T's and R's") can be injected and produces an effect similar to that of heroin mixed with cocaine.

Butorphanol tartrate (Stadol NS) is a mixed agonist-antagonist (agonist at κ-opioid receptors and a mixed agonist-antagonist at μ-opioid receptors) that offers the flexibility of intranasal administration. In general, it has not been widely used by physiatrists, but rather has been most widely used in the general surgical setting as a preoperative sedative and analgesic, as a supplement to balanced anesthesia, for conscious sedation, for suppression of postanesthesia shaking, control of postoperative pain, as well as in obstetrics for analgesia during labor and relief of moderate postpartum pain. In addition, butorphanol has been used for migraine headache treatment. Although it has been studied for use in opioid detoxification programs as it was thought to have a low-addiction potential, cases of butorphanol addiction have been reported and a highly publicized lawsuit against the manufacturer has been filed (209). There is scant literature on its use in musculoskeletal pain (210,211).

Relevant Side Effects and Drug Interactions

The overall side-effect profile for narcotic analgesics is relatively favorable, especially in the elderly. There is, however, ongoing confusion regarding tolerance, addiction, and physical dependence. *Tolerance* is defined as the phenomenon of more drug being needed to produce a given effect. *Addiction* is the habitual use of a substance in order to achieve a certain effect (usually euphoria) that the patient perceives as pleasurable. *Dependence* is the onset of withdrawal symptoms when the drug is abruptly removed. Confusion among these terms has led to bias against the use of narcotic analgesics, particularly for nonmalignant pain.

In particular, fear of addiction is perhaps the major reason why physicians tend to under-prescribe narcotics. Although there is controversy as to whether psychological addiction actually develops in patients with chronic pain without a past history of substance abuse, it is generally believed that the rate is low.

One may need to explain tolerance to patients and their families in order to quell the anxiety that often develops when a patient's narcotic dosage requirement increases after they have been on the medication for approximately 1 month. Specifically, although tolerance probably begins to occur after the first dose, it does not become apparent until 2 to 3 weeks after the medication is begun and it generally lasts 1 to 2 weeks after the medication is removed. In contrast, some feel that if the medication doses are matched closely with the patient's needs, then tolerance never develops because no excess medication is present to cause euphoria. An advantage of tolerance is that it also occurs with essentially all narcotic side effects (except constipation). Since there is incomplete cross-tolerance among the different narcotics, better analgesia can often be obtained by simply switching to another agent.

Physical dependence refers to the fact that withdrawal symptoms occur if the opioid is suddenly stopped. The onset and duration of withdrawal symptoms correlate with the half-life of the drug. Like addiction, some feel that if the medication doses are matched closely with the patient's needs, then physical dependence never develops. However, most patients who take opioids for more than 1 month develop at least some degree of physical dependence. In order to avert withdrawal symptoms in physically dependent patients, guidelines have been developed for weaning patients off an opioid (212). If withdrawal should still develop, autonomic symptoms can be blunted with the use of oral or transdermal clonidine at a dose of 0.1 to 0.2 mg per day. Since a patient going through withdrawal might only complain of relatively mild nonspecific muscle aches, withdrawal should be considered as a possibility when patients are taken off opiates.

Constipation is the most common narcotic side effect. Unlike most other narcotic side effects, tolerance does not develop to constipation. Since constipation can have such a profound adverse effect, patients who are begun on narcotics should be considered for prophylactic bowel stimulants or osmotic agents, and if constipation still develops, it should be treated aggressively.

Other GI side effects include nausea and vomiting. In contrast to constipation, prophylaxis against nausea is not routinely given since tolerance to nausea usually develops. If nausea should develop, treatment depends upon its underlying etiology. For example, if the nausea is actually due to constipation associated with the narcotic, then the constipation should be treated. In contrast, if nausea is due to a primary effect of the medication (i.e., stimulation of the chemotrigger zone), then prochlorperazine is generally regarded as the first-line agent. If the patient is still nauseous, then other agents such as haloperidol could be considered. If the patient is nauseous and agitated, chlorpromazine would be an appropriate second-line agent of choice due to its strong sedative effects. Since nausea can also be due to gastric outlet obstruction from the antimotility effect of opioids, metoclopramide can be tried. In terms of adjuvant analgesics in a patient who is nauseous from narcotics, an agent with a nonoral administration route may be better. Examples are indomethacin (pr) or ketorolac (i.m.).

Potential CNS side effects include sedation and euphoria. While sedation can be countered using CNS stimulants such as caffeine, dextroamphetamine, and methylphenidate, euphoria is more potentially troublesome as it is the basis behind psychological addiction. Sensorineural hearing loss has been rarely described with chronic opioid analgesic use (213,214).

Cardiopulmonary adverse effects include orthostatic hypotension to a degree that can create considerable difficulty in rehabilitation patients who are undergoing transfer and ambulation training. Another CNS side effect is respiratory depression which can be severe enough to cause respiratory arrest. Tolerance develops to this side effect however and explains the well-known phenomenon of why a large narcotic dose that would be fatal to a narcotic-naïve patient is well tolerated by a habitual user. Prior to developing tolerance to the respiratory effects of narcotics, patients often have diminished respiratory rates and thus relative hypoxia, hypercapnia, and blunted respiratory responses to exercise, which may or may not be clinically important.

TRAMADOL HCL (ULTRAM); TRAMADOL HCL AND ACETAMINOPHEN (ULTRACET)

Relevance to Physiatry

Tramadol is a synthetic analgesic with FDA-approval for moderate to severe pain. Despite binding to opioid receptors with a codeinelike affinity, it is not classified as a controlled substance.

It also has a TCA-like action. Given its dual mechanism, it offers the physiatrist an analgesic for both nociceptive and neuropathic pain. It has shown some efficacy in diabetic neuropathy and other peripheral neuropathies (215). For chronic nociceptive pain, the American College of Rheumatology (ACR) recommends it in its medical management guidelines for knee and hip OA (3). Tramadol has also been studied in acute dental and surgical pain. In acute dental pain models, the 50 mg dose provided analgesia superior to codeine sulfate 60 mg, but it was not as effective as the combination of ASA 650 mg and codeine phosphate 60 mg. In single-dose pain models after surgery, it provided analgesia equal to APAP 650 mg with propoxyphene.

Ultracet is a relatively new combination of tramadol (37.5 mg) and acetaminophen (325 mg). Its exact role in pain management is unclear but it does offer the potential advantage of a combination medication with potentially synergistic analgesia via a total of three mechanisms of action but no apparent synergistic side effects. In a randomized multicenter study involving adults with chronic nonmalignant low back pain or OA pain, it was as effective as APAP with codeine (300 mg per 30 mg) and better tolerated (216).

Mechanism of Action and Pharmacokinetics

Tramadol has two complementary analgesic mechanisms including binding of μ-opioid receptors and pain impulse transmission modification via weak inhibition of norepinephrine and serotonin reuptake. It can therefore be thought of as a combination of a synthetic opioid and a TCA. Tramadol has an analgesic onset within 1 hour and a mean peak plasma concentration within 1.5 to 2 hours. Once in the serum, there is low protein binding and extensive first-pass hepatic metabolism. It is converted to several metabolites, one of which may have some efficacy. Eventually the unchanged drug and metabolites are renally excreted. Tramadol has a half-life of 6 hours and steady-state is achieved within 2 days when it is taken qid.

Preparations and Dosing

Tramadol is available in the U.S. in 50 mg tablets or oral drops. In Europe it is also available as i.v., i.m., s.c. and pr preparations. It can dosed at 50 to 100 mg q 4 to 6 hours, with a maximum recommended 400 mg total daily dose. Dosing adjustments are recommended for people older than 75 (no more than 300 mg per day), in those with creatinine clearance less than 30 mL per minute (q 12 hour dosing and maximum daily dose of 200 mg), and in hepatic cirrhosis. In order to decrease the possibility of nausea or dizziness related to initiation of treatment, it is recommended in some patients with nonacute pain that it be administered in a titrated fashion starting at 50 mg every day and increasing by one 50 mg dose every 3 days until a maximum of 100 mg qid.

When used to treat acute pain, it is recommended that an initial 50 mg dose be administered followed by another 25 to 50 mg dose if inadequate analgesia is achieved within the first 60 minutes. An alternative strategy is to begin with an initial 100 mg dose.

Relevant Side Effects and Drug Interactions

Nausea and dizziness are the most common side effects, while the next most frequent are sedation, dry mouth, and sweating. Respiratory depression is possible, but uncommon (217). Constipation, a traditional opioid side effect is also rare. Psychological addiction is extremely unlikely since euphoria is not common. Although withdrawal due to physical dependence can be seen, it is not as severe as with opioids. Finally, there is a low probability of tolerance to the analgesic effect as shown by two long-term safety studies in chronic, nonmalignant pain (218, 219). Serious and rarely fatal anaphylactoid reactions have occurred, usually following the first dose. Those with a history of anaphylactoid reactions to opioids may be at higher risk. As with opioids, pruritus is also possible. Caution should be exercised if tramadol is used in those with epilepsy, a seizure history, or seizure risk factors (such as TBI, metabolic disorders, alcohol and drug withdrawal, CNS infections).

Medication interactions include seizure threshold lowering, CNS depression if used with other CNS depressants, death if used with MAOIs, and enhanced tramadol metabolism. Carbamazepine so markedly induces tramadol's metabolism that up to twice the usual tramadol dose might be needed. In addition, it should be avoided in patients taking TCAs and tricyclic compounds such as cyclobenzaprine.

TRANSDERMAL ANALGESIC MEDICATIONS

The skin can be used to deliver medications locally to a target tissue or systemically. Depending upon the medication, delivery can be via an exogenous disposable transdermal (TD) delivery system or simply by the application of a cream or an ointment. For example, exogenous TD delivery systems are used for local lidocaine delivery via the lidocaine patch whereas systemic fentanyl delivery can be achieved using the fentanyl patch. Topical NSAIDs are an example of TD medication administration via a formulation consisting of TD vehicles and enhancers, which essentially pull the drug through the skin.

TD medication delivery has become increasingly popular as it provides the major advantage of medication delivery without reliance on GI tract absorption or hepatic first-pass metabolism. It has also been shown for TD medications that they achieve tissue concentrations under the application site that are significantly higher than serum medication levels. This can be particularly important for focal tissue pathology. It is likely that an increasing number of medications will be delivered via this route as TD delivery systems have evolved from first-generation reservoir systems to second-generation matrix systems. Both share the common advantages of the maintenance of constant drug-plasma levels, extension of drug activity for those with short half-lives, and improved patient compliance by increasing the dosing interval. Unfortunately, TD delivery is not suitable for all medications and contact dermatitis can occur.

Disadvantages of TD medication delivery in general include the relatively short shelf-life of some topical medications (especially topical NSAIDs), thus making mass production difficult. Another disadvantage is the multiplicity of factors that determine their efficacy. For example, in the case of compounded medications, the skill of the compounding pharmacist is of paramount importance. Rational medication selection can also be challenging yet very important. In particular, the target tissue needs to be considered in medication selection. For example, if the target tissue is synovial fluid, then the medication must be suitable in aqueous vehicles.

The physiatrist should become familiar with this mode of delivery as many of these medications are applicable to physiatrics. This list is only a partial one as many other medications from various classes are also available and include antibiotics, anticholinergics, antiemetics, and hormones. In addition, other medications can be delivered via mucous membranes including intranasal sprays, ophthalmologic solutions, and suppository medications. Many TD medications are not available by usual prescription but instead via compounding pharmacies. There is also a relative lack of placebo-controlled compounded

medication trials for the treatment of various musculoskeletal conditions. In the case of topical NSAIDs, there have been European studies but these have not passed FDA scrutiny in the United States.

Individual Agents

EMLA, lidocaine, and fentanyl patches are discussed previously in this chapter.

CAPSAICIN (ZOSTRIX, ZOSTRIX-HP)

Relevance to Physiatry
Capsaicin is used by physiatrists to manage localized pain states such as focal neuropathic pain and joint arthralgias such as knee and finger OA. Its use in OA is discussed in greater detail elsewhere in this text (see Chapter 31). There is scant literature on its successful use in chronic nonspecific low back pain and neuropathic pain states such as diabetic neuropathy and postherpetic neuralgia (220–222). A literature review on pharmacologic management of neuropathic pain found that its NNT was higher than that of oral medications (215). In addition to the clinical trials noted earlier, isolated case reports and case series have also been published. In the physiatric literature, management with capsaicin has been noted with complex regional pain syndrome type I and traumatic amputee neurogenic residual limb pain (223,224).

Not all the literature has found capsaicin to be effective. For example, capsaicin did not help with pain due to HIV-associated peripheral neuropathy, nor was it superior to placebo in a double-blind, placebo-controlled study of chronic distal painful polyneuropathy (225,226).

Studies on the combined use of capsaicin and other topical medications have also been performed. For example, the combination of capsaicin (0.25%) and topical 3.3% doxepin was found to be more efficacious than either agent alone in neuropathic pain (18).

In addition to its use in clinical practice, capsaicin has also become a part of basic science pain management research (227–229). An oral capsaicin pain model has been developed based upon the production of burning pain when it is applied to the tongue (230). Basic science research suggests that an endogenous capsaicin-like substance is released in inflamed tissues and produces nociceptive neural impulses by acting on capsaicin receptors on sensory neurons (231).

Capsaicin has been studied for a variety of conditions that have less direct physiatric application. For example, it has been used to manage some painful urological conditions, to manage orofacial pain states such as trigeminal neuralgia and temporomandibular joint pain, to prophylax against cluster headaches, to treat chemotherapy-induced mucositis, to treat nasal hyperreactivity, and to treat psoralen and long-wave ultraviolet radiation (PUVA)-induced skin pain (232–237).

Mechanism of Action and Pharmacokinetics
Capsaicin is a naturally occurring reversible neurotoxin that has been extracted from Solanaceae family plants (i.e., "hot" chili peppers) and is therefore classified as a capsaicinoid. Analgesia occurs via binding to the vanilloid receptor-1 followed by the localized depletion and prevention of reaccumulation of substance P (SP), an endogenous neuropeptide made by small-diameter, primary, sensory "pain" fibers and involved in pain impulse transmission from peripheral nociceptors and stimulates lymphocytes and mast cell activity (238). In addition to SP depletion, there is blockade of SP transport and *de novo* synthesis. Inflammation is also indirectly inhibited as the neu-

rons affected by capsaicin, besides generating pain sensations, participate through antidromic activation of nerve fibers leading to inflammation (neurogenic inflammation) (239). This concept of neurogenic inflammation is based on SP and related peptides released by an axon reflex mechanism. In rheumatic diseases, SP may enhance inflammatory joint reactions. For example, high synovial fluid SP levels were found in rheumatoid arthritis (240).

Overall, capsaicin causes a reversible chemical sensory denervation that leads to pain desensitization (220). Other details of capsaicin's analgesic effect are being studied (241,242).

Preparations and Dosing

Capsaicin has been formulated into a cream that is applied transdermally and is available in 0.025% (Zostrix) and 0.075% (Zostrix-HP) concentrations. It should be applied tid to qid. In order to maximize the probability that the patient will not prematurely discontinue it due to the initial application site stinging (see below), it is best to begin with the 0.025% concentration.

Relevant Side Effects and Drug Interactions

Transient application site stinging or burning is common, particularly with the high potency formulation as capsaicin stimulates nociceptors. (Capsaicin, in fact, is the active ingredient in "pepper sprays.") Application site stinging usually remits after the first few days as SP becomes depleted at that site but can be intense enough to cause patients to self-discontinue it. No adverse effect upon nerve function and no drug interactions have been found (243).

ANTICOAGULANTS

Relevance to Physiatry

These medications are primarily used as prophylaxis against excessive clot formation. In general, they affect the function and synthesis of clotting factors, thus reducing the tendency toward clot propagation and the risk of developing or extending a deep venous thrombosis (DVT), or pulmonary/cerebral embolus. Patients at risk for developing thromboembolic phenomena are frequently encountered in the rehabilitative setting, and include those with SCI, stroke, multiple trauma, as well as hip and knee arthroplasties. Risk reduction, including anticoagulation and conservative means to stimulate blood flow in the legs, such as with external compression devices, is warranted in appropriate patients. Patients who have suffered a cerebral thromboembolic event, and those with proximal DVT and pulmonary emboli are generally treated similarly (244–248).

Anticoagulants can be classified into heparin and coumarin groups. The heparin group is administered parenterally and includes unfractionated heparin (UFH), low-molecular-weight heparin (LMWH), and heparinoids. Traditionally, intravenous full-dose UFH has been used for acute thromboembolic phenomena, whereas subcutaneous fixed low-dose UFH and LMWH have been more commonly used for prophylaxis. LMWH is more effective than fixed low-dose UFH and is associated with a lower risk of hemorrhage (249,250). However, there is an increasing acceptance of treating acute thromboembolic events, such as DVT, pulmonary embolus (PE), as well as unstable angina and non-Q-wave MI, initially with subcutaneous LMWH instead of intravenous UFH (245–248,251–256). Heparinoids are used as thromboembolism prophylaxis in those with a history of heparin-induced thrombocytopenia (257–259).

Warfarin is by far the most commonly used coumarin medication. Its use in DVT prophylaxis following hip or knee arthroplasty has been well established (249,260). Although its efficacy in preventing DVT in orthopedic patients may be somewhat less than that of LMWH, it is the mainstay of maintenance treatment of thromboembolism following initial heparin treatment. Another important indication for oral anticoagulation is stroke prophylaxis, especially in the presence of atrial fibrillation (AF) (260–262). Specifically, it has been shown that oral anticoagulation is associated with a significant reduction of stroke risk, and that it is more efficacious than ASA in preventing stroke in the setting of AF (262).

Whenever an anticoagulated patient is undergoing physical or occupational therapy, it is prudent to include this information in the therapy prescription so that the therapist can take appropriate precautions to prevent falls and injuries. This also alerts the therapist to monitor closely and report potential signs of bleeding, such as a newly swollen joint, as this may represent a hemarthrosis.

Mechanism of Action and Pharmacokinetics

Heparin and its derivatives affect key reactions involved with thrombosis and stable clot formation. Low-dose UFH and LMWH primarily prevent the conversion of prothrombin to thrombin (factor II) via inactivation of factor Xa. At higher doses, heparin can prevent fibrinogen to fibrin conversion by inactivation of thrombin and also prevents stable fibrin clot formation. After subcutaneous injection, activity onset is rapid, with peak plasma levels at about 4 hours. Metabolism occurs in the liver and the reticulo-endothelial system.

Warfarin interferes with vitamin K by inhibiting hepatic coagulation factor II, VII, IX, and X synthesis. Its effect is detectable once the baseline level of these factors already in circulation starts to be depleted by metabolic degradation. After oral administration, the maximal plasma concentration is between 1 to 9 hours. Almost all of the medication (97%) is bound to plasma albumin. The initial effect is apparent in 24 hours, but the peak effect occurs between 3 to 4 days and lasts for 4 to 5 days. It is metabolized in the liver and has a half-life of around 2.5 days.

Preparations and Dosing

Both UFH and LMWH are mucopolysaccharides derived from porcine intestinal mucosa. LMWH is derived from UFH by depolymerization and possesses a higher ratio of antifactor Xa to antifactor IIa activity than pure UFH. Therefore, it is purported to have a lower incidence of bleeding complications than UFH. The molecular size of both heparin classes does not permit oral administration as they would not be readily absorbed from the GI tract. Therefore they are currently administered either by deep subcutaneous injection or intravenously. Modified, orally active forms of heparin are being studied (263). During standard, prophylactic, fixed low-dose UFH and LMWH therapy, it is not necessary to monitor the activated partial thromboplastin time (aPTT), since this index is essentially unaffected. However, this monitoring is required during full-dose intravenous UFH therapy, which is commonly used during the initial treatment of acute thromboembolic conditions including PE, proximal DVT, nonhemorrhagic stroke, and MI. In this instance, UFH is given initially as a bolus followed by continuous infusion. Subsequently, the aPTT is monitored at frequent intervals, and the heparin infusion rate is adjusted to maintain the value

TABLE 56-18.   Heparin and Heparin Derivatives Administered Subcutaneously

Generic (Trade) Name	Type	Typical Dosage and Indications (FDA Approved and Not Approved)
Heparin sodium	UFH	DVT prophylaxis: 5,000 units q 8–12 h; lower doses in geriatric patients
Dalteparin (Fragmin)	LMWH	DVT prophylaxis: 5,000 units qd following orthopedic surgery (FDA approved only for THA); 2,500 units qd for other conditions (not FDA approved); DVT treatment (not FDA approved): 200 units/kg qd or 100–120 units/kg bid
Enoxaparin (Lovenox)	LMWH	DVT prophylaxis: 30 mg q 12 h (approved for THA/TKA; not approved for SCI and MT) or: 40 mg qd (approved alternate dosing following THA or immobilization because of medical illness). DVT/PE treatment: 1 mg/kg q12h, or 1.5 mg/kg qd
Tinzaparin (Innohep)	LMWH	DVT/PE treatment: 175 anti-Xa units/kg qd until therapeutic anticoagulation with warfarin. Also not approved indication for DVT prophylaxis: 4,500 units qd following orthopedic surgery or 3,500 units qd following general surgery
Danaparoid (Orgaran)	Heparinoid	DVT prophylaxis: 750 anti-Xa units q12h (approved for THA; not approved for other surgeries and medical conditions). Also not approved indication for intravenous anticoagulation in presence of heparin-induced thrombocytopenia
Fondaparinux (Arixtra)	Synthetic factor Xa inhibitor	DVT prophylaxis: 2.5 mg qd (approved for THA/TKA and hip fracture surgeries)

between 1.5 and 2.5 times the control value (264). Several other approaches used for dosing heparin intravenously have also been described (264–267). It is important to note that therapeutic dosages of LMWH affect the aPTT and can therefore be used in monitoring.

These medications are generally used short term, typically in inpatient settings, although the trend for outpatient treatment using subcutaneous heparins is increasing (253,255,268). For prophylaxis, heparins are used very variably based upon diagnosis or until risk of thromboembolism has diminished. In the event of acute PE or DVT, they are administered at therapeutic doses concomitantly with warfarin, which is initiated within the first 3 days. Once a therapeutic INR is achieved, typically within 5 to 7 days, heparin is discontinued, while warfarin therapy is maintained for a variable time period depending on the underlying condition. In certain CVAs or MIs, antiplatelet agents are used in lieu of warfarin. Dosages and indications for subcutaneous administration of heparins and derivatives are shown in Table 56-18.

Warfarin sodium (Coumadin, Panwarfin) is the most commonly used oral anticoagulant. In those rare cases when oral administration is not feasible, warfarin may be given intravenously. Dosage is individualized and based on monitoring its efficacy by regular prothrombin time (PT) assessment. Because of significant variability in thromboplastin reagents used in making these assessments among laboratories, a common standardized scale, the INR, was developed to allow for more comparable monitoring of efficacy regardless of the reagents used. An INR of 2.0 to 3.0 is generally recommended for both prophylaxis and thromboembolism treatment. The effectiveness of anticoagulation within this range is essentially equivalent to that of higher dosages, yet with fewer hemorrhagic events (269). In contrast to biological heart valve replacement, a higher INR (2.5 to 3.5) is suggested for mechanical heart valves.

Warfarin's usual starting dose is from 5 to 10 mg qd. Larger loading doses should be avoided, given the increased risk for hemorrhage. It is also prudent to start with lower loading doses in the elderly or debilitated or in those who are known to be sensitive to warfarin. Oral anticoagulation is usually initiated at the time of heparin treatment, is overlapped with it for about 4 to 5 days in order for the INR to increase to 2.0 to 3.0, and is then continued alone. For instance, the common practice in treating orthopedic patients is to discontinue the anticoagu-

lant before discharge home or when the patient is fully ambulatory. However, there is evidence that supports longer treatment in order to further reduce DVT risk (244,270).

If oral anticoagulants are used concomitantly with heparin, the PT should be checked at least 5 hours following the last intravenous dose and 24 hours following the last subcutaneous heparin dose. This is recommended because heparin itself can prolong the one-stage PT.

Relevant Side Effects and Drug Interaction

Adverse effects of greatest concern with anticoagulants are hemorrhage, most commonly presenting as bruising, petechiae, epistaxis, GI, or urinary tract bleeding. Extreme caution should be exercised in those at increased risk for bleeding, including those that are already taking antiplatelet agents.

A potential problem specific to heparin is heparin-induced thrombocytopenia which occurs from either a direct effect on platelets or by an immunologic response. Thus, it is important to monitor CBCs, especially at the start but also at regular intervals during treatment. Also, there have been reports of spinal epidural hematomas with ensuing paralysis following use of LMWH in patients that have or very recently had epidural catheters or punctures. Therefore, the manufacturers of LMWH have issued warnings against administering these drugs within specific times before and following procedures involving epidural invasion. Other adverse effects that may occur include local irritation (especially with deeper injections; thus the need to avoid intramuscular injection) and hypersensitivity reactions, especially with pork allergies.

A relatively rare but potentially hazardous reaction associated with warfarin use is skin necrosis, which may develop in susceptible individuals such as those patients with protein C deficiency, because there is normally local thrombosis that occurs within the first few days of initiating the drug. The concurrent administration of heparin for the first 5 to 7 days of anticoagulation reduces the risk of this reaction.

Many drugs can alter the therapeutic efficacy of warfarin. Those that may increase the PT include APAP, amiodarone, ASA, NSAIDs, phenytoin, sulfonamides, and thyroid supplements. Those that can decrease the PT include adrenocorticoids, antacids, antihistamines, carbamazepine, haloperidol, and vitamin C. Others, including diuretics and H2 blockers, may cause either an increase or decrease in the PT.

TABLE 56-19.   Antiplatelet Agents

Generic (Trade) Name	Mechanism of Action	Dosing (mg)	Other Properties, Relevant Side Effects and Drug Interactions
Aspirin (ASA)	Inhibits thromboxane A-2 synthesis and thus ability of platelet aggregation	81–325 po qd	Regular, buffered, and enteric-coated; avoid using with ticlopidine
Ticlopidine (Ticlid)	Interferes with platelet membrane function, reducing aggregation by impeding ADP-induced platelet-fibrinogen binding. Effect persists for the life of the platelet.	250 po bid (as with ASA, higher doses associated with greater likelihood of adverse effects, but antithrombotic effect is the same) (289)	Risk of severe hematological reactions such as neutropenia, agranulocytosis, or thrombotic thrombocytopenic purpura (TTP), especially . in the first 3 months of therapy. Need to monitor CBC biweekly during this time. Should not be used in severe liver impairment. Phenytoin and propranolol levels might be increased by ticlopidine
Dipyridamole (DP) (Persantine)	Increases platelet cAMP, thus less adherence, aggregation and enzymatic activity	75–100 po qid	Vasodilation, thus caution in those with hypotension; diarrhea, vomiting, flushing, or pruritus
Aggrenox (DP+ASA)	See above	1 cap (200 mg DP/ 25 mg ASA) po bid	
Clopidogrel (Plavix)	Interferes with platelet membrane function, reducing aggregation by impeding ADP-induced platelet-fibrinogen binding. Effect persists for the life of the platelet.	75 po daily	May cause TTP, usually in first 2 weeks
Cilostazol (Pletal)	Phosphodiesterase III inhibitor	100 po bid	Contraindicated in CHF; reduce dose when used with cytochrome P450 3A4 and 2C19 inhibitors

ANTITHROMBOTICS

Relevance to Physiatry

Antithrombotics (i.e., antiplatelet drugs, because of their primary effect of inhibiting platelet aggregation) have widespread use in CVA and cardiac patients. The most widely used agent in this group is ASA, which in appropriate patients, has been associated with significant reductions in stroke and MI risks (271). It has also been suggested that ASA given early after ischemic CVA onset can help to reduce morbidity and mortality (272,273). However, other antithrombotic drugs such as clopidogrel, cilostazol, ticlopidine, and dipyridamole play an important and expanding role. In fact, there is evidence that they can be more effective than ASA in stroke prevention. This was demonstrated over 10 years ago with ticlopidine, but the risk of potentially serious adverse effects has limited its use (274). In contrast, clopidogrel, a drug similar to ticlopidine, has been reported to be as effective yet with a better safety profile (275–280). The combined use of dipyridamole and ASA is superior for stroke prevention compared to either of these equally efficacious agents alone (271,281–284). Cilostazol is a phosphodiesterase III inhibitor which improves walking distance and exercise tolerance in patients with peripheral vascular disease and may also improve lipid profiles (285–288).

Mechanism of Action and Pharmacokinetics; Preparations and Dosing; Relevant Side Effects; and Drug Interactions

See Table 56-19.

ANTIHYPERLIPIDEMIC MEDICATIONS

Relevance to Physiatry

The importance of antihyperlipidemics in treating CV disease has become evident in recent years. It is widely accepted that serum lipid reduction, including cholesterol and triglycerides, is associated with decreased cardiac morbidity from atherosclerotic CV disease. More recent evidence suggests that these medications can reduce ischemic stroke risk in the presence of CV risk factors and may also play a neuroprotective role during CVA (290–294).

Mechanism of Action and Pharmacokinetics

These drugs can be classified into "fibrates" and HMG-CoA reductase inhibitors, known popularly as the "statins". The latter primarily lower serum low-density lipoprotein (LDL) cholesterol levels, whereas the fibrates lower serum triglyceride and very low-density lipoprotein (VLDL) cholesterol levels. All of these medications have the beneficial effect of elevating serum high-density lipoprotein (HDL) cholesterol.

Preparations and Dosing

See Table 56-20.

TABLE 56-20.   Antihyperlipidemic Medications

Generic (Trade) Name	Typical Oral Dose (mg)
HMG-CoA Reductase Inhibitors	
Atorvastatin (Lipitor)	10 qd, max 80 qd
Fluvastatin (Lescol, Lescol XL)	20 H/S, max 80 qd (XL), or 40 bid
Lovastatin (Mevacor)	20 q p.m., max 80 qd
Pravastatin (Pravachol)	10 qd, max 40 qd
Simvastatin (Zocor)	20 q p.m., max 80 qd
"Fibrate" Medications	
Clofibrate (Atromid-S)	1,000 bid
Fenofibrate (Tricor)	67 qd, max 200 qd; taken with a meal
Gemfibrozil (Lopid)	600 bid before meals

Relevant Side Effects and Drug Interactions

Potential concerns associated with these drugs include myopathy and rhabdomyolysis, especially when both classes are used together, and liver dysfunction. The fibrates in particular can also elevate PT results in patients receiving warfarin.

CARDIOVASCULAR MEDICATIONS

Medications that affect the CV system are frequently encountered in the rehabilitative setting, especially in the elderly. It is not uncommon for the physiatrist to adjust these medications, especially while the patient is on an inpatient rehabilitation unit. Because these medications can have such a profound impact on the patient's medical status and general well-being, it is important for the physiatrist to have a basic knowledge of the types of medications used, their indications, and their effects.

Alpha Blockers: Alpha-1-Adrenergic and Alpha-2-Adrenergic Antagonists

RELEVANCE TO PHYSIATRY

Although HTN and prostate-related bladder outlet obstruction are the primary general medical uses of α-blockers, especially α_1-adrenergic blockers, they are also used for the control and prevention of vascular manifestations of autonomic dysreflexia (295). A nonselective α-blocker such as phenoxybenzamine can also be effective in RSD because it affects both types of α-receptors, thus leading to a chemical sympathectomy. It is usually best to initiate these drugs at bedtime given the frequent occurrences of orthostatic hypotension and reflex tachycardia during the first few days of initiating treatment (i.e., the first-dose phenomenon) and the fact that postural hypotension can also occur following rapid increases in dosage, during the established use of these medications, or following the addition of a second antihypertensive.

Alpha-2 selective blockers [e.g., yohimbine (Yocon)] might help with erectile dysfunction, diabetic neuropathy, and postural hypotension (296,297).

MECHANISM OF ACTION AND PHARMACOKINETICS

These medications block α_1- and α_2-adrenergic receptors. Selective α_1-receptor blockers inhibit vasoconstriction, resulting in decreased peripheral vascular resistance and a subsequent decrease in BP. They also reduce resistance to urinary outflow by inhibiting smooth muscle contractions at the base of the urinary bladder. In contrast, selective α_2-blockers and nonselective blocking agents indirectly cause the release of norepinephrine from peripheral sympathetic nerve endings, thus increasing overall sympathetic outflow, and leading to subsequent elevations in HR (heart rate) and BP.

PREPARATIONS AND DOSING; RELEVANT SIDE EFFECTS; AND DRUG INTERACTIONS
See Table 56-21.

Alpha-2 Agonists

RELEVANCE TO PHYSIATRY; MECHANISM OF ACTION; AND PHARMACOKINETICS

These medications are indicated for hypertension, either alone or in combination with other medications. They may be used in acute autonomic dysreflexia refractory to other measures and also in the prevention of its recurrence (295). Because of their centrally acting mechanism (stimulation of α_2-adrenergic receptors), they may cause drowsiness, a definitely untoward effect when attempting to objectively monitor the progress of a patient with altered mental status (e.g., early TBI or CVA) and therefore can interfere with rehabilitation. Clonidine and especially the newer α_2-agonist tizanidine (Zanaflex), are also useful in treating spasticity in various patients, including those with SCI, TBI, multiple sclerosis, and CVA (298–304). Transdermal or intrathecal clonidine may be of benefit in RSD pain (305,306).

PREPARATIONS AND DOSING
See Table 56-21.

RELEVANT SIDE EFFECTS AND DRUG INTERACTIONS

Dry mouth, sedation, various GI symptoms, and orthostatic hypotension are the most common side effects of these medications. Rebound hypertension may occur with their sudden discontinuation. Major drug interactions include potentiation of the action of CNS depressants, attenuation of the hypotensive effect of TCAs, and additive CV side effects with other CV medications.

TABLE 56-21. Cardiovascular Medications Acting on the Sympathetic Nervous System

Generic (Trade) Name	Typical Dose (mg)	Other Properties & Side Effects
[Alpha agonists]		
Clonidine hydrochloride (Catapres, Catapres-TTS)	oral: 0.1 bid–2.4 mg/d patch: 0.1–0.3/d—change q wk	Renally metabolized; also used to blunt autonomic symptoms from narcotic withdrawal
Guanfacine hydrochloride (Tenex)	0.5–1.0 po/d–3.0/d	Taken @ H/S to avoid daytime somnolence; renal metabolism
Guanabenz acetate (Wytensin)	4 po bid and increased prn by 4/d up to 32/d	Hepatically metabolized
Methyldopa (Aldomet)	250 po bid up to 2,000/d	First metabolized in the brain to methyl-norepinephrine, which activates alpha-2 receptors; parenteral form also available
Tizanidine (Zanaflex)	4–8 po q6–8h, max of 36 per 24 h for spasticity control	Reported to have a much less tendency than clonidine for lowering of blood pressure, thus not used for HTN
[Alpha-1 antagonists]		
Doxazosin (Cardura)	Start 1 po qd; max. 16 po qd	
Prazosin (Minipress)	Start 1 po bid–tid; max. 40 po qd	If peripheral edema, can switch to Minizide (prazosin/polythiazide), 1 tab po bid
Tamsulosin (Flomax)	Benign prostatic hypertrophy (BPH): 0.4 po qd; max. 0.8 po qd	Reportedly less postural hypotension compared to the other alpha blockers
Terazosin (Hytrin)	Start 1 po q H/S; max. 20 po qd	Not available in combination with a diuretic

Angiotensin-Converting Enzyme Inhibitors and Angiotensin II Receptor Blockers

RELEVANCE TO PHYSIATRY

These medications are commonly encountered in hypertensive or cardiac rehabilitation patients. Angiotensin-converting enzyme inhibitors (ACEIs) exert a renal-protective effect in diabetics and are believed to reduce the risk of recurrent CVA (307–309). They are usually indicated for HTN and CHF. Angiotensin II receptor blockers (ARBs) have been introduced more recently and are indicated for HTN (310). An advantage of these classes of medications is their relative lack of CV side effects compared to other agents.

MECHANISM OF ACTION AND PHARMACOKINETICS

ACEIs prevent the conversion of angiotensin I to angiotensin II, a potent vasoconstrictor and adrenal stimulator. The overall effect is a reduction in systemic vascular resistance with subsequent lowering of BP and cardiac output improvement. The hypotensive effects of ARBs occur via selective blocking of the binding of angiotensin II to specific receptors, especially in vascular smooth muscles and adrenal glands. Medications of this class are well absorbed from the GI tract and are well tolerated. They vary in onsets, peaks, and durations of action, which is reflected in their recommended dosage.

PREPARATIONS AND DOSING

See Table 56-22.

RELEVANT SIDE EFFECTS AND DRUG INTERACTIONS

These medications are generally well tolerated with rare serious adverse reactions. Side effects can include skin rash, neutropenia, impaired renal function (especially if there is preexisting impairment), GI discomfort, and a nonproductive cough due to an alteration in bradykinin production. Renal function should be monitored, especially in the elderly with poor oral fluid intake. ACEIs can act synergistically with diuretics or other antihypertensives. Hyperkalemia can occur when drugs that can elevate serum potassium concentrations (such as potassium supplements or potassium-sparing diuretics) are used with ACEIs and ARBs. Adverse effects of ARBs are generally minor and rare.

ANTIARRHYTHMIC MEDICATIONS

Relevance to Physiatry

This group is likely to be encountered in patients undergoing cardiac rehabilitation or those who have a pertinent cardiac history and are undergoing inpatient rehabilitation.

Preparations and Dosing

See Table 56-23.

Relevant Side Effects and Drug Interactions

The most common antiarrhythmic medication side effects include cardiac rhythm disturbances, hypotension, and GI disturbance. Since various drug interactions are possible, it is important for the physiatrist to consider this whenever a new medication is added.

TABLE 56-22.   Angiotensin Converting Enzyme Inhibitors and Angiotensin II Receptor Blockers

Generic (Trade) Name	Oral Dose (mg)
Angiotensin Converting Enzyme Inhibitors	
Benazepril (Lotensin)	HTN: 10 qd, up to 80 daily
Captopril (Capoten)	HTN: 25 bid–tid, up to 450 daily
	CHF: 6.25–12.5 tid
Enalapril (Vasotec)	HTN: 5 qd/bid, up to 40 daily
	CHF: 2.5 qd/bid, up to 40 daily
Fosinopril (Monopril)	HTN: 10 qd, up to 80 daily
Lisinopril (Prinivil, Zestril)	HTN: 10 qd, up to 40 daily
	CHF: 5 qd, up to 20 daily
Moexipril (Univasc)	HTN: 7.5 qd, up to 30 daily
Perindopril (Aceon)	4 qd up to 16 daily
Quinapril (Accupril)	HTN: 10 qd, up to 80 daily
	CHF: 5 bid, up to 20–40 daily
Ramipril (Altace)	HTN: 2.5 qd, up to 20 daily
Trandolapril (Mavik)	HTN: 1 qd, up to 4 daily
Angiotensin II Receptor Blockers[a]	
Candesartan (Atacand)	16 qd, max 32 qd
Eprosartan (Teveten)	600 qd, max. 800 qd (in single or divided bid)
Irbesartan (Avapro)	150 qd, max. 300 qd
Losartan (Cozaar)	50 qd, max. 100 qd
Telmisartan (Micardis)	40 qd, max. 80 qd
Valsartan (Diovan)	80 qd, max. 320 qd

[a]All preparations indicated for HTN; starting dosage should be ½ in volume-depletion.

TABLE 56-23. Antiarrhythmic Medications

Class I_A	Electrophysiologic Effect: Blockage of Sodium Channels
Examples	**Typical Oral Dosages (mg) and Arrhythmia Indications**
Quinidine gluconate (Quinaglute, Quinalan, Quinate); quinidine sulfate (Quinidex, Quinora); procainamide (Procanbid, Pronestyl); disopyramide (Norpace, Norpace CR); moricizine (Ethmozine)	Prevention of AF/flut and PVCs, 324–648 q8–12h; AF/flut, 200–400 q6–8h (IR) or 300–600 q8–12h (ER); ventricular dysrhythmias, 250–625 q3h (IR) or 500–1,250 q6h (SR) or 500–1,000 q12h (Procanbid); ventricular dysrhythmias 400–800 per 24 h (q6h if IR or q12h if ER); 200 q8h, max of 900 per 24 h
Class I_B	**Electrophysiologic Effect: Blockage of Sodium Channels**
Lidocaine (Xylocaine, Xylocard); mexiletene (Mexitil); tocainide (Tonocard)	V tach/VF, monitored i.v. dosage; ventricular dysrhythmias, 200 q8h, max. 400 per 24 h; ventricular dysrhythmias, 400 q8h, max. 2,400 per 24 h
Class I_C	**Electrophysiologic Effect: Blockage of Sodium Channels**
Flecainide (Tambocor); propafenone (Rythmol)	PSVT or PAF: 50 q12h, max. 300 per 24 h or sustained V tach: 100 q12h, max. 400 per 24 h; PSVT, PAF, sustained V tach: 150 q8h, max. 300 q8h
Class II	**Electrophysiologic Effect: Blockage of Beta Adrenergic Receptors**
Acebutolol (Sectral); propranolol (Inderal, Inderal LA); sotalol (Betapace, Betapace AF)	Ventricular dysrhythmias, 200 bid, max. 1,200 bid; 10–30 tid–qid; ventricular dysrhythmias (Betapace) or AF/flut (Betapace AF), 80 bid, max. 640 per 24 h
Class III	**Electrophysiologic Effect: Prolongation of Membrane Depolarization**
Amiodarone (Cordarone, Pacerone); bretylium (Bretylol); dofetilide (Tikosyn); sotalol (see above)	Ventricular dysrhythmias, 800–1,600 qd for 1–3 wks, then 600–800 qd for 1 mo, then 400 qd; monitored i.v. dosage; AF/flut, 0.5 bid; see above
Class IV	**Electrophysiologic Effect: Blockade of Calcium Channels**
Verapamil (Calan, Calan SR, Covera-HS, Isoptin)	PSVT or RVR in AF, 240–480 per 24 h divided tid–qid

BETA-BLOCKERS

Relevance to Physiatry
The physiatrist should understand the reason(s) for which a patient is on a β-blocker. This is especially important following MI or with cardiac arrhythmias. During the second phase of a three-phase cardiac rehabilitation program, a therapeutic exercise program of appropriate intensity for a patient on β-blockers is based on a percentage of the symptom-limited heart rate or on the maximum work load performed on an exercise stress test rather than being based on absolute heart rate (311). Beta-blockers tend to impair a patient's exercise tolerance.

Beta-blockers are especially used for HTN, angina pectoris, and arrhythmias. More recently, some of the β-blockers have been used in selected patients with compensated CHF (312, 313). In addition, β-blockers are also used for migraine headaches, heightened metabolic turnover states, such as thyrotoxicosis, tremors of various etiologies, and may be of benefit in treating aggression such as that associated with TBI (314–319).

Mechanism of Action
These medications bind with varying affinities to β₁- and β₂-adrenergic receptors. Those having a predominant β₁-receptor affinity are referred to as β₁-selective, or cardioselective, as this receptor is primarily cardiac. The therapeutic effect therefore is to decrease heart rate and myocardial contractility, which contributes to decreasing myocardial oxygen demand in coronary artery disease and leads to BP reduction in certain hypertensive patients. Others β-blockers are nonselective since they demonstrate essentially equal affinities for both β₁- and β₂-receptors. There are also β₂-selective compounds, however they are not clinically relevant because blockade of the β₂-receptors (mostly located in bronchiolar smooth muscles), causes bronchoconstriction. Some also possess mild β-mimetic or α₁-antagonistic activity, which facilitates cardiac stimulation while blocking systemic effects of excess catecholamines.

Preparations and Dosing
See Table 56-24.

Relevant Side Effects and Drug Interactions
Adverse effects that can interfere with rehabilitation include orthostatic hypotension, bradycardia, and chronic obstructive pulmonary disease (COPD), asthma, or CHF exacerbation. Fatigue, sleep disturbance, and depression may also occur. Sudden medication discontinuation may exacerbate angina because of increased catecholamine sensitivity that may develop during prolonged treatment.

NSAIDs, phenytoin, and phenobarbital can alter the effects of β-blockers. Antihypertensives and antiarrhythmics should be used cautiously if given with β-blockers.

CALCIUM CHANNEL BLOCKERS

Relevance to Physiatry
Calcium channel blockers (CaCBs) are commonly encountered in the physiatric setting given their efficacy and convenient

TABLE 56-24.   Beta Blockers

[Beta-Blocker Class] Generic (Trade) Name	Oral Dose (mg)	Indications and Unique Properties
[Beta-1 selective]		
Acebutolol (Sectral)	200 bid–1200 qd	HTN, also angina (off-label); mild intrinsic beta-mimetic properties
Atenolol (Tenormin)	50 qd–100 qd	i.v. dosing available for acute MI
Betaxolol (Kerlone)	10 qd–20 qd	HTN
Bisoprolol (Zebeta)	5 qd–20 qd	HTN
Metoprolol (Lopressor)	50 bid –450 daily	Angina, HTN, compensated CHF; i.v. dosing available for acute MI
(Toprol XL)	50–100 qd–400 daily	
[Beta (nonselective)]		
Carteolol (Cartrol)	2.5 qd up to 10 qd	HTN; mild intrinsic beta-mimetic activity
Carvedilol (Coreg)	3.125 bid–50 bid, if over 85 kg	Compensated CHF; exerts alpha-1 antagonistic effect
Labetalol (Trandate, Normodyne)	100 bid–2,400 daily	HTN; alpha-1 antagonistic properties; i.v. dosing available for hypertensive emergencies
Nadolol (Corgard)	40 qd–320 daily	HTN; ventricular arrhythmias (off-label)
Penbutolol (Levatol)	20 qd–80 daily	HTN; mild intrinsic beta-mimetic activity
Pindolol (Visken)	5 bid–60 daily	HTN; also angina (off-label); mild intrinsic beta-mimetic activity
Propranolol (Inderal) (Inderal-LA)	40 bid–640 daily	HTN, angina, cardiac arrhythmias, MI, migraine prophylaxis
Sotalol (Betapace, Betapace AF)	80 bid–640 daily	Ventricular arrhythmias, AF/flut
Timolol (Blocadren)	10 bid–60 daily	HTN, post-MI, migraine headaches; angina (off-label)

dosing (especially the controlled- and sustained-release preparations) for hypertension and angina. The immediate-release forms, although useful in various clinical situations, have become less popular because of adverse outcomes reportedly related to their use (320). This especially applies to SCI patients with autonomic dysreflexia for which nifedipine had been commonly given sublingually, a practice that should be avoided. Predominant side effects include orthostatic hypotension, peripheral edema, and headache. The physiatrist should be careful in ordering physical therapy modalities (e.g., whirlpool or Hubbard tank) that can accentuate the vasodilation in a patient taking a CaCB or other vasodilator. Concomitant use of other antihypertensives or antiarrhythmic should be done cautiously. Although grapefruit juice can enhance the effect of CaCBs, this is not usually of clinical significance unless the patient is on the previously popular grapefruit fad diet.

Mechanism of Action and Pharmacokinetics
These drugs inhibit the entry of Ca2+ ions into the myocardial, sinoatrial, atrioventricular, and vascular smooth muscle cells by binding to specific voltage-sensitive channels in the cell membrane. This results in multiple CV effects. One of these is to reduce the strength of myocardial contraction. Another is to relax the arterial smooth muscles in the coronary arteries and peripheral arterioles. This leads to improved coronary blood flow and decreased peripheral vascular resistance with systemic BP reduction. Finally, pacemaker cell depolarization is impaired with a resultant slowing of cardiac conduction.

Preparations and Dosing
See Table 56-25.

Relevant Side Effects and Drug Interactions
Side effects most commonly relate to vasodilation and include dizziness, orthostatic hypotension, reflex tachycardia, headache, and edema. Coughing, GI disturbances, and bradyarrhythmias (especially in diseases affecting sinoatrial and atrioventricular nodes) can occur. Concomitant use with β-blockers is usually well tolerated, but sometimes leads to hypotension, CHF, or cardiac dysrhythmias. CaCBs may elevate serum digoxin and levels of other medications metabolized via the cytochrome P450 system.

CARDIAC GLYCOSIDES

Relevance to Physiatry
Cardiac glycosides include digitalis, digoxin, digitoxin, and deslanoside, and are primarily used for mild to moderate CHF and ventricular rate control in atrial fibrillation. Although digoxin is most commonly used, the group is often referred to as digitalis, the prototype agent. As potentially lethal side effects can occur, one should have a high index of suspicion for early signs of digoxin toxicity and the lowest effective dose should be used. Periodic monitoring of its efficacy and serum medication and electrolyte levels is wise.

Mechanism of Action and Pharmacokinetics
Digitalis increases myocardial contractile force via increased intracellular Ca2+ concentration, which enhances myofilament cross-bridging. Digitalis also slows cardiac impulse conduction. This is related to changes in cellular ion transport and concentrations that affect the rates and degree of transmembrane potentials.

GI absorption of digoxin varies depending on the preparation, thus it is important to familiarize yourself with a specific preparation. After oral dosage, peak plasma concentration occurs in 2 to 3 hours and maximum effect in 4 to 6 hours. The half-life is 1 to 2 days, and steady-state plasma concentration may require 1 week of regular dosage, unless a loading dose is given initially. Increased extracellular potassium (K+) concentrations decrease its tissue binding. Elimination is renal, thus dose adjustments should be made if there is renal dysfunction.

Preparations and Dosing
Maintenance digoxin (Lanoxin, Lanoxicap, Digitek) doses are generally 0.125 to 0.25 mg every day.

Relevant Side Effects and Drug Interactions
Digitalis toxicity is a frequent occurrence, especially with unmonitored dosing and lack of a high enough index of suspicion

TABLE 56-25.   Calcium Channel Blockers

Generic (Trade) Name	Typical Oral Dose (mg)	Indications
Amlodipine (Norvasc)	2.5–5 qd–10 qd	HTN, stable and variant angina
Bepridil (Vascor)	200 qd–400 qd	Stable angina; rarely used because of proarrhythmic effects
Diltiazem (Cardizem)	30 qid–360 qd	HTN (extended preparations), stable and variant angina
(Cardizem CD; Dilacor,	60–120 bid–360 qd	Can be use i.v. for rapid AF
Dilacor CR, Tiazac)	180–240 qd–540 qd	
Felodipine (Plendil)	5 qd–10 qd	HTN
Isradipine (DynaCirc, DynaCirc CR)	2.5 bid (or 5 qd of CR) –20 qd	HTN; i.v. form for HTN emergencies
Nicardipine (Cardene)	20 tid–120 qd	HTN (SR form), stable angina; i.v. form available for hypertensive emergencies
(Cardene SR)	30 bid–120 qd (SR)	
Nifedipine (Procardia, Adalat)	10 tid–120 qd (IR)	Angina
(Procardia XL, Adalat CC)	30–60 qd–120 qd (ER)	HTN
		(Excessive decline in BP or even stroke may occur if IR form taken Sublingual [SL])
Nimodipine (Nimotop)	60 q4h for 21 d	Only indicated for reduction of cerebral vasospasm following subarachnoid hemorrhage; must start within 96 h of the bleed
Nisoldipine (Sular)	10–40 qd	HTN
Verapamil		HTN; can also be used i.v. for treatment of SVT, although adenosine is preferred for this indication
(Isoptin, Calan)	80 tid–360 qd	
(Isoptin SR, Calan SR, Verelan, Covera HS)	240 qd–480 qd Covera HS: 180–480 @ H/S	

for early signs and symptoms of toxicity. These signs often include anorexia, GI disturbances (nausea, vomiting, or diarrhea), fatigue, headache, drowsiness, and visual disturbances. Cardiac abnormalities can also occur, and with increasing toxicity, the risk for severe or even fatal rhythm disturbances increases. In fact, digitalis toxicity can mimic essentially any rhythm disturbance, particularly premature atrial or ventricular beats, paroxysmal atrial tachycardia, ventricular tachycardia, or high-degree atrioventricular block.

Many drugs may affect the efficacy of digitalis. Certain diuretics and other medications may cause hypokalemia, which increases toxicity risk. Quinidine, verapamil, diltiazem, and amiodarone, cause increased plasma digitalis concentrations. Beta-adrenergic agonists may increase the risk of cardiac arrhythmias. In addition, drugs that induce hepatic microsomal enzyme activity may increase digitalis metabolism.

DIURETICS

Relevance to Physiatry

Although diuretics are primarily used for hypertension and certain forms of edema, other physiatric uses have included the acute treatment of immobilization hypercalcemia (e.g., in SCI) (321). Diuretics may also facilitate fluid mobilization in early lymphedema but should not be used for chronic treatment of this condition (322). Diuretic-associated orthostatic hypotension is a potential problem, particularly for transfer and gait training.

Mechanism of Action

Diuretics in general act by decreasing the volume of extracellular fluid by enhancing urinary excretion through sodium resorption. Because this increases the tubular osmotic gradient, water also is resorbed into the tubules and subsequent diuresis occurs. Each of the three most frequently used diuretic classes specifically act in different areas of the tubules to achieve this effect. The thiazides and high-ceiling (or "loop diuretic") classes are more vigorous in their diuretic, natriuretic, and potassium-wasting effects. Potassium-sparing diuretics are less vigorous in action and because they interfere with the normal sodium-potassium exchange in the distal tubule, potassium

tends to be spared from increased secretion into the urine. A less commonly used class is the carbonic anhydrase inhibitors. These alkalinize the urine through increased bicarbonate concentration and, as a result, cause sodium and potassium ions to be excreted. Additional agents with diuretic properties include osmotic agents such as mannitol, and methylxanthines (e.g., theophylline).

Relevant Side Effects and Drug Interactions

See Table 56-26.

Potential medication interactions should be considered. These include cardiac toxicity from digitalis due to diuretic-induced hypokalemia, decreased renal lithium clearance, interference with oral hypoglycemics, and increased risk of NSAID-induced renal failure.

NITRATES

Relevance to Physiatry

Organic nitrates are commonly used in inpatient rehabilitative settings where there are many patients with coronary artery disease. In addition to their use in angina and in certain patients with CHF, oral or transdermal nitrates may help to reduce acute BP elevations, such as in autonomic dysreflexia. The physiatrist should also be well aware of possible deleterious effects in those undergoing intensive rehabilitation. In particular, it is important to prevent orthostatic hypotension and tachycardia through measures such as gradual position changes, especially in the morning, and having patients avoid prolonged standing if lower extremity strength is diminished.

Mechanism of Action and Pharmacokinetics

After being converted into nitrous oxide within the body, organic nitrates cause smooth muscle relaxation. This occurs by stimulation of intracellular synthesis of 3',5'-cyclic guanosine monophosphate (cGMP), which leads to myosin dephosphorylation and loss of smooth muscle contractility.

After oral ingestion, organic nitrates undergo first pass hepatic inactivation via hydrolysis. Sublingual administration of organic nitrates leads to an onset of action in 1 to 2 minutes and a rapid decrease in effects thereafter. When given orally, higher

TABLE 56-26. Commonly Prescribed Diuretics

[Class] Generic (Trade) Name	Dose (mg)	Other Characteristics & Side Effects
Thiazide		Avoid in patients with allergies to sulfonamide-containing drugs
Chlorothiazide (Diuril)	250–500 po qd/bid	Available in a suspension form
Chlorthalidone (Hygroton)	25–100 po qd	Rarely used
Hydrochlorothiazide (HCTZ, Esidrix, Oretic, Hydrodiuril)	25–200 po qd	Lower doses effective in antihypertensive combinations; can be used less frequently than daily for maintenance edema management
Indapamide (Lozol)	1.25–5.0 po qd	An indoline; main use is for HTN
Methyclothiazide (Enduron, Aquatensen)	2.5–10 po qd	Maintenance dosage for edema may be qod or 3–5 d/wk
Metolazone (Zaroxolyn)	5–20 po qd	Used with loop diuretics in edema refractory to loop diuretics alone
Loop		Used for rigorous diuresis and in edema with decreased renal function.
Bumetanide (Bumex)	0.5–2.0 po qd, 0.5–1 IV/i.m.	1 mg equivalent to 40 mg Lasix
Ethacrynic acid (Edecrin)	25–100 po qd/bid, 0.5–1 mg/kg i.v. up to 50	
Furosemide (Lasix)	20–80 po qd/bid, 1 mg/kg i.v. up to 20–40	Most commonly used loop diuretic
Torsemide (Demadex)	5–20 po/i.v. qd	Equal efficacy with oral or i.v. doses
Potassium-sparing		Possible hyperkalemia, especially if used with ACE inhibitors or ARBs
Amiloride (Midamor)	5–10 po qd	Rarely used; lack mineralocorticoid side effects
Spironolactone (Aldactone)	25–50 po qd/bid	Aldosterone antagonist
Triamterene (Dyrenium)	100 po bid	Rarely used; lack mineralocorticoid side effects

doses must be used to saturate the hepatic metabolism and prevent their degradation. Subsequently, they have a slow onset of action, with peak effects occurring at 60 to 90 minutes, and a duration lasting from 3 to 6 hours. In contrast, transdermal application, either by ointment or patch, allows for gradual absorption and prolonged delivery. With the former, the initial effects occur within 60 minutes and last 4 to 8 hours. In dosing by patch, peak effects are achieved after 1 to 2 hours and can last up to 24 hours. It is important to note however, that long-term continuous use of organic nitrates can lead to the development of tolerance to them. This can be avoided by ensuring a nitrate-free interval for short periods of time (e.g., removing a nitrate patch daily at bedtime and reapplying a new one in the morning).

The efficacy of nitrates in relieving angina pectoris lies in their ability to decrease venous return to the heart (preload) and systemic peripheral resistance (afterload), thereby reducing myocardial oxygen demand. Because they also affect nonvascular smooth muscle, they may relieve atypical chest pain, which can occur in spasmodic conditions of the esophagus or bile ducts.

Dosage and Preparations
Multiple organic nitrate preparations exist. Sublingual, intravenous, and inhalant preparations are used in acute anginal episodes, whereas buccal and sustained-released oral tablets, ointments, and patches are preferred for prophylaxis against anginal episodes.

Relevant Side Effects and Drug Interactions
The most common side effect is vascular headache which can occasionally be severe. It usually improves however with reduction of the dosage and continued use. Postural hypotension may occur but can be relieved by maneuvers that increase central venous return, such as lying supine with leg elevation or with true Trendelenburg positioning. Concomitant use of nitrates with alcohol or antihypertensives can lead to significant hypotension.

Preparations and Dosing
See Table 56-27.

TABLE 56-27. Nitrates

Generic (Trade) Name	Dose
Isosorbide dinitrate	
• Tablets (Isordil, Sorbitrate)	10–40 mg po at least 6 h apart
• Sublingual tablets (Isordil, Sorbitrate)	1 tab (2.5–10 mg) SL prn
• Sustained release (Isordil Tembids, Dilatrate SR)	5–40 mg tid; max of 80 mg po bid
Isosorbide mononitrate	
• Tablets (ISMO, Monoket)	20 mg po bid at least 7 h apart
• Extended release (Imdur)	30–240 mg po qd (start with 30–60 po qd)
Nitroglycerin	(15 mg/inch)
• Ointment 2% (Nitro-Bid, Nitrol)	0.5 inch q8h, maintenance 1–2 inches q8h; max. 4 inches q4–6h
• Spray (Nitrolingual)	1–2 SL sprays prn
• Sublingual (Nitrostat, NitroQuick)	0.4 mg SL prn
• Transdermal (Deponit, Minitran, Nitro-Dur, Nitrodisc, Transderm-Nitro)	1 patch (doses of 0.1–0.8 mg/h) 12–14 h daily

TABLE 56-28. Antiemetics

Medication Class and Mechanism of Action	Generic (Trade) Name	Typical Dose (mg)	Other Properties & Side Effects
Phenothiazine derivatives: act at the chemoreceptor trigger zone (CTZ) and the vomiting center	Prochlorperazine (Compazine)	5–10 po/i.m. tid–qid 25 pr q12h i.v. dosing possible	Antidopaminergic: extrapyramidal reactions and neuroleptic malignant syndrome possible
	Promethazine (Phenergan)	1/kg up to max. 25–50 po/i.m./pr q4–6h	H-1 receptor blocker, therefore antihistaminergic; much less effect on dopamine; i.v. form also available
	Thiethylperazine (Torecan)	10 po/i.m. q8h	Same as for prochlorperazine
Antihistamines: act at the CTZ and the vomiting center	Dimenhydrinate (Dramamine)	50 po/i.m./IV q4–6h	Sedating; transdermal preparation no longer commercially available
Other: act at the CTZ and vomiting center	Trimethobenzamide (Tigan)	250 po q6–8h 200 i.m./pr q6–8h	Hypersensitivity and Parkinson-like symptoms have been reported
	Scopolamine (Transderm Scop)	One patch behind ear, change after 3 d prn	Belladonna alkaloid, therefore anticholinergic side effects
Cannabinoids: complex CNS effects, including sympathomimetic	Dronabinol (Marinol)	Dosage varies	Chemotherapy-related nausea or anorexia associated with AIDS
Selective serotonin 5-HT$_3$ receptor inhibitors: blocks receptors in peripheral vagus nerve terminals and CTZ	Dolasetron (Anzemet)	Up to 100 po single dose (alternate i.v. dosing)	Prevention of chemotherapy-related or post-op nausea
	Granisetron (Kytril)	1 po bid × 1 d 2 po single dose (alternate i.v. dosing)	Prevention of chemotherapy-related or oradiation therapy-related nausea
	Ondansetron (Zofran)	8 po before and 8h after 8 po tid (alternate i.v. dosing)	Prevention of chemotherapy-related, radiation therapy-related and post-op nausea

GASTROINTESTINAL MEDICATIONS

Antiemetics

RELEVANCE TO PHYSIATRY
Nausea is a troublesome symptom that frequently prevents patients from meaningfully participating in a rehabilitation program. It can be particularly prevalent in patients enrolled in cancer rehabilitation programs who are receiving chemotherapy. Nausea should always evoke suspicion of early digoxin toxicity in patients taking cardiac glycosides. Nausea can be treated with agents from several medication classes, each with their own mechanisms, pharmacokinetic principles, side effects, and drug interactions (Table 56-28).

Medications That Act by Affecting Gastrointestinal Motility

RELEVANCE TO PHYSIATRY
Abnormally slow GI transit can especially occur in diabetic patients. Since physiatrists commonly manage patients who also have diabetes, knowledge of promotility agents is important. The two most commonly used agents are metoclopramide (Reglan) and cisapride (Propulsid). Use of the latter is limited because of many drug interactions and potentially fatal cardiac dysrhythmias. Metoclopramide is dosed for gastroesophageal reflux and diabetic gastroparesis at 10 to 15 mg orally 30 minutes before meals and sleep, and should be reduced to 5 mg in elderly patients. It can be used for prevention of chemotherapy-induced emesis and is available for i.v. or i.m. dosing. Because it is a dopamine-receptor antagonist, CNS side effects and extrapyramidal reactions can occur.

MECHANISM OF ACTION AND PHARMACOKINETICS
These drugs enhance acetylcholine release and action at the myenteric plexus, thereby stimulating upper GI peristalsis.

This leads to reflux reduction and gastric emptying. Metoclopramide undergoes hepatic conjugation, but otherwise little hepatic metabolism.

Antidiarrheal Drugs

RELEVANCE TO PHYSIATRY
Hospitalized patients commonly complain of diarrhea. This condition obviously can interfere with rehabilitation. Therefore, medications are often used for short-term management of acute, nonspecific diarrhea and may also be used for chronic inflammatory bowel disease-associated diarrhea. They should be avoided, however, when diarrhea is suspected to be the result of obstructive jaundice, fecal impaction, or infection with toxin production. If diarrhea is not controlled within 48 hours, further workup is warranted.

The two most commonly used antidiarrheal agents for hospitalized patients are loperamide (Imodium) and diphenoxylate or its principal metabolite difenoxin, combined with atropine (Lomotil and Motofen, respectively).

MECHANISM OF ACTION AND PHARMACOKINETICS
As they are opioid-derived, these agents directly inhibit intestinal smooth muscle peristalsis.

PREPARATIONS AND DOSING
See Table 56-29.

SIDE EFFECTS AND DRUG INTERACTIONS
As is expected from medications that impair intestinal motility, abdominal discomfort and nausea can occur. In addition, opioidlike side effects such as fatigue, drowsiness, or dry mouth can occur. Lomotil and Motofen are chemically related to the narcotic analgesic meperidine (Demerol) and are combined with atropine. They may therefore interact with MAOIs and

TABLE 56-29. Antidiarrheal Agents

Agent	Dosage
Imodium[a]	4 mg initially, then 2 mg s/p loose bowel movement to a maximum of 16 mg/24 h
Lomotil	2 tablets qid or 10 cc qid
Motofen	2 tabs initially, then 1 tab prn to a maximum of 8 tabs/24 h

[a]Also available OTC.

are likely to cause sedation when used with other CNS depressants. Lomotil and Motofen may also prolong the biological half-lives of drugs for which the elimination rate is dependent upon microsomal drug metabolizing enzyme systems. Although Imodium is somewhat chemically similar to meperidine, it is not combined with atropine and therefore has a safer side-effect profile and less drug interactions.

Medications That Reduce Gastric Acid Secretion

RELEVANCE TO PHYSIATRY
Besides their use in the prevention and treatment of NSAID-induced GI pathology (see the NSAID section of this chapter and Chapter 31), these medications are also used for idiopathic gastric and duodenal ulcers, as well as for gastroesophageal reflux disease. They are also often used to prevent stress ulcers and are thus encountered in patients undergoing rehabilitation for stroke, TBI or SCI. Other than cimetidine, which can cause CNS changes in the elderly, they are usually well tolerated and do not interfere with rehabilitation.

MECHANISM OF ACTION AND PHARMACOKINETICS; PREPARATIONS AND DOSING; RELEVANT SIDE EFFECTS AND DRUG INTERACTIONS
See Table 56-30.

Laxatives

RELEVANCE TO PHYSIATRY
As is true for diarrhea, constipation can also have a significant negative impact upon rehabilitation. Laxatives can facilitate or restore regular bowel movements in constipated patients. Some are used as part of a bowel program in neurologically impaired patients, especially those with SCI (323,324). Many preparations are available (Table 56-31) and their effects range from mild (bulking agents) to more aggressive (hyperosmolar preparations). Caution should be exercised in those with nausea, vomiting, or unexplained abdominal pain.

MECHANISM OF ACTION AND PHARMACOKINETICS; PREPARATIONS AND DOSING; RELEVANT SIDE EFFECTS AND DRUG INTERACTIONS
See Table 56-32.

HYPNOTICS

Relevance to Physiatry
Insomnia is frequently associated with major stressors such as injury or illness or conditions such as fibromyalgia, myofascial pain syndromes, and chronic fatigue syndrome (325). It can significantly interfere with rehabilitation due to resultant daytime lethargy, irritability, difficulty with concentration, and so forth. Hence, treatment of insomnia with hypnotics can play an important role in overall patient management. Hypnotics are

TABLE 56-30. Medications That Act by Reducing Gastric Secretion

Medication Class: Mechanism	Generic (Trade) Name	Usual Oral Dose (mg)	Unique Characteristics & Side Effects
H2 Blockers: Block H2 receptors of gastric acid-producing parietal cells	Cimetidine (Tagamet)	800 @ H/S or 400 bid	Because of the change in gastric fluid acidity due to H2 blockers, GI absorption of various drugs can be altered i.v. form also available; replaced by newer agents due to side effects (esp. in older adults and in impaired renal function) and medical interactions
	Famotidine (Pepcid)	40 @ H/S or 20 bid	i.v. form also available
	Nizatidine (Axid)	300 @ H/S or 150 bid	
	Ranitidine (Zantac)	300 @ H/S or 150 bid	i.v. form also available
Proton pump inhibitors: decrease gastric acid secretion by inhibiting the parietal cell membrane enzyme that actively transports hydrogen ions out of the cell			Numerous indications, including gastroesophageal reflux disease, gastritis, peptic ulcer disease, erosive esophagitis, and prevention/treatment of NSAID or ASA-induced ulcers. Well tolerated but sometimes nausea, diarrhea, headache, dizziness, and possible gastric bacterial colonization from elevation of gastric fluid PH. Inhibition of metabolism of medications processed by cytochrome P-450 system.
	Esomeprazole (Nexium)	20–40 qd	
	Lansoprazole (Prevacid)	15–30 qd	
	Omeprazole (Prilosec, Losec)	20–40 qd	
	Pantoprazole (Protonix, Pantoloc)	40 qd	
	Rabeprazole (Aciphex)	20 qd	
Prostaglandin analogue: mucosal protection and reduces gastric acid secretion	Misoprostol (Cytotec)	100–200 µg qid (depending on indication)	Diarrhea very common; not to be used in women of child-bearing age due to abortifactant properties from smooth muscle contraction; no known drug interactions

TABLE 56-31.   Laxatives

Medication Class: Mechanism	Generic (Trade) Name	Common Doses	Unique Characteristics & Side Effects
Bulking agents: contain natural fiber, which increases fecal H_2O capacity and enhances bacterial floral growth	Psyllium (Metamucil, Fiberall); methylcellulose (Citrucel); polycarbophil (FiberCon, Fiberall)	1 tsp po qd–tid; 1 tb po qd–tid; 1 g po qid prn	Gritty texture prohibits use in some patients
Colonic stimulants: ("irritant cathartics") act on colonic and rectal sensory nerve endings upon mucosal contact. Peristalsis, and subsequent purging then occurs by parasympathetic reflexes.	Bisacodyl (Dulcolax); castor oil (Purge); sodium bisphosphonate (Fleet enema, Fleet Phospho-soda, Fleet Bisacodyl supp., Fleet Bisacodyl tabs); senna (Senokot) tablets (8.6 mg/tab) or syrup (8.8 mg tsp)	5–15 mg po/pr prn; 325 mg or 5 mL po qd; 15–30 mL po qd; 1 pr; 45 mL; 1 pr; 4 tabs; 2–4 tabs po qd–bid; 10–15 mL po qd	Dulcolax affects fluid and electrolyte absorption throughout the intestine; Senokot act on the large intestine, so there is a delayed effect of approximately 8 h and may cause urine discoloration; castor oil intestinally hydrolyzed to a cathartic (ricinoleic acid)
Combination products:	Docusate/casanthranol (Peri-Colace) senna/docusate (Senokot-S tabs) Milk of Magnesia-Cascara	1–2 caps qd 2, max. 4 po qd 15–30 mL qd	Peri-Colace capsule, 100 mg docusate/ 30 mg casanthranol Peri-Colace liquid, 60 mg docusate/30 mg casanthranol per 15 mL
Hyperosmolar agents: ("bulk cathartics") cause H_2O secretion into the colon and rectum, leading to loosening and facilitated expulsion of feces	Magnesium citrate soda; magnesium hydroxide (Milk of Magnesia); MiraLax	200–300 mL po; 15–60 mL po 17 g (about 1 heaping tb) of powder/d in 8 oz of water	Because of their osmotic concentration, hyperosmolar agents should be avoided in acute congestive heart failure and used with caution with impaired renal function, heart disease, and electrolyte imbalances; Fleet products usually used as bowel preps 3 h before a procedure
Miscellaneous agents:	Glycerin suppositories; lactulose (Chronulac); mineral oil	1 pr; 15–30 mL or 10–20 g powder qd; 15–45 mL po or 120 mL pr	Glycerin stimulates rectal contraction within 15–30 min via hyperosmotic and irritant actions; lactulose is a synthetic disaccharide converted by colonic bacteria to short-chain organic acids that cause colonic fluid accumulation; mineral oil softens and lubricates stool and is useful for fecal impaction; MiraLax
Stool softeners: surfactant, thus increases stool H_2O absorption as it descends the lower GI tract	Docusate sodium (Colace) [capsules or syrup/liquid]; docusate calcium (Surfak)	100 mg po qd–tid; 240 mg po qd	May not see the effect until 1–3 d; begin with the highest dose and then reduce when the first bowel movement occurs

commonly used in hospitalized patients in acute care, in rehabilitation units, and rehabilitation hospitals.

Mechanism of Action and Pharmacokinetics

Benzodiazepines (BNZs) exert hypnotic and anxiolytic effects by binding nonselectively to the GABA-BZ receptor complex, particularly in the limbic system, thalamus, and hypothalamus. In doing so, they reduce delta sleep. They are well absorbed, undergo very little first-pass metabolism, are highly metabolized by the liver, are excreted with short elimination half-lives, and their metabolites do not accumulate.

Zolpidem-tartrate (Ambien) is structurally unrelated to other hypnotics. It preferentially binds to the ω_1-subunit of the GABA-BZ receptor complex, which is the purported reason for its selective hypnotic effect yet lack of anticonvulsant, anxiolytic, and muscle relaxant properties seen with BNZs. Sleep architecture is relatively preserved in both healthy patients and in those with acute or chronic insomnia. It is rapidly absorbed and has a mean elimination half-life of 2.5 hours. It does not accumulate if used short-term and thus is less likely to cause daytime sedation.

Preparations and Dosing

See Table 56-32.

TABLE 56-32.   Hypnotic Medications

Medication Class	Generic (Trade) Name	Usual Oral Dose (mg)	Unique Characteristics & Side Effects
Benzodiazepine	Estazolam (ProSom)	1–2 @ H/S, 0.5 (older adults)	Medium $t_{1/2}$ of 10–15 h
	Flurazepam (Dalmane)	15–30 @ H/S	Long $t_{1/2}$ of 70–90 h
	Lorazepam (Ativan)	2–4 @ H/S	Medium $t_{1/2}$ of 10–20 h
	Temazepam (Restoril)	7.5–30 @ H/S	One of the most widely used agent in this class; $t_{1/2}$ of 8–25 h
	Triazolam (Halcion)	0.125–0.25 @ H/S, max. 0.5 qd	Less popular; significant interactions reported with "conazole" antifungals, macrolides, and cimetidine; short $t_{1/2}$ of 2–3 h
Zolpidem (Ambien)		Dosage: 5–10 @ H/S	

Relevant Side Effects and Drug Interactions

Daytime drowsiness, headache, and fatigue are the most frequently reported side effects in controlled clinical studies involving bedtime BNZ use. Dependence and rebound insomnia can develop, particularly if used regularly for more than a few weeks. These drugs should be used with caution in patients taking other CNS depressants.

Ambien's side-effect profile is superior but still includes daytime drowsiness, usually during short-term use and dizziness or "drugged" feelings with long-term use. As with BNZs, it should be used cautiously in patients taking other CNS depressants.

HYPOGLYCEMICS

Relevance to Physiatry

A physiatrist often manages patients who have diabetes mellitus as a comorbid medical condition. Proper glucose control is important both acutely, in order to avoid uncontrolled blood sugar elevations or hypoglycemia, and chronically in order to avoid long-term complications (326,327). The effects of exercise on blood glucose levels must be taken into account, especially in patients who have not previously exercised regularly.

INSULIN

Mechanism of Action and Pharmacokinetics

Insulin is a large polypeptide, secreted by pancreatic beta cells, that lowers blood glucose concentrations by inhibiting hepatic gluconeogenesis and by increasing peripheral glucose uptake and metabolism. It also affects lipid, ketone, and protein metabolism by reducing glycerol and free fatty acid blood concentrations, reducing ketone body formation, and increasing protein synthesis in muscles and other tissues. Insulin's various effects are exerted via interaction with highly specific receptor's on target cell membranes. This interaction leads to intracellular mechanisms that produce target cell-specific end-organ effects. Exogenous insulin preparations can be of human, porcine, or bovine origin. The latter two differ from human insulin by one and three amino acids, respectively, within the peptide chain.

Preparations and Dosing

As shown in Table 56-33, insulin preparations can be classified as short-acting, intermediate-acting, and long-acting. Most dosing regimens involve a mixture of short- and intermediate-acting insulin preparations given at fixed dosages prior to breakfast and dinner. Another method of dosing insulin is fre-

quent monitoring of blood glucose levels and adjusting insulin dosage with each administration accordingly. This is known as intensive insulin therapy and has been shown to reduce long-term complications of diabetes (302,303).

Side Effects and Drug Interactions

The most common side effect of hypoglycemic therapy is hypoglycemia, as a result of excessive dose, reduced, delayed or omitted meals, or factors that reduce insulin requirements, such as exercise. Hypoglycemia is also more common in the elderly and in patients with impaired hepatic or renal function who take longer-acting preparations. The early signs of hypoglycemia may be blunted in patients chronically treated with insulin.

Hypersensitivity may also occur and can range from local skin reactions to more generalized systemic ones, and even injection-site subcutaneous fat atrophy. This occurs more commonly with the beef and pork insulin preparations; however, it can also occur during treatment with human insulin. Switching the type of preparation and rotation of the injection site may help to reduce these effects.

Many medications can affect blood sugar levels in patients receiving insulin. Those that may cause hypoglycemia include β-adrenergic antagonists, salicylates, and some NSAIDs. In contrast, corticosteroids, oral contraceptives, CaCBs, and some diuretics can blunt the effect of insulin by increasing blood glucose levels.

ORAL HYPOGLYCEMICS

Mechanism of Action and Pharmacokinetics

Although the exact mechanisms of action vary somewhat according to chemical class as shown in Table 56-34, all depend upon a certain degree of endogenous insulin production, thus they are not effective in treating type I diabetes. All are well absorbed from the GI tract.

Preparations and Dosing; Relevant Side Effects and Drug Interactions

See Table 56-34.

RESPIRATORY MEDICATIONS

Decongestants, Expectorants, and Mucolytics

RELEVANCE TO PHYSIATRY

Respiratory tract disorders and infections are commonly encountered in patients undergoing rehabilitation. Various med-

TABLE 56-33. Insulin Preparations				
		Pharmacokinetic Properties		
Insulin Class	Generic (Trade) Name	Onset	Peak Effect	Duration
Rapid-acting	Insulin aspart (Novolog)	15 min	45 min	3–5 h
	Insulin lispro (Humalog)	0–15 min	30–90 min	6–8 h
	Regular; Semilente	30–60 min	2–4 h	8 h
Intermediate-acting	NPH; Lente	1–2 h	6–12 h	18–24 h
Long-acting	Insulin glargine (Lantus)	Slow absorption, with consistent concentration over 24 h		
	protamine zinc insulin suspension;			
	Ultralente	4–6 h	10–30 h	>36 h

TABLE 56-34. Oral Hypoglycemic Agents

Class: Mechanism of Action	Generic (Trade) Name	Usual Oral Dose (mg) (Starting Dose/ Maximum)	Unique Characteristics & Side Effects
Sulfonylureas (first generation): stimulate insulin release from pancreatic beta-cells and increase the insulin sensitivity of various peripheral tissues	Chlorpropamide (Diabenese); tolbutamide (Oramide, Orinase); tolazamide (Tolamide, Tolinase);	100–250/1,000 qd; 250–500/3,000 qd (daily or divided into 2 doses); 100–250/1,000 qd	Chlorpropamide has a very long duration (up to 24 h), making it relatively dangerous, esp. in older adults; tolbutamide has a duration up to 10 h
Sulfonylureas (2nd generation): same mechanism as above	Glimepiride (Amaryl); glipizide (Glucotrol, Glucotrol XL); glyburide (DiaBeta, Micronase, Glynase)	1–2/8 qd; 5/40 qd (divided into 2 daily doses if more than 15/d is required, max. dose of XL 20 qd); 2.5–5/20 qd	Starting doses of glipizide and glyburide 2.5 and 1.25, respectively, recommended in older adults; duration up to 10 h
Biguanides: improve glucose tolerance in patients with NIDDM without inducing hypoglycemia; lower both basal and postprandial glucose levels by decreasing hepatic glucose production, decreasing intestinal glucose absorption, and improving insulin sensitivity	Metformin (Glucophage, Glucovance, Glucophage XL)	500 qd or bid/2,550 qd (higher doses usually divided into bid or tid)	May cause potentially serious lactic acidosis in those with abnormal renal or hepatic function, thus it is contraindicated in these patients and should be temporarily held in patients undergoing radiologic studies involving injectable contrast agents and in those who are dehydrated
Glucosidase inhibitors: decrease the digestion of ingested carbohydrates, thereby reducing postprandial hyperglycemia; possess no systemic effects	Miglitol (Glyset); acarbose (Precose)	Both started at 25 tid; individualized dosing to max of 100 tid	Metabolized in the GI tract; contraindicated in patients with inflammatory bowel disease or intestinal obstruction
Meglitinide: stimulates insulin release	Repaglinide (Prandin)	0.5–2 tid/max. of 16 qd in divided doses (tid)	Most common adverse effect is hypoglycemia
Other agent, amino acid derivative having similar action to meglitinide	Nateglinide (Starlix)	120 tid	Most common adverse effect is hypoglycemia; to be used with caution in presence of liver dysfunction
Thiazolidinediones: decrease insulin resistance in peripheral tissues by stimulating the peroxisome proliferator-activated receptor	Pioglitazone (Actos); rosiglitazone (Avandia)	15–30/45 qd; 4/8 qd	May cause fluid retention, thus to be used cautiously in patients with CHF or edema; liver function should be monitored

ications are used in managing these conditions (Table 56-35). Decongestants treat upper respiratory congestion and the increased mucosal secretion that occurs in colds, seasonal allergies, or infections. Particularly when combined with postural drainage and percussion, expectorants and mucolytics are useful in facilitating pulmonary toilet through improving the quality and expulsion of mucus. Selective β_2-adrenergic agonists are useful in the treatment of reversible airway obstruction in bronchial asthma or COPD. Their use in exercise-induced asthma also has direct physiatric application. Anticholinergic medications can be of benefit in relieving bronchoconstriction, particularly in COPD. Finally, inhaled glucocorticoids and leukotriene inhibitors, a newer medication class, are effective in maintenance therapy of asthma.

TRAUMATIC BRAIN INJURY MEDICATIONS

See Table 56-35.

Each year more than 1.5 million Americans survive a TBI, among which 80,000 to 90,000 are left with permanent disability (328). Currently there are no medications that are FDA-approved to treat the early or late sequelae of TBI. The complex nature of the injury and recovery, along with previous research

failures, has created pharmaceutical industry apathy. Medications used to treat the behavioral and cognitive consequences of TBI are often based on success in other disorders with similar symptoms. Most TBI population neuropharmacology studies are just case reports.

The TBI manifestations for which medications are most commonly used include disorders of arousal, attention, concentration, initiation, and behavior. Before drug therapy is started, a careful review of the patient's current medications is warranted since medications commonly used for other medical conditions may cause or exacerbate the TBI manifestation (see Table 56-36). In general, noncentrally acting medications should be used since these are less likely to have their own cognitive side effects as well as interactions with medications likely to be employed for TBI manifestations. Only after eliminating medications with these unwanted side effects and potential medication interactions should initiation of new drugs be considered.

Cognitive and behavioral impairment in the patient with TBI results from neurochemical alterations. These alterations are caused by shear injury of the ascending and descending cortical pathways to the brain stem, along with hypoxic lesions, contusions, and hemorrhages (329). More specific understanding of the pathophysiology of TBI on a cellular and

TABLE 56-35.   Respiratory Medications

Medication Class (Mechanism)	Generic (Trade) Names	Dose	Unique Characteristics & Side Effects
Anticholinergics: relieve bronchoconstriction via antagonism of muscarinic cholinergic receptors	Ipratropium bromide (Atrovent)	2 puffs (by metered-dose inhaler) qid, up to 12 puffs per 24 h; maximal clinical effects in 30–90 min and last for 4 h	Most cause significant systemic side effects because of easy absorption; fewer side effects with ipratropium because very little respiratory or GI absorption
Decongestants (alpha-1 adrenergic agonists): nasal mucosa blood vessel vasoconstriction, thus decreased secretion and congestion	Ephedrine, epinephrine, naphazoline, oxymetazoline, phenylephrine, phenylpropanolamine, pseudoephedrine (Sudafed), tetrahydrozoline, and xylometazoline	Depends upon the particular preparation	Decreases secretions and congestion, also used in combination with agents such as expectorants, antitussives, or antihistamines; side effects, headaches, dizziness, increased BP, and palpitations
Expectorants: not clearly understood how they enhance respiratory tract secretion production, but make it easier to advance sputum upward	Guaifenesin (Robitussin, Humibid LA, Guiatuss, Fenesin, Guaifenex LA), terpin hydrate	100–400 mg po q4h or 600–1,200 mg po q12h (releaser)	Usually given orally, either alone or in combination with other respiratory agents; GI distress, especially in high doses; in extended usage, those containing iodide may cause iodism, hypothyroidism, or hypersensitivity
Mucolytics: decrease mucus viscosity by splitting mucoprotein disulfide bonds	Acetylcysteine (Mucomyst, Mucosol)	6–10 cc 10% or 3–5 cc 20% solution; nebulized form q6–8h	Possible nausea and vomiting, stomatitis, or rhinorrhea
Inhaled steroids: inhibit inflammatory cells and mediators		Adverse effects are similar to those that occur with systemic glucocorticoids; adrenal suppression is not as common as with systemic use, except for the more potent inhaled forms or if used at higher than recommended dosages; oral candidiasis may occur; caution needs to be exercised when changing to inhaled steroids from systemic dosage; not intended to alleviate acute asthma	
	Beclomethasone (Beclovent, Vanceril)	2 puffs (84 µg) tid–qid, max. 20 puffs/24 h;	Flunisolide is the most potent of these inhaled drugs; fluticasone inhaler available in strengths of 44 µg, 110 µg, 220 µg
	Budesonide (Pulmicort)	200 µg/puff, 1–2 puffs bid, max 4 puffs bid;	
	Flunisolide (AeroBid)	250 µg/puff, 2 puffs bid, max. 4 puffs bid;	
	Fluticasone (Flovent)	2–4 puffs bid, max of 880 mcg bid;	
	Triamcinolone (Azmacort)	2 puffs (200 µg) tid–qid or 4 puffs bid, max 16 puffs/24 h	
Leukotriene inhibitors: block leukotriene receptors found in the lung airways (montelukast and zafirlukast) or inhibit the formation of certain leukotrienes (LTB_4, LTC_4, LTD_4, LTE_4) by specifically inhibiting 5-lipoxygenase (zileuton)	Montelukast (Singulair); zafirlukast (Accolate); zileuton (Zyflo)	10 mg q p.m. 20 bid 600 qid	Common side effects are headache, abdominal discomfort, and cough; also, zafirlukast and zileuton may elevate pro times in patients on warfarin; also, zileuton may augment the effects of propranolol and may cause elevated liver enzymes
Selective beta-2-adrenergic agonists: affinity for beta-2 adrenergic receptors in bronchiolar smooth muscles	Albuterol (Proventil, Ventolin, Volmax), bitolterol (Tornalate), formoterol (Foradil), isoetharine (Bronkosol, nebulized; Bronkometer, inhaled), levalbuterol (Xopenex), metaproterenol (Alupent, Metaprel, ProMeta), pirbuterol (Maxair), salmeterol (Serevent), terbutaline (Brethine, Bricanyl)	Response rate varies with administration mode: rapid response to aerosol inhalation or subcutaneous injection; delayed but longer if given orally	Tachycardia, arrhythmias, and myocardial ischemia, especially with underlying cardiac disease

neurochemical level will allow clinicians to tailor the pharmacologic treatment to individual patients. The following will describe those agents more commonly used in the patient with TBI.

Selective Serotonin Reuptake Inhibitors

In addition to their use in neuropathic pain and depression discussed elsewhere in this text, SSRIs are also used in the setting of TBI to treat sleep disturbance, agitation, affective disorders, emotional incontinence, aggression, and impaired arousal (330–332). SSRIs are preferred to TCAs in the TBI population since they have fewer cognitive side effects. The use of SSRIs in TBI is directly related to serotonin's multiple roles in brain functioning including sleep initiation, sexual response, movement, mood, aggression, anxiety, appetite, and addictive behaviors (333).

Trazodone

Trazodone is specifically used in TBI patients for agitation (dosed 50 to 100 mg q 6 hours around the clock or prn) and for sleep disturbance (initiated at 50 mg at bedtime and titrated up to 300 mg to achieve 6 to 8 hours of sleep). Its role in sleep disorders is particularly important as insomnia occurs in more than 50% of TBI patients both early and late after injury and may exacerbate disability by further impairing arousal, attention, and increasing one's susceptibility to confusion and agitation (334,335).

Fluoxetine, Sertraline, and Paroxetine

These SSRIs are commonly used for other cognitive/behavioral manifestations besides sleep disturbance. Their dosages are the same as recommended for depression. Slow titration and clinical monitoring is necessary to avoid apathy, an SSRI side effect.

Agents That Act on Catecholamines

Cerebral catecholamines are produced in the sympathetic ganglia from the amino acid tyrosine. Dopamine (DA) is enzymatically converted to norepinephrine (NE) and then to epinephrine. An increase in any one of the catecholamines increases the others. DA cell bodies are primarily in the substantia nigra and hypothalamus. There are five types of DA receptors, each with specialization of action. DA neuronal connections have important effects on attention, arousal, and memory (336). Norepinephrine CNS cell bodies are found in the locus ceruleus. Although this small nucleus contains only several hundred neurons, it sends axons to all CNS regions. Catecholamines are thought to play an important, although not fully defined role in recovery after brain TBI. Catecholamine antagonists should therefore be minimized to avoid the risk of detrimental effects on functional outcomes. A detrimental effect from haloperidol and a beneficial effect of dextroamphetamine on motor recovery in an animal model has been observed (337). Significantly poorer motor and functional outcomes in CVA patients exposed to catecholamine antagonists was then reported (338). Finally, a longer duration of posttraumatic amnesia in those treated with haloperidol for posttraumatic agitation was found in a retrospective review of rehabilitation outcomes in severe TBI (339).

In contrast, catecholamine agonists have a beneficial effect on motor control and executive function, with a resultant improvement in arousal, attention, processing speed, and depression (336). A beneficial effect of a single dose of amphetamine in the motor function of CVA patients was demonstrated (340). Catecholamine agonist side effects include hallucinations, GI upset, orthostasis, and dyskinesias.

Carbidopa/Levodopa

This presynaptic DA agonist is used in Parkinson's disease and is reported to improve cognition in TBI patients with persistent deficits and to increase arousal after TBI and encephalitis (341–344). It is used at 25 to 100 mg tid up to 25 to 250 mg 8 times per day.

Bromocriptine (Parlodel)

This DA agonist has been reported in case studies to enhance functional recovery in vegetative TBI patients (345). It is initi-

ated at 2.5 mg every morning, with slow titration up to 60 mg every day in divided doses with careful monitoring for nausea.

Amantadine (Symmetrel)

Amantadine facilitates DA action at pre- and postsynaptic receptors and is thought to have neuroprotective properties by acting as an NMDA-receptor antagonist (346). It has been reported to improve arousal, attention, concentration, and decrease agitation but can lower the seizure threshold (347–349). Dosing is 100 to 400 mg divided once a day to twice a day.

Methylphenidate (Ritalin)

Ritalin blocks presynaptic DA and NE reuptake (336). It is most commonly used for impaired initiation, concentration, and attention. To avoid insomnia, it should be given early in the day at 5 to 60 mg in divided doses. Although anorexia, arrhythmias, and hypertension are potential side effects, studies have not supported that it increases seizure risk and have consistently reported a low side-effect incidence and subject drop out (350). Studies of Ritalin for attention and concentration have shown mixed results (351–353). It has been inferred from studies that methylphenidate's action may be more pronounced early after TBI and that its efficacy on attention and concentration in acute TBI may increase therapy participation and thus speed functional recovery (336,351,352).

Agents That Affect Acetylcholine

Acetylcholine (Ach) is primarily produced in the nucleus basalis of Meynert and is the neurotransmitter most involved with memory (330). Cholinergic fiber loss is thought to play a key role in attention and memory deficits in Alzheimer's disease and TBI (354). The Ach system has therefore been targeted for pharmacologic modulation to enhance memory. Older cholinergic agents, such as physostigmine and tacrine had limited use due to systemic side effects and short half-lives. More recently a new class of acetylcholinesterase inhibitors has been FDA-approved for dementia and has been studied in TBI. Specifically, beneficial effects of donepezil (Aricept) have been reported in an open label study of 4 severe TBI subjects who were more than 2 years' postinjury and showed significant improvement in both memory and behavior during 12 weeks of treatment (354). No significant side effects were reported. Randomized trials are needed.

Agents Used to Treat Agitation

Agitation is a common occurrence in the TBI recovery period (334). Before considering an agent to treat this, any medication that may potentiate agitation by impairing cognition should be minimized (Table 56-36), environmental modifications should be instituted to minimize unnecessary stimuli and assist with orientation, and disordered sleep-wake cycles should be treated as needed. Pharmacologic treatment for agitation spans a broad range of medications including anticonvulsants, antidepressants, antihypertensives, antipsychotics, benzodiazepines, buspirone, stimulants, and amantadine (334). Treatment choice is based on type and frequency of target behaviors. Optimally, the medication should minimize agitation without impairing arousal and cognition. When possible, a medication should be chosen that also treats a coexisting condition. Careful monitoring of target behaviors and side effects is critical for successful treatment.

TABLE 56-36.   Medications That Can Impair Cognition

aminophylline
anticholinergic agents (e.g., Benadryl)
anticonvulsants
antiemetics
antipsychotics
barbiturates
β-blockers
benzodiazepines
central-acting antihypertensive agents (e.g., Clonidine)
gastric motility agents (e.g., metoclopramide)
cardiac glycosides
H2 blockers
hypnotics
opiates

Miscellaneous Agents: Modafinil

Hypoarousal and fatigue are common complaints after TBI and can lead to poor cognitive and physical functioning. Stimulants can be effective in some patients. Modafinil (Provigil) is approved to treat narcolepsy. Its mechanism of action has not been fully elucidated, but it does not appear to work through any of the aforementioned neurotransmitter systems. Modafinil was reported to reduce fatigue in multiple sclerosis and was well tolerated at 200 mg qd (355). No published studies to date have been done in the TBI population, but trials on fatigue and cognitive impairment are warranted (356).

REFERENCES

1. Ross E. Moving towards rational pharmacological management of pain with an improved classification system of pain. *Expert Opin Pharmacother* 2001;2(10):1529–1530.
2. Wallace MS. Pharmacologic treatment of neuropathic pain. *Curr Pain Headache Rep* 2001;5(2):138–150.
3. Altman R, Hochberg M, Moskowitz R, et al. Recommendations for the medical management of osteoarthritis of the hip and knee: 2000 update. *Arthritis & Rheumatism* 2000;43(9):1905–1915.
4. Flower RJ and Vane JR. Inhibition of prostaglandin synthetase in brain explains the anti-pyretic action of paracetamol (4-acetamidophenol). *Nature* 1972;240:410.
5. Batchlor EE, Paulus HE. *Principles of drug therapy.* In: Moskowitz RW, Howell DS, Goldberg VM, eds. *Osteoarthritis: diagnosis and medical/surgical management.* Philadelphia: WB Saunders, 1992.
6. Benison H, Kaczynski J, Wallerstedt S. Paracetamol medication and alcohol abuse: a dangerous combination for the liver and the kidney. *Scand J Gastroenterol* 1987;22:701–704.
7. Jones AF, Vale JA. Paracetamol poisoning and the kidney. *J Clin Pharm Ther* 1993;18:5–8.
8. Henrich WL, Agodaoa LE, Barret B, et al. Analgesics and the kidney: summary and recommendations to the Scientific Advisory Board of the National Kidney Foundation from an Ad Hoc Committee of the National Kidney Foundation. *Am J Kidney Dis* 1996;27:162–165..
9. Hylek EM, Heiman H, Skates SJ, et al. Acetaminophen and other risk factors for excessive warfarin anticoagulation. *JAMA* 1998;279(9):657–662.
10. Fitzmaurice DA, Murray JA. Potentiation of anticoagulant effect of warfarin. *Postgrad Med J* 1997;73:439–440.
11. Max MB. Thirteen consecutive well-designed randomized trials show that antidepressants reduce pain in diabetic neuropathy and postherpetic neuralgia. *Pain Forum* 1995;4(4): 248–253.
12. Onghena P, Van Houdenhove B. Antidepressant-induced analgesia in chronic non-malignant pain: a meta-analysis of 39 placebo-controlled studies. *Pain* 1992;49: 205–219.
13. McQuay HJ, Tramer M, Nye BA, et al. A systematic review of antidepressants in neuropathic pain. *Pain* 1996;68:217–227.
14. Sullivan MJL, Reesor K, Mikail S, et al. The treatment of depression in chronic low back pain: review and recommendations. *Pain* 1992;50:5.
15. McQuay HJ, Carroll D, Glynn CJ. Low dose amitriptyline in the treatment of chronic pain. *Anesthesia* 1992;47:646.
16. Kishore-Kumar R., Max MB, Schafer SC, et al. Desipramine relieves postherpetic neuralgia. *Clin Pharmacol Ther* 1990;47:305–312.
17. Max MB, Lynch SA, Muir J, et al. Effects of desipramine, amitriptyline, and fluoxetine (Prozac) on pain in diabetic neuropathy. *N Engl J Med* 1992;326:1250–1256.
18. McCleane G. Topical application of doxepin hydrochloride, capsaicin and a combination of both produces analgesia in chronic human neuropathic pain: a randomized, double-blind, placebo-controlled study. *Br J Clin Pharmacol* 2000;49(6):574–579.
19. Finestone DH, Ober SK. Fluoxetine and fibromylgia. *JAMA* 1990;264:2869–2870.
20. Wolfe F, Cahtey MA, Hawley DJ. A double-blind placebo controlled trial of fluoxetine in fibromyalgia. *Scand J Rheumatol* 1994;23:255–259.
21. Goldenberg D, Mayskiy M, Mossey C, et al. A randomized, double-blind crossover trial of fluoxetine and amitriptyline in the treatment of fibromyalgia. *Arthritis Rheum* 1996;39:1852–1859.
22. Sindrup SH, Gram LF, Bronsen K, et al. The selective serotonin reuptake inhibitor paroxetine is effective in the treatment of diabetic neuropathy symptoms. *Pain* 1990;42:135–144.
23. Sindrup SH, Bjerre U, Dejgaard A, et al. The selective serotonin reuptake inhibitor citalopram relieves the symptoms of diabetic neuropathy. *Clin Pharmacol Ther* 1992;52(5):547–552.
24. Goodnick PJ, Jimenez I, Kumar A. Sertraline in diabetic neuropathy: preliminary results. *Ann Clin Psychiatry* 1997;9:255–257.
25. Jung AC, Staiger T, Sullivan M. The efficacy of selective serotonin reuptake inhibitors for the management of chronic pain. *J Gen Intern Med* 1997;12:384–389.
26. Ciaramella A, Grosso S, Poli P. Fluoxetine versus fluvoxamine for treatment of chronic pain. *Minerva Anestesiol* 2000;66(1–2):55–61.
27. Manna V, Bolino F, Di Cicco L. Chronic tension-type headache, mood depression and serotonin: therapeutic effects of fluvoxamine and mianserine. *Headache* 1994;34(1):44–9.
28. Brannon GE, Stone KD. The use of mirtazapine in a patient with chronic pain. *J Pain Symptom Manage* 1999;18(5):382–385.
29. Brannon GE, Stone KD. Potentiation of opioid analgesia by the antidepressant nefazodone. *Eur J Pharmacol* 1992;211(3):375–381.
30. Lynch ME. Antidepressants as analgesics: a review of randomized controlled trials. *J Psychiatry Neurosci* 2001;26(1) 30–36.
31. Wilson RC. The use of low-dose Trazodone in the treatment of diabetic neuropathy. *J Am Podiatr Med Assoc* 1999;89(a): 468–471.
32. Sumpton JE, Moulin DE. Treatment of neuropathic pain with venlafaxine. *Ann Pharmocother* 2001;35(5):557–559.
33. Lithner F. Venlafaxine in treatment of severe painful peripheral diabetic neuropathy. *Diabetes Care* 2000;23(11):1710–1711.
34. Pernia A, Mro JA, Calderon E, Torres, LM. Venlafaxine for the treatment of neuropathic pain. *J Pain Symptom Manage* 2000;19(6):408–410.
35. Markowitz JS, Petrick KS. Venlafaxine-tramadol similarities. *Med Hypotheses* 1998;51(2):167–168.
36. Kiayias JA, Vlachou ED, Lakka-Papadodima E. Venlafaxine HCl in the treatment of painful peripheral diabetic neuropathy. *Diabetes Care* 2000;23:699.
37. Pernia A, Mico JA, Calderon E, et al. Venlafaxine for the treatment of neuropathic pain. *J Pain Symptom Manage* 2000;19:408–410.
38. Davis JL, Smith RL. Painful peripheral diabetic neuropathy treated with venlafaxine HCl extended release capsules. *Diabetes Care* 1999;22(11):1909–1910.
39. Songer DA, Schulte H. Venlafaxine for the treatment of chronic pain. *Am J Psychiatry* 1996;153(5):737.
40. Galer BS. Neuropathic pain of peripheral origin: advances in pharmacological treatment. *Neurology* 1995;45[Suppl 9]:S17–S25.
41. Nutt D, Johnson FN. Potential applications of venlafaxine. *Rev Contemp Pharmacother* 1998;9:321–331.
42. Semenchuk MR, Davis B. Double-blind, randomized trial of bupropion SR for the treatment of neuropathic pain. *Neurology* 2001;57(9):1583–1588.
43. Clayton AH, Pradko JF, Croft HA, et al. Prevalence of sexual dysfunction among newer antidepressants. *J Clin Psychiatry* 2002;63(4):357–366.
44. Zajecka J, Tracy KA, Mitchell S. Discontinuation symptoms after treatment with serotonin reuptake inhibitors: a literature review. *J Clin Psychiatry* 1997;58(7):291–297.
45. Medina CA. Clitoral priapism: a rare condition presenting as a cause of vulvar pain. *Obstet Gynecol* 2001;94[4 Suppl]:S26–S27.
46. Green SM, ed. *The 1997 Tarascon pocket pharmacopoeia.* Loma Linda, CA: Tarascon Publishing, 1997.
47. Lennard TA. *Physiatric procedures in clinical practice.* Philadelphia: Hanley & Belfus, Inc.
48. American Medical Association Department of Drugs, Division of Drugs and Technology. *Drug evaluations,* 6th ed. Chicago: American Medical Association, 1986.
49. Trentin L, Visentin M. The predictive lidocaine test in treatment of neuropathic pain. *Minerva Anestesiol* 2000;66(3):157–161.
50. Galer BS, Dworkin RH. Pharmacologic treatment of neuropathic pain. In: Galer BS, Dworkin RH, eds. *A clinical guide to neuropathic pain.* Minneapolis: McGraw-Hill Co, 2000:53–83.
51. Kalso E, Tramer MR, McQuay HJ, et al. Systemic local-anaesthetic-type drugs in chronic pain: a systematic review. *Eur J Pain* 1998;2(1):3–14.
52. Chabal C, Jacobson L, Mariano A, et al. The use of oral mexiletine for the treatment of pain after peripheral nerve injury. *Anesthesiology* 1992;76(4):513–517.

53. Stracke H, Meyer U, Schumacher H, et al. Mexiletine in treatment of painful diabetic neuropathy. *Med Klin* 1994;89(3):124–131.
54. Oskarsson P, Ljunggren JG, Lins PE. Efficacy and safety of mexiletine in the treatment of painful diabetic neuropathy. The Mexiletine Study Group. *Diabetes Care* 1997;20(10):1594–1597.
55. Stracke H, Meyer UE, Schumacher HE, et al. Mexiletine in the treatment of diabetic neuropathy. *Diabetes Care* 1992;15(11):1550–1555.
56. Dejgard A, Petersen P, Kastrup J. Mexiletine for treatment of chronic painful diabetic neuropathy. *Lancet* 1988;1(8575–6):9–11.
57. Nishiyama K, Sakuta M. Mexiletine for painful alcoholic neuropathy. *Intern Med* 1995;34(6):577–579.
58. Davis RW. Successful treatment for phantom pain. *Orthopedics* 1993;16(6):691–695.
59. Ando K, Wallace MS, Braun J, et al. Effect of oral mexiletine on capsaicin-induced allodynia and hyperalgesia: a double-blind, placebo-controlled, crossover study. *Reg Anesth Pain Med* 2000;25(5):468–474.
60. Awerbuch GI, Sandyk R. Mexiletine for thalamic pain syndrome. *Int J Neurosci* 1990;5(2–4):129–133.
61. Okada S, Kinoshita M, Fujioka T, et al. Two cases of multiple sclerosis with painful tonic seizures and dysesthesia ameliorated by the administration of mexiletine. *Japan J Med* 1991;30(4):373–375.
62. Kemper CA, Kent G, Burton S, et al. Mexiletine for HIV-infected patients with painful peripheral neuropathy: a double-blind, placebo-controlled, crossover treatment trial. *J Acquir Immune Defic Syndr Hum Retrovirol* 1998;19(4):367–372.
63. Chio-Tan FY, Tuel SM, Johnson JC, et al. Effect of mexiletine on spinal cord injury dysesthetic pain. *AMJPMR* 1996;75(2):84–87.
64. Pascual J, Berciano J. Failure of mexiletine to control trigeminal neuralgia. *Headache* 1989;29(8):517–518.
65. Wallace MS, Magnuson S, Ridgeway B. Efficacy of oral mexiletine for neuropathic pain with allodynia: a double-blind, placebo-controlled, crossover study. *Reg Anesth Pain Med* 2000;25(5):459–467.
66. Ando K, Wallace MS, Braun J, et al. Effect of oral mexiletine on capsaicin-induced allodynia and hyperalgesia: a double-blind, placebo-controlled, crossover study. *Reg Anesth Pain Med* 2000;25(5):468–474.
67. Peraire M. Diagnosis and treatment of the patient with trigeminal neuralgia. *Neurologia* 1997;12(1):12–22.
68. Jackson CE, Barohn RJ, Ptacek LJ. Paramyotonia congenita: abnormal short exercise test, and improvement after mexiletine therapy. *Muscle & Nerve* 1994;17(7):763–768.
69. Hayashi T, Ichiyama T, Tanaka H, et al. Successful treatment of incontinence of feces in myotonic muscular dystrophy by mexiletine. *No to Hattatsu [Brain & Development]* 1991;23(3):310–312.
70. Kwiecinski H, Ryniewicz B, Ostrzycki A. Treatment of myotonia with antiarrhythmic drugs. *Acta Neurol Scand* 1992;86(4):371–375.
71. Puniani TS, Bertorini TE. Tocainide therapy in muscle cramps and spasms due to neuromuscular disease. *Muscle Nerve* 1991;14(3):280–285.
72. Hahn AF, Parkes AW, Bolton CF et al. Neuromyotonia in hereditary motor neuropathy. *J Neurol Neurosurg Psychiatry* 1991;54(3):230–235.
73. Guieu R, Mesdjian E, Rochat H, et al. Central analgesic effect of valproate in patients with epilepsy. *Seizure* 1993;2(2):147–150.
74. Tremont-Lukats IW, Megeff C, Backonja MM. Anticonvulsants for neuropathic pain syndromes: mechanisms of action and place in therapy. *Drugs* 2000;60(5):1029–1052.
75. Block F. Gabapentin zur schmerztherapie [Gabapentin for therapy of neuropathic pain]. *Schmerztherapie* 2001;15(4):280–288.
76. Backonja MM. Gabapentin monotherapy for the symptomatic treatment of painful neuropathy: a multicenter, double-blind, placebo-controlled trial in patients with diabetes mellitus. *Epilepsia* 1999;40[Suppl 6]:S57–S59; discussion S73–S74.
77. Backonja M, Beydoun A, Edwards KR et al. Gabapentin for the symptomatic treatment of painful neuropathy in patients with diabetes mellitus: a randomized controlled trial. *JAMA* 1998;280(21):1831–1836.
78. Rowbotham M, Harden N, Stacey B et al. Gabapentin for the treatment of postherpetic neuralgia: a randomized controlled trial. *JAMA* 1998;280(21):1837–1842.
79. Rice AS, Maton S, the Postherpetic Neuralgia Study Group (UK). Gabapentin in postherpetic neuralgia: a randomized, double blind, placebo-controlled study. *Pain* 2001;94:215–224; *Pain* 2002;96(3):411–412.
80. Priebe MM, Sherwood AM, Graves DE, et al. Effectiveness of gabapentin in controlling spasticity: a quantitative study. *Spinal Cord* 1997;35(3):171–175.
81. Jensen TS. Anticonvulsants in neuropathic pain: rationale and clinical evidence. *Eur J Pain* 2002;6[Suppl A]:61–68.
82. di Vadi PP, Hamann W. The use of lamotrigine in neuropathic pain. *Anaesthesia* 1998;53 (8):808–809.
83. Zakrzewska JM. Trigeminal neuralgia. *Prim Dent Care* 1997;4(1):17–19.
84. Simpson DM, Olney R, McArthur JC, et al. A placebo-controlled trial of lamotrigine for painful HIV-associated neuropathy. *Neurology* 2000;54(11):2115–2119.
85. Vestergaard K, Andersen G, Gottrup H, et al. Lamotrigine for central post-stroke pain: a randomized controlled trial. *Neurology* 2001;56(2):184–190.
86. Backonja MM. Anticonvulsants (antineuropathics) for neuropathic pain syndromes. *Clin J Pain* 2000;16[2 Suppl]:S67–S72.
87. McCleane G. 200 mg daily of lamotrigine has no analgesic effect in neuropathic pain: a randomised, double-blind, placebo controlled trial. *Pain* 1999;83(1):105–107.
88. Comment in: *Pain* 2000;86(1–2):211–212.
89. Sindrup SH, Jensen TS. Pharmacotherapy of trigeminal neuralgia. *Clin J Pain* 2002;18(1):22–27.
90. Rabinovich A, Fang J, Scrivani S. Diagnosis and management of trigeminal neuralgia. *Columbia Dental Rev* 2000;5:4–7.
91. Beydoun A, Kutluay E.Oxcarbazepine. *Expert Opin Pharmacother* 2002;3(1):59–71.
92. Gonzalez-Darder JM, Ortega-Alvaro A, Ruz-Franzi I, et al. Antinociceptive effects of phenobarbital in "tail-flick" test and deafferentation pain. *Anesth Analg* 1992;75(1):81–86.
93. Ipponi A, Lamberti C, Medica A, et al. Tiagabine antinociception in rodents depends on GABA(B) receptor activation: parallel antinociception testing and medial thalamus GABA microdialysis. *Eur J Pharmacol* 1999;368(2–3):205–211.
94. Novak V, Kanard R, Kissel JT, et al. Treatment of painful sensory neuropathy with tiagabine: a pilot study. *Clin Auton Res* 2001;11(6):357–361.
95. Meldrum BS, Chapman AG. Basic mechanisms of Gabitril (tiagabine) and future potential developments. *Epilepsia* 1999;40[Suppl 9]:S2–S6.
96. Martinez-Salio A, Porta-Etessam J, Berbel-Garcia A, et al. Antiepileptic drugs and neuropathic pain. *Rev Neurol* 2001;32(4):345–350.
97. Bajwa ZH, Sami N, Warfield CA, et al. Topiramate relieves refractory intercostal neuralgia. *Neurology* 1999;52(9):1917.
98. Canavero S, Bonicalzi V, Paolotti R. Lack of effect of topiramate for central pain. *Neurology* 2002;58(5):831–832.
99. Rozen TD. Antiepileptic drugs in the management of cluster headache and trigeminal neuralgia. *Headache* 2001;41[Suppl 1]:25–33.
100. Davies AN. Sodium valproate in cancer-related neuropathic pain. *J Pain Symptom Manage* 2002;23(1):1.
101. Ekbom K, Hardebo JE. Cluster headache: aetiology, diagnosis and management. *Drugs* 2002;62(1):61–69.
102. Hardy JR, Rees EA, Gwilliam B, et al. A phase II study to establish the efficacy and toxicity of sodium valproate in patients with cancer-related neuropathic pain. *J Pain Symptom Manage* 2001;21(3):204–209.
103. Drewes AM, Andreasen A, Poulsen LH. Valproate for treatment of chronic central pain after spinal cord injury. A double-blind cross-over study. *Paraplegia* 1994;32(8):565–569.
104. Grafova VN, Danilova EI, Reshetniak VK. The action of sodium valproate in central pain syndromes. *Eksp Klin Farmakol* 1994;57(2):8–11.
105. Martin C, Martin A, Rud C, et al. Comparative study of sodium valproate and ketoprofen in the treatment of postoperative pain. *Ann Fr Anesth Reanim* 1988;7(5):387–392.
106. Campostrini R, Paganini M, Boncinelli L, et al.[Alterations of the state of consciousness induced by valproic acid: 6 case reports]. *Riv Patol Nerv Ment* 1983;104(1):23–34.
107. Kito M, Maehara M, Watanabe K. Mechanisms of T-type calcium channel blockade by zonisamide. *Seizure* 1996;5(2):115–119.
108. Okada M, Kaneko S, Hirano T, et al. Effects of zonisamide on dopaminergic system. *Epilepsy Res* 1995;22(3):193–205.
109. Devers A, Galer BS. Topical lidocaine patch relieves a variety of neuropathic pain conditions: an open-label study. *Clin J Pain* 2000;16(3):205–208.
110. Argoff CE. New analgesics for neuropathic pain: the lidocaine patch. *Clin J Pain* 2000;16[2 Suppl]:S62–S66.
111. Relieving the pain of postherpetic neuralgia with lidocaine patch 5%. *Drugs & Therapy Perspectives* 2000;16(9):1–3.
112. Christopher R, Buchanan L, Begalia K. Pain reduction in local anesthetic administration through pH buffering. *Ann Emerg Med* 1988;17:117–120.
113. McKay W, Morris R, Mushlin P. Sodium bicarbonate attenuates pain on skin infiltration with lidocaine, with or without epinephrine. *Anesth Analges* 1987;66:572–574.
114. Friedman PM, Mafong EA, Friedman ES, et al. Topical anesthetics update: EMLA and beyond. *Dermatol Surg* 2001;27(12):1019–1026.
115. Galinkin JL, Rose JB, Harris K, et al. Lidocaine iontophoresis versus eutectic mixture of local anesthetics (EMLA®) for IV placement in children. *Anesth Analg* 2002;94(6):1484–1488.
116. Galer BS. Topical lidocaine patch relieves a variety of neuropathic pain conditions: an open-label pilot study. Paper presented at: American Academy of Neurology; May 6–13, 1995; Seattle.
117. Lycka B, Watson CPN, Nevin K, et al. EMLA cream for treatment of pain caused by postherpetic neuralgia: a double-blind controlled study. In: Proceeding of American Pain Society meeting; November 14–17, 1996; Washington, DC. 1996:A111 (abstract).
118. Attal N, Brasseur L, Chauvin M, et al. Effects of single and repeated applications of a eutectic mixture of local anesthetic (EMLA) cream on spontaneous and evoked pain in post-herpetic neuralgia. *Pain* 1999;81:203–209.
119. Lidoderm (lidocaine patch 5%) prescribing information. Endo Pharmaceuticals, Inc., Chadds Ford, PA.
120. Galer BS, Rowbotham MC, Perander J, et al. Topical lidocaine patch relieves postherpetic neuralgia more effectively than a vehicle topical patch: results of an enriched enrollment study. *Pain* 1999;80:533–538.
121. Data on file. Endo Pharmaceuticals, Inc., Chadds Ford, PA.
122. Ciccone CD. Pharmacology in rehabilitation. In: *Skeletal muscle relaxants*, 2nd ed. Philadelpha: F.A. Davis Co, 200X:, 162.
123. Browning R, Jackson JL, O'Malley PG. Cyclobenzaprine and back pain: a meta-analysis. *Arch Intern Med* 2001;161(13):1613–1620.
124. Weber C. NMDA-receptor antagonist in pain therapy. *Anasthesiol Intensivmed Notfallmed Schmerzther* 1998;33(8):475–483.

125. Medrik-Goldberg T, Lifschitz D, Pud D, et al. Intravenous lidocaine, aman-tadine, and placebo in the treatment of sciatica: a double-blind, randomized, controlled study. *Reg Anesth Pain Med* 1999;24(6):534–540.

126. Rabben T, Skjelbred P, Oye I. Prolonged analgesic effect of ketamine, an N-methyl-D-aspartate receptor inhibitor, in patients with chronic pain. *J Pharmacol Exp Ther* 1999;289(2):1060–1006.

127. Mercadante S, Lodi F, Sapio M, et al. Long-term ketamine subcutaneous continuous infusion in neuropathic cancer pain. *J Pain Symptom Manage* 1995;10(7):564–568.

128. Berger JM, Ryan A, Vadivelu N, et al. Ketamine-fentanyl-midazolam infu-sion for the control of symptoms in terminal life care. *Am J Hosp Palliat Care* 2000;17(2):127–134.

129. Mercadante S, Arcuri E, Tirelli W, et al. Analgesic effect of intravenous keta-mine in cancer patients on morphine therapy: a randomized, controlled, double-blind, crossover, double-dose study. *J Pain Symptom Manage* 2000; 20(4):246–252.

130. Lauretti GR, Lima IC, Reis MP, et al. Oral ketamine and transdermal nitro-glycerin as analgesic adjuvants to oral morphine therapy for cancer pain management. *Anesthesiology* 1999;90(6):1528–1533.

131. Mercadante S. Ketamine in cancer pain: an update. *Palliat Med* 1996;10(3): 225–230.

132. Mizuno J, Sugimoto S, Ikeda M, et al. Usefulness of epidural administration of ketamine for relief of postherpetic neuralgia. *Masui* 2001;50(8):904–907.

133. Kishimoto N, Kato J, Suzuki T, et al. A case of RSD with complete disappear-ance of symptoms following intravenous ketamine infusion combined with stellate ganglion block and continuous epidural block. *Masui* 1995;44(12): 1680–1684.

134. Le DA, Lipton SA. Potential and current use of N-methyl-D-aspartate (NMDA) receptor antagonists in diseases of aging. *Drugs Aging* 2001;18 (10):717–724.

135. Parsons CG. NMDA receptors as targets for drug action in neuropathic pain. *Eur J Pharmacol* 2001;429(1–3):71–78.

136. Gottschalk A, Schroeder F, Ufer M, et al. Amantadine, an N-methyl-D-aspar-tate receptor antagonist, does not enhance postoperative analgesia in women undergoing abdominal hysterectomy. *Anesth Analg* 2001;93(1):192–196.

137. Helmy SA, Bali A. The effect of the preemptive use of the NMDA receptor antagonist dextromethorphan on postoperative analgesic requirements. *Anesth Analg* 2001;92(3):739–744.

138. Yeh CC, Ho ST, Kong SS, et al. Absence of the preemptive analgesic effect of dextromethorphan in total knee replacement under epidural anesthesia. *Acta Anaesthesiol Sin* 2000;38(4):187–193.

139. Himmelseher S, Ziegler-Pithamitsis D, Argiriadou H, et al. Small-dose S(+)-ketamine reduces postoperative pain when applied with ropivacaine in epidural anesthesia for total knee arthroplasty. *Anesth Analg* 2001;92(5): 1290–1295.

140. Wadhwa A, Clarke D, Goodchild CS, et al. Large-dose oral dextromethor-phan as an adjunct to patient-controlled analgesia with morphine after knee surgery. *Anesth Analg* 2001;92(2):448–454.

141. Weinbroum AA, Rudick V, Paret G, et al. The role of dextromethorphan in pain control. *Can J Anaesth* 2000;47(6):585–596.

142. *http://www.usdoj.gov/dea/concern/ketamine.htm.*

143. Eisenberg E, Pud D. Can patients with chronic neuropathic pain be cured by acute administration of the NMDA receptor antagonist amantadine? *Pain* 1998;74(2–3):337–339.

144. Kunzelmann V. Oral combination therapy of zoster neuralgia. Pain reduc-tion by 1-adamantanaminesulfate and carbamazepine per os. *FortschrMed* 1993;111(27):423–425.

145. Tolbert D. Predicted versus actual steady-state plasma levels for oxaprozin, a new nonsteroidal anti-inflammatory drug. *Drug Therapy* 1993(March) [Suppl]:47–51.

146. Singh G, Ramey DR, Morfeld D, et al. Gastrointestinal tract complications of nonsteroidal anti-inflammatory drug treatment in rheumatoid arthritis. *Arch Intern Med* 1996;156:1530–1536.

147. Product information. In: Sifton DW, ed. *Physician's desk reference.* Montvale, NJ: Medical Economics Company, 2002.

148. Muscara MN, Wallace JL. Nitric oxide. V. Therapeutic potential of nitric oxide donors and inhibitors. *Am J Physiol* 1999;276(6 Pt 1):G1313–1316.

149. Bensen WG. Anti-inflammatory and analgesic efficacy of COX-2 specific in-hibition: from investigational trials to clinical experience. *J Rheumatol Suppl* 2000;60:17–24.

150. Bombardier C, Laine L, Reicin A, et al. Comparison of upper intestinal toxic-ity of rofecoxib and naproxen in patients with rheumatoid arthritis. *N Engl J Med* 2000;343:1520–1528.

151. Silverstein F, Faich G, Goldstein J, et al. Gastrointestinal toxicity with cele-coxib vs. nonsteroidal anti-inflammatory drugs for osteoarthritis and rheumatoid arthritis. The CLASS Study: a randomized controlled trial. *JAMA* 2000;284:1247–1255.

152. DuBois RN, Abramson SB, Crofford L, et al. Cyclooxygenase in biology and disease. *FASEB* 1998;12:1063–1073.

153. Brater D. Effects of non-steroidal anti-inflammatory drugs on renal function: focus on cyclooxygenase-2-selective inhibition. *Am J Med* 1999;107:65S–71S.

154. Perazella M, Eras J. Are selective COX-2 inhibitors nephrotoxic? *Am J Kidney Dis* 2000;35(5):937–940.

155. Vioxx prescribing information, 2002.

156. Stevenson DD, Simon RA. Sensitivity to aspirin and nonsteroidal anti-inflammatory drugs. In: Middleton E, Reed CE, Ellis EF, et al., eds. *Allergy principles and practice*, 4th ed. St. Louis: Mosby, 1993.

157. Frishman WH. Effects of nonsteroidal anti-inflammatory drug therapy on blood pressure and peripheral edema. *Am J Cardiol* 2002;89(6A):18D–25D.

158. Mukherjee D, Nissen S, Topol E. Risk of cardiovascular events associated with selective Cox-2 inhibitors. *JAMA* 2001;286:954.

159. Greenberg H, Gottesdiener K, Huntington M, et al. A new cyclooxygenase-2 inhibitor, rofecoxib (Vioxx®), did not alter the antiplatelet effects of low-dose aspirin in healthy volunteers. *J Clin Pharmacol* 2000;40:1509–1515.

160. Leese P, Hubbard R, Karim A, et al. Effects of celecoxib, a novel cyclooxyge-nase-2 inhibitor, on platelet function in healthy adults; a randomized, con-trolled trial. *J Clin Pharmacol* 2000;40:124.

161. Catella-Lawson F, Reilly M, Kapoor S, et al. Cyclooxygenase inhibitors and the antiplatelet effects of aspirin. *N Engl J Med* 2001;345:1809–1817.

162. Saper JR, Winner PK, Lake AE 3rd. An open-label dose-titration study of the efficacy and tolerability of tizanidine hydrochloride tablets in the prophy-laxis of chronic daily headache. *Headache* 2001;41(4):357–368.

163. Delzell JE Jr, Grelle AR. Trigeminal neuralgia. New treatment options for a well-known cause of facial pain. *Arch Fam Med* 1999;8(3):264–268.

164. Fromm GH, Aumentado D, Terrence CF. A clinical and experimental investi-gation of the effects of tizanidine in trigeminal neuralgia. *Pain* 1993;53(3): 265–271.

165. Vorobeichik IAM, Kukushkin ML, Reshetniak VK, et al. The treatment of phantom pain syndrome with tizanidine. *Zh Nevropatol Psikhiatr Im S S Kor-sakova* 1997;97(3):36–39.

166. Kukushkin ML, Ivanova AF, Ovechkin AM, et al. Differential combined drug therapy of phantom pain syndrome after amputation of extremity. *Anesteziol Reanimatol* 1996; (4):39–42.

167. Sos I, Kiss N, Csorba J, et al. Tizanidine in the treatment of acute withdrawal symptoms in heroin dependent patients. *Orv Hetil* 2000;141(15):783–786.

168. Hennies OL. A new skeletal muscle relaxant (DS 103–282) compared to di-azepam in the treatment of muscle spasm of local origin. *J Int Med Res* 1981;9(1):62–68.

169. Berry H, Hutchinson DR. A multicenter placebo-controlled study in general practice to evaluate the efficacy and safety of tizanidine in acute low-back pain. *J Int Med Res* 1988;16(2):75–82.

170. Berry H, Hutchinson DR. Tizanidine and ibuprofen in acute low-back pain: results of a double-blind multicentre study in general practice. *J Int Med Res* 1988;16(2):83–91.

171. Smith TR. Low-dose tizanidine with nonsteroidal anti-inflammatory drugs for detoxification from analgesic rebound headache. *Headache* 2002;42(3): 175–177.

172. Murros K, Kataja M, Hedman C, et al. Modified-release formulation of ti-zanidine in chronic tension-type headache. *Headache* 2000;40(8):633–637.

173. Fogelholm R, Murros K. Tizanidine in chronic tension-type headache: a placebo controlled double-blind cross-over study. *Headache* 1992;32(10): 509–513.

174. Zanaflex prescribing information.

175. Smith HS, Barton AE. Tizanidine in the management of spasticity and mus-culoskeletal complaints in the palliative care population. *Am J Hosp Palliat Care* 2000;17(1):50–58.

176. Portenoy R. Opioid therapy for chronic nonmalignant pain: a review of the critical issues. *J Pain Symptom Manage* 1996;11:203–217.

177. Cherny NI. Opioid analgesics: comparative features and prescribing guide-lines.

178. Ripamonti C, Dickerson ED. Strategies for the treatment of cancer pain in the new millennium. *Drugs* 2001;61(7):955–977.

179. Kefalianakis F, Kugler M, van der Auwera R, et al. Opioid rotation in pain therapy. Case report. *Anaesthesist* 2002;51(1):28–32.

180. Mercadante S. Opioid rotation for cancer pain: rationale and clinical aspects. *Cancer* 1999;86(9):1856–1866.

181. Likar R, Schafer M, Paulak F et al. Intraarticular morphine analgesia in chronic pain patients with osteoarthritis. *Anesth Analg* 1997;84(6):1313–1317.

182. Stein A, Yassouridis A, Szopko C, et al. Intraarticular morphine versus dex-amethasone in chronic arthritis. *Pain* 1999;83(3):525–532.

183. Peloso PM, Bellamy N, Bensen W, et al. Double blind randomized placebo control trial of controlled release codeine in the treatment of osteoarthritis of the hip or knee. *J Rheumatol* 2000;27(3):764–771.

184. Perin ML. Problems with propoxyphene. *Am J Nurs* 2000;100(6):22.

185. Marquardt KA, Tharratt RS, Musallam NA. Fentanyl transdermal (Duro-gesic, Janssen). *Intensive Crit Care Nurs* 1995;11(6):360–361.

186. Jeal W, Benfield P. Transdermal fentanyl. A review of its pharmacological properties and therapeutic efficacy in pain control. *Drugs* 1997;53(1):109–138.

187. Gourlay GK. Treatment of cancer pain with transdermal fentanyl. *Lancet Oncol* 2001;2(3):165–172.

188. Allan L, Hays H, Jensen NH, et al. Randomised crossover trial of transder-mal fentanyl and sustained release oral morphine for treating chronic non-cancer pain. *BMJ* 2001;322(7295):1154–1158.

189. Donner B, Zenz M. Transdermal fentanyl: a new step on the therapeutic lad-der. *Anticancer Drugs* 1995;6[Suppl 3]:39–43.

190. Flannagan LM, Butts JD, Anderson WH. Fentanyl patches left on dead bod-ies—potential source of drug for abusers. *J Forensic Sci* 1996;41(2):320–321.

191. Zambaux M, Bonneaux F, Du H, et al. Validation of a method to inactivate fentanyl in the used devices of Durogesic. *Ann Pharm Fr* 2000;58(3):176–179.

192. Marquardt KA, Tharratt RS. Inhalation abuse of fentanyl patch. *J Toxicol Clin Toxicol* 1994;32(1):75–78.

193. Frolich MA, Giannotti A, Modell JH, et al. Opioid overdose in a patient using a fentanyl patch during treatment with a warming blanket. *Anesth Analg* 2001;93(3):647–648.
194. Newshan G. Heat-related toxicity with the fentanyl transdermal patch. *J Pain Symptom Manage* 1998;16(5):277–278.
195. Mancuso G, Berdondini RM, Passarini B. Eosinophilic pustular eruption associated with transdermal fentanyl. *J Eur Acad Dermatol Venereol* 2001;15 (1):70–72.
196. Quigley C. Hydromorphone for acute and chronic pain. *Cochrane Database Syst Rev* 2002;(1):CD003447.
197. Angst MS, Drover DR, Lotsch J et al. Pharmacodynamics of orally administered sustained- release hydromorphone in humans. *Anesthesiology* 2001;94 (1):63–73.
198. Latta KS, Ginsberg B, Barkin RL. Meperidine: a critical review. *Am J Ther* 2002;9(1):53–68.
199. Altier N, Dion D, Boulanger A, et al. Successful use of methadone in the treatment of chronic neuropathic pain arising from burn injuries: a case-study. *Burns* 2001;27(7):771–775.
200. Makin MK, Ellershaw JE. Substitution of another opioid for morphine. Methadone can be used to manage neuropathic pain related to cancer. *BMJ* 19984;317(7150):81.
201. Gagnon B, Bruera E. Differences in the ratios of morphine to methadone in patients with neuropathic pain versus non-neuropathic pain. *J Pain Symptom Manage* 1999;18(2):120–125.
202. Bruera E, Sweeney C. Methadone use in cancer patients with pain: a review. *J Palliat Med* 2002;5(1):127–138.
203. Bergmans L, Snijdelaar DG, Katz J, et al. Methadone for phantom limb pain. *Clin J Pain* 2002;18(3):203–205.
204. Bruera E, Neumann CM. Role of methadone in the management of pain in cancer patients. *Oncology (Huntingt)* 1999;13(9):1275–1282.
205. Wasserman S. States respond to growing abuse of painkiller. *State Legis* 2001;27(9):33–34.
206. Stambaugh JE, Reder RF, Stambaugh MD, et al. Double-blind, randomized comparison of the analgesic and pharmacokinetic profiles of controlled- and immediate-release oral oxycodone in cancer pain patients. *J Clin Pharmacol* 2001;41(5):500–506.
207. Hale ME, Fleischmann R, Salzman R, et al. Efficacy and safety of controlled-release versus immediate-release oxycodone: randomized, double-blind evaluation in patients with chronic back pain. *Clin J Pain* 1999;15(3):179–183.
208. Likar R. Buprenorphine TTS—A new transdermal therapeutic system [meeting abstract]. Presented at a symposium entitled: Buprenorphine TTS—A Well Proven Substance in a New Guise.
209. Glatt W. A new method for detoxifying opioid-dependent patients. *J Subst Abuse Treat* 1999;17(3):193–197.
210. Wolford R, Kahler J, Mishra P, et al. A prospective comparison of transnasal butorphanol and acetaminophen with codeine for the relief of acute musculoskeletal pain. *Am J Emerg Med* 1997;15(1):101–103.
211. Scott JL, Smith MS, Sanford SM, et al. Effectiveness of transnasal butorphanol for the treatment of musculoskeletal pain. *Am J Emerg Med* 1994; 12(4):469–471.
212. Max MB, Payne R, Edwards WT, et al. *Principles of analgesic use in the treatment of acute pain and cancer pain*, 3d ed. Skokie, IL: American Pain Society, 1993.
213. Harell M, Shea JJ, Emmett JR. Total deafness with chronic propoxyphene abuse. *Laryngoscope* 1978;88(9 Pt 1):1518–1521.
214. Oh AK, Ishiyoma A, Baloh RW. Deafness associated with abuse of hydrocodone/acetaminophen. *Neurology* 2000;54(12):2345.
215. Sindrup SH, Jensen TS. Efficacy of pharmacological treatments of neuropathic pain: an update and effect related to mechanism of drug action. *Pain* 1999;83(3):389–400.
216. MullicanWS, Lacy JR. TRAMAP-ANAG 06 Study Group. Tramadol/acetaminophen combination tablets and codeine/acetaminophen combination capsules for the management of chronic pain: a comparative trial. *Clin Ther* 2001;23(9):1429–1445.
217. Houmes RJM, Voets MA, Verkaaik A, et al. Efficacy and safety of tramadol versus morphine for moderate and severe postoperative pain with special regard to respiratory depression. *Anesth Analg* 1992;74:520–514.
218. Osipova NA, Novikov GA, Beresnev VA, et al. Analgesic effect of tramadol in patients with chronic pain: a comparison with prolonged action morphine sulfate. *Curr Ther Res* 1991;50:812–821.
219. Rodrigues N, Rodrigues PE. Tramadol in cancer pain. *Curr Ther Res* 1989; 46:1142–1148.
220. Keitel W, Frerick H, Kuhn U, et al. Capsicum pain plaster in chronic nonspecific low back pain. *Arzneimittelforschung* 2001;51(11):896–903.
221. Jensen PG, Larson JR. Management of painful diabetic neuropathy. *Drugs Aging* 2001;18(10):737–749.
222. Alper BS, Lewis PR. Treatment of postherpetic neuralgia: a systematic review of the literature. *J Fam Pract* 2002;51(2):121–128.
223. Ribbers GM, Stam HJ. Complex regional pain syndrome type I treated with topical capsaicin: a case report. *Arch Phys Med Rehabil* 2001;82(6):851–852.
224. Cannon DT, Wu Y. Topical capsaicin as an adjuvant analgesic for the treatment of traumatic amputee neurogenic residual limb pain. *Arch Phys Med Rehabil* 1998;79(5):591–593.
225. Paice JA, Ferrans CE, Lashley FR, et al. Topical capsaicin in the management of HIV-associated peripheral neuropathy. *J Pain Symptom Manage* 2000;19(1): 45–52.
226. Low PA, Opfer-Gehrking TL, Dyck PJ, et al. Double-blind, placebo-controlled study of the application of capsaicin cream in chronic distal painful polyneuropathy. *Pain* 1995;62(2):163–168.
227. Harding LM, Murphy A, Kinnman E, et al. Characterization of secondary hyperalgesia produced by topical capsaicin jelly—a new experimental tool for pain research. *Eur J Pain* 2001;5(4):363–371.
228. Malisza KL, Docherty JC. Capsaicin as a source for painful stimulation in functional MRI. *J Magn Reson Imag* 2001;14(4):341–347.
229. May A, Buchel C, Turner R, et al. Magnetic resonance angiography in facial and other pain: neurovascular mechanisms of trigeminal sensation. *J Cereb Blood Flow Metab* 2001;21(10):1171–1176.
230. Ngom PI, Dubray C, Woda A, et al. A human oral capsaicin pain model to assess topical anesthetic-analgesic drugs. *Neurosci Lett* 2001;316(3):149–152.
231. Kwak JY, Jung JY, Hwang SW, et al. A capsaicin-receptor antagonist, capsazepine, reduces inflammation-induced hyperalgesic responses in the rat: evidence for an endogenous capsaicin-like substance. *Neuroscience* 1998;86 (2):619–626.
232. Barbanti G, Maggi CA, Beneforti P, et al. Relief of pain following intravesical capsaicin in patients with hypersensitive disorders of the lower urinary tract. *Br J Urol* 1993;71(6):686–691.
233. Fusco BM, Marabini S, Maggi CA, et al. Preventative effect of repeated nasal applications of capsaicin in cluster headache. *Pain* 1994;59(3):321–325.
234. Burrows NP, Norris PG. Treatment of PUVA-induced skin pain with capsaicin. *Br J Dermatol* 1994;131(4):584–585.
235. Filiaci F, Zambetti G, Ciofalo A, et al. Local treatment of aspecific nasal hyperreactivity with capsaicin. *Allergol Immunopathol (Madr)* 1994;22(6):264–268.
236. Epstein JB, Marcoe JH. Topical application of capsaicin for treatment of oral neuropathic pain and trigeminal neuralgia. *Oral Surg Oral Med Oral Pathol* 1994;77(2):135–140.
237. Hersh EV, Pertes RA, Ochs HA. Topical capsaicin-pharmacology and potential role in the treatment of temporomandibular pain. *J Clin Dent* 1994;5(2): 54–59.
238. Tominaga M, Julius D. Capsaicin receptor in the pain pathway. *Jpn J Pharmacol* 2000;83(1):20–24.
239. Fusco BM, Giacovazzo M. Peppers and pain. The promise of capsaicin. *Drugs* 1997;53(6):909–914.
240. Menkes CJ, Renoux M. Substance P and rheumatic diseases. *RevPract* 1994; 44(12):1569–1571.
241. Minami T, Bakoshi S, Nakano H, et al. The effects of capsaicin cream on prostaglandin-induced allodynia. *Anesth Analg* 2001;93(2):419–423.
242. Yang K, Kumamoto E, Furue H, et al. Capsaicin induces a slow inward current which is not mediated by substance P in substantia gelatinosa neurons of the rat spinal cord. *Neuropharmacology* 2000 23;39(11):2185–2194.
243. Forst T, Pohlmann T, Kunt T, et al. The influence of local capsaicin treatment on small nerve fibre function and neurovascular control in symptomatic diabetic neuropathy. *Acta Diabetol* 2002;39(1):1–6.
244. Trowbridge A, Boese CK, Woodruff B, et al. Incidence of posthospitalization proximal deep vein thrombosis after total hip arthroplasty: a pilot study. *Clin Orthop*; 299:203–208.
245. Tait RC. Anticoagulation in patients with thromboembolic disease. *Thorax* 2001;56 [Suppl 2]:ii30–37.
246. Merli GJ. Treatment of deep venous thrombosis and pulmonary embolism with low molecular weight heparin in the geriatric patient population. *Clin Geriatr Med* 2001;17(1):93–106.
247. Hyers TM, Agnelli G, Hull RD, et al. Antithrombotic therapy for venous thromboembolic disease. *Chest* 2001;119[1 Suppl]:176S–193S.
248. Merli GJ. Low-molecular-weight heparins versus unfractionated heparin in the treatment of deep vein thrombosis and pulmonary embolism. *Am J Phys Med Rehabil* 2000;79(5 Suppl):S9–S16.
249. Geerts WH, Heit JA, Clagett GP, et al. Prevention of venous thromboembolism. *Chest* 2001;119[1 Suppl]:132S–175S.
250. Collins R, Scrimgeour A, Yusuf S, et al. Reduction in fatal pulmonary embolism and venous thrombosis by perioperative administration of subcutaneous heparin: an overview of results of randomized trials in general, orthopedic, and urologic surgery. *N Engl J Med* 1988;318:1162–1173.
251. Antman EM, Kereiakes DJ. Antithrombotic therapy in unstable angina/non-ST elevation myocardial infarction: the evolving role of low-molecular-weight heparin. *J Invasive Cardiol* 2000;12[Suppl E]:E1–E4.
252. Davidson BL. DVT treatment in 2000: state of the art. *Orthopedics* 2000;23[6 Suppl]:S651–S654.
253. Yeager BF, Matheny SC. Low-molecular-weight heparin in outpatient treatment of DVT. *Am Fam Physician* 1999;59(4):945–952.
254. Cohen M. The role of low-molecular-weight heparin in the management of acute coronary syndromes. *Curr Opin Cardiol* 2001;16(6):384–389.
255. Wells PS. Outpatient treatment of patients with deep-vein thrombosis or pulmonary embolism. *Curr Opin Pulm Med* 2001;7(5):360–364.
256. Aguilar D, Goldhaber SZ. Clinical uses of low-molecular-weight heparins. *Chest* 1999;115(5):1418–1423.
257. Acostamadiedo JM, Iyer UG, Owen J. Danaparoid sodium. *Expert Opin Pharmacother* 2000;1(4):803–814.
258. Hirsh J. New anticoagulants. *Am Heart J* 2001;142[2 Suppl]:S3–S8.
259. McKeage K, Plosker GL. Argatroban. *Drugs* 2001;61(4):515–522.
260. Imperiale TF, Speroff T. A meta-analysis of methods to prevent venous thromboembolism following total hip replacement. *JAMA* 1994;271:1780–1785. [Erratum, *JAMA* 1995;273:288].
261. Chimowitz MI, Kokkinos J, Strong J, et al. The warfarin-aspirin asymptomatic intracranial disease study. *Neurology* 1995;45:1488–1493.

262. Stroke Prevention in Atrial Fibrillation Investigators. Warfarin compared to aspirin for prevention of thromboembolism in atrial fibrillation. *Lancet* 1994;343:687–691.

263. Pineo GF, Hull RD, Marder VJ. Orally active heparin and low-molecular-weight heparin. *Curr Opin Pulm Med* 2001;7(5):344–348.

264. Ginsberg JS. Management of venous thromboembolism. *N Engl J Med* 1996;335:1816–1828.

265. Raschke RA, Reilly BM, Guidry JR, et al. The weight-based heparin dosing nomogram compared with a standard care nomogram: a randomized controlled trial. *Ann Intern Med* 1993;119:874–881.

266. Cruickshank MK, Levine MN, Hirsh J, et al. A standard heparin nomogram for the management of heparin therapy. *Arch Intern Med* 1991;151:333–337.

267. Hull RD, Raskob GE, Rosenbloom D, et al. Oral anticoagulants: mechanism of action, clinical effectiveness, and optimal therapeutic range. *Chest* 1992;102[Suppl]:312S–325S.

268. Hull RD, Pineo GF, Stein PD, et al. Extended out-of-hospital low-molecular-weight heparin prophylaxis against deep venous thrombosis in patients after elective hip arthroplasty: a systematic review. *Ann Intern Med* 2001;135 (10):858–869.

269. Hirsh J, Dalen JE, Deykin D, et al. Oral anticoagulants: mechanism of action, clinical effectiveness, and optimal therapeutic range. *Chest* 1992;102[Suppl]: 312S–325S.

270. Bergqvist D, Benoni G, Bjorgell, O, et al. Low-molecular-weight heparin (Enoxaparin) as prophylaxis against venous thromboembolism after total hip replacement. *N Engl J Med* 1996;335:696–700.

271. Antiplatelet Trialists' Collaboration. Collaborative overview of randomised trials of antiplatelet therapy. I: Prevention of death, myocardial infarction, and stroke by prolonged antiplatelet therapy in various categories of patients. *Br Med J* 1994;308:81–106.

272. CAST: randomised placebo-controlled trial of early aspirin use in 20,000 patients with acute ischaemic stroke. CAST (Chinese Acute Stroke Trial) Collaborative Group. *Lancet* 1997;349(9066):1641–1649.

273. The International Stroke Trial (IST): a randomised trial of aspirin, subcutaneous heparin, both, or neither among 19,435 patients with acute ischaemic stroke. International Stroke Trial Collaborative Group. *Lancet* 1997;349 (9065):1569–1581.

274. Easton JD. What have we learned from recent antiplatelet trials? *Neurology* 1998;51[3 Suppl 3]:S36–S38.

275. Barer D. CAPRIE trial. *Lancet* 1997;349(9048):355–356.

276. A randomised, blinded, trial of clopidogrel versus aspirin in patients at risk of ischaemic events (CAPRIE). CAPRIE Steering Committee. *Lancet* 1996; 348(9038):1329–1339.

277. Sharis PJ, Cannon CP, Loscalzo J. The antiplatelet effects of ticlopidine and clopidogrel. *Ann Intern Med* 1998;129(5):394–405.

278. Bhatt DL, Kapadia SR, Yadav JS, et al. Update on clinical trials of antiplatelet therapy for cerebrovascular diseases. *Cerebrovasc Dis* 2000;10[Suppl 5]:34–40.

279. Paciaroni M, Bogousslavsky J. Clopidogrel for cerebrovascular prevention. *Cerebrovasc Dis* 1999;9(5):253–260.

280. Majid A, Delanty N, Kantor J. Antiplatelet agents for secondary prevention of ischemic stroke. *Ann Pharmacother* 2001;35(10):1241–1247.

281. Grotta JC, Norris JW, Kamm B. Prevention of stroke with ticlopidine: who benefits most? *Neurology* 1992;42:111–115.

282. Sacco RL, Elkind MS. Update on antiplatelet therapy for stroke prevention. *Arch Intern Med* 2000;160(11):1579–1582.

283. Diener HC, Cunha L, Forbes C, et al. European Stroke Prevention Study. 2. Dipyridamole and acetylsalicylic acid in the secondary prevention of stroke. *J Neurol Sci* 1996;143(1–2):1–13.

284. Sivenius J, Cunha L, Diener HC, et al. Second European Stroke Prevention Study: antiplatelet effect is effective regardless of age. ESPS2 Working Group. *Acta Neurol Scand* 1999;99(1):54–60.

285. Shah H, Gondek K. Aspirin plus extended-release dipyridamole or clopidogrel compared with aspirin monotherapy for the prevention of recurrent ischemic stroke: a cost-effectiveness analysis. *Clin Ther* 2000;22(3):362–370.

286. Lee TM, Su SF, Hwang JJ, et al. Differential lipogenic effects of cilostazol and pentoxifylline in patients with intermittent claudication: potential role for interleukin-6. *Atherosclerosis* 2001;158(2):471–476.

287. Dawson DL, Cutler BS, Hiatt WR, et al. A comparison of cilostazol and pentoxifylline for treating intermittent claudication. *Am J Med* 2000;109(7): 523–530.

288. Beebe HG, Dawson DL, Cutler BS, et al. A new pharmacological treatment for intermittent claudication: results of a randomized, multicenter trial. *Arch Intern Med* 1999;159(17):2041–2050.

289. Dawson DL, Cutler BS, Meissner MH, et al. Cilostazol has beneficial effects in treatment of intermittent claudication: results from a multicenter, randomized, prospective, double-blind trial. *Circulation* 1998;98(7):678–686.

290. Callahan A. Cerebrovascular disease and statins: a potential addition to the therapeutic armamentarium for stroke prevention. *Am J Cardiol* 2001;88(7B): 33J–37J.

291. Vaughan CJ, Delanty N, Basson CT. Statin therapy and stroke prevention. *Curr Opin Cardiol* 2001;16(4):219–224.

292. Amarenco P. Hypercholesterolemia, lipid-lowering agents, and the risk for brain infarction. *Neurology* 2001;57[5 Suppl 2]:S35–S44.

293. Delanty N, Vaughan CJ, Sheehy N. Statins and neuroprotection. *Expert Opin Invest Drugs* 2001;10(10):1847–1853.

294. Fenton JW Jr, Shen GX. Statins as cellular antithrombotics. *Haemostasis* 1999;29(2–3):166–169.

295. Braddom RL, Rocco JF. Autonomic dysreflexia. *Am J Phys Med Rehabil* 1991;70:234–241.

296. Tam SW, Worcel M, Wyllie M. Yohimbine: a clinical review. *Pharmacol Ther* 2001;91(3):215–243.

297. Reid D, Morales A, Harris C, et al. Double-blind trial of yohimbine in treatment of psychogenic impotence. *Lancet* 1987;2:421–423.

298. Schapiro RT. Management of spasticity, pain, and paroxysmal phenomena in multiple sclerosis. *Curr Neurol Neurosci Rep* 2001;1(3):299–302.

299. Burchiel KJ, Hsu FP. Pain and spasticity after spinal cord injury: mechanisms and treatment. *Spine* 2001;26[24 Suppl]:S146–S160.

300. Nance PW. Alpha adrenergic and serotonergic agents in the treatment of spastic hypertonia. *Phys Med Rehabil Clin N Am* 2001;12(4):889–905.

301. Meythaler JM, Guin-Renfroe S, Johnson A, et al. Prospective assessment of tizanidine for spasticity due to acquired brain injury. *Arch Phys Med Rehabil* 2001;82(9):1155–1163.

302. Gelber DA, Good DC, Dromerick A, et al. Open-label dose-titration safety and efficacy study of tizanidine hydrochloride in the treatment of spasticity associated with chronic stroke. *Stroke* 2001;32(8):1841–1846.

303. Elovic E. Principles of pharmaceutical management of spastic hypertonia. *Phys Med Rehabil Clin N Am* 2001;12(4):793–816, vii.

304. Remy-Neris O, Denys P, Bussel B. Intrathecal clonidine for controlling spastic hypertonia. *Phys Med Rehabil Clin N Am* 2001;12(4):939–951, ix.

305. Kingery WS. A critical review of controlled clinical trials for peripheral neuropathic pain and complex regional pain syndromes. *Pain* 1997;73(2): 123–139.

306. Rauck RL, Eisenach JC, Jackson K, Young LD, Southern J. Epidural clonidine treatment for refractory reflex sympathetic dystrophy. *Anesthesiology* 1993;79 (6):1163–1169.

307. Lewis E, Hunsicker L, Bain R, et al. The effect of angiotensin-converting-enzyme inhibition on diabetic nephropathy. *N Engl J Med* 1993;329:1456–1462.

308. Vivian EM, Goebig ML. Slowing the progression of renal disease in diabetic patients. *Ann Pharmacother* 2001;35(4):452–463.

309. Alberts MJ. Secondary prevention of stroke and the expanding role of the neurologist. *Cerebrovasc Dis* 2002;13[Suppl 1]:12–16.

310. Mimran A, Ribstein J. Angiotensin receptor blockers: pharmacology and clinical significance. *J Am Soc Nephrol* 1999;10[Suppl 12]:S273–S277.

311. Flores AM. Hospital based cardiac rehabilitation. In: Halar E, ed. Cardiac rehabilitation. Part II. *PM&R Clin North Am*. Philadelphia: WB Sanders, 1995: 243–261.

312. Goldstein S. Benefits of beta-blocker therapy for heart failure: weighing the evidence. *Arch Intern Med* 2002;162(6):641–648.

313. Foody JM, Farrell MH, Krumholz HM. beta-Blocker therapy in heart failure: scientific review. *JAMA* 2002;287(7):883–889.

314. Marjama-Lyons J, Koller W. Tremor-predominant Parkinson's disease. Approaches to treatment. *Drugs Aging* 2000;16(4):273–278.

315. Louis ED. A new twist for stopping the shakes? Revisiting GABAergic therapy for essential tremor. *Arch Neurol* 1999;56(7):807–808.

316. Uitti RJ. Medical treatment of essential tremor and Parkinson's disease. *Geriatrics* 1998;53(5):46–48, 53–57.

317. Fava M. Psychopharmacologic treatment of pathologic aggression. *Psychiatr Clin North Am* 1997;20(2):427–451.

318. Haspel T. Beta-blockers and the treatment of aggression. *Harv Rev Psychiatry* 1995;2(5):274–281.

319. Bell KR, Cardenas DD. New frontiers of neuropharmacologic treatment of brain injury agitation. *NeuroRehabilitation* 1995;5:223–244.

320. Grossman E, Messerli FH, Grodzicki T, et al. Should a moratorium be placed on sublingual nifedipine capsules given for hypertensive emergencies and pseudoemergencies? *JAMA* 1996;276:1328–1331.

321. Maynard FM. Immobilization hypercalcemia following spinal cord injury. *Arch Phys Med Rehabil* 1986;67:41–44.

322. Ernst CB, Stanley JC, ed. *Therapy in vascular surgery*, 2nd ed. Philadelphia: BC Decker, 1991.

323. Amir I, Sharma R, Bauman WA, et al. Bowel care for individuals with spinal cord injury: comparison of four approaches. *J Spinal Cord Med* 1998;21(1): 21–24.

324. Frisbie JH. Improved bowel care with a polyethylene glycol based bisacodyl suppository. *J Spinal Cord Med* 1997;20(2):227–229.

325. Moldofsky H, Lue FA, Mously C, et al. The effect of zolpidem in patients with fibromyalgia: a dose ranging, double blind, placebo controlled, modified crossover study. *J Rheumatol*;23;3:529–533.

326. Reichard P, Nilsson B-Y, Rosenquist U. The effect of long-term intensified insulin treatment on the development of microvascular complications of diabetes mellitus. *N Engl J Med* 1993;329:304.

327. The Diabetes Control and Complications Trial Research Group. The effect of intensive treatment of diabetes on the development and progression of long-term complications in insulin-dependent diabetes mellitus. *N Engl J Med*;329:977.

328. Centers for Disease Control and Prevention, National Center for Injury Prevention and Control: Traumatic Brain Injury in the United States: A Report to Congress. Atlanta: CDC, 1999. Available at http://www.cdc.gov/ncipc/pub-res/tbicongress.htm. Accessed February 24, 2004.

329. Gualtieri CT. Review: pharmacotherapy and the neurobehavioral sequelae of traumatic brain injury. *Brain Injury* 1998;2:101–129.

330. Scharf MB. Sachais BA. Sleep laboratory evaluation of the effects and efficacy of trazodone in depressed insomniac patients. *J Clin Psychiatry* 1990;51[Suppl]:13–17.

331. Mysiw WJ, Sandel ME. The agitated brain injured patient. Part 2: pathophysiology and treatment. *Arch Phys Med Rehabil* 1997;78:213–220.

332. Nahas Z, Arlinghaus KA, Kotrla KJ, et al. Rapid response of emotional incontinence to selective serotonin reuptake inhibitors. *J Neuropsychiatry Clin Neurosci* 1998;10:453–455.

333. Stahl SM. *Essential psychopharmacology: neuroscientific basis and practical applications.* Cambridge, UK: Cambridge University Press, 2000.

334. Beetar JT, Guilmette TJ, Sparadeo FR. Sleep and pain complaints in symptomatic traumatic brain injury and neurologic populations. *Arch Phys Med Rehabil* 1996;77:1298–1302.

335. Fichtenberg NL, Zafonte RD, Putnam S, et al. Insomnia in a post-acute brain injury sample. *Brain Injury* 2002;16:197–206.

336. Challman TD, Lipsky JJ. Methylphenidate: its pharmacology and uses. *Mayo Clin Proc* 2000;75:711–721.

337. Feeney DM, Gonzalez A, Law WA. Amphetamine, haloperidol and experience interact to affect the rate of recovery after motor cortex injury. *Science* 1982;217:855–857.

338. Goldstein LB, Matchar DB, Morgenlander JC, et al. Influence of drugs on the recovery of sensorimotor function after stroke. *J Neurol Rehabil* 1990;4: 137–144.

339. Rao N, Jellnick M, Woolstion D. Agitation in closed head injury: haloperidol effects on rehabilitation outcomes. *Arch Phys Med Rehabil* 1985;66:30–34.

340. Chrisostomo EA, Duncan PW, Propst MA, et al. Evidence that amphetamine with physical therapy promotes recovery of motor function in stroke patients. *Ann Neurol* 1988;23:94–97.

341. Zafonte RD, Lexell J, Cullen N. Possible applications for dopaminergic agents following traumatic brain injury: Part 1. *J Head Trauma Rehabil* 2000;15:1179–1182.

342. Krause MF, Maki P. The combined use of amantadine and L-dopa/carbidopa in the treatment of chronic brain injury. *Brain Injury.* 1997;11:455–460.

343. Haig AJ, Ruess JM. Recovery from vegetative state of six months' duration with Sinemet (levodopa/carbidopa). *Arch Phys Med Rehabil* 1990;71:1081–1083.

344. Chandra B. Treatment of disturbances of consciousness caused by measles encephalitis with levodopa. *Eur Neurol.* 1978;17:265–270.

345. Passler MA, Riggs RV. Positive outcomes in traumatic brain injury—vegetative state: patients treated with bromocriptine. *Arch Phys Med Rehabil* 2001;82:311–315.

346. Zafonte RD, Lexell J, Cullen N. Possible applications for dopaminergic agents following traumatic brain injury: part 2. *J Head Trauma Rehabil* 2001;16:112–116.

347. Gaultieri CT, Evans RW. Stimulant treatment for the neurobehavioral sequelae of traumatic brain injury. *Brain Injury* 1988;2:273–290.

348. Zafonte RD, Watanabe T, Mann NR. Amantadine: a potential treatment for the minimally conscious state. *Brain Injury* 1998;12:617–621.

349. Chandler M, Barnhill J, Gualtieri C. Amantadine for the agitated head-injured patient. *Brain Injury* 1988;2:309–311.

350. Wroblewski BA, Leary JM, Phelan AM, et al. Methylphenidate and seizure frequency in brain injured patients with seizure disorders. *J Clin Psychiatry.* 1982;53:86–89.

351. Kaelin DL, Cifu DX, Matthies B. Methylphenidate effect on attention deficit in the acutely brain-injured adult. *Arch Phys Med Rehabil* 1996;77:6–9.

352. Plenger PM, Dixon CE, Castillo RM. Subacute methylphenidate for moderate to moderately severe traumatic brain injury: a preliminary double-blind placebo-controlled study. *Arch Phys Med Rehabil* 1996;77:536–540.

353. Speech TJ, Rao SM, Osmon DC. A double-blind controlled study of methylphenidate treatment in closed head injury. *Brain Injury* 1993;7:333–338.

354. Masanic CA, Bayley MT, vanReekum R. Open-label study of donepezil in traumatic brain injury. *Arch Phys Med Rehabil* 2001;82:896–901.

355. Rammohan KW, Rosenberg JH, Lynn DJ. Efficacy and safety of modafinil (Provigil) for the treatment of fatigue in multiple sclerosis: a two centre phase 2 study. *J Neurol Neurosurg Psychiatry* 2002;72:179–183.

356. Elovic E. Use of Provigil for underarousal following TBI. *J Head Trauma Rehabil* 2000;15:1068–1071.

CHAPTER 57

Medical Emergencies in Rehabilitation Medicine

Keith M. Robinson, Deborah J. Franklin, and William H. Shull

An emergency is a perilous situation that arises suddenly and threatens the life or welfare of a person or a group of people, as a natural disaster, medical crisis, or trauma situation (1). This definition must be broadened within the context of rehabilitation, in which medical emergencies include life-threatening episodes, events that interfere with potential therapeutic functional effects of rehabilitation treatments, and the potentially deleterious effects of rehabilitation treatments.

EMERGENCIES SHOULD BE EXPECTED

Emergencies should be expected in rehabilitation because of the nature of the patient populations who are being treated under circumstances of increasing financial restraint. Older and more medically complex patients are being treated in rehabilitation programs (2). The prospective payment reimbursement formulae for inpatient and home rehabilitation programs potentially encourage rehabilitation specialists to treat patients in a more compressed temporal context (3–7).

Although the biological life span of the human species has not been extended, more American people will continue to survive into old age, particularly beyond the age of 80 (8,9). Normal aging has been biologically characterized as a linear decrease in adaptive or reserve capacity across organ systems. The experience of acute illness and related medical and surgical treatments, including rehabilitation treatments such as therapeutic exercise, can be viewed more precariously as people grow older (10). Aging is associated with more medical comorbidity and higher levels of functional disability (11–13). Furthermore, aging in this country does not exclude exposure to highly technological, expensive, lifesaving treatments, despite increased vulnerability to undesirable complications from these treatments (14–16).

Rehabilitation specialists in all treatment settings are encountering more medically complex patients, including those who have spinal cord and traumatic brain injuries, multiple organ system trauma, cerebrovascular and neurodegenerative diseases, organ transplantations, cancer, and end-stage manifestations of chronic diseases, such as severe heart failure, renal failure, and obstructive/restrictive pulmonary diseases. Such patients are being treated with expensive chemotherapeutic agents and surgical procedures in critical care settings and are

surviving (17–19). The social expectation of continued costly investment in life-continuing treatments encompasses rehabilitation. Moreover, exposure to rehabilitation treatments has become more compressed as cost-cutting efforts have been continued with the 1997 Balanced Budget Act. Medicare-directed prospective payment for acute hospitalization, inpatient rehabilitation and home care, and managed-care health insurance plans are limiting treatment contacts by rehabilitation specialists. The impact of "across the board" service compression in treating more medically complex patients remains unclear, but several positive and negative influences can be postulated. On the positive side, decreasing hospital lengths of stay may promote earlier remobilization and less deconditioning, however, there may be fewer therapeutic contacts by rehabilitation specialists to direct, monitor, and sustain early remobilization efforts in hospital and home-care settings. This potentially places the responsibility of reinforcing treatments that enhance and maintain activity levels on to the patient and/or the caregivers. An empowered patient/consumer theoretically emerges from rehabilitation therapeutic contacts that emphasize developing/teaching treatment programs with/to their clients, rather than performing "hands-on" treatment. On the negative side, less time is spent by rehabilitation specialists closely observing responses to a progression of rational treatments, allowing fewer opportunities to individualize treatment programs as directed by spontaneous recovery and to troubleshoot during treatment, and then to intervene before complications evolve into more severe problems that require emergent interventions (5,7).

THE ROLE OF THE PHYSIATRIST

When medically managing patients who are receiving rehabilitation interventions, the physiatrist can be viewed as a multidimensional gatekeeper. As a gatekeeper, the physiatrist coordinates medical care in the roles of both general medical provider and medical specialist. During inpatient rehabilitation, the physiatrist provides frontline management of patients' medical problems, often in collaboration with other medical and surgical specialists (20). The physiatrist must anticipate and troubleshoot life-threatening events. This general medical management role involves resuming or continuing all previous

---

TABLE 57-1.   Guidelines for Requesting Specialty Consultation in Rehabilitation

1. Ask a specific question.
2. Assess the patient before calling the consultant to develop an empiric database of symptoms, signs, and laboratory and radiographic studies.
3. Communicate directly with the consultant over the telephone or in person.
4. Collaborate with the consultant as a comanager and educational resource.
5. Ask for one specialty consultation at a time to minimize conflicting advice.

From Goldman L, Lee T, Rudd P. Ten commandments for effective consultations. *Arch Intern Med* 1983;143:1753–1755.

---

treatments, whether they are medications or therapeutic precautions recommended by other medical and surgical specialists. A common example of performing this role includes transitioning diabetic patients during the postsurgical period from sliding scale insulin regimens back toward their usual doses of NPH/regular insulin and/or oral agents, as their diet is advanced and as their activity increases, using blood glucose via scheduled finger sticks for guidance. This general medical role involves coordinating recommendations made by an array of consultants in a rational manner. Appropriate consultation with nonphysiatric colleagues assumes that the physiatrist is anticipating that minor medical problems can evolve toward life-threatening events and that early consultation should be requested for treatment advice to prevent such events from occurring. For example, consulting a nephrologist to assess a well-hydrated patient with heart failure whose serum creatinine is increasing without clear reasons seems reasonable. Guidelines for requesting nonphysiatric consultation as a general medical provider in rehabilitation settings are summarized in Table 57-1 (20,21).

As the medical specialist in disability, the physiatrist is the best physician to prescribe, monitor, triage, and revise rehabilitation services in all treatment settings. It is the responsibility of the physiatrist to incorporate medical information into the rehabilitation plan, usually by articulating therapeutic guidelines and precautions. Common examples include establishing heart rate and blood pressure parameters at rest and during activity for patients with cardiovascular diseases to define when treatment should be held or interrupted, and requesting monitoring of hemoglobin-oxygen saturation levels via pulse oximetry at rest and during exercise in oxygen-dependent patients to guide weaning of supplemental oxygen. Other medical and surgical specialists expect that the physiatrist operationalize this role. Nonmedical rehabilitation specialists similarly expect that the physiatrist perform this role in a collaborative and nonhierarchical manner.

COMORBIDITY IN REHABILITATION

Higher levels of medical complexity and comorbidity that often is aging related predicts the occurrence of medical emergencies when patients are participating in rehabilitation programs. Common comorbid conditions include amputation, cerebrovascular diseases, dementia, chronic obstructive pulmonary disease, heart failure, peripheral neuropathy, and other end-organ manifestations of diabetes mellitus—all being examples of later-stage disease processes associated with com-

promised physiologic reserves to handle stress. Patients with such conditions may appear medically stable during periods of inactivity, but medical instability can become unmasked during therapeutic exercise and activities during rehabilitation.

Death is rare during inpatient rehabilitation. The overall annual mortality rate on inpatient rehabilitation services is at most 3%. The annual rate of transfer back to acute medical/surgical services because of medical instability ranges from 5% to 20%, despite screening for severe medical conditions that would preclude reasonable participation in rehabilitation programs (20, 22–26). Many inpatient rehabilitation programs continue to be comfortable treating medical complications when the potential interference with participation is minimal, such as urinary tract infections with or without sepsis, pneumonias requiring supplemental oxygen, nebulized bronchodilators provided by respiratory therapists and intravenous antibiotics, deep venous thrombosis requiring heparin and a few days of bed rest, and delirium that is slowly resolving. Felsenthal and colleagues have characterized the quantity and severity of medical complications of elderly patients who participated in inpatient rehabilitation: a mean of 3.7 indications for medical interventions per patient was reported, and most were easily handled by the physiatrists (20). Siegler and colleagues have described the degree of comorbidity of patients who participated in inpatient rehabilitation: a mean of 1.8 comorbid conditions per patient was reported, and more comorbid conditions and lower functional status were predictive of medical complications. Furthermore, this study reported that these medical complications necessitated program interruption in more than half of the studied patients and that almost 90% of these patients had at least one complication (25). In both of these studies, mortality rate was less than 1% from cardiovascular and pulmonary embolic sources. Common complications defined in both studies are summarized in Table 57-2. It is clear that physiatrists, particularly those who are increasingly identified as "hospitalists" must be prepared to manage a broad range of medical conditions. Finally, a relationship between a higher level of comorbidity and a lower level of function should be expected in patients who participate in rehabilitation (27,28).

MEDICAL EMERGENCIES COMMONLY SEEN IN REHABILITATION

What is idiosyncratic about medical emergencies when they occur in rehabilitation? Rehabilitation treatments, particularly strengthening and endurance types of therapeutic exercise, can

---

TABLE 57-2.   Common Medical Complications Seen in Rehabilitation

Infectious	Urinary tract infections, pneumonia
Cardiovascular	Heart failure, supraventricular arrhythmias
Thromboembolic	Deep venous thrombosis, pulmonary embolism
Orthopedic	Wound infections, hip prosthesis dislocation
Gastrointestinal	Pseudomembranous enterocolitis, gastroesophagitis
Neurologic	Delirium, new focal findings
Rheumatologic	Acute gouty arthritis, septic arthritis
Renal/metabolic:	Dehydration, worsening renal function with oliguria, electrolyte imbalances

From Felsenthal G, Cohen S, Hilton B, et al. The physiatrist as primary physician for patient on an in-patient rehabilitation unit. *Arch Phys Med Rehabil* 1984;65:375–378; and Goldman L, Lee T, Rudd P. Ten commandments for effective consultations. *Arch Intern Med* 1983;143:1753–1755.

be viewed as physiologically stressful when applied during the recovery phase of illness. This necessitates close monitoring and anticipation that emergencies are likely. Although the differential diagnosis for any presenting symptom or sign is the same in every medical setting, including rehabilitation, the nature of the impairments that results in the activity limitations that are being treated in rehabilitation shift certain diagnostic possibilities higher. For example, shoulder pain in the hemiparetic limb of a patient recovering from a stroke can be caused by a number of common diagnostic possibilities, including osteoarthritis, tendonitis, trauma, myocardial ischemia, and cervical radiculopathy. However, stroke-associated phenomena—such as glenohumeral subluxation associated with poor tone development, sympathetically mediated pain, or imbalance of muscle tone development between anterior and posterior muscle groups—deserve more serious consideration. Furthermore, the nature of the patient population in rehabilitation settings lends to a lack of specificity during clinical symptom/sign presentation. Those patients who are elderly, who are cognitively impaired, and who have sensory deficits are particularly vulnerable because of an inability to experience physiologically the expected somatic warnings and/or communicate these to care providers in a focused manner. For example, hemiparetic lower-limb swelling associated with cellulitis or venous thrombosis in the diabetic stroke patient recovering from a delirium cannot be experienced readily, because of multifactorial sensory system compromise, until later in its natural progression and potentially closer to the event, becoming catastrophic.

All rehabilitation providers should have access to current medical information to facilitate providing background information and direction on how to handle emergencies and to assist in formulating questions to address consultants. This medical information could be obtained through Internet search engines such as MedLine and through purchase of resource textbooks in internal medicine, general surgery, orthopedic surgery, neurology, geriatric medicine, emergency medicine, and pharmaceuticals. Often useful are abridged handbooks of medical and neurologic therapeutics, emergency treatments, and basic and advanced cardiopulmonary life support.

Autonomic Dysreflexia

Traditionally, autonomic dysreflexia has evolved as the prototype of a medical emergency managed in rehabilitation. Its consequences are life threatening and include hypertensive crisis, stroke, and/or seizures. Its treatments are often common-sensical and simple. However, they require education of patients at risk, their care providers, and health-care personnel unfamiliar with complications of cervical and high thoracic spinal cord injuries. For example, a discussion with the 35-year-old pregnant patient with tetraparesis, her partner, obstetrician, and anesthesiologist during the pregnancy, labor, delivery, and postpartum phase about the warning symptoms/signs and treatments of autonomic dysreflexia could be lifesaving to this patient and infant. There are several normal pregnancy-related events that the compromised nervous system could interpret as noxious stimuli, including uterine contractions before and after delivery, an inflamed episiotomy scar, and breast-feeding. An algorithm, as depicted in Figure 57-1, can be applied to guide treatment (29).

Among the population with spinal cord injury with lesions at or above the midthoracic level, the symptoms and signs of autonomic dysreflexia can indicate an array of underlying disorders, such as urinary tract infection, venous thrombosis, and pneumonia. Because of fundamental disturbances in autonomic feedback systems that control reflex physiologic re-

sponses to acute illnesses including fever, tachycardia, tachypnea, and appreciation of pain, these medical entities may not be recognized clinically until they have advanced to the level of hemodynamic instability (29–31).

Pancytopenia in the Immunocompromised Patient

Cytopenia is a common finding in patients with cancer. It occurs for a variety of reasons and can affect all cell lines: erythrocytes, granulocytes, and platelets. Bone marrow failure is the most common cause of cytopenia. Marrow failure may be caused by marrow metastases—e.g., melanoma, kidney, adrenal, or thyroid cancers—or by fibrosis in hemoproliferative disorders. Radiation therapy and chemotherapies can suppress bone marrow, although the cytopenic effects of chemotherapy are more likely to reverse over time. The duration of suppression and the time to lowest counts (nadir) is known for specific drugs. Most myelosuppressive regimens produce a nadir within 10 days after administration with recovery by 3 to 4 weeks. The nadir associated with nitrosoureas may not occur until the fifth week. Cytopenia in cancer patients may result from increased cell destruction or from splenic sequestration.

Granulocytopenia carries a risk of bacterial infection, and, if prolonged, of fungal infection. The risk of infection and subsequent sepsis begins to increase as the absolute neutrophil count falls below 1,000/µL and becomes more pronounced below 500/µL. Prolonged neutropenia creates the greatest risk of infection (32). A single, isolated, oral temperature greater than 38.3°C (101°F) or a fever of 38.0°C (100.4°F) lasting 1 hour in a patient with granulocytopenia must be regarded as a serious infection until proven otherwise (33). Endogenous bacteria are the most common cause of infection in neutropenic patients, with 75% caused by gram-negative organisms. Thorough clinical examination, with attention to indwelling catheter sites, oral and rectal areas, skin, and sinuses is essential. Surveillance blood cultures are mandatory. Urine, sputum, and stool cultures and a chest x-ray are often necessary as well. Emergent, empirical treatment with broad-spectrum third-generation cephalosporins with or without aminoglycoside synergy may be started, and the treating oncology and infectious disease services should be consulted immediately. Febrile neutropenic patients should be transferred to an acute medical setting. Colony-stimulating factors, such as filgrastim, are being used prophylactically in patients who have experienced neutropenic fevers during previous chemotherapy cycles, but have not been shown to reduce infection in patients who are already neutropenic (34,35). They should not be given within the first 24 hours after chemotherapy. The efficacy of stringent isolation precautions or a neutropenic diet avoiding uncooked fruits and vegetables has not been proven in controlled studies (36).

There is no formal contraindication against exercise in asymptomatic patients with granulocytopenia, but exertion is discouraged in patients with significantly elevated temperatures because of their increased respiratory and heart rates, poor exercise tolerance, and increased platelet consumption.

Thrombocytopenia may also result from the primary disease process or following chemotherapy. Little risk of spontaneous bleeding has been demonstrated in patients whose platelet counts remain greater than 20,000/mm (34). Unrestricted aerobic exercise is generally permitted for patients with platelet counts between 30,000/mm and 50,000/mm, but resistance work should be avoided because of the concern that isometric contraction can elevate systemic blood pressure and cause intracranial hemorrhage (34). High-impact activities are also discouraged, as they can result in intramuscular or intraarticular hemorrhage. Patients requiring repeated platelet trans-

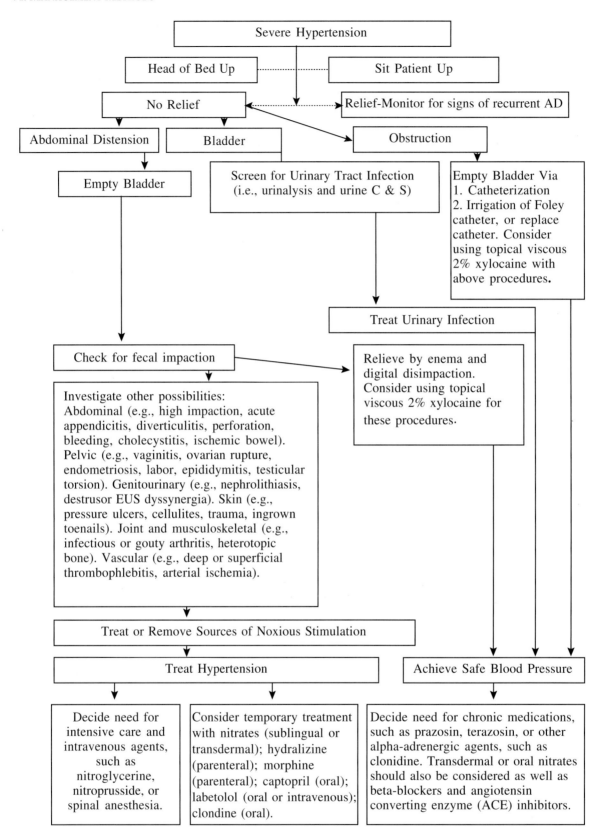

Figure 57-1. Algorithm for managing severe hypertension in automatic dysreflexia (AD) in spinal cord injury. C & S, culture and sensitivity; EUS, external urethral sphincter. (Adapted from McGuire TJ, Kumar VN. Autonomic dysreflexia in the spinal cord injured. *Postgrad Med* 1986;80:87–89; Abdelwahab W, Frishman W, Landau A. Management of hypertensive urgencies and emergencies. *J Clin Pharmacol* 1995;35:747–762; and Consortium for Spinal Cord Medicine. *Acute management of autonomic dysreflexia: individuals with spinal cord injury presenting to health care facilities.* Washington, DC: Paralyzed Veterans of America, 2001.

fusions for prolonged or symptomatic thrombocytopenia should have human lymphotropic antigen (HLA)–matched single donor platelets, as they will become refractory to random donor platelets (37).

Anemia can be treated with transfusion of packed red blood cells if the patient is symptomatic or if hemoglobin concentration falls below 7–8g/dl (38). Patients with coronary artery disease should be maintained above 9g/dl (38). Subcutaneous erythropoietin injections have been shown to decrease transfusion requirements in patients with chemotherapy-induced anemia (39).

Therapy should not be entirely discontinued when blood counts require restricted activity. Gentle range of motion should be pursued in order to minimize contractures; brief standing exercises can be performed to prevent gastrocnemius-soleus shortening; and breathing exercises should be encouraged to reduce atelectasis and the risk of pneumonia, and to optimize ventilation. Patients who undergo marrow ablative procedures, such as bone-marrow transplantation or stem-cell transplantation, are encouraged to participate in conservative endurance programs, e.g., upright or recumbent stationary bicycling. Contraindications for conservative exercise programs in the cytopenic patient are summarized in Table 57-3 (34,39).

Thromboembolic Diseases

The threat of deep venous thrombosis and pulmonary embolism in patients who are participating in rehabilitation is ubiquitous because of their inactivity (40). For example, in the stroke population, deep venous thrombosis has been reported in as many as 50% of patients in the paretic or plegic lower limbs and in as many as 10% in the uninvolved limbs (41,42). In patients who are receiving prophylactic anticoagulation after total hip arthroplasty, deep venous thrombosis has been reported to occur in about 1% and pulmonary embolism about 0.05% (43). Screening all patients who are admitted to inpatient rehabilitation programs with venous Doppler or duplex ultrasonography has received little support. Screening may be viewed as potentially cost-saving in high-risk patients when compared with the projected expense of treating thromboembolism, but the risks and costs of the complications of prophylactic anticoagulation have not been factored into these discussions (44).

DIAGNOSIS

Clinical examination continues to be inadequate to diagnose deep venous thrombosis and must at least be supplemented with noninvasive investigation, such as lower-limb venous compression ultrasonography (sensitivity 90% to 100%; specificity 90% to 100%) when suspected in the legs, and spiral computerized tomography or magnetic resonance imaging (sensitivity 100%, specificity 95% to 100%) when suspected in the pelvic and calf vessels (45–49). Laboratory studies, such as measurement of plasma fibrin D-dimers (that is, cross-linked fibrin derivatives), are being explored; however, this is highly sensitive but poorly specific (50). Yet, when used in combination with ultrasonography, finding negative results in both studies is thought to be highly negatively predictive, justifying holding anticoagulant therapy in a clinically suspicious limb (50). Venography should be rarely necessary for confirmatory purposes. Similarly, clinical presentation is inadequate to diagnose pulmonary embolism, and noninvasive radiographic investigation must be pursued with ventilation-perfusion scanning or spiral computerized tomography (90% to 95% sensitivity and specificity), which is replacing the need for pulmonary angiography as a confirmatory study. Spiral computer-

---

TABLE 57-3. Contraindications for Exercise in the Cytopenic Patient

1. Symptomatic (e.g., fever, shortness of breath tachypnea) patient with absolute neutrophil count less than 1000/μL.
2. Platelet count less than 20,000/mm. Avoid isometric strengthening and isotonic/isokinetic strengthening with resistance when platelet count is between 20,000 and 50,000/mm.
3. Hemoglogin level less than 7 g/dL in an asymptomatic patient without coronary heart disease; hemoglobin level less than 9 g/dL in a symptomatic patient (e.g., dizziness, shortness of breath) without coronary heart disease; hemoglobin level less than 9 g/dL in any patient with coronary heart disease.

From Oppenheim B, Heather A. Management of febrile neutropenia in low risk cancer patients. *Thorax* 2000;55(Suppl 1):S63–S69; and Rizzo JD, et al. Use of epoetin in patients with cancer: evidence-based clinical practice guidelines of the American Society of Clinical Oncology and the American Society of Hematology. *Blood* 2002;100:2303–2320.

---

ized tomography is best for detecting the presence of large emboli; thus, ventilation-perfusion scanning may be preferred with smaller emboli (51,52).

PROPHYLAXIS

There is little consensus as to the preferred prophylactic intervention in patients during remobilization in rehabilitation (53,54). Available treatment options include unfractionated heparin (UH), low molecular weight heparin (LMWH), Coumadin, aspirin, intermittent pneumatic compression, and inferior vena cava filter. In stroke patients, subcutaneous UH and intermittent pneumatic compression of the lower limbs have been reported as comparable (55). Ideally, the use of UH to achieve prophylaxis requires achieving a partial thromboplastin time (PTT) of between 30 and 40. Using adjustable doses in the range of 8,000 to 10,000 units subcutaneously every 8 to 12 hours is reported to be the recommended dose to achieve this goal (55). However, it is not common practice to use adjustable dose UH or to monitor the PTT when it is used for thromboembolic prophylaxis. LMWH has demonstrated to be at least as effective as UH for thromboembolic prophylaxis in nonorthopedic populations and probably more effective in orthopedic (total joint arthroplasty, fracture) populations. LMWH prophylactically is usually given as a fixed dose subcutaneously, once or twice daily, for example, enoxaparin 40 to 60 mg daily or 30 mg every 12 hours (56–60). In orthopedic populations, Coumadin, maintaining the international numerical ratio (INR) in the range of 1.5 to 2.0, continues to be accepted practice, particularly in anyone with a history of thromboembolism. However, this requires daily phlebotomy for monitoring the INR and continuation of prophylactic treatment for up to 6 weeks after total joint arthroplasty. Aspirin (325 mg twice daily) is increasingly being used as a prophylactic agent in orthopedic patients with uncomplicated histories after total joint arthroplasty and after surgical interventions to reduce/fixate lower-limb fractures; however, it continues to require a large-scale prospective and comparative study to show its efficacy (61). The use of an inferior vena cava filter as a prophylactic intervention should be limited to patients who have major lower-limb or pelvic trauma associated with a high risk for bleeding. Its placement is protective of pulmonary embolism but not venous thrombosis. As bleeding risk decreases, use of prophylactic anticoagulation should be considered in addition to intermittent venous compression (62).

TREATMENT

Despite prophylaxis, thromboembolic events continue to occur. In its early stages, pulmonary embolism should usually be treated in an acute care setting and in a critical care setting if there is any demonstration or risk of hemodynamic compromise. Treatment of venous thromboembolism during inpatient rehabilitation depends on the resources of each program and the patterns of relationships of comanaging consultants. Use of LMWH to treat venous thrombosis has decreased the need for laboratory monitoring but not clinical monitoring in these patients (58). When UH, then Coumadin, are used to treat thromboembolism, those rehabilitation programs that treat such patients must be able to administer intravenous UH, must have access to laboratory services for at least daily monitoring of the PTT and the INR, and must have the flexibility to tolerate dose adjustments of UH up to several times daily and of Coumadin once daily.

Cardiovascular Complications

As comorbid conditions, cardiovascular diseases have associated with them disabilities that augment the functional compromise associated with the underlying disorder primarily being treated in rehabilitation. Amputation and stroke, discussed below, are excellent examples of a potential negative synergistic effect on functional status when coupled with cardiovascular diseases. Among general rehabilitation populations, cardiovascular diseases commonly are thought to influence the course of treatment. However, when these populations have been screened clinically—or noninvasively, using electrocardiographic techniques such as 24-hour Holter monitoring—the screening methods have demonstrated to be poorly predictive for identifying patients at high risk for life-threatening cardiovascular events (63).

CARDIAC DISEASE AND AMPUTATION

When dysvascular amputees have been screened for cardiovascular complications that occur during physical therapy, a broad range of abnormalities that require medical interventions, such as a change in medications, have been demonstrated, including extreme increases in blood pressure, angina, heart failure, and arrhythmias. In screening for such complications in amputees, the use of continuous noninvasive electrocardiographic monitoring seemed to add little when combined with clinical monitoring of symptom experience by therapists: the sensitivity of history alone was reported to be 83% for predicting a worrisome cardiovascular event (64). When modified upper-extremity exercise testing has been used to assess cardiovascular risk in dysvascular amputees, baseline electrocardiographic abnormalities have been observed in all of these patients, and as many as 25% of these patients were observed to have ST segment depression during the exercise testing. Regardless, cardiovascular events seemed to interfere minimally with achieving successful prosthetic use (65).

How can these series of observations be rationalized? It has been well established among dysvascular amputees that the higher the level of the amputation and the more lower limbs that are amputated, the higher the myocardial energy consumption during ambulation per unit distance (66). However, it has not been demonstrated that a higher level of amputation, or that having more limbs amputated, is associated with more cardiovascular complications. Moreover, those with above-knee amputations have been demonstrated to ambulate with prostheses more slowly, and the associated myocardial energy consumption per unit time is comparable to that consumed by below-knee amputees (66). Thus, amputees decrease their walking speed to accommodate their cardiovascular system's ability to support prosthetic ambulation. Such compensatory behavior can be offered to explain the observation of low cardiovascular events among dysvascular amputees during pre-prosthetic and prosthetic use.

CARDIAC DISEASE AND STROKE

There is a stronger argument that comorbid cardiac disease is more influential on recovery and rehabilitation after stroke than after amputation. Myocardial infarction is recognized both as causal of stroke and as an associated event after stroke. Large myocardial infarctions and myocardial infarctions that present with heart failure are predisposing factors for stroke, presumably from cerebral embolism and hypoperfusion (67). Stroke has been associated with an array of cardiovascular findings newly realized after the event, including electrocardiographic changes, such as ST segment depression, T wave inversion, and QT interval prolongation; transient arrhythmias, such as atrial fibrillation, premature ventricular contractions, and ventricular tachycardia; left ventricular hypertrophy; and myocardial damage with creatine phosphokinase elevations reported in up to 30% of studied stroke populations, with true myocardial infarction occurring in about 5% of stroke patients at the time of presentation. Patients who have cerebral infarctions have more evidence of myocardial damage and have more arrhythmias than patients who have brainstem infarctions. Elevations in creatine phosphokinase appear to continue beyond 48 hours when they typically peak after myocardial infarction. A myonecrosis phenomenon has been postulated to explain these cardiac events after stroke. A release of sympathetic adrenergic neurotransmitters from the damaged brain tissue is thought to elevate their levels, systemically inducing myocardial damage during the immediate poststroke period. Ischemic electrocardiographic changes, elevations in serum creatine phosphokinase and plasma norepinephrine, and arrhythmias have been observed clinically. Moreover, autopsy data in acute stroke patients who have died has documented myocytolysis (68–70).

Cardiovascular diseases are the most common comorbidities associated with stroke, being symptomatic in as many as 30% of patients at the onset of the event, and their presence independently influences negatively functional outcome after stroke based on prospective data generated from the Mayo Clinic and the Framingham databases (71,72). Cardiovascular diseases are the most common cause of death after stroke. Among stroke survivors, the prevalence of these comorbid conditions has included hypertension (67%), hypertensive heart disease (53%), coronary heart disease (32%), and heart failure (18%) (71–75).

How should patients with known cardiovascular diseases be managed by the physiatrist during rehabilitation? Comanagement with patients' internists or cardiologists is essential for a number of reasons. These consultants presumably are knowledgeable about patients' idiosyncratic clinical presentations during cardiac events. Acknowledging their usual symptom experience and realizing when this pattern changes can indicate a more serious or life-threatening event that requires closer monitoring, further investigation with electrophysiologic studies, coronary angiography, medication changes, or procedural interventions, such as electrophysiologic ablation, coronary angioplasty, or surgical bypass. These consultants can also advise on restarting cardiovascular medications that have been discontinued during surgical procedures and unstable periods associated with acute illness.

Monitoring heart rate, blood pressure, and hemoglobin-oxygen saturation at rest and their responses during graduated therapeutic exercises provides fundamental data indicating physiologic adaptations during stress, as well as the efficacy of medications being used to control hypertension, myocardial oxygen consumption, and arrhythmias. Delineating heart rate and blood pressure parameters that define boundaries of when not to treat or of when to interrupt treatment provides therapists with relatively safe guidelines in which to operationalize their interventions. The standard formulae for defining submaximal exercise intensities using age-associated maximal predicted heart rate are generally not useful to define heart rate parameters because many patients are so severely deconditioned that they have resting tachycardias, or a tachycardia is easily achieved with minimal submaximal activity. Moreover, the intended therapeutic effect of some cardiac medications—for example, beta blockers—is to disallow an increase in heart rate into the range that requires adrenergic stimulation, that is, greater than 120 beats per minute. One pragmatic approach is to keep their submaximal exercise intensity within 20 beats of their resting heart rate, monitoring closely for symptoms.

Hypertension can be unmasked during therapeutic exercise programs, particularly isometric strengthening and submaximal endurance activities. Using the expected physiologic increases in systolic and diastolic blood pressure during exercise can provide a starting place to define blood pressure parameters. At rest, it should be defined what is the upper limit of the normal range for specific patients. For example, elderly and poststroke patients may be allowed to start exercise programs at systolic pressures as high as 160 mm Hg to facilitate better cerebral perfusion because of carotid/vertebrobasilar disease or because of cerebral autoregulatory dysfunction. During exercise, systolic pressure should increase within 50 mm Hg over resting levels, and diastolic pressure should not increase more than 5 mm Hg because of peripheral vasodilatation. A pragmatic approach here is to hold treatment for resting pressures higher than 160/100 mm Hg and to interrupt treatment for pressures higher than 200/105 mm Hg (76). Needless to say, a decrease in systolic blood pressure during activity indicates a lowering of cardiac output possibly because of myocardial ischemia. Treatment should be stopped and held until further consultation with cardiology. General guidelines for monitoring heart rate and blood pressure in sick patients during rehabilitation are offered in Table 57-4.

Aspiration

Aspiration encompasses a spectrum of situations, from laryngeal penetration of ingested or refluxed substances to frank pneumonia. Laryngeal penetration and microaspiration can be viewed as serious predisposing factors to aspiration pneumonia. Macroaspiration involves entry of bacterial and nonbacterial oral and gastric contents into the airways and usually induces pneumonia. Aspiration pneumonia can involve segmental or lobar areas of the lung and can evolve to a more diffuse pulmonary inflammatory reaction, as well as systemic illness with bacteremia, sepsis, and end-organ consequences of hypoxia (77,78). Aspiration, in its full-blown form as pneumonitis, is life threatening and costly, sometimes requiring mechanical ventilation and critical care: Up to 40% mortality has been reported to result from aspiration pneumonia, with more than 50% of those who died requiring mechanical ventilation (79). Aspiration is associated with swallowing dysfunction or dysphagia and upper-gastrointestinal disorders causing reflux. It can be associated with central and peripheral neurologic disorders and peripheral and mechanical obstructive diseases. Aspiration can be both an indication for enteral forms of nutritional support and hydration and a complication of these alternative forms of feeding. More-

---

TABLE 57-4. Guidelines for Monitoring Heart Rate and Blood Pressure in Sick Patients during Rehabilitation

1. Do not treat if resting heart rate is greater than 120 beats per minute or resting blood pressure is greater than 160/100 mm Hg.
2. Do not treat if resting heart rate is less than 50 beats per minute or resting systolic blood pressure is less than 80 mm Hg.
3. During exercise or functional activities, maintain heart rate response to resting plus 20 beats per minute. For example, if resting heart rate is 100 beats per minute, then during a graduated exercise program, keep heart rate less than 120 beats per minute during activity.
4. During exercise or functional activities, maintain systolic blood pressure response to resting systolic pressure plus 50 mm Hg, and maintain diastolic pressure to resting diastolic pressure plus 5 mm Hg. For example, if resting blood pressure is 140/100 mm Hg, then during a graduated exercise program, keep blood pressure less than 190/105.
5. Stop exercise if systolic blood pressure decreases during activity.

---

over, enteral nutrition may alkalinize the gastric contents, promoting bacterial overgrowth (80, 81). Aspiration pneumonia is viewed as preventable by a clearer definition of the anatomy and pathophysiology of oropharyngeal and esophageal dysphagia; through a clinical swallowing evaluation performed by a speech therapist and otorhinolaryngologist; and through radiographic studies, such as modified barium or videofluoroscopic swallowing study, performed jointly with the speech therapist and radiologist (82–85).

Dysphagia associated aspiration is associated with a broad range of diseases treated in rehabilitation. Three major mechanisms can be delineated to categorize these diseases:

1. *Neuromuscular*—This includes central and peripheral neurologic diseases that can result in dysphagia and reflux. Any central neurologic condition that impairs the basic cognitive skills of self-awareness and attention of orally presented foods and handling of secretions, suppresses protective gag and cough reflexes, and alters voluntary oral motor control and a coordinated pharyngeal reflex is included, for example, stroke, head injury, brain tumors, cerebral infections, and neurodegenerative diseases (such as Parkinson's disease, multiple sclerosis, motor neuron diseases, and muscular dystrophies). Additionally, peripheral neural disorders that result in dysmotility of the esophagus, stomach, and small bowel associated with reflux are included, such as achalasia, diabetes and other causes of autonomic peripheral neuropathies, hiatal hernia, and gastroesophageal reflux disease (86–89).
2. *Mechanical*—Anatomic interruption of the swallowing mechanism can predispose to aspiration. This encompasses a variety of causes, including inflammatory, (e.g., retropharyngeal or submandibular infections), structural (e.g., Zenker's diverticulum or tracheoesophageal fistula, blunt and penetrating trauma), and oncologic (e.g., pharyngeal or esophageal tumors).
3. *Iatrogenic*—This includes enteral feeding, endotracheal intubation, tracheostomies, general anesthesia, and radiation treatment directed toward the head/neck/upper chest (90).

Among those disorders mentioned above, dysphagia has been best studied in stroke, and what we learn from this literature can be used to provide clinical guidance when managing other patient populations. Dysphagia has been reported to occur in at least 50% of stroke survivors, and silent aspiration is reported in up to 75% of these patients (86,89). Silent aspiration not appreciated during swallowing examination is observed in less than one-half of patients who prove to aspirate on radiographic studies (86,89). Predicting aspiration in stroke is problematic. Lesion site, bilateral lesions, and dysphagia-related symptoms, such as coughing after food ingestion, are poorly predictive. The absence of a gag reflex is not predictive, and its presence is not protective of dysphagia and aspiration (91). One useful "bedside" screening test reported for dysphagia is the presence of an involuntary cough up to 1 minute after being challenged to drink and swallow 3 ounces of water without interruption (92). An adequate voluntary cough does not indicate an effective protective cough. The absence of a voluntary cough should preclude further oral intake until further clinical assessment is performed by speech therapy (91).

Decision making about dysphagia and managing enteral feedings is common during rehabilitation programs. These involve clinical management issues that often place the physiatrist in the gate-keeping role among the speech therapist, occupational therapist, nutritionist, nurse, otorhinolaryngologist, gastroenterologist, radiologist, and surgeon. Among hospitalized patients on medical and surgical services, about 25% of enterally fed patients who were dysphagic were reported to develop aspiration pneumonia (93). Being fed with a large-bore nasogastric/nasoduodenal tube was reported to be particularly problematic when compared with other access methods, such as gastrostomy and jejunostomy (93). When comparing access methods, neither intermittent nor continuous feeding schedules, and neither gastric nor duodenal distal tube sites, seemed to matter (94). The presence of a tracheostomy tube was also a serious predisposing factor in the general hospitalized population (93,94). One practical management suggestion inferred from these studies was that nasogastric and gastrostomy tubes should be avoided in patients with esophageal dysfunction (reflux), gastric atony, and any degree of gastric outlet obstruction when documented during dynamic radiographic assessment. In these patients, a distal duodenal tube site is thought to be safer theoretically because there are two potential protective valves anatomically, the pyloric and the gastroesophageal, to prevent reflux (90,93,94).

A multidisciplinary approach is essential during dysphagia management and aspiration prevention. For example, the clinical assessment by the speech therapist is often best to determine the usefulness of laryngoscopic examination by the otorhinolaryngologist and the need for a modified barium swallow. If an obstructive lesion is being suspected, direct laryngoscopy is mandatory. The modified barium swallow is best performed jointly by the speech therapist and radiologist in that the feeding of different food consistencies and the use of different protective head and neck positions for each food texture can be assessed. Based on their observations, occupational therapists, nurses, and nutritionists and family caregivers can operationalize optimal feeding and nutritional intake (82). As the gatekeeper in rehabilitation, the physiatrist must synthesize information from multiple sources, operationalize management decisions, and educate other rehabilitation team members and family caregivers in a rational manner regarding feeding and nutritional support. When recommended, the patient's/caregiver's choice to use a specific protective strategy or to opt for enteral nutrition can be difficult. Choosing not to follow through with the team's recommendations should be allowed, and the choice not to comply with the team's recommendations assumes that the risks have been articulated to, and understood by, the patient and caregivers. The physiatrist's role in this kind of decision making is key. Guidelines for aspiration prevention and management in the dysphagic patient are summarized in Table 57-5.

TABLE 57-5.   Guidelines for Preventing and Managing Aspiration in Dysphagic Patients

1. Know those disorders commonly associated with dysphagia.
2. Integrate into the functional history screening questions for dysphagia (e.g., coughing or choking after drinking/eating, drooling, nasal regurgitation, difficulty clearing secretions, "wet voice"). Include screening maneuvers as part of the physical examination (e.g., imitation of oral motor maneuvers to screen for apraxia, lingual/buccal sensory testing, and observing for the above symptoms for up to a minute after drinking a small amount of a thin liquid).
3. When dysphagia is clinically suspected, hold oral intake held until a clinical swallowing assessment can be performed by the speech therapist.
4. Order calorie counts by the nutritionist to monitor if daily caloric requirements are being met when oral feeding is recommended.
5. Integrate the recommended compensatory feeding and positioning strategies and supervision requirements into nursing and dietary care plans, and advance these as patients receive swallowing treatments by the speech therapist.
6. Order the appropriate radiographic studies, and make sure they are executed with the appropriate parties involved, for example, both radiologist and speech therapist performing a modified barium swallow.
7. Refer to other medical specialists when appropriate:
   - *Otorhinolaryngologist* for direct visualization of the oropharynx when obstructive/mechanical lesions and vocal cord paralysis are suspected
   - *Gastroenterologist* for endoscopic evaluation when gastroesophageal dysmotility disorders, particularly reflux and mechanical lesions, are suspected, as well as when enteral feeding tubes are sought to be placed percutaneously using endoscopic guidance in appropriate patients
   - *Surgeon* when enteral feeding tube placement requires an open surgical procedure, for example, in patients who have had previous adhesion-producing bowel surgery or who have unusual gastrointestinal anatomy (94,95)

Seizures and Epilepsy

A seizure is a paroxysmal event, caused by abnormal, excessive, hypersynchronous discharges from central nervous system neurons ranging in presentation (96,97). Approximately 5% to 10% of the population will have at least one seizure during their lifetime, most likely in early childhood and late adulthood (99). Seizures may be preceded by an array of phenomena, including abdominal sensations, light-headedness/dizziness, nausea, chest discomfort, visual hallucinations, olfactory hallucinations, déjà vu, flushing, limb jerking, fear, paresthesias, and minor tonic-clonic movements. Postseizure (postictal) symptoms include complex hallucinations, prolonged tonic or clonic movements, tongue or cheek biting, lethargy, confusion, myalgias, and headache.

Epilepsy is a disorder characterized by the occurrence of at least two unprovoked seizures. The lifetime likelihood of experiencing one seizure is about 9%, and the lifetime likelihood of being diagnosed as having epilepsy is slightly less than 3% (96).

CLASSIFICATION

There are several classification systems of epileptic seizures based on clinical symptoms and electroencephalographic (EEG) findings (100). The main characteristic that distinguishes the different categories is whether the seizure activity is partial (localized or focal) or generalized. EEG findings and epilepsy classifications are reviewed in more detail elsewhere (101).

Partial seizures occur within discrete regions of the brain. Simple partial seizures cause motor, sensory, autonomic, or behavioral symptoms without an alteration in consciousness. In some patients, the abnormal movements begin in a restricted region (e.g., fingers) and gradually progress to a larger portion of the extremity, known as a Jacksonian march. Patients may experience a localized paresis in the involved extremity for minutes to days after the seizure, a phenomenon called Todd paralysis (101).

Complex partial seizures are characterized by a focal seizure activity associated with a transient impairment in consciousness. In this case, the patient is unable to appropriately respond to visual or auditory commands and has amnesia during the ictal phase. The start of the ictal phase is often a sudden behavioral event accompanied by involuntary movements, called automatisms, such as chewing, lip smacking, swallowing, picking, or emotional behaviors (101).

Generalized seizures arise from both cerebral hemispheres simultaneously, without any detectable focal onset clinically or electroencephalographically. There are several subtypes. Absence (i.e., petit mal) seizures are characterized by a sudden, brief alteration of consciousness without loss of postural control. Tonic-clonic (i.e., grand mal) seizures are the most common seizure type, resulting from metabolic derangements. The initial tonic phase is characterized by contraction of muscles throughout the body, impaired respiration, oropharyngeal pooling of secretions, mandibular contraction with tongue lacerations, and increased sympathetic tone (tachycardia, hypertension, and pupillary dilatation). The clonic phase follows with superimposed muscle relaxation, followed by the ictal phase. Unresponsiveness, muscle flaccidity, stridorous breathing, and sometimes bowel/bladder incontinence characterize the postictal phase (101).

Atonic seizures are characterized by a sudden loss of postural muscle tone lasting seconds with brief loss of consciousness but usually no postictal confusion. They are often associated with falls and have an increased risk for bony and head injury. Myoclonic seizures are manifested by a sudden, brief muscle contraction that involves one or more body parts. Commonly observed while falling asleep, they are also associated with hypoxic brain injury (97).

Psychogenic seizures (i.e., not true seizures) are nonepileptic behaviors that resemble seizures typically precipitated by underlying psychosocial stress and often a component of a conversion reaction. The diagnosis can often be difficult, and EEG and video-EEG monitoring may be necessary (102).

CAUSES AND BASIC MECHANISMS

The most common causes of seizures occur in disorders causing physical, cognitive-linguistic, and behavioral impairment, thus they should be expected during rehabilitation. In young adults, the most common causes are trauma, alcohol withdrawal, illicit drug use, brain tumor, and idiopathic (97). In a patient with traumatic brain injury (TBI) who has penetrating trauma, depressed skull fracture, intracranial hemorrhage, prolonged coma, or prolonged posttraumatic amnesia, there is a 40% to 50% risk of developing a seizure (103). Mild TBI (GCS score = 13–15) is not associated with an increased risk of epilepsy, unless there was presence of intracranial hemorrhage, although many physiatrists upgrade TBI classifications to "moderate" in the presence of any hemorrhage on head computerized tomography regardless of GCS score (103,104).

In the elderly, the most common causes of seizures are cerebrovascular diseases, followed by brain tumor, TBI, toxic metabolic disorders, and degenerative diseases (105). Immediate seizures at the time of the stroke are seen more often with embolic rather than hemorrhage or thrombotic strokes (105).

Initiation of seizures is associated with a complex interplay among an influx of extracellular calcium, increased flow of sodium ions through voltage-dependent sodium channels, and generation of repetitive action potentials. Hyperpolarization of gamma amino butyric acid receptors, potassium channels, and in some cases N-Methyl-D-aspartate subtype of amino acid receptors also occurs. Many factors control neuron excitability, including conductance of ion channels, membrane receptors, cytoplasmic buffering, second-messenger systems, protein expression, amount/type of neurotransmitters present at the synapse, synaptic input, and nonneural cells (e.g., astrocytes, oligodendrocytes) (105).

TREATMENT

During or shortly after a seizure, the priority is to monitor vital signs and provide respiratory and cardiovascular support. Central nervous system infection, metabolic abnormality, or drug toxicity should be investigated with appropriate laboratory studies (e.g., complete blood count, electrolytes, calcium, magnesium, glucose, liver and renal function tests, urinalysis, toxicology screen) while waiting for neurologic or neurosurgical consultation. If the patient is currently on antiepileptic drugs, serum levels should be evaluated. A lumbar puncture is indicated if there is any suspicion of meningitis or encephalitis and is mandatory in all patients who are seropositive for human immune virus (HIV) antibody. The EEG will help establish the diagnosis of epilepsy, classify the seizure type, and help direct pharmacologic intervention. Most patients should also undergo brain imaging with computerized tomography or magnetic resonance imaging to rule out structural abnormality (98).

Status epilepticus refers to continuous seizures or repetitive, discrete seizures with impaired consciousness during the interictal period. Although the duration has been traditionally defined as 15 to 30 minutes, starting aggressive interventions at 5 minutes has been advised (106,107). In the first few minutes, establish basic life support, intravenous access, and oxygenation. Send blood tests as previously described. Administer glucose in a 50% concentration (50 mL intravenous bolus) and thiamine (10 mg intravenous bolus). More recent recommendations are encouraging intravenous phenytoin at this point (20 mg per kg of body weight at 50 mg/min) as opposed to the benzodiazepines (107). The reasoning is that benzodiazepines sedate consciousness and depress respiration (107). Phenobarbital (20 mg/kg intravenously at 50–75 mg/min) is given if seizures continue after the phenytoin infusion. General anesthesia should be administered if phenobarbital fails.

Maintenance therapy for epilepsy involves treating the underlying condition, avoidance of precipitating factors, and suppression of recurrent seizures by using antiepileptic medications. This is often managed best by an epileptologist. However, physiatrists are often managing neurologically impaired patients who have seizure disorders or who are using medications for seizure prophylaxis, so knowledge of antiepileptic medications is essential. These medications are reviewed elsewhere (see Chapter 56) (108,109).

Delirium and Psychiatric Emergencies

Changes in mental status are a common presentation of serious underlying medical problems. In rehabilitation settings, patients' abilities to attend to and articulate their somatic experience commonly can be limited because of an array of reasons, including medications, their underlying comorbidities, and environmental effects. Changes in mental status include "internal" disturbances in cognition (e.g., attention, memory, language, visuoperception, executive functions), perception (e.g., example, illusions, hallucinations), thought content (e.g., delusions), mood/affect (e.g., depression, anxiety, anger), and personality (e.g., aggressive/passive, obsessive). They may manifest as "external" displays of behavior that can be counterproductive vis-à-vis the current treatments (110,111).

The terms *change in mental status* and *delirium* often are used interchangeably; however, this is appropriate when the change in mental state from a clearly defined baseline fulfills other syndrome criteria of delirium. This should include that the change occurs over a short period of time (i.e., hours to days), that the behavioral disturbances fluctuate during the course of the day (such as disturbed sleep/wake cycles and extremes of psychomotor agitation or retardation), and that there is objective evidence to support that an underlying physiologic disturbance is the cause. Furthermore, delirium is transient with resolution occurring over days to weeks. In its more severe form, it is unlikely that patients will be able to participate in a therapeutic program of rehabilitation without pharmacologic treatment. As resolution occurs, incremental reengagement of treatment is possible with gradual reduction of neuromodulating medications. Delirium is likely to lengthen the time period of need for treatments because of associated compromise in learning abilities and decline in functional abilities below a predelirium baseline. Delirium is likely to increase the burden of care required by caregivers both in hospitals and at home, and can challenge a previously expected and well-planned home discharge and recovery (112–114).

Data that estimate the incidence of delirium on acute medical and surgical services can influence what to expect in rehabilitation settings, despite screening efforts to delay the entry of patients with delirium into structured rehabilitation programs. In fact, delirium should not be surprising in elderly postsurgical patients, for example, after knee/hip arthroplasty or after coronary artery grafting, at the time of initiating rehabilitation interventions. This occurs with the shared expectation of concurrent resolution of interfering symptoms, along with medical treatments of these symptoms (i.e., minimizing narcotic analgesics, equilibrating fluids and electrolytes, treating infections) and accelerating therapy participation. Moreover, increased dependence on protocols that move patients from acute medical/surgical services to rehabilitation settings in an effort to shorten hospital lengths of stay and keep hospital beds open reinforces that delirium should be expected. On general medical and surgical services, the incidence of delirium is as high as 15% overall, 35% in the elderly, 30% after open heart procedures, and 50% after fractures requiring open fracture reduction and fixation (115,116). Risk factors that predispose to delirium in hospitalized patients include stroke, brain tumor, neurovascular degenerative diseases, impaired hearing and vision, aging-related changes in metabolizing and eliminating drugs, sleep deprivation, and pain (115,116). When delirium does not resolve as expected and persists beyond several weeks, it is thought the experience of an acute illness or surgical procedure requiring general anesthesia may have unmasked a dementia that existed before the delirium. The belief is that dementia was not likely fully recognized or was in its early phases before the illness/surgery (117).

Managing delirium requires a prompt diagnostic investigation seeking reversible factors to explain its behavioral manifestations. Management guidelines are presented in Table 57-6 (118).

TABLE 57-6. Guidelines for Managing Delirium in Rehabilitation

1. Perform a thorough medication review to identify those agents having psychotropic side effects.
2. Perform a complete physical examination, including cognitive screening, especially looking for infectious sources and neurologic focality that is new.
3. Monitor and document cognition and behavior serially.
4. Monitor sleep/wake cycles, paying attention to factors that interfere with sleep, such as unnecessary wake-ups to dispense medications and obtain vital signs.
5. Order screening laboratory tests: complete blood count; serum electrolytes, glucose, blood urea nitrogen, creatinine, liver profile, thyroid profile, calcium, magnesium, phosphorus, B_{12}, folate; serologies to screen for syphilis and Lyme disease (in high risk areas).
6. Order an electrocardiogram, hemoglobin-oxygen saturation via pulse oximetry, a urine culture, a sputum culture and chest radiograph if pneumonia is suspected, abdominal radiographs if fecal impaction is suspected, and a brain computerized tomography or magnetic resonance imaging.
7. Consult geriatrician/internist or neurologist if an explanation is not readily elucidated.

From Conn DK. Delirium and other organic mental disorders. In: Sadavoy J, Lazarus LW, Jarvik LF, eds. *Comprehensive review of geriatric psychiatry.* Washington, DC: American Psychiatric Press, 1991:311–336.

As the diagnostic process is initiated, treatment interventions must be simultaneously initiated empirically based on removing likely causes/aggravating factors, and then modified based on the results of the diagnostic database, feedback from consultants and rehabilitation providers, and patient response. Commonsensical interventions include restoring fluids and electrolytes; stopping unnecessary medications, particularly those with psychotropic side effects, minimizing doses, and simplifying dosing regimens; regulating sleep/wake cycles by reducing wake-ups during nighttime, creating a nighttime environment that facilitates sleep, and using a low-dose, short-acting benzodiazepine derivative temporarily at bedtime; controlling pain with standing doses of nonnarcotic substances if safe to use, for example, acetaminophen 1,000 mg every 8 hours or ibuprofen 600 mg every 8 hours (with a histamine-2 blocker); reversing constipation with emollients and cathartics; close behavioral tracking, including vital signs, by rehabilitation personnel with courteous reorientation, and one-on-one surveillance when necessary; use of pharmacologic agents to control agitation, including low-dose benzodiazepines, such as lorazepam 0.5 mg every 6 to 8 hours (beware of disinhibition) or low-dose bedtime neuroleptics, such as risperidone 0.5 to 1 mg; using supplemental oxygen and bronchodilating treatments when indicated; and starting appropriate antibiotics empirically to treat a suspected infection and until culture results and radiographs are available to verify an infectious process by a specific organism.

When does a change in mental status evolve to become a psychiatric emergency? The fundamental issues here are whether the displayed behaviors are potentially harmful to the patient and others in the immediate environment—for example, threatened or real self-injury, aggression, and psychosis (e.g., hallucinations, paranoid delusions)—and whether the delirium is worsening without a clear explanation. Moreover, if the patient's behaviors are interfering with a reasonable diagnostic investigation or threatening to interrupt appropriate treatments, particularly if the patient is threatening to leave against medical advice, then the patient's abilities to recognize the consequences of treatment, or lack of treatment, and to make rational medical/health decisions must be explored. Psychiatric consultation to define competence must be pursued, a proxy decision maker for the patient must be defined, and involuntary psychiatric admission may be necessary (119,120).

Aggression, violence, and assaultive behaviors should not be tolerated. These behaviors should be treated quickly and decisively by removing from the immediate environment all items that could be injurious and then physically and/or chemically restraining and secluding the patient. If this latter intervention is necessary, seeking immediate assistance from the local security forces or police may be necessary. Never act alone; recruit additional personnel before interviewing. Intramuscular benzodiazepines (lorazepam 1 to 2 mg) or neuroleptics (haloperidol 2 to 5 mg) should be administered in repeated doses until the patient deescalates. The treating physician is expected to take the lead in directing such treatment or until the patient can receive appropriate psychiatric care. Behaviors that can warn rehabilitation personnel about impending violence include verbal threats, hyperactivity, mania, possession of weapons, autonomic arousal, abuse of nonprescribed substances, paranoia, antisocial behaviors, panic reactions, and disinhibition (121).

Other less dramatic behaviors that can be categorized as psychiatric emergencies include severe loss reactions, including depression, self-neglect, panic reactions, and caregiver abuse/neglect. Severely depressed patients, particularly those with a known history of depression with or without suicidality, must have their suicidal potential assessed and monitored. Suicidal ideation has been reported in up to 7% of patients who participate in inpatient rehabilitation (122). Other suicide risk factors include previous substance abuse, including alcohol, a history of chronic pain, and antisocial and psychotic behaviors. Articulation of suicidal intention and demonstration of self-injurious behaviors must be explored as attention-seeking versus an actual plan to act. One-to-one nursing surveillance is essential when suicide is suspected, and psychiatric consultation to consider possible psychiatric admission is mandatory.

More passive behaviors, such as poor participation or compliance with a rehabilitation treatment plan, should be explored as self-injurious as well (121,123). Panic and other extreme manifestations of anxiety are an appropriate physiological response to myocardial (ischemia or arrhythmias with lowered cerebral perfusion) and ventilatory (hypoxemia) compromise, thyrotoxicosis, and noradrenergic-secreting tumors. Compromise of vision and hearing can interfere with comprehension and communication, resulting in extreme anxiety when participating in a structured program requiring goal-directed progress in response to treatments. The physiologic contribution to panic and anxiety and the situational/interpersonal/environmental precipitants must be identified for appropriate behavioral and pharmacologic treatments to be applied (124).

Caregiver abuse and neglect is often not recognized until caregiver education is incorporated into the treatment program, until an explicit discharge or continuing care plan contingent on caregiver participation is offered, or until the patient is discharged from the hospital and receiving home services. When family meetings are missed and caregiver education sessions resisted by caregivers, this can indicate that they are overwhelmed emotionally or are ambivalent about their relationship with the patient. Poor operationalization of essential preventive/maintenance therapeutic programs will likely result. Mental illness or substance abuse in the household should increase vigilance about a potentially abusive situation. Psy-

chological and social service assessments should be sought to explore the range of motives (altruistic, financial), or the lack thereof, underpinning such caregiver-patient relationships. The limits of a caregiver's tolerance of disability should be made explicit. Relationships that have been historically difficult and role reversals that occur when one's partner becomes disabled should be reasons to invite the involved parties into counseling. Home-care services can unobtrusively monitor and provide emotional support to caregivers. Surrogate caregivers through the extended family, community, and church groups should be sought to decompress those who have the primary responsibility of managing the daily lives of disabled patients. Admissions to skilled nursing facilities for respite on a regular basis should be explored.

REFERENCES

1. Anderson DM (chief lexographer). *Mosby's Medical, Nursing and Allied Health Dictionary*, 6th ed. St Louis: Mosby Inc, 2002:588.
2. Hanks RA, Lichtenberg PA. Physical, psychological and social outcomes in geriatric rehabilitation patients. *Arch Phys Med Rehabil* 1996;77:783–792.
3. Centers for Medicare and Medicaid Services, Health and Human Services. Medicare programs: prospective system for inpatient rehabilitation facilities. Final rule. *Fed Regist* 2001;66(152):41315–41430.
4. Gage B. Impact of the Balance Budget Act on post-acute utilization. *Health Care Financ Rev* 1999;20(4):103–126.
5. Melvin JL. Impact of Health Care Financing Administration changes on stroke rehabilitation. *Phys Med Rehabil Clin N Am* 1999;19(4):943–955.
6. Rovinsky M. Provisions of the Balanced Budget Act challenge integrated delivery systems (IDSs) care coordination patterns. *Health Financ Manage* 1999;53(8):31–34.
7. Schulmerich SC. Public policy and the crisis in home care. *Caring* 2000;19(9):42–45.
8. Day JC. *Current Population Reports: Population projections of the United States by age, sex, race and Hispanic origin: 1993–2050.* Washington, DC: US Bureau of the Census, 1993:25–1104.
9. Fries JF. Aging, cumulative disability, and the compression of morbidity. *Compr Ther* 2001;21(4):322–329.
10. Rowe JW. Health care of the elderly. *N Engl J Med* 1985;312:827–835.
11. Crimmins EM, Hayward MD, Salto Y. Changing mortality and morbidity rates and the health status and life expectancy of the older population. *Demography* 1994;31(1):159–175.
12. McNeil, *Current Population Reports*: Americans with Disabilities 1991—92. Washington, DC: US Bureau of the Census, 1993:70–133.
13. Health United States: 2001. *Current Population Reports, American with Disabilities, 1997,* Washington, DC: US Bureau of the Census and the National Center on Health Statistics,, 2001:70–73.
14. Edmunds LH, Stephenson LW, Edie RN, et al. Open heart surgery in octogenarians. *N Engl J Med* 1988;319:131–136.
15. Patterson C, Crescenzi C, Steel K. Hospital use by the extremely elderly (nonagenarians): a two year study. *J Am Geriatr Soc* 1984;32:350–352.
16. Steel K. Iatrogenic disease on a medical service. *J Am Geriatr Soc* 1984;32:445–449.
17. Conraads VM, Beckers PJ, Vorlat A, et al. Importance of physical rehabilitation before and after cardiac transplantation in a patient with myotonic dystrophy: a case report. *Arch Phys Med Rehabil* 2002;83:724–726.
18. Mercer TH, Crawford G, Gleeson NP, et al. Low volume exercise rehabilitation improves functional capacity and self-reported functional status of dialysis patients. *Am J Phys Med Rehabil* 2002;81:162–167.
19. Modawal A, Candadai NP, Mandell KM, et al. Weaning success among ventilator-dependent patients in a rehabilitation facility. *Arch Phys Med Rehabil* 2002;83:154–157.
20. Felsenthal G, Cohen S, Hilton B, et al. The physiatrist as primary physician for patient on an in-patient rehabilitation unit. *Arch Phys Med Rehabil* 1984;65:375–378.
21. Goldman L, Lee T, Rudd P. Ten commandments for effective consultations. *Arch Intern Med* 1983;143:1753–1755.
22. Marciniak CM, Heinemann AW, Monga T. Changes in medical stability upon admission to a rehabilitation unit. *Arch Phys Med Rehabil* 1993;74:1157–1160.
23. Stineman M, Brody SJ, Shelton B, et al. Severe medical complications during rehabilitation pre- and post-introduction of acute care prospective payment. *Arch Phys Med Rehabil* 1986;67:650 (abst).
24. Wright RE, Smith RM, Harvey RF. Risk factors for death and emergency transfer in acute and subacute rehabilitation. *Arch Phys Med Rehabil* 1996;77:1049–1055.
25. Siegler EL, Stineman MG, Maislin G. Development of complications during rehabilitation. *Arch Intern Med* 1994;54:2185–2190.
26. Deutsch A, Fiedler RC, Granger CV, et al. The Uniform Data System for Medical Rehabilitation report of patients discharged from comprehensive

medical rehabilitation programs in 1999. *Am J Phys Med Rehabil* 2002;81: 133–142.

27. Patrick L, Knoefel F, Gaskowski P, et al. Medical co-morbidity and rehabilitation efficiency in geriatric inpatients. *J Am Geriatr Soc* 2001;49(11): 1471–1477.

28. Giaquinto S, Palma E, Maiolo I, et al. Importance and evaluation of comorbidity in rehabilitation. *Disabil Rehabil* 2001;23(7):296–299.

29. Abdelwahab W, Frishman W, Landau A. Management of hypertensive urgencies and emergencies. *J Clin Pharmacol* 1995;35:747–762.

30. Silver JR. Early autonomic dysreflexia. *Spinal Cord* 2000;38(4):220–233.

31. Karlsson AK. Autonomic dysreflexia. *Spinal Cord* 1999;39(11):805.

32. Galpin J. Infectious complications. In: Casciato D, Lowitz B. eds. *Manual of clinical oncology,* 4th ed.Philadelphia: Lippincott Williams and Wilkins, 2000: 638.

33. Pizzo P. Management of fever in patients with cancer and treatment-induced neutropenia. *N Engl J Med* 1993;328:1323–1332.

34. Oppenheim B, Heather A. Management of febrile neutropenia in low risk cancer patients. *Thorax* 2000;55[Suppl 1]:S63–S69.

35. Mangi MH, Newland AC. Febrile neutropenia: prophylactic and therapeutic use of GM-CSF. *Eur J Cancer* 1999;35[Suppl 3]:S4–S1.

36. Nauseef WM, Maki DG. A study of the value of simple protective isolation in patients with granulocytopenia. *N Engl J Med* 1981;304(8):448–453.

37. Casciato DA. Hematologic complications. In: Casciato D, Lowitz B., eds., *Manual of clinical oncology,* 4th ed. Philadelphia: Lippincott Williams and Wilkins, 2000:615–637.

38. Shulman L, Braunwald E, Rosenthal D. Hematological-oncological disorders and heart disease. In: Braunwald E, ed. *Heart disease: a textbook of cardiovascular medicine.* Philadelphia: WB Saunders, 1997:1786–1808.

39. Rizzo JD, et al. Use of epoetin in patients with cancer: evidence-based clinical practice guidelines of the American Society of Clinical Oncology and the American Society of Hematology. *Blood* 2002;100:2303–2320.

40. Gans BM. Rehabilitation care settings and deep vein thrombosis. *Am J Phys Med Rehabil* 2000;79[Suppl 5]:S1–S2.

41. Warlow C, Ogston D, Douglas AS. Deep venous thrombosis of the legs after stroke. *BMJ* 1976;1178–1183.

42. Gibberd FB, Gould SR, Marks P. Incidence of deep venous thrombosis and leg oedema in patients with stroke. *J Neurol Neurosurg Psychiatry* 1976;39: 1222–1225.

43. Borghi B, Casati A, Rizzoli Study Group on Orthopaedic Anesthesia. Thromboembolic complications after total hip replacement. *Int Orthop* 2002; 26(1):44–47.

44. Meythaler JM, DeViro MJ, H Hayne JB. Cost effectiveness of routine screening for proximal deep venous thrombosis in acquired brain injury patients admitted to rehabilitation. *Arch Phys Med Rehabil* 1996;77:1–5.

45. Kennedy D, Setnik G, Li J. Physical examination findings in deep venous thrombosis. *Emerg Med Clin North Am* 19(4):869–876.

46. Jacobson AF. Diagnosis of deep venous thrombosis: a review of radiographic, radionuclide, and non-imaging methods. *Q J Nucl Med* 45(4):324–333.

47. Mustafa BO, Rathbun SW, Whitsett TL, et al. Sensitivity and specificity of ultrasonography in the diagnosis of upper extremity deep vein thrombosis: a systematic review. *Arch Intern Med* 2002;162(4):401–404.

48. Fraser DGW, Moody AR, Morgan PS, et al. Diagnosis of lower limb deep venous thrombosis: a prospective blinded study of magnetic resonance direct thrombosis imaging. *Arch Intern Med* 2002;136:89–98.

49. Rosen CL, Tracy JA. The diagnosis of lower extremity deep venous thrombosis. *Emerg Med Clin North Am* 2001;19(4):895–912.

50. Kelly J, Rudd A, Lewis RR, et al. Plasma D-dimers in the diagnosis of venous thromboembolism. *Arch Intern Med* 2002;162(7):747–756.

51. Wood KE. Major pulmonary embolism: review of a pathophysiological approach to the golden hour of hemodynamically significant pulmonary embolism. *Chest* 2002;121(3):877–905.

52. Bounameaux H. Integrated diagnostic approach to suspected deep vein thrombosis and pulmonary embolism. *Vasa* 2002;31(1):15–21.

53. Burke DT. Prevention of deep venous thrombosis: overview of available therapy options for rehabilitation patients. *Am J Phys Med Rehabil* 2000;79 [Suppl 5]:S3–S8.

54. Della V, Mirzabeigi E, Zuckerman JD, et al. Thromboembolic prophylaxis for patients with a fracture of the proximal femur. *Am J Orthop* 2002; 31(1):16–24.

55. Pambianco G, Orchard T, Landau D. Deep venous thrombosis: prevention in stroke patients during rehabilitation. *Arch Phys Med Rehabil* 1995;76:324–330.

56. Leizorovicz A, Haugh MC, Chapnis F-R, et al. Low molecular weight heparin in the prevention of perioperative thrombosis. *BMJ* 1992;305:913–920.

57. Geerts WH, Code KI, Jay RM, et al. A prospective study of venous thromboembolism after major trauma. *N Engl J Med* 1994;331:965–968.

58. Merli GJ. Low molecular weight heparins versus unfractionated heparin in the treatment of deep vein thrombosis and pulmonary embolism. *Am J Phys Med Rehabil* 2000;79[Suppl 5]:S16–S19.

59. Routledge PA, West RR. Low molecular weight heparin. *BMJ* 1992;305:906.

60. Bergqvist D. Enoxaparin: a pharmacoeconomic review of its use in the prevention and treatment of venous thromboembolism and in acute coronary syndromes. *Pharmacoeconomics* 2002;20(4):225–243.

61. Brookenthal KR, Freedman KB, Lotke PA, et al. A meta-analysis of thromboembolic prophylaxis in total knee arthroplasty. *J Arthroplasty* 2001;16:293–300.

62. Brenner C, Molloy M, McEnuff N. Use of inferior vena cava filters in thromboembolic disease: two case reports with a literature review. *Ir Med J* 2001;94(9):267–268.

63. Siegler EL, Taylor L, Norris R, et al. Silent ischemia can be detected in rehabilitation patients, but it has limited clinical utility. *Arch Phys Med Rehabil* 1992;73:730–734.

64. Roth EJ, Weisner S, Green D, et al. Dysvascular amputee rehabilitation: the role of continuous noninvasive cardiovascular monitoring during physical therapy. *Am J Phys Med Rehabil* 1987;69:16–22.

65. Cruts HEP, deVries J, Zivold G, et al. Lower extremity amputees with peripheral vascular disease: graded exercise testing and results of prosthetic training. *Arch Phys Med Rehabil* 1987;68:14–19.

66. Gonzalez, EG, Edelstein, JE. Energy expenditure during ambulation. In: Gonzalez ED, chief ed. *Downey and Darling's physiological basis of rehabilitation,* 3rd ed. Boston: Butterworth, Heinemann 2001:417–447.

67. Meltzer RS, Visser CA, Fuster V. Intracardiac thrombi and systemic embolization. *Ann Intern Med* 1986;104:689–698.

68. Dimant, J, Grob, D. Electrocardiographic changes and myocardial damage in patients with acute cerebrovascular accidents. *Stroke* 1997;8:448–455.

69. Myers MS, Norris JW, Hachinski VC, et al. Cardiac sequelae of acute stroke. *Stroke* 1982;13:838–842.

70. Norris JW. Effects of cerebrovascular lesions on the heart. *Neurol Clin* 1983;1:98–101.

71. Dombovy ML, Basford JR, Whisnant JP, et al. Disability and use of rehabilitation services following stroke in Rochester, Minnesota 1975–1979. *Stroke* 1987;18:830–836.

72. Gresham GE, Phillips TF, Wolf PA, et al. The epidemiologic profile of long term stroke disability: the Framingham study. *Arch Phys Med Rehabil* 1978;60:487–491.

73. Roth EJ, Mueller K, Green D. Stroke rehabilitation outcome: impact of coronary artery disease. *Stroke* 1988;19:47–49.

74. Roth EJ. Heart disease in patients with stroke: incidence, impact and implications for rehabilitation. Part 1: classification and prevalence. *Arch Phys Med Rehabil* 1993;74:752–760.

75. Roth EJ. Heart disease in patients with stroke. Part 2: impact and implications for rehabilitation. *Arch Phys Med Rehabil* 1994;75:94–101.

76. Lim PO, McFadyen RJ, Clarkson PBM, et al. Impaired exercise tolerance in hypertensive patients. *Ann Intern Med* 1996;124:41–55.

77. Pennza PT. Aspiration pneumonia, necrotizing pneumonia, and lung abscess. *Emerg Med Clin North Am* 1989;7:279–307.

78. Robinson KM, Zorowitz RD. Mechanisms of aspiration disorders. In: Fishman AP, ed. *Pulmonary diseases and disorders,* 3rd ed. New York: McGraw Hill, 1998:1211–1214.

79. Cohen B, Malik N, Robinson KM. A multidisciplinary swallowing team for prevention of aspiration pneumonia. *Arch Phys Med Rehabil* 1991;72: 793(abst).

80. Pingleton SK. Enteral nutrition as a risk factor for nosocomial pneumonia. *Eur J Clin Microbiol Infect Dis* 1989;8:51–55.

81. Kohn CL, Keithley JK. Enteral nutrition: potential complications and patient monitoring. *Nurs Clin North Am* 1989;23:339–342.

82. Logemann JA. The role of the speech language pathologist in the management of dysphagia. *Otolaryngol Clin North Am* 1988;21:783–788.

83. O'Neill PA. Swallowing and prevention of complications. *Br Med Bull* 2000;56(2):457–465.

84. Shapiro J. Evaluation and treatment of swallowing disorders. *Compr Ther* 2000;26(3):302–309.

85. Eibling DE, Carrau RL. Detection, evaluation, and management of aspiration in rehabilitation hospitals: role of the otolaryngologist—head and neck surgeons. *J Otolaryngol* 2001;30(4):235–241.

86. Horner J, Massey EW. Silent aspiration following stroke. *Neurology* 1988;38:317–319.

87. Ogorek CP, Fisher RS. Detection and treatment of gastroesophageal reflux disease. *Gastroenterol Clin North Am* 1989;18:293–313.

88. Bushman M, Dobmeyer SM, Leeker L, et al. Swallowing abnormalities and their response to treatment in Parkinson's disease. *Neurology* 1989;39: 1309–1314.

89. Johnson ER, McKenzie SW, Sievers A. Aspiration pneumonia in stroke. *Arch Phys Med Rehabil* 1993;74:973–976.

90. Sitzmann JV. Nutritional support of the dysphagic patient: methods, risks and complications of therapy. *J Parent Ent Nutr* 1990;14:60–63.

91. Pennington GR, Kratsch JA. Swallowing disorders: assessment and rehabilitation. *Br J Hosp Med* 1990;44:17–20.

92. DePippo KL, Holas MA, Reding MA. The Burke dysphagia screening test: validation of its use in patients with stroke. *Arch Phys Med Rehabil* 1994;745:1284–1286.

93. Flynn KT, Norton LC, Fisher RL. Enteral tube feeding: indications, practices and outcomes. *Image J Nurs Scholar* 1987;19:16–19.

94. Llaneza PP, Menendez AM, Roberts R, et al. Percutaneous endoscopic gastrostomy: clinical experience and follow up. *South Med J* 1988;321–324.

95. Mamel JJ. Percutaneous endoscopic gastrostomy. *Am J Gastroenterol* 1989;84:703–710.

96. Cavazos JE. Seizures and epilepsy overview and classification. *Med J Neurol* 2002;3(1):1–25.

97. Lowenstein D. Diseases of the central nervous system: seizures and epilepsy. In: Braunwald E, et al., eds. *Harrison's on line.* Columbus: McGraw-Hill, 2001–2002;360:1–22.

98. Schemer ML, Pedley TA. The evaluation and treatment of seizures. *N Engl J Med* 1990;323:1468–1474.
99. Hauser WA. Seizure disorders: the changes with age. *Epilepsia* 1992;33 [Suppl 4]:S6–S14.
100. Commission on Classification and Terminology of the Internal League against Epilepsy. Proposal for revised clinical and electroencephalographic classification of epileptic seizures. *Epilepsia* 1981;22:489–501.
101. Mosewich RK, So EL. A clinical approval to the classification of seizures and epileptic syndromes. *Mayo Clin Proc* 1981;71(4):405–414.
102. Chabolle DR, Krahn LE, So EL, et al. Psychogenic nonepileptic seizures. *Mayo Clin Proc* 1996;71(5):493–500.
103. Salenzer AM, Tabbari B, Vance SC, et al. Epilepsy after penetrating head injury. *Neurology* 1985;35:1406–1414.
104. Lee ST, Lui TN. Early seizures after mild closed head injury. *Neurosurgery* 1992;76:435–439.
105. Thomas R. Seizures and epilepsy in the elderly. *Arch Intern Med* 1997;157 (6):605–617.
106. Epilepsy Foundation of America's Working Group on Status Epilepticus. Treatment of convulsive status epilepticus: recommendations of the Epilepsy Foundation of America's Working Group on Status Epilepticus. *JAMA* 1993;270:854–859.
107. Lowenstein DH, Alldredge GN. Status epilepticus. *N Engl J Med* 1998;338: 970–976.
108. Brodie MJ, Dichter MA. Anti-epileptic drugs. *N Engl J Med* 1996;334(3): 168–175.
109. Dichtle MA, Brodie MJ. New anti-epileptic drugs. *N Engl J Med* 1996;334(24): 1583–1590.
110. Lipowski ZJ. Update on delirium. *Psychiat Clin North Am* 1992;15(2): 335–346.
111. Lerkoff SE, Evans DA, Lipzin B, et al. Delirium. *Arch Intern Med* 1992;152: 334–340.
112. Murray AM, Lerkoff SE, Wetle TT, et al. Acute delirium and functional decline in hospital elderly patients. *J Geront* 1993;48(5):M181–M186.
113. Francis J, Kapoor WN. Prognosis after hospital discharge of older medical patients with delirium. *J Am Geriatr Soc* 1992;40:601–606.
114. McCusker J, Cole M, Dendukuri N, et al. Delirium in older medical inpatients and subsequent cognitive and functional status: a prospective study. *CMAJ* 2001;165(5):575–583.
115. Lipowski ZK. *Delirium: acute confusional states.* New York: Oxford University Press, 1990.
116. Beresin EV. Delirium in the elderly. *J Geriatr Psychiatry Neurol* 1988;1:127–143.
117. Pfitzenmeyer P, Musat A, Lenfant L, et al. Post operative cognitive disorders in the elderly. *Presse Med* 2001;30(13):648–652(abst).
118. Conn DK. Delirium and other organic mental disorders. In: Sadavoy J, Lazarus LW, Jarvik LF, eds. *Comprehensive review of geriatric psychiatry.* Washington, DC: American Psychiatric Press, 1991:311–336.
119. Applebaum PS, Grisso T. Assessing patients' capacities to consent to treatment. *N Engl J Med* 1988;319:1636–1638.
120. Applebaum PS, Roth LH. Clinical issues in the assessment of competence. *N Engl J Med* 1981;138:1462–1466.
121. Tueth MJ. Diagnosing psychiatric emergencies in the elderly. *Am J Emerg Med* 1994;12:964–396.
122. Kishi Y, Robinson RG, Kosier JT. Suicidal ideation among patients during the rehabilitation period after life threatening physical illness. *J Nerv Ment Dis* 2001;189(9):623–628.
123. Kennedy GJ, Lowinger R. Psychogeriatric emergencies. *Clin Geriatr Med* 1993;9(3):641–653.
124. Tueth MJ. Management of behavioral emergencies. *Am J Emerg Med* 1995;13: 344–350.

CHAPTER 58

Nutrition in Physical Medicine and Rehabilitation

Faren H. Williams and Barbara Hopkins

Good nutrition can optimize rehabilitation efforts in both the acute care and the long-term care settings. A wide variety of nutritional problems are seen in the rehabilitation setting because many diverse diseases and injuries can result in disabilities. There are patients with congenital problems and others with acquired disabilities as a result of trauma or aging. This chapter discusses some of the special nutritional needs of disabled persons. Basic nutritional principles are discussed, and special needs for different groups of disabled people are identified.

BASIC PRINCIPLES OF NUTRITION MANAGEMENT

Nutritional science involves the study of food, the nutrients that food contains, and the way in which food supports health and life. The goal of nutrition management is to ensure that an individual has a diet containing all the necessary substances in the amounts appropriate for that person and is accessible and acceptable to the person.

Malnutrition exists when a person has a poor nutritional status. Historically, malnutrition has been considered primarily to be the result of a lack of one or more nutrients in the diet. The problems of excessive and unbalanced nutrient intake, however, have become evident as life expectancy increased, food supplies in the developed nations of the world have stabilized at abundant levels, and the metabolic bases of chronic disease states have been identified. Thus, any one of three conditions can result in suboptimal function secondary to malnutrition:

1. Nutrient deficiency (undernutrition). This condition develops when insufficient amounts of one or more nutrients are taken in to meet metabolic needs.
2. Nutrient excess (overnutrition). This condition is the result of an excessive intake of one or more nutrients.
3. Nutrient imbalance. This condition develops when a person consumes a diet that is not balanced in nutrients. Therefore, some nutrients might be consumed in excessive amounts and others in insufficient amounts.

The development of malnutrition follows a continuum that initially develops as body stores of a nutrient are changed from a condition of balance to one of imbalance, involving depletion or excess of one or more nutrients. Further imbalance of nutrient intake then leads to alterations of metabolism at the biochemical level. If the imbalance continues, overt disease will result.

FOOD COMPOSITION

Food is made up of chemical substances. Those that must be consumed by living organisms to sustain life are known as nutrients. Other substances that may affect health and function are present in some foods. An adequate diet is achieved by balancing the substances in food in amounts appropriate for a given person.

Nutrients

Nutrients include six major categories of chemical compounds:

1. Water
2. Proteins
3. Carbohydrates
4. Fats
5. Vitamins
6. Minerals.

The specific categories of nutrients are based on their chemical composition. Water is the most basic compound essential for life, comprising more than 50% of total body mass, and is an integral part of cell structures and the basic medium for body fluid. Protein, carbohydrates, and fats share the function of supplying energy. In addition, each has a unique chemical composition and, thus, they serve different functions in areas of body composition, cell structure, and metabolic activity. Vitamins are divided into two categories, based on their solubility in fat or water. Many of the vitamins function primarily as cofactors for enzymatic reactions to support metabolic needs of the body. The fat-soluble and some of the water-soluble vitamins are stored in the body to some extent, so that not all vitamins must be obtained daily to maintain balanced nutrition. Minerals include inorganic elements, classified according to the relative quantities required for health (Table 58-1).

Although all nutrients are considered essential to life, the amounts of some nutrients necessary for health are variable be-

TABLE 58-1.   Vitamins and Minerals

Nutrient	Major Function(s)
Water-soluble vitamins	
Thiamin (B_1)	Coenzyme in carbohydrate metabolism; nerve function
Riboflavin (B_2)	Coenzyme in citric acid cycle, fat metabolism, and electron transport chain
Niacin (B_3)	Coenzyme in citric acid cycle, fat metabolism, and electron transport chain
Biotin	Coenzyme in glucose production and fat synthesis
Pyridoxine	Coenzyme in protein metabolism, neurotransmitter and hemoglobin synthesis
Pantothenic acid	Coenzyme in citric acid cycle and fat metabolism (synthesis and beta-oxidation)
Folate	Coenzyme in RNA and DNA synthesis
Vitamin B_{12}	Coenzyme in folate metabolism, nerve function
Vitamin C	Collagen synthesis; hormone and neurotransmitter synthesis; antioxidant
Fat-soluble vitamins	
Vitamin A (retinoids and provitamin A carotenoids)	Vision; growth; cell differentiation; immunity; antioxidant
Vitamin D	Absorption of calcium and phosphorus; bone maintenance
Vitamin E	Antioxidant
Vitamin K	Blood clotting
Major minerals (>100 mg/day)	
Calcium	Bone and tooth structure; blood clotting; muscle contractions; nerve transmission
Phosphorus	Bone and tooth structure; intermediary metabolism; membrane structure; ATP
Sodium	Major extracellular cation; nerve transmission; regulate fluid balance
Potassium	Major intracellular cation; nerve transmission
Magnesium	Bone structure; enzyme function; nerve and muscle function; ATP
Chloride	Major extracellular anion; nerve transmission
Sulfur	Part of vitamins and amino acids; acid–base balance
Minor minerals (<20 mg/day)	
Iron	Part of hemoglobin and myoglobin; immunity
Cobalt	Part of vitamin B_{12}
Manganese	Functions in carbohydrate and fat metabolism; superoxide dismutase
Molybdenum	Cofactor for several enzymes
Fluoride	Strengthens tooth enamel
Copper	Iron metabolism; superoxide dismutase; nerve and immune function; lipid metabolism; collagen
Zinc	Cofactor in hundreds of enzyme systems; protein synthesis; growth; immunity; superoxide dismutase; alcohol metabolism
Iodine	Synthesis of thyroid hormone
Selenium	Antioxidant function as component of glutathione paroxidase
Chromium	Glucose tolerance

ATP, adenosine triphosphate; DNA, deoxyribonucleic acid; RNA, ribonucleic acid.

cause functions overlap. An example of this variability is the proportion of protein, fats, and carbohydrates needed for health. Because all share the function of providing energy to the body, the proportions of these three nutrients in the diet can vary. However, protein and fats have unique roles. There is a basic essential requirement for these substances in the diet not reflected in energy requirements because the body is unable to make the basic components of protein (specific essential amino acids) and of fats (specific essential fatty acids) (1,2). But when amino acids are used for energy they must be modified chemically in the liver to remove the nitrogen. This process requires more calories, and the ability to remove nitrogen and excrete it has finite limits, which if exceeded may lead to increased ammonia in the body. Therefore, protein can be harmful if it is the only source of energy. Optimal ratios of these three substances should be achieved with a balanced diet.

Another major factor affecting the requirements of various nutrients is the body's ability to store them. Fats and any other excess energy from carbohydrates or proteins are stored as adipose tissue, except for minimal quantities of carbohydrate stored as glycogen. The glycogen must be produced from absorbed food substances or from the glycerol component of fat stores. Excess protein results in the conversion of carbon skeletons to fat, and when protein in the diet is limited, the protein of skeletal muscle will be broken down to meet the metabolic requirements of life-sustaining functions (3).

Other Components of Food

Interest in the role of human gut flora in the maintenance of good health has led to the study of the effects of prebiotics and probiotics on human microbiota (4). Probiotics are microbial foods or supplements that prevent or reduce the colonization of pathogenic flora and reestablish normal gut flora (4). The microbial strains that prove to be the most beneficial are *Lactobacillus* and *Bifidobacterium*. There are several clinical applications for probiotics which include treatment of antibiotic-associated diarrhea, urinary tract infections, and *Candida* vaginitis, reduction in *Clostridium difficile*, the management of hepatic encephalopathy, and the reduction in serum cholesterol levels (4–7). Potential benefits may also include management of inflammatory bowel disease and the prevention of cancer. Food sources of probiotics consist of dairy products with live microorganisms such as yogurt and culture-added milks. Other forms of probiotics are capsules, tablets, and powders but the amount of viable bacteria is often lower than what the label claims.

Prebiotics are nondigestible food ingredients that stimulate the growth or activity of specific bacteria in the colon (5). The major prebiotics are transgalactosylated disaccharides, fructooligosaccharides (FOSs), xylooligosaccharides, and soybean oligosaccharides . The most well-known prebiotic is FOS. FOSs resist enzyme hydrolysis by the small intestine and arrive in the colon completely intact. While in the colon bacteria ferment them, producing energy, short chain fatty acids, and various gases. Fermentation allows an increased production of *Bifidobacterium*, which proves to be beneficial to the health of the host. Increased levels of *Bifidobacterium* have shown to increase calcium absorption and decrease the growth of potential pathogens (5,6). Foods with a high FOS content include chicory, onions, and bananas. In addition, FOSs have been added to beverages and dietary supplements (e.g., they appear as inulin or FOS on the ingredient list on food labels).

FIBER

Fiber refers to carbohydrates and related substances in the diet that are not digestible; therefore, it is not classified as a nutrient. However, fiber does perform several physiological functions in the gastrointestinal (GI) system (8). The primary properties of fiber in the gut seem to be (a) its hydrophilic capacity, which increases stool bulk and decreases transit time, (b) its ability to bind other dietary substances, so that changes in the fiber in the gut seem to be its hydrophilic capacity, which increases stool bulk and decreases transit time, and (c) its ability to bind other dietary substances, so that changes in the fiber content of the diet will alter absorption and bioavailability of both nutrients and toxins. These functions may sound simple, but the overall impact of fiber in the diet is diverse and varies with the type of fiber consumed. The physiological consequences have been shown to affect the control of diabetes mellitus, disorders of lipid metabolism, and obesity. Fiber content of the diet may also affect the incidence of some cancers.

Another positive aspect of fiber ingestion is fiber fermentation. All fibers, except lignin, can be fermented by the gut bacteria and produce components known as short-chain fatty acids (SCFAs). The three most common fatty acids produced are propionate, acetate, and butyrate. Each of these provides energy to the colonocytes, but only butyrate has trophic effects on the colonocytes. The more soluble the fiber (pectins, gums, mucilages), the greater is the SCFA production.

CHOLESTEROL

Cholesterol is a member of the sterol group of organic compounds. It is derived from fats and can be synthesized endogenously in quantities sufficient to meet metabolic demand. It is an integral part of cell structures and a precursor of some hormones and vitamin D. Cholesterol is present in some foods and is absorbed during the process of digestion. Dietary sources of cholesterol may be associated with the development of atherosclerosis, but it is not known whether disabled people are affected to the same extent.

DIETARY STANDARDS

Dietary standards serve as guidelines for the amounts of essential nutrients that should be consumed to ensure optimal health. The dietary standards used in the United States are the Dietary Reference Intakes (DRIs). They are used in assessing and planning diets. The DRIs have been established by the Food and Nutrition Board of the National Academy of Sciences and replace and expand the 1989 Recommended Dietary Allowances. The DRIs are a set of four nutrient-based reference values, which include the Estimated Average Requirement (EAR), the Recommended Dietary Allowances (RDA), Adequate Intake (AI), and the Tolerable Upper Intake Level (UL) (9–12) (Table 58-2).

- EAR is the estimated nutrient intake that meets the requirement for 50% of the healthy individuals in a specific life stage and gender group.
- RDA EAR is the average dietary intake level to meet the requirement of 97% to 98% of the healthy individuals in a specific life stage and gender group.
- AI is a recommended intake level that is assumed to be adequate and is used when there are not enough scientific data to estimate an EAR or an RDA.
- UL refers to the highest daily nutrient intake for most individuals that will not have adverse health effects.
- DRIs are grouped according to particular life stages and gender.

DIETARY RECOMMENDATIONS

The purpose of dietary recommendations is to translate the information about nutrients required for health and the nutrient composition of food into the amount and type of food that should be consumed to meet nutritional needs. Two commonly used methods are the Dietary Guidelines for Americans (Fig. 58-1) and the Food Guide Pyramid (Fig. 58-2). Both of these methods are designed to promote good health and disease prevention. The Dietary Guidelines offer suggestions for food choices and emphasize the importance of variety and moderation. The Food Guide Pyramid recommends a diet plan based on servings from five food groups.

Assessment of Nutritional Status

The assessment of nutritional status helps determine the presence of malnutrition or risk for malnutrition. It involves the gathering and interpretation of data from which the effect of disease, injury, other stressors, and nutritional intervention can be monitored over time. Screening is used to identify individuals who need full nutrition assessment. For comprehensive nutrition assessment, there needs to be direct measurement or estimation of food and nutrient intake and the use of subjective and objective measures of the clinical, anthropometric, biochemical, and physiological status of the person. Appropriate assessment techniques may vary depending on the goals of the assessment.

Screening for Nutritional Risk

In daily clinical practice it is necessary to be able to identify subjects at risk for malnutrition. There is a tendency to focus on the specifics of food intake alone, but the development of malnutrition is multifactorial, and one needs to identify all the potential factors to successfully treat it (Fig. 58-3). People are at risk of going from well nourished to malnourished when any one of these factors is altered. Screening is important to determine which people need more intensive nutritional assessment and intervention.

For routine screening a simple checklist can rapidly identify those with new risk factors and serve as a guide for referral to a registered dietitian, who can do a more detailed assessment and make recommendations to prevent further nutritional problems (Fig. 58-4).

Evaluation of Food/Nutrient Intake

A record of food intake is necessary to determine the nutrient content of the food actually consumed. The nutrient intake is

TABLE 58-2. Dietary Reference Intakes

Macronutrients / Vitamins

Life Stage Group	Protein (g/d)	Carbohydrate (g/d)	Fiber (g/d)	Fat (g/d)	A (µg/d)*	C (mg/d)	D (µg/d)	E (mg/d)	K (µg/d)	Thiamin (mg/d)	Riboflavin (mg/d)	Niacin (mg/d)	B6 (mg/d)	Folate† (µg/d)	B12 (µg/d)	Pantothenic Acid (mg/d)	Biotin (µg/d)	Choline (mg/d)
Infant																		
0–6 mo	9.1	60	ND	31	400	40	5	4	2.0	0.2	0.3	2	0.1	65	0.4	1.7	5	125
7–12 mo	13.5	95	ND	30	500	50	5	5	2.5	0.3	0.4	4	0.3	80	0.5	1.8	6	150
Children																		
1–3 y	13	130	19	ND	300	15	5	6	30	0.5	0.5	6	0.5	150	0.9	2	8	200
4–8 y	19	130	25	ND	400	25	5	7	55	0.6	0.6	8	0.6	200	1.2	3	12	250
Males																		
9–13 y	34	130	31	ND	600	45	5	11	60	0.9	0.9	12	1.0	300	1.8	4	20	375
14–18 y	52	130	38	ND	900	75	5	15	75	1.2	1.3	16	1.3	400	2.4	5	25	550
19–30 y	56	130	38	ND	900	90	5	15	120	1.2	1.3	16	1.3	400	2.4	5	30	550
31–50 y	56	130	38	ND	900	90	5	15	120	1.2	1.3	16	1.3	400	2.4	5	30	550
51–70 y	56	130	30	ND	900	90	10	15	120	1.2	1.3	16	1.7	400	2.4	5	30	550
>70 y	56	130	30	ND	900	90	15	15	120	1.2	1.3	16	1.7	400	2.4	5	30	550
Females																		
9–13 y	34	130	26	ND	600	45	5	11	60	0.9	0.9	12	1.0	300	1.8	4	20	375
14–18 y	46	130	26	ND	700	65	5	15	75	1.0	1.0	14	1.2	400	2.4	5	25	400
19–30 y	46	130	25	ND	700	75	5	15	90	1.1	1.1	14	1.3	400	2.4	5	30	425
31–50 y	46	130	25	ND	700	75	5	15	90	1.1	1.1	14	1.3	400	2.4	5	30	425
51–70 y	46	130	21	ND	700	75	10	15	90	1.1	1.1	14	1.5	400	2.4	5	30	425
>70 y	46	130	21	ND	700	75	15	15	90	1.1	1.1	14	1.5	400	2.4	5	30	425
Pregnancy																		
14–18 y	71	175	28	ND	750	80	5	15	75	1.4	1.4	18	1.9	600	2.6	6	30	450
19–30 y	71	175	28	ND	770	85	5	15	90	1.4	1.4	18	1.9	600	2.6	6	30	450
31–50 y	71	175	28	ND	770	85	5	15	90	1.4	1.4	18	1.9	600	2.6	6	30	450
Lactation																		
14–18 y	71	210	29	ND	1200	115	5	19	75	1.4	1.4	17	2.0	500	2.8	7	35	550
19–30 y	71	210	29	ND	1300	120	5	19	90	1.4	1.4	17	2.0	500	2.8	7	35	550
31–50 y	71	210	29	ND	1300	120	5	19	90	1.4	1.4	17	2.0	500	2.8	7	35	550

Recommended Dietary Allowances (RDAs) are in bold type and Adequate Intakes are in ordinary type. ND: not determined; * as retinal activity equivalents (RAE)–1 RAE = 1 µg retinal, 12 µg β-carotene. † Dietary folate equivalent (DFE); 1 DFE = 1 µg food folate, = 0.6 µg folic acid from fortified food or supplement consumed with food, = 0.5 µg of a supplement taken on an empty stomach

Elements

Life Stage Group	Calcium (mg/d)	Chromium (µg/d)	Coppers (µg/d)	Fluoride (mg/d)	Iodine (µg/d)	Iron (mg/d)	Magnesium (mg/d)	Manganese (mg/d)	Molybdenum (µg/d)	Phosphorus (mg/d)	Selenium (µg/d)	Zinc (mg/d)
Infant												
0–6 mo	210	0.2	200	0.01	110	0.27	30	0.003	2	100	15	2
7–12 mo	270	5.5	220	0.5	130	11	75	0.6	3	275	20	3
Children												
1–3 y	500	11	340	0.7	90	7	80	1.2	17	460	20	3
4–8 y	800	15	440	1	90	10	130	1.5	22	500	30	5
Males												
9–13 y	1300	25	700	2	120	8	240	1.9	34	1250	40	8
14–18 y	1300	35	890	3	150	11	410	2.2	43	1250	55	11
19–30 y	1000	35	900	4	150	8	400	2.3	45	700	55	11
31–50 y	1000	35	900	4	150	8	420	2.3	45	700	55	11
51–70 y	1200	30	900	4	150	8	420	2.3	45	700	55	11
>70 y	1200	30	900	4	150	8	420	2.3	45	700	55	11
Females												
9–13 y	1300	21	700	2	120	8	240	1.6	34	1250	40	8
14–18 y	1300	24	890	3	150	15	360	1.6	43	1250	55	9
19–30 y	1000	25	900	3	150	18	310	1.8	45	700	55	8
31–50 y	1000	25	900	3	150	18	320	1.8	45	700	55	8
51–70 y	1200	20	900	3	150	8	320	1.8	45	700	55	8
>70 y	1200	20	900	3	150	8	320	1.8	45	700	55	8
Pregnancy												
14–18 y	1300	29	1000	3	220	27	400	2.0	50	1250	60	12
19–30 y	1000	30	1000	3	220	27	350	2.0	50	700	60	11
31–50 y	1000	30	1000	3	220	27	360	2.0	50	700	60	11
Lactation												
14–18 y	1300	44	1300	3	290	10	360	2.6	50	1250	70	13
19–30 y	1000	45	1300	3	290	9	310	2.6	50	700	70	12
31–50 y	1000	45	1300	3	290	9	320	2.6	50	700	70	12

Recommended Dietary Allowances (RDAs) are in bold type and Adequate Intakes are in ordinary type.

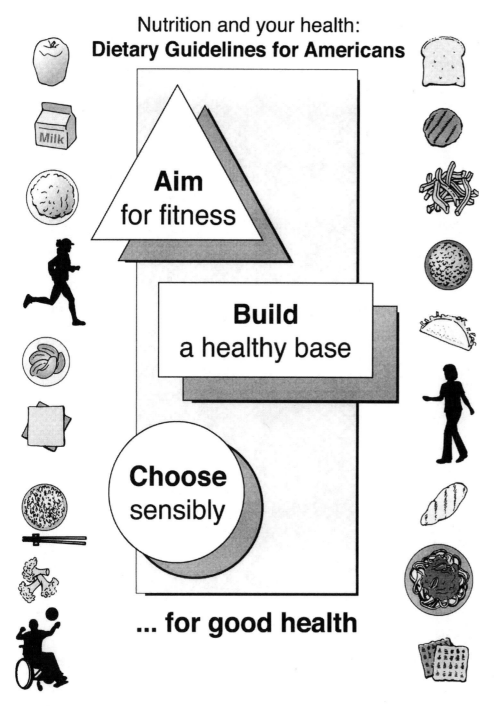

Figure 58-1. Dietary guidelines for Americans. (From U.S. Department of Agriculture, U.S. Department of Health and Human Services, 1995.)

compared with standards so that adequacy of the diet can be determined. Various methods exist for obtaining this information, all of which have advantages and limitations (13–15).

Collection Methods

Several of the more common collection methods are reviewed here, with the intention of concentrating on both their strengths and weaknesses. Information of this type is crucial to selecting the type of data collection needed to meet the need of any given patient care situation (14).

TWENTY-FOUR–HOUR FOOD RECALL
The registered dietitian, trained dietetic technician, or family member interviews the patient to determine what foods and fluids have been consumed in the previous 24 hours. This is an extremely easy method, but the assumption is that one's intake is "typical" of every day. Possible errors include lack of memory, inability to estimate portions, and inaccurate reporting.

FOOD RECORD DIARY
The food and fluid consumed over several days (usually 3 to 7 days) can be recorded. Because food habits vary, especially between weekdays and weekends, it is important to know what specific days have been included. Records are kept by each patient or by the patient's caregiver. Accuracy is increased if portions are measured or weighed as prepared and waste is subtracted.

FOOD FREQUENCY RECORD
The frequencies with which major groups of foods are consumed (i.e., daily, weekly, monthly, sporadic, or never) can be

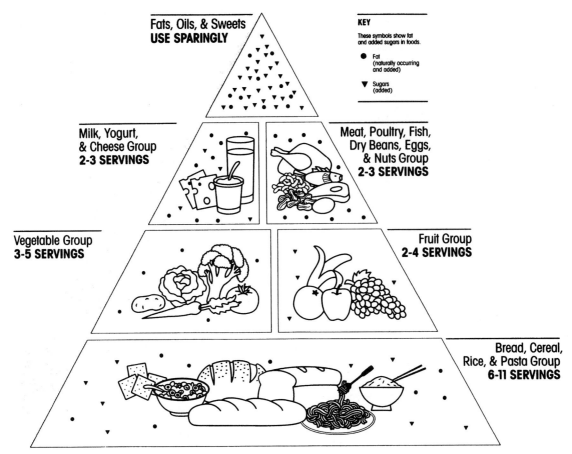

Figure 58-2. The food guide pyramid is a general guideline to what a person should eat each day in order to get needed nutrients as well as the right amount of calories to maintain a healthy weight. It emphasizes foods from the five food groups as shown in the three lower sections of the pyramid. (From U.S. Department of Agriculture and U.S. Department of Health and Human Services.)

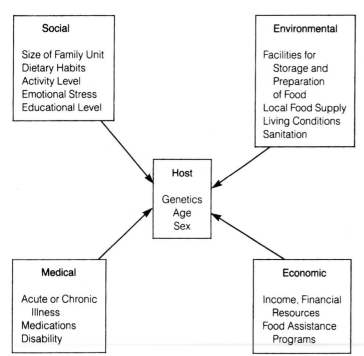

Figure 58-3. Multifactorial etiology of malnutrition. (From Frankel DL. Nutrition. In: DeLisa JA, Gans BM, et al., eds. *Rehabilitation medicine: principles and practice*, 2nd ed. Philadelphia: JB Lippincott Co, 1993:599.)

Has there been a change in any of the following?

1. Income   _____
2. Living Situation   _____
3. Source of Food   _____
4. Medical Condition   _____
5. Physical Activity   _____
6. Transportation   _____
7. Employment Status   _____
8. Eating Habits   _____

Figure 58-4. Screening for risk of malnutrition. If there is a change in any of these factors since the patient was last evaluated, there is a new risk of malnutrition, and further screening of nutritional status should be undertaken. (From Frankel DL. Nutrition. In: DeLisa JA, Gans BM, et al., eds. *Rehabilitation medicine: principles and practice*, 2nd ed. Philadelphia, JB Lippincott Co, 1993:599.)

surveyed. A standard portion size provides the base against which the number of portions for a given time interval is determined. Information is obtained through a questionnaire or interview. It is often used with a 24-hour recall.

OBSERVATION OF FOOD INTAKE

Alcohol and Other Food Supplements

It is important to obtain information on alcohol consumption and use of nutritional supplements as part of the survey. It may be helpful to have information about minerals in the water supply. Sodium content of the diet may be highly variable, even within communities, because of variations in the water supply or use of water softeners. If supplements are consumed, it is important to get information on their nutrient content directly from packaging material or the manufacturer because combinations and amounts of ingredients vary among brands.

The reliability of any of the methods will increase with repetition. Through the use of a combination of food intake survey methods, increased reliability can be achieved (16).

By combining a food intake survey with the measurement of related biochemical parameters, it is possible to validate the accuracy of the dietary intake information. This approach has been applied successfully to the study of dietary protein intake (17).

Adequacy of Food/Nutrient Intake

The dietary information collected by methods such as those reviewed previously must be translated into information about nutrient composition to determine the adequacy of intake. Methods that assess frequency of food or food group intakes usually are evaluated for nutrient content by comparing the patient's diet pattern with standard intake patterns, as mentioned earlier. If a significant imbalance is evident, there is indication of possible malnutrition, which may be related to poor dietary habits.

When actual food intake is recorded or recalled, it may be compared against patterns of food intake with food surveys, or specific nutrient/energy content may be calculated by information available from food composition tables (18–20). Historically, this was a tedious task, but computer software now transforms food intake data into nutrient intake. There are some potential sources of error. These include nutrient content differences depending on where the food was produced and how it was stored and prepared. Information in food composition tables is based on average data from small samples; therefore, one must use some caution in interpreting the data. If one conducts metabolic balance studies, then nutrient analysis is done on the actual food being consumed.

BALANCE STUDIES

Another method for determining the adequacy of food/nutrient intake is that of energy/nutrient balance studies. The assumption is that the optimally nourished person is in a state of equilibrium, with the amount of energy/nutrients used or lost in daily metabolic activity being replaced by energy/nutrients in the diet. When a person is in a physiological stage of growth or tissue repair, it is necessary for the balance to become positive, taking in a greater amount of energy/nutrients. For healthy weight loss, it is necessary for energy balance to become negative, but without loss of lean body mass. Balance for energy and nutrients fluctuates with time, but over a given period, a day or week, the dietitian can assess the overall direction of balance. The measures of energy, nitrogen, and fluid balance have multiple direct clinical applications in the day-to-day nutrition management of a patient.

Energy Balance

Energy is necessary for all activities of life, including the internal work of metabolic processes for maintenance and repair of bodily tissues and the external work done by a person on the environment. The optimal state of nutrition with regard to energy is one of equilibrium. In the person who is growing, either naturally or recovering from an injury to body tissue, energy balance must be positive. If the energy (caloric) intake is inadequate, then body tissues will be metabolized for transformation into energy. Conversely, consumption of excessive amounts of energy (calories) will lead to excess adipose tissue.

The major sources of energy in the diet are carbohydrates, protein, and fat (Table 58-3).

Ethanol, too, is a source of energy and may provide significant calories for some individuals. The traditional unit for expression of energy content of foods and energy requirements is the kilocalorie (kcal), commonly referred to as a calorie. It is the amount of heat necessary to raise the temperature of 1 kg of water from 15°C to 16°C. The energy content of foods and nutrients has been determined through calorimetric techniques and is used to calculate the energy value of food consumed (18–20). A reasonable estimate of energy sources in the diet is necessary to prevent insufficient or excessive energy intake.

TABLE 58-3. Sources of Energy in the Diet	
	kcal/g (average)
Carbohydrates	4.0
Protein	4.0
Fat	9.0
Ethanol	7.1

Adapted from Silberman H, Eisenberg D. Evaluation of nutritional status. In: Silberman H, Eisenberg D, eds. *Parenteral and enteral nutrition for the hospitalized patient.* Norwalk, CT: Appleton-Century-Crofts, 1982;37.

The estimate needs to be made in the context of the clinical situation to avoid underfeeding or overfeeding.

In a steady state, energy requirements can be determined by weighing someone over time and using predictive equations. If the weight remains stable, then one's energy needs can be calculated. If the person is gaining or losing weight, then the energy intake is either excessive or deficient, respectively. Routine weights are helpful for management of long-term dietary goals and for educational purposes. Body weight also reflects hydration status, with 1 L being equivalent to approximately 2 lbs. When weight gain is too fast or too excessive, then fluid shifts should be suspected and appropriate labs checked. Adjustments should be made by closely monitoring the clinical situation and nutrition management (i.e., amount of calories and nutrients being provided to the patient).

It is ideal to have a direct measurement tool. For basic research, direct calorimetry is the most accurate method for the determination of energy expenditure. It requires that the patient be in an insulated chamber. The amount of heat given off directly is determined by temperature measures. The heat removed by vaporization of water from the body surface is calculated from information obtained by measuring the amount of moisture added to the air in the chamber (21). This is too cumbersome, expensive, and demanding for clinical applications.

The technique of indirect calorimetry allows the calculation of energy expenditure through the estimation of heat production from measures of gaseous exchange (i.e., oxygen consumed or carbon dioxide produced) during normal respiration (22,23). With the development of portable equipment for gaseous sampling and analysis, it is possible to apply this technique clinically, as an aid to direct determination of energy expenditure in both the acutely ill patient and the patient with chronic disability, during rest and activity (23–35). Indirect calorimetry is applied mostly in the determination of resting energy expenditure (REE), with additional calories added to cover the demands of both metabolic and physical activity by estimation and clinical monitoring.

Nitrogen Balance

Nitrogen balance reflects the protein status equilibrium of the body and therefore provides useful information for monitoring the adequacy of nutrition support. It is most important in patients with high rates of metabolic activity, such as those with head trauma, and patients requiring supplemental feedings.

To assess nitrogen balance, the clinician measures the nitrogen content of the diet plus supplements and the nitrogen content of material lost from the body (through urine and feces), then determines the difference between intake and output. Measures of nitrogen intake can be determined accurately in the hospital setting for patients on total enteral or parenteral feedings because the amount of substrate administered and its protein or nitrogen content are known. However, it is more difficult to accurately determine the amount of nitrogen for patients eating regular meals, and extremely difficult to calculate nitrogen losses. Twenty-four-hour urine collections are needed to do nitrogen balance studies. The urinary urea nitrogen content can be measured, and a correction factor applied for non-urea nitrogen. Additional estimates are used for approximation of the non-urea nitrogen losses in feces and skin. These formulas will be inaccurate in patients with protein-losing enteropathy and those with burns, decubitus ulcers, or abscesses. Those patients lose protein and nitrogen secondary to fluid exudates or necrotic tissue sloughs, and those losses are hard to calculate. There are some nitrogen balance equations that can be helpful.

Fluid Balance

Fluid balance is monitored in the acute hospital by measuring fluid intake, urine output, and body weight. A clinical assessment for edema and dehydration is also helpful. With diarrhea, vomiting, or fever, fluids in excess of output may be required. Fluid balance is affected by hepatic and renal function through the role of plasma proteins and electrolytes in the distribution of body fluid between body compartments. When patients have a neurogenic bladder, fluid intake needs to be spread out during the day so fluid shifts are minimized. Having patients chart their fluid intake may be helpful.

CLINICAL EVALUATION

The clinical history and examination are extremely valuable in identifying people with nutritional problems. Baker (36) studied general surgical patients and found a high correlation between clinical assessment and nutritional status (37).

Historical Information

Much information regarding nutritional status can be obtained from questions asked as part of the general medical history. Of particular concern is information about the following:

- Change in body weight, especially if this was not the result of specific dietary intervention
- Change in appetite or eating habits
- Change in activity level
- Change in GI function
- Presence of acute or chronic medical-surgical problems
- Specific feeding or swallowing problems
- Regular medication or supplement use.

A sample of questions is presented in Figure 58-4. There are several examples of historical surveys in the literature that either stand by themselves or are used in conjunction with objective data (16,38–40).

Physical Examination

Specific physical changes associated with nutrient deficiencies are rarely seen in developed countries, but there are abnormalities on physical examination that should alert the clinician to the potential for malnutrition. The physical consequences of specific nutrient deficiency may be seen most frequently in patients on long-term nutritional support with manufactured nutritional supplements or elemental formulations (40).

The physiological manifestations of specific nutrient excesses have been identified in people who take large amounts of nutritional supplements. An awareness of specific findings is important. Some of these specific findings are given in Table 58-4.

Physical findings can reflect three different stages in the development of malnutrition. First, the integrity of body tissues with a rapid turnover, such as skin and mucous membranes, reflects the adequacy of recent nutrition support. Second, the condition of body tissues that have developed over time, such as hair and nails, may reflect changes in nutritional status during variable growth periods. Third, the proportions of body tissues that serve as reservoirs of nutrients, such as skeletal muscle and adipose tissue, reflect chronic nutritional status. With severe malnutrition, the physician may find changes in the size or function of specific organ systems that can be observed on clinical examination.

TABLE 58-4. Nutrition Assessment: Physical Findings

Clinical Findings	Possible Nutritional Causes
Hair	
Dyspigmentation (flag sign)	Protein deficiency
Easily plucked	Protein deficiency
Sparse	Protein, biotin, zinc deficiency
Corkscrew hairs	Vitamin C deficiency
Nails	
Spoon nails (koilonychia)	Iron deficiency
Brittle nails	Iron deficiency; excess vitamin A
Transverse ridging	Protein deficiency
Skin	
Scaling	Vitamin A, essential fatty acid, zinc deficiency
Follicular hyperkeratosis	Vitamin A deficiency
Petechiae	Vitamin A, C deficiency
Purpura	Vitamin C, K deficiency
Yellow coloration	Excess carotene
Pellagrous dermatitis	Niacin deficiency
Cellophane appearance	Protein deficiency
Eyes	
Night blindness	Vitamin A deficiency
Bitot spots	Vitamin A deficiency
Papilledema	Vitamin A excess
Pale conjunctivae	Iron deficiency
Mouth	
Angular stomatitis	Riboflavin, niacin, pyridoxine deficiency
Chailosis	Riboflavin, niacin, pyridoxine deficiency
Tongue	
Pale, atrophic	Iron deficiency
Atrophic lingual papillae	Riboflavin, niacin, folate, vitamin B_{12}, protein, iron deficiency
Glossitis (scarlet)	Riboflavin, niacin, folate, vitamin B_{12}, pyridoxine deficiency
Hypogeusia	Zinc deficiency
Gums	
Spongy, bleeding	Vitamin C deficiency
Musculoskeletal	
Beading of ribs	Viamin D deficiency
Muscle wasting	Protein-calorie malnutrition
Tenderness	Vitamin C deficiency
Neurologic	
Confusion	Thiamin, niacin, vitamin B_{12} deficiency
Ophthalmoplegia	Thiamin, phosphorus deficiency
Peripheral neuropathy	Thiamin, pyridoxine, vitamin B_{12} deficiency
Tetany	Calcium deficiency
Other	
Cardiomegaly	Thiamine deficiency
Cardiomyopathy	Selenium deficiency
Hepatomegaly	Protein malnutrition
Edema	Protein, thiamin deficiency
Thyroid enlargement	Iodide deficiency

Adapted from Lee RD, Nieman DC, *Nutritional assessment, 2nd ed.* St. Louis: CV Mosby, 1996; and Whitney EN, Cataldo CB, Rolles SR. *Understanding normal and clinical nutrition.* New York: West Publishing, 1994.

Anthropometric Measures

Body mass index (BMI) is a useful tool to assess the degree of adiposity and the potential health risks of overweight status (41–43). BMI compares weight to height and can be calculated using either of the following equations:

$$BMI = \frac{weight\ (kg)}{height\ (m^2)} \quad or \quad BMI = \frac{weight\ (kg)}{height\ (in.)} \times 705$$

The classification for obesity and its association to health risk is presented below.

Risk of Associated Disease According to BMI and Waist Size

BMI		Waist less than or equal to 40 in. (men) or 35 in. (women)	Waist greater than 40 in. (men) or 35 in. (women)
18.5 or less	Underweight	—	N/A
18.5–24.9	Normal	—	N/A
25.0–29.9	Overweight	Increased	High
30.0–34.9	Obesity (class 1)	High	Very high
35.0–39.9	Obesity (class 2)	Very high	Very high
40 or greater	Extreme obesity (class 3)	Extremely high	Extremely high

Source: National Heart, Lung, and Blood Institute

Measures of body size, weight, and proportions all are anthropometric techniques useful in assessing and following nutritional status. The most widely recognized measures are those of height and weight. These measurements should be routinely obtained and recorded. Other anthropometric techniques include skinfold thickness measures, from which one can calculate estimates of total body fat stores; bony measures, such as elbow breadth, arm span, and leg length to estimate frame size, stature, or skeletal mass; and limb circumference, which can be combined by a formula with skinfold thickness to yield an estimate of muscle mass. These techniques allow the health care provider to obtain objective measures with relatively simple, low-risk, noninvasive, low-cost techniques. These techniques may appear deceptively simple, but there is significant potential for erroneous data collection if meticulous attention is not paid to anatomic detail and if the average of repeated measurements is not used (43–46,48–52).

The information gained from anthropometric measures can be used in the nutritional management of patients in several ways (53):

1. It can provide the basis for comparing a person with a group normal standard, classifying a person as to his or her relative position within a group (i.e., patient weighs less than the average person of the same gender and height).
2. It is theoretically possible to estimate the size of specific body compartments, such as skeletal muscle mass and subcutaneous fat tissue. However, the formulas for extrapolation are less than perfect and have been derived primarily from information gained from studies of physiologically normal people (44–49).
3. It can provide baseline information from which to monitor change over time and, thus, the effectiveness of nutritional intervention and long-term nutrition management (i.e., patient has gained 2 lbs in the past month).

The clinician must recognize potential sources of error when using anthropometric data. It is important to understand factors that affect anthropometric measures. Changes in body weight with time will reflect hydration status, total body tissue mass, or both. Edema secondary to venous stasis, hypoalbuminemia, or both can result in falsely increased skinfold thickness and limb girth measures. Conversely, relative dehydration

TABLE 58-5A.   Objective Biochemical Measurement of Nutrition Status: Assessment of Protein Status

Protein Marker	Reference Range	Half-Life	Remarks
Albumin	3.5–5.0 g/dl Clinical significance: Mild depletion: 2.8–3.49 g/dl Moderate depletion: 2.1–2.79 g/dl Severe depletion: <2.1 g/dl days	20	Decreased in protein malnutrition, metabolic stress, liver disease, overhydration, nephrotic syndrome, protein-losing enteropathies; increased in dehydration
Transferrin	200–300 md/dl Clinical significance Mild depletion: 150–200 mg/dl Moderate depletion: 100–150 mg/dl Severe depletion: <100 mg/dl	8 days	Decreased in protein malnutrition, chronic infections, acute catabolic states, protein-losing enteropathies, nephropathy; increased in iron-deficiency anemia, pregnancy, acute hepatitis
Transthyretin (prealbumin)	16–35 mg/dl Clinical significance Mild depletion: 10–15 mg/dl Moderate depletion: 5–10 mg/dl Severe depletion: <5 mg/dl	48 hr	Decreased in acute catabolic states, protein-losing enteropathies; increased in chronic renal failure
Retinol-binding protein	3.0–6.0 mg/dl	5–7 hr	Decreased in vitamin A deficiency, acute catabolic states, postsurgery; increased in chronic renal failure
Insulin-like growth factor (IGF-1)	0.01–0.04 mg/dl	2 hr	Decreased with starvation and quickly responds to re-feeding
Fibronectin	22–40 mg/dl	15 hr	Possible role during nutrition repletion

Adapted from Lee RD, Nieman DC. *Nutritional assessment, 2nd ed.* St Louis: CV Mosby, 1996; and Heymsfield SB, Tighe A, Wang ZM. Nutrition assessment by anthropometric and biochemical methods. In: Shils ME, Olson JA, Shike M, eds. *Modern nutrition in health and disease, 8th ed.* Philadelphia: Lea & Febiger, 1994.

may falsely decrease these values. In the presence of abnormal tissue, such as heterotopic ossification, the basic assumptions regarding the meaning of the data no longer apply, so results can be misleading. With control of these variables, repetitive measures can be of value in assessing changes over time. It is necessary to understand the basic assumptions made in establishing the standards against which results are compared (44–53).

Other Methods

Standard laboratory techniques for estimating body composition include measures of body density by underwater weighing, air displacement, estimates of specific body compartment sizes by multiple isotope dilution techniques, radiographic estimates of fatty tissue layers and bony sizes, creatinine-height index, whole-body liquid scintillation counting to determine total body potassium content, and bioelectric impedance (53–57). Body composition can be studied with ultrasound and computerized tomographic scanners to determine sizes of specific body tissue layers and organs (58). Other techniques under assessment include infrared interactance (59), dual-photon absorptiometry (60), dual-energy x-ray absorptiometry (57), and neutron inelastic scattering (61).

BIOCHEMICAL DATA

The assessment of nutrition status includes the use of several protein markers (Table 58-5A). Although they have limitations, they provide some objective data on protein status and clinical outcome. Heme protein is useful in determining the presence of anemia. Additional tests confirm the presence of a nutritional anemia (Table 58-5B).

One type of physiological functional assessment technique that seems of particular interest is applying measures of skeletal muscle function to the assessment of nutritional status. Both the force of contraction with rapid repetitive stimuli and the maximal relaxation rate of the abductor pollicis brevis have been studied for this purpose. Suboptimal performance was found in malnourished patients with chronic renal failure (62). In a small group of obese patients, skeletal muscle function became abnormal during a 2-week period of a very low-calorie diet (400 kcal/day) and persisted during an additional 2 weeks of fasting. Function returned to normal after a 2-week period of refeeding. Standard parameters of nutritional status, including serum albumin and transferrin values, creatinine-height index, anthropometric measures, and total body nitrogen and potassium levels, did not change during this study (63). One study has shown grip strength to be a more sensitive indicator of general nutritional status in surgical patients than standard anthropometric measures or serum albumin (64). These studies describe innovative methods for assessing nutritional status.

TABLE 58-5B.   Objective Biochemical Measurement of Nutrition Status: Nutrition-Related Anemias

Nutritional Anemia	Parameters
Iron deficiency	↓RBC, ↓Hgb, ↓MCV, ↓MCH, ↓MCHC, ↑Transferrin, ↑TIBC, ↓Ferritin
Macrocytic Folate deficiency	↓RBC, ↓Hgb, ↑MCV, ↑MCH, nl MCHC, ↓Serum folate, ↓Red cell folate
Vitamin B_{12}	↓RBC, ↓Hgb, ↑MCV, ↑MCH, nl MCHC, ↓Serum B_{12}

Hgb, hemoglobin; MCH, mean corpuscular hemoglobin; MCHC, mean corpuscular hemoglobin concentration; MCV, mean corpuscular volume, nl, normal; RBC, red blood cell; TIBC, total iron-binding capacity.

APPLICATION OF PRINCIPLES OF NUTRITION MANAGEMENT IN THE PRACTICE OF REHABILITATION MEDICINE

Risk of Nutrition Problems

Disability results from physiological alterations of the physical or mental capacity or function of the patient. Thus, by definition, people with new onset of disability, through illness or injury, are at risk for the development of malnutrition (Fig. 58-5).

The need for specific attention to nutritional status and nutritional support in patients admitted to rehabilitation units has been studied. Those patients with abnormal nutrition assessments have increased morbidity and mortality (65). As the patients with disabilities become more chronic, it cannot be assumed that nutrition status and requirements for nutrients stabilize. The homeostatic balance in people living with chronic disability is more precarious than that in able-bodied individuals. With musculoskeletal and neurologic abnormalities, there are changes in body composition. Other factors affecting the person's nutrition are acute or chronic illness and use of medication.

Acute or Chronic Illness

Acute or chronic illnesses may affect nutritional status by altering the body's metabolic activity, changing the bioavailability of nutrients, changing body composition, or changing the activity level (66–69).

Some conditions are seen more frequently in disabled people. One is skin ulcerations. With decubiti, there is an increased loss of nutrients through dead tissue and seepage of body fluids. It is not possible to measure these losses clinically, but the needs for increased nutrition for healing are well documented. Respiratory tract and urinary tract infections are commonly seen in the disabled. Energy requirements are greater as body temperature rises. Please refer to Table 58-6 for effects of infection on nutrient requirements.

GI tract symptoms of anorexia, early satiety, bloating, and constipation are reported in more than 50% of people with chronic obstructive pulmonary disease (COPD) (69). One survey of people with spinal cord injury demonstrated that 23% had at least one hospital admission for GI complaints after recovery from the acute injury, and 27% had recurrent symptoms sufficient enough to require chronic treatment or alter lifestyle (70). Gastroesophageal reflux is encountered frequently in children with developmental disability (28,71,72).

TABLE 58-6. Effects of Infection on Nutrient Requirements

1. Nutrient losses: most nutrients, especially intracellular minerals and nitrogen. Exception is retention of water and salt after initial losses.
2. Increased metabolic rate from fever.
3. Decreased food intake seconary to anorexia.
4. Functional nutrient loss secondary to overuse, diversion, and sequestration of nutrients.
5. Hypermetabolism and accelerated use of cellular energy with phagocytosis.

From Biesel WR. Infectious diseases. In: Schneider HA, Anderson CE, Coursi DB, eds. *Nutritional support of medical practice, 2nd ed.* Philadelphia: JB Lippincott, 1983;443–457.

Check if answer to question is yes. Nutrition risk increases as the number of checks increases.

1. Are you on a special diet? _____

2. Have you had a change in your eating habits? _____

3. Has your weight changed? _____

4. Do you have any cravings or desires for specific foods, liquids, or other substances to eat or drink? _____

5. Has your appetite changed? _____

6. Do you eat most of your food away from home? _____

7. Are you experiencing any of the following?
    a. Difficulty seeing at night? _____
    b. Dry skin or rashes? _____
    c. Nausea or vomiting? _____
    d. Constipation or diarrhea? _____
    e. Swelling of legs? _____
    f. Change in hair color, texture, or thickness (other than chemically or mechanically induced by hair care)? _____
    g. Yellow skin or eyes? _____
    h. Easy bruising? _____
    i. Swollen, tender joints? _____
    j. Poor healing of minor cuts or scratches? _____

8. Have you been ill or had surgery? _____

9. Are you taking any medicines or supplements? _____

10. Do you avoid any foods, liquids, or additives because of allergies or bad reactions? _____

Figure 58-5. Historical information suggesting nutritional risk. (From Frankel DL. Nutrition. In: DeLisa JD, Gans BM, et al., eds. *Rehabilitation medicine: principles and practice,* 2nd ed. Philadelphia: JB Lippincott Co, 1993: 602.)

Use of Medication

Patients with disabilities are often on medications. Food intake, nutritional status, and efficacy of pharmaceutical agents are interrelated. Food and nutrients can interact with drugs to alter absorption, metabolism, or drug excretion. Drugs can affect nutritional status by their effect on appetite, GI function, emotions, renal metabolism, and hepatic metabolism.

Information about drug-nutrient interactions can be obtained from a pharmacist or registered dietitian (73). Other good sources of information are the *Physician's Desk Reference* or drug information sheets. There are an increasing number of references pertaining to this topic (74–79). One may need to change the medication if there is a potential interaction. Other changes may include administering the drug at a different time, altering the diet, adding nutrition supplements, or a combination of these.

Other Nutrition Problems

With chronic disease or disability, there may be reduced reserves in the body to tolerate other stresses. Functional disability from chronic disease may be aggravated by other factors, some of which may be partially controlled through dietary means. People with mobility impairment may expend fewer calories and be more prone to excessive weight gain. The resulting obesity may add to the mobility impairment.

The multidisciplinary rehabilitation team can assist with nutritional support by identifying each patient's individual needs. It is helpful to have a dietitian who attends weekly rehabilitation conferences as an integral member of the team.

Because of the decreased length of acute hospital stays, there may be more nutritional problems identified among rehabilitation patients. It is important to identify these problems early so nutrition intervention can occur as soon as possible, thereby decreasing mortality and morbidity (67,69,80–92).

People with chronic disease and disability may turn to alternative treatment regimens, which often foster charlatans and quacks. The focus is often on nutrition "supplementation" or "diet" therapy. Although supplementation may be beneficial, excessive supplements may cost patients precious dollars and provide little benefit. In some cases, nutritional imbalances may be caused by some of these additional therapies (93). The health care provider should ask patients about alternative therapies and demonstrate a willingness to work with patients who choose to explore other options. This allows the medical practitioner to maintain his or her rapport with the patient and may result in the patient receiving the most optimal nutrition therapy.

Food Accessibility

Many factors are involved in optimizing nutritional status (see Fig. 58-3). Changes in any of these factors can change one's access to food, which can affect one's nutritional status significantly. Rehabilitation involves maximizing one's level of independence physically, emotionally, and economically. With transportation, access to shopping, kitchen modifications, adaptive utensils, and more prepared foods available, the disabled person can achieve more independence. Some people will continue to need help with shopping or food preparation, but with that assistance they can live independently.

Nonphysiological Factors

Nonphysiological factors are influenced by disability and can be instrumental in the development of malnutrition. Although the primary physiological reason for eating is to meet the metabolic requirements of the body, actual food consumed is affected by the factors discussed below.

ECONOMIC STATUS

People in developed countries purchase most of their food. With disability, there is often a loss of income and an increase in medical expenses. Because quality of diet may be directly related to income, there may be a change in the variety of nutritious food available for consumption. Limited finances could also limit transportation, resulting in reduced opportunity for shopping. When there are competing financial obligations, one may compromise the variety and quality of food purchased.

ENVIRONMENT

Temperature and humidity extremes have an impact on nutrition requirements. In very hot or cold climates, one's nutritional requirements change. The same is true when one is using an air-fluidized mattress system for prevention or healing of skin decubiti. With the increased temperature and constant flow of air, one's fluid requirements are increased. Patients using these mattresses are often debilitated and malnourished, so it is even more imperative that they have all of the nutrients required for promotion of health and healing.

PLACE OF RESIDENCE

When a person lives in a private residence, his or her proximity and access to stores, as well as facilities for food storage and preparation influence the food intake. If an attendant is required to care for someone at home, it is important that the attendant be included in discharge education. Nutrition status of dependent persons correlates with the nutrition knowledge and resources of the family (94,95). Education and social interventions may be needed to achieve optimal nutrition.

If a person lives in an institution, the food presentation and taste, as well as the dining facilities and congeniality of other individuals in the environment may influence how well one eats. Regulations include attention to providing balanced meals and evaluation of one's functional status and health maintenance. Despite these regulations, there are variabilities in nutrition management in these settings (96). The support staff responsible for feeding patients in institutions needs to understand basic nutrition principles to maintain optimal nutrient intake for disabled patients. Nutrition education for institutional staff has been shown to have a positive effect on the resident's nutritional status (97,98).

SOCIAL FACTORS

Food and beverages, including alcohol, are present at most social gatherings. Choices are based on taste, convenience, and cost, resulting in a relative abundance of foods high in fat, salt, and sugar. Thus, a more active social life may promote poor nutrition habits, with consumption of foods high in calories but with low nutrient density. Conversely, people who are alone and associate eating with socialization may not eat adequately.

Massive advertising campaigns for food products influence food intake, encouraging the consumption of more manufactured foods with variable nutrition content. Food is sometimes used as a reward for good behavior, or it may be seen as a punishment for people with significant feeding disorders. Values are then attributed to food and may have a significant impact on food consumption.

When patients become more dependent because of acute or chronic illness or a severe handicap, they may have decreased appetite and reduced food choices. Food may become the object of a power struggle rather than a basic need for health. Some problems related to food and nutritional status can be prevented by allowing the disabled person to have a choice in food selection or preparation. In some cases, a more comprehensive behavioral management approach to nutrition management is required (99,100).

PHYSIOLOGICAL FACTORS

The major physiological factors contributing to food accessibility include mobility, upper extremity function, communication skills, cognitive function, and oral-motor/swallowing skills. Losing the ability to feed oneself has major implications for liv-

ing independently. The rehabilitation team helps to evaluate all of the physiological factors and tries to address them to the extent possible.

Upper extremity function is necessary for self-feeding (refer to Table 58-7). When one loses some function, there are multiple ways to compensate (101,102). Loss of fine motor coordination and ataxia may compromise independence in self-feeding. Environmental control systems and robotic technology may help resolve some feeding problems related to upper extremity impairment. These devices may have limited application in the patient with tremors or ataxia. Devices also must be as discreet and cosmetic as possible (103).

TABLE 58-7. Motions of the Upper Extremity Necessary for Self-Feeding

Body Part	Motion	Purpose	Substitution	Loss	Device Used to Compensate
Hand	Palmar prehension	Pick up and hold utensil	1. Lacing spoon between fingers 2. Adduction of fingers 3. Hook grasp	Minimal	1. Utensil interlaced in fingers (some shaping may be necessary) 2. Moleskin or tape over handle to prevent slipping
	Lateral prehension to middle finger (modified lateral pinch)			Moderate	3. Build-up handle (wood, sponge, or other material) 4. Grip-shaped handles 5. Handle with horizontal and vertical dowels (pegged handle) 6. Handle with finger rings
				Severe	7. Warm Spring–type short opponents with C-bar and utensil attachment 8. Plastic and metal holder

				Complete	9. ADL (universal) cuff
					10. Prehension orthosis
					  • Manually operated
					  • Power operated

Wrist	Stabilization (slight flexion and exension of radial and ulnar deviation normally used depending on whether grasp is hook or pinch)	Positioning of hand for optimal function (to prevent wrist flexion)	1. Use of finger or thumb extensors	Partial stability	1. ADL wrist support dorsal (leather with sprint steel insert) 2. Flexible, adjustable nylon wrist support or Klenzac joints
				Complete	3. Tubular spring-clip (ADL) orthosis 4. Cock-up splint, rigid palmar 5. Warm Springs–type long opponents
Forearm	Pronation	Place food on utensil	1. Shoulder abduction and internal rotation 2. Raise forearm to vertical position and then rotate	Partial or complete	1. Swivel spoon 2. Bent fork or spoon
	Supination	Keep utensil level while putting food in mouth to avoid spill	3. Should adduction and external rotation		1. Swivel spoon 2. Placing fork or spoon over thumb, use thumb extensors
Elbow	Flexion of forearm	Raising hand to mouth	1. Use of knee 2. Shoulder abduction 3. Trunk flexion	Partial or complete	1. Balanced forearm orthosis (ball-bearing feeder) 2. Overhead sling with feeder attachment
	Extension	Lowering hand to plate	4. Rock forearm to edge of table		3. Overhead sling with built-up lapboard 4. Long-handled utensil 5. Functional arm orthosis
Shoulder	Stabilization against hyperextension and internal rotation in position of • Slight flexion • Slight abduction	Provides positioning and assists in raising hand to level of mouth	1. Trunk flexion 2. Prop elbow on table	Partial or complete	1. Pillow behind upper arm 2. Overhead sling 3. Balanced forearm orthosis 4. Functional arm orthosis 5. Hyperextension stop

ADL, activities of daily living.
From Zimmerman ME, Activities of daily living. In: Willard HS, Spackman GS, eds. *Occupational therapy*, 4th ed. Philadelphia: JB Lippincott, 1971;228.

Oral-motor/swallowing function must be intact for eating and requires integrity of anatomic structures, appropriate control of oral musculature, and coordinated peristaltic action in the esophagus. A comprehensive evaluation includes observation of the oral/pharyngeal phase of swallowing, evaluation of body position, assessment of primitive reflexes, and a feeding trial with foods of different consistencies. The latter should help determine the patient's aspiration risk. It is important to record length of time required to eat a meal, as a patient may be able to swallow adequately but tire too quickly to consume adequate nutrients and calories within a reasonable time (104–107). The major complications of oral-motor/swallowing dysfunction include undernutrition and aspiration pneumonia, both of which can compromise the outcome of rehabilitation efforts.

Patients may perceive feeding problems or deny having any problems. Either situation may affect nutritional status (107). Signs and symptoms of dysphagia include difficulty articulating words, decreased tongue mobility, facial weakness, weak or hoarse cough, decreased gag reflex, impaired sensitivity in the mouth or face, coughing and choking during or after meals, a wet or gurgled voice quality, pockets of food in the mouth, unexplained weight loss or lack of interest in eating, and chart notes that indicate the need for total assistance with feeding.

Feeding management systems are only as successful as their acceptance for those using them (the disabled person and others involved with his or her care). Try to feed patients foods they like but that are modified appropriately in consistency. Let patients experience all the flavors of foods served by feeding each item separately, not all mixed together.

The economic, social, and psychological status of the disabled person must be given equal consideration and related to the physical or cognitive disabilities present. A high-tech feeding device must be accepted and affordable. For some individuals, especially those who live alone, having a personal assistant for feeding may be more optimal as that person can provide needed socialization.

Alternate Feeding Routes

People who cannot take in sufficient nutrients orally may need to be fed by an alternate route, either enteral or parenteral, or a combination. Both physiological and psychological factors contribute to decisions regarding alternate feeding routes. Some patients may have a decreased appetite or feeding disturbances related to psychological factors. These routes allow for adequate nutrients and calories and may be a partial or complete means of nutritional support. Alternate feeding routes may be used to provide excess nutrients needed for additional demands or to prevent malnutrition in a person with severe feeding or GI function disturbances.

The importance of alternate feeding routes in patients with major trauma or burns is well established (24,28,31,33,35,92, 108–115). The effectiveness of alternate feeding routes in patients who have started to recover or have more chronic problems is not as well studied (116–119).

Enteral feeding is an integral part of the nutrition management of children with severe neurological impairments (104,120–122). In children and teenagers with cystic fibrosis, enteral feeding supplements improve total body nitrogen (123).

There are some risks associated with alternate feeding routes. These routes bypass the homeostatic control mechanisms of the body that regulate food and fluid intake. Objective monitors must be used routinely to assess the adequacy of nutritional support to avoid overfeeding or underfeeding (81).

Monitoring should include daily records of intake and output, frequent weight checks, and monitoring of vital signs. Nitrogen balance, fluid balance, serum electrolytes, glucose, blood urea nitrogen, creatinine, and hepatic enzyme levels may need to be evaluated regularly. Indirect calorimetry has improved the ability to provide appropriate calories for people dependent on alternative feeding routes.

Any decisions regarding alternate feeding routes are multifactorial and include the needs and wants of the patient and family and the capacity of the health care delivery system. An in-house nutrition support team is very helpful to implement specific guidelines and protocols for providing nutrition through alternative feeding methods. Some nutrition support teams are available for consultation after discharge from the hospital. The team greatly enhances the success of this technology while decreasing the complications (32,81,92,111,124–130).

Enteral Feeding

Enteral feeding uses the GI tract as the site of food intake but bypasses any proximal obstacles to feeding that might exist. Pureed food, liquid nutritional supplements, or elemental nutrient solutions are delivered directly to either the stomach or the small intestine. Enteral routes include nasogastric, nasoenteric, esophagogastric, gastrostomy, and jejunostomy. When oral feeding is impossible or limited, or one cannot move food through proximal structures of the GI tract despite normal oral function, enteral feeding should be considered. It allows safe administration and absorption of dietary substances, provided there is sufficient GI function. Enteral feeding is the least expensive alternate feeding route, has lower risks of complications from access or induced metabolic abnormalities, and provides the most physiological approach to alternative feeding.

Products for enteral feeding are numerous, and appropriate formula selection requires knowledge about the specific nutritional needs of the patient, awareness of digestive and absorptive capabilities, and knowledge about the potential effects of formulas on GI, metabolic, and immunological functions. Formulas can be classified according to specific characteristics. Because protein is the most significant formula component, it seems reasonable to classify formulas according to the type of protein present, with subcategories describing formula characteristics. Types of protein include intact, hydrolyzed, and amino acids.

The primary risk for tube feedings is aspiration. With a depressed gag reflex or impaired swallow, there is no natural protective mechanism to prevent aspiration pneumonia, especially with gastroesophageal reflux or proximal placement of the tube.

The direct gastrostomy or jejunostomy routes are considered most desirable when tube feedings will be needed for a prolonged time. These routes may decrease some of the problems associated with gastroesophageal reflux and are more cosmetic. Other techniques for placement or small tubes are percutaneous (110,126,131). The advantages of percutaneous insertion are the ability to start tube feedings less than 24 hours after surgery and avoidance of general anesthesia with its risks. Large-bore tubes placed surgically (e.g., Janeway gastrostomy, esophagogastrostomy procedures), with the creation of a permanent stoma, have the advantage of being easily inserted and removed, so the tube needs to be in place only during mealtimes (126,132). Placement of the tube through a jejunostomy minimizes the risk of aspiration. The disadvantages of more distal placement of the feeding tubes are related to the decreased absorptive capacity of the remaining gut, including less tolerance of high-osmolar loads and less absorption of some pharmaceutical agents and nutrients.

The rate of administration may be intermittent bolus or continuous drip and depends on the needs and tolerance of the patient, the staff, and the equipment available. Continuous drip requires a mechanical pump to control flow rate, which may limit activity to some extent. Activity tolerance may be limited by the physiological response to a full stomach. Bolus feedings can be problematic because of limited gastric capacity and delayed gastric emptying. When possible, continuous drip feedings, limited to the late evening and night, provide a means of minimizing complications while maximizing patient freedom. Patients receiving gastric feedings while in bed should have the head elevated. One complication is the potential for shear forces, which may compromise skin care.

PARENTERAL FEEDING

Parenteral feeding uses the venous system for direct delivery of elemental forms of nutrients to the body. It is generally done through a central venous access line, which allows for the administration of the entire day's nutrient requirements, but peripheral venous access may be used in limited circumstances. Total parenteral nutrition (TPN) is indicated when the gut is nonfunctional or must be free of food for extended periods of time. Parenteral supplementation is indicated when GI function is temporarily interrupted or in the presence of hypermetabolic states that require nutrients in excess of the absorptive capacity of the gut.

Nutrients are delivered in elemental forms. Initial estimates of nutrient requirements were extrapolated from the RDAs, which were established based on administration of food through the gut. Bypassing the gut means the loss of nutrients made by GI bacteria and absence of first-pass hepatic metabolism of nutrients, which normally are absorbed from the gut into the portal vein and delivered directly to the liver with oral and enteral feedings. Therefore, patients dependent on parenteral feeding require close observation and frequent monitoring of nutritional status. Complications from nutrient deficiency and nutrient excess have been identified in patients receiving parenteral feeding. The optimal elemental composition of parenteral solutions varies widely, and recommendations are modified on a regular basis as research and experience with parenteral nutrition continue (31,41,125,129,130, 133).

Risks are associated with the delivery of parenteral alimentation through a central venous line. With catheter insertion, there is the risk of pneumothorax. Routine use of the catheter may result in infection or contaminated substrate. Fluid and electrolyte balance must be closely monitored. The optimal ratio of carbohydrate and protein must be achieved so that nitrogen retention is optimized without placing excessive metabolic demands on the liver and kidneys for amino acid metabolism and elimination of nitrogenous waste products. The requirement of sufficient lipid to supply essential fatty acids has been recognized for several years, but the value of lipids in relatively significant quantities is still a subject of research (133,134). The ratio of the basic nutrients that provide energy affects the amount of substrate and fluid required because lipids are a more concentrated source of calories than carbohydrates or protein. Carbohydrate metabolism is associated with greater carbon dioxide production than lipid metabolism, a factor recognized to contribute significantly to carbon dioxide levels, and may affect respiratory drive in some patients with respiratory compromise (83,38,135). Severely burned patients

have an increased incidence of sepsis when receiving nutrition solely through parenteral access. This problem may be the result of loss of gut integrity from disuse, with subsequent movement of intestinal bacteria into the circulation (136,137).

Complications

Often it is impossible to deliver a full day's nutrient requirements through a peripheral line. Peripheral venous supplementation is indicated in specific situations, such as a temporary interruption of oral feeding (129).

The psychological impact of the long-term use of alternate feeding routes in cancer patients has been reviewed (138). Enteral routes are less problematic than parenteral ones. Psychological problems associated with enteral feeding include gustatory deprivation, dry mouth, and tube-related discomforts. With parenteral feeding, problems have been identified in regard to the loss of normal eating ability and associated body image changes as well as depression and decreased sexual activity. For some there is stress associated with fear of the apparatus, its maintenance, and its function.

Transitional Feeding

At some point it may be desirable to reintroduce oral feedings. Several factors (139) have been identified when this step is considered. One is resolution of the medical problem for which the tube feeding was introduced; others are adequate oral-motor/swallowing skills to support oral food intake and the patient and caregiver readiness.

Children who have been enterally fed from birth have had feeding problems associated with the change from enteral to oral feeding (140). These children may not have developed chewing skills. To prevent these problems, children should receive oral-motor/swallowing stimulation even while receiving all their nutrition enterally.

A gradual transition period from enteral to oral food intake ensures more success. This includes:

1. Normalize tube feedings to approximate meals/snacks
2. Alter feeding schedule to promote hunger
3. Reduce tube feeding by 25% of calories
4. Provide adequate fluids
5. Decrease tube feedings as oral intake increases.

When moving patients from TPN to enteral feedings, Winkler et al. found that patients were able to maintain body weight and continue to improve plasma protein with TPN after tolerating 60% of caloric requirements by the oral/enteral route (141).

Assessment and Nutritional Status in the Rehabilitation Population

FOOD/NUTRIENT INTAKE

Because there are changes in metabolic demand and activity with disability, current reference standards for food (RDAs) are not entirely appropriate for the diverse problems seen in this population group.

The food/nutrient intake of children with disabilities has been extensively studied. There are similarities in various studies, indicating that food/nutrient intake varies widely. Poor diets may be related to the disability itself or to associated feeding difficulties (94,95,104). Other factors such as family income

(84), educational level of the parents (95), and quality of the food offered to children living in institutions (142) are significant in determining the adequacy of food/nutrient intake. Level of dietary supplements (95,143) and amount of salty, high-fat, and sweet foods consumed will affect diet quality (143). These same factors affect the diets of healthy children; thus, a physical or mental disability alone does not result in poor dietary habits.

There are wide individual variations in caloric and nutrient intake of disabled adults, as identified by dietary surveys (144–147). People with physically disabling chronic illness (148,149) consume relatively fewer calories, whereas adults with mental retardation take in more calories (150). Litchford and Wakefield (98) identified a strong correlation between the knowledge of caregivers and the adequacy of diets of mentally retarded adults. Dysgeusia and xerostomia are significant factors in the adequacy of diets (151,152).

Bowman and Rosenberg have summarized multiple dietary surveys of the elderly (153). Average energy intakes are below two-thirds of the RDAs, but fewer than 10% have intakes of calcium, iron, vitamin A, and water-soluble vitamins below two-thirds of the RDAs. In a study of elderly veterans, dietary adequacy was correlated to a greater extent with the self-perception of chewing problems than with clinically determined dental status or the degree of social isolation (118).

FOOD/NUTRIENT REQUIREMENTS

Food/nutrient requirements vary with the effects of multiple factors, including body size, body composition, activity level, environmental conditions, presence of illness or injury, medication usage, metabolic activity, body temperature regulation, and amount of specific types of body tissues (23,66). The effect of disability on energy balance has been studied more than its effect on any specific nutrient requirement.

With sudden traumatic changes, such as amputation, there may be a dramatic change in body size or metabolism. Slower changes in body composition may occur after some problems, such as spinal cord injury, related to the amount of muscle atrophy. To estimate the effect of altered body size on energy requirements one must consider:

1. The time period during which the body is undergoing physiological adaptation to the disability condition
2. The time period after physiological adaptation required for body size to stabilize at a new level.

The onset of disability often affects the metabolic activity of the body. After acute trauma, there is an increase in metabolic requirements associated with the body's stress reaction. There is a catabolic phase with negative nitrogen balance, which may not be entirely reversible even with optimal nutritional support (28,35,92,111,131,149). In the hypermetabolic patient, it is important to avoid iatrogenic stress from exogenous protein loads that exceed the metabolic capacity of the body for anabolic purposes. The optimal level of protein support in the initial stages after severe trauma or acute illness has yet to be determined (26,31,109,114,115). Barbiturate therapy in acute head injury has been shown in one study to decrease nitrogen excretion (30). Clifton et al. have demonstrated that use of a standard correction factor may underestimate total urinary nitrogen excretion when a major catabolic insult has occurred (28); therefore, accuracy in determining nitrogen balance in such cases requires the direct measurement of non-urea nitrogen in the urine. Acutely, it may not be possible to achieve positive energy and nitrogen balance.

After the acute injury, there is an adaptive period during which further adjustments of energy consumption and metabolism occur. This adaptation is followed by a period of relative stability when the steady state of body composition and activity has been achieved (49,142,154,155).

Disabled and healthy people have variable levels of physical activity. Patients with spinal cord injury also have variable activity levels, but they may be further affected by the presence or absence of spasticity. A paraplegic able to walk expends more energy than one who is wheelchair-dependent. Energy expenditure may vary with different types of prosthetic devices or orthoses (32).

Children with cerebral palsy may have spasticity, which inhibits purposeful movement and results in lower activity levels, whereas those with athetoid forms may have higher activity levels (156–158). To assess energy needs in stable disabled children, it is important to consider requirements for normal growth. These energy requirements are related to both height and physical mobility status (158).

Formulas have been used to estimate the energy needs of disabled people, both acutely after injury (29,154) and at later stages in recovery (116,144–146). Critical assessments of these formulas demonstrate a significant variation from actual energy expenditure, as determined by direct and indirect measures (22,159). Errors are significant with traumatic injuries, such as spinal cord injury (160), head injury (28,), and burns (47,161).

Indirect calorimetry measures are being used more frequently. It is practical and provides better accuracy than formulas, especially acutely (24–35). For more chronic patients, it is more feasible to rely on formulas to estimate caloric and nutrient requirements. Because of the inaccuracies, close clinical monitoring is indicated.

NUTRITION STATUS PARAMETERS

One's nutritional status needs to be assessed to determine the appropriate nutrition intervention. The traditional parameters of nutritional status may not be applicable to persons with disability. It is not clear whether physiological adaptations to disability result in changes of body composition or biochemical function because of the specific disability/illness or as a result of malnutrition. Finally, one needs to investigate whether altered measures of nutritional status in the disabled reflect an imbalance of diet or a change in absorption, metabolism, or excretion related to the disability.

Currently, information obtained regarding nutritional status measures only where the disabled person stands in relation to standards for able-bodied persons. These standards are not applicable to a patient with a spinal cord injury who loses muscle mass in the paretic muscles or to an amputee who loses part of his or her body mass. Thus, serum creatinine is lowered but may not reflect impairment of renal function. To accurately assess renal function, one needs a creatinine clearance measurement. The implications for determining appropriate dosages of medications with renal elimination and potential for renal impairment are significant.

Changes in body composition alter the physiological activity of some pharmaceutical agents. Water-soluble medications are distributed throughout the total-body water compartment; fat-soluble medications are stored in fat. As a result of altered body composition, there may be changes in both the half-life and the effective serum levels of a medication. The further body composition moves from "normal" the more important it is to monitor dosages of medications, with serum levels or astute clinical observations to monitor for potential activity.

Measurements of serum albumin reflect plasma oncotic pressure, which affects the distribution of body fluids and the active level of drugs that bind to albumin.

MEASURES OF BODY COMPOSITION

The "ideal" body composition for persons with disability has not been defined, and such a definition may be difficult because of the multitude of problems that result in disability. The main clinical use for body composition in nutrition management of the disabled is to define baseline and monitor overall clinical condition and function. Studies of body composition in persons with spinal cord injuries (155,162–164) have shown the following:

- There is generally a depletion of lean body mass.
- There is a tendency toward an increased proportion of body fat.
- There is an increase in total body fluid.
- There is a high degree of intersubject variability.

Initially, patients with spinal cord injuries lose weight, but there is significant variability of the weight at which patients stabilize (144,146,154,155,165). Some have recommended that these patients weigh less than their ideal weight by 10 to 20 lbs to facilitate improved mobility (166). Others have suggested that those with spinal cord injuries who weigh less than 10% below the mean for ideal body weight are at risk for malnutrition (146,165). There are no studies to support these conclusions, and the optimal weight-for-height standard after spinal cord injury has not yet been determined. It will probably vary depending on the degree of paralysis and extent of spasticity, which helps to maintain some muscle tone and mass. In paraplegics, there will be a disproportionate increase in muscle mass in the more exercised upper extremities.

Some have concluded that patients with amyotrophic lateral sclerosis (ALS) who have lost more than 10% of their body weight are underweight and at nutritional risk (149). But it is natural that with loss of functioning muscle, as in ALS or spinal cord injury, there will be loss of weight unless there is an increase in body fat or water. The latter would result in an imbalance of lean body mass relative to other body compartments, which is consistent with a poorer nutritional status.

Determining height requires alternate measures in people with contractures or other physical deformities (167).

Combining serial weights with arm circumference and skinfold thickness allows the clinician to follow changes in the proportion of lean body mass compared with fat. Body weight is easily measured, but there is potential for error with patients being weighed at different times of the day, by different individuals using slightly different techniques, or with different scales. All scales need to be calibrated routinely.

Some innovative techniques to determine body composition have helped to evaluate the effects of chronic illness on body composition. Dual-photon absorptiometry has been used to measure the distribution and time course of changes in bone mineral content after paraplegic spinal cord injury. Bone mass was lost, initially, in the proximal tibia and femoral neck, stabilizing at a lower level 2 years postinjury. No change was seen in the spine or distal forearm bones (168). Bioelectric impedance has been shown to be more effective in estimating fat-free mass than skinfold thickness in people with COPD (169). Other work with cancer and renal patients is ongoing (57,170,171).

Children with myelomeningocele have been studied. They have normal body composition until age 3; but after age 4 there is a significant depletion of body cell mass and total body water and an increased percentage of body fat. The total body water is present disproportionately in the extracellular compartment.

BIOCHEMICAL AND PHYSIOLOGICAL MEASURES

Of the static biochemical measures, albumin has consistently been a predictor of outcome for acute medical management and rehabilitation (172–174). Other functional measures need to be evaluated for this population.

Clinical Application of Nutrition Management in Selected Disabilities

CHRONIC OBSTRUCTIVE PULMONARY DISEASE

Donahoe and Rogers have summarized the research investigating the role of nutrition in health and longevity of people with COPD (68). The most consistent nutritional predictor of mortality is a body weight less than 90% of the ideal. By indirect calorimetry, it has been shown that the REE as a percentage of predicted metabolic requirements in the underweight group is greater than that in the normal-weight group. (25,165). The reason for inadequate dietary intake remains obscure. It is possible that many of the symptoms associated with COPD (e.g., anorexia, early satiety, dyspnea, fatigue, bloating, constipation, dental problems) contribute to dietary inadequacy (175,176). Demonstrations of successful refeeding rule against impaired nutrient utilization (119,176). Weight gain can be achieved with close attention to nutritional intake. With adequate calories for energy expenditure, there does not seem to be a problem with variations in carbon dioxide production as a consequence of the ratio among dietary fat, protein, and carbohydrates (68). It is difficult to maintain this weight gain, as losses can occur rapidly during exacerbations of the disease. There is a decrease in respiratory muscle strength with undernutrition (129,177), which reverses with short-term refeeding and weight gain (129). Improved immune function with refeeding after recent weight loss has been reported in nine patients with COPD (176). Peak exercise performance and ventilatory muscle strength are reduced in COPD patients who weigh less than 90% ideal body weight (177). Walking distance was found to be proportional to serum albumin and creatinine-height index (178). Because these studies involved a small number of subjects, other more definitive studies on larger populations need to be done before generalizations can be made.

CEREBRAL PALSY

Growth failure, defined as decreased height and weight for age, is seen in most children with cerebral palsy (71,122). Multiple factors contribute to poor food intake in these children. These include poor dentition, refusing food, oral motor dysfunction (including involuntary tongue thrust and delayed or absent initiation of the swallowing reflex), vomiting, rumination, and GI reflux because of abnormal peristalsis and lower esophageal sphincter dysfunction. Mechanical oral-motor problems cannot always be overcome, especially if the feeding time needed to consume adequate calories becomes excessive (104). With enteral feedings as supplementation, these children can achieve more normal growth (122), although optimal growth parameters for these children have not been established. Nutrition supplements should be started within 1 year of central nervous system (CNS) insult. When children are within 8 years of the CNS insult and significantly small for their age, they can achieve within 90% of ideal height with the addition of enteral feedings. After 8 years, weight may increase, but height will not change as significantly (121). This speaks to the need for early aggressive nutritional support. Some caregivers, however, may prefer that the children remain smaller because of the mobility dependence and physical care issues.

Nutritional Implications of Specific Clinical Problems

URINARY TRACT STONES

Patients with a neurogenic bladder have an increased incidence of urinary tract stones. The causes of these stones are multifactorial (179–181). The increased rate of calcium loss from bone after spinal cord injury and immobilization is well known and difficult to control (182–185). Diet may be critical in some instances. Recommendations for dietary modification include a low-calcium diet (400 to 500 mg/day), a low-sodium diet, and the combination of thiazides and a low-calcium diet (179,186). Some postulate that a high-protein diet, which helps control the adverse effects of nitrogen depletion, may increase calcium excretion in the urine (187). There is no conclusive evidence that control of hypercalciuria will decrease the incidence of stone formation.

There has been concern about the potential for oxalate stone formation in the urinary tract of patients taking in large amounts of vitamin C (i.e., several grams). The increase in urinary oxalate excretion associated with high vitamin C intake may be an artifact induced by the laboratory assay (188,189). Patients with neurogenic bladders continue to use vitamin C supplementation, but without conclusive evidence regarding its benefit.

Sufficient fluid intake to support adequate urine volume (2 to 2.5 L/day) will keep the urine dilute and decrease the tendency of substances to crystallize out because of high concentration (190). This fluid output is difficult to maintain in patients managed with intermittent catheterization. Thus, the tendency to form stones is only one factor in deciding optimal fluid intake for patients with neurogenic bladders.

The pH of the urine can be manipulated to reduce the tendency to form stones. It is best controlled with medication, as it is difficult to change the urine pH with dietary methods (65).

CONSTIPATION

Standard bowel programs used on rehabilitation units are excellent in controlling neurogenic bowel syndromes. One important aspect is having a regular source of fiber in the diet or as a supplement (e.g., psyllium). Up to 30 g/day of fiber may be needed to control constipation in disabled people, especially if there is a combination of immobility and previous laxative abuse (191). Successful alteration of fiber intake in the diet generally requires individual dietary instruction.

Some patients fail a bowel program. In these cases, the failure may be related to inadequate fluid intake. Increasing fluid intake to 1.5 to 2 L/day will usually help the bowel problems but may make management of a neurogenic bladder more difficult.

DECUBITI (ULCERS)

Skin breakdown continues to be a significant cause of morbidity and is an expensive complication of disability. There are multiple studies pertaining to this problem, but prevention is difficult to achieve. The immediate cause of decubiti is excess pressure on the skin surface, but cells break down because of inability to sustain metabolism. The latter occurs because of poor delivery of nutrients and poor removal of waste products. Thus, local cellular nutrition imbalance is a significant factor that contributes to this problem.

Nutritional needs are increased for healing of a decubitus ulcer, since fluid containing proteins, vitamins, and minerals is continuously lost through the open wound surface. It is important that these patients' nutritional status be monitored closely, with adjustments made in the diet as indicated. Other factors such as smoking, diabetes, anemia, and steroids may impede the wound healing process, and need to be controlled or corrected to the extent possible (192–194).

EDEMA

When there is decreased muscle activity, edema from venous pooling occurs in dependent limbs. It is important to determine whether the edema is related to venous pooling versus decreased plasma oncotic pressure. In the latter case, one's serum albumin will be low.

Nonpharmacologic treatment of edema involves elevation of the dependent extremities or compression with elastic stockings. Some clinicians give diuretics or decrease sodium intake to help control edema. There are two problems with these methods:

1. Patients with flaccid paralysis and decreased lean body mass have a decreased total body potassium. With use of potassium-wasting diuretics, the levels of potassium depletion may be dangerous. Serum potassium levels need to be monitored closely when diuretics are used.
2. Decreased plasma volume may also aggravate the tendency toward orthostatic hypotension, especially in patients with poor cardiovascular response to postural changes.

OBESITY

Obesity is often a problem among the disabled with a significant decrease in activity level or if there is a brain insult with associated cognitive impairment, such as decreased initiation for eating or altered satiety levels. Successful nutritional intervention may require application of behavioral techniques to control food intake as well as a general understanding of the caloric content of foods and how to modify them in one's diet.

Obesity is a common form of malnutrition among the elderly, and malnutrition may occur in association with obesity. The risk of myocardial infarction, stroke, hypertension, non-insulin-dependent diabetes mellitus, osteoarthritis, and some types of cancer is increased with obesity.

ELDERLY

The elderly may have impairments in their functional activities of daily living, which may limit their access to different types of food. Limited finances and social isolation may lead to decreased nutrient intake. Many elderly may be overweight, have dietary lipid intakes above recommended levels, and have decreased calcium and folic acid intakes. Accurate information regarding food intake is essential in evaluating the nutritional status of this group. Special services such as Meals on Wheels-type resources may help to optimize nutrition intake.

REFERENCES

1. Jackson AA. Aminoacids: essential and non-essential? *Lancet* 1985;1:1034–1037.
2. Lands WEM. Renewed questions about polysaturated fatty acids. *Nutr Rev* 1986;44:189–195.

3. Pike RL, Brown ML. *Nutrition: an integrated approach*, 2nd ed. New York: John Wiley & Sons, 1975.

4. Gibson GR, Roberfroid MB. Dietary modulation of the human colonic microbiota: introducing the concept of prebiotics. *J Nutr* 1995;125:1401–1412.

5. Roberfroid MB. Prebiotics and probiotics: are they functional foods? *Am J Clin Nutr* 2000;71:1682S–1687S.

6. Chow J. Probiotics and prebiotics: a brief overview. *J Renal Nutr* 2002; 12:76–86.

7. Marteau P. Nutritional advantages of probiotics and prebiotics. *Br J Nutr* 2002;87:S153–S157.

8. Vahouny GV. Conclusions and recommendations of the Symposium on Dietary Fibers in Health and Disease, Washington D.C., 1981. *Am J Clin Nutr* 1982;35:152–156.

9. Barr S, Murphy SP, Poos MI. Interpreting and using the dietary reference intakes in dietary assessment of individuals and groups. *J Am Diet Assoc* 02; 102:780–788.

10. Institute of Medicine. *Dietary reference intakes for calcium, phosphorus, magnesium, vitamin d, and fluoride*. Washington, DC: National Academy Press, 1997.

11. Institute of Medicine. *Dietary reference intakes for thiamin, riboflavin, niacin, vitamin B6, folate, vitamin B12, pantothenic acid, biotin, and choline*. Washington, DC: National Academy Press, 1998.

12. Institute of Medicine. *Dietary reference intakes for vitamin C, vitamin E, selenium, and carotenoids*. Washington, DC: National Academy Press, 2000.

13. Smicklas-Wright H, Guthrie HA. Dietary methodologies: their uses, analyses, interpretations, and implications. In: Simko MD, Cowel C, Gilbride JA, eds. *Nutrition assessment: a comprehensive guide for planning intervention*. Rockville, MD: Aspen Systems, 1984:119–138

14. Wotecki CE. Improving estimates of food and nutrient intake: applications to individuals and groups. *J Am Diet Assoc* 1985;85:295–296.

15. Wotecki CE. Dietary survey data: sources and limits to interpretation. *Nutr Rev* 1986;44[Suppl]:204–213.

16. Kalisz K, Kevall S. A nutritional interview for clients with development disorders. *Ment Retard* 1984;22:279–288.

17. Bingham SA, Cummings JH. Urine nitrogen as an independent validatory measure of dietary intake: a study of nitrogen balance in individuals consuming their normal diet. *Am J Clin Nutr* 1985;42:1276–1289.

18. Adams CF. Nutritive value of American foods in common units. Agriculture Handbook No. 456, United States Department of Agriculture. Washington DC: U.S. Government Printing Office, 1975.

19. Pennington JAT, Church HN. *Bowes Church's food values of portions commonly used*, 15th ed. Philadelphia: JB Lippincott Co, 1989.

20. Watt BK, Merrill AL. Composition of foods: raw, processed, prepared. Agriculture Handbook No. 8, United States Department of Agriculture. Washington DC: U.S. Government Printing Office, 1975.

21. Goodhart RS, Shils ME, eds. *Modern nutrition in health and disease*, 6th ed. Philadelphia: Lea & Febiger, 1980.

22. Silberman H. *Parenteral and eternal nutrition*, 2nd ed. Norwalk, CT: Appleton-Century-Crofts, 1982.

23. Shils ME. Food and nutrition related to work, exercise, and environmental stress. In: Goodhart RS, Shils ME, eds. *Modern nutrition in health and disease*, 6th ed. Philadelphia: Lea & Febiger, 1980:814–851.

24. Cunningham JJ, Lyndon MK, Russell WE. Calorie and protein revision for recovery from severe burns in infants and young children. *Am J Clin Nutr* 1990;51:553–557.

25. Moore R, Najarian MP, Konvolinka CW. Measure energy expenditure in severe head trauma. *J Trauma* 1989;29:1633–1636.

26. Saffle JR, Larson CM, Sillivan J. A randomized trial of indirect calorimetry-based feeding in thermal injury. *J Trauma* 1990;30:776–783.

27. Allard JP, Pichard C, Hoshino E, et al. Validation of a new formula for calculation of the energy requirements of burn patients. *J Parent Ent Nutr* 1990;14:115–118.

28. Clifton GL, Robertson CS, Contant CF. Eternal hyperalimentation in head injury. *J Neurosurg* 1985;62:186–193.

29. Dickerson RN, Guenter PA, Gennearelli TA, et al. Brief communication: increased contribution of protein oxidation to energy expenditure in head-injured patients. *J Am Coll Nutr* 1990;9:86–88.

30. Fried RC, Dickerson RN, Guenter PA, et al. Barbiturate therapy reduced nitrogen excretion in acute head injury. *J Trauma* 1989;29:1558–1564.

31. Kelly K. Advances in perioperative nutritional support. *Med Clin North Am* 1993;77(2):465–475.

32. Merkel KD, Miller NE, Merritt JL. Energy expenditure in patients with low-, mid-, and high-thoracic paraplegia using Scott-Craig knee-ankle-foot orthoses. *Mayo Clin Proc* 1985;60:165–168.

33. Saffle JR, Medina E, Raymond J, et al. Use of indirect calorimetry in the nutritional management of burned patients. *J Trauma* 1985;25:32–39.

34. Schols AMWJ, Soeters PB, Mostert R, et al. Energy balance in chronic obstructive pulmonary disease. *Am Rev Respir Dis* 1991;243:1248–1252.

35. Turner WW. Nutritional considerations in the patient with disabling brain disease. *Neurosurgery* 1985;16(25):32–39.

36. Baker JP, Detsky AS, Wesson ED, et al. Nutritional assessment: a comparison of clinical judgment and objective measurements. *N Engl J Med* 1982;306: 969–972.

37. Shils ME. Nutrition assessment in support of the malnourished patient. In: Simko MD, Cowell C, Gilbride JA, eds. *Nutrition assessment: a comprehensive guide for planning intervention*. Rockville, MD: Aspen, 1984.

38. Christensen KS, Gstundiner KM. Hospital-wide screening improves basis for nutrition intervention. *J Am Diet Assoc* 1985;83:704–406.

39. Hunt DR, Maslovitz, A. Rowlands BJ, et al. A simple nutrition screening procedure for hospital patients. *J Am Diet Assoc* 1985;85:332–335.

40. Webb P, Sangal S. Sedentary daily expenditure: a base for estimating individual energy requirements. *Am J Clin Nutr* 1991;53:606–611.

41. Evans MJ. The role of total parenteral nutrition in critical illness: guidelines and recommendations. *AACN Clin Issues Crit Care Nurs* 1994;5(4):476–484.

42. Gilmore J. Body mass index and health. *Health Reports* 1999;11:31–43.

42a. Bray GA. Clinical evaluation of the overweight patient. *Endocrine* 2000;13: 167–186.

43. Heymsfield SB, Wang J, Lictman S, et al. Body composition in elderly subjects: a critical appraisal of clinical methodology. *Am J Clin Nutr* 1989;50: 1167–1175.

44. Johnston FE. Relationships between body composition and anthropometry. *Hum Biol* 1982;54:221–245.

45. Mackie A, Hannan WJ, Tothill P. An introduction to body composition models used in nutritional studies. *Clin Phys Physiol Meas* 1989;10:297–310.

46. Williams SR. *Nutrition and diet therapy*, 5th ed. St. Louis: CV Mosby, 1985.

47. Barlett HI, Puhl SM, Hodgson, JL, et al. Fat-free mass in relation to stature: ratios of fat-free mass to height in children, adults, and elderly subjects. *Am J Clin Nutr* 1991;53:1112–1116.

48. Dixon JK. Validity and utility of anthropometric measurements. A survey of cancer outpatients. *J Am Diet Assoc* 1985;85:439–444.

49. Himes JH, ed. *Anthropometric assessment of nutritional status*. New York: Wiley-Liss, 1991.

50. Abernathy RP. Body mass index: determination and use. *J Am Diet Assoc* 1991;91:843.

51. Frisancho AR. New standards of weight and body composition by frame size and height for assessment of nutritional status of adults and the elderly. *Am J Clin Nutr* 1984;40:808–819.

52. Willet WC, Stampfer M, Manson JA, et al. New weight guidelines for Americans: justified or injudicious? *Am J Clin Nutr* 1991;53:1102–1103.

53. Bistrian BR, Blackbrn CI, Sherman J, et al. Therapeutic index of nutritional depletion in hospitalized patients. *Surg Gynecol Obstet* 1975;14:312–316.

54. Forbes GB, Bruining GI. Urinary creatinine excretion and lean body mass. *Am J Clin Nutr* 1976;29:1359–1366.

55. Grande F, Keys A. Body weight, body composition and calorie status. In: Goodhart RS, Shils MD, eds. *Modern nutrition in health and disease*, 6th ed. Philadelphia: Lea & Febiger. 1980:3–34.

56. Szeluga DJ, Stuart RK, Utermohlen V, et al. Nutritional assessment by isotope dilution analysis of body composition. *Am J Clin Nutr* 1980;40:847–854.

57. Svendsen OI, Haarbo J, Heitmann BI, et al Measurement of body fat in elderly subjects by dual-energy x-ray absorptiometry, bioelectrical impedance, and anthropometry. *Am J Clin Nutr* 1991;53:1117–1123.

58. Heymsfield SB, McManus CB. Tissue components of weight loss in cancer patients: a new method of study and preliminary observations. *Cancer* 1985;55:238–249.

59. Conway JM, Norris KH, Bodwell CE. A new approach for the estimation of body composition: infrared interactance. *Am J Clin Nutr* 1984;40;1123–1130.

60. Mazess RB, Peppler WW, Gibbons M. Total body composition by dual-photon (153Gd) absorptiometry. *Am J Clin Nutr* 1984;40:834–839.

61. Kehayias JJ, Heymsfeld SB, LoMonte AF, et al. In vivo determination of body fat by measuring total body carbon. *Am J Clin Nutr* 1991;53:1339–1344.

62. Berkelhammer CH, Leiter LA, Jeejeebhoy KN, et al. Skeletal muscle function in chronic renal failure: an index of nutritional status. *Am J Clin Nutr* 1985;42:845–854.

63. Russell DmcR, Leiter LA, Whitwel J, et al. Skeletal muscle function during hypocaloric diets and fasting: a comparison with standard nutritional assessment parameters. *Am J Clin Nutr* 1983;37:133–138.

64. Hunt DR, Rowlands BJ, Johnston D. Hand grip strength: a simple prognostic indicator in surgical patients. *J Parent Ent Nutr* 1985;9:701–704.

65. Baugh E. Actions to improve nutrition care on a general rehabilitation unit. *J Am Diet Assoc* 1985;85:1632–1634.

66. Food and Nutrition Board. *Recommended dietary allowances*, 10th ed. Washington DC: National Academy Press, 1989.

67. Dickerson JWT. Vitamin requirements in different clinical conditions. *Bibl Nutr Diets* 1985;35:44–52.

68. Donahoe M, Rogers RM. Nutritional assessment and support in chronic obstructive pulmonary disease. *Clin Chest Med* 1990;11:487–504.

69. Wretlind A. Nutrient requirements in various clinical conditions. *Bibl Nutr Diets* 1985;35:31–43.

70. Stone JM, Nino-Murcia M, Wolfe AV, et al. Chronic gastrointestinal problems in spinal cord injury patients: a prospective analysis. *Am J Gastroenterol* 1990;85:1114–1119.

71. Fee MA, Charney EB, Robertson WW. Nutritional assessment of the young child with cerebral palsy. *Infants Young Child* 1988;1:33–40.

72. Morris MJ, Ingram DH, Howison M, et al. The disabled child. In: Gines DJ, ed. *Nutrition management in rehabilitation*. Rockville, MD: Aspen Publications, 1990:109–137.

73. Murray JJ, Healy MD. Drug-nutrient interactions: a new responsibility for the hospital dietitian. *J Am Diet Assoc* 1991;92:66–73.

74. Awad AG. Diet and drug interactions in the treatment of mental illness: a review. *Can J Psychiatry* 1984;29:609–613.

75. Hansten PD. *Drug interactions*, 5th ed. Philadelphia: Lea & Febiger, 1985.

76. O'Brien RY. Spinal cord injury. In: Gines DJ, ed. *Nutrition management in rehabilitation*. Rockville, MD: Aspen Publications, 1990:159–174.

77. Roe DA. *Drug-induced nutritional deficiencies*, 2nd ed. Westport, CT: Avi Publishing, 1985.

78. Roe DA. *Diet and drug interactions.* New York: Van Nostrand Reinhold, 1989.

79. Wolman PG. Arthritis. In: Gines DJ, ed. *Nutrition management in rehabilitation.* Rockville, MD: Aspen Publications, 1990;245–270.

80. Grant JP, Custer PB, Thurlow J. Current techniques of nutritional care. *Surg Clin North Am* 1981;64:437–463.

81. MacBurney M, Wilmore DW. Rational decision making in nutrition care. *Surg Clin North Am* 1981;61:571–582.

82. Solomon NW, Allen LH. The functional assessment of nutritional status: principles, practice and potential. *Nutr Rev* 1983;41:33–50.

83. Caldwell MD, Kennedy, Caldwell C. Normal nutritional requirements. *Surg Clin North Am* 1981;61:489–507.

84. Barton RG. Nutrition support in critical illness. *Nutr Clin Pract* 1994;9(4):127–139.

85. Haider M. Haider SQ. Assessment of protein-calorie malnutrition. *Clin Chem* 1984;30:1286–1299.

86. Hannaman KN, Penner SF. A nutrition assessment tool that includes diagnosis. *J Am Diet Assoc* 1985;85:607–609.

87. Jensen TG, Long JM III, Dudrick SJ, et al. Nutritional assessment indications of postburn complications. *J Am Diet Assoc* 1985;85:68–72.

88. Kaminski MV Jr, Blumeyer TH. Metabolic and nutritional support of the intensive care patient. Ascending the learning curve. *Crit Care Clin* 1993;9(2):363–376.

89. Blackburn GL, Thornton, PA. Nutritional assessment of the hospitalized patient. *Med Clin North Am* 1979;63:1103–1115.

90. Burton BT, Foster WR. Health implications of obesity; an NIH consensus development conference. *J Am Diet Assoc* 1985;85:1117–1121.

91. Dickhaut SC, DeLee JC, Page CP. Nutritional status: importance in predicting wound healing after amputation. *J Bone Joint Surg* 1984;66:71–75.

92. Kudsk KA, Stone JM, Sheldon GF. Nutrition in trauma and burns. *Surg Clin North Am* 1982;62:183–192.

93. Sibley WA. *Therapeutic claims in multiple sclerosis,* 2nd ed. New York: Demos Publications, 1988.

94. Bryan AH, Anderson EL. Dietary and nutritional problems of crippled children in five rural counties of North Carolina. *Am J Public Health* 1965;55:1545–1554.

95. Gouge AL, Ekwall SW. Diets of handicapped children: physical, psychological, and socioeconomic correlations. *Am J Ment Defic* 1975;80:149–157.

96. Cunningham K, Gibney MJ, Kelly A, et al. Nutrient intakes in long-stay mentally handicapped persons. *Br J Nutr* 1990;64:3–11.

97. Magnus MH, Roe DA. Computer instruction in drug-nutrient interactions in long term care. *J Nutr Educ* 1991;23:10–17.

98. Hull MA, Kidwell J. Feeding skills and weight gain in institutionalized adults with severe handicaps. *Dietet Dev Psychiatr Dis* 1988;7(2).

99. White W, Kamples G. Dietary noncompliance in pediatric patients in the burn unit. *J Burn Care Rehabil* 1990;11:167–174.

100. McCarran MS, Andrasik F. Behavioral weight-loss for multiple handicapped adults: assessing caretaker involvement and measures of behavior change. *Addict Behav* 1990;15:13–20.

101. Loosen BM. Self-help aids. In: Redfore JB, ed. *Orthotic etcetera,* 2nd ed. Baltimore: Williams & Wilkins, 1980;650–681.

102. Zimmerman ME. Activities of daily living. In: Willard HS, Spackman GS, eds. *Occupational therapy,* 4th ed. Philadelphia: JB Lippincott Co, 1971:228.

103. Broadhurst MI, Stammers CW. Mechanical feeding aids for patients with ataxia: design consideration. *J Biomed Eng* 1990;12:209–214.

104. Gisel EG, Patrick J. Identification of children with cerebral palsy unable to maintain a normal nutritional state. *Lancet* 1988;1:283–285.

105. Stratton M. Behavioral assessment scale of oral functions in feeding. *Am J Occup Ther* 1981;35:719–721.

106. Kenny DJ, Koheil RM, Greenberg J, et al. Development of a multidisciplinary feeding profile for children who are dependent feeders. *Dysphagia* 1989;4:16–28.

107. Gordon SR, Kelley SI, Sybyl JR, et al. Relationship in very elderly veterans of nutritional status, self-perceived chewing ability, dental status, and social isolation. *J Am Geriatr Soc* 1985;33:334–339.

108. Pfisterer M, Leisire H, Kleine R, et al. Caloric requirements in burned patients. *Acta Anaesthesiol Belg* 1989;40:187–194.

109. Dominioni L, Trochi O, Fang CH, et al. Enteral feeding in burn hypermetabolism: nutritional and metabolic effects of different levels of calorie and protein intake. *J Parent Ent Nutr* 1985;9:269–279.

110. Gay F, et Nawar A, Van-Gossum A. Percutaneous endoscopic gastrostomy. *Acta Gastroenterol Belg* 1992;55(3):285–294.

111. Kudsk KA, Stone JM, Sheldon GF. Nutrition in trauma. *Surg Clin North Am* 1981;61:671–679.

112. Rapp RP, Young B, Twyman D, et al. The favorable effect of early parenteral feeding on survival in head-injured patients. *J Neurosurg* 1983;58:906–912.

113. Twyman D, Young AB, Ott L, et al. High protein enteral feedings: a means of achieving positive nitrogen balance in head injured patients. *J Parent Ent Nutr* 1985;9:679–684.

114. Enzi G, Casadei A, Sergi G, et al. Metabolic and hormonal effects of early nutritional supplementation after surgery in burn patients. *Crit Care Med* 1990;18:719–721.

115. Chiarelli A, Enzi G, Casadei A, et al. Very early nutrition supplementation in burned patients. *Am J Clin Nutr* 1990;51:1035–1039.

116. Bildsten C, Lamid S. Nutritional management of a patient with brain damage and spinal cord injury. *Arch Phys Med Rehabil* 1983;64:382–383.

117. Newmark SR, Simpson S, Daniel P, et al. Nutritional support in an inpatient rehabilitation unit. *Arch Phys Med Rehabil* 1981;62:634–637.

118. O'Gara JA. Dietary adjustments and nutritional therapy during treatment of oral-pharyngeal dysphagia. *Dysphagia* 1990;4:109–112.

119. Whittaker JS, Ryan CF, Buckley PA, et al. The effects of refeeding on peripheral and respiratory muscle function in malnourished chronic obstructive pulmonary disease patients. *Am Rev Respir Dis* 1990;142:283–288.

120. Isaacs JS. Neurologically impaired children fed by gastrostomy. *Diet Dev Psychiatr Dis* 1991;9:1–3.

121. Sanders, KD, Cox K, Cannon R, et al. Growth response to enteral feeding by children with cerebral palsy. *J Parent Ent Nutr* 1990;14:23–26.

122. Shapiro BK, Green P, Krick J, et al. Growth of severely impaired children: neurological versus nutritional factors. *Dev Med Child Neurol* 1986;28:720–733.

123. Gaskin KJ, Waters DL, Baur LA, et al. Nutritional status, growth and development. I: children undergoing intensive treatment for cystic fibrosis. *Acta Paediatr Scand (Suppl)* 1990;366:106–110.

124. Taylor, KB, Anthony LE. *Clinical nutrition.* New York: McGraw-Hill, 1983.

125. Mattox TW, Bertch KE, Mirtallo JM, et al. Recent advances: parenteral nutrition support. *Ann Pharmacother* 1995;29(2):174–180.

126. Boyes, RJ, Kruse JA. Nasogastric and nasoenteric intubation. *Crit Care Clin* 1992;8(4):865–878.

127. Moore MC, Greene HL. Tube feeding of infants and children. *Pediatr Clin North Am* 1985;32:401–417.

128. Rombeau HL, Caaldwell MD. *Clinical nutrition: enteral and tube feeding,* 2nd ed. Philadelphia: WB Saunders, 1990.

129. Driscoll DF, Bistrian BR. Special considerations required for the formulation and administration of total parenteral nutrition therapy in the elderly patient. *Drugs Aging* 1992;2(5):395–405.

130. Wesley JR, Coran AG. Intravenous nutrition for the pediatric patient. *Semin Pediatr Surg* 1992;1(3):212–230.

131. DiLorenzo J, Dalton B, Miskovitz P. Percutaneous endoscopic gastrostomy. *Postgrad Med* 1992;9(1):277–281.

132. Tealey AR. Percutaneous endoscopic gastrostomy in the elderly. *Gastroenterol Nurs* 1994;16(4):151–157.

133. Fleming CR. Hepatobiliary complications in adults receiving nutrition support. *Dig Dis* 1994;12(4):191–198.

134. Bell SJ, Mascioli EA, Bistrian BR, et al. Alternative lipid sources for enteral and parenteral nutrition: long- and medium-chain triglycerides, structured triglycerides, and fish oils. *J Am Diet Assoc* 1991;91:74–78.

135. Irwin MM, Openbrier DR. A delicate balance: strategies for feeding ventilated COPD patients. *Am J Nurs* 1985;85:274–280.

136. Alexander JW, Gottschlich MM. Nutritional immomodulation in burn patients. *Crit Care Med* 1990;18[Suppl]:149–153.

137. Lipman TO. Bacterial translocation and enteral nutrition in humans: an outsider looks in. *J Parent Ent Nutr* 1995;9(2):156–165.

138. Padilla GV, Grant MM. Psychological aspects of artificial feeding. *Cancer* 1985;55:301–304.

139. Glass RP, Lucas B. Making the transition from tube feeding to oral feeding. *Nutr Focus* 1990;5:1–6.

140. Illingworth RS, Lister J. The critical or sensitive period, with special reference to certain feeding problems in infants and children. *J Pediatr* 1964;65:839–847.

141. Winkler MF, Pomp A, Caldwell MD, et al. Transitional feeding: the relationship between nutritional intake and plasma protein concentrations. *J Am Diet Assoc* 1989;89:969–970.

142. Berg K. Somatic adaptation in cerebral palsy: summary and general discussion. *Acta Raediatr Scand (Suppl)* 1971;204:81–93.

143. Brown JE, Davis E, Flemming PL. Nutritional assessment of children with handicapping conditions. *Ment Retard* 1979;17:129–132.

144. Barboriak JJ, Rooney CB, El Ghatit AZ, et al. Nutrition in spinal cord injury patients. *J Am Paraplegia Soc* 1983;6:32–36.

145. Newmark SR, Sublett D, Black J, et al. Nutritional assessment in a rehabilitation unit. *Arch Phys Med Rehabil* 1981;62:279–282.

146. Peiffer SC, Bluse P, Leyson JFJ. Nutritional assessment of the spinal cord injured patient. *J Am Diet Assoc* 1981;78:501–505.

147. Hodges P, Sauriol D, Man SFP, et al. Nutritional intake of patient with cystic fibrosis. *J Am Diet Assoc* 1984;84:664–669.

148. Hewson DC, Phyillips MA, Simpson KE, et al. Food intake in multiple sclerosis. *Hum Nutr Appl Nutr* 1984;38A:355–367.

149. Slowie LA, Paige MS, Antel JP. Nutritional considerations in the management of patients with amyotrophic lateral sclerosis (ALS). *J Am Diet Assoc* 1983;83:44–47.

150. Green EM, McIntosh EN. Food and nutrition skills of mentally retarded adults: assessment and needs. *J Am Diet Assoc* 1985;85:611–613.

151. Mattes-Kulig DA, Henkin RI. Energy and nutrient consumption of patient with dysgeusia. *J Am Diet Assoc* 1985;85:611–613.

152. Rhodus NL, Brown J. The association of xerostomia and inadequate intake in older adults. *J Am Diet Assoc* 1990;90:1688–1692.

153. Bowman BB, Rosenberg IH. Assessment of the nutritional status of the elderly. *Am J Clin Nutr* 1982;35:1141–1142.

154. Cos SAR, Weiss SM, Posuniak EA, et al. Energy expenditure after spinal cord injury: an evaluation of stable rehabilitating patients. *J Trauma* 1985;25:419–423.

155. Greenway RM, Houser HB, Lindan O, et al. Long-term changes in gross body composition of paraplegic and quadriplegic patients. *Paraplegia* 1969;7:301–318.

156. Berg K, Olsson R. Energy requirements of school children with cerebral palsy as determined from indirect calorimetry. *Acta Paediatr Scand J Suppl* 1971;240:71–80.

157. Culley WJ, Middleton TO. Caloric requirements of mentally retarded children with and without motor dysfunction. *J Pediatr* 1969;75:380–384.
158. Eddy TP, Nicholson AH, Wheeler DF. Energy expenditures and dietary intake in cerebral palsy. *Dev Med Neurol* 1965;7:377–386.
159. Daly JM, Meysfield SB, Head CA, et al. Human energy requirements: overestimation by widely used prediction equation. *Am J Clin Nutr* 1985;42:1170–1174.
160. Kearns PJ, Pipp TL, Quick M, et al. Nutritional requirements in quadriplegics. *J Parent Ent Nutr* 1982;6:577(abstr).
161. Turner WW, Ireton CS, Hunt JL, et al. Predicting energy expenditures in burned patients. *J Trauma* 1985;25:11–16.
162. Chantraine A, Delwaide PA. Hydroelectrolytic determination in paraplegics. *Paraplegia* 1976;14:138–145.
163. Claus-Walker J, Halstead LS. Metabolic and endocrine changes in spinal cord injury: I. The nervous system before and after transaction of the spinal cord. *Arch Phys Med Rehabil* 1981;62:595–601.
164. Kuhlemeier KV, Milelr JM III, Nepomuceno CS. Insensible weight loss in patients with spinal cord transaction. *Paraplegia* 1976;14:195–201.
165. Mirahmadi MK, Barton CH, Vaziri ND, et al. Nutritional evaluation of hemodialysis patients with and without spinal cord injury. *Am J Paraplegia* 1983;6:36–40.
166. Pierce DS, Nickel VH. *The total care of spinal cord injuries.* Boston: Little, Brown, & Co., 1977.
167. Feucht S. Assessment of growth. *Nutr Focus* 1989;4:1–8.
168. Biering-Sorensen F, Bohr JJ, Schaadt OP. Longitudinal study of bone mineral content in the lumbar spine, the forearm and the lower extremities after spinal cord injury. *Eur J Clin Invest* 1990;20:330–335.
169. Schols AMWJ, Wouters, EFM, Soeters PB, et al. Body composition by bioelectrical-impedance analysis compared with deuterium dilution and skinfold anthropometry inpatients with chronic obstructive pulmonary disease. *Am J Clin Nutr* 1991;53:421–424.
170. Panzetta F, Guerra J, d'Angelo A, et al. Body composition and nutritional status in patients on continuous ambulatory peritoneal dialysis (CAPD). *Clin Nephrol* 1985;23:18–25.
171. Shizgal HM. Body composition of patients with malnutrition and cancer: summary of methods of assessment. *Cancer* 1985;55:250–253.
172. Foster MR, Heppenstall RB, Friedenberg ZB, et al. A prospective assessment of nutritional status and complications in patients with fractures of the hip. *J Orthop Trauma* 1990;4:49–57.
173. Sullivan DH, Patch GA, Walls RC, et al. Impact of nutrition status on morbidity and mortality in a select population of geriatric rehabilitation patients. *Am J Clin Nutr* 1990;51:749–758.
174. Sullivan DH, Walls RC, Lipschitz DA. Protein-energy undernutrition and the risk of mortality within 1 y of hospital discharge in a select population of geriatric rehabilitation patients. *Am J Clin Nutr* 1991;53:599–605.
175. Wilson DO, Donahoe M, Rogers RM, et al. Metabolic rate and weight-loss in chronic obstructive lung disease. *J Parent Ent Nutr* 1990;14:7–11.
176. Fuensalida CE, Petty TL, Jones ML, et al. The immune response to short-term nutritional intervention in advanced chronic obstructive pulmonary disease. *Am Rev Respir Dis* 1990;142:49–56.
177. Gray-Donald K, Gibbons L, Shapiro SH, et al. Effect of nutritional status on exercise performance in patients with chronic obstructive pulmonary disease. *Am Rev Respir Dis* 1990;142:49–56.
178. Rutan RL, Herndon DN. Growth delay in postburn pediatric patients. *Arch Surg* 1990;125:392–395.
179. Abraham PA, Smith CL. Medical evaluation and management of calcium nephrolithiasis. *Med Clin North Am* 1984;68:281–299.
180. DeVivo MJ, Fine PR, Cutter GR, et al. The risk of renal calculi in spinal cord injury patients. *J Urol* 1984;131:857–860.
181. Robertson WG, Peacock M. Metabolic and biochemical risk factors in renal stone disease. *Contrib Nephrol* 1984;37:1–4.
182. Claus-Walker J, Spencer WA, Caraeter RE, et al. Bone metabolism in quadriplegia: dissociation between calciuria and hydroxyprolinuria. *Arch Phys Med Rehabil* 1975;56:327–332.
183. Kaplan PE, Grandhavadi B, Richards L, et al. Calcium balance in paraplegic patients: influence of injury duration and ambulation. *Arch Phys Med Rehabil* 1978;59:447–450.
184. Maynard FM, Imai K. Immobilization hypercalcemia in spinal cord injury. *Arch Phys Med Rehabil* 1977;58:16–24.
185. Naftchi NE, Viau AT, Sell GH, et al. Mineral metabolism in spinal cord injury. *Arch Phys Med Rehabil* 1908;61:139–142.
186. Lamid S, El Ghati AZ, Melvin JL. Relationship of hypercalcuria to diet and bladder stone formation in spinal cord injury patients. *Am J Phys Med* 1984;63:182–187.
187. Fellstrom B, Danielson BG, Karlstrom B, et al. Urinary composition and supersaturation on a high protein diet. *Contrib Nephrol* 1984;37:27–30.
188. Fituri N, Allawi N, Bentley M, et al. Urinary and plasma oxalate during ingestion of pure ascorbic acid: a reevaluation. *Eur Urol* 1983;9:312–315.
189. Hoffer A. Ascorbic acid and kidney stones [Letter]. *Can Med Assoc J* 1985;132:320.
190. Power C, Barker DJP, Nelson M, et al. Diet and renal stones: a case-control study. *Br J Urol* 1984;46:456–459.
191. Burr M, Alton M. Constipation in immobile patients. *Med J Aust* 1984;1:446–447.
192. Pontieri-Lewi, V. The role of nutrition in wound healing. *Med Surg Nurs*; 6:187–192.
193. Flanigan KH. Nutritional aspects of wound healing. *Adv Wound Care* 1997; 10(3):48–52.
194. *Clinical Practice Guideline: Treatment of pressure ulcers.* Rockville, MD: US Dept of Health and Human Services; 1994, Guideline #15.

CHAPTER 59

Wheelchairs

Michael L. Boninger, Rory A. Cooper, Mark Schmeler, and Rosemarie Cooper

The ability to maneuver unfettered in an environment is a basic component of human independence. In the Institute of Medicine model on the enablement/disablement process (1), a wheelchair and its components are fundamental for altering the interaction with the user and the environment, therefore leading to independence. Not surprisingly, studies in various populations and nations have repeatedly shown that mobility is closely tied to quality of life (2–7). It is therefore critical that the physiatrist take an active role in the wheelchair prescription process. Fundamental to this role is knowledge related to the complex components that make up seating and wheelchairs.

Seating and wheelchair technology has become increasingly complex and of much greater variety. In this chapter, the reader will find information to help gain an understanding for differentiation among various types of manual and power wheelchairs, and seating systems. In addition, we will discuss newer hybrid wheelchairs, such as power add-on units. The importance of the wheelchair-user interface, ride comfort, durability, proper selection of wheelchair accessories, and powered-wheelchair access devices will also be stressed. The reader will be introduced to wheelchair and seating measurements, and a variety of cushions and postural supports.

PRESCRIPTION PROCESS

Team Approach

The complexity of wheelchair and seating components combined with the nuances of individuals and various disease processes make it virtually impossible for a single clinician to act independently when prescribing assistive technology for mobility. For this reason, it is important to involve an interdisciplinary team in the decision-making process (8–9). The most important team member is the patient. The interaction of the patient with the team is critical to success and must be varied based on the level of knowledge of the individual. Some patients have been using a wheelchair for years and know exactly what they are looking for. For these individuals, team members act to provide unbiased information. Alternatively, a novice patient may have little knowledge of what is available and the tradeoffs of each decision. For this individual, the team will need to be more directive. The family and caregiver should also provide input, as they will be the next most affected by the choice of wheelchair.

The assessment team usually consists of a variety of rehabilitation professionals (Table 59-1). The physician is usually responsible for signing the prescription for the wheelchair. An occupational or physical therapist conducts the evaluation process and works closely with a rehabilitation engineer or a professional certified in rehabilitation technology by RESNA (Rehabilitation Engineering and Assistive Technology Society of North America), including an assistive technology practitioner (ATP), assistive technology supplier (ATS), or certified rehabilitation supplier (CRTS, National Association of Rehabilitation Technology Suppliers). Those involved in the wheelchair selection process should have knowledge about the technology available on the market. Magazine articles and commercial database sources such as ABLEDATA (http://www.abledata.com/) or WheelchairNet (www.wheelchairnet.org) are good places to research devices, or to direct patients who want to educate themselves. People choose their seating and mobility devices based on the features available that will facilitate activities or address needs (10), therefore it is important to be aware of the user's preferences and the features of various devices.

Assessment

The assessment process involves obtaining critical information about the user and his or her environment. The assessment process usually involves a structured interview with the patient and then a physical motor assessment. It is important to establish the diagnosis that requires the wheelchair and to assure that there are no ongoing medical problems or complications that are not being adequately addressed. These types of problems need to be clarified because they can impact the wheelchair prescription and the patient's health.

To properly specify a wheelchair, it is important to understand both the intentions and the abilities of the user (11). The best wheelchair prescription will not be successful if rejected by the user. Most people's activities can be placed into one of three categories: basic and instrumental activities of daily living, vocational and educational activities, and leisure activities. Access to a range of heights might be important to reach objects in the home and other environments. To support vocational needs, specific requirements may exist for mobility within a laboratory, operating room, courtroom, or machine shop. Leisure activities, pursued in such places as community centers, restaurants, movie theaters, and recreational environments, often place the most demands on the wheelchair. For some users, many of the desired tasks may be accomplished simply

TABLE 59-1. Members of the Seating and Assessment Team

- Patient
- Rehabilitation Engineer
- Occupational Therapist
- Physical Therapist
- Rehabilitation Technology Supplier
- Speech and Language Pathologist
- Rehabilitation Physician

and with existing off-the-shelf technology. Others will require custom products, and some will not be able to achieve all of their goals with any existing technology.

Additional necessary information includes type of insurance, methods of transportation, and physical capabilities. Also, if the patient has been using a chair, historical information about their current chair should be addressed, including current problems they may be having. The wheelchair model chosen should also be compatible with the public and private transportation options available to the wheelchair user, such as a bus, train, car, or van. If the wheelchair user plans to travel by air, modular wheelchairs that operate on sealed gel batteries should be considered. This type of battery has become the standard.

In all environments, the surface conditions may impose restrictions on the type of wheelchair that is most appropriate. The regularity of the surface and its firmness and stability are important in determining the tire size, drive wheel location, and wheel diameter. The performance of the wheelchair is often dictated by the need to negotiate grades, as well as height transitions, such as thresholds and curbs. The clearance widths in the environment will determine the overall dimensions of the wheelchair. A scooter may not fit around a corner in an average person's home but might perform well outdoors on a sidewalk. The need to be able to operate in snow, rain, changing humidity and temperature levels, and other weather conditions are important considerations as well.

Physical Examination

With an understanding of the individual's need or desire to perform different activities, the next step is examining the user. The history likely provided significant insight related to their physical abilities. To verify this, a physical examination should focus on aspects of the patient that will (a) help justify the wheelchair and seating system, (b) help determine the most appropriate wheelchair and seating system, and (c) assure that medical issues are appropriately addressed. Based on the interview of the patient, it may be possible to omit some portions of the examination listed below.

Often individuals require a wheelchair because of cardiopulmonary disease. For these individuals it is important to document a heart and lung examination. Attention should be paid to dyspnea on exertion and changes in vital signs with activity. Other common reasons for requiring a wheelchair are musculoskeletal and neurologic deficits. The clinician should document the neurologic and musculoskeletal deficits in a methodical fashion. In a patient who has sustained a cerebral vascular accident, for instance, an examination to check for neglect or visual field deficit is important because it will impact on the ability to independently drive a chair.

Obvious examination items include strength and range of motion. For individuals with chronic arthritis problems and pain, the examination should document the painful, swollen, or malaligned joints. When no strength deficit is seen, it is important to document issues with coordination, tone, and proprioception. A recent article found that many individuals with multiple sclerosis were unable to effectively propel a manual wheelchair despite a normal standard sensory and motor upper extremity examination (12). This same study found that simple questions related to the ability to button a shirt were related to the ability to propel a chair.

While completing the examination, the physician should be thinking about how the individual will control the wheelchair. If there is poor hand coordination, then a foot joystick may be possible. Alternatively, head control or switch control may be needed. For some individuals, the examination and history will not necessarily establish a clear need for a wheelchair. In these cases, it is important to consider alternative options that meet the individual's functional needs. The bottom line, however, should be function. If from the history and examination it is determined that the deficit will be transient, then a rental chair may be appropriate. If during the history and physical examination medical issues that require intervention are identified, it may be appropriate to delay wheelchair prescription so that changes in the patient status do not necessitate changes in the prescription.

Once the examination documents the medical need for the wheelchair, the remainder of the examination can focus on the appropriate technology. Key components of this section of the examination include postural stability, skin, posture, and size. Stability can be assessed by observing the individual in the current wheelchair or by asking him or her to sit unsupported on a mat table. Ask the patient to perform simple reaching tasks to determine the lateral and forward stability of the trunk, hand and arm strength, and hand fine motor skills. Appropriate seating can enhance reach and stability, thus improving the performance of manual activities from the wheelchair.

The presence of kyphosis, scoliosis, or other fixed deformities should be determined. Critical points to evaluate are hip and knee range of motion because contractures may need to be accommodated in the wheelchair. Poor stability usually indicates the need for special attention with respect to seating and position. It is well known that various groups of wheelchair users will develop kyphosis or scoliosis over time (13). What is less well known is whether spinal deformities can be prevented with appropriate seating. Even if prevention is not a goal, accommodation is needed for comfortable seating.

Finally, a thorough check of the individual's skin is important. This may not be needed for individuals with cardiopulmonary disease, but it is essential for individuals with neurologic deficits or those with any previous history of pressure sores. The examination should include not only the buttocks, but also the feet and calves, which can be affected by pressure against a leg rest. Attention should be paid to bony prominences and previous scars. This examination will help with cushion selection and wheelchair set up. Large, previously untreated ulcers are sometimes discovered, ultimately leading to treatment before seating plans can be implemented.

For many people, a few simple measurements can be used to determine the proper dimensions for a wheelchair (14). Body measurements are typically made with the consumer in the seated position. Probably the most obvious body measurements are the consumer's height and weight. The consumer's weight is critical to obtaining a wheelchair that is sufficiently strong. Many manufacturers claim that their wheelchairs are rated to hold up to 250 pounds. The height of the wheelchair user provides information about the person's size and can be used to check the final wheelchair measurements. For example, the sum of the sitting height, sitting depth, and lower-leg length should be close to the person's supine height. Additional measurements and definitions are used when specialized seating and postural support systems are required.

Documentation

Providing quality wheelchairs is paperwork intensive. At the very least, a prescription and various insurance forms must be provided. For more expensive interventions, a letter of medical necessity (LMN) is frequently required. This letter describes the person's disability, problems with existing equipment or method of mobility, evaluation procedures, conclusions, explanation of why lower-cost alternatives will not work, risks of not providing the equipment, and a line-item justification for each of the various components being recommended. Other clinicians, such as occupational and physical therapists, can assist in preparing a letter; however, the letter must be reviewed and cosigned by a physician. Often wheelchair vendors can play a helpful role in completing the documentation and in letting patients try different types of mobility devices. However, it is important that physicians and therapists be actively involved in the process, as vendors may allow concern for profit, or easy reimbursement, to influence selection. It is not appropriate for a physician to sign an LMN for a patient if he or she has not evaluated the patient for the device prescribed.

FUNDING

For many individuals, funding can present a major limitation to the type and quality of the wheelchair they can receive through their health insurance. It is tempting as a practitioner to determine the wheelchair that insurance will cover and then work from this limitation. This path can be poor for the patient and in the long term will not lead to changes in policy. Therefore, it is important that the clinician working with the patient determine what is the optimal mobility device. After making this determination, the team can then assess what is the best way to convince insurance that the device is medically necessary and should be covered.

Having stated this, it is helpful to know current policies and their impact on patients. The section below is focused on the United States of America. Across the world there are widely varying policies related to wheelchair coverage, including no coverage at all in many developing countries. In the United States, wheelchairs and seating systems are covered in whole or part by health insurance plans, including Medicare Part B, state Medicaid programs, commercial insurance, and managed care plans, unless the policy clearly stipulates no durable medical equipment coverage. Other funding sources also exist, such as state vocational rehabilitation programs, if the device is needed for work-related activities.

In order for any health insurance provider to approve coverage for a wheelchair and seating system, the practitioner must establish medical necessity. Each funding source may have its own definition of "medically necessary," however; in general, when it comes to wheelchairs, it is necessary to accommodate or replace a malfunctioning body part (i.e., paralysis or weakness of the lower extremities) or to reduce or manage disability. The funding sources also require the recommended intervention to be the least costly, reasonable alternative. Therefore, as part of an evaluation, it is helpful to document that lower-cost alternatives have been tried and were unsuccessful, and to cite specific reasons for the higher-cost choice. It is also helpful to document that the device was chosen based on a clinical trial or simulation, as well as describing the potential outcomes if the

person is not provided with the equipment. Examples of these risks include falls and fractures, development of pressure sores, joint contractures and musculoskeletal deformities, increased pain and discomfort, loss of function, and ultimately being more restricted to a bed or chair.

Medicare has specific requirements for payment of wheelchairs that includes completion of a certificate of medical necessity. Many other health insurers have adopted the Medicare standard. Unfortunately, the standards were developed in the early 1980s and are viewed by many experts in the field as being antiquated based on today's available wheelchair technology and research findings. There is much activity under way to change these policies, and perhaps some may be implemented by the time one reads this text.

The qualifying criteria for the various types of wheeled mobility devices are as follows:

The device is required for use in the home. This is a very restrictive criteria that can be interpreted as for use only within the interior of the home. It derives from the fact that wheelchairs are classified under Medicare as home medical equipment. Some people have interpreted this to mean that a person who can ambulate short distances on flat surfaces inside the home, but requires the device for outdoor and community mobility, will not receive coverage. Medicare has not provided an operational definition of "home," therefore practitioners should assess the person's situation when defining "home." The home can include one's house, yard, neighborhood, and community. If a person's illness or disability prohibits them from accessing these entities, then a wheeled mobility device is certainly indicated for their medical as well as psychological and social wellbeing. Funding sources are also interested in the person's required instrumental and basic activities of daily living and how the equipment will facilitate participation in these activities regardless of where they are performed.

The patient is unable to ambulate. For this section, it is usually sufficient to explain that an individual can only ambulate short distances or is unsafe ambulating. Placing these limitations in the context of their current living situation and usual activities can help persuade payers of the need.

Lightweight and Ultralightweight Wheelchairs. To qualify for either of these wheelchairs, it necessary to document that the person is unable to propel a lower-cost alternative standard wheelchair. It also helps to document the person's lifestyle situation and how the wheelchair will facilitate their ability to engage in activities.

Power Wheelchairs and Power-Operated Vehicles. To qualify for a power wheelchair or power-operated vehicle (or scooter), one must document that the person cannot effectively propel any type of manual wheelchair. For individuals with upper-extremity paralysis, it is obvious that they cannot propel a manual chair. However, many other individuals can require a power wheelchair. People with upper-extremity pain that limits propulsion meet this criterion, because pain and risk of aggravating injury may make them incapable of propelling a manual chair. This is also true for individuals with cardiopulmonary disease or obesity. Both of these conditions make functional manual wheelchair propulsion difficult and, in some cases, impossible. These deficits and risks should be documented and explained in the LMN.

MANUAL WHEELCHAIRS

Manual wheelchairs have developed rapidly in recent years. Only a few years ago, there was only one style of wheelchair, and it came in one color: chrome. Now, there are numerous types of wheelchairs to choose from, and they come in a wide range of colors. Wheelchairs have moved from being chairs with wheels designed to provide some minimal mobility to advanced orthotic support systems designed to meet the mobility demands of the user (11). The proper selection and design of a wheelchair depends on the abilities of the user and on the intended uses (15). Thus, specialized wheelchairs have been and continue to be developed to yield better performance (16).

Manual wheelchairs offer many advantages over powered mobility. Manual wheelchairs are much easier to transport because of their lighter weight. No special equipment is needed to place a manual wheelchair in a backseat, and individuals with paraplegia and tetraplegia are often capable of transporting their wheelchairs independently. In addition, manual wheelchairs generally require less maintenance than power devices, and there are no concerns related to batteries or controllers. Finally, manual wheelchairs offer a degree of physical exercise that can benefit the wheelchair user. Unfortunately, this same physical exertion can lead to upper-limb injuries and pain. Recent research suggests that it may be possible to prevent these injuries through the appropriate selection and configuration of the wheelchair and with the appropriate training of the user (17,18).

Depot and Attendant-Propelled Wheelchairs

The depot or institutional wheelchair is essentially the same wheelchair that was produced in the 1940s. This type of chair corresponds to the Medicare category of K0001 and, despite its numerous shortcomings, is the default chair for many insurance companies and Medicare. Some depot wheelchairs may be a bit lighter than the 1940s models, but the basic frame design is unchanged. Depot wheelchairs are intended for institutional use, where several people may use the same wheelchair. These wheelchairs are typically used in airports, hospitals, and nursing care facilities. They are inappropriate for active people who use wheelchairs for personal mobility, including older persons in nursing homes. Depot wheelchairs are designed to be inexpensive, to accommodate large variations in body size, to be low maintenance, and to be attendant propelled. Unlike the attendant-propelled chairs described below, depot chairs are not designed for the comfort of the person being transported, nor for the person pushing the chair. A typical depot wheelchair will have swing-away footrests, removable armrests, a single cross-brace frame, and solid tires (Fig. 59-1). Depot wheelchairs have sling seats and back supports, which

are uncomfortable and provide little support. Swing-away footrests add weight to the wheelchair; however, they make transferring into and out of the wheelchair easier. Armrests provide some comfort and stability to the depot wheelchair user and can aid in keeping clothing off the wheels. Depot chairs typically fold to reduce the area for storage and transportation. Solid tires are commonly used to reduce maintenance. Solid tires typically dramatically reduce ride comfort, increase rolling resistance, and add weight. There is very little, if anything, that can be adjusted to fit the user on a depot chair. Typically, only the leg-rest length is adjustable. Depot chairs are available in various seat widths, seat depths, and backrest heights.

Attendant-Propelled Chairs

Not all wheelchairs are propelled by the person sitting in the wheelchair. In many hospitals and long-term care facilities, wheelchairs are expected to be propelled by attendants. In addition, some individuals with severe disabilities are unable to propel a wheelchair or control a power wheelchair. For children who use attendant-propelled chairs, it is necessary to continually reassess if they may be able to use independent mobility. The primary consideration in the attendant-propelled chair is that the wheelchair has two users: the rider and the attendant. If the wheelchair is propelled solely by attendants with no assistance from the rider, then there may be no need for the larger drive wheels (Figure 59-2). If the occupant will be sitting in the chair for prolonged periods of time, then attention must be paid to comfort. For this reason, attendant-propelled chairs often have tilt-in-space as an option.

A variant of the attendant-propelled wheelchair is sometimes called a "Gerry" chair in reference to geriatric users. This type of attendant-propelled wheelchair is typically designed to minimize the independent mobility of the rider. The rider is seated in a large recliner-type wheelchair. The soft padding, reclined position, small wheels, and large size make it impossible for the rider to move the wheelchair and difficult for most riders to exit the wheelchair. This helps long-term care facility to exercise control over their clients with cognitive dysfunction. There has been considerable discussion about the appropriate use of attendant-propelled chairs that significantly restrain the rider's mobility.

Lightweight and Ultralight Wheelchairs

The terms *lightweight* and *ultralight wheelchairs* are derived from the Medicare categories K0004 and K0005, respectively. K0004 wheelchairs must weigh less than 34 pounds without footrests or armrests, and K0005 must weigh less than 30 pounds without foot or arm supports. K0004 wheelchairs have very limited adjustability (Figure 59-3). Like depot chairs, they can be sized to the user, but many of these chairs do not offer features such as adjustable axle plates, quick-release wheels, or a method to change the seat to back angle of the wheelchair. Because of the way Medicare reimbursement works, both depot and lightweight chairs have primarily been engineered for low cost. Manufacturers have attempted to build the best wheelchair possible under a certain Medicare reimbursable cost. This has not led to the best-designed chairs.

The ultralight wheelchair is the highest-quality chair that is designed specifically as an active mobility device. These chairs, which can easily cost more than $2,000, are usually highly adjustable and incorporate numerous design features made to enhance the ease of propulsion and increase the comfort of the wheelchair user. At present, it is necessary to justify the need

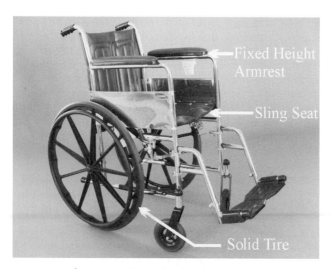

Figure 59-1. K0001 depot-style wheelchair.

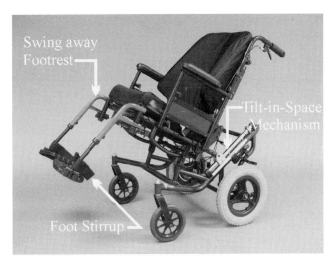

Figure 59-2. Attendant-propelled wheelchair with tilt-in-space.

for a K0004 or K0005 wheelchair instead of a standard K0001. Unfortunately, prior authorization—meaning the vendor is guaranteed ahead of time to be reimbursed for the wheelchair—is not possible. As a result, vendors are unwilling to take the risk that a $2,000 item will be rejected by Medicare and become their problem. As of press time, Medicare is pilot testing a program that allows for preauthorization of these chairs.

Ultralight wheelchairs usually have a number of options and adjustments that can be made to appropriately fit the user. Following is list of many of the components of chairs and options that are available. Some of these options are also available on lightweight and depot type chairs. It is important to note that the components used on ultralight chairs are generally better in quality.

FRAMES

There are two basic frame types: folding and rigid. Within these two frame types, there are a number of different varieties. The most common type of manual wheelchair frame is the folding cross-brace frame (see Figure 59-3). The cross-brace folding mechanism consists of two frame members connected in the middle and attached to the bottom of a side-frame member on one side of the chair and to the seat upholstery above the top side-frame member on the opposite side. The cross members are hinged at the bottom and pinned together in the middle. When viewed from the back of the frame, the cross members form an X. The chair is folded by pulling upward on the seat upholstery. Cross-member folding mechanisms are simple and easy to use. However, the wheelchair may collapse when tilted sideways, and the frame becomes taller when folded. Some chairs incorporate snaps or over-center locking mechanisms to reduce the problem of frame folding while on a side slope.

The most common rigid chair is the box frame. The box frame is named for its rectangular shape and the frame tubes that form a "box" (11). Box frames can be very strong and very durable. These frames can also be collapsed to relatively small dimensions. The backrest usually folds forward, and when used with quick-release wheels, the chair becomes a rather compact shape. An alternative to the box frame is the frame that can act as suspension (i.e., there is some flexibility purposely built into the frame). These cantilever frames may also have fewer tubes and fewer parts and thus be more aesthetically pleasing (Figure 59-4).

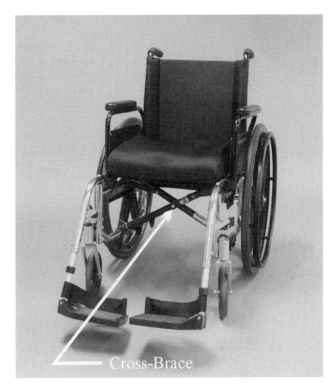

Figure 59-3. K0004 lightweight wheelchair with folding cross-brace design.

A number of manufacturers have recently added suspension elements to the frame. This is in part a response to evidence that vibration exposure in wheelchair users is excessive (19). Hinges are placed at the front of the seat, and elastic elements are placed at the back of the seat. The elastic elements act to provide some suspension. The flexible element for the suspension can use either metal springs or polymer dampeners (see Figure 59-4). Recent work has shown that these elastic elements have not necessarily resulted in lower levels of vibration being transmitted to the user (20). In addition, the shock absorption can result in lost energy during propulsion. Therefore, the decision to purchase a suspension wheelchair should depend on whether the patient prefers the drive, feel, and comfort of the wheelchair.

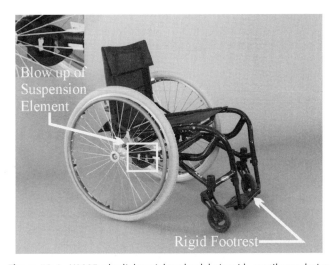

Figure 59-4. K0005 ultralightweight wheelchair with cantilever design and suspension element.

FOOTRESTS

Most wheelchair users require support for their feet and lower legs. This support is provided by footrests. Footrests may be fixed, folding, swing away (see Figure 59-2), or elevating. The footrests must provide sufficient support for the lower legs and feet, and must hold the feet in proper position to prevent foot drop or other deformities. It is essential to assess limitations in knee and foot range of motion. Some users have very tight hamstrings, requiring that the feet be positioned closer to or under the front edge of the seat. This is difficult to accomplish in most configurations. Extending the knees out to accommodate the standard design of the footrest position in front of the seat results in a sitting posture with a posterior pelvic tilt and a tendency to slide forward in the seat. This is commonly seen in elderly people in nursing homes using depot-type wheelchairs.

The feet must remain on the footrests at all times during propulsion, and therefore some type of cradle is recommended. Some wheelchairs (primarily those with swing-away footrests) use foot stirrups behind the heels of each foot (see Figure 59-2). However, for other wheelchairs, it is best to use a continuous strap behind both feet because the rider's feet sometimes come over stirrups during active use. The feet should not be pinched, trapped, or scratched by the footrests during normal driving activities or when transferring. The frame should be selected and configured so that the feet sit firmly upon the footrests, with shoes on, without lifting the upper legs from the seat cushion. Care must be taken that sufficient ground clearance is maintained. The footrests are commonly placed between 25 and 50 mm (1–2 in.) from the ground. Often, the footrests are the first part of the chair to come in contact with an obstacle (such as a door, wall, or another chair), so they must be durable.

Rigid wheelchairs often use simple tubes across the front of the wheelchair. By using a tubular rigid footrest, the wheelchair becomes stiffer and stronger (see Figure 59-4). Rigid footrests are used during sports activities and work well for people who are very active in their wheelchair. Forward antitip rollers can be mounted to rigid footrests. This is helpful for playing court sports and reducing the risk of some forward-tipping accidents. Rigid footrests may be used on folding wheelchairs. This prevents them from folding. However, for people who like to use one wheelchair for daily use and one for recreational use, two sets of leg rests (e.g., one rigid and one split) may help to accomplish this. Folding wheelchairs often use footrests that fold up and leg rests that swing out of the way to ease in transfers. Swing-away leg rests are not as durable as rigid ones. In some cases, manufacturers design swing-away leg rests that will flexibly bend on impact. This helps to absorb the energy of the impact and possibly prevent serious injury to the wheelchair rider. Elevating leg rests can be used for people who can not maintain a 90-degree knee angle or who need their legs elevated for venous return. Elevating leg rests make the wheelchair longer and heavier. This also has the effect of making the wheelchair less maneuverable by increasing the turning radius. Therefore, if elevating leg rests are needed, a power wheelchair should strongly be considered.

ARMRESTS AND CLOTHING GUARDS

Armrests provide a form of support and are convenient handles to hold onto when the rider leans to one side or the other. Armrests are also helpful when attempting to reach higher places. For example, some people use their removable armrests as a tool to nudge items off high shelves. Armrests are commonly used to perform a "push-up" to assist with seat pressure relief. By placing a forearm or hand on each armrest and pushing upward, some wheelchair users are capable of lifting their buttocks from the seat. This helps to improve blood flow to the lower extremities and reduces the risk of developing a pressure ulcer.

There are three basic styles of armrests: wraparound, full-length, and desk-length. Wraparound armrests mount at the back of the wheelchair onto the frame below the backrest in most cases. The armrest comes up along the back of the backrest supports and wraps around to the front of the wheelchair. The major advantage of this design is that the armrest does not increase the width of the wheelchair like the other types of armrests. Wraparound armrests are popular among active wheelchair users. The most significant drawback of this design is that the armrest does not serve as a side guard to keep the rider's clothing away from the wheels.

Full-length and desk-length armrests are similar in design, the main difference being the length of the armrest. Full-length armrests provide support for nearly the entire upper arm. They are popular on electric-powered wheelchairs because they provide a convenient and functional location for a joystick or other input device. Full-length armrests make it difficult to get close to some tables and desks. This is why manufacturers produce shorter desk-length armrests. Both of these types of armrests include clothing guards to protect clothing from the wheels. These types of armrests are mounted to the side of the wheelchair and may add as much as 5 cm (2 in.) to the width of the wheelchair.

Armrests can be fixed or height adjustable. Height-adjustable armrests may move up and down to accommodate the length of the rider's trunk and arms. Most armrests can be moved in order to provide clearance for transferring in and out of the wheelchair, and to allow a person to lean over the sides of the wheelchair. Armrests are either removed or flipped back. Both styles commonly use a latch, which is operated by the user. It is important to have secure latches on the armrests because armrests form convenient places for people to hold onto when attempting to provide assistance. If the armrests and latches are designed properly, two people can lift the rider and wheelchair by holding onto the armrests. In some cases, armrests are designed to pull out if any upward force is applied to them. These are not intended to be used for lifting the chair. It should be noted that armrests could alter the way in which a person propels a wheelchair. The hands and arms must clear the armrest in order to reach the push rim. This can force the user into excessive abduction at the shoulder, which could be a risk factor for injury.

WHEEL LOCKS

Wheel locks act as parking brakes to stabilize the wheelchair when the rider transfers to other seats and when the rider wishes to remain in a particular spot. When locked, they keep the wheelchair stable to allow the rider to push things from the chair. There are a variety of wheel locks used to restrain wheelchairs when transferring or parking. High-lock brakes, which are located near the front corner of the seat, are most common, however, location can vary. High-lock brakes require the least dexterity to operate. Extension levers can be added for people with limited reach or minimal strength. Other wheel locks allow selection of the braking force; these are sometimes called sweeper brakes, as the wheelchair can still be pushed in some positions, which allow the user to push and then sweep a broom to clean a floor. Wheel locks are standard equipment on wheelchairs, and they are simple to mount if the wheelchair does not come equipped with locks from the manufacturer.

Wheel locks may be push to lock or pull to lock. Most people prefer push to lock because wheel locks are more difficult to engage than to disengage. Riders often find it easier to push with the palm than pull with the fingers. High wheel locks are often mounted to the upper tube of the wheelchair's side frame. Low wheel locks are usually mounted to the lower tube of the wheelchair's side frame. Low wheel locks require more mobility to operate. They also alleviate the common problem that is seen with high wheel locks of the user hitting his or her thumb against the lock. This problem can be addressed for high wheel lock users by selecting retractable (i.e., scissors or butter-fly) wheel locks. The retractable type of wheel lock helps to prevent jamming the thumbs and can also accommodate a wide variety of camber angles. The major drawback of re-tractable wheel locks is that they are more difficult to use than other types of wheel locks. The wheel lock must be positioned properly with respect to the wheel in order to operate effec-tively. If the wheels are repositioned, then the wheel locks must be repositioned. Tire pressure also affects the locking grip of these wheel locks.

TIRES

A variety of options exist with respect to tires. The most com-mon type of tire is pneumatic. These tires are lightweight and provide cushioning against impact and vibration from rolling over surfaces. This cushioning may increase rider comfort and improve wheelchair durability. Pneumatic tires are recom-mended for outdoor usage. The main downside of pneumatic tires is that they require maintenance and they can puncture. Tire pressure needs to be kept at a predetermined level because it is critical to rolling resistance, which can be related to risk of secondary injury associated with manual wheelchair use. Clin-icians involved with wheelchair users should squeeze their pa-tients' tires to assure they are keeping up with this important regular maintenance issue.

An alternative to pneumatic tires is solid inserts. These foam inserts fit into the pneumatic tire and replace the air-filled inner tube that would normally be there. They add some weight to the chair and may slightly worsen performance but are a good alternative for individuals who do not want to be responsible for maintenance of air pressure. A less viable alternative is solid tires. These tires require no maintenance and are low in cost. Unfortunately, they make for an uncomfortable ride as all ground shocks are transmitted to the wheelchair user.

ADDITIONAL FEATURES

Many additional features are available that are unique to man-ual wheelchairs.

Antitippers

Antitippers are often placed on wheelchairs to assure they do not tip over backward. These can inhibit the ability to climb curbs, but they do offer a measure of safety. It is suggested that these be ordered for all wheelchairs and then have the user take them off when they are comfortable with the stability of the chair.

Push Rims

A number of different push rims are currently available, and new styles are likely to be introduced into the market. An-odized aluminum rims are the current standard on most K0004 and K0005 chairs. Less expensive chairs may come with plastic push rims. For individuals with difficulty gripping the rim, al-ternative rims should be considered. These can include vinyl-coated rims, rims with projections (Figure 59-5), and rims wrapped with surgical tubing. All of these rims have the ad-vantage of increased friction, making it easier to push the chair forward. Unfortunately, this increased friction can lead to burns when the wheelchair user attempts to slow down the

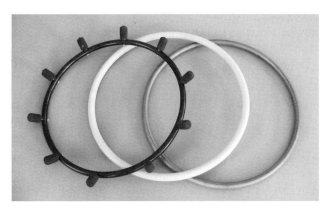

Figure 59-5. Wheelchair push rims: **(left)** quad-knob or projection rim. **(center)** vinyl-coated rim, **(right)** anodized aluminum rim.

chair. There is ongoing research into advanced ergonomic push-rim designs that allow for easier propulsion as well as braking (21).

Wheels

The standard wheels on lightweight and ultralightweight wheelchairs have spokes. Plastic wheels can be used on low-end chairs. These increase weight and decrease performance. High-end wheels are now available with flexible spokes or with graphite and composite materials. These wheels can be easier to maintain than standard spokes and also offer im-proved aesthetics.

Caster Wheels

Caster wheels are available in a variety of shapes and sizes. Pneumatic wheels are larger than solid casters and may inter-fere with the footrests when turning. Pneumatics offer the ad-vantage of easier propulsion over rough terrain and increased shock absorption. Many wheelchair users are using narrow Rollerblade type wheels, which can get caught in sewer grates. These wheels reduce rolling resistance and allow quicker turns. Adding "frog-legs" can provide shock adsorption. This device adds an elastomer shock absorber in series with the caster as a means of reducing vibration exposure (Figure 59-6).

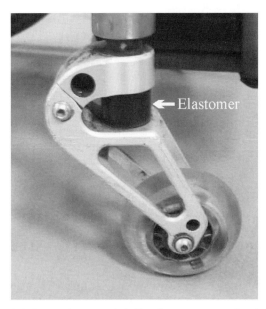

Figure 59-6. Suspension caster fork. The elastomer acts to absorb shocks.

Push Handles

Push handles, also known as canes, are attached to the back of the chair with the primary purpose of making it easier for an assistant to propel the wheelchair. Canes can also be used by the wheelchair occupant to help with pressure relief. The wheelchair user can hook the arm around the cane and pull to raise the contralateral hip, even in the absence of strong triceps muscles. Canes can also be used to hang a book bag or backpack onto the back of the chair.

Grade-Aids

Grade-Aids are devices that attach to the wheel and allow it to roll forward, but not back. In this manner, they can make it easier to roll up a hill. These should be considered for individuals who have upper-limb weakness and who must negotiate hills.

Manual Wheelchair Selection and Set-up

As stated previously, a number of the features described above and the adjustments described below will not be available without an ultralightweight wheelchair. Best practice dictates that any individual who will propel a wheelchair as a primary means of mobility should receive this type of chair. The chair should be as narrow as possible without causing undue pressure on the thighs. Rear axle position should be adjustable to fit the user, as it can affect caster flutter, rolling resistance, stability, and control and maneuverability. With a longer wheel base or more rearward axle position, the chair becomes more stable (22); however, rolling resistance is increased (16,23), caster flutter is increased, and downward turning on side slopes is increased. These changes are primarily related to the proportion of the weight that is placed onto the back, or larger, wheels. As the rear wheels are moved backward, more weight is placed on the front casters. These smaller-diameter wheels have higher rolling resistance. The cadence of the propulsive stroke is also higher, with a more rearward axle position. This has been implicated in relating to risk of repetitive strain injury (17). Given these issues, the axle should be as far forward as possible, providing that the wheelchair user still feels stable. Most wheelchairs come in a factory-set position, with the axle most rearward. This should be gradually adjusted forward to maximize performance of the chair. Typically, active users prefer control over the chair to stability.

Axle height, or the distance between the shoulder and the axle, is also an important parameter. If the seat is too high, the wheelchair user will not be able to reach much of the push rim, and so they will push with shorter strokes and a faster cadence. If the seat is too low, the user will be forced to abduct at the shoulder during the propulsive stroke, which may cause rotator cuff impingement. In general, while sitting upright with the hands resting on the top of the wheels, the elbow angle should be between 100 and 120 degrees for optimal mobility (23,24). Alternatively, if the arms are left to hang freely at the side while sitting in the chair, the fingertips should be very close to the axle of the wheel.

Camber is the vertical angle of the wheel with respect to the chair. Increasing camber has several advantages: the footprint of the chair is widened, creating greater side-to-side stability; it allows quicker turning; it helps to protect the hands by having the bottom of the wheels scuff edges, preventing them from hitting the area where the hands are in contact with the push rims; and it positions the push rims more ergonomically for propulsion (it is more natural to push down and out) (25). In addition, adding camber to the rear wheels reduces effective stiffness between the rolling surface and frame, thus reducing the vibration exposure of the user. The width of the chair depends on the width of the frame and the camber angle. Generally, for daily use, the chair should be as narrow as possible without substantially diminishing the handling characteristics. The wheels should be offset enough from the seat to avoid rubbing against the clothing or body. Narrow chairs are easier to maneuver in an environment made for walking. There are many other aspects of a wheelchair that can be adjusted to improve fit and performance. Some of these adjustments are discussed in the seating section that follows.

Alternative Manual Wheelchairs

Two alternatives worth mentioning are chairs for amputees and chairs for individuals with hemiparesis. Wheelchairs for individuals with amputations are typically designed with the rear axle set far behind the user. This is needed because the absence of a leg causes the body's center of gravity to be further back, thus reducing rearward stability. As stated above, a more rearward axle increases stability. Unfortunately, all of the negative aspects of a rearward axle are present. An alternative can be to add weight to front of the wheelchair. Unfortunately, increased weight means increased rolling resistance. There is no simple answer as to what is best, and individual patients should make this decision for themselves.

For individuals with hemiparesis or other disability that makes propulsion with a leg or both legs superior to propulsion with the arms, a "hemiheight" chair is an alternative. In this chair, there is typically one footrest or none at all, and the seat is low enough to the ground so that the feet can reach the floor. For an individual with hemiparesis, the use of the uninvolved arm and leg can provide limited, but functional, propulsion.

Another alternative for an individual with hemiparesis is a one-arm drive chair. This chair has two push rims on one side that control separate wheels. One-arm drives are heavier than standard chairs and can be difficult to control. These limitations make them less than ideal for an elderly stroke patient. For some individuals with cerebral palsy and hemiparesis, a power chair should be strongly considered.

Although not popular in the United States, lever-drive wheelchairs are seen in Europe. These chairs offer a mechanical advantage by using a lever to make propulsion more efficient. Unfortunately, they do not offer the direct proprioceptive feedback of hand rim contact and can be difficult to maneuver in tight spaces and when traveling backward. Lever-drive chairs are heavier and often wider than standard chairs.

Manual Wheelchair Propulsion Technique

In recent years, much has been learned about the most appropriate way to propel a wheelchair. This has been learned by studies that have found an association between upper-limb injuries and wheelchair propulsion biomechanics. Manual wheelchair users should propel with long smooth strokes that minimize the cadence with which they push and maximize the length of the stroke or contact angle (17,18). The wheelchair user should attempt to impact the rim smoothly and match the speed of the hand to the rotating speed of the push rim. During the recovery stage of the propulsive stroke, the user should let the hand drop below the push rim and stay below the push rim until he or she is ready to begin propulsion again (26) (Figure 59-7). The user should attempt to minimize the component of the force directed toward the axle of the wheel, as this force acts equally and opposite to drive the head of the humerus into the acromioclavicular arch. However, a recent study has shown that teaching a user to propel their chair with only a force tan-

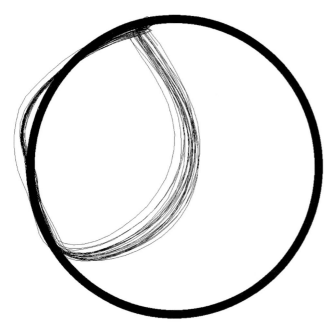

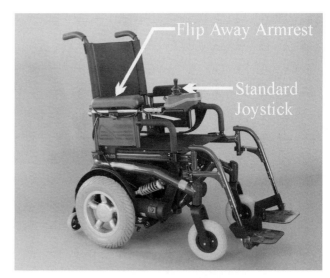

Figure 59-8. Rear-wheel-drive power wheelchair.

Figure 59-7. Recovery pattern. This represents data from a wheelchair user. The dark circle is the push rim. The thinner lines are from a marker placed on the wrist. This recovery pattern was found to provide the best efficiency. Direction of travel is left.

gential to the wheel may not improve efficiency (27). Optimal methods to train wheelchair users remain to be determined.

POWER WHEELCHAIRS

There is strong evidence in the literature to indicate that the use of powered mobility facilitates independence, improves occupational performance, and is correlated with a higher sense of quality of life for people who cannot ambulate or propel a manual wheelchair effectively (2, 3, 6). However, there are some disadvantages to powered mobility devices that need to be factored into the decision of powered versus manual wheelchair mobility (Table 59-2). Power wheelchairs come in a number of configurations. Two types are those with a power base and those with integrated seating systems. In general, wheelchairs with integrated seating systems are less expensive and offer less with respect to seating options. Integrated systems are often rear-wheel drive. However, front wheel drive and mid wheel drive chairs are available (see below).

TABLE 59-2.   Powered Versus Manual Wheelchair Mobility

Advantages of Manual Wheelchairs	Advantages of Power Wheelchairs
Transportation: Easy to transport; can travel with friends without special vehicles	Distance: Can travel long distances without fatigue
Maintenance: Can be worked on independently	Speed: Can travel at higher speed without fatigue
Exercise: Theoretical benefit to the user from using own force to propel	Terrain: May be able to traverse rougher terrain
Aesthetics: Less appearance of disability	Protect the arm: Avoid repetitive strain injuries that are due to manual wheelchair propulsion

Power Bases

The power base is the lower portion of a power wheelchair that houses the motors, batteries, drive wheels, casters, and electronics to which a seating system is attached (Figure 59-8). The base allows for the mounting of any variety or combination of different seating systems and seat functions, including tilt-in-space, reclining back, and seat elevator.

Drive Classification

Power wheelchair bases can be classified as rear-wheel drive (RWD), midwheel drive (MWD), or front-wheel drive (FWD). The classification of these three drive systems is based on the drive wheel location relative to the system's center of gravity. The drive wheel position defines the basic handling characteristic of any power wheelchair. Each system has unique driving and handling characteristics. In RWD power bases (see Figure 59-8), the drive wheels are behind the user's center of gravity, and the casters are in the front. RWD systems are the traditional design, and therefore many long-term power wheelchair users are familiar with their performance and prefer them to other designs. A major advantage of a RWD system is its predictable drive characteristic and stability. A potential drawback to a RWD system is its maneuverability in tight areas because of a larger turning radius.

In MWD power bases (Figure 59-9) , the drive wheels are directly below the user's center of gravity and generally have a set of casters or antitippers in front and rear of the drive wheels. The advantage of the MWD system is a smaller turning radius to maneuver in tight spaces. A disadvantage is a tendency to rock or pitch forward, especially with sudden stops or fast turns. When transitioning from a steep slope to a level surface (like coming off a curb cut), the front and rear casters can hang up, leaving less traction on the drive wheels in the middle.

A FWD power base (Figure 59-10) has the drive wheels in front of the user's center of gravity, and the rear wheels are casters. The advantage of a FWD system is that it tends to be quite stable and provides a tight turning radius. FWD systems may climb obstacles or curbs more easily as the large front wheels hit the obstacle first. A disadvantage is that a FWD system has more rearward center of gravity; therefore, the system may tend to fishtail and be difficult to drive in a straight line, especially on uneven surfaces.

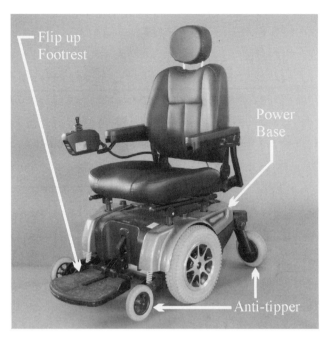

Figure 59-9. Mid-wheel-drive power wheelchair with power base. The seating system can be removed and replaced with a different seating configuration.

Controls

The primary function of an access device is the control of the powered mobility system. Secondary applications are for use with environmental control systems and computer access. By using the same control interface for both the power wheelchair and the secondary systems, the seating position and control selection can be optimized for multiple functional purposes. The majority of input controls are programmable, allowing changes in speed and the amount of movement to determine the direction of the wheelchair. Many power wheelchair users brace some portion of their hand against the control box and use their hand and arm coordination to operate the joystick. Gross arm function, in many cases, can be used to operate a joystick.

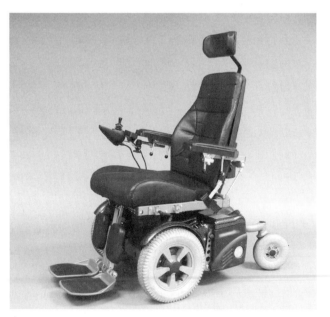

Figure 59-10. Front-wheel-drive power wheelchair.

If the user does not have the hand function or coordination to operate a joystick input device, other options are available. Other parts of the body, such as the chin or foot, can operate a modified joystick.

As the physical and functional abilities of the user decrease, the cognitive abilities required to operate an alternative control typically increase. Visual skills, including sight accuracy and depth perception, are also important for safe operation of a powered wheelchair. Programmable wheelchair controllers allow reduction of the maximum velocity and modification of the acceleration and deceleration rates of the wheelchair (28). To assist persons with more severe cognitive or visual limitations, technologies are being developed that enable the wheelchair to follow walls, navigate through doorways, and stop when other objects are contacted. For persons with spasticity, particularly tremor in the hand, modern controllers have filters that can be adjusted to give smoother wheelchair control. Positioning technology enables the joystick to be placed in a variety of locations to optimize the user's ability to operate it.

JOYSTICKS

Joysticks are the most common access devices for powered wheelchair systems. The majority of joysticks are proportional, meaning the control's speed output to the wheelchair from the joystick is in proportion to how far the joystick is pushed from the center position. Digital joysticks based on a new standard called M3S are being introduced, especially in the European market. These joysticks may offer improved immunity to interference from sources such as police radios, cellular phones, ham radios, and even the electric motors of the wheelchair itself. Joysticks can be fitted with a template that only allows motion in certain directions. This is useful for people with poor motor control, such as can be seen in athetoid cerebral palsy.

The end of the joystick can also be modified for easier grip. One common modification is a goalpost shaped attachment (T-bar) with the upright section of the joystick on either side of the hand. Alternatively, a simple tennis ball cut to fit over a traditional joystick can make gripping easier.

SIP-AND-PUFF

Sip-and-puff switches are used primarily by people with tetraplegia. A Sip-and-puff access device consists of a replaceable straw located near the mouth. Pulling and pushing air through the straw with the mouth controls the wheelchair. These systems can be set up in a variety of configurations. Generally, the user will sip a specific number of times to indicate a direction and puff to confirm the choice and activate the movement of the wheelchair. It is common for an auxiliary visual display to be used with sip-and-puff to provide feedback to the user. Sip-and-puff is becoming somewhat antiquated now that microproportional joysticks, head array sensors, and gyroscopic-based joysticks are available.

SWITCHES AND BUTTONS

An array of switches or a single switch can be used to control a chair. The more switches, the greater the motor control needed to operate the equipment. Using scanning, a single switch can control a wheelchair. In scanning, choices are presented to the user on the wheelchair controller. When the desired choice is presented, the user activates the switch to select that command. Two switches can fully control a wheelchair in a fashion similar to the one described above for sip-and-puff systems. An array of switches can be used for quicker control. There is no proportional control of the wheelchair's speed with switched control. Thus, users are forced to travel at the same, rather slow velocity at all times.

Many of the input devices described in this section can be used for more than the control of powered wheelchairs. Two common additional uses are environmental control and computer access. In some cases, the computer is mounted to the wheelchair, but often it is at a fixed site. A critical consideration when selecting or designing a user interface is that the ability of the user to accurately control the interface is heavily dependent on the stability of the user within the wheelchair. Often custom seating and postural support systems are required for a user interface to be effective. The position and stability of the user interface are also critical to its efficacy as a functional access device.

Considerations in Selection of Electric-Powered Mobility

There are many considerations in defining the correct power wheelchair for a given individual. Factors that are important include the means of transportation, surface conditions the chair must negotiate, need to negotiate thresholds and curbs, and clearance widths in the environment. In addition, subject preference is important, as well as maximum speed and range. Because of these considerations, it is important to allow the user to test drive various wheelchairs, preferably in the home environment. This is when a good relationship with a wheelchair dealer can be helpful, as they are often willing to allow the user to test devices in the home before purchase. This type of home assessment is almost always indicated for a person considering a power wheelchair for the first time. For all users, regardless of functional ability, skills need to be developed and tuned to enable safe operation. Typically a wheelchair will be used all day, 7 days a week, for all major life activities—such as activities of daily living, work, school, recreation, and sports—for a useable life expectancy of 3 to 5 years.

SEATING AND POSITIONING

Seating systems can be organized into three general categories: off-the-shelf systems, modular systems, and custom-molded systems. Overlap exists between the categories, and a given seating system should be prescribed and designed specific to the user's medical, functional, and personal preference needs. The simplest form of seating system is a linear seating system. A linear seating system refers to a planar seat and back with fixed angles and orientations.

Medically, a system should address issues of soft-tissue management, comfort, reducing the potential for or accommodating orthopedic deformities, and maintaining vital organ capacity. Functionally, the system should address the movements and supports the user needs to reach or access objects, transfer, get under tables, and perform activities of daily living. The chair must become an extension of the user's body, much like an orthosis. This requires careful matching of critical chair dimensions to body dimensions, user abilities, and intended uses. The user's preference as to one system over another should be paramount in the prescription process. For example, a user may choose to forgo pressure relief and comfort for a firmer seating system that provides greater stability and allows him or her to slide off the seat for transfers.

Soft-Tissue Management

Soft-tissue management is a concern for all people who sit for prolonged periods of time and who have compromised sensation or the inability to perform weight shifts. The cost of treat-

ment or repair of a pressure ulcer is substantial. External causes of skin breakdown or pressure sores include excessive prolonged pressure over bony prominences, friction and shear, as well as heat and moisture. Intrinsic factors include the inability to move, poor nutrition, vascular problems, and the loss of soft-tissue elasticity (29). The loss of sensation is a key factor because discomfort is the usual trigger for shifting and moving. Because the causes of pressure ulcer vary, the choice of seat cushion will vary based on the client's risk factors and the characteristics of the cushion.

The fit of the wheelchair also contributes to pressure distribution. Footrests mounted too high lever more force into the buttocks region. Properly adjusted arm rest height allows weight to be distributed through the upper extremities. The angle of the back, relative to the seat, affects how much a person will slouch, and the slouch posture affects pressure over the sacrococcygeal regions.

MATERIAL PROPERTIES OF SEATING SYSTEMS

Cushions are chosen based on their characteristics, which are related to the properties of the materials used in their construction. Materials specific to those used in the design and manufacture of seating systems have certain characteristics, as shown in Table 59-3. Manufacturers make cushions that possess these qualities using flat and contoured foams, air-filled bladders, combinations of air and foam, flotation, viscous fluids, contoured plastic honeycombs, custom-contoured foam, and alternating pressure systems. These cushions vary in efficacy of pressure distribution, provision of postural stability, ability to insulate or conduct heat, and the reliability of their performance over time. Finding a cushion with good airflow and pressure distribution would be important for an immobile client who perspires heavily or is incontinent. Alternately, for a client prone to pressure ulcers, a practitioner would identify cushions with optimal redistribution of peak pressures. Active manual wheelchair users may not like an air-filled cushion because it does not provide a stable base for propulsion-related activities. If all the needed features cannot be found in one cushion, tradeoffs are necessary. Research evidence supports that a properly fitted pressure-reducing cushion, in contrast to

---

TABLE 59-3. Characteristics of Materials Used in the Design and Manufacture of Seating Systems

Property	Application
Density: The ratio of mass or quantity of material to the volume of the cushion	A cushion composed of air will be much lighter than one composed of gel. Weight may be a problem for someone who has to lift it or propel a manual wheelchair.
Stiffness: The strength of the resistance to compression	Foam has low stiffness and doesn't resist body weight compared with a solid seat base. A solid surface provides greater pelvic stabilization; foam may allow better pressure distribution.
Thermal characteristics: The ability of the material to insulate or conduct heat	Dense foam cushions retain body heat. Honeycomb-designed cushions hold less heat. Gel and fluids tend to pull heat away from the body.
Friction: The ability to maintain position and to reposition if needed	Cushions with solid bases and slick covers make sliding in lateral transfers easier but may promote sacral sitting.

a low-cost foam cushion, reduces the probability of a pressure sore (30).

PRESSURE MAPPING

Pressure-mapping technology estimates interface pressure. A thin mat with pressure sensors is placed between the client and the seating surface. The mat connects to a computer and presents data in both graphic and numeric forms. As part of a skilled clinical assessment, it can be predictive of potential risk for pressure sores (31). This technology can help a clinician decide which cushion provides the best pressure distribution for a particular client. It is important to remember that pressure-mapping devices do not measure shear forces, heat, moisture, postural stability, or maintenance of the cushion. These factors must also be considered.

CUSTOM-CONTOURED SEATING

Custom-contoured seating systems are necessary when all available off-the-shelf or modular seating systems cannot address the needs of the individual. This may occur in individuals with moderate to severe fixed and semiflexible structural deformities of the spine and extremities. In addition, individuals who require significant off-loading of soft tissue because of pressure sore issues may need a custom-contoured seat.

Custom-contoured seating involves a process of capturing a specific mold of a person's body. The mold can be obtained through several methods, including liquid foam in place or plaster molds. More current technology allows these seating systems to be produced through Computer Aided Design/Computer Aided Manufacturing (CAD/CAM) with greater control and accuracy. The process usually involves the use of a seating simulator composed of bead bags for the seat and backrest supports. The bead bags are manually and gravitationally contoured around the shape of the person's deformities or pressure points, followed by vacuum evacuation of the air from the bags to produce a rigid mold. This mold is then scanned, using sensors that send data to a robotic milling machine for the production of a positive mold.

Custom-molded systems are not capable of correcting deformities. Careful skin inspections should be performed, and pressure-mapping systems should be used as appropriate to verify that the custom-molded seat contours are applied properly. Inappropriately applied contours can lead to pressure sores. Careful consideration of transfer technique is needed with these seating systems because proper positioning in the seat is essential to performance, and the custom contours usually make transfers more difficult.

BACK SUPPORT

A back support should conform to the normal spinal curvature while allowing movement as required by the user. The typical back support in a folding-frame wheelchair is sling upholstery, not because it is good back support, but because it bends to allow the chair to fold. Sling seats provide little in the way of support. The sling-back support stretches before an effective force is applied to the rim, resulting in inefficiencies during wheelchair propulsion. In individuals with tetraplegia, the stretching of the sling back can mean that the wheelchair user adopts a more posterior tilt of the pelvis, and this may contribute to a kyphotic spine (13). Like cushions, wheelchair backs are chosen based on the client's seating goals. For clients with muscle weakness in the trunk, the stability from a contoured backrest with or without modular lateral supports is needed to maintain head and neck position. Some clients may only need the soft contouring of an adjustable tension sling backrest, whereas others with significant kyphoscoliosis may

need a custom-molded backrest to enable sitting in a more upright posture. Clients with this level of weakness or deformity will most likely use this seating in a powered mobility base or an attendant-operated base.

RECLINE AND TILT-IN-SPACE

Recline and tilt-in-space technologies relieve pressure, manage posture, provide comfort, and help with personal care activities. Recline helps to stretch hip flexors and also assists with attending to catheters, toileting, and dependent transfers. Because reclining the seat back creates shear, the user often shifts in the wheelchair into a sacral-seated position. For a patient who is unable to reposition without help, adding tilt may help the user reposition independently. Tilt-in-space keeps the hip and knee angles constant when tilting the client back. Unlike reclining systems, the position of the user is maintained in the tilt seating system. Subjects unable to independently shift weight, or with pain as a result of prolonged sitting, need to be considered for this option. It is unnatural to sit in the same position for extended periods of time, and the majority of power wheelchair users are in their chairs more than 12 hours a day. Tilt-in-space should be strongly considered in individuals with progressive disorders. An individual with amyotrophic lateral sclerosis may find it easy to perform weight shift and repositioning at an initial evaluation, but this can change quickly, leading to the need for modifications. Tilt and recline are also available in manual wheelchairs. For the most part, these chairs are only used for patients who require attendant control. As in recline, tilt-in-space greatly reduces pressure on the ischial tuberosities by shifting the pressure to the back. Research supports the combination of these interventions (32).

OTHER POSITIONING SYSTEMS

Stand-up wheelchairs are a costly alternative that deserves mention. The benefits of standing for individuals normally unable to do so may include decreased bladder infections, reduced osteoporosis, and decreased spasticity (33). In addition, there are likely psychological benefits that result from the feeling of upright posture and the ability to interact at eye level. Certain people cannot use a stand-up wheelchair because they do not have adequate joint range of motion. Some of the benefits of a stand-up wheelchair can be obtained by using a variable-seat-height wheelchair. The most common function of variable-seat-height wheelchairs is to provide seat elevation. Seat elevation can assist an individual in reaching high objects. In addition, seat elevation is sometimes critical for transfers, as it permits an individual to transfer downhill. Finally, some newer chairs offer lateral tilt-in-space. This feature allows the user to be leaned to either side and offers an alternative for people with difficult pressure sore or pain issues.

Seating Set Up

Setting up the wheelchair is critical to optimizing performance. A therapist or rehabilitation supplier working with the clinic commonly performs this. Seat height can be adjusted on most chairs. The seat height is dependent on the total body length of the user. Users with longer leg lengths will require higher seat heights to achieve sufficient clearance for the footrests. There is some flexibility when selecting seat height, even for taller individuals, because most active users prefer some seat angle or dump. By tilting the seat down toward the backrest (decreasing the seat-to-back angle), the user fits more securely into the chair, which will increase the user's trunk stability and make the chair more responsive to the user's body movements. Seat depth is determined from the length of the upper legs. Gener-

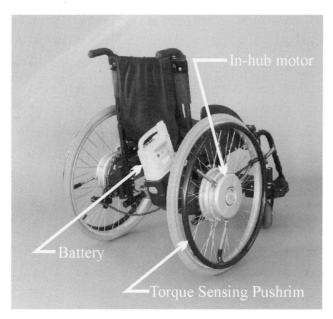

Figure 59-11. Power-assist wheelchair.

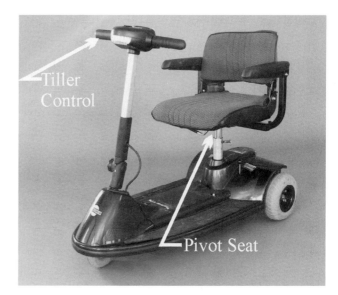

Figure 59-12. Scooter.

ally no more than a 75 mm (3 in.) gap should be between the front of the seat and the back of the knees when the person is in the wheelchair. This will help to ensure broad distribution of the trunk weight over the buttocks and upper legs, without placing undue pressure behind the knee. Some gap is required to allow the user some freedom to adjust their position. Seat width is determined from the width of the person's hips, the intended use, and whether the person prefers to use side guards (a rigid material placed between the seat and rear wheels to prevent clothing from rubbing on the rear wheels). Generally, the wheelchair should be as narrow as possible; thus, a chair about 1 inch wider than the user's hips is desirable.

Power-Assisted Wheelchairs

A developing class of wheelchairs provides a power assist when desired, but allows the user to push the wheelchair as one would with a manual wheelchair. Power-assisted wheelchairs (Figure 59-11) have force/moment-sensing push rims that provide an additional torque to the rear axle proportional to the applied moment. Such devices have potentially important benefits, such as enabling people normally provided with power wheelchairs to self-propel a wheelchair despite obstacles such as steep ramps. These potential benefits were recently demonstrated in a study of a power-assist device (34). Using power assists, subjects demonstrated significantly lower oxygen consumption and heart rate. Subjects completed some tasks significantly faster than with their personal wheelchair, but they encountered difficulty transferring from the chair equipped with power assist and in disassembling the power-equipped chair for transport. For individuals with upper-limb pain or tetraplegia, the power-assisted wheelchair may prove to be a good compromise between a manual wheelchair and a power wheelchair.

Scooters

Scooters (Figure 59-12) are a good option for certain individuals. These devices typically have a single front wheel for steering and two drive wheels in the back. Possibly because scooters are available to help shoppers in many large department stores, they seem to have a greater degree of social acceptability than wheelchairs. This leads many clients to request these devices. Steering is accomplished via hand bars that are intuitive to users who have previously used a bicycle. Seating is provided in a chair having foam padding typical of a car seat. The backrest height ends at the level of the shoulder blades, which allows for unencumbered rotation of the trunk.

Scooters have a number of advantages and disadvantages that must be critically considered when prescribing this device (Table 59-4). In general, scooters are a reasonable option for individuals who retain some ability to ambulate, such as those with cardiopulmonary disease limiting the ability to walk. Scooters are a poor option for individuals with progressive neuromuscular disorders because they have few options to accommodate progressive disability. They are also a poor choice if one needs to stay in the chair all day because seating options are limited.

Power Wheelchair Training

Before individuals ride away in their new powered mobility, they should go through a wheelchair-training program. Training is particularly important for younger children. Wheelchair users can first practice basic maneuvers in controlled environments that meet Americans with Disabilities Act (ADA) Accessibility Guidelines (35). They should practice negotiating uneven surfaces and slope transitions (i.e., level to sloped surfaces) in both the uphill and downhill directions and maneuvering through tight environments. Once these skills are

TABLE 59-4. Scooters	
Advantages	**Disadvantages**
Lower cost	Less stability
Easier to assemble and disassemble for transportation	Require greater arm strength and control to drive
Better than some chairs at rough terrain	Fewer seating options
Less perceived stigma of disability	Poor turning radius
	Must transfer out of chair for many activities

mastered, they should gradually tackle more challenging environments, such as steep grades and step transitions that exceed ADA Accessibility Guidelines. The rider should always practice with an appropriate lap belt (36) and chest support in place, and a spotter (therapist) to assist if needed. The wheelchair user should also be given an opportunity to experience the limits of the technology he or she is using. By setting up and practicing in safe environments, users can experience the limits of the lateral stability, as well as the front and rear stability, of their chair so that they have a better understanding of its performance limits.

PEDIATRICS

In many ways, the seating and mobility needs of children with disabilities are similar to those of adults. Children seek comfort, stability, and function, and there is no one perfect position for every activity or situation. There is a tendency to be aggressive with children and force them to sit upright with many postural supports in the hope of preventing or delaying deformities. This tendency in the design of the seating system may force postures that are not tolerated or desired over time. It is important to seek out input from both the child and the caregivers who will be dealing with the seating system on an hourly basis. Several variables in system design need to be considered with children, including developmental status, mobility, growth, age-appropriate activities, school, therapies, the environment, and family issues. Children not only change in size, but their disability often changes as they grow, even in nonprogressive disorders such as cerebral palsy.

Pediatric Seating Systems

Pediatric seating systems can be classified similar to those for adults as stated in the previous section, with off-the-shelf, modular, and custom-molded systems available. The issue of growth should not be overvalued over function or other points of concern. There are some systems that can accommodate growth to a certain degree; however, these modular systems tend to be heavier and bulkier than the lighter, more compact, off-the-shelf systems that cannot change with growth. The weight and bulkiness of a system can have negative impacts for a child who is capable of self-propulsion or other functions. Pediatric clinicians often fall into this dilemma by prescribing seating and mobility systems that provide growth because of the fear that they won't be able to justify a new system in less than 3 to 5 years, when other, lighter systems are more appropriate. Consider the analogy of forcing a child to wear an adjustable pair of shoes or a bulky lower extremity prosthesis that has 3 to 5 years of growth factored into the design.

In certain cases, such as when a child lacks muscle control, modular systems can offer advantages. Trunk lateral supports may need to be removed while the child is engaged in a dynamic reaching activity or in therapy working on trunk control, but replaced to sit more passively when he or she fatigues. A child should also be allowed to passively sit when focused on other activities, such as schoolwork, or relaxing while riding in a vehicle or watching television. If the child has to focus all his or her energy on balance and stability, then he or she will have no energy to focus on the task at hand. If a seating system is too confining or restrictive with multiple supports, the child may fight the system to be able to move and be dynamic. Thus the pediatric seating specialist must find a balance between appropriate amounts of support without overly restricting movement. An anterior chest harness or support may be needed for stabilization during transportation but removed to engage in schoolwork. It is important to educate all parties as to when a certain support is appropriate and when it is inappropriate. Inappropriate use of chest harnesses has resulted in strangulation when the child slid down in the seat because he was becoming uncomfortable and trying to fight the restrictions of the seating system. It is often difficult to find a balance between providing enough support while still allowing for some freedom of movement. Having systems that are more modular and flexible, as well as educating caregivers, can help find this balance.

Custom-molded systems essentially accommodate to the shape of a child's posture and are indicated when a child's postural deformities are so severe that they cannot be supported by a modular or off-the-shelf seating system. Custom-molded systems are not as common with children as they are with adults, as children's deformities tend not to be as severe. As with off-the-shelf systems, custom-molded systems have no growth capabilities.

Wheelchairs and their seating systems are also often used as passenger seats in vehicles, especially on school buses and family vehicles. School buses are required to use a separate passenger restraint system from what is incorporated in the design of the seating system. This includes both a tested tie-down system for the mobility base and another vehicle-mounted restraint system for the passenger. Many families do not restrain their child in their wheelchairs in a vehicle to these standards because of financial and burden-of-care issues. Practitioners need to be cognizant of this and counsel clients, families, and caregivers.

Mobility

Mobility is the precursor to all childhood development. Children need to explore their environment to know where things are and how to get them. The need for specific types of mobility bases, such as strollers, self-propelled systems, and powered systems, will depend on the age and the physical, developmental, and functional capabilities of the child, as well as the environmental and transportation resources of the family. Very young children may need a seating system that can be transferred and attached to a variety of bases for different activities. For play, children want to be close to the floor near their toys and peers. For eating, they need to be up where a caregiver can have access. Some manufacturers make seating systems that can be transferred to various mobile and stationary bases that are height adjustable. For example, one seating system can be transferred between a folding-style stroller type base, a higher eating base, and a power-wheelchair base, and can also serve as crash-tested car seat.

There has been a historical tendency to push children with disabilities to ambulate with braces and other aids. Upright ambulation may not always be the most effective method of mobility, and it often requires greater energy expenditure. The practitioner needs to consider the mobility demands of the child, including the expected surfaces and distances. A manual or power wheelchair may be more efficient and actually provide greater independence. Children often abandon cumbersome upright ambulation in favor of a wheelchair when they are able to make their own choice. Consider a child with cerebral palsy in school trying to ambulate with braces and crutches as well as carry a bag full of books through a crowded hallway. Manual wheelchairs are sometimes a useful option for children; however, the weight of the chair may be an issue. Even an ultralightweight manual wheelchair weighing 20 pounds is going to be heavy for a 30- to 40-pound child. Proper chair selection and training are essential to the long-term health of the child.

Powered mobility is important for children who cannot effectively self-propel a manual system; however, families often do not have the resources or psychological readiness either to make the necessary home modifications or to purchase an accessible vehicle that can accommodate a powered system. Research and clinical intuition indicate that children without cognitive disability should be offered mobility devices such as power wheelchairs or adapted ride-on power toys as early as 12 to 18 months—about the time able-bodied children begin moving on their own (4,37,38). Even with a power wheelchair, there is often the need for a transportable folding supportive stroller-type base, as described previously, for use in family outings.

Psychosocial and Family Issues

There are many psychosocial and family-related issues practitioners need to be cognizant of and respect. Having a child with a birth or acquired disability can devastate a family. Initially, there tends to be focus on the search for a cure to the problem, especially given the advanced medical resources in society. Therefore, they may be a reluctant to accept use of a wheelchair, place a ramp in front of the home, or purchase a van with a ramp. The practitioner needs to counsel the family regarding the realistically expected short- and long-term outcomes of the child's situation. There is also a tendency to "care for" a child with a disability, especially in certain cultures and religions. It is common for children with disabilities to develop learned helplessness and for parents to develop a codependency in the relationship with their child (39). Later in life, this can result in lack of ability to make decisions or function in society. Children with disabilities need to experience the same stages of development—including successes as well as failures—as their able-bodied peers within the norms and values of that culture. Practitioners again need to counsel families so that they can effectively use this equipment to facilitate development and promote active participation by the child as appropriate based on their current and potential capabilities.

STANDARDS AND DURABILITY

International standards are applied to mobility devices. The standards are formulated by: ISO, the International Standards Organization; the American National Standards Institute; and by RESNA (40). The standards concern many aspects of wheelchairs, including electrical systems, durability, dimensions, flammability, strength of arm rests, ability to withstand an impact, and stability, to name a few. These standards can be requested from the manufacturer and can serve as a method of comparing classes of wheelchair as well as individual wheelchairs to each other. Wheelchair users should be confident of the structural integrity of their wheelchair. Failure of any component is more than an inconvenience for the wheelchair user—it is the limitation of their mobility and can be life-threatening.

Tests included in the standards protocol include the curb drop and double drum. In the curb drop, the wheelchair and a 70 kg test dummy are lifted 5 cm and dropped to the ground. In the double-drum test, the wheelchair and test dummy are placed on two independent rollers (rear wheels on one roller and the front on the other). Each roller has two 1 cm high by 2 cm wide slats that simulate door thresholds. The standards require that the chair survive 200,000 cycles on the double drum and 6,666 drops. A study by Fitzgerald et al. (41) compares the results of ISO standards testing on three classifications of manual wheelchairs. The classes followed Medicare definitions of K0001, depot or hospital-type (42); K0004. lightweight (43); and K0005, ultralight (44). Using ISO equivalent number of testing cycles, curb-drop and double-drum tests were expressed as a single variable, and Kaplan-Meier survival curves were determined. The fatigue life of ultralight wheelchairs was significantly greater than both the lightweight or hospital-type wheelchairs. Because ISO testing is based on a 5-year life cycle, it was concluded that lightweight and hospital-type wheelchairs might not last the typical 3- to 5-year period expected by health insurers. A better investment was shown to be the ultralight, despite its initial high cost. This analysis did not take into account the other advantages of ultralight wheelchairs described in this chapter. More recent studies have also shown differences in power wheelchairs.

SECONDARY INJURY/ACCIDENTS

Unfortunately, wheelchair users are at risk for other injuries as direct result of their wheelchair use. Kirby and Ackroyd-Stolarz (45) used the databases of the Food and Drug Administration for insights into the nature and causes of such problems. There were 368 injuries, 21 of which were fatal. Fractures were the most common injury seen in 45% of reported cases. The proportion of incidents related to the use of scooters, powered wheelchairs, and manual wheelchairs were 52.8%, 24.6%, and 22.6%, respectively. Four broad classes of contributing factors, often acting in combination, were implicated: engineering (60.5%), environmental (25.4%), occupant (9.6%), and system (4.6%). Of the tips and falls, those in the forward direction were most common in incidents affecting manual or powered wheelchairs, but the sideways direction was most common in scooters.

Another important area of concern is transportation. Most wheelchairs are not crashworthy for use as seats in motor vehicles. The seat belts and other seating components of wheelchairs are not designed to withstand forces occurring in motor vehicle accidents. The seating system keeps the patient comfortable in the wheelchair but should not be considered as a passenger restraint. Using seating systems and wheelchairs in this manner can lead to injury. Additional seat belts and tie downs must be used to individually hold both the patient and the wheelchair secure. Clinicians should be aware of this and discuss transportation directly with the patient.

Possibly the most important area of concern for manual wheelchair users are repetitive strain injuries of the upper extremities. These injuries are so significant that some researchers have gone so far as to say that damage to the upper limbs may be functionally and economically equivalent to a spinal cord injury of a higher neurologic level (46). The two most common areas of injury are the shoulder, with rotator cuff disease (47) and degenerative arthritis (48), and the wrist, in the form of carpal tunnel syndrome (49,50). These studies have found injury rates as high as 70%. Recent work has found a direct link between manual wheelchair propulsion and injury at both the shoulder and wrist (17,18). Clinicians must be aware that an appropriately prescribed and set-up wheelchair, which is propelled in an appropriate manner, can reduce the risk of injury. In addition, for some individuals, it may be appropriate to discuss power assist or power wheelchairs as a means for preserving the upper limb for activities such as transfers.

THE REAL WORLD

As can be seen from the text, the prescription of wheelchairs is a complex and time-consuming task. Many parties need to be involved, and technology is constantly changing. In an ideal world, all wheelchairs would be prescribed using all the members of the team described earlier in this chapter, and clinicians would be reimbursed at a level that allowed for appropriate evaluation and training. Unfortunately, wheelchair clinics are costly to run; therefore, the team approach described may not be the case in many settings. It is essential, however, that the physician signing the prescription understand the equipment well enough to explain the choices made. Just like a medication prescription, the doctor should know the tradeoffs, limitations, and safety issues related to the chair and make sure that the consumer is educated and able to make informed choices.

For a solo clinician without a clinic, it is still possible to provide good care. The best approach is to find a therapist in the rehabilitation team who has an interest in wheelchairs. If possible, the therapist should attend meetings such as RESNA (www.resna.org), the International Seating Symposium (www.iss.pitt.edu), or Medtrade (www.medtrade.com) to learn about new technology. In addition, the therapist should consider taking the ATP examination for certification. This can be sold to the hospital as a value-added service that their institution has and others do not. The other key team member then becomes the dealer. As the doctor and therapist team, you should request (or require) that the dealer become a CRTS. You can also ask the dealer to support the team by having equipment available for trials and by visiting the patient's house. This team can be very effective at wheelchair delivery and can improve the function and quality of life of their patients.

FUTURE

New and exciting products are placed on the market each day. Maybe the most exciting recent development has been the interest of huge companies such as Yamaha Motor Corporation and Johnson & Johnson. These companies bring substantial research and development budgets to this important area. As mobility products improve, the line between needing the device because of a disability and wanting the device because it enhances mobility can become blurred. This blurring is a great thing for wheelchair users. It expands the market and lowers costs. In addition, it blurs the line between disability and normal function. The future is likely to see more blurring to the point that everyone has a personal mobility device, such as Segway, and the only difference between individuals with disabilities and individuals without impairments is that individuals with disabilities always use their vehicle. With these advances it will be important for health-care professionals to continue to lobby on behalf of their patients to increase funding for wheelchairs so that function dictates the prescription.

REFERENCES

1. Brandt EN, Pope AM. *Enabling America: assessing the role of rehabilitation science and engineering.* Washington, D.C.: National Academy Press, 1997.
2. Miles-Tapping C. Power wheelchairs and independent lifestyles. *Canadian Journal of Rehabilitation* 1996;10(2):137–145.
3. Evans R. The effect of electrically powered indoor/outdoor wheelchairs on occupation: a study of users' views. *British Journal of Occupational Therapy* 2000;63(11):547–553.
4. Frank AO, Ward J, Orwell NJ, et al. Introduction of a new NHS electric-powered indoor/outdoor chair (EPIOC) service: benefits, risks and implications for prescribers. *Clin Rehabil* 2000;14(6):665–673.
5. Bottos M, Bolcati C, Sciuto L, et al. Powered wheelchairs and independence in young children with tetraplegia. *Dev Med Child Neurol* 2001;43(11):769–777.
6. Buning ME, Angelo JA, Schmeler MR. Occupational performance and the transition to powered mobility: a pilot study. *Am J Occup Ther* 2001;55(3):339–344.
7. Aronson KJ. Quality of life among persons with multiple sclerosis and their caregivers. *Neurology* 1997;48(1):74–80.
8. Chase J, Bailey DM. Evaluating potential for powered mobility. *Am J Occup Ther* 1990;44(12):1125–1129.
9. Cooper RA, Cooper R. Electric powered wheelchairs on the move. *Physical Therapy Products* 1998;July/August:22–24.
10. Mills T, Holm MB, Trefler E, et al. Development and consumer validation of the Functional Evaluation in a Wheelchair (FEW) instrument. *Disabil Rehabil* 2002;24(1–3):38–46.
11. Cooper RA. *Rehabilitation engineering applied to mobility and manipulation.* Bristol, England: Institute of Physics, 1995.
12. Ambrosio F, Boninger ML, Fay B, et al. A fatigue analysis during wheelchair propulsion in patients with multiple sclerosis. *Proceedings of the 25th Annual RESNA Conference.* Minneapolis, MN: RESNA, 2002:282–284.
13. Boninger ML, Saur T, Trefler E, et al. Postural changes with aging in tetraplegia. *Arch Phys Med Rehabil* 1998; 79(12): 1577–1581.
14. Grieco A. Sitting posture: an old problem and a new one. *Ergonomics* 1986; 29:345–362.
15. Brubaker CE. Wheelchair prescription: an analysis of factors that affect mobility and performance. *J Rehabil Res Dev* 1986;23(4):19–26.
16. Cooper RA. A perspective on the ultralight wheelchair revolution. *Technology and Disability* 1996;5:383–392.
17. Boninger ML, Cooper RA, Baldwin MA, et al. Wheelchair pushrim kinetics: body weight and median nerve function. *Arch Phys Med Rehabil* 1999; 80(8):910–915.
18. DiCianno BE, Boninger ML, Towers JD, et al. Wheelchair propulsion forces and MRI evidence of shoulder injury. Abstract. *Am J Phys Med Rehabil* 2001; 80(4):311–312.
19. Van Sickle DP, Cooper RA, Boninger ML, DiGiovine CP. Analysis of vibrations induced during wheelchair propulsion. *J Rehabil Res Dev* 2001;38(4):409–421.
20. Kwarciak AM, Cooper RA, Wolf E. Effectiveness of rear suspension in reducing shock exposure to manual wheelchair users during curb descents. *Proceedings of the 25th Annual RESNA Conference.* Minneapolis, MN: RESNA, 2002:365–367.
21. Baldwin MA, Boninger ML, Koontz AM, et al. Comparison of propulsion kinetics and forearm EMG between two wheelchair pushrim designs. *Proceedings 21st Annual IEEE/EMBS International Conference, Atlanta, GA,* 1999, CD-ROM.
22. Kirby RL, Sampson MT, Thoren FA, MacLeod DA. Wheelchair stability: effect of body position. *J Rehabil Res Dev* 1995;32(4):367–372.
23. Boninger ML, Baldwin MA, Cooper RA, et al. Manual wheelchair pushrim biomechanics and axle position. *Arch Phys Med Rehabil* 2000;81(5):608–613.
24. van der Woude LHV, Veeger DJ, Rozendal RH, Sargeant TJ. Seat height in handrim wheelchair propulsion. *J Rehabil Res Devel* 1989;26:31–50.
25. Veeger D, Van der Woude LHV, Rozendal RH. The effect of rear wheel camber in manual wheelchair propulsion. *J Rehabil Res Devel* 1989;26(2):37–46.
26. Boninger ML, Souza AL, Cooper RA, et al. Propulsion patterns and pushrim biomechanics in manual wheelchair propulsion. *Arch Phys Med Rehabil* 2002;83:718–723.
27. de Groot S, Veeger HE, Hollander AP, van der Woude LH. Consequence of feedback-based learning of an effective hand rim wheelchair force production on mechanical efficiency. *Clin Biomech* 2002;17(3):219–226.
28. Brown KE, Inigo RM, Johnson BW, An adaptable optimal controller for electric wheelchairs. *J Rehabil Res Devel* 1987;24(2):87–98.
29. Byrne DW, Salzberg CA. Major risk factors for pressure ulcers in the spinal cord disabled: a literature review. *Spinal Cord* 1996;34:255–263.
30. Geyer MJ, Brienza DM, Karg P, et al. A randomized control trial to evaluate pressure-reducing seat cushions for elderly wheelchair users. *Advances in Skin and Wound Care* 2001;14(3):120–129.
31. Brienza DM, Karg PE, Geyer MJ, et al. The relationship between pressure ulcer incidence and buttock-seat cushion interface pressure in at-risk elderly wheelchair users. *Arch Phys Med Rehabil* 2001;82(4):529–533.
32. Sprigel S, Sposato B. Physiologic effects and design considerations of tilt and recline wheelchairs. *Orthopedic Physical Therapy Clinics of North America* 1997;6(1):99–122.
33. Dunn RB, Walter JS, Lucero Y, et al. Follow-up assessment of standing mobility device users. *Assist Technol* 1998;10(2):84–93.
34. Cooper RA, Fitzgerald SF, Boninger ML, et al. Evaluation of a pushrim-activated, power-assisted wheelchair. *Arch Phys Med Rehabil* 2001;82:702–708.
35. Davies TD, Beasley KA. *Fair housing design guide for accessibility.* Washington, D.C.: Paralyzed Veterans of America, 1992.

36. Cooper RA, Dvorznak MJ, O'Connor TJ, et al. Braking electric powered wheelchairs: effect of braking method, seatbelt, and legrests. *Arch Phys Med Rehabil* 1998;79(10):1244–1249.
37. Butler C. Effects of powered mobility on self-initiated behaviors of very young children with locomotor disability. *Dev Med Child Neurol* 1986;28(3):325–332.
38. Tefft D, Guerette P, Furumasu J. Cognitive predictors of young children's readiness for powered mobility. *Dev Med Child Neurol* 1999;41(10):665–670.
39. Holmbeck GN, Johnson SZ, Wills KE, et al. Observed and perceived parental overprotection in relation to psychosocial adjustment in preadolescents with a physical disability: the mediational role of behavioral autonomy. *J Consult Clin Psychol* 2002;70(1):96–110.
40. Axelson P, Minkel J, Chesney D. *A guide to wheelchair selection: how to use the ANSI/RESNA wheelchair standards to buy a wheelchair.* Washington, D.C.: Paralyzed Veterans of America, 1994.
41. Fitzgerald SG, Cooper RA, Boninger ML, Rentschler AJ. Comparison of fatigue life for three types of manual wheelchairs. *Arch Phys Med Rehabil* 2001;82(10):1484–1488.
42. Cooper RA, Robertson RN, Lawrence B, et al. Life-cycle analysis of depot versus rehabilitation manual wheelchairs. *J Rehabil Res Dev* 1996;33(1):45–55.
43. Cooper RA, Gonzalez J, Lawrence B, et al. Performance of selected lightweight wheelchairs on ANSI/RESNA tests. *Arch Phys Med Rehabil* 1997;78(10):1138–1144.
44. Cooper RA, Boninger ML, Rentschler A. Evaluation of selected ultralight manual wheelchairs using ANSI/RESNA standards. *Arch Phys Med Rehabil* 1999;80(4):462–467.
45. Kirby RL, Ackroyd-Stolarz SA. Wheelchair safety—adverse reports to the United States Food and Drug Administration. *Am J Phys Med Rehabil* 1995;74(4):308–312.
46. Sie IH, Waters RL, Adkins RH, Gellman H. Upper extremity pain in the postrehabilitation spinal cord injured patient. *Arch Phys Med Rehabil* 1992;73:44–48.
47. Escobedo EM, Hunter JC, Hollister MC, et al. MR imaging of rotator cuff tears in individuals with paraplegia. *AJR* 1997;168:919–923.
48. Boninger ML, Towers JD, Cooper RA, et al. Shoulder imaging abnormalities in individuals with paraplegia. *J Rehabil Res Dev* 2001;38(4):401–408.
49. Gellman H, Chandler DR, Petrasek J, et al. Carpal tunnel syndrome in paraplegic patients. *J Bone Joint Surg Am* 1988;70:517–519.
50. Davidoff G, Werner R, Waring W. Compressive mononeuropathies of the upper extremity in chronic paraplegia. *Paraplegia* 1991;29:17–24.

CHAPTER 60

Assistive Technology

Cathy Bodine and Dennis Matthews

HISTORICAL BACKGROUND AND PERSPECTIVE ON ASSISTIVE TECHNOLOGY

Humans have used tools to accomplish everyday tasks in many cultures throughout history (and prehistory), but the perception remains that the use of technology as a tool for persons with disabilities is a fairly recent phenomenon. In fact, James and Thorpe describe any number of assistive devices used as early as the sixth or seventh century B.C. (1). Their descriptions include partial dentures, artificial legs and hands, and drinking tubes or straws. The earliest documented account of optical and lens technologies, or eyeglasses, came from Venice around A.D. 1300 (2). The term *assistive technology* (AT) to describe devices used to facilitate the accomplishment of everyday tasks by persons with disabilities is actually the more recent development (3).

In 1988, Public law 100–407 defined assistive technology as "Any item, piece of equipment or product system whether acquired commercially off the shelf, modified, or customized that is used to increase or improve functional capabilities of individuals with disabilities." This definition also included a second component defining AT services as any service that directly assists an individual with a disability in the selection, acquisition, or use of an AT device. This includes:

1. The evaluation of the needs of an individual with a disability, including a functional evaluation of the individual in their customary environment;
2. Purchasing, leasing, or otherwise providing for the acquisition of AT by persons with disabilities;
3. Selecting, designing, fitting, customizing, adapting, applying, retaining, repairing, or replacing AT devices;
4. Coordinating and using other therapies, interventions, or services with AT devices, such as those associated with existing education and rehabilitation plans and programs;
5. Training or technical assistance for the person with a disability or, if appropriate, their family; and
6. Training or technical assistance for professionals (including individuals providing education or rehabilitation services), employers, or other individuals who provide services to, employ, or are otherwise substantially involved in the major life functions of children with disabilities (4).

This definition has also been included in other federal legislation authorizing services or supports for persons with disabilities, including the Rehabilitation Act (5) and the Individuals with Disabilities Act (6).

So what is AT? In short, AT is *a tool* used by someone with a disability to perform everyday tasks such as getting dressed, moving around, or controlling his or her environment, learning, working, or engaging in recreational activities. As a tool, AT is no different than using a hammer when the human hand would otherwise be unable to drive a nail. Fewer than 30 years ago, there were fewer than 100 devices commercially available. Today, more than 29,000 assistive devices are listed on the AbleData website (www.abledata.com). AT use often begins as early as birth and continues throughout the life span of individuals with disabilities.

Included within this textbook are chapters on wheelchairs and other mobility aids, recreational therapies, orthotics and prosthetics, and many other rehabilitation devices or tools. The devices described by the authors of these chapters also fall within the definition of AT. This chapter covers basic information on various categories of AT products, evaluation, prescription and funding for AT, use of a team approach, and outcomes measurement in the field of AT devices and services. Readers will be referred to the appropriate chapter for more in-depth information on those devices covered elsewhere in the textbook.

AT tends to be divided into two major categories: low technology and high technology. Low-technology or "low-tech" devices tend to be simple, non-electronic devices, such as dressing aids, pencil grips, picture-based communication boards for persons who are nonspeaking, and items such as a magnifier for persons with visual impairments. High-technology or "high-tech" devices are typically described as sophisticated, electronic devices such as power wheelchairs, computers, or augmentative and alternative communication (AAC) devices that provide synthetic voice output for persons who are nonspeaking. These devices are usually fairly expensive and often require extensive training to ensure they are used to their fullest potential by persons with disabilities (7).

There are a number of myths surrounding the provision of AT that tend to reflect common misperceptions about both the technology and individuals with disabilities. These myths include:

1. AT is the "be all and end all."
2. AT is complicated and expensive.
3. Persons with the same disability benefit from the same devices.
4. Professionals are the best source of information for AT.
5. AT descriptions are always accurate and helpful.
6. A user's AT requirements need to be assessed just once.

7. AT devices will always be used.
8. Individuals with disabilities want the latest, most expensive device.
9. AT is a luxury.
10. Only people with certain types of disabilities find AT useful.

Although AT does hold a great deal of promise for persons with disabilities who would like to pursue the everyday tasks that most of us take for granted, myths such as these have a tendency to cause practitioners and those they serve to disregard the potential utility of assistive devices. Tasks such as navigating freely throughout the community, talking with a loved one, or writing a letter are often out of reach for persons with disabilities. Proper prescription of assistive technologies can enable persons with disabilities to learn, work, and play, just like everyone else. Dispelling the myths surrounding AT will also do much to ensure those who can benefit from assistive devices and services will receive the appropriate supports.

ASSISTIVE TECHNOLOGY AND ABANDONMENT

It is important to recognize that not everyone with a disability enjoys using technology, however useful it might appear to practitioners. Depending on the type of technology, nonuse or abandonment can be as low as 8% or as high as 75%. On average, one-third of more *optional* ATs are abandoned, most within the first 3 months after the device is acquired. To date, research has not been done to ascertain the number of individuals who must continue to use devices they are not pleased with simply because they cannot abandon the technology without severe consequences (8,9). For example, an individual who has just received a new wheelchair that does not meet expectations simply cannot stop using the chair to navigate independently within their community. Rather, they must wait until third-party funding becomes available again (often as long as 3 to 6 years) or engage in potentially difficult and unproductive discussions with the vendor who has more than likely provided the chair as it was prescribed by the assessment team.

Research does tell us the number-one reason individuals with disabilities choose not to use assistive devices is because practitioners failed to consider their opinions and preferences during the device selection process. In other words, the person with a disability was not included as an active member of the team during the evaluation process (8).

HUMAN FACTORS AND ASSISTIVE TECHNOLOGY

A growing body of research in the field of human factors is being applied to the design and development of AT devices for persons with disabilities. Analysis of human factors in a global sense is concerned with how humans interact with various technologies. When you sit in a new car and notice how comfortable it is—how well the seat contours with your body and how accessible the controls are for the stereo system—you have experienced the growing information derived from human factors research.

Dr. Thomas King (10), a professor at the University of Wisconsin–Eau Claire, has expanded key points found in the literature on human factors and applied them to research and development in AT. He tells us that human factors in AT must be concerned with how human beings who have special needs, limitations, or disabilities interact with devices and tools that may support, supplement, or replace some process or ability that has been lost or impaired by illness or injury. We must be concerned not only with how the user interacts with the devices, but also with how the family or other close care providers react to the use of tools and devices in their settings. The interaction of the AT user alone with the technology introduced into his or her life does not tell us the whole story because persons who use assistive technologies must interact closely and frequently with or depend on others more than do general consumers for daily care and other aspects of their lives. The larger impact on those around the user must also be considered because they are key players in implementation of any AT in the user's life. Across all component areas of AT, human factors must be concerned with how the potential user—as well as his or her family, personal care providers, education and therapy aides, teachers, and clinicians—interacts with the assistive devices and technological systems.

Analysis of human factors in AT is concerned with finding out the special needs, capabilities, and limitations of users and then matching devices and controls to each individual user. Heterogeneity and individualization are primary considerations in dealing with persons who have special needs; however, mass-produced technologies (such as computers) must be designed for mass-market users, rather than for unique individuals. Flexibility and adaptability of technology to a wide range of user characteristics is critically important.

Human factors considerations in AT are especially focused on reducing the user's exertion, stress, and fear of use. We all have a bit of "technophobia" when it comes to use of new tools and devices—especially complex, high-tech devices. This fear and stress, particularly when they relate to devices that may be difficult to set up or require a great deal of exertion to use, can be deleterious to the AT user. Persons relying on AT typically already have some type of limitation or disability. The expectation that the individual will become skilled in additional tools, devices, or technology can be highly stressful to users and their caregivers because it simply adds complexity to their life.

Human factors also focuses on reducing danger caused by the device to the user and persons around them. AT professionals should also strive to reduce the possibility of failure during use, which can lead to rejection or abandonment of the device for future use, even when the system has considerable merit for the person with a disability (10).

ASSISTIVE TECHNOLOGY AND THE INTERNATIONAL CLASSIFICATION OF IMPAIRMENT, DISABILITIES, AND HANDICAPS

Disability itself is not precise and quantifiable. The concept of disability is not always agreed on by persons who self-identify as having a disability, persons who study disability, or the general public (11). This lack of agreement creates obstacles for studies focused on disability and to the equitable and effective administration of programs and policies intended for persons with disabilities. To facilitate agreement about the concept of disability, the World Health Organization (WHO) has developed a global common health language—one that is understood to include physical, mental, and social well-being. The WHO first published the International Classification of Impairment, Disabilities, and Handicaps (ICIDH) in 1980 as a tool for classification of the "consequences of disease."

The newest version, International Classification of Functioning, Disability and Health, known as ICF (2001), like its most recent predecessor ICIDH-2, moves away from a "consequences of diseases" classification (1980 version) to a "components of health" classification. This latest model is designed to provide a common framework and language for the description of health domains and health-related domains. Using the common language of the ICF can help health-care professionals to communicate the need for health-care and related services, such as the provision of AT for persons with disabilities (12).

In the context of health, the following language is used:

- *Body functions* are the physiologic and psychological functions of body systems.
- *Body structures* are anatomic parts of the body, such as organs, limbs, and their components.
- *Impairments* are problems in body function or structure, such as significant deviation or loss.
- *Activity* is the execution of a task or action by an individual.
- *Participation* is involvement in a life situation.
- *Activity limitations* are difficulties an individual may have in executing activities.
- *Participation restrictions* are problems an individual may experience in involvement in life situations.
- *Environmental factors* make up the physical, social, and attitudinal environments in which people live and conduct their lives (12).

Application of the WHO global common health language makes possible the definition of the need for health-care and related services; defines health outcomes in terms of body, person, and social functioning; provides a common framework for research, clinical work, and social policy; ensures the cost-effective provision and management of health-care and related services; and characterizes physical, mental, social, economic, or environmental interventions that will improve lives and levels of functioning. Provision of AT for persons with disabilities is an intervention that has the potential to diminish activity limitations and participation restrictions and in turn, improve the quality of life of individuals with disabilities. Throughout this chapter, the use of the WHO common health language is used to discuss the potential impact of appropriate AT.

ASSISTIVE TECHNOLOGY FOR MOBILITY IMPAIRMENTS

Individuals with mobility impairments often present with unique needs and abilities. Some may demonstrate only lower-body impairment, such as a spinal cord injury or spina bifida, with no other complications. AT solutions might include crutches, a scooter, or a wheelchair. Simple modifications or adaptations to the environment, such as removing physical barriers to access (wide doorway or a ramp instead of stairs), may be all that is needed. For others, automobile hand controls, adapted saddles for horseback riding, sit skis for downhill skiing, or even placing bricks under a desk or table to allow the wheelchair user to work comfortably at a workstation can do the trick.

Other adaptive equipment for persons with mobility impairments might include a van with an attached lift. Many individuals who use wheelchairs drive a wide range of motor vehicles as well as bicycles using specially customized hand controls for turning and braking (Fig. 60-1). Chapter 59, Wheelchairs, and Chapter 65, Gait Restoration and Gait Aids, provide in-depth discussions of a wide range of assistive technologies for persons with mobility impairments that interfere with ambulation and other activities of daily living.

For someone with upper-body mobility impairment, such as poor hand control or paralysis, assistive devices might include alternate keyboards or other input methods to access a computer. Alternate keyboards come in many shapes and sizes. There are expanded keyboards, such as the Intellikeys™ (Fig.

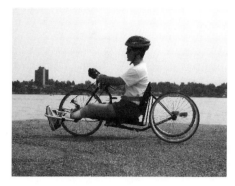

Figure 60-1. Assistive technology for mobility impairments. (Courtesy of Marlin Cohrs, Assistive Technology Partners, Department of Rehabilitation Medicine, University of Colorado Health Sciences Center.)

60-2), which provides a larger surface area than a standard keyboard, larger letters with a contrasting yellow background, and options such as a delayed response of the activated key for individuals who have difficulty either initiating touch or removing their finger after they have activated the key. For individuals who have never used a standard QWERTY keyboard layout, the letters on this keyboard can be arranged alphabetically. This key arrangement is often helpful for young children who are developing literacy skills, as well as for adults who have cognitive or visual impairments that necessitate additional supports for using literacy skills.

There are also small keyboards, such as the Tash Mini Keyboard™ (Fig. 60-3), that are designed in what is called a "frequency of occurrence" layout. Individuals who are one-handed typists, or who use a head stick or mouth stick to type, frequently prefer a smaller-sized keyboard. The home row (middle row) consists of the most frequently occurring letters in the English alphabet, with the letters a, e, and the space bar placed in the center of the keyboard for easy access. All other characters, numbers, and functions (including mouse control) fan from the center of the keyboard based on how frequently they need to be used by the average computer operator.

For individuals who are unable to use any type of keyboard or other device that requires hand or stick mobility, there are a wide range of switches available that provide access not only to the computer, but also to battery-operated electric toys and

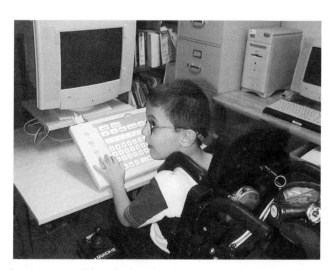

Figure 60-2. Intellikeys keyboard. (Courtesy of Jim Sandstrum, Assistive Technology Partners, Department of Rehabilitation Medicine, University of Colorado Health Sciences Center.)

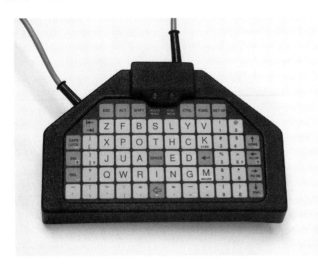

Figure 60-3. Tash Mini keyboard. (Courtesy of Marlin Cohrs, Assistive Technology Partners, Department of Rehabilitation Medicine, University of Colorado Health Sciences Center.)

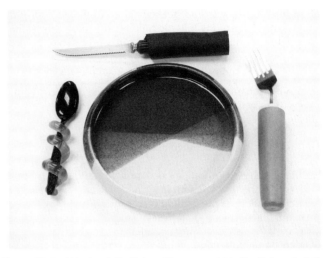

Figure 60-5. Aids for daily living. (Courtesy of Marlin Cohrs, Assistive Technology Partners, Department of Rehabilitation Medicine, University of Colorado Health Sciences Center.)

home-based or work appliances. These switches may be as simple as a "rocking lever" switch (Fig. 60-4) designed to be activated through a gross motor movement that involves touching or hitting the switch with the head, hand, arm, leg, or knee. Other switches can be activated by tongue touch, sipping and puffing on a straw, or through very fine movements, such as an eye blink or a single muscle twitch.

Fairly recent developments include eye gaze switches that calibrate intentional eye movement patterns and select targets such as individual keys on an on-screen keyboard, and also brain wave technology (Eye and Muscle Operated Switch, or EMOS™) that responds to excitation of alpha waves to trigger the selection. Other input methods for the computer include devices such as the Head Mouse™ and Tracker 2000™. These devices also rely on an on-screen keyboard visible on the computer monitor. The user wears a reflective dot on his or her forehead or other head mounted signaling device to tell the computer what key or command they wish to activate. With these and many other high tech control devices, individuals with disabilities, even those with the most severe motor impairments, can monitor and control an unlimited array of home, work, and school activities.

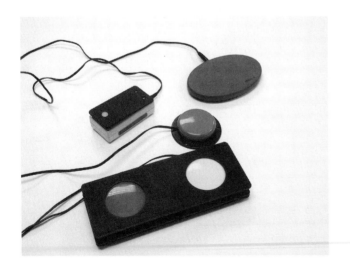

Figure 60-4. Switches. (Courtesy of Marlin Cohrs, Assistive Technology Partners, Department of Rehabilitation Medicine, University of Colorado Health Sciences Center.)

There are thousands of lower-tech assistive devices available for persons with motor impairments. Commonly referred to as aids for daily living, these devices include such things as weighted spoons, scoop plates, and other devices used to facilitate eating (Fig. 60-5); aids for personal hygiene, such as bath chairs and long-handled hairbrushes; adapted toys for play; built-up pencil grips for writing and drawing tasks; items for dressing, such as sock aids and one-handed buttoners; and many others. Prices and availability cover a wide range for items such as these. Many low-tech mobility aids can be hand-made for just a few dollars, whereas others, such as an adult bath chair, may cost several hundred dollars. All share the common goal or utility of reducing activity limitations and increasing participation in daily life activities.

ASSISTIVE TECHNOLOGY FOR COMMUNICATION DISORDERS

For individuals with severe expressive communication impairments, there is a wide range of AT devices available. For persons who have reduced phonation or breath support and speak very quietly, there are a number of portable amplification systems available that work much like a sound system in a large lecture hall. There is also a device available that clarifies speech for individuals with dysarthria. Called the Speech Enhancer™, it consists of a headset attached to a portable device and is worn much like a shoulder bag (Fig. 60-6). The individual using this system speaks into the microphone, and the sound is processed and then projected via speakers attached to the unit. Although not for everyone, this device has proven effective for a number of individuals struggling to be understood when communicating with medical personnel, family members, and others in the community.

For individuals who are unable to talk at all or who have such severe expressive communication difficulties that only their most intimate associates understand them, there are a wide range of AAC systems available. These devices range from very simple picture books to high-end sophisticated electronic communication devices with digitally recorded or synthetic speech output. Children and adults with severe expressive communication impairments can benefit academically, vocationally, emotionally, and socially from the provision of a device that allows them to communicate their thoughts, learn

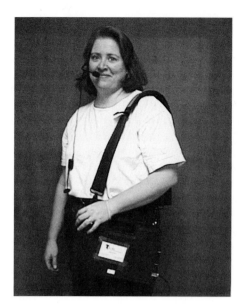

Figure 60-6. Speech Enhancer. (Courtesy of Marlin Cohrs, Assistive Technology Partners, Department of Rehabilitation Medicine, University of Colorado Health Sciences Center.)

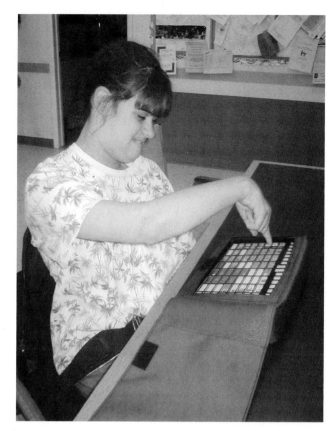

Figure 60-7. Using an augmentative and alternative communication device. (Courtesy of Jim Sandstrum, Assistive Technology Partners, Department of Rehabilitation Medicine, University of Colorado Health Sciences Center.)

and share information and ideas, and otherwise participate in life activities.

It is important to note these AAC devices, although extremely useful and important to the lifestyles of many individuals who are nonspeaking, do not replace natural speech. Instead they *augment* or provide an *alternate* form of communication. Other communicative modalities, such as vocalizations, gestures, sign language systems, eye gaze, etc., remain valid and acceptable forms of communication and should be encouraged to develop along with the facility to communicate out loud using an AAC device.

Congenital conditions such as autism, cerebral palsy, mental retardation, developmental verbal apraxia, and developmental language disorders can result in severe expressive communication impairments, necessitating the need for AAC interventions (13). Acquired disorders for which AAC is often used include traumatic brain injury, stroke, amyotrophic lateral sclerosis, tetraplegia, multiple sclerosis, and laryngectomy that is due to cancer (7,14). Augmentative communication systems (Fig. 60-7) have also been used successfully for individuals who are temporarily nonspeaking as a result of ventilator dependence (15).

There are two common myths surrounding the use of AAC. The first is that individuals who are nonspeaking must demonstrate certain developmental prerequisites before the prescription of an AAC device. On the contrary, there are no strict sets of cognitive or physical prerequisites to the use of AAC devices. Specific AAC techniques that match the individual's needs and abilities are chosen on the basis of a comprehensive evaluation by a qualified team of clinicians, family members, teachers, and others. The second myth is that the use of an AAC device will stifle or preclude the development or return of natural speech. However, the research tells us that use of an AAC device can actually support improved speech production and it in no way creates barriers to the development or return of natural speech (16).

Low-tech picture and alphabet boards are often used as either a preliminary step before purchasing an electronic voice output system, or as back-up systems, should an electronic device break or its use not be convenient (e.g., during swim lessons). These low-tech systems (Fig. 60-8) can be made from picture library software available through commercial vendors

(BoardMaker™, PCS Symbols™) or can be handmade using digital photographs, pictures from catalogs or books, or by simply using a marker to write or draw letters, words, phrases, or pictures. Adults with progressive diseases such as amyotrophic lateral sclerosis (ALS) or multiple sclerosis (MS) frequently use low-tech picture or alphabet boards to clarify their meaning as communication abilities decrease or as they fatigue during the day.

Figure 60-8. Low-tech augmentative and alternative communication device. (Courtesy of Marlin Cohrs, Assistive Technology Partners, Department of Rehabilitation Medicine, University of Colorado Health Sciences Center.)

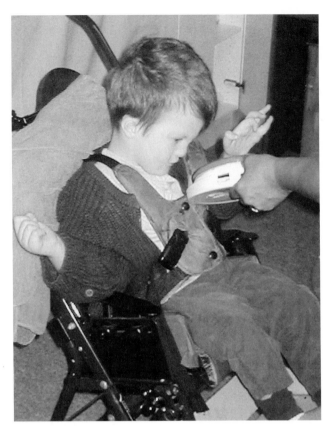

Figure 60-9. Using the Big Mac. (Courtesy of Diane Brians, Assistive Technology Partners, Department of Rehabilitation Medicine, University of Colorado Health Sciences Center.)

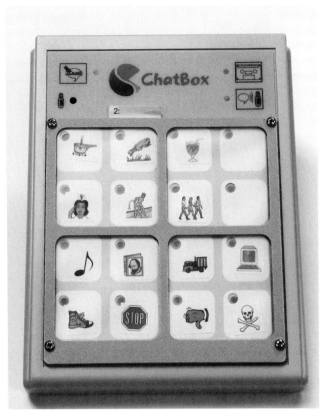

Figure 60-10. The Chatbox. (Courtesy of David Hershberger, Saltillo Corporation, Millersburg, Ohio.)

There are a number of low-tech voice output AAC devices available that are simple to program and use. The One Step™, Step by Step™, and Big Mac™ communication devices all use digital speech output (Fig. 60-9). Digital speech devices work much like a tape recorder. The person setting up the device simply holds down a button and records live voice into the microphone. The speech is digitized or recorded within the device. When the end-user chooses to speak, they simply press to activate the device. It then speaks the prerecorded message. The good news is these devices are simple and fairly inexpensive to purchase. It is important to bear in mind, however, that they are intentionally designed to communicate quick, simple messages, such as "hi," "let's play," or "leave me alone." These devices are not appropriate for individuals who have more than a few things to say or who have the ability to generate complex thoughts and feelings.

There are a number of more sophisticated digital devices available as well. These include the Dynamo™, Chatbox™ (Fig. 60-10), Springboard™, and others. These devices have the capacity to encode several minutes of live voice and are often used by individuals who are not yet literate, have developmental disabilities, or simply wish to have a simpler device to use when going to the store or out to eat.

At the high end of AAC systems are the text-to-speech devices (Fig. 60-11). These voice output systems use built-in speech synthesis to speak messages that have been typed and previously stored into the device. They are capable of encoding several thousand words, phrases, and sentences. AAC devices such as these are also designed to provide an alternate access to the computer and control appliances such as TVs, door openers, and other electrical items found in many environments. Three popular text-to-speech devices are the Pathfinder™, LightWriter™

(Fig. 60-12) and the Dynamyte™. It is important to note that these AAC systems have the capacity to serve as sophisticated communication systems and that they are expensive ($6,000 to $9,000). They also form a critical link to the world for individuals with severe expressive communication impairments.

All of the AAC devices on the market can be activated through direct selection using either a finger or other pointing device, such as a head or mouth stick. A large number of the digital and text-to-speech devices can be activated using either

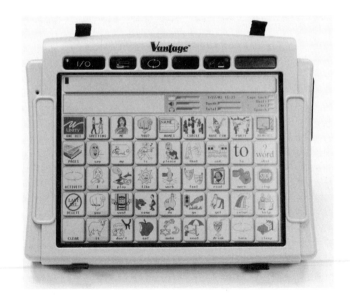

Figure 60-11. The Vantage Communication Device. (Courtesy of Barry Romich, Prentke Romich Company, Wooster, Ohio.)

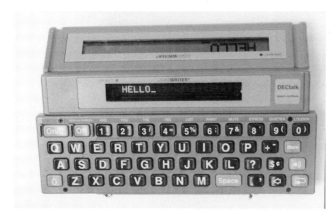

Figure 60-12. Using the LightWriter. (Courtesy of Marlin Cohrs, Assistive Technology Partners, Department of Rehabilitation Medicine, University of Colorado Health Sciences Center.)

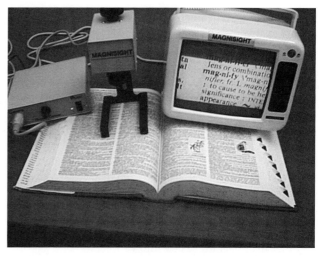

Figure 60-13. Low-tech magnification. (Courtesy of Marlin Cohrs, Assistive Technology Partners, Department of Rehabilitation Medicine, University of Colorado Health Sciences Center.)

direct selection or an alternate input mode. Alternate input includes all of the switches described above, as well as other additional infrared and wireless switches currently on the market. When an individual with a severe motor impairment and a severe expressive communication impairment chooses to use a switch to access the AAC device, the device can be preset to scan. The most commonly used switch access method is called row column scanning. In this instance, the end user starts by activating a switch to begin the scan. When the correct row is highlighted, the end user hits the switch again to start the lights scanning across the row (hence column). When the correct button is highlighted, the end user hits the switch again to activate the chosen button. As can be surmised, using a scanning system to activate an AAC device can be a slow and tedious process. For many individuals, however, this method provides the only available access to spoken and written communication, and for those select persons it is highly prized as a window to the world.

One of the more vigorous debates within the field of AAC centers around the encoding or mapping strategies used to represent language on a communication device. Currently available systems vary greatly in vocabulary storage and retrieval methods, but all systems are based on communication symbols, whether orthographic or pictographic. Symbols vary in their transparency (guessability) and translucency (learnability). In order to select a set of symbols for an individual's communication system, it is important to match these factors with the individual's cognitive and perceptual abilities.

Additionally, the world of technology moves at a very rapid pace. AAC devices currently on the market have been designed using today's technologies. As more and more innovations become available, such as wireless global positioning systems, the capabilities and flexibility of these devices will change. As with all technologies, it is important that clinicians and practitioners remain current on these and future technology developments.

ASSISTIVE TECHNOLOGY FOR VISUAL IMPAIRMENTS, INCLUDING BLINDNESS

The term *visual impairment* technically encompasses all degrees of permanent vision loss, including total blindness, which affects a person's ability to perform the usual tasks of daily life. *Low vision* refers to a vision loss that is severe enough to impede performance of everyday tasks but still allows some useful visual discrimination. Low vision cannot be corrected to normal by regular eyeglasses or contact lenses.

For individuals with visual impairments, there are a variety of AT devices and strategies available to assist them to perform daily activities such as reading (Fig. 60-13), writing, daily care, mobility. and recreational activities. Among the low-tech solutions are simple handheld magnifiers, the use of large print, or mobility devices (e.g., long cane) for safe and efficient travel. High-contrast tape or markers can be used to indicate what an item is or where it is located within a physical plant.

Other low-tech devices include items such as wind chimes to facilitate direction finding, using easily legible type fonts such as Verdana (16 point or larger), and using vanilla- or beige-colored paper rather than white to improve visibility of text. For children and adults interested in recreational activities, solutions include beeper balls, three-dimensional puzzles, and "Braille Trails" specifically designed to improve access to wilderness and other outdoor activities (Fig. 60-14).

Many restaurants now provide large-print, Braille, and picture-based menus for customers with a variety of abilities. Books on tape are another readily available resource for individuals with severe visual impairments. Libraries that provide

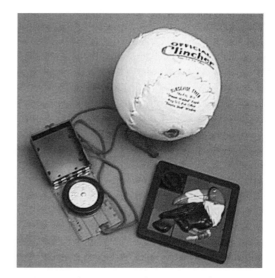

Figure 60-14. Low-tech recreation aids. (Courtesy of Marlin Cohrs, Assistive Technology Partners, Department of Rehabilitation Medicine, University of Colorado Health Sciences Center.)

TABLE 60-1. Resources: American Federation for the Blind (AFB)	
Resource	**Contact Information**
American Federation of the Blind Information Center	(800) AFB-LINE, (800) 232–5463 E-mail afbinfo@afb.net
AccessWorld Solutions	(800) 824–2184 E-Mail awsolutions@afb.net
Journal of Visual Impairment and Blindness and Access World	(800) 232–3044 or (412) 741–1398 E-mail afbsub@abdintl.com
National Technology Center	(212) 502–7642 E-mail techctrn@afb.net

print materials in alternate formats for persons who have visual and learning impairments can arrange to have textbooks and other materials translated into various formats. For more information, contact the American Federation for the Blind (Table 60-1).

High-tech solutions for persons with visual impairments can include a computer outfitted with a speech synthesizer and software that allows text, software menus, and other writing on the computer screen to be heard aloud by the person unable to see well enough to read the computer screen (Jaws™, Outspoken™). Brailled text, although somewhat less popular than in years past as a result of technology advances, is still the first choice of many individuals to facilitate reading of print materials.

For individuals with some degree of visual ability, screen magnification software is available for computers. Zoomtext™ and Zoomtext Xtra™ (Fig. 60-15) are two of the more popular versions of screen magnification programs. These softwares enable the end user to choose the amount and type of magnification he or she prefers for optimal computer access.

A recent addition to the screen magnification software list is one called Bigshot™. This software is less expensive ($199) and provides fewer features. However, it appears to be a nice alternative for computer users who do not need access to the more sophisticated computer functions, and it is affordable for public facilities such as libraries that wish to provide reasonable accommodations for customers accessing information databases.

Chapter 86 provides additional information on low vision rehabilitation.

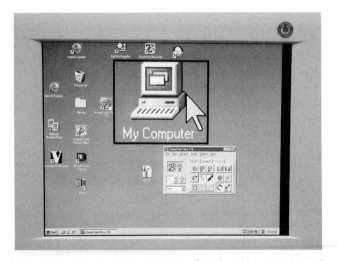

Figure 60-15. Zoomtext Xtra. (Courtesy of Marlin Cohrs, Assistive Technology Partners, Department of Rehabilitation Medicine, University of Colorado Health Sciences Center.)

ASSISTIVE TECHNOLOGY FOR LEARNING AND COGNITION

Children and adults can present with a variety of learning and cognitive impairments resulting from either acquired or developmental disabilities. Not only can AT provide important accommodations for those with disabilities of all types, it can also become a critical tool to be used during the recovery or acquisition of functional skill sets. For those with learning disabilities, there are a wide range of behaviors and abilities that may benefit from an AT solution.

For example, many children with learning and cognitive impairments struggle with developing literacy skills. Fortunately, there are a number of both low- and high-technology solutions available to assist them. Many benefit from the use of specially designed software programs that *predict* the word or phrase they are trying to spell as they type the first letter(s) of a word (Co:Writer™). Other software programs provide highlighted text and voice output so they are able to hear the words that they are generating (Write Outloud™, Kurzweil 3000™) on the computer. Individuals who are unable to read print materials often use some of the software solutions mentioned in the previous section, such as Jaws™ for voice output or books on tape.

Voice recognition has become a popular request both for persons with mobility impairments who are unable to type using their hands and for individuals whose learning disabilities are so significant they are unable to develop literacy skills. Voice recognition software enables an individual to speak into a microphone in order to input words, phrases, and sentences into standard computer word processing programs such as Microsoft Word™. Although a bit trickier, voice recognition can be used for input and control functions for other softwares, such as database programs and Windows.

Although voice recognition software is a rapidly developing technology, it is important to remember that it takes a fifth- to sixth-grade reading ability to train the standard software, simply because the individual's voice file cannot be developed unless they use the standard training package that comes with the software, and that requires being able to read. Dragon Systems has developed a version for children, but its success rate for children with learning and other cognitive disabilities has not yet been published. In addition, ambient noise, such as in a typical classroom, as well as fluctuating vocal abilities (e.g., fatigue) found in many individuals with disabilities will have an impact on the accuracy of the voice recognition. In general, it takes more than 20 hours to train the software to an acceptable level of accuracy (greater than 90%). Although caution is in order when prescribing this type of software, the rapid pace of development bodes well for future use of this type of software for persons with disabilities.

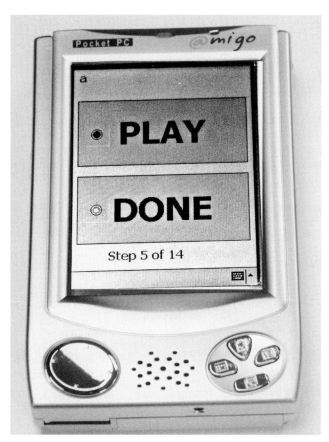

Figure 60-16. The PocketCoach. (Courtesy of Dan Davies, AbleLink Technologies, Inc. Colorado Springs, Colorado.)

Simple solutions for persons with learning and/or cognitive impairments can include colored highlighter tape, pencil grips, enlarged text, and other easy-to-provide adaptations, such as using a copy holder to hold print materials for easy viewing. Reminder lists with important times, places, and activities highlighted with a marker are often useful for individuals who need a subtle memory prompt to be in the right place at the right time.

Recent technology developments include the handheld personal digital assistants or PDAs. AT software developers (AbleLink Technologies, Inc.) have taken this technology a step further by developing a software application named Pocket-Coach™ (Fig. 60-16) that provides auditory prompts for individuals with cognitive disabilities. This software can be set up to remind someone what step they need to take next. It can be used for something as simple as a vocational task, such as mopping a floor, all the way to the complexity of prompting someone through the steps of a math problem. The latest edition of this software combines voice prompts with visual prompts (Visual Assistant™). The individual setting up the system can simply take a picture with the accompanying digital camera and combine the pictures with digitally recorded voice prompts to further facilitate memory and cognition.

A number of software packages are available for these populations that focus on a range of topics, including academics, money management, personal skills development, behavior training, development of cognitive skills, memory improvement, problem solving, time concepts, safety awareness, speech and language therapy, telephone usage, recreation, and games. For individuals with cognitive and learning impairments, a number of simple techniques can be kept in mind when evaluating or designing activities and materials for use by persons with cognitive and learning impairments. Table 60-2 includes some components of accessible interfaces to keep in mind.

TABLE 60-2. Components of Accessible Interfaces

Simplicity of layout, operation, and appearance
- Is the interface crowded, complex, or otherwise overwhelming?
- Does the interface require complex mouse actions or keystroke combinations?
- Is the language level of the interface too complex for the user?

Consistency of critical elements in the interface
- Are interface elements and controls located consistently throughout the application?
- Are interface elements and controls activated in the same manner throughout the application?

Saliency of active elements
- Is the user directed visually or otherwise toward the central content of the interface?
- Is key information highlighted?
- Is there a minimum of competing information?
- Is it clear to the user when actions or changes occur in the interface?

Intuitive operation
- Is the operation of the software obvious to the user?
- Is the selection of user interface components simple and direct?
- Is it clear to the user that the interface is responding to their input?
- Is there clear feedback when the application is busy completing a task?

Organization
- Are similar functions grouped logically together?
- Does the organization of the interface make sense visually?

Adaptability
- Does the interface offer a choice of modalities for the user (e.g., can on-screen text be read aloud)?
- Can interface elements be added or removed easily to adjust to a user's abilities?
- Does the interface offer context-sensitive help, such as tool tips?
- Are on-screen instructions provided?
- Are cues provided automatically to the user if they wait for assistance?
- Is there a timed response?

Recoverability
- Can the user easily recover from an error?
- Is clear warning provided if an action cannot be undone?
- Can the user explore the interface safely without causing instability?

ASSISTIVE TECHNOLOGY FOR HEARING

For an individual who is deaf or hard of hearing, there are two major effects of hearing loss: lack of auditory input and compromised ability to monitor speech output. AT devices, such as hearing aids and FM systems, can often be used to facilitate both auditory input and speech output. Other types of AT devices provide a visual representation of the auditory signal. These include flashing lights to indicate an emergency alarm (fire, tornado), the phone ringing, or someone at the door.

Low-technology solutions or technology-free solutions might include use of sign language or other visual representation of the spoken word or providing information in a print format. Another recent adaptation is computer-assisted translation. Referred to by the acronym CART (Computer Assisted Realtime Translation or Communication Access Realtime Technology), this solution involves a specially trained typist who captures or types the discourse of the speaker(s) on a computer that is then projected onto a monitor or other display. A variation of CART is computer-assisted note taking (CAN), when the primary purpose is to provide a written record for a student or employee.

Environmental adaptations can frequently support individuals who are deaf or hard of hearing. For example, when speaking to someone who has difficulty hearing, do not stand in front of a light source (windows, lamps, etc.), and do not over exaggerate lip movements, but do include gestures, which can be helpful. For individuals who wear hearing aids, there are a number of additional technologies that can facilitate hearing in large rooms or in crowded environments, such as a restaurant. The Conference Mate™ and Whisper Voice™ are two products especially designed for this issue. The person with the hearing loss wears a neck loop (it looks much like a bolo tie). In the case of the Conference Mate™, a small octagonal device is placed on a convenient table. This device picks up voices within the room that are transmitted to the neck loop and then to the hearing aid for better reception. Although it may sound cumbersome, it can be an excellent solution for office- and school-based environments. The Whisper Voice™ works much the same way, except the device contains a small microphone and is portable. It can be passed from speaker to speaker with sound transmitted to the neck loop and then to the hearing aid for amplification. Chapters 45 and 87 contain additional information on hearing loss and auditory rehabilitation.

ASSISTIVE TECHNOLOGY FOR ERGONOMICS AND PREVENTION OF SECONDARY INJURIES

A rapidly growing area of concern for AT practitioners is the development of repetitive motion disorders. For many persons with disabilities, the use of computer keyboards and other technology presents an opportunity for secondary injuries to occur. Computer desks, tables, and chairs used in computer labs, classrooms, and at the office do not always match the physical needs of the end user. When those with disabilities (and those without) are not positioned properly and then spend hours repetitively performing the same motor movement, they can and do develop (incur) injuries.

An entire industry of AT has developed over the past few years dealing with repetitive motion disorders. Potential solutions for someone demonstrating this type of impairment include raising or lowering a chair or desk for the appropriate fit, implementing routine breaks within activities for the individual to move about or do something different, lumbar and other supports, specially designed ergonomic keyboards, and other ATs.

Many of the ATs described in earlier sections, such as voice recognition software, alternate and specially designed ergonomic keyboards, and strategies designed to minimize keystrokes and other repetitive movements can also provide useful solutions for individuals with repetitive stress injuries. There are a number of Internet-based resources available that target ergonomic issues, such as those found in Table 60-3.

ELECTRONIC AIDS TO DAILY LIVING

Electronic Aids to Daily Living (EADLs), also described as environmental control units, provide alternative control to devices within the environment. These devices may include the TV, VCR, stereo, lights, appliances, telephone, door, electric bed, and more. EADLs are designed to improve independence in these activities of daily living. EADLs are primarily used in the home, but can also be used at work and school.

Who Can Benefit from This Technology?

EADLs provide alternative control and are designed for persons who are unable to use standard controls such as light switches or other electronic or battery-operated appliances and fixtures. EADLs can be helpful for persons with physical and

TABLE 60-3. Internet-Based Resources

Resource	What It Is	Web Address
Occupational Safety and Health Administration (OSHA)	Definitions and explanations of ergonomic safety issues, resources, and links	http://www.usemomics.com/hf.html
Human Factors and Ergonomics	Links to search engines, metasites, research studies, and educational training	http://www.safetyoffice.uwaterloo.ca/hspm/documents/office_ergo/ergo/vdt.html
MacWorld—Parent's Guide to Ergonomics	Intricacies of computer ergonomics for parents and kids as well as proper seating techniques	http://www.findarticles.com/cf d1s/mOMCW/10_17/65018479/p1/articlejhtml
Library of Ergonomic Articles—Mead-Hatcher, Inc.	Collection of useful ergonomic articles for tips on how to create a healthy and comfortable work space	http://www.meadhatcher.com/artcls.php3
Typing Injury FAW: Alternative Keyboards and Accessories	Source of information on alternative keyboards with links to manufacturers	http://www.cs.princeton.edu/-dwallach/tifaq/keyboards.html
UCLA Ergonomics	Guide to the field of ergonomics, including discussions, resources, links, and definitions	http://ergonomics.ucla.edu/

cognitive disabilities. For example, a person who has aphasia and motor impairments that are due to stroke may not be able to easily move from the couch to the TV to change channels. This person may benefit from a solution as simple as a standard TV remote control.

A person with cerebral palsy may have difficulty with the small buttons on a remote control. This person may benefit from an EADL that is accessed by a switch to scan choices. Persons of all ages can benefit from this technology as well. For example, entry level EADLs provide alternative control of toys for very young children.

How Are These Systems Controlled?

EADLs are controlled by three different access methods: direct, switch, and voice. Direct access is generally finger-to-button, as on a standard remote control. Some EADLs have enlarged buttons or keyguards to assist direct access. Enlarged buttons can also make the buttons easier to see. Typically, individuals who use direct EADLs have fair to good fine motor control and vision.

In switch access, any type of switch can be placed at the best location for activation by the person. The first switch activation begins a scan of choices, usually of general categories (i.e., TV, lights, phone). The second switch activation chooses one of these categories. Choices within that category are now scanned (i. e., channel up, channel down, mute). A third switch activation selects the desired function, and the signal is sent to the TV. Most of these systems have visual displays with small text in English (although some EADLs are available in other languages) and no speech feedback. The person generally must have good sequencing skills and vision and be able to read.

Voice-operated EADLs respond to verbal commands. For example, if the user says "TV on," a signal is immediately sent to the TV to turn it on. The individual using the device needs to have a consistent, understandable voice to operate these EADLs. They must also remember the available commands or be able to read a list to remind themselves. A person with a high-level spinal cord injury is a typical patient who could benefit from this type of device.

Many augmentative communication devices are capable of sending signals to control devices within the home environment. This can be advantageous for several reasons. First, because the EADL capability is built in, no additional funding is needed. Second, these AAC devices allow the use of larger text, graphics, and auditory scanning. Auditory scanning verbally announces each choice as it is scanned. Depending on the AAC device, these auditory prompts can even be recorded in another language. This can be very helpful for individuals with low or no vision, who need prompts to assist with memory or sequencing challenges, or who do not read (or do not read English). If they are already using a communication device, these features can be easily programmed to increase independence in the home. Some individuals who do not require an AAC device still use one solely for the EADL features because of the visual and cognitive advantages. AAC devices can be accessed directly by switch scanning, mouse control, or joystick.

Finally, software and hardware are available for computers to provide control of devices within the environment. Typically, this technology is designed for computer users who are interested in automating their home. These EADLs are not designed for persons with disabilities and can be challenging to use both cognitively and via motor control. Whatever method a person is using to access their computer (i.e., keyboard) is what is used to access the EADL features.

Safety

People must both feel and be safe in their home, especially if they are left alone for any period of time. Primary safety concerns are control of the telephone and door opener. The person with a disability must have independent access to both, if at all possible. The telephone is crucial for calling emergency personnel (i.e., medical emergency, possible burglary), calling when an attendant does not show up, and calling when a caregiver becomes incapacitated. Of course, phone access is also dependent on their ability to judge an emergency appropriately and call emergency services when warranted. The phone must have battery backup, as some emergencies are linked to power outages.

If the person is mobile and the home entrance is accessible, a power door opener may be necessary. However, if the individual has cognitive limitations affecting judgment and should not leave the home without supervision, independent control of the door may not be appropriate. Independent control of a door opener is crucial for leaving the home in an emergency such as a fire and letting in caregivers and visitors so safety and security are not compromised.

Considerations in EADL Selection

Features that are essential to consider in EADL selection are (a) portability, (b) whether the client needs to use the EADL from their bed, and (c) safety. A portable device is very important for an individual who is mobile within the home (i.e., driving a power wheelchair) and for people who need to use the EADL from more than one position, such as from a wheelchair and also from bed. A portable EADL can be moved from one location to another.

Accessing the EADL from bed is very important for many persons with disabilities. Alerting a caregiver of a need in the night, controlling an electric bed, turning on a light, and turning on some quiet music to help someone go to sleep are just some of the reasons. Motor control can change dramatically from sitting to lying down, which may require a different access method in general or two different access methods (i.e., hand switch in the wheelchair and head switch in bed).

There are a number of important questions to be discussed during the EADL selection process. These include:

1. What environments will the person be in, and how much time is spent in each setting?
2. What appliances or devices need to be accessed?
3. Will the users needs and abilities be changing?
4. What are the individual's cognitive and sensory abilities? (17)

AT specialists should assess for the most appropriate EADL based on what devices the person would like to control, as well as motor, cognitive, and sensory skills. The AT specialist or the AT supplier or vendor can also assist with procuring funding, installing equipment in the home, and training the end user and caregivers in its use.

Appropriately prescribed EADLs result in a more productive and satisfying lifestyle. In the hospital setting, EADLs allow patients to experience greater independence and can decrease the level of required nursing supervision and support. In the home, an EADL allows an individual more independence and flexibility while demonstrating the cost benefit of decreased home health care and assistance.

TABLE 60-4.	Credentialing Specialties in Assistive Technology
Specialty	**Definition**
Rehabilitation engineering technologist	Person who applies engineering principles to the design, modification, customization, and/or fabrication of assistive technologies for persons with disabilities
Assistive technology practitioner (ATP)	Service provider primarily involved in analysis of a consumer's needs and training in use of a particular device
Assistive technology supplier (ATS)	Service provider involved in the sales and service of commercially available devices

TEAMING AND ASSISTIVE TECHNOLOGY

"Teaming means you work together, no matter what. You do it because you'll come up with better ideas. And, if (or when) you disagree, you just figure it out—without fighting" (18). Equal participation in the collaborative teamwork process by the consumer, family members, and service providers is critical for individuals to achieve their goals. As it is in so many areas of physical medicine and rehabilitation, AT services are delivered in a wide variety of settings, including comprehensive medical rehabilitation centers, university-affiliated clinics, state agency-based AT programs, private rehabilitation engineering and technology firms, and nonprofit disability organizations (19). Because AT is a relatively new field and preservice and inservice preparation is just beginning to register an impact, persons with disabilities may encounter difficulty locating experienced and credentialed professionals to deliver AT services.

A transdisciplinary model of service delivery is preferred as it provides a larger pool of resources and expertise. The team may include occupational and physical therapists, rehabilitation engineers, speech language pathologists, physiatrists, case managers, and other professionals identified as important to meeting the individualized goals of the person with a disability. It is critical that the team include as *recognized members* the person with the disability(s), and his or her family and significant others when appropriate. It is also critical that at least one member of the team have some background knowledge and training in the field of AT. There are a number of university and online courses available for professionals to build expertise as well as resources in the field of AT.

The field of AT, like many other growing professions, is working to develop standards of practice and credentialing opportunities. The Rehabilitation Engineering and Assistive Technology Society of North America (RESNA), an interdiscipli-

nary association for the advancement of rehabilitation and AT, has developed guidelines and credentialing examinations for three categories of specialists in AT (Table 60-4).

For more information about the credentialing process and criteria for credentialing, contact RESNA at http://www.resna.org. A number of universities throughout the United States and Canada offer training in AT for a wide range of audiences. Table 60-5 lists only a few of the available options. For more information, visit the Web and type *assistive technology training* into the search engine.

ASSESSMENT USING A TEAM APPROACH

The goal of any AT evaluation is to determine whether the individual receiving this service has the potential, and the desire, to benefit from AT devices and services at home, school, work, or play. Other outcomes of an AT evaluation include providing a safe and supportive environment for the person with a disability and their family to learn about and review available assistive devices; identifying necessary AT services such as training, modification, etc., that may be necessary for the equipment to be effective; and developing a potential list of recommended devices for trial usage before a final determination is made. Also, the individual and family, as well as the involved professionals, should specify exactly what they hope to achieve as a result of the evaluation (i.e., equipment ideas, potential success with vocational or educational objectives).

When selecting team members to conduct an AT evaluation, appropriate disciplines should be chosen based on the identified needs of the person with the disability. For example, if the individual presents with both severe motor and communication impairments, then an occupational or physical therapist with expertise in AT, as well as a speech-language pathologist

TABLE 60-5.	Sample of Available University-Based Training Programs in Assistive Technology
University	**Web Site**
California State University-Northridge	http://www.csun.edu/codtraining
University of Southern Maine	http://vatu.usm.maine.edu/courses.htm
Washington Assistive Technology Alliance	http://www.wata.org/wata/
American Occupational Therapy Association	http://www.aota.org/nonmembers/area3/links/linkO8i.asp
George Mason University	http://chd.gse.gmu.edu/chdinfo/training.htm
University of Colorado Health Sciences Center	http://www.uchsc.edu/atp
University of Kentucky	http://www.ukv.edu/

with a background in working with persons with severe communication impairments and alternative forms of communication, should be included as members of the team. If a cognitive impairment has been identified during the intake process, someone versed in learning processes such as a psychologist, neurolinguist, teacher, or special educator might be appropriate members of the team. If there is an ergonomic issue (i.e., carpal tunnel syndrome), an evaluator with training in ergonomic assessment or a background in physical or occupational therapy is a necessary component for a successful experience.

It is *not* appropriate for an AT vendor to be called in to perform the AT evaluation. Although vendors can and should be considered as identified members of the team, it must be recognized that they have an inherent conflict of interest. They are there to sell products. When requested by the team, vendors *should* demonstrate their products, discuss pertinent features, and assist in setting up the equipment for evaluation and trial usage. However, other team members, including the end user and their family, should carry out the actual evaluation and make the final recommendation(s).

Phase I of the Assessment Process

Knowledge within the field of AT continues to grow and change, sometimes on a daily basis. As this evolution continues, a number of important variables are being identified that directly impact whether the AT recommended by the assessment team will be used or abandoned by the consumer (9,20). As a result of this information, the evaluation process continues to be refined. Many researchers are working to develop standardized AT measurement tools (9,21,22), but the fact remains that there are few available resources to guide practitioners who have not received formalized training in AT.

As mentioned earlier in this chapter, the number-one reason AT is abandoned is because the needs and preferences of the consumer were not taken into account during the evaluation process. Other reasons cited for abandonment of devices include:

- Changes in consumer functional abilities or activities
- Lack of consumer motivation to use the device or do the task
- Lack of meaningful training on how to use the device
- Ineffective device performance or frequent breakdown
- Environmental obstacles to use, such as narrow doorways
- Lack of access to and information about repair and maintenance
- Lack of sufficient need for the device functions
- Device aesthetics, devices, weight, size, and appearance (8)

Careful review of these factors suggests that many of these issues can be considered during the evaluation process. At the University of Colorado Health Sciences Center, the assessment protocol has evolved from a group of practitioners trying any number of devices with the individual to a team process that starts by leaving the technology out of sight. The process about to be described may sound laborious and cumbersome. With practice, we have reduced the time necessary for the evaluation process and have increased the likelihood that the individual who will be using it selects the appropriate technology. In addition, this process has decreased both installation and follow-up training time and has resulted in improved outcomes for end users.

Phase I of the assessment process is initiated once a referral is received. Standard intake information is collected, usually over the phone, that provides the name, primary diagnosis, age, reason for referral, etc. In the majority of cases, cognitive, motor, vision, and other standard clinical assessments have already been performed, and a release of information is requested from the individual or their caregivers for this information to be forwarded to the team. If it has not previously occurred, these evaluations are scheduled as a component of Phase II of the assessment process.

Based on the preliminary information, an appropriate team of professionals is assembled and a date chosen for the evaluation. The team leader takes responsibility for ensuring that the individual with the disability, their family, and any other significant individuals are invited to the evaluation. It is not unusual to vary the schedule to meet the needs of the family rather than the professionals.

When the time arrives for the evaluation, team members are invited to gather and spend some time getting to know the individual. Using methods described by Cook and Hussey (22) and Galvin and Scherer (8), the team first identifies the life roles of the consumer (e.g., student, brother, musician, etc.). Then the specific activities engaged in by the individual to fulfill that life role are identified. For example, if they are a brother, then that means he may play hide and seek with a sibling, squabble over toys, or otherwise engage in brotherly activities. If he is a musician, then he may want or need to have access to musical instruments, sheet music, or simply a radio.

Next, the team identifies any problems that may occur during these activities. For example, the musician may not have enough hand control to play the piano or may experience visual or cognitive difficulties with sheet music. Specific questions are asked regarding where and when these difficulties occur (activity limitations). Perhaps problems occur when the individual is tired, or not properly positioned, or when he or she tries to communicate with others. The individual is also asked to describe instances of success with these activities and to discuss what made them successful (prior history with and without technology). Interestingly enough, the team by now is usually able to recognize patterns of success and failure from the individual's perspective as common themes across environments emerge.

Finally, we ask the team to prioritize the order in which we can address identified barriers to participation, and a *specific* plan of action is developed. Within the specific plan of action, "must statements" are also developed. For example, the device *must* have a visible display in sunlight, or the technology chosen *must* weigh less than 2 pounds. In one instance, the must statement read, "It *must* be purple."

It is at this point that the team may be reconfigured. For example, if the individual is not properly seated and positioned, they are referred first to the occupational or physical therapist for a seating and positioning evaluation before any other technology issues being addressed. At all times, the configuration of the team includes the individual being assessed and the caregivers as the primary members to be consulted.

In many instances, various members of the team in collaboration with others determine that further assessment from their perspective is not warranted for the technology component to proceed. In other situations, it is determined that additional team members who were not previously considered should be invited to participate (e.g., vision specialist).

Phase II of the Assistive Technology Assessment

Once the team has agreed on the specific plan of action and those things that must occur, Phase II of the assessment process begins. The person with the disability and/or their caregivers are asked to preview any number of assistive devices that may serve to reduce activity limitations and increase participation in their chosen environments. These ATs are tried with the individual, and various adaptations, modifications, and setups are explored to ensure an appropriate match of the technology to the individual is made.

It is at this point that the AT skill sets of the clinician become critical. If trial devices are not properly configured or if the wrong information is given to the consumer, then they will be unable to make an appropriate selection. Because so many devices require extensive training and follow-up, it is also critical that realistic information regarding training issues (including learning time) is provided and appropriate resources within the local community be identified.

In a number of instances, the technology that appears to be optimal for an individual does not carry with it the appropriate community supports. In those cases, it is often advantageous to work first to identify local resources or local AT professionals willing to receive additional training before sending the device home with the end user. At all times, the end user and their families should be informed and updated so that they can make the final decision regarding when and where they wish the equipment to be delivered.

With very few exceptions, the wise course of action involves borrowing or renting the equipment before a final purchase decision. For many individuals with disabilities, the actual use of various technologies on a day-to-day basis elicits new problems that must be resolved. Unexpected benefits, including changes in role and status, also occur as a result of improved functioning. In some cases, these *unexpected benefits* create an entirely new set of problems that must be addressed. For most, these disruptions can be resolved with time and energy. Others decide that they either prefer the old way of doing things, or that they are interested in adding or changing the technology once they have had a chance to experiment with it in different settings.

Writing the Evaluation Report

When writing the evaluation report for an AT assessment, it is important to ensure that a number of items are included. First and foremost, case managers, educators, and others unfamiliar with assistive technologies appreciate layman's terms when discussing the need for AT and what it will accomplish.

In cases in which medical insurance is being used to purchase the technology, it is critical to document the actual medical necessity for the device(s). For example "Mrs. Smith will use this device to communicate her health-care needs and to meet the functional goals outlined in the attached report." In instances when the evaluation was requested to determine educational or vocational benefit with assistive devices, it is important to document how these specific needs will be met with the prescribed equipment.

It is extremely important that all components of the assistive devices be included (e.g., cables, ancillary peripherals, or consumable supplies) in the list of recommended equipment. In many instances, devices are recommended for purchase as a "system." When this occurs, acquisition and implementation can be delayed for months because an item was not included in the initial list. It is also important to include contact information for the various vendors who sell the equipment. Many purchasers are unfamiliar with these companies, and acquisition can be delayed for months if this information is not included in the report.

FUNDING ASSISTIVE TECHNOLOGY

The funding sources for AT fall into several basic categories (Table 60-6). One source to be investigated is private or government medical insurance. Medical insurance defines AT as medical equipment necessary for treatment of a specific illness or injury. A physician's prescription is usually required. When writing a prescription for an AT device, it is important that the physician is aware of the costs and benefits of the devices they are prescribing and is prepared to justify their prescriptions to third-party payors. Funding includes not only the initial cost of the device, but the expense involved in equipment maintenance and patient education, as well as the potential economic benefits it provides to the patient (e.g., return to work).

According to a publication sponsored by the American Medical Association (23), the following items (reprinted with permission) should be taken into account when prescribing AT and certifying medical necessity:

1. The physician must provide evidence of individual medical necessity.

TABLE 60-6.   Potential Funding Sources for Assistive Technology

Public Programs	Alternative Financing	U.S. Tax Code
Medicare	Private insurance	Medical care expense deduction
Medicaid—Early and Periodic Screening, Diagnosis, and Treatment (EPSDT)	Private foundations	Business deductions
State grants	State loan programs	Americans with Disabilities Act credit for business
Individuals with Disabilities Education Act (Part B and Part C)	Employee accommodation programs	Charitable contributions deduction
Vocational rehabilitation state grants, including Title VH, Chapter 2	Corporate-sponsored loans	Targeted jobs tax credit
The Developmental Disabilities state grants	Community reinvestment programs	
Workers Compensation Programs	Family and friends	
Social Security Supplemental Security Income PASS Program	Religious organizations	
CHAMPUS/TRI-CARE	Community groups	
Department of Veterans Affairs	Service clubs and advocacy organizations	

2. An "appropriate" prescription is one that takes into consideration the comprehensive assessment process, including motivation and availability of training, the potential patient functional outcome, and the cost/benefit of available products.

3. Physicians should be prepared to provide sufficient information to insurance companies to ensure approval. Dialogue is often necessary to show medical necessity of complex assistive technologies (power wheelchairs, computer-based environmental control systems).

4. Basic knowledge of AT reimbursement for patient and physician includes familiarity with established medical necessity forms and prior authorization procedures.

5. Avoid making static decisions on a dynamic problem; anticipate future need.

6. Base decision on both expected performance and durability of the device.

Documentation in the Medical Record

In addition to prescribing and certifying medical necessity on various forms, physicians must be sure to maintain complete patient records that include the following information:

- Patient diagnosis or diagnoses
- Duration of the patient's condition
- Expected clinical course
- Prognosis
- Nature and extent of functional limitations
- Therapeutic interventions and results
- Past experience with related items
- Consultations and reports from other physicians, interdisciplinary team, home health agencies, etc.
- Complete listing of all assistive devices the patient is using, including copies of prescriptions and certification forms or letters
- Tracking system for device performance, including follow-up assessment schedules and lists of professional and vendor names to contact if problems occur

Letters of Medical Necessity

These letters should include the following areas:

1. Diagnoses ICD-10-CM codes
2. Functional limitation(s) (a partial list of disabilities as examples follows):
   a. Balance disorder
   b. Developmental delay
   c. Hypotonia
   d. Joint deformity or instability
   e. Hemiparesis
   f. Side affected or bilateral
   g. Diaparesis
   h. Paraparesis
3. "Because of the patient's functional limitation, he/she is unable to . . . "
   a. Perform
      i. Activities of daily living (ADLs)
      ii. Instrumental ADLs
      iii. ADLs and functional mobility
      iv. Functional mobility
      v. Work activities
   b. Communicate
      i. Verbally
      ii. In writing
      iii. Independently over the phone
4. Use of equipment "The use of the equipment will/allow the patient to . . . "
   a. Function independently
   b. Function independently with the device/equipment
   c. Perform independent wheelchair mobility in the home
   d. Perform independent wheelchair mobility in the home and community
   e. Return home
   f. Be required as a lifetime medical need (if shorter duration, explain need)
   g. Improve the patient's functional ability
5. Description of equipment (a partial list as examples follows):
   a. Wheelchair
   b. Wheelchair frame
      i. Electric
      ii. Manual
      iii. Manual backup
      iv. One-arm drive
      v. Lightweight
      vi. Nonstandard
      vii. Reclining
      viii. Miscellaneous
   c. Other
      i. Bathing aids
      ii. Toileting aids
      iii. High-technology vision enhancers
      iv. Other hearing assistive devices
      v. Hospital bed
      vi. Stander
6. Rationale (a partial list as examples follows):
   a. Safety or safe positioning for an activity
   b. Cost effectiveness in prevention of secondary complications (e.g., pressure sores)
   c. Mobility restrictions preventing independent activity
   d. Access to areas in home, such as bathroom and kitchen
   e. Access to workplace, school
   f. Duration of expected use
   g. Past experience, interventions, and results (failure of less expensive solutions)
   h. Duration of expected use
   i. Goals and benefits to patient

AT is usually covered under policy provisions for durable medical equipment, orthotics and prosthetics, or daily living and mobility aids. With private insurance, AT providers request funding under the specific provisions of the individual policy, appealing any denials (an inevitable) and offering medical justification for coverage. With government insurance policies, such as Medicaid and Medicare, coverage is based on existing law and regulations. In 2002, regulations were promulgated by Medicare to include coverage of AAC devices (24).

Information on covered services and how to request funding is available from the Medicaid programs in individual states and from the regional offices for Medicare. AT professionals and other health-care providers should continually advocate for adequate coverage of AT in all health-care plans.

Funding of AT is also available from other federal and state government entities, such as the Veterans Administration, State Vocational Rehabilitation, Rehabilitation Services Administration, State Independent Living Rehabilitation Centers, and State Education Services. Local school districts may fund educational-related AT for children. Each agency or program sets criteria for the funding of AT based on the mission of the agency and the purpose of the technology. For example, vocational rehabilitation agencies generally pay for devices to facilitate gainful employment, and education program funding is directed toward enhancing the client's performance in school.

Private funding is often available through subsidized loan programs, churches, charitable organizations, and disability-related nonprofit groups. The AT provider must keep abreast of the requirements of various funding sources in order to direct the client to appropriate organizations. Often a combination of funding from several sources is needed to reduce personal out-of-pocket costs. Because funding for replacement of AT devices is also difficult to obtain, careful selection of the initial device is required. Providers can also assist clients by considering funding when making equipment recommendations by including both low- and high-cost alternatives with their relative advantages. Funding is generally available for AT, but persistence and advocacy by the AT provider are required for success (25,26).

MEASURING OUTCOMES IN ASSISTIVE TECHNOLOGY

The study of the impact of AT devices for individuals with disabilities poses a challenge in outcomes research. The field itself is a multidisciplinary area of study encompassing medicine, rehabilitation, psychology, education, engineering, and biotechnology specialties, and involves physical, cognitive, psychosocial, sensory, and physiological effects. Consequently, there is a lack of consistency in what has been studied, how the outcomes have been measured, and where the results have been recorded. In the field of AT, there is also a paucity of outcomes measurement research in general (27).

In 1995, Frank DeRuyter of the Rancho Los Amigos Medical Center in Downey, California, stated that "evaluating assistive technology services to demonstrate quality or to measure outcomes is the ethical obligation of the entire AT community" (28, p. 3). He went on to remind us that the systematic application of outcomes management research within AT has been fragmented and limited at best, and suggested it is incumbent upon all stakeholders in the AT community to evaluate the value and outcomes in all aspects of services delivery. In 1996, RESNA dedicated an entire issue to AT outcomes. In his editorial, Larry Trachtman again reminded AT professionals to develop a methodology for measuring and reporting outcomes. He argued that no accepted way exists to collect data in order to verify trends or to support or refute practices. As a field, there is little or no agreement on the measures, data collections points, or even the desired outcomes (27, pp. 67–68).

Persons with functional limitations and the AT devices provided by professionals do not operate in a vacuum. They exist on a broad continuum and are impacted by such things as environmental and psychosocial issues, family finances, cultural differences, and other contextual factors. Services are often fragmented, with many consumers receiving interventions from any number of teams and facilities. It is not unusual to hear families talk about their school team, hospital team, and any number of private therapists as independent service providers who do not interact. Rarely are discussions held regarding appropriateness of devices across environments, cost-effectiveness, or prevention of secondary conditions. General agreement within the field suggests that outcome measurement is a critical, unmet need. But a conceptual framework for developing measurement tools and measurement research has remained elusive (28–32). Studies of the treatment efficacy of

AT devices and services have typically been relegated to single case study reports and occasional multiple case reports showing changes from baseline (33,34).

AT traditionally includes the prescription and implementation of devices for sensory augmentation (speech, hearing, vision, etc.), but in recent years, the concept of AT has been broadened to encompass any technology that can improve a person's function (35). This is an important distinction, because it places nonoperative rehabilitation interventions, such as orthotics, prosthetics, electrical stimulation, and functional neuromuscular stimulation, in the realm of AT.

The application of technology to improve human function has long been the goal of the AT professional. In many cases, clinicians working in AT have been the most successful at crossing traditional clinical boundaries to reach out to their health-care partners who may be less familiar with AT, producing collaborations that are both innovative and productive. The AT specialist has the hands-on clinical experience to see what works and understands those factors leading to technology abandonment. Typical clinical practice, however, does not lend itself to the development of experimental methodologies to objectively evaluate patient performance with AT devices and services. Moreover, most AT clinicians do not have the resources to actively participate in a sustained program of research, nor are these behaviors emphasized as a component of clinical intervention in most training programs.

Despite this limitation, AT professionals and the AT service delivery model have been effective in getting technology into the hands of the people who need it, creating a foundation for rehabilitation intervention service delivery in general. Because the AT specialist functions across disciplines, he or she is often the first to notice the impact of other treatment modalities. For example, it is typical for a child with an acquired disability to enter rehabilitation services with a variety of needs and assignments to various disciplines for treatment. It is often the AT specialist who notices incompatibilities between systems, such as a seating system with a lap tray that interferes with a child in development of an alternate access method to a computer used to complete educational tasks.

In recent years, the National Institute on Disability and Rehabilitation Research and the National Institutes of Health's National Center for Medical Rehabilitation Research have begun to fund various research activities devoted to developing standardized outcomes measurement systems in order to determine the efficacy of various AT devices and services. The plan for these activities calls for the dissemination of information to individuals with disabilities, their families, caregivers, funding sources, and manufacturers. The field of AT is one of growth and excitement. Results from studies such as these are a welcome and necessary component for the continued development of this discipline.

ACKNOWLEDGEMENTS

Funding for this chapter is due in large part to NIDDRR grant # H224A940014–01: Colorado Assistive Technology Project, State Grants for Technology Related Assistance.

Special thanks are also due to staff of Assistive Technology Partners, Department of Physical Medicine and Rehabilitation, University of Colorado Health Sciences Center, including Maureen Melonis, Jim Sandstrum, Pat McAleese, Marlin Cohrs, Julia Beems, Diane Brians, and Brian Simms. The authors also wish to thank Dr. Thomas W. King, Department of Communication Disorders, University of Wisconsin–Eau Claire; Department of Geriatric Health, American Medical Association; Michelle Lange for her work on the EADL section; and the previous assistive technology chapter authors.

REFERENCES

1. James P, Thorpe N. *Ancient inventions.* New York: Ballentine Books, 1994.
2. Trease G. *Timechanges: the evolution of everyday life.* New York: Warmick Press, 1985.
3. Public Law 100–407. The Technology-Related Assistance Act for Individuals with Disabilities of 1988. 1988; 34CFR 300.5.
4. Public Law 100–407. The Technology-Related Assistance Act for Individuals with Disabilities of 1988. 1988; 19 34CFR 300.6.
5. Public Law 102–569. Reauthorization of the Rehabilitation Act of 1973, 1992.
6. Public Law 94–142. Reauthorization of the Individuals with Disabilities Education Act (IDEA), 1991.
7. Beukelman DR, Mirenda P. *Augmentative and alternative communication: management of severe communication disorders in children and adults,* 2nd ed. Baltimore: Paul H. Brookes, 1998.
8. Galvin JC, Scherer MJ. *Evaluating, selecting and using appropriate assistive technology.* Gaithersburg, MD: Aspen Publications, 1996.
9. Scherer MJ. *Living in the state of stuck: how technologies impact the lives of people with disabilities.* 3rd ed. Cambridge, MA: Brookline Books, 2000.
10. King TW. *Assistive technology: essential human factors.* Boston: Allyn and Bacon, 1999:40–42.
11. LaPlante MP. The demographics of disability. *Milbank Q* 1991;69:55–77.
12. World Health Organization. *International classification of function, disability, and health.* Geneva: WHO, 2001.
13. Miranda P, Mathy-Laikko P. Augmentative and alternative applications for persons with severe congenital communication disorders: an introduction. *Augmentative Alternative Communication* 1989;5:3–13.
14. Fried-Oken M, Howard JM, Stewart SR. Feedback on AAC interventions from adults who are temporarily unable to speak. *Augmentative Alternative Communication* 1988;4:21.
15. Blake D, Bodine C. Assistive technology and multiple sclerosis. *J Rehabil Res Dev* 2002;39(2):299–312.
16. Kangas K, Lloyd L. Early cognitive skills and prerequisites to augmentative and alternative communication: what are we waiting for? *Augmentative Alternative Communication* 1988;4:21.
17. Swenson JR, Barnett LL, Pond B, et al. Assistive technology for rehabilitation and reduction of disability. In: DeLisa J, Gans B, eds. Rehabilitation medicine: principles and practice, 3rd ed. Philadelphia: Lippincott-Raven Publishers, 1998:745–762.
18. Rainforth B, York-Barr J. *Collaborative teams for students with severe disabilities: integrating therapy and educational services.* Baltimore: PH Brookes, 1997.
19. Hobson DA. RESNA: Yesterday, today, and tomorrow. *Assistive Technology* 1996;8:131.
20. Phillips B, Zhao H. Predictors of assistive technology abandonment. *Assistive Technology* 1993;5:36–45.
21. Demers L, Ska B, Giroux F, Weiss-Lambrou R. Stability and reproducibility of the Quebec User Evaluation of Satisfaction with assistive technology (QUEST). *Journal of Rehabilitation Outcomes Measures* 1999;3(4):42–52.
22. Cook. A, Hussey S. *Assistive technology: principles and Practice.* St. Louis: Mosby Press, 1995.
23. Schwartzberg J,Kakavas K, Malkind S, et al. *Guidelines for the use of assistive technology: evaluation, referral, prescription.* Chicago: American Medical Association, 1996:37–41.
24. Golinker L. AAC and Medicare Funding Guidelines, 2002. Ithaca NY: Assistive Technology Law Center.
25. Hoffman A. How you can make it work. In: Coston C, ed. *Planning and implementing augmentative communication service delivery: proceedings of the national planners conference on assistive device service delivery.* Washington, DC: RESNA, 1988:64–74.
26. Wallace J. Creative financing of assistive technology. In: Flippo KF, Inge KJ, Barcus JM, eds. *Assistive technology: a resource for school, work, and community.* Baltimore: Paul H. Brookes Publishers, 1995:245–268.
27. Trachtman L. Measuring and documenting assistive technology outcome. *Assistive Technology* 1996;8(2):67–70.
28. DeRuyter F. Evaluating outcomes in assistive technology: do we understand the commitment? *Assistive Technology* 1995;7(1):3–8.
29. Cushman LAS. Measuring the relationship of assistive technology use, functional status over time, and consumer-therapist perceptions of ATs. *Assistive Technology* 1996;8(2):103–109.
30. DeRuyter F. The importance of outcome measures for assistive technology service delivery systems. *Technology and Disability* 1997;6:89–104.
31. Jutai J, Ladak N, Schuller R, et al. Outcomes measurement of assistive technologies: an institutional case study. *Assistive Technology* 1996;8(2):110–120.
32. Merbitz C. Frequency measures of behavior for assistive technology and rehabilitation. *Assistive Technology* 1996;8(2):121–130.
33. Oldridge N. Outcomes measurement: health related quality of life. *Assistive Technology* 1996;8(2):82–93.
34. Smith R.. Measuring the outcomes of assistive technology: challenge and innovation. *Assistive Technology* 1996;8(2):71–81.
35. Gray DB, Quatrano LA, Lieberman ML. *Designing and using assistive technology: the human perspective.* Baltimore: Paul H. Brookes, 1998.

CHAPTER 61

Upper and Lower Extremity Prosthetics

Andrew Gitter and Gordon Bosker

Major limb amputation influences multiple aspects of an individual's life: body image, self-care activities, mobility, psychosocial health, vocational, and avocational opportunities. Successful rehabilitation allows the individual with an amputation to return to their highest level of activity and function. Assuring that, the most comfortable, cosmetic, and functional prosthesis is a major goal in the rehabilitation process. Tempering expectations with reality, balancing the use of prosthetic technology with the individual's perceived needs, physical and cognitive capabilities, social support network, and financial resources is an essential feature of rehabilitative care.

Advances in the care and prosthetic restoration of the individual with an amputation have always come from multiple arenas: development in new surgical techniques, improvements in the preoperative and postoperative management, advances in prosthetic technology, and better understanding of the psychosocial implications of limb loss. In the past decade, the greatest advances have occurred in the areas of prosthetic technologies, fabrication techniques for prosthetic sockets, and improved components that more effectively replace the lost function of the extremity. Organized teams of health care providers in regional centers who treat a large number of the individuals with an amputation are able to provide optimal prosthetic rehabilitation because of their combined experience (1). While such integrated teams are ideal, a less formal coordination of efforts between surgeons, physiatrists, prosthetists, and therapists in the community can provide effective care to most individuals with an amputation who lack access to specialized centers.

In this chapter, the causes of amputation, basic surgical issues, and the overall approach to the medical and physiatric care of the individual with an amputation are reviewed. An expanded discussion of the prosthetic management of amputation at different levels in both the lower and upper limbs follows to aid the practitioner in organizing the myriad options available for restoring the function of the lost limb. Finally common problems, medical complications, and special issues in pediatric amputation are discussed.

INCIDENCE AND ETIOLOGY

Acquired Amputation

The etiology of limb loss influences the clinical treatment, management, and functional expectations of the individual with an amputation. Data from the Agency for Healthcare Research and Quality (AHRQ) and the Veterans Health Administration (VHA) from the late 1980s to the late 1990s estimates that a total of 140,000 amputations are performed yearly in the United States (2,3). Acquired amputation accounts for 96% to 99% of all limb loss with the remaining 1% to 4% related to congenital causes.

The distributions of upper and lower extremity amputation by level are shown in Figure 61-1. In the lower extremity (LE), 75% to 93% of acquired amputations are the result of vascular disease (diabetic vascular disease, atherosclerosis, immunologic, and idiopathic). Diabetes is a major risk factor for amputation contributing to two-thirds of all LE amputations (2,3). Approximately 6% to 10% of acquired LE amputations result from traumatic injuries to the extremities with the remainder due to benign or malignant tumors. While accounting for a smaller overall percentage of LE amputation, trauma is the most common cause for LE amputation in the second and third decades of life. Among those between the ages of 10 to 20 years, tumor is the most frequent cause of all amputations (4–6).

In the upper extremity (UE), trauma is the leading cause of limb loss accounting for 80% of amputations. The vast majority of traumatic UE amputations are limited to the digital amputations. There are an estimated 10,000 to 15,000 upper limb amputations at the transradial level and above yearly in the United States (Table 61-1) (7). Most of these occur in individuals between the ages of 20 and 40. As in the LE, tumor is the most common cause of UE amputation in children.

From 1988 to 1996, the rates of trauma- and cancer-associated amputations declined by more than 40% (2,8). This decline likely reflects improved surgical reconstruction techniques for trauma, limb-sparing management of musculoskeletal tumors, and greater prevention through improved occupational safety awareness. In contrast to the reduction in tumor- and trauma-related limb loss, dysvascular amputation rates have increased 10% to 19% over the past several decades. The increase in dysvascular-related amputation has occurred despite considerable evidence that comprehensive management of the diabetic foot at risk can substantially reduce or delay amputation. Factors that account for this adverse trend include the difficulty of implementing systematic comprehensive management strategies for the diabetic foot coupled with an increasing prevalence of diabetes, smoking, hypertension, and hypercholesteremia placing more individuals at risk (2,9,10).

Percentages of Upper and Lower Amputations

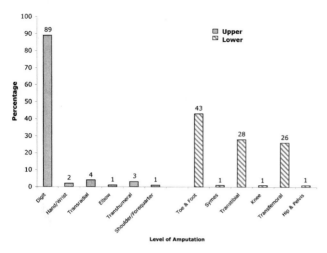

Figure 61-1. Showing percentage and level of amputations. [Data taken from the Agency for Healthcare Research and Quality (AHRQ) and the Veterans Health Administration (VHA).]

Congenital Amputation

The absence of part or all of an extremity at birth is more appropriately referred to as a congenital skeletal deficiency rather than a congenital amputation. The Birth Defects Monitoring Program, a national program monitoring congenital malformations for the United States, reports the incidence of congenital upper and lower limb skeletal deficiency at 2.41 per 10,000 births (upper limb, 1.58 per 10,000 births; lower limb, 0.83 per 10,000 births) (11). Although a few genetically determined syndromes, such as Holt-Oram, Fanconi, thrombocytopenia, absent radius and drugs (e.g., thalidomide) have been associated with skeletal deficiencies (12–14), no etiology can be determined for most congenital limb loss.

Multiple systems for classifying congenital limb deficiencies have been proposed in both Europe and North America, but no one system has been universally accepted. A commonly used and preferred system is based on the International Society for Prosthetics and Orthotics recommendations which classify congenital limb loss as either a transverse or longitudinal skeletal deficiency. Transverse limb deficiency, also referred to as terminal deficiency, is defined as the loss of all skeletal components distal to a particular transverse axis level (e.g., transverse forearm or transverse radial limb deficiency). Longitudinal limb deficiency, also referred to as intercalary limb loss, is defined as the loss (complete or partial) of one or more skeletal elements within the long axis of the limb, with preservation of some or all of the more distal skeletal elements. Classification of congenital limb deficiencies often is confused further when congenital deficiencies are described in the same terms used for acquired amputations, such as "transradial" or "transtibial." The use of similar terminology occurs either because the congenital deficiency appears similar to an acquired amputation or because a congenital skeletal deficiency has undergone a surgical conversion to accommodate appropriate prosthetic restoration. Surgical conversion has been estimated to be necessary in the management of 50% of LE congenital deficiencies and 8% of UE deficiencies (15).

Amputation Surgery

The underlying principle in choosing the level of amputation is to preserve as much limb length as possible that is consistent with wound healing, an acceptable soft-tissue envelope, and functional prosthetic fitting. While in principle, decision making is straightforward, in practice many issues must be weighed including the severity of the underlying disease process, tissue viability, overall medical condition of the patient,

TABLE 61-1. Numbers and Adjusted Rates of Limb Loss by Etiology and Level (7)			
Level	Dyvascular NO. (%) 1988–1996	Trauma-Related NO. (%) 1988–1996	Cancer-Related NO. (%) 1988–1996
Lower limb (Total)	953,367 (97)	61,605 (31)	8,351 (76.1)
Toe	309,589 (31.5)	27,233 (13.9)	1,466 (13.4)
Foot	102,872 (10.5)	4,483 (2.3)	482 (4.4)
Ankle	7,478 (0.8)	823 (0.4)	164 (1.5)
Transtibial	271,550 (27.6)	14,244 (7.3)	1,501 (13.7)
Through-Knee	4,237 (0.4)	921 (0.5)	133 (1.2)
Transfemoral	253,145 (25.8)	10,821 (5.5)	2,499 (22.8)
Hip disarticulation	3,554 (0.4)	418 (0.2)	726 (6.6)
Pelvic	469 (0.1)	52 (0.03)	1,369 (12.5)
Bilateral	0 (0)	1,504 (0.8)	0 (0)
Upper limb (Total)	29,426 (3)	134,421 (68.6)	2,617 (23.9)
Thumb	2,344 (0.2)	24,325 (12.4)	352 (3.2)
Finger(s)	21,427 (2.2)	100,316 (51.2)	529 (4.8)
Hand	1,255 (0.1)	983 (0.5)	92 (0.8)
Wrist	514 (0.1)	415 (0.2)	21 (0.2)
Transradial	1,626 (0.2)	4,001 (2.0)	212 (1.9)
Through-elbow	385 (0.04)	346 (0.2)	123 (1.1)
Transhumeral	1,511 (0.2)	3,008 (1.5)	488 (4.4)
Shoulder	236 (0.02)	154 (0.1)	365 (3.3)
Bilateral	0 (0)	462 (0.2)	0 (0)
Forequarter	132 (0.01)	15 (0.01)	439 (4)

the morbidity associated with limb salvage, and the expected functional level after amputation. In patients with vascular disease, noninvasive vascular studies can assist in predicting wound healing; an absolute ankle Doppler blood pressure of 70 mm Hg or greater, an ankle-brachial index of 0.5 or greater, and transcutaneous oxygen pressure of greater than 20 to 30 mm Hg are all suggestive of a greater likelihood of healing at the transtibial level. Other nonvascular factors associated with compromised wound healing include poor nutritional status (albumin below 3.5 g/dL) or immunocompromised status (total lymphocyte count <1,500). Despite these identified predictive factors, the final choice of amputation level in the vascular patient often cannot be made until the time of surgery, when the amount of blood flow in the relevant tissues can be observed (8,16–18). In most medical centers, the physiatrist plays a limited role in presurgical planning. In centers where multidisciplinary teams are used, the physiatrist can offer useful insights into the likelihood of achieving various functional goals at differing levels of amputation. This information allows the health care team and the patient to weigh surgical options when uncertainty exists.

The decision between amputation and limb salvage following trauma is a complex one. Early or immediate amputation may be required in life-threatening multiple trauma situations when the physiologic demands associated with repeated surgery to salvage a limb would not be tolerated. The presence of preexisting medical conditions such as peripheral vascular disease (PVD) or neurologic injury that adversely affect function of the residual limb may also favor immediate amputation. However, when the injuries are not immediately life-threatening, the decision to amputate versus attempting limb salvage must be based on an assessment of the approach that will most effectively restore function and return the individual to his or her preinjury activities. Extensive soft-tissue loss, proximal arterial injuries, multiple arterial injuries, and sciatic or tibial nerve damage are poor prognostic indicators for successful limb salvage (17,19). In general, limb salvage of the LE requires more surgeries, involves longer hospital stays, delays weight bearing, and slows the return to preinjury activities compared to amputation. (19). Because the functional demands of the UE are different from the LE, a bias toward limb salvage has developed in UE trauma surgery. The lack of weight-bearing forces, the ability to function with partial sensation, and the limited functionality of UE prostheses are reasons cited for greater effort directed toward limb salvage and reimplantation (20,21).

Amputation surgery must be approached as a reconstructive procedure. Bones are beveled to minimize sharp edges that can cause tissue trauma and pain with weight bearing. The nerves are sharply transected and allowed to retract into proximal soft tissues so that they do not become adherent in scar or remain in a location subjected to high loading forces from a prosthesis. Appropriate myofascial closure of the muscle or myodesis provides for good control of the remaining bone in the residual limb, and appropriate placement of the skin incision line avoids bony prominences and adherence to underlying bone. Such attention to detail will result in a well-shaped residual limb that can be effectively fit with a prosthesis. Ilizarov techniques or free fibular grafts (22–24) have been used to lengthen short residual limbs, though the indications for their use and their success are highly individualized. Skin grafts and myocutaneous free flaps (25,26) have been used successfully to preserve length in nonvascular individuals with an amputation, but in general the presence of skin grafts or insensate skin in the residual limb often results in recurring skin breakdown. When recurring skin breakdown occurs, stump re-

vision, use of tissue expanders, and creative approaches to prosthetic design may be needed. The preferred levels of amputation are as follows.

Lower Extremity

- Toe amputations
- Ray resections
- Transmetatarsal amputations
- Syme amputation (i.e., ankle disarticulation)
- Transtibial amputation (between the junction of the middle and distal thirds of the leg)
- Knee disarticulation
- Transfemoral amputation (8 cm or more proximal to the level of the knee joint)
- Hip disarticulation (short transfemoral amputation at or proximal to the greater trochanter is functionally a hip disarticulation)
- Hemipelvectomy

Upper Extremity

- Finger or thumb amputation
- Ray resection
- Transmetacarpal resection
- Wrist disarticulation
- Transradial amputation
- Elbow disarticulation
- Transhumeral amputation (i.e., 6.5 cm or more proximal to the elbow joint)
- Shoulder disarticulation
- Forequarter amputation (interscapulothoracic disarticulation)

LOWER EXTREMITY AMPUTATION

General Principles of Lower Extremity Amputation Management

The interaction of the health care team working with the patient to achieve the goal of prosthetic restoration and rehabilitation is referred to as prosthetic management (27). The process of prosthetic rehabilitation can be organized into a four-phase process: preprosthetic management, postoperative care, prosthetic fitting and training, and long-term follow-up care. This staging permits the rehabilitation physician to assess the individual with an amputation and organize the rehabilitation program.

PREPROSTHETIC PATIENT EVALUATION AND MANAGEMENT
Preprosthetic management begins when the decision to perform an amputation is made, when a patient initially is evaluated after a traumatic amputation, or when a child is born with a congenital skeletal deficiency. It ends with the fitting of a prosthesis. Optimal care is ensured when members of the prosthetic team can evaluate the patient before amputation, but often the events surrounding an amputation delay the rehabilitation assessment until the postoperative period.

The preprosthetic evaluation, whether performed pre- or postoperatively, should focus on identifying factors that will affect the ultimate functional status of the patient and limit prosthetic fitting. Issues that need evaluation include assessing the premorbid functional status, identifying coexisting musculoskeletal, neurologic, and cardiopulmonary disease that will

TABLE 61-2.   Goals of Post Operative Management of the Amputee

- Successful healing of the amputation
- Pain control
- Maintaining range of motion in the remaining proximal joints of the amputated extremity
- Strengthening of residual muscle groups needed for biomechanical compensation
- Preparation of the residual limb for prosthetic fitting
- Achieving independence in ADL's and mobility without a prosthetic limb
- Education about the process of prosthetic limb fitting and expected functional outcome.
- Psychosocial support for the adaptations resulting from the amputation.

influence rehabilitation potential, determining the available social support network, and understanding the patient's goals and expectations postamputation. Education of the patient and family about the functional consequences of amputation and the steps involved in prosthetic rehabilitation will help allay some of the fears the patient may have about his or her future. Therapy programs for range of motion, conditioning exercises, correct positioning of the residual limb, ambulation with gait aids, relaxation techniques, and activities of daily living (ADLs) should be started as soon as medically appropriate. The patient is often better able to absorb and comply with a therapy program during the preoperative period than during the early postoperative period, when incisional pain, medication, or apprehension may interfere with the ability to participate.

POSTOPERATIVE CARE

The goals that direct the postoperative, preprosthetic management of the individual with an amputation are outlined in Table 61-2. During the immediate postoperative period, general medical care focuses on optimizing control of underlying disorders that can interfere with rehabilitation: diabetes, coronary artery disease, congestive heart failure, renal disease. Maintaining nutritional status is frequently neglected, yet it plays a critical role in ensuring wound healing (8) and in facilitating the muscular strength adaptations needed for prosthetic mobility. The principles guiding residual limb care are based on ensuring primary wound healing, controlling pain, minimizing edema, and preventing contractures.

Options for wound management include soft dressings, semi-rigid dressings (Unna casts), rigid dressings (plaster or fiberglass casts), and air splints. Each option has advantages and disadvantages that have influenced its use. Soft dressings are typically used with an elastic bandage wrap (i.e., Ace bandage) or a compressive stockinette. Soft dressings have the advantage of being readily available, quickly applied, and allowing frequent wound inspection. However, they do not provide protection from external trauma and only have a limited ability to control edema. If poorly applied, elastic wraps can lead to tourniquet effect. Elastic bandages require considerable cooperation, skill, and attention on the part of the patient, family, and medical staff because the wraps need to be reapplied frequently and carefully to be successful. In practice their use is problematic enough that alternatives such as compressive stockinettes, elastic stump shrinkers, or roll-on gel liners are often a better choice of edema management. Despite a number

of limitations, soft dressings remain the most commonly used wound care approach (28) following amputation.

Rigid dressings have been reported to reduce wound-healing time and lead to more rapid and improved rehabilitation (29,30). The primary concerns surrounding rigid dressings are the inability to inspect the wound and the potential increase in wound breakdown from incorrect application or early weight bearing in dysvascular individuals with an amputation. In spite of these limitations, postoperative rigid dressings may be the preferred method of wound care especially for the transtibial individual with an amputation, but their clinical use and acceptance has been limited by the lack of expertise in their application. Rigid dressings can be fabricated as a removable rigid dressing that resembles a transtibial prosthetic socket or as a nonremovable cast that extends to the midthigh level. The rigid dressing is most commonly made using standard orthopedic cast materials but commercially available prefabricated devices are also available. A nonremovable rigid dressing is typically applied during or shortly after surgery and replaced every 7 to 14 days. The midthigh length of the dressing prevents knee flexion contractures and is continued until adequate wound healing has occurred so that concerns over future contracture development are minimized. Subsequent dressings are fabricated as removable rigid dressings that can be taken off whenever the wound needs to be inspected. Rigid dressings have been predominantly used in the individuals with a traumatic amputation because of lessened concern over wound healing or residual limb injury from the dressing. While rigid dressings can be used simply as a wound care strategy, they can also be used with a pylon attachment to which components can be attached, creating a preparatory prosthesis that enables immediate or early weight bearing.

Because little objective data exist that clearly identify a superior wound dressing strategy, the choice of wound management appears to be driven largely by practice conventions, availability of skilled staff, and the personal experience of the surgeon. Greater attention to optimizing and facilitating rapid wound healing is needed especially in the individual with a dysvascular amputation in whom the effects of prolonged immobilization may substantively complicate rehabilitation effects. The preprosthetic phase of management, before preparatory prosthetic fitting, can typically last 6 to 10 weeks for the individual with a dysvascular LE amputation, a considerably shorter period of time for the individual with a traumatic amputation, and 3 to 6 weeks for the individual with a UE (12).

Muscle imbalance and postoperative positioning to facilitate comfort leads to the development of knee flexion contracture in the transtibial residual limb and to hip flexion and abduction contractures in the individual with a transfemoral amputation. Contractures are preventable through a postoperative therapy program that emphasizes range of motion exercises and early remobilization. Strengthening of muscle groups that biomechanically substitute for the lost function of the limb is needed. In the individual with an LE amputation, the hip extensors (gluteus maximus and hamstrings), gluteus medius, hip flexors, and the contralateral ankle plantar flexors all contribute to restoring ambulation ability (31,32). In the individual with a UE amputation, proximal shoulder girdle muscle strengthening should be taught, emphasizing the trapezius, serratus anterior, pectoralis major, as well as any residual deltoid and biceps functions.

The response to amputation has been compared to the grieving process that variably includes identifiable stages of denial, anger, depression, coping, and acceptance. Not every person ultimately adapts to limb loss. The individual's ultimate response to the psychosocial impact of limb loss is determined by many factors, including the cause of the amputation, personal life experience and inner strengths, the available social support system, the care provided by the prosthetic team, and the functional outcome that is achieved through rehabilitation.

PROSTHETIC FITTING AND TRAINING

An understanding of functional needs of the individual with an amputation, their interest and motivation in pursuing prosthetic fitting, and an assessment of their ambulatory potential are required to set realistic goals for prosthetic fitting and training. Not all the individuals with an amputation are candidates for prostheses. Although the factors that predict success in prosthetic use are incompletely understood, a number of factors have been associated with a poor outcome in returning the individual with an amputation to functional ambulation at household or community levels. Negative prognostic factors include a delay in wound healing, the presence of joint contractures, dementia or cognitive disorders, medical comorbidities, and higher levels of limb amputation (transfemoral) (33–35). Age has inconsistently been identified as a predictor of prosthetic success, implying that unless advanced age is present (>80 to 85 years) other factors play a more important role in determining the rehabilitation potential of the individual with an amputation.

As a result of the uncertainty in identifying prosthetic candidates, considerable clinical judgment is required. Some general guidelines can be followed. An individual with an amputation should have reasonable cardiovascular reserve, adequate wound healing, and good soft-tissue coverage, range of motion, muscle strength, motor control, and learning ability to achieve useful prosthetic function. Individuals with an LE amputation who can walk with a walker or crutches without a prosthesis usually possess the necessary balance, strength, and cardiovascular reserve to walk with a prosthesis. Examples of poor candidates for functional prosthetic fitting would be an individual with a dysvascular LE amputation with an open or poorly healed incision, an individual with a transfemoral amputation with a 30-degree flexion contracture at the hip, or an individual with a transradial amputation with a flail elbow and shoulder. Generally, individuals with a bilateral, short, transfemoral amputation over the age of 45 years are considered unlikely candidates for full-length prosthetic fitting. Additional medical problems such as severe coronary artery disease, pulmonary disease, severe polyneuropathy, or multiple-joint arthritis may result in an individual with an amputation who could be fitted with a prosthesis but who may not be a functional prosthetic user. Patients in whom prognosis is poor, life expectancy is short, or with a disease that results in significant fluctuations in body weight are not good candidates. In borderline cases, it may be necessary to proceed with actual prosthetic fitting to determine eventual prosthetic function. The use of a less costly removable rigid dressing with pylon and foot or a preparatory prosthesis is appropriate before a decision is made about fitting such a person with a more costly definitive prosthesis. The overall success rate in restoring functional ambulation in the individual with a lower limb amputation varies approximately from 36% to 70%. Amputation resulting from vascular disease is a manifestation of a severe systemic vasculopathy. The early mortality following major LE amputation is 15% to 20%, largely related to myocardial infarction. Overall, the individuals with dysvascular amputation have a 3- to 5-year 50% mortality, which underlies the importance of successful early rehabilitation to allow for an improved quality of life in their remaining years.

The timing of prosthetic fitting for the individual with an LE amputation remains controversial, reflecting the clinical uncertainty over early versus delayed weight bearing. Because the majority of LE amputations occur as the result of peripheral vascular disease, primary wound healing at the amputation site is of paramount importance. When the rigid dressing was introduced on a wide scale in the 1970s, it was used to implement immediate postoperative prosthesis (IPOP) (a rigid dressing with a pylon and foot) as a means to speed rehabilitation for individuals with LE amputation (36). Problems with wound healing and residual limb trauma from poorly fabricated devices and a lack of experienced teams to manage this approach to early postoperative care led to abandoning their use in the individual with a dysvascular amputation. Despite these problems, in selected centers with adequate experience and a process to monitor closely the residual limb, an immediate or early postoperative prosthesis fabricated several weeks after surgery has been used safely in individuals with a dysvascular amputation (37). Immediate fitting in the younger patient with traumatic amputation has been more successful and is a reasonable method of treatment. Immediate and early postoperative prostheses are in effect a removable rigid dressing with a pylon and foot attached. This device is used to achieve limited partial to full weight bearing, reduce edema, and accomplish initial gait training. Because the fit of these devices is always suboptimal compared to a custom-molded socket, they are not recommended for extended use.

When concern over wound healing dominates clinical care in the postoperative period, prosthetic fitting is delayed until the residual limb has healed adequately to allow unrestricted weight bearing. Providing a prosthesis is typically performed in two stages: a preparatory prosthetic limb phase is followed by the provision of a definitive prosthesis. The preparatory prosthesis is often of simple design, lower performance, and is more accommodating to changes in residual limb volume then is the definitive limb. It allows the individual with an amputation to gain skill and confidence in walking with prosthesis, facilitates residual limb maturation, and affords the rehabilitation team the opportunity to better define the ultimate functional level of the individual. When stump maturation has occurred, a definitive prosthesis is prescribed to meet all of the anticipated needs of the individual with an amputation. Stump maturation is an imprecisely defined concept that occurs when the volume of the residual limb has stabilized, soft-tissue atrophy has occurred, and the residual limb has been molded into a cylindrical shape that optimizes prosthetic fitting. This can usually be determined when the individual with an amputation reports a plateau in the number of sock plies worn by clinical exam that shows edema resolution. Residual limb maturation typically takes about 4 months (38) but may extend substantially longer depending on the activity level, amount of prosthetic limb use, and coexisting medical disease. After stump maturation occurs, a definitive prosthesis is prescribed to specifically meet the ADLs and vocational and avocational needs of the individual with an amputation. In the case of young children, the prosthesis prescription must also meet any needs related to the development of age-appropriate motor milestones. Although a two-stage approach (preparatory followed by definite limb) is commonly used, financial considerations are becoming increasingly important with many health insurance programs allowing for only a single limb. Under these situations, the prosthetic team may elect to prescribe as the initial prosthesis a limb that is projected to meet all the long-term needs of the individual with an amputation. Patients who are not candidates for functional prosthetic use may choose to have a cosmetic prosthesis. These cosmetic prostheses can be fabricated to have an appearance similar to that of the opposite limb.

GAIT TRAINING

After completing the final prosthetic evaluation, the individual with a new amputation will require a period of gait training to learn how to function with the prosthesis. This training takes place under the supervision of the physical therapist. The individual with an amputation is instructed in how to put on and take off the prosthesis, how to determine the appropriate number of limb socks to be worn, when and how to check the skin for evidence of irritation, and how to clean and care for the prosthesis. For the individual with a new amputation it is best if the initial gait training occurs while the prosthesis is still capable of being adjusted to permit alignment or length changes that may become apparent during gait training. Gait training often occurs on an outpatient basis and may last from weeks to months. The more proximal levels of amputation require lengthier gait training.

Gait training begins with weight shifting and balance activities while still in the parallel bars. Once weight shifting and balance activities have been mastered, a program of progressive ambulation begins in the parallel bars and progresses to the most independent level of ambulation possible with or without gait aids. Specific training should focus on transfers, gaining knee stability, equal step lengths, and avoiding lateral trunk bending. Following mastery of ambulation on flat, level surfaces, techniques for managing uneven terrain, stairs, ramps, curbs, and falling and getting up off the ground are learned. Moving from a walker to less cumbersome gait aids can be achieved for most individuals with an LE amputation. For higher functioning individuals with an amputation, prosthetic training should include instruction and practice in driving, recreation, and vocational pursuits. Developing the optimal benefit from a prosthesis must take into account the specific mechanical attributes of the components used. For example, using a dynamic response (i.e., energy-storing) prosthetic foot requires loading the prosthetic toe during midstance and late stance to capture energy for push off assistance or to activate a prosthetic knee to initiate swing phase.

Wearing tolerance for the prosthesis gradually must be increased. Initially, the individual with an amputation will wear the prosthesis only for 15 to 20 minutes, removing it to check the condition of the skin. As tolerance to weight bearing increases, the length of wearing time is gradually increased. Several weeks may be required before the individual with an amputation is able to wear the prosthesis full-time. The individual with an amputation may take the prosthesis home when safe and independent ambulation has been demonstrated and residual limb skin checks are assured. Common gait deviations and their causes are highlighted in Table 61-3.

LOWER EXTREMITY PROSTHETIC FOLLOW-UP

During the initial 6 to 18 months, most individuals with an amputation will experience continued loss of residual limb volume, resulting in a prosthetic socket that will be too large. During this period, return visits should occur frequently enough to ensure that this loss of residual limb volume is being compensated for by the use of additional limb socks or by appropriate modifications of the prosthetic socket. It is usual for an individual with a new amputation to require replacement of the prosthetic socket during this time because of the significant loss of soft-tissue volume. During follow-up clinic visits the condition of the residual limb, the prosthesis, the individual's gait, and the level of function are reviewed (39). Appropriate medical treatment, prosthetic modifications, or additional therapies are prescribed as needed. When the residual limb volume has stabilized sufficiently and the patient is doing well with the prosthesis, yearly visits to the amputee clinic are appropriate. Once the residual limb has stabilized, the average life expectancy for an LE prosthesis before replacement should be 3 to 5 years.

Lower Extremity Prostheses

The LE prosthetic prescription must balance the individual's need for stability, mobility, durability, and cosmesis with available resources and financial sponsorship. Understanding the role and importance of prosthetic ambulation in achieving the mobility goals of the individual with an amputation is essential for correctly prescribing a prosthetic device. Prosthetic ambulation is usually the primary mode of mobility for the younger individual with an amputation as well as for other patients across a wider age range when the amputation is at the transtibial and more distal levels. For the elderly, with dysvascular amputation above the knee and more proximal level, prosthetic ambulation is often limited to transfers, indoors, or short community distances. The prescription of the LE prosthesis is based on several guiding principles: maximizing comfort, matching specific components to the mobility needs of the individual with an amputation, and providing acceptable cosmesis. Comfort is the most critical aspect of any prosthesis and depends on achieving an appropriate distribution of forces between the residual limb and the socket. A poorly fitting or uncomfortable socket will limit mobility and often leads to rejection of the prosthesis. Once comfort has been established, the appropriate choice of components facilitates achieving maximal independence and function during sitting, standing, transferring, walking, and running. Lastly, cosmetic concerns are considered. Cosmesis is influenced by personal preferences and psychosocial dynamics but is usually satisfactorily achieved using contoured foam and a nylon or rubber skin tone cover. Some individual's with an amputation prefer not to have their prosthesis covered because of the possible interference with prosthetic component function.

Medicare, a major funding source for prosthetic limbs in the United States, requires that the functional level of the individual with an amputation be taken into account when prescribing a prosthesis. The functional index is referred to as the Medicare "K" code and limits the components that can be used when fabricating the prosthesis. Although only required for Medicare, the "K" code classification is a simple but useful hierarchical framework for classifying the mobility potential of all individuals with an LE amputation (Table 61-4).

Lower Extremity Prosthetic Components

The continual introduction of new component designs and the overlap in functional features of components from various manufacturers makes it very difficult for the typical physiatrist to stay abreast of available prosthetic options. Clinical collaboration between health care providers (physician, prosthetist, and therapist) is essential in developing an appropriate, individualized limb prescription. Seldom is there a single correct choice of components for a prosthesis, rather most individuals with an amputation can be successfully fit using components that span a reasonable range of mechanical and functional characteristics. Because objective data linking prosthetic component characteristics to the demographics of individuals with

TABLE 61-3.   Transtibial Amputee Gait

Gait Cycle	Observed Gait Abnormality	Possible Cause	Suggested Modifications
Initial contact to loading response	Abrupt heel contact, rapid knee flexion	Excessive heel lever[a]	Realign posthetic foot, change heel stiffness
	Prolonged heel contact, knee remains fully extended	Inadequate heel lever[a] or heel worn out Improper socket flexion Learned gait pattern, quadriceps weakness	Increase heel stiffness Realign prosthesis, Gait training and strengthening
	Jerky knee motion	Socket loose, poor alignment, inadequate suspension	
Mid stance	Medial or lateral socket thrust, lateral trunk shift over prosthesis	Foot too far outset or inset, socket loose	Realign prosthesis, replace socket or adjust socks
	Pelvis drops or elevates	Prosthesis too short/too long	Adjust prosthetic length
Mid stance to terminal stance	Early knee flexion or "drop off"	Inadequate toe lever[a]	Realign prosthesis, replace foot
Terminal stance	Heel off too early	Excessive toe lever,[a] too much socket extension	Realign prosthesis
	Heel off excessively delayed	Inadequate toe lever, too much socket flexion	Realign prosthesis
Swing phase	Prosthetic foot drags	Prosthesis too long, inadequate suspension	Shorten limb, modify suspension
Successive double support	Uneven step length	Hip flexion contracture, gait insecurity Uncomfortable socket	Physical therapy Adjust socket fit

Transfemoral Amputee Gait

Gait Cycle	Observed Gait Abnormality	Possible Cause	Suggested Modifications
Initial contact to loading response	Foot rotation at heel strike	Poor socket fit/rotation	Adjust socket fit, add belt for rotation control
		Heel too firm	Reduce heel stiffness
	Knee buckling	Excessive heel lever Incorrect prosthetic knee alignment Weak hip extensors	Realign limb, reduce heel stiffness Realign TKA relationship Gait training and strengthening
Mid stance	Lateral trunk bend or shift over prosthesis	Prosthetic limb abducted:	
		Too much socket abduction, foot too far outset	Realign prosthesis
		Prosthesis too long	Shorten prosthesis
		Medial groin pain	Adjust socket fit
		Poor medial-lateral prosthetic control	
		Poor socket fit	Adjust socket fit
		Weak hip abductors	Gait training and strengthening
		Short residual limb	Accept, possibly add hip joint
		Prosthesis too short	Adjust prosthetic length
Initial swing	Uneven heel rise	Knee friction too tight or loose Knee extension	Adjust knee friction or damping
Swing phase	Circumduction or prosthetic limb	Inadequate knee flexion, knee too stiff Prosthesis too long, inadequate suspension Poor gait pattern	Adjust knee friction or damping Adjust prosthesis length Physical therapy
	Whips	Improper knee rotational alignment Excessive socket rotation	Realign prosthesis Adjust socket fit
Successive double support	Uneven step length	Hip flexion contracture Insufficient socket flexion	Physical therapy Realign prosthesis

[a]Causes of excessive heel lever—Foot dorsiflexed too much, foot too far posterior, heel cushion too hard, shoe heel too hard
Causes of inadequate heel lever—Foot plantarflexed too much, foot too far anterior, heel cushion too soft
Causes of excessive toe lever—Foot plantarflexed too much, foot too far anterior, foot keel too stiff
Causes of inadequate toe lever—Foot dorsiflexed too much, foot too far posterior, foot keel too soft/flexible

an amputation are limited, empiric approaches and experience play a major role in limb prescription. The prescription for an LE prosthesis should include the Medicare "K" code, diagnosis, type of prosthesis (with modifiers), socket type, liner, suspension method, foot, knee and hip systems (as required by amputation level), diagnostic or check socket, and supplies.

PROSTHETIC FEET
All prostheses for amputations at or proximal to the ankle require the use of a prosthetic foot. The selection of an appropriate prosthetic foot is complicated by the wide range of foot de-

signs, marketing-driven claims of performance, and the limited availability of objective data comparing the relative biomechanical and functional advantages of different feet. In the clinical setting, the selection of a prosthetic foot is largely empirically based on the conceptual goal of matching the functional characteristics of the foot to the expected activity needs of the individual with an amputation (40–45). Within this approach it is useful to group feet by their major functional feature(s) as belonging to rigid keel, flexible keel, single/multiaxial, or dynamic response (or energy-storing) categories. It is acceptable for the prescribing physician to define the functional features

TABLE 61-4.   Medicare Guidelines for Functional Classification of Patients with Prosthesis

K Code Level	Functional Level	Activity Level
K0	Not a potential user for ambulation or transfer	Does not have the ability or potential to ambulate or transfer safely with or without assistance and a prosthesis does not enhance their quality of life or mobility
K1	A potential household ambulator including transfers	Has the ability or potential to use a prosthesis for transfer or ambulation on level surfaces at fixed cadence. Typical of the limited and unlimited household ambulator.
K2	A potential limited community ambulatory	Has the ability or potential for ambulation with the ability to traverse low level environmental barriers such as curbs, stairs or uneven surfaces. Typical of the limited community ambulator
K3	Community ambulator using variable cadence including therapeutic exercise or vocation	Has the ability or potential for ambulation with variable cadence. Typical of the community ambulator who has the ability to traverse most environmental barriers and may have vocation, therapeutic, or exercise activity that demands prosthetic utilization beyond simple locomotion.
K4	High activity user which exceeds normal ambulation skills	Has the ability or potential for ambulation that exceeds basic ambulation skills, exhibiting high impact, stress, or energy levels. Typical of the prosthetic demands of the child, active adult, or athlete.

Source DMERC medicare Advisory Bulletin, Columbia SC, 1994;12:95–145

desired in the foot and to rely on the prosthetist who typically has a better working understanding of the commercially available feet to select the specific manufacturer and foot within the desired functional class. This multidisciplinary approach is increasingly important as foot designs become more sophisticated, more costly, and combine different functional characteristics into a single foot. Occasionally another characteristic of a foot such as an adjustable heel height, cosmesis, or being waterproof is the primary determinate in its selection.

The solid ankle cushion heel (SACH) foot (Fig. 61-2) is the least expensive and most commonly prescribed prosthetic foot. It is durable and lightweight, which accounts in part for its usefulness. The SACH foot has no moving parts and consists of a

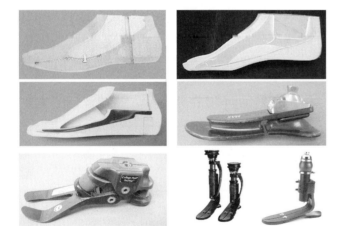

Figure 61-2. Prosthetic feet from the Single Axis Cushion Heel (SACH) and stationary-and-flexible endoskeletal (Safe II flexible keel) foot **(top)**. The Carbon Copy II Lite Foot (dynamic response) and Luxon Max (dynamic response with multi-axis) **(middle)**. The College Park TruStep (dynamic response, with some inversion, eversion, and transverse motion); the FlexFoot VSP (vertical shock pylon, dynamic response, multi-axis); and the Ceterus (vertical shock pylon, dynamic response, multi-axis, and transverse motion) **(bottom)**. The prosthetic manufacturers have numerous feet available for a wide range of patients, from homebound to paralympic. (Courtesy of Kingsley, Ohio Willow Wood, Otto Block, CPI, and Ossur. See Web Site listings.)

wooden or composite keel with a compressible foam heel and toes that flex under load allowing limited simulation of the effects of the heel and forefoot rocker mechanisms of the normal foot. A SACH foot is appropriate for individuals with an amputation who have a lower activity level (K1-K2), with ambulation primarily limited to level surfaces. It can be used in a wide range of individuals with an amputation for the preparatory prosthesis and upgraded as the individual with an amputation progresses to a higher activity level. For a juvenile with an amputation, the SACH foot is often the most cost-effective foot due to the need for frequent foot changes because of rapid growth.

The flexible keel foot (see Fig. 61-2) is designed to mimic the motion of the forefoot rocker mechanism by replacing the rigid keel of the SACH foot with a flexible keel. The keel bends with controlled stiffness as the foot moves from midstance through preswing. Several versions of flexible keel feet are commercially available, each with different construction but sharing similar function. The stationary-ankle-flexible endoskeletal (SAFE) II foot is a commonly used flexible keel foot. The flexible keel foot allows some inversion and eversion and gives a smoother rollover than a SACH foot, making it appropriate for general mobility needs in the individual with an amputation with a low to moderate activity level. However, the more active individual with an amputation may perceive the flexible keel foot as being too soft, especially for fast walking or running activities.

Articulating prosthetic feet include both single axis and multiaxis designs. The single axis foot allows controlled movement in the sagittal plane (plantar-flexion and dorsiflexion), adjusted by using different durometer bumpers. The primary advantage of the single axis foot is its ability to reduce knee-bending moments during limb loading, thus improving knee stability. Disadvantages include a greater weight than many other feet and more maintenance to ensure correct function. This foot is primarily used in the individual with a proximal amputation that requires better knee stabilization, such as the elderly individual with a transfemoral amputation or the individual with a transfemoral amputation and a short residual limb.

Multiaxial foot designs allow for varying degrees of controlled movement in the sagittal, coronal, and transverse planes (plantar/dorsiflexion, inversion/eversion, some degree of transverse rotation). Multiaxis feet can use mechanical joints to supply motion such as the Greissinger foot or the College Park foot (see Fig. 61-2), but increasingly rely on the inherent flexibility of rubber and polymer materials to provide multiaxial motion. Using flexible materials improves durability and reduces both weight and maintenance compared to mechanical jointed feet. Multiaxis "ankle" motion can be integrated into the foot (e.g., Endolite foot, Luxon) or added to other feet through the use of separate multiaxial ankle components (e.g., EarthWalk Ankle, Ohio Willow Wood, Mt. Sterling, OH). Multiaxis capabilities are appropriate for the individual with an amputation who needs improved ankle motion to accommodate uneven terrain and for the active individual with an amputation who requires greater ankle movement to adjust to different speeds or for cutting and pivoting quickly.

Dynamic response (i.e., energy-storing) prosthetic feet incorporate elastic (springlike) elements that store energy in the foot during limb loading and midstance as the elastic material compresses or flexes. Energy is returned at the time of push-off as the spring component of the foot returns to its normal shape or configuration. Examples include the Flex-Foot, the Springlite feet, Seattle foot, and the Carbon Copy II feet (see Fig. 61-2). The dynamic energy characteristics of these feet make them particularly suitable for individuals with an amputation involved in activities requiring running and jumping. Many individuals with an amputation believe that they are more functional with a dynamic response foot. Dynamic elastic response (DER) feet were expected to make ambulation more efficient by reducing the oxygen consumption of individuals with an amputation but the results of objective studies have been mixed (44,46). The metabolic benefits of DER designs are limited and primarily seen at faster walking speeds.

Prosthesis by Level of Amputation

PARTIAL FOOT AMPUTATIONS

Toe amputations, ray resections, and transmetatarsal amputations are highly functional amputations that require minimal prosthetic/orthotic intervention. At the more distal foot amputation levels and for the less active individual with a transmetatarsal amputation, accommodative shoes with custom insoles, arch supports, and toe fillers are usually adequate. More active individuals with a transmetatarsal amputation may benefit from orthotic modifications that better substitute for the lost anterior foot lever arm. Options include the addition of carbon fiber or spring steel sole shanks, rocker soles, or short ankle foot orthosis. Partial foot amputations at the tarsal-metatarsal and transtarsal levels (e.g., Lisfranc, Chopart) are relatively uncommon and have historically been associated with equinovarus contracture of the hindfoot, increasing the likelihood of skin breakdown over the plantar surface of the foot. However, improved surgical techniques that include Achilles tendon lengthening/resection and anterior tibialis and peroneus tendon transfers have reduced equinovarus deformities and result in a functional and useful amputation level (47, 48). Prosthetic/orthotic devices for the individual with a proximal partial foot amputation need to supply medial-lateral stabilization of the hindfoot and substitute for the lost forefoot lever. Options include: (a) an extra-depth shoe with toe filler, steel shank, and rocker bottom modifications; (b) custom posterior leaf-spring ankle-foot orthosis with toe filler; or (c) a custom prosthetic foot with a self-suspending rear-opening split socket (47,48). A major advantage of all partial foot amputa-

tions is the ability to be fully end-bearing, allowing ambulation without any devices.

SYME AMPUTATION

Similar to the hindfoot amputation, the Syme (tibiotarsal disarticulation) amputation is capable of full weight end bearing. The heel flap is anchored to the distal end of the tibia and fibula, and following healing, allows short distance ambulation without a prosthesis. The substantial leg length discrepancy makes long distance ambulation impractical. Over time, posterior migration of the distal heel pad occurs in some individuals with a Syme amputation leading to problems with skin breakdown and difficulty in prosthetic fitting (49–51). The relatively bulbous distal end of the residual limb has the advantage of enabling the use of self-suspending prosthetic designs, however it also contributes to the major disadvantage of the Syme amputation—poor cosmesis due to the bulkiness of the prosthesis around the ankle joint. There are several different types of prostheses available for individuals with a Syme amputation.

The most common prosthetic style uses a total contact socket with a removable medial window (Fig. 61-3). The distal removable medial window allows the bulbous portion of the residual to slip easily into the socket, which is then held in place by closing and securing the window with Velcro straps. The major disadvantages to this prosthesis style are the poor cosmesis and the reduced strength of the socket due to the window. A second option uses a fixed posterior opening socket. The type of prosthesis is used for a very bulbous residual limb. This prosthesis is prone to breakage at the ankle joint and is not recommended for heavy-duty users.

Alternative designs to windowed sockets use a flexible socket wall or liner to allow donning the prosthesis around the distal bulbous end of the residual limb. In the "stovepipe" design, a pelite or similar liner is used that is built up proximal to the ankle area, creating a cylindrical stovepipe-shaped inner liner. To don the prosthesis the patient slips the distal bulbous residual past the narrow center of the liner that then can be easily inserted into the socket. This style of prosthesis is somewhat bulky but can be easily modified and is durable, making it suitable for use as a preparatory prosthesis or in active or obese patients.

The expandable wall prosthesis uses a double-wall socket that has a flexible, expandable inside liner and a rigid outer frame. The inner wall is made of silicone or other elastomers that are flexible enough to allow the bulbous residual limb to slide into the prosthesis. This prosthesis is typically difficult to modify but has the advantage of being very strong and useful

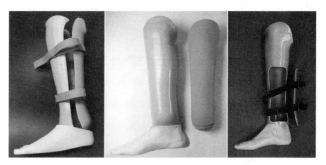

Figure 61-3. From left to right: The posterior opening Symes for bulbous distal end; patella tendon-bearing (PTB) Symes with Pelite liner; Canadian-type Syme prosthesis as modified by the Veterans Administration Prosthetic Center. (Courtesy of PSL Fabrication, Fulton, MO.)

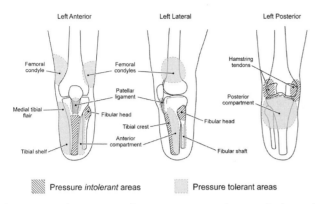

Figure 61-4. Showing areas that are pressure intolerant and tolerant for modification and fabrication of a specific weight-bearing (SWB) or patella tendon-bearing (PTB) socket.

for active users or obese patients and is generally easy to don and doff, making it suitable for individuals with upper limb impairment or cognitive impairment.

Low-profile feet are needed for Syme prosthesis due to the limited space available beneath the socket. Acceptable foot options range from the rigid keel SACH feet through multiaxial and dynamic response feet.

TRANSTIBIAL AMPUTATIONS

Transtibial amputations are the most common amputation level seen in the general practice. Considerable effort over the past several decades has gone into designing components to address the needs of individuals with transtibial amputations. The large number of options available increases uncertainty when choosing components but if approached systematically, straightforward reasoned decisions can be used to generate a prosthetic prescription. The following discussion of transtibial prosthetic components is organized to parallel a recommended approach for prescribing prostheses. Initially the socket and liner system that is anticipated to optimize comfort and skin

protection is determined. Next, the suspension system is chosen and finally pylon and foot/ankle components are selected.

The patella tendon-bearing (PTB) total contact socket has been the internationally accepted standard transtibial socket since the 1960s (52). The PTB total contact socket is fabricated from a cast of the residual limb which has been modified to direct weight bearing to specific regions that are pressure tolerant and correspondingly modified to decrease pressure over bony prominences such as the tibia crest, fibula, and distal portion of the tibia (Fig. 61-4).

The standard PTB total contact design has several variations (53–55). The PTB total contact-supracondylar (PTB-SC) socket has high medial and lateral sidewalls that extend above and over the femoral condyles, providing enhanced mediolateral stability and self-suspension of the prosthesis. The PTB total contact-supracondylar/suprapatellar (PTB-SCSP) socket further extends the PTB-SC socket concept by also extending the anterior aspect of the socket so that the patellar is encompassed within the socket. The PTB-SCSP gives additional stiffness to the mediolateral walls and applies force proximal to the patella during stance to provide sensory feedback to limit genu recurvatum. Both the PTB-SC and PTB-SCSP are primarily used in individuals with an amputation with short residual limbs to improve varus/valgus control and to provide greater surface area for weight distribution (Fig. 61-5).

An alternative socket design for individuals with a transtibial amputation is the total surface-bearing (TSB) socket made practical by the development of gel and elastomeric liner systems (discussed below). The TSB socket is made from a cast of the residual limb that has minimal modifications. When used with gel liners the TSB socket is believed to distribute pressure more uniformly within the socket. The relative advantages and disadvantages of TSB versus PTB total contact sockets remain poorly understood. When a comfortable fit cannot be achieved with one style of socket, empirically switching to the other can be successful.

Socket fit coupled with the choice of a liner are key considerations in assuring comfort and acceptance of the prosthetic limb. The liner functions as the primary interface between the residual limb and the remainder of the prosthesis. In this role it

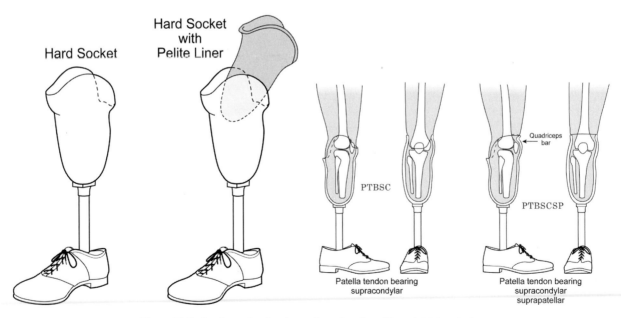

Figure 61-5. Patella tendon-bearing style sockets (specific weight- bearing).

must complement socket fit to ensure optimal pressure distribution while also eliminating harmful shear forces and providing a favorable moisture, heat, and chemical environment that prevents skin breakdown. PTB total contact sockets can be fit as hard sockets that do not use a liner or more commonly use a liner made from closed cell foam such as pelite for improved comfort. Using PTB total contact sockets and pelite liners are often an advantage in the preparatory prosthesis because of the relative ease with which the liner can be modified to accommodate changes in residual limb volume (52,55,56). Roll-on silicone or elastomeric gel liners are another option that can be used with a PTB total contact socket but are generally recommended for use with TSB socket designs. Gel liners are thought to enhance comfort and reduce shear, making them the initial choice for residual limbs with scarring or skin grafts that compromise skin integrity (52,56). Gel liners result in more sweating and are generally tolerated less in warm climates than other liners. Contraindications to the use of gel liners are residual limbs with open wounds, poor hygiene, or a history of contact dermatitis.

The suspension system for the transtibial prosthesis must securely attach the limb during all anticipated activities, minimize pistoning, and be comfortable when sitting. When working with individuals with an amputation who run, play sports, or are involved in climbing activities, ensuring effective suspension is especially important. Suspension systems can be grouped into categories that include straps, sleeves, gel liners with locking mechanisms, and suction (Fig. 61-6). A commonly used suspension system is the supracondylar cuff strap. Several variants exist, all of which consist of a multipart strap that attaches to sidewalls of the socket and encircles the distal thigh using the normal anatomic flare of the supracondylar portion of the femur to maintain suspension. The supracondylar strap is inexpensive, easily applied, and is comfortable during sitting. It supplies adequate suspension for the low-to- moderate activity-level individual with an amputation and is often the best option when impaired hand function limits grip strength and coordination. Waist belts with an anterior fork strap that attaches to the socket are a rarely used suspension option. This type of suspension is most commonly used in conjunction with a PTB total contact socket with side joint and a high corset. The weight and bulk of the resulting limb makes it a poor initial choice for a contemporary prosthetic limb, but it does remain a useful option for long-term users of this style of prosthesis.

Other individuals with an amputation that may benefit from this type of limb are those with a short transtibial amputation who require maximal medial-lateral stability for outdoor or work activities. This type of limb may also be preferred when coexisting ligamentous instability of the knee is present, or to partially off load a painful or weight-intolerant residual limb.

Sleeve suspension systems consist of rubber, neoprene, or elastic sleeves that are pulled up onto the distal thigh after donning the prosthesis (56). Sleeves are a general purpose suspension system that is inexpensive and effective for individuals with an amputation across a wide spectrum of activity levels. The primary disadvantages are related to excessive heat or sweating, the need for good grip strength to pull the sleeve up, and the occasional occurrence of contact dermatitis, especially with the use of neoprene-based sleeves. Silicone and elastomeric gel liners are prosthetic sock-shaped sleeves made from a variety of silicone and urethane elastomeric compounds that are rolled onto the residual limb. They function as both an interface and suspension method. The suspension function requires either a metal pin attached to the distal end of the liner which inserts into a locking mechanism in the bottom of the socket or by a Velcro lanyard strap that passes through a slot in the socket and mates with its counterpart attached to the outside of the socket. The suspension pin or lanyard securely anchors the liner to the socket, and the subsequent friction and suction that develops between the liner and the residual limb supplies the force required for suspension (Fig. 61-7). This approach provides excellent suspension for a wide range of activities and is increasingly being used as a general purpose suspension system. The main disadvantages to gel liners are their high cost compared to straps or sleeves and their limited durability, which necessitates replacement of the liners every 6 to 12 months. In the presence of loose or excessive soft tissue in the residual limb, elongation and stretching of the distal tissues during swing phase can occur that may lead to pain.

The last option for suspension of the transtibial prosthesis uses suction. By combining a one-way air valve ported to the bottom of the socket with an airtight sleeve, a partial vacuum is created within the socket, effectively suspending the prosthesis during swing phase (57). The vacuum needed to hold the residual limb can be generated through a pistoning action of the residual limb within the socket or by vacuum pump built into the prosthetic shank that is activated at heel strike. This latter

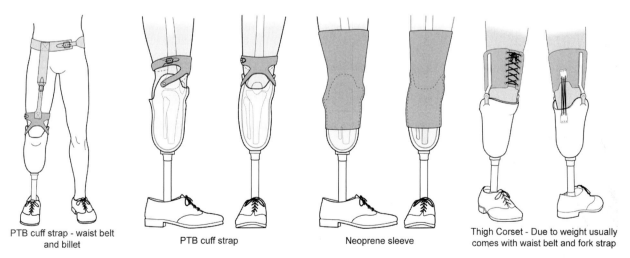

PTB cuff strap - waist belt and billet

PTB cuff strap

Neoprene sleeve

Thigh Corset - Due to weight usually comes with waist belt and fork strap

Figure 61-6. Showing suspension systems used for the transtibial prosthesis.

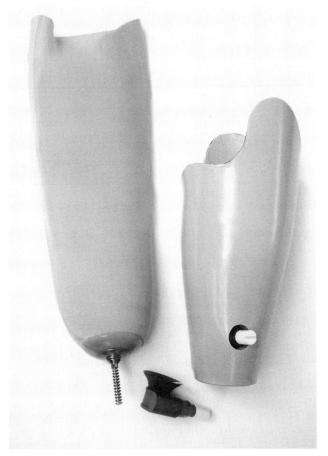

Figure 61-7. Total surface-bearing (TSB) socket with gel liner and pin system. If pin or lanyard system is not being used then the socket will be held on by a suspension sleeve.

option is known as vacuum-assisted socket suspension (VASS) (Fig. 61-8).

Most contemporary prostheses are endoskeletal in design. Using an endoskeletal pylon allows alignment changes after prosthetic fabrication and enables the use of additional components that can absorb forces or allow motion between the socket and the remainder of residual limb. Commonly used

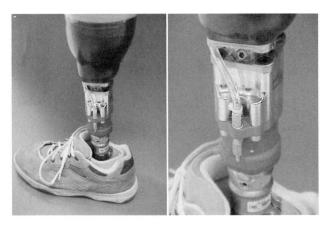

Figure 61-8. Vacuum-assisted socket suspension (VASS) works by use of a vertical shock pylon that acts like a vacuum pump and continually withdraws air from the sealed socket while ambulating. (Courtesy of Otto Bock, see Web site listing)

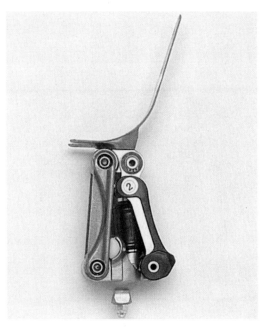

Figure 61-9. The 3R46 modular polycentric knee joint for knee disarticulation. (Courtesy of Otto Bock, see Web site listing.)

components include transverse rotators that reduce axial torques and vertical shock absorbers that cushion impact loading and may reduce oxygen consumption (46,58). The selection of a prosthetic foot completes the transtibial prosthesis prescription.

KNEE DISARTICULATION

Knee disarticulation (KD) amputations share some of the same advantages and disadvantages as the Syme amputation (ankle disarticulation) (59). Similar to the Syme amputation, full weight bearing on the distal end of the KD residual limb is usually possible and the anatomic flare of the femoral condyles can be used for self-suspension of the prosthesis. Because of the improved distal weight bearing, the KD amputation does not require an ischial weight-bearing socket leading to enhanced comfort and sitting tolerance as does a transfemoral amputation. The KD has a bulbous distal end, which compromises prosthetic cosmesis. Compared to the individual with a transfemoral amputation, the long length of the KD residual improves prosthetic control and allows a greater degree of dynamic muscular stability. However, the long residual limb limits the choice of prosthetic knee units that can be used to maintain symmetric knee centers between the amputated and nonamputated side. Advances in the design and development of the four-bar linkage knee units (Fig. 61-9) offer good biomechanical function and acceptable limb cosmesis. KD, while an uncommon amputation level, is reemerging as an alternative to the transfemoral amputation when wound healing concerns are acceptable because of the improved sitting balance, reduced energy cost of walking, and better acceptance rate than that for a transfemoral amputation (60).

TRANSFEMORAL AMPUTATIONS

The development of new technology, materials, and prosthetic components over the past decade has arguably had the greatest impact on the care of the individual with an amputation at the transfemoral level. The following discussion of transfemoral prosthetic components is organized to parallel a reasonable approach to prescribing a prosthesis. Initially the socket style is

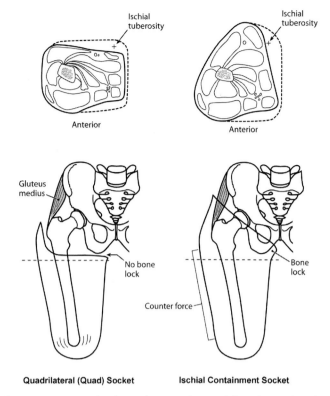

Figure 61-10. Note the shapes between the quadrilateral (Quad) socket and the ischial containment socket (ICS). Also note the ischium sits inside the ICS socket rather than the socket brim (as does the quad socket).

specified. Next the residual limb interface/liner and suspension system are determined. Because liner and suspension options are closely linked at the transfemoral level, they are discussed together. Following selection of socket and suspension, the knee unit is selected and finally pylon and foot/ankle components are chosen.

The quadrilateral socket introduced following World War II had been the standard socket design for transfemoral prostheses until the emergence of a new socket design, the ischial containment socket (ICS) during the past 15 years. The quadrilateral socket, named for its quadrilateral shape as viewed in the transverse plane, is designed for ischial weight bearing on the posterior brim. Quadrilateral sockets are still used for long-term wearers who have become accustomed to its weight-bearing and control characteristics but also remain an option for the individual with a transfemoral amputation with a long residual limb and for individuals who require UE aids for trunk stability (61) (Fig. 61-10). However, for the majority of individuals with new transfemoral amputations, the ICS is believed to provide a more normal anatomic alignment of the femur inside the prosthesis. This is accomplished by extending the socket trimlines proximal and contouring the medial aspect of the socket to capture the ischial tuberosity inside the socket rather than allowing the tuberosity to sit on the posterior brim as in the quadrilateral socket. The ICS allows more effective hip and pelvic stabilizing forces to be developed during stance phase (61–63) which improve medial-lateral control of the trunk. While the ICS is useful for all individuals with transfemoral amputations, the improved stability is especially beneficial for those with a short residual limb.

Several variants of the ICS have been introduced that include the normal shape-normal alignment, contoured adducted trochanter-controlled alignment method, the Sabolich,

and the Northwestern ICS (61–65). These options vary somewhat in contour details but all retain the basic functional characteristics of the ICS. No clear consensus has emerged favoring one-design variant over the others but all require considerable skill to fabricate correctly. Both ISC and quadrilateral sockets can be fabricated as a rigid socket or by using a flexible thermoplastic inner socket supported by graphite-reinforced, laminated open framework (66,67). The advantages of the rigid frame-flexible liner type of socket designs are flexible walls that increase comfort especially at the proximal brim, improved proprioception, accommodation of minor volume changes, less heat buildup, and enhanced suspension as the inner socket warms during use, increasing its flexibility and improving the intimacy of the fit (63).

A number of interface liner systems and suspension options exist for the transfemoral prosthesis (Fig. 61-11) (56). The simplest liner system uses a hard socket with wool or cotton socks adjusted in plies to achieve a comfortable fit. Suspension for this type of prosthesis most commonly uses a Silesian belt or total elastic suspension (TES) belt. The Silesian belt attaches to the anterior and lateral portions of the proximal prosthetic socket and passes over the opposite iliac crest. The TES belt is made of the same neoprene material used for transtibial suspension sleeves. It slips over the outside of the prosthetic socket and surrounds the waist above the iliac crests to provide suspension. Both Silesian and TES suspension systems are simple to don, can be adapted for use by individuals with impaired hand function, and usually provide acceptable prosthetic limb suspension for low activity-level patients. Disadvantages include some inevitable pistoning of the prosthesis, reduced comfort due to bandage pressure, and heat or occasional dermatitis, especially with the TES belt. The TES and Silesian suspension systems can be used as a primary suspension system or coupled with other suspension options (discussed below) as an axillary suspension system when additional suspension security or rotation control is needed. Other suspension belt options include the pelvic band and hip joint. This option uses a single-axis hip joint integrated into the lateral socket wall, which is attached to a pelvic band and belt closely contoured about the iliac crest. The side joint and band discourage rotation of the prosthesis and extend the lateral lever arm stabilizing the prosthesis, making it especially useful for the short residual transfemoral prosthesis.

Suction socket suspension is the second major type of suspension for the individual with a transfemoral amputation and, whenever feasible, is generally the preferred option (56). Suction sockets are total contact sockets worn directly against the skin of the residual limb that incorporate a one-way air valve in the distal socket. To don the prosthesis, the individual with an amputation has to pull the residual limb into the socket. This can be accomplished using an elastic stockinette, an Ace bandage, or an "EZ pull" sock made from a thin slippery nylon fabric. An alternative method to pull socks uses a "wet fit" process in which a liquid powder is applied to the residual limb, temporarily lubricating the skin, which can then be slipped into the socket. Once the socket is donned, the suction valve is installed and the remaining air expelled through the valve, creating a small vacuum that holds the socket on the limb. For most users, suction suspension provides a very secure and comfortable suspension effect free from external belts or straps. Suction suspension requires a stable residual limb volume, and as a result is not a good option for preparatory prostheses when rapid limb shrinkage is expected. The presence of scar tissue can compromise the ability to maintain suction and may be poorly tolerated by the inherent high skin friction present in the socket. Prostheses that use suction sockets

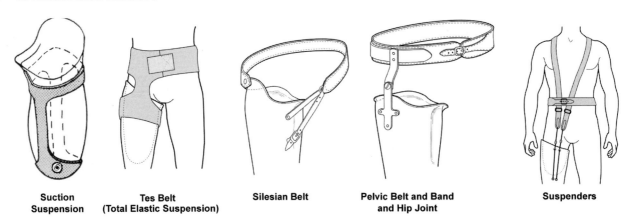

Suction Suspension   **Tes Belt (Total Elastic Suspension)**   **Silesian Belt**   **Pelvic Belt and Band and Hip Joint**   **Suspenders**

Figure 61-11. Showing possible suspensions that could be used for the transfemoral amputee.

must be donned while standing and require both good balance and adequate hand strength and coordination to manipulate the pull sock and to install the valve. Difficulty with consistently pulling all of the proximal soft tissues of the thigh into the socket can lead to an adductor roll (a compression of the soft tissues of the medial groin between the proximal socket and the pelvis) that is painful and can lead to skin breakdown. Correcting this problem may require socket modifications, changes to the donning technique, or the use of external vacuum pumps to help elongate the tissue of the residual limb to promote a better fit (68).

A variant of the hard socket uses hypobaric socks, conventional limb socks with an impregnated silicone band near the proximal end of the sock. The silicone band provides a seal to prevent air leak, allowing for a partial suction suspension effect that, when coupled with an auxiliary Silesian suspension or TES, is an alternative option to the standard suction socket that can accommodate changing residual limb volume secondary to limb shrinkage or weight change.

Similar to a transtibial prosthesis, silicone and elastomeric gel suspension liners with a lanyard strap or pin attachment can be used to provide a beltless pseudosuction type of suspension. This suspension system provides good suspension, minimal pistoning, effective control of adductor rolls, and good comfort across a wide range of activity levels. Socks can be added over the suspension liner to accommodate for volume change of the residual limb. Effective use of gel liners can be problematic in the residual limb with excess or loose soft tissue because of difficulties in consistently donning the liner, excessive traction on soft tissue during swing, and poor rotational control of the prosthesis. The use of auxiliary TES or Silesian suspension may be needed in this situation.

During the last decade, a wide variety of prosthetic knee joints have been designed, fabricated, and made commercially available. A recent survey cataloged over 200 knee units that were used over the past decade, ranging from the simple single-axis knee joints to the completely computerized knee unit. The primary purposes of the prosthetic knee are to provide stability during stance (to prevent knee buckling), either through alignment or mechanical means, knee motion during swing to permit clearance of the toe, and adequate flexion to allow the knee to bend when sitting. The knee unit should control the heel rise of the shank, assisting or resisting the acceleration and deceleration of the shank during swing phase. The selection of an appropriate knee unit is primarily based on matching the stance phase stability features and the swing control aspects of the knee to the anticipated activity level and usage of the prosthesis (69–71). Hydraulic or pneumatic knee units are used for

the K3 and K4 individual with an amputation and provide either swing phase control or swing and stance phase control for individuals who change their cadence frequently. For the K1 or K2 individual with an amputation who has difficulty maintaining knee stability during stance, locking knees and weight-activated–stance control knees are available. The four-bar, five-bar, and six-bar knee units are becoming increasingly popular due to the moveable centroid (Fig. 61-12), which gives better stabil-

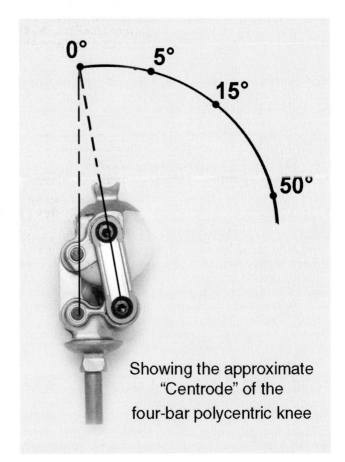

Showing the approximate "Centrode" of the four-bar polycentric knee

Figure 61-12. The approximate instant center of rotation (centrode) of the 3R36 polycentric knee joint. Once the knee starts to bend, the centrode moves anterior making the knee easier to bend. The more posterior and proximal the centrode, the more stable the knee becomes. Most four bar knees can be adjusted for different amputee requirements. (Courtesy of Otto Bock, see Web site listing.)

TABLE 61-5. General Information on Prosthetic Knees and Usage

Type of Knee	Advantage	Disadvantage	Possible Usage
Single axis constant friction	Simple Durable Low-maintenance	Only constant swing phase control. No stance control Single Cadence	Excellent for pediatrics Having good voluntary control of swing and stance phase but single cadence
Polycentric (not fluid control)	Varying stability through stance. Shortens shank during swing for better toe clearance. While sitting some give natural and better cosmetic appearance.	Increased weight and bulk Complex mechanism Single Cadence	Knee disartics Long transfemoral for appearance and short transfemoral for knee stability Weak hip extensors
Weight-activated– stance control	Do not have adequate control to manage a bending knee or good enough hip control to stabilize Braking mechanism if weight applied with knee flexed 0–20 degrees Helpful to slower clients.	Requires regular maintenance. Not very responsive for active walker. Gail modified to unload knee Single Cadence	Geriatrics Short residual limb General debility Uneven surfaces
Manual lock	Total stability in stance phase.	No swing phase flexion, resulting in stiff knee gait Awkward in sitting	Patient requires mechanical stability in stance Last resort
Fluid Control			
Single axis pneumatic control	Responds to changing gait speeds.	Higher cost May need more maintenance Heavier	From pediatrics to adults with go control
Single axis hydraulic control	Swing respond to changing gait speeds. If Stance phase has hydraulic resistance to knee flexion during weight bearing	Higher cost May need more maintenance Heavier	From pediatrics to adults with go control Excellent reliability. For the more active amputee
Polycentric & multi-axis fluid control	Varying stability through stance. Shortens shank during swing for better toe clearance. While sitting some give natural and better cosmetic appearance. Variable cadence	Higher cost May need more maintenance Heavier	Knee disartics Long transfemoral for appearance and short transfemoral for knee stability Range from homebound to highly active amputee
Microprocessor Control			
Single axis or multi-axis fluid control	On board computer adjusting knee for variable gait cycles. Energy saving	Highest cost Heavy Unproven track record for dependability	For the more active patients. Some computerized knees use a computer-regulated valve to adjust the swing phase resistance of a pneumatic cylinder. Some use the computer to control swing phase function and stance phase stability. Some systems using multiple sensors to send messages about changes walking back to the microchip 50 times a second.

ity of the knee. Table 61-5 outlines the major types of knee joints and their advantages and disadvantages.

The same pylon components (vertical shock pylons and rotators) that are available for the individual with an amputation at the transtibial level are also available at the transfemoral level. In addition, a thigh rotator can be added for the individual with a transfemoral amputation who has a need to cross the prosthetic leg for ADLs (i.e., riding in a car, donning and doffing clothing or shoes, etc.) (Fig. 61-13).

HIP DISARTICULATION/HEMIPELVECTOMY
Individuals with a transfemoral amputation with less than 5 cm of residual femur usually are fitted at hip disarticulation level. The standard prosthesis for a hip disarticulation is the Canadian hip disarticulation prosthesis (Fig. 61-14). The socket of this prosthesis encloses the hemipelvis on the side of the amputation and extends around the hemipelvis of the nonamputated side, leaving an opening for the nonamputated LE. There is a flexible anterior wall with an opening that allows the prosthesis to be donned. Weight is borne on the ischial tuberosity of the amputated side. Endoskeletal prosthetic components are preferred for this level of amputation to reduce the overall weight. The endoskeletal hip joint has an extension assist, as does the knee unit, which usually is a constant-friction knee. Endoskeletal components may be made from aluminum, titanium, or carbon graphite composite materials. Traditionally, a single-axis or SACH foot with a soft heel has been the most common choice for the prosthetic foot. The newer lightweight

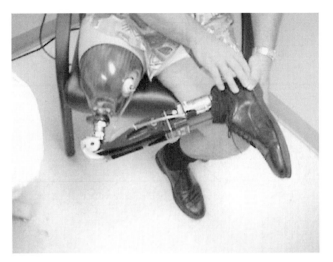

Figure 61-13. Showing rotator adaptor for rotation to allow better access for donning and doffing clothing or comfort while in a vehicle. (Courtesy of Otto Bock, see Web site listing.)

foot/ankle combination such as the Endolite foot/ankle complex or the Endolite ankle with a Seattle Lite foot may be a better option for this level. A cosmetic cover completes the prosthetic prescription. If necessary, locking hip or knee joints can be used.

The prosthesis for a hemipelvectomy resembles that for the hip disarticulation except in the interior configuration of the

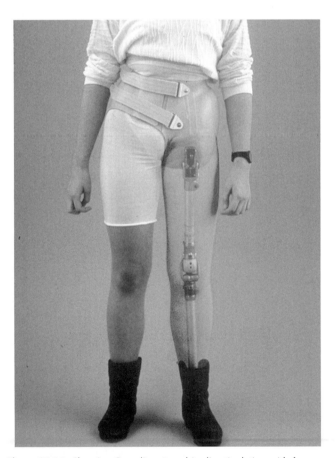

Figure 61-14. Showing Canadian stype hip disarticulation with free motion hip joint and four bar knee with outline of cover. (Courtesy of Otto Bock, see Web site listing.)

socket. In the hemipelvectomy, most of the weight is borne by the soft tissues on the amputated side, with some of the weight being borne by the sacrum, the rib cage, and the opposite ischial tuberosity.

Hemicorporectomy

Although rare, the hemicorporectomy (HCP), or translumbar amputation, has the most significant physiologic and psychologic implications. During this procedure the bony pelvis, pelvic contents, lower extremities, and external genitalia are removed following disarticulation of the lumbar spine and transection of the spinal cord. HCP is usually a last resort for patients with life-threatening conditions such as advanced pelvic tumors, pelvic osteomyelitis, crushing pelvic trauma, or intractable decubiti in the pelvic region. Once the amputation site is adequately healed then a prosthetist should begin fabrication of the prosthesis.

The prosthesis is bucket-shaped with two cut apertures to accommodate the patient's colostomy and ileostomy sites. This type of prosthesis is similar to those used in other cases of HCP (72). When first using the prosthesis the patient must be limited in the use and allow frequent checks for skin breakdown for the next several weeks. At first, the base of the prosthesis is attached to a flat board to provide a level seating surface and possibly later replaced with a rocker type board for greater mobility when transferring to and from a wheelchair and promoting easier wheelchair use.

UPPER EXTREMITY AMPUTATION

General Principles of Upper Extremity Amputation Management

The general approach to the care of the individual with a UE amputation parallels that used in treating a lower limb amputation outlined earlier in this chapter. The main differences will be highlighted and areas of unique management discussed.

PREPROSTHETIC PATIENT EVALUATION AND MANAGEMENT
The preprosthetic evaluation, whether performed preoperatively or postoperatively, should focus on identifying factors that will interfere with rehabilitation and prosthetic fitting. Of particular importance is the presence of coexisting musculoskeletal or neurologic compromise such as significant shoulder range of motion loss or brachial plexus injury that would seriously compromise or prevent the successful use of a prosthesis. Initial education about the rehabilitation process, prosthetic options, and a discussion of realistic expectations should occur during this stage.

POSTOPERATIVE CARE
The options for postoperative care of the residual limb are similar to those used in the LE. Soft dressings along with stump shrinkers or elastic compressive stockinettes are the most commonly used wound care approach. In centers with experience in the application of removable rigid dressings (RRDs), their use in the immediate and early postoperative period is advocated because of presumed benefits of better residual limb protection, edema control, and pain reduction. RRDs work best at the transradial amputation level because of the ease in suspending the cast. An additional advantage of RRDs is the ability to implement immediate or early postprosthetic fitting by attaching a hook, harness, and control system to the cast. Early

prosthetic fitting is particularly important for the individual with a bilateral UE amputation to avoid the potentially profound psychology consequences resulting from the complete dependence that accompanies the loss of both UEs.

PROSTHETIC FITTING

Even more so than in the individual with an LE amputation, an understanding of the individual's vocational and avocational needs, motivation in pursuing prosthetic fitting, availability of a supportive social network, and cosmetic concerns are critical in goal setting and decision making regarding prosthetic prescription. There are no fixed guidelines for deciding which individual with an upper limb amputation will benefit from a prosthetic limb. Factors that often prevent successful fitting and training include significant cognitive deficits, upper motor neuron syndromes that impair volitional coordination of the residual limb, plexopathies or peripheral nerve injuries, significant sensory loss, hyperpathia of the residual limb, or range of motion loss in the shoulder. The typical sequence of prosthetic rehabilitation involves initial fitting and training with a body-powered preparatory prostheses followed by a definite prosthesis when residual limb maturation has occurred 3 to 6 months postsurgery. Advantages of using a body-powered preparatory prosthesis include the greater ease of fitting, greater adaptability to changes in residual limb volume, early training in ADLs, and a lower cost compared to external powered devices. Since it is difficult to predict either the likelihood of long-term acceptance of an upper limb prosthesis or an individual's preferred type of prosthetic system (body or external powered), the preparatory prosthetic phase should be used to explore various prosthetic options. Different types of terminal devices should be tried and the individual with a UE amputation given enough time to explore the advantages and disadvantages of using the prosthesis in a variety of home, work, and social settings. This type of clinical trial allows more informed decision making and participation of the patient at the time of definitive prosthetic prescription.

The overall acceptance and continued use of a prosthetic limb is influenced by a number of factors (73–76). Similar to the LE, as the amputation level moves more proximal, the prosthetic rejection rate increases. The majority of individuals with an amputation at the shoulder disarticulation or forequarter level ultimately reject prostheses. Approximately 40% of individual with a transhumeral amputation become long-term users of a prosthetic limb. At the transradial amputation level, approximately 90% of individuals continue to use a prosthesis at least on an occasional basis. More distal amputations in the hand have a lower rate of prosthetic limb acceptance, typically because of the greater preserved function of the residual limb. Individuals with bilateral amputations at all levels tend to have a higher acceptance rate for prosthetic limb use. Early work by Malone (73) indicated that early fitting within 30 days postoperatively was associated with higher long-term acceptance. More recent studies (74,75) have not shown as strong a correlation, suggesting that even delayed fitting can be successful. Common reasons for rejecting a prosthetic limb include limited usefulness, excessive weight, residual limb pain, and poor durability (myoelectric prosthesis).

FINAL PROSTHETIC EVALUATION AND CONTROL TRAINING

Prosthetic training is an important component of the rehabilitation process and affects the successful use and acceptance of the prosthesis (77). General strengthening and range of motion exercises for the proximal residual limb started in the preprosthetic phase should continue. After the prosthesis has been fabricated, it should be checked by the members of the prosthetic team to make sure that the fit is comfortable and that the control system is properly adjusted for maximum functional operation. During initial use and training, the prosthesis should be removed every 15 to 30 minutes to check for signs of excessive pressure or irritation that may occur with poor socket fit or overuse. As skin tolerance increases, wearing time is gradually increased during the first few days of wear and thereafter more quickly. With a well-fitting prosthesis, an individual with a UE amputation can wear the limb for an entire day within a week or two of receiving it.

Specific training involves instruction in how to put on and remove the prosthesis, adjusting the number of sock plies, and how to clean and care for the residual limb and prosthesis. Initial skills are acquired to control the terminal device and to activate position and lock the elbow in the individual with a transhumeral amputation. Grasping and releasing objects, transferring objects, and positioning of the terminal device for functional activities should be practiced under the guidance and feedback of an experienced therapist. ADLs, homemaking, and occupational and recreational activities should be undertaken and simulated in the training sessions. Successful prosthetic users rely on basic skills learned in therapy, which are supplemented and polished by practice at home during everyday tasks. The individual who is long-term experienced in the use of the upper limb often has very specific use patterns and preferences for components, harness type, and control cable adjustments. It is prudent to incorporate the desires of the individual into the decision-making and prescription process.

Control training for externally powered prostheses is more complex than for body-powered UE prostheses. The same goals as outlined for conventional prostheses are appropriate for myoelectric controlled prostheses. In addition, the individual must learn to separate, modulate, and sustain voluntary muscle contractions in the muscles selected to control the powered functions of the prosthesis. Training with an externally powered (electric) prosthesis often requires more time than with a body-powered prosthesis because more exacting individual muscle motions and quantity of muscle contraction are required for control of the prosthesis.

Adults and older children can be expected to practice specific tasks and routines both in therapy and at home as outlined by the therapist to achieve the necessary skills for independent function. The training time in a young child with a UE prosthesis will be significantly longer than that for an adult or older child.

UPPER EXTREMITY PROSTHETIC FOLLOW-UP

The routine follow-up visits for an individual with a new amputation should occur initially 4 to 6 weeks after delivery of the prosthesis, then every 2 to 6 months until a definite prosthesis is prescribed. Once clinically stable in a definitive prosthesis, yearly clinic visits or whenever a problem arises is usually adequate. At these follow-up visits, the individual's use and function with the prosthesis should be reviewed, any difficulties or problems resolved, the fit and condition of the prosthesis evaluated, and the condition of the residual limb noted. If necessary, additional therapy may be suggested, repairs to the prosthesis made, medical problems with the residual limb addressed, and a new prosthesis prescribed if indicated. With average use, an UE prosthesis can be expected to be worn for 3 to 5 years before total replacement is necessary. The socket itself may need to be replaced more frequently than the other components.

Although our emphasis has been on prosthetic restoration, the focus of rehabilitation should remain on the individual with the UE amputation and his or her desired lifestyle following limb loss. Many individuals with a UE amputation do well without the aid of a prosthesis and should not be viewed as having failed if they choose not to wear a prosthesis.

BILATERAL UPPER EXTREMITY AMPUTATIONS

The individual with a bilateral UE amputation is immediately faced with the loss of ability to perform almost every ADL. Early restoration of any ADL is important. Providing a utensil cuff, which can be attached to a residual arm, can assist the patient with feeding and tooth brushing. In the individual with a bilateral UE amputation, early prosthetic fitting should be accomplished, even with temporary or preparatory prostheses. In the individual with a bilateral amputation, the longer residual limb usually assumes dominance. Special component considerations apply in this case. Wrist flexion units, at least on the dominant side or perhaps bilaterally, will permit midline activities such as shirt buttoning, belt buckling, and toileting. Also wrist rotator units, which provide terminal device positioning, provide for easier bilateral prosthetic use. Special toileting techniques must be taught for patient independence. In addition, foot skills should be reviewed, and LE mobilizing exercises should be performed.

Upper Extremity Prostheses

A UE prosthesis attempts to replace very complex functions. The hand is able to perform a wide range of functional activities ranging from fine dexterity tasks requiring light prehensile forces to gross grasping movements with great prehensile forces, all under the guidance of sensory feedback. To accomplish these tasks in the dynamic world around us, the coordinated movements of the proximal muscles and joints of the UE must position the hand for functional activities. The prosthetic

replacement for the UE is a limited substitute for the lost body part. With practice, it can replace several of the simple grasping and manipulating functions of the hand through a mildly to moderately restricted sphere of functional reach. A critical limitation of all UE prosthetic limbs is the severe restriction in sensory feedback from the terminal device relegating its use to that of simply assisting bimanual activities. The limited ability of the prosthetic limb to replace normal hand function typically results in a shift in hand dominance with amputation of the dominant hand.

UE prostheses can be divided into three groups: conventional or body-powered, external powered or electric, and passive or cosmetic. The advantages and disadvantages for each of the three general types of upper limb prostheses are presented in Table 61-6.

Body-Powered Prostheses: Components

Since the majority of individuals with UE amputation first learn to use a body-powered limb, an initial discussion of the function of various components (78,79) used in this type of prosthetic limb follows. Understanding the role, use, and limitations of body-powered prosthetic limbs forms the framework for subsequent discussions of externally powered devices. All conventional body-powered UE prostheses have these component parts:

- Socket
- Suspension
- Control cable system
- Terminal device
- Interposing joints (wrist, elbow, shoulder) as needed by the level of amputation.

TABLE 61-6.   Various Upper Limb Prostheses

Type	Pros	Cons
Cosmetic	Most lightweight	High cost if custom made
	Best cosmesis	Least function
	Less harnessing	Low-cost glove stains easily
Body Powered	Moderate cost	Most body movement to operate
	Moderately lightweight	Most harnessing
	Most durable	Least satisfactory appearance
	Highest sensory feedback	Increased energy expenditure
	Variety of prehensors available for various activities	
Battery powered (Myoelectric and/or switch controlled)	Moderate or no harnessing	Heaviest
	Least Body movement to operate	Most expensive
	Moderate cosmesis	Most maintenance
	More function-proximal areas	Limited sensory feedback
	Stronger grasp in some cases	Extended therapy time
Hybrid (cable to elbow or TD and battery powered)	All-cable excursion to either elbow or TD	
If excursion to elbow and battery powered TD	All-cable excursion to elbow	Battery powered TD weights forearm (Harder to lift but good for elbow disarticulation or long THA)
	Increased TD pinch	
If excursion to TD and battery powered elbow	All-cable excursion to TD	Lower pinch for TD and least cosmetic
	Low effort to position TD	
	Low maintenance TD	

TD, terminal device; THA, transhumeral amputation

SOCKETS

Traditionally UE prostheses have used a dual-wall socket design fabricated from lightweight plastic or graphite composite materials. In dual wall designs, a rigid inner socket is fabricated from a custom mold of the residual limb and is the primary interface between the user and the prosthesis. Comfort and function are directly tied to the quality of the fit of the inner socket. The outer socket wall is fabricated to have the general shape, length, and contour of the normal arm or forearm, serves both a cosmetic function, and supplies the foundation for the mounting of required components. This type of socket is durable and easily accommodates variation in residual limb volume using socks to adjust the fit.

An alternative approach to the design of the socket parallels the rigid frame, flexible liner approach used in lower limb prostheses. An inner socket is fabricated from flexible plastic materials to provide a total contact fit and is optimized for the use of suction suspension. Surrounding the inner socket is a rigid frame that provides the structural integrity of the socket. Windows in the outer socket allow for movement of the muscles of residual limb to enhance comfort.

SUSPENSION

The suspension system must hold the prosthesis securely to the residual limb and accommodate and distribute the forces associated with the weight of the prosthesis and any superimposed lifting loads. Suspension systems can be classified as harness-based, self-suspending sockets, or suction. Table 61-7 outlines the types of harnesses and their suggested uses, advantages, and disadvantages.

The most commonly used suspension for body-powered prostheses are variants of the harness-based system. The most commonly used harness is the figure-8 strap (Fig. 61-15). On the intact side, the harness loops around the axilla anchoring the limb and providing the counterforce for suspension and control cable forces. On the prosthetic side, the anterior strap carries the major suspending forces to the prosthesis by attaching directly to the socket (transhumeral) or indirectly through an intermediate Y-strap and triceps pad (transradial). The posterior strap on the prosthetic side attaches to the control cable. For heavier lifting activities or when axillary pressure from a figure-8 harness is unacceptable, a shoulder saddle with chest strap system is a useful alternative suspension system. A leather or flexible plastic saddle is positioned over the prosthetic side shoulder and is secured using a chest strap that wraps around the intact chest wall in an infraaxillary location. The suspension of the prosthesis occurs through an inverted U-shaped cable or strap that is anchored to the top of the saddle and drapes downward to attach to the front and back of the prosthetic socket (transhumeral) or triceps pad (transradial). The control cable attaches to the posterior aspect of the chest strap.

Self-suspending socket designs are used when the bony configuration of the residual limb allows suspension, similar to the effect used in Syme amputations. Self-suspending sockets are largely limited to wrist and elbow disarticulations. In both harness and self-suspending systems, socks can be worn to optimize fit and improve comfort.

Suction suspension sockets are similar those available to the individual with an LE amputation and use either a total contact socket with a one-way air valve or a roll-on silicone gel sleeve with a locking pin. Suction sockets are appropriate primarily for the transhumeral residual limb with good soft-tissue envelope, an absence of invaginated scarring, and a stable volume. Donning the suction socket with air valve involves the use of water-based lubricants or a pull sock to seat the residual limb into the socket. The one-way air valve creates a negative pressure inside of the socket, maintaining suspension. When using a silicone gel (or similar polymer materials) sleeve with a distal attachment pin, the sleeve is rolled onto the residual limb and inserted into the socket where the pin mates with a locking mechanism. Suspension is accomplished through a combination of suction and skin friction.

TABLE 61-7. Upper Extremity Prosthetic Suspension Options

Suspension		Indications	Advantages	Disadvantages
Harness	Figure-8	Transradial Transhumeral Light to normal duty activities	Simple, durable, adjustable.	Axillary pressure reduces discomfort.
	Shoulder saddle and chest strap	Transradial Transhumeral Heavy lifting	Greater lifting ability, more comfortable than Figure-8	Difficult to adjust in women because straps cross breasts. Reduced control compared to Figure-8 harness
Self-suspending	Muenster Northwestern Supracondylar	Wrist disarticulation Elbow disarticulation Short transradial Myoelectric transradial	Ease of use	Limited lifting capacity compared to harness systems, compromised cosmesis, reduced elbow flexion
Suction	Suction socket with air valve	Transhumeral with good soft tissue cover	Secure suspension, elimination of suspension straps	Requires stable residual volume, harder to don than other suspension systems
	Gel sleeve with locking pin	Transradial Transhumeral Compromised limbs with scarring or impaired skin integrity.	Accommodate limb volume change with socks. Reduced skin shear.	Greater cleaning and hygiene requirements. Can be uncomfortable in hot climates

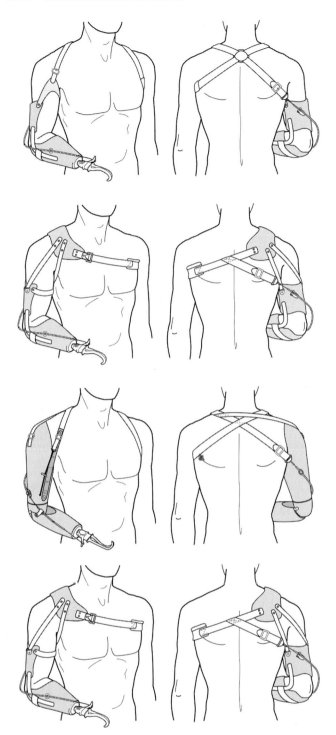

Figure 61-15. The transradial amputee has two types of harnessing. **Top:** The figure 8 harness. and the next shows the shoulder saddle and chest strap harness. The terminal device is activated by arm flexion or by bi-scapular abduction. **Bottom:** For the transhumeral amputee, the same motion stated above will move the elbow and operate the terminal device once the elbow is in locked position. To lock or unlock the elbow the amputee must simultaneously use arm extension, shoulder depression, and arm abduction. Figure 8 and shoulder saddle for the transradial and transhumeral body powered harness. Shoulder saddle harnessing is used for the heavier lifting activities or axillary pressure cannot be tolerated.

CONTROL CABLE MECHANISM

Body-powered prosthetic limbs use cables to link movements of the shoulder and humerus to activation of the terminal device and elbow. The movements that are captured for control include scapular abduction, shoulder depression and abduction, and humeral flexion. Control cables used to activate a single prosthetic component such as the terminal device are known as single-control cables or Bowden cables. Dual-control cable systems use the same cable to control two prosthetic functions, typically elbow flexion and terminal device opening in the transhumeral prosthesis. The control cable is attached to the figure-8 or chest strap harness used for suspension of the prosthesis. When a body-powered prosthesis incorporates a self-suspending socket design or suction suspension, a simple figure-9 harness strap system is required to allow control functions to be performed.

TERMINAL DEVICES

Terminal devices for body-powered prostheses can be hooks, functional or active hands, cosmetic or passive hands, or special terminal devices designed for specific activities (e.g., bowling ball terminal device, golf club holder). Hook-style terminal devices provide the equivalent of a lateral pinch grip while active hand terminal devices provide a three-point chuck action (80). The most commonly used active terminal device is the voluntary-opening hook. While different voluntary-opening hook designs are available for various applications, the most commonly prescribed for general use is the Dorrance 5X, 5XA, and 7 (Hosmer Dorrance, Campbell, CA) (Fig. 61-16). With voluntary-opening devices, the individual with a UE amputation provides power through a cabling system to open the terminal device and relies on springs or rubber bands to provide the closing prehensile force. Typical closing forces range from 5 to 10 lbs. Voluntary-opening active hands are available and in general are more cosmetic, but are heavier, interfere with visualizing the object being grasped, and provide lower prehensile forces. Voluntary-closing terminal devices allow the individual to provide a variable prehensile force transmitted through the control cable to the terminal device. Voluntary closing devices are capable of providing larger prehensile forces up to 20 to 25 lbs and provide indirect sensory feedback through the force exerted on the control cable. A significant disadvantage of voluntary-closing devices is the need for a constant pull on the control cable during prolonged grasping, a skill that is difficult to accomplish during dynamic tasks. Passive (cosmetic) hands are lighter than active hands and can be passively positioned but provide little if any function. A cosmetic glove tinted to approximate the individual's skin color covers both of these hands.

WRIST UNITS

Wrist units provide a receptacle for connecting the terminal device to the prosthesis and permit pre-positioning of the terminal device for functional activities (i.e., rotation for all units and flexion if the appropriate unit is used). Wrist rotation is performed using the intact hand or by pushing the terminal device against a firm surface and is held in place with either friction or a mechanical lock. Friction control wrist units are easily positioned but can slip when lifting heavier loads. A locking wrist unit enhances the use of the terminal device with heavier objects or where leverage with the terminal device is important for function. A wrist flexion unit allows the terminal device to be positioned in flexion, enhancing the ability to perform activities close to the body, a feature that is important for the individual with a bilateral UE amputation. A quick-disconnect op-

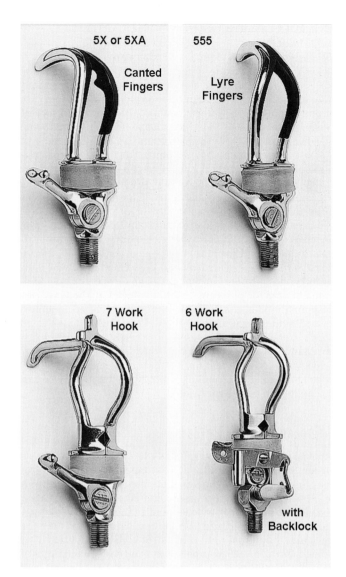

Figure 61-16. Most common terminal devices. (Courtesy of Hosmer-Dorrance, see Web site listing.)

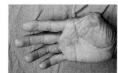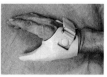

Figure 61-17. Thumb prosthesis set in position to allow for grasping and object manipulation.

tion permits the easy interchange of different terminal devices, such as a hook for a hand.

Additional details regarding components, sockets, suspension, and control systems are discussed where appropriate in the following sections relating to specific levels of amputation.

Prostheses by Level of Amputation

PARTIAL HAND

For partial hand amputations (e.g., phalanges, ray resections, transmetacarpal), a prosthesis may not be necessary. To be functionally useful, the residual hand needs to be able to provide a rudimentary grasp. This requires two opposing posts that can be moved into contact with each to provide a prehensile force. When possible, surgical reconstruction of the remaining partial hand is often the preferred approach to preserving or enhancing function while maintaining sensation. When only one movable digit remains, as in a transmetacarpal amputation of digits 2 through 5, either an open or mitt-shaped prosthetic opposition post can be used to provide a stable surface for opposition with

the thumb. In general, the substantial variability in the anatomy of the remaining partial hand requires creative custom solutions to optimize function (Fig. 61-17). At times, an individual with a UE amputation may require several devices customized for specific activities. A cosmetic prosthesis is frequently provided for this level of amputation. Long-term usage varies but the majority of individuals continue to wear them at least occasionally for social situations (81)

TRANSRADIAL AMPUTATIONS/WRIST DISARTICULATION

The length of the bony forearm measured from the medial epicondyle classifies transradial amputations: very short (<35%), short (35% to 55%), and long (55% to 90%). Longer residual limb length enhances the forearm lever, making lifting easier, and allows capturing residual pronation-supination motion of the forearm. Long transradial residual limbs retain from 60 to 120 degrees of supination-pronation, which decreases to less than 60 degrees in short transradial residual limbs. For short and long transradial amputations, a dual-wall socket is attached to a triceps pad with flexible elbow hinges (straps) to allow pronation-supination. The triceps pad helps to distribute suspension forces and is needed to anchor the control cable. Most commonly, a figure-8 harness system is used for suspension and control. For very short transradial amputation levels, rigid hinges generally are used to provide greater stability of the socket on the residual limb. With transradial amputations, in which range of motion is limited at the elbow, polycentric elbow joints or a split socket with step-up hinges can be used to provide additional flexion. The additional flexion gained with the use of these elbow hinges is offset by a loss of elbow flexion power and lifting ability.

The wrist disarticulation (WD) prosthesis is a variant of the transradial prosthesis. Because wrist disarticulation spares the distal radial-ulnar joint, full forearm supination-pronation is preserved. Socket designs for the WD level are flattened distally to form an oval to capture supination-pronation, allowing active rotational positioning of the terminal device during activities. The distal flare of the residual limb can be taken advantage of to fabricate a self-suspending socket but this usually leads to a bulbous, cosmetically compromised appearance similar to that occurring in the LE Syme amputation. The long residual limb necessitates the use of a special thin wrist unit to minimize the overall length of the prosthesis. If cosmesis is of primary importance to the patient, a long transradial amputation may be a more appropriate amputation level.

An example for the prescription of a transradial/wrist disarticulation limb could read: *dual-wall total contact socket, flexible elbow hinges, triceps pad, figure-8 harness, single control cable, constant friction wrist unit with quick disconnect, 5XA hook, and cosmetic hand.*

TRANSHUMERAL AMPUTATIONS/ELBOW DISARTICULATION

The length of the residual humerus measured from the acromion classifies transhumeral amputations: humeral neck (<30%), short transhumeral (30% to 50%), standard transhumeral (50% to 90%), and elbow disarticulation (90% to 100%). For short and standard transhumeral residual limb lengths, the traditional dual-wall socket extends to just below the acromion and attaches to either a figure-8 or a shoulder saddle and chest strap harness for suspension. With shorter residual limbs, securing the socket to the residual, especially under load, is more difficult. To accommodate this problem, the socket extends proximal and medial to the acromion, creating a partial shoulder cap. This socket design often can be suspended with only a chest strap, but other harness systems can be used for additional security or to improve control functions. Suction socket suspension systems are becoming the preferred system for individuals with a transhumeral amputation because of the improved suspension and greater ability to position the limb for activities. Even when suction suspension systems are used, an axillary harness is needed for control and can augment suspension, especially when lifting larger loads. Suction suspension, when used with externally powered myoelectric components, can result in a self-suspending prosthesis free of any harness.

The standard elbow component for the transhumeral prosthesis is the internal elbow joint. Internal elbow units allow for 135 degrees of flexion and can be manually locked into a number of preset flexed positions. The standard internal elbow unit incorporates a turntable that allows passive internal or external rotation of the forearm. Elbow spring-lift assist units are available and are generally recommended for internal elbow units to help counterbalance the weight of the forearm, making elbow flexion easier for the individual with an amputation. The standard elbow unit requires approximately 5 cm of length. If the level of amputation is less than 5 cm proximal to the epicondyles, then an internal elbow unit cannot be used unless an asymmetric elbow position compared to the intact limb is cosmetically acceptable. When the internal elbow unit cannot be used, locking external elbow joints are available but these are less durable and less cosmetic.

The control system for the transhumeral prosthesis uses two separate cables: a dual control cable that controls the elbow and terminal device and a secondary elbow locking cable. To control the prosthetic limb, the individual with the amputation uses scapular protraction and humeral flexion to flex the elbow into the desired position. The elbow is locked using the secondary control cable. Once locked, the same shoulder movements that powered the elbow are now available to activate the terminal device. Locking the elbow is typically accomplished by using a control cable that is routed along the anterior aspect of the socket and attaches to the front of the harness. Shoulder depression and humeral extension movements are used to lock-unlock the elbow.

An elbow disarticulation prosthesis is a variant of the transhumeral prosthesis. The socket is flat and broad distally to conform to the anatomic configuration of the epicondyles of the distal humerus. This design provides some self-suspension and allows the individual with an amputation active rotation of the prosthesis (internal and external rotation of the humerus). The length of the residual limb requires the use of external elbow joints, with a cable-operated locking mechanism. The harness is either a figure-8 or a shoulder saddle and chest strap. The control system for this level is the same as for the individual with a more proximal transhumeral amputation.

Example prescription for a short transhumeral prosthetic limb: *flexible wall/rigid frame suction socket, figure-8 axillary suspension and control harness, dual-control cable, internal locking elbow with turntable and flexion assist, lightweight forearm shell, constant friction wrist unit with quick disconnect, 5XA hook, and cosmetic hand.*

SHOULDER DISARTICULATION/FOREQUARTER AMPUTATION

For shoulder disarticulation and forequarter amputation, the socket extends onto the thorax to suspend and stabilize the prosthesis. The portion of the thorax covered by the socket is more extensive for the forequarter amputation. In some cases, an open-frame socket rather than a plastic laminated socket is chosen for these levels to reduce prosthetic weight and to minimize heat buildup by reducing the amount of skin coverage.

Prosthetic components are similar to those for the transhumeral prosthesis with the addition of a shoulder unit, which allows passive positioning of the shoulder joint in flexion-extension and abduction-adduction. Chest straps are attached to the anterior and posterior socket for suspension. The loss of ipsilateral shoulder motion for control purposes severely compromises the use of the prosthesis. A harness and control cable system that uses three individual cables can be used. Individual cables use intact side humeral flexion for prosthetic elbow control, chest expansion for terminal device control, and a manual nudge or pull cable for elbow locking. The body-powered prosthesis is cumbersome to don, has limited functionality, and is often used mainly for cosmesis. The difficulty in providing suitable body-powered prostheses at these proximal amputation levels argues against their routine use. For many individuals, a cosmetic limb is sufficient. For the highly motivated individual, externally powered prostheses may be more functional and can be considered.

Externally Powered Prostheses

External powered prosthetic limbs use small electric motors incorporated into the prosthetic component to control its function. Reliable external power units are available for terminal device operation, wrist rotation, and elbow flexion-extension. Myoelectric signals or switches control these electric motors. It is often difficult to predict the preferred prosthetic limb for a particular individual until trial use of both has occurred. Compared to body-powered prostheses, external powered prostheses are typically heavier, more costly, and less durable, especially if manual labor activities are frequently performed. Important advantages of external-powered prostheses compared to body-powered devices include improved comfort due to the reduced harness needs, better control, and lifting capacity for short transhumeral and shoulder disarticulation amputation levels, and the greater terminal device grip force of electric hooks and hands. In the case of the transradial level amputation, the prosthesis can use a self-suspending socket that eliminates the need for a harness (Fig. 61-18).

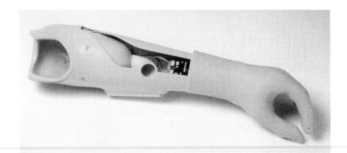

Figure 61-18. Otto Bock self-suspending transradial myoprosthesis and the internal placement of the electronic components. (Courtesy of Otto Bock, see Web site listing.)

The preferred control system for external-powered prostheses is myoelectrical control. Myoelectrical control uses surface electrodes embedded in the prosthetic socket that make contact with the skin and detect muscle action potentials from voluntarily contracting muscles in the residual limb. The myoelectric signal controls an electric motor to provide a function (e.g., terminal device operation, wrist rotation, elbow flexion). Prior to the prescription and fitting of a myoelectric prosthesis, the individual's ability to reliably contract and relax at least one muscle group in the residual limb should be ascertained. This can be accomplished using electromyographic biofeedback equipment or a myoelectric tester to identify the most appropriate electrode control location(s). Several different types of myoelectric controllers are available depending on the number of prosthetic functions that need to be controlled and the number of useful electrode sites identified. The dual-electrode system uses two sets of electrodes positioned over antagonist muscles allowing natural and intuitive myoelectric control to occur. For example, at the transradial level, activation of the forearm flexor muscles closes the terminal device while activation of the forearm extensors opens the terminal device. Most contemporary myoelectric control systems use proportional control so that the speed or strength of terminal device activation varies with the intensity of muscle contraction. When there are an inadequate number of usable electrode sites available to control all desired functions of the prosthesis, alternative control strategies can be used. Single-site controllers use the strength of voluntary contraction from a single electrode (i.e., amplitude of the myoelectric signal) to control which motion will occur (i.e., a weak contraction will close the terminal device and a strong contraction will open the terminal device) (81). Sequential or multistate controllers use the same electrode pair to control several functions (e.g., terminal device control and elbow activation). This type of controller uses a brief co-contraction to switch between control modes. Any of the alternative control schemes take longer to learn and are not consistently mastered by all individuals with an amputation.

When myoelectric control is not available or there are not enough electrode sites available, switches incorporated into the prosthetic socket or the harness can be used to implement or augment the control of various components. Simple on-off switches can be used to implement basic control of a powered component. More sophisticated servo control techniques based on position or force switches in the harness systems can be used to provide proportional control (83).

Myoelectric prosthetic components are available and sized to fit a wide range of people, from infants to adults. Most myoelectric terminal devices are hands, but some electric hook designs are available. Myoelectrically controlled prostheses can and have been fit immediately after surgery (84), but it is generally recommended that myoelectric fitting be delayed until the residual limb is healed and the limb volume has stabilized. A stable limb volume is needed to ensure a consistent socket fit and reproducible electrode position and skin contact. Myoelectric components have been combined with body-powered components to result in a hybrid prosthesis, which may provide better function for some individuals with an amputation than either myoelectric or body-powered control used alone.

Cosmetic Prosthesis

A conventional body-powered or myoelectric prosthesis with a hand terminal device supplies adequate cosmesis for many individuals with an amputation. Using custom covers that are color and texture matched to the skin of the intact side can enhance cosmesis. These covers are expensive and have a limited life expectancy if used during functional activities. When an individual with an amputation is not a candidate for an active prosthetic limb, a passive, cosmetic prosthetic can be fabricated using lightweight components that can be passively positioned to create a symmetric body image while wearing clothing.

SPECIAL ISSUES IN THE CARE OF INDIVIDUALS WITH AN AMPUTATION

Pain

Pain is a common problem following amputation. Identifying the etiology of a pain complaint is often challenging because of the limited ability to examine the residual limb during prosthetic use and overlapping symptoms from different pain sources. The initial decision required in addressing pain complaints is to differentiate phantom limb pain from residual limb pain.

PHANTOM SENSATION AND PHANTOM PAIN
Phantom sensation, defined as the awareness of a nonpainful sensation in the amputated part of the limb, occurs in nearly all acquired amputations (84–86). Phantom sensation is most prominent immediately after amputation and gradually fades over time, often in a telescoping fashion. The most vivid sensations are typically in the distal portion of the limb. Phantom limb sensations may persist indefinitely but in general do not require treatment. An occasionally problem with phantom sensation occurs when individuals are confused by the phantom sensation and attempt to walk without using a prosthesis.

Phantom pain is pain perceived in the amputated portion of the extremity. The incidence of phantom pain has been difficult to determine with reported frequency ranging from 4% to 80% (70,85,86). Like phantom sensation, phantom pain is most common early after amputation and usually becomes less frequent, less intense, and shorter in duration over time. Persistent phantom pain requiring treatment occurs in approximately 5% of individuals with an amputation. Phantom pain is often described as burning, cramping, stabbing, or squeezing but is sometimes reported as bizarre contortions of the limb. The pain may be generalized but more commonly it is experienced mainly in the distal parts of the missing limb. The cause and underlying physiology of phantom pain remain poorly understood but the incidence of phantom pain has been associated with the presence of preamputation pain, phantom sensation, and residual limb pain. The correlation between preamputation pain and the subsequent development of phantom pain has led to attempts at preventing phantom pain by controlling periamputation limb pain with continuous epidural or peripheral nerve anesthesia. These attempts have shown mixed effectiveness (86). Once established, the successful treatment of phantom pain can be difficult and many therapeutic modalities have been tried (70,87–90). Although convincing evidence-based algorithms for the treatment of phantom pain do not exist, empiric clinical guidelines are frequently used. Medication is usually the first line of treatment employing tricyclic antidepressants and anticonvulsants (e.g., carbamazepine, gabapentin) either alone or in combination. Other drugs that have been used with some success include mexiletine, calcitonin, N-methyl-D-aspartate (NMDA) receptor antagonists, and opioids. Evaluation and correction of any coexisting residual limb pain or prosthetic fit problems is also an important component of the initial management of phantom pain. Range-of-motion exercises, relaxation exercises, residual limb massage, transcutaneous electrical nerve stimulation (TENS), compressive stocking, and encouraging prosthesis use have little risk and may be useful adjuncts to medical management. Since problematic phantom pain often occurs only intermittently and is typically short-lived, the patient's participation in decision making is essential to weigh possible benefits of drug trials with the inconvenience and possible side effects of medications that need to be taken on a regular, continuous basis. Surgical treatments have not been shown to provide lasting pain relief and are rarely used.

RESIDUAL LIMB PAIN

In contrast to phantom limb pain, residual limb pain is pain perceived as originating in and affecting the residual portion of the limb. Persistent residual limb pain occurs in up to 70% of individuals with lower limb amputation with about half reporting the pain as moderately to severely bothersome (85–88). Residual limb pain is commonly described as aching, sharp, throbbing, and burning in character. The underlying causes of residual limb pain can be classified as intrinsic or extrinsic.

Intrinsic residual limb pain is caused by changes or complications in the underlying neurovascular, bony, or soft tissues of the residual limb. Neuromas develop in all residual limbs after amputation but may only become problematic when entrapped in scar or positioned such that they are exposed to external mechanical loading. Diagnosing an underlying neuroma as the cause of pain can be difficult. When present, neuropathic symptoms including typical dysesthetic pain descriptors, radiation of pain in a specific nerve distribution, and the presence of pain when not using a prosthesis are helpful diagnostic aids but at times the pain location and description is nonspecific. Neuroma-related pain may be precipitated by tapping (Tinel's sign), direct compression from manual palpation or socket pressure, or traction on an adherent scarred nerve. Larger neuromas can be imaged with magnetic resonance imaging (91). When prosthetic use exacerbates neuroma pain, initial treatment interventions should include prosthetic modifications that attempt to reduce loading of pressure-sensitive areas. Useful approaches include the use of gel socks or liners to better distribute loads and to reduce shearing of adherent tissues, flexible sockets, or socket modification to relieve sensitive areas. Infiltration of the perineuromal region with local anesthetics combined with steroids can be a useful diagnostic and therapeutic procedure. If the injection relieves the pain, a series of similar injections over several months can be attempted to try to achieve lasting relief. When neuroma pain persists and limits function, surgery to resect and move the neuroma to a more protected location can often be helpful. However, following the neuroma resection, the neuroma will reform and, on occasion, again become symptomatic.

Bony overgrowth from the distal end of the residual limb skeletal elements occasionally occurs in adults but is primarily a problem that occurs in children with an amputation. Heterotopic bone can form in the soft tissues of the residual limb and may follow trauma, hematoma, or fracture of the residual limb. Poorly contoured bone edges following surgery can lead to regions of high-pressure concentration. In any of these situations, the abnormal bone leads to localized tissue compression, pain, and tenderness that can progress to the development of adventitial bursa or soft-tissue ulceration. Diagnosis is made with plain radiographs of the residual limb. Management is focused on prosthetic socket modifications to offload painful areas but achieving a lasting comfortable fit can be difficult. When prosthetic approaches fail, surgical revision is typically needed.

Osteomyelitis, tumor recurrence, stress fractures, and persistent limb ischemia may cause more generalized residual limb pain and require medical and surgical management.

Extrinsic residual limb pain is caused by a mismatch between residual limb tissue tolerance and prosthetic loads imposed on the soft tissues. Poor socket fit or limb malalignment are the main causes. The coexistence of a compromised residual limb from intrinsic pathology reduces the margin of safety between tissue tolerance and prosthetic socket loads, making it more difficult to achieve and maintain a comfortable fit. The ability to attain a comfortable socket fit is one of the most important aspects of prosthetic acceptance and function. Most contemporary prosthetic sockets are designed for total contact with modifications to the socket shape to preferentially load weight-tolerance tissues. Socket fit is inevitably compromised with body weight changes or residual limb soft-tissue atrophy over time. Clinical manifestations of poor fit or excessive local tissue loading include a gradual onset of pain while using a previously comfortable prosthesis, erythema persisting more than 15 to 20 minutes after wearing the limb, or the development of blisters, bursas, calluses, or skin ulceration. Changing the number of sock plies, adding pads to the socket, relieving high-pressure areas, or substituting a gel liner for socks can often restore a comfortable fit and prolong the useful life of a socket. When minor modifications fail, a replacement socket will need be to be fabricated.

Malalignment of lower limb prostheses can create abnormally high or prolonged loading forces in the residual limb leading to pain even when the socket fit is acceptable. In the individual with a transtibial amputation, sagittal plane alignment problems most commonly affect the distal tibia region while frontal plane malalignment primarily affects loading forces along the fibula. In the individual with a transfemoral amputation, distal femur pain is often seen with alignment problems.

CHOKE SYNDROME

A specific socket fit problem almost exclusively seen in the individual with an LE amputation is the choke syndrome. A choke syndrome develops when there is a simultaneous impairment of venous return from a prosthetic socket that is too tight proximally and a lack of total contact between the residual limb and the socket. Edema develops in the residual limb where total contact is lost. Most commonly, this occurs in the distal aspect of the transtibial residual limb as atrophy takes place over time and additional socks are used to fill in for the loss of soft-tissue volume. Because there is not a corresponding volume change in the proximal bony aspect of the limb, the fit becomes too tight and constricts venous return. Initially, a circumscribed indurated region develops while wearing the prosthesis. If significant edema develops acutely, there can be associated weeping or blistering of the skin. The area of choke is tender to palpation and is prone to developing cellulitis. As the choke syndrome becomes chronic, the tissues become increasingly thickened and indurated, verrucous hyperplasia develops, and skin becomes hyperpigmented because of hemosiderin deposition. Choke syndromes are treated by relieving the proximal constriction and restoring total contact between the residual limb and the socket (90,92). When the choke syndrome is mild, reducing the number of socks to decrease proximal residual limb constriction and adding or modifying the distal end pad may be adequate but typically a new total contact socket is needed.

Dermatologic Disorders

Dermatologic problems are common, particularly in the individual with an LE amputation, with surveys estimating that 30% to 50% of individuals with amputations experience one or more skin problems because of a prosthesis (91–94). Dermatologic complaints can be classified as related to hyperhidrosis, physical effects of prosthetic use, contact dermatitis, and infection.

Hyperhidrosis, while not indicative of underlying disease, is one of the most common skin- related complaints and has become more common with the introduction of silicone liners in the 1990s. An increase in sweating is reported by about half of the patients with the use of silicone liners. Over several weeks, adaptation typically occurs and excessive sweating resolves in many of these patients. Persistent hyperhidrosis makes it more difficult to maintain hygiene, increases the likelihood of skin maceration, and may contribute to the development of contact dermatitis (92–94). When using suction sockets, suspension effectiveness can be compromised. Problematic sweating can be controlled by using concentrated antiperspirants, such as Drysol (Person & Covey, Glendale, CA), on the residual limb or by changing to a liner system that allows the individual with an amputation to wear socks directly against the skin.

The skin of the residual limb is subjected to repeated shear, frictional, and loading forces. The physical effects of these repetitive loads can lead to keratin plugging of sebaceous glands and follicular hyperkeratosis leading to the development of epidermoid cysts, folliculitis, and dermal granulomas. Cysts are frequently very tender and can spontaneously break open or become secondarily infected. Commonly affected areas are those that are subjected to high loading and shearing forces such as the groin region in the individual with a transfemoral amputation and the medial tibial flare and popliteal fossa in the individual with a transtibial amputation. Treatment is directed at local skin care as well as prosthetic modifications to reduce mechanical skin forces. Meticulous hygiene needs to be encouraged to keep skin, socks, and liner clean. Cosmetic or acne scrub pads can be used to help keep skin pores open. Warm compresses to promote drainage and oral antibiotics are useful in managing folliculitis and infected cysts. Larger and more persistent sebaceous cysts may require surgical drainage or excision. Concurrent with medical management, a review of prosthetic fit and alignment to ensure that loading of the affected region is optimized should be undertaken. Recurring problems can be helped with the use of prosthetic components that reduce residual limb shear and loading forces. These include gel liners, rotators, vertical shock pylons, and multiaxis ankle/foot devices.

Allergic or contact dermatitis accounts for approximately 20% of prosthetic-related dermatoses (93). Clinical symptoms range from mild lichenification or scaling to weeping eczema. A wide variety of offending agents has been identified. Detergents, scented emollients, creams, and talcs used for skin care should be considered as possible allergens and discontinued or changed. The use of gel sheaths and liners may result in contact dermatitis. The exact allergen is difficult to identify and is probably residual soap used in cleaning or chemical additives used in liner manufacturing rather than the hypoallergenic silicone material itself. If continued use of gel-type liners is needed, it is reasonable to switch to a different manufacturer or change to a different liner base material (e.g., silicone to urethane) to empirically attempt to resolve the rash. Neoprene, resins used in socket fabrication, and dyes and tanning agents used in leather are also potential allergens. If empiric trials of different materials cannot identify the allergen, patch testing for 24 to 48 hours with a small piece of the suspected material on the forearm may be helpful.

The use of gel sheaths, liners, and suspension sleeves can create a moist warm environment that may contribute to contact dermatitis, bacterial, and fungal skin infections. Attention to proper skin care and liner cleansing can minimize skin disorders. At times, wearing natural fiber socks or a nylon sheath between the liner and residual limb can absorb or wick away moisture and reduce skin problems.

Pediatric Limb Deficiency or Amputation

When amputations are performed in children for disease, tumor, or trauma or to surgically convert a congenital skeletal deficiency to a level more appropriate for prosthetic fitting, a disarticulation-level amputation is preferred rather than an amputation through a long bone when the resulting level of function with a prosthesis will be similar. Approximately 12% of children with acquired amputations experience a condition known as bony overgrowth. Bony overgrowth is the appositional deposition of bone to the end of the amputated long bone. This bone growth results in a spikelike formation at the end of the bone that has a thin cortex and no medullary canal. The bone frequently grows faster than the overlying skin and soft tissues; a bursa may develop over the sharp end, or the bone actually may protrude through the skin with subsequent development of cellulitis and osteomyelitis. Overgrowth is seen most frequently in the humerus, fibula, tibia, and femur, in that order. It has been reported in the congenital limb deficiencies, but rarely. Several treatment approaches have been advocated for the management of this problem, all with limited

TABLE 61-8. Guidelines for Pediatric Prosthetic Fitting

Amputation Level	Age for Prosthetic Fitting	Developmental Milestones	Prosthetic Prescription
Transradial	6–7 months	Sitting balance, reaches across midline for bimanual object manipulation	Body-powered—passive mitt, self suspending socket
	9–15 months		Externally powered for greater grip strength, single control site (voluntary opening, auto close)
	24–36 months		Change to two site control for voluntary opening and closing
Transhumeral	6–7 months	Same as for transradial	Body-powered—passive mitt and elbow, activate elbow at 18 months.
	24–48 months		Externally powered terminal device, when terminal device control mastered activate the elbow.
Transtibial	9–12 months	Child pulls to stand	PTB, supracondylar strap
Transfemoral	9–12 months	Child pulls to stand	Ischial containment socket, belt suspension, no knee unit until ages 3–4.

TABLE 61-9.   Children vs. Adult

General		
Dynamic (growing)	vs.	Adynamic (decelerates-aging)
Dependent	vs.	Independent
Untrained (life disciplines)	vs.	Trained
Nonresponsible	vs.	Responsible
Malleable	vs.	Less malleable

Physical		
Growing	vs.	Static
Immature	vs.	Mature
Longitudinal growth	vs.	Non-longitudinal growth
Circumferential growth	vs.	Circumferential growth (dietary)
Circulation & tissue tolerance are ideal	vs.	Circulation & tolerance vary with age and health
	Influences surgical indications, site of amputation and goals of training	

Social		
Member of family group	vs.	Independent person
Few independent social responsibilities	vs.	Variable responsibilities; depends on age, marriage, parenthood, etc.
Adjustment relatively easy	vs.	Adjustment less easy because of fixed social environment

Economic		
By family	vs.	By patient
Not self-supporting	vs.	Self-supporting or at least contribute to economic welfare of family
Amputation not of economic importance	vs.	Amputation may interfere with established economic status

Education		
Process of obtaining basic education	vs.	Usually completed
Advanced education can be planned to include handicap and its limitation and needs	vs.	Age often makes long re-education and training difficult, if not impossible

Vocational		
Not selected or established	vs.	Established
Oriented around handicap	vs.	Must re-orient vocationally because of handicap

Psychological		
Because of immaturity of development, may not have the profound changes sometimes seen in the adult. Usually reflects family (parental) reaction to the amputation or deformity. In general, is not a great problem in a stable family situation.	vs.	Great variation. All the way from profound psychoneurosis to mature, reasonable acceptance of the disability. The impact of the amputation on the socio-economic areas of the patient's existence are generally profound.

success. The technique proposed by Marquardt in which the distal end of the bone is capped with a cartilage epiphysis is the best of the surgical options available to manage this problem (15).

For the child with a congenital skeletal deficiency, the initial prosthesis for the UE usually is fitted when the child has attained independent sitting balance, or at approximately 6 months of age (96–99) (Table 61-8). For the LE, the initial pros-

thesis is fitted when the child begins to pull to a stand, which generally is between 9 and 14 months. Young children and infants usually learn to use their prostheses by incorporating them as part of play activities rather than through specific exercises. Prosthetic training periods for children may last only for several minutes at a time because of limited attention span, and they may require much longer periods of free play interspersed between actual training sessions. It is important that parents be instructed in techniques to help their children attain the necessary prosthetic skills because much of the training in the use of the prosthesis will occur in the home rather than in the clinic. It is also important to understand when working with children who have a limb deficiency or amputation of the UE that the prosthesis becomes an aid rather than a replacement (Table 61-9). If the child cannot habilitate with the prosthesis then it will be discarded.

The age at which to fit children with a myoelectric prosthesis is a controversial and complex issue beyond the scope of this chapter. This subject is reviewed in detail elsewhere (12,96,97).

PROSTHETIC PRESCRIPTION EXAMPLE CASES

The prosthetic prescriptions presented for these cases are as examples only. They do not represent the standard or typical prosthetic prescriptions for these levels of amputation. We want to be clear that a specific prosthetic prescription must be tailored to meet the specific needs of an individual with an amputation. The examples presented here serve to highlight the decision process that might be followed to arrive at an appropriate prosthetic prescription.

Case 61-1: Transradial Amputation
A 24-year-old, right-handed man sustains a work-related crush injury to his right hand, resulting in a long transradial level of amputation. He plans to return to work operating a drill press.

Possible prosthetic prescriptions include:

- Body power
  - Double-wall plastic laminate socket
  - Quick-change locking wrist unit
  - No. 7 (heavy duty, "Farmer's hook") terminal device
  - Flexible elbow hinges
  - Triceps pad
  - Figure-8 harness for suspension
  - Bowden single-control cable
- External power
  - Double-wall plastic laminate socket with self-suspending design
  - Otto Bock Greifer (myoelectric hook) terminal device

In this person, body power will be lightest in weight, most durable, and least expensive. If more than 6 to 7 lbs of pinch force are necessary from the terminal device for functional activities, the Greifer will provide up to 35 lbs of pinch force.

Case 61-2: Transhumeral Amputation
A 35-year-old, right-handed female homemaker sustains a short transhumeral level of amputation following a motor vehicle accident. Possible prosthetic prescriptions include:

- Body power
  - Double-wall plastic laminate socket
  - Constant-friction wrist unit
  - No. 5XA (lightest weight) terminal device
  - Internal, alternating locking elbow with turntable
  - Figure-8 harness

  - Bowden double-control cable
- External power
  - Double-wall plastic laminate socket
  - Otto Bock myoelectric hand
  - Utah myoelectric elbow
  - Figure-8 harness

In this woman, because of the short residual limb, external power may be more comfortable and functional but will be heavier and much more expensive than body power.

Case 61-3: Transtibial Amputation
A 72-year-old-retired man with type II diabetes and peripheral vascular disease has a transtibial amputation for an infected nonhealing ulcer and gangrenous foot. Possible prosthetic prescriptions include:

- Provisional
  - Total contact PTB thermoplastic socket
  - Foam liner (soft insert)
  - Neoprene sleeve suspension
  - Lightweight alignable shank
  - SACH foot
- Definitive
  - Exoskeletal design prosthesis
  - Total-contact laminated PTB socket
  - Silicone suction suspension (3-S)
  - Lightweight multiaxial foot

The provisional prosthesis is a lightweight design that provides a stable support base on which to learn to walk with a prosthesis. The soft liner will make modifications for changes in residual limb volume that are expected to be easier to accomplish. An exoskeletal design with multiaxis foot was chosen for the definitive prosthesis in consideration of the individual's desire to return to his gardening activities, which required a prosthesis that was more durable and stable on uneven ground with a secure suspension system that would not be torn up when kneeling with the prosthesis.

Case 61-4: Transfemoral Amputation
A 28-year-old female day care teacher sustained an open comminuted distal femur fracture while mountain climbing and ultimately had a midthigh level transfemoral amputation after developing osteomyelitis. Possible prosthetic prescriptions include:

- Provisional
  - Total contact thermoplastic ischial containment socket
  - TES belt suspension
  - Hydraulic knee unit
  - Lightweight dynamic-response foot
  - Cosmetic foam cover
- Definitive
  - Total-contact carbon fiber, reinforced ischial containment suction frame socket with Thermoflex liner
  - Thigh rotator
  - Swing and stance phase-control hydraulic knee unit
  - Split-toe Flex-Foot
  - Cosmetic foam cover

The provisional prosthesis, an endoskeletal design with a nonsuction socket, belt suspension, and hydraulic knee unit, was chosen to allow easy accommodation for anticipated major changes in residual limb volume that were expected to occur quickly with prosthetic use while at the same time recognizing this individual's high level of physical activity. The cosmetic cover was added to the provisional prosthesis, not usually done, recognizing her work with small children and her desire not to scare them with the prosthesis. The changes in the definitive prosthesis reflected the individual's desire to eliminate the belt suspension, achieve a more secure suspension, and accommodate her recreational and competitive sports activities. The thigh rotator was added so that she could sit on the floor and work with the children in her class.

IN MEMORY OF ANDREW J. GITTER, MD (1957–2003)

Dr. Gitter was appointed as an associated professor at the University of Texas Health Science Center in rehabilitation medicine on February 7, 1997, having previously served on the faculty of the University of Washington Medical School. Dr. Gitter was awarded tenure in September 2001.

Dr. Gitter received his B.S., magna cum laude, in computer engineering from Rochester University in 1979, and he received his M.D., cum laude, from the University of Michigan Medical School in 1980. After completing his residency and an NIDRR Research Fellowship at the Department of Rehabilitation Medicine at the University of Washington, he joined their faculty.

Dr. Gitter was the University of Washington, Department of Rehabilitation Medicine Faculty Teacher of the Year in 1991, and in 1999 he was honored as The University of Texas Health Science Center at San Antonio, Department of Rehabilitation Medicine Faculty Teacher of the Year. He received the American Board of PM & R Earl C. Elkins Award in 1991 for the highest written board exam score. In 1992, Dr. Gitter won the PM & R Education and Research Foundation Award for Best Scientific Paper Published by a Physiatrist in Practice Less Than 5 Years, and in 1996 he won the PM & R Education and Research Foundation Award for Best Scientific Paper Published by a Physiatrist in Practice More Than 5 Years.

Dr. Gitter was the Chief of Rehabilitation Medicine at the Audie L. Murphy Memorial Veterans Hospital and he also served on the staff of Reeves Rehabilitation Center at University Hospital. Dr. Gitter was actively involved with prosthetic research and he was known worldwide for his expertise in gait analysis. He established the first Gait Analysis Laboratory at the Veterans Hospital. Dr. Gitter had an active medical practice and he was particularly revered by his patients from the amputee clinic.

Dr. Gitter is survived by his wife Brenda, and daughters Anna Caitlin, Maria Sofya Catherine, and Yulia Katrina; parents, Richard and Elizabeth Gitter; in-laws, Harlan and Lorena Green; brothers and their wives, Joseph and Linda Gitter, Theodore and Nancy Gitter, Thomas and Karen Gitter; and sisters and their husbands, Diane and Thomas Mueller, Carol and Kenneth Casolari.

Dr. Gitter was the consummate physician, teacher, researcher, husband, father, and friend. He will be missed by all those who respected and loved him.

WEB Site Listings

COMPANY WEBSITES

Otto Bock	www.ottobockus.com
Ossur	www.ossur.com
CPI	www.college-park.com
Becker	www.beckerorthopedic. com
Endolite	www.endolite.com
Kingsley	www.kingsleymfg.com
Living Skin	www.livingskin.com
TRS	www.oandp.com/products/trs
Hosmer	www.hosmer.com
Motion Control	www.utaharm.com
Liberating Technologies	www.liberatingtechnologies.com
Animated Prosthetics	www.animatedprosthetics.com
IPOS	www.ipos-orthopedics.com
Ohio Willow Wood	www.owwco.com
Daw Industries	www.daw-usa.com

RESOURCES ON THE WEB FOR AMPUTEE ATHLETES

Disabled Sports USA	www.dsusa.org
Challenged Athletes Foundation	www.challengedathletes.org/caf/
Active Amp.org	www.activeamp.org
International Paralympics Committee	www.paralympic.org
Limbs for Life	www.limbsforlife.org
American Amputee Soccer Assoc.	www.ampsoccer.org

OTHER INTERESTING SITES

Amputee Resource Foundation of America, Inc	www.amputeeresource.org
International Society for Prosthetics and Orthotics	www.i-s-p-o.org
American Academy of Orthotists and Prosthetists	www.oandp.org
Barr Foundation	www.oandp.com/resources/ organizations/barr
National Limb Loss Information Center	www.amputee-coalition.org/ nllic_about.html
Amputee Coalition of America	www.amputee-coalition.org

REFERENCES

1. Malone JM, Moore WS, Goldstone J, et al. Therapeutic and economic impact of a modern amputation program. *Ann Surg* 1979;189:798–802.
2. Dillingham TR, Pezzin LE, MacKenzie EJ. Limb amputation and limb deficiency: epidemiology and recent trends in the United States. *South Med J* 2002;95:875–883.
3. Mayfield JA, Reiber GE, Maynard C, et al. Trends in lower limb amputation in the Veterans Health Administration, 1989–1998. *J Rehabil Res Dev* 2000;37: 1:23–30.
4. Kay HW, Newman JD. Relative incidences of new amputations: statistical comparisons of 6,000 new amputees. *Orthot Prosthet* 1975;29:3–16.
5. Sanders GT. *Lower limb amputations: a guide to rehabilitation*. Philadelphia: FA Davis, 1986.
6. Glattly HW. A statistical study of 12,000 new amputees. *South Med J* 1964;57: 1373–1378.
7. Dillingham TR, Pezzin LE, Mackenzie EJ. Limb amputation and limb deficiency—epidemiology and recent trends in the United States. *South Med J* 2002;95(8):875–883.
8. Pinzur MS. Current concepts: amputation surgery in peripheral vascular disease. *Instruct Course Lect* 1997;46:501–509.

9. Pohjolainen T, Alaranta H. Epidemiology of lower limb amputees in Southern Finland in 1995 and trends since 1984. *Prosthet Orthot Int* 1999;23(2): 88–92.

10. Holstein P, Ellitsgaard N, Bornefeldt Olsen B, et al. Decreasing incidence of major amputations in people with diabetes. *Diabetologia* 2000;43:844–847.

11. Edmonds LD, James LM. Temporal trends in the prevalence of congenital malformations at birth based on the birth defects monitoring program: United States, 1979–1987. *CDC Surveil Summ Morbid Mortal Weekly Rep* 1990; 39(S4):19–23.

12. Atkins DJ, Meier RH, eds. *Comprehensive management of the upper-limb amputee.* New York: Springer-Verlag, 1989.

13. Jain S. Rehabilitation in limb deficiency. 2. The pediatric amputee. *Arch Phys Med Rehabil* 1996;77:S9–S13.

14. Setoguchi Y. The management of the limb deficient child and its family. *Prosthet Orthot Int* 1991;15:78–81.

15. Bowker JH, Michael JW. *Atlas of limb prosthetics: surgical, prosthetic, and rehabilitation principles,* 2nd ed. American Academy of Orthopedic Surgeons. St. Louis: CV Mosby, 1992.

16. Murdoch G, Wilson AB. *Amputation surgical practice and patient management.* Boston: Butterworth-Heinemann, 1996.

17. Wutschert R, Bounameaux H. Determination of amputation level in ischemic limbs. *Diabetes Care* 1997;20:315–1318.

18. Burgess EM, Matsen FA III. Determining amputation levels in peripheral vascular disease. *J Bone Joint Surg [Am]* 1981;63A:1493–1497.

19. Tornetta P, Olson SA. Amputation versus limb salvage. *Instruct Course Lect* 1997;46:511–518.

20. Trautwein LC, Smith DG, Rivera FP. Pediatric amputation injuries: etiology, cost, and outcome. *J Trauma Injury Infect Crit Care* 1996;41:831–838.

21. Graham B, Adkins P, Tsai TM, et al. Major replantation versus revision amputation and prosthetic fitting in the upper extremity: a late functional outcome study. *J Hand Surg* 1998;23A:783–791.

22. Kour AK, Seo JS, Pho RW. Combined free flap, Ilizarov lengthening and prosthetic fitting in the reconstruction of a proximal forearm amputation—a case report. *Ann Acad Med* 1995;24[Suppl]:135–137.

23. Vavylov VN, Kalakutsky NV, Agrachyova IG. Reconstruction of very short humeral stumps. *Ann Plast Surg* 1994;32:145–147.

24. Stricker SJ. Ilizarov lengthening of a posttraumatic below elbow amputation stump. A case report. *Clin Orthop* 1994;306:124–127.

25. Kasabian AK, Glat PM, Eidelman Y, et al. Salvage of traumatic below-knee amputation stumps utilizing the filet of foot free flap: critical evaluation of six cases. *Plast Reconstr Surg* 1995;96:1145–1153.

26. Rees RS, Nanney LB, Fleming P, et al. Tissue expansion: its role in traumatic below-knee amputations. *Plast Reconstr Surg* 1986;77:133–137.

27. Coletta EM. Care of the elderly patient with lower extremity amputation. *J Am Board Fam Pract* 2000;13:23–34.

28. Choudhury SR, Reiber GE, Pecoraro JA, et al. Postoperative management of transtibial amputation in VA hospitals. *J Rehabil Res Dev* 2001;38:3:293–298.

29. Wong CK, Edelstein JE. Unna and elastic postoperative dressings: comparison of their effects on function of adults with amputation and vascular disease. *Arch Phys Med Rehabil* 2000;81:1191–1198.

30. Vigier S, Casillas JM, Dulieu V, et al. Healing of open stump wounds after below-knee amputation: plaster cast socket with silicon sleeve versus elastic compression. *Arch Phys Med Rehabil* 1999;80:1327–1330.

31. Gitter A, Czerniecki JM, DeGroot DM. Biomechanical analysis of the influence of prosthetic feet on below knee amputee walking. *Am J Phys Med Rehabil* 1991;70:142–148.

32. Seroussi RE, Gitter A, Czernieeki JM, et al. The mechanical work adaptations of amputee ambulation. *Arch Phys Med Rehabil* 1996;27:1209–1214.

33. Cutson TM, Bongiorini DR. Rehabilitation of the older lower limb amputee: a brief review. *J Am Geriatr Soc* 1996;44:1388–1393.

34. Fletcher DD, Andrews KL, Butters MA, et al. Rehabilitation of the geriatric vascular amputee patient: a population-based study. *Arch Phys Med Rehabil* 2001;82:776–779.

35. Predictive factors for successful early prosthetic ambulation among lower-limb amputees. *J Rehabil Res Dev* 2001;38:4:379–384.

36. Burgess EM, Romano RL, Zetti JH. The management of lower extremity amputations. Washington, DC: US Government Printing Office, 1969.

37. Folsom D, King T, Rubin JR. Lower-extremity amputation with immediate postoperative prosthetic placement. *Am J Surg* 1992;164:320–322.

38. Liljia M, Oberg T. International forum: proper time for permanent prosthetic fitting. *JPO* 1997;9:90–95.

39. Czerniecki JM. Rehabilitation in limb deficiency. 1. Gait and motion analysis. *Arch Phys Med Rehabil* 1996;77:S3–S8.

40. Hafner BJ, Sanders JE, Czerniecki JM, et al. Transtibial energy storage and return prosthetic devices: a review of energy concepts and a proposed nomenclature. *J Rehabil Res Dev* 2002;39:1–11.

41. Edelstein JE. Current choices in prosthetic feet. *Crit Rev Phys Rehabil Med* 1991;2:213–226.

42. Esquenazi A, Torres MM. Prosthetic feet and ankle mechanisms. *Phys Med Rehabil Clin* 1991;2:299–309.

43. Nassan S. The latest designs in prosthetic feet. *Phys Med Rehabil Clin North Am* 2000;11:609–625.

44. Czerniecki JM, Gitter A. Prosthetic feet: a scientific and clinical review of current components. *Phys Med Rehabil: State of the Art Rev* 1994;8:109–129.

45. Romo HD. Specialized prostheses for activities. *Clin Orthop* 1999;361:63–70.

46. Klute GK, Kallfelz CF, Czerniecki J. Mechanical properties of prosthetic limbs: adapting to the patient. *J Rehabil Res Dev* 2001;38:3:299–397.

47. Early JS. Transmetatarsal and midfoot amputation. *Clin Orthop* 1999;361:85–90.

48. Philbin TM, Leyes M, Sferra JJ, et al. Orthotic and prosthetic devices in partial foot amputations. *Foot Ankle Clin* 2001;6:215–228.

49. Stuck RM. Syme's ankle disarticulation. *Clin Pod Med* 1997;14:763–773.

50. Pinzur M. Restoration of walking ability with Syme's ankle disarticulation. *Clin Orthop* 1999;361:71–75.

51. Hudson JR, Yu GV, Marzano R, Vincent AL. Syme's amputation. Surgical technique, prosthetic considerations, and case reports. *J Am Podiatr Med Assoc* 2002;92(4):232–246.

52. Feragson J, Smith DG. Socket considerations for the patient with a transtibial amputation. *Clin Orthop* 1999;361:76–84.

53. Kahle JT. Conventional and hydrostatic interface comparison. *JPO* 1999; 11:85.

54. Hachisuka K, Dozono K, Ogata H, et al. Total surface bearing below-knee prosthesis: advantages, disadvantages, and clinical implications. *Arch Phys Med Rehabil* 1998;79:783–789.

55. Kahle JT. Conventional and hydrostatic interface comparison. *JPO* 1999; 11:85–90.

56. Kapp S. Suspension systems for prostheses. *Clin Orthop* 1999;361:55–62.

57. Board WJ, Street GM, Caspers C. A comparison of trans-tibial amputee suction and vacuum socket conditions. *Prosthet Orthot Int* 2001;25(3):202–209.

58. Buckley JG, Jone SF, Birch KM. Oxygen consumption during ambulation: comparison of using a prosthesis fitted with and without a tele-torsion device. *Arch Phys Med Rehabil* 2002;83(4):576–80.

59. Pinzur MS, Bowker JH. Knee disarticulation. *Clin Orthop* 1999;361:23–28.

60. Function after through knee compared with below knee and above knee amputation. *Prosthet Orthot Int* 1992;Dec 16(3):168–173.

61. Schuch CM, Pritham CH. Current transfemoral sockets. *Clin Orthop* 1999; 361:48–54.

62. Gottschalk FA, Stills M. The biomechanics of transfemoral amputation. *Prosthet Orthot Int* 1994;18:12–17.

63. Pritham CH. Biomechanics and shape of the above knee and above knee amputation, *Prosthetic Orthotic International* 1992;Dec 16(3):9–21.

64. Long IA. Normal shape-normal alignment (NSNA) above-knee prosthesis. *Clin Prosthet Orthot* 1985;9:168–173.

65. Sabolich J. Contoured adducted trochanteric-controlled alignment method (CAT-CAM): introduction and basic principles. *Clin Prosthet Orthot* 1985;9: 15–26.

66. Kristinsson O. Flexible above-knee socket made from low-density polyethylene suspended by a weight-transmitting frame. *Prosthet Orthot* 1983;37: 25–27.

67. Pritham CH. Biomechanics and shape of the above-knee socket considered in light of the ischial containment concept. *Prosthet Orthot Int* 1990;14:9–21.

68. Layton H. A vacuum donning procedure for transfemoral suction suspension prostheses. *JPO* 1998;10(1):21–24.

69. van de Veen PG. Above knee prosthetic technology. Consultancy: The Netherlands, 2001.

70. Esquenazi A, Meier RH. Rehabilitation in limb deficiency. 4. Limb amputation. *Arch Phys Med Rehabil* 1996;77:S18–S28.

71. Michael JW. Modern prosthetic knee mechanisms. *Clin Orthop* 1999;361: 39–47.

72. Smith J, Tuel SM, Meythaler JMet al. Prosthetic management of hemicorporectomy patients: new approaches. *Arch Phys Med Rehabil* 1992;73(5):493–497.

73. Malone JM, Fleming LL, Robenson J, et al. Immediate, early, and late postsurgical management of upper-limb amputation. *J Rehabil Res Dev* 1984;21: 3–41.

74. Wright TW, Hagen AD, Wood MB. Prosthetic usage in major upper extremity amputations. *J Hand Surg* 1995;20A619–622.

75. Crandall RC, Tomhave W. Pediatric unilateral below-elbow amputees: retrospective analysis of 34 patients given multiple prosthetic options. *J Pediatr Orthop* 2002;22:380–383.

76. Silcox DH, Rooks MD, Vogel RR, et al. Myoelectric prostheses: a long-term follow-up and a study of the use of alternate prostheses. *JBJS* 1993;75-A: 1781–1789.

77. Lake C. Effects of prosthetic training on upper-extremity prosthesis use. *JPO* 1997;9:3–9.

78. Meier RH. Upper limb amputee rehabilitation. *Phys Med Rehabil STAR* 1994;8(1):165–185.

79. Millsten S, Heger H, Hunter A: Prosthetic use in adult upper limb amputees: a comparison of the body powered and electrically powered prosthesis. *Prosthet Orthot Int* 1986;10:27–34.

80. LeBlanc M. Use of prosthetic prehensors. *Prosthet Orthot Int* 1988, 12(3): 152–154.

81. Leow ME, Pho RWH, Pereira BP. Esthetic prostheses in minor and major upper limb amputations. *Hand Clin* 2001;17:489–497.

82. Michael JW. Upper limb powered components and controls: current concepts. *Clin Prosthet Orthot* 1986;10:66–77.

83. Uellendahl JE. Upper extremity myoelectric prosthetics. *Phys Med Rehabil Clinic North Am* 2000;11:639–652.

84. Malone JM, Childers SJ, Underwood J, et al. Immediate postsurgical management of upper extremity amputation: conventional, electric, and myoelectric prostheses. *Orthot Prosthet* 1981;35:1–9.

85. Nikolajsen L, Jenson TS. Phantom limb pain. *Br J Anaesth* 2001;87:107–116.

86. Hill A. Phantom limb pain: a review of the literature on attributes and potential mechanisms. *J Pain Symptom Manage* 1999;17:125–142.

87. Halbert J, Crotty M, Camerson ID. Evidence for the optimal management of acute and chronic phantom pain: a systematic review. *Clin J Pain* 2002;18:84–92.

88. Sherman RA. Published treatments of phantom limb pain. *Am J Phys Med* 1980;59:232–244.

89. Sherman RA, Sherman CJ, Gail NA. Survey of current phantom limb treatment in the United States. *Pain* 1980;8:85–99.

90. Spire MC, Leonard JA. Prosthetic pearls: solutions to thorny problems. *Phys Med Rehabil Clinics North Am* 1996;7:509–526.

91. Boutin RD, Pathria MN, Resnick D. Disorders in the stumps of amputee patients: MR imaging. *AFR* 1998;171:497–501.

92. Levy SW. *Skin problems of the amputee.* St. Louis: Warren H Green, 1983.

93. Lyon CC, Kulkarni J, Zimerson E, et al. Skin disorders in amputees. *J Am Acad Dermatol* 2000;42:501–507.

94. Lake C, Supan TJ. The incidence of dermatologic problems in the silicone sleeve user. *JPO* 1997;9:97–106.

95. Hachisuka K, Nakamura T, Ohmine S, et al. Hygiene problems of residual limb and silicone liners in transtibial amputees wearing the total surface bearing socket. *Arch Phys Med Rehabil* 2001;82:1286–1290.

96. Shaperman J, Landsberger SE, Setoguchi Y. Early upper limb prosthesis fitting: when and what do we fit. *J Prosthet Orthot* 2003;15:11–17.

97. Scott RN. *Myoelectric prostheses for infants*, 4th ed. Fredrickton, NB: University of New Brunswick, 1992.

98. Jain S. Rehabilitation in limb deficiency. 2. The pediatric amputee. *Arch Phys Med Rehabil* 1995;77:S9–S13.

99. Cummings DR. Pediatric prosthetics. *Phys Med Rehabil Clinic North Am* 2000;11:653–679.

100. Nagarajan R, Neglia JP, Clohisy DR, et al. Education, employment, insurance, and marital status among 694 survivors of pediatric lower extremity bone tumors: a report from the childhood cancer survivor study. *Cancer* 2003;97(10):2554–2564.

CHAPTER 62

Spinal Orthotics

Ferne Pomerantz and Eva Durand

An orthosis is a mechanical device that applies forces to the body in an effort to support, limit, and stabilize moving parts, assist and improve motion, correct and align deformities, and prevent and protect susceptible areas. The location, direction, and magnitude of these forces vary with the components and design of the orthosis. The word orthotic is derived from the Greek word "orthos", meaning straight, normal, or true. Orthotics, also called braces or splints, have been described since ancient Egypt. Their use continues today; however, changes and advances in materials and techniques of fabrication, interrelated with newer surgical procedures and medical treatments, have expanded their applications.

An orthotist is a professional who designs, makes, and, with the referring physician, helps prescribe the proper orthosis for a patient. Orthoses can be prefabricated to fit a large variety of patients or custom molded to a specific patient. Their effectiveness is directly dependent upon the proper fit and alignment of the components as well as proper use and compliance by the patient. The physician and orthotist should prepare a detailed prescription together in order to avoid deliveringthe wrong device. Once delivered each should be present to "check out" the device in order to ensure proper fit.

The prescription of an orthosis requires an understanding of the pathology of the disorder to be treated and must take into account the goals to be achieved. Knowledge of anatomy, biomechanics, and kinesiology, as well as an understanding of the indications (positive effects) and limitations (negative effects) of the orthosis are paramount when prescribing such devices.

One should not get confused by the myriad classifications and names for orthoses. Some are named for their founder, others for the location where they were developed, and still others for the parts of the body to which they are applied. The most standard way to name an orthosis is by the joints that it encompasses and the motion it controls (1). In this chapter we review the different types of spinal orthotics, indications for their use, positive and negative effects, and problems that may interfere with the ongoing rehabilitation of the patient. Braces for scoliosis and osteoporosis are not covered in this chapter.

MECHANISM OF ACTION

Spinal orthotics are prescribed for a variety of reasons (Table 62-1). They are designed to protect the spinal column and supporting structures (ligaments and muscles) from loads and stresses that can cause pain or progression of angular and translational deformity. The physiologic mechanisms responsible for this protection are control of motion, trunk support, and spinal alignment (2).

Control of Motion

The control of motion varies by the flexibility of the device. Numerous studies have attempted to quantify the degree of motion restriction. The most minimal limitation in gross movement likely occurs because the device acts as a physical and kinesthetic reminder to the patient not to move in harmful ways. Braces such as soft collars or lumbar corsets are examples of these. These types of devices also serve to provide warmth and heat to the patient, which may reduce spasm and pain. More restrictive braces act to limit intersegmental spinal motion and further yet, inhibit flexion-extension, lateral bending, and axial rotation.

Trunk Support

Trunk support is achieved by an increase in intraabdominal pressure. An increase in the thoracoabdominal pressure reduces the demand on the spinal extensor musculature and the vertical loading on the thoracolumbar spine.

Spinal Alignment

Spinal alignment is achieved by the application of the three-point force system inherent in all bracing. The corrective component ideally is located midway between the opposing forces above and below it. These systems shift forces from diseased areas to more healthy segments and prevent unopposed forces from causing deformity.

At each spinal level, orthoses require different designs to achieve their desired function. The desired physiologic effect must be decided upon when prescribing an orthosis so that the least restrictive device capable of completing the job is ordered. For example, if trunk support by thoracoabdominal containment is sufficient to reduce compressive forces on the spinal column and stress on the musculature, then joint motion stabilization should not be required (2).

Before prescribing an orthosis, one must begin with the indication and develop a goal; then decide which orthosis will achieve the desired goal. Once that goal has been achieved and the device is no longer needed, it should be discarded. Considerable diversity and controversy can surround the choice of an

TABLE 62-1.   Indications for Spinal Orthotics

Stabilize spine after fracture (with or without neurological deficit)
Limit spinal motion in cases of pain or sprain
Support posture and prevent deformity after paralysis
Postsurgical stabilization (with or without fracture)

TABLE 62-3.   Effects of Cervical Collars on Percent Mean Motion Permitted

	Flexion/ Extension	Lateral Flexion	Rotation	Source
Soft collar	74.2	92	83	Johnson (3)
	91	91	89	Sandler (4)
	92	92	91	Carter (5)
Philadelphia	29	67	44	Johnson
	58/53	78	52	Lunsford (6)
	60	89	73	Sandler
Miami J	41	—	20	Richter[a] (7)
	52/62	65	52	Lunsford (6)
Malibu	47/43	59	39	Lunsford
Newport	63/62	73	51	Lunsford
Minerva	46		14	Richter[a]
SOMI	28	66	34	Johnson
	39	82	82	Sandler
Halo	4	4	1	Johnson

[a]Richter only studied the upper cervical spine.

orthosis and the length of time needed for immobilization. Specific guidelines are generally lacking.

Spinal orthotics are divided into groups by the joints they encompass. Within each group there are many different designs (Table 62-2). They may further be differentiated by the motion they restrict or allow.

It is essential to be aware of the negative effects of bracing. Weakness, atrophy, and contracture, may follow restriction of motion and muscular activity. Skin irritation from poor fit, hygiene, and pin site shear and pressure can result in ulceration, pain, and infection. Impaired ambulation and balance can result from the limitation in motion and weight of the device such as with the halo, which in turn, may make an individual more dependant in their activities of daily living. Eating and swallowing may become compromised due to the position of the head and neck. There can be a decrease in pulmonary capacity due to the restricted chest wall motion and an increase in energy consumption. Psychological dependence on the brace can develop as well. This should all be taken into account when prescribing these braces because patients with certain medical conditions (e.g., neuromuscular disease), body types, and personalities may not be able to tolerate them.

Effective spinal bracing, therefore, is a complicated procedure and needs to take into account multiple factors. It is contingent upon correct fit, patient compliance, body habitus, the ability to restrict gross and segmental vertebral motion as well as the ability to minimize and prevent the negative side effects. Compliance is dependent on the patient's understanding of the condition, willingness to tolerate a snug fitting appliance, and overall comfort. Discomfort may be related to strap tightness, complaints of confinement, or increased perspiration caused by the brace. With patients who can volitionally adjust the straps, the effectiveness of the brace may be compromised if they loosen the straps. Individuals with a short stout neck and no chin are harder to fit with a cervical collar. Pendulous breasts, short trunk, thoracic kyphosis, or an obese abdomen make it difficult to comfortably fit cervicothoracic or thoracolumbosacral appliances. Two braces may need to be given to the patient so that one can be washed on a regular basis in order to maintain hygiene. Skin under the brace needs to be checked and washed daily. While in the brace, an exercise program needs to be implemented, if possible. Once the brace is discontinued a more aggressive strengthening and stretching program is initiated in order to prevent the negative effects of disuse. In addition, the patient or caregiver must be instructed

TABLE 62-2.   Categories of Orthoses

Cervical (CO) – soft or rigid head cervical (Philadelphia, Aspen, Miami, Newport)
Cervicothoracic (CTO) – Halo, SOMI, Minerva
Thoracolumbosacral (TLSO) – custom-molded body jacket, CASH, Jewitt,
Lumbosacral (LSO) – chairback, Knight, corsets/binders
Sacroiliac (SO) – trochanteric belt, sacral belt, sacral corset

in the donning and doffing of the orthosis, its wearing schedule, advice such as whether or not the patient needs to sleep and shower in the brace, and the length of time the orthosis is recommended. Follow-up of its continued use is required both for the physician and patient.

CERVICAL ORTHOSES

Cervical bracing can be categorized in several different manners. In general these devices can be subdivided into two broad categories: cervical and cervicothoracic. Cervical devices encircle the cervical spine; whereas cervicothoracic braces extend into the thoracic spine. When adding a thoracic extension piece, the cervical orthosis provides greater motion control of the lower cervical spine. To limit extension and hyperextension of the cervical spine an intimate fit under the occiput must be achieved.

With cervical appliances, the ability to control cervical motion varies significantly from the soft collar that provides minimal control to the halo that offers significant reduction in movement. Several studies have examined the effects of various orthoses on mean cervical range of motion (3–7). Many of these studies used different methods to quantify the amount of restriction (e.g., radiographic analysis, goniometric assessment, and computerized spinal motion analysis). In addition the sample size and characteristics varied from study to study (i.e., healthy spines verses injured spine). Table 62-3 outlines motion restriction (3–7).

Cervical Biomechanics

The cervical spine is a highly mobile structure allowing flexion, extension, lateral flexion, and rotation; thus, motion occurs in three planes: sagittal, frontal, and transverse. The atlantooccipital joint primarily permits flexion and extension with minimal axial rotation and lateral flexion. Functionally, this synovial joint enables an individual to nod their head. At the atlantoaxial (C1-C2) joint, the predominant motion is rotation. Having no vertebral body or disc, the atlas rotates around the odontoid axis. Cervical rotation begins first at this articulation and then proceeds caudally. Approximately 50% of the total rotation achieved by the cervical vertebral column occurs at this joint.

Between C4-C7, maximum flexion and extension occurs, with the greatest motion occurring at C5-C6. During flexion the vertebral foramina open and with extension close. Lateral flexion (lateral side bending), however, occurs between C2-C7 in the coronal plane. Given the configuration of the articulating facets, lateral flexion and rotation are coupled motions; as right rotation occurs, it initiates right lateral flexion and as left cervical rotation occurs, it initiates left lateral flexion. Sagittal motion occurring at C2-C7 is uncoupled.

Soft Cervical Collars

A soft cervical collar is prefabricated foam rubber with a cotton stockinette covering and Velcro closures (Fig. 62-1). These closures are worn posteriorly. Depending on the patient's dexterity and upper extremity range of motion, some can only fasten the closures anteriorly and rotate the collar around their neck while others leave the Velcro closures in the front. The manufacturer's intention was to have these collars worn with the closures facing posteriorly. Collars range in size from small to extra large. To identify the correct size, circumferential neck measurements are taken. This measure corresponds with predetermined sizes. Patients tolerate this device very well. Carter and associates reported that the degree of motion restriction achieved with the soft collar was dependent on Velcro closure position (5). If the intent is to limit flexion then the collar should be worn in the reverse position with the tabs facing anteriorly. The explanation for this is a function of the starting position of the head. Given its soft material construction, the soft collar can only provide warmth, psychological reassurance, and kinesthetic reminders to limit cervical range of motion; it cannot provide structural support. Its use may be appropriate to treat mild muscular spasms associated with arthritic changes and mild soft-tissue injuries.

These collars are often prescribed for the early management of whiplash injuries. A study evaluating their effectiveness on reducing the duration and intensity of the patient's pain following a whiplash (8) showed that test patients wearing a soft collar and control patient not wearing a soft collar reported persistent pain for at least 6 weeks postinjury. Patients should be advised that wearing a soft collar may or may not reduce the duration or intensity of their pain. Considerations regarding the negative effects of brace wearing (i.e., psychological dependency, muscle atrophy, etc.) should be weighed against pain management in this condition.

Hard Cervical Collars

These rigid prefabricated orthoses are used for prehospital trauma immobilization or for long-term patient management in an ambulatory setting. Each of these devices is radiolucent. Examples of collars used for emergency stabilization are the Philadelphia (Philadelphia Cervical Collar Company, Thorofare, NJ), Stifneck (Laerdal Medical, Wappinger Falls, NY), and the NecLoc (Jerome Medical, Moorestown, NJ). These collars are either a one- or two-piece design. The Philadelphia orthoses also may be used for long-term patient management. Newer brands of collars used for long-term application are the Miami J (Jerome Medical, Moorestown, NJ), Aspen (Aspen Medical Products, Long Beach, CA), Newport (California Medical Products, Long Beach, CA), and Malibu. The Newport orthosis has been replaced by the Aspen collar. The Philadelphia collar is a latex-free, two-piece design constructed from closed cell Plastizote foam with molded chin and occipital supports. Anteriorly it extends from the mandible to the sternum and posteriorly it extends from the occiput to the upper thoracic

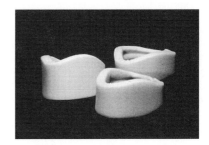

Figure 62-1. Soft cervical collars.

spine. The Miami J, Newport, and Aspen collars are two-piece polyethylene shells with internal padding. The Miami J collar offers greater customization; the anterior and posterior shells permit angle adjustability around the chin and occiput allowing for individual differences in bony anatomy. The Newport collar has superior and inferior adjustable supporting tabs that distribute the load along the occiput, upper thoracic spine, sternum, and upper trapezius. Each of these collars has an anterior opening to accommodate a cricothyrotomy/tracheotomy.

When prescribing cervical collars with removable padding, a second set of replacement pads should be included. The patient will need a second set to replace soiled odorous pads, to allow moist pads to air dry after patient showering or perspiring, and when the pads show wear. Since these pads can be cleaned, it is not necessary to discard them. For specific cleaning directions, have the patient consult the manufacturer's guide. Proper cleaning prevents skin irritation. Patients with long hair should be advised to wear their hair outside the collar to prevent irritation.

Typically, these devices are prescribed for midcervical bony or ligamentous injuries as well as postoperative stabilization or post-halo removal. In cases of spinal instability, these rigid devices are contraindicated. Recently, however, these appliances are being used as the first line of treatment over traditional halo devices for the conservative management of stable upper cervical fractures (9–13), including: Jefferson, (fracture of C1) (9,11), Hangman (traumatic spondylolisthesis of the axis-C2 on C3) (10,11,13), and certain types of odontoid fractures (10–12). Studies analyzing patient outcomes in the aforementioned situations showed stable fracture healing, and no increased disability or neurologic compromise on follow-up examination (9,11, 13). In addition these devices are cost-effective, easily applied, and do not have the increased risks associated with the use of the halo. Frequent radiographic monitoring to detect instability is recommended.

When assessing fit or proper donning of the brace, look at the patient's face to determine if the chin is centered in the anterior piece. If the chin extends beyond the collar edge it is too small. If the chin falls inside the collar it is too large. These visual markers indicate whether or not the device is sized or donned correctly. Patients should be familiar with proper donning and doffing procedures.

Pressure ulcer formation is a potential complication of rigid collar use. Fragile or insensate skin is particularly vulnerable to ulceration. Common areas susceptible to damage are the occipital protuberance, mental protuberance of the mandible (chin) clavicles, and ears. These wounds may be the result of pressure, shear, or moisture accumulation. A poorly fitting orthotic could exert an external pressure greater than the acceptable skin pressure of 25 to 32 mm Hg; when this occurs tissue ischemia ensues, resulting in an ulcer. In addition, shearing forces can arise due to facial hair and skin sliding over the collar surface, or from positional changes. For example, when a patient moves from supine to a semi-Fowler position in preparation for getting out of bed, or if the patient slides down toward the foot of the bed, shear forces can develop. Since beards increase shear forces, it is suggested that patients shave regularly. Since constant collar wearing increases local skin temperature, excessive perspiration in and around the area can occur. Constant moisture macerates the skin, inducing breakdown. Jirika and colleagues found that patients with moist skin were four times more likely to develop skin breakdown compared to those with dry skin (14). Provisions should be made to keep the skin clean, dry, and cool.

To assess for skin breakdown remove the anterior shell to inspect the chin and clavicles, then refasten the straps before log rolling the patient onto his or her side. Remove the posterior portion and inspect the occipital protuberance and ear lobes. When removing or applying the collar or a portion of it, the physician must maintain proper neck alignment to prevent injuring the cervical spine. Prior to discharge, patients should be advised to contact their physician if they notice any redness or sores.

Plasier and colleagues conducted a study evaluating craniofacial pressures when using different hard cervical collars: Stifneck, Philadelphia, Newport, and Miami J (15). The study found that the Newport and Miami J collars had lower skin capillary closing pressures, and their open-cell foam material prevented moisture accumulation. In supine and upright positions, the Philadelphia collar exerted high capillary closing pressures leaving the tissues susceptible to injury. In another study, occipital pressure, skin temperature, and humidity were compared when wearing the Philadelphia and Aspen collars (16). Measurements were taken at two separate time intervals, zero and 30 minutes. Using paired t-tests the authors found no difference in pressure or skin temperature with the two collars. Skin humidity, however, was higher when wearing the Philadelphia collar. Skin humidity relates to perspiration; perhaps the closed cell materials used in the Philadelphia collar caused the subjects to perspire more. For patients predisposed to excessive perspiration, the materials used in the collar's construction should be considered in order to optimize patient comfort, compliance, and minimize ulcer formation. Additional but uncommon complications associated with the use of hard collars have included marginal mandibular nerve palsy (17), dysphagia (18), changes in intracranial pressure (19), reduction in tidal volume (20), and tetraparesis (21).

Cervicothoracic Orthosis

Several prefabricated hard collars (i.e., Philadelphia, Miami, and Aspen) can be made available with an extension piece to transform them into cervicothoracic orthoses. These devices can be ordered to restrict middle and lower cervical motion. Other examples of these include the SOMI and Minerva. The SOMI is named for its body attachments: sternum, occiput, mandible, immobilizer (Fig. 62-2). If the mandibular support interferes with the patient's ability to chew, or a pressure sore develops, or the patient has a prominent chin, a forehead strap attaching to the occipital support can be substituted. The Minerva is a total contact orthosis with fixation points at the chin, occiput, sternum and thorax, and a forehead strap. The jacket is made of polyethylene and lined with an open cell material. In addition to controlling the middle and lower cervical spine it can be used for the upper cervical spine below C2. Benzel and colleagues found that when comparing the halo to the Minerva the average movement from flexion to extension was 3.7 degrees plus or minus 3.1 for the halo and 2.3 degrees plus or minus 1.7 for the Minerva suggesting that the Minerva should be considered over the halo in injuries below C2 (22). Between the occiput and C1 the halo provided better stabilization (23). When comparing the rigid Miami J collar to the Minerva, the

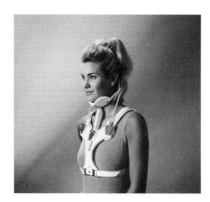

Figure 62-2. SOMI. The SOMI is named for its body attachments: sternum, occiput, mandible immobilizer.

Minerva did not provide better control of the upper cervical spine. (7) Greene and associates recommend using either a rigid collar or a SOMI for stable upper C-spine fractures (10). There has been a published case report of the Minerva brace causing dysphagia with resultant aspiration pneumonia (24). The report outlined several mechanisms placing the patient at risk for aspiration pneumonia: head elevation, slight cervical extension, and limited chin tuck. These combined factors interfere with the swallowing mechanism in some patients.

Halo Orthosis

The halo cervicothoracic orthosis provides triplanar cervical vertebral motion control. While it offers significant restriction, intersegmental vertebral "snaking" has been described (25). "Snaking" is defined as flexion of one vertebral segment with extension of the adjacent vertebral body. It has been blamed for motion occurring while immobilized. Koch and Nickel found motion for individuals wearing a halo averaged 31% of normal in the lower cervical spine with the greatest motion at C4-C5 (25). Johnson and colleagues reported 4% sagittal and frontal motion and 1% transverse motion (3). Lind and associates also detected motion ranging from 2 to 17 degrees with an average of 9 degrees between C2-C6; the largest movement occurred between the occiput and C1 (26). One study attempted to reduce this intersegmental motion by inserting a posterior pad (27). Using 30 healthy volunteers wearing a halo with and without a posterior pad attachment, spinal motion measurements were taken in supine and upright positions. The results revealed that the posterior pad did not prevent segmental motion.

The halo has been used postoperatively as an adjunct to internal fixation as well as the primary method for fracture stabilization. Although it is the most restrictive appliance, it does not guarantee alignment or fusion. It does have several advantages: it provides immediate cervical spinal stability in patients sustaining an acute fracture or subluxation; it is a nonsurgical alternative for patients refusing operative care or for whom surgical intervention is contraindicated; and it permits early mobilization without risk of compromising spinal alignment.

The basic halo vest components include a rigid open or closed back stabilizing ring fixed to the cranium by four skeletal traction pins with supporting rods and a superstructure that connects the ring to a fleece-lined plastic vest (Fig. 62-3). All parts and vest designs are compatible with diagnostic imaging: magnetic resonance, computed tomography, or x-ray. In cases where emergency access to the thoracic cavity is required, such as to administer cardiopulmonary resuscitation, the vest can be opened. To open the vest, some designs require a specialized tool while others have quick release buckles or an integrated

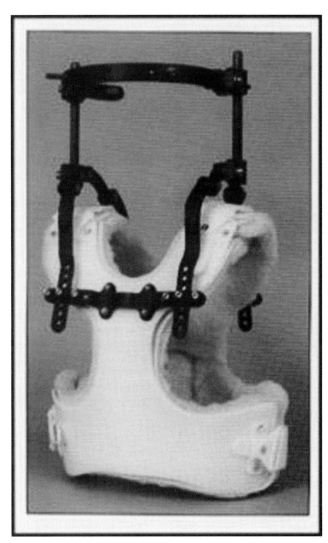

Figure 62-3. Halo vest.

cles, scapula or abdomen thus improving patient comfort and reducing the incidence of pressure sore development. Fukui and colleagues found that the distraction loads were less than the "standard" vest type.

When identifying precautions for the halo vest, the physician should instruct the therapist to limit the patient's shoulder abduction to 90 degrees and avoid shoulder shrugging (26). Apparently, large distraction forces are generated with these therapeutic exercises. Such forces may pose a danger to the injured vertebral segment (26). In general, ample space should exist between the shoulders and the shoulder vest straps to prevent excessive distraction forces on the cervical spine. When this space is reduced, the shoulders press against the straps and changes in forces are created.

Care must be taken not to lift, turn, or move the patient by pulling on the plastic vest, the rods, or the superstructure. External forces applied to these areas could affect spinal alignment and loosen pins. In the literature pin loosening is defined as a visible pin tip or the actual pin is manually rotated (31). In addition to external forces affecting tightness, there appears to be a natural decrease in compressive pin force over the duration of use (32). Subjectively, the patient may report clicking/grating/creaking sounds, a sensation of looseness, pain at the pin site, headache, or halo vest movement. Since pin loosening is the most frequent complication, all members of the rehabilitation team should be aware of these signs and symptoms.

Loose pins are either retightened or removed and reinserted elsewhere. Initially, the preferred pin placement is anterolateral above the orbital rim and posterolateral below the largest diameter of the skull (33). These positions prevent piercing the temporalis muscle and the frontal and temporal fossa, as well as injury to the cranial nerves. If the temporalis muscle is penetrated, the patient will complain of increased pin site pain during mastication. Patients with a cranioplasty may be more susceptible to pin penetration and alternative safe positions for the pins may need to be identified prior to their insertion (34). A case report identified a patient who sustained an epidural abscess as a result of pin penetration through the temporal cranioplasty. In another case report, 11 years after the halo was removed, the patient developed tonic-clonic seizures (35). On investigation of the etiology, it was determined that the epileptic focus was the scar tissue caused by the pin penetration. Vertullo and colleagues recommend tightening pins 24 to 48 hours after insertion and at 1 week (31). He found that it was a safe and effective method to decrease pin site complications.

Pin site infection is another common complication. To prevent infection, careful inspection for acute signs and symptoms of infection and prophylactic treatment should be ordered for the rehabilitation nurses. Olson recommends cleansing the sites using sterile cotton-tip applicators with antimicrobial soap and normal saline (36). Other topical cleansing agents such as povidone-iodine (Betadine), hydrogen peroxide, and alcohol have been associated with pin corrosion, interference with bacterial autolysis, ineffective infection reduction, and disruption of the healing process (36). Topical ointments can obstruct fluid drainage and increase the risk of infection; hence, prophylactic use is discouraged (37). Crusts surrounding the pins should be gently removed with a saline-soaked cotton-tip applicator. If left alone these crusts could cause fluid buildup predisposing the wound for infection (37). Pin site care should be performed daily. When crusts or drainage are present, it should be done more frequently (36). If drainage or erythema is present then laboratory testing for culture and sensitivity should be ordered to evaluate for an infectious organism.

In a case study by Rosenblum and Ehrlich (38), a 26-year-old man was treated with a halo secondary to a C6 burst fracture. One week after admission to rehabilitation his right rear halo

hinge system. The rehabilitation team should be familiar with how to open the vest. Laterally, the vest has straps that adjust the amount of tightness across the torso. One study found that the strap tension influenced the degree of spinal motion (28). Increasing strap tension decreased motion especially in lateral bending. No detectable differences were noted for extension. Clinically, the straps should be examined periodically to ensure adequate fit between the vest and thorax. Over the course of rehabilitation changes in the person's body habitus are expected; for example, weight loss due to diuresis, or changes in appetite affect chest circumference and strap adjustments may be indicated. Failure to monitor vest thorax fit could compromise cervical stability offered by this external device. Trunk deformities may interfere with the patient's ability to tolerate such an intimate vest fit. Patients and caregivers should be discouraged from arbitrarily manipulating these straps without consulting the physician.

A recent design variation to the standard whole torso vest is an adjustable four-pad (4PAD) thoracic vest (29). Instead of a two-piece vest, this orthotic consists of two lateral pads, one sternal and one thoracic spine pad. These pads move independent of one another. This design does not use shoulder straps. Fuki and colleagues evaluated this new product and found that it compared favorably in terms of patient outcomes and in its ability to immobilize the cervical spine despite its reduced torso contact (30). These pads do not interface with the clavi-

TABLE 62-4.   Complications Associated with Halo Vest Use
• Loss of spinal reduction while wearing a halo • Failure to develop spinal stability after the wearing the halo • Pressure sore development • Pin loosening • Pin site pain • Pin tract infection • Brain abscess • Local osteoporosis • Acute equilibrium impairments • Forehead scarring • Dysphasia • Pin penetration of the skull • Halo ring migration • Cranial nerve palsy • Brachial plexopathy • Reduction in vital capacity

pin loosened and it was retightened. Pin care orders were for hydrogen peroxide three times a day. Four weeks later the right pin was loose with mild crusting. Subsequently the patient presented with signs and symptoms consistent with psychosis. Magnetic resonance imaging (MRI) results were consistent with a brain abscess at the temporal-parietal junction. Bone and brain biopsy revealed *Staphylococcus aureus*. The patient was treated with systemic antibiotics. His psychosis resolved. This illustrates that changes in mentation may be a possible indicator of brain abscess in patients wearing a halo. Furthermore other signs and symptoms such as scalp/pin cellulitis, headache, eye pain, fever, and seizures should alert the physician to consider brain abscess due to halo pins in their differential diagnosis.

A prospective study evaluating bone mineral density changes in the cervical spine for patients wearing a halo found that the vest produced local osteoporosis in the immobilized vertebra (39). The reduction in bone mineral density however was not related to the level or type of cervical injury, age, or gender of the patient. At the 5- to 6-month follow-up, the local vertebral osteoporosis was mostly reversible.

In preparation for discharging a patient to the community with a halo vest, the patient and caregivers should be aware that the halo has an effect on balance. In a study evaluating balance impairments in young healthy subjects wearing a halo, the authors discovered that their subjects' balance was compromised (40). This certainly has implications for geriatric patients who frequently have underlying equilibrium impairments. In fact, their cervical injury could have been a result of a fall. Intrinsic and extrinsic factors related to prevention of falls should be explored prior to discharge. Home modifications to eliminate potential fall hazards should be discussed (e.g., removal of scatter rugs, installation of stair rails, wearing proper footwear, etc.). A home visit conducted by the inpatient rehabilitation team or a home care therapist can evaluate the discharge environment and make safety recommendations to prevent falls.

Numerous other complications have been associated with the use of the halo device (33–43). Table 62-4 outlines complications associated with the halo orthoses.

THORACOLUMBOSACRAL ORTHOSES

The thoracolumbosacral orthosis (TLSO) is a spinal orthosis that provides fixation at the extremes of the pelvis and the shoulders in an attempt to immobilize the thoracolumbar spine in varying directions. All trunk orthoses produce their desired effect by applying anterior abdominal compression, restricting trunk/intervertebral motion, or supporting/aligning the spine, as previously discussed. The abdominal compression results in increased intracavity pressure, which leads to a reduction in the lumbar lordosis and a decreased load on the vertebrae and intervertebral discs. The ability of different devices to produce a desired effect depends on how restrictive they are in design and in materials. The effectiveness in limiting intersegmental motion of the thoracic, lumbar, and sacral spine in all three planes has been studied repeatedly though not as extensively as that of cervical orthoses. Dorsky and associates found various types of orthoses effective in controlling lateral side-bending as compared to flexion-extension motion (44). The custom-molded TLSO resulted in the most gross body motion restriction and the corset resulted in the least (45). All TLSOs have been shown to be more effective in reducing motion at the upper levels than at the lower levels, with greatest motion at the lumbosacral joints (46–48). With three-column injuries, none of these braces were able to adequately limit motion (49). Myoelectric activity of erector spinae muscles has been investigated with inconsistent results. Lantz and colleagues compared the lumbosacral corset, the chairback, and a molded TLSO. Overall, the TLSO reduced myoelectric signal activity the most (50). Nachemson showed the same reduction in intradiscal pressures by 25% with a corset and a rigid brace. (51)

The TLSOs can be divided into categories based on the direction of motion they control: flexion, flexion-extension, flexion-extension-lateral, and flexion-extension-lateral-rotary control orthoses.

Thoracic and Lumbosacral Spine Biomechanics

The thoracic spine can be thought of best by dividing into upper (T1-T4), middle (T5–8), and lower (T9-T11) segments and the lumbar spine as the thoracolumbar junction (T12-L1), midlumbar (L2–4) segment, and the lumbosacral junction (L5-S1). The 12 thoracic vertebrae are limited in motion in all directions by their attachment to the ribs and orientation of the facet joints; they are further limited in extension by overlapping of their spinous processes. As one goes in a craniocaudal direction, the range of sagittal plane flexion extension motion increases. The coronal plane (lateral) flexion-extension motion and axial rotation increases to the maximum degree at the lower thoracic and thoracolumbar junction and then decreases again. At the thoracolumbar junction the curvatures of kyphosis and lordosis change direction, the facet joints change direction from frontal to sagittal plane, the gravity line bisects the T12-L1 disc and there is the weakest muscular protection. As a result, this area is considered the most mobile segment and is prone to traumatic injuries. The lower lumbar segments, L4-L5 and L5-S1, are more susceptible to herniated discs and spondylolisthesis (52).

Flexion Control Orthosis

The flexion control orthosis is also referred to as an anterior hyperextension brace, which functions to extend the thoracolumbar region. It is prefabricated and lightweight. The Jewett and cruciform anterior spinal hyperextension (CASH) braces are examples of this type of orthosis (Figs. 62-4 and 62-5). Both use a three-point pressure system without any abdominal compression. The Jewett brace consists of a metal anterior and lateral frame. Attached to the frame are two lateral pads, a sternal pad, a suprapubic pad, and a posterior thoracolumbar pad. The pads exert pressures over a small area and therefore may cause discomfort. The CASH orthosis consists only of an ante-

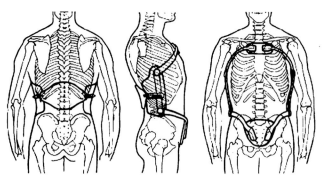

Figure 62-4. Jewett brace.

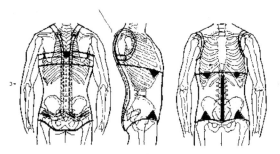

Figure 62-6. Taylor brace.

rior metal frame that is shaped like a cross with the pads attached at the ends. The horizontal bar is attached at the midpoint. It is easier to don and doff than the Jewett and is better tolerated. Both are designed to prevent flexion only and do not limit lateral and rotary movements. They have been used to aid in the treatment of osteoporosis and anterior compression fractures. However they have not been found to decrease kyphosis and have been found to cause excessive hyperextension forces on the posterior elements, inducing fracture. They are contraindicated in unstable fractures or in cases where extension must be prohibited, such as spondylolisthesis.

Flexion-Extension Control Orthosis

The Taylor brace designed in 1863 for the treatment of Pott's disease, consists of two thoracolumbosacral posterior uprights attached inferiorly to a pelvic band and superiorly to an interscapular band that also serves as an attachment for axillary straps (Fig. 62-6). Anteriorly, there is a corset for abdominal compression. The axillary straps extend over the shoulders and pass under the axillae, buckling at each end of the interscapular band. This brace limits trunk extension primarily in the mid-to-lower thoracic and upper lumbar areas with a compensatory increase in motion at the upper thoracic, lower lumbar, and lumbosacral junction. The straps must be tight in order for the brace to be effective and thereby may cause shoulder pain limiting the patient's compliance. In addition the straps may restrict end-range shoulder motion.

Flexion-Extension-Lateral Control Orthosis

The Knight-Taylor brace is a combination of the Knight (described later) and the Taylor brace (described above). It adds a pair of lateral uprights to the design in an attempt to limit lateral trunk motion (Fig. 62-7).

Flexion-Extension-Lateral-Rotary Control Orthosis

This is similar to the Knight-Taylor except that the interscapular band is extended anteriorly and superiorly, and subclavicular pads are added. Called the cowhorn orthosis, it has the added benefit of limiting trunk rotation and flexion in the thoracic and upper lumbar spine; however, it can also cause a compensatory increase in motion at the lower lumbar spine and lumbosacral junction.

Plastic Body Jacket

The custom-molded plastic body jacket is the orthotic apparatus of choice when maximum immobilization is necessary (Fig. 62-8). Fabricated from polypropylene through a plaster cast taken of the patient, body jackets provide total contact to soft tissues and reliefs over bony prominences, thereby distributing forces over a large area for greater comfort, support, and motion control. The superior and inferior portions of the anterior section restrict flexion in the thoracolumbar and lumbosacral segments. The superior and inferior forces from the posterior shell and the forces from the abdominal area in the anterior component resist extension. The upper and lower portions of the lateral aspects of the jacket limit lateral trunk motion. And lastly, these forces combine to limit thoracolumbar rotation. Abdominal compression also alleviates pressure on the vertebrae and discs and reduces myoelectric activity of erector spinae musculature.

Proper fit requires that the inferior border of the anterior shell rest one-half inch above the pubic symphysis, the trim follows the inguinal fold when the patient is sitting, and the superior border encompasses the sternal notch. If the anterior-inferior border is too long, the patient will have difficulty sitting forward and performing sit-to-stand transfers, as the brace would block the forward motion required to transfer. If during transfer training, as the therapist attempts to guide and position the trunk forward in preparation to transfer, the patient complains of pain in and around the pubis, the orthotist must

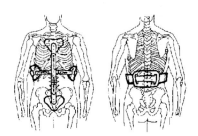

Figure 62-5. Cash brace.

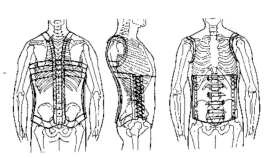

Figure 62-7. Knight-Taylor brace.

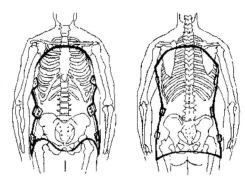

Figure 62-8. Custom-molded body jacket.

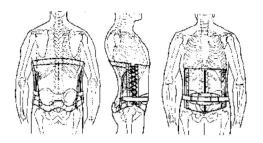

Figure 62-10. Williams brace.

be contacted to trim the brace. Posteriorly, the shell should extend from the spine of the scapula to the sacrococcygeal junction with the upper gluteal mass contained and the axillae and trochanter free (53). Extra precautions must be taken when fitting a jacket to an insensate patient; however, since the jackets are total contact in design, they are better tolerated. Plastizote lining and ventilation holes make the jackets still more comfortable and breathable. They can be washed and modified as needed; they can even be modified to accommodate a drain. The jackets can be made into lumbosacral orthoses (LSOs) and cervical thoracolumbosacral orthoses (CTLSOs) when the upper thoracic spine needs immobilization. They should be worn at all times when on an incline greater that 30 degrees, though this is often modified by the surgeon (e.g., to allow the patient to shower). Restrictions of activity and brace wearing must be individualized for each patient's needs.

LUMBOSACRAL ORTHOSES

The lumbosacral orthosis (LSO) may be either flexible or rigid. The flexible LSOs refer to corsets, belts and binders. While not effective in restricting motion to a significant degree, they can elevate intraabdominal pressure, thereby unloading the spine and supporting structures, as well as provide inhibitory kinesthetic feedback and warmth. The rigid LSOs are categorized in the same fashion as the TLSOs are, namely by the motion they control; in this case flexion-extension, flexion-extension-lateral and extension-lateral.

Flexion-Extension Control Orthosis

The chairback brace is a rigid LSO that consists of two posterior uprights attached to a pelvic band inferiorly and a thoracic band superiorly with an abdominal support fastened to the posterior uprights with straps. The thoracic band should rest

just below the inferior border of the scapula and the pelvic band at the sacrococcygeal junction. Its forces serve to restrict flexion and extension as well as provide abdominal compression when the abdominal support is tight.

Flexion-Extension-Lateral Control Orthosis

The Knight brace further limits motion with lateral uprights added to the chairback brace (Fig. 62-9). The lateral bars pass over the iliac crests so they must be fitted carefully to avoid pressure on these bony prominences.

Extension-Lateral Control Orthosis

The Williams orthosis limits extension and lateral motion but encourages flexion (Fig. 62-10). Its effect is to reduce the lumbar lordosis. It consists of pelvic and thoracic bands joined by a pair of lateral uprights (no posterior uprights), which decreases the lateral motion. The thoracic and lateral bars are directly attached to each other but the pelvic band is attached to the lateral upright with oblique lateral bars that pivot at the top but secure rigidly at the bottom. The abdominal support is elastic and an adjustment strap between the pairs of uprights acts as a lever to pull the oblique uprights more posterior and decrease the lordosis.

Corsets and Binders

When treating low back pain, flexible LSOs are the most prescribed spinal orthoses. These are garments made of fabric, typically prefabricated, that close in the front with Velcro or laces and encircle the lumbar and abdominal areas. Designs vary and include the lumbar/abdominal binder, the Warm-N-Form, and the lumbosacral corset (Fig. 62-11 and Fig. 62-12).

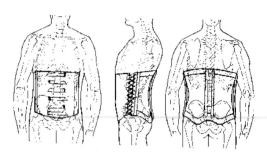

Figure 62-9. Knight brace.

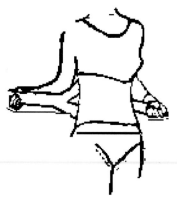

Figure 62-11. Lumbar binder.

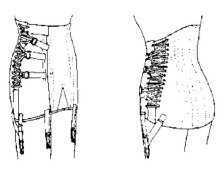

Figure 62-12. Lumbosacral corset.

TABLE 62-5. Orthotic Treatment of Clinical Conditions
Sciatica
Degenerative disc disease
Herniated nucleus pulposus
Radiculopathy
Spondylolisthesis – congenital and degenerative
Spondylosis
Osteoarthritis – facet joint arthritis
Traumatic fractures – compression, burst, fracture-dislocation
Osteoporosis – kyphosis, compression fracture
Spinal fusion
Laminectomy or discectomy
Inflammatory arthritis – rheumatoid arthritis, psoriatic arthritis, ankylosing spondylitis
Infectious diseases – spinal osteomyelitis and abscess, tuberculosis
Spinal tumors
Paralysis – tetraplegia, paraplegia
Spina bifida
Scoliosis
Cervical and lumbar sprain
Torticollis
Whiplash

The latter can be further modified to include posterior stays and shoulder straps.

The binder is elastic and must be wrapped tightly around the lumbar and lower abdominal area in order to elevate intraabdominal pressure. A common error in donning the binder is placing it above the diaphragm. The addition of a thermoplastic insert (Warm-N-Form) molded to the patients' lumbar curve and inserted into a posterior pocket may provide increased support and feedback.

The lumbosacral corset is longer than the binder, with the anterior-superior border extending to just below the xiphoid process and the inferior border to just above the pubic symphysis. Posteriorly, the borders go from below the scapula to just below the gluteal fold for women and gluteal bulge for men. The garment needs to fit all body contours snugly. As with other spinal orthoses, continued use will result in weakness and atrophy of trunk muscles and an exercise program needs to be given to the patient concomitantly. It addition to its use for pain relief, it provides postural, vasomotor, and respiratory support in cases of paralysis. In patients with paralysis and respiratory insufficiency, it places the diaphragm in a superior position and can assist the patient with increased diaphragmatic expansion.

SACROILIAC ORTHOSES

Sacroiliac orthoses include trochanteric belts, sacral belts, and sacral corsets. They are prefabricated devices that wrap around the pelvis between the iliac crests and greater trochanters. They are differentiated by the height of their superior borders, their adjustability, and materials. They may have perineal straps attached to prevent upward displacement and a sacral pad to apply pressure over the sacrum (Fig. 62-13). While not effective in restricting motion, they may increase intraabdominal pressure and provide kinesthetic feedback to maintain a neutral pelvis. These devices can help to stabilize the sacroiliac joint, support pelvic fractures and traumatic sacroiliac joint separations, and decrease sacroiliac joint and postpartum pain.

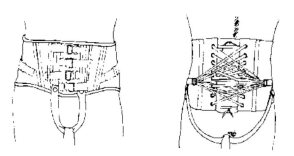

Figure 62-13. Sacroiliac corset.

CLINICAL USES FOR SPINAL ORTHOTICS

Spinal bracing is a common modality used for treatment in a variety of conditions affecting the spine (Table 62-5). There are no definitive recommendations when choosing a particular orthosis for a given condition and considerable variability exists among practitioners. An in-depth discussion of each condition identified above goes well beyond the scope of this chapter. Nevertheless, certain general principles apply.

If motion restriction for pain relief is the goal, and stability in not in question, as in cases of arthritis, sprain, strain, degenerative disc disease, osteoporosis, and even tumors or infections without neurologic impairment or instability, then corsets, collars, and binders may be adequate. This must be balanced with mobilization and proper exercise. The length of its use must be discussed with the patient and tailored based on variables such as age, concomitant conditions, and chronicity of complaints.

In cases requiring orthoses for spinal stability, flexible devices will not be adequate. In cases of vertebral fracture and trauma, spinal level and degree of injury must be ascertained. Treatments may include surgical stabilization, bracing, or both. Controversy in treatment exists in deciding which fractures have enough stability to be treated in an orthosis alone and in which surgical stabilization is needed. Denis described instability in 1984 (54,55) based on the three-column spine with instability defined as it relates to the integrity of the middle column. While some base their evaluation of stability on the presence of injury to the posterior elements (56,57) and others on the structural integrity of the middle column's bony as well ligamentous structures (58), Denis' theory was supported by Panjabi and colleagues in 1995 (59) and is generally accepted. Other conditions considered unstable generally follow these same principles with variability due to needs of the specific patient.

First-degree instability (Denis type I) is seen in compression fractures. In these cases, only the anterior column is affected. The middle column's structural integrity remains intact and is therefore considered a stable fracture. There exists, however, a subset of these lesions that can become progressive and lead to a posttraumatic kyphosis. According to Ferguson and Allen (60), this occurs when the compression is greater than 50% of the original body height and is the result of posterior ligamentous injury. Conservative treatment will suffice in the majority of these injuries and tends to include hyperextension bracing. Frequent monitoring is required. When the compression is 30% or less, no external support is required, and early ambulation was reported to be as effective as bracing intervention (61).

Second-degree instability is typical of the burst fracture (Denis type II), a compression injury of the anterior and middle columns. These fractures may behave more like fracture/dislocation injuries making categorization in terms of "burst" variable. This has resulted in considerable controversy in treating these fractures. Nevertheless, the two-column instabilities are usually treated conservatively with a Jewett, CASH, or custommolded TLSO appliance (62) depending upon severity. Fractures with posterior element instability will likely require surgery.

Seat belt injuries (Denis type III) may heal with a hyperextension TLSO if the fracture line passes through bone, the socalled Chance fracture (63) (about 50% of these injuries). However, if the fracture passes through the soft tissues, known as a slice fracture, then surgery is required.

Fracture/dislocation injury (Denis type IV) is an unstable fracture and frequently results in paralysis. This always requires surgery unless there are other contraindications (49).

Following surgery, a rigid brace may be required for 6 to 12 weeks until the fusion heals, or if no surgery is performed, perhaps longer. This will depend upon the type and location of the fracture, the procedure performed, and the personal views of the surgeon. In cervical injuries, the rigid cervical, cervicothoracic, or halo orthoses are used. For high-level thoracic fractures (T1-T6), some believe that a CTLSO is required (64). For lower level fractures of the thoracic and lumbar spine, various TLSOs have been used without the literature being specific about the most restrictive.

In any of these cases, the patient may participate, if needed, in a rehabilitation program to address mobility, activities of daily living, and community reentry. The patient should also be instructed in any restrictions of activity, donning and doffing of the brace, cleaning of the brace, and proper skin care. A T-shirt should be worn under the TLSO to protect the skin, and the orthosis must be donned tightly, otherwise the stabilizing effect is diminished (49). It is usually best to don a TLSO while in the supine position in order for it to be aligned properly.

REFERENCES

1. Harris EE. A new orthotics terminology—a guide to its use for prescription and fee schedules. *Orthot Prosthet* 1973;27(2):6–19.
2. Berger N, Edelstein J, Fishman S, et al. *Spinal orthotics*, rev. ed. New York: New York University Medical Center Post-Graduate Prosthetics & Orthotics, 1987:37–38.
3. Johnson RM, Hart DL, Simmons EF, et al. Cervical orthosis: a study comparing their effectiveness in restricting cervical motion in normal subjects. *J Bone Joint Surg (Am)* 1977;59:332–339.
4. Sandler AJ, Dvorak J, Humke T, et al. The effectiveness of various cervical orthoses: an in vivo comparison of the mechanical stability provided by several widely used models. *Spine* 1996;21(14):1624–1629.
5. Carter VM, Fasen JM, Roman J, et al. The effect of a soft collar used normally recommended or reversed on three planes of cervical range of motion. *J Orthop Sports Phys Ther* 1996;volume 23:209–215.
6. Lunford, TR, Davidson M, Lunsford BR et al. The effectiveness of four contemporary cervical orthoses in restricting cervical motion. *JPO* 1994;6(4):93–99.
7. Richter D, Latta LL, Milne, et al. The stabilizing effects of different orthoses in the intact and unstable upper cervical spine: a cadaver study. *J Trauma* 2001;50:848–854.
8. Gennis P, Miller L, Gallagher EJ, et al. The effect of soft cervical collars on persistent neck pain in patients with whiplash injury. *Acad Emerg Med* 1996; 3(6):563–564.
9. Lee T, Green B, Petrin D, et al. Treatment of stable burst fractures of the atlas (Jefferson fracture) with rigid cervical collar. *Spine* 1998;23:1963–1967.
10. Greene K, Dickman C, Marciano F, et al. Acute axis fractures. Analysis of management and outcome in 340 conservative cases. *Spine* 1997;22:1843–1852.
11. Cosan TE, Tel E, Arslantas A, et al. Indications of Philadelphia collar in the treatment of upper cervical injuries. *Eur J Emerg Med* 2001;8(10):33–37.
12. Chiba K, Fujimura Y, Toyama Fuji E, et al. Treatment protocol for fractures of the odontoid process. *J Spinal Disord* 1996;9:267–276.
13. Coric D, Wilson JA, Kelly DL Jr, et al. Treatment of traumatic spondylolisthesis of the axis with non-rigid immobilization: a review of 64 cases. *J Neurosurg* 1996;85(4):550–554.
14. Jirika M, Ryan R, Carvalho M, et al. Pressure ulcer risk factors in an ICU population. *Am J Crit Care* 1995;4:361–367.
15. Plasier B, Gabram SG, Schwartz RJ, et al. Prospective evaluation of craniofacial pressure in four different cervical orthoses. *J Trauma* 1994;37(5):714–720.
16. Black CA, Buderer NM, Blaylock B, et al. Comparative study of risk factors for skin breakdown with cervical orthotic devices: Philadelphia and Aspen. *J Trauma Nurs* 1998;5(3):62–66.
17. Rodgers JA, Rodgers WB, et al. Marginal mandibular nerve palsy due to compression by a cervical collar. *J Orthop Trauma* 1995;9(2):177–179.
18. Houghton DJ, Curley JW, et al. Dysphagia caused by a hard cervical collar. *Br J Neurosurg* 1996;10(5):501–502.
19. Raphael JH, Chotai R, et al. Effects of the cervical collar on cerebral spinal fluid pressure. *Anesthesia* 1994;49:437–439.
20. Dodd FM, Simon E, Mckeown D, et al. The effect of a cervical collar on the tidal volume of anaesthetised adult patients. *Anesthesia* 1995;50:961–963.
21. Papadopoulos MC, Chakraborty A, Waldron G, et al. Exacerbating cervical spine injury by applying a hard collar. *BMJ* 1999;319:171–172.
22. Benzel EC, Haden TA, Saulsberg CM, et al. A comparison of the Minerva and halo jackets for stabilization of the cervical spine. *J Neurosurg* 1989; 70:411–414.
23. Sharpe KP, Rao S, Ziogas A, et al. Evaluation of the effectiveness of the Minerva cervicothoracic orthosis. *Spine* 1995;20:1475–1479.
24. Odderson R, Lietzow D. Dysphagia complications of the Minerva brace. *Arch Phys Rehabil* 1997;78:1386–1388.
25. Koch RA, Nickel VL, et al. The halo vest: an evaluation of motion and forces across the neck. *Spine* 1978;3:103–107.
26. Lind B, Sihlbom H, Nordwall A, et al. Forces and motions across the neck in patients treated with Halo vest. *Spine* 1988;13:162–167.
27. Glaser JA, Myers MA, McComis GP, et al. Cervical motion after adding a posterior pad to the halo vest. *Am J Orthop* 2000;29(7):557–562.
28. Mirza SK, Moquin RR, Anderson PA, et al. Stabilizing properties of the Halo apparatus. *Spine* 1997;22(7):727–733.
29. Tomonaga T, Krag MH, Novotny JE, et al. Clinical, radiographic and kinematic results from an adjustable four-pad halo vest. *Spine* 1997;22(11):1199–1208.
30. Fuki Y, Krag M, Huston D, et al. Halo dynamic loads. Full crossover comparison of three vest types. *Spine* 2002;27(3):241–249.
31. Vertullo CJ, Duke PF, Askin GN, et al. Pin site complications of the halo thoracic brace with routine in re-tightening. *Spine* 1997;22(21):2514–2516.
32. Fleming BC, Krag MH, Huston DR, et al. Pin loosening in a halo-vest orthosis. A biomechanical study. *Spine* 2000;25(11):1325–1331.
33. Botte MJ, Byrne TP, Abrams RA, et al. The halo skeletal fixator: current concepts of application and maintenance. *Orthopedics* 1995;18:463–471.
34. Papagelopoulos PJ, Sapakas GS, Kateros KT, et al. Halo pin intracranial penetration and epidural abscess in a patient with a previous cranioplasty. case report and review of the literature. *Spine* 2001;26(19):E463–467.
35. Nottmeier EW, Bondurant CP, et al. Delayed onset of tonic clonic seizures as a complication of halo orthosis. Case report. *J Neurosurg* 2000;92[2 Suppl]:233–235.
36. Olson RS. Halo skeletal traction pin site care: toward developing a standard of care. *Rehabil Nurs* 1996;21:243–246.
37. Celeste S, Folick M, Dumas K, et al. Identifying a standard for pin site care using the quality assurance approach. *Orthop Nurs* 1984;3:17–24.
38. Rosenblum D, Ehrlich V. Brain abscess and psychosis as a complication of a halo orthosis. *Arch Phys Med Rehabil* 1995;76(9):865–867.
39. Korovessis P, Konstantinou D, Piperos G, et al. Spinal bone mineral density changes following halo vest immobilization for cervical trauma. *Eur Spine J* 1994;3(4):206–208.
40. Richardson JK, Ross AD, Riley B, et al. Halo vest effect on balance. *Arch Phys Med Rehabil* 2000;81(3):255–257.
41. Lind B, Bake B, Lundqvist C, et al. Influence of halo vest treatment on vital capacity. *Arch Phys Med Rehabil* 1986;Nov:449–452.
42. Glaser JA, Whitehill R, Stamp WG, et al. Complications associated with the halo vest. *J Neurosurg* 1986;65:762–769.
43. Garfin SR, Botte MJ, Waters RL, et al. Complications in the use of the halo fixation device. *J Bone Joint Surg* 1986;68A:320–325.
44. Dorsky S, Buchalter D, Kahanovitz N, et al. A three dimensional analysis of lumbar brace immobilization utilizing a noninvasive technique. In: Proceedings of the 33rd Annual Meeting, Orthopedic Research Society; 1987; San Francisco.
45. Lantz SA, Schultz AB, et al. Lumbar spine orthosis wearing—I. Restriction of gross body motions. *Spine* 1986a;11(8):834–837.
46. Norton PL, Brown T. The immobilizing efficiency of the back braces: their effect on the posture and motion of the lumbosacral spine. *J Bone Joint Surg* 1957;39A:111–139.
47. Lumsden RM, Morris JM, et al. An in vivo study of axial rotation and immobilization at the lumbosacral joint. *J Bone Joint Surg* 1968;50A:1591.

48. Miller RA, Hardcastle P, Renwick SE, et al. Lower spinal mobility and external mobilization in the normal and pathologic condition. *Orthop Rev* 1992; 21(6):753–757.
49. Patwardhan AG, Li S, Gavin TM, et al. Orthotic stabilization of thoracolumbar injuries—a biomechanical analysis of the Jewett hyperextension orthosis. *Spine* 1990;15(7):654–661.
50. Lantz SA, Schultz AB, et al: Lumbar spine orthosis wearing—II. Effect on trunk muscle myoelectric activity. *Spine* 1986b;11(8):838–842.
51. Nachemson AL. Disc pressure measurements. *Spine* 1981;6:93–97.
52. Anderson CW, Bedford JB. Orthotic treatment for injuries and diseases of the spinal column. *Phys Med Rehabil: State of the Art* 2000;14(3):471–484.
53. Berger N, Edelstein J, Fishman S, et al. *Spinal orthotics*, rev. ed. New York: New York Univeristy Medical Center Post-Graduate Prosthetics & Orthotics, 1987:9–17.
54. Denis F. Spinal instability as defined by the three-column spine concept in acute spinal trauma. *Clin Orthop* 1984;189:65–70.
55. Denis F. The three column spine and its significance in the classification of acute thoracolumbar spinal injuries. *Spine* 1983;8(6):817–831.
56. McAfee PC, Yuan HA, Lasda NA, et al. The unstable burst fracture. *Spine* 1982;7(4):363–373.
57. Slosar PJ Jr, Patwardhan AG, Lorenz M, et al. Instability of the lumbar burst fracture and limitations of transpedicular instrumentation. *Spine* 1992;20 (13):1452–1461.
58. Farcy JPC, Weidenbaum M, Glassman SD, et al. Sagittal index in management of thoracolumbar burst fractures. *Spine* 1990;15(9):958–965.
59. Panjabi MM, Oxland TR, Kifune M, et al. Validity of the three-column theory of thoracolumbar fractures: a biomechanic investigation. *Spine* 1995;20(10): 1122–1127.
60. Ferguson RL, Allen BL, et al. A mechanistic classification of thoracolumbar spine fractures. *Clin Orthop* 1984;189:77–88.
61. Ohana N, Sheinis D, Rath E, et al. Is there a need for lumbar orthosis in mild compression fractures of the thoracolumbar spine? A retrospective study comparing radiographic results between early ambulation with and without a lumbar orthosis. *Spinal Discord* 2000;13(4):305–308.
62. Cantor JB, Lebwohl NH, Garvey T, et al. Nonoperative management of stable thoracdumbar burst fractures with early ambulation and bracing. *Spine* 1993;18(8):971–976.
63. Chance GO. Note on a type of flexion fracture of the spine. *Br Radiol* 1948; 21:452–453.
64. Meyer PR. Fractures of the thoracic spine: T1-T10. In: Meyer PR Jr, ed. *Surgery of spine trauma*. New York: Churchill Livingstone, 1989:525–571.

CHAPTER 63

Upper Extremity Orthotics

Heikki Uustal

This chapter will enlighten and educate the practicing clinician on the prescription, fabrication, and use of upper extremity orthoses. Historically, upper extremity orthotic prescription has been complicated by a lack of universal nomenclature, and a multitude of methods used to obtain orthoses (occupational therapist, a certified orthotist, or simply ordered direct from a catalog and custom-fitted to a patient by any medical professional). This chapter will help clarify the common uses and designs of upper extremity orthoses, and promote the use of universal terminology for the prescription of these devices.

DEFINITIONS AND NOMENCLATURE

The term *orthosis* refers to a device that is externally applied to the body to support or improve the function of that segment. Over the past decade, there has been a strong effort to name all orthoses by the joints they cross, and then specifying any design features related to those joints. Unfortunately, over the past 50 years, upper limb orthoses have been named after the designer or facility at which they were developed. The better universal terminology would simply include the five common joints of the upper extremity including finger, hand, wrist, elbow, and shoulder. The options or control features at each joint could simply be described in a fashion similar to that currently used in lower limb orthotics. The common options for a joint include fixing the joint in one position, flexion/extension block, flexion/extension traction, and flexion/extension assist. The term "block" refers to a limitation in range of motion of the joint created by the orthosis. The term "traction" refers to an external force applied across a joint for the purpose of stretching soft tissues (e.g., contracture). The term "assist" refers to an external force applied across a joint to substitute for weak muscles. This is certainly easy to understand as it relates to finger, metacarpophalangeal (MCP) joint, and elbow where we primarily have a hinged joint design. Additional design features will need to describe thumb positioning due to its unique function in opposing the other fingers for both gross grasp and fine motor skills. These design features have been previously described as an opponens bar (for palmar abduction) and C-bar (to maintain first web space). The wrist also requires special attention to address adduction and abduction positioning, or pronation and supination control. The shoulder is a very flexible joint allowing mobility in multiple planes, and potentially leading to challenging nomenclature for positioning. Fortunately, the vast majority of upper extremity orthoses incorpo-

rating the shoulder are designed to fix the shoulder in a predetermined position following surgery or trauma. There are upper extremity orthoses which stabilize a bony segment following fracture or surgery, but do not cross any joint. These orthoses can be named by the segment involved. All the features described here can be incorporated into a prescription template as shown in Figure 63-1.

All upper extremity orthoses can be classified into one of three categories: static, dynamic, or hybrid. *Static orthoses* have no movable joints incorporated into the design. However, a static orthosis may allow active joint motion in one direction, but block motion in another direction (static with block). A static orthosis may also be changed or adjusted to alter the motion allowed or alter the pressure across a joint for stretching purposes (progressive static).

Dynamic orthoses have movable joints that can limit motion (block), increase motion through traction, or substitute for weak muscles using supplemental force (assist).

Hybrid orthoses will incorporate features of both static and dynamic orthoses into one device. This type of orthosis will cross multiple joints with the intention of limiting or stopping motion at some joints, but allowing or augmenting motion at other joints.

Therefore, a proper prescription for an upper extremity orthotic device should include the simple definition of the basic platform by the joints or segments that are involved, followed by special design features controlling each of those joints. The prescription should also include materials for each of these components and any special padding indicated. As with any good orthotic prescription, the diagnosis, disability, prognosis, and duration of need should be indicated on the prescription. There should always be communication between the prescribing physician and the professional that fabricates or fits the upper extremity orthotic device to ensure clear understanding of the goals of the device.

UPPER EXTREMITY ORTHOTIC GOALS

The primary purpose of all upper extremity orthoses, and the rehabilitation program related to their prescription, is to regain or to preserve prehension of the hand. The upper extremity is vastly different from the lower extremity, because of the unique and critical functioning of the hand. The lower extremity simply maintains our body weight as we move through space, and lower extremity orthoses primarily prevent us from falling. Conversely, it is the role of the shoulder, elbow, and wrist to po-

Upper Extremity Orthosis Prescription

Patient Name: _____   Prescribing Physician: _____
Diagnosis: _____   Vendor: _____
Disability: _____   Orthosis Common Name: R   L _____
Duration of Need: _____   Materials/Padding _____

☐ Finger   2   3   4   5   (circle as needed)

☐ DIP / ☐ PIP	☐ Static at ___ / ☐ Dynamic	☐ Flexion block at ___ / ☐ Extension block at ___	☐ Flexion traction / ☐ Extension traction	☐ Flexion assist / ☐ Extension assist

☐ Thumb   ☐ Static in opposition / ☐ Dynamic   ☐ Flexion block at ___ / ☐ Extension block at ___   ☐ Flexion traction / ☐ Extension traction   ☐ Flexion assist / ☐ Extension assist

☐ MCP   ☐ Static at ___ / ☐ Dynamic   ☐ Flexion block at ___ / ☐ Extension block at ___   ☐ Flexion traction / ☐ Extension traction   ☐ Flexion assist / ☐ Extension assist

☐ Hand   ☐ Circumferential / ☐ Dorsal / ☐ Volar

☐ Wrist   ☐ Static at ___ / ☐ Dynamic   ☐ Flexion block at ___ / ☐ Extension block at ___   ☐ Flexion traction / ☐ Extension traction   ☐ Flexion assist / ☐ Extension assist

☐ Forearm   ☐ Circumferential / ☐ Dorsal / ☐ Volar

☐ Elbow   ☐ Static at ___ / ☐ Dynamic   ☐ Flexion block at ___ / ☐ Extension block at ___   ☐ Flexion traction / ☐ Extension traction   ☐ Flexion assist / ☐ Extension assist

☐ Humerus   ☐ Circumferential / ☐ Dorsal / ☐ Volar

☐ Shoulder   ☐ Static at ___ / ☐ Dynamic   ☐ Flexion block at ___ / ☐ Extension block at ___   ☐ Flexion traction / ☐ Extension traction   ☐ Flexion assist / ☐ Extension assist

Special designs:
☐ Tenodesis   ☐ BFO   ☐ Universal cuff

_____   _____
Physician Signature   Date

Figure 63-1. Upper extremity prescription template.

sition the hand properly in space to provide the essential function of gross motor grasp and fine motor skills. It is the preservation or restoration of this hand function that we strive for with upper extremity orthotics. With this in mind, there are five common goals for upper extremity orthotics:

1. Substitute for weak or absent muscles
2. Protect damaged or diseased segments by limiting load or motion
3. Prevention of deformity
4. Correction of contracture
5. Attachment of other assistive devices.

The first goal is a very common indication for upper extremity orthotics. In this case, we are *substituting for weak or absent muscles* at the wrist, elbow, or shoulder that fail to properly position the hand, or we are substituting for weak musculature within the hand itself, which fails to provide proper prehension. Common clinical examples would include cervical spinal injury, brachial plexus injury, or peripheral nerve injury to the median, ulnar, or radial nerves.

The second goal is to *protect damaged or diseased segments* such as those commonly seen in surgical repairs, trauma, or rheumatoid arthritis. With trauma or surgical repair, the orthosis is designed to control loading across damaged bony segments or sprained/strained soft tissues, in order to promote proper healing. This goal is commonly achieved through a series of progressive static or dynamic orthoses, each allowing increasing loads or movements across a joint. In the case of rheumatoid arthritis and other progressive diseases, such as scleroderma, loads or motions are controlled with the goal of slowing the progression or natural course of this disease. In these conditions, orthoses are also used as an adjunct in pain control when inflamed joints must be temporarily immobilized and then slowly progressed over time.

The third goal of upper extremity orthoses is the *prevention of deformity*. There are many clinical situations of upper and lower motor neuron disease or injury (brain injury, stroke,

spinal cord injury, brachial plexus injury, peripheral nerve injury) where proper positioning of the upper extremity is critical to prevent contracture or deformity. In these cases, there is no actual disease or injury to the segment included in the orthosis, but there has been proximal neurological injury creating the risk of deformity or contracture.

The fourth goal of upper extremity orthoses is the *correction of contracture*, which may have occurred as a result of disease or immobilization. Very commonly, clinicians are forced to immobilize upper extremity segments or joints following a fracture or other significant injury to promote soft-tissue and bony healing. Subsequently, normal range-of-motion at these joints must be regained through progressive stretching orthoses. This can be achieved through a series of progressive static orthoses or dynamic orthoses that are modified on a regular basis. The aggressiveness of the orthotic treatment program is determined by the degree and duration of contracture, and appropriate identification of the soft tissue involved.

The fifth goal of upper extremity orthoses is to provide a base for *attachment of other assistive devices*. The simplest example of this would be a universal cuff, which wraps around the hand to provide positioning of a spoon, fork, or other eating utensils. Universal cuffs have also been commonly used for writing or keyboard devices or other grooming devices. On the opposite extreme, the clinician should recognize that the balanced forearm orthosis (BFO) is simply a wheelchair-mounted accessory, which then attaches to a forearm trough. The BFO provides enormous assistance to the patient with spinal cord injury to carry out activities of daily living (ADLs), such as feeding, grooming, and even access to household technologies (light switch, telephone, television remote control).

BIOMECHANICAL PRINCIPLES

There are five critical concepts that must be understood to appreciate the proper design and fabrication of upper limb or-

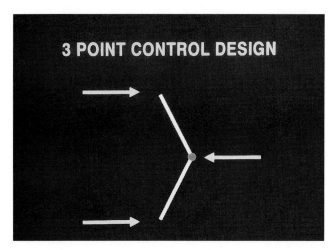

Figure 63-2. Three-point control concept. A strong force is applied at a joint to control motion, and a counter force is applied proximal and distal to the joint.

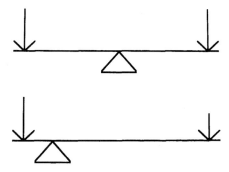

Figure 63-3. Lever force. Less force is needed with a longer lever distance.

thoses. Failure to understand and integrate these principles into the upper extremity orthosis may produce less than optimum functional outcome or even injury to the patient. The five principles include:

1. Three-point control concept
2. Tissue tolerance to compression forces and shear forces
3. The biomechanics of levers and forces
4. Selection of materials
5. Static versus dynamic control.

The *three-point control concept* is the basis of nearly all upper and lower extremity orthotic designs (Fig. 63-2). Generally, a strong force is applied at a joint and a counterforce is applied proximal and distal to that joint. The location of the force and counterforces may be clearly identified as a specific loop or bar in the orthotic design. However, in many instances the force and counter forces may be obscurely hidden into the design of the orthotic device. The precise point of application and the magnitude of the force and counterforce are critical to achieve the goal of controlling that joint.

The *tissue tolerance to both compressive forces and shear forces* must be understood if the orthosis is to be designed and fabricated safely. There are more than 30 pressure-sensitive bony prominences in the wrist, hand, and fingers alone. Avoiding prolonged, excessive pressure over these bony prominences will preserve skin integrity and patient comfort. Pressure duration curves adopted from other rehabilitation fields (such as seating systems) have indicated that higher pressures of 100 to 300 mm Hg are tolerated for only 2 to 4 hours, whereas lower pressures of 20 to 50 mm Hg are tolerated for up to 12 hours a day. If high pressures are anticipated at a joint or bony prominence, then a proper wearing schedule should clearly delineate the duration of time and the frequency of use throughout the day or night. Although a longer stretching time will reduce a contracture more rapidly, the risk of skin breakdown increases steadily with wearing duration. The clinician should also remember that distribution of pressure over a larger surface area is better tolerated than a small focused pressure. It is also important to remember the natural position of the transverse and longitudinal arches of the hand, especially in static positioning orthoses.

The *biomechanical forces* applied in upper extremity orthotics are most analogous to a class one lever, commonly known as a seesaw. Most individuals recognize that a seesaw has a force applied at both ends with a central fulcrum. Rehabilitation spe-

cialists should also understand that a relationship exists between the magnitude of the pressure applied (force) and the distance to the fulcrum (lever). In essence, the farther one is from the fulcrum or from the joint, the less pressure one needs to apply to generate a fixed force across the joint. If tissue tolerance is a concern due to the required magnitude of pressure, one can simply move the point of pressure application farther from the joint in order to decrease the magnitude of the applied pressure. In other words, by increasing the lever distance, less pressure can generate the same force across the joint (Fig. 63-3). The angle of pull of force is also very important to produce effective control of the identified joint, and to prevent damage to collateral ligaments. If the angle of pull is not perpendicular to the joint, the orthosis may overstretch collateral ligaments and create mediolateral instability at the joint. As an example, stretching a flexion contracture across the MCP joint or interphalangeal (IP) joint requires a direction of pull perpendicular to the finger. If the pull is at an angle to the finger, then less effective stretching of the flexor tendon is achieved and the unwanted stretching of collateral ligaments may occur (Fig. 63-4). The clinician must also understand that forces will impact the design of the device and help determine the materials that will be used to provide structural stability to the orthosis. For example, a long outrigger attached to a small platform on the dorsum of the hand may provide an inadequate base of support and lead to bending or deformity of the outrigger or the orthosis. A more stable outrigger and longer base of support will provide good biomechanical stability to the orthosis and provide the adequate stretch necessary.

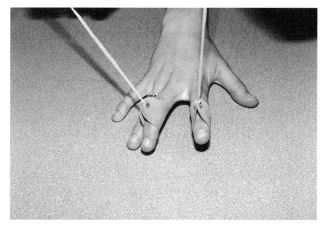

Figure 63-4. Traction angle. The angle of pull is correct on the index finger, but incorrect on the middle finger, because it is not perpendicular to the metacarpophalangeal joint.

The *selection of materials* for upper extremity orthoses depends on the flexibility, strength, and durability of the material necessary to achieve the proper outcome. Most upper extremity orthoses now use thermoplastics for most of the structural design. Low-temperature thermoplastics are commonly used because they can be easily shaped or formed to the patient's limb without the need for high-temperature ovens. They can also be easily modified by a common heat gun. However, these devices may also deform under exposure to common heat sources such as the sun or radiators. High-temperature thermoplastics may be indicated for certain longer-term or high-stress devices. Various metals are still used for parts of upper extremity orthoses where a lightweight, strong, and compact design is indicated. This includes aluminum frames, joints, and spring wire materials. Ultimately, carbon fiber materials can be used for very strong and very light designs, but manufacturing these orthoses requires specialized equipment and training. Foam materials are commonly used as padding to improve tissue tolerance in high-pressure areas.

Finally, the overall biomechanics of any upper extremity orthosis can be defined as static, dynamic, or hybrid. A traditional static orthosis will simply stabilize or fix one or multiple joints. Generally, a static positioning splint for a flaccid limb will create very low tissue pressures and very low forces at joints. This is tolerated well and can be worn nearly continuously without concern of skin breakdown. However, static positioning splints for an upper extremity with increased tone will certainly generate much higher tissue pressures and the design should incorporate additional padding in these situations. A wearing schedule is also much more important when increased tone is encountered. A dynamic orthosis allows or enhances movement across a joint, and generally will have fairly low tissue pressures unless external forces are applied such as stretching of a contracture, or in the case of abnormal increased tone from upper motor neuron injury. In these cases of a dynamic orthosis with an external force applied, the biomechanical stresses within the orthosis will be high and the tissue compression forces will be high.

ANATOMICAL PRINCIPLES

Proper upper extremity positioning requires an understanding of multiple anatomical issues, particularly when a joint will be immobilized. The wrist should be immobilized in slight extension and neutral pronation/supination. This position facilitates hand prehension activities to reach the face and midline trunk for ADLs.

The IP joints of the fingers should be immobilized in extension, but the MCP joints should be immobilized in flexion to maintain the length of the collateral ligaments. The IP and MCP joints should be mobilized as soon as possible to prevent contracture and adhesions of the long flexor and extensor tendons.

The thumb should be immobilized opposite the fingers in palmar abduction and extension. The web space should be maximized to maintain both gross grasp and fine motor pinch (Fig. 63-5).

The hand itself has two transverse arches (proximal and distal metacarpals) with two different radii. These arches must be preserved to maintain proper finger positioning. As each finger is flexed individually, its fingertip points to the scaphoid bone, because of the distal arch. An orthosis that provides traction in finger flexion must also follow this same angle to the scaphoid. As mentioned earlier, traction across a finger or any segment

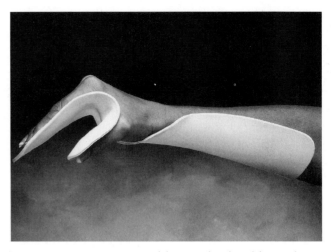

Figure 63-5. Proper positioning of the wrist, hand, and finger when immobilized. (Courtesy of North Coast Medical.)

should be perpendicular to that segment and follow the anatomical angle of the joint involved.

COMMON UPPER EXTREMITY ORTHOTIC DESIGNS

Finger and Thumb Orthoses

Simple static orthoses for the fingers or thumb are commonly used to treat fractures, collateral ligament sprains, and burns of the digits. These can be partial or complete circumferential designs providing both flexion-extension control and mediolateral stability across the IP joints. Static positioning of the IP joints should be in extension to maintain the full functional length of collateral ligaments. Static finger orthoses with a flexion or extension block allow motion in one direction, but not the other. The best example of this is the finger ring orthoses, commonly used in rheumatoid arthritis (Fig. 63-6). The boutonniere's deformity creates flexion at the proximal interphalangeal joint (PIP) joint and hyperextension at the distal interphalangeal (DIP) joint. This can be controlled using the ring orthoses to block flexion at the PIP joint. The swan-neck deformity causes hyperextension at the PIP and flexion at the DIP

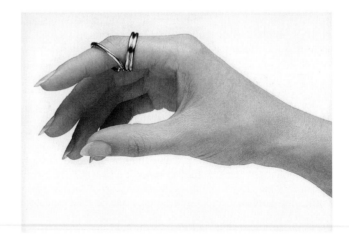

Figure 63-6. Static finger ring orthosis. (Courtesy of North Coast Medical.)

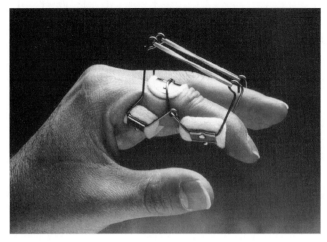

Figure 63-7. Dynamic finger orthoses. (Courtesy of North Coast Medical.)

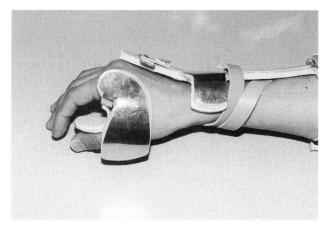

Figure 63-9. Opponens orthosis metal design with C-bar and opponens bar to stabilize thumb.

joint. The same ring orthoses can be reversed to encourage flexion and block extension at the PIP. A variety of dynamic orthoses across the IP joints of the fingers are used for the purpose of stretching flexion contracture at the IP joint (Fig. 63-7). Traction is placed across the contracted joint using spring wire or rubber bands. A progressive static orthotic program can accomplish the same result with regular adjustment or alteration of a static orthosis to stretch contracture across an IP joint. This can be accomplished through tightening of the screw, adjusting of a thermoplastic design, or altering a Velcro strap (Fig. 63-8).

Hand-Finger Orthosis

The most common reason for fabricating hand-finger orthoses is to gain control of the MCP joint of the fingers or thumb. Historically, the traditional static hand-finger orthosis consisted of a short opponens orthosis fabricated from metal, which wrapped around the medial or lateral side of the hand, preserving the arch of the hand. This would then act as a platform for outriggers or additional features, which would control the thumb, the MCP joints, or the fingers. A traditional short opponens orthosis would include a C-bar to maintain the web space between the thumb and the other fingers, and an opponens bar to position the thumb opposite the fingers for gross grasp and fine motor pinch (Fig. 63-9). This is most commonly used for median nerve injuries where control of the thumb and opposi-

tion are lost. An MCP extension block can also be incorporated into this orthosis to prevent MCP hyperextension (claw-hand deformity) which occurs in both median and ulnar nerve injuries. This modification allows the remaining intrinsic hand muscles to function as effectively as possible. The same short opponens design can be replicated using plastics with a circumferential design to maintain the transverse arches of the hand, place the thumb in opposition, and act as a platform for other attachments (Fig. 63-10). The term "thumb spica" refers to a hand-finger orthosis, which is based on the hand and extends circumferentially around the thumb to fix the thumb in opposition (Fig. 63-11). This is most commonly used for inflammatory conditions of the thumb such as rheumatoid arthritis, osteoarthritis, or de Quervain's tenosynovitis. This can also be used for fracture of the first metacarpal to maintain the thumb in a functional position. Other static hand-finger orthoses are commonly used for rheumatoid arthritis to control or prevent MCP subluxation and ulnar drift (Fig. 63-12). These would still allow long flexor and extensor tendons to activate finger control while still maintaining stability at the MCP joints.

Dynamic hand-finger orthoses are most commonly used for flexion or extension contracture across the MCP joints. The three-point control concept is again used with a force applied close to the MCP joint and opposing counterforces proximal and distal. The common "knuckle-bender orthosis" is used to

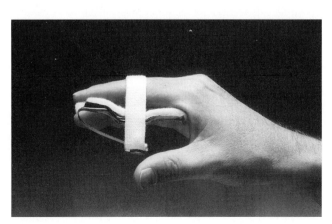

Figure 63-8. Progressive static finger orthosis. (Courtesy of North Coast Medical.)

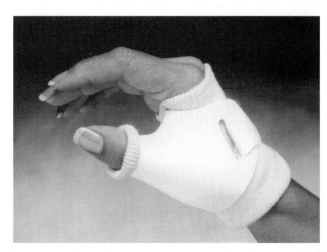

Figure 63-10. Plastic short opponens. (Courtesy of North Coast Medical.)

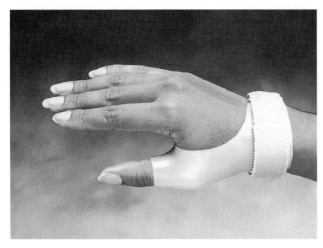

Figure 63-11. Thumb spica. (Courtesy of North Coast Medical.)

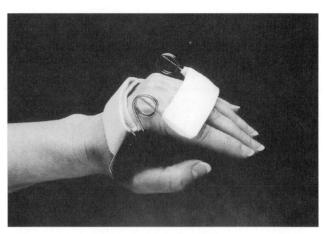

Figure 63-13. "Knuckle-bender" orthosis. Dynamic design to promote flexion at metacarpophalangeal joint. (Courtesy of North Coast Medical.)

stretch extension contracture at the MCP joints when collateral ligaments have been allowed to shorten due to immobilization (Fig. 63-13). Dynamic hand-finger orthoses can also be used for more vigorous stretching of flexion contracture at the PIP joints. These orthoses would incorporate a thermoplastic circumferential platform at the hand with attachment of MCP block to prevent hyperextension, and an outrigger to create extension stretch across the PIP joint (Fig. 63-14). Once again, it is important to remember that the direction of pull must be perpendicular to the segment and that the angle of pull must follow the joint motion. As the flexion contracture improves, the positioning of the outrigger must be adjusted to accommodate for this change. Failure to provide MCP extension block may simply create hyperextension across the MCP and failure to stretch the PIP contracture.

Wrist-Hand-Finger Orthosis

Today, static wrist-hand orthoses are most commonly used for the treatment of carpal tunnel syndrome. This orthosis includes wrist positioning in 0 to 20 degrees of extension and allows full freedom of thumb and finger movement (Fig. 63-15). Carpal tunnel syndrome commonly results from overuse of the wrist and hand causing inflammation within the carpal tunnel. Therefore, immobilization of the wrist for part or all of the day and night often helps to resolve symptoms. Other uses of static wrist-hand orthoses include traumatic wrist sprain, or wrist inflammation due to diseases such as rheumatoid arthritis. Static wrist-hand-finger orthoses are also commonly used as the first step following injury or repair to flexor or extensor tendons of the hands. A short period of immobilization is often followed by limited motion to prevent adhesions of flexor and extensor tendons, and joint contracture. With flexor tendon repair, the wrist is commonly positioned in neutral or flexion position. The MCP joints are blocked in flexion and the IP joints may be allowed to go to full extension. Often, flexion traction is applied across the fingers to promote a protective positioning of the finger and eliminate tension across the repair (Fig. 63-16). As healing progresses, the MCP block is eliminated to allow further motion without allowing full extension at the wrist until the repair is completely healed. The wrist-hand-finger orthosis for extensor tendon repair includes a similar but opposite design where the wrist is positioned statically at neutral or

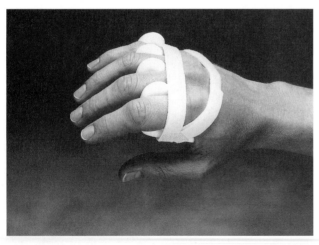

Figure 63-12. Hand-finger orthosis. Plastic design to control metacarpophalangeal subluxation in rheumatoid arthritis. (Courtesy of North Coast Medical.)

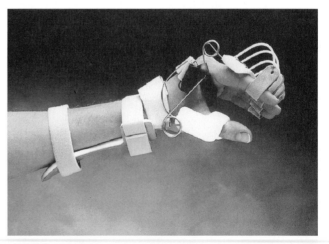

Figure 63-14. Dynamic wrist-hand-finger orthosis with metacarpophalangeal block and active extension stretch across proximal interphalangeal joints using an outrigger. (Courtesy of North Coast Medical.)

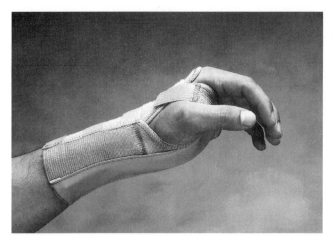

Figure 63-15. Static wrist-hand orthosis. (Courtesy of North Coast Medical.)

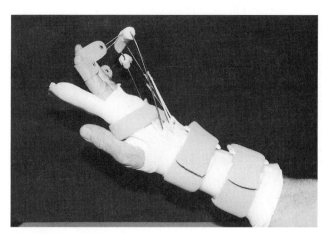

Figure 63-17. Dynamic wrist-hand-finger orthosis with flexion block at metacarpophalangeal joint and fingers, and traction at fingers.

extension position with a flexion block at the MCP and IP joints of the involved fingers. Often extension traction is applied across the MCP and IP joints to alleviate tension across the repair site (Fig. 63-17). As healing progresses, further flexion is allowed at the MCP and IP joints. Finally, full wrist flexion is allowed once healing is complete.

Radial nerve injury also requires a wrist-hand-finger orthoses to assist wrist extension and finger extension. This is accomplished with a dynamic orthosis with rubber bands or spring wire providing extension at the wrist and outriggers with rubber bands providing extension at the fingers. An outrigger or C-bar must also be incorporated to maintain the thumb in opposition (Fig. 63-18).

The tenodesis prehension orthosis or flexor hinge orthosis is a dynamic wrist-hand-finger orthosis incorporating active wrist extension movement to regain gross grasp and fine motor pinch of the thumb and fingers. This is used in C6-level quadriplegia where some wrist extension strength is maintained with little or no long finger flexor strength or intrinsic muscle strength of the hand. The Rehabilitation Institute of Chicago design incorporates a nonelastic cord, which crosses the wrist, hand, and MCP joint to facilitate three-jaw chuck pinch with

active wrist extension (Fig. 63-19). The more traditional, and more elaborate, flexor hinge design uses an adjustable rigid rod that facilitates prehension. The size of the opening of the hand is adjustable through changes in the length of the rigid rod (Fig. 63-20).

Finally, simple static wrist-hand-finger orthoses can be used for positioning of the hand following stroke, brain injury, or brachial plexus injury. As mentioned previously, the MCP joints should be positioned near full flexion and the IP joints in full extension to prevent contracture of the collateral ligaments. The thumb should also be positioned opposing the fingers and maintaining the web space (see Fig. 63-5).

Elbow Orthoses

Dynamic elbow orthoses are commonly used for flexion or extension contracture across the elbow due to immobilization. If burn scars are involved, this should include total contact across the burn scar area for compression treatment of the burn. Various spring-loaded elbow orthoses are commercially available, which can be easily adjusted by the patient or therapist to steadily increase tension across the elbow as stretching pro-

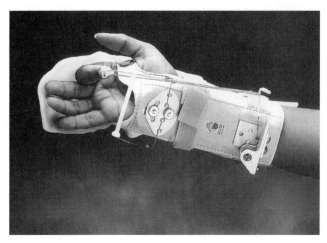

Figure 63-16. Dynamic wrist-hand-finger orthosis with extension block at metacarpophalangeal joint and fingers, and dynamic traction at index finger. (Courtesy of North Coast Medical.)

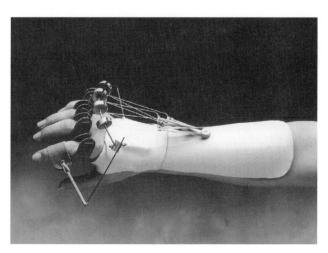

Figure 63-18. Dynamic wrist-hand-finger orthosis with stabilization of the wrist and extension of the fingers and thumb following radial nerve injury. (Courtesy of North Coast Medical.)

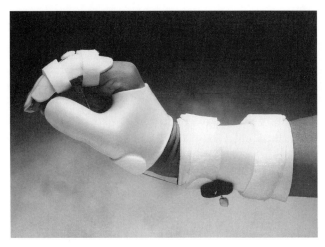

Figure 63-19. Dynamic wrist-hand-finger orthosis using Rehabilitation Institute of Chicago design for prehension. (Courtesy of North Coast Medical.)

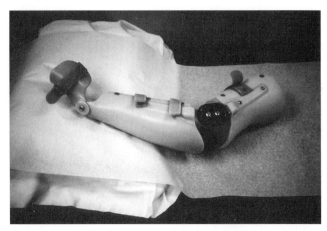

Figure 63-22. Elbow-wrist orthosis with adjustable lock at elbow and controlled motion at wrist.

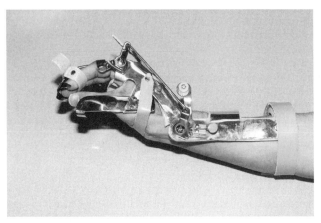

Figure 63-20. Dynamic wrist-hand-finger orthosis with traditional metal flexor hinge design.

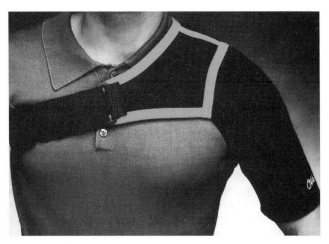

Figure 63-23. Flexible shoulder orthosis used to control humeral subluxation. (Courtesy of North Coast Medical.)

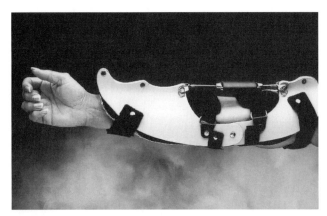

Figure 63-21. Dynamic elbow orthosis. (Courtesy of North Coast Medical.)

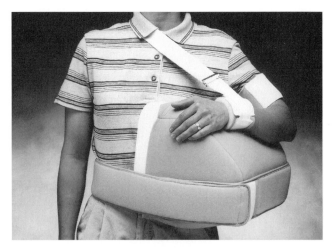

Figure 63-24. "Airplane splint" for static humeral abduction positioning. (Courtesy of North Coast Medical.)

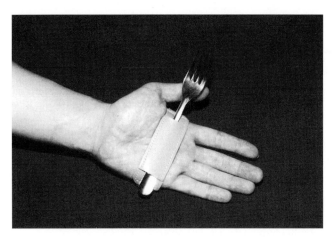

Figure 63-25. Universal cuff with fork inserted.

gresses (Fig. 63-21). Spring-assisted elbow orthoses are also used to augment elbow flexion when weakness or paralysis of the biceps muscle exists. Static circumferential orthoses across the elbow are often used for fractures at or near the elbow. Fractures of the radius and ulna should incorporate the elbow, wrist, and hand to control pronation and supination. An adjustable lock such as the dial lock can be incorporated into the elbow-wrist-hand orthosis to steadily progress motion at the elbow in flexion or extension, and still control pronation and supination (Fig. 63-22). Humeral fracture management may include a circumferential orthosis across the entire humeral segment and forearm. This would initially start as a static orthosis and slowly progress movement at the elbow as healing of the humeral fracture occurs.

Shoulder Orthoses

Flexible arm slings of various sorts have been used for a variety of problems including clavicular fracture, acromio-clavicular joint injury, proximal humeral fracture, and glenohumeral subluxation due to hemiparesis. These do not clearly fit into the categorization of static or dynamic design due to their inherit lack of identifiable joints or rigid design features. These orthoses commonly consist of fabrics and straps that encompass the mid- to proximal humerus, and then extend across the shoulder anteriorly and posteriorly to the opposite axilla (Fig. 63-23). The primary goal is to maintain glenohumeral integrity and to limit motion across the AC and glenohumeral joints. A true static shoulder-elbow-wrist-hand orthosis, such as the airplane splint or arm abduction orthosis, can prevent movement across the glenohumeral joint by stabilizing the arm in abduction (Fig. 63-24). This is done for shoulder dislocation, shoulder surgery (e.g., rotator cuff repair) and some proximal fractures. Care must be taken to mobilize the glenohumeral joint as soon as possible to prevent adhesive capsulitis.

Other specialized orthoses in this category include the BFO for patients with C5-level spinal injury. This device includes a forearm trough which is suspended on a series of brackets and swivels mounted on the wheelchair. This eliminates the weight of the arm and allows the patient to use elbow flexion and shoulder adduction/abduction for feeding and limited ADLs. A universal cuff or hand orthosis is used to attach a swivel spoon or other device, which would then allow independent feeding by the patient (Fig. 63-25). Finally, a combination of prosthetic and orthotic components can be used for the patient with brachial plexus injury to create a shoulder-elbow-wrist-hand

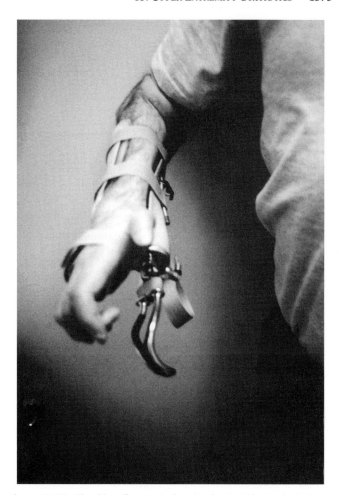

Figure 63-26. Shoulder-elbow-wrist-hand orthosis with prosthetic hook for prehension.

orthosis to regain some limited prehension at the hand once the elbow is locked and stabilized. A dual control cable to a figure-8 harness can use biscapular abduction to position the elbow and activate a prehension orthosis at the wrist and hand when there is complete paralysis at the elbow and hand. If the hand is not usable due to contracture, then a can be applied at the palmar surface of the hand to obtain prehension (Fig. 63-26). The elbow can be locked in place using an additional strap which is activated with shoulder movements or by reaching across with the opposite hand. The paralyzed limb can then be used as a helper or stabilizer for the remaining functional arm.

As you can see, most common upper limb orthotic designs can be appropriately described using universal terminology and a prescription template, rather than abstract names. Any new or unique design features or materials can be added to this same template. Communication between the prescribing physician, patient, and therapist/orthotist will ensure fabrication and fit of a proper upper limb orthosis. Adequate instruction to the patient, and appropriate therapy and follow-up will help to prevent complications and achieve a favorable outcome.

SUGGESTED READINGS

Ader PB, Nadel E, Wingate L. A survey of postoperative elbow immobilization approaches. *J Burn Care Rehabil* 1992;13(3):365–370.
Aoki M, Manske PR, Pruitt DL, et al. Tendon repair using flexor tendon splints: an experimental study. *J Hand Surg [Am]* 1994;19 (6):984–990.

Bain GI, Mehta JA, Heptinstall RJ. The dynamic elbow suspension splint. *J Shoulder Elbow Surg* 1998;7(4):419–421.

Boozer JA, Sanson MS, Soutas-Little RW, et al. Comparison of the biomedical motions and forces involved in high-profile versus low-profile dynamic splinting. *J Hand Ther* 1994;7(3);171–182.

Callinan NJ, Mathiowetz V. Soft versus hard resting hand splints in rheumatoid arthritis; pain relief, preference, and compliance. *Am J Occup Ther* 1996;50(5): 347–353.

Chao RP, Braun SA, Ta KT, et al. Early passive mobilization after digital nerve repair and grafting in a fresh cadaver. *Plast Reconstr Surg* 2001;108(2):386–391.

Colditz JC. The biomechanics of a thumb carpometacarpal immobilization splint: design and fitting. *J Hand Ther* 2000;13(3):228–235.

Crimmins CA, Jones NF. Stenosing tenosynovitis of the extensor carpi ulnaris. *Ann Plast Surg* 1995;35(1):105–107.

Falconer J. Hand splinting in rheumatoid arthritis. A perspective on current knowledge and directions for research. *Arthritis Case Res* 1991;4(2):81–86.

Fess EE, Philips CA, eds. *Hand splinting principles and methods*, 3rd ed. St. Louis: Mosby, 2001.

Hannah SD, Hudak PL. Splinting and radial nerve palsy: a single-subject experiment. *J Hand Ther* 2001;14(3):195–201.

Ip WY, Chow SP. Results of dynamic splintage following extensor tendon repair. *J Hand Surg [Br]* 1997;22(2):283–287.

Landsman JC, Seitz WH Jr, Froimson AI, et al. Splint immobilization of gamekeeper's thumb. *Orthopedics* 1995;18(12):1161–1165.

Lester B, Jeong GK, Perry D, et al. A simple effective splinting technique for the mallet finger. *Am J Orthop* 2000;29(3):202–206

Lindner-Tons S, Ingell K. An alternative splint design for trigger finger. *J Hand Ther* 1998;11(3):206–208.

Osterhout BM. Postoperative splinting of the pediatric upper extremity. *Hand Clin* 1990;6(4):693–695.

Pagnotta A, Baron M, Korner-Bitensky N. The effect of a static wrist orthosis on hand function in individuals with rheumatoid arthritis. *J Rheumatol* 1998;25 (5):879–885.

Peterson-Bethea D. A static progressive splint for Dupuytren's release. *J Hand Ther* 1997;10 (4):312–323.

Redford, JB. *Orthotics et cetera*. Baltimore: Williams & Wilkins, 1986.

Rempel D, Manojlovic R, Levinsohn DG, et al. The effect of wearing a flexible wrist splint on carpal tunnel pressure during repetitive hand activity. *J Hand Surg [Am]* 1994;19(1):106–110.

Reswick JB, ed. *Bedsore biomechanics*. London: The McMillan Press, Ltd, 1976.

Rose H. MP/PIP adjustable digit blocking splint. *J Hand Ther* 1996;9(3):247–248.

Schanzer D. Static progressive end-range proximal interphalangeal/distal interphalangeal flexion splint. *J Hand Ther* 2000;13(4):310–312.

Scheker LR, Chesher SP, Netscher DT, et al. Functional results of dynamic splinting after transmetacarpal, wrist, and distal forearm replantation. *J Hand Surg [Br]* 1995;20(5):584–590.

Sirotakova M, Elliot D. Early active mobilization of primary repairs of the flexor pollicis longus tendon. *J Hand Surg [Br]* 1999;24(6):647–653.

Slater RR Jr, Bynum DK. Simplified functional splinting after extensor tenorrhaphy. *J Hand Surg [Am]* 1997;22 (3):445–451.

Smrcka V, Dylevsky I. Treatment of congenital swan neck deformity with dynamic tenodesis of proximal interphalangeal joint. *J Hand Surg [Br]* 2001;26 (2):165–167.

Spoorenberg A, Boers M, van der Linden S. Wrist splints in rheumatoid arthritis: what do we know about efficacy and compliance? *Arthritis Care Res* 1994;7(2): 55–57.

Swezey RL. Trigger finger splinting. *Orthopedics* 1997;22(2):180.

Swigart CR, Eaton RG, Glickel SZ, et al. Splinting in the treatment of arthritis of the first carpometacarpal joint. *J Hand Surg [Am]* 1999;24(1):86–91.

Tilley W, McMahon S, Shukalak B. Rehabilitation of the burned upper extremity. *Hand Clin* 2000;16(2):303–318.

Van Alphen JC, Oepkes CT, Bos KE. Activity of the extrinsic finger flexors during mobilization in the Kleinert splint. *J Hand Surg [Am]* 1996;21(1):77–84.

Van Straten O, Sagi A. "Supersplint": a new dynamic combination splint for the burned hand. *J Burn Care Rehabil* 2000;21(1 Pt 1): 71–73; discussion 70.

Weiss ND, Gordon L, Bloom T, et al. Position of the wrist associated with the lowest carpal-tunnel pressure: implication for splint design. *J Bone Joint Surg [Am]* 1995;77(11):1695–1699.

Weiss S, LaStayo P, Mills A, et al. Prospective analysis of splinting the first carpometacarpal joint: an objective, subjective, and radiographic assessment. *J Hand Ther* 2000;13(3):218–226.

CHAPTER 64

Lower Extremity Orthotics, Shoes, and Gait Aids

Kristjan T. Ragnarsson

Orthotics is the systematic pursuit of straightening and improving function of the body or body parts by the application of an orthosis to the outside of the body. The term "orthosis" may refer to a number of devices with a more restricted or specific meaning, such as braces, splints, calipers, and corsets. Depending on the design, an orthosis may totally immobilize a joint or body segment, restrict movement in a given direction, control mobility, assist with movement, or reduce weight-bearing forces. In the presence of weak or paralyzed muscles, orthotic immobilization of a joint or an entire limb provides support. In the presence of unbalanced muscle forces, an orthosis prevents the generation of a deformity or joint contracture. In the presence of inflamed or injured musculoskeletal segments, an orthosis reduces pain and allows healing. Extension of an orthosis to a healthy body part can transfer or redistribute the weight-bearing forces, thereby reducing the actual load on a long bone or whole limb. This may help to relieve pain and allow healing of injured parts. The primary principle behind the prescription of an orthosis is the improvement of function.

PRESCRIPTION CONSIDERATIONS

Before an orthosis is prescribed, the precise functions it is meant to improve must be determined. The physician needs to know the indications for prescribing a specific orthosis, the anatomy and neuromuscular function of the relevant body regions, and the functional and biomechanical deficits present. The physician must also thoroughly understand the mechanical principles of orthotic application, the materials used in fabrication, the various designs that are available, and the training that the patient must receive, both before and after receiving the orthosis. Finally, the physician needs to be aware of the cost of the orthosis and the patient's financial means, carefully judging whether the benefits to be obtained will justify the cost.

Whereas the indications for prescribing and using an orthosis may be obvious, contraindications are more subtle. The use of an orthosis should be discontinued when it causes pain, reduces function, worsens posture or gait, causes emotional distress, or when more effective results may be achieved by physical therapy or relatively minor surgical procedures. Allergy to

the orthotic materials, restriction of peripheral circulation, or development of pressure sores requires immediate alteration or adjustment of the orthosis. Although an orthosis may significantly improve mobility and self-sufficiency, it also is a visible reminder of a lasting or permanent disability. Cosmetic appearance and comfort of the orthosis are two factors that will ease the patient's adjustment to the disability and facilitate acceptance of the device.

MATERIALS AND MECHANICS

A wide variety of materials have been used to fabricate orthotic appliances. Some have been used for centuries, such as metal, rubber, leather, and canvas, whereas others have been developed more recently, such as plastics and synthetic fabrics. When the appropriate materials are selected for an orthotic device, their strength, durability, flexibility, and weight need to be carefully considered. The orthotic design should be simple, inconspicuous, comfortable, and as cosmetic as possible. It should adhere to the basic principle of distributing forces over a sufficiently large surface area. Parts that are in contact with the body should be accurately contoured and padded.

The choice of orthotic material depends on the clinical purpose and the characteristics of the patient. Traditional orthotic devices use metals to provide strength and durability with straps and padding made of leather (Fig. 64-1). The metals primarily used are steel and aluminum, mostly in alloy forms with various other metals to further increase the strength of the orthosis and to resist corrosion. Although metal orthoses are heavy and are cosmetically unappealing, their adjustability allows them to accommodate for growth and the changing needs of the patient.

Orthoses that are made of plastic (Fig. 64-2) generally are somewhat lighter and closer fitting because they can be molded directly to the body or over a plaster replica of the body part. The close fit of the plastic orthosis provides wider distribution of the corrective forces than is possible with a metal orthosis. Comfort may be increased by adding foam liners on the inside of the orthosis. Based on the weight of the patient, the use of the orthosis, the specific type of plastic used, and the design of the orthosis, plastic materials generally pro-

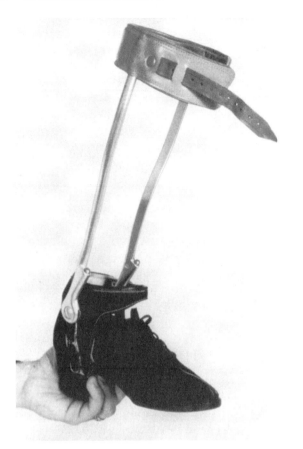

Figure 64-1. Klenzak ankle-foot orthosis with a medial T-strap to control vagus.

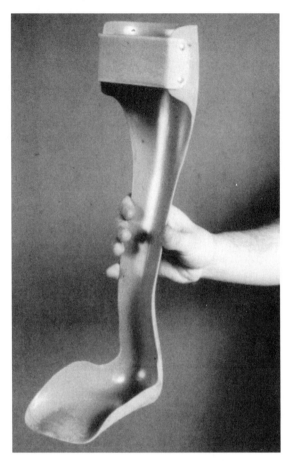

Figure 64-2. Plastic leaf-spring ankle-foot orthosis (PLSO).

vide adequate strength and durability. Plastic orthoses generally are not adjustable in length, but some materials allow reshaping when heated to accommodate or provide relief at pressure points. Plastic orthoses are usually fitted with metal joints or flexible spring-loaded plastic bars because plastic joints are not as durable.

Two major types of plastic materials are used in orthotics: thermosetting and thermoplastic materials. Thermosetting plastics include formaldehyde, epoxy, and polyester resins that are typically used as laminates in a laminated form. They require heat to harden but do not soften with subsequent heating. Thermoplastics soften when they are heated, making the material moldable. Subsequent heating will soften the material for further molding, and lowering the temperature hardens the material once again. Low-temperature thermoplastics, such as Orthoplast and Plastazote, become workable at temperatures that are just above the body temperature. This allows quick fabrication and molding directly on the body. Unfortunately, these materials lack strength and durability and therefore are not indicated for long-term use. The high-temperature thermoplastics, such as polyethylene, polypropylene, copolymers, ortholene, and vinyl polymers, require heating to 150°F or more to make them workable. Fabrication of an orthosis made of any of these materials requires an exact plaster replica of the body part. The heated plastic is then applied to the replica for proper molding. These materials generally are strong and durable, and they have a "good memory," returning to their original position after flexible deformation. The orthosis provides support and may also give a spring-action assist force. Most plastic orthoses designed for long-term use are made of high-temperature thermoplastics.

TERMINOLOGY

In the past, the lexicon of terms used to describe orthotics was very confusing; often, clinicians used different terms to describe even the most basic device. Devices or parts of orthoses were given names that might describe their purpose, the body part to which they were applied, the inventor of the device, or where they were developed. To facilitate communication and minimize the use of acronyms, a logical, easy-to-use system of standard terminology was developed. This system uses the first letter of each joint that the orthosis crosses in correct sequence, with the letter "O" for orthosis at the end. Thus, the more common orthoses would be named AFO (ankle-foot orthosis), KAFO (knee-ankle-foot orthosis), and KO (knee orthosis). A properly written orthotic prescription does not just state the name of the orthosis, it also is necessary to state the desired function to be obtained, the specific material from which the device is to be made, and the specific design and construction that is to be employed.

SHOES AND FOOTWEAR

The basic function of commercial shoes is to protect the feet from rough walking surfaces, the weather, and the environment as well as to provide support for the feet during standing and walking. To improve comfort and function, special shoes are commercially available for certain unusual or abnormal foot activities, mostly for recreational use and for pathologic foot conditions. The clinician frequently fails to appreciate the importance of comfortable and well-fitting shoes. Foot prob-

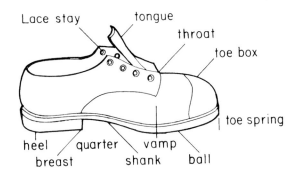

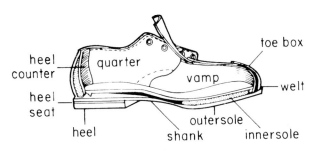

Figure 64-3. Shoe components.

lems that easily could be corrected by prescription of proper shoes or shoe modifications often interfere with optimum functional performance.

Components

The parts of a shoe (Fig. 64-3) consist of the sole, the heel, the upper, the linings, and reinforcements. Each component can be made of a wide variety of materials and designs, depending on the quality and specific use of the shoe.

The sole is the bottom part of the shoe. It is divided into the outer sole, or the surface that touches the ground, and the inner sole, the part closest to the foot and to which the upper and the outer sole are attached. Sometimes compressible filler made of cork or latex separates the inner from the outer soles. It is preferable that both the inner and the outer soles be made of leather of variable thickness. Leather soles best maintain proper fit and are particularly indicated if shoe modifications are required. Rubber soles make modifications more difficult and have the additional drawback of eliminating a large ventilating surface, which may result in excessive sweating and skin problems. The greater friction coefficient of rubber soles may also cause the shoe to stop abruptly on heel strike, thrusting the foot forward into the forepart of the shoe. The widest part of the sole is at the metatarsal heads and is called the ball. The narrowest part of the sole, between the heel and the ball, is called the shank. The shank usually is reinforced by a strip of metal, leather, fiberboard, or other firm material. The external heel seat is the posterior part of the sole to which the heel is secured. The toe spring is attached to the outer surface, between the outer sole and the floor. The purpose of the toe spring in the design of the shoe is to cause a rocker effect during push-off and to reduce wrinkling of the upper.

The heel is attached to the outer sole under the anatomic heel and is made of leather, wood, plastic, rubber, or metal. The heel block, which is fastened to the heel seat, is made of a firm material, but the plantar surface is usually made of hard rubber. The anterior surface of the heel is called the breast. The

height of the heel is measured in eighths of an inch at the breast. The height and design of the heel vary greatly. The flat heel has a broad base and measures 0.75 to 1.25 inches in height. A Thomas heel is flat and has a medial extension to support a weak longitudinal foot arch. A military heel has a slightly narrower base and measures 1.25 to 1.375 inches in height. A Cuban heel has a still narrower base but is higher. Heels up to 2 to 3 inches high are available, but they are mainly used for fashionable appearance rather than for extended walking. Shoes with lower heels, no heels, or negative heels also exist. A spring heel, which has a heel height of only ⅛ to 3/16 of an inch, is placed under the outer sole and thus eliminates the heel breast. This type of heel is common on shoes for infants and children up to 3 years of age. Many athletic shoes, including running shoes, have no heels because one can run faster without heels. The negative heel popularized on the earth shoe provided comfort for some people. The clinician needs to be aware that the height of the heel affects foot and ankle positions as well as the general posture of the trunk. Heel height may thus be a factor in certain clinical conditions, such as shortening of gastrocnemius and low back pain. High heels, especially those with a tapered, narrow striking point, make the ankle and foot more unstable and thereby contribute to ankle injuries and falls.

The upper is that part of the shoe that is above the sole. It is most commonly made of leather, although any soft and durable material may be used. Leather is found to be most comfortable because it allows evaporation and absorption of moisture and molds well to the shape of the foot. The upper consists of the vamp, quarters, and lace stay. The vamp is the anterior portion of the upper, which covers the toes and the instep. The tongue, a strip of leather lying under the laces, and the throat, the opening at the base of the tongue, are parts of the vamp. Anteriorly, the vamp has a reinforced toe box or toe cap to maintain appearance and to protect the toes against trauma. The lace stay, or the portion containing the eyelets for laces, is usually part of the vamp, but it may be part of the quarters.

The two quarters make up the posterior part of the shoe. The quarters usually are reinforced by the heel counter, which stabilizes the foot by supporting the calcaneus and gives structural stability to the shoe. The counter usually extends anteriorly to the heel breast, but it may extend further forward or upward on specially made shoes. Similar to the toe box, it is made of firm leather or synthetic material. Laterally, the quarter is cut lower to avoid infringing on the lateral malleolus. Sometimes a band of leather, referred to as a collar, is stitched to the top of the quarters to reduce pistoning or to prevent the shoe from falling off. The linings are made of leather, cotton, or canvas and should be used in all portions of the shoe that are in contact with the foot to absorb perspiration and smooth the contact area, thus providing added comfort.

Fabrication

Shoes are built around a positive model or replica of the weight-bearing foot, which is called a last (1). The last, which is made of solid rock maple or plastic materials, determines the fit, walking comfort, appearance, and style of the shoe. Usually the last has a slight forefoot in-flare. Other common lasts include the broad-toe last with a straight medial border that extends from the heel to the toe; the juvenile symmetric straight last, which can be bisected into nearly equal right and left halves; and the orthopedic last with special features designed to accommodate various structural and anatomic problems (e.g., varus, valgus).

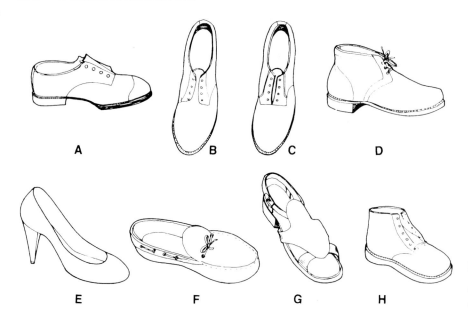

Figure 64-4. Shoe types and styles. **A:** Oxford or low quarter. **B:** Blucher-type Oxford. **C:** Bal-type Oxford. **D:** Chukka or high quarter. **E:** Pump. **F:** Moccasin. **G:** Sandal. **H:** Childs.

During fabrication, the insole is nailed to the last, the lining is tucked to the inner sole rim, and the reinforcements (i.e., counter, toe box) are attached. The upper of the shoe is softened by humidity for easier molding and fitted snugly to the last to adapt to its every detail and then nailed or glued to the inner sole. Finally, the outer sole and heel are attached. The Goodyear welt construction of shoes is a method used in production of high-quality shoes in which the upper is sewn to the sole. This method provides a perfectly smooth inner surface, comfort, and a strong shoe that retains its shape and is easy to modify and repair. Unfortunately, these shoes tend to be bulky, heavy, and less flexible.

Types and Styles

There are innumerable shoe types and styles (Fig. 64-4), although basic designs are relatively few. The basic designs are mainly determined by the shape of the upper, particularly the design of the toe and the height of the quarters. On low-quarter shoes, or the oxford, the quarters extend approximately 1-inch below the malleoli and do not restrict ankle or subtalar motions. In high-quarter shoes, the quarters may cover the malleoli, either just barely, as in the chukka shoe, or by 2 inches or more, as in boots. This style prevents piston action during walking and back-and-forth sliding of the foot. In addition, it provides medial-lateral stability at the ankle and subtalar joints and resistance to plantar flexion. The most common throat style is the blucher type, in which the lace stay is not directly fastened to the vamp. This style gives a wide opening for the foot for easy insertion and greater adjustability over the midfoot. The bal-type (Balmoral) throat, which has the face stay attached directly to the vamp, does not provide such easy foot access. A lace-to-toe shoe, often referred to as a surgical shoe, allows exposure of the entire foot by opening up to the toes. Shoe closure usually is accomplished by cotton laces, which thread through two or more pairs of eyelets, although closure also can be achieved by buckles, zippers, Velcro flaps, or elastics.

Athletic shoes (Fig. 64-5) have changed dramatically in design and materials that have been introduced and used in their fabrication in recent years. Except for their sporty appearance, modern athletic shoes have little in common with old-fash-ioned sneakers, which were made primarily of a canvas upper and a rubber sole and provided little foot support. Different sports may require different shoe design features for optimal performance and comfort. The sole of a good athletic shoe is stiff at the heel and at the shank but very flexible at the forefoot, where it should bend easily at the ball. The outer sole usually is made of highly durable rubber compounds that provide a good grip on the ground, whereas the inner sole is designed to fit the contours of the foot closely. Between the outer and inner soles, gel- or foamlike materials are placed for cushioning to dampen shocks to the foot. The outer sole often is designed to flare out laterally at the heel and toward the midfoot to improve mediolateral stability at the ankle and to ensure the foot is flat as it strikes the ground in the normal, slightly supinated position. Rising up from the rear sole to a height of approximately 0.5 inches is a heel cradle, which further increases mediolateral motion control and hind foot stability. The rigid and noncompressible heel counter provides added stability, but for athletes with a tendency to recurrent ankle sprains, there is the option of using high-top shoes. The upper is reinforced in the midfoot area for maximum stability and to resist excessive side-to-side motion. Such reinforcement is obtained by adding bands, stabilized lacing systems, and motion control straps. In addition to their use in various sports, athletic shoes frequently are used by the elderly and people with gait disorders because they are lightweight and provide excellent foot stability.

Children's shoes (see Fig. 64-4) generally are designed similarly to those for adults. During infancy, shoes are important primarily for foot protection and therefore should be lightweight, flexible, and quadrangularly shaped to conform to the normal foot shape. The soles should be soft and flexible for the crawling child to allow easy bending and to minimize forced inversion or eversion of the foot. Rigid shoes are not necessary for normal development of feet. Children who habitually go barefoot usually have healthy feet that are supple, flexible, and mobile (2). Toddlers up to 3 years of age usually are fitted with shoes that are somewhat more rigid than infants' shoes, although these still must be flexible to permit foot mobility and light in weight to reduce energy cost. The upper should be made of soft leather or permeable fabric to allow evaporation; the toe box should be broad, the medial border relatively straight, and the heel counter firm and snug. The sole should be firm and rein-

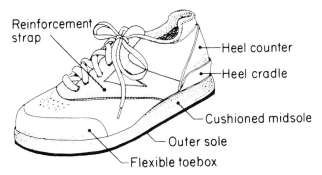

Reinforcement strap

Heel counter

Heel cradle

Cushioned midsole

Outer sole

Flexible toebox

Figure 64-5. Components of an athletic shoe.

forced at the shank, and its friction should be similar to that of the bare foot (i.e., it should be neither slippery nor slide-resistant). The heel should be flat or of the low-spring type. A high-top design may be helpful to keep the shoe from slipping off during running and jumping. For the remainder of the growing years, proper footwear clearly continues to be of great importance. At least a half-inch of space should be allowed between the shoe and the longest toe on weight bearing, whereas the heel of the shoe upper should fit snugly and comfortably without excessive gaping. Excessively worn or ill-fitting children's shoes should be discarded, and other people's shoes (i.e., hand-me-downs) should not be used.

Fitting

The first requirement of a shoe is that it fits and does not cause pain, skin problems, or deformities. Both feet should be measured, and the shoes tried on both feet in case of size discrepancy, in which case the shoe size should be chosen that is most comfortable for the larger foot. Footwear preferably should be purchased at the end of the day, when the feet often are slightly swollen. When shoes are fitted, each shoe should be judged individually in a fully weight-bearing position. The shoe should fit snugly enough not to fall off but be loose enough to adapt to the size and shape of the foot, which changes with climate, ambient temperature, time of day, body position, and weight bearing whether the person is lying, sitting, or standing. Because the foot expands with weight bearing, shoes initially should be carefully tested for fit, both in length and width, not only by standing but by walking or running several steps and stopping short. The real proof of fit, however, is if the shoe is comfortable after hours of continuous wear or walking. An old piece of advice is to find a comfortable pair of shoes and then take one size larger.

In length, the shoes should extend at least a half-inch beyond the longest toe, usually the hallux or the second toe. The heel-to-ball distance of the foot and the shoe should be equal. Thus, the first metatarsal joint should be located at the inner curve of the shoe, and on toe dorsiflexion, the shoe should bend easily and the toe break should run directly across the ball. The widest part of the shoe, the ball, should coincide with the broadest part of the foot, leaving enough free space medial and lateral to the heads of the first and fifth metatarsal bones, respectively. The transverse arch of the foot should function normally, weight should be evenly distributed, and no sliding of the forefoot within the shoe should occur. The medial and lateral quarters should not gap, and the heel counter should close around the heel bone without bulges, allowing only a small amount of pistoning. Some pistoning usually is unavoidable in a shoe with a rigid sole and heel counter. The height of

the vamp should be adequate to prevent pressure or irritation over the toes and the instep. The height of the quarters should be sufficient to hold the shoe securely on the foot. If the quarters are too high, they can cause irritation of the malleoli.

Different shoe sizes are commercially available and are marked by numbers to indicate length and by letters to indicate width. The numbers used in the United States and Europe are different, as are the numbers used to indicate the sizes of men's, women's, and children's feet. Sizes often vary from one manufacturer to another. In the United States, the smallest shoe is infant size 000, and the largest is men's size 16. Most shoe stores, however, carry only men's shoe sizes up to 14 or 15 and women's sizes up to 12 or 13. Larger sizes are available in specialty shoe stores, or they may be special ordered. The shoe widths measured at the ball are available in different sizes, ranging from A, which is narrow, to E, which is wide. Each size represents a 0.25-inch increase in width. Few shoe stores stock shoes of extreme width. Shoe depth is not fabricated in different sizes, although extra-depth shoes and shoes with adjustable insoles are available to accommodate foot abnormalities and shoe inserts.

If there is loss of sensation in the feet, new shoes should be worn for 2 hours only, after which shoes and socks should be removed and the feet carefully inspected. Before donning, each shoe should be carefully checked on the inside with the hands for irregularities, foreign objects, and so forth, which could damage the feet.

Modifications

Stock shoes may require minor or major modifications by various methods to support the abnormal foot during weight bearing, to reduce pressure on painful areas, and to limit motion of weak, unstable, or painful joints. For these purposes, the clinician may select a special type of shoe, order certain alterations in the construction of the shoe, or apply corrections directly to the foot. The clinician needs to make an accurate diagnosis of the problem, have a clear understanding of why corrections are needed, and write a specific prescription that is best accompanied by a simple drawing to clarify the request. Although certain simple external modifications may be applied easily to many types of commercial shoes, welt shoes are more suitable to work with, especially for major internal modifications, because the shoe structure is not altered by removing and reattaching the sole to the upper. Orthopedic shoes are welt shoes made of good leather, with relatively thick soles, a high and wide toe box, extended medial heel counter, rigid wide steel shank, and a Thomas heel. They are the most frequently prescribed shoes for foot problems requiring shoe modification, and they also are regarded as high-quality footwear for normal feet. Extra-depth orthopedic shoes are made commercially and are widely available. They offer removable insoles, which allow the placement of most foot orthoses (FOs) without compromising fit or comfort. Moldable shoes have uppers that are constructed from thermoplastic materials that can be reshaped when heated to accommodate minor and moderate foot deformities.

A fixed deformity needs accommodation, using the shoe to bring the weight-bearing surface to the foot, whereas a flexible deformity may be actively corrected. Adults usually have relatively fixed deformities requiring passive stabilization, but young children have flexible deformities that may be corrected actively by proper shoe prescription if they are minor or moderate. In more severe cases, serial plaster cast and surgical operations may be required.

Internal Modifications

Shoe modifications can be classified as either internal (i.e., those that are inserted into the inner surface of the shoe or sandwiched between shoe components) or external (i.e., those that are attached to the sole or heel). Internal modifications are mechanically more effective. Although they generally are made of soft materials, they are less well tolerated because they reduce the size of the shoe and distort the inner sole. They may be removable or built in as an integral part of the shoe. Internal shoe corrections include steel shanks, cookies (e.g., scaphoid and metatarsal pads), interior heel lifts and wedges, extended or reinforced heel counters, and protective metal toe boxes. Steel shanks can be used to support a weak longitudinal arch, but if this is insufficient, a cookie made of firm materials, such as leather or rubber, may be placed along the medial border of the insole at the talonavicular joint. Scaphoid pads also provide additional longitudinal arch support but are made of compressible material. They are prescribed for people who cannot tolerate the firmness of a cookie. The longitudinal arch support of a cookie or scaphoid pad is improved further by insertion of a long medial counter made of rigid leather. Metatarsal pads, which are commercially available in many sizes, may be positioned inside the shoe just proximal to the metatarsal heads to protect and reduce pressure on the second, third, and fourth metatarsal heads by transferring force to their bone shafts. A sesamoid or dancer's pad is thicker and broader, and extends medially to the proximal part of the first metatarsal head. Thus, it provides greater support for more severe cases of metatarsalgia. Heel elevations of more than ¼-inch should be placed externally. Interior heel wedges of ¹⁄₁₆- to ⅛-inch in height may be placed on either the medial or lateral half of the interior heel.

External Modifications

External shoe modifications (Fig. 64-6) include sole and heel wedges, flanges and elevations, metatarsal and rocker bars, and different types of heel designs. Wedges are constructed of leather and positioned under the outer sole or heel. Sole and heel wedges usually are placed medially, but occasionally they are placed laterally to shift the body weight from that side of the foot to the other. Flanges or flare-outs are ¼-inch–wide medial or lateral extensions of the sole or heel that provide stability. A lateral flange provides a lever arm, which ensures a foot flat in the presence of excessive inversion or varus deformity.

Such small lateral flanges are seen on most commercially available running shoes, where they are intended to prevent inversion sprains.

Elevations (i.e., lifts) of the sole and heel are prescribed for leg-length discrepancies. Leg-length discrepancies of less than ½-inch generally do not require a shoe modification, but a greater discrepancy should be corrected to make the pelvis level. It may not be necessary or even desirable to provide an elevation for the total leg length to be equal on both sides. If an elevation of more than ¼-inch is required, these should be applied externally. Elevations up to 1 inch in height can be added exclusively to the heel. When elevation of greater than 1 inch is indicated, it has to be applied to both the heel and sole of the shoe. The height of the elevation must be greatest at the heel and taper off from the ball of the shoe to the toe. Elevations greater than 1 inch should be made of lightweight materials, such as layered cork.

A metatarsal bar (i.e., anterior heel) made of leather or rubber may be attached transversely to the outer sole immediately proximal to the metatarsal heads to relieve pressure on them and to reduce pain. A rocker bar is similarly placed but extends distally beyond the metatarsal heads. It also relieves pressure on the metatarsal heads and reduces metatarsal phalangeal flexion on push-off by providing a smooth plantar roll to toe-off. It thus may improve gait when painful or paralytic conditions prevent good push-off. A Denver bar is placed under the metatarsal bones to support the transverse arch extending from the metatarsal heads anteriorly to the tarsal-metatarsal joints posteriorly.

Several kinds of external heel modifications are available. Already mentioned are heel elevations, wedges, and flanges. The Thomas heel (see Fig. 64-6) or the orthopedic heel is similar in design and material to the regular flat heel but has an anteromedial extension to provide additional longitudinal arch support. This extension may be of variable length, depending on the extent of support required, and its effect may be augmented further by a medial wedge or a Thomas heel wedge. A reverse Thomas heel is an anterolateral extension to support a weak lateral longitudinal arch, but this variety is rarely used. Occasionally, compressible, resilient materials are inserted into the heel (i.e., solid ankle cushion heel), usually in conjunction with a rocker bar for a cushioning effect on heel strike. The result is a simulation of plantar flexion with minimal ankle movement, while the rocker bar provides smooth push-off. Thus, a more natural gait may be obtained in certain clinical conditions despite relative immobilization of the foot and ankle.

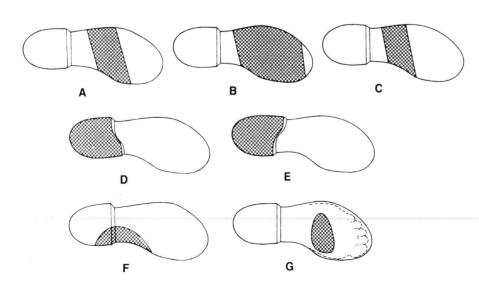

Figure 64-6. Common shoe modifications (plantar views). **A:** Metatarsal bar. **B:** Rocker bar. **C:** Denver bar. **D:** Thomas heel. **E:** Reverse Thomas heel. **F:** Scaphoid (navicular) pad insert. **G:** Metatarsal pad insert.

LOWER EXTREMITY ORTHOSES

Foot Orthoses

Foot orthoses (FOs) are removable foot supports made of variable materials placed inside the shoe to manage different foot symptoms and deformities. They have the advantage over shoe modifications in that they can be transferred from shoe to shoe, may be modified without disturbing the shoe, and are more durable than the modified shoe. Although commercially available arch supports exist, such devices are relatively ineffective. Therefore, custom-made FOs are preferred when maintenance of a specific foot alignment over long periods of time is indicated. The usual clinical indications for FOs are to relieve pressure on areas that are painful, ulcerated, scarred, or calloused, to support weak or flat longitudinal or transverse foot arches, and to control foot position and thus affect the alignment of other lower limb joints.

Soft or flexible FOs are made from leather, cork, rubber, soft plastics, and plastic foam. Many of these are commercially available and used for simple problems, but they are a poor choice for more severe conditions. The soft FOs are usually fabricated in full length from heel to toe with increased thickness where weight bearing is indicated and relief where no or little pressure should occur. Rubber FOs are generally least acceptable because of poor permeability for evaporating perspiration, lack of molding properties, and excessive compression on weight bearing. Materials that provide best cushioning tend to wear out fast and therefore may require frequent replacement. Numerous varieties of thermoplastic polyethylene foams, such as Plastazote, are available in different densities and thicknesses. They are commonly used for ischemic, insensitive, ulcerated, or arthritic feet. After heating, some of these materials can be molded conveniently directly on the foot, but others with high, specific heat require the use of a positive model of the foot. The softer-grade materials tend to bottom out early and may require a latex cork backing to prolong usefulness. Some of these materials have a high friction coefficient and may have to be covered on the foot side with softer material to reduce shear.

The semi-rigid and rigid FOs come in a variety of materials such as leather, cork, and metals, but most commonly they are made of solid plastics, which allow minimal flexibility. Optimal fabrication requires applying a plaster-of-Paris cast on the patient's feet, removing it, and making a positive replica of the foot on which the orthosis can be accurately molded. These orthoses generally extend from the posterior end of the heel to the metatarsal heads (i.e., three-quarter length) and may have medial and lateral flanges. They are molded to provide support under the longitudinal arch and metatarsal area and to provide relief for painful or irritated areas. The most rigid FOs are made of metal, usually steel or duraluminum, covered with leather, and molded on a positive cast of the patient's foot (e.g., Whitman, Mayer, and Shaffer plates; Boston arch support).

MANAGEMENT OF FOOT CONDITIONS

Numerous clinical foot problems and deformities are managed best by modification of shoes or fabrication of an FO. The most common of these conditions are listed in Table 64-1 with the suggested shoe modifications. No single remedy or combination of remedies can serve for all cases and instances. Each case has to be judged individually, and other shoe modifications and different interventions considered. Very frequently, a custom-made FO or AFO may negate the necessity for shoe modification, and surgery may be required to obtain optimal correction. Strappings, paddings, and appliances may be applied directly to the foot and toes to correct deformities and protect tender areas, such as corns, calluses, ulcers, nails, and bony outgrowths from excessive friction or pressure. Before padding, excess corns, calluses, and nails should be removed.

The clinician prescribing shoes, shoe modifications, and FOs needs to be thoroughly familiar with the normal anatomy, biomechanics, and development of the foot, diagnosis and management of pathologic conditions affecting the foot, as well as the terminology, mechanisms, and manufacture of shoes, their components, and modifications. The clinician needs to educate the patient with foot disorders about foot care and footwear needs. Before and after shoe modifications are applied and periodically thereafter, the shoe and the foot should be examined carefully to ensure proper fit, comfort, and mechanics.

Loss of sensation in the feet often occurs in persons with diabetes mellitus and polyneuropathy. This may result in poor sensory feedback regarding plantar pressures during standing and walking, which in turn may lead to tissue breakdown, ulcer formation, and eventual limb loss (3). Plantar pressures recorded under the posterior and anterior heels and the first metatarsal region of insensate feet have been found to be greater than those in sensate feet (3). Plantar ulcers in diabetic persons have been noted to develop consistently at the site of maximum plantar loading (4–7), and therefore, it is of great importance to provide proper and even redistribution of the plantar pressures through use of therapeutic shoes and custom-molded insoles (8,9). Modestly priced athletic shoes have been found to be more effective in reducing plantar pressures in diabetic persons than the more expensive leather-soled oxford shoes (10). Prevention and care of diabetic foot ulcers must emphasize patient education, glycemic control, and careful daily foot hygiene in addition to providing appropriate footwear (11), but therapeutic shoes and inserts in persons without severe foot deformity but with history of foot ulcer have not been shown to reduce incidence of ulcers (12). The use of FOs and external modifications of athletic or prescription shoes is an important component of the prevention and management of foot and ankle injuries in sports (13) and in the elderly. Athletes are not only at a greater risk of injury than the general population but also have a tendency to self-treat, look for quick and easy solutions, resume activity before healing is complete, and disregard pain as a symptom of reinjury (13). For the elderly, painful foot problems frequently make walking difficult, and diminished foot proprioception may contribute to the high frequency of falls in this age group (14). Appropriate footwear and provision of good foot care may do much to keep the elderly population safely ambulating.

Ankle-Foot Orthoses

Ankle-foot orthoses (AFOs) are most commonly prescribed for muscle weakness affecting the ankle and subtalar joints (15), including weakness of dorsal and plantar flexors, invertors, and evertors. Such AFOs also can be prescribed for prevention or correction of deformities of the foot and ankle and reduction of weight-bearing forces. In addition to having mechanical effects on the ankle, the AFOs may also affect the knee stability by varying the degree of ankle plantarflexion or dorsiflexion. An ankle fixed in dorsiflexion will provide a flexion force at the knee and thus may help to prevent genu recurvatum; a fixed plantarflexion will provide an extension force that may help to support a weak knee during the stance phase of gait.

Although traditional metal orthoses are still prescribed, plastic AFOs have become more common. They may be fabri-

TABLE 64-1.   Clinical Foot Condition and Suggested Modifications of the Orthopedic Shoe

Clinical Condition	Objectives of Modifications	Modifications

Limb shortening	Provide symmetric posture
	Improve gait
		Heel elevation:
		  If <½ in: internal
		  If >½ in: external
		Heel and sole elevation (if >1 in)
		Rocker bar
		High-quarter shoe

Arthritis, fusion, or instability of ankle and subtalar joints	Support and limit joint motion Accommodate deformities Improve gait	High-quarter shoe Reinforced counters Long steel shank Rocker bar SACH heel

Pes plano-valgus	Reduce eversion
	Support longitudinal arch
		For children:
		  High-quarter shoe with broad heel, long medial counter, and medial heel wedge
		For adults:
		  Thomas heel with medial high wedge
		  Medial longitudinal arch support with cookie or scaphoid pad

Pes equinus (fixed)	Provide heel strike Contain foot in shoe Reduce pressure on MT head Ease putting on of shoe Equalize leg length	High-quarter shoe, especially for children Heel elevation Heel and sole elevation on other shoe Modified lace stay for wide opening Medial longitudinal arch support Rocker bar, occasionally
Pes varus	Obtain realignment for flexible deformity Accommodate a fixed deformity Increase medial and posterior weight bearing on foot	High-quarter shoe Long lateral counter Reverse Thomas heel Lateral sole and heel wedges for flexible deformity Medial wedges for fixed deformity Lateral sole and heel flanges Medial longitudinal arch support
Pes cavus	Distribute weight over entire foot Restore anteroposterior foot balance Reduce pain and pressure on MT heads	High-quarter shoe High toe box Lateral heel and sole wedges Metatarsal pads or bars Molded inner sole Medial and lateral longitudinal arch support
Calcaneal spurs	Relieve pressure on painful area	Heel cushion Inner relief in heel and fill with soft sponge
Metatarsalgia	Reduce pressure on MT heads Support transverse arch	Metatarsal or sesamoid pad Metatarsal or rocker bar Inner sole relief
Hallux valgus	Reduce pressure on 1st MTP joint and big toe Prevent forward foot slide Immobilize 1st MTP joint Shift weight laterally	Soft vamp with broad ball and toe Relief in vamp with cut-out or balloon patch Low heel Metatarsal or sesamoid pad Medial longitudinal arch support Soft vamp
Hallus rigidus	Reduce pressure and motion of 1st MTP joint Improve push off	Long steel spring in sole Sesamoid pad Metatarsal or rocker bar Medial longitudinal arch support
Hammer toes	Relieve pressure on painful areas Support transverse arch Improve push off	Soft-vamp, extra-depth shoe with high toe box or balloon patch Metatarsal pad
Foot shortening (unilateral)	Fit shoe to foot	Extra inner sole and padded tongue for difference of less than one size Shoes of split sizes or custom-made
Foot fractures	Immobilize fractured part	Long steel shank Longitudinal arch support Metatarsal pad Metatarsal or rocket bar

MT, metatarsal; MTP, metatarsophalangeal; SACH, solid ankle cushion heel.

cated from either thermoplastic or thermosetting materials, depending on the required function. Inexpensive, ready-to-use AFOs are widely available and useful for minor or temporary deficits, but custom-made orthoses molded on a replica of the foot, ankle, and leg are indicated for more severe and permanent deficits. Plastic AFOs are worn inside the shoe and consist of the footplate, an upright component, and a Velcro calf strap. The shoe that attaches the orthosis to the foot has to have secure closures. Although these orthoses can be changed from shoe to shoe, it is important that all shoes worn have the same heel height to provide equal biomechanical effects at the ankle and knee. The footplate in a custom-made AFO may be accurately molded to provide all the functions of a molded FO; at the least, it should always support the metatarsal and longitudinal foot arches.

The upright components on plastic AFOs vary in design, depending on the desired function, but often these extend from the footplate without a joint mechanism to the upper calf approximately 1 to 2 inches below the head of the fibula. A plastic AFO can be fabricated to control plantarflexion, dorsiflexion, or inversion or eversion of the ankle, depending on the design, built-in position of the orthosis, thickness of the material used, and location of the trim lines. A plastic leaf-spring orthosis (PLSO) is probably the most commonly prescribed type of AFO (see Fig. 64-2). It substitutes for weakness of ankle dorsiflexors and provides some mediolateral stability. An associated strong tendency for ankle inversion, as often seen in persons with hemiplegia, may be counteracted by increasing the rigidity of the upright component at the ankle and increasing the lateral support at the calf. Severe spasticity of the ankle may require prescription of a solid-ankle plastic AFO (Fig. 64-7). Most

ready-to-wear AFOs are of the PLSO or solid-ankle varieties. A plastic spiral AFO may be prescribed effectively for concomitant weakness of both the ankle dorsiflexors and plantarflexors when spasticity is absent or insignificant. In recent years, plastic AFOs have been fabricated in the more traditional design with double uprights and a foot plate, with ankle joint mechanism and anterior/posterior stops.

Metal AFOs usually have both medial and lateral uprights with an ankle joint mechanism. The uprights are attached to the shoe by a stirrup and secured to the calf by a padded leather-covered calf band, leather strap, and a buckle. Sturdy shoes, such as orthopedic shoes, are required for metal orthoses. The stirrups usually are attached directly to the shoe between the sole and the heel, although a footplate inside the shoe occasionally is used. The upper end of the stirrup connects with the uprights at the ankle joint. The solid stirrup is used most commonly and provides the most rigid and least bulky shoe attachment. The split stirrup allows removal of the uprights from the caliper plate which is attached to the shoe, and insertion of another shoe with similar caliper plate.

Different ankle joint mechanisms allow fixed, limited, or full dorsiflexion or plantarflexion. The Klenzak ankle joint orthosis (see Fig. 64-1) permits ankle dorsiflexion assistance by inclusion of a spring. A plantarflexion stop can induce knee flexion, whereas a dorsiflexion stop induces a knee extension force during the stance phase of gait. The round caliper is a design that attaches uprights without ankle joints to the shoe by a metal plate, but the uprights are easily detachable from the shoe. Motion occurs where the uprights are inserted into the sole of the shoe at a considerable distance from the axis of the anatomic ankle joint. The round caliper often is prescribed for children with cerebral palsy who have difficulty putting on an orthosis. T-straps (see Fig. 64-1) may be attached to the shoe medially or laterally to control valgus (i.e., eversion) or varus (i.e., inversion) and are buckled around the contralateral upright to apply a counteracting force.

A variety of prefabricated AFOs are available for prevention of foot and ankle deformities. Such AFOs are frequently prescribed for neurologic conditions when there is a risk of Achilles tendon shortening, but they may also be helpful in the management of plantar fasciitis and heel pain (16). They are usually worn at night only and are not designed for weight bearing.

Standard Knee-Ankle-Foot Orthoses

Below the knee, the components of the standard knee-ankle-foot orthoses (KAFOs) are the same as those of metal or plastic AFOs, except that the uprights extend to the knee joint, where they join the thigh uprights (Fig. 64-8). Although the anatomic knee joint has a changing axis of rotation, polycentric designed knee joints have few clinical applications because during ambulation the orthotic knee joint usually is locked. A free knee joint is indicated when mediolateral instability or genu recurvatum is present but knee extension strength is adequate for weight bearing.

If knee extensors are weak, and buckling occurs, a knee lock or offset joint is indicated. The drop-ring lock is used most commonly. It is placed on the lateral upright bar and drops over the joint when it is fully extended. A spring-loaded pull rod may be added to the ring to ease locking and unlocking, especially when the patient is unable to reach the knee. A cam lock with a spring-loaded cam that fits into a groove in full extension is easier to release but still gives good stability and may

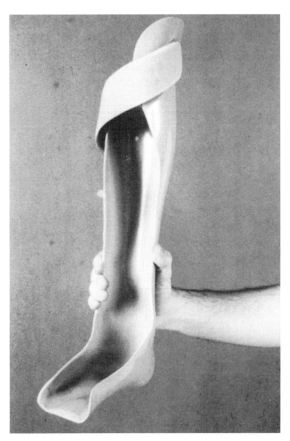

Figure 64-7. Plastic solid ankle-foot orthosis.

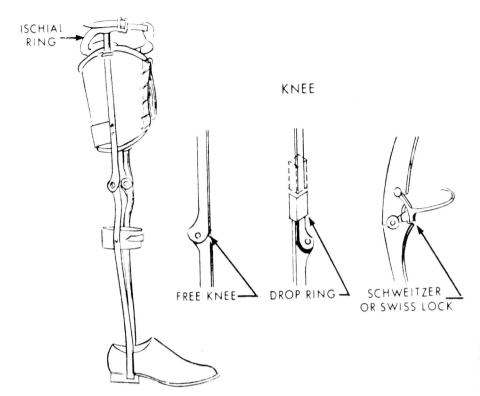

ISCHIAL RING

KNEE

FREE KNEE — DROP RING — SCHWEITZER OR SWISS LOCK

Figure 64-8. Conventional knee-ankle-foot orthosis with variations of knee locks. (From American Academy of Orthopedic Surgeons. *Atlas of orthotics.* St. Louis: CV Mosby, 1975.)

be used in severe spasticity. A bail lock (i.e., Swiss lock) is a lever bow that snaps into locked position on full extension and unlocks automatically when pressed upward against an object such as a chair. In the presence of a knee flexion contracture, an adjustable knee joint may be indicated using either a fan or dial lock. In the absence of knee flexion spasticity or contracture, a posteriorly offset knee joint provides a stable knee during stance but allows flexion during the swing phase.

Even when mechanically locked, the knee with weak extensors would bend on weight bearing if not stabilized by straps above and below the patella or by a patellar strap, a soft leather pad covering the kneecap and fastened with four adjustable straps to the uprights. The thigh uprights are connected by a rigid, padded upper thigh band with an anterior soft closure. This band should be 1.5 inches below the ischium, unless ischial rest is prescribed. Usually, a second, rigid lower thigh band also is used with soft anterior straps.

The Scott-Craig orthosis eliminates the lower thigh and calf bands, which makes it easier to put on and remove (Fig. 64-9) (17). It consists of two uprights with four rigid connections: posterior rigid upper thigh band, bail-type knee lock, rigid anterior upper tibial band with soft posterior strap, and at the lower end, a stirrup with a rigid sole plate built into the shoe extending to the metatarsal heads. It is connected to the uprights by double-stop (Becker) ankle joints that are adjusted to place the orthosis in 5° of dorsiflexion for optimum balance (18). The shoe sole is perfectly flat from the heel to the metatarsal bar, where it becomes slightly rounded to the toe. Properly adjusted, the orthosis should stand balanced on its own. It is a stable orthosis that biomechanically functions as the standard KAFO.

Modified Knee-Ankle-Foot Orthoses

Plastic laminated knee-ankle-foot orthoses KAFOs may incorporate standard ankle and knee components, but the uprights

and bands are made of lightweight skin-colored laminated plastic that closely fits the limb (Fig. 64-10). The thigh piece is a quadrilaterally shaped posterior thigh shell with or without an ischial weight-bearing seat closed anteriorly by a plastic band and a Velcro strap. A suprapatellar or pretibial shell provides knee extension force, which eliminates the need for patellar strap and provides mediolateral knee stability. At the lower end, the uprights are connected to a molded plastic footplate to be worn inside a shoe.

A plastic laminated supracondylar KAFO is indicated for patients who lack knee and ankle muscle power but have normal hip extensors, full knee extension, and no spasticity (18). A molded footplate and a solid ankle design immobilize the foot and ankle in equinus, which produces a knee extension force during stance. Genu recurvatum is controlled by a supracondylar anterior shell and a counteracting popliteal shell posteriorly. The absence of a mechanical knee joint allows free knee flexion during swing phase with better gait pattern and reduced energy cost.

Lightweight modular KAFOs have been designed for quick and easy assembly and provided for children with Duchenne muscular dystrophy in order to extend their walking ability (19). Such a KAFO consists of a plastic thigh piece and an AFO, both available in several prefabricated sizes. The two components are joined at the knee by a metal joint system with an automatic ring or bail locks.

Knee Orthoses

Knee orthoses (KOs) are prescribed to prevent genu recurvatum and to provide mediolateral stability. As such they may be used during sports and other physical activities to provide functional support for unstable knees or during the rehabilitation phase following injury or surgery on the knee. The use of KOs for the prevention of knee injury in athletes is controversial (20). Numerous designs of KOs are available, a develop-

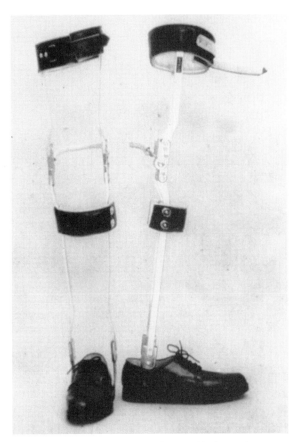

Figure 64-9. The Scott-Craig knee-ankle-foot orthosis.

ment enhanced by the growing field of sports medicine. Most KOs consist of two uprights, free or adjustable knee joints, and thigh and calf cuffs. The Swedish knee cage (Fig. 64-11) prevents recurvatum but permits flexion. The three-way knee stabilizer orthosis looks similar and gives good control of structural knee instability in the lateral, medial, and posterior directions and is indicated for genu valgum, varus, and recurvatum. The standard KOs have short lever arms and may not be effective when strong forces are required for control. They also have a tendency to slip down, or migrate during movement. Numerous KO designs with longer lever arms and, often, derotational components have been commercially fabricated and prescribed for advanced physical activities and athletics.

Hip-Knee-Ankle-Foot Orthoses

Hip-knee-ankle-foot orthoses (HKAFOs) consist of the same components as described for the standard AFOs and KAFOs, with the addition of an attached lockable hip joint and a pelvic band to control movements at the anatomic hip joint. The hip joint usually has a ring drop lock. The pelvic band, which may be unilateral or bilateral, encompasses the pelvis between the iliac crest and greater trochanter laterally, curves down over the buttocks, and then passes up again over the sacrum. The indications for prescribing a pelvic band have been controversial because several studies indicate that it increases lumbar excursion and displacement of gravity during ambulation, and thus energy cost may be greater. For most persons with paraplegia, pelvic bands probably are not necessary, although they may improve standing balance, especially if spasticity is severe.

The Louisiana State University reciprocating gait orthosis (Fig. 64-12) provides bilateral KAFOs with posterior offset knee joints, knee locks, posterior plastic ankle-foot and thigh pieces,

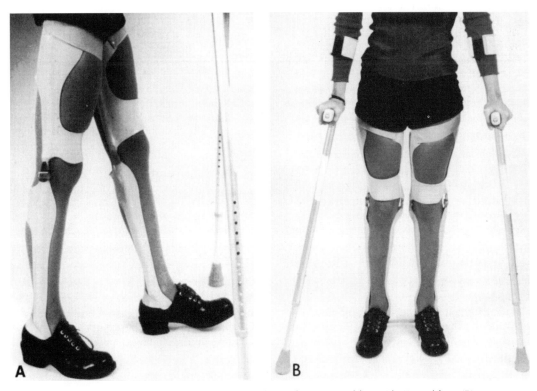

Figure 64-10. Plastic-laminated knee-ankle-foot orthoses viewed from side **(A)** and front **(B)**.

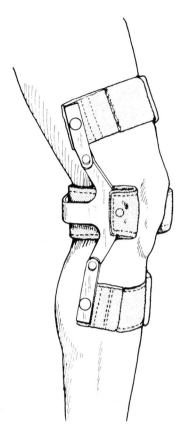

Figure 64-11. The Swedish knee cage is an example of a knee orthosis (KO).

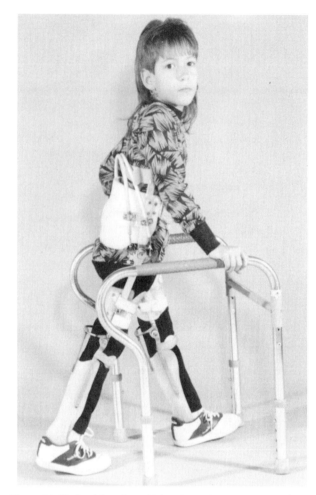

Figure 64-12. Louisiana State University reciprocating gait orthosis.

a custom-molded pelvic girdle, and special thrust-bearing hip joints, coupled together with a cable and conduit, and a thoracic extension with Velcro straps (21,22). The cable coupling mechanism provides hip stability by preventing simultaneous bilateral hip flexion, yet allows free hip flexion coupled with reciprocal extension of the contralateral hip when a step is attempted. Using two crutches, persons with paraplegia are able to ambulate with a four-point gait pattern. This orthosis also has been tested and used in conjunction with a functional electric stimulation system to facilitate ambulation by persons with paraplegia.

Fracture Orthoses

Orthoses of different designs have been used in the management of fractures (23). By definition, a plaster-of-Paris cast applied to a fractured limb is an orthosis that provides rigid immobilization while healing occurs. The term "fracture orthosis," however, refers to a concept of management based on the hypothesis, supported by considerable clinical evidence, that mobilization of adjacent joints does not impede healing of fractures, that functional activity stimulates osteogenesis, and that rigid immobilization of fractures is not a prerequisite for healing. Even when this management concept is applied, all fractures initially are immobilized either by traction or in conventional casts while the acute pain and swelling associated with the injury subsides and early healing takes place. Such immobilization should be maintained for at least 3 weeks, but no more than 6 weeks, before the fracture orthosis is applied. The initial immobilization is done to minimize leg shortening, but the lowest incidence of leg shortening has been found in those patients who have had fracture orthoses applied 2 to 4 weeks postinjury.

Problems associated with fracture orthoses are increased angulation of the bone and refracturing, both of which are rare. Fracture orthoses have been used most often to treat fractures of the shafts of the tibia and femur when internal fixation is unnecessary, contraindicated, or refused by the patient and when healing is significantly delayed or does not occur. Fracture orthoses are contraindicated when satisfactory alignment of the fracture cannot be obtained or maintained.

Initial efforts to use orthotic devices for lower extremity fractures were inspired by prostheses for lower extremity amputees. Three basic components are required for fabrication of a fracture orthosis: a cylinder, footplate, and joint mechanisms. The cylindrical component closely fits the fractured limb to provide a hydraulic mechanism that will promote stability for the bony structures and resist shortening. The vertical load of weight bearing is offset by lateral and oblique forces from an essentially incompressible fluid chamber that is created by the encasing cylindrical orthotic component. Most proximally on the orthosis, a weight-bearing surface may be provided, such as a patellar tendon-bearing socket or ischial seat, to reduce further the pressure on the fracture site. This mechanism is far less important in the distribution of weight-bearing pressures than the hydraulic mechanism mentioned. The cylindrical components usually are made of plaster-of-Paris cast or low-temperature thermoplastics (Orthoplast). The second major component of a fracture orthosis is a footplate, which is to be worn inside a shoe. The footplate usually is prefabricated and

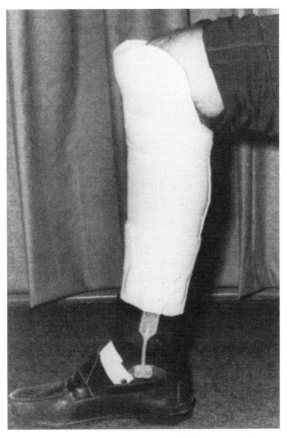

Figure 64-13. Orthosis for fracture of the tibia. (From American Academy of Orthopedic Surgeons. *Atlas of orthotics.* St. Louis: CV Mosby, 1975.)

made of plastic, although custom-made footplates occasionally are made. The footplate usually is attached to the cylindrical component by simple plastic hinges rather than metallic joints. Similar joint mechanisms may be used for the knee, connecting the above- and below-knee pieces.

Appropriately designed and fitted, fracture orthoses allow functional ambulation with progressively increasing weight bearing. Absence of pain, good callus formation, and lack of gross motion at the fracture site indicate that the fracture is stable. The fracture is considered healed when full weight-bearing is tolerated and radiographs show that the fracture is obliterated with evidence of good callus formation and consolidation. Fractures of the tibial shaft generally do not require surgical intervention and heal spontaneously. After 2 to 4 weeks of immobilization in a long leg cast, most patients with closed tibial fractures are ready for active range of motion of the knee and ambulation with increased weight bearing. Fractures of the distal tibia can be treated with a below-knee orthosis with a patellar tendon indentation for weight bearing (Fig. 64-13). Fractures of the proximal tibia, especially those involving the knee joint, generally require a thigh piece that is connected to the leg portion with a polycentric knee joint. Closed transverse fractures of the midfemoral shaft generally are best treated with intramedullary nailing, but for some open, severely comminuted, or oblique femoral fractures, management with fracture orthoses may present a better approach (24). Fractures of the mid- or distal femoral shaft are managed more successfully with fracture orthoses than are fractures of the proximal femoral shaft because of the latter's strong tendency to produce varus angulation and malalignment. The thigh component of the orthosis resembles that of the quadrilateral above-knee prosthesis with an ischial seat and a three-point fixation contour that resists varus angulation (Fig. 64-14). The thigh component is connected to the calf piece by freely moving

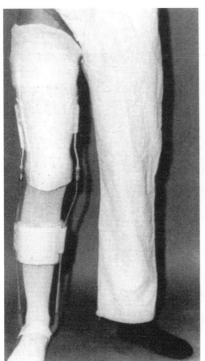
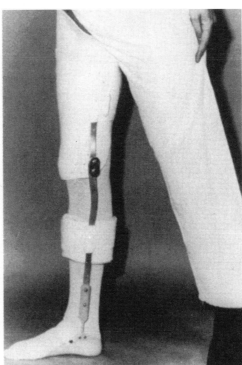
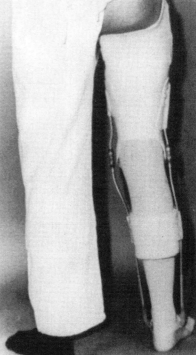

A　　　　　　　　　　　　　　　　　　　　　　　　　　　　　　　**B,C**

Figure 64-14. Front (**A**), side (**B**), and rear (**C**) views of an orthosis for fracture of the distal femur. (From American Academy of Orthopedic Surgeons. *Atlas of orthotics.* St. Louis: CV Mosby, 1975.)

metal or plastic joints. The calf piece is attached to a footplate by joints, as seen in the tibial fracture orthosis (see Fig. 64-13).

Occasionally, fracture orthoses are used in the management of fractures of the forearm and wrist as a therapeutic alternative to other means of external or internal fixation. A cylindrical forearm component is attached by a joint mechanism to a handpiece. Active use of muscles and joints is encouraged, although weight bearing generally is not indicated because it may not be necessary.

GAIT AIDS

Canes

Canes, when properly used, will increase base of support, decrease loading and demand on the lower limb and skeletal structures, provide additional sensory information, and assist with acceleration and deceleration during locomotion. Canes are prescribed for various disabilities to improve balance, to decrease pain, to reduce weight-bearing forces on injured or inflamed structures, to compensate for weak muscles, and to scan the immediate environment. Pathologic conditions affecting the upper limbs may interfere with the use of canes and crutches or warrant prescription of specially designed gait aids.

The total length of a properly measured cane should equal the distance from the upper border of the greater trochanter to the bottom of the heel of the shoe. The patient should be able to stand with the cane with the elbow flexed at 20° to 30° and both shoulders level. The patient should be instructed in the proper use of the cane, to hold the cane in the hand opposite the affected limb, and to advance the cane and the affected leg in a three-point gait pattern. When ascending stairs the good leg is advanced first, but when descending, the cane and the affected leg lead.

Canes are most commonly made of hardwood or aluminum but can vary in design (Fig. 64-15). All canes should be fitted with a deeply grooved 1- to 2-inch-wide rubber tip for good traction and safety, and the clinician should check these regularly for wear. The common C handle or crook-top cane is inexpensive, but this type of handle may be uncomfortable and difficult to grasp, especially for those with hand problems. Additionally, the weight-bearing line falls behind the shaft of the cane, thus reducing its supportive value. A functional handle that fits the grip, conforms to the natural angle of the hand, and is more centered over the shaft of the cane is more comfortable and provides better support. Wide-based canes made of metal provide a wider area of support. These designs consist of three or four short legs attached to a single upright shaft with a molded or wooden handle. Several base widths are available, and the length of the shaft is adjustable. Wide-based canes are prescribed for persons with greater degrees of impaired balance, preferably only for temporary use, because these canes often are heavy and awkward in appearance.

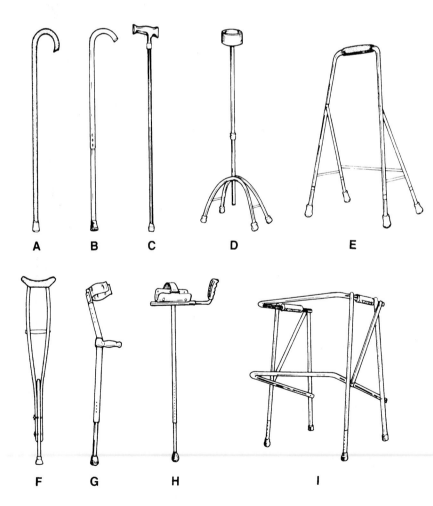

Figure 64-15. Canes, crutches, and walkers. **A:** C-handle or crook-top cane. **B:** Adjustable aluminum cane. **C:** Functional grip cane. **D:** Adjustable wide-base quad cane. **E:** Hemiwalker. **F:** Adjustable wooden axillary crutch. **G:** Adjustable aluminum Lofstrand crutch. **H:** Forearm support or platform crutch. **I:** Walker or walkerette.

Crutches

The indications for prescribing a pair of crutches are similar to those for canes, but the clinical deficits usually are greater. Good strength of the upper limbs usually is required because persons needing crutches tend to require them more for weight bearing and propulsion than for balancing or as sensory aids. For effective crutch walking, the upper limb joints should have good range of motion, and the key muscle groups (i.e., shoulder flexors and depressors, elbow and wrist extensors, finger flexors) should be strong. Axillary crutches (see Fig. 64-15) are the most commonly prescribed crutches in the United States. The wooden axillary crutch is easily adjustable and made of hardwood with two upright shafts connected by a padded axillary piece on top, a handpiece in the middle, and an extension piece below. The extension piece and shafts have numerous holes at regular intervals so the total length of the crutch and the height of the handles may be adjusted. A large, soft rubber suction tip is attached to the extension piece to allow total contact with the floor. Metal axillary crutches consist of a single contoured tubular structure, which can be adjusted by telescoping and push-button positions. A functional handle is adjustable in height.

When a person is measured for axillary crutches, the total length of the crutch and the height of the handle are the two main dimensions to be considered. The handle height is measured in the same manner as with canes, but the total length of the crutch should be equal to the distance from the anterior fold of the axilla to either a point 6 inches anterolaterally from the foot or to the bottom of the heel, plus 1 or 2 inches.

The popular Lofstrand crutch (see Fig. 64-15) consists of a single aluminum tubular shaft, adjustable in length, a molded handpiece, and a forearm piece bent posteriorly just above the handpiece. The forearm piece, also adjustable in length, extends to 2 inches below the elbow, where a forearm cuff with a narrow anterior opening is attached. This crutch is lightweight, easily adjustable, and gives freedom for hand activities because the handpiece can be released without loosing the crutch. It requires, however, greater skills than the axillary crutch, good strength of the upper limbs, and adequate trunk balance for safe ambulation.

The Canadian elbow extensor crutch (i.e., triceps crutch) has a single aluminum upright shaft attached to bilateral uprights, which extend to above the elbow. These are connected by a handle and two half cuffs, one below and one above the elbow. This crutch rarely is prescribed but may benefit those with triceps weakness.

Forearm support (i.e., platform) crutches (see Fig. 64-15) may be prescribed when clinical conditions of the forearm, wrist, or hands prevent safe or comfortable weight bearing, such as in the presence of arthritis of the elbow, wrist, or hand, fractures of forearm or hand, or weakness of triceps or grasp.

Walkers

Walkers provide a wider and more stable base of support than do either canes or crutches (see Fig. 64-15). They may be prescribed for patients requiring maximum assistance with balance, the elderly, the fearful, and the uncoordinated. The patient must have good grasp and arm strength bilaterally, although forearm supports can be used as described previously. Walkers are conspicuous in appearance and interfere with development of smooth reciprocal gait patterns. Although they are very useful during rehabilitation, care should be taken that the patient does not become emotionally dependent on the balance stability provided by the walker. Walkers are available in various sizes, are adjustable in height, and come in different designs, such as folding, rolling, reciprocal, or stair walkers.

REFERENCES

1. Zamosky I, Licht S, Redford JB. Shoes and their modifications. In: Redford JB, ed. *Orthotics et cetera.* Baltimore: Williams & Wilkins, 1980:368–431.
2. Staheli LT. Shoes for children: a review. *Pediatrics* 1991;88:371–375.
3. Zhu H, Wertsch JJ, Harris GF, et al. Sensate and insensate in-shoe plantar pressures. *Arch Phys Med Rehabil* 1993;74:1362–1368.
4. Stokes IAF, Fairs IB, Hutton WC. The neuropathic ulcer and loads on the foot in diabetic patients. *Acta Orthop Scand* 1975;46:839–847.
5. Cavanagh PR, Hennig EM, Rodgers MM, et al. The measurement of pressure distribution on the plantar surface of diabetic feet. In: Whittle M, Harris D, eds. *Biomechanical measurements in orthopaedic practice.* Oxford: Clarendon Press, 1985:159–166.
6. Duckworth T, Boulton AJM, Betts RP, et al. Plantar pressure measurements and the prevention of ulceration in the diabetic foot. *J Bone Joint Surg* 1985; 67B:79–85.
7. Boulton AJM, Betts RP, Franks CI, et al. The natural history of foot pressure abnormalities in neuropathic diabetic subjects. *Diabetic Res* 1987;5:73–77.
8. Lord M, Hosein R. Pressure redistribution by molded inserts in diabetic footwear: a pilot study. *J Rehabil Res Dev* 1994;31:214–221.
9. Chen RCC, Lord M. A comparison of trial shoe and shell shoe fitting techniques. *Prosthet Orthot Int* 1995;19:181–187.
10. Perry JE, Ulbrecht JS, Derr JA, et al. The use of running shoes to reduce plantar pressures in patients who have diabetes. *J Bone Joint Surg* 1995;77a:1819–1828.
11. Birrer RB, Dellacorte MP, Grisafi PJ. Prevention and care of diabetic foot ulcers. *Am Fam Physician* 1996;53:601–611.
12. Reiber GE, Smith DG, Wallace C, et al. Effect of therapeutic footwear on foot reulceration in patients with diabetes: a randomized controlled trial. *JAMA* 2002;287:2552–2558.
13. Janisse DJ. Indications and prescriptions for orthoses in sports. *Orthop Clin North Am* 1994;25:95–107.
14. Robbins S, Waked E, McClaran J. Proprioception and stability: foot position awareness as a function of age and footwear. *Age Aging* 1995;24:67–72.
15. Lehmann JF. Biomechanics of ankle foot orthoses: prescription and design. *Arch Phys Med Rehabil* 1979;160:200–207.
16. Ryan J. The use of posterior night splints in the treatment of plantar fasciitis. *Am Fam Physician* 1995;52:891–898.
17. O'Daniel WE, Hahn HR. Follow-up usage of the Scott-Craig orthosis in paraplegia. *Paraplegia* 1981;19:373–378.
18. Lehneis HR. New developments in lower limb orthotics through bioengineering. *Arch Phys Med Rehabil* 1972;53:303–310.
19. Taktak DM, Bowker P. Lightweight modular knee-ankle-foot orthosis for Duchenne muscular dystrophy: design, development and evaluation. *Arch Phys Med Rehabil* 1995;76:1156–1162.
20. Podesta L, Sherman MF. Knee bracing. *Orthop Clin North Am* 1988;19:737–745.
21. Douglas R, Larson PF, D'Ambrosia R, et al. The LSU reciprocation-gait orthosis. *Orthopedics* 1983;6:834–839.
22. Durr-Fillauer Medical, Inc. *LSU reciprocating gait orthoses: a pictorial description and application manual.* Chattanooga, TN: Durr-Fillauer Medical, Inc., 1983.
23. Sarmiento A, Sinclair WF. *Atlas of orthotics: biomechanical principles and application.* St. Louis: Mosby, 1975:245–254.
24. St Pierre RK, Holmes HE, Flemming LL. Cast bracing of femoral fractures. *Orthopedics* 1982;5:739–745.

CHAPTER 65

Gait Restoration and Gait Aids

Ross A. Bogey and Sue Ann Sisto

GAIT TRAINING—PRINCIPLES

The major emphasis in training for independent walking is on methods of training support and propulsion of the lower limbs, balance of the body mass over one or both feet, and control of the foot and knee paths throughout swing. Gait training is typically accomplished through a combination of weight bearing, stretching techniques, and walking practice. While several neuromuscular techniques foster specific hand contacts to facilitate desired movement, sometimes the use of the hands should be discouraged to enable the restoration of dynamic balance (1).

The essential components of gait have been described for the stance and swing phases (1). The stance phase should include extension of the hip with dorsiflexion of the ankle to move the body forward. There is a lateral shift of the pelvis, to the stance phase side. Flexion of the knee should occur at heel contact, followed by extension, then flexion again just prior to pre-swing. The knee is flexed at the start of the swing phase, then extended in preparation for the subsequent ipsilateral heel strike. Similar to the knee, there are two flexion-extension epochs per gait cycle. The ankle is plantarflexed from initial contact to the start of single limb support, then dorsiflexed for the remainder of the single support phase (1). There is substantial plantarflexion in pre-swing, and then the ankle is dorsiflexed to neutral (or slightly beyond) to assure foot clearance during swing (1).

Intervention strategies for gait training should take into account the importance of eliciting and strengthening synergistic muscle activity and task-related practice. For example, individuals with upper motor neuron lesions have difficulty with support, propulsion, and balance. Training to improve force generation and speed of muscular contraction are usually needed. Functional improvement depends on regaining the appropriate timing of segmental rotations that require practice of walking (2).

BALANCE TRAINING

Therapy aimed at improving balance is necessary prior to resuming gait after central nervous system (CNS) insult. However, there is no direct correlation between improved dynamic or static balance and improvement in gait variables. Winstein and colleagues examined standing balance and locomotor performance in 21 stroke survivors (3). They found that while standing balance and locomotor control mechanisms were highly interrelated, a reduction in standing balance asymmetry did not necessarily lead to reduced gait asymmetry. Wolf and colleagues (4) showed that a short individualized exercise program, including balance training, led to short-term improvement. However, gains were not maintained one year after completing training. While balance is an essential component of gait recovery, it is not statistically related to improvements in gait performance variables.

TECHNIQUES TO GAIT TRAINING

Several types of therapy intervention are in common use today. A generally accepted classification of these methods differentiates between the conventional versus the neurofacilitory treatment approaches. The conventional approach to the treatment of a patient's neurological deficits involves training such patients to use their remaining motor capabilities to compensate for those that were lost.

Conventional Approach

From the standpoint of gait training using conventional treatment approaches, the goal would be to use the stronger limbs to compensate for the weaker. The weaker leg would be maximally braced with a lower limb orthosis to provide maximal stability and avoid collapse. By relying on the support of the brace, the patient may never learn to facilitate the use of the weaker limb. Additionally, a cane may be employed where the patient would lean toward the cane for support, thereby restricting shifting of the body weight and center of mass toward the weaker side. Finally, the patient may wear a sling supporting the upper limb by affixing it to the body. This restriction, although sometimes necessary, limits natural arm swing that contributes to a normal gait pattern.

Neurofacilitory Approaches

In contrast to the conventional methods, neurofacilitory approaches focus on rejuvenation of the lost motor capabilities. In that sense, Voss (5) referred to "hidden potentials for recovery" and Bobath (6) referred to "some untapped potential for more highly organized activity." In the late 1950s and early 1960s, neurofacilitation techniques developed and resulted in dramatic clinical changes in the treatment of patients with neurological diseases (7). These techniques developed due to clinicians' dissatisfaction with the muscle reeducation techniques employed during the polio era. For the most part, clinicians still use neurofacilitory approaches to assess and treat neurological patients.

Neurofacilitory techniques primarily focus on retraining motor control by facilitating or inhibiting movement patterns. Desirable movement patterns for gait would be facilitated while massed patterns or synergies would be inhibited because these stereotypical movements, resulting from a neurological injury or disease, are not functional. Neurofacilitory techniques include the Bobath approach, the Brunnstrom approach, and proprioceptive neuromuscular facilitation (PNF). All approaches are based primarily on assumptions of reflex and hierarchical theories of motor control.

Karl and Berta Bobath developed the Bobath approach for the care of patients with cerebral palsy. Bobath (6) states that it is possible to get a great deal of normal activity out of the affected side by a systematic treatment designed to prepare that side for functional use. However, functional improvement has been found to be possible only in those patients who have little or no sensory deficit. During the acute stage, the emphasis on treatment is placed on developing the functional potential of the affected side.

Bobath's technique is based on the idea that a normal automatic postural reflex mechanism is the basis for normal motion patterns (humans move *only* in motion patterns, *never* in single motions). This means that every motion has its own postural adaptations. In brain injury, the supraspinal inhibitory control of the patient's motor functions is reduced. Reflexes are liberated and show themselves as spastic patterns throughout all of the affected side. Motions, which demand a constantly changing background of postural control and adaptation, are thus hindered, the hemiplegic patient being locked within a few stereotyped positional and motion patterns, including flexor- and extensor-synergies.

According to this approach, treatment goals for gait training must therefore be to change the stereotyped postural background to stimulate more normal motions. Conventional strength training of spastic, abnormal patterns are generally thought to worsen and sustain the pathological reflex activity, because the activity of a spastic muscle may not necessarily produce functional movements as a result of strength training. However, additional research is needed to determine if spasticity must be inhibited or reduced before implementing strengthening exercises.

The Bobath concept differs from other neurofacilitation techniques in that normal postural tone is considered to be the basis for any normal motion. Tone must be regulated. Hypertonicity must be inhibited, low tone increased, and unstable tone must be stabilized. Muscles are typically treated in a proximal-to-distal manner.

Muscle tone is regulated using the Bobath approach of normalizing muscle tone by positioning the limb "out of synergy." The reflex inhibitory movement patterns are opposite to the typical hemiplegia synergy patterns and are performed without resistance. This means that if a typical synergistic pattern during the swing phase of gait is flexion and external rotation of the hip, then specific manual guidance techniques, either as pre-gait activities in a recumbent position or in stance, would foster hip extension and internal rotation. If the leg were in an extensor synergy, it would be positioned in hip adduction, internal rotation, knee extension, plantar flexion, and inversion. Recumbent or standing pre-gait activities would focus on hip extension with abduction and external rotation using the Bobath approach.

During training, any time an abnormal pattern is evident, the task is terminated or modified to a less challenging movement pattern. For example, if an abnormal synergy were present such as knee extension with ankle inversion during the swing phase of gait, treatment, using the Bobath approach, would be adjusted to avoid ambulation training and focus on pre-gait activities. These activities might include facilitation of swing with the knee in more flexion and the ankle in neutral and dorsiflexion using manual contacts while the patient is supported in the parallel bars, with an assistive device, or even in the sitting or supine position. One assumption that you "wait" for recovery of normal movement before practicing walking (until muscle tone is normal) is common despite evidence that such assumptions are in error (8).

Although the Bobath approach is widely used in the gait rehabilitation of hemiparetic patients, especially in Europe, there is little neurophysiological evidence for its presumed effects on gait symmetry and facilitation of paretic muscles during the therapeutic intervention. Hesse and associates (9) evaluated the immediate effects of therapeutic facilitation on the gait of 22 hemiparetic patients using gait entrainment or repetitive practice aimed at gait symmetry and facilitation of paretic muscles by five Bobath trained therapists. The study confirmed a more balanced walking pattern, in conjunction with facilitation of more weight-bearing muscles based on electromyogram (EMG). The authors attributed these gait changes to a prolonged single stance period of the affected leg, unobstructed hip movement and faster gait, due to the Bobath-based therapy.

The Bobath approach has been examined for its application to gait and has been compared to interventions directed toward nonneurological patients such as the geriatric population. Since 1990, the Bobath approach has changed (10). Using a focus group design, peer-nominated therapists discussed topics related to neurology or elderly care based on published literature. All therapists agreed that the analysis of normal movement, the control of muscle tone, and the facilitation of movement defined the Bobath approach. Neuroplasticity was described as the primary rationale of the Bobath approach to target the damaged CNS. Motor learning was a primary theme of the Bobath focus group, whereas in the geriatric group, patient-focused goals related to function were discussed.

Lennon and associates (11) conducted a survey of over 1,000 senior level physiotherapists in the United Kingdom, where questions about theoretical beliefs about gait reeducation were asked. Approximately two-thirds of the therapists preferred the Bobath approach with one-third preferring a more eclectic approach. The consensus view of the theoretical beliefs underlying the current practice of Bobath for gait training was identified. In general there was a substantial difference in these beliefs compared to the eclectic therapists where the Bobath therapists considered the need for normal tone and movement patterns to perform functional tasks. The training of these tasks was delayed if abnormal tone or movement would be reinforced by practice. Still the conclusion was made that Bobath therapists need to make the translation into function more automatic, in the way activities are practiced and performed outside of therapy. However, since the practice of gait using the Bobath approach is closer to the actual functional task of walking, there is less controversy over this approach than for other Bobath approaches, such as those directed toward recovery of arm function. Due to differences in reimbursement systems between the United States and the United Kingdom, though, most U.S. Bobath trained therapists incorporate an eclectic approach when providing gait therapy due to the limited number of sessions allowable and the need to focus on functional recovery regardless of normalcy of movement patterns.

Langhammer and Stanghelle (12) studied the difference between a Bobath or motor relearning program in acute stroke rehabilitation using a randomized control design. The motor relearning approach focuses on functional recovery without an emphasis on the sequential return of normal movement patterns from proximal to distal underlying the Bobath approach. The authors found no difference between the groups for motor, functional, or quality of life scores except the motor relearning group demonstrated greater improvement in activities of daily living (ADLs) than did the Bobath group. These results may point to the need to focus more on functional recovery in acute neurological patients. The health care reimbursement system allows for a very limited inpatient stay. This limitation requires rehabilitation specialists to be sure that patients are functional, even if it means independent function using abnormal movement patterns.

Proprioceptive Neuromuscular Facilitation

Proprioceptive neuromuscular facilitation (PNF) uses resistance to facilitate movement (13). The therapist provides maximal resistance to the stronger muscle components of specific diagonal patterns. The assumption is that functional movements occur across more than one joint and incorporate three planes of movement. The application of PNF incorporates only enough resistance so as not to facilitate abnormal movement patterns, and can be applied with impairments such as in hypotonia.

One common facilitating component to PNF is the application of a quick stretch of the agonist before maximal contraction (13). In the instance of gait training, while a patient is standing with support, the swing limb could be stretched into hip extension, thereby facilitating hip flexion contraction to promote hip flexion during swing. Surburg (14) compared PNF with and without resistance to weight training in a sports medicine sample and found no difference between groups in reaction time, response time, and movement time. These results may point to the PNF approach being less applicable to the neurologically intact individual.

Even treatment methods that are purportedly based on neurophysiological principles do not have a fully comprehensive and experimentally proven neurophysiological basis. Dickstein and colleagues (15) examined the recovery of 196 persons after stroke. Patients were randomly assigned to one of three groups: conventional therapy, Bobath, and PNF. Dependent measures included the functional independence measure (FIM), Ashworth scale, isolated motor control status, and ambulatory status. No significant differences were observed in improvement in ADLs, muscle tone, active range of motion (ROM), or walking ability.

Brunnstrom Method

Twitchell described six stages of motor recovery in hemiplegia, progressing from complete flaccidity, through spasticity and gross synergistic movements to the return or normal isolated and coordinated joint movements (16). The Brunnstrom approach uses resistance, associated reactions, and primitive postural reactions to facilitate gross synergistic movements and the return of muscle tone (17). Incorporated into gait training, the Brunnstrom approach might include a gentle push in the anterior direction of a standing stroke patient to facilitation of a reflex stepping pattern, and theoretically, to improve automatic gait. During later stages of recovery, the development of iso-

lated movement and control are emphasized (18). Like PNF, the Brunnstrom method is advocated to help normalize tone in a hemiparetic patient with persistent flaccidity.

The Brunnstrom approach is often used as a classification schema rather than a treatment approach. For example, Higashi and colleagues (19) compared the excitability of motor neuron pools of hemiplegic patients assessing Brunnstrom recovery stages using H reflex and M responses. These electrophysiological responses were shown to better match the bell-shaped pattern of the Brunnstrom stages of recovery than conventional measures. Wagennar and associates (20) found that walking velocity progressed according to both the Brunnstrom and neurodevelopmental technique stages after 5 weeks of either Bobath or Brunnstrom methods of treatment, but there was no generalization to the Barthel Index or neurological or neuropsychological measures.

Rood Method

The Rood method uses tactile stimulation such as fast brushing or stroking or icing to facilitate specific muscle groups to promote functional activity (21). Rood describes four stages of recovery and the selection of which muscle groups to facilitate depends on the stage of recovery that the patient has achieved. These stages of neurophysiological mobility include: (a) development of functional mobility, (b) development of stability, (c) development of stability and mobility, and (d) development of skilled movement (22). Level one involves activities such as rolling over. Levels two and three involve the development of stability in preparation for weight bearing and include such positions as quadruped and standing. Level four includes skilled movement such as walking (18). It becomes clear why many of these neurofacilitory techniques are referred to as neurodevelopmental techniques (NDT) as they follow the progression or normal physical development. Rood techniques can be used to facilitate muscles that are hypotonic or to reduce spasticity in muscles that are hypertonic (Table 65-1).

Biofeedback

The literature on the efficacy of biofeedback has suggested that its application (particularly to stroke patients) can enhance recovery of motor function and may supplement physiotherapeutic techniques. Biofeedback is the technique of using electronic equipment to reveal instantaneously to patient and therapist certain physiological events and to teach the patient to control these otherwise involuntary events by manipulating the displayed signals. The production of consistently reproducible behavior augmented by biofeedback suggests that with practice and training, patients rely more on internal versus external cues. Biofeedback should not be a substitute for motor training but considered an adjunct by providing additional information to increase learning and improve performance (23). In rehabilitation, EMG, position, or force feedback is most commonly provided. Visual and auditory displays are supplied instantaneously based on information of specified transducers. As learning occurs, patients rely less on visual feedback, then auditory feedback which should be gradually withdrawn by the clinician. Eventually, success is determined based on the relearning of internal cues for movement. Providing feedback about performance, such as success at reaching a target threshold, is referred to knowledge of results (KR). Providing KR periodically rather than continuously has been demonstrated to enhance learning and retention (24). In contrast to the viewpoint of most clinicians, verbal feedback can delay the relearn-

TABLE 65-1.   Comparison of Foci and Treatment Elements for Common Neuromuscular Facilitation Techniques

	Bobath	Brunnstrom	PNF[a]	Rood
Key treatment element	Position limb out of synergy	Resistance and postural reactions	Strengthening	Tactile stimulation
Focus of treatment	Proximal-to-distal	General-to-isolated movements	Multi-joint movement	Muscle selection based on recovery stage
Means to establish more normal movement	Reestablish automatic postural reflexes	Synergistic patterns (early)	"Diagonal" pattern development	Gross motor, progressing to skilled movements
Tone adjustment	Correct hypertonia and hypotonia prior to treatment	Attenuates hypotonia	Attenuates hypotonia	Attenuates hypotonia and hypertonia

[a] Proprioceptive neuromuscular facilitation.

ing process because it lacks information specificity (25). One practical advantage of biofeedback is that the patient can practice motor tasks without the need for one-to-one supervision.

The most common techniques supply information from muscle contractions (EMG feedback) in the muscle reeducation of patients with CNS disease. Biofeedback practitioners currently quantify more functional, limb-specific activities rather than emphasizing individual muscle responses (26). In locomotor impairments, techniques that combine knowledge of body movements plus EMG during walking are increasingly used.

Basmajian and colleagues (27) and Brudney and colleagues (28) found that biofeedback techniques that augmented the recruitment of ankle dorsiflexors while simultaneously inhibiting plantar flexors allowed stroke patients to walk with fewer or no assistive devices. Wolf and colleagues (29) showed that proprioception and cognitive integrity were critical to maximize independent walking. Biofeedback need not be limited to muscle signals. Electrogoniometer signals indicating joint angles and pressure or force signals can also be used. Center of pressure is an example of force feedback that has been used for balance assessment and training patients to control postural sway. However, there has been limited evidence indicating the control of balance carries over to functional tasks such as gait. There is also limited evidence that control of balance trained through force platforms relates to the reduction of falls, most likely because balance training is bipedal and falls usually occur in single limb support (30). Gait training techniques such as walking slowly to increase time in single limb support may have a greater effect on the prevention of falls.

Petrofsky (31) used EMG biofeedback to decrease the magnitude of Trendelenburg gait in patients with incomplete spinal cord lesions. Five patients wore a two-channel EMG biofeedback training device at home. Therapy consisted of strengthening and gait training. The device provided warning tones giving feedback of improper gait through bilateral assessment of the use of the hip abductor muscles. The group that received EMG biofeedback had a 28% decrease in hip rotation, a significant reduction compared to the control group. The small sample size (N = 5) and limited patient type (incomplete spinal cord injury), however, makes generalization difficult.

Force feedback during gait using a shoe insole has been demonstrated to improve symmetry of gait in a variety of conditions (stroke, hip arthroplasty). Force feedback allows for better quantification and control of weight bearing. Gauthier-Gagnon and colleagues (32) found that force feedback could enhance the control of leg amputees. Flowers and associates (33) used biofeedback in gait training of transfemoral am-

putees, and demonstrated increased hip extension after biofeedback. Poor hip extension and insufficient weight bearing are two common characteristics in the gait of amputees. Montoya and colleagues (34) used a single gait parameter (stride length) as feedback in individuals undergoing gait retraining after stroke. Step length was increased on the hemiparetic side, and stride characteristics such as time of single support were also improved.

Another application of force feedback for gait training is the instrumentation of strain gauges on a cane or other assistive device. Auditory feedback can be provided to produce a tone when the force generated exceeds a preset threshold (35). This feedback encourages patients to rely less on the assistive device and place more weight on the limbs.

Thaut and colleagues (36) used rhythmic auditory stimulation (RAS) for gait training for patients with Parkinson's disease. Training consisted of the use of a gait pacemaker during a 3-week home-based program. Stride parameters and gait EMG were the dependent measures. Patients with Parkinsons who trained with RAS significantly improved their gait velocity, stride length, and step cadence. Carryover to other diseases, such as stroke, with marked side-to-side differences in step time and step length remains to be determined. In a subsequent study, Thaut and colleagues (37) employed this same therapy to persons after acute stroke. Rehabilitative procedures that involve highly repetitive, rhythmically patterned movement training have been shown to be particularly effective, possibly facilitating long-term potentiation in the sensorimotor cortex as a mechanism for motor learning. They noted a significant difference in the recovery rate in persons with RAS training. This resulted in increased stride length, increased stance time on the weaker limb, and increased walking velocity. RAS produced a noticeable improvement in stride symmetry compared to the control group. An important finding was the large degree of swing symmetry after the RAS training. Asymmetry is a persistent feature in gait patterns of stroke patients, and is very resistant to rehabilitation efforts (38,39). RAS may act more on central facilitating mechanisms, since the symmetry of stride times as well as stride length have been shown to improve with RAS. The data suggested that auditory rhythmic timekeepers might enhance more regular motor unit recruitment patterns. Hurt and associates (40) used RAS in gait training of eight individuals after acquired brain injury. They noted that an important aspect of well-coordinated movement involved proper timing. RAS enhances the timing of gait movements, which could improve gait velocity, cadence, stride length, and symmetry. Walking velocity, cadence, and stride length showed statistically significant improvement in the study group. A trend toward improvement in stride symmetry was noted.

Despite these findings, the efficacy of biofeedback remains unclear. Meta-analyses of EMG biofeedback in stroke rehabilitation produced conflicting results of the effectiveness of biofeedback for stroke rehabilitation. Schleenbaker and Mainous (41) found an overpositive pooled effect size for this modality. Glanz and colleagues (42) indicated that the available evidence did not support the use of EMG biofeedback to restore joint motion in hemiplegic patients. Statistically wide confidence intervals may have masked the clinical benefit (type II error). Mooreland and colleagues found more substantial effect sizes for muscle strength and gait symmetry (43). Bradley and associates (44) randomly assigned patients to EMG biofeedback or control groups. The intervention consisted of adding EMG biofeedback to conventional physical therapy in patients after acute stroke. Patients were encouraged to facilitate or attenuate abnormal muscle tone via auditory or visual signals transmitted from surface electrodes. There were no significant differences between the EMG and control groups in the rate of improvement after stroke. There was little clinical evidence to support using biofeedback to improve gait in the acute phase after stroke. However, EMG values themselves may not be conclusive in confirming the efficacy of treatment. Combined with other measures such as ROM, torque or time to peak torque, or time to complete a task may help to complete the clinical picture (25). In summary, the effect(s) of biofeedback remain inconclusive.

Functional Electrical Stimulation

Functional electrical stimulation (FES) may be defined as the application of electrical currents to neuronal tissue for the purpose of restoring control of body functions. The idea behind FES to restore walking is simple: artificial stimulation is used to replace lost descending control. The goal of FES as it relates to gait is to manipulate the individual's movement control so that learning occurs and function improves. Preservation of the entire lower motor neuron is essential for FES because the stimulation requirements may be painful and even dangerous. FES systems are designed to deliver pulses of electrical currents at predetermined frequencies and amplitudes to the nerves or myoneural junctions. Most systems are external to the body with surface skin electrodes and the stimulator and power source carried by the user. More recently, implanted electrodes are being used with an external power source.

In classical muscle mechanics, researchers usually examine and model the relation between stimulation and force in an isolated muscle. In FES, researchers usually examine and model the relation between stimulation and angular displacement of a joint, or, less frequently, its joint moment (torque). Thus, the properties of limbs rather than muscle properties can dominate the relation of stimulation to displacement.

Like the other therapies, there are a substantial number of questions to be answered prior to the selection of therapy type. This is particularly important when considering FES as a therapy intervention. In principle, artificial stimulation of the muscles can produce upright, unencumbered walking. The most basic task is to define the goal of FES for walking. Is it to be a replacement for a wheelchair? An adjunct to wheelchair use? Must the gait look "normal"? How rapid must gait be? These questions must be answered before embarking on the design elements of an FES system. If slow or short distance walking is the goal, then changes in muscle properties with time can be ignored. On the other hand, if "normal"-appearing gait is the

goal then the associated muscle models will have to include length-tension, force-velocity, and a series of elasticity elements, all of which change with onset of fatigue. The complexity of the associated rules increases dramatically, and in some cases the prospect with FES may become impractical.

An important consideration is the level of complexity required to meet the needs of the patient. Complexity has costs—it complicates analysis, hinders customization to the patient, and requires expensive and bulky sensors. It may not be needed, if one can accept a slow walk with restricted ROM. Initial use of FES was limited to augmenting foot clearance during the swing phase of gait. A therapist regulated gait-ankle dorsiflexion during gait by using a hand switch or a heel pressure switch (45). With careful selection of stimulation ramping and on/off cycles, the system was timed to match the gait cycle. Taylor and colleagues (46) studied the use of a drop-foot stimulator on the speed and effort of walking of stroke and multiple sclerosis patients. There was a 93% compliance rate with treatment, a 27% increase in walking speed, and 31% reduction of the physiological cost index using the stimulation.

Reported benefits of FES include: (a) reduction in muscle tone (i.e., spasticity), (b) increase in voluntary muscle strength, (c) decrease in the physiological cost of gait, and (d) increase in stride length. Despite promising laboratory results of the benefits of FES systems and the promotion of gait in spinal cord injury (SCI), only one commercially available system has been introduced in the United States with no paraplegic patient reporting the use of it as the primary means of locomotion.

Some form of sensors is required in all FES systems. Two common uses for sensors in lower limb FES have been reported. These include: (a) detection of gait events such as stance and swing detection and the detection of knee buckling, and (b) the continuous monitoring of a joint angle, most commonly the knee-flexion angle. A neural prosthesis could use or require both gait events and joint angle positioning for controlling motion.

The artificial sensors that have been typically used for FES lower limb control include electrogoniometers, pressure insoles, foot switches, and inclinometers. Difficulty in donning and doffing devices, calibration, migration, and resistance to mechanical failure continue to be adverse issues related to external sensors. In proposing a sensor system for FES control, size, encumbrance, and convenience of use must be considered. Ideally the sensors would be situated in the presently used architecture of an FES system and allow the patient to don or doff the sensory system in conjunction with the FES system. The components of a sensor system must be able to monitor nongait events as well, such as the mechanics of sit-to-stand. Natural sensors have been proposed for control of FES. Stance and swing detection by analysis of epineural potentials, and closed loop control of ankle motion in an acute animal study using infrafascicular electrodes has been demonstrated. Williamson and Andrews (47) combined analog accelerometers and rate gyroscopes. The combination led to successful detection of many gait events, but large errors were detected in the transitions from mid-stance to terminal stance and terminal stance to pre-swing.

Functional neuromuscular stimulation is a promising rehabilitation tool for restoring motor control. However, FES systems with surface electrodes are impractical. Thus, indwelling stimulating electrodes are required. Current implantable electrode designs raise concerns of failure rate, invasiveness of the placement procedure, and electrode migration away from the motor point. Daly and colleagues (48) designed a percutaneous electrode to address at least some of these concerns. The electrode survival rate was high, and delivered a comfortable stimulus. Marsolais and Kobetic (49) had a higher failure rate for implanted electrodes in an earlier study. They noted a 35% failure rate within 4 months after implantation. To address the potential problems associated with using a significant number of surface electrodes Daly and colleagues (50) developed a system of functional neural stimulation with intramuscular electrodes. They developed a gait template for each subject, modified and tailored to the needs of each patient and specific muscle function. They noted improved FIM scores, and that the patients tolerated the procedure well, with no adverse effects. The small sample size (N = 5) and timing of the intervention (acute stroke) support the possibility that spontaneous recovery could potentially explain some of the observed improvement. In a later study Daly and Ruff (51) examined the functional response to surface and intramuscular electrical stimulation after stroke in a single-subject design. They noted statistically significant differences between conventional and intramuscular functional neural stimulation therapy. Compared with other types of rehabilitation techniques, the most important advantage of the electrical stimulation technique for motor learning after stroke is that it directly stimulates a muscle and produces a desired muscle contraction in muscles that are otherwise not activated at all, abnormally activated, or abnormally responding. All FES systems for patients with SCI require arm support from canes, crutches, or walkers since ambulation balance cannot be provided. Spinal cord injury FES systems are hybrid systems, as they include orthotic support to provide joint stability, prevent injuries, reduce oxygen consumption, and ultimately reduce the number of stimulation parameters required. Marsolais and colleagues (52) studied six people with paraplegia who were trained to use a reciprocating gait orthosis plus electrical stimulation. Walking distance was two times greater with the combination of stimulation plus orthosis, compared with stimulation alone. Additionally, patients reported less perceived exertion.

FES systems can be of either an "open" or "closed" loop design. Most clinically available systems use "open loop" control. This control does not use a muscle model at all. Instead, the controller delivers a preset stimulus pattern that does not vary. The algorithm does not compensate for changes in muscle length, contraction velocity, peripheral fatigue, or task changes (such as walking on uneven terrain). Open loop control is relatively simple, and it does not need sensors or transducers. However, it also does not adapt. If the muscle fatigues or aspects of the environment force the stride to begin from a novel position, the same stimulation is still supplied.

In theory, classical "closed loop" control can give a predictable, consistent output with little or no model of the neuromuscular system. If the feedback "gain" (ratio of degrees of joint motion to pulse-width duration) can be made high enough muscle properties become irrelevant. FES systems can either use no muscle model or just a simple one. Closed loop control is simple, well understood, and powerful. It controls muscle force well. However, it does not control limb displacement well because the limb tends to become unstable. One approach has been to use machine-learning techniques to "teach" a closed loop system to control a limb. Alternatively, several groups have used a feed-forward control, which requires a good muscle model. The controller sets the stimulation by reversing the usual analysis technique, that of relating stimulation (dynamic EMG) to muscle force or movement. That is, it works backward from the desired output to the stimulation needed to produce that output. The model typically includes moment-angle, moment-velocity, and activation dynamics relations. If the model is accurate, the control is good. The difficulty lies in finding simple relations that are accurate for all conditions, including fatigue. In theory, the problems of feed-forward control can be overcome by allowing the parameters of the model to change with time, or by adding closed-loop feedback to correct for errors. In practice, this has not been successfully demonstrated.

The swing limb trajectory is modified considerably from that used for normal level-ground locomotion when we are forced to step over an obstacle in our travel path. The criteria used by the CNS to produce the observed movement pattern are unknown. During level ground locomotion, researchers have used various single criterion optimization methods to explain the specific recruitment of muscles validating the predicted muscle recruitment profiles based on experimentally measured muscle activity profiles. Lack of agreement between predicted muscle recruitment with the muscle activity profiles have led researchers to speculate that perhaps more than one aspect is optimized during locomotion. Stepping over obstacles is a prime example where several objectives have to be simultaneously satisfied. The limb must be elevated over the obstacle to prevent tripping, yet also achieve controlled landing to avoid slipping. Control of the limb trajectory over obstacles encountered during early swing is relatively simpler, as fewer objectives have to be satisfied (53).

FES has been combined with other forms of therapy, with mixed results. Isakov and associates (54) examined the synergistic effect of applying FES to SCI individuals attempting to walk with the aid of a reciprocating gait orthosis (RGO). Unfortunately, this combination was only of functional benefit in "very fit," young, low-level paraplegics, with coincident spasticity. The authors' noted that the energy cost of gait with the FES-RGO combination was much greater than wheelchair propulsion, and subjects self-selected wheelchair propulsion as their preferred mode of locomotion.

For gait, the prime mover of the RGO system is the hip extensor of the stance limb, which results in propulsive hip flexion of the contralateral swing limb. Going from sit-to-stand, the RGO knee joints are locked, and the subject is required to pull and push his or her entire body weight over a walker. Conversely, standing up and sitting down, by FES, is accomplished by stimulation of the hip extensor (gluteus maximus) and knee extensor (quadriceps) muscles of both legs. By adding FES with the RGO system, important biomechanical advantages could theoretically be obtained. The hybrid system (FES plus RGO) does not appear to assist in gait, but may be a useful adjunct to transfers. The patients did experience a subjective decrease in effort, despite the relatively small changes in gait performance that were observed.

Solomonow and colleagues (55) studied the physiological effects of the reciprocating gait orthosis with electrical stimulation (RGO II) in 70 paraplegic patients. The heart rate at the end of a 30-meter walk showed that the RGO II required only a moderate level of exertion that was found to be the lowest among the other mechanical and muscle stimulation orthoses available to paraplegics. The authors concluded that a limited but reasonable level of functional gain is provided by the RGO II and associated general improvements in physiological conditioning could be obtained if used a minimum of 3 to 4 hours per week. Yet, Sykes and colleagues (56) did not find a substantial benefit in energy expenditure using the RGO II when walking continuously for 5 minutes. They suggested that the hybrid orthosis might be of more benefit during prolonged walking.

Phillips (57) tested a similar FES plus RGO combination. Phillips noted that patient acceptance of this device may be a problem, where a substantial number of surface electrodes (14) had to be applied to the body. The application of the electrodes is cumbersome. Good positioning over motor points is important for optimal performance of the system.

Complexity of the system, stimulator size, number and position of electrodes, and muscle selectivity are disadvantages known to surface stimulation with FES. Fatigue is a problem common to FES with both surface and intramuscular stimulation. The large number of muscles involved in the control of locomotor behavior theoretically provides the CNS with a large number of options, and most FES systems use recruitment to activate muscles. They control the force by varying the width of the stimulus pulse ("pulse-width modulation"), although amplitude may be varied as well. This differs from the body's stimulation algorithm, where rate coding is used to vary muscle force output. Varying pulse width, rather than frequency, may be advantageous, because it produces a given force with fewer stimuli and less fatigue. However, grading muscle force by varying pulse width recruits motor units in reverse order—larger, faster (type II) units first. To date, no form of artificial stimulation can match natural activation for precision or fatigue resistance, although some forms of activation can mimic the normal recruitment order (58).

Conclusions

Before FES systems for SCI are more widely used, electrodes must be more reliable, safe, and implantable. They must allow for more automatic gait and address problems of muscle atrophy and spasticity. As more patients with SCI are left with residual motor function, FES systems will need to be highly adaptable to varying levels of natural recovery.

SUPPORTED WALKING

Finch and colleagues suggested the concept of treadmill training combined with body weight support in the mid-1980s (59). Supported walking has been used in the therapy for many neurological conditions, including SCI (60) and stroke (61–63).

This form of therapy is well tolerated. This fact is particularly important in the recovery of walking after stroke, as most of these individuals will have coincident cardiovascular disease. Malouin and associates (64), in a trial with acute stroke patients, showed good compliance, and patients were able to withstand nearly 45 minutes of treadmill walking, on average. Cardiovascular comorbidity in stroke patients is an important clinical factor affecting both rehabilitation and long-term health outcomes. Generalized fatigue, and not fatigue in the hemiparetic leg, is often the limiting exercise factor. Thus, physical deconditioning rather than strength in the paretic limb per se appears to be the most important factor limiting peak exercise capacity in this population.

Studies show that gait recovery after ischemic stroke appears to plateau within several months (65). This is consistent with the time frame of conventional stroke rehabilitation, which emphasizes therapies for optimizing recovery of ADLs in the post-stroke period. Aerobic exercise is not routinely prescribed for stroke patients, the majority of whom are elderly. There is substantial evidence that this population is physically deconditioned and has a high prevalence of cardiovascular disease risk factors potentially modifiable by exercise therapy (66). This may be a consequence of practitioners' concerns for fall risk, injury from repetitive exercise, or lack of evidence to date that exercise training can reduce the high energy expenditure or cardiovascular demands of walking in the chronic hemiparetic condition. Early studies recognized the high-energy expenditure of hemiparetic gait after stroke. The energy expenditure required to perform self-selected speed walking is increased by 50% to 100% in hemiparetic stroke patients (66,67), compared to age-matched healthy individuals. Hemiparetic individuals, particularly those of advanced age, are often unable to maintain their most efficient walking speed comfortably, indicating that the elevated energy demands of walking and poor endurance further compromise functional mobility.

Macko and colleagues examined the cardiac response of individuals after stroke, during treadmill training (68). Exclusion criteria included symptomatic congestive heart failure (CHF), unstable angina, inability to participate in a cardiac stress test [according to American College of Sports Medicine (ACSM) criteria], peripheral or occlusive vascular disease, dementia, depression, or aphasia. Exercise testing was begun with an initial treadmill tolerance test at 0° incline, to assess gait safety and to select the target walking velocity for subsequent peak-effort treadmill testing. Training consisted of three 40-minute sessions weekly (Monday-Wednesday-Friday) of treadmill walking at 60% of heart rate reserve (HRR), where HRR was determined according to the Karvonen formula. Maximum oxygen consumption increased 9% (15.4 to 17.0 mL/kg/minute), and there was decreased oxygen demand at submaximal effort. The economy of gait reached a plateau by 3 months, while peak ambulatory workload capacity progressively increased by 39% over 6 months. A follow-up study by the same group (69) examined the hypothesis that older persons with gait velocity limited by stroke-related hemiparesis could still achieve exercise intensities adequate for cardiopulmonary assessment using a treadmill at progressive workloads by increasing inclines. Stroke patients achieved a mean of 85% predicted maximum heart rate. Previous work (70) with a modified supine bicycle ergometry test found that only 2 out of 11 subjects could achieve greater than 85% predicted maximum heart rate. These findings suggest that a customized, graded treadmill is a more effective modality for exercise testing in older, paretic patients.

After stroke multiple factors contribute to functional disability. These include reduced cardiovascular fitness, elevated energy expenditure during locomotion, poor motor control, deficient lower limb strength, disuse atrophy, and abnormal gait biomechanics. Gait deviations secondary to hemiparesis also contribute to increased fall risk, further promoting a sedentary habitus and physical deconditioning. Silver and colleagues (71) examined 5 male stroke patients two or more years after their most recent stroke. The men performed thrice-weekly treadmill exercise over a period of 3 months. Exercise intensity was advanced as tolerated, to 40 minutes duration at 60% to 70% maximum heart rate. An improvement in a modified "Get-Up-and-Go" test was reported. The authors found a trend toward a more "normalized" gait, but were not able to separate gains due to cardiovascular improvement from improved neuromotor control. Their findings suggested that treadmill locomotion represents a biomechanical stimulus that may lead over time to improved motor control of locomotion in individuals with chronic hemiparesis.

Supported walking is based on sound physiological principles. The performance of complete gait movements on a treadmill with partial body weight support as a task-oriented approach has been shown to restore gait of nonambulatory patients in less time than gait recovery in patients who received "conventional" therapy (72). Modern concepts of motor learning favor a task-specific repetitive training (i.e., "the patient who wants to relearn walking has to walk") (73).

Hesse and colleagues have extensively examined the biomechanics of supported walking. In addition, they have developed a machine-controlled gait trainer (discussed subsequently). An early study with nine hemiparetic patients showed independent gait after 25 treadmill sessions with body-weight support (74). In a subsequent study Hesse and colleagues (75) trained seven individuals with body-weight support (BWS) after middle cerebral artery (MCA)-distribution ischemic stroke. The individuals were 7 months' postinfarct but still in an inpatient setting. A control group received "conventional" therapy. The authors demonstrated improvement in gait temporal variables (velocity, symmetry) in the body weight support (BWS) group, but no change in gait after conventional therapy. Volitional muscle force was assessed via functional tests (Rivermead Motor Score, Motricity Index). Gait was improved, although there was no improvement in strength reported. Treadmill training might have stimulated the presumed spinal central pattern generators (76). In addition, intact supraspinal centers, via the ipsilateral descending motor pathways, might have also contributed to the observed treatment effect. An important finding was that spasticity, as measured by Ashworth scores, was not increased.

Recently Hesse and colleagues examined the potential of augmenting recovery with machine-controlled gait (73). They assessed 14 hemiplegic patients (9 MCA, 5 intracranial hemorrhage (ICH)), none of whom could walk independently. Gait training was divided between partial body-weight–supported treadmill training and therapy using an instrumented gait trainer. Objective measures (foot switch patterns, EMG) failed to show a distinct advantage for the gait trainer versus supported walking.

Balance training is an important part of the return of walking after SCI or stroke. The relationship between static balance and ability to walk, however, is not intuitive. Winstein and colleagues (3) reported that balance training while standing could improve balance (symmetry) but not gait symmetry in hemiparetic patients.

GAIT AIDS

Canes, crutches, and walkers are often prescribed to assist in walking in persons with joint, muscle, and sensory functional losses (Figs. 65-1–65-3).

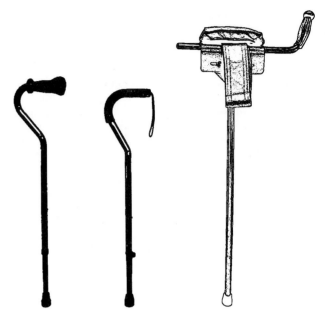

Figure 65-2. Depicted from left to right: single point cane with Sure-Grip handle, single point cane with curved handle, and platform crutch.

Canes serve many functions. They are an important component in treating persons with balance deficits. Cane use can increase the anteroposterior and mediolateral base of support. They provide an important safety-related function, providing information related to the position of the limb in space, and an assist to individuals who are vision-impaired such that they can scan the environment. Increased joint reaction (contact) force magnitude has been associated with increases in subjec-

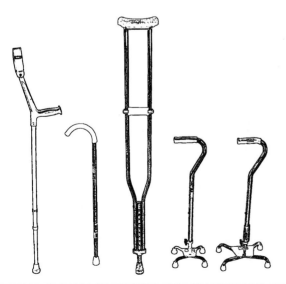

Figure 65-1. Depicted from left to right: Lofstrand (forearm) crutch, single point cane with curved handle, axillary crutch, narrow-based quad-point cane, and wide-based quad-point cane.

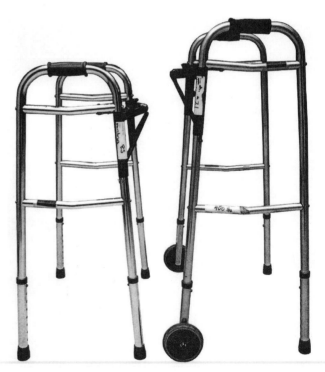

Figure 65-3. Depicted from left to right: foldable walker and foldable front-wheel walker.

tive discomfort at the joint. A cane, when properly positioned, can decrease the amount of muscle force necessary to stabilize a joint. This in turn leads to attenuation of joint reaction forces and decreased pain symptoms. Muscle weakness may also be offset with cane use, where gait deficits such as excessive knee or hip flexion may be overcome. They may also assist with acceleration or deceleration during walking. Pathological conditions affecting the upper limbs may interfere with the use of canes or crutches, and may warrant the prescription of specially designed gait aids.

The cane should be held in the less-affected hand with hemiplegia, and the patient should advance the cane and weaker leg simultaneously in a three-point gait pattern. When ascending stairs (with hemiplegia) the less-affected (stronger) leg is advanced first. The opposite pattern is recommended when descending stairs, with the weaker limb plus cane leading. When treating joint pain, the cane should be held opposite the side with greatest amount of joint pain.

Canes consist of a handle, shaft, and base. Of course, improper fit severely diminishes the effectiveness of the device. The total length should equal the length from the base of the heel to the upper border of the greater trochanters (77). Canes are most commonly made of hard woods or aluminum. Designs vary, but all should be fitted with a deeply grooved 2- to 5-cm rubber tip for safety. Several types of tips are available to be attached to the cane shaft. A single-point cane weighs less, which is important for individuals with decreased functional reserves. It is less intrusive, and may be easier to negotiate in cramped spaces. Where stability is compromised, a wide-based cane may provide a greater base of support. These designs consist of three or four short legs attached to a single upright. Three- or four-prong canes stay upright when they are released, which can be an advantage. These canes are often heavy and awkward to use, and temporary use is thus preferred. Cosmesis may also be an important consideration with wide-based cane use.

The most common handle is the "C"-type. It is inexpensive, but this type of handle may be uncomfortable to use and difficult to grasp for individuals with hand pathology. Additionally, the line of support differs from the cane's line of action, which produces a bending moment that must be overcome with muscular effort. An alternative approach is a "functional" handle. A functional handle conforms to the natural angle of the hand and is centered over the cane shaft (no bending moment). This type is perceived as more comfortable and provides better support. However, functional handles increase the cost of the device.

The rationale for crutch prescription is similar to canes. The clinical deficits however are usually more pronounced. Good upper extremity strength, joint integrity, and ROM are essential to maximize benefit with crutch use. Shoulder flexors and depressors, elbow and wrist extensors, and finger flexors must have good strength (four out of five). Most commonly crutches are prescribed to decrease loading, with muscle weakness or joint pain. Where "push-off" is limited in locomotion, crutch use may aid in propulsion. Crutches provide sensory feedback and increase the base of support. Yet they are less commonly prescribed for balance deficits compared to canes.

Crutch types include axillary, Lofstrand, Canadian elbow extensor (i.e., triceps crutch), and forearm support (platform crutch). Axillary crutches are the most common. They are typically made of hardwood or aluminum, with two upright shafts and a series of connecting links. Connections include a padded upper support, middle hand piece, and lower extension. The extension piece and shaft, have numerous, regularly spaced holes for height adjustment. A soft, rubber tip (similar to canes) is attached at the bottom to increase crutch contact surface area and provide additional stability. Again, proper fit is essential. Total length and handle height are the main considerations. Axillary crutch length should approximate the distance from anterior fold of axilla to: (a) bottom of heel (plus 3 to 5 cm) or (b) a point 6 inches in front of the anterolateral border of the foot. Drawbacks include increased assistive device mass and restriction of hand use. Some patients may have trouble coordinating gait with crutches. Additionally, patients who lean on the axillary crutches may experience neurological injury in the hand due to nerve compression (i.e., crutch palsy).

The Lofstrand crutch consists of a molded hand piece, a molded forearm piece bent posteriorly just above the hand piece, and a single, length-adjustable aluminum tubular shaft. The forearm piece extends 4 to 5 cm below the elbow. A forearm cuff with a narrow anterior opening is attached at this site. Lofstrand crutches are typically lightweight, and the hand piece can be released without losing the crutch. The result is that the hands are freed up to perform other activities, which is a significant advantage. Good upper extremity strength and adequate trunk balance are minimum requirements for safe use of Lofstrand crutches.

The triceps crutch extends just above the elbow, and has a single aluminum upright attached to bilateral uprights. This crutch is rarely prescribed, but may be of benefit in individuals with triceps weakness. Forearm support (platform) crutches may be prescribed when clinical conditions involving the hands, wrists, or forearms prevent safe or comfortable weight bearing. Examples include weakness of triceps or grasp, or arthritic conditions involving the upper extremity joints.

A walker is a device with a frame that is inherently stable. There are a number of different types of walker, the most common of which is made of aluminum, has four posts, and may have small front or rear wheels. The person pushes or lifts the walker in front of himself or herself while walking. Walkers have advantages and disadvantages, and each should be considered when prescribing a walker as an assistive device. There are no absolute indications for the use of walkers.

Walkers provide a wider base of support than either canes or crutches. They may be prescribed for patients requiring maximum assistance for balance. This may include severe sensory deficits, ataxic conditions, and persons with substantial fear during gait.

They may be useful during rehabilitation, but care should be taken to assure that the patient does not become too reliant or emotionally dependent on the balance stability provided by the walker. Proper use requires bilateral grasp and arm strength. They are bulky in appearance, may be difficult to maneuver in tight quarters, and interfere with the development of reciprocal gait. A heavy walker is generally awkward and not particularly useful for most patients. Thus, the use of a walker may tax the endurance of the user. To cope with fatigue four-wheeled walkers are often outfitted with a seat to make it possible to travel longer distances with intermediate rest periods. This practice is not risk-free, and the dangers of sitting on a parked walker are well known.

This suggests that minimizing the weight of the walker is advantageous. While generally true, most walkers are too light for individuals with incoordination coupled with good upper extremity strength. Weight may be added to this type of walker to attenuate this problem.

Walkers can be instrumented with wheels to promote better gait timing without having to stop each cycle to advance the walker. Wheels help patients with incoordination or weakness of the upper extremity, where lifting crutches or walkers and placing them forward may be difficult. The rolling (wheeled) walker does not require as much strength and balance to maneuver, compared to nonwheeled walkers, as the user does not have to lift it from the floor. However, the instability introduced by the wheels may prove dangerous.

REFERENCES

1. Perry J. Gait analysis: normal and pathological function. New York: McGraw-Hill, Inc., 1992.
2. Carr J, Shepherd R. Walking. In: *Neurological rehabilitation: optimizing motor performance*, 2nd ed. Oxford: Butterworth-Heinemann, 1998:107–125.
3. Winstein C, Gradner E, McNeal D, et al. Standing balance training: effects on balance and locomotion in hemiparetic adults. *Arch Phys Med Rehabil* 1989;70:755–762.
4. Wolf B, Feys H, De Weerdt V, et al. Effect of a physical therapeutic intervention for balance problems in the elderly: a single-blind, randomized, controlled multicentre trial. *Clin Rehabil* 2000;15:624–636.
5. Voss D. Proprioceptive neuromuscular facilitation. *Am J Phys Med Rehabil* 1967;46:S38–S98.
6. Bobath B. Treatment of adult hemiplegia. *Physiotherapy* 1977;63:310–313.
7. Gordon J. Assumptions underlying physical therapy intervention: theoretical and historical perspectives. In: Carr J, Shepherd R, Gordon J, eds. *Movement science: foundations for physical therapy rehabilitation*. Rockville, MD: Aspen Publishers, 1987.
8. Hesse S, Jahnke M, Schreiner B, et al. Gait symmetry and functional walking performance in hemiparetic patients prior to and after a 4-week rehabilitation programme. *Gait Posture* 1993;1:166–171.
9. Hesse S, Jahnke M, Schaffrin A, et al. Immediate effects of therapeutic facilitation on the gait of hemiparetic patients as compared with walking with and without a cane. *Electroencephalograph Clin Neurophysiol* 1998;109:515–522.
10. Lennon S, Ashburn A. The Bobath concept in stroke rehabilitation: a focus group study of the experienced physiotherapists' perspective. *Disabil Rehabil* 2000;22:665–674.
11. Lennon S, Baxter D, Ashburn A. Physiotherapy based on the Bobath concept in stroke rehabilitation: a survey within the UK. *Disabil Rehabil* 2001;23:254–262.
12. Langhammer B, Stanghelle J. Bobath or motor relearning programme? A comparison of two different approaches of physiotherapy in stroke rehabilitation: a randomized controlled study. *Clin Rehabil* 2000;14:361–369.
13. Knott M, Voss D. *Proprioceptive neuromuscular facilitation: patterns and techniques*, 2nd ed. New York: Harper & Row, 1968.
14. Surburg S. Interactive effects of resistance and facilitation patterning upon reaction and response times. *Phys Ther* 1979;59:1513–1517.
15. Dickstein R, Hocherman S, Pillar T, et al. Three exercise therapy approaches. *Phys Ther* 1986;66:1233–1237.
16. Twitchell T. The restoration of motor function following hemiplegia in man. *Brain* 1951;74:443–480.
17. Brunnstrom S. *Movement therapy in hemiplegia. a neurophysiological approach*. New York: Harper and Row, 1970.
18. Frontera W, Moldover J, Borg-Stein J, et al. Exercise. In: Gonzalez E, Myers S, Edelstein J, et al., eds. *Physiological basis of rehabilitation medicine*, 3rd ed. Boston: Butterworth-Heinemann, 2001:379–396.
19. Higashi T, Funase K, Kusano K, et al. Motoneuron pool excitability of hemiplegic patients: assessing recovery stages by using H-reflex and M response. *Arch Phys Med Rehabil* 2001;82:1604–1610.
20. Wagenaar R, Meijer O, Wieringen PV, et al. The functional recovery of stroke: a comparison between neuro-developmental treatment and the Brunnstrom method. *Scand J Rehabil Med* 1990;22:1–8.
21. Rood M. Neurophysiological reactions as a basis for physical therapy. *Phys Ther Rev.* 1954;34:444–449.
22. Dewald J. Sensorimotor neurophysiology and the basis of neurofacilitory therapeutic techniques. In: Brandstater M, Basmajian J, eds. *Stroke rehabilitation*. Baltimore: Williams & Wilkins, 1987.
23. Mulder T, Hulstijn W. From movement to action: the learning of motor control following brain damage. In: Meijer O, Roth K, eds. Complex movement behaviour: the motor-action controversy. New York: Elsevier Science, 1988:247–259.
24. Winstein C, Schmidt R. Reduced frequency of knowledge of results enhances motor skill learning. *J Exp Psychology, Learning, Memory, Cognition* 1990;10:677–691.
25. Wolf S. Biofeedback. In: Gonzalez E, Myers S, Edelstein J, et al., eds. *Physiological basis of rehabilitation medicine*. 3rd ed. Boston: Butterworth-Heinemann, 2001:747–759.
26. LeCraw D, Wolf S. Contemporary perspectives on electromyographic feedback for rehabilitation clinicians. In: Gersh M, ed. *Electrotherapy*. Philadelphia: FA Davis, 1991.
27. Basmajian J, Kukulka C, Narayan M. Biofeedback treatment of foot-drop after stroke compared with standard rehabilitation technique: effects on voluntary control and strength. *Arch Phys Med Rehabil* 1975;56:231–236.
28. Brudney J, Korein J, Grynbaum B, et al. Sensory feedback therapy as a modality of treatment in central nervous system disorders of voluntary movement. *Neurology* 1974;24:925–932.
29. Wolf S, Baker M, Kelly J. EMG biofeedback in stroke: effect of patient characteristics. *Arch Phys Med Rehabil* 1979;60:96–102.
30. Pavol M, Owings T, Foley K, et al. The sex and age of older adults influence the outcome of induced trips. *J Gerontol* 1999;54:103–108.
31. Petrofsky J. The use of electromyogram biofeedback to reduce Trendelenburg gait. *Eur J Appl Physiology* 2001;85:491–495.
32. Gauthier-Gagnon C, St. Pierre D, Drouin G, et al. Augmented sensory feedback in the early training of standing balance of below-knee amputees of below-knee amputees. *Physiother Canada* 1986;38:136–142.
33. Flowers W, Cullen C, Tyra K. A preliminary report on the use of a practical biofeedback device for gait training of above-knee amputees. *J Rehabil Res Dev* 1986;23:7–18.
34. Montoya R, Dupui P, Pages B, et al. Step-length biofeedback device for walk rehabilitation. *Med Biol Eng Comp* 1994;32:416–420.
35. Baker M, Hudson J, Wolf S. A "feedback" cane to improve the hemiplegic patient's gait. *Phys Ther* 1979;59:170–171.
36. Thaut M, McIntosh G, Rice R, et al. Rhythmic auditory stimulation in gait training for Parkinson's disease patients. *Movement Disord* 1996;11:193–200.
37. Thaut M, McIntosh G, Rice R. Rhythmic facilitation of gait training in hemiparetic stroke rehabilitation. *J Neurolog Sci* 1997;151:207–212.
38. Kramers de Quervain I, Simon S, Luergans S, et al. Gait pattern in the early recovery period after stroke. *J Bone Joint Surg* 1996;78-A:1506–1514.
39. Gronley J, Mulroy S, Newsam C, et al. Lower extremity strength and gait performance in the acute stroke patient. *Gait Posture* 1997;5:159.
40. Hurt C, Rice R, McIntosh G, et al. Rhythmic auditory stimulation in gait training for patients with traumatic brain injury. *J Music Ther* 1998;XXXV:228–241.
41. Schleenbaker R, Mainous A. Electromyographic biofeedback for neuromuscular re-education in the hemiplegic stroke patient: a meta-analysis. *Arch Phys Med Rehabil* 1993;74:1301–1304.
42. Glanz M, Klawansky S, Stason W, et al. Biofeedback therapy in post-stroke rehabilitation: a meta-analysis of the randomized controlled trials. *Arch Phys Med Rehabil* 1995;76:508–515.
43. Mooreland J, Thomson M, Fuoco A. Electromyographic biofeedback to improve lower extremity function after stroke: a meta-analysis. *Arch Phys Med Rehabil* 1998;78:506–515.
44. Bradley L, Hart B, Mandana S, et al. Electromyographic biofeedback for gait training after stroke. *Clin Rehabil* 1998;12:11–22.
45. Liberson W, Holmquest H, Scot D, et al. Functional electrotherapy: stimulation of the peroneal nerve synchronized with the swing phase of gait of hemiplegic patients. *Arch Phys Med Rehabil* 1961;42:101–105.
46. Taylor P, Burridge J, Dunkerley A, et al. Clinical use of the Odstock dropped foot stimulator: its effect on the speed and effort of walking. *Arch Phys Med Rehabil* 1999;80:1577–1583.
47. Williamson R, Andrews B. Sensor systems for lower limb functional electrical stimulation (FES) control. *Med Eng Phys* 2000;22:313–325.
48. Daly J, Kollar K, Debogorski A, et al. Performance of an intramuscular electrode during functional neuromuscular stimulation for gait training post stroke. *J Rehabil Res Dev* 2001;38:513–526.
49. Marsolais E, Kobetic R. Implantation techniques and experience with percutaneous intramuscular electrodes in the lower extremities. *J Rehabil Res Dev* 1986;23:1–8.
50. Daly J, Ruff R, Haycook K, et al. Feasibility of gait training for acute stroke patients using FNS with implanted electrodes. *J Neurolog Sci* 2000;179:103–107.
51. Daly J, Ruff R. Electrically induced recovery of gait components for older patients with chronic stroke. *Am J Phys Med Rehabil* 2000;79:349–360.
52. Marsolais E, Kobetic R, Polando G, et al. The Case Western Reserve University hybrid gait orthosis. *J Spinal Cord Med* 2000;23:100–108.
53. Armand M, Huissoon J, Patla A. Stepping over obstacles during locomotion: insights from multi-objective optimization on set of input parameters. *IEEE Trans Rehabil Eng* 1998;6:43–53.
54. Isakov E, Douglas R, Berns P. Ambulation using the reciprocating gait orthosis and functional electrical stimulation. *Paraplegia* 1992;30:239–245.
55. Solomonow M, Reisin E, Aguilar E, et al. Reciprocating gait orthosis powered with electrical stimulation (RGO-II). Part II: medical evaluation of 70 paraplegic patients. *Orthopedics* 1997;20:411–418.
56. Sykes L, Campbell I, Powell E, et al. Energy expenditure of walking for adult patients with spinal cord lesions using the reciprocating gait orthosis and functional electrical stimulation. *Spinal Cord* 2000;34:659–665.
57. Phillips C. Electrical muscle stimulation in combination with a reciprocal gait orthosis for ambulation by paraplegics. *Phys Ther* 1989;11:338–344.
58. Baratta R, Solomonow M. The dynamic performance model of skeletal muscle. *Crit Rev Biomed Eng* 1992;19:419–454.
59. Finch L, Barbeau H, Arsenault B. Influence of body weight support on normal human gait: development of a gait retraining strategy. *Phys Ther* 1991;71:842–855.
60. Dobkin B, Harkema S, Requejo P, et al. Modulation of locomotor-like EMG activity in subjects with complete and incomplete spinal cord injury. *J Neurolog Rehabil* 1995;9:183–190.
61. Laufer Y, Dickstein R, Chefez Y, et al. The effect of treadmill training on the ambulation of stroke survivors in the early stages of rehabilitation: a randomized study. *J Rehabil Res Dev* 2001;38:69–78.

62. Macko R, Smith G, Dobrovolny C, et al. Treadmill training improves fitness reserve in chronic stroke patients. *Arch Phys Med Rehabil* 2001;82:879–884.

63. Sullivan K, Knowlton B, Dobkin, B. Step training with body weight support: effect of treadmill speed and practice paradigms on poststroke locomotor recovery. *Arch Phys Med Rehabil* 2002;83:683–691.

64. Malouin F, Potvin M, Prevost J, et al. Use of an intensive task-oriented gait training program in a series of patients with acute cerebrovascular accidents. *Phys Ther* 1992;72:781–793.

65. Jorgensen H, Nakayama H, Raaschou H, et al. Recovery of walking function in stroke patients: the Copenhagen stroke study. *Arch Phys Med Rehabil* 1995; 76:27–32.

66. Waters R, Mulroy S. The energy expenditure of normal and pathological gait. A review. *Gait Posture* 1999;9:207–231.

67. Waters R, Yakura J. The energy expenditure of normal and pathological gait. *Clin Rev Phys Rehabil Med* 1989;1:183–209.

68. Macko R, DeSouza C, Tretter L, et al. Treadmill aerobic exercise training reduces the energy expenditure and cardiovascular demands of hemiparetic gait in chronic stroke patients. *Stroke* 1997;28:326–330.

69. Macko R, Katzel L, Yataco A, et al. Low-velocity graded treadmill stress testing in hemiparetic stroke patients. *Stroke* 1997;28:988–992.

70. Moldover J, Daum M. Cardiac stress testing of hemiparetic patients with a supine bicycle ergometer: preliminary study. *Arch Phys Med Rehabil* 1984;65: 470–473.

71. Silver K, Macko R, Forrester L, et al. Effects of aerobic treadmill training on gait velocity, cadence, and gait symmetry in chronic hemiparetic stroke: a preliminary report. *Neurorehabil Neural Repair* 2000;14:65–71.

72. Wernig A, Muller S. Laufband locomotion with body weight support improved walking in persons with severe spinal cord injuries. *Paraplegia* 1992; 30:229–238.

73. Hesse S, Uhlenbrock D, Sarkodie-Gyan T. Gait pattern of severely disabled hemiparetic subjects on a new controlled gait trainer as compared to assisted treadmill walking with partial body weight support. *Clin Rehabil* 1999;13: 401–410.

74. Hesse S, Bertelt C, Schaffrin A, et al. Restoration of gait in nonambulatory hemiparetic patients by treadmill training with partial body weight support. *Arch Phys Med Rehabil* 1994;75:1087–1093.

75. Hesse S, Bertelt C, Jahnke M, et al. Treadmill training with partial body weight support compared with physiotherapy in nonambulatory hemiparetic patients. *Stroke* 1995;26:976–981.

76. Grillner S, Zangger P. On the central generation of locomotion in the low spinal cat. *Experimental Brain Research* 34:241–261,1979.

77. Knott M, Voss D. *Proprioceptive neuromuscular facilitation: patterns and techniques*, 2nd ed. New York: Harper and Row, 1968.

CHAPTER 66

Functional Neuromuscular Stimulation

John Chae, Ronald J. Triolo, Kevin L. Kilgore,
Graham H. Creasey, and Anthony F. DiMarco

Neuromuscular electrical stimulation (NMES) can be broadly categorized as therapeutic or functional. Therapeutic neuromuscular stimulation is defined as the use of repetitive stimulation of paralyzed muscles to minimize specific impairments such as limited range of motion, motor weakness, spasticity, and cardiovascular deconditioning. While therapeutic NMES may, and hopefully will lead to functional improvements, the electrical stimulation does not directly provide function. In this chapter, functional neuromuscular stimulation (FNS) is defined as the use of NMES to activate paralyzed muscles at a precise sequence to assist in the performance of activities of daily living (ADLs) or to provide stability to a joint to maintain biomechanical integrity and therefore function. Devices or systems that provide FNS are also appropriately called *neuroprostheses*.

This chapter focuses on the application of FNS in tetraplegia and paraplegia secondary to traumatic spinal cord injury (SCI), and hemiplegia secondary to stroke. The physiology of NMES is reviewed. The components of FNS systems and their evolution in design are presented. The clinical implementation of FNS is discussed with respect to upper and lower extremity function for persons with SCI and stroke, and with respect to bladder and pulmonary function for persons with SCI. Finally, perspectives on future developments and directions are presented.

PHYSIOLOGY OF NEUROMUSCULAR ELECTRICAL STIMULATION

Excitation of Nervous Tissue by Neuromuscular Electrical Stimulation

The action potential produced by NMES is identical to the action potential produced by natural physiologic means. The lowest level of charge that will generate an action potential is defined as the stimulus threshold. Large diameter α-motor neurons, which are associated with large motor units have the lowest thresholds for stimulation (1,2) and are activated first, followed by activation of smaller diameter α-motor neurons, which are associated with smaller motor units and have higher threshold for stimulation. This property of NMES is referred to as the reverse recruitment order, which is the reverse of the physiological size principle (3) where normally, small diameter axons are recruited initially, and then larger diameter axons.

The stimulus current diminishes as a function of the distance from the stimulating source (2,4). Therefore, neurons furthest away from an electrode are least likely to receive stimulation at a level above threshold. The threshold for direct muscle fiber excitation is about 100 to 1,000 times higher than the threshold for nerve stimulation (2). Therefore, it is unlikely that direct muscle stimulation occurs as a result of any of the electrical stimulation paradigms described in this chapter. Although FNS systems are often described as involving stimulation of a "muscle," technically they are referring to stimulation of the nerves innervating the muscle, resulting in muscle contraction.

Muscle Response to Neuromuscular Electrical Stimulation

Muscle fibers are divided into three groups based on their contractile properties (Table 66-1). At one end of the spectrum are the fast twitch glycolytic (type II) fibers, which generate high levels of force, but fatigue rapidly (4,5). At the other end of the spectrum are the slow twitch oxidative (type I) fibers, which generate lower forces, but are fatigue-resistant (4,5). Fatigue resistance is probably the most desirable quality for most NMES applications involving the skeletal muscle. However, because large fibers have lower threshold for stimulation, large type II fibers are recruited preferentially by NMES. Furthermore, disuse atrophy tends to convert type I to type II fibers (6). Fortunately, this muscle atrophy with the concomitant change in fiber type can be reversed with chronic NMES (7). Human studies have demonstrated that cyclic NMES of paralyzed muscles can increase muscle bulk and stimulated joint torques (8,9). All current neuroprostheses applications use some form of muscle conditioning patterned after these studies. Successful stimulation of muscle for functional purposes requires that the lower (alpha) motor neuron (LMN) be intact, and therefore, extensive LMN damage is a contraindication for NMES.

In order to maintain smooth contraction and maximize fatigue resistance, the ideal stimulation frequency ranges between 12 to 16 Hz for upper extremity applications and 18 to 25 Hz for lower extremity applications. As the duration or amplitude of a stimulus pulse is increased, the stimulus threshold will be reached for neurons further away from the stimulating electrode leading to activation of more neurons and greater force generation. Factors external to stimulation parameters that influence force generation include movement of the electrode with respect to the target nerve (10,11), inherent length-

TABLE 66-1. Characteristics of Skeletal Muscle Fibers Based upon Their Metabolic and Mechanical Properties

	Slow Oxidative (Type I)	Fast Oxidative-Glycolytic (Type IIa)	Fast Glycolytic (Type IIb)
Muscle fiber diameter	Small	Large	Intermediate
Muscle color	Red	Red	White
Motor unit strength	Low	High	High
Contractile speed	Slow	Fast	Fast
Rate of fatigue	Slow	Intermediate	Fast
Major source of ATP	Oxidative phosphorylation	Oxidative phosphorylation	Glycolysis
Oxidative capacity	High	Intermediate	Low
Glycolytic capacity	Low	Intermediate	High

tension characteristics of muscle, changes in the tendon moment arm as a function of joint angle, and volume conduction of current that may recruit muscles beyond the target muscle.

Safe Stimulation of Living Tissue

The parameters for safe stimulation and materials for safe electrodes for implanted systems have been experimentally established (2). Improper stimulation can result in electrochemical changes in the electrode material, leading to corrosion or dissolution of metal ions. Therefore, balanced biphasic stimulation should always be used with intramuscular stimulation to avoid this phenomenon. Tissue damage is also related to the charge per unit area of stimulation, not the voltage of the stimulus. In implanted systems, the contact area of the electrode is assumed to remain constant. In order to ensure that the stimulus charge is maintained below safe levels, electrical stimulation should be current-controlled (current is the charge delivered per unit time). Therefore, for implanted electrodes, it is safer to use a stimulator that controls current rather than voltage because the former provides more direct control of the charge density.

However, there are other factors to consider when transcutaneous electrodes are used. The electrode-tissue contact area is generally not constant as electrodes often pull away from the skin, which significantly decreases the electrode-tissue contact area. When constant current stimulation is used, this will lead to high current densities, which can burn the underlying tissue. When using constant voltage stimulation, the increased resistance will result in decreased current delivered to the tissue. Although this may be safer, it results in variations in the stimulation delivered to the muscle, changing the force output. However, even with good electrode-skin contact, burning of the tissue can occur if the current densities are too high. Therefore, transcutaneous stimulation should be used with caution and with frequent examination of the skin when applied to patients with impaired sensation or cognition.

Intramuscular electrodes eliminate the risk of direct skin reaction to the applied stimulus, but have the risk of muscle tissue damage if the stimulus is improperly applied. Safe stimulation parameters with this type of electrode are biphasic pulses with amplitude of 20 mA and pulse duration of 200 μs. Frequency is typically in the range of 10 to 50 Hz, although frequency is not a factor in adverse tissue response to stimulation. Intramuscular NMES using these parameters has been applied for human use for over 15 years without any evidence of current related muscle damage (12).

Most direct nerve stimulation is accomplished using a nerve cuff electrode that encompasses the nerve trunk. Nerve tissue damage can occur through the same electrochemical mechanism as muscle tissue damage, but it can also occur through mechanical movement of the cuff relative to the nerve. In addition, tissue growth around nerve cuff electrodes can result in compression of the nerve leading to secondary damage (13). Despite these potential problems, nerve cuffs have been used safely in many applications (14–16). Stimulation of nerves typically requires about one-tenth of the current necessary for intramuscular stimulation. Although intramuscular stimulation activates nerves and not muscles directly, higher current is required because electrodes are still some distance away from the motor point.

SYSTEM COMPONENTS AND EVOLUTION IN DESIGN

FNS systems can be completely external or implanted. Implantable systems offer the advantages of placing the stimulating electrodes in close proximity to nerves, thus greatly increasing the selectivity and efficiency of activation while reducing the current required. For long-term clinical application, implanted systems provide major advantages over other systems including improved convenience, cosmesis, reliability, and repeatability (17). Most clinically available electrodes fall into three broad classes: transcutaneous electrodes applied to the skin, muscle-based electrodes, and nerve-based electrodes. Electrode leads are classified as external, percutaneous, or implanted. All transcutaneous electrodes use external leads, while muscle- and nerve-based electrodes are connected to either percutaneous or implanted lead wires.

Transcutaneous electrodes are applied to the surface of the skin over the "motor point," the location exhibiting the best contraction from the target muscle at the lowest levels of stimulation. NMES with transcutaneous electrodes offers several distinct advantages: (a) the electrodes are generally easy to apply and remove, (b) the stimulation technique is noninvasive and therefore reversible, (c) the use of transcutaneous electrodes can be easily learned and applied in the clinic, and (d) stimulators and transcutaneous electrodes are relatively inexpensive and commercially available. Stimulation with transcutaneous electrodes is the most widely used technique for therapeutic applications (18), and has been successfully employed to produce standing, stepping, and grasping motions and to assist with respiratory function (17,19–21). However, in spite of their apparent convenience when applied individually in small numbers, transcutaneous electrodes have several disadvantages: (a) they cannot produce isolated contractions of small muscles, (b) daily doffing and donning can complicate use, especially if electrode positions vary slightly from day to day, and (c) in many cases, cutaneous pain receptors are excited, and patients with preserved or heightened sensation may find it difficult to tolerate.

Muscle-based electrodes bypass both the high resistance of the skin and the cutaneous sensory fibers. They require significantly lower currents, exhibit greater muscle selectivity, and are better tolerated than transcutaneous stimulation. Intramuscular electrodes can be introduced either percutaneously (8,22) or in an open surgical procedure (23) and allow access to deep nerves and muscles. Early movement of the electrode tip away from the target nerve within the first 6 weeks postimplantation is the most frequently observed failure mode (24). Epimysial electrodes are sutured directly to the epimysium or fascia to eliminate this early movement and provide immediate and permanent fixation (25).

Nerve-based electrodes have a more intimate contact with neural structures and therefore require even less current than muscle-based electrodes. They take the form of epineural electrodes, which are sutured to the connective tissue surrounding a motor nerve, cuff electrodes which envelope the nerve, and penetrating intraneural probes, which are still laboratory-based investigational tools. Epineural and nerve cuff designs have both been employed as stimulating electrodes in FNS systems to restore motor function in patients with SCI or who have experienced a stroke (16,26). Cuff electrodes have also been configured to record from afferent nerves in attempts to use the natural sensors in the body to provide feedback signals (27).

Electrodes are connected to stimulating or recording circuitry through lead wires. Percutaneous leads are designed to connect chronically indwelling electrodes to circuitry external to the body while maintaining a barrier to infection. However, percutaneous leads must be cleaned, dressed, and properly inspected and maintained in order to reduce the risk of complications. Although the electrode failure rate due to breakage is low during the first few months postimplantation, the cumulative 1-year failure rate can vary between 56% and 80% (28,29), which limits the use of percutaneous electrodes to short-term applications (<3 months). Other potential complications include formation of granulomas from retained electrode fragments and electrode-related infections, which are treated with oral antibiotics or minor outpatient surgical procedure. Implanted leads generally have larger dimensions than percutaneous lead wires because they need to be more robust and resistant to failure, and are not required to cross the skin. To allow repair or revision of implanted FNS systems, provisions have been made in several designs to isolate system subcomponents from each other via high reliability implantable connectors (30). In-line connectors permit the surgical removal and repositioning of individual electrodes with minimal dissection and without extensive exposure of larger implanted circuit packages. Implantable electronic components can also be designed as passive devices, which derive their power from the radiofrequent signals providing the communication channels to external command or control processors. Systems using this configuration eliminate the need for additional surgery to replace internal batteries.

UPPER EXTREMITY NEUROPROSTHESES

Spinal Cord Injury

OBJECTIVES OF UPPER EXTREMITY SYSTEMS

FNS has been used to provide grasp and release for individuals with an SCI at the cervical level (17,31–33). The objectives of these neuroprostheses are to reduce the need of individuals to rely on assistance from others, reduce the need for adaptive equipment, reduce the need to wear braces or other orthotic devices, and reduce the time it takes to perform tasks. Neuroprostheses make use of the patient's own paralyzed musculature to provide the power for grasp and the patient's voluntary musculature to control the grasp. Typically, patients use the neuroprosthesis for such tasks as eating, personal hygiene, writing, and office work. These systems are now available clinically, providing a rehabilitation treatment option that can enable cervical-level SCI patients to gain a new level of independence.

CANDIDATE SELECTION

The majority of upper extremity neuroprostheses have been targeted for individuals with C5 and C6 motor levels. For these patients, the provision of grasp opening and closing using FNS provides an obvious functional benefit. At the C4 motor level, control of elbow flexion and shoulder stability must be provided by stimulation of the biceps or brachialis, or by a mechanical or surgical means. FNS has been applied to a limited extent to these individuals, but there are no clinically deployed systems for this population to date. For individuals with C7 or C8 motor level function, there are other treatment options (such as tendon transfers) that can provide considerable function. For this latter population, neuroprostheses will need to become simpler to use before they can be considered to be a good treatment alternative.

Electrical stimulation is delivered to intact LMNs, as described earlier in this chapter, and is not used to directly activate denervated muscle. For C5 and C6 spinal cord injuries, the muscles most likely to sustain LMN damage are the wrist extensors. Peckham and Keith (34) found that between 80% and 100% of the muscles necessary for grasp had sufficient intact innervation to generate functional levels of force. In many cases, other paralyzed muscles can be used to substitute for the function that is not available (35).

FNS can be applied at any time postinjury, but it is typically applied after neurological stability has been achieved. Joint contractures must be corrected or functional ability will be limited. Spasticity must be under control. Individuals who are motivated and desire greater independence are the best candidates for neuroprostheses. In addition, most current neuroprosthetic systems still require assistance in donning the device, so it is necessary for the individual to have good attendant support.

OPERATING PRINCIPLES

All existing upper extremity neuroprosthetic systems consist of a stimulator that activates the muscles of the forearm and hand and an input transducer and control unit. The control signal for grasp is derived from an action that the user has retained voluntary control over, which can include joint movement (31, 36–40), muscle activity (41–44), respiration (45), or voice control (31,32,46). A coordinated stimulation pattern is developed so that the muscles are activated in a sequence that produces a functional grasp pattern. The user typically has control over grasp opening and closing, but does not have direct control over the activation of each muscle, thus simplifying the control task required by the user.

CLINICALLY EVALUATED APPLICATIONS

Three commercially available neuroprosthetic systems are designed to provide upper extremity muscle conditioning and function for persons with SCI: Handmaster® (NESS Ltd., Ra'anana, Israel), FESMate® (NEC Medical Systems, Tokyo), and Freehand® (NeuroControl Corp., Valley View, OH) (47). The primary technical distinction between these systems is their relative invasiveness. The Handmaster uses transcutaneous stimulation, FESMate uses percutaneous electrodes, and the

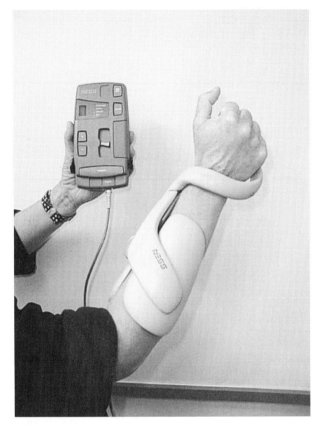

Figure 66-1. The Handmaster system, which consists of an arm splint with built-in transcutaneous electrodes and a control unit.

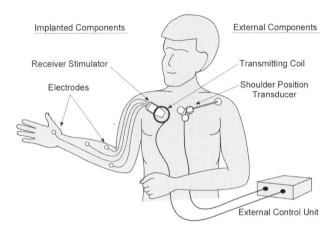

Figure 66-2. The FreeHand system, which consists of an implanted stimulator and electrodes, an external power and control unit, and a shoulder position sensor.

Freehand system uses implanted electrodes and an implanted stimulator.

Transcutaneous Neuroprosthesis. Nathan (32,33) has developed a splint, which incorporates transcutaneous electrodes for grasp, called the Handmaster (Fig. 66-1). The brace fixes the wrist in neutral, making it applicable primarily to C5 level tetraplegic individuals who do not have a tenodesis grasp. A clinical study of the Handmaster was done by Snoek and colleagues (33). Ten C5/C6 quadriplegic individuals were evaluated for fitting of the neuroprosthesis, and four participated in the functional training. Each user underwent 2 weeks of muscle conditioning using the stimulator, and then 6 to 12 weeks of functional training. Functional performance was assessed in at least four tasks, which included pouring water from a can, opening a jar, opening a bottle, and inserting and removing a video tape. The results show that all four of the subjects could perform at least two tasks independently using the Handmaster that they could not perform without assistance using their hand with a splint. Three of the subjects demonstrated improvement in pouring from a can and opening a bottle. Other improved tasks included shaving, putting on socks, and handling a hammer. In this group, only one subject continued to use the Handmaster at home. Evaluation of a similar transcutaneous stimulation unit demonstrated a significant therapeutic benefit from the stimulation (48). The Handmaster has the European Community (CE) mark in Europe and is approved by the Food and Drug Administration (FDA) as a therapeutic device in the United States.

Percutaneous Neuroprosthesis. The FESMate system uses up to 30 percutaneous electrodes to provide palmar, lateral, and parallel extension grasp patterns, and was developed by Handa and colleagues (22,45,49). Percutaneous systems were developed to address the problems of specificity and repeatability encountered with transcutaneous stimulation systems (34,42,50,51). The implantation is minimally invasive, requiring needle insertion only, with no surgical exposure. Grasp opening and closing is controlled by a switch operated by the opposite arm or by respiration using a sip/puff type of control. This system is primarily available in Japan. A formal assessment of outcomes with respect to disability and user satisfaction has not been reported.

Implanted Neuroprosthesis. An implanted upper extremity neuroprosthesis was first implanted in 1986 by Peckham and colleagues and is now known as the FreeHand system (Fig. 66-2) (12,17). The FreeHand system consists of eight implanted electrodes and an implanted receiver-stimulator unit (52), providing lateral and palmar grasp to persons with C5 and C6 tetraplegia. A radiofrequency inductive link provides the communication and power to the implant receiver-stimulator. The proportional control of grasp opening and closing is achieved using shoulder motion, which is measured using an externally worn joystick on the chest and shoulder (37). The FreeHand system has FDA approval in the United States and the CE mark in Europe as a neuroprosthesis providing hand function for SCI.

A multicenter study was conducted to evaluate the safety, effectiveness, and clinical impact of the implanted neuroprosthesis on 50 individuals with C5 or C6 SCI (17,53).The results showed that the neuroprosthesis produced increased pinch force in every patient. In a test of grasp and release ability using six objects of different size and weight (54,55), 49 of the 50 participants (98%) moved at least one more object with the neuroprosthesis than they could without it. The direct impact of the neuroprosthesis in the performance of ADLs was tested in 28 patients. Each participant was tested in 6 to 15 tasks, which included eating with a fork, drinking from a glass, writing with a pen, dialing a phone, inserting and removing a computer diskette, and brushing teeth. All 28 (100%) participants improved in independence in at least one task, and 78% were more independent using the neuroprosthesis in at least three tasks tested. Satisfaction and daily use of the neuroprosthesis at home was measured through surveys and device data logging (56). More than 90% of the participants were satisfied with the neuroprosthesis, and most use it regularly. Follow-up surveys indicate that usage patterns are maintained at least 4 years postimplant. Adverse events due to the implanted components and surgical installation were few. The infection rate was less than 2%. There were no cases of neuroprosthesis failure and less than 1% lead failures.

Summary of Upper Extremity Clinical Neuroprosthetic Applications. Neuroprostheses have been demonstrated to provide increased independence for C5- and C6-level SCI individuals. The different commercially available neuroprosthetic systems provide the patient and clinician with a variety of choices, depending on the individual's needs and goals. If the primary goal is muscle conditioning and contracture prevention, transcutaneous stimulation provides a noninvasive option that is relatively easy and inexpensive to implement. If the individual wants to maximize functional capability, implanted systems, in conjunction with surgical reconstruction, provide the greatest functional potential and have shown the greatest long-term use. For those individuals who are unwilling to undergo surgery, or who have not yet achieved neurologic stability postinjury, percutaneous or even transcutaneous stimulation systems may provide the individual with an opportunity to evaluate the function provided by neuroprostheses.

CURRENT RESEARCH IN UPPER EXTREMITY NEUROPROSTHESES

Current research in the application of neuroprosthetics to the upper extremity in SCI include the provision of additional function through the stimulation of more muscles, evaluation of new methods of control, new technological advancements, and the development of systems for C3- and C4-level SCI.

Additional Function. All three commercially available neuroprosthetic systems focus on the provision of grasp and release, but it has been shown that stimulation of additional muscles can provide even more function. Overhead reach can be provided by stimulation of the triceps muscle and subjects can combine triceps activation with stimulated grasp function to gain improved functional abilities (32,57–59). Stimulation of the pronator quadratus muscle can develop adequate pronation that can be opposed by voluntarily generated supination (60). Stimulation of the finger intrinsic muscles can improve grasp function (61).

New Control Methods. A number of alternative methods for controlling a neuroprosthesis have been pursued. The use of wrist position to control grasp has been shown to be a better method of control for some patients when compared to control of grasp using shoulder position (40). Activation of voluntary antagonists has been used to control elbow angle and forearm supination/pronation (59,60). The use of the myoelectric signal from either forearm or neck muscles has been shown to be a viable method of control (40,41,43,44).

Technological Advances. Technological advancements include implanted control transducers (62,63), new electrode technology (27,64) and use of devices that minimize surgical invasiveness (65). A second-generation implanted neuroprosthetic system has undergone clinical feasibility testing in four subjects (66). This system consists of an implanted stimulator-telemeter, 10 implanted electrodes, and an implanted wrist position sensor. This neuroprosthesis provided increased independence for each subject, including grasp and release, elbow extension, and forearm pronation for C6-level SCI.

Application to C3/C4 Spinal Cord Injury. Neuroprosthetic applications for high-level tetraplegia have been demonstrated clinically (32,45,46,49,67). Transcutaneous or percutaneous stimulation has been used to provide hand and elbow motion. Braces are used to support the shoulder. User control of both hand and arm function is provided through voice command, sip-puff control, or through voluntary shoulder movements. Functional ability has been demonstrated in activities such as eating, drinking, and writing.

Stroke

SHOULDER SUBLUXATION AND PAIN

Shoulder pain is a common complication in hemiparesis (68). Many causes of shoulder pain in hemiparesis are postulated including adhesive capsulitis, impingement syndrome, complex regional pain syndrome, brachial plexopathy, and spasticity. One of the most commonly cited causes of shoulder pain in hemiparesis is shoulder subluxation (68–70). Shoulder subluxation occurs due to the paralysis of active restraints, which plays a critical role in maintaining glenohumeral joint integrity, and is more likely to occur in patients with flaccid hemiparesis within the first 3 weeks after stroke (71). Shoulder subluxation is common in hemiparesis and an incidence of 50% is reported in one of the largest series of hemiparetic subjects followed longitudinally for an average of 11 months (68).

Although frequently hypothesized, the relationship between shoulder subluxation and shoulder pain in hemiparesis remains controversial (72). However, documented correlations between subluxation and other types of painful shoulder pathology suggest that subluxation plays a role in their genesis (68–70). Thus, despite the uncertain relationship between shoulder subluxation and pain, treatment of subluxation continues to be the standard of care in many rehabilitation facilities.

Transcutaneous Systems. Unfortunately, the available options for preventing or treating shoulder subluxation and pain are limited. However, FNS of the supraspinatus and deltoid muscles is a promising treatment option under investigation. Five controlled trials that evaluated shoulder pain have been published in the literature. Three studies evaluated FNS as a treatment modality (73–75), one evaluated prevention (76), and one evaluated a combination of treatment and prevention (77). The stroke onset to study entry ranged between less than 48 hours in one study (76) to as late as 37 weeks in another (73). All studies demonstrated reduction of subluxation at least in the short-term, although reduction in pain was less consistent.

Baker and Parker (73), Chantraine and associates (74), and Wang and associates (75) investigated FNS as a treatment modality. Baker and Parker reported significant reduction in subluxation at the end of 6 weeks of treatment, but without significant effect on pain reduction. In contrast, Chantraine and associates reported significant reduction in subluxation and pain for up to 24 months posttreatment. Wang and associates reported significant improvement in reduction and pain-free range of motion for acute subjects, but not for chronic subjects. The differences in results may be due to differences in methodology, especially subject population. Wang and associates demonstrated that FNS has significant benefit for those with acute hemiparesis, but not with chronic hemiparesis.

Faghri and associates (77) reported results of a randomized, controlled trial in 26 acute hemiparetic subjects with flaccid shoulder muscles. Neither shoulder subluxation nor shoulder pain was included in the inclusion criteria. Nevertheless, some subjects had shoulder subluxation at baseline and some had pain. Whether some had both is unclear. The study is best described as a mix of both treatment and prevention. The authors reported improvement in shoulder subluxation in the FNS group compared to controls. They also reported improvements in shoulder pain. However, this improvement was demonstrated only through pretest, posttest analysis of each group separately. The authors did not report results of analysis across groups, suggesting the possibility that the differences are not significant compared to the control group.

Linn and associates (76) assessed the efficacy of NMES in preventing shoulder subluxation and pain among acute stroke survivors with less than antigravity strength in the upper limb. The study randomized acute stroke survivors with no evidence of subluxation or pain to a treatment group, which received 4 weeks of treatment with FNS, or to a control group, which did not receive FNS treatments. Statistically significant differences between groups were not seen for any measures after 4 weeks or after 8 weeks of follow-up. However, there was a trend toward less subluxation in the treatment group at 4 weeks.

Intramuscular Systems. Despite the evidence for clinical benefit, the clinical use of transcutaneous FNS for shoulder subluxation and pain in hemiplegia is limited for several reasons. First, stimulation of cutaneous nociceptors cannot be avoided resulting in stimulation-induced pain that limits tolerance and compliance. Second, activation of deep muscles cannot be achieved without stimulation of more superficial muscles. Third, stimulated muscle contraction cannot be precisely titrated. Fourth, clinical skill is required to place the electrodes and adjust stimulation parameters to provide optimal and tolerable treatment.

A potential solution is intramuscular FNS systems, which can be placed percutaneously or injected into the target muscle. Intramuscular stimulation has multiple advantages over transcutaneous stimulation. First, intramuscular stimulation is less painful than surface stimulation (78), which may enhance patient compliance with treatment. Second motor points do not need to be located with each treatment session, which eases donning and doffing of the device, ensures repeatability and reliability of stimulation, and minimizes need for skilled care. Finally, because of the focal nature and reliability of intramuscular stimulation, the best muscles to stimulate can be identified and current intensity on multiple channels can be titrated to provide optimal reduction.

Intramuscular stimulation systems under investigation include a percutaneous electrode system with external stimulator and an injectable neuromuscular stimulator system with an external antenna. The components of the percutaneous system (StIM™, NeuroControl Corp., Valley View, OH) include helical intramuscular electrodes, which are percutaneously placed, a "beeper"-sized stimulator, which is worn on a belt, and a connector, which connects the electrodes to the stimulator. The electrodes are removed by gentle traction after completion of treatment. A pilot study of the percutaneous system among eight chronic stroke survivors with shoulder subluxation and pain demonstrated significant improvement in shoulder subluxation and pain that was maintained for up to 3 months after completion of treatment (79). Long-term follow-up of one of the patients demonstrated sustained pain relief for up to 3 years posttreatment (80). The percutaneous system is presently undergoing a multicenter randomized clinical trial. Injectable neuromuscular stimulators (Bion®, Advanced Bionics Corp., Valencia, CA) are microminiature, single-channel stimulators that are percutaneously placed without external lead wires exiting the skin. They receive power and individually addressed commands from an external magnetic field via a garment antenna. Preliminary results from a randomized clinical trial demonstrate reduction in shoulder subluxation and increase in the thickness of the stimulated muscles (81). The duration of

therapeutic effect for either system is unknown at this time. The potential advantage of the injectable neuromuscular stimulator system, however, is that the stimulators are permanently implanted and, if shoulder subluxation or pain recurs, additional treatments can be provided without further implantation. However, the system also requires a large antenna that must be worn, which may compromise clinical acceptance.

Summary. Shoulder subluxation and pain are common complications in hemiparesis. Although the relationship between subluxation and pain remains controversial, subluxation may result in traction injury to neurovascular and musculoskeletal structures predisposing hemiparetic persons to the development of painful shoulder pathology. Painful hemiparetic shoulder is often refractory to treatment. The use of FNS reduces shoulder subluxation, at least in the short-term, and may reduce shoulder pain and facilitate motor recovery. However, additional studies are needed to more definitively address the question of clinical efficacy. Future studies should be large, multicenter, blinded, randomized clinical trials. Subject population should be clearly defined as acute or chronic, and their stroke characteristics and potential confounds should be presented. The object of the study should be clearly defined as "treatment" or "prevention." In order to remain clinically relevant, reduction or prevention of pain should be the principal goal in these studies. For "treatment" interventions, subjects should have both shoulder subluxation and pain at study entry. For "prevention," acute stroke patients who already have shoulder subluxation, but have not yet developed pain, are probably the best candidates. Valid and reliable measures of radiographic subluxation, pain, impairment, and disability should be used with follow-up of at least 6 months. As with all randomized trials, appropriate power analyses, description of randomization method, analyses of potential confounds, and intention-to-treat analyses should be included. Finally, future studies should elucidate optimal stimulation parameters for the "treatment" and "prevention" interventions.

HAND NEUROPROSTHESIS

Transcutaneous Systems. In view of the success of the hand neuroprosthesis in tetraplegia (53), it is reasonable to apply the technology to persons with hemiplegia. However, there are only two full-length articles in English language peer-review journals that evaluate the effectiveness of a hand neuroprosthesis for enhancing the function of stroke survivors. Both studies used open-label designs with performance evaluation with and without the neuroprostheses.

In 1973 Rebersek and Vodovnik (82) published the first paper on the use of a hand neuroprosthesis in hemiplegia. Transcutaneous FNS opened the hand while closing was mediated by termination of the stimulation and the subject's own volitional ability. The intensity of stimulation was proportionally controlled with a position transducer mounted on the contralateral nonparalyzed shoulder. With training, subjects demonstrated progressive improvements in the number of hand positions they can maintain and the extent of hand opening using the device. A subset of subjects demonstrated progressive improvements in the number of plugs and baskets they can manipulate with the device. The authors noted that without the stimulation, subjects performed less than 10% of the tasks. The feasibility of the device in enhancing upper extremity–related ADLs was not assessed.

In 1975 Merletti and associates (83) evaluated a similar transcutaneous hand neuroprosthesis system. The device provided hand opening, but subjects again provided hand closure without the assist of the FNS. Subjects were trained to move a small plastic basket or bottle from one defined area to another and back again using the shoulder-mounted position, transducer-controlled stimulation. All subjects were able to perform the tasks with triceps and hand stimulation, although with varying degrees of success. However, none of the enrolled subjects could perform the assigned tasks without the stimulation, or with hand stimulation only. The authors noted that the functional tasks required a considerable amount of mental concentration. In several cases voluntary effort to control the paretic limb produced tremors, spasticity, and erratic shoulder movement, which resulted in reduced performance.

These exploratory studies suggested that it might be possible to develop a hand neuroprosthesis system to provide hand function for persons with hemiplegia. Because of their exploratory nature, statistical analyses were not performed and outcomes were limited to simulated hand tasks without evaluations of everyday ADLs. Nevertheless, the results were encouraging and should have led to promising developments. However, since these early reports there have been no additional studies on the functional efficacy of hand neuroprostheses systems in hemiplegia. There is no evidence in the literature that these devices were further developed or clinically implemented.

Intramuscular Systems. In view of these earlier studies and the recent success of implanted systems for tetraplegia (53), Chae and associates (84) explored the feasibility of a percutaneous intramuscular hand neuroprosthesis system in hemiplegia. Due to the limitations of transcutaneous stimulation as described in earlier sections, Merletti and associates (83) suggested that an implanted system would best meet the clinical needs of persons with hemiplegia. Six subjects with chronic hemiplegia were implanted with percutaneous intramuscular electrodes to demonstrate adequacy of intramuscular FNS for hand opening and closing, identify control strategies that reliably open and close the hand under subject control, and demonstrate functional use.

Various muscles of the paretic hand and forearm were stimulated in order to demonstrate the effectiveness of percutaneous, intramuscular FNS for hand opening and closing. With the proximal arm supported and the entire arm in a resting state, full hand opening was achieved via stimulation of the extensor digitorum communis, extensor indices proprius, and extensor pollicis longus. In three subjects, dorsal interosseous muscles were also stimulated due to the "intrinsic minus" posture assumed by the hand during stimulation of extensor digitorum communis in the face of finger flexor spasticity. As long as the subjects remained relaxed the spastic hand could be opened and closed using simple switches, potentiometers, shoulder and wrist position transducers, and electromyography-mediated controllers. However, when subjects tried to assist the NMES to open and close the hand during functional tasks, marked tremor and spasticity of the distal arm and hand were generated, which prevented the completion of the task. When subjects were able to grasp an object firmly, they often had difficulty releasing the object even with the stimulation due to the onset of marked finger flexor spasticity. Pharmacological interventions were generally ineffective in sufficiently decreasing finger flexor tone. In view of these limitations, formal functional assessment of the percutaneous hand neuroprosthesis system was not pursued.

Summary. In summary, transcutaneous and intramuscular FNS are able to open a spastic hemiparetic hand as long as subjects remain relaxed and do not assist the electrical stimulation. However, when subjects try to assist the electrical stimulation

or to use the system for functional tasks, significant decline in performance may occur. A recent study demonstrated increased ability of transcutaneous electrical stimulation for opening spastic hemiparetic hands by decreasing the tenodesis effect at the wrist (85). However, subjects in this study were relaxed with proximal arm supported, subjects did not assist the stimulation, and functional tasks were not attempted. Similarly, Hines and associates (86) reported that surface stimulation was able to open a spastic hemiparetic hand. However, as soon as the subject voluntarily tried to assist the system in hand opening, significant flexor spasms were noted with reduction in electrically induced finger extension moment.

A clinically viable hand neuroprosthesis system must demonstrate that persons with hemiparesis are able to perform bilateral tasks and are able to perform these tasks faster and more efficiently compared to the usual single-handed approach. The system must provide proximal as well as distal function. The system must have sufficient miniaturization and robustness to allow ambulation. The control paradigm must allow smooth, volitionally controlled functional movement of the impaired upper extremity without compromising the function of the intact extremities. Once functional efficacy is reasonably assured, a fully implanted system should be developed to increase cosmesis and "user friendliness" and minimize the potential for complications surrounding electrode skin interfaces.

In order to meet these specifications a number of techniques are worthy of further development. Weakness is only of one of several features of motor control dysfunction in hemiparesis and, as noted earlier, delay in the initiation and termination of muscle activation, co-contraction of antagonist muscles. and co-activation of synergistic muscles are also prominent manifestations. In view of the complex nature of motor control in upper extremity hemiparesis, a neuroprosthesis system must be able to "turn off" overactive muscles just as well as it is able to "turn on" weak muscles. Several methods are under investigation to electrically block nerve conduction that may be rapidly modulated. Specific techniques include collision block (87,88), hyperpolarization block (89), and subthreshold depolarization block (90). The lack of an appropriate control paradigm is another major barrier to the clinical implementation of a hand neuroprosthesis system in hemiparesis. Alternatives to the traditional shoulder control that require further development include ipsilateral wrist control (40), myoelectric control (43), prediction of intent from shoulder motion (91), and cortical control (61).

LOWER EXTREMITY NEUROPROSTHESES

Spinal Cord Injury

FNS can provide individuals paralyzed by thoracic or low cervical SCI with the ability to perform many activities that were previously impossible or difficult from the wheelchair, including standing, transfers, stepping short distances, and simple mobility functions such as side and back stepping (92–94). Preliminary clinical trials of lower extremity neuroprostheses suggest that continuous open-loop stimulation of the trunk, hip, and knee extensors can allow people with paraplegia to overcome physical obstacles, negotiate architectural barriers, and exert a greater control over their environment by affording them the ability to reach and manipulate objects that are otherwise inaccessible from the wheelchair (95–97).

NEUROPROSTHESES FOR STANDING AND TRANSFERS
Multichannel transcutaneous stimulation systems have been successful at producing standing and stepping movements in

people with SCI in both laboratory and clinical settings with relatively simple systems consisting of two to six channels of continuous stimulation (20,93,98,99). Lower extremity FNS systems employing percutaneous intramuscular electrodes have also been successful in providing simple mobility and one-handed reaching tasks while standing to individuals with paraplegia using 16 or fewer channels (100,101). Percutaneous approaches to most muscles of the lower extremities have been defined, allowing the generation of more complex movements than with transcutaneous stimulation alone (102). More recently, totally implanted pacemaker-like neuroprostheses for standing after SCI have undergone feasibility and initial clinical testing. Exercise and standing have been reported with a cochlear implant that was modified to stimulate motor neurons (103), and 12-channel system for activation of the L2-S2 motor roots has been applied to a handful of volunteers (104). For long-term clinical application, implanted systems such as these provide major advantages over transcutaneous and percutaneous stimulation including improved convenience, cosmesis, reliability, and repeatability.

Figure 66-3 shows individuals with complete motor paraplegia using implanted neuroprostheses for standing based on

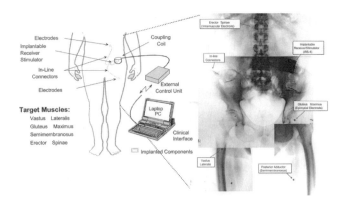

Figure 66-4. System level diagram of the standing neuroprosthesis (**left**) and composite x-ray showing implanted components.

the Case Western Reserve University (CWRU)/Veterans Affair (VA) eight-channel receiver-stimulator (52). In a single surgical procedure, epimysial electrodes are installed bilaterally in the vastus lateralis, semimembranosus or posterior portion of the adductor magnus, and gluteus maximus, while intramuscular electrodes are inserted at L1/L2 to activate the lumbar spinal roots for the erector spinae muscles (97). A system-level diagram of the standing system, and a composite x-ray of the internal components of the neuroprosthesis are shown in Figure 66-4.

After a critical period of bed rest and restricted activity to promote healing immediately postimplantation and completion of a reconditioning exercise program, patterns of stimulation are constructed for the sit-to-stand and stand-to-sit transitions. Rehabilitation for the system user progresses from standing in parallel bars to a walker, to standing pivot transfers and swing-to gait. Balance training includes stand-to-retrieve tasks and releasing a hand to manipulate the controls of a wearable external control unit.

Neuroprostheses recipients interact with the system through a series of buttons on the enclosure of the external controller, or via remote switches worn on a ring or attached to the walker, crutch, or other support device. Users or their assistants select a preprogrammed pattern of stimulation for exercise or function from a series of menu options. To stand, a single activation of one switch initiates the stimulation sequence to raise the body from the seated position. After a short delay to allow the user to comfortably position their hands on an assistive device, stimulation to the trunk, hip, and knee extensors is increased to levels sufficient to raise the body from the seated position and maintained continuously to keep the body upright during standing. Another depression of the switch reverses the process and lowers the user to a seated position in a controlled fashion.

Continuous stimulation to the extensor musculature braces the body against collapse while the hands are used for balance. Stepping can be achieved with 16 channels of stimulation through the addition of a second implant to activate the hip flexors and ankle dorsiflexors (105,106). Multicenter clinical trials for FDA approval of the implanted neuroprosthesis for standing are underway (107). Long-term follow-up of at least 12 months has been completed on 10 subjects, and at least 2 years on 5 volunteers. Preliminary results indicate that stimulation thresholds are stable and internal components are reliable with survival rates of epimysial electrodes in the extremities approaching 95% (108,109).

Initial results from the clinical trials of the implanted standing systems show that the stimulated responses of the knee,

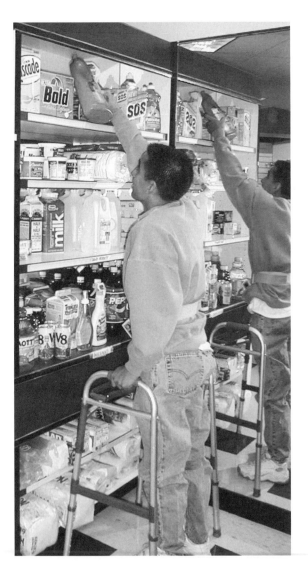

Figure 66-3. Standing with continuous stimulation to the trunk, hip, and knee extensors with an eight-channel implanted neuroprosthesis. Balance must be maintained by one extremity on an assistive device.

hip, and trunk extensors are sufficiently strong and fatigue-resistant for functional use. After completing the program of reconditioning exercise, American Spinal Cord Injury Association (ASIA) total motor scores with stimulation are 16% to 37% (mean of 20) greater than without FNS. Subjects who completed the exercise protocols were able to stand for sufficient lengths of time to complete various activities ranging from standing transfers to working at a counter. The amount of practice and training, body size, hip and trunk extensor strength, and quadriceps endurance appear to be important influences on standing duration, which can vary from 2 to greater than 40 minutes. Users and their assistants report a preference for FNS-assisted transfers over conventional methods when moving to and from high surfaces, while conventional pivot or sliding transfers were still the method of choice for level transfers (110). Transfers to heights impossible to perform by conventional lifting transfers required moderate effort or assistance with the neuroprosthesis.

All lower extremity FNS systems still require assistive devices, such as crutches, walkers, or additional bracing to provide supplemental support or allow the upper extremities to inject the corrective forces necessary to maintain a stable upright posture. The magnitudes of these corrective forces can be quite small—on the order of 10% of body weight or less (107). They can be produced routinely by a single extremity without undue exertion, freeing the other hand to perform reaching tasks or other functions, as illustrated in Figure 66-3. FNS can readily generate the muscle forces and joint moments required for rising from a chair into a standing posture with minimal assistance from the upper extremities. Producing the postural corrections necessary to maintain balance in the presence of intrinsic (voluntary motions) or extrinsic (unanticipated environmental perturbations) destabilizing disturbances, however, remains a major challenge to the designers of FNS systems. Practical and robust control systems to provide standing balance (i.e., the maintenance of standing posture), even for the brief periods of time typically required for completing simple reaching activities, has been an elusive goal and is still an active area of research.

Although the upper extremity corrective forces required for balance with open-loop stimulation can be quite small, on the order of the weight of the arms themselves, this is not true for all users of currently available standing neuroprostheses, a group that exhibits a great deal of variability in their standing performance. The support forces imposed on the arms while upright depend on many variables, including postural alignment and the stimulated moment produced at the joints. Increasing stimulated hip extension consistently decreases the vertical support forces placed on the upper extremities; the same hip extension moment is more effective at decreasing the forces on the arms at more erect standing postures. At more erect postures (5 and 10 degrees of hip flexion), small amounts of active stimulated hip extension moment produce large decreases in arm support forces. At more flexed postures (15 to 25 degrees), much more hip extension is required to reduce the arm support forces by similar amounts (111). These results indicate that strong stimulated hip extension, and the ability to assume an erect posture, will be prerequisites for advanced systems providing postural corrections to destabilizing events.

The metabolic energy consumption associated with quiet standing with continuous FNS is less than three times the basal metabolic rate during able-bodied standing (112), or standing with knee-ankle-foot orthoses. This is a level comparable to tub bathing, piano playing, or fishing (113), and is due primarily to the stimulated activity of the lower extremity musculature rather than from upper extremity exertion. Control strategies

that minimize high levels of continuous stimulation to prepare for, or respond to, a change in postural demand need to be considered to keep energy expenditures at reasonable levels.

NEUROPROSTHESES FOR AMBULATION

Functional Neuromuscular Stimulation-only Systems

Pioneering work in the application of FNS for restoration of standing and walking function to individuals with complete and incomplete SCIs was conducted in the 1970s and 1980s and continues to be employed in many laboratories and clinics around the world (93,114). Using as few as two transcutaneous stimulation channels per leg, standing and reciprocal walking are produced by activation of the quadriceps muscles and the triggering of a flexion-withdrawal reflex. A pair of transcutaneous electrodes is placed over the quadriceps on the anterior thigh. A second pair of electrodes is located distally over the dermatomes of the peroneal, sural, or saphenous sensory nerves. Standing is achieved by simultaneously activating the quadriceps bilaterally in response to a command input, such as the simultaneous depression of switches on the handles of a rolling walker or crutches. A stride is produced by maintaining activation to the quadriceps of the stance leg while initiating a flexion withdrawal in the contralateral limb. Depression of the crutch- or walker-mounted switch on the swing leg stimulates the afferent sensory fibers and triggers a spinal reflex arc that causes hip, knee, and ankle flexion. To complete the stride, activation of the knee extensors on the swinging leg is initiated while the reflex is still active and flexing the hip. The stimulus producing the flexion reflex is then removed, leaving the user in double-limb support once again with bilateral quadriceps stimulation. Some paralyzed subjects have been reported to walk at speeds approaching one-fourth of normal, and ascend a curb or step with transcutaneous stimulation. These implementation procedures for standing and stepping with transcutaneous stimulation have been successfully transferred to clinical practice and have received FDA approval (Parastep®, Sigmedics, Inc., Fairborn, OH) (20,21).

Complicating issues with this system include active flexion generated by the rectus femoris when the quadriceps is stimulated with transcutaneous electrodes. This makes erect standing difficult and results in an anterior pelvic tilt with compensatory lordosis, or excessive weight on the arms to maintain an upright posture. Not all patients will exhibit a flexion withdrawal reflex that is strong or repeatable enough to be used for stepping. Because it is a mass flexion pattern resulting from synergistic activity of a group of muscles triggered by a single stimulus, the swing limb motion is difficult to control. Reflex stepping can be effective in well-selected individuals, although it tends to be jerky and the reflex can habituate with repeated activation, limiting the number of steps that can be taken at one time.

With the help of FNS, many with neurologically incomplete spinal cord lesions can become functional walkers since some degree of motor, sensory, and proprioception function has been preserved. Voluntary strength can improve with exercise and therapy augmented with electrical stimulation. In these cases, increased stride length and reduced physiological cost index during walking can be achieved. Alternatively, the quality of stimulated responses can improve while volitional function remains unchanged, necessitating a neuroprosthetic application of FNS. In some patients an exaggerated extensor tone can provide safe standing, but they are unable to initiate a step. In those patients peroneal stimulators may be useful to inhibit extensor tone and help initiate a step (115,116). Hip abductors, hamstrings, and trunk extensors are included in stimulation patterns when needed (117). But the high variability of the incomplete SCI population requires caution in the application of FNS.

These approaches have been extended through the use of implanted electrodes for personal mobility functions such as transfers, standing, stepping, and stair ascent and descent. This approach involves individual activation of a number of muscles (typically eight or more) rather than the use of synergistic patterns such as the flexion-withdrawal reflex, or extensive bracing. Complex lower extremity motions have been synthesized by activating up to 48 separate muscles with chronically indwelling, helically coiled, fine-wire intramuscular electrodes with percutaneous leads under the control of a programmable microprocessor-based external stimulator. Some well-trained subjects are able to walk 300 meters repeatedly at 0.5 meters per second with this system (118). All components are worn by the user, freeing him or her from cabling to a walker or other assistive device. Freely articulating ankle-foot orthoses are used to protect the ligaments and structure of the foot and ankle. The quality of the motions produced by FNS with this system depend on the availability, strength and endurance of paralyzed muscles, the ability of the therapist or engineer to specify patterns of stimulation for ambulation, and the subject's experience with the device.

Hybrid Systems Combining Functional Neuromuscular Stimulation and Orthoses

One method to achieve ambulation after SCI involves combining FNS with conventional bracing (119–122). The energy required to operate these hybrid systems is less than braces alone, but increases rapidly with walking velocity at the same rate as braces alone. This is due primarily to an increased reliance on the arms and trunk musculature to move the body forward with increasing speed. The need to overcome mechanical constraints on step length imposed by the orthoses contributes to this phenomenon. Faster walking speeds are usually achieved by increasing both step length and cadence (steps per minute). Braces restrict step length, lock the knee, and define a fixed ratio of ipsilateral hip extension to contralateral hip flexion, which forces their users to rely only on increased cadence and increased upper body exertion to achieve higher walking velocities. Taking short steps at higher rates is less energy-efficient than simultaneously modulating both step length and cadence because of the work required by the upper body to lift the mass of the body to clear the floor with the swinging limb with the knees locked.

At slow to moderate speeds, energy consumption for both braces and hybrid brace-FNS modes of walking is still less than with FNS alone. However, energy cost for FNS walking decreases modestly as walking speed increases, suggesting that as velocities approach normal, the differences between walking modalities will be minimized or reversed (with brace-walking requiring more energy than FNS). The slight decline in energy consumption with FNS is probably due to shorter stimulation times for the major leg and hip muscles with faster walking velocities, while upper extremity effort remains relatively constant since the body is being propelled by the contracting lower extremity musculature rather than by contortions of the arms and torso. The energy-saving effect of hybrid systems is primarily due to their ability to constrain the motions of the joints, reduce the degrees of freedom of movement, and provide mechanical stability. For static activities such as quiet standing, individuals with paraplegia can assume a stable posture with little or no muscular exertion by locking the knees of a brace and hyperextending the hips, thus avoiding the fatigue associated with continuous stimulation. FNS is quite effective at introducing large impulsive forces into the biomechanical system

through activation of large lower extremity muscles, which reduces the upper extremity exertion required for walking in conventional braces. Combining FNS and bracing in a hybrid orthosis takes advantage of the positive aspects of each technology and minimizes the potential shortcomings.

Hybrid systems of various types employing various brace and stimulation components have been fitted to patients with complete or incomplete thoracic or low-level cervical injuries at research and clinical centers in North America and Europe (123). One design combines a Louisiana State University Reciprocating Gait Orthosis (LSU-RGO) with a four-channel transcutaneous stimulator and a flexible copolymer electrode cuff. Since walking is accomplished with the knees locked, stimulating the hamstrings extends the hip, and flexes the contralateral hip through the action of the reciprocating mechanism. Conversely, the rectus femoris actively flexes the hip and assists with contralateral hip extension via the reciprocating mechanism. Rectus femoris and contralateral hamstrings are activated simultaneously to initiate a step on the depression of a walker-mounted switch. Follow-up studies on RGO-based hybrid orthoses have shown that up to 41% of system recipients used it for gait (124), while 66% used it for exercise (125).

Hybrid systems are reliable and simple to implement in clinical environments with orthotic and prosthetic fabricating capacity. Standing with the knee joints of the brace locked allows all stimulation to be removed, thus postponing the onset of fatigue. The orthotic component of these may also protect the insensate joints and osteoporotic bones of users with long-standing SCI from possible damage resulting from the loads applied during weight bearing and ambulation. However, the bracing employed by hybrid systems can potentially encumber individuals in the execution of ADLs for which they were not designed. For example, locking the knees can hinder the completion of more complex movements useful for personal mobility, such as stair climbing. Similarly, the thoracic component can prohibit lateral bending and trunk rotation while sitting in the wheelchair. The devices are usually worn outside the clothing, and donning, doffing, and cosmetic aspects are similar to conventional braces.

Metabolic Costs of Functional Neuromuscular Stimulation Ambulation Systems

The study of energy consumption during locomotion with hybrid or FNS-only neuroprostheses is complicated by several factors that make generalization difficult. Most reports involve a small number of subjects with varying experience with the technology, and well-controlled or randomized trials are almost impossible to perform since raters and subjects alike can not be blinded to the status of their neuroprosthesis system. Furthermore, energy efficiency during ambulation is highly correlated to the frequency of use of a neuroprosthesis (126). Therefore, direct comparisons between different systems on the same volunteers would require them to have comparable amounts of practice with each device, which is often impractical. In addition, methodologies vary and almost uniformly require subjects to achieve a steady state metabolic response for validity, which is not always possible with FNS-assisted ambulation. Nevertheless, several small-scale studies of the metabolic costs of walking with transcutaneous-stimulation systems and hybrid orthosis systems have been reported.

The energy expenditure required for experienced users to walk distances up to 200 feet with surface stimulation has been reported to be approximately equivalent to a 1.5-mile walk at 3 miles per hour for an able-bodied adult (127). The Physiological Cost Index (PCI), which is the ratio of change in heart rate from baseline (beats per minute) to steady state velocity (meters per minute) has been used as a measure of energy costs during normal walking (128) as well as ambulating with transcutaneous stimulation and hybrid orthoses. The PCI has been shown to be an indicator of energy costs in disabled individuals (129) and applied as a measure of gait efficiency with different assistive devices after SCI (130). A wide range of PCI values were observed in four of five fully trained users of surface stimulation systems for ambulation with mid- to low-thoracic level injuries. Physiological cost indices ranging from 2.3 to 6.3 beats per meter, and walking velocities ranging from approximately 5 to over 24 meters per minute have been reported (126), which are comparable to walking in a conventional RGO (131). Just as with other upright mobility devices for individuals with SCIs, walking with surface stimulation systems is slower and less energy-efficient than normal walking, which exhibits a PCI ranging between 0.11 and 0.51 beats per meter (with a mean of 0.21) at self-selected speeds (126). However, it provides reasonable upright mobility at velocities and energy costs that appear to be within the physiological capacities of people with paraplegia (132). With energy costs similar to long leg braces, transcutaneous FNS systems may be better suited as a means of providing the documented physical benefits of exercise than as a daily mode of personal transportation (133–136).

Oxygen consumption (VO$_2$), heart rate, and velocity during walking with an RGO alone, and with a hybrid FNS-RGO system have also been documented. Lower PCI values and slightly faster velocities are possible with a hybrid FNS-RGO system than with the brace alone. The addition of FNS to the reciprocating orthosis appeared to decrease mean PCI from 2.55 beats per meter to 1.54 beats per meter at average self-selected velocities of approximately 24 and 25 meters per minute, respectively (130). These results are at the upper limits of performance reported for other studies of walking with FNS or RGOs alone, but the statistical significance of any apparent differences cannot be determined and care should be taken when comparing the results from studies involving small series of patients and varying experimental conditions. In a well-controlled study of oxygen consumption during ambulation with the LSU-RGO and the hybrid FNS-RGO system, a 16% reduction in rate of energy consumption (kcal/kg/minute) was observed at all walking speeds with the hybrid FNS-RGO system as compared to the orthosis alone (137). When expressed in terms of energy consumed per meter walked (kcal/kg/m), a similar 16% to 18% reduction in energy costs was observed with the hybrid system at velocities slower than the self-selected pace of 21 meters per second, although these advantages diminished rapidly with increasing walking speed. Like ambulation systems using surface stimulation alone, these values are still considerably larger than those reported for able-bodied ambulation, indicating that hybrid systems may also be most useful as an effective mode of exercise for individuals SCIs (125) rather than a means of transportation.

The true value of lower extremity FNS systems in their current forms lies in their ability to facilitate or provide options for short-duration mobility-related tasks such as overcoming physical obstacles or architectural barriers in the vicinity of the wheelchair. Exercise, standing, standing transfers, and one-handed reaching are all possible with relatively simple transcutaneous or surgically implanted FNS systems without extensive external bracing. The functional impact of lower extremity neuroprosthetic applications of FNS on the ability to complete ADLs is still an active area of research. It is clear from preliminary work, however, that exercise and standing with FNS can improve tissue viability and overall health, facilitate standing transfers by eliminating the heavy lifting and lowering re-

quired by an assistant, and allow selected individuals with SCI to regain access to objects, places, and opportunities impossible or exceedingly difficult from the wheelchair. FNS can augment and extend the function of the wheelchair and may prove to be a valuable option to enhance the well-being and independence of persons with disabilities. All this can be achieved with reliable implanted components that maximize cosmesis, personal convenience, and long-term use. From the reports in the literature to date, walking with FNS appears to be a promising form of exercise rather than an alternative to wheelchair locomotion. Acceptable energy levels for long-term activities are dependent on an individual's maximal aerobic capacity (normal walking requires approximately 30% of maximal aerobic capacity). Oxygen supply to tissue and capacity of the aerobic energy-producing mechanisms are usually sufficient to satisfy energy requirements in untrained individuals during activities requiring 50% of the maximal aerobic capacity, which has been proposed as a threshold for acceptability of brace, FNS, and hybrid systems for ambulation after SCI (138). The metabolic energy currently required to walk with FNS is too high to make it a truly practical alternative to the wheelchair for long distance transportation over level surfaces, although this remains a worthwhile and achievable long-term goal.

Stroke

The principal functional goal of a lower extremity neuroprosthesis for hemiplegia is to provide a symmetric, energy-efficient safe gait for community ambulation. During the swing phase of gait, diminished ankle dorsiflexion, knee flexion, or hip flexion can result in inability to clear the floor with the affected limb. In such a case, one or more of several compensatory strategies can be adopted, including circumducting the affected limb, dragging the affected limb, and vaulting over the unaffected limb in order to clear the floor with the affected limb. A neuroprosthesis may be used to stimulate insufficiently or inappropriately active limb flexor musculature so that a more normal-appearing swing phase results. Likewise, diminished control of weight-bearing muscles can result in gait deficits during the stance phase of gait. Gait deficits can include stance phase genu recurvatum, hyperflexion of the knee during stance, and deficient weight shifting to the affected limb. Neuroprostheses may be used to retrain weight-bearing muscles and improve stance phase limb control.

ANKLE DORSIFLEXION
The initial application of NMES in hemiplegia focused on transcutaneous stimulation for ankle dorsiflexion. In 1961 Lieberson and associates (139) described a single-channel peroneal nerve stimulator to provide ankle dorsiflexion during the swing phase of gait. Since then, other investigators have reported similar findings using open label with and without stimulation designs with outcome measures ranging from qualitative observations to metabolic cost indices (140–142). However, not all subjects experienced a clear neuroprosthetic effect and when neuroprosthetic effect was present there was often evidence of a motor relearning effect as well.

In the only study of transcutaneous peroneal nerve stimulators employing an experimental design, Burridge and associates (143) randomized 32 chronic stroke survivors to treatment versus control. Both groups received a course of 10 one-hour physiotherapy sessions during the first 4 weeks of the trial. The treatment group presumably used the stimulator for everyday ambulation, although this is not explicitly stated. All subjects were assessed at 4 and 12 weeks after onset of the trial. Subjects in the treatment groups were assessed with and without the stimulation. Subjects were trained to regularly adjust the stimulus intensity to accommodate changing skin impedance, condition of electrodes, fatigue, and changing resistance in dorsiflexion due to changing spasticity. Subjects were also trained to adjust the electrode position as the optimal position varied from person to person and sometimes within subjects from day to day. At the end of the 12-week study, the treatment group exhibited significantly greater increase in walking velocity with the stimulation than the control group. A similar finding was noted with the physiologic cost index. There were no differences between groups when the treatment group did not use the stimulator. The study suggests clinically relevant improvements in ambulation function for subjects using the transcutaneous peroneal stimulator.

In order to address the limitations of transcutaneous stimulation reported by early investigators, the feasibility of implantable peroneal stimulators was evaluated in two studies. Waters and associates used a single-channel implantable system to correct foot drop (144). Statistically significant increases were seen in walking velocity, stride length, and step frequency with the stimulation compared to preimplantation. However, after surgery, differences in outcome with and without the NMES were not statistically significant as improvements were seen even without the stimulation compared to baseline due to a probable motor relearning effect. Technical limitations included inability to balance inversion and eversion due to use of a single channel, lack of an in-line connector, which required removal of the entire implant in the event of component failure, and poor reliability of early version heel-switch and foot-floor contact transmitters. In another case series, Kljajic and associates evaluated 19 of 35 chronic stroke survivors implanted with single-channel peroneal nerve stimulators (145). Using an ordinal measure, the authors reported statistically significant neuroprosthetic improvements with the stimulation compared to without the stimulation. As in the Waters study, several subjects demonstrated motor relearning effects. Nearly half the subjects in this series required reimplantation due to electrode displacement or failure. Randomized controlled trials of implantable peroneal stimulators have not been reported.

MULTICHANNEL SYSTEMS

Since gait deviation in hemiplegia is not limited to ankle dysfunction, several studies have also investigated multichannel transcutaneous stimulation systems. Stanic and associates (146) reported significant improvements in qualitative and quantitative measures of gait using a six-channel transcutaneous FNS system, which provided ankle dorsiflexion, eversion and plantarflexion, knee flexion and extension, and hip extension and abduction. Bogataj and associates (147) reported similar findings with their six-channel FNS system, which provided ankle dorsiflexion and plantarflexion, knee extension and flexion, and hip extension. There was sufficient carryover effect to allow all subjects to continue with gait training without the stimulation and continue to improve. Bogataj and associates (148) also carried out the only controlled trial of multichannel transcutaneous FNS system, which also provided ankle dorsiflexion and plantarflexion, knee extension and flexion, and hip extension during ambulation. They reported significantly greater improvements in gait performance and motor function in subjects treated with 3 weeks of FNS compared to those receiving conventional therapy.

Summary

Although the development of lower extremity FNS systems is further along than upper extremity systems, numerous issues presently limit their clinical implementation. First, transcutaneous stimulation systems, which make up the majority of published reports, are limited by pain of stimulation, poor patient compliance, poor muscle selectivity, lengthy time required to place and remove multi-electrode systems, poor reproducibility of muscle contraction, and limited accessibility to deep muscles. Percutaneous and fully implanted systems may address these issues, but these potential benefits must be tempered with the risks and costs associated with an invasive procedure. Second, the indications for the level of complexity required for a specific individual remain undefined. Some individuals will require complex multichannel systems that stimulate multiple muscles, while simple dorsiflexion assist devices will suffice for others. Third, it remains unclear as to when motor relearning ends and neuroprosthetic needs begin. The intent of the studies reviewed in this section was clearly to develop and evaluate neuroprostheses. However, nearly all studies reported evidence of motor relearning to at least some degree, even among chronic stroke survivors. Finally, clinical efficacy must be more firmly established. Future studies should employ more rigorous experimental designs, namely randomized designs with appropriate blinding of evaluations. Subject population should be more clearly defined. Short- and long-term outcomes should be documented with close attention to patient compliance using valid and reliable outcome measures. Clinical relevance must be established by evaluating the effects of the intervention on physical disability, handicap, and quality of life. Despite these issues, there are sufficient data to justify pursuit of large multicenter, randomized clinical trials to demonstrate the clinical efficacy of simple ankle dorsiflexion assist devices. The development of more sophisticated systems that activate multiple muscles during ambulation should also be pursued.

BLADDER AND BOWEL NEUROPROSTHESES

Patients with suprasacral cord lesions can have electrical stimulation applied to the surviving sacral nerves or nerve roots to produce effective micturition and improve bowel function, significantly reducing complications and costs of bladder and bowel care (149–156). An implantable device for this purpose (Fig. 66-5) has been used by over 2,000 patients in at least 20 countries.

Operating Principles

MICTURITION

Contraction of the detrusor muscle of the bladder can be produced by electrical activation of the sacral parasympathetic preganglionic neurons. Their axons usually travel in the S3 and sometimes S4 or S2 anterior roots and nerves, and are closely accompanied for much of their course by somatic efferent axons to the external sphincter and pelvic floor. The somatic axons, being of larger diameter than the parasympathetic axons, have a lower threshold for electrical activation, and it is therefore difficult to produce contraction of the detrusor without contraction of the external sphincter. However, micturition can be produced by the technique of post-stimulus voiding, which uses the fact that the detrusor muscle of the bladder relaxes more slowly than the striated muscle of the external sphincter. Bladder pressure can be built up by a series of bursts of electrical stimulation, each lasting a few seconds, and is maintained between the bursts; the external sphincter contracts strongly during bursts but relaxes rapidly for a few seconds between bursts, allowing urine to flow. It was initially thought by

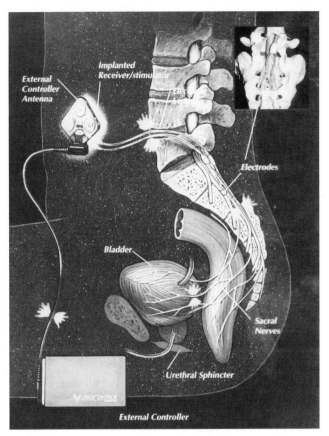

Figure 66-5. The Vocare system, which consists of an implanted stimulator and electrodes, and an external power and control unit.

injection are often needed. Reflex ejaculation, too, is not always effective but seminal emission can be produced from a high proportion of men with SCI by rectal-probe electrostimulation, and other techniques for obtaining viable sperm are available. These alternative techniques for assisting with erectile function or fertility can still be used after posterior rhizotomy, and the implant itself may produce erection when S2 roots are stimulated, an effect that appears to be potentiated by sildenafil. A decision about rhizotomy should therefore be made on a case by case basis. However, the advantages of posterior rhizotomy are such that since the mid-1980s it has generally been carried out when a bladder stimulator is implanted, thereby improving both micturition and continence.

Candidate Selection

Micturition by electrical stimulation requires intact parasympathetic neurons to the detrusor. The function of these neurons can be demonstrated by reflex detrusor contractions on a cystometrogram. Other sacral reflexes such as ankle tendon reflexes, the bulbocavernosus reflex, anal skin reflex, and reflex erection are confirmatory. Subjects can be implanted at any time after reaching neurological stability. They should also have a degree of emotional and social stability. Frequent urinary tract infection and problems with catheters or anticholinergic medication are further indications. In the United States the procedure is approved by the FDA as a humanitarian use device for subjects with complete SCI, although subjects with incomplete lesions have received the implant in other countries.

Female paraplegics with persistent reflex incontinence are often particularly grateful for the continence produced by posterior rhizotomy, because of the lack of satisfactory urine collecting devices for females. Paraplegic and low tetraplegic males often wish to dispense with a urine collection bag whereas males with higher tetraplegia may choose to continue to wear a condom collection device for convenience. If a tetraplegic male plans to use condom drainage with electrical stimulation it is wise to check preoperatively that the condom can be retained satisfactorily. It is also advisable to discuss options for sexual function and to offer a trial of various techniques for erectile function.

Technique

Electrodes may be placed either intradurally on the sacral anterior nerve roots in the cauda equina via a lower lumbar laminectomy, or extradurally on the mixed sacral nerves in the sacral canal via a laminectomy of S1–3. The intradural approach has been more widely used in Europe but extradural electrodes are usually used in the U.S. because the technique of implanting them carries less risk of trauma to the nerves or cerebrospinal fluid leakage. Intraoperative electrical stimulation and recording of bladder pressure is used to confirm the identity of the nerves supplying the bladder. Leads from the electrodes are tunneled subcutaneously to a radio-receiver/stimulator placed under the skin of the abdomen or chest, and powered and controlled by a battery-powered remote control operated by the patient.

Posterior rhizotomy is best done intradurally where the sensory and motor roots can be more easily separated. If intradural electrodes are being implanted the rhizotomy can be done at the cauda equina. If extradural electrodes are used, the rhizotomy is usually done at the conus medullaris through a separate laminectomy, though it can also be done within the lower end of the dural sac, which is preferable if there has been a fracture or internal fixation at the thoracolumbar junction.

some that the intermittent contraction of the sphincter during voiding might produce harmful pressures in the bladder leading to ureteric reflux or hydronephrosis, but these fears have not been borne out in long-term follow-up.

CONTINENCE
The major cause of incontinence in subjects with suprasacral SCI is detrusor hyperreflexia. Research is in progress evaluating reflex inhibition of the detrusor by electrical stimulation of large afferent neurons in the sacral dermatomes, a process known as neuromodulation, which shows some benefit in ablebodied subjects with urge incontinence (157,158). Similar inhibition can be observed following SCI, using the same implant as above; however, hyperreflexia of the external urethral sphincter can persist and may hamper voiding (159,160). Hyperreflexia of the sphincter and of the detrusor can be abolished by surgical division of the sacral sensory nerve roots, a procedure known as posterior rhizotomy. This produces a dramatic abolition of reflex incontinence; it also reduces the risk of damage to the upper urinary tracts by lowering the pressure at which urine is stored in the bladder, and may result in some improvement in reflux or hydronephrosis if these have already occurred. It abolishes the autonomic hyperreflexia and potentially dangerous rises in blood pressure, which can otherwise result from sacral afferent input when the bladder or bowel is distended. However, it also abolishes other potentially useful sacral reflexes, such as reflex erection and reflex ejaculation, as well as sacral sensation and orgasm from sacral stimulation if these were preserved after the SCI. Reflex erection is not always effective after SCI, though it may be improved by oral sildenafil, and alternative techniques such as intracavernosal

Postoperatively, urodynamic studies are used to guide the setting of stimulus parameters to give an acceptable voiding pressure and rate and pattern of flow. The patient can usually be discharged within a week of surgery with a working device. The stimulus program should be checked between 1 and 3 months after the operation since the response of the bladder may change with repeated use; thereafter review is recommended at least annually, monitoring lower and upper urinary tract function.

Clinical Outcomes

The majority of patients with an implanted bladder stimulator use it routinely for producing micturition four to six times per day. Residual volume in the bladder following implant-driven micturition is usually less than 60 mL and often less than 30 mL (155,161). A substantial decrease in symptomatic urine infection has been reported by many groups following the use of the implant (150,155,162,163).

Continence is achieved in over 85% of patients (164–166). This is largely attributable to the abolition of detrusor hyperreflexia and increase in bladder compliance that follow posterior sacral rhizotomy, and which persist long-term provided the rhizotomy is complete from S2 caudally. About 10% to 15% of patients report some stress incontinence of urine following implantation of the stimulator and posterior rhizotomy (167). It is not always clear whether this stress incontinence was formerly masked by more profound reflex incontinence or whether it results from the abolition of spasticity in the external urethral sphincter. However, being of small volume it is usually more manageable than reflex incontinence, which may require a change of clothing, and is managed in some subjects by low-level stimulation of the external urethral sphincter. Urodynamic studies show that there are substantial increases in bladder capacity and compliance following posterior rhizotomy (167,168). Typically bladder capacity is greater than 400 mL with a storage pressure less than 40 cm water. Voiding pressure can be controlled by adjusting the parameters of electrical stimulation and, while it is sometimes greater than in non-SCI subjects, this does not appear to be harmful to the upper tracts (149,150, 162,168,169).

Several centers in Europe have followed patients long-term, particularly with regard to the upper tracts (151,155,161,168). This experience indicates that trabeculation, ureteric reflux, and hydronephrosis tend to decrease in patients who undergo implantation and posterior rhizotomy. It appears likely in these patients that any harmful effects from transient high pressure during micturition are outweighed by the beneficial effects of low-pressure storage of urine during the majority of each day. There also is a reduction in the incidence of autonomic dysreflexia due to the interruption of afferent fibers from the bladder, lower bowel, and the perineum by posterior sacral rhizotomy. This outcome is particularly beneficial to tetraplegic males formerly dependent on an indwelling catheter prone to blockage from frequent infection. The ability to micturate on demand and improved continence of urine both contribute to a reduction in use of intermittent and indwelling catheterization. Most users become free of urine collection bags but some male tetraplegics with impaired ability to handle clothing or a urine bottle choose to continue to wear a condom drainage system for convenience. Reduction of urinary tract infection results in substantially less use of antibiotics. The abolition of detrusor hyperreflexia by posterior rhizotomy allows patients to discontinue anticholinergic medication, which in turn reduces constipation and other side effects such as a dry mouth, blurred vision, and drowsiness.

Regular stimulation of the sacral parasympathetic nerves contributes to transport of stool through the distal colon into the rectum, and most users report a reduction in constipation and reduced need for laxatives and stool softeners. Some users are able to defecate by a pattern of intermittent stimulation similar to that used for micturition but with longer intervals between bursts of stimulation to allow passage of stool (170). However, most patients also check with a finger in the rectum whether there is stool remaining after this procedure and if so, remove it manually. The frequency of bowel emptying increases toward the preinjury pattern and the overall time spent on bowel management is greatly reduced.

Studies in Europe and the U.S. indicate that the use of the implanted stimulator together with posterior sacral rhizotomy results in substantial savings in the cost of bladder and bowel care, particularly from reduction in supplies needed for bladder care, medications, and visits to physicians for management of complications (171–173). Savings in bladder and bowel care exceed the cost of purchasing and implanting the stimulator after 5 to 8 years, and thereafter are expected to result in progressive savings to the health care payer.

Complications

Infection of these implants is rare, occurring in only 1% of the first 500 implants. Infection is usually introduced at surgery or through a subsequent break in the skin. A technique of coating the implants with antibiotics was introduced in 1982 and reduces the infection rate (174). Technical faults in the implanted equipment are uncommon, occurring on average once every 19.6 implant-years (156). The most common sites for faults are in cables, which can usually be repaired under local anesthesia.

Summary and Conclusions

Electrical stimulation of the sacral parasympathetic nerves can restore effective micturition to people with suprasacral spinal cord damage, reducing urine infection and the use of catheters. It is often combined with posterior sacral rhizotomy to abolish reflex incontinence. The rhizotomy also reduces the risk of renal damage and autonomic dysreflexia, and reduces the use of anticholinergic medication and urine collection devices; however, it also abolishes reflex erection and reflex ejaculation, which may need to be provided by alternative techniques. Overall, these interventions can dramatically improve bladder and bowel function, reduce complications and costs, and increase quality of life after SCI.

RESPIRATORY MUSCLE STIMULATION

Following cervical SCI, a significant number of individuals suffer from chronic respiratory insufficiency requiring mechanical ventilation (175,176). Since the average age at time of injury is 32 years, these patients are usually maintained on mechanical ventilation for 20 to 25 years or longer (177–179).

Unfortunately, mechanical ventilation is associated with substantial morbidity, mortality, inconvenience, physical discomfort, fear of disconnection, difficulty with speech, and reduced mobility. Activation of the diaphragm by electrical stimulation of the phrenic nerve eliminates many of these problems and provides a more natural form of artificial ventilation, more closely mimicking spontaneous breathing.

Phrenic nerve pacing has now been applied in more than 1,200 patients worldwide and has become a clinically accepted technique to provide artificial ventilatory support in patients with trauma with respiratory failure secondary to cervical SCI injury (180–185). Although there may be significant patient variability, most patients describe an improved level of comfort, reduced anxiety and embarrassment, increased mobility, improved speech, and greater sense of well being and overall health as most important benefits compared to mechanical ventilation (179,184,186–189). However, various factors have limited more widespread use of diaphragm pacing. Many of these patients have suffered damage to the phrenic motor neuron pools in the spinal cord or to the phrenic nerves directly precluding successful pacing. Moreover, this technique requires a major surgical procedure, which is quite expensive.

Stimulation Devices

Three phrenic nerve pacing systems are commercially available. Each system has a similar configuration. Stimulation electrodes, radiofrequency receivers, and attached wiring must be surgically implanted and comprise the internal components. A radiofrequency transmitter, wires and antenna constitute the external components. The stimulating electrodes are implanted directly on each phrenic nerve. Small wires tunneled subcutaneously connect the electrodes to radiofrequency receivers which are implanted in an easily accessible area over the anterior portion of the thorax. External antennas connect to the transmitter. The transmitter generates a radiofrequency signal, which is inductively coupled to the implanted receivers. The signal is demodulated by the receivers, converting it to electrical signals, which are delivered to the stimulating electrodes.

Bilateral phrenic nerve stimulation results in descent of each diaphragm and fall in intrathoracic pressure resulting in inspiration. Cessation of stimulation results in diaphragm relaxation, an increase in intrathoracic pressure, and exhalation. To provide a normal level of ventilation, this pattern is repeated 8 to 14 times per minute. Stimulus amplitude and frequency, and train rate can be adjusted by the operator to alter tidal volume and respiratory rate, respectively. Inspiratory time and inspiratory flow rate can be varied, in tandem, by changing the duration of stimulation.

The technical characteristics of each currently available pacing systems are presented in Table 66-2. The Avery system (Avery Laboratories, Inc., Commack, NY) is FDA-approved and is the most widely used system worldwide. Monopolar electrodes are used to activate the phrenic nerves. The Atrotech

system (Atrotech OY, Tampere, Finland) is commercially available in most developed countries and is currently being used under an investigational device exemption from the FDA in the U.S. There is some evidence that the four-pole electrode system and stimulation paradigm reduces the stimulation frequency of individual axons to about one-fourth of that with unipolar stimulation. This technique is thought to provide greater time for recovery, decrease risk of fatigue, and shorten the reconditioning process (190). The MedImplant system (MedImplant Biotechnisches Labor, Vienna, Austria) has limited availability, predominantly in Austria and Germany. It is not available in the U.S. This system uses a four-electrode array positioned around each nerve. As with the Atrotech device, only a portion of the nerve is stimulated, and consequently, only a portion of the diaphragm is activated at any given time.

Patient Evaluation and Assessment

In patients who remain ventilator-dependent following cervical SCI, the success of phrenic nerve pacing is dependent upon the integrity of the phrenic nerves. The amplitude of the phrenic nerve response is roughly proportional to the number of axons available to stimulate. Therefore, phrenic nerve function must first be assessed to determine the presence or absence of a response, and if response is present, to determine the phrenic nerve conduction time. In adults (age range: 18 to 74 years), mean onset latency is 7.5 ± 0.6 milliseconds with an upper limit of 9.0 milliseconds (191,192). Successful pacing in adults has been achieved with mild prolongation of conduction velocity up to 14 milliseconds. Other indicators of adequate phrenic nerve function include diaphragm descent of at least 3 to 4 cm during supramaximal tetanic stimulation and transdiaphragmatic pressures of approximately 10 cm H_2O with a single shock stimulation to either phrenic nerve.

Candidates for phrenic nerve pacing must be free of significant lung disease or primary muscle disease because factors may preclude successful pacing. Implantation of the device requires a major surgical procedure with associated potential complications. Therefore, patients must be carefully screened. Following careful evaluation, some patients with sufficient inspiratory muscle strength may be better suited for noninvasive means of ventilatory assistance. In these patients, intermittent mouth-positive pressure ventilation may be an effective alternative to conventional mechanical ventilation.

TABLE 66-2. Technical Features of Phrenic Nerve Stimulation Systems

Device/Manufacturer	Avery Laboratories Inc., USA		Atrotech OY, Finland	Medimplant Inc., Austria
Transmitter (stimulus generator)	S-232G	Mark IV	PX 244	Medimplant 8-channel stimulator
Size (mm)	179 × 114 × 97	146 ×140 × 25	185 × 88 × 28	170 × 130 × 51
Transmitter/battery weight (kg)	3.6	0.54	0.45 + 0.6 (12V) 0.45 + 0.045 (9V)	1.42
Rate (breaths/min)	10–50	6–24	8–35	5–60
Pulse width (μs)	150	150	200	100–1000
Battery life (hr)	160	400	160–320 (12V) 8 (9V)	24
Sigh possible	yes	yes	yes	yes
Antenna	902A	902A	TC 27-250/80	RF transmission coil
Receiver	Model I-170A	Model I-110A	RX 44-27-2	implantable receiver
Size (mm)	46 (diam) × 16	30 (diam) × 8	49 (diam) × 8.5	56 × 53 × 14
Electrodes	Monopolar, bipolar	Monopolar, bipolar	Quadripolar	Quadripolar
No. of receivers to stimulate both hemidiaphragms	2	2	2	1

Patient psychosocial conditions are also important considerations in assessing the potential success of phrenic nerve pacing. Before any technical assessment, therefore, a critical evaluation of the motivation of both the patient and family members is mandatory. Phrenic nerve pacing is most likely to be successful in home situations in which the patient and family members are anxious to improve the overall health, mobility, social interaction, and occupational potential of the patient. The patient should also have a clear understanding of the potential benefits to be achieved.

Surgical Implantation

Electrodes may be positioned around the phrenic nerve in either the cervical region or within the thorax (180,182,193). The thoracic approach requires a thoracotomy, which has significant associated risks including hemothorax and pneumothorax, and which requires chest tube placement and intensive postoperative care. The cervical approach is limited by potential lack of excitation of the entire nerve (nerve to branches which join the nerve in the thoracic region), activation of other nerves, and risk of mechanical stress resulting from movement of the neck. The thoracic approach, therefore, is the preferred method of electrode placement (194,195). Although there are a number of acceptable surgical approaches for thoracic electrode placement, the second intercostal space is most commonly used (193,196). It is critical that the phrenic nerves are manipulated with extreme care to avoid mechanical trauma to the nerve and its blood supply. A radiofrequency receiver is positioned in a subcutaneous pocket on the anterior chest wall; wires from the electrode are passed through the third or fourth interspace and connected to the receiver.

The pacing system should be tested prior to closure of the surgical incisions. Threshold currents of each electrode should be determined by gradually increasing stimulus amplitude until a diaphragm twitch is observed. Threshold current should range between 0.1 and 2.0 mA. Suprathreshold current should result in a forceful, smooth diaphragm contraction. If threshold values are high or the difference between the lowest and highest thresholds exceeds 1 mA, the electrode leads may need to be repositioned around the phrenic nerve. We prefer to place the receivers over the lower anterior rib cage just above the costal margin. In thin people, however, the anterior abdominal wall may be preferable to avoid pressure injury. The receivers in the Avery and Atrotech systems, both of which require two receivers, should be placed at least 15 cm apart.

Pacing Schedules

Phrenic nerve pacing is usually initiated about 2 weeks after surgery to allow adequate time for all surgical wounds to begin healing and for inflammation and edema around the electrode site to resolve (196). The diaphragm must be gradually reconditioned to improve strength and endurance. During the initial trials of phrenic nerve pacing, minute ventilation necessary to maintain normal values of P_{CO_2} (35 to 45 mm Hg) over 5- to 10-minute periods should be determined. Respiratory rate is usually set at 8 to 12 breaths per minute; tidal volume is adjusted by altering stimulation frequency to maintain the desired level of ventilation.

General recommendations to initiate pacing are to provide phrenic nerve pacing for 10 to 15 minutes each hour initially and to increase this gradually, as tolerated. Although the conditioning phase may take 8 to 10 weeks or longer, it is possible to bring some patients up to full-time support within 4 weeks. After full-time pacing is achieved during waking hours, pacing is provided during sleep and gradually increased until full-time pacing is achieved. During the conditioning phase, the patient must be carefully monitored for signs of fatigue, which is usually manifested by the patient's complaint of shortness of breath or reduction in inspired volume. Higher levels of stimulation may be required in the sitting compared to supine posture as a result of shorter diaphragm length during sitting. This can be alleviated to a significant degree, however, by the use of a snug-fitting abdominal binder, which reduces the change in abdominal girth.

Complications

While a number of complications have been reported since phrenic nerve pacing was first introduced, technical developments and patient experience have markedly reduced their incidence (187,197). With careful patient selection, appropriate use of stimulus parameters, adequate patient monitoring, and involvement of experienced professionals, the incidence of complications should be very low. Nonetheless, complications do arise and appropriate precautions must be taken and remedial action instituted promptly, when necessary. All patients require a backup mechanical ventilator in the event of pacemaker failure.

There are several factors that may result in insufficient ventilatory support during diaphragmatic pacing. Low battery charge is one of the most common causes of failure, which is easily prevented by regular battery changes or recharging schedules. Breakage of antenna wires at connection points is also a common cause of failure. Receiver failure was a common occurrence with older systems but is much less common with current systems due to improvement in housing materials. Iatrogenic injury to the phrenic nerve may occur during implantation, but can be prevented by meticulous dissection technique. After implantation, adverse tissue reaction and scar tissue formation can lead to gradual reduction in inspired volume and may require surgical intervention. A more serious, but fortunately less common, complication is the development of infection of the implanted materials, which necessitates removal of all implanted components (188,193,198). Diaphragm contraction without coincident contraction of the upper airway muscles results in collapse of the upper airway or obstructive apneas. This complication is completely preventable by maintaining a patent tracheostomy, especially nocturnally when risk is the highest.

In children, paradoxical motion of the rib cage may be substantial due to its high compliance, resulting in reduced inspired volume generation. Because compliance gradually decreases between 10 and 15 years of age, the performance of the pacing system can be expected to improve over time (197). Because the diaphragm has a very small percentage of type I, fatigue-resistant fibers in small children, a much longer period of conditioning may be required to achieve full-time ventilatory support compared to adults (182).

Patient Outcomes

Phrenic nerve pacing is clearly an effective means of providing ventilatory support with significant advantages over mechanical ventilation (180–182). However, earlier analyses of large patient groups describe significant numbers of individuals in whom successful ventilatory support could not be achieved. In one retrospective analysis, about half of the patients who were deemed failures should not have been selected for phrenic nerve pacing. It is also important to note that this study and others were performed at a time when the technology of phrenic nerve pacing and methods of patient-selection were not fully developed. Unfortunately, there are few recent analyses of modern-day success rates and incidence of side effects and complications. Long-term follow-up of 14 tetraplegic patients who used bilateral low-frequency stimulation recorded using the device successfully for as long as 15 years with a mean use of 7.6 years (197).

When applied in appropriate candidates, there is some evidence that improved electrode and receiver design is associated with a low incidence of pacer malfunction and high success rates. The outcome of 64 patients (45 tetraplegic patients) who underwent phrenic nerve pacing with the Atrotech system since 1990 was recently evaluated (198). The duration of pacing averaged 2 years. The incidence of electrode and receiver failure was quite low at 3.1% and 5.9%, respectively. These values are lower than those previously reported with monopolar and bipolar systems. In this group, four patients developed infections, but none occurred in the tetraplegic group. In order to determine the actual success rate of this technique, ongoing analyses, perhaps in the form of an international registry, are badly needed. The true incidence of side effects and complications could then also be determined.

Although there are no controlled studies, it is conceivable that phrenic nerve pacing may improve life expectancy in patients with tetraplegia. Carter reported only 63% survival at 9 years in patients on positive-pressure ventilation (176). In contrast, all 12 tetraplegic patients who completed the Yale phrenic nerve pacing protocol were alive after 9 years. It is possible that mechanical ventilation is associated with a higher incidence of respiratory infections and mechanical problems related to the mechanical ventilator, tubing, and tracheostomy.

Future Directions

Phrenic pacing can provide important health and lifestyle benefits compared to mechanical ventilation (184,199,200). However, existing systems continue to have limitations and require further refinement. For example, many patients with ventilator-dependent tetraplegia cannot be offered phrenic nerve pacing due to partial or complete injury of one of the phrenic nerves. Combined intercostal and unilateral diaphragm pacing may be a useful therapeutic modality in selected patients with only unilateral phrenic nerve function (Fig. 66-6) (201–204). Conventional placement of phrenic nerve electrodes carries the risk of phrenic nerve injury and generally requires a thoraco-

tomy, which is a major surgical procedure with associated risk, inpatient hospital stay, and high cost. Preliminary results suggest that intramuscular diaphragm pacing can provide similar benefits as conventional phrenic nerve pacing without the need for an invasive surgical procedure and less risk of phrenic nerve injury (205). The laparoscopy-guided procedure can be performed on an outpatient basis and therefore at much lower overall cost. The development of a fully implantable system would eliminate the need for the application of devices on the body surface and the risk of decoupling between the transmitter and receiver.

CONCLUSIONS

The principal goal of rehabilitation management of persons with upper motor neuron paralysis is to maximize quality of life. While quality of life is clearly influenced by a wide range of variables including social, emotional, psychological, vocational, and educational factors, the persistent neurological impairment after injury to the central motor system remains a powerful reminder and determinant of one's ability to function in society. FNS systems bypass the injured central circuitry to activate neural tissue and contract muscles to provide function to what is otherwise a nonfunctioning limb or structure. Recent advances in clinical medicine and biomedical engineering have made the clinical implementation of FNS systems to enhance the mobility and function of the paralyzed person more feasible. Hand neuroprosthesis systems can significantly enhance the upper extremity ADLs of persons with tetraplegia. The application of this technology for persons with hemiplegia is in its infancy and must await further technical and scientific developments if it is to be applicable to the broader stroke population. However, the use of FNS for treatment of shoulder subluxation and pain in hemiplegia is ready for large scale multicenter clinical trials to confirm clinical efficacy. Several lower extremity systems with and without bracing are being investigated for the purpose of functional transfers and standing, and to a lesser degree for ambulation for patients with paraplegia. While multichannel FNS systems for hemiplegia are still under development, the foot-drop stimulator is ready for large-scale multicenter clinical trials. The bladder FNS system can provide catheter-free micturation for persons with either paraplegia or tetraplegia. Finally, phrenic pacing systems can provide artificial ventilatory support for patients with ventilator-dependent tetraplegia.

After decades of development, the clinical use of FNS systems is finally becoming realized. However, in view of the dynamic nature of the present health care environment, the future of FNS technology is still difficult to predict. By necessity, scientists and clinicians must continue to explore new ideas and improve upon the present systems. Components will be smaller, more durable, and more reliable. The issues of cosmesis and ease of donning and doffing will require systems to be fully implantable. Control issues will remain central, and the implementation of cortical control will dictate the nature of future generations of FNS systems. Future developments will be directed by consumers. In the present health care environment where cost has become an overwhelming factor in the development and implementation of new technology, the consumer will become one of technology's greatest advocates. Finally, the usual drive toward greater complexity will be tempered by the practical issues of clinical implementation where patient and clinician acceptances are often a function of a tenuous balance between the "burden of cost" associated with using a system and the system's impact on the user's life.

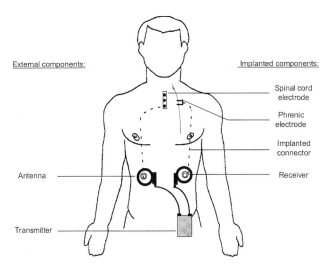

Figure 66-6. Combined intercostals and diaphragm pacing system.

ACKNOWLEDGMENTS

This work was supported in part by grants from the National Center for Medical Rehabilitation Research of the National Institutes of Child Health and Human Development, the Neuroprosthesis Program of the National Institutes of Neurological Diseases and Strokes, the Food and Drug Administration, and the Veterans Affairs Functional Electrical Stimulation Center of Excellence.

CONFLICT OF INTEREST

Dr. Chae serves as a consultant to NeuroControl Corporation, which has a direct financial interest in the subject matter and materials discussed in this chapter.

REFERENCES

1. McNeal R. Analysis of a model for excitation of myelinated nerve. *IEEE Trans Biomed Eng* 1976;23:329–337.
2. Mortimer JT. Motor prostheses. In: Brookhart JM, Mountcastle VB, eds. *Handbook of physiology—the nervous system II*. Bethesda, MD: American Physiological Society, 1981:155–187.
3. Henneman E. Relation between size of neurons and their susceptibility to discharge. *Science* 1957;126:1345–1347.
4. Burke RE. Motor units: anatomy, physiology, and functional organization. In: Brookhart JM, Mountcastle VB, eds. *Handbook of physiology—the nervous system II*. Bethesda, MD: American Physiological Society, 1981:345–422.
5. Sweeney JD. Skeletal muscle response to electrical stimulation. In: Reilly JP, ed. *Electrical stimulation and electropathology*. New York: Cambridge University Press, 1992:391–398.
6. Riley DA, Allin EF. The effects of inactivity, programmed stimulation, and denervation of the histochemistry of skeletal muscle fiber types. *Exp Neurol* 1973;40:391–398.
7. Peckham PH, Mortimer JT, Marsolais EB. Alteration in the force and fatigability of skeletal muscle in quadriplegic humans following exercise induced by chronic electrical stimulation. *Clin Orthop* 1976;114:326–334.
8. Marsolais E, Kobetic R. Functional walking in paralyzed patients by means of electrical stimulation. *Clin Orthop* 1983;175:30–36.
9. Kagaya H, Shimada Y, Sato K, et al. Changes in muscle force following therapeutic electrical stimulation in patients with complete paraplegia. *Paraplegia* 1996;34:24–29.
10. Grandjean PA, Mortimer JT. Recruitment properties of monopolar and bipolar epimysial electrodes. *Ann Biomed Eng* 1986;14:53–66.
11. Kilgore KL, Peckham PH, Keith MW, et al. Electrode characterization for functional application to upper extremity FNS. *IEEE Trans Biomed Eng* 1990;37:12–21.
12. Keith MW, Peckham PH, Thrope GB, et al. Implantable functional neuromuscular stimulation in the tetraplegic hand. *J Hand Surg [Am]* 1989;14:524–530.
13. Naples GG, Mortimer JT, Scheiner A, et al. A spiral nerve cuff electrode for peripheral nerve stimulation [see Comments]. *IEEE Trans Biomed Eng* 1988;35:905–916.
14. Glenn WWL, Phelps ML. Diaphragm pacing by electrical stimulation of the phrenic nerve. *Neurosurgery* 1985;14:53–66.
15. Kim JH, Manuelidis EE, Glen WW, et al. Diaphragm pacing: histopathological changes in the phrenic nerve following long-term electrical stimulation. *J Thorac Cardiovasc Surg* 1976;72:602–608.
16. Waters R, McNeal D, Faloon W, et al. Functional electrical stimulation of peroneal nerve for hemiplegia. *J Bone Joint Surg* 1985;67:792–793.
17. Kilgore KL, Peckham PH, Keith MW, et al. An implanted upper-extremity neuroprosthesis. Follow-up of five patients. *J Bone Joint Surg Am* 1997;79:533–541.
18. Benton LA, Baker LL, Bowman BR, et al. *Functional electrical stimulation: a practical clinical guide*. Downey, CA: Ranchos Los Amigos Medical Center, 1981.
19. Bajd T, Kralj A, Turk R, et al. The use of a four channel electrical stimulator as an ambulatory aid for paraplegic patients. *Phys Ther* 1983;63:1116–1120.
20. Graupe D, Kohn K. *Functional electrical stimulation for ambulation by paraplegics*. Malabar, FL: Krieger Publishing Co, 1994.
21. Gallien P, Brissot R, Eyssette M, et al. Restoration of gait by functional electrical stimulation for spinal cord injured patients. *Paraplegia* 1995;33:660–664.
22. Handa Y, Hoshimiya N, Iguchi Y, et al. Development of percutaneous intramuscular electrode for multichannel FES system. *IEEE Trans Biomed Eng* 1989;36:706–710.
23. Memberg W, Peckham PH, Keith MH. A surgically implanted intramuscular electrode for an implantable neuromuscular stimulation system. *IEEE Trans Rehabil Eng* 1994;2:80–91.
24. Scheiner A, Polando G, Marsolais EB. Design and clinical application of a double helix electrode for functional electrical stimulation. *IEEE Trans Biomed Eng* 1994;41:425–431.
25. Waters RL, Campbell JM, Nakai R. Therapeutic electrical stimulation of the lower limb by epimysial electrodes. *Clin Orthop* 1988:44–52.
26. Holle J, Frey M, Gruber H, et al. Functional electrostimulation of paraplegics. Experimental investigations and first clinical experience with an implantable stimulation device. *Orthopaedics* 1984;7:1145–1160.
27. Haugland MK, Hoffer JA, Sinkjaer T. Skin contact force information in sensory nerve signals recorded by implanted cuff electrodes. *IEEE Trans Rehabil Eng* 1994;2:18–28.
28. Memberg WD, Peckham PH, Thorpe GB, et al. An analysis of the reliability of percutaneous intramuscular electrodes in upper extremity FNS applications. *IEEE Trans Rehabil Eng* 1993;1:126–132.
29. Smith BT, Betz RR, Mulcahey MJ, et al. Reliability of percutaneous intramuscular electrodes for upper extremity functional neuromuscular stimulation in adolescents with C5 tetraplegia. *Arch Phys Med Rehabil* 1994;75:939–945.
30. Letechipia JE, Peckham PH, Gazdik M, et al. In-line lead connector for use with implanted neuroprosthesis. *IEEE Trans Biomed Eng* 1991;38:707–709.
31. Handa Y, Hoshimiya N. Functional electrical stimulation for the control of the upper extremities. *Med Prog Technol* 1987;12:51–63.
32. Nathan RH, Ohry A. Upper limb functions regained in quadriplegia: a hybrid computerized FNS system. *Arch Phys Med Rehabil* 1990;71:415–421.
33. Snoek GJ, Ijzerman MJ, in't Groen FA, et al. Use of the NESS Handmaster to restore hand function in tetraplegia. *Spinal Cord* 2000;38:244–249.
34. Peckham PH, Keith MW. Motor prostheses for restoration of upper extremity function. In: Stein RB, Peckham PH, Popovic DB, eds. *Neural prostheses: replacing motor function after disease or disability*. New York: Oxford University Press, 1992:162–190.
35. Keith MW, Kilgore KL, Peckham PH, et al. Tendon transfers and functional electrical stimulation for restoration of hand function in spinal cord injury. *J Hand Surg [Am]* 1996;21:89–99.
36. Buckett JR, Peckham PH, Thrope GB, et al. A flexible, portable system for neuromuscular stimulation in the paralyzed upper extremity. *IEEE Trans Biomed Eng* 1988;35:897–904.
37. Johnson MW, Peckham PH. Evaluation of shoulder movement as a command control source. *IEEE Trans Biomed Eng* 1990;37:876–885.
38. Perkins TA, Brindley GS, Donaldson ND, et al. Implant provision of key, pinch and power grips in a C6 tetraplegic. *Med Biol Eng Comput* 1994;32:367–372.
39. Scott TR, Peckham PH, Keith MW. Upper extremity neuroprostheses using functional electrical stimulation. In: Brindley GS, Rushton DN, eds. *Baillieres clinical neurology*. Vol 4. London: Bailliere Tindall, 1995:57–75.
40. Hart RL, Kilgore KL, Peckham PH. A comparison between control methods for implanted FES hand-grasp systems. *IEEE Trans Rehabil Eng* 1998;6:208–218.
41. Vodovnik L, Long C, Reswick JB, et al. Myo-electric control of paralyzed muscles. *IEEE Trans Biomed Eng* 1965;12:169–172.
42. Peckham PH, Mortimer JT, Marsolais EB. Controlled prehension and release in the C5 quadriplegic elicited by functional electrical stimulation of the paralyzed forearm musculature. *Ann Biomed Eng* 1980;8:369–388.
43. Saxena S, Nikolic S, Popovic D. An EMG-controlled grasping system for tetraplegics. *J Rehabil Res Dev* 1995;32:17–24.
44. Solomonow M, Barrata R, Shoji H, et al. The myoelectric signal of electrically stimulated muscle during recruitment: an inherent feedback parameter for a closed-loop control scheme. *IEEE Trans Biomed Eng* 1986;33:735–745.
45. Hoshimiya N, Naito A, Yajima M, et al. A multichannel FES system for the restoration of motor functions in high spinal cord injury patients: a respiration-controlled system for multijoint upper extremity. *IEEE Trans Biomed Eng* 1989;36:754–760.
46. Handa Y, Handa T, Nakatsuchi Y, et al. [A voice-controlled functional electrical stimulation system for the paralyzed hand]. *Iyodenshi To Seitai Kogaku* 1985;23:292–298.
47. Triolo R, Nathan R, Handa Y, et al. Challenges to clinical deployment of upper limb neuroprostheses. *J Rehabil Res Dev* 1996;33:111–122.
48. Popovic D, Stojanovic A, Pjanovic A, et al. Clinical evaluation of the bionic glove. *Arch Phys Med Rehabil* 1999;80:299–304.
49. Handa Y, Handa T, Ichie M, et al. Functional electrical stimulation (FES) systems for restoration of motor function of paralyzed muscles—versatile systems and a portable system. *Front Med Biol Eng* 1992;4:241–255.
50. Peckham PH, Mortimer JT. Restoration of hand function in the quadriplegic through electrical stimulation. In: Reswick JB, Hambrecht FT, eds. *Functional electrical stimulation: applications in neural prosthesis*. New York: Marcel Dekker, Inc, 1977:83–95.
51. Peckham PH, Marsolais EB, Mortimer JT. Restoration of key grip and release in the C6 tetraplegic patient through functional electrical stimulation. *J Hand Surg [Am]* 1980;5:462–469.
52. Smith B, Peckham PH, Keith MW, et al. An externally powered, multichannel implantable stimulator for versatile control of paralyzed muscle. *IEEE Trans Biomed Eng* 1987;34:499–508.
53. Peckham PH, Keith MW, Kilgore KL, et al. Efficacy of an implanted neuroprosthesis for restoring hand grasp in tetraplegia: a multicenter study. *Arch Phys Med Rehabil* 2001;82:1380–1388.

54. Wuolle KS, Van Doren CL, Thrope GB, et al. Development of a quantitative hand grasp and release test for patients with tetraplegia using a hand neuroprosthesis. *J Hand Surg [Am]* 1994;19:209–218.

55. Smith BT, Mulcahey MJ, Betz RR. Quantitative comparison of grasp and release abilities with and without functional neuromuscular stimulation in adolescents with tetraplegia. *Paraplegia* 1996;34:16–23.

56. Wuolle KS, Van Doren CL, Bryden AM, et al. Satisfaction and usage of a hand neuroprosthesis. *Arch Phys Med Rehabil* 1999;80:206–213.

57. Grill JH, Peckham PH. Functional neuromuscular stimulation for combined control of elbow extension and hand grasp in C5 and C6 quadriplegics. *IEEE Trans Rehabil Eng* 1998;6:190–199.

58. Bryden AM, Memberg WD, Crago PE. Electrically stimulated elbow extension in persons with C5/C6 tetraplegia: a functional and physiological evaluation. *Arch Phys Med Rehabil* 2000;81:80–88.

59. Crago PE, Memberg WD, Usey MK, et al. An elbow extension neuroprosthesis for individuals with tetraplegia. *IEEE Trans Rehabil Eng* 1998;6:1–6.

60. Lemay MA, Crago PE, Keith MW. Restoration of pronosupination control by FNS in tetraplegia—experimental and biomechanical evaluation of feasibility. *J Biomech* 1996;29:435–442.

61. Lauer RT, Peckham PH, Kilgore KL. EEG-based control of a hand grasp neuroprosthesis. *Neuroreport* 1999;10:1767–1771.

62. Johnson MW, Peckham PH, Bhadra N, et al. Implantable transducer for two-degree of freedom joint angle sensing. *IEEE Trans Rehabil Eng* 1999;7:349–359.

63. Smith B, Tang Z, Johnson MW, et al. An externally powered, multichannel, implantable stimulator-telemeter for control of paralyzed muscle. *IEEE Trans Biomed Eng* 1998;45:463–475.

64. Grill WM, Jr., Mortimer JT. Quantification of recruitment properties of multiple contact cuff electrodes. *IEEE Trans Rehabil Eng* 1996;4:49–62.

65. Loeb GE, Zamin CJ, Schulman JH, et al. Indictable microstimulator for functional electrical stimulation. *Med Biol Eng* 1991;29:NS13–NS19.

66. Peckham PH, Kilgore KL, Keith MW, et al. An advanced neuroprosthesis for restoration of hand and upper arm control using an implantable controller. *J Hand Surg [Am]* 2002;27:265–276.

67. Betz RR, Mulcahey MJ, Smith BT, et al. Bipolar latissimus dorsi transposition and functional neuromuscular stimulation to restore elbow flexion in an individual with C4 quadriplegia and C5 denervation. *J Am Paraplegia Soc* 1992;15:220–228.

68. Van Ouwenaller C, Laplace PM, Chantraine A. Painful shoulder in hemiplegia. *Arch Phys Med Rehabil* 1986;67:23–26.

69. Pinzur MS, Hopkins GE. Biceps tenodesis for painful inferior subluxation of the shoulder in adult acquired hemiplegia. *Clin Orthop* 1986;206:100–103.

70. Dursun E, Dursun N, Ural CE, et al. Glenohumeral joint subluxation and reflex sympathetic dystrophy in hemiplegic patients. *Arch Phys Med Rehabil* 2000;81:944–946.

71. Chaco J, Wolf E. Subluxation of the glenohumeral joint in hemiplegia. *Am J Phys Med Rehabil* 1971;50:139–143.

72. Zorowitz RD, Hughes MB, Idank D, et al. Shoulder pain and subluxation after stroke: correlation or coincidence? *Am J Occup Ther* 1996;50:194–201.

73. Baker LL, Parker K. Neuromuscular electrical stimulation of the muscles surrounding the shoulder. *Phys Ther* 1986;66:1930–1937.

74. Chantraine A, Baribeault A, Uebelhart D, et al. Shoulder pain and dysfunction in hemiplegia: effects of functional electrical stimulation. *Arch Phys Med Rehabil* 1999;80:328–331.

75. Wang RY, Yang YR, Tsai MW, et al. Effects of functional electric stimulation on upper limb motor function and shoulder range of motion in hemiplegic patients. *Am J Phys Med Rehabil* 2002;81:283–290.

76. Linn SL, Granat MH, Lees KR. Prevention of shoulder subluxation after stroke with electrical stimulation. *Stroke* 1999;30:963–968.

77. Faghri PD, Rodgers MM, Glaser RM, et al. The effects of functional electrical stimulation on shoulder subluxation, arm function recovery, and shoulder pain in hemiplegic stroke patients. *Arch Phys Med Rehabil* 1994;75:73–79.

78. Yu DT, Chae J, Walker ME, et al. Comparing stimulation-induced pain during percutaneous (intramuscular) and transcutaneous neuromuscular electric stimulation for treating shoulder subluxation in hemiplegia. *Arch Phys Med Rehabil* 2001;82:756–760.

79. Yu DT, Chae J, Walker ME, et al. Percutaneous intramuscular neuromuscular electric stimulation for the treatment of shoulder subluxation and pain in patients with chronic hemiplegia: a pilot study. *Arch Phys Med Rehabil* 2001; 82:20–25.

80. Chae J, Yu D, Walker M. Percutaneous, intramuscular neuromuscular electrical stimulation for the treatment of shoulder subluxation and pain in chronic hemiplegia: a case report. *Am J Phys Med Rehabil* 2001;80:296–301.

81. Dupont A-C, Bagg SD, Creasey JL, et al. Clinical trials of BION Injectable neuromuscular stimulators. Paper presented at: 6th Annual Conference of the International Functional Electrical Stimulation Society; June 16–20, 2001; Cleveland, OH.

82. Rebersek S, Vodovnik L. Proportionally controlled functional electrical stimulation of hand. *Arch Phys Med Rehabil* 1973;54:378–382.

83. Merletti R, Acimovic R, Grobelnik S, et al. Electrophysiologic orthosis for the upper extremity in hemiplegia: feasibility study. *Arch Phys Med Rehabil* 1975;56:507–513.

84. Chae J, Kilgore K, Triolo R, et al. Neuromuscular stimulation for motor neuroprosthesis in hemiplegia. *Crit Rev Phys Rehabil Med* 2000;12:1–23.

85. Cameron T, McDonald K, Anderson L, et al. The effect of wrist angle on electrically evoked hand opening in patients with spastic hemiplegia. *IEEE Trans Rehab Eng* 1999;7:109–111.

86. Hines AE, Crago PE, Billian B. Hand opening by electrical stimulation in patients with spastic hemiplegia. *IEEE Trans Rehabil Eng* 1995;3:193–205.

87. Sweeney JD, Mortimer JT. An asymmetric two electrode cuff for generation of unidirectionally propagated action potentials. *IEEE Trans Biomed Eng* 1986;33:541–549.

88. Sweeney JD, Mortimer JT, Bodner DR. Acute animal studies on electrically induced collision block of pudendal nerve motor activity. *Neurol Urodyn* 1989;8:521–536.

89. Rijkhoff NJ, Hendrikx LB, van Kerrebroeck PE, et al. Selective detrusor activation by electrical stimulation of the human sacral nerve roots. *Artif Organs* 1997;21:223–226.

90. Grill WM, Mortimer JT. Inversion of the current-distance relationship by transient depolarization. *IEEE Trans Biomed Eng* 1997;44:1–9.

91. Au AT, Kirsch RF. EMG-based prediction of shoulder and elbow kinematics in able-bodied and spinal cord injured individuals. *IEEE Trans Rehabil Eng* 2000;8:471–480.

92. Marsolais EB, Kobetic R. Functional electrical stimulation for walking in paraplegia. *J Bone Joint Surg [Am]* 1987;69:728–733.

93. Kralj A, Bajd T. *Functional electrical stimulation: standing and walking after spinal cord injury.* Boca Raton, FL: CRC Press, 1989.

94. Jaeger RJ. Lower extremity applications of functional neuromuscular stimulation. *Assist Technol* 1992;4:19–30.

95. Triolo RJ, Reilley B, Freedman W, et al. Development and standardization of a clinical evaluation of standing function. *IEEE Trans Rehab Eng* 1993;1: 18–25.

96. Moynahan M, Mullin C, Cohn J, et al. Home use of a functional electrical stimulation system for standing and mobility in adolescents with spinal cord injury. *Arch Phys Med Rehabil* 1996;77:1005–1013.

97. Davis JA, Triolo RJ, Uhlir C, et al. Performance of a surgically implanted neuroprosthesis for standing and transfers. In: *Proceedings of the 5th Annual Conference of the International Functional Electrical Stimulation Society Meeting.* Aalborg, Denmark, 2000.

98. Jaeger RJ, Yarkony GM, Smith RM. Standing the spinal cord injured patient by electrical stimulation: refinement of a protocol for clinical use. *IEEE Trans Biomed Eng* 1989;36:720–728.

99. Yarkony GM, Jaeger RJ, Roth E, et al. Functional neuromuscular stimulation for standing after spinal cord injury. *Arch Phys Med Rehabil* 1990;71:201–206.

100. Kobetic R, Marsolais EB. Synthesis of paraplegic gait with multichannel functional neuromuscular stimulation. *IEEE Trans Biomed Eng* 1994;2:66–67.

101. Triolo RJ, Bieri C, Uhlir J, et al. Implanted FNS systems for assisted standing and transfers for individuals with cervical spinal cord injuries. *Arch Phys Med Rehabil* 1996;7:1119–1128.

102. Marsolais EB, Kobetic R. Implantation technique and experience with percutaneous intramuscular electrodes in the lower extremities. *J Rehab R D* 1986;23:1–8.

103. Davis R, Eckhouse R, Patrick JF, et al. Computer-controlled 22-channel stimulator for limb movement. *Acta Neurochirurgica* 1987;39S:117–120.

104. Donaldson N, Rushton D, Tromans T. Neuroprostheses for leg function after spinal cord injury. *Lancet* 1997;350:711.

105. Sharma M, Marsolais EB, Polando G, et al. Implantation of a 16-channel functional electrical stimulation walking system. *Clin Orthop* 1998:236–242.

106. Kobetic R, Triolo RJ, Uhlir JP, et al. Implanted functional electrical stimulation system for mobility in paraplegia: a follow-up case report. *IEEE Trans Rehabil Eng* 1999;7:390–398.

107. Triolo RJ, Bogie K. Lower extremity applications of functional neuromuscular stimulation after spinal cord injury. *Topics in SCI Rehab* 1999;5:44–65.

108. Davis JA, Triolo RJ, Uhlir JP, et al. Clinical performance of a surgically implanted neuroprostheses for exercise, standing, transfers and upright mobility. *J Spinal Cord Med* 2000;23:3(abst).

109. Uhlir JP. Performance of implanted epimysial electrodes in the lower extremities of individuals with spinal cord injury. Paper presented at: 2nd National Meeting VA Rehabilitation Research and Development; 2000; Washington, DC.

110. Bieri C, Triolo RJ, Danford GS, et al. A functional performance measure for effort and assistance required for sit-to-stand and standing pivot transfer maneuvers. *J Spinal Cord Injury Medicine* 2000;23:4(abst).

111. Triolo R, Wibowo M, Uhlir J, et al. Effects of stimulated hip extension moment and position on upper-limb support forces during FNS-induced standing—a technical note. *J Rehabil Res Dev* 2001;38:545–555.

112. Miller P, Kobetic R, Lew R. Energy costs of walking and standing using functional electrical stimulation. In: *Proceedings of the 13th Annual RESNA Conference.* Washington DC, 1990.

113. Glaser RM. Physiologic aspects of spinal cord injury and functional neuromuscular stimulation. *Central Nervous System Trauma* 1986;3:49–61.

114. Bajd T, Kralj A, Turk R. Standing up of a healthy subject and a paraplegic patient. *J Biomech* 1982;15:1–10.

115. Bajd T, Kralj A, Stefancic M, et al. Use of functional electrical stimulation in the lower extremities of incomplete spinal cord injured patients. *Artif Organs* 1999;23:403–409.

116. Kralj A, Bajd T, Kvesic Z, et al. Electrical stimulation of incomplete paraplegic patients. In: *Proceedings of the 4th Annual RESNA Conference.* Washington DC, 1981.

117. Granat MH, Ferguson AC, Andrews BJ, et al. The role of functional electrical stimulation in the rehabilitation of patients with incomplete spinal cord injury—observed benefits during gait studies. *Paraplegia* 1993;31:207–215.

118. Kobetic R, Marsolais EB, Samane P, et al. The next step: artificial walking. In: Rose J, Ganble JG, eds. *Human walking*. Baltimore: Williams & Wilkins, 1994: 225–252.

119. Solomonow M, Baratta RV, Hirokawa S. The RGO generation II: muscle stimulation powered orthosis as a practical walking system for paraplegics. *Orthopaedics* 1989;12:1309–1315.

120. Solomonow M. Biomechanics and physiology of a practical functional neuromuscular stimulation powered walking orthosis for paraplegics. In: Stein RB, Peckham PH, Popovic DP, eds. *Neural prostheses: replacing motor function after disease or disability*. New York: Oxford University Press, 1992:202–232.

121. Marsolais EB, Kobetic R, Chizeck HJ, et al. Orthoses and electrical stimulation for walking in complete paraplegics. *J Neuro Rehabil* 1991;5:13–22.

122. Kantor C, Andrews BJ, Marsolais EB, et al. Report on a conference on motor prostheses for workplace mobility of paraplegic patients in North America. *Paraplegia* 1993;31:439–456.

123. McClelland R, Andrews BJ, Patrick JH, et al. Augmentation of the Oswestry Parawalker orthosis by means of surface electrical stimulation: gait analysis of three patients. *Paraplegia* 1987;25:32–38.

124. Franceschini M, Baratta S, Zampolini M, et al. Reciprocating gait orthosis: a multicenter study of their use by spinal cord injured patients. *Arch Phys Med Rehabil* 1997;78:582–586.

125. Solomonow M, Reisin E, Aguilar E, et al. Reciprocating gait orthosis powered with electrical muscle stimulation (RGO II). Part II: Medical evaluation of 70 paraplegic patients. *Orthopedics* 1997;20:411–418.

126. Winchester P, Carollo JJ, Habasevich R. Physiologic costs of reciprocal gait in FES assisted walking. *Paraplegia* 1994;32:680–686.

127. Graupe D, Kohn K. Clinical results and observations over 12 years of FES-based ambulation. In: *Functional electrical stimulation for ambulation by paraplegics*. Malabar, FL: Kreiger Publishing Co, 1994:136.

128. MacGregor J. The evaluation of patient performance using long-term ambulatory monitoring technique in the domiciliary environment. *Physiotherapy* 1981;67:30–33.

129. Rose J, Gamble JG, Medeiros JM. Energy cost of walking in normal children and those with cerebral palsy: comparison of heart rate and oxygen uptake. *J Pediatr Orthop* 1989;9:276–279.

130. Isakov E, Douglas R, Berns P. Ambulation using the reciprocating gait orthosis and functional electrical stimulation. *Paraplegia* 1992;30:239–245.

131. Bowker P, Messenger N, Ogilvie C, et al. Energetics of paraplegic walking. *J Biomed Eng* 1992;14:344–350.

132. Chaplin E. Functional neuromuscular stimulation for mobility in people with spinal cord injuries. The Parastep I System. *J Spinal Cord Med* 1996;19: 99–105.

133. Klose KJ, Jacobs PL, Broton JG, et al. Evaluation of training program for persons with SCI paraplegia using the Parastep 1 ambulation system: Part 1. Ambulation performance and anthropometric measures. *Arch Phys Med Rehabil* 1997;78:789–793.

134. Guest RS, Klose KJ, Needham-Shropshire BM, et al. Evaluation of a training program for persons with SCI paraplegia using the Parastep 1 ambulation system: part 4. Effect on physical self-concept and depression. *Arch Phys Med Rehabil* 1997;78:804–807.

135. Jacobs PL, Nash MS, Klose KJ, et al. Evaluation of a training program for persons with SCI paraplegia using the Parastep 1 ambulation system: part 2. Effects on physiological responses to peak arm ergometry. *Arch Phys Med Rehabil* 1997;78:794–798.

136. Nash MS, Jacobs PL, Montalveo BM, et al. Evaluation of a training program for persons with SCI paraplegia using the Parastep 1 ambulation system: Part 5. Lower extremity blood flow and hyperemic responses to occlusion are augmented by ambulation training. *Arch Phys Med Rehabil* 1997;78:806–814.

137. Hirokawa S, Grimm M, Le T, et al. Energy consumption in paraplegic ambulation using the reciprocating gait orthosis and electrical stimulation of the thigh muscles. *Arch Phys Med Rehabil* 1990;71:687–694.

138. Waters RL, Lunsford BR. Energy cost of paraplegic locomotion. *J Bone Joint Surg Am* 1985;67:1245–1250.

139. Lieberson W, Holmquest H, Scot D, et al. Functional electrotherapy: stimulation of the peroneal nerve synchronized with the swing phase of the gait of hemiplegia patients. *Arch Phys Med Rehabil* 1961;42:101–105.

140. Merletti R, Andina A, Galante M, et al. Clinical experience of electronic peroneal stimulators in 50 hemiparetic patients. *Scand J Rehabil Med* 1979;11: 111–121.

141. Granat MH, Maxwell DJ, Ferguson AC, et al. Peroneal stimulator; evaluation for the correction of spastic drop foot in hemiplegia. *Arch Phys Med Rehabil* 1996;77:19–24.

142. Takebe K, Kukulka C, Narayan M, et al. Peroneal nerve stimulator in rehabilitation of hemiplegic patients. *Arch Phys Med Rehabil* 1975;56:237–240.

143. Burridge JH, Taylor PN, Hagan SA, et al. The effects of common peroneal stimulation on the effort and speed of walking: a randomized controlled trial with chronic hemiplegic patients. *Clin Rehabil* 1997;11:201–210.

144. Waters R, McNeal D, Perry J. Experimental correction of footdrop by electrical stimulation of the peroneal nerve. *J Bone Joint Surg* 1975;57A:1047–1054.

145. Kljajic M, Malezic M, Acimovic R, et al. Gait evaluation in hemiparetic patients using subcutaneous peroneal electrical stimulation. *Scand J Rehabil Med* 1992;24:121–126.

146. Stanic U, Acimovic-Janezic R, Gros N, et al. Multichannel electrical stimulation for correction of hemiplegic gait. *Scand J Rehabil Med* 1978;10:75–92.

147. Bogataj U, Gros N, Malezic M, et al. Restoration of gait during two to three weeks of therapy with multichannel electrical stimulation. *Phys Ther* 1989; 69:319–327.

148. Bogataj U, Gros N, Kljajic M, et al. The rehabilitation of gait in patients with hemiplegia: a comparison between conventional therapy and multichannel functional electrical stimulation therapy. *Phys Ther* 1995;76:490–502.

149. Arnold EP, Gowland SP, MacFarlane MR, et al. Sacral anterior root stimulation of the bladder in paraplegia. *Aust N Z J Surg* 1986;56:319–324.

150. Brindley GS, Polkey CE, Rushton DN, et al. Sacral anterior root stimulators for bladder control in paraplegia: the first 50 cases. *J Neurol Neurosurg Psychiatry* 1986;49:1104–1114.

151. Robinson LQ, Grant A, Weston P, et al. Experience with the Brindley anterior sacral root stimulator. *Br J Urol* 1988;62:553–557.

152. Brindley GS, Rushton DN. Long-term follow-up of patients with sacral anterior root stimulator implants. *Paraplegia* 1990;28:469–475.

153. Madersbacher H, Fischer J. Sacral anterior root stimulation: prerequisites and indications. *Neurourol Urodyn* 1993;12:489–494.

154. Creasey GH. Electrical stimulation of sacral roots for micturition after spinal cord injury. *Urol Clin North Am* 1993;20:505–515.

155. Van Kerrebroeck PE, Koldewijn EL, Debruyne FM. Worldwide experience with the Finetech-Brindley sacral anterior root stimulator. *Neurourol Urodyn* 1993;12:497–503.

156. Brindley GS. The first 500 patients with sacral anterior root stimulator implants: general description. *Paraplegia* 1994;32:795–805.

157. Bosch JL, Groen J. Sacral (S3) segmental nerve stimulation as a treatment for urge incontinence in patients with detrusor instability: results of chronic electrical stimulation using an implantable neural prosthesis. *J Urol* 1995; 154:504–507.

158. Ishigooka M, Hashimoto T, Hayami S, et al. Electrical pelvic floor stimulation: a possible alternative treatment for reflex urinary incontinence in patients with spinal cord injury. *Spinal Cord* 1996;34:411–415.

159. Kirkham AP, Shah NC, Knight SL, et al. The acute effects of continuous and conditional neuromodulation on the bladder in spinal cord injury. *Spinal Cord* 2001;39:420–428.

160. Kirkham AP, Knight SL, Craggs MD, et al. Neuromodulation through sacral nerve roots 2 to 4 with a Finetech-Brindley sacral posterior and anterior root stimulator. *Spinal Cord* 2002;40:272–281.

161. van der Aa HE, Alleman E, Nene A, et al. Sacral anterior root stimulation for bladder control: clinical results. *Arch Physiol Biochem* 1999;107:248–256.

162. Madersbacher H, Fischer J, Ebner A. Anterior sacral root stimulator (Brindley): experience especially in women with neurogenic urinary incontinence. *Neurourol Urodyn* 1988;7:593–601.

163. Colombel P, Egon G. [Electrostimulation of the anterior sacral nerve roots]. *Ann Urol Paris* 1991;25:48–52.

164. Madersbacher H, Fischer J. Anterior sacral root stimulation and posterior sacral root rhizotomy. *Akt Urol* 1993;24[Suppl]:32–35.

165. Van Kerrebroeck PE, Koldewijn EL, Rosier PF, et al. Results of the treatment of neurogenic bladder dysfunction in spinal cord injury by sacral posterior root rhizotomy and anterior sacral root stimulation. *J Urol* 1996;155:1378–1381.

166. Egon G, Barat M, Colombel P, et al. Implantation of anterior sacral root stimulators combined with posterior sacral rhizotomy in spinal injury patients. *World J Urol* 1998;16:342–349.

167. MacDonagh RP, Forster DM, Thomas DG. Urinary continence in spinal injury patients following complete sacral posterior rhizotomy. *Br J Urol* 1990;66:618–622.

168. Van Kerrebroeck PEV, Kolewijn EL, Wijkstra H, et al. Urodynamic evaluation before and after intradural posterior sacral rhizotomies and implantation of the Finetech-Brindley anterior sacral root stimulator. *Urodinamica* 1992;1:7–12.

169. Cardozo L, Krishnan KR, Polkey CE, et al. Urodynamic observations on patients with sacral anterior root stimulators. *Paraplegia* 1984;22:201–209.

170. MacDonagh RP, Sun WM, Smallwood R, et al. Control of defecation in patients with spinal injuries by stimulation of sacral anterior nerve roots. *BMJ* 1990;300:1494–1497.

171. Wielink G, Essink-Bot ML, van Kerrebroeck PE, et al. Sacral rhizotomies and electrical bladder stimulation in spinal cord injury. 2. Cost-effectiveness and quality of life analysis. Dutch Study Group on Sacral Anterior Root Stimulation. *Eur Urol* 1997;31:441–446.

172. Creasey GH, Kilgore KL, Brown-Triolo DL, et al. Reduction of costs of disability using neuroprostheses. *Assist Technol* 2000;12:67–75.

173. Creasey GH, Dahlberg JE. Economic consequences of an implanted neuroprosthesis for bladder and bowel management. *Arch Phys Med Rehabil* 2001;82:1520–1525.

174. Rushton DN, Brindley GS, Polkey CE, et al. Implant infections and antibiotic-impregnated silicone rubber coating. *J Neurol Neurosurg Psychiatry* 1989; 52:223–229.

175. National Spinal Cord Injury Statistical Center, University of Alabama at Birmingham, Annual Statistical Report 1997. Birmingham: University of Alabama, 1997.

176. Carter RE, Donovan WH, Halstead L, et al. Comparative study of electrophrenic nerve stimulation and mechanical ventilatory support in traumatic spinal cord injury. *Paraplegia* 1987;25:86–91.

177. DeVivo MJ, Ivie CS 3rd. Life expectancy of ventilator-dependent persons with spinal cord injuries. *Chest* 1995;108:226–232.

178. Esclarin A, Bravo P, Arroyo O, et al. Tracheostomy ventilation versus diaphragmatic pacemaker ventilation in high spinal cord injury. *Paraplegia* 1994;32:687–693.
179. Whiteneck GG, Charlifue SW, Frankel HL, et al. Mortality, morbidity, and psychosocial outcomes of persons spinal cord injured more than 20 years ago. *Paraplegia* 1992;30:617–630.
180. Glenn WW, Hogan JF, Loke JS, et al. Ventilatory support by pacing of the conditioned diaphragm in quadriplegia. *N Engl J Med* 1984;310:1150–1155.
181. Glenn WW, Hogan JF, Phelps ML. Ventilatory support of the quadriplegic patient with respiratory paralysis by diaphragm pacing. *Surg Clin North Am* 1980;60:1055–1078.
182. Glenn WW, Sairenji H. Diaphragm pacing in the treatment of chronic ventilatory insufficiency. In: Roussos C, Macklem PT, eds. *The thorax: lung biology in health and disease.* Vol 29. New York: Marcel Dekker, Inc, 1985:1407.
183. Hunt CE, Brouillette RT, Weese-Mayer DE, et al. Diaphragm pacing in infants. Technique and results. *Pacing Clin Electrophysiol* 1988;11:2135–2141.
184. Ilbawi MN, Idriss FS, Hunt CE, et al. Diaphragmatic pacing in infants: techniques and results. *Ann Thorac Surg* 1985;40:323–329.
185. Thoma H, Gerner H, Holle J, et al. The phrenic pacemaker: substitution of paralyzed functions in tetraplegia. *Trans Am Soc Artif Intern Organs* 1987;33:472–479.
186. Chen CF, Lien IN. Spinal cord injuries in Taipei, Taiwan, 1978–1981. *Paraplegia* 1985;23:364–370.
187. Dobelle WH, D'Angelo MS, Goetz BF, et al. 200 cases with a new breathing pacemaker dispels myths about diaphragm pacing. *Trans Am Soc Artif Intern Organs* 1994;40:244–252.
188. Glenn WW, Phelps ML, Elefteriades JA, et al. Twenty years of experience in phrenic nerve stimulation to pace the diaphragm. *Pacing Clin Electrophysiol* 1986;9:780–784.
189. Hackler RH. A 25-year prospective mortality study in the spinal cord injured patient: comparison with the long-term living paraplegic. *J Urol* 1977;117:486–488.
190. Oda T, Glenn WW, Fukuda Y, et al. Evaluation of electrical parameters for diaphragm pacing: an experimental study. *J Surg Res* 1981;30:142–153.
191. McKenzie DK, Gandevia SC. Phrenic nerve conduction times and twitch pressures of the human diaphragm. *J Appl Physiol* 1985;58:1496–1504.
192. McLean IC, Mattoni TA. Phrenic nerve conduction studies: a new technique and its application in quadriplegic patients. *Arch Phys Med Rehabil* 1981;62:70–73.
193. Glenn WW, Holcomb WG, Hogan J, et al. Diaphragm pacing by radiofrequency transmission in the treatment of chronic ventilatory insufficiency. Present status. *J Thorac Cardiovasc Surg* 1973;66:505–520.
194. Fodstad H. The Swedish experience in phrenic nerve stimulation. *Pacing Clin Electrophysiol* 1987;10:246–251.
195. Vanderlinden RG, Epstein SW, Hyland RH, et al. Management of chronic ventilatory insufficiency with electrical diaphragm pacing. *Can J Neuro Sci* 1988;15:63–67.
196. Glenn WW, Phelps ML. Diaphragm pacing by electrical stimulation of the phrenic nerve. *Neurosurgery* 1985;17:974–984.
197. Glenn WW, Brouillette RT, Dentz B, et al. Fundamental considerations in pacing of the diaphragm for chronic ventilatory insufficiency: a multi-center study. *Pacing Clin Electrophysiol* 1988;11:2121–2127.
198. Weese-Mayer DE, Silvestri JM, Kenny AS, et al. Diaphragm pacing with a quadripolar phrenic nerve electrode: an international study. *Pacing Clin Electrophysiol* 1996;19:1311–1319.
199. Biering-Sorensen F, Jacobsen E, Hjelms E, et al. [Diaphragm pacing by electric stimulation of the phrenic nerves]. *Ugeskr Laeger* 1990;152:1143–1145.
200. Marcus CL, Jansen MT, Pousen MK, et al. Medical and psychosocial outcome of children with congenital central hypoventilation syndrome. *J Pediatr* 1991;119:888–895.
201. DiMarco AF, Altose MD, Cropp A, et al. Activation of the inspiratory intercostal muscles by electrical stimulation of the spinal cord. *Am Rev Respir Dis* 1987;136:1385–1390.
202. DiMarco AF, Budzinska K, Supinski GS. Artificial ventilation by means of electrical activation of the intercostal/accessory muscles alone in anesthetized dogs. *Am Rev Respir Dis* 1989;139:961–967.
203. DiMarco AF, Supinski GS, Petro J, et al. Artificial respiration via combined intercostal and diaphragm pacing in a quadriplegic patient. *Am Rev Respir Dis* 1994;149:A135.
204. DiMarco AF, Kowalski KE, Petro JA, et al. Evaluation of intercostal and diaphragm pacing to provide ventilatory support in tetraplegic patients. Paper presented at: ATS International Conference; 2001; San Francisco.
205. DiMarco AF, Mortimer JT, Stellato T, et al. Bilateral phrenic nerve pacing via intramuscular electrodes in tetraplegic patients. Paper presented at: ATS International Conference; 2001; San Francisco.

CHAPTER 67

Spasticity and Movement Disorder

Elie Elovic and Ross Bogey

INTRODUCTION

Spasticity is derived from the Greek word *spasticus*, which means "to pull." The treatment team involved in its management may find it one of the most challenging issues confronting them in the care of patients with neurologic disability. Spasticity is a component of the upper motor neuron syndrome (UMNS). The upper motor neuron syndrome is caused by a lesion proximal to the anterior horn cell; in the spinal cord, brainstem, or brain. It has both positive and negative components. Weakness, paralysis, and fatigue are the negative signs of the syndrome, whereas spasticity, athetosis, hyperreflexia, release of primitive reflexes, and dystonia are the positive. Hyperreflexia, spread of reflexes beyond muscles stimulated, hypertonicity, clonus, and rigidity are often seen in association with spasticity (1).

Neuroanotomy of Neuronal Control

To facilitate the discussion of spasticity pathophysiology, it is useful to discuss normal motor control. To function effectively, the motor system must be able to integrate sensory feedback, control reflex activity, and coordinate volitional movement. It is critical for the controller to have information concerning the position of muscles and joints in addition to muscle velocity. It is also critical for the system to be able to respond rapidly to the outside, to control and respond to reflex activity, and to initiate and stop motor activity. Feedback must exist among the many pathways that pass through the cortical, subcortical, brainstem, spinal cord, peripheral nerve, and muscle. The most distal unit involved in motor control is the motor unit, a part of the peripheral nervous system that is critical for control based on excitation and inhibition of muscle fibers.

THE MOTOR UNIT

The motor unit was first described by Sherrington (2). It is comprised of the α motor neuron and all the muscle fibers that are innervated by it. Not all the units are the same, as they differ in recruitment patterns and their rates of firing. This is a result of the different demands and purposes of individual motor units. The units also differ by the types of muscle fibers that comprise them. There are two major fiber types: type I and type II. Type I fibers are small, red, and oxidative, and they fatigue slowly. Motor unit function reflects the fibers that they contain. Motor units full of type I fibers are responsible for the baseline tonic muscle activity. Type II fibers, on the other hand, are large,

white, and anaerobic. These muscles are more powerful and can deliver greater speed and velocity than type I; however, they can fatigue easily. These units are brought in to increase the force or speed of a contraction. Other motor units are a hybrid of the two fiber types (3,4). When working properly, motor units fire with coordination of agonist and antagonists system, normal patterns of recruitment and decruitment (5). Katz et al. reported the problems that can be created by co-contraction of muscles and muscles firing out of phase or at angles different from their normal areas of activity. This loss of the normal recruitment and decruitment pattern may play a key role in spasticity (6).

MOTOR UNIT REGULATION

The motor control system uses a feedback loop, integrating information about muscle activity, position, and velocity. This enables the motor system to control and coordinate the stimulation of agonist and antagonist muscles around a joint as part of the kinetic chain. Critical information required by the control system includes muscle length, velocity, muscle tension, and joint position. This is mediated by a combination of immediate monosynaptic reflexes and more complicated higher-level activities involving spinal and supraspinal polysynaptic activity. This activity can either increase or inhibit activity at the motor unit level. Units fire when the net excitation minus inhibition reaches threshold (4).

MUSCLE SPINDLE AND GOLGI TENDON ORGANS

The muscle spindle plays a critical role in control and the provision of necessary information for proper motor control. It is attached in parallel to the main muscle mass, and it contains afferent type Ia and II fibers that communicate information concerning position and rate of change of a muscle to the spinal column. It would be difficult for the spindle to provide accurate information throughout a muscle's range of motion (ROM), as the spindle would be under less tension as the muscle contracts. This is a situation analogous to a volleyball net being supported by two poles. The muscle contracting would be similar to the poles being brought closer together. It is crucial for the spindle to deliver accurate information throughout the ROM. Somehow the tension must be maintained. The γ motor neuron that is an integral component of the muscle spindle saves the day. The γ motor unit co-activates with the α motor neuron and maintains the spindle tension and efficiency (4). When a sudden stretch, such as tapping on the knee, is applied, the knee jerk reflex is triggered. It is a monosynaptic reflex, which is mediated by the firing of the Ia afferent in response to stretch, which in turn prompts the α motor neuron to fire. During normal movement this stretch reflex must be suppressed. Some suppression of muscle activity is mediated through the Golgi tendon organs. Found within the muscle tendons, through the Ib fibers and their related interneurons, the Golgi tendon organs limit muscle contraction by facilitating antagonists and inhibiting agonists. Thus, they serve to impose a ceiling effect on muscle contraction and prevent musculotendinous injury (7).

SPINAL INTERNEURONS

The spinal interneurons play a critical role in normal motor control and spasticity. The effects of the Ia and Ib fibers mentioned earlier are often mediated through and with the help of interneurons called Ia and Ib interneurons, respectively. Other interneurons, including the Renshaw cell and the propriospinal interneurons, also are an important part of the control process. As mentioned earlier, the Golgi tendon organs generate a ceiling effect for maximum muscle tension. The Ib afferents from these organs connect to their respective Ib interneurons. These interneurons also receive supra- and propriospinal influences from above that facilitate antagonists and inhibit the firing of agonist (4,6). The type Ia interneurons receive activation from the type Ia neurons from the muscle spindle. When activated they facilitate agonist activity and reciprocally inhibit antagonist muscles, preventing the futility of co-contraction. They are also under supraspinal influence, and this plays a critical role in strengthening of reciprocal inhibition by the type Ia interneuron. The loss of this influence on the Ia interneurons plays a critical role in co-contraction and cerebral origin spasticity (8).

The process of recurrent inhibition involves the Renshaw cell, which receives input directly from the α motor neuron. This process shuts off agonist activity by its direct effect on the α motor neuron, in addition to facilitation of antagonist's function mediated via the antagonist's Ia interneuron (9). Tight motor control requires the function of the Renshaw circuit, and a loss of its function may greatly complicate some of these movements (6). Like many other neurons, spinal and supraspinal input influence Renshaw cell function. Renshaw cell inhibition is increased in spinal cord injury (SCI) (10).

SUPRASPINAL INFLUENCES

The supraspinal influences play a major role in both volitional movement and the pathophysiology of spasticity. Rothwell et al. (11) demonstrated cortico-motoneuronal pathways. These pathways were specific for specialized coordinated functions such as truncal balance or the initiation of fine coordinated hand movements and originate from the primary motor cortex. Loss of these fibers leads more to a functional deficit than to spasticity. Reducing tone from the hands may improve passive and gross hand function but does not greatly improve fine movement (12).

The corticospinal tract, the major motor tract, originates from many areas within the brain. This includes the extrapyramidal cells from the prefrontal region, supplementary motor region, the cingulate gyrus, and the postcentral gyrus of the parietal lobe. The pontine medial reticulospinal and lateral vestibulospinal are the main extensor pathways within the brain. The pontine system facilitates the α and γ motor neurons of the extensors of the limb muscles with some input into the system from the sensorimotor cortex. The lateral vestibular is found in the ventromedial portion of the cord and terminates at the spinal cord motor neurons. Stimulating this tract affects the motor neurons of the flexor muscles differently from the extensors, with the α and γ motor neurons of the flexors inhibited and those of the extensors facilitated. The nucleus of the cerebellum also has an excitatory influence on extensor pathways (13).

Several pathways facilitate flexion. The medullary lateral reticular formation (MLRF) inhibits extensor pathways. The cortex facilitates its action, and cortical injury can lead to net overactivity of the lower-extremity extensor system. The medullary lateral reticular formation demonstrates its effect through its connections to the motor neurons, type Ia interneurons, and type Ib system. In cats the corticospinal, corticoreticulospinal, and corticorubrospinal all show significant flexor facilitation. Through interneurons, the corticorubrospinal tract excites flexor motor neurons and inhibits extensors. In addition, the medullary reticulospinal tract is a predominant part of a largely flexor-oriented system (14).

Pathophysiology of Spasticity

So from where does spasticity come? Dietz and Berger have suggested that intrinsic properties of the muscle itself could explain the changes seen with spasticity (15). Based on work from animal models, the concept of "gamma rigidity" was raised. With overfiring of the γ motor neuron, the spindle would be too taut and the Ia interneurons would be hyperexcitable. Efforts at identifying this with microneurography failed to confirm this hypothesis (16). Delwaide felt that spasticity resulted from a loss of loss of descending, facilitatory, inhibitory influences that act on Ia interneuron inhibition (17). This loss would make it impossible for the inhibitory influence of the interneuron to shut off antagonist muscles, with resultant increased velocity-dependent resistance to movement mediated by the muscle spindle. The concept of a hyperexcitable motor neuronal pool has been recently raised. In essence these neurons would be hypervigilant and initiation of firing would occur with less excitation. This may result from a loss of tonic inhibition secondary to a loss of supraspinal influences. Some have expressed the belief that the ionic properties of the membrane itself are changed as well. Other theories that may explain spasticity include central collateral sprouting (18), presynaptic disinhibition (17), and denervation hypersensitivity (19). Neurotransmitters may also play some role in spasticity. Some suspects include serotonin and substance P. In animal literature, serotonin has been noted to prolong responses and facilitate extensor responses (20).

MANAGEMENT

An integrated team is required to successfully mange spasticity. Under the direction of a physician who is skilled in the management of spasticity, the team should be able to deliver the entire continuum of services. The remainder of this chapter will concern itself with the indications and benefits of the different treatment modalities (Table 67-1). How do clinicians decide what treatment to offer? Often the question is answered by the skills of the treating clinician, in that a man with a hammer sees everything as a nail. A physician skilled in chemoneurolysis is far more likely to perform a nerve block than one less comfortable with the procedure. Physicians may be more inclined to prescribe an oral pharmacologic agent than to prescribe serial casting or splinting. Therefore, it is important for the treatment team to communicate effectively and access to needed surgical consultations as appropriate. It is important to

TABLE 67-1. Indications for Spasticity Intervention

Passive	Active
Improved hygiene	Improvement of transfers
Ease of care	Improvement in ADL's
Positioning	Improved mobility
Facilitate casting or splinting	Decrease spasms
Reduce pain	Release inhibition of antagonists

keep in mind that not all spasticity is dysfunctional. Some women with spasticity use their elbow flexor tone to hold their pocketbooks, whereas lower-extremity tone may assist in transfers, standing, and ambulation. Optimizing function should be the primary outcome parameter in the treatment of spasticity. The entire treatment team must observe for efficacy and adverse effects that result from their treatment and adjust treatment as required. Only in this fashion can one maximize the quality of life for the patients undergoing treatment (Table 67-2).

Functional Approaches

Overall, spasticity and the upper motor neuron syndrome are a result of an irreversible process within the central nervous system (CNS). By itself, they are not a disease state and treatment decisions should be made based on the functional limitations that they create. Specific impairments or functional deficits such as pain, problems with position, hygiene, or mobility are the specific issues that therapy should address. Gans and Glenn (21) divided treatment goals into two categories. The first is the management of passive function, such as reduction of pain, positioning, hygiene, splint wearing, and prevention of contracture. The second is related to functional activities. As they described it, "Dimished capacity of the patient to accomplish useful work with the motor system." The goals of these treatment interventions are to improve volitional purposeful movement. Some examples include unmasking functional movement that is inhibited by antagonist spasticity, improved transfers, ambulation, and performance of activities of daily living (ADLs).

REDUCTION OF NOXIOUS STIMULATION

The first step in any program to manage spasticity is the reduction of noxious stimulation. Spasticity and muscle overactivity have been shown to be increased as a result of this input (22). Stimulation of the flexor reflex afferents may lead to an increase in pathologic activity (23). The term *noxious stimulation* encompasses a wide variety of conditions such as pressure ulcers, ingrown toenail, contracture, kinked catheter, urolithiasis, urinary tract infection, DVT, heterotopic ossification, fecal impaction, sepsis, and fracture. This is just a partial list. Addressing these conditions should almost always be the first approach in spasticity management.

POSITIONING

Proper positioning is an extremely important component of spasticity management. Poor positioning can result in an increase in spasticity and in in decreased ROM, contractures, increased noxious stimulation, pain, and exacerbation of a vicious cycle that can lead to worsening spasticity (24). This is especially true in the ICU and acute hospital (22). Proper goals for a positioning program include improvement in body alignment and greater symmetry. Benefits include easing of nursing care, facilitation of therapy, and maximization of a patient's function. Postures that should be avoided include a scissoring posture (bilateral hip extension, adduction, internal rotation), windswept position (hip flexion, abduction, external rotation on one side and relative hip extension, adduction, and internal rotation on the other), and frog-leg position, which can exacerbate the problem. Positioning is also important in the wheelchair. Tone can be minimized by placing the patient with the hips and knees at 90 degrees and by maintaining good torso position (24).

STRETCH

As a result of the upper motor neuron syndrome, muscles can be shortened for several reasons. One, is the immobilization of paralyzed muscles in shortened positions. This resultant decrease in longitudal tension (muscle unloading) can predispose to contracture. Other factors include a reduction in protein synthesis in immobilized muscles, which promotes atrophy (25). Spasticity and muscle overactivity also play a part in muscle shortening (26). This can in turn result in an increase in spindle activity and sensitivity (27). Gracies et al. (22) have discussed the need to promote the commencement of stretch early in the

TABLE 67-2. Comparisons of Different Treatment Modalities for Spasticity

Spasticity Treatment	Indications	Advantages	Disadvantages
Modalities	Should be used prior to other interventions	Minimal side effects	Short duration of effect
Oral Medications	Generalized tone, spasms, no focal region of spasticity	Systemic administration, can treat large area of spasticity	Systemic side effects such as sedation, metabolic load
Botulinum Toxins	Focal area of spasticity	Can treat spastic area without systemic side effects	Expensive, 3-month duration when procedure needs to be repeated
Phenol	Focal area of spasticity	Can treat spastic area without systemic side effects, much cheaper than Botulinum toxins and longer duration	Requires considerable skill of injector, risk of dysestesias, pain procedure
Orthopedics Procedure	Potential improvement in passive or active ADL's. Stable neurologically	Can be long term repair	Surgical risk, loss of motor strength
Intrathecal Baclofen	Significant tone not responsive to other treatments ? time post	Baclofen gets to spinal cord with minimal systemic absorption	Surgical procedure, pump and catheter will eventually need replacement, high cost, risk of catheter dislodgement or kink

treatment of any neurologic condition. Stretch has the advantage of being a focal treatment that can combat the development of the previously mentioned muscle shortening and increase in spindle sensitivity (25).

Schmidt et al. have demonstrated the benefit of a relatively brief stretch in the management of spasticity (28). However, the benefit is very short lived, as the tone returns after a single contraction (29). Therefore, stretch needs to be applied for a longer period of time to have potential functional benefit. A study involving the use of a Lycra garment that provided a stretch of 3 hours demonstrated both an improvement in spasticity and good patient tolerance (30). Stretch has been shown to be useful in volitional movement in both agonist (31) and antagonist muscles (32). Chronic stretch via casting or splints changes reflexive activity and reduces the stretch reflex (33–35). In summary, stretching activities have the advantage of being a local treatment, with limited risk that has demonstrated proven effect in the management of spasticity.

PHYSICAL MODALITIES

Physical modalities (see Chapter 11) can play a critical role in the management of spasticity. Like stretching, they have the benefit of being a benign intervention that has the potential to treat locally. The use of these agents will most likely remain a part of a spasticity treatment program. Used correctly the physical modalities can have an important role in spasticity management.

Cooling of muscles is beneficial in the management of spasticity (36,37). It both inhibits the monosynaptic stretch reflexes and lowers receptor sensitivity after it is removed (38,39). Cooling can be used in different ways. The quick icing technique, with ice applied with a light striking movement, results in facilitation of α and γ motor neurons and is used to facilitate antagonist function (40), whereas prolonged cooling can result in decreased conduction velocity and a reduction in the maximal motor CMAP (36,41–43). The issue of cooling and muscle elasticity was addressed in a study that found a 3% to 10% decrease in elastic stiffness after a 30-minute ice cooling over the calf muscles (44). However, the effect lasted less than 1 hour. Other methods of delivering include the use of a cooling evaporating spray, such as ethyl chloride (45).

Heat is another modality that can be applied in various forms. Ultrasound, paraffin, fluidotherapy, superficial heat, and whirlpool are some of the most common ways heat is applied. Heat's effect is short lived (46) and, like cold, its application should be followed immediately by stretching and exercise. The effects of heat on spasticity have been studied in only a limited way. Its major effect seems to be related to an increase in elasticity that may assist in stretching activities (47).

Deeper heating modalities have also been used in the management of spasticity. Wessling et al. (48) demonstrated that 1.5 watts./cm^2 in combination with stretch resulted in a 20% greater distensibility than stretch alone.

ELECTRICAL STIMULATION

Electrical stimulation is another modality that can help spasticity management. Transcutaneous electrical nerve stimulation (TENS) units have been shown to be useful in the management of pain. Through its nociceptive action and resultant reduction in pain it was felt that it could reduce spasticity. Specifically, by reducing the flexor reflex afferents that are facilitated by nociceptive stimulation (23), Bajd et al. (49) demonstrated a reduction in SCI-related spasticity in three of six patients in a dermatomal pattern, while a group applying TENS in an acupuncture method demonstrated a substantial reduction in spasticity that was partially reversed by co-administration of naloxone (50).

Other potential mechanisms of action for spasticity reduction include inhibition or fatiguing of spastic muscles and possible activation of antagonist muscles through the Ia interneurons (51).

MASSAGE

Massage is a therapy that is often desired by patients and their families. However, a review of the literature does not reveal any strong scientific evidence that supports its efficacy and utility (40,52,53).

Pharmacologic Treatments

Four common methods are currently being used in the delivery of pharmacologic agents. The oldest method is delivery though the enteral system, either by mouth or via g-tube. Agents such as baclofen, benzodiazepines, or tizandine are delivered in this fashion. These agents undergo systemic absorption and demonstrate an effect throughout the entire body. A second method, which is closely related to enteral delivery, is the use of a transdermal system. An example of this is Catapress TTS. Medications administered in this fashion are also absorbed systemically and demonstrate their effects throughout the body. They differ from the enteral methods by having a more steady-state blood drug level throughout the day with less fluctuation. Intrathecal administration of active agents is a third method of drug delivery. By placing the medications closer to their site of action, systemic side effects are reduced and clinical efficacy is obtained with lower total doses. Baclofen, morphine, and clonidine are some of the more common medications that are delivered in this manner. Local injection of chemodenervation agents is the fourth method of drug delivery. Agents such as phenol and ethanol classically and now in the last decade the botulinum toxin products fall in this category. This last mode of administration is the one that can be used best to treat a focal issue with a minimum of systemic effect, though some systemic absorption is still detectable.

SPECIFIC COMPONENTS OF SPASTICITY: PHARMACOLOGIC DECISION PROCESS

The decision as to which pharmacologic agent to use in a particular patient is based on many factors. A partial list includes etiology, time since onset of medical issue, prognosis, accessibility to medical services, personal support system, concurrent medical problems, cognitive status, and financial resources. All these items are important. A brilliantly planned intervention that the patient cannot afford is of no value. Similarly, an aggressive outpatient therapy program is of no value if transportation cannot be obtained for the patient.

Spasticity Etiology

Despite the fact that spasticity from different etiologies may present similarly, spasticity resulting from different etiologies may respond very differently to interventions. As an example, enteral pharmacologic agents have been shown to be of great efficacy in the management of spasticity resulting from spinal cord injury or multiple sclerosis (54–58), whereas the benefit in spasticity caused by traumatic brain injury or stroke is far less apparent. A further complicating factor in cerebral origin spasticity is the potential for impairment of recovery secondary to treatment (59), or a potentially intolerable cognitive side effect profile even when the agent may be effective (60).

Time Since Onset

As a general rule, more aggressive spasticity interventions are tried later in the course of an event. Medications that may impair recovery are less likely to be used early in recovery. For patients that are low-level post traumatic brain injury (TBI), physicians are less likely to prescribe sedating antispasticity agents. Phenol neurolysis is rarely used early in recovery, as the scarring of muscle and nerve and long duration of action may be undesirable in a recovering patient. Orthopedic interventions are almost never offered early on, as there needs to be stabilization of the neuromuscular structures before the performance of any permanent surgical interventions. Relative to intrathecal baclofen (ITB) there is now some controversy as to what is considered too early. A recent report from France demonstrated that intrathecal baclofen may be beneficial when initiated in the first month of injury when spasticity was recalcitrant (61).

Functional Prognosis

When a patient's prognosis for motor and functional recovery is very guarded, this may lead clinicians to attempt more aggressive, permanent interventions such as a rhizotomy. The need to assist in care may be preeminent over efforts to promote an unlikely recovery.

Support System

Can medication administration be supervised in the cognitively impaired patient? A family member or other caregiver may be critical for the physician to safely prescribe medications. Is supervision and assistance available for transportation to therapy or assistance in safe utilization of splinting devices? Will the patient be able to follow up for intrathecal baclofen pump refills or will there be the risk of withdrawal if the pump goes dry?

Cognitive Status

It is important to assess a patient's cognitive ability when prescribing treatment. The clinician must address the patient's ability to be compliant and remain safe while using a treatment modality. Will the patient be noncompliant with a medication and risk withdrawal seizures? Will there be a risk of skin breakdown with the use of a splint or serial cast?

Concurrent Medical Problems

The overall medical condition of the patient being treated must be considered. Patients with hypotension, syncope, balance disturbances, or ataxia may be unable to tolerate the side effect profile of certain agents. Would an oral agent cause hypotension and resultant syncope, exacerbate ataxia, coordination or balance disturbance? Does the patient have chronic infections that would increase the risk of development of an infection with an indwelling catheter or intrathecal baclofen system?

Distribution of Spasticity

How diffuse is the area that needs treatment? Is there a focal or segmental area that needs treatment or is throughout the entire body? If there is discrete region, chemodenervation may be most appropriate. If the condition is systemic, then treatment that is more global will be necessary.

Financial Issues

Intrathecal baclofen and botulinum toxin injections cost thousands of dollars. Paying out of pocket for some modalities is not realistic and the physician, patient, and family have to deal with third-party payers. Some insurance companies are requiring trials with less expensive agents such as oral antispasticity agents before approving toxin injections. The clinicians are often placed in the position of needing to justify their decisions and recommendations.

Oral and Transdermal Medications

Oral and transdermal medications are commonly used in the treatment of spasticity. Table 67-3 summarizes the usage of these medications.

BENZODIAZEPINES

The benzodiazepines were the first agents used in the management of spasticity. Of this class, diazepam (Valium) is most commonly used, and other members of this family that have also been used in spasticity management include clorazepate (Tranxene) and clonazepam (Klonipin). Ketazolam (Loftran) is another class member that has been trialed for spasticity that is available in Canada but not in the United States (62). The benzodiazepines' mechanism of action is central in origin, acting on the brainstem reticular formation and spinal polysynaptic pathways (63). The benzodiazepines demonstrate their effect via $GABA_A$ (γ-aminobutyric acid), which opens the membranes Cl^- channels with resultant hyperpolarization. The net effect is

TABLE 67-3. Commonly Used Oral Medications

Medication	Daily Dosage (range)	Mechanism of Action	Comments
Baclofen	10–300 mg	Presynaptic inhibition of $GABA_B$ receptors. Is active both pre and post synaptically. Hyperpolarizes cell membrane	Risk of withdrawal seizures and hallucinations. Dose must be adjusted with renal disease
Diazepam	4–60 mg	Facilitates post-synaptic effects of $GABA_A$ by opening chloride channels in membranes resulting in increased presynaptic inhibition secondary to hyperpolarization	Oldest class of medications used for spasticity that is still in common use. Can have very long half life
Dantrolene	25–400 mg	Interferes with calcium release from sarcoplasmic reticulum	Only truly peripherally acting or agent. LFT's must be watched carefully
Clonidine	Oral 0.05 mg bid — 0.4 mg/day Or 1–6 patch/wk	Alpha-2 agonist. Decreases tonic facilitation via locus coeruleus and in spinal cord enhances presynaptic inhibition	Primary use in SCI population. Theoretical limitation to use in ABI secondary to interference with recovery
Tizanidine	1–36 mg	Alpha-2 agonist. Blocks release or excitatory neurotransmitters and facilitates inhibitory neurotransmitters. Antinociceptive and reduces spinal reflexes	Now available in 2 and 4 mg tablets. Slow titration reduces sedation side effect that is major limiting factor

a reduction of mono- and polysynaptic reflexes and an increase in presynaptic inhibition (62). Initial dosing is 2 mg bid or 5 mg at bedtime with a gradual titration upward to a maximum of 60 mg a day. After enteral administration it is well absorbed, peaking at 1 hour. It has a relatively long half-life of between 20 and 80 hours, if one includes its active metabolites. The side effect profile can be quite problematic and includes problems with addiction and withdrawal, ataxia, weakness, cognitive impairment, memory dysfunction, poor coordination, fatigue, and CNS depression that can be potentiated by alcohol. Research with diazepam has demonstrated improvements in painful spasms, hyperreflexia, and passive ROM. Evidence concerning functional improvement is hard to find.

Clorazepate is another benzodiazepine that may have a more favorable side effect profile than diazepam. In clinical trials it was noted to have fewer problems with sedation and memory (64,65). Its half-life is relatively short but its active metabolite, desmethyldiazepam, has a half-life of up to 70 hours. In obese patients it can be more than 200 hours (66). Doses of 5 mg bid have been used in clinical trials.

Benzodiazepines in SCI
The greatest benefit for diazepam has been demonstrated in the SCI population. A double-blind crossover study with 22 patients with SCI-related spasticity demonstrated efficacy (67), whereas another study with 21 patients with multiple sclerosis or SCI showed that diazepam is superior to placebo in treating spasticity. Whether the benzodiazepines are better in complete or incomplete lesions is still open to debate. Some authors suggest that they are effective only in incomplete lesions. Whyte and Robinson (68) suggest that they are effective only incomplete lesions, but this is still controversial (69,70). A survey performed at Veterans Administration SCI programs showed that 70% of prescribers routinely give benzodiazepines to their patients (71).

Benzodiazepines in Multiple Sclerosis
Studies performed in patients with multiple sclerosis have compared the efficacy and side effect profile of the benzodiazepines to those of baclofen. The two agents had very comparable efficacies and tolerance. Sedation was found more often with the benzodiazepines, whereas the baclofen group had a more varied list of side effects (72–74).

Benzodiazepines in Acquired Brain Injury
Benzodiazepines are rarely used in the acquired brain injury population because of their potential for cognitive side effects as well as their potential to compromise motor recovery (59).

Benzodiazepines in Cerebral Palsy
Engle (75) conducted a double-blind crossover study that demonstrated the efficacy of diazepam in the management of patients with cerebral palsy. However, there was some question if the improvements were behavioral in origin. Nogen (76) studied diazepam and dantrolene in patients with cerebral palsy and found benefit for both agents. The literature is quite sparse concerning the issue with no recent studies performed.

BACLOFEN
Baclofen (Lioresal) is another agent that mediates its activity through the GABA system. It differs from the benzodiazepines by mediating its effect via $GABA_B$ rather than by $GABA_A$ and is active both pre- and postsynaptically. Its action presynaptically is to bind to the GABA interneuron, where it causes hyperpolarization of the membrane that prevents the influx of calcium and resultant release of neurotransmitter. When it binds post-

synaptically, it hyperpolarizes the cell membrane by acting on the Ia afferents. As a result, baclofen is inhibitory on both the mono- and polysynaptic reflex pathways. Baclofen is eliminated via the kidney, and its half-life is roughly 3.5 hours (62).

When initiating treatment, 5 mg bid to tid is recommended, and this can be increased 5 to 10 mg/day/week. The PDR suggests a maximum dose of 80 mg/day, but while not routinely recommended, doses as high as 300 mg/day have been used safely (53). Baclofen-related side effects reported include sedation, fatigue, weakness, nausea, dizziness, paresthesias, hallucinations, and lowering of seizure threshold. The patient is at greatest risk when the agent is abruptly discontinued, as hallucinations and withdrawal seizures have been reported (68). Since baclofen primarily undergoes renal clearance, dosing may need to be adjusted with kidney-related issues (77). When one switches from oral baclofen to V, one must be wary of potential withdrawal-related issues. This is based on the efficiency of localization that results from V, as there is a relatively low dose of baclofen in the brain as compared with the lumbar cord region.

Baclofen in SCI and Multiple Sclerosis
It is appropriate to combine those with SCI and multiple sclerosis, since much of the baclofen literature combines these populations, although some differences will be highlighted (55, 77–80). Feldman et al. (79) reported that the use of baclofen in patients with multiple sclerosis demonstrated a significant reduction in spasticity as well as reducing painful flexor spasms. Flexor spasms in the SCI population also responded to baclofen administration (55,81–85). It is far more difficult to find studies that demonstrate functional improvement, as studies were unable to demonstrate improvements in ADLs and ambulation with administration of baclofen (83,85). Orsnes et al. (86) more recently studied patients with multiple sclerosis treated with baclofen but again found no functional improvement. Nielsen et al. (87,88) studied the effect of oral baclofen on the soleus muscle. Treatment with baclofen reduced ankle stiffness and increased soleus response latency. However, it also was found to increase the weakness in soleus function, which may explain the lack of functional improvement.

Baclofen in Acquired Brain Injury
There is limited literature that has noted positive effect with oral baclofen in the acquired brain injury population (89–91). A double-blinded study in the elderly stroke population was discontinued because of treatment-related sedation (92).

Baclofen in Cerebral Palsy
Milla and Jackson (93) conducted the one blinded crossover trial in the cerebral palsy literature that demonstrated efficacy. Actual functional benefits were not seen, but decreased scissoring and improvements in ROM were noted. The authors reported few side effects and recommended dosing of a total of 5 to 10 mg total per day in divided doses for children 2 to 7 years of age.

DANTROLENE SODIUM
Unlike many other agents, dantrolene (Dantrium) is an enteral medication that acts peripherally, at the level of the muscle itself. Its mechanism of action is to inhibit calcium release from the sarcoplasmic reticulum during muscle contraction. Rather than stopping neuronal activation, it blocks the strength of contraction. In addition to its action on the muscle extrafusal fibers, it reduces muscle spindle's sensitivity by action on the γ motor neuron (53). Dantrolene's primary action is on fast-twitch fibers, and parameters affected by it include easier ROM

and tone. Starting dose is 25 mg bid and can be increased weekly by 25 to 50 mg to a maximum of 400 mg/day (94). Dantrolene's enteral half-life is approximately 15 hours and is given bid to qid (62). Dantrolene is probably best known for its potential liver toxicity; however, it is overall a rare occurrence, with a rate of only 1.8% (95) when administered for more than 60 days. Even when discovered it is usually reversible. It is found most commonly in women over the age of 30, especially if they had been on high doses for a long period of time. Fatal liver failure has been reported in 0.3% of those who received the medication. Therefore, it is critical for clinicians to follow liver function tests when prescribing dantrolene. Blood draws should be weekly the first month, monthly the first year, and four times a year after that. In addition to liver toxicity, other problems associated with dantrolene include weakness, paresthesias, nausea, and diarrhea (62).

Dantrolene in SCI

Since dantrolene is associated with weakness, there have been few trials reported with its use. Glass and Hannah (96) reported that it was more effective than diazepam in controlling spasticity; however, it also was associated with greater weakness. Studies have demonstrated improvements in ROM and tone but no functional improvement (97,98). Two other cases are reported in the literature where SCI patients responded to dantrolene when treated for baclofen withdrawal (99,100).

Dantrolene in Multiple Sclerosis

There is limited literature describing the use of dantrolene in patients with multiple sclerosis. Again, this may well be due to a poor tolerance for additional muscle weakness. The two studies performed demonstrated improvement in tone and ROM. However, the benefits were more than overwhelmed by the clinical weakness that was found while on the medication (101,102). Its use in patients with multiple sclerosis cannot be recommended from the literature.

Dantrolene in Acquired Brain Injury

Whyte and Robinson (68) have recommended dantrolene for use in the treatment of acquired brain injury–related spasticity. Chyatte et al. (103) reported on nine patients with cerebrovascular accident–related spasticity. Although they demonstrated no functional improvements in ADLs and mobility, they noted improved ROM, deep tendon reflexes (DTRs), and some upper-extremity function. Ketel and Kolb (104) reported that in their selected population of dantrolene responders, there was an exacerbation with clinical deterioration when they were placed on placebo.

Dantrolene in Cerebral Palsy

While reviewing the data concerning the use of dantrolene in patients with cerebral palsy, Krach (105) reported on four studies that demonstrated efficacy. Haslam et al. (106) reported decreases in DTRs and scissoring. Dosing in the pediatric population has been up to 12 mg/kg.

CLONIDINE

Clonidine(Catapress) is an imidazoline derivative that is primarily an antihypertensive agent. It is a α_2-adrenergic agonist that has been shown to demonstrate some efficacy in spasticity management, primarily in SCI. It peaks in 3 to 5 hours when taken orally and has a usual half-life of 5 to 19 hours. However, it can be as high as 40 hours with persons with renal impairment. Clonidine's clearance is primarily renal, with half of it first metabolized by the liver. Clonidine has two distinct mechanisms of action. First, it acts directly on the locus ceruleus and

decreases tonic facilitation (62). It also has a spinal mechanism, acting to enhance α_2-mediated presynaptic inhibition (107–109). Clonidine doses as low as 0.1 mg orally are often effective in treating spasticity (108). Clonidine can also be administered via a transdermal system that allows for more uniform blood levels and easier administration. There have been two separate reports demonstrating its potential efficacy in the SCI population (110,111). Side effects reported with clonidine include bradycardia, depression, lethargy, syncope, and hypotension (108,112). At this time there is no literature that describes clonidine usage in patients with multiple sclerosis or cerebral palsy.

Clonidine in SCI

As mentioned earlier, clonidine has been used most effectively in the SCI population. Nance et al. (109) showed that resistance to stretch was reduced in her small series of four patients treated with 0.2 mg/day, who had reduced resistance to stretch and spasms on 0.2 mg/day. Donovan et al. (107) reported on the use of clonidine as an adjunct to baclofen in spasticity management. They reported an overall 56% response rate, with improvements noted in paraplegics and quadriplegics, complete and incomplete lesions. The authors reported that three patients who had been responsive had to be discontinued secondary to postural hypertension.

Clonidine in Acquired Brain Injury

Clonidine can impair motor recovery (59), thus making its use in these patients somewhat controversial. There are two publications, one a case report concerning brainstem origin spasticity (113), the other a six-patient case series (114). Further work needs to be done to clarify clonidine's place as an antispasticity agent.

TIZANIDINE

Like clonidine, tizanidine (Zanaflex)is an imidazoline derivative with α_2-agonist effects and is the newest, widely used antispasticity agent. Its onset is rapid, 1 hour, and it has a very short 2.5-hour half-life and may require frequent dosing. It is cleared via liver metabolism and then is excreted by the kidneys. One mechanism of action is mediated through its effect on neurotransmitters. Tizanidine blocks the release of the excitatory amino acids, glutamate and aspartate, in addition to facilitating the inhibitory neurotransmitter glycine (62). Animal research reveals other potential mechanisms of action that include antinociceptive activity (115–117), in addition to an ability to reduce spinal cord reflex activity (116,118).

The side effects of tizanidine can be quite troubling, with close to 15% of participants discontinuing them during clinical trials (119). Drowsiness is reported in up to 50% of patients on clinical trials (119–121). The work of Meythaler et al. (60) may be most telling, as patients who were obtaining benefit from tizanidine's antispasticity effect were lowering the dose, despite a lower clinical efficacy. Another major side effect is dry mouth (119–121), with up to 11% of people complaining of it. Other complaints included fatigue and dizziness. Hypotension has also been reported with tizanidine (122). Other side effects reported include muscle weakness, nausea, and vomiting. There is a potential for liver damage, and liver function tests should be evaluated before medication initiation, 1, 3, and 6 months after initiating treatment. Initial dosing begins at 2 to 4 mg at hour of sleep and can be increased to a maximum of 36 mg/day (62).

Tizanidine in SCI

Tizanidine has been well studied in this population (57,123). It has been shown to be effective with an acceptable side effect profile. There was also no weakness noted in this population, and the agent is considered safe and effective in this population.

Tizanidine in Multiple Sclerosis

Tizanidine has been well studied in this population and several studies have demonstrated its efficacy in patients with multiple sclerosis (119,121,124–129). In work from the UK Tizanidine Trial Group (124) an improvement in clonus and spasms was seen but not in tone or function. The work by Lapierre et al. demonstrated improvement in clonus and DTRs, but again no functional changes could be detected (121). Two studies compared tizanidine to baclofen and revealed that tizanidine was as effective as baclofen and better tolerated (119,126).

Tizanidine in Acquired Brain Injury

Despite being a relatively new agent, tizanidine has undergone the most rigorous testing in acquired brain injury and may turn out to be the most effective agent. Meythaler et al. (60) reported on a series of 17 patients treated with an escalating dose of tizanidine. When they had reached their maximal dose the patients demonstrated statistically significant decreases in their upper- and lower-extremity Ashworth scores and lower-extremity spasm scores. The changes were not significant in upper-extremity spasms or any of the reflex scores. The side effect profile in general—and more specifically, primarily sedation—was problematic. The original plan was to have the dose up to 36 mg by 4 weeks; however, the maximal dose reached was a mean of 25.2 mg/day. This was lowered by an average of 2 mg later in the trial, when the patients were able to self-select dosing. Once again there was no evidence of improved function, with the FIM and the Craig Handicap Assessment and Reporting Technique (CHART) showing no change with treatment. Bes et al. (120) performed a study that compared tizanidine to diazepam in the management of patients with chronic spastic hemiplegia. They reached their maximal level for each medication by week 6, and they underwent evaluation at week 8. Improvements in nonfunctional measures duration such as stretch, duration of muscle contraction, and reduction of clonus were noted with both agents. However, only tizanidine demonstrated a functional improvement, as noted in walking distance on flat ground. They also reported that tizanidine was better tolerated than diazepam.

Tizanidine in Cerebral Palsy

There are no clinical trials published in the English literature that have tested the use of tizanidine in the management of patients with cerebral palsy. A review article reported that it can be safely used in this population if the tablets are divided (105). The new 2-mg tablet may aid in its use. A study from Russia (130) reported that a dose of 1 mg three times a day for children under 10 and 2 mg three times for children older had significant benefit. However, the outcome measures in this study are quite broad and clearly further research is needed.

OTHER MEDICATIONS

Since spasticity is a significant and recalcitrant problem, the list of medications that have been tried in its treatment is endless. It would be impossible to list them all. Instead the authors will mention a few medications that have potential benefit or are undergoing further investigation. Piracetam is a GABA and baclofen analog that is available in Europe and is used as a cognitive enhancer (62). Although not available in the local pharmacy, it can be obtained via a compound pharmacy or via the Internet. One well-designed study was performed in the 1970s. Piracetam was tested against placebo in a double-blinded crossover design. With a minimal side effect profile the patients demonstrated improved passive range, hand function, and ambulation (131). Gracies et al. (62) have recommended further evaluation. The cannaboids have been shown to have efficacy in neurologic populations and are currently under study (132,133). Gabapentin's potential in spasticity management has been examined in several studies in patients with multiple sclerosis and spinal cord injury (134–138). These studies suggested that at doses of 400 mg tid, gabapentin reduced spasticity with a benign side effect profile. Another anticonvulsant tiagbine, a GABA analog, was noted to decrease spasticity in an open-label trial (139). The drug was being used to treat spasticity. In their evaluation of outcome, the investigators noted a 50% reduction in tone on the modified Ashworth score improvement in strength, coordination, and ROM. Finally, an open-label trial with the antinarcolepsy drug modafinil was noted to improve spasticity in seven out of nine patients with cerebral palsy treated with the drug (140).

Nerve Blocks, Motor Points, and Chemical Denervation

It was mentioned earlier that when the symptoms of spasticity are focal, segmental, or regional, they can be treated with chemical neurolysis or chemical denervation (CD). In simple terms, chemical neurolysis is the process of a clinician treating spasticity and the upper motor neuron syndrome by creating a lesion to the lower motor neuron. This is true regardless of the agent used, be it phenol, ethanol, or one of the botulinum toxins. Treatment goals are very straightforward: focally treat the area of muscle overactivity with the most beneficial side effect profile. First some working definitions.

Nerve block: the application of a chemical to a nerve to impair function, either temporally or permanently.

Chemical neurolysis or *chemodenervation:* a type of nerve block where there is actual destruction of nerve tissue to give a longer-lasting block.

Motor point block: the condition that occurs when a portion of a nerve lower down on the nerve trunk (hopefully, below the sensory branches) is blocked to create a motor block with a more limited sensory involvement (141).

What are some of the indications for chemical denervation? Autti-Ramo et al. (142) suggested that chemical denervation should be performed as part of the planning process before performing any orthopedic hand surgery. Chemical denervation can be beneficial when one chooses realistic, obtainable goals that will benefit from local intervention and includes the planning and performance of appropriate follow-up services. In a skilled clinician's hand it can improve quality of life, reduce pain, increase ROM, break synergy patterns, and improve positioning and hygiene (141,143).

AGENTS AVAILABLE FOR CHEMICAL DENERVATION

Phenol and ethanol were the original agents used for chemical denervation. For chemical denervation, phenol should be used in a concentration of between 5% and 7%. At that concentration, it has an immediate anesthetic effect with a subsequent neurolytic effect that matures within 2 days. Ethanol, on the other hand, should be used in concentrations ranging from 45% to 100% to create a neurolytic effect. When comparing the two agents, one will find much more literature describing the use of phenol than alcohol. However, alcohol is less toxic and is easier for clinicians to obtain. The typical duration of effect of chemical denervation with either agent is between 3 and 9 months, but it may last as long as 12 to 18 months (141,143).

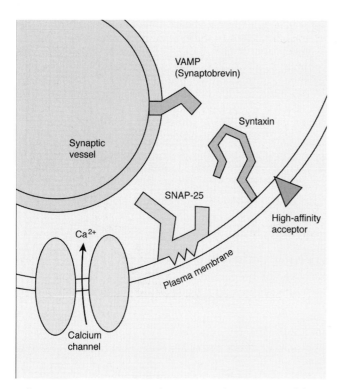

Figure 67-1. Representation of SNARE complex at motor endplate

Now an additional class of chemical denervation agents is available, the botulinum toxins. Toxin type A has been available in the United States since 1989 under the trade name Botox. Its approved indications are strabismus, hemifacial spasm and blephrospasm, dystonia, and now cosmesis. A large percentage of the product is for off-label usage (144). There is now a second type of botulinum toxin, toxin type B, which is being marketed by Elan Pharaceuticals under the trade name Myobloc.

MECHANISMS OF ACTION FOR THE CHEMICAL DENERVATION AGENTS

Ethanol and phenol's action are mediated via their ability to denature protein. It is a crude process that can demonstrate an effect on both motor and sensory fibers, as the action is on the nerve itself (22,141,145). In contrast the 144 "botulinum toxins" act on the neuromuscular junction, where they inhibit the release but not the production of acetylcholine (ACh). Acetylcholine exocytosis is an important component of transmission at the neuromuscular junction with the SNARE complex critical for this process. The different toxins act as proteolytic agents at different sites of the SNARE complex (Fig. 67-1). Toxin A is active on Snap-25 (25-kD synaptosomal associated protein), whereas the B works on Synaptobrevin (also called VAMP), a protein attached to the ACh vesicle (146).

CHEMICAL DENERVATION WITH PHENOL AND ALCOHOL

Numerous publications describe the efficacy of phenol and alcohol chemical denervation. Khalili et al. (147), Halpern et al. (148), deLateur (149), and Awad (150) are just some of the original authors who are early publishers of work showing the efficacy of phenol nerve blocks. Kong and Chua (151–153) have demonstrated efficacy of alcohol chemical denervation. This technique has been used in various patient populations, including adult stroke, traumatic brain injury, and cerebral palsy (154–157).

SIDE EFFECTS AND COMPLICATIONS OF NERVE BLOCK

Chemical denervation with phenol and alcohol can be a source of side effects even when performed correctly. Some of these include pain at time of injection, excessive weakness, change in kinesiologic pattern, and loss of protective reflexes and beneficial spasticity. Other, less frequent complications include bleeding, edema, swelling, pain, and deep venous thrombosis. The risk of dysesthesias with nerve blocks has been reported in 3% to as many as 32% of patients. Factors associated with this effect include injector skill, agent concentration, and the nerve that is blocked. When nerves like the median, which has rich sensory branches, are blocked, dysesthesias are more likely. When nerves with limited sensory components such as the obturator and the musculocutaneous are injected, the risk is much less. Treatment of dysesthesias includes therapy modalities and membrane-stabilizing anticonvulsants or antidepressants. If it is resistant to initial treatment, reblockade will usually relieve the symptoms (141,143).

BOTULINUM TOXIN THERAPY

Van Ermengem isolated the *Clostridium botulinum* after musicians developed a paralytic syndrome after eating raw ham at a wedding. There are seven serotype toxins produced by the bacteria, named A through G. Allergan markets the toxin type A under the trade name Botox. In 1989 the toxin was licensed by the Food and Drug Administration (FDA) as an orphan drug in the treatment of strabismus, hemifacial spasm, and blephrospasm. It has since been approved for dystonia, but its use in spasticity remains off label. For years Botox was the only botulinum toxin available in the United States. In December 2000 the FDA approved the Elan Pharmaceuticals botulinum toxin B under the trade name MyoBloc.

All seven serotypes demonstrate their action at the neuromuscular junction, where they inhibit the release but not the production of acetylcholine (ACh) via proteolytic cleavage of a membrane or soluble protein of the system involved in ACh exocytosis called the (SNAP—soluble N-eythyl-maleimide sensitive factor attachment protein Receptor complex) SNARE complex. The SNARE complex has three critical components: synaptobrevin, a protein attached to the ACh vesicle, SNAP-25 (25-kD synaptosomal associated protein), and syntaxin, which are attached to the cell membrane. Toxins B, D, F, and G cleave synaptobrevin, whereas toxins A, C, and E cleave SNAP-25. Toxin C cleaves syntaxin as well.

As biologic agents the toxins are measured by their toxic potencies. A unit of toxin is the LD_{50} for an IP injection of toxin into a 18 GM Swiss-Webster Mouse. There are interspecies differences, so the effect on humans of 1 mouse unit of A toxin is not the same that of 1 mouse unit of B toxin. There is no simple formula for converting a toxin A dose to a toxin B dose (52, 53,144).

BOTULINUM TOXIN A (BOTOX)

Botulinum toxin A comes packaged in a frozen lyophilized form of purified botulinum toxin A and is the most potent in humans. In contrast to phenol, botulinum toxin will be transported to the nerve terminals, and electromyography (EMG) or electrical localization is needed only to identify the muscles injected (158,159).

There has been an enormous amount of literature describing the efficacy of botulinum toxin A in various conditions. Yablon et al. (160) reported on toxin A efficacy in an open-label fashion on 21 patients after they failed conservative measures. Wilson et al. (161) demonstrated an improvement in parameters related to gait symmetry in addition to gait velocity using a single case design. Richardson et al. (162) reported on a double-blinded study in a mixed neurologic population and reported improvement 3 to 12 weeks after injection. The first large-scale multicenter randomized, double-blind, placebo-controlled trial treating chronic stroke-induced upper-extremity spasticity demonstrated significant tone reduction in both the elbow and the wrist with botulinum toxin A injection (163). This work has been recently been replicated in another randomized double-blind placebo-controlled stroke study where botulinum toxin A was superior to placebo in ROM, tone, and improvement in self-chosen and reported disability (164). Repeated injection with botulinum toxin type A has been shown to be safe and efficacious (165).

Chemical denervation with botulinum toxin does lead to occasional side effects. Systemic absorption does occur and antibody formation is a real concern in the dystonia literature (166,167). No study has yet addressed this problem with spasticity. Yablon (160) noted a very benign side effect profile (<2%) with no long-term sequelae. Headache, weakness, swelling, and flulike syndrome have been reported. The large multicenter studies also reported no increase in serious adverse events between placebo and treatment groups (163,164).

The maximal therapeutic doses have been increasing as more information relative to safety has been obtained. It is most likely safe to begin adult dosing at 400 units. There still is a wide window for therapeutic versus fatal doses. For the primate, a lethal dose is 40 units/kg, or roughly 3,000 units for a 70-kg man (168).

BOTULINUM TOXIN B MYOBLOC

In December 2000, the FDA approved Elan Pharmaceutical's botulinum toxin type B product, under the trade name Myobloc for the indication of cervical dystonia (169). Therefore, similar to Allergan's botulinum toxin A product, Botox, its use for spasticity will be off label. At the time of this chapter being written there are no published studies with Myobloc being used to treat spasticity. However, there are some abstracts suggesting safety and efficacy in the management of spasticity. Be-Dell et al. (170) reported on a single case of severe spastic quadriplegia that was managed effectively with 12,000 units of Myobloc without difficulty. Hecht et al. (171) reported on an open-label trial of 10,000 to 12,000 units of Myobloc injected into the subscapularis and pectoralis major for the treatment of shoulder pain and internal rotation spasticity. Jayasooriya et al. (172) reported on their series of 11 patients with acquired brain injury that had their upper-extremity spasticity treated with between 4,250 and 17,500 units of botulinum toxin B. Six of their patients complained of dry mouth and tone returned to baseline 12 weeks post injection. Moberg-Wolff and Walke (173) performed a retrospective chart review of 125 children who were treated with botulinum toxin B. Their doses ranged from 80 units to more than 24,000. The average dosing was approximately 15,000 or 500 to 600 units per kg. They reported that four of their patients had "reversible side effects" and that the approximate conversion ratio from Myobloc to Botox was 30/1. The two most quoted studies concerning botulinum toxin Bc are two multicenter cervical dystonia papers for both A-resistant and A-responsive patients (174,175). On the whole the studies seem quite safe, with self-limited dysphagia and dry mouth reported to be of higher incidence in the treatment group.

In summary, chemical denervation is a valuable treatment modality in the management of spasticity. Phenol and alcohol treatment requires considerable skill to perform effectively, but clearly this method still has a place in the management of focal spasticity. Botulinum toxin A has a long record of success in the treatment of spasticity. The B toxin is still new, and the jury is

out regarding its place in the treatment armamentarium. There is no large-scale study that has demonstrated safety and efficacy in spasticity management. The authors are unable to answer at this time which toxin is more effective or antigenic than the other. There is no evidence that suggests that alternating agents will delay antibody formation. Each company's science officers are happy to point their finger at their competition. Those answers will have to be deferred to some time in the future. There also is no fixed ratio of conversion when switching toxins, as they are different related drugs, in the same fashion as calcium channel blockers. At this time the clinician's skill and judgment will be an important factor in the dosing decision.

Surgical Techniques

INTRATHECAL MEDICATIONS

One of the first reports on the efficacy of intrathecal baclofen was by Penn et al. (176), who reported on its benefit in severe spasticity in patients with multiple sclerosis and spinal cord injury. The authors demonstrated that intrathecal baclofen was beneficial, acutely via a double-blinded placebo intrathecal baclofen injection over 3 days. They also were able to demonstrate a long-term treatment effect in an open-label follow-up study of between 10 and 32 months' duration after pump insertion. In 1993 Albright et al. (177) demonstrated that intrathecal baclofen was also useful in the management of cerebral palsy–related spasticity. Intrathecal baclofen has been shown to be useful in the treatment of other neurologic populations, including those suffering from TBI (178), anoxia (179), and stroke-related spastic hemiplegia (180,181).

Potential candidates for intrathecal baclofen undergo screening for potential efficacy. Their spasticity is evaluated at baseline and they are then given an intrathecal bolus of 50 µg of baclofen. If there is a substantial improvement in their spasticity, the screen is considered successful and the patient is offered insertion of an intrathecal baclofen system. If the initial trial does not demonstrate improvement, it is repeated with an escalation of the dose up to a maximum bolus of 100 µg. If any of the above trials prove successful, the patient is still offered the intrathecal baclofen system, with the starting dose often set at twice the effective bolus dose per 24 hours. Therefore if the patient responded to a 100-µg bolus, the intrathecal baclofen system is set to run at 200 µg per 24 hours. The advantage of the intrathecal baclofen system is that it delivers a continuous supply of baclofen through a catheter that is directly connected to the subarachnoid space. As a result, there is a demonstration of reduced spasticity at a dose that is substantially lower than that required via oral administration (52). Dralle et al. (182) reported that required dosing was roughly 1% of that needed for oral administration. As a result, the CNS side effects that are commonly seen with oral antispasticity agents are greatly reduced with intrathecal baclofen (183). The placement of intrathecal baclofen should not be taken lightly. The system requires a commitment to a surgical procedure and the insertion of a foreign object that will have to be replaced in 3 to 7 years, based on today's technology. In addition, there are problems associated with its use. They include the system's high cost (184), infection risk (185), seizures (186), baclofen overdose, pump dysfunction, withdrawal (187,188), and kinking or disconnection of the catheter tubing (189). Originally, the most cephalad placement of the catheter was between the levels of T8 to T10 (190). More recently, surgeons have been placing it higher (178,191) and reported significant improvement in spasticity in both the upper and lower extremities. Broseta et al.

(192) reported on the safe administration of intrathecal baclofen with the catheter placed as high as C4.

Baclofen is not the only medication that has been used intrathecally. Other pharmacologic agents that have been administered intrathecally, either alone or in combination with baclofen, include clonidine, midazalom, morphine, lidocaine, and fentanyl (193–197). Fentanyl has even been shown to be effective after the patient had developed resistance to baclofen (193). Midazalom has been used intrathecally for the management of spasticity. Work in animals has shown that the agent can work as a CNS depressant, analgesic, anticonvulsive, and myorelaxant (62). There is substantial risk of toxicity, with past animal studies showing potential toxicity on the blood–brain barrier, neurons, and the myelin sheath (198,199). As a result, questions about its use in humans have been raised (62,200, 201). It use is also limited by its sedating effects, and a careful review of the literature did not find any report of its use since 1988 (62).

Morphine has also been used intrathecally in the management of spasticity, with reduction in tone noted with boluses of 1 to 2 mg (202) and doses of 2 to 4 mg administered daily in the treatment of SCI-induced spasticity (203). The authors also reported that only one of the 12 patients who had responded to treatment had become resistant after 3 years of treatment. The use of intrathecal morphine is complicated by a significant side effect profile that includes development of tolerance, itching, GI disturbances, hypotension, and urinary retention (62). Lydon et al. (204) reported on problems with gastric emptying, whereas Glass (205) reported that an intrathecal bolus dose of 0.4 mg induced respiratory depression. Itching is the most common side effect with intrathecal morphine, whereas respiratory depression, common with doses of 1 to 2.5 mg, is the most troubling. As a result, the place of intrathecal morphine in the management of spasticity is not yet clear (62).

Intrathecal clonidine has also been used in the management of spasticity (196), especially in spinal cord patients (195). Remy-Neris et al. (206) reported that the use of intrathecal clonidine on patients with incomplete SCI showed significant electrophysiologic changes, in addition to three of of eight patients demonstrating improvements in gait velocity. It has also been shown to demonstrate decreases in the stretch reflex in this population. The functional results of intrathecal clonidine are mixed. In the previously mentioned trial, three participants did indeed demonstrate an increase in their preferred walking speed, and three others demonstrated a decrement in their performance (loss of their ability to stand), most likely as a result of the functional benefits of their tone. This loss of the ability to stand was not dose related (195). Another potential benefit of intrathecal clonidine is its ability to reduce detrusor hyperreflexia in the SCI population (207,208).

The side effect profile for intrathecal clonidine is potentially problematic. In addition to the functional loss reported earlier, there are the cardiac problems (hypotension, bradycardia, and decreased cardiac blood flow) (195,209), besides the problems of dry mouth and sedation. In particular, the homodynamic side effect of intrathecal clonidine may be the most limiting factor in its use (62).

NEUROSURGICAL PROCEDURES

In addition to intrathecal administration of pharmacologic agents, other neurosurgical procedures do have their place in the management of spasticity. Dorsal root rhizotomy is a procedure that has demonstrated efficacy in the management of spasticity. This procedure should be considered when the patient's condition has been recalcitrant to other, more conservative measures, or where financial or compliance issues may direct treatment interventions. Much of the literature concerning rhizotomy that has demonstrated efficacy is found in the cerebral palsy literature (210–213). It has been shown to be useful in other populations, such as those with multiple sclerosis (214, 215). A radiofrequency rhizotomy was performed by Kasdon and Lathi in 1974, and the authors reported significant improvement in 24 out of the 25 patients who had been treated (216). Initially, rhizotomy was not that selective with motor and sensory roots ablated. The idea of interrupting just a limited number of the most pathologic sensory rootlets was derived later. The idea was to remove the most pathologic nerve rootlets. This would lessen the chance of anesthesia and leave the motor system intact and is called a selective dorsal root rhizotomy (SDR). Much work concerning this subject has been published by Sindou and his colleages (215,217,218). Recent studies have shown that the selective dorsal root rhizotomy procedure demonstrates benefit years after surgery. Gul et al. (211) showed that 5 years after injury, their patients still maintained their improvements in tone and muscle strength. Mital et al. (219) demonstrated that fine motor improvement that was seen at 1 year was still maintained at 3- and 5-year follow-up.

Numerous complications have been reported as a result of selective dorsal root rhizotomy. They include bronchospasm, aspiration pneumonia, urinary retention, ileus, sensory loss, hypotonia, and bowel dysfunction, though many of these problems are transient (220–222). These authors all concluded that the benefits of the procedure far outweighed the potential complications.

There has been some controversy over how many rootlets should be ablated and how they should be chosen. Mittal et al. (223) stated that using electrophysiologic stimulation to identify nerve rootlets was very effective in choosing pathologic rootlets for ablation. They also reported the rootlet scoring was 93% reproducible and felt their technique resulted in great reduction in tone with only very limited loss of strength. On the other hand, Sacco et al. (224) reported that they had similar results to selective dorsal root rhizotomy when they performed nonspecific dorsal root rhizotomy on 10 patients.

One final comment regarding selective dorsal root rhizotomy is the work of Bertelli et al. (225), who reported on a new method in the treatment of spasticity that involved the upper extremity. They performed a brachial plexus dorsal root rhizotomy and reported reduction in tone without any sensory difficulties. For patients who have not benefited from any of the previous interventions, some aggressive modalities, such as myelotomy or cordotomy, are available. Bischoff has advocated the use of this procedure as being of value in severely spastic patients; however, it is controversial because it may cause dysfunction of the bowel and bladder (52).

ORTHOPEDIC PROCEDURES

Although the preceding discussion highlights the numerous pharmacologic and therapeutic modalities available in the management of spasticity, sometimes orthopedic interventions are still necessary that directly act on the muscle and tendons. Rhizotomy, oral agents, and intrathecal agents are still unable to target a particular site, the way a chemoneurolytic or orthopedic procedure can. This may be especially true in the management of childhood-related spasticity (226), where orthopedic surgical intervention can be effective in improving both function and the limitation of complications.

Orthopedic procedures are often irreversible and physicians sometimes experience resistance from patients and their family. As a consequence, realistic goal setting is critical and requires that the family, health-care providers, and patients all be on the same page. Another critical factor is the need for the treatment team to understand the pathophysiology, kinesiology, and overall patient function. Improper preprocedure planning can result in limited benefit or even a worsening of the patient's function and quality of life. When planned, executed, and given appropriate follow-up, orthopedic interventions such as improved positioning or hygiene can play a major role in active functioning tasks such as ambulation.

In the limited space available here it is impossible to discuss all surgical options. Here the goal is to assist the reader in developing general principles that he or she can generalize. As mentioned earlier, careful planning is critical before any operation. If available, dynamic EMG can be exceptionally beneficial in the decision-making process (52). When this is not available, in addition to clinical evaluation, previous results from chemoneurolysis and temporary nerve blocks may assist in the decision process. The evaluation should look for muscles cocontracting or firing out of phase. These muscles may benefit from lengthening or a transfer of distal attachment site.

An example is a brachioradialis muscle that fires during attempted extension. Transferring the muscle's distal insertion to the extensor surface will allow it be of assistance rather than a hindrance. Another example is foot inversion during gait. This movement can be caused by a host of muscles, such as the gastrocsoleus complex, tibialis anterior, tibialis posterior and flexor digitorum longus, and flexor and extensor hallicus longus. Dynamic EMG (227) or selective botulinum toxin injection may help identify the offending muscle or muscles.

Based on these tests and clinical evaluation, surgery can be planned and performed with the best chance for functional benefit. Increased activity involving elbow flexion may require the treatment of one, two, or all three elbow flexors that can be treated with lengthening procedures (228). The tibialis anterior is best known for its critical function related to ankle dorsiflexion. It can also, when overfiring, cause inversion of the foot during swing phase. The SPLATT procedure, which divides the tendon's distal attachment on the medial service and anchors it into the medial and lateral aspect of the foot, removes its inverting quality with limited loss of strength as a dorsiflexor (229). Both passive and sometimes functional improvement can be seen when hyperactivity and knee flexion contractures are treated with a release of the hamstrings with positional improvement (230). When there is shortening of the Achilles tendon, the performance of a Z-plasty procedure that lengthens the tendon may be of benefit. However, there may be some loss of strength at the ankle joint as a result. Keenan et al. (231) showed that transfer of the flexor hallicus and the digitorum longus to the os calus improved ankle strength and reduced the need for long-term use of a brace. An iliopsoas tenotomy may be necessary when there is significant spasticity or a hip flexor contracture of greater than 20 degrees after the application of more conservative measures (230). In patients with severe spasticity from multiple sclerosis or cerebral palsy, the problem of hip subluxation may be encountered. This can be treated with adductor myotomies, or if not successful, femoral osteotomy (52).

As often is the case, patients with severe spasticity receive multiple treatments, with orthopedic surgery contemplated in combination with intrathecal baclofen. Gerszten et al. (232) reviewed the cerebral palsy literature. They found that 18 out of 28 patients who were to undergo orthopedic procedures after intrathecal baclofen placement did not require it, as their spasticity had substantially improved. Grabb and Doyle (226) generally agree with this recommendation for their ambulatory patients with spasticity and structural issues, as they perform intrathecal baclofen or rhizotomy before orthopedic intervention. Their exception was the lower-level ambulator, where they feel the tone is a functional benefit to ambulation and they are more likely to perform soft-tissue release first. For the nonambulatory patient they recommend intrathecal baclofen before orthopedic intervention.

Specific Movement Disorder Management

The movement observed and treated often classifies movement disorders. Specific movement disorders are compared in Table 67-4.

DYSTONIA

Dystonia is not a single disease. Instead it is a movement disorder that is "characterized by sustained muscle contractions" (233). It can result from many different condition and causes. The contraction can be sustained or intermittent and can be exacerbated by a particular movement or task and worsened by stress (233). There are numerous methods to classify dystonias, including age of onset, areas of involvement (234,235), and etiology (234).

When classifying dystonia by age, 26 years has been chosen arbitrarily as the line of demarcation. When presentation occurs before 26 years of age, it is called an early onset; when it occurs after 26, it is considered late onset (233). When anatomy is used to classify a dystonia it is called *focal* when one area is involved, *segmental* when it involves two or more adjacent areas, *multifocal* when it involves two or more noncontinuous, *generalized* when both legs and an arm are involved, and *hemidystonic* when one side of the body is involved (233–235).

Fahn divides dystonia into five separate categories based on etiology (234). A primary dystonia is one where dystonia is the only symptom without injury or other disease. The second category is dystonia plus, when the dystonia is associated with other symptoms, such as myoclonus or parkinsonian. The third group is secondary dystonias, which includes the cases where the condition develops after brain injury, peripheral trauma, or stroke. The fourth group includes neurodegenerative disorders such as Parkinson's disease, multiple system atrophy, Wilson's disease, and mitochondrial disorders. The final group is psychogenic dystonia (233,234).

The most common form of primary dystonia is the idiopathic variety (236,237). It is a diagnosis of exclusion after all the known etiologies are excluded. There are a number of dystonias that have a genetic origin and they are designated by the abbreviation DYT and an assigned number; however, the actual genetic defect is not always identified (233). As an example, DYT1 is caused by a three base pair deletion in the TORIA gene (238). It has been found commonly in the Askenazi Jewish population (239) as well in the non-Jewish population (240). DYT5, also known as Segawa's syndrome, is an example of a dystonia plus. Its onset is normally in childhood, but it can present as an adult (241) and is responsive to dopamine replacement.

Secondary dystonia can be caused by a variety of insults. It can be seen after brain injury (242,243), cancer chemotherapy (244), peripheral trauma and SCI (245), and dental procedures (246). It can occur as a response to a wide variety of medications, including anticonvulsants, antidepressants, buspirone, ergots (233), and antipsychotics (247–249), including atypicals (250,251). Hereododegenerative disorders such as Parkinson's disease (252), Huntington's chorea (253), and Wilson's disease (254) can be a source of dystonia.

Treatment for dystonia is often symptomatic, with Segawa's syndrome (241) and Wilson's disease (233) being the excep-

TABLE 67-4. Comparison of Different Movement Disorders

Motor Disorder	Movement Observed	Common Treatment	Common Medications Used
Spasticity	Velocity dependent Resistance to movement	Modalities, casting, splinting, oral medications, chemodenervation, ITB, orthopedic intervention	Dantrolene, valium, baclofen, tizanidine, botulinum toxin
Dystonia	Sustained muscle contractions	Oral medications, botulinum toxin injection, ITB, ramisectomy, thalmotomy, intracranial electrical stimulation	Dopamine agonists, anticholinergics, baclofen, atypical antipsychotics and botulinum toxin
Tremor	An involuntary, rhythmic oscillation of reciprocally innervated, antagonistic muscle groups	Oral medications, thalmotomy and intracranial electrical stimulation	Depends on etiology Anticholinergics, dopamine agonists, primidone, β-blockers and isoniazid
Chorea	Irregular, rapid, flowing, non-stereotyped and random involuntary movement	Oral medications	Valproate, carbamazepine, clonazepam, typical and atypical antipsychotics
Myoclonus	Sudden, shock like, brief involuntary movements	Oral medications	Valproate, carbamazepine, clonazepam, anticonvulsants, anticholinergics and 5-hydroxytryptophan

tions. Dopamine agonists can be useful in the treatment of up to 20% idiopathic dystonias (255). In the majority of patients who do not respond to dopamine agonists, anticholinergic agents may be of some value (256,257). Secondary to their high side effect profile, these agents should be started low but often require titration to high levels (233). Other medications that have been tried as well in the management of dystonia include baclofen, clonazepam, and anticonvulsants (258). More recently, the atypical antipsychotics have been used in treating dystonia (259–262).

It is fair to say that the use of botulinum toxin injections has revolutionized the treatment of focal dystonia (263). Two different botulinum toxins are now available. The A toxin's efficacy has been demonstrated in too many studies to list here (264,265). There have also been studies that have demonstrated efficacy for the B toxin in cervical dystonia in both A-responsive (174) and A-resistant patients (175). The duration of effect for these treatments is approximately 3 to 4 months, and patients require reinjection to maintain clinical benefit.

There are also surgical options in dystonia management that may be critical for patients who are toxin resistant or unresponsive to pharmacologic intervention. Intrathecal baclofen has been used with some benefit in patients with dystonia (266–268). Albright et al. reported that there was greater improvement when the catheter was placed at T4 or higher (266). However, benefit has not always been demonstrated with studies of its use (269). Other procedures have been used in treating dystonia. Ford et al. (270) reported on the use of ramisectomy on 16 patients with cervical dystonia who were resistant to the botulinum toxins. Six of them had near normal neck function 5 years after surgery. Thalamotomy is a surgical procedure that was developed in the 1960s for the treatment of dystonia. It is an effective procedure but has problems with speech and swallowing function, especially when performed bilaterally (271). Andrew et al. (272) reported on his results with 55 patients who underwent sterotaxtic thalamotomy. They found significant complications, including a 15% rate of hemiparesis, and felt that the procedure should be used in hemidystonias, where it should be performed unilaterally only. Early results have shown bilateral pallidotomy to be of benefit in the management of dystonia (273,274). Electrical pallidal and thalamic stimulation has also been used in the treatment of dystonia (275–278). Kraus et al. (278) reported on their results with eight patients with dystonia treated with pallidal stimulation and re-

ported significant improvement in dsytonia severity, disability, and pain. Further work needs to be performed with larger populations before definitive opinions can be developed.

CHOREA

Syndemham was the first to describe the condition that is now known as chorea. He wrote about a syndrome that developed after an infection and called it St. Vitus dance (279). In 1872 Huntington reported a chorea that was transmitted via heredity (280), which further focused attention on the area. Chorea, which means "dance" in Greek, is a movement disorder that is characterized by "irregular, rapid, flowing, nonstereotyped and random involuntary movements" (281). Chorea can be caused by a variety of different etiologies, including hereditary, infectious, endocrinologic, drug side effect, and vascular (281).

Of the hereditary causes of chorea, Huntington's may be the most notorious. It is an autosomal dominant disorder that in addition to the movement component also presents with cognitive and psychiatric symptoms (282). The typical onset is in the third or fourth decades of life (281,282). Other, rarer genetic causes of chorea include neuroacanthocytois, dentatorubropallidolusysian atrophy, benign hereditary chorea, paroxysmal chorea, and Wilson's disease (281).

There are of course numerous nonhereditary choreas. Sydenham's chorea is correlated with a previous group A strep infection and is usually self-limited (283). Lupus can be associated with chorea in approximately 1% of patients with the condition (281) and can be part of the antiphosolipid syndrome (284). Chorea has also been found in women during pregnancy (285), in those with polycythemia vera (286), and as a result of hyperthyroidism (287). Other noniatrogenic causes of chorea include stroke and AIDs (281). Pharmacologic agents can also be a source of chorea. The dopamine antagonists that are used to treat psychosis have been linked to numerous movement disorders, including chorea (288,289), which may not improve after stopping the agent (288). The atypical antipsychotics may have an advantage over the classic antipsychotics because of their diverse areas of activity (290).

Treatment of chorea has been disappointing (281). Clearly, removing the offending agent is important. Both valproate and carbamazepine have been shown to be safe and efficacious in Syndenham's chorea (291). Caviness has recommended initiating treatment with clonazepam as a first step for all choreas (292).Tetrabenazine, a dopamine receptor blocker, and monamine depleter have been trialed with some success (293). Typical (292) and atypical antipsychotics have also been used in the management of chorea (292 294).

TREMOR

Tremor is defined as an involuntary, rhythmic oscillation of reciprocally innervated, antagonistic muscle groups, causing movement of a body part about a fixed plane in space (295–297). It is its rhythmicity that distinguishes tremor from other movement disorders (295). Tremors can be classified by their oscillation frequencies. They are called slow when they occur at a rate of 3 to 5 Hz, intermediate when they are 5 to 8 Hz, and rapid when they occur at 9 to 12 Hz (298). The tremors can also be described as fine, medium, or coarse, based on the amount of movement that the tremor causes (298). Finally and most important, tremors are classified by a person's activity when he or she experiences the tremor. A postural tremor is one that occurs as the person tries to maintain his or her posture. A resting tremor is one that occurs when the body part is being held at rest. An action tremor occurs when intentional movement is attempted (296,298).

Tremor can be symptom in a variety of neurologic disorders. Treatment is primarily symptomatic and varies according to etiology (297). In Parkinson's disease, the tremor occurs at rest, has a frequency of 4 to 6 Hz, and has medium amplitude. The tremor most commonly affects the hand in the classically known "pill rolling." However, especially as the disease progresses, it can also be seen in other body parts, including the head, trunk, jaw, and lips (296,298). A resting tremor can also be found in the similar, related neurodegenerative diseases, multiple-systems atrophy, and progressive supranuclear palsy. However, the tremor from these disorders is not as prominent as the one secondary to Parkinson's disease (297). The disease is a result of degeneration in the substantia nigra that causes the dopamine fibers that project to the striatum to be affected. They are part of the extra-pyramidal system that is critical in motor control (299). As a result of this degeneration, the ventral intermediate nucleus of the thalamus becomes overactive. The neurons in this nucleus fire at a rate that matches the parkinsonian tremor, suggesting that it is the source (300). Treatment for Parkinson's disease involved the use of the classic dopamine-based antiparkinsonian regimen of L-dopa, carbidopa–levodopa, bromocriptine, pergolide, ropinirole, and pramipexole. In addition, the anticholinergic agents trihexyphenidyl and benztropine may be particularly effective when tremor is a major symptom (297,301).

Essential tremor is the most common movement disorder (296,298 302,303). It is a postural tremor with a frequency of between 4 and 11 Hz, which most commonly affects the upper extremities (303). The tremors that involve the more proximal body parts, the head, have a lower frequency than those affecting the more distal, such as the hand. In addition to the hand, the head, tongue, and legs can be affected (296,298,303). Its prevalence increases with age, with onset beginning anywhere from teenage years until 60 years of age (302), and its course is one of slow progression (298). Its pathophysiology is unknown, and it can appear in a sporadic or genetically inherited form. The transmission pattern appears to be autosomally dominant, with a variable penetration (304). Unlike Parkinson's, there is no clear agent that is clearly superior to any other. Many different pharmacologic agents have been used in the management of essential tremor. The most commonly used agents in the management of essential tremor are propanolol and primidone (297). Other β-blockers have also been tried and include metoprolol and naldol (296). Essential tremor also is improved with alcohol ingestion (298). Charles et al. (297) have stated that primidone and propranolol are equally effective and that patients who do not respond to one agent for a few weeks should be switched to the other.

Many tremors originate from the cerebellum. Most cerebellar origin tremors are of the action variety. Pathology in the lateral cerebellar nuclei or superior cerebellar peduncle or one of its related circuits is the source of the tremor (297). Another tremor, commonly found in multiple sclerosis (MS), is a cerebellar postural tremor that is an action and is postural (304). Treatment options for cerebellar tremor are quite limited, with isoisoniazid in combination with pyridoxine being used for severe MS cases (304).

Tremor can also be found when a patient is experiencing alcohol withdrawal. It is similar to essential tremor with a few small differences. The frequency of the tremor is one means to differentiate, with the frequency of alcohol withdrawal tremor higher than that of essential tremor. Koller et al. (305) reported that three-fourths of those with alcoholic withdrawal tremor had a frequency greater than 8 Hz, whereas the essential patients had a slower rate. They also found that the severity of disability and family history of tremor was much less in the group than was true with essential tremor. A final means to differentiate the tremors is localization. With alcohol withdrawal it is primarily restricted to just the hands, whereas in essential tremor more areas are involved.

Although less frequent, there are other tremors that can be seen by physicians who treat them. These include psychogenic, orthostatic and tremors that originate from peripheral neuropathies. Psychogenetic tremors are often complex and can occur at rest, during action, or as a postural variant. The examination can be inconsistent. Changes in frequency and amplitude can be seen with distraction and are normally poorly responsive to classic antitremor medications (297,306). An orthostatic tremor occurs at a frequency of 13 to 18 Hz and is a postural tremor that involves the legs as a patient stands up. It is improved when the patient sits or ambulates (307). Several medications have been used successfully in the treatment of orthostatic tremor. They include cloanazepam (308,309), chlordiazepoxide (308), and valproate (309). Finally, tremors that are associated with peripheral neuropathy can appear very similar to essential tremor. Some of the peripheral neuropathies that can be associated with tremor include Charcot-Marie-Tooth disease, diabetes mellitus, uremia, and porphyria (296).

When pharmacologic options fail, there are surgical alternatives. Stereotactic thalamotomy can be useful in the management of essential tremor. It can also be of value in the treatment of drug-resistant Parkinson's (310,311). For Parkinson's disease an alternative procedure, pallidotomy, has also been used with some success (312). The preceding procedures involve the placement of a surgical placed lesion, are irreversible, and have the potential for cognitive side effects. The relatively new procedure of programmable thalamic and subthalamic stimulation with an implanted electrical electrode may turn out to be extremely effective and may have a better risk–benefit ratio than the destructive procedures mentioned previously for tremor of various etiologies (313,314).

MYOCLONUS

Myoclonus is a neurologic condition that is characterized by sudden, shocklike, brief involuntary movements. They can result from a contraction of a muscle (positive myoclonus) or inhibition of a muscle (negative myoclonus) (315–317). Like spasticity, myoclonus is not a diagnosis but is more of a description term (316). Myoclonus is classified in many different fashions, including anatomic, temporal, activation patterns, etiology, and underlying pathophysiology. Examples of anatomic classification include focal, multifocal, segmental, or generalized. Myoclonic activity is considered focal when it is found in one region of the body and is called multifocal when two or more areas are involved that are not adjacent. The activity is described as segmental when it involves one area, such as a limb, and it is called generalized when multiple muscle groups are involved (318). Myoclonus has also been described in terms of its temporal factors. It can be described as rhythmic or irregular, or it can be portrayed as sporadic or repetitive (316). The behavior seen in proximity to myoclonus is another method of classification. When myoclonus occurs without an antecedent it is called spontaneous. If it occurs as a response to a specific stimulus, it is called reflexive, and when it occurs with volitional movement it is called action or intentional if it is a specific movement (316,318).

Marsden et al. (319) were the first to propose a method of classification based on etiology. Under their schema, myoclonus is called *physiologic* when no other abnormality is found on examination and there is no disability, *essential* when the condition is isolated and causing minimal disability, *epileptic* when associated with a seizure disorder, and *secondary* or *symptomatic* when it is a result of another neurologic condition (316).

Essential myoclonus is divided into two categories. The first is *hereditary essential myoclonus*; the second is *sporadic essential myoclonus*. The hereditary variant has a dominant inheritance pattern and an onset before age 20. The clinical course is benign, often involves the upper extremities, and is associated with no other neurologic condition or EEG abnormality. Those with the condition have a fairly normal life span and quality of life (320). On the other hand, the sporadic essential variant is more heterogeneous. It is a wastebasket diagnosis for all the myoclonic conditions that do not fit into other categories. A major study of this condition revealed patients with the condition ranging in age from age 2 to 64, with patients having no specific age of onset, clinical presentation, or region affected (321). It has been proposed that the diagnosis is made either because of false negatives in family history or diagnostic categories not yet identified (316).

Myoclonus can be associated with seizures and is called *epileptic myoclonus*. It can be found either at the start or near the end of a generalized tonic–clonic seizure (316) or can be the only part of a seizure that has myoclonus as its only presentation. Epilepsia partialis continua is a condition where myoclonus can be seen for periods that can range from hours to possibly weeks. The patient will have periods where for up to 10 seconds myoclonus is evident in one part of the body (322). Myoclonus can be a part of an absence seizure (323) or can be the main component in myoclonic seizures (324).

Secondary myoclonus can be found as a symptom of many other conditions that include genetic storage diseases, such as Tay-Sachs disease (325). It can also be found in a variety of neurodegenerative diseases such as cerebellar myoclonic syndrome (326), multiple system atrophy (327), Creutzfeldt–Jakob disease (328), and Alzheimer's disease (329). Burkhardt et al. (330) reported that myoclonus can be found in up to 15% of people with diffuse Lewy body disease. Lance and Adams (331) described the presence of spontaneous myoclonus after severe anoxic injury. Myoclonus can also be a result of toxic or metabolic disturbances. The best-known example of this is asterixis, which is frequently seen with metabolic encephalopathies (332). Myoclonus is also seen as a result of exposure to

toxin or pharmacologic agents. A partial list includes aluminum, mercury, oven cleaner, marijuana, antidepressants, lithium, and typical and atypical antipsychotics (316). Finally, myoclonus has been identified to be a result of a focal lesion in the nervous system. They can arise from focal lesions in the cortex (333), brainstem (334,335), spinal cord (336,337), and even the peripheral nervous system (335).

The treatment of myoclonus is based on its etiology. If its source is a metabolic abnormality or a response to a medication, treating the former or removing the latter may be all that is needed. Although physiologic, myoclonus requires no treatment at all (316). When the myoclonus arises associated with a seizure disorder, the use of anticonvulsants and especially valproic acid and clonazepam is appropriate (338). Valproic acid and clonazepam are overall the most effective agents in the treatment of symptomatic myoclonus (338). 5-hydroxytryptophan has been shown to be beneficial in the treatment of postanoxic myoclonus (339,340). Other agents that have been trialed in the treatment of myoclonus include piracetam (341), anticholinergic agents (342), anticonvulsants (316), benzodiazepines (343), tetrabenazine (344), opiates, and dopaminergic agents (345).

REFERENCES

1. Gans BM, Glenn MB. Introduction. In: Glenn MB, Whyte J, eds. *The practical management of spasticity in children and adults.* Philadelphia: Lea & Febiger, 1990:1–7.
2. Sherrington CS. On plastic tonus and proprioceptive reflexes. *Q J Exp Neurol* 1909;2:109–156.
3. Henneman E. Skeletal muscle: the servant of the nervous system. In: Mountcastle VB, ed. *Medical physiology.* St Louis: CV Mosby, 1980:674–702.
4. Whitlock JA. Neurophysiology of spasticity. In: Glenn MB, Whyte J, eds. *The practical management of spasticity in children and adults.* Philadelphia: Lea & Febiger, 1990:8–33.
5. AAPMR, ed. *Spasticity management in the patient with brain injury.* Orlando: American Academy of PM&R, 1995.
6. Katz R, Pierrot-Deseilligny E. Recurrent inhibition of alpha-motoneurons in patients with upper motor neuron lesions. *Brain* 1982;105(Pt 1):103–124.
7. Moore JC. The Golgi tendon organ: a review and update. *Am J Occup Ther* 1984;38:227–236.
8. Hultborn H, Illert M, Santani I. Convergence on interneurons mediating the reciprocal Ia inhibition of motor neurones. *Acta Physiol Scand* 1976;96:193–201.
9. Brooks VB. *The neural basis of motor control.* New York: Oxford University Press, 1986.
10. Shefner JM, Berman SA, Sarkarati M, et al. Recurrent inhibition is increased in patients with spinal cord injury. *Neurology* 1992;42:2162–2168.
11. Rothwell JC, Thompson PD, Day BL, et al. Stimulation of the human motor cortex through the scalp. *Exp Physiol* 1991;76:159–200.
12. Turton A, Fraser C, Flament W, et al. Organization of cortico-motorneuronal projections from the primary motor cortex: evidence for task related function in monkey and in man. In: Thrilmann AF, Burke DJ, Rymer WZ, eds. *Spasticity: mechanisms and management.* Berlin: Springer, 1993:8–24.
13. Brodal A. *Neurological anatomy in relationship to clinical medicine.* New York: Oxford University Press, 1981.
14. Magoun HW, Rhines R. An inhibitory mechanism in the bulbar reticular formation. *J Neurophysiol* 1946;9:165–171.
15. Dietz V, Berger W. Normal and impaired regulation of muscle stiffness in gait: a new hypothesis about muscle hypertonia. *Exp Neurol* 1983;79:680–687.
16. Hagbarth KE. Exteroceptive, proprioceptive and sympathetic activity recorded with microelectrodes from human peripheral nerves. *Mayo Clin Proc* 1979;54:353–364.
17. Delwaide PJ. Human monosynaptic reflexes and presynaptic inhibition. In: Esmedt JE, ed. *New developments in electromyography and clinical neurophysiology.* Basel: Karger, 1973:508–522.
18. McCouch GP. Sprouting as a cause of spasticity. *J Neurophysiol* 1958;21:205–216.
19. Cannon WB, Haimovici H. The sensitization of motor neurons by partial denervation. *Am J Physiol* 1939;126:731–740.
20. Willis WD. The raphe–spinal system. In: Barnes CD, ed. *Brainstem control of spinal cord function.* New York: Academic, 1984:141–214.
21. Gans BM, Glenn MB. Introduction. In: Glenn MB, Whyte J, eds. *The practical management of spasticity in children and adults.* Philadelphia: Lea & Febiger, 1990:1–7.

22. Gracies JM, Elovic E, McGuire J, et al. Spasticity: traditional pharmacologic treatments part I: local treatments. In: Mayer NH, Simpson DM, eds. *Spasticity: etiology, evaluation, management and the role of botulinum toxin.* New York: We Move, 2002:44–64.

23. Lund S, Lundberg A, Vyklicky L. Inhibitory action from the flexor reflex afferents on transmission to Ia afferents. *Acta Physiol Scand* 1965;64:345–355.

24. Zafonte RD, Elovic E. Spasticity and abnormalities of muscle tone. In: Grabois M, Garrison SJ, Hart KA, et al, eds. *Physical medicine and rehabilitation: the complete approach.* Malden, MA: Blackwell Science, 2000:848–858.

25. Gracies JM. Pathophysiology of impairment in patients with spasticity and use of stretch as a treatment of spastic hypertonia. *Phys Med Rehabil Clin N Am* 2001;12:747–768, vi.

26. Ranson SW, Dixon HH. Elasticity and ductility of muscle in myostatic contracture caused by tetanus toxin. *Am J Physiol* 1928;86:312–319.

27. WIlliams RG. Sensitivity changes shown by spindle receptors in chronically immobilized skeletal muscle. *J Physiol* 1980;306:26–27.

28. Schmidt BD, Dewald JP, Rymer WZ. Stretch reflex adaptation in elbow flexors during repeated passive movements in unilateral brain injured patients. *Arch Phys Med* Rehabil 2000;81:269.

29. Wilson LR, Gracies JM, Burke D, et al. Evidence for fusimotor drive in stroke patients based on muscle spindle thixotropy. *Neurosci Lett* 1999;264(1–3):109–112.

30. Gracies JM, Marosszeky JE, Renton R, et al. Short-term effects of dynamic Lycra splints on upper limb in hemiplegic patients. *Arch Phys MedRehabil* 2000;81:1547–1555.

31. Tremblay F, Malouin F, Richards CL, et al. Effects of prolonged muscle stretch on reflex and voluntary muscle activations in children with spastic cerebral palsy. *Scand J Rehabil Med* 1990;22:171–180.

32. Carey JR. Manual stretch: effect on finger movement control and force control in stroke subjects with spastic extrinsic finger flexor muscles. *Arch Phys Med Rehabil* 1990;71:888–894.

33. Brouwer B, Davidson LK, Olney SJ. Serial casting in idiopathic toe-walkers and children with spastic cerebral palsy. *J Pediatr Orthop* 2000;20:221–225.

34. Hill J. The effects of casting on upper extremity motor disorders after brain injury. *Am J Occup Ther* 1994;48:219–224.

35. Otis JC, Root L, Kroll MA. Measurement of plantar flexor spasticity during treatment with tone-reducing casts. *J Pediatr Orthop* 1985;5:682–686.

36. Lightfoot E, Verrier M. Neurophysiological effects of prolonged cooling of the calf in patients with complete spinal cord transection. *Physiotherapy* 1976;62:114–117.

37. Weiss M, Duma-Drzewinska A. [Cooling as a method of reducing spasticity]. *Neurol Neurochir Pol* 1976;10:335–343.

38. Knutsson E. On effects of local cooling upon motor functions in spastic paresis. *Prog Phys Ther* 1970;1:124–131.

39. Knutsson E. Topical cryotherapy in spasticity. *Scand J Rehabil Med* 1970;2:159–163.

40. Gracies JM. Physical modalities other than stretch in spastic hypertonia. *Phys Med Rehabil Clin N Am* 2001;12:769–792, vi.

41. Bell KR, Lehmann JF. Effect of cooling on H- and T-reflexes in normal subjects. *Arch Phys Med Rehabil* 1987;68:490–493.

42. Douglas WW, Malcom JL. The effect of localized cooling on conduction in cat nerves. *J Physiol* 1955;130:53.

43. Lee JM, Warren MP. Ice, relaxation and exercise in reduction of muscle spasticity. *Physiotherapy* 1974;60:296–302.

44. Price R, Lehmann JF. Influence of muscle cooling on the viscoelastic response of the human ankle to sinusoidal displacements. *Arch Phys Med Rehabil* 1990;71:745–748.

45. Travell J. Ethyl chloride spray for painful muscle spasms. *Arch Phys Med Rehabil* 1952;33:291.

46. Lehmann JF, de Lateur BJ. Diathermy and superficial heat and cold therapy. In: Krusen F, ed. *Handbook of physical medicine.* Philadelphia: WB Saunders, 1996.

47. Warren CG, Lehmann JF, Koblanski JN. Heat and stretch procedures: an evaluation using rat tail tendon. *Arch Phys Med Rehabil* 1976;57:122.

48. Wessling KC, DeVane DA, Hylton CR. Effect of static stretch versus static stretch and ultrasound combined on triceps surae muscle extensibility in healthy women. *Phys Ther* 1987;67:674.

49. Bajd T, Gregoric M, Vodovnik L, et al. Electrical stimulation in treating spasticity resulting from spinal cord injury. *Arch Phys Med Rehabil* 1985;66:515–517.

50. Han JS, Chen XH, Yuan Y, et al. Transcutaneous electrical nerve stimulation for treatment of spinal spasticity. *Chin Med J (Engl)* 1994;107:6–11.

51. Walker WC. Retraining the neuromuscular system: biofeedback and neuromuscular electrical stimulation. In: Grabois M, Garrison SJ, Hart KA, et al., eds. *Physical medicine and rehabilitation: the complete approach.* Malden, MA: Blackwell Science, 2000:513–529.

52. Elovic E, Zafonte RD. Spasticity management in traumatic brain injury. *State Art Rehabil* 2001;15:327–348.

53. Elovic E. Principles of pharmaceutical management of spastic hypertonia. *Phys Med Rehabil Clin N Am* 2001;12:793–816, vii.

54. Kirshblum S. Treatment alternatives for spinal cord injury related spasticity. *J Spinal Cord Med* 1999;22:199–217.

55. Duncan GW, Shahani BT, Young RR. An evaluation of baclofen treatment for certain symptoms in patients with spinal cord lesions. A double-blind, cross-over study. *Neurology* 1976;26:441–446.

56. Hudgson P, Weightman D. Baclofen in the treatment of spasticity. *Br Med J* 1971;4:15–17.

57. Nance PW, Bugaresti J, Shellenberger K, et al. Efficacy and safety of tizanidine in the treatment of spasticity in patients with spinal cord injury. *Neurology* 1994;44[11 Suppl 9]:S44–S51.

58. Groves L, Shellenberger MK, Davis CS. Tizanidine treatment of spasticity: a meta-analysis of controlled, double-blind, comparative studies with baclofen and diazepam. *Adv Ther* 1998;15:241–251.

59. Goldstein LB. Common drugs may influence motor recovery after stroke. *Neurology* 1995;45:865–871.

60. Meythaler JM, Guin-Renfroe S, Johnson A, et al. Prospective assessment of tizanidine for spasticity due to acquired brain injury. *Arch Phys Med Rehabil* 2001;82:1155–1163.

61. Francois B, Vacher P, Roustan J, et al. Intrathecal baclofen after traumatic brain injury: early treatment using a new technique to prevent spasticity. *J Trauma* 2001;50:158–161.

62. Gracies JM, Elovic E, McGuire J, et al. Spasticity: traditional pharmacologic treatments part II: systemic treatments. In: Mayer NH, Simpson DM, eds. *Spasticity: etiology, evaluation, management and the role of botulinum toxin.* New York: We Move, 2002:65–93.

63. Tseng TC, Wang SC. Locus of action of centrally acting muscle relaxants, diazepam and tybamate. *J Pharmacol Exp Ther* 1971;178:350–360.

64. Lossius R, Dietrichson P, Lunde PK. Effect of clorazepate in spasticity and rigidity: a quantitative study of reflexes and plasma concentrations. *Acta Neurol Scand* 1985;71:190–194.

65. Scharf MB, Hirschowitz J, Woods M, et al. Lack of amnestic effects of clorazepate on geriatric recall. *J Clin Psychiatry* 1985;46:518–520.

66. Abernethy DR, Greenblatt DJ, Divoll M, et al. Prolonged accumulation of diazepam in obesity. *J Clin Pharmacol* 1983;23:369–376.

67. Corbett M, Frankel HL, Michaelis L. A double blind, cross-over trial of Valium in the treatment of spasticity. *Paraplegia* 1972;10:19–22.

68. Whyte J, Robinson KM. Pharmacologic management. In: Glenn MB, Whyte J, eds. *The practical management of spasticity in children and adults.* Philadelphia: Lea & Febiger, 1990:201–226.

69. Verrier M, Ashby P, MacLeod S. Diazepam effect on reflex activity in patients with complete spinal lesions and in those with other causes of spasticity. *Arch Phys Med Rehabil* 1977;58:148–153.

70. Cook JB, Nathan PW. On the site of action of diazepam in spasticity in man. *J Neurol Sci* 1967;5:33–37.

71. Broderick CP, Radnitz CL, Bauman WA. Diazepam usage in veterans with spinal cord injury. *J Spinal Cord Med* 1997;20:406–409.

72. Cartlidge NE, Hudgson P, Weightman D. A comparison of baclofen and diazepam in the treatment of spasticity. *J Neurol Sci* 1974;23:17–24.

73. From A, Heltberg A. A double-blind trial with baclofen (Lioresal) and diazepam in spasticity due to multiple sclerosis. *Acta Neurol Scand* 1975;51:158–166.

74. Roussan M, Terrence C, Fromm G. Baclofen versus diazepam for the treatment of spasticity and long-term follow-up of baclofen therapy. *Pharmatherapeutica* 1985;4:278–284.

75. Engle HA. The effect of diazepam (Valium) in children with cerebral palsy: a double–blind study. *Dev Med Child Neurol* 1966;8:661–667.

76. Nogen AG. Medical treatment for spasticity in children with cerebral palsy. *Childs Brain* 1976;2:304–308.

77. Basmajian JV. Lioresal (baclofen) treatment of spasticity in multiple sclerosis. *Am J Phys Med* 1975;54:175–177.

78. Nance PW. A comparison of clonidine, cyproheptadine and baclofen in spastic spinal cord injured patients. *J Am Paraplegia Soc* 1994;17:150–156.

79. Feldman RG, Kelly-Hayes M, Conomy JP, et al. Baclofen for spasticity in multiple sclerosis: double-blind crossover and three-year study. *Neurology* 1978;28:1094–1098.

80. Hedley DW, Maroun JA, Espir ML. Evaluation of baclofen (Lioresal) for spasticity in multiple sclerosis. *Postgrad Med J* 1975;51:615–618.

81. Hudgson P, Weightman D. Baclofen in the treatment of spasticity. *Br Med J* 1971;4:15–17.

82. Ashby P, White DG. "Presynaptic" inhibition in spasticity and the effect of beta(4-chlorophenyl)GABA. *J Neurol Sci* 1973;20:329–338.

83. Basmajian JV, Yucel V. Effects of a GABA-derivative (BA-34647) on spasticity. Preliminary report of a double-blind cross-over study. *Am J Phys Med* 1974;53:223–228.

84. Jones RF, Burke D, Marosszeky JE, et al. A new agent for the control of spasticity. *J Neurol Neurosurg Psychiatry* 1970;33:464–468.

85. Pedersen E, Arlien-Soborg P, Grynderup V, et al. GABA derivative in spasticity. (Beta-(4-chlorophenyl)-gamma-aminobutyric acid, Ciba 34.647-Ba). *Acta Neurol Scand* 1970;46:257–266.

86. Orsnes GB, Sorensen PS, Larsen TK, et al. Effect of baclofen on gait in spastic MS patients. *Acta Neurol Scand* 2000;101:244–248.

87. Nielsen JF, Anderson JB, Sinkjaer T. Baclofen increases the soleus stretch reflex threshold in the early swing phase during walking in spastic multiple sclerosis patients. *Mult Scler* 2000;6:105–114.

88. Nielsen JF, Sinkjaer T. Peripheral and central effect of baclofen on ankle joint stiffness in multiple sclerosis. *Muscle Nerve* 2000;23:98–105.

89. Jones RF, Lance JW. Baclofen (Lioresal) in the long-term management of spasticity. *Med J Aust* 1976;1:654–657.

90. Pedersen E. Clinical assessment and pharmacologic therapy of spasticity. *Arch Phys Med Rehabil* 1974;55:344–354.

91. Pinto OS, Polikar M, Debono G. Results of international clinical trials with Lioresal. *Postgrad Med J* 1972;48:Suppl-25.
92. Hulme A, MacLennan WJ, Ritchie RT, et al. Baclofen in the elderly stroke patient its side-effects and pharmacokinetics. *Eur J Clin Pharmacol* 1985;29:467–469.
93. Milla PJ, Jackson AD. A controlled trial of baclofen in children with cerebral palsy. *J Int Med Res* 1977;5:398–404.
94. Katz RT, Campagnolo DI. Pharmacologic management of spasticity. In: Katz RT, ed. *Spasticity: state of the arts review.* Philadelphia: Hanley & Belfus, 1994: 473–480.
95. Utili R, Boitnott JK, Zimmerman HJ. Dantrolene associated hepatic injury: incidence and character. *Gastroenterology* 1977;72:610.
96. Glass A, Hannah A. A comparison of dantrolene sodium and diazepam in the treatment of spasticity. *Paraplegia* 1974;12:170–174.
97. Weiser R, Terenty T, Hudgson P, et al. Dantrolene sodium in the treatment of spasticity in chronic spinal cord disease. *Practitioner* 1978;221:123–127.
98. Monster AW. Spasticity and the effect of dantrolene sodium. *Arch Phys Med Rehabil* 1974;55:373–383.
99. Mandac BR, Hurvitz EA, Nelson VS. Hyperthermia associated with baclofen withdrawal and increased spasticity. *Arch Phys Med Rehabil* 1993;74:96–97.
100. Khorasani A, Peruzzi WT. Dantrolene treatment for abrupt intrathecal baclofen withdrawal. *Anesth Analg* 1995;80:1054–1056.
101. Gelenberg AJ, Poskanzer DC. The effect of dantrolene sodium on spasticity in multiple sclerosis. *Neurology* 1973;23:1313–1315.
102. Tolosa ES, Soll RW, Loewenson RB. Letter: treatment of spasticity in multiple sclerosis with dantrolene. *JAMA* 1975;233:1046.
103. Chyatte SB, Birdsong JH, Bergman BA. The effects of dantrolene sodium on spasticity and motor performance in hemiplegia. *South Med J* 1971;64:180–185.
104. Ketel WB, Kolb ME. Long-term treatment with dantrolene sodium of stroke patients with spasticity limiting the return of function. *Curr Med Res Opin* 1984;9:161–169.
105. Krach LE. Pharmacotherapy of spasticity: oral medications and intrathecal baclofen. *J Child Neurol* 2001;16:31–36.
106. Haslam RH, Walcher JR, Lietman PS, et al. Dantrolene sodium in children with spasticity. *Arch Phys Med Rehabil* 1974;55:384–388.
107. Donovan WH, Carter RE, Rossi CD, et al. Clonidine effect on spasticity: a clinical trial. *Arch Phys Med Rehabil* 1988;69(3 Pt 1):193–194.
108. Nance PW, Shears AH, Nance DM. Clonidine in spinal cord injury. *Can Med Assoc J* 1985;133:41–42.
109. Nance PW, Shears AH, Nance DM. Reflex changes induced by clonidine in spinal cord injured patients. *Paraplegia* 1989;27:296–301.
110. Weingarden SI, Belen JG. Clonidine transdermal system for treatment of spasticity in spinal cord injury. *Arch Phys Med Rehabil* 1992;73:876–877.
111. Yablon SA, Sipski ML. Effect of transdermal clonidine on spinal spasticity. *Am J Phys Med Rehabil* 1993;72:154–157.
112. Rosenblum D. Clonidine-induced bradycardia in patients with spinal cord injury. *Arch Phys Med Rehabil* 1993;74:1206–1207.
113. Sandford PR, Spengler SE, Sawasky KB. Clonidine in the treatment of brainstem spasticity. *Am J Phys Med Rehabil* 1992;71:301–303.
114. Dall JT, Harmon RL, Quinn CM. Use of clonidine for treatment of spasticity arising from various forms of brain injury: a case series. *Brain Inj* 1996;10: 453–458.
115. Kameyama T, Nabeshima T, Sugimoto A, et al. Antinociceptive action of tizanidine in mice and rats. *Naunyn Schmiedebergs Arch Pharmacol* 1985;330: 93–96.
116. Davies J, Johnston SE. Selective antinociceptive effects of tizanidine (DS 103–282), a centrally acting muscle relaxant, on dorsal horn neurones in the feline spinal cord. *Br J Pharmacol* 1984;82:409–421.
117. Davies J, Johnston SE, Hill DR, et al. Tizanidine (DS103–282), a centrally acting muscle relaxant, selectively depresses excitation of feline dorsal horn neurones to noxious peripheral stimuli by an action at alpha 2-adrenoceptors. *Neurosci Lett* 1984;48:197–202.
118. Newman PM, Nogues M, Newman PK, et al. Tizanidine in the treatment of spasticity. *Eur J Clin Pharmacol* 1982;23:31–35.
119. Bass B, Weinshenker B, Rice GP, et al. Tizanidine versus baclofen in the treatment of spasticity in patients with multiple sclerosis. *Can J Neurol Sci* 1988;15:15–19.
120. Bes A, Eyssette M, Pierrot-Deseilligny E, et al. A multi-centre, double-blind trial of tizanidine, a new antispastic agent, in spasticity associated with hemiplegia. *Curr Med Res Opin* 1988;10:709–718.
121. Lapierre Y, Bouchard S, Tansey C, et al. Treatment of spasticity with tizanidine in multiple sclerosis. *Can J Neurol Sci* 1987;14[3 Suppl]:513–517.
122. Johnson TR, Tobias JD. Hypotension following the initiation of tizanidine in a patient treated with an angiotensin converting enzyme inhibitor for chronic hypertension. *J Child Neurol* 2000;15:818–819.
123. Mathias CJ, Luckitt J, Desai P, et al. Pharmacodynamics and pharmacokinetics of the oral antispastic agent tizanidine in patients with spinal cord injury. *J Rehabil Res Dev* 1989;26:9–16.
124. A double-blind, placebo-controlled trial of tizanidine in the treatment of spasticity caused by multiple sclerosis. *Neurology* 1994;44[11 Suppl 9]:S70–S78.
125. Smith C, Birnbaum G, Carter JL, et al. Tizanidine treatment of spasticity caused by multiple sclerosis: results of a double-blind, placebo-controlled trial. *Neurology* 1994;44[11 Suppl 9]:S34–S42.
126. Eyssette M, Rohmer F, Serratrice G, et al. Multi-centre, double-blind trial of a novel antispastic agent, tizanidine, in spasticity associated with multiple sclerosis. *Curr Med Res Opin* 1988;10:699–708.
127. Bass B, Weinshenker B, Rice GP, et al. Tizanidine versus baclofen in the treatment of spasticity in patients with multiple sclerosis. *Can J Neurol Sci* 1988; 15:15–19.
128. Lapierre Y, Bouchard S, Tansey C, et al. Treatment of spasticity with tizanidine in multiple sclerosis. *Can J Neurol Sci* 1987;14[Suppl]:513–517.
129. Smith C, Birnbaum G, Carter JL, et al. Tizanidine treatment of spasticity caused by multiple sclerosis: results of a double-blind, placebo-controlled trial. *Neurology* 1994;44[Suppl 9]:S34–S42.
130. Brin IL, Kurenkov AL, Gotlib VI. [The use of sirdalud in cerebral palsy in children]. *Zh Nevrol Psikhiatr Im S S Korsakova* 1999;99:30–33.
131. Maritz NG, Muller FO, Pompe van Meerdervoort HF. Piracetam in the management of spasticity in cerebral palsy. *S Afr Med J* 1978;53:889–891.
132. Baker D, Pryce G, Croxford JL, et al. Cannabinoids control spasticity and tremor in a multiple sclerosis model. *Nature* 2000;404:84–87.
133. Petro DJ, Ellenberger C, Jr. Treatment of human spasticity with delta 9-tetrahydrocannabinol. *J Clin Pharmacol* 1981;21[Suppl]:413S–416S.
134. Cutter NC, Scott DD, Johnson JC, et al. Gabapentin effect on spasticity in multiple sclerosis: a placebo-controlled, randomized trial. *Arch Phys Med Rehabil* 2000;81:164–169.
135. Dunevsky A, Perel AB. Gabapentin for relief of spasticity associated with multiple sclerosis. *Am J Phys Med Rehabil* 1998;77:451–454.
136. Gruenthal M, Mueller M, Olson WL, et al. Gabapentin for the treatment of spasticity in patients with spinal cord injury. *Spinal Cord* 1997;35:686–689.
137. Mueller ME, Gruenthal M, Olson WL, et al. Gabapentin for relief of upper motor neuron symptoms in multiple sclerosis. *Arch Phys Med Rehabil* 1997; 78:521–524.
138. Priebe MM, Sherwood AM, Graves DE, et al. Effectiveness of gabapentin in controlling spasticity: a quantitative study. *Spinal Cord* 1997;35:171–175.
139. Holden KR, Titus MO. The effect of tiagabine on spasticity in children with intractable epilepsy: a pilot study. *Pediatr Neurol* 1999;21:728–730.
140. Hurst DL, Lajara-Nanson W. Use of modafinil in spastic cerebral palsy. *J Child Neurol* 2002;17:169–172.
141. Glenn MB. Nerve blocks. In: Glenn MB, Whyte J, eds. *The practical management of spasticity in the adult and child.* Philadelphia: Lea & Febiger, 1990:227–258.
142. Autti-Ramo I, Larsen A, Peltonen J, et al. Botulinum toxin injection as an adjunct when planning hand surgery in children with spastic hemiplegia. *Neuropediatrics* 2000;31:4–8.
143. Glenn MB. Nerve blocks for the treatment of spasticity. In: Katz RT, ed. *Spasticity: state of the arts review.* Philadelphia: Hanley & Belfus, 1994:481–505.
144. Glenn MB, Elovic E. Chemical denervation for the treatment of hypertonia and related disorders: phenol and botulinum toxin. *J Head Trauma Rehabil* 1997;12:40–62.
145. Glenn MB, Elovic E. Chemical denervation for the treatment of hypertonia and related disorders:phenol and botulinum toxin. *J Head Trauma Rehabil* 1997;12:40–62.
146. Setler P. The biochemistry of botulinum toxin type B. *Neurology* 2000;55 [Suppl 5]:S22–S28.
147. Khalili AA, Harmel MH, Forster S, et al. Management of spasticity by selective peripheral nerve block with dilute phenol solutions in clinical rehabilitation. *Arch Phys Med Rehabil* 1964;45:513–419.
148. Halpern D, Meelhuysen FE. Phenol motor point block in the management of muscular hypertonia. *Arch Phys Med Rehabil* 1966;47:659–664.
149. deLateur BJ. A new technique of intramuscular phenol neurolysis. *Arch Phys Med Rehabil* 1972;53:179–185.
150. Awad EA. Phenol block for control of hip flexor and adductor spasticity. *Arch Phys Med Rehabil* 1972;53:554–557.
151. Chua KS, Kong KH. Clinical and functional outcome after alcohol neurolysis of the tibial nerve for ankle–foot spasticity. *Brain Inj* 2001;15:733–739.
152. Chua KS, Kong KH. Alcohol neurolysis of the sciatic nerve in the treatment of hemiplegic knee flexor spasticity: clinical outcomes. *Arch Phys Med Rehabil* 2000;81:1432–1435.
153. Kong KH, Chua KS. Outcome of obturator nerve block with alcohol for the treatment of hip adductor spasticity. *Int J Rehabil Res* 1999;22:327–329.
154. Koman LA, Mooney JF III, Smith BP. Neuromuscular blockade in the management of cerebral palsy. *J Child Neurol* 1996;11[Suppl 1]:S23–S28.
155. Garland DE, Lucie RS, Waters RL. Current uses of open phenol nerve block for adult acquired spasticity. *Clin Orthop* 1982;217–222.
156. Moore TJ, Anderson RB. The use of open phenol blocks to the motor branches of the tibial nerve in adult acquired spasticity. *Foot Ankle* 1991;11: 219–221.
157. Spira R. Management of spasticity in cerebral palsied children by peripheral nerve block with phenol. *Dev Med Child Neurol* 1971;13:164–173.
158. O'Brien C. Clinical pharmacology of botulinum toxin. In: O'Brien C, Yablon S, eds. *Management of spasticity with botulinum toxin.* Littleton, CO: Postgraduate Institute for Medicine, 1995:6.
159. Jankovic J, Brin MF, Comella CL. Botulinum toxin: chemistry, pharmacology, toxicity and immunology. In: Jankovic J, Brin MF, Comella CL, eds. *Botulinum toxin treatment of cervical dystonia.* New York: Churchill Livingstone, 1994:6–19.
160. Yablon SA, Agana BT, Ivanhoe CB, et al. Botulinum toxin in severe upper extremity spasticity among patients with traumatic brain injury: an open-labeled trial. *Neurology* 1996;47:939–944.

161. Wilson DJ, Childers MK, Cooke DL, et al. Kinematic changes following botulinum toxin injection after traumatic brain injury. *Brain Inj* 1997;11:157–167.

162. Richardson D, Sheean G, Werring D, et al. Evaluating the role of botulinum toxin in the management of focal hypertonia in adults [In Process Citation]. *J Neurol Neurosurg Psychiatry* 2000;69:499–506.

163. Simpson DM, Alexander DN, O'Brien CF, et al. Botulinum toxin type A in the treatment of upper extremity spasticity: a randomized, double-blind, placebo-controlled trial. *Neurology* 1996;46:1306–1310.

164. Brashear A, Gordon MF, Elovic E, et al. Intramuscular injection of botulinum toxin for the treatment of wrist and finger spasticity after a stroke. *N Engl J Med* 2002;347:395–400.

165. Lagalla G, Danni M, Reiter F, et al. Post-stroke spasticity management with repeated botulinum toxin injections in the upper limb. *Am J Phys Med Rehabil* 2000;79:377–384.

166. Green P, Fahn S, Diamind B. Development of resistance to botulinum toxin type A in patients with torticollis. *Mov Disord* 1994;9:213–217.

167. Zuber M, Sebald M, Bathien N, et al. Botulinum antibodies in dystonic patients treated with type A botulinum toxin: frequency and significance. *Neurology* 1993;43:1715–1718.

168. Scott BA, Suzuki D. Systemic toxicity of botulinum toxin by intra-muscular injection in the monkey. *Mov Disord* 1988;3:333–335.

169. Myobloc Package Inset, 2000.

170. BeDell K, Plant K, Forcier S. Use of botulinum toxin type B for the treatment of spasticity in a child with severe spastic quadriplegic cerebral palsy: a case report. *Arch Phys Med Rehabil* 2002;83:1675(abst).

171. Hecht JS, Preston LA, McPhee S. Effects of botulinum toxin type B on shoulder pain, hyperonia and function in adults with spastic hemiparesis. *Arch Phys Med Rehabil* 2002;83:1690(abst).

172. Jayasooriaya SM, Francisco GE, Healy W. Early experience with the use of Myobloc (botulinum toxin type b) for the treatment of upper limb spastic hypertonia. *Arch Phys Med Rehabil* 2002;83:1677(abst).

173. Moberg-Wolff EA, Walke K. Use of botulinum toxin type B in the pediatric population. *Arch Phys Med Rehabil* 2002;83:1673(abst).

174. Brashear A, Lew MF, Dykstra DD, et al. Safety and efficacy of NeuroBloc (botulinum toxin type B) in type A—responsive cervical dystonia. *Neurology* 1999;53:1439–1446.

175. Brin MF, Lew MF, Adler CH, et al. Safety and efficacy of NeuroBloc (botulinum toxin type B) in type A-resistant cervical dystonia. *Neurology* 1999;53:1431–1438.

176. Penn RD, Savoy SM, Corcos D, et al. Intrathecal baclofen for severe spinal spasticity. *N Engl J Med* 1989;320:1517–1521.

177. Albright AL, Barron WB, Fasick MP, et al. Continuous intrathecal baclofen infusion for spasticity of cerebral origin. *JAMA* 1993;270:2475–2477.

178. Meythaler JM, Guin-Renfroe S, Grabb P, et al. Long-term continuously infused intrathecal baclofen for spastic–dystonic hypertonia in traumatic brain injury: 1-year experience. *Arch Phys Med Rehabil* 1999;80:13–19.

179. Becker R, Alberti O, Bauer BL. Continuous intrathecal baclofen infusion in severe spasticity after traumatic or hypoxic brain injury. *J Neurol* 1997;244:160–166.

180. Gwartz BL. Intrathecal baclofen for spasticity caused by thrombotic stroke. *Am J Phys Med Rehabil* 2001;80:383–387.

181. Meythaler JM, Guin-Renfroe S, Brunner RC, et al. Intrathecal baclofen for spastic hypertonia from stroke. *Stroke* 2001;32:2099–2109.

182. Dralle D, Muller H, Zierski J, et al. Intrathecal baclofen for spasticity. *Lancet* 1985;2:1003.

183. Bucholz RD. Management of intractable spasticity with intrathecal baclofen. In: Katz RT, ed. *Spasticity: state of the arts review*. Philadelphia: Hanley & Belfus, 1994:565–578.

184. Steinbok P, Daneshvar H, Evans D, et al. Cost analysis of continuous intrathecal baclofen versus selective functional posterior rhizotomy in the treatment of spastic quadriplegia associated with cerebral palsy. *Pediatr Neurosurg* 1995;22:255–264.

185. Teddy P, Jamous A, Gardner B, et al. Complications of intrathecal baclofen delivery. *Br J Neurosurg* 1992;6:115–118.

186. Kofler M, Kronenberg MF, Rifici C, et al. Epileptic seizures associated with intrathecal baclofen application. *Neurology* 1994;44:25–27.

187. Green LB, Nelson VS. Death after acute withdrawal of intrathecal baclofen: case report and literature review. *Arch Phys Med Rehabil* 1999;80:1600–1604.

188. Reeves RK, Stolp-Smith KA, Christopherson MW. Hyperthermia, rhabdomyolysis, and disseminated intravascular coagulation associated with baclofen pump catheter failure. *Arch Phys Med Rehabil* 1998;79:353–356.

189. Penn RD. Intrathecal baclofen for spasticity of spinal origin: seven years of experience. *J Neurosurg* 1992;77:236–240.

190. Ivanhoe CB, Tilton AH, Francisco GE. Intrathecal baclofen therapy for spastic hypertonia. *Phys Med Rehabil Clin N Am* 2001;12:923–929, ix.

191. Grabb PA, Guin-Renfroe S, Meythaler JM. Midthoracic catheter tip placement for intrathecal baclofen administration in children with quadriparetic spasticity. *Neurosurgery* 1999;45:833–836.

192. Broseta J, Garcia-March G, Sanchez-Ledesma MJ, et al. Chronic intrathecal baclofen administration in severe spasticity. *Stereotact Funct Neurosurg* 1990;54–55:147–153.

193. Chabal C, Jacobson L, Terman G. Intrathecal fentanyl alleviates spasticity in the presence of tolerance to intrathecal baclofen. *Anesthesiology* 1992;76:312–314.

194. Chabal C, Jacobson L, Schwid HA. An objective comparison of intrathecal lidocaine versus fentanyl for the treatment of lower extremity spasticity. *Anesthesiology* 1991;74:643–646.

195. Remy-Neris O, Denys P, Bussel B. Intrathecal clonidine for controlling spastic hypertonia. *Phys Med Rehabil Clin N Am* 2001;12:939–951, ix.

196. Middleton JW, Siddall PJ, Walker S, et al. Intrathecal clonidine and baclofen in the management of spasticity and neuropathic pain following spinal cord injury: a case study. *Arch Phys Med Rehabil* 1996;77:824–826.

197. Muller H, Gerlach H, Boldt J, et al. [Spasticity treatment with spinal morphine or midazolam. In vitro experiments, animal studies and clinical studies on compatibility and effectiveness]. *Anaesthesist* 1986;35:306–316.

198. Malinovsky JM, Cozian A, Lepage JY, et al. Ketamine and midazolam neurotoxicity in the rabbit. *Anesthesiology* 1991;75:91–97.

199. Erdine S, Yucel A, Ozyalic S, et al. Neurotoxicity of midazolam in the rabbit. *Pain* 1999;80:419–423.

200. Malinovsky JM. Is intrathecal midazolam safe? *Can J Anaesth* 1997;44:1321–1322.

201. Bahar M, Cohen ML, Grinshpoon Y, et al. An investigation of the possible neurotoxic effects of intrathecal midazolam combined with fentanyl in the rat. *Eur J Anaesthesiol* 1998;15:695–701.

202. Erickson DL, Blacklock JB, Michaelson M, et al. Control of spasticity by implantable continuous flow morphine pump. *Neurosurgery* 1985;16:215–217.

203. Erickson DL, Lo J, Michaelson M. Control of intractable spasticity with intrathecal morphine sulfate. *Neurosurgery* 1989;24:236–238.

204. Lydon AM, Cooke T, Duggan F, et al. Delayed postoperative gastric emptying following intrathecal morphine and intrathecal bupivacaine. *Can J Anaesth* 1999;46:544–549.

205. Glass PSA. Respiratory depression following only 0.4 mg of intrathecal morphine. *Anesthesiology* 1984;60:256–257.

206. Remy-Neris O, Barbeau H, Daniel O, et al. Effects of intrathecal clonidine injection on spinal reflexes and human locomotion in incomplete paraplegic subjects. *Exp Brain Res* 1999;129:433–440.

207. Chartier-Kastler E, Azouvi P, Yakovleff A, et al. Intrathecal catheter with subcutaneous port for clonidine test bolus injection. A new route and type of treatment for detrusor hyperreflexia in spinal cord-injured patients. *Eur Urol* 2000;37:14–17.

208. Denys P, Chartier-Kastler E, Azouvi P, et al. Intrathecal clonidine for refractory detrusor hyperreflexia in spinal cord injured patients: a preliminary report. *J Urol* 1998;160(6 Pt 1):2137–2138.

209. Kroin JS, McCarthy RJ, Penn RD, et al. Intrathecal clonidine and tizanidine in conscious dogs: comparison of analgesic and hemodynamic effects. *Anesth Analg* 1996;82:627–635.

210. Boscarino LF, Ounpuu S, Davis RB III, et al. Effects of selective dorsal rhizotomy on gait in children with cerebral palsy. *J Pediatr Orthop* 1993;13:174–179.

211. Gul SM, Steinbok P, McLeod K. Long-term outcome after selective posterior rhizotomy in children with spastic cerebral palsy. *Pediatr Neurosurg* 1999;31:84–95.

212. Wright FV, Sheil EM, Drake JM, et al. Evaluation of selective dorsal rhizotomy for the reduction of spasticity in cerebral palsy: a randomized controlled trial. *Dev Med Child Neurol* 1998;40:239–247.

213. Hodgkinson I, Berard C, Jindrich ML, et al. Selective dorsal rhizotomy in children with cerebral palsy. Results in 18 cases at one year postoperatively. *Stereotact Funct Neurosurg* 1997;69(1–4 Pt 2):259–267.

214. Morrison G, Yashon D, White RJ. Relief of pain and spasticity by anterior dorsolumbar rhizotomy in multiple sclerosis. *Ohio State Med J* 1969;65:588–591.

215. Sindou M, Millet MF, Mortamais J, et al. Results of selective posterior rhizotomy in the treatment of painful and spastic paraplegia secondary to multiple sclerosis. *Appl Neurophysiol* 1982;45:335–340.

216. Kasdon DL, Lathi ES. A prospective study of radiofrequency rhizotomy in the treatment of posttraumatic spasticity. *Neurosurgery* 1984;15:526–529.

217. Sindou M, Mifsud JJ, Boisson D, et al. Selective posterior rhizotomy in the dorsal root entry zone for treatment of hyperspasticity and pain in the hemiplegic upper limb. *Neurosurgery* 1986;18:587–595.

218. Sindou M, Mifsud JJ, Rosati C, et al. Microsurgical selective posterior rhizotomy in the dorsal root entry zone for treatment of limb spasticity. *Acta Neurochir Suppl (Wien)* 1987;39:99–102.

219. Mittal S, Farmer JP, Al Atassi B, et al. Impact of selective posterior rhizotomy on fine motor skills: long-term results using a validated evaluative measure. *Pediatr Neurosurg* 2002;36:133–141.

220. Abbott R. Complications with selective posterior rhizotomy. *Pediatr Neurosurg* 1992;18:43–47.

221. Kim DS, Choi JU, Yang KH, et al. Selective posterior rhizotomy in children with cerebral palsy: a 10-year experience. *Childs Nerv Syst* 2001;17:556–562.

222. Steinbok P, Schrag C. Complications after selective posterior rhizotomy for spasticity in children with cerebral palsy. *Pediatr Neurosurg* 1998;28:300–313.

223. Mittal S, Farmer JP, Poulin C, et al. Reliability of intraoperative electrophysiological monitoring in selective posterior rhizotomy. *J Neurosurg* 2001;95:67–75.

224. Sacco DJ, Tylkowski CM, Warf BC. Nonselective partial dorsal rhizotomy: a clinical experience with 1-year follow-up. *Pediatr Neurosurg* 2000;32:114–118.

225. Bertelli JA, Ghizoni MF, Michels A. Brachial plexus dorsal rhizotomy in the treatment of upper-limb spasticity. *J Neurosurg* 2000;93:26–32.

226. Grabb PA, Doyle JS. The contemporary surgical management of spasticity in children. *Phys Med Rehabil Clin N Am* 2001;12:907–922, viii.

227. Mayer NH, Esquenazi A, Wannstedt G. Surgical planning for upper motor neuron dysfunction: the role of motor control evaluation. *J Head Trauma Rehabil* 1996;11:37–56.
228. Keenan M, Ahearn R, Lazarus M, et al. Selective release of spastic elbow flexors in the patient with brain injury. *J Head Trauma Rehabil* 1996;11:57–68.
229. Keenan MA. Surgical decision making for residual limb deformities following traumatic brain injury. *Orthop Rev* 1988;17:1185–1192.
230. Keenan MA, Ure K, Smith CW, et al. Hamstring release for knee flexion contracture in spastic adults. *Clin Orthop* 1988;Nov:221–226.
231. Keenan MA, Lee GA, Tuckman AS, et al. Improving calf muscle strength in patients with spastic equinovarus deformity by transfer of the long toe flexors to the Os calcis. *J Head Trauma Rehabil* 1999;14:163–175.
232. Gerszten PC, Albright AL, Johnstone GF. Intrathecal baclofen infusion and subsequent orthopedic surgery in patients with spastic cerebral palsy. *J Neurosurg* 1998;88:1009–1013.
233. Friedman J, Standaert DG. Dystonia and its disorders. *Neurol Clin* 2001;19: 681–705, vii.
234. Fahn S, Bressman SB, Marsden CD. Classification of dystonia. *Adv Neurol* 1998;78:1–10.
235. Fahn S. Concept and classification of dystonia. *Adv Neurol* 1988;50:1–8.
236. Nutt JG, Muenter MD, Aronson A, et al. Epidemiology of focal and generalized dystonia in Rochester, Minnesota. *Mov Disord* 1988;3:188–194.
237. Muller J, Kiechl S, Wenning GK, et al. The prevalence of primary dystonia in the general community. *Neurology* 2002;59:941–943.
238. Bressman SB, De Leon D, Raymond D, et al. The role of the DYT1 gene in secondary dystonia. *Adv Neurol* 1998;78:107–115.
239. Bressman SB, De Leon D, Kramer PL, et al. Dystonia in Ashkenazi Jews: clinical characterization of a founder mutation. *Ann Neurol* 1994;36:771–777.
240. Ozelius LJ, Hewett JW, Page CE, et al. The early-onset torsion dystonia gene (DYT1) encodes an ATP-binding protein. *Nat Genet* 1997;17:40–48.
241. Segawa M, Hosaka A, Miyagawa F, et al. Hereditary progressive dystonia with marked diurnal fluctuation. *Adv Neurol* 1976;14:215–233.
242. Krauss JK, Mohadjer M, Braus DF, et al. Dystonia following head trauma: a report of nine patients and review of the literature. *Mov Disord* 1992;7:263–272.
243. Lee MS, Rinne JO, Ceballos-Baumann A, et al. Dystonia after head trauma. *Neurology* 1994;44:1374–1378.
244. Brashear A, Siemers E. Focal dystonia after chemotherapy: a case series. *J Neurooncol* 1997;34:163–167.
245. Jankovic J. Can peripheral trauma induce dystonia and other movement disorders? Yes! *Mov Disord* 2001;16:7–12.
246. Jankovic J. Atypical and typical cranial dystonia following dental procedures. *Mov Disord* 2000;15:366.
247. Burke RE, Fahn S, Jankovic J, et al. Tardive dystonia: late-onset and persistent dystonia caused by antipsychotic drugs. *Neurology* 1982;32:1335–1346.
248. Chiu H, Shum P, Lau J, et al. Prevalence of tardive dyskinesia, tardive dystonia, and respiratory dyskinesia among Chinese psychiatric patients in Hong Kong. *Am J Psychiatry* 1992;149:1081–1085.
249. Gunal DI, Onultan O, Afsar N, et al. Tardive dystonia associated with olanzapine therapy. *Neurol Sci* 2001;22:331–332.
250. Tachikawa H, Suzuki T, Kawanishi Y, et al. Tardive dystonia provoked by concomitantly administered risperidone. *Psychiatry Clin Neurosci* 2000;54: 503–505.
251. Dunayevich E, Strakowski SM. Olanzapine-induced tardive dystonia. *Am J Psychiatry* 1999;156:1662.
252. Albanese A. Dystonia in parkinsonian syndromes. *Adv Neurol* 2003;91:351–360.
253. Louis ED, Lee P, Quinn L, et al. Dystonia in Huntington's disease: prevalence and clinical characteristics. *Mov Disord* 1999;14:95–101.
254. Svetel M, Kozic D, Stefanova E, et al. Dystonia in Wilson's disease. *Mov Disord* 2001;16:719–723.
255. Lang AE. Dopamine agonists in the treatment of dystonia. *Clin Neuropharmacol* 1985;8:38–57.
256. Lang AE, Sheehy MP, Marsden CD. Anticholinergics in adult-onset focal dystonia. *Can J Neurol Sci* 1982;9:313–319.
257. Fahn S. High-dosage anticholinergic therapy in dystonia. *Adv Neurol* 1983; 37:177–188.
258. Jankovic J. Medical therapy and botulinum toxin in dystonia. *Adv Neurol* 1998;78:169–183.
259. Adityanjee, Estrera AB. Successful treatment of tardive dystonia with clozapine. *Biol Psychiatry* 1996;39:1064–1065.
260. Burbaud P, Guehl D, Lagueny A, et al. A pilot trial of clozapine in the treatment of cervical dystonia. *J Neurol* 1998;245(6–7):329–331.
261. Jaffe ME, Simpson GM. Reduction of tardive dystonia with olanzapine. *Am J Psychiatry* 1999;156:2016.
262. Lucetti C, Bellini G, Nuti A, et al. Treatment of patients with tardive dystonia with olanzapine. *Clin Neuropharmacol* 2002;25:71–74.
263. Jankovic J. Botulinum toxin in movement disorders. *Curr Opin Neurol* 1994;7:358–366.
264. Berardelli A, Formica A, Mercuri B, et al. Botulinum toxin treatment in patients with focal dystonia and hemifacial spasm. *Ital J Neurol Sci* 1993;14: 361–367.
265. Blitzer A, Brin MF, Stewart CF. Botulinum toxin management of spasmodic dysphonia (laryngeal dystonia): a 12-year experience in more than 900 patients. *Laryngoscope* 1998;108:1435–1441.
266. Albright AL, Barry MJ, Fasick P, et al. Continuous intrathecal baclofen infusion for symptomatic generalized dystonia. *Neurosurgery* 1996;38:934–938.
267. Ford B, Greene PE, Louis ED, et al. Intrathecal baclofen in the treatment of dystonia. *Adv Neurol* 1998;78:199–210.
268. Hou JG, Ondo W, Jankovic J. Intrathecal baclofen for dystonia. *Mov Disord* 2001;16:1201–1202.
269. Ford B, Greene P, Louis ED, et al. Use of intrathecal baclofen in the treatment of patients with dystonia. *Arch Neurol* 1996;53:1241–1246.
270. Ford B, Louis ED, Greene P, et al. Outcome of selective ramisectomy for botulinum toxin resistant torticollis [see comments]. *J Neurol Neurosurg Psychiatry* 1998;65:472–478.
271. Cooper IS. 20-year followup study of the neurosurgical treatment of dystonia musculorum deformans. *Adv Neurol* 1976;14:423–452.
272. Andrew J, Fowler CJ, Harrison MJ. Stereotaxic thalamotomy in 55 cases of dystonia. *Brain* 1983;106(Pt 4):981–1000.
273. Lai T, Lai JM, Grossman RG. Functional recovery after bilateral pallidotomy for the treatment of early-onset primary generalized dystonia. *Arch Phys Med Rehabil* 1999;80:1340–1342.
274. Iacono RP, Kuniyoshi SM, Lonser RR, et al. Simultaneous bilateral pallidoansotomy for idiopathic dystonia musculorum deformans. *Pediatr Neurol* 1996;14:145–148.
275. Chang JW, Choi JY, Lee BW, et al. Unilateral globus pallidus internus stimulation improves delayed onset post-traumatic cervical dystonia with an ipsilateral focal basal ganglia lesion. *J Neurol Neurosurg Psychiatry* 2002;73: 588–590.
276. Ghika J, Villemure JG, Miklossy J, et al. Postanoxic generalized dystonia improved by bilateral Voa thalamic deep brain stimulation. *Neurology* 2002;58: 311–313.
277. Krauss JK, Pohle T, Weber S, et al. Bilateral stimulation of globus pallidus internus for treatment of cervical dystonia. *Lancet* 1999;354:837–838.
278. Krauss JK, Loher TJ, Pohle T, et al. Pallidal deep brain stimulation in patients with cervical dystonia and severe cervical dyskinesias with cervical myelopathy. *J Neurol Neurosurg Psychiatry* 2002;72:249–256.
279. Haller JS Jr. Etiology, pathology and treatment of chorea in the nineteenth century. *Trans Stud Coll Physicians Phila* 1972;40:55–63.
280. Huntington G. On chorea. *Med Surg Reporter* 1872;26:317–321.
281. Higgins DS, Jr. Chorea and its disorders. *Neurol Clin* 2001;19:707–722, vii.
282. Harper PS. The epidemiology of Huntington's disease. *Hum Genet* 1992;89: 365–376.
283. Harel L, Zecharia A, Straussberg R, et al. Successful treatment of rheumatic chorea with carbamazepine. *Pediatr Neurol* 2000;23:147–151.
284. Levine SR, Welch KM. Antiphospholipid syndrome. *Ann Neurol* 1989;26: 386–389.
285. O'Brien CF, Kurlan R. Movement disorders in pregnancy. In: Goldstein PJ, Stern BJ, eds. *Neurologic disorders of pregnancy.* Mount Kisco, NY: Futura Publishing, 1992:181–201.
286. Bruyn GW, Padberg G. Chorea and polycythaemia. *Eur Neurol* 1984;23: 26–33.
287. Yen DJ, Shan DE, Lu SR. Hyperthyroidism presenting as recurrent short paroxysmal kinesigenic dyskinesia. *Mov Disord* 1998;13:361–363.
288. Jimenez-Jimenez FJ, Garcia-Ruiz PJ, Molina JA. Drug-induced movement disorders. *Drug Saf* 1997;16:180–204.
289. Hyde TM, Hotson JR, Kleinman JE. Differential diagnosis of choreiform tardive dyskinesia. *J NeuroPsychiatry Clin Neurosci* 1991;3:255–268.
290. Elovic EP, Lansang R, Li Y, et al. The use of atypical antipsychotics in traumatic brain injury. *J Head Trauma Rehabil.* 2003;(In Press).
291. Genel F, Arslanoglu S, Uran N, et al. Sydenham's chorea: clinical findings and comparison of the efficacies of sodium valproate and carbamazepine regimens. *Brain Dev* 2002;24:73–76.
292. Caviness JN. Primary care guide to myoclonus and chorea: characteristics, causes, and clinical options. *Postgrad Med* 2000;108:163–172.
293. Ondo WG, Tintner R, Thomas M, et al. Tetrabenazine treatment for Huntington's disease-associated chorea. *Clin Neuropharmacol* 2002;25:300–302.
294. Jimenez Jimenez FJ, De Toledo M, Puertas I, et al. [Olanzapine improves chorea in patients with Huntington s disease]. *Rev Neurol* 2002;35:524–525.
295. Adams RD, Victor M, Ropper AH. Tremor, myoclonus, focal dystonias and tics. In: Adams RD, Victor M, Ropper AH, eds. *Principles of neurology.* New York: McGraw-Hill, 1997:94–113.
296. Anouti A, Koller WC. Tremor disorders: diagnosis and management. *West J Med* 1995;162:510–513.
297. Charles PD, Esper GJ, Davis TL, et al. Classification of tremor and update on treatment. *Am Fam Physician* 1999;59:1565–1572.
298. Sandroni P, Young RR. Tremor: classification, diagnosis and management. *Am Fam Physician* 1994;50:1505–1512.
299. Burchiel KJ. Thalamotomy for movement disorders. *Neurosurg Clin N Am* 1995;6:55–71.
300. Lenz FA, Normand SL, Kwan HC, et al. Statistical prediction of the optimal site for thalamotomy in parkinsonian tremor. *Mov Disord* 1995;10:318–328.
301. Cutson TM, Laub KC, Schenkman M. Pharmacological and nonpharmacological interventions in the treatment of Parkinson's disease. *Phys Ther* 1995; 75:363–373.
302. Louis ED, Ottman R, Hauser WA. How common is the most common adult movement disorder? estimates of the prevalence of essential tremor throughout the world. *Mov Disord* 1998;13:5–10.
303. Britton TC. Essential tremor and its variants. *Curr Opin Neurol* 1995;8:314–319.

304. Hallett M. Classification and treatment of tremor. *JAMA* 1991;266:1115–1117.

305. Koller W, O'Hara R, Dorus W, et al. Tremor in chronic alcoholism. *Neurology* 1985;35:1660–1662.

306. Koller W, Lang A, Vetere-Overfield B, et al. Psychogenic tremors. *Neurology* 1989;39:1094–1099.

307. Britton TC, Thompson PD, van der KW, et al. Primary orthostatic tremor: further observations in six cases. *J Neurol* 1992;239:209–217.

308. Gates PC. Orthostatic tremor (shaky legs syndrome). *Clin Exp Neurol* 1993;30:66–71.

309. McManis PG, Sharbrough FW. Orthostatic tremor: clinical and electrophysiologic characteristics. *Muscle Nerve* 1993;16:1254–1260.

310. Jankovic J, Hamilton WJ, Grossman RG. Thalamic surgery for movement disorders. *Adv Neurol* 1997;74:221–233.

311. Jankovic J, Cardoso F, Grossman RG, et al. Outcome after stereotactic thalamotomy for parkinsonian, essential, and other types of tremor. *Neurosurgery* 1995;37:680–686.

312. Laitinen LV. Pallidotomy for Parkinson's disease. *Neurosurg Clin N Am* 1995;6:105–112.

313. Benabid AL, Benazzouz A, Hoffmann D, et al. Long-term electrical inhibition of deep brain targets in movement disorders. *Mov Disord* 1998;13[Suppl 3]:119–125.

314. Benabid AL, Koudsie A, Pollak P, et al. Future prospects of brain stimulation. *Neurol Res* 2000;22:237–246.

315. Fahn S. Hypokinesia and hyperkinesia. In: Goetz CG, Pappert EJ, eds. *Textbook of clinical neurology.* Philadelphia: WB Saunders, 1999:267–284.

316. Caviness JN. Myoclonus. *Mayo Clin Proc* 1996;71:679–688.

317. Fahn S, Marsden CD, Van Woert MH. Definition and classification of myoclonus. *Adv Neurol* 1986;43:1–5.

318. We Move. Myoclonus. http://www.wemove.org/. 2002. Accessed 12–18–2002.

319. Marsden CD, Hallett M, Fahn S. The nosology and pathophysiology of myoclonus. In: Marsden CD, Fahn S, eds. *Movement disorder.* London: Butterworths, 1982:196–248.

320. Mahloudji M, Pikielny RT. Hereditary essential myoclonus. *Brain* 1967; 90:669–674.

321. Bressman SB, Fahn S. Essential myoclonus. *Adv Neurol* 1986;43:287–294.

322. Obeso JA, Rothwell JC, Marsden CD. The spectrum of cortical myoclonus: from focal reflex jerks to spontaneous motor epilepsy. *Brain* 1985;108(Pt 1):193–24.AQ1

323. Lockman LA. Absence seizures and variants. *Neurol Clin* 1985;3:19–29.

324. Proposal for revised clinical and electroencephalographic classification of epileptic seizures. From the Commission on Classification and Terminology of the International League Against Epilepsy. *Epilepsia* 1981;22:489–501.

325. Rapin I. Myoclonus in neuronal storage and Lafora diseases. *Adv Neurol* 1986;43:65–85.

326. Lance JW. Action myoclonus, Ramsay Hunt syndrome, and other cerebellar myoclonic syndromes. *Adv Neurol* 1986;43:33–55.

327. Wenning GK, Ben Shlomo Y, Magalhaes M, et al. Clinical features and natural history of multiple system atrophy. An analysis of 100 cases. Brain 1994;117(Pt 4):835–845.

328. Shibasaki H, Motomura S, Yamashita Y, et al. Periodic synchronous discharge and myoclonus in Creutzfeldt-Jakob disease: diagnostic application of jerk-locked averaging method. *Ann Neurol* 1981;9:150–156.

329. Hallett M, Wilkins DE. Myoclonus in Alzheimer's disease and minipolymyoclonus. *Adv Neurol* 1986;43:399–405.

330. Burkhardt CR, Filley CM, Kleinschmidt-Demasters BK, et al. Diffuse Lewy body disease and progressive dementia. *Neurology* 1988;38:1520–1528.

331. Lance JW, Adams RD. The syndrome of intention or action myoclonus as a sequel to hypoxic encephalopathy. *Brain* 1963;86:111–136.

332. Young RR, Shahani BT. Asterixis: one type of negative myoclonus. *Adv Neurol* 1986;43:137–156.

333. Kuzniecky R, Berkovic S, Andermann F, et al. Focal cortical myoclonus and rolandic cortical dysplasia: clarification by magnetic resonance imaging. *Ann Neurol* 1988;23:317–325.

334. Lapresle J. Palatal myoclonus. *Adv Neurol* 1986;43:265–273.

335. Obeso JA, Artieda J, Marsden CD. Different clinical presentations of myoclonus. In: Jankovic J, Tolosa ES, eds. Parkinson's disease and movement disorder. Baltimore: Urban & Schwarzenberg, 1988:263–274.

336. Bussel B, Roby-Brami A, Azouvi P, et al. Myoclonus in a patient with spinal cord transection: possible involvement of the spinal stepping generator. *Brain* 1988;111:1235–1245.

337. Brown P, Thompson PD, Rothwell JC, et al. Axial myoclonus of propriospinal origin. *Brain* 1991;114:197–214.

338. Pranzatelli MR, Snodgrass PJ. The pharmacology of myoclonus. *Clin Neuropharmacol* 1985;8:99–130.

339. Lhermitte F, Peterfalvi M, Marteau R, et al. Analyse pharmacologique d'un cas de myoclonies d'intention et d'action post-anoxiques. *Rev Neurol* 1971; 124:21–31.

340. Growdon JH, Young RR, Shahani BT. L-5-hydroxytryptophan in treatment of several different syndromes in which myoclonus is prominent. *Neurology* 1976;26:1135–1140.

341. Obeso JA, Artieda J, Rothwell JC, et al. The treatment of severe action myoclonus. *Brain* 1989;112(Pt 3):765–777.

342. Jabbari B, Rosenberg M, Scherokman B, et al. Effectiveness of trihexyphenidyl against pendular nystagmus and palatal myoclonus: evidence of cholinergic dysfunction. *Mov Disord* 1987;2:93–98.

343. Vincent FM, Vincent T. Lorazepam in myoclonic seizures after cardiac arrest [letter]. *Ann Intern Med* 1986;104:586.

344. Silfverskiold BP. Rhythmic myoclonias including spinal myoclonus. *Adv Neurol* 1986;43:275–285.

345. Krueger BR. Restless legs syndrome and periodic movements of sleep. *Mayo Clin Proc* 1990;65:999–1006.

CHAPTER 68

Immobility and Inactivity: Physiological and Functional Changes, Prevention, and Treatment

Eugen M. Halar and Kathleen R. Bell

The adverse effects of prolonged bed rest and immobility have become well recognized over the past five decades. Bed rest and immobilization were widely used before 1950 in the management of trauma and acute illness, before their physiologic effects were well understood. It was generally assumed that rest fostered healing of the affected part of the body. What was not appreciated was that physical inactivity could be harmful to the unaffected parts of the body. For example, the immobilization of long bones with a rigid cast has a beneficial effect on bone healing after fractures. However, it may also result in undesirable effects, such as joint contracture and atrophy of the healthy muscles and bones.

Clinical studies on enforced bed rest in normal subjects and on astronauts in microgravity conditions (in which their bodies rest from the effects of gravity) have shown significant undesirable effects that may override the therapeutic effects of bed rest in subacute and chronic conditions, impacting complexity and cost of medical treatment as well as functional outcome. Fortunately, many of these complications are easily prevented or, if they occur, easily treated once they are recognized.

A recent review of randomized controlled trials on the effects of bed rest and early mobilization did not demonstrate improvement or better outcome of primary medical conditions for those on extended periods of bed rest. In many cases, worsening occurred if early mobilization was not provided (1). Persons who are chronically sick, aged, or disabled are particularly susceptible to the adverse effects of immobility. For example, a healthy subject placed on prolonged bed rest will develop shortening in the musculature of the back and legs, especially those muscles that cross the hip and knee joints. In similar circumstances, a patient with motor neuron disease and its accompanying limb weakness or spasticity would be expected to develop the same musculoskeletal complications but at a much accelerated rate. The degree to which each of these hypothetical patients is affected is quite different. The healthy subject may only show some degree of atrophy, weakness, stiffness, and discomfort, whereas the neurologically impaired subject will likely also lose a significant amount of independent functioning. Therefore, the prevention of such complications should be one of the basic principles of any rehabilitation management plan (2).

The effects of immobility are rarely confined to only one body system (Table 68-1). Immobility reduces the functional reserve of the musculoskeletal system, resulting in weakness, atrophy, and poor endurance. Metabolic activity and oxygen extraction in muscle are reduced, which negatively influence the functional capacity of the cardiovascular system (i.e., cardiac output and work capacity). In addition, postural hypotension and deep venous thrombosis (DVT) are commonly encountered in bedridden patients. Immobilization osteoporosis is yet another complication that has been well documented in the studies of astronauts and individuals exposed to prolonged bed rest. Over time, clinical experience has dictated a move toward earlier mobilization, with a resulting decrease in the length of hospitalization and in the incidence of major morbidity associated with prolonged immobility (3).

Deleterious effects of immobility may be grouped together under the general term "deconditioning," which is defined as reduced functional capacity of musculoskeletal and other body systems. It should be considered a distinct diagnosis from the original condition that led to a curtailment of normal physical activity (4) (Fig. 68-1).

This chapter will describe the widespread effects of immobility and physical inactivity, review therapeutic and prophylactic approaches to counteract these complications, and direct attention to the benefits of physical activity and exercises in maintaining good health and independence.

MUSCULOSKELETAL EFFECTS OF IMMOBILITY AND INACTIVITY

Freedom to move the body and limbs in the environment is an important physical function requiring that the muscles, nerves, bones, and joints be in an optimal physiologic state. Disuse weakness and reduction of free joint motion can cause minimal functional limitations that can be easily overlooked or neglected. However, advanced contractures and disuse weakness can cause a loss of mobility and decrease in activities of daily living functions (5).

TABLE 68-1. Adverse Effects of Immobility

System(s)	Effect(s)
Musculoskeletal	Contractures
	Muscle weakness and atrophy
	Immobilization osteoporosis
	Immobilization hypercalcemia
Cardiovascular and pulmonary	Redistribution of body fluids
	Orthostatic hypotension
	Reduction of cardiopulmonary functional capacity
	Thromboembolism
	Mechanical resistance to breathing
	Hypostatic pneumonia
Genitourinary and gastrointestinal	Urinary stasis, stones, and urinary infections
	Loss of appetite
	Constipation
Metabolic and endocrine	Electrolyte alterations
	Glucose intolerance
	Increased parathyroid hormone production
	Other hormone alterations
Cognitive and behavioral	Sensory deprivation
	Confusion and disorientation
	Anxiety and depression
	Decrease in intellectual capacity
	Impaired balance and coordination

For the neurologically impaired or multiple trauma victim, considerations such as preserving functional range of motion (ROM) may seem trivial; however, neglect of these simple factors can be responsible for prolonging hospital stays, increasing the use of health-care resources, and prolonging dependency in mobility and the activities of daily living (6).

Three main types of effects from immobilization are found in the musculoskeletal system: muscle atrophy and weakness, joint contracture, and immobilization osteoporosis (see Table 68-1).

EFFECTS OF IMMOBILITY AND INACTIVITY ON SKELETAL MUSCLE

Physiological Impairments

DISUSE ATROPHY

Decrease in the size of muscle fibers and reduction of muscle mass is the hallmark of muscle atrophy. In a lower motor neu-

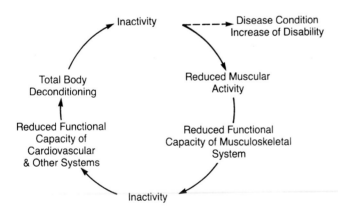

Figure 68-1. Inactivity, immobility, and prolonged bed rest influence total body functioning.

ron lesion, the atrophy is regional and related to the particular nerve or root. Atrophy associated with muscle disease is more pronounced in the proximal muscles. The atrophy of disuse is generalized or localized to the immobilized limb(s) and more prominent in the antigravity muscles. It is a consequence of the limited physical activity and musculoskeletal loading that occurs during immobilization, immobility, bed rest, or exposure to microgravity during space flight. As a general rule, increased muscular activity leads to hypertrophy, whereas limited physical activity leads to disuse atrophy and weakness.

Disuse atrophy is defined as an alteration of muscle cell homeostasis in response to muscle inactivity. During and after bed rest, disuse atrophy is more prominent in the lower limbs than in the upper limbs (7). Recent studies indicate that muscle protein synthesis as well as whole body protein production is significantly reduced during immobility and is considered the main contributor to muscle atrophy. The rate of muscle weight loss during bed rest is slow during the first day or two but becomes rapid thereafter. By 10 days, it reaches 50% of eventual muscle weight loss. Similarly, muscle protein synthesis is reduced to 50% of the baseline level at 14 days of immobilization and then gradually tapers off to reach a new steady state (8,9). The mean cross-sectional area of dark adenosine triphosphatase (ATPase) and light ATPase fibers are reduced by 46% and 69% respectively (9).

Muscle thickness and fascicle angulations from the aponeurosis can be reliably measured in some muscle by ultrasound scanning. Using this technique, the reduction of muscle thickness is on average −2.1% to −4.4% and varies significantly for different muscles of the lower limbs (10). However, magnetic resonance imaging (MRI) studies have revealed much greater atrophy of the muscles in the lower limbs with the same duration of bed rest. A consecutive MRI study of thigh and calf muscles revealed that cross-sectional area and muscle volume of the gastrocnemius and soleus muscles were reduced to a greater extent than knee extensors and flexors (−9.4% to −10.3% versus −5.1% to −8.0%) after 20 days of bed rest (11). Atrophy of type I muscle fibers is more prominent than type II fibers during immobility. The mean size of type I fibers in human soleus muscle decreased by 12% and 39%, at 2 and 4 months of bed rest, respectively. This reduction could be prevented by simulated gravity loading for 10 hours a day during bed rest (12).

Along with muscle atrophy, the synthesis of collagen fibers is also reduced, although this reduction is much less than the reduction of muscle protein. This leads to a temporary or permanent relative increase of muscle collagen content and changes in its mechanical properties (13). The increase in muscle stiffness and alteration in viscoelastic properties of plantar flexors during space flight correlated with the duration of the flight, but the changes were less prominent than those found during immobilization or bed rest (14). In both situations, weight bearing is eliminated, but joint motion is free and abundant during space flights. In healthy subjects, the main resistance to excessive elongation of muscle fiber is via myofibrils and in a lesser part to the sarcolemma itself. Titin, a myofibrillar protein, appears to have a major role in providing resistance to passive elongation and is increased in immobility. When titin is chemically removed, this resistance to passive stretch is significantly diminished (15).

Prominent histochemical changes occur in muscle during bed rest and immobility. Serum creatine kinase isomer and fibroblast growth factor release after myofiber injury are both reduced during bed rest; this decrease is proportional to muscle fiber size reduction. Resistive exercises during bed rest significantly increase the level of these factors and prevent muscle fiber atrophy, indicating that myofiber wound-mediated fibroblast growth factor may play an important role in disuse atrophy (16). Myostatin, a newly discovered growth factor-beta protein, which inhibits muscle synthesis, is increased during bed rest. As a result, the total lean body mass declines by an average of 2.2 kg, and plasma myostatin-immunoreactive protein level increases 12% after 25 days of bed rest. It is speculated that suppression of myostatin may prevent muscle atrophy during space flight (17). At this time, the only proven way to prevent and treat disuse atrophy is with exercise and remobilization.

The muscle mass and strength loss associated with aging is called sarcopenia. It is a major cause of disability and frailty in the elderly population. Inactivity is one of the many factors responsible for development of sarcopenia, along with decline in number of alpha-motor neurons, reduction in growth hormone, inadequate protein intake, and overproduction of catabolic cytokines. High-intensity resistive exercise can reverse sarcopenia, indicating that physical inactivity is a major risk factor (18). Many articles have been written about the functional decline in hospitalized and nursing-home older patients. General deconditioning is the most frequent cause of this functional decline, along with primary disease and the adverse effects of treatment. The reconditioning process takes much longer in the elderly in comparison with the younger population.

Although the primary reason for atrophy is reduction of muscle protein synthesis, an increased nitrogen loss is also found during immobility despite the fact that the major energy sources during rest are primarily derived from carbohydrates and fat. It is believed that the early decline of mitochondrial function results in protein breakdown. Decrease in muscle and whole body protein synthesis is aggravated by gastrointestinal mechanisms, such as loss of appetite and reduced intestinal absorption of protein. Although daily loss of nitrogen for an immobilized healthy person may reach 2 g/day, a nutritionally depleted person may lose as much as 12 g/day. Increased nitrogen loss usually begins on the fifth day of recumbency, with the peak loss occurring at the end of the second week (19). Urinary excretion of creatine is minimal under normal conditions, except in pregnancy and infancy. The excretion of creatine is greater in starvation, diabetes, muscular dystrophy, hyperthyroidism, and fever, as well as during immobility. Prolonged bed rest and weightlessness causes a significant increase in the excretion of both creatine and creatinine, the mechanism of which is not well understood (20).

LOSS OF STRENGTH

Muscle weakness, leading to reduced endurance and tolerance to work, is the functional consequence of muscle atrophy. The maximal strength of a muscle can fall to 25% to 40% of baseline level without sufficient exertion (7). During strict bed rest, muscles may lose 10% to 15% of their original strength per week and, over 5 weeks, 35% to 50%. The loss of strength is rapid after the first day of immobilization and reaches its maximum 10 to 14 days later (21). Resistive leg exercises performed above 50% of maximum every second day in healthy subjects on bed rest can maintain muscle protein synthesis at the same level as in healthy subjects engaged in normal activity (22). A recent study on dynamic leg-press training in healthy subjects during bed rest demonstrated maintenance of cross-sectional area and strength for the knee extensors and flexors but not for ankle plantar and ankle dorsiflexors. Actual locomotion is necessary to preserve strength in the ankle plantar and dorsiflexors (23).

As in disuse atrophy, the loss of strength is more prominent in the lower limbs than the upper limbs. Loss of muscle power reaches −20% to −44% in knee flexors and extensors, but the loss in the upper limbs does not reach a significant level (−5%) during immobilization. The decrease in maximal muscle tension of knee flexors and extensor ranges from −19% to −26%, far more than the reduction in cross-sectional area of these muscles (−7%), indicating that loss of strength and power is greater than reduction in size of the respective muscles (24). However, the number of myofibrils per fiber volume is reduced, contributing to the loss of strength in disuse atrophy subjects (12).

In addition, maximal instantaneous muscular power is reduced to a greater extent than cross-sectional areas for bed-rest subjects than for those who live in a prolonged high-altitude setting. Although the loss of strength in immobility has long been well documented, the loss of explosive muscle power as measured by a maximal jump with both feet on a force plate was only recently demonstrated. After 45 days of bed rest, instantaneous muscular power was reduced 24%, and recovery required one and one-half months of remobilization (25). These findings indicate that specific training in instantaneous power should be considered during space flight or prolonged bed rest to preserve functions such as standing up, transfers, and initial ambulation in order to maintain muscular and neural control.

Decline in muscle twitch and tetanic tension parallels the decline in muscle strength (26). In rats, maximal tension obtained by electrical stimulation in the soleus muscle declined significantly after 6 weeks of immobilization (27). Changes in contractile forces of immobilized muscle are the result of diminished levels of muscle protein as well as qualitative changes in muscle composition. Thom et al. demonstrated that 10 days of leg-cast immobilization causes a reduction of sarcoplasmic reticulum calcium ion uptake, but not of the rate of its release and ATPase activity, and results in decreased quadriceps cross-sectional area and strength (28).

LOSS OF ENDURANCE

Multiple studies have demonstrated that prolonged immobility or inactivity causes a significant and progressive reduction in muscle endurance. Unexercised muscle demonstrates a reduction of adenosine triphosphate (ATP) and glycogen storage, and rapid depletion after resumption of activity. Reduction of muscle protein synthesis and oxidative enzyme function, and early triggering of anaerobic energy production with rapid accumulation of lactic acid, are important factors leading to fatigability and reduced endurance (29). Additionally, alteration in shape and size of the motor endplates and dysfunction of acetylcholine receptors are partly responsible for the loss of strength and endurance of a disused muscle (30).

Metabolic and enzymatic alterations in unexercised muscle result from reduced demand for oxygen and changes in the blood supply. Initially after bed rest, succinate dehydrogenase enzyme activity per muscle fiber increases, but the overall amount is reduced significantly with prolonged immobilization (31). Oxidative enzyme activity and content as well as the number and size of mitochondria are all reduced during immobility (32). Unexercised muscle also shows decreased ability to utilize fatty acids when compared with trained subjects.

Ferretti et al. studied peripheral and central factors that contribute to the decline of VO_{2max} after 42 days of bed rest. VO_{2max} is reduced by 16%, cardiac output by 30%, and oxygen delivery by 40%, which parallels the reduction in muscle cross-sectional area of 17%, volume density of mitochondria −16%, and total mitochondria volume in the magnitude of −28%. Oxidative

TABLE 68-2.   Effect of Immobility on Skeletal Muscle

Component	Characteristic Effect[a]
SDH (succinyl dehydrogenase and other oxidative enzymes)	Decreased aerobic function
Glycogen	Depleted storage levels
CK (creatine kinase)	Depleted storage levels
Sarcomeres	Decreased number in series
Type I and II fiber atrophy	Decreased strength and endurance
Myofibrils	Decreased number
	Slowed twitch contraction time
	Reduced maximum twitch and tetanic force
Na-ATPase, K-ATPase	Decreased concentrations of Na and K pumps
VO_2max	Progressive reduction of VO_2max and fitness

[a]The significance of some of these changes remains unclear.

enzyme activity falls by 11%. The greatest changes are found in oxygen delivery. This study and others have demonstrated a significant contribution of the peripheral and central factors in causing decline in $VO_{2\,max}$, confirming a close interrelationship between the muscular and cardiovascular systems (29).

In conclusion, prolonged reduction of muscle contractions below 50% of maximum and global inactivity alters muscle protein homeostasis, decreases energy storage of glycogen and ATP, causes a reduction of oxidative enzymes, and reduces mitochondrial function and microvascular circulation, muscle metabolic activity, strength, and endurance. As a result, the oxygen supply is attenuated, and the extraction of oxygen from blood is diminished, further negatively affecting VO_{2max} and cardiovascular reserve (Table 68-2).

Functional Limitation Resulting from Unexercised Muscles

MOBILITY AND ACTIVITIES OF DAILY LIVING

The progressive weakness and reduced stamina resulting from inactivity negatively impacts the ability to perform the basic physical functions of mobility and activities of daily living. In the lower limbs, type I muscle fibers, which are active during ambulation, are especially affected with a rapid reduction in endurance. If the quadriceps muscle is immobilized in an extended position, the deep layer of vastus intermedius, which has predominantly type I fibers, will show the greatest histochemical changes (33). This accelerated rate of atrophy and weakness was noted especially in quadriceps, hip, and back extensors, decreasing endurance for walking and causing backache (34).

PAIN AND STIFFNESS

Back pain during bed rest has been frequently reported in the literature. The cause of this pain is still not fully understood. Recent studies in which spine length and degree of movement were determined by miniature ultrasound transmitters have demonstrated that back pain is much more prominent in cases in which the trunk movement was limited in a supine position. It is speculated that localized, prolonged, isometric muscle contractions of low intensity cause this pain. Back pain could be averted in these subjects by slow stretching exercises (35).

Limb muscle pain is not frequently encountered during generalized immobility but may occur during specific limb immobilization, especially with swelling. A limb kept in a nonphysiologic position for a week or more will be stiff and painful during remobilization. Intermittent stretching can prevent the loss of sarcomeres in series when the limb is placed in such conditions (36). Spector and colleagues have shown that the position in which a joint is immobilized has a significant influence on the number of sarcomeres present in a single muscle fiber. Immobilization in a shortened position can cause a muscle fiber to lose 40% of its sarcomeres (37). If extensor muscles are kept in full joint extension, or if flexors are kept shortened in full flexion during immobilization, the number of sarcomeres in series declines, contributing to weakness and muscle stiffness (33,36). Whether the reduction in sarcomeres in single muscle fibers contributes to stiffness is not fully known.

Direct Effects of Muscle Disuse on Cardiovascular and Other Systems

Diminished functioning of the musculoskeletal system can adversely affect the cardiovascular and other systems. Chronic inactivity impairs the function of both the musculoskeletal and cardiovascular systems, leading to a significant reduction of maximal oxygen consumption, cardiovascular reserve, and fitness. In only 3 weeks of bed rest, VO_{2max} can decline by 25%, reducing significantly cardiovascular fitness (38). Individuals with an inactive lifestyle and a low level of fitness are more prone to develop coronary artery disease and are at a higher risk of suffering myocardial infarction and death. A number of epidemiologic studies have demonstrated a dose-response relationship between higher physical activity and lower mortality from coronary artery disease (39). Sedentary lifestyle and limited physical activity, for example, have been found to increase morbidity and mortality of coronary heart disease (40). Multiple possible mechanisms have been implicated for this association. The changes that occur in skeletal muscles that are due to chronic limited physical activity, such as reduced oxidative metabolism and blood supply, may lead to endothelial dysfunction and alteration in nitric oxide response. This is a very simplified explanation of this complex relationship (41). However, it is well proven that a daily regimen of 30 to 45 minutes of aerobic activity will reduce the risk of developing coronary heart disease, as well as non–insulin-dependent diabetes, hypertension, and colon cancer. The physiatrist is thus obliged to teach how to avoid inactivity and to prescribe fitness exercises and aerobic leisure activity for his/her own patients (42).

When inactivity is combined with other factors, the catabolic changes in muscle are aggravated. When the fact is considered that VO_{2max} already declines with age, immobility can be especially detrimental to the aged. Even minor trauma combined with strict bed rest can accelerate the loss of muscle strength. A similar aggravation is found in protein breakdown. This effect is due to the catabolism of muscles caused by the hypercortisolemia associated with acute trauma. If hydrocortisone is given intravenously to an immobilized person, catabolism of muscle is enhanced threefold when compared with subjects placed on bed rest only (43). In incomplete upper or lower motor neuron conditions, in addition to the affected limbs and muscles, unaffected muscle may also undergo disuse wasting with associated decline in strength, endurance, and fitness. These effects of bed rest can be prevented by exercises in the supine position if the patient is not ambulatory or by early mobilization. A study has shown that muscle weakness and protein synthesis reduction during bed rest can be prevented by leg exercise if done three times a week (44).

Prevention and Treatment

PRINCIPLES

- Identify clinical and subclinical alterations in strength, endurance, and physical function.
- Determine if atrophy and weakness are caused by inactivity alone or in a combination with other conditions, such as acute trauma or chronic disease.
- Ascertain the reasons that a person is immobilized, bedridden, or inactive, and determine if the treatment can be altered.
- Correlate patient's situation with the factors known to cause disuse atrophy.
- Consider that the absence of symptoms may not indicate optimal muscle function.

STRATEGIES

- Prevent inactivity by prescribing progressive resistive exercises and activity programs.
- Quickly recognize the side effects of inactivity that can be treated effectively.
- Use a combination of two or three specific exercises, such as flexibility exercise, exercise for strength, and exercise for endurance and fitness.
- Functionally remobilize the patient as quickly as possible.

FLEXIBILITY EXERCISE

Stretching to maintain optimal resting length of the muscle belly as well as viscoelastic properties are important factors in the maintenance of normal muscle function. Recent animal studies indicate that passive stretching of striated muscle is associated with muscle hypertrophy, increase in muscle fiber area, and muscle fiber proliferation. Undifferentiated, quiescent myoblasts residing on the sarcolemma of muscle fibers (satellite cells) are activated and by their own fission are believed to be responsible for this stretch-induced muscle hypertrophy. Passive stretch is also a potent mechanical stimulus to influence gene expression and muscle proliferation. For example, myogenin mRNA per microgram RNA was significantly increased after 3, 6, 14, and 21 days of stretch overload in avian latissimus dorsi, and the cross-sectional area was significantly larger after 6 days of stretch overloading (45). Stiffness of a muscle occurs through the reduction of the elongation properties of elastic, collagen, and muscle fibers. It is also a result of structural changes that occur in the muscle, such as muscle fiber angulations, reduction of sarcomeres in series, and rearrangement of collagen fibers. Daily stretching of a muscle for a half hour can prevent the loss of sarcomeres in series of the immobilized muscle (46). Even a relative increase in muscle connective tissue may lead to muscle stiffness and reduction of joint motion. Two-jointed muscles like hamstrings, gastrocnemius, and long back extensors are particularly prone to become stiff, even in healthy subjects, with limited physical activity. In immobilized and inactive persons, however, this process is accelerated because naturally occurring stretch is lacking. Stiffness and subsequent muscle belly shortening of two-jointed muscles drastically interfere with functional walking. Hip flexion contracture at 35 degrees as a result of iliopsoas muscle tightness causes a 60% increase in energy consumption per unit distance during ambulation (6,47).

STRENGTHENING EXERCISE

Prevention

First, resumption of normal activities is encouraged, and then a prescription for resistance exercise should be added. Daily muscle contraction at 30% to 50% of one repetition maximal strength for 2 to 5 minutes, three times a week, should suffice to prevent muscle loss and weakness. Muscle weakness can also be prevented by the use of electrical stimulation (48). For example, applying local stimulation to the quadriceps while in a long leg cast may help preserve muscle bulk and strength and also may shorten rehabilitation time, a factor that may be particularly important in an athlete. A typical program consists of three sessions per day for 30 minutes, using rectangular biphasic pulse stimulation (49). During space flight, astronauts are exposed to microgravity and develop muscle atrophy similarly to the healthy subjects who are placed on prolonged bed rest. It was found that electrical stimulation can prevent atrophy when applied 6 hours/day, with 1 second on and 2 seconds off stimulation at 20% to 30% of maximum tetanic force applied to the two pair of agonist-antagonist muscles in the legs (50).

In cases in which extensive immobilization is required but stretching and strengthening is not provided, profound weakness and contractures may result. The need for prolonged strengthening and stretching is necessary for several months, and return of strength may not be complete (34).

Treatment

Prescription for a typical resistance exercise program includes intensity, frequency, duration, and goal.

- Establish one repetition maximum for each muscle group.
- Select initial and later intensity of 50% to 80% of that maximum.
- Repetition is performed 10 to 15 times, twice per session for each muscle group, three times per week.
- Include the large muscle groups of the lower and upper limbs and, if indicated, back and abdominal muscles.
- Focus on antigravity muscles, agonists. and antagonists.
- Reestablish the new one-repetition maximum, as well the intensity and duration after 2 to 3 weeks of training.

If resistance exercises are performed on a regular basis for 8 weeks or more, improvements in endurance, VO_{2max}, and cardiovascular fitness can be expected as demonstrated by several studies (38). Resistance to fatigue and functional performance after 8 weeks of immobilization in persons with ankle fracture has been shown to require 10 weeks of supervised physical therapy, indicating that more time is needed to restore endurance and functional performance than to create it (51).

EXERCISES FOR ENDURANCE AND FITNESS

These exercises should be prescribed for physically inactive individuals with history of prolonged bed rest, immobility, or limited physical activity regardless of age and sex. Convertino found that decline in VO_{2max} is progressive and parallels the duration of bed rest as the level of preimmobility fitness, but it occurs independently of age, sex, and the presence of any other disease (52). Thus, physical inactivity is considered an independent risk factor for the loss of cardiovascular fitness, and exercise can effectively prevent it. Daily endurance exercises at 60% to 80 % of $VO_{2\,max}$ or at a target heart rate are required to maintain or improve aerobic capacity ($VO_{2\,max}$) in persons with deconditioning. Daily resistive exercise to the muscles in the lower and upper limbs should be prescribed in such cases to restore and increase endurance and fitness (53).

Several studies have demonstrated that exercises can prevent, attenuate, or reverse the process of deconditioning of the musculoskeletal and other systems during inactivity. For example, high-intensity and short-duration isotonic ergometer exercises maintained work capacity and plasma and red-cell volume, reversed negative body water balance, and decreased the quality of sleep and concentration when compared with a no-exercise group during bed rest. High-intensity short duration isokinetic exercises could only attenuate the decrease in peak $VO_{2\,max}$ and the loss of red-cell volume but not plasma volume, reverse negative water balance, and have no effect on quality of sleep and concentration (54). This study points out that different training protocols are required to restore or prevent the adverse effects of inactivity.

Changes in motor unit recruitment and force of contraction with decreased tolerance to fatigue are other undesired effects of prolonged immobility, thus contributing to loss of endurance and easy fatigability of these subjects (55). It should be emphasized that loss of muscle mass leads to reduction of muscle strength and endurance, which creates a vicious circle of events, such as reduced muscle blood flow, reduced red blood cell delivery, reduction of oxidative enzyme activity with reduction of oxygen extraction and utilization in the muscle, decline in arteriolar and venous oxygen difference, and reduction in $VO_{2\,max}$ leading to a loss of musculoskeletal and cardiovascular functional reserve to low or dangerous levels. Although in most otherwise healthy individuals these effects are easily reversible, they may be functionally devastating for those with preexisting neurologic or musculoskeletal disease. Aerobic fitness, not just strength of a muscle, is related to the improvement of cardiovascular functional capacity and coronary artery disease prevention.

CONNECTIVE TISSUE CHANGES AND JOINT CONTRACTURE

Joint contractures most frequently result from two or more processes that include pathologic changes in the joint and adjacent tissue and immobility imposed by pathology or some other extrinsic factors. A variety of conditions may limit joint movement, including joint pain, paralysis, capsular or periarticular tissue fibrosis, or primary muscle damage. The single factor that contributes most frequently to the occurrence of fixed contractures, however, is the lack of joint mobilization throughout the full allowable range. Prolonged joint immobilization—e.g., in a flexed position—will cause reduction of resting flexing muscle length and capsular or soft-tissue tightness with resultant fixed joint contracture (56).

Many factors, such as limb position, duration of immobilization, and preexisting pathology and joint restrictions, affect the rate of contracture development. Edema, ischemia, bleeding, and other alterations to the microenvironment of muscle and periarticular tissue can precipitate the development of fibrosis. Advanced age also must be considered; both muscle fiber loss and a relative increase in the proportion of connective tissue in the body occur in the elderly (57). In addition, the microvascular changes and relative ischemia found in diabetes mellitus predispose to contractures, especially of the hand (58). Contractures that are precipitated by pathologic changes in the joints or muscles may be classified into three groups (Table 68-3): arthrogenic, myogenic, and soft tissue. It is important to remember that all tissues surrounding a joint may become secondarily involved in joint contracture regardless of the initiating disease process.

Mechanical Properties of Connective Tissues

Connective tissue is subdivided into five major groups: (a) loose connective tissue, (b) dense connective tissue (i.e., ligaments), (c) cartilage, (d) bone, and (e) blood vessels. Loose and dense connective tissues are complex, dynamic structures that

TABLE 68-3. Anatomical Classification of Contractures

Type of Contracture	Causes
Arthrogenic	Cartilage damage, joint incongruency (e.g., congenital deformities), inflammation, trauma, degenerative joint disease, infection, immobilization
	Synovial and fibrofatty tissue proliferation (e.g., inflammation) pain, effusion
	Capsular fibrosis (e.g., trauma, inflammation, immobilization)
Soft and dense tissue	Periarticular soft tissue (e.g., trauma, inflammation, immobilization)
	Skin, subcutaneous tissue (e.g., trauma, burns, infection, systemic sclerosis)
	Tendon and ligaments (e.g., tendinitis, bursitis, ligamentous tear and fibrosis)
Myogenic Intrinsic, structural	Trauma (e.g., bleeding, edema, immobilization)
	Inflammation (e.g., myositis, polymyositis)
	Degenerative changes (e.g., muscular dystrophy)
	Ischemic (e.g., diabetes, peripheral vascular disease, compartment syndrome)
Extrinsic	Spasticity (e.g., strokes, multiple sclerosis, spinal cord injuries and other upper motor neuron diseases)
	Flaccid paralysis (e.g., faulty position, muscle imbalance)
	Mechanical (e.g., faulty position in bed or chair, immobilization and lack of stretch)
Mixed	Combined arthrogenic, soft tissue and muscle contractures noted in a single joint

are important for structural support, stabilization, and movement. It is not always well appreciated that these are living, changeable tissues that can adapt both structure and composition in response to a change in environment, particularly to changes in the applied mechanical stresses. An appreciation of the anatomic design is important to fully understand the mechanical properties of both loose and dense connective tissues and their relationship to passive stretch. Both loose and dense connective tissues are composed of cells (fibroblasts) and intercellular macromolecules surrounded by polysaccharide gel, also called extracellular matrix. The intercellular substances, or collagen, impact the mechanical properties of the tissue, whereas the cells are important for homeostasis, adaptation, and repair functions (59).

COLLAGEN

There are two types of intercellular substances in connective tissues: collagen fibers and proteoglycans. Fibers in tendons, ligaments, joint capsules, and endomysium and perimysium in the muscle are predominantly of the collagen type, although there is a significant population of elastic fibers in tendons. This is consistent with their function in that tendons have great tensile strength and some elasticity to allow a joint complex to move through both muscle contraction and relaxation. Ligaments, on the other hand, are relatively inelastic and are composed primarily of collagen fibers. Collagen is the most abundant protein in the body and accounts for more than 20% of total body mass. At least 12 different collagens have been identified so far. Each type represents different aggregations of specific polypeptide products of more than 20 different collagen genes (60).

The terminology used in describing the organization and aggregation of collagen molecules is inconsistent and confusing. All collagen molecules have a unique protein conformation known as the triple helix, a result of three constituent polypeptide chains of the collagen molecule coiled together. The synthesis of these chains from amino acids, known as pro-alpha-chains, occurs in the rough endoplasmic reticulum of the fibroblast. The precise sequence of amino acids differs between the different types of collagens and accounts for the tissue-specific properties. When the collagen molecules (monomers) are subsequently secreted from the cell, enzymatic cleavage of part of the molecule occurs, and the molecules aggregate in a systematic manner to form fibrils in the extracellular space (60). Collagen fibrils, visible with the electron microscope, are grouped into fibers that are visible with the light microscope. Cross-linking between collagen fibrils is another important structural feature that varies with location and function. The type and strength of collagen cross-linking is the key to tensile strength and is probably altered, depending on the direction and magnitude of applied mechanical loads. The fibers aggregate into fiber bundles that are grouped together into fascicles. A large number of fascicles form the whole tendon or ligament (61). In striated muscle, collagen fibers form endomysium around the muscle bundles and perimysium around the muscle fascicles. These are covered with thin films of loose or dense connective tissues surrounding collagen fiber bundles (endotendon or endoligament), fascicles (peritendon or periligament), and the whole tendon or ligament (epitendon or epiligament). The epitendon and epiligament, as well as endomysium, are thought to be critically important in responding to mechanical loads and injury (62).

In tendons and ligaments, type I collagen predominates, although types III, IV, and VI also have been found. Important variations in collagen diameter have been found in association with site, age, activity level, and repair. Investigations in several animal models and humans alike have demonstrated that changes in collagen diameter, density, and orientation follow Wolff's law; connective tissues orient themselves in form and mass to best resist extrinsic forces. This has been established in response to physiologic conditions (e.g., immobilization or exercise) as well as in response to injury. Changes in collagen are mediated by fibroblasts that are sensitive to mechanical stimuli, enzymes (collagenase and tissue inhibitor of metalloproteinases), and growth factors. These factors shift the dynamic equilibrium toward synthesis or degradation, depending on environmental factors (63). If the extrinsic factors, such as stretch or weight-bearing, are limited, or if a joint is immobilized in a foreshortened position, collagen fiber density and mass will be readjusted to new positions or new loads, reducing the previous full ROM of that joint (64).

PROTEOGLYCANS

Although proteoglycans make up only about 1% of the dry weight of ligaments and tendons, their functions of lubrication, spacing, and gliding are essential (65). Proteoglycans also impact viscoelastic properties of dense connective tissues. There are several different types of proteoglycans (e.g., hyaluronic acid, chondroitin sulfate, decorin, aggrecan, biglycan) that are specific to site and function. An examination of different regions of a tendon as it traverses around a bony pulley is an excellent example of adaptation of proteoglycans by dense connective tissues. The proximal region of the tendon (at a distance from the bony pulley) is only exposed to tensional forces and contains a scant amount of decorin providing some lubrication to the surrounding collagen fibers. In contrast, the region of tendon that is in contact with bone (and subjected to compression, gliding, and tension) contains approximately 10-fold more proteoglycan, most of which is chondroitin sulfate.

In other words, the tissue is more like fibrocartilage in the area of compression to withstand the mechanical forces in that region. Work in animal models has demonstrated that these proteoglycan levels may adjust to environmental factors and be reduced in immobility (65).

Morphologic Changes

After trauma or inflammation of connective tissue, undifferentiated mesenchymal cells start to migrate to the site of injury and gradually change into mature fibroblasts. The fibroblasts travel along fibrin layers, multiply, and develop collagen-producing organelles (60). These new collagen fibers are either arranged randomly in the loose connective tissue or packed and oriented in the direction of force and stretch in dense connective tissue. Hence, the mechanical property of newly formed connective tissue is the result of the type and amount of collagen produced, as well as bonding and orientation of the collagen fibers (56,61).

The balance between synthesis and degradation is disturbed by physical factors, such as the lack of stretch that is seen in prolonged immobilization and immobility. Trauma with bleeding into the soft tissue and muscle, inflammation, degeneration, or ischemia could all trigger an increased synthesis of collagen. In these conditions, additional lack of stretch and mobility may cause the collagen fibers to become more tightly packed and randomly arranged (61).

The collagen in muscle connective tissue provides important functions, such as linking muscle cells and tendons, and is a supportive structure that holds muscle fibers and fascicles together. The synthesis of collagen tissue in the muscle is influenced by tension produced by muscular contraction, weight bearing, and stretching imposed by these activities. Hence, collagen synthesis in the muscle is greater during activity and reduced during immobility. Immobilization for 1 week causes 21% and 65% decreases in activity of the enzymes prolyl 4-hydroxylase and galactosylhydroxylase glucosyl transferase in nontrained and trained experimental animals, respectively (61,63). Collagen synthesis is reduced during immobility, but proportionally less than muscle protein synthesis, and both can be reversed by resistance exercise (7,44). Passive stretch alone can prevent contracture but not muscle atrophy, which can explain why contractures are less frequent in microgravity than during bed rest or limb immobilization. Daily clinical observations suggest that multiple factors play a part in development of joint contractures. The initial muscle stiffness and tightness in contracture formation is due to myofibrils protein titin, sarcolemma (containing collagen IV), and possible reduction of sarcomeres in series, as well as changes in the angulations of muscle fibers in respect to their origin and insertion. In the early stages of fixed contracture development, the connective tissues in the muscle, joints, and soft tissue become randomly oriented, tightly packed, and shortened in their length (36, 66,67).

Myogenic Contracture

Myogenic contracture is a shortening of resting muscle length that is due to intrinsic or extrinsic causes, limiting full ROM and causing abnormal positioning of the limbs or body. Intrinsic changes are structural and may be associated with inflammatory, degenerative, or traumatic processes. Extrinsic muscle contracture is secondary, resulting from neurologic abnormalities or mechanical factors. The diagnosis of muscle contracture should be made only after careful physical examination, which should include an evaluation of active and passive ROM. Observing limitation of active ROM alone can lead to an erroneous conclusion of fixed contracture; such limitation also could be due to muscle weakness.

Muscular dystrophy is an example of an intrinsic degenerative process in the muscle. The most significant histologic changes in this condition are muscle fiber loss, segmental necrosis, and increased amounts of lipocytes and fibrosis. The replacement of functional muscle fibers with collagen and fatty tissue in concert with chronically shortened resting muscle length results in contracture (68). In the inflammatory myopathies, muscle fibers are replaced by increasing amounts of collagen and connective tissue in association with lymphocytic infiltration (36,69). Direct muscle trauma also can result in fibrosis. After hemorrhage into a muscle, fibrin deposition occurs. Within 2 to 3 days, the fibrin fibers are replaced by reticular fibers, which then assemble into a loose connective tissue network. If the muscle is kept immobilized, this network rapidly progresses in density and resists stretching. After trauma, external factors such as immobilization result in increases in serum creatine kinase activity, local vascular permeability, swelling, and, eventually, soft-tissue contracture (69).

Among the processes that may also cause intrinsic muscle shortening is heterotopic ossification. This is most commonly noted after trauma, joint surgery(especially of the hip), spinal cord injury, or other central nervous system injury. The actual initiating factor is unknown. An alteration in local metabolism or blood flow, in connection with the systemic alteration in calcium metabolism that occurs with immobility, may be responsible for initiating this process. Although no truly effective treatment exists, ROM should be aggressively maintained. Surgical resection of the bone may be considered after the bone matures. Surgery for immature heterotopic ossification is often associated with a rebound phenomenon that worsens the extent of previous bone deposition. Prophylaxis can be accomplished through the use of disodium etidronate, a diphosphonate compound that prevents the calcification of ground substance, along with nonsteroidal antiinflammatory drugs and early mobilization (70).

Extrinsic myogenic contracture is the most common type occurring after multiple injuries and chronic illness, as well as in individuals with disabilities. In planning a therapeutic approach, it is useful to identify the cause of an extrinsic contracture as paralytic, spastic, or biomechanical. If a paralyzed muscle cannot provide adequate resistance to its antagonist muscle across a joint, then the stronger muscle will eventually become shortened. A common example of this is the shortened triceps surae seen in persons with chronic peroneal nerve palsy or in patients with plantar-flexor spasticity. Stretch applied to the muscle is essential to prevent contracture in these situations; strengthening of the weak muscle and proper positioning are also vital.

Similarly, in the presence of spasticity, a dynamic imbalance of muscle control exists across one or more joints. The resting length of spastic muscle is reduced because of increased muscle tone, which encourages faulty joint positioning (Fig. 68-2). It is often clinically difficult to identify the actual onset of structural secondary changes. If full ROM is unobtainable even after prolonged stretch and tension, then an intrinsic shortening also must be present. Treatment is directed at stretching the abnormal muscle; other antispasticity measures also may be of use, including pharmacological agents and local nerve or motor point blocks. Animal studies have indicated that in the neurologically normal rat, 2 weeks of hind-limb immobilization did not result in fixed contracture. However, immobilization for 6 weeks resulted in a 70% reduction of ROM. Five times greater than normal tension was required to achieve end range motion (67).

Mechanical factors also can cause extrinsic muscle contracture. Some degree of muscle shortening is present even in healthy persons who are sedentary, especially in those muscles that cross multiple joints. Two joint muscles in the lower extremities are naturally stretched during ambulation; during bed rest, this does not occur. The back and hamstring muscles are the most commonly shortened; the iliopsoas, rectus femoris, tensor fascia lata, and gastrocnemius are next most likely to shorten. In the upper limbs, the internal rotators of the shoulder are the most frequently contracted. The below-knee amputee with prolonged knee flexion while sitting will develop decreased knee extension as a result of tight hamstrings and contracted soft tissue behind the knee. On the other hand, the below-knee amputee treated with a rigid postoperative dressing in full knee extension may develop quadriceps muscle tightness that prevents full flexion of the knee.

Patients with muscular dystrophy provide yet another example of contracture aggravated by biomechanical factors. In muscular dystrophy, hip extensors often are very weak, forcing the patient into excessive lumbar lordosis to thrust the center of gravity behind the hip and in front of the knee joints; the patient tends to walk on his or her toes. Walking on the toes in full ankle plantar flexion prevents natural stretching of the triceps surae from occurring during the stance phase of gait, encouraging muscle shortening. If a clinician does not recognize this sequence of events, he or she might assume that weakness and fibrosis are the only reasons for a plantar-flexion contracture. A surgical lengthening of the Achilles tendon in such a case will not give the expected improvement. The lengthening of the tendon will actually shorten the muscle belly, decreasing plantar-flexor strength and diminishing the ability of these patients to walk on their toes. Because walking on the toes is the only feasible method of ambulation, the result of an ill-advised tendon lengthening may be a wheelchair-dependent patient (68).

Arthrogenic Contracture

Pathologic processes involving joint components, such as degeneration of cartilage, congenital incongruency of joint surfaces, or synovial inflammation, can lead to capsular tightness and fibrosis. Synovial inflammation and effusion are accompanied by pain that predisposes to limited joint motion, leading eventually to capsular or soft-tissue contractures. In experimentally induced acute crystalline arthritis, exercises aggravate synovitis, whereas a short period of immobilization helps to reduce inflammation (71). In chronically induced experimental arthritis, however, joints immobilized for several weeks showed much greater destruction of joint cartilage than freely mobilized joints (72). Short-term immobilization is indicated in acute arthritis because of the presence of interleukin-1 in inflammatory synovial fluid. Studies indicate that passive ROM during acute arthritis may increase the release of interleukin-1, promoting interleukin-1 penetration into cartilage and binding to the receptors on the chondrocyte membranes, and inhibiting the production of proteoglycans necessary for protection of cartilage (72,73). However, a study by van den Ende et al. clearly demonstrated that intensive dynamic exercise performed in addition to ordinary physical therapy in active rheumatoid arthritis patients did not induce worsening of the disease process, but rather, physical functioning in these patients was significantly improved. The authors concluded that an intensive exercise program is more effective than a conservative exercise program in improving the strength and functional capacity, and did not worsen activity of the disease (74).

The cartilage loss and pain associated with muscle splinting leads to decreased movement of the joint and a loss in ROM (75). That fact that pain, not the loss of cartilage, is responsible

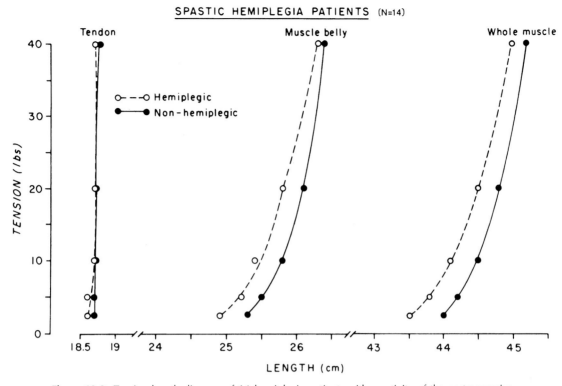

Figure 68-2. Tension-length diagram of 14 hemiplegic patients with spasticity of the gastrocnemius-soleus muscles. The curve for spastic muscle is shifted to the left; the resting length of muscle belly, but not tendon, is reduced. At 2.5, 5, 10, 20, and 40 pounds of tension, the amount of elongation of spastic and unaffected muscles is not different. This indicated that elongation characteristics are essentially unchanged for spastic muscle, although the resting length of muscle is reduced. The gastrocnemius-soleus muscle belly elongates about 1.5 cm during full dorsiflexion. (From Halar EM, Stolov WC, Venkatesh B, et al. Gastrocnemius muscle belly and tendon length in stroke patients and able-bodied persons. *Arch Phys Med Rehabil* 1978;59:476–484, with permission)

for the development of contracture is illustrated by patients with Charcot joint. These patients lack both pain sensation and proprioception but maintain relatively well-preserved ROM or even hypermobility of the involved joints in the presence of severe destruction of cartilage and joint surfaces.

The joint capsule also can lose extensibility as a consequence of collagen fiber shortening which is a result of inadequate joint stretching and positioning in flexion (66,75). If entire capsule is involved, ROM is compromised in all directions of movement. In the later stages of arthrogenic contracture, the periarticular tissue also may undergo histochemical changes (65). If repeated trauma with pain are combined swelling and prolonged immobilization, periarticular tissue contracture will occur. In these situations, proteoglycan content is also decreased, leading to joint stiffness and fixed joint contractures (65).

The shoulder and hip joint capsules are more prone than others to contracture. Initiating factors may include bicipital tendonitis, subdeltoid bursitis, rotator cuff damage, spasticity, or poor positioning coupled with immobility. The posterior knee capsule is another common site for capsular shortening as a consequence of the prolonged flexion seen in patients who use wheelchairs (76) (Fig. 68-3).

Soft-Tissue Contracture

Cutaneous, subcutaneous, and loose connective tissue around the joint also may become contracted with immobility. Trauma to soft tissue with bleeding, for example, can initiate fibrosis, which may progress to contracture if stretching is not pro-

vided. In this situation, collagen fibers usually proliferate and are laid down in random arrangements. In contrast to capsular tightness, soft-tissue shortening usually will limit movement in only one plane or axis. Burned skin is particularly susceptible to contracture. During recovery, burns that cross any joint must be ranged diligently and positioned to oppose the shortening forces of scarred tissue.

Topical steroid and vitamin E applications have failed to reduce soft-tissue contracture or postoperative scar formation after reconstructive joint surgeries. Vigorous active and passive ROM exercises, placement of the joint in a functional resting position, and use of compressive garments should be considered to prevent contractures in burn patients. Here again, adequate stretch and mobilization are important factors in the prevention of fixed contractures.

Ligaments also show biomechanical and biochemical changes during immobility. They become weaker and break easily. In experimental animals, the rate of growth, length of ligament, and elongational characteristics are influenced by tension applied to the ligament, growth hormones, size of underlying bones, and possibly other unknown factors (76,77). A study by Dahner et al. showed that in young, skeletally immature rabbits, the lateral collateral ligament of the knee elongated significantly (140%) when tension was applied for 6 weeks (77). This and other studies indicate that physiologic stretch and tension are important factors in helping both growing and mature ligaments to elongate and to withstand the stresses of weight bearing and mobility. Newton et al. found that ligaments become significantly weaker after prolonged immobilization because of decreased collagen synthesis. In addition, the ligament in-

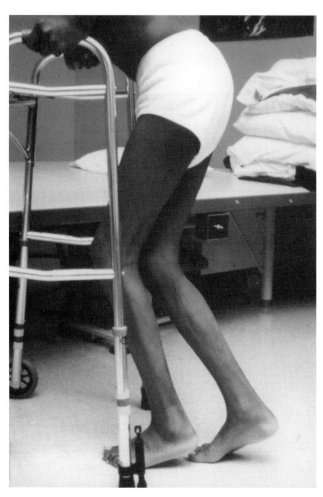

Figure 68-3. A sequence of contracture development occurred from hip down to knee in a patient with traumatic hip fracture treated operatively with the pins. As a result of hip flexion contracture and immobility, the hamstring and eventually posterior capsule with neurovascular soft tissue of the knee became tight and contracted, causing knee flexion contracture. With these contractures, a person must walk on his or her toes, which increases energy expenditure.

sertion sites on bone show an increase in osteoclastic activity. During immobility, the fibroblasts of the cruciate ligament may assume a spindle shape with multiple cytoplasmic extensions and demonstrate reduced production of collagen fibrils; resistance to ligament breakage is reduced (76). In a study by Klein et al., the atrophy of collateral and cruciate ligaments was prevented completely with active ROM exercise in non–weight-bearing limbs. However, this exercise could not prevent significant bone loss in the femur and tibia of the same experimental animal. This study indicates that active joint motion could prevent ligamentous atrophy, but that for full prevention of osteoporosis, weight bearing and exercise of appropriate duration and intensity are important factors (78,79).

Loss of Physical Function

Contractures interfere with mobility, with the basic activities of daily living, and with nursing care of skin. Lower-extremity contractures alter the gait pattern and, in extreme cases, can prevent ambulation (see Fig. 68-3). A hip-flexion contracture, for example, reduces hip extension, shortens stride length, and requires the patient to walk on the ball of the foot with increased lumbar lordosis and increased energy consumption. For biomechanical reasons, hip-flexion contractures cause the

hamstring muscles to shorten, which in turn flexes the knee. It is not uncommon to see a patient with hip contracture develop progressive knee and ankle joint contractures, especially if the joints are not aggressively mobilized. Plantar-flexion contractures will cause an absence of heel strike and abnormal push-off, resulting in decreased momentum of forward progression. Hip-extension contractures are not frequently encountered. Wheelchair ambulation is impaired by advanced hip and knee extension contractures. Car transfers also may be difficult with the knee fixed in extension. Limitations in upper-extremity ROM may lead to impaired reaching, dressing, grooming, eating, and performance of fine motor tasks (6). Multiple joint contractures can severely interfere with bed positioning, standing upright, and mobility, making perineal hygiene and skin care difficult. In addition, joint contractures tend to accentuate areas of increased pressure on skin, which may be impossible to prevent without first correcting the contracture. Advanced hip-flexion contracture may increase energy consumption 60% or more during ambulation. The mean oxygen consumption of walking with an immobilized knee in extension increases by 22.7%, and, when knee and upper limb are immobilized, the consumption is increased to 24.7%. This suggests that arm immobilization (as occurs in stroke patients) minimally increases energy consumption, whereas a spastic leg with equinovarus positioning and knee extension will significantly increase it (80).

Low Back Pain

Clinical observations have provided ample support for the theory that prolonged bed rest may cause low back pain, especially after resumption of mobility. This pain is related to several factors, including tightness of the back and hamstring muscles and/or weakness of the back and abdominal muscles. Any shortening of these muscles will alter spinal alignment and posture, increasing spinal curvature and weight bearing on the small apophyseal lumbar joints. Abdominal muscle strengthening exercises as well as strengthening and sensible stretching of paraspinal and hamstring muscles, along with general conditioning, may prevent these complications of immobility.

Acute low back pain has been treated with bed rest; however, the therapeutic value of prolonged bed rest has been disproven. In a well-controlled and randomized study, Deyo et al. have shown that patients with acute and chronic low back pain who were prescribed 2 days of bed rest subsequently lost less time from work than did patients who received 1 week of bed rest (81). There was no difference between the two groups in functional outcome. This study reinforces the principle that prolonged bed rest should not be considered a therapeutic tool in the treatment of low back pain syndrome.

Management of Contractures

ANALYSIS

The basis for initiating treatment for contractures is a careful determination of the predisposing factors, as well as knowledge of what joint components or tissues are actually involved. An observant neuromuscular examination emphasizing active and passive ROM is essential. Particular attention should be directed to those muscles crossing two joints. In patients with severe uncontrolled spasticity, it may be necessary to obtain accurate ROM measurements with the use of regional or local nerve anesthesia; this is particularly helpful when surgery to repair a decubitus ulcer is contemplated. Of course, the best treatment is prevention, so a careful analysis of positioning and ROM

TABLE 68-4. Basic Principles in the Prevention and Treatment of Contractures

Prevention
    Proper positioning in bed, resting splints
    Range-of-motion exercises (active or passive)
    Early mobilization and ambulation
    CPM (continuous passive motion)
Treatment
    Passive range-of-motion exercises with terminal stretch
    Prolonged stretch using low passive tension and heat
    Progressive (e.g., dynamic) splinting, casting
    Treatment of spasticity; pharmacologic, motor point or nerve
    blocks using phenol, injection of botulinum toxin A
    Surgical interventions (e.g., tendon lengthening, osteotomies, joint
    replacement) (see Table 44-5)
    Pain management

---

should be undertaken with any patient who is immobilized by disease or by the treatment of disease.

STRETCH AND RESTORATION OF RANGE OF MOTION PRINCIPLES

Once a contracture has developed, the sine qua non for treatment is active and passive ROM exercise combined with a sustained terminal stretch at least twice a day (Table 68-4) (36, 60,61). For mild contracture, a shorter sustained or intermittent stretching for 20 to 30 minutes may be effective. Prolonged stretches of 30 minutes or more combined with appropriate positioning and splinting are necessary for more severe contractures. This generally is more successful when used in combination with the application of heat to the musculotendinous junction or joint capsule. Ultrasound is the most popular heat source for large joints; its properties allow local heating in the presence of metallic implants and rapid increase of tissue temperature to the therapeutic level. Heating of the tissue to 40° C to 43° C will increase the viscous properties of connective tissue and maximize the effect of stretching.

When applying terminal stretch to a joint, the proximal body part should be well stabilized. In many cases, slight distraction of the joint during stretch will prevent joint compression and possible soft-tissue impingement, particularly in the small joints of the hand. The shoulder is commonly a site of contracture, particularly in the adducted and internally rotated position. In this position, the normal downward sliding and rotation of the humeral head on the glenoid fossa does not occur; forced abduction will therefore simply cause painful impingement of the rotator cuff tendon against the acromion. Stretch applied in forward flexion and external rotation will restore some of this motion and should be attempted before abduction.

Sustained stretch lasting 2 hours or more can be obtained by the use of splinting. Serial casting is the application of plaster or polymer bandages with careful padding over bony prominences. The cast is applied immediately after the use of heat and manual stretch to obtain maximal ROM. The cast can be reapplied every several days or weekly. Serial casting is particularly useful for plantar flexion, knee flexion, and elbow contractures. In patients with spasticity, chemical denervation before casting may improve tolerance and decrease the occurrence of skin breakdown.

Dynamic splinting provides tension in the desired direction with the use of springs or elastic bands. This type of splinting is often used in the hand and arm because it allows a measure of function while providing stretch. Another way to provide a form of sustained stretch is to use a continuous passive mobilization (CPM) device. The use of these devices has become rel-

atively routine for providing postoperative ROM stretching of the knee, and they have been adopted for use on other joints. CPM is recommended for the early mobilization of infected joints, synovectomized knees and hips, knee fractures, ligamentous repairs, total knee joint replacement, or any incipient arthrogenic contractures. A study of periosteal joint autografts with postoperative CPM demonstrated a 63% increase in hyaline cartilage formation compared with autograft joints that were immobilized without use of CPM (82). Early passive mobilization with CPM has been shown to promote the exchange of joint fluid, reduce the need for pain medication after surgery, and prevent contractures in high-risk patients. During CPM therapy, muscles around the joint remain relaxed, and pain is usually minimal. CPM is typically prescribed for 8 to 12 hours a day for a total of 3 to 5 days after surgery. When used alone, CPM is not effective in the treatment of fixed contractures.

To achieve optimal joint position, it sometimes is necessary to lengthen tendons by surgical means (Table 68-5). The benefits and risks of tendon lengthening should be considered carefully. It must be remembered that the muscle belly will remain shortened even though the tendon is longer; therefore, full active ROM may not be restored. Tendon lengthening combined with muscle transfer procedures in spastic or paralytic contractures may give better results because the process attempts to restore equilibrium around the joint; this method is particularly effective at the ankle, using the tibialis posterior muscle. Electromyographic analysis of muscle function before tendon transfer will optimize results by assuring the transferred muscle is innervated. In other situations, such as hip adductor contractures secondary to spasticity, tenotomy may be combined with obturator nerve neurolysis to obtain optimal results. In a chronic fixed joint contracture that interferes with the patient's basic physical functions, the selection of the appropriate surgical procedure is of great importance. Table 68-5 provides the surgical options for different joint contracture management and their surgical treatment (83–85).

PREVENTION AND TREATMENT OF CONTRACTURES

Prevention of contracture in a bed-bound patient starts with the selection of an adequate bed and mattress, proper bed positioning, and a bed mobility training program. The patient should be moved out of bed as soon as his or her medical condition allows. If bed rest is unavoidable, then bed positioning and bed mobility are incorporated into the patient's nursing management program. To assist a patient in turning side to side or in sitting up, partial side rails for grasp should be a standard part of bed equipment. An overhead trapeze is useful for patients with impaired bed mobility, allowing them to use their upper extremities to help them roll from side to side, scoot up and down, attain a sitting position, and transfer into and out of bed.

For the patient with immobility that is due to paralysis or with compromised extremity function, a variety of assistive devices are used to keep the joints in functional positions. In addition, active or passive ROM should be provided for at least 15 to 20 minutes daily to prevent contracture formation. Provision of daily ROM and flexibility exercises are essential for prevention and treatment of any type of contractures.

One of the major areas to be considered in the prevention and treatment of contractures is the maintenance and restoration of function. Encouraging the use of the limb for ambulation or other activities will help maintain the function of uninvolved joints and improve ROM and function of the affected joints. Muscle strengthening should be a primary concern in order to obtain a balance of forces across joints, especially the muscles that oppose progression of contracture. The elimina-

TABLE 68-5. Surgical Treatment of Contractures

Joint	Contracture	Procedure	Comments
Shoulder	Adduction, internal rotation	Subscapularis, pectoralis major tenotomy or lengthening	Postoperative stretching is necessary
Elbow	"Simple" flexion	Open or arthroscopic capsulectomy, biceps tendon lengthening, brachialis myotomy	Compound joint surgery generally not recommended for contractures <30% loss ROM
	Flexion/pronation	Myotomy of brachioradialis combined with z lengthening of biceps tendon	
Wrist and hand	Flexion (may include thumb-in-pain deformity)	Tenotomy of deep and superficial tendons at wrists (transfer of flexor carpi ulnaris to the extensor carpi radialis brevis or extensor carpi radialis longus with pronator releases)	
	"Windblown hand" (flexion contracture and sublaxation of MCP joints)		
	Pronation/wrist flexion		
Hip	Flexion	Psoas tenotomy or z lengthening	
	Adduction	Adductor myotomy	
	Pediatric hip dislocation (hip flexors and adductors)		
Knee	Flexion	Distal hamstring lengthening	May combine with distal rectus femoris transfer
		Posterior capsulotomy, proximal hamstring tenotomy	
		Total knee arthroplasty	
Ankle and foot	Plantar flexion	Lengthening Achilles tendon	Separation of lengthening of gastrocnemius and soleus may preserve strength
	Equinovarus calcaneus deformity	Soft-tissue release, triple arthrodesis	Resection or temotomy of anterior tibial tendon, posterior transfer of anterior tibialis muscle
		Release of long toe flexors, IP joint arthrodeses	

IP, interphalangeal; MCP, metacarpophalangeal; ROM, range of motion.

tion of poor habits in ambulation and posture, and the use of strength and endurance programs, are necessary to prevent recurrent joint contractures (47).

DISUSE OSTEOPOROSIS

Maintenance of skeletal mass depends largely on mechanical loading applied to bone by tendon pull and the force of gravity. Bone mass will increase with repeated loading stresses and will decrease with the absence of muscle activity or with the elimination of gravity (86–88). Certain populations are more susceptible to the effects of muscle inactivity or reduced weight bearing, such as the aging adult or the person with a spinal cord injury (89). Even in the healthy aging adult, the rate of bone loss exceeds the rate of new bone formation, leading to some degree of osteopenia (90). It has been well documented in the literature that bed rest, microgravity, immobility, and a lack of muscle activity can significantly reduce bone mineral density. Accelerated bone loss of tibia, for example, is found in the subjects on prolonged bed rest, and their losses of bone mineral density are similar to those seen in persons treated with chronic corticosteroids or who have osteoporosis that is due to menopause. Non–weight bearing over several weeks can cause a significant trabecular and endosteal (and later cortical) mineral bone loss in the tibia, which requires 1 to 1.5 years to return to baseline level with normal activity (91). Bone mass begins to decline in the fourth and fifth decades of life, occurring most rapidly in women in the first 5 to 7 years after menopause (92,93), and the addition of inactivity and non–weight bearing definitely aggravates bone mineral loss.

After spinal cord injury, a mismatch also occurs between bone growth and bone loss. Soon after initial injury, osteoblastic activity diminishes, and a rapid loss of bone occurs, result-ing in severe osteopenia in the paralyzed region of the body (94). Even relatively minor muscle dysfunction can result in bone loss regionally. Persons with rotator cuff ruptures have been shown to have significantly decreased bone mineral density as compared with controls and with bone density proportional to the remaining shoulder function (95). Immobilization of forearms and wrists for a period of almost 5 weeks resulted in significant loss of bone mineral density in both men and women, which was not ameliorated after almost 5 weeks of remobilization and hand therapy (96).

Immobilization or immobility primarily decreases bone formation, specifically in the zones of high turnover rate (primary spongiosa). When coupled with other risk factors, bone mineral loss is significantly worsened. Animal studies showed that immobilization, estrogen, and calcium deficiency each alone reduce cancellous bone density. When combined, greater losses in bone volume and density are found, although estrogen and calcium deficiencies result in higher rates of bone resorption rather than the decreased bone formation seen in the first weeks of immobility (97).

In a study of stroke patients with paralysis and immobility, the serum and urine indices of bone resorption did not decline with time from onset of stroke but rather actually continued during the period of immobility. This suggests that osteopenia resulting from combined immobility and paralysis is not self-limiting and that immobility is an important factor in osteopenia in such patients (98). A study of identical twins with one of each pair having spinal cord injury demonstrates that the bone mass of the pelvis and legs continues to decline over time regardless of age and gender (99). Immobilization osteopenia is also a risk factor for hip fracture, especially in elderly patients (93).

Osteopenia that is due to immobilization is characterized by a loss of calcium and hydroxyproline from the cancellous portion of long bone, epiphyses, metaphyses, and cortical bone near the marrow cavity. To what degree an increase in bone resorption plays a part in the process of disuse osteoporosis needs further research. However, during 12 weeks of bed rest, it has been found that bone resorption and osteoclastic activity became a later factor in the bone mineral loss because of immobility (80,81,100).

Studies indicate that with longer duration of immobility, an increasingly long time is required to restore bone density to the preimmobility level. In animal experiments, full body recumbency resulted in a loss of both trabecular and compact bone, which remained below baseline even 2 months after free activity was allowed (88).

Prevention and Physical Modality Treatment

The importance of exercise in overcoming inactivity-induced osteopenia should not be overlooked. Disuse osteoporosis can be minimized by the regular use of isometric or isotonic exercises. Ambulation, or at least standing on a tilt table or in a standing frame, may retard the loss of calcium. Bourrin and associates (101) studied the effect of controlled exercise on rats immobilized by tail suspension. In all the rats thus treated, there were significant decreases in bone density and bone formation. Abnormalities were especially seen in trabecular bone. Animals who received specific limb exercise in addition to normal remobilization not only recovered bone mass parameters but also had improvement in the trabecular patterns; nonexercised animals had persisting trabecular alterations (101,102).

In patient groups at highest risk for significant osteopenia—those either with paralysis or with hormonally based osteoporosis—care should be taken when exercising to prevent fracture. Despite this risk of pathologic fracture, weight-bearing exercise is particularly important to these groups to prevent progression of bone loss. Additionally, in the elderly, exercise targeted at strengthening limb-girdle muscles and lessening the chance of falls is an important adjunct (89,91,93).

PRINCIPLES AND FRAMEWORK
- Understand and recognize immobility and the lack of loading as a risk factor either by itself or in combination with other factors.
- Understand the musculoskeletal adaptability to weight bearing, muscle contraction, and mechanical loading in the development of disuse osteopenia.
- Understand the value of remobilization, weight bearing, and physical activity, including resistance exercises, in prevention and treatment (103,104).

RESISTANCE EXERCISES FOR OSTEOPOROSIS
There is great deal of evidence that resistive exercise can increase bone mass. Studies have demonstrated that there is a significant correlation between muscle strength and bone mineral density. For example, the strength of paraspinal muscles correlates with mineral density of the lumbar spine (105). Reduced back extensor muscle strength is associated with a higher incidence of vertebral fractures, thus suggesting that immobility plays an important role in development of osteoporosis in women. Low mineral density of the spine can be improved with back extensor exercises (106).

TYPICAL PRESCRIPTION
- Progressive resistive strengthening exercise training for back extensors, hip extensors and abductors, and shoulder girdle muscles

- Posture training and ambulation
- Avoidance of flexion exercise of lumbar spine or high-impact exercises (e.g., jogging, step aerobics), especially when vertebral fractures or advanced osteoporosis are suspected

Immobilization Hypercalcemia and Hypercalciuria

Despite a normal serum calcium level, immobilized patients are markedly hypercalciuric. However, adolescent boys after acute spinal cord injury may show a significant hypercalcemia as well. Symptoms of hypercalcemia include anorexia, abdominal pain, nausea, vomiting, constipation, confusion, and, ultimately, coma (107,108). Treatment of immobilization hypercalcemia relies on achieving adequate calcium excretion through hydration with normal or one-half normal saline and diuresis with furosemide. Patients with the end-stage renal disease on maintenance hemodialysis can develop an acute hypercalcemia when placed on bed rest even for 3 days, which is difficult to treat with the standard approach but can be improved with mobilization (109). For immobilized healthy persons, urinary calcium excretion increases above normal levels on the second and third days of recumbency. Maximum loss occurs during the fourth or fifth week, when urinary calcium excretion is double the level of the first week; on the average, calcium loss is 1.5 g/week (104,110). This decrease in total calcium continues even after resumption of physical activity. Three weeks after physical activity is resumed, calcium losses of as much as 4.0 g have been measured. This negative calcium balance can last for months and even years (90).

Negative calcium balance can be induced even by decreased physical activity without actual confinement to bed. The sedentary person tends to progressively lose calcium from bone. Several well-controlled studies have shown that normal subjects on a year-long program of exercises will increase their bone mass compared with those who are inactive. Protracted negative balance can lead to secondary complications, such as hip and vertebral bone fractures after minimal trauma or ectopic calcification around the large joints (91,93,106,110).

Some newer developments in treating or preventing bone loss may have some application for rehabilitating patients. The bisphosphonates are analogues of a naturally occurring bone chemical that inhibit bone resorption in addition to inhibiting calcium phosphate crystal formation and dissolution (111,112). Pamidronate and clodronate are now used to treat Paget disease, immobilization-induced hypercalcemia, metastatic bone disease, and other malignancies affecting bone (110,113). One bisphosphonate compound, tiludronate, has been used in paraplegic patients with some efficacy in maintaining bone volume without impairing bone formation. Salmon calcitonin is another compound that has demonstrated some success in maintaining bone density and may be particularly helpful in patient populations that cannot be adequately mobilized (114).

EFFECT OF IMMOBILITY AND INACTIVITY ON CARDIOVASCULAR AND PULMONARY FUNCTIONS

Cardiovascular Alteration

Cardiovascular hemodynamic responses to bed rest, upright position, and mobility are related to body fluid distribution, appropriate vasoconstriction of blood vessels upon assuming an upright position, and the pumping effect of the gastrocnemius and soleus muscles in moving venous blood toward the heart during ambulation. The vertical column of arterial blood exerts significant pressure on the lower part of the arterial tree, provoking norepinephrine release and vasoconstriction, thus preventing hypoperfusion of the brain upon arising. When standing, there is a shift of 500 cc of venous blood from the thorax and upper limbs to the legs, causing an increase in venous pressure to 80–100 mm Hg (115). Even a short bout of leg exercise will reduce the venous blood volume and venous pressure to 25 mm Hg. During ambulation, the increased need for oxygen will enhance cardiac and pulmonary responses and local vasodilatation in the muscles. These mechanisms can be significantly altered in subjects who lose mobility function because of paralysis, prolonged bed rest, or immobility for any reason. Normal response of the cardiopulmonary system to musculoskeletal demands requires the endothelial vascular system and blood components to function normally. Immobility and inactivity will alter the erythrocyte and platelet enzymatic antioxidant defense mechanisms, increase serum triglycerides, and decrease high-density lipoproteins and apolipoprotein AI, all of which may contribute to development of atherosclerosis (116,117).

During prolonged recumbency, the resting heart rate increases by one beat per minute every 2 days, leading to immobilization tachycardia at rest and abnormal increases in heart rate on submaximal exercise and workloads. This abnormal response of heart rate on resumption of physical activity correlates to duration of bed rest. Three days after strict bed rest, heart rate increases 32% above the pre–bed-rest response when resuming submaximal activity, 62% after 7 days, and 89% after 21 days of recumbency (118,119).

Assuming an upright position also provokes a significant increase in pulse rate, and the extent of this response is related to the duration of bed rest, too. A healthy, active person's heart rate increases 13% on getting up from a supine position (119, 120). Saltin and coworkers found a pulse rate response on submaximal exercise of 129 beats per minute for active healthy persons, compared with 165 beats per minute at the same level of exercise intensity after bed rest of 3 weeks (121).

Other cardiovascular functions also have been found to change with prolonged bed rest. Stroke volume may decrease 15% after 2 weeks of bed rest, a response that may be related in part to blood volume reduction. Although heart rate response to submaximal exercise increases progressively, cardiac output is reduced (119,120). The alterations of cardiovascular function induced by immobility are frequently referred to as cardiovascular adaptation syndrome (CAS). Diminished cardiac output coupled with reduced peripheral oxygen utilization can cause a significant decline in maximal oxygen consumption (VO_{2max}). After 20 days of bed rest, VO_{2max} may decline by 27%. If a patient with coronary artery disease develops CAS, cardiac ischemia may be aggravated. For example, orthostatic hypotension may precipitate the onset of angina in patients with coronary artery disease. One way of preventing CAS is to encourage early ambulation and graded activity. In the 1950s, patients with myocardial infarction were kept in bed for 2 to 3 weeks; today they are encouraged to start walking on the second day. For those patients who, for some reason, cannot be mobilized, electrical stimulation of muscles can partially prevent the negative side effects of prolonged immobility. Quinttan et al. have demonstrated that electrical stimulation of thigh muscles in patients with refractory congestive heart failure significantly improved the strength and cross-sectional muscle area of the stimulated muscle as well as measures of quality of life (122).

IMPAIRED CARDIOVASCULAR PERFORMANCE AND FITNESS

The efficiency of the cardiopulmonary response to muscle demand depends on the frequency with which the maximal work capacity of muscle is approached. Because of interaction between these two systems, the maximal cardiovascular capacity gradually declines with reduced physical activity (119,123). This decline of cardiovascular function is enhanced in chronically ill and disabled individuals who are immobile.

After 3 weeks of bed rest, the resting pulse increases 10 to 12 beats per minute, and the pulse rate increases an average of 35 to 45 beats above normal response after 30 minutes of walking at 3.5 miles per hour up a 10% grade. This represents a 25% decrease in cardiovascular performance (124). There is a gradual elevation of the systolic blood pressure in response to increased peripheral vascular resistance. In addition, the absolute systolic ejection time is shortened, and the diastolic filling time reduced, resulting in stroke volume reduction. Work capacity, which is derived from left ventricular pressure and force of ventricular contraction, is also reduced. Overall declines in cardiac output and left ventricular function with prolonged immobility have been reported in several studies (119,121,124).

Furthermore, reduced physical activity and fitness is associated with a twofold increase in risk of cardiovascular mortality and morbidity (125,126). Increase in physical activity and mobility, on the other hand, increases cardiovascular performance (127). The cardiovascular risk of reduced physical activity is similar to that of hypertension, diabetes, and high cholesterol, and it is dose related. A number of studies have found a dose-response relationship between higher physical activity and lower mortality from cardiovascular disease (126). Physical activity and exercise (even of moderate intensity) have a beneficial effect on the other cardiovascular risk factors such as hypertension, type 2 diabetes, and obesity (127,128). Regular physical activity and appropriate diet can reduce risk of type 2 diabetes development by 58%. This percentage is even higher in people older than 60, who have a nearly one-in-five chance of developing type 2 diabetes. It has also been documented that even low levels of physical activity have a beneficial effect on cardiovascular fitness (129). Current international guidelines suggest that 30 minutes per day or 3–4 hours per week of exercise should be performed to maintain fitness and prevent cardiovascular deconditioning. Only 1–2 hours of this activity needs to be of higher intensity (42).

Inactivity is a widespread chronic health problem. At least 25 % of the U.S. population is not physically active at all and is at risk for development of cardiovascular and musculoskeletal complications (123). In addition to the effect on nonexercisers, people who are active can benefit even more by increasing the intensity and duration of their activity (123). Many benefits of exercise training, however, can be lost within 2 weeks if physical activity is substantially reduced. These benefits are completely lost within 2–8 weeks if physical activity is not resumed.

Pulmonary Alterations

The respiratory complications of immobility are known to be life threatening. Initial pulmonary alterations result from restricted movement of the chest in the supine position and gravity-induced changes in the perfusion of blood through different parts of the lung. When venous and hydrostatic pressures that are due to gravity are increased in different parts of the lung, then perfusion is also increased. The balance between perfusion and ventilation is altered during recumbency (130). A change of position from upright to supine results in a 2% reduction in vital capacity, a 7% reduction of total lung capacity, a 19% reduction in residual volume, and a 30% reduction in functional residual capacity (131). Vital capacity and functional reserve capacity may be reduced by 25% to 50% after prolonged bed rest. Mechanisms responsible for this may include diminished diaphragmatic movement in the supine position, decreased chest excursion, progressive decrease in ROM of costovertebral and costochondral joints, and shallower breathing with a subsequent increase in respiratory rate (132).

Clearance of secretions is more difficult in a recumbent position. The dependent (i.e., usually posterior) lobes accumulate more secretions, whereas the upper parts (i.e., anterior) become dry, rendering the ciliary lining ineffective for clearing secretions and allowing secretions to pool in the lower bronchial tree. The effectiveness of coughing is impaired because of ciliary malfunction and abdominal muscle weakness. Regional changes in the ventilation perfusion ratio in dependent areas occur when ventilation is reduced and perfusion is increased. This may lead to significant arteriovenous shunting with lowered arterial oxygenation. Atelectasis and hypostatic pneumonia may be the ultimate result of these alterations.

The intercostal and axillary respiratory muscles for deep breathing gradually lose their strength and overall endurance. Treatment or prevention involves early mobilization, frequent respiratory toileting, and frequent position changes. A patient in a recumbent position should be persuaded to perform regular pulmonary toileting and deep breathing and coughing exercises, and to maintain adequate hydration. An incentive spirometer, chest percussion, and postural drainage with oropharyngeal suctioning can prevent aspiration and atelectasis. The presence of preexisting pulmonary disease requires the use of bronchodilators.

REDISTRIBUTION OF BODY FLUIDS

Normally, 20% of total blood volume is contained within the arterial system, 5% in the capillaries, and 75% in the venous system. Immediately upon lying down, 500 mL of blood shifts to the thorax, heart rate decreases, and cardiac output increases by 24%. Estimated myocardial work is increased by approximately 30%. During lengthy periods of bed rest, there is a progressive decline in blood volume, with the maximum reduction on day 14 and with reduction of cardiac output. This reduction in blood volume is due to a reduced hydrostatic blood pressure and decreased secretion of antidiuretic hormone. Plasma volume decreases more than red-cell mass, leading to increased blood viscosity and, possibly, to thromboembolic phenomena. The loss of plasma volume after 24 hours is 5%, whereas after 6 and 14 days, the loss is 10% and 20%, respectively, of the pre–bed-rest level (133). Extracellular fluid volume remains unchanged, although longer periods of bed rest will produce a decrease (134). For normal subjects on bed rest, the reduction of plasma volume can be diminished by exercise. Therapeutic isotonic exercises are almost twice as effective as isometric exercises in preventing plasma volume reduction (135).

In addition, a reduction of plasma proteins is noted after prolonged bed rest. Although short periods of intensive exercise produce a small loss of plasma proteins, sustained submaximal exercise actually induces a net gain in plasma protein, which contributes to the stabilization of the plasma volume depletion (135). Hypovolemia, along with circulatory stasis that is due to bed rest, are important precipitating factors in thrombogenesis.

ORTHOSTATIC INTOLERANCE

One of the most dramatic effects of prolonged bed rest is the impaired ability of the cardiovascular system to adjust to the upright position. After several days of bed rest, if a healthy person stands up from a supine position, the usual shift of 500 mL of blood from the thorax into the legs causes blood pooling problems because of impaired venous response. Venous return to the heart is reduced as a result of intravascular volume depletion, change in venous compliance, and venous pooling. The end result is decreased stroke volume and cardiac output, and a significant decrease in the systolic blood pressure on rising. In normal situations, blood pressure decrease is prevented by immediate activation of the adrenergic sympathetic system. Baroreceptors in the right atrium, carotid arteries, and aortic arch trigger adrenergic reflexes, releasing norepinephrine. The increase in plasma norepinephrine levels influences the release of renin and angiotensin II, which in return potentiate the sympathetic response, resulting in an immediate increase in pulse rate and restoration of blood pressure along with vasoconstriction of lower limb and mesenteric blood vessels (136,137).

During prolonged recumbency, the circulatory system is also unable to maintain a stable blood pressure and, for unknown reasons, is unable to mount an adequate sympathetic vasopressive response. Although plasma renin and aldosterone levels remain normal, vasoconstriction is inadequate. The recent study by Kamiya et al., however, revealed that 6 days of bed rest in a 6-degree head-down position caused decrease in plasma norepinephrine level, but sympathetic nerve activity was actually increased (138). This decrease in venous return along with the rapid heart rate prevents optimal ventricular filling during end diastole. Stroke volume, which depends on diastolic filling, may be insufficient to maintain adequate cerebral perfusion (139,140). The clinical signs and symptoms of postural hypotension are tingling, burning in the lower extremities, dizziness, lightheadedness, fainting, vertigo, increased pulse rate (more than 20 beats per minute), decreased systolic pressure (more than 20 mm Hg), and decreased pulse pressure. In patients with coronary artery disease, anginal symptoms may be caused by the decreased coronary blood flow that accompanies inadequate diastolic filling (141).

In healthy people, adaptation to the upright position may be completely lost after 3 weeks of bed rest. A significant increase in heart rate and decrease in systolic pressure may even occur after several days of recumbency in those with sepsis, major trauma, major medical illness, or advanced age. The process of restoring the normal postural cardiovascular responses can take 20 to 72 days. Older people take much longer to restore normal blood pressure and heart rate during remobilization.

As a group, patients with tetraplegia are quite susceptible to orthostatic hypotension. When tilted up, they show a significant decrease in mean arterial pressure and an increase in heart rate. Both sympathetic and plasma renin activities, as measured by serum dopamine-beta-hydroxylase and plasma renin radioimmunoassay, are normal or slightly increased. Two possible mechanisms may account for orthostatic hypotension in patients with spinal cord injury. First, the normal increase in plasma norepinephrine that occurs on tilting is delayed in patients with tetraplegia. Second, the successful use of compressive antigravity suits in treating patients with quadriplegia and postural hypotension indicates that venous pooling may play an important role in the occurrence of orthostatic hypotension (142,143).

Early mobilization is the most effective way to counter orthostatic hypotension and should include ROM exercises, strengthening exercises in supine and upright positions, and progressive ambulation. Abdominal strengthening and isotonic/isometric exercises involving the legs are optimal for reversing venous stasis and pooling. Elevating leg rests and reclining backs or tilt-in-space wheelchairs are used to assist patients during the reconditioning process. Occasionally a tilt table may be necessary, with the goal of tolerating 20 minutes at 75 degrees of tilt. Supportive garments such as elastic bandage wraps, full-length elastic stockings, and a variety of abdominal binders are used regularly. Ephedrine and phenylephrine are sympathomimetic agents that help to maintain blood pressure; fludrocortisone (Florinef, Apothcon), a mineralocorticoid, is the next choice of drug to use. Maintaining an adequate salt and fluid intake will prevent any worsening of hypotension secondary to blood volume contraction (136,143). Infusion of saline solution is also indicated when fluid volume and dehydration cannot be corrected by ordinary methods (144).

IMMOBILITY AND DEEP VENOUS THROMBOSIS

Immobility exposes the patient to two factors that are contained in Virchow's triad and contribute to clot formation: venous stasis and increased blood coagulability. The third factor, injury to the vessel wall, is all that is required to further increase the patient's risk for thromboembolism (145). Paralysis and trauma to the lower limbs or pelvis may add to the risk for development of DVT. A direct relationship between the frequency of DVT and the length of bed rest has been observed (146).

In stroke patients, DVT is 10 times more common in the involved extremities than in the uninvolved extremities. In nonambulatory stroke patients, DVT is five times more frequent than in patients who can walk more than 50 feet (147,148). Although the first week of immobilization is the most frequent time for development of DVT, it may occur later during remobilization. When stasis is present, thrombus formation usually starts behind the valve cusp of the deep veins. Stasis may contribute to anoxia and damage of the endothelial cells in the valve pocket, thus adding the third factor for initiating the onset of DVT. Whether stasis alone can result in DVT is not fully confirmed. However, several studies suggest that stasis may lead to increased formation of thrombin, which then leads to platelet aggregation and thrombosis (149). DVT mostly commonly forms in the veins in the calf. Usually, such thrombi will attach to the wall of the vein within 1 week; however, 20% of calf thrombi extend to popliteal and thigh veins, and half of these will embolize to the lungs, posing a serious threat to the patient's life (150).

Venous stasis in the lower extremities is mainly due to decreased pumping activity of the calf muscles and increased orthostatic pressure. Other factors that can contribute to stasis are surgery, age, obesity, and congestive heart failure, all of which can lead to abnormal blood flow mechanics. The incidence of DVT in postoperative patients published in 1979 was 29% for those who had general surgery and 44% for those who had hip surgery (146). Also contributing to the likelihood of DVT occurrence in the patient confined to bed is a hypercoagulable state, produced by decreased blood volume and increased blood viscosity and associated with many conditions, such as malignancy.

Clinical detection of DVT begins with the observation of signs and symptoms, including edema, tenderness, hyperemia, venous distention, and Homans' sign. When DVT is suspected on clinical grounds, one or more of these additional diagnostic studies should be considered:

- *Doppler ultrasound study* may be 95% accurate, depending on the skill of the examiner, but cannot be used to detect thrombi reliably above the level of the femoral vein.
- *Radionuclide venography* is both sensitive and specific for thrombi above the knee, but cannot detect calf thrombi or distinguish between old and new disease unless the patient has a previous study available for comparison.

- *Contrast venography* remains the standard for diagnosis. However, it is invasive, time consuming, painful, and irritating to the venous lining.

Pulmonary emboli are manifested by a sudden onset of dyspnea, tachypnea, tachycardia, or chest pain and often are associated with a preexisting DVT. Diagnosis rests on arterial blood gases, ventilation/perfusion scans, and pulmonary angiography.

The most common means of preventing thromboembolic complications is to use low-dose subcutaneous injections of heparin (5,000 units twice a day) (151). Low-molecular-weight heparins (LMWHs), however, are more effective in prevention of DVT than subcutaneous injection of heparin after hip and knee surgery. Lovenox is a commonly used LMWH in a prophylactic dose of 30 mg subcutaneously every 12 hours or 40 mg once a day starting 12 hours postoperatively. Prevention of DVT in stroke or spinal cord injury patients can effectively be accomplished by LMWHs. The treatment of DVT without or with pulmonary emboli is also effective with LMWHs. Lovenox in the dose of 1.0 mg/kg subcutaneously every 12 hours or 1.5mg/kg every 24 hours is used for inpatient treatment of DVT and for outpatient treatment, 1.0 mg/kg every 12 hours, until anticoagulation with oral agents is achieved. However, intravenous heparin is the treatment of the choice for femoral or pelvic thrombosis and pulmonary embolism. The usual intravenous dose is load of 5.000 units; mix 25,000 units in 250 mL D5W (100 units per mL), then infuse in the rate 11 mL/hour. The dose is monitored by activated partial thromboplastin time. For chronic treatment of DVT, warfarin (Coumadin) is a standard approach. The dose is monitored by the prothrombin time and the standardized international ratio, which should be in 2.0–3.0 range (152).

After the diagnosis of DVT is made and treatment with heparin and warfarin is initiated, ambulation can be permitted on the second or third day if the partial thromboplastin time is within the therapeutic range. Recent literature supports the conclusion that 5 to 7 days of bed rest is not necessary for DVT if a therapeutic level of anticoagulation is achieved (153–155). Other preventive measures include external intermittent leg compression, elastic leg wrappings, active exercise, and early mobilization. After anticoagulation is established, the patient is remobilized and allowed to participate in activities of daily living and mobility functions. Early remobilization will reduce swelling and pain in the calf muscle but will not completely eliminate danger of pulmonary emboli, especially in the patients with a proximal part of the thrombus freely flattering and unattached to the wall of a vein (155).

GASTROINTESTINAL AND GENITOURINARY SIDE EFFECTS

Genitourinary Alteration

Many compromises occur in the physical and metabolic functions of the urinary tract system. Prolonged bed rest contributes to increased incidence of bladder or renal stones and urinary tract infections. Hypercalciuria is a frequent finding in persons who are immobilized. Other important factors include an altered ratio of citric acid to calcium and an increased urinary excretion of phosphorus. In the supine position, urine must flow uphill from the renal collecting systems to be drained through the ureters. Patients often find it difficult to initiate voiding while supine, a situation that is not ameliorated by reduced intraabdominal pressure secondary to abdominal muscle weakness and deconditioning. Studies have demonstrated less complete voiding occurs in immobilized animals, leading to urinary retention (156).

Incomplete bladder emptying (e.g., in patients with spinal cord injury or diabetes mellitus) puts the patient at greater risk for stone formation (157). The most common types of stones are struvite and carbonate appetite, found in 15% to 30% of immobilized patients. Bladder stones allow bacterial growth and decrease the efficacy of standard antimicrobial treatment. Irritation and trauma to the bladder mucosa by stones can encourage bacterial overgrowth and infection. Urea-splitting bacteria then increase the urine pH, leading to further precipitation of calcium and magnesium (156).

Treatment of these problems lies first in prevention, which includes adequate fluid intake to reduce bacterial colonization, use of the upright position for voiding, and scrupulous avoidance of bladder contamination during instrumentation. Other therapeutic approaches might include acidification of the urine through the use of vitamin C, urinary antiseptics, and, in those populations at highest risk for stone formation, a urease inhibitor. Treatment of stones after they have formed may require surgical removal or the use of ultrasonic lithotripsy. Appropriate antibiotic selection based on urine cultures and sensitivity trials is required to eliminate urinary tract infection. If retention is suspected, postvoiding residual volumes should be measured several times a day with ultrasound scanning devices. After stroke or spinal cord injury, removal of the Foley catheter and initiation of voiding trails should coincide with sitting and ambulation training. A dysfunctional urinary bladder with poor contractility of the detrusor muscle and deficient sphincter coordination will aggravate the adverse effects of immobility.

Gastrointestinal Alterations

Gastrointestinal alterations that are due to immobility are easily overlooked. Loss of appetite, slower rate of absorption, and distaste for protein-rich foods all lead to nutritional hypoproteinemia. Passage of food through the esophagus, stomach, and small bowel is slowed in the supine position. An upright position increases the velocity of the esophageal waves and shortens the relaxation time of the lower esophagus (158). Thus, sleeping on two or three pillows with the upper trunk elevated in bed has therapeutic implications in preventing and treating reflux esophagitis. The transit of food through the stomach is 66% slower and gastric acidity is higher in the supine position than when a person is upright (159). Peristalsis and passage of food through the small bowel is reduced with prolonged bed rest. Absorption of food is also reduced. For example, calcium absorption during normal activity is 31% of intake and decreased to 24% during bed rest, although calcium excretion through the bowels is increased from average 797 mg/day to 911 mg/day (160). Constipation is a common complication that results from the interaction of multiple factors. Immobility causes increased adrenergic activity, which inhibits peristalsis and causes sphincter contraction (160). The loss of plasma volume and dehydration aggravate constipation. In addition, the use of a bedpan for fecal elimination places the patient in a nonphysiological position, and the desire to defecate is reduced by social embarrassment. The end result can be fecal impaction, which requires enemas, manual removal, or, in extreme cases, surgical intervention (161,162).

Prevention of constipation requires an adequate intake of an appealing, fiber-rich diet, including raw fruits and vegetables, and of liberal amounts of fluids. Stool softeners and bulk-forming agents are helpful in maintaining bowel function. The use of narcotic agents should be limited because they slow peristalsis. Limited use of glycerin or peristalsis-stimulating supposi-

tories, in combination with a regularly timed bowel program, will further assist in the prevention of impaction (163).

METABOLISM AND ENDOCRINE SYSTEM ALTERATIONS RESULTING FROM IMMOBILITY

Daily human energy needs include basal metabolic activity, thermogenesis of food, and the activities of daily living and locomotion. It is unclear whether basal metabolism changes during bed rest; this uncertainty stems from inadequate scientific studies on control of factors that could influence the basal metabolic rate during prolonged bed rest. Lean body mass decreases during bed rest, and an equal gain in body fat maintains constant total body weight (164). The reduced lean body mass is associated with muscle atrophy and decreased metabolic activity of muscle, diminished utilization of oxygen and glucose, increased insulin resistance and reduction of maximal oxygen consumption, with further deterioration of the functional capacity of the musculoskeletal system (165,166).

Electrolyte Balance

Prolonged immobility, especially if associated with posttraumatic electrolyte changes, will cause an alteration in the metabolic balance of sodium, sulfur, phosphorus, and potassium. A decrease in total body sodium occurs in tandem with the diuresis seen early during bed rest. However, serum sodium levels do not correlate well with the severity of orthostatic hypotension. Hyponatremia is manifested especially in the elderly by lethargy, confusion and disorientation, anorexia, and seizures. Potassium levels progressively decrease during the early weeks of bed rest as well (163). Immobility alone rarely causes serious electrolyte disturbances, aside from the high calcium levels seen in immobilization hypercalcemia (94). Nevertheless, patients with multiple medical illnesses may be seriously affected by even slight electrolyte abnormalities (Fig. 68-4).

Hormonal Disorders

A lack of physical activity can cause altered responsiveness of hormones and enzymes. Although they may be clinically undetected during early immobility, numerous changes have been demonstrated to occur in the endocrine system. Significant car-

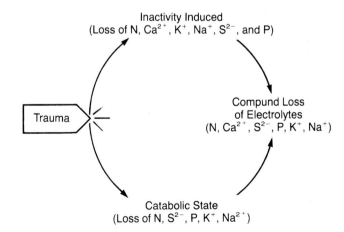

Figure 68-4. Metabolic imbalance and endocrine changes induced by trauma can be aggravated by immobility, resulting in a prolonged recovery of primary disease or in development of wide variety of physiological and functional impairment and disease conditions.

bohydrate intolerance has been noted as early as the third day of immobility, and peripheral glucose uptake may decline 50% after 14 days (165). The duration of immobility correlates proportionally with the degree of carbohydrate intolerance. The glucose intolerance induced by bed rest can be improved by isotonic, but not isometric, exercises of the large muscle groups (166,167). The reason for this intolerance is not lack of insulin, but rather increased resistance to the action of insulin, resulting in hyperglycemia and hyperinsulinemia. Possible explanations include a reduction in number or affinity of insulin receptors or postreceptor changes in the target cells. Inactivity appears to cause a reduction in insulin-binding sites, predominantly on the muscle membrane (168,169).

There are several other hormonal effects, including an increase in serum parathyroid hormone, which is related to hypercalcemia from immobility, although its precise mechanism is unknown (170). Tri-iodothyronine (T3) blood levels are also elevated during immobility (171). In addition, alterations have been reported in androgen levels and spermatogenesis, in growth hormone response to hypoglycemia, in levels of adrenocorticotropic hormone, and in catecholamine secretion from the sympathomedullary system (172,173). Measurements of serum corticosteroid levels during bed rest have been inconclusive. Although the excretion of urinary cortisol is increased, the adrenal gland response to the stimulus of the adrenocorticotropic hormone is reduced after prolonged bed rest. Studies of bed rest for periods of 1 month or more have found that adrenocorticotropic hormone levels were three times higher than baseline and required about 20 days of physical activity to return to normal (173). In contrast, prolonged exercise has been shown to increase plasma hydrocortisone levels and decrease plasma norepinephrine levels (174). Total cholesterol levels are also increased with lower high-density lipoprotein levels during protracted immobility.

THE NERVOUS SYSTEM AND IMMOBILITY

Sensory deprivation is a silent hazard of prolonged bed rest. Healthy subjects placed on strict bed confinement for 3 hours and required to wear gloves, goggles, and earplugs to reduce sensory input experience hallucinations and disorientation. During prolonged bed rest, exposure to social and chronological cues, such as time of day and movement through space, is reduced (175,176). Social isolation alone with preserved mobility can cause emotional lability and anxiety but usually does not cause any intellectual alterations. However, prolonged bed rest and social isolation together produce much greater alterations in mental concentration, orientation to space and time, and other intellectual functions. Restlessness, anxiety, decreased pain tolerance, irritability, hostility, insomnia, and depression may occur during 2 weeks of recumbency and social isolation. Furthermore, judgment, problem solving and learning ability, psychomotor skills, and memory all may be impaired. Perceptual impairment can be altered even after only 7 days of immobility (177,178).

Lack of concentration and motivation, depression, and reduced psychomotor skills may drastically affect the patient's ability to achieve the highest possible level of functioning and independence. These behavioral effects of immobility may result in a lack of motivation and diminish the patient's ability to attain optimal healing and restoration of function. Balance and coordination also are impaired after prolonged immobility, and this effect appears to be due to altered neural control rather than muscle weakness (179,180).

An important strategy in the prevention and treatment of these complications is to apply appropriate physical and psychosocial stimulation early in the course of illness. Options for the treatment of these effects include group therapy sessions, attention to socialization, encouragement of family interaction and avocational pursuits during evenings and weekends, as well as participation in regular physical activity and exercise. In a multicenter, prospective study of older, noninstitutionalized women tested over 6 to 8 years, greater intensity of physical activity was associated with smaller declines in cognitive function, even when age, estrogen use, and other comorbidity was controlled for. The authors concluded that physical activity prevents decline in cognitive function in older women (181).

CONCLUSION

In 1862, the English surgeon John Hilton advocated bed rest as a basic physiologic approach in the treatment of human illness. Since that time, bed rest has often been used indiscriminately in the treatment of acute and chronic illnesses. The complications of prolonged bed rest have been increasingly recognized and reported since the mid-1940s. After World War II, clinical investigators, starting with Deitrick and colleagues in 1948, have shown that prolonged bed rest may cause multiple adverse effects in a number of organs and systems (182). During the 1960s and 1970s, studies on astronauts greatly advanced our knowledge of the deleterious effects of bed rest and weightlessness, making clinicians more aware of a wide range of adverse effects associated with prolonged bed rest and immobility. As a result, a great number of new epidemiologic and randomized studies in the last three decades have been conducted which in a great preponderance have demonstrated significant benefits of physical activity and exercises on cardiopulmonary, musculoskeletal, and total body functions.

A new era of advocating exercise and cardiovascular conditioning has begun. Studies have indicated that prolonged bed rest and sedentary lifestyles have negative effects on human body functioning. These effects are magnified in persons with neurologic disease or in the elderly. The principles advocated by rehabilitation medicine have contributed significantly to the current philosophy on the use and misuse of immobility.

REFERENCES

1. Allen C, Glasziou P, Del Mar C. Bed rest: a potential harmful treatment needing more careful evaluation. *Lancet* 1999;354(9186):1229–1233. Comments in *Lancet* 2000;355(9206):844.
2. Harper CM, Lyles YM. Physiology and complications of bed rest. *J Am Geriatr Soc* 1988;36:1047–1054.
3. Downey RJ, Weissman C. Physiological changes associated with bed rest and major body injury. In Gonzales EG, Meyers SJ, eds. *Physiological basis of rehabilitation medicine*, 3rd ed. Wobury, MA: Butterworth-Heinemann, 2001:449–484.
4. Hoenig HM, Rubenstein LZ. Hospital-associated deconditioning and dysfunction. *J Am Geriatr Soc* 1991;39:220–222.
5. Clark LP, Dion DM, Barker WH. Taking to bed: rapid functional decline in an independently mobile older population living in an intermediate-care facility. *J Am Geriatr Soc* 1990;38:967–972.
6. Kottke FJ. The effects of limitation of activity upon the human body. *JAMA* 1966;196:117–122.
7. Berg HE, Dudley GA, Haggmark T, et al. Effect of lower limb unloading on skeletal muscle mass and function in humans. *J Appl Physiol* 1991;70:1882–1885.
8. Ferrando AA, Lane HW, Stuart CA, et al. Prolonged bed rest decreases skeletal muscle and whole body protein synthesis. *Am J Physiol* 1996;270:E627–E663.
9. Haggmark T, Eriksson E, Lanssom E. Muscle fiber type changes in human skeletal muscle after injury and immobilization. *J Orthopaedics* 1986;9(2):181–185.

10. Abe T, Kawakami Y, Suzuki Y, et al. Effect of 20 days bed rest on muscle morphology. *Journal of Gravitational Physiology* 1997;4(1):S10–14.
11. Akima H, Kuno S, Suzuki Y, et al. Effects of 20 days of bed rest on physiological cross-sectional area of human thigh and leg muscles evaluated by magnetic resonance imaging. *Journal of Gravitational Physiology* 1997;4(1): S15–21.
12. Ohira Y, Yoshinaga T, Ohara M, et al. Myonuclear domain and myosin phenotype in human soleus after bed rest with or without loading. *J Appl Physiol* 1999;87(5):1776–1785.
13. Savolainen J, Vaanen K, Vihko V, et al. Effect of immobilization on collagen synthesis in rat skeletal muscles. *Am J Physiol* 1987; 252:R883–888.
14. Goubel F. Changes in mechanical properties of human muscle as a result of space flights. *Int J Sports Med* 1997; 18[Suppl.4]:S285–S287.
15. Lowey S, Wallers GS, Trybus KM. Function of skeletal muscle myosin heavy and light chain isoforms by an in vitro motility assay. *J Biol Chem* 1993;268: 20414–20418.
16. Clarke MS, Bamman MM, Feeback DL. Bed rest decreases mechanically induced myofiber wounding and consequent wound-mediated FGF release. *J Appl Physiol* 1998;85(2):593– 600.
17. Zachwieja JJ, Smith SR, Sinka-Hikim I, et al. Plasma myostatin-immunoreactive protein is increased after prolonged bed rest with low-dose T3 administration. *Journal of Gravitational Physiology*1999;6(2):11–15.
18. Rubinoff R. Sarcopenia: a major modifiable cause of fragility in the elderly. *J Nutr Health Aging* 2000;4(3):140–142.
19. Mack PB, Montgomery KB. Study of nitrogen balance and creatine and creatinine excretion during recumbency and ambulation of five young adult human males. *Aerospace Medicine* 1973;44:739–746.
20. Zorbas YG, Andreyev VG, Popescu LB. Fluid-electrolyte metabolism and renal function in men under hypokinesia and physical exercise. *International Urology and Nephrology* 1988;20:215–223.
21. Muller EA. Influence of training and of inactivity on muscle strength. *Arch Phys Med Rehabil* 1970;51:449–462.
22. Ferrando AA, Tipton KD, Bamman MM, Wolfe RR. Resistive exercise maintains skeletal muscle protein synthesis during the bed rest. *J Appl Physiol* 1997;82(3):807–810.
23. Akima H, Kubo K, Imai M, et al. Inactivity and muscle: effect of resistance training during bed rest on muscle size in the lower limb. *Acta Physiol Scand* 2001;172(4):269–278.
24. Funato K, Matsuo A, Yata Y, et al. Changes in force-velocity and power output of upper and lower extremity musculature in young subjects following 20 days bed rest. *Journal of Gravitational Physiology* 1997;4(1):S22–30.
25. Ferretti G. The effect of prolonged bed rest on maximal instantaneous muscle power and its determinants. *Int J Sports Med* 1997;18(4):S287–S289.
26. Witzmann FA, Kim DH, Fitts RH. Effect of hindlimb immobilization on the fatigability of skeletal muscle. *J Appl Physiol* 1983;54:1242–1248.
27. Booth FW. Physiologic and biochemical effects of immobilization on muscle. *Clin Orthop* 1987;219:115–120.
28. Thom JM, Thompson MW, Ruell PA, et al. Effect of 10-days cast immobilization on sarcoplasmic reticulum calcium regulation in humans. *Acta Physiol Scand* 2001;172(2):141–147.
29. Ferretti G, Antonutto G, Denis C, et al. The interplay of central and peripheral factors in limiting maximal O2 consumption in men after prolonged bed rest. *Journal of Physiology (Lond)* 1997;501:677–686.
30. Pestronk A, Drachmann B, Griffin IW. Effect of muscle disuse on acetylcholine receptors. *Nature* 1976;260:352–353.
31. Henriksson R, Reitman JS. Time course of changes in human skeletal muscle succinate dehydrogenase and cytochrome oxidase activities and maximal uptake with physical activity and inactivity. *Acta Physiol Scand* 1977;99: 91–97.
32. Appell HJ. Muscular atrophy following immobilization: a review. *Sports Med* 1990;10:42–58.
33. Michelsson JE, Aho HJ, Kalimo H, et al. Severe degeneration of rabbit vastus intermedius muscle immobilized in shortened position. *APMIS* 1990;98: 336–344.
34. Rutherford OM, Jones DA, Round JM. Long-lasting unilateral muscle wasting and weakness following injury and immobilization. *Scand J Rehabil Med* 1990;22:33–37.
35. Baum K. Essfeld D. Origin of back pain during bed rest: a new hypothesis. *Eur J Med Res* 1999;4(9):389–393.
36. Williams PE. Use of intermittent stretch in the prevention of serial sarcomere loss in immobilized muscle. *Ann Rheum Dis* 1990;49:316–317.
37. Spector SA, Simard CP, Fournier SM, et al. Architectural alterations of rat hind limb skeletal muscle immobilized at different lengths. *Exp Neurol* 1982;76:94–110.
38. Wannamethee SG, Sharper AG, Walker M. Physical activity and mortality in older men with diagnosed coronary heart disease. *Circulation* 2000;102(12): 1358–1363.
39. Sesso AD, Paffenbarger RS, Lee IM. Physical activity and coronary heart disease in men: the Harvard Alumni Health Study. *Circulation* 2000;102(9): 975–980.
40. Bair SN, Kampert JB, Kohl HW Jr, et al. Influence of cardiorespiratory fitness and other precursors on cardiovascular disease and all-cause mortality in men and women. *JAMA* 1996;276:205–210.
41. DeSouza CA, Shapiro LF, Clevenger CM, et al. Regular aerobic exercise prevents and restores age-related declines in endothelial-dependent vasodilatation in healthy men. *Circulation* 2000;102(12):1351–1357.
42. U.S. Department of Health and Human Services. Physical activity and health: a report of the Surgeon General. Atlanta, GA: Centers for Diseases Control and Prevention, National Center for Chronic Disease Prevention and Health Promotion: 1996.
43. Ferrando AA, Stuart CA, Shefield-Moore M, Wolfe RR. Inactivity amplifies the catabolic response of skeletal muscle to cortisol. *J Clin Endocrinol Metab* 1999;84(10):3515–3521.
44. Ferrando AA, Tipton KD, Bamman MM, Wolfe RR. Resistance exercise maintains skeletal muscle protein synthesis during bed rest. *J Appl Physiol* 1997;8(3):807–810
45. Carlson JA, Booth FW. Myogenin mRNA is elevated during rapid, slow, and maintenance phases of stretch-induced hypertrophy in chicken slow-tonic muscle. *Pflugers Arch* 1998;435(part 6):850..
46. Holly RG, Barnett CR, Ashmoore CR, et al. Stretch induced growth in chicken wing muscle: a new model of stretch hypertrophy. *Am J Physiol* 1980;238:C62–71.
47. Baker JH, Matsumoto DE. Adaptation of skeletal muscle to immobilization in a shortened position. *Muscle Nerve* 1988;11:231–244.
48. Gould N, Donnermeyer D, Pope M, Ashikaga T. Transcutaneous muscle stimulation as a method to retard disuse atrophy. *Clin Orthop* 1982;164: 215–220.
49. Davies CTM, Rutherford IC, Thomas DO. Electrically evoked contractions of the triceps surae during and following 21 days of voluntary led immobilization. *Eur J Appl Physiol* 1987;56:306–312.
50. Mayr W, Bijak M, Girsh W, et al. Myostim-FES to prevent muscle atrophy in microgravity and bed rest: preliminary report. *Artif Organs* 1999;23(5):428–431.
51. Shaffer MA, Okereke E, Esterhai JL Jr, et al. Effects of immobilization on plantarflexion torque, fatigue resistance, and functional ability following an ankle fracture. *Phys Ther* 2000;80(8):769–780.
52. Covertino VA. Cardiovascular consequences of bed rest: effect on maximal oxygen uptake. *Med Sci Sports Exerc* 1997;29(2):191–196.
53. Converetino VA, Bloomfield SA, Greenleaf JE. An overview of the issue: physiological effects of bed rest and restricted physical activity. *Med Sci Sports Exerc* 1997;29(2):187–190.
54. Greenleaf JE. Intensive exercise training during bed rest attenuates deconditioning. *Med Sci Sports Exerc* 1997;29(2):207–215.
55. Robinson GA, Enoka RM, Stuart DG. Immobilization-induced changes in motor unit force and fatigability in the cat. *Muscle Nerve* 1991;14:563–573.
56. Amiel D, Woo SL-Y, Harwood FL, et al. The effect of immobilization of collagen turnover in connective tissue: a biochemical-biomechanical correlation. *Acta Orthop Scand* 1982;53:325–332.
57. Garcia-Bunuel L, Garcia-Bunuel VM. Connective tissue metabolism in normal and atrophic skeletal muscle. *J Neurol Sci* 1980;47:69–77.
58. Campbell RR, Hawkins SJ, Maddison PJ, et al. Limited joint mobility in diabetes mellitus. *Ann Rheum Dis* 1985;44:93–97.
59. Alberts B, Bray D, Lewis J, et al. *Molecular biology of the cell.* New York: Garland, 1983:673–715.
60. Bornstein P, Byers PH. Collagen metabolism: current concepts (pamphlet). Kalamazoo, MI: Upjohn, 1980.
61. Karpakka J, Vaananen K, Orava S, et al. The effects of preimmobilization training and immobilization on collagen synthesis in rat skeletal muscle. *Int J Sports Med* 1990;11:484–488.
62. Jozsa L, Kannus P, Thoring I, et al. The effect of tenotomy and immobilization on intramuscular connective tissue. *J Bone Joint Surg Br* 1990;72:293–297.
63. Harper J, Amiel D, Harper E. Collagenases from periarticular ligaments and tendon: enzyme levels during the development of joint contracture. *Matrix* 1989;9:200–205.
64. Karpakka J, Vaananen K, Vinanen P, et al. The effects of remobilization and exercise on collagen biosynthesis in rat tendon. *Acta Physiol Scand* 1990;139: 139–145.
65. Saamanen AM, Tammi M, Jurvelin J, et al. Proteoglycan alterations following immobilization and remobilization in the articular cartilage of young canine knee (stifle) joint. *J Orthop Res* 1990;8:863–873.
66. Akeson WH, Garfin S, Amiel D, et al. Para-articular connective tissue in osteoarthritis. *Semin Arthritis Rheum* 1989;18(suppl 2):41–50.
67. Reynolds CA, Cummings GS, Andrews PD. Effect of non-traumatic immobilization on ankle dorsiflexion stiffness in rats. *J Orthop Sports Phys Ther* 1996;23:27–33.
68. Johnson EW. Pathokinesiology of Duchenne muscular dystrophy: implications for management. *Arch Phys Med Rehabil* 1977;54:4–7.
69. Stuart CA, Shangraw RE, Prince MJ, et al. Bed-rest-induced resistance occurs primarily in muscle. *Metabolism* 1988;37:802–806.
70. Chappard D, Alexandre C, Palle S, et al. Effects of a bisphosphonate (1-hydroxy ethylidene-1, 1 bisphosphonic acid) on osteoclast number during prolonged bed rest in healthy humans. *Metabolism* 1989;38:822–825.
71. Fam AG, Schumacher HR Jr, Clayburne G, et al. Effect of joint motion on experimental calcium pyrophosphate dihydrate crystal induced arthritis. *J Rheumatol* 1990;17:644–655.
72. Van Lent PLEM, van den Bersselaar L, van de Putte LBA, et al. Immobilization aggravates cartilage damage during antigen-induced arthritis in mice. *Am J Pathol* 1990;136:1407–1416.
73. Van Lent PLEM, Wilms FHA, Van Den Berg WB. Interaction of polymorphonuclear leucocytes with patellar cartilage of immobilized arthritic joints: a scanning electron microscopic study. *Ann Rheum Dis* 1989;48:832–837.

74. Van den Ende CHM, Breedveld FC, la Cessie S, et al. The effect of intensive exercised on patients with active rheumatoid arthritis: a randomized clinical trial. *Ann Rheum Dis* 2000;59:615–621.

75. Behrens F, Krah EL, Oegema TR Jr. Biochemical changes in articular cartilage after joint immobilization by casting or external fixation. *J Orthop Res* 1989;7:335–343.

76. Newton PO, Woo SL-Y, Kitabayashi LR, et al. Ultrastructural changes in knee ligaments following immobilization. *Matrix* 1990;10:314–319.

77. Dahner DE, Sky KE, Muller PR. A study of the mechanisms influencing ligament growth. *J Orthop Res* 1989;12:1569–1572.

78. Klein L, Heiple KG, Torzilli PA, et al. Prevention of ligament and meniscus atrophy by active joint motion in a non-weight bearing model. *J Orthop Res* 1989;7:80–85.

79. Inoue M, Woo SL-Y, Gomez MA, et al. Effects of surgical treatment and immobilization on the healing of the medial collateral ligament: a long-term multidisciplinary study. *Connect Tissue Res* 1990;25:13–26.

80. Hanada E, Kerrigan DC. Energy consumption during level walking with arm and knee immobilized. *Arch Phys Med Rehabil* 2001;82 (9):1251–1254.

81. Deyo RA, Diehl AK, Rosenthal M. How many days of bed rest for acute low back pain? *N Engl J Med* 1986;315:1064–1092.

82. Salter RB, Bell RS, Keeley FW. The protective effect of continuous passive motion on living articular cartilage in acute septic arthritis: an experimental investigation in the rabbit. *Clin Orthop* 1981;159:223–247.

83. Nene AV, Evans GA, Patrick JH. Simultaneous multiple operations for spastic diplegia: outcome and functional assessment of walking in 18 patients. *J Bone Joint Surg* Br. 1993 May;75(3):488–494.

84. Moreno-Alvarez MJ, Espad G, Maldonado-Cocco JA, Gagliardi SA. Long term follow up of hip and knee soft tissue release in juvenile chronic arthritis. *J Rheumatol* 1992;19:1608–1610.

85. Delp SL, Statler K, Carroll NC. Preserving planter flexion strength after surgical treatment for contracture of the triceps surae: a computer simulation study. *J Orthop Res* 1995;13:96–104.

86. Van-Loon JJ, Bervoets DJ, Burger EH, et al. Decreased mineralization and increased calcium release in isolated fetal mouse long bones under near weightlessness. *J Bone Miner Res* 1995;10:550–557.

87. Gross TS, Rubin CT. Uniformity of resorptive bone loss induced by disease. *J Orthop Res* 1995;13:708–714.

88. Cann CE, Genant HK, Young DR. Comparison of vertebral and peripheral mineral losses in disuse osteoporosis in monkey. *Radiology* 1980;134:525–559.

89. Lips P, van Ginkel FC, Netelenbos JC, et al. Lower mobility and markers of bone resorption in the elderly. *Bone and Mineral* 1990;9:49–57.

90. Leblanc AD, Schneider VS, Evans HJ. Bone mineral loss and recovery after 17 weeks of bed rest. *J Bone Miner Res* 1990;5:843–850.

91. Ito M, Matsumoto T, Enomoto H, et al. Effect of non-weight bearing on tibial bone density measured by QCT in patient with hip surgery. *J Bone Min Metab* 1999;17(1):45–50.

92. Avioli LV. Hormonal alterations and osteoporotic syndromes. *J Bone Miner Res* 1993;2[Suppl]:511–514.

93. Perloff JJ, McDermott MT, Perloff KG, et al. Reduced bone mineral content is a risk factor for hip fractures. *Orthop Rev* 1991;20:690–698.

94. Uebelhart D, Demiaux-Domenech G, Roth M, Chantraine A. Bone metabolism in spinal cord injured individuals and in others who have prolonged immobilization: a review. *Paraplegia* 1995;33:669–673.

95. Kannus P, Leppala J, Lehto M, et al. A rotator cuff rupture produces permanent osteoporosis in the affected extremity, but not in those with whom shoulder function has returned to normal. *J Bone Miner Res* 1995;10:1263–1271.

96. Houde JP, Schulz LA, Morgan WJ, et al. Bone mineral density changes in the forearm after immobilization. *Clin Orthop* 1995;317:199–205.

97. Shen V, LianXG, Birchman R, et al. Short-term immobilization-induced cancellous bone loss is limited to regions undergoing high turnover and/or modeling in nature rats. *Bone* 1997;21(1)71–78.

98. Fiore CE, Pennisi P, Ciffo F, et al. Immobilization-dependent bone collagen breakdown appear to increase with the time: for a lack of new bone equilibrium in response to reduced load during prolonged bed rest. *Horm Metab Res* 1999;31(1):31–36.

99. Bauman WA, Spungen AM, Wang J, et al. Continuous loss of bone during chronic immobilization: a monozygotic twin study. *Osteoporos Int* 1999;10(2):123–127.

100. Zerweekh JE, Ruml LA, Gottschalk F, Pak CY. The effects of twelve weeks of bed rest on bone histology, biochemical markers of bone turnover, and calcium homeostasis in eleven normal subjects. *J Bone Miner Res* 1998;13(10):1954–1601.

101. Bourrin S, Palle S, Gentry C, Alexandre C. Physical exercise during remobilization restores abnormal bone trabecular network after tail suspension-induced osteopenia in young rats. *J Bone Miner Res* 1995;10:820–828.

102. Sinaki M, Offord KP. Physical activity in post-menopausal women: effect on back muscle strength and bone mineral density of the spine. *Arch Phys Med Rehabil* 1988;69:277–280.

103. Marcus R. Relationship of age-related decreases in muscle mass and strength to skeletal status [Review]. *J Gerontol* 1995;50:86–87.

104. Schneider VS, McDonald J. Skeletal calcium homeostasis and counter measures to prevent disuse osteoporosis. *Calcif Tissue Int* 1984;36:151–154.

105. Sinaki M, Wahner HW, Bergstralh EJ, et al. Three year controlled randomized trial of the effect of dose-specific loading and strengthening exercises on bone mineral density of spine and femur in nonathletic physically active women. *Bone* 1996;19(3):233–244.

106. Sinaki M, Wollan PC, Scott RW, Gelczer RK. Can strong back extensors prevent vertebral fractures in women with osteoporosis? *Mayo Clin Proc* 1996;71:951–956.

107. Andrews PL, Rosenberg AR. Renal consequences of immobilization in children with fractured femurs. *Acta Paediatr Scand* 1990;79:311–315.

108. Gallacher SJ, Ralston SH, Dryburgh FJ, et al. Immobilization related hypercalcemia: a possible novel mechanism and response to pamidronate. *Postgrad Med J* 1990;66:918–922.

109. Gopal H, Sklar AH, Sherrard DJ. Symptomatic hypercalcemia in a patient with end-stage renal disease. *Am J Kidney Disease* 2000;35(5):969–972.

110. Minaire P. Immobilization osteoporosis: a review. *Clin Rheumatol* 1989;8 [Suppl 2]:95.

111. Singer FR, Minoofar PN. Bisphosphonates in the treatment of disorders of mineral metabolism. *Advances in Endocrinology and Metabolism* 1995;6:259–288.

112. Fleisch H. Bisphosphonates in osteoporosis: an introduction. *Osteoporos Int* 1999;3[Suppl]:3–5.

113. Chappard D, Minaire P, Privat C, et al. Effects of tiludronate on bone loss in paraplegic patients. *J Bone Miner Res* 1995;10:112–118.

114. Tsakalakos N, Magiasis B, Tsekoura M, Lyritis G. The effect of short-term calcitonin administration on biochemical bone markers in patients with acute immobilization following hip fracture. *Osteoporos Int* 1993;3:337–340.

115. Flue MW. Disorders of veins. In Sabiston DC, e). *Textbook of surgery.* Philadelphia: WB Saunders, 1986:1709–1730.

116. Pawlak W, Kedziora J, Zolynski K, et al. Effect of long term bed rest in men on enzymatic antioxidative defense and lipid peroxidation in erythrocytes. *Journal of Gravitational Physiology*1998;5(1):P163–164.

117. Yanagibori R, Suzuki Y, Kawakubo K, et al. The effect of 20 days bed rest on serum lipids and lipoprotein concentrations in healthy young subjects. *Journal of Gravitational Physiology* 1997;4(1) S 82–90.

118. Green DJ, O'Driscoll JG, Blanksby BA, Taylor RR. Effect of casting on forearm resistance vessel in young men. *Med Sci Sports Exerc* 1997;29(10): 13251331.

119. Taylor HL. The effects of rest in bed and of exercise on cardiovascular function. *Circulation* 1968;38:1016–1017.

120. Convertino VA, Doerr DF, Eckberg DL, et al. Carotid baroreflex response following 30 days exposure to simulated microgravity. *Physiologist* 1989;32 [Suppl]:67–68.

121. Saltin B, Blomqvist G, Mithcell JH, et al. Response to exercise after bed rest and after training. *Circulation* 1968;38[Suppl VII]:1–78.

122. Quinttan M, Wiesinger GF, Sturm B, et al. Improvement of thigh muscles by neuromuscular electrical stimulation in patients with refractory heart failure: a single-blind, randomized, controlled trial. *Am J Phys Med Rehabil* 2001; 80(3):206–214; quiz. 215–216, 224.

123. Booth FW, Gordon SE, Carson CJ, Hamilton MT. Waging war on modern chronic disease. *J Appl Physiol* 2000;88:774–787.

124. Demida BF, Machinski I. Use of rehabilitation measures for restoration of human physical work capacity after the prolonged limitation of motor activity. *Kosmicheskaia biologiiai aviakosmichcskaia meditsina* 1979;13:74–75.

125. Blair SN, Kohl HW III, Paffengerger RS, et al. Physical fitness and all-cause mortality: a prospective study of healthy men and women. *JAMA* 1989;262: 1395–2410.

126. Kujala UM, Kaprio J, Sarna S, Koskenvuo M. Relationship of leisure-time physical activity and mortality: the Finish twin cohort. *JAMA* 1998;279:440–444.

127. Blair SN, Kampert, Kohl WH III, et al. Influence of cardiorespiratory fitness and other precursors on cardiovascular disease and all-cause mortality in men and women. *JAMA* 1998;276:205–210.

128. Dunn AL, Marcus BH, Kampert JB, et al. Comparison of lifestyle and structured interventions to increase physical activity and cardiovascular fitness: a randomized trial. *JAMA* 1999;281:327–334.

129. Manson JE, Hu FB, Rich-Edwards JW, et al. A prospective study of waking compared with vigorous exercise in the prevention of coronary heart disease in women. *N Engl J Med* 1999;341:650–658.

130. Svanberg L. Influence of posture on the lung volumes ventilation and circulation in normals. *Scand J Clin Lab Invest* 1957;9[Suppl 25]:1–195.

131. West JB. *Ventilation blood flow and gas exchange,* 3rd ed. Philadelphia: JB Lippincott, 1977.

132. Craig DB, Wahba WM, Don HF. Airway closure and lung volume in surgical positions. *Can Anaesth Soc J* 1971;18:92–99.

133. Van Beaumont W, Greenleaf JE, Juhos L. Disproportional changes in hematocrit, plasma volume, and proteins during exercise and bed rest. *J Appl Physiol* 1972;33:55–61.

134. Greenleaf JE, Van Beaumont W, Brock PJ, et al. Plasma volume and electrolyte shifts with heavy exercise in sitting and supine positions. *Am J Physiol* 1979;236:206–214.

135. Greenleaf JE, Bernauer EM, Young HL, et al. Fluid and electrolyte shifts during bed rest with isometric and isotonic exercise. *J Appl Physiol* 1977; 42:59–66.

136. Greenleaf JE, Wade CE, Leftheriotis G. Orthostatic responses following 30-day bed rest deconditioning with isotonic and isokinetic exercise training. *Aviat Space Environ Med* 1989;60:537–542.

137. Melada GA, Goldman RH, Luetscher JA, et al. Hemodynamics, renal function, plasma renin and aldosterone in man after 5 to 14 days of bed rest. *Aviat Space Environ Med* 1975;46:1049–1055.

138. Kamiya A, Iwase S, Sugiyama Y, et al. Vasomotor sympathetic nerve activity in men during bed rest on orthostasis after bed rest. *Aviat Space Environ Med* 2000;71(2):142–149.

139. Stremel RW, Convetino VA, Bernauer EM, Greenleaf JE. Cardiorespiratory deconditioning with static and dynamic leg exercise during bed rest. *J Appl Physiol* 1976;41:905–909.
140. Robinson BF, Ebstein SE, Beiser GD, et al. Control of heart rate by automatic system: studies in man on the interrelation between baroreceptor mechanism and exercises. *Circ Res* 1966;19:400–411.
141. Fareeduddin K, Abelmann WH. Impaired orthostatic tolerance after bed rest in patients with myocardial infarction. *N Engl J Med* 1969;280:345–350.
142. Vallbona C, Spencer WA, Cardus D, Dale JW. Control of orthostatic hypotension in quadriplegic patients with the use of a pressure suit. *Arch Phys Med Rehabil* 1963;44:7–18.
143. Vogt FB. Effect of intermittent leg cuff inflation and intermittent exercise on the tilt table response after ten days' bed recumbency. *Aerospace Medicine* 1966;37:943–947.
144. Haruna Y, Takenaka K, Suzuki Y, et al. Effect of acute saline infusion on the cardiovascular deconditioning after 20-days head down tilt bed rest. *Journal of Gravitational Physiology* 1998;(1):P45–46.
145. Gibbs NM. Venous thrombosis of the lower limbs with particular reference to bed rest. *Br J Surg* 1957;191:209–235.
146. Kudsk KA, Fabian TC, Baum S, et al. Silent deep vein thrombosis in immobilized multiple trauma patients. *Am J Surg* 1989;158:515–519.
147. Warlow C, Ogston D, Douglas AS. Deep venous thrombosis of the legs after strokes: Part I. incidence and predisposing factors. Part II. natural history. *Br Med J* 1976;1:1178–1183.
148. Miyamoto AT, Miller LS. Pulmonary embolism in stroke: prevention by early heparinization of venous thrombosis detected by iodine-125 fibrinogen leg scans. *Arch Phys Med Rehabil* 1980;61:584–587.
149. Malone PC, Hamer JD, Silver IA. Oxygen tension in venous valve pockets. *Thromb Haemost* 1979;42:230.
150. Hume M, Sevitt S, Thomas LP. *Venous thrombosis and pulmonary embolism.* Cambridge, MA: Harvard University Press, 1977.
151. Pini M, Pattacini C, Quintaralla R, et al. Subcutaneous vs. intravenous heparin in the treatment of deep venous thrombosis: a randomized clinical trial. *Thromb Haemost* 1990;64:222–226.
152. Nance PW, ed. *Rehabilitation pharmacotherapy: physical medicine and rehabilitation clinics of North America.* Philadelphia: WB Saunders, 1999.
153. Hirsh I. Heparin. *N Engl J Med* 1991;324:1565–1574.
154. Hull RD, Raskob GE, Rosenbloom D, et al. Heparin for 5 days as compared with 10 days in the initial treatment of proximal venous thrombosis. *N Engl J Med* 1990;322:1260–1264.
155. Blattler W. Ambulatory care for ambulant patients with deep vein thrombosis. *J Mal Vasc* 1991;16(2):137–141.
156. Anderson RL, Lefever FR, Francis WR, et al. Urinary and bladder responses to immobilization in male rats. *Food Chem Toxicol* 1990;28:543–545.
157. Leadbetter WF, Engster HE. Problems of renal lithiasis in convalescent patients. *J Urol* 1957;53:269.
158. Dooley CP, Schlossmacher B, Valenzuela JE. Modulation of esophageal peristalsis by alterations of body position: effect of bolus viscosity. *Dig Dis Sci* 1989;34:1662–1667.
159. More JG, Datz FL, Christin PE, et al. Effect of body posture on radionuclide measurements of gastric emptying. *Dig Dis Sci* 1988;33:1592–1595.
160. LeBlank A, Schneider V, Spector E, et al. Calcium absorption, endogenous excretion, and endocrine changes during and after long-term bed rest. *Bone* 1995;16(4):330IS–3304S.

161. Evans DF, Foster GE, Harcastle JD. Does exercise affect small bowel motility in man? *Gut* 1989;10–12.
162. Moses FM. The effect of exercise on gastrointestinal tract. *Sports Med* 1990;9:159–172.
163. Zorbas YG, Merkov AB, Nobahar AN. Nutritional status of men under hypokinesia. *J Environ Pathol Toxicol Oncol* 1989;9:333–342.
164. Krebs JM, Schneider VS, Evans H, et al. Energy absorption, lean body mass, and total body fat changes during 5 weeks of continuous bed rest. *Aviat Space Environ Med* 1990;61:314–318.
165. Stuart CA, Shangraw RE, Prince MJ, et al. Bed rest-induced insulin resistance occurs primarily in muscle. *Metabolism* 1988;37:802–806.
166. Lipman RL, Schnure Jl, Bradley EM, Lecocq FR. Impairment of peripheral glucose utilization in normal subjects by prolonged bed rest. *J Lab Clin Med* 1970;76:221–230.
167. Dolkas CB, Greenleaf JE. Insulin and glucose responses during bed rest with isotonic and isometric exercise. *J Appl Physiol* 1977;43:1033–1038.
168. Mikines KJ, Dela F, Tronier B, Galbo H. Effect of 7 days of bed rest on dose-response relation between plasma glucose and insulin secretion. *Am J Physiol* 1989;257:43–48.
169. Seider MJ, Nicholson WF, Booth FW. Insulin resistance for glucose metabolism in disused skeletal muscle of mice. *Am J Physiol* 1982;242:E12–18.
170. Lerman S, Canterbury JM, Reiss E. Parathyroid hormone and the hypercalcemia of immobilization. *J Clin Endocrinol Metab* 1977;45:425–488.
171. Balsam A, Leppo LE. Assessment of the degradation of thyroid hormones in man during bed rest. *J Appl Physiol* 1975;38:216–219.
172. Cockett AT, Elbadawi A, Zemjanis R. The effects of immobilization on spermatogenesis in subhuman primates. *Fertil Steril* 1970;21:610–614.
173. Varnikos-Danellis J, Winget CM, Leach CS. *Circadian endocrine and metabolic effects of prolonged bed rest: two 56-day bed rest studies.* NASA Technical Bulletin, No. Tm V-3051. Washington, D.C.: United States National Aeronautic and Space Administration, 1974.
174. Takayama H, Tomiyama M, Managawa A, et al. The effect of physical exercise and prolonged bed rest on carbohydrate, lipid and amino acid metabolism. *Japanese Journal of Clinical Pathology* 1974;22[Suppl]:126–136.
175. Banks R, Cappon D. Effects of reduced sensory input on time perception. *Percept Mot Skills* 1962;14:74.
176. Ryback RS, Lewis OF, Lessard CS. Psychobiologic effects of prolonged bed rest (weightlessness) in young healthy volunteers (study 11). *Aerospace Medicine* 1971;42:529–535.
177. Downs FS. Bed rest and sensory disturbances. *Am J Nurs* 1974;74:434–438.
178. Smith MJ. Changes in judgment of duration with different patterns of auditory information for individuals confined to bed. *Nurs Res* 1975;24:93–98.
179. Haines RF. Effect of bed rest and exercise on body balance. *J Appl Physiol* 1974;36:323–327.
180. Trimble RW, Lessard CS. *Performance decrement as a function of seven days of bed rest.* USAF School of Aerospace Medicine Technical Report 70–56. Alexandria, VA: Aerospace Medical Association, 1970.
181. Yaffe K, Barnes D, Nevitt M, et al. A prospective study of physical activity and cognitive decline in elderly women. *Arch Intern Med* 2001;161:1703–1708.
182. Deitrick JE, Whedon GD, Shorr E. Effect of immobilization upon various metabolic and physiologic functions of normal men. *Am J Med* 1948;4:3–32.

CHAPTER 69

Primary Care for Persons with Disability

William L. Bockenek, Gerben DeJong, Indira S. Lanig,
Michael Friedland, and Nancy Mann

The issue of providing quality medical care to all persons has been brought to the forefront with the current changes in medicine and health-care reform. Terms such as "cost containment," "appropriate utilization of resources," and "quality management" are heard by practicing physicians on a daily basis concerning their patient-care interactions. The impetus to make changes in our current health-care system has also been influenced by economic issues (1). Health-care costs have increased exponentially in recent years, and even though these costs have risen significantly, patients' health outcome and satisfaction have not risen proportionately. When the United States was compared with numerous other countries with respect to health outcomes and satisfaction in relation to cost, the United States ranked lowest of the nations studied, compared with countries such as The Netherlands, which is among the best (1). When the same countries were compared with respect to their percentage of primary care physicians, the results were similar, with the United States having the smallest percentage of primary care physicians and the countries with greatest satisfaction having the greatest percentage of primary care physicians. When the cost factor is eliminated, however, health-care quality in the United States is among the finest in the world. Unfortunately, it is not accessible and available to all. Because of lack of income, lack of insurance, isolation, language, culture, or physical disability, millions still face barriers to quality health care. The Health Resources and Services Administration's number-one goal is the expansion of quality health care for all Americans. The 2002 budget for this organization approximates 6.2 billion dollars, some of which is allotted to those with disabilities. The Bureau of Primary Health Care within the Health Resources Service Administration is allotted 1.48 billion dollars for 2002 (2).

Although there is great consensus in the United States and abroad that primary care is a critical component of any health-care system, there is considerable imbalance between primary and specialty care in the United States (3). The proportion of specialists in the United States is more than 70% of all patient-care physicians, whereas in other industrialized countries, 25% to 50% of physicians are specialists (3). Furthermore, fewer than one-fourth of recent medical school graduates are choosing to enter primary-care specialties (4).

Further work has shown that based on staffing patterns in classic health maintenance organizations (HMOs), there are about 3.1 times more pathologists, 2.5 times more neurosurgeons, 2.4 times more general surgeons, 2.0 times more cardiologists and neurologists, 1.9 times more gastroenterologists, 1.8 times more ophthalmologists, and 1.5 times more radiologists in the nation than would be needed (3). Although it is clear that there is a plethora of specialists and a need for greater primary-care services, considerable room for debate remains on its true impact on health-care costs and quality of patient care.

Beginning in the late 1980s and continuing to the present, recognition of the difficulties that persons with disabilities face in accessing quality health care has become apparent. Persons with disabilities represent approximately 10% of the world's population, yet they are among the most underserved groups (5). Although the medical literature is relatively sparse on this issue, multiple conferences and publications have addressed this topic. The Association of Academic Physiatrists and the American Academy of Physical Medicine and Rehabilitation have both developed position statements on the provision of primary-care services to persons with disabilities, lending their support to physiatrists who choose to provide these services, however, there is a variety of opinions among practitioners as to how these services are best provided (6,7).

This chapter provides an overview of the primary-care issue, with special emphasis on persons with disabilities, as well as a discussion of issues on health promotion in this population. A practical approach to primary medical care in a general population that can easily be adapted to persons with disabilities follows. The chapter concludes with a review of several models of primary care and describes management issues more specific to those with disabilities.

DEFINITIONS OF PRIMARY CARE

The Health Resources and Services Administration has defined primary care based on the following three anchoring principles: (a) the routine medical care and services people receive on first contact with the health-care system for a particular health incident, i.e., prevention, maintenance, diagnosis, limited treatment, management of chronic problems, and referral; (b) assumption of longitudinal responsibility for the patient regardless of the presence or absence of disease (i.e., all of a person's health-care needs—physical, psychological, and social—are met); and (c) integration of other health resources when necessary (gatekeeper function) (8).

The Institute of Medicine (9) has provided a definition as well, which states that primary care is the provision of integrated, accessible health-care services by clinicians who are accountable for addressing a large majority of personal health-care needs, developing a sustained partnership with patients, and practicing in the context of family and community. "Integration" includes comprehensive, coordinated and continuous services. "Accessibility" refers to eliminating geographical, financial, and cultural barriers to seeing the caregiver. "Health-care services" includes hospitals, nursing homes, office, school, home, and intermediate care facilities. "Clinicians" can be physicians, nurse practitioners, physician assistants, or similar health-care practitioners. "Accountable" refers to the clinician being responsible for quality of care, patient satisfaction, efficient use of resources, and ethical behavior. "Majority of personal health-care needs" describes the full spectrum of physical, mental, emotional, and social concerns. "Sustained partnership" is a long-term relationship that includes health promotion, disease prevention, and the management of disease itself. "Context of family and community" includes an understanding of the patient's social background and support systems.

Another approach at defining primary care is from the patients perspective (10). A primary-care physician is a trusted physician who (a) performs all preventive care necessary to safeguard health; (b) diagnoses and treats self-limiting conditions; (c) diagnoses serious conditions and either treats those for which he or she has expertise or refers the patient to the best available expert for treatment. A strength of this functional patient-oriented definition is that it delineates the three tiers of health care provided by all primary-care physicians.

Primary care may be distinguished from specialty care by the time, focus, and scope of services provided to the patients (3). Primary care as noted above is first-contact care on entry into the health-care system. Specialty care generally follows primary care upon referral from the primary-care provider. Whereas primary care addresses the person as a whole, specialty care usually focuses on specific diseases or organ systems. Because primary-care providers see patients at their initial interface with the health-care system, they are presented with a variety of symptoms and concerns that may represent early stages of disease that are not yet easily classified into specific diseases or organ systems. Through the various roles of the primary-care provider, but especially the gatekeeper function, referral to specialty care occurs when organ- or diagnostic-specific disease is identified that is beyond the scope of services provided by the primary-care provider. Although primary care is comprehensive in scope and is present throughout the continuum of care, specialty care tends to be limited to specific illness episodes, the organ system involved, or the disease process identified.

PRIMARY CARE ISSUES IN GRADUATE MEDICAL EDUCATION

Three specialties typically are thought of as primary-care fields. The largest is general internal medicine, followed by general pediatrics and family practice. Obstetrics and gynecology, although regarded by the American College of Obstetrics and Gynecology and the American Medical Association as a primary-care provider for women, does not traditionally fulfill this role because it does not meet the "whole body" medicine criterion often cited as the standard for judging whether a specialty offers primary care (11). Nevertheless, it is clear that many women consider their gynecologist to be their primary care provider (12).

In its third report (13), the Council on Graduate Medical Education (COGME) stated that generalist physicians are trained, practice, and receive continuing education in a broad set of competencies to care for the entire population in office, hospital, and residential settings; provide comprehensive age- and sex-specific preventive care; evaluate and diagnose common symptoms; treat common acute conditions; provide ongoing care for chronic illnesses and behavior problems; and seek appropriate consultation for other needed specialized services. Given these required competencies, COGME concluded that family physicians, general internists, and general pediatricians are properly trained to function as generalist physicians. Although other physicians provide elements of primary care, COGME also noted that physicians who are broadly educated as generalist physicians provide more comprehensive and cost-effective care than do other specialists and subspecialists (14).

The recent emphasis on health-care system reform has sparked the decades-old debate as to whom is a generalist physician and has reemerged with important implications for physician work-force policy and medical education (14). In its third report (13), COGME recommended that the nation set a goal that at least 50% of all physicians be practicing generalist physicians. The Association of American Medical Colleges recommended that a majority of graduating medical students be committed to generalist careers (15). Both COGME and the Association of American Medical Colleges define generalist physicians as residents who complete a 3-year training program in either family medicine, internal medicine, or pediatrics and who do not subspecialize. Given the enhanced role and growing prestige of the generalist physician and the increased emphasis on primary care, other physician groups, including physical medicine and rehabilitation (PM&R) have suggested that they be included in this category (6,14). In its fourth report (16), COGME stated that the designation of a specialty being included as primary care should be based on an objective analysis of training requirements in disciplines that provide graduates with broad capabilities for primary-care practice. In an analysis of the training requirements of numerous specialties, including those typically thought of as primary-care specialties (family practice, internal medicine, pediatrics) and several that have proposed inclusion as a primary-care specialty (emergency medicine and obstetrics and gynecology), only the previously established primary-care fields actually prepared their residents in the broad competencies required for primary-care practice (14). Although PM&R was not included in the analysis, based on the current training requirements and a similar analysis, it would not fulfill the necessary training needs.

The ability to provide effective primary care or appropriate treatment for life-threatening illnesses not only depends on adequate training but a continued interest in the area of concern, as well as continued experience based on an appropriate number of cases (10). A recent emphasis in organized medicine for physician competency and maintenance of certification beyond initial board certification sheds additional light on the requirements to maintain expertise in primary-care activities. It is not enough to be adequately trained during residency in specific aspects of primary care or the treatment of a serious disease or high-risk procedure because this training quickly becomes outdated in the face of the rapid advances in clinical medicine. The individual choosing to be a primary-care provider needs to remain current in the management of any condition that is diagnosed and is needing treatment (10).

In its eighth report (17), COGME evaluated five models that attempted to determine projections for the number of physicians needed for the current century. The differences in the five models lie in the degree to which historic increases in the demand for specialists are assumed to continue in the increasingly competitive managed-care setting. COGME hypothesized that market forces will at least balance increasing demand for specialty services resulting from new technology. Consequently, increasing demand for specialists were not as anticipated. The ultimate requirement for generalists and specialists will depend on the configuration of future health-care systems. COGME anticipated increased utilization of nurse practitioners and physician assistants, both in specialty care and in primary care. The overall trend, however, was felt to be an increased emphasis on generalists within managed systems of care, thus reducing the demand for specialists.

GENERALIST VERSUS SPECIALIST

Although it is well accepted that there is an imbalance between primary and specialty care, numerous arguments have been advanced by advocates of both the generalist and specialist perspectives (3,13,18). The generalist perspective points to the research that supports the efficacy of primary care and indicates that generalists have broader medical knowledge and skills; are better trained in psychosocial, preventive, and community aspects of care; and provide less costly care and are more accessible, factors that make them preferable to specialists as primary-care providers (18). In addition, the generalists' cross-disciplinary skills provide for more efficient referral patterns when using their gatekeeper function.

Specialists, on the other hand, assert that their training before subspecialization is equivalent to generalists, allowing them to deal with primary-care issues (similar to generalists) as well as manage problems within their specialty (that generalists might have to refer elsewhere) (18). Numerous studies support the specialist viewpoint that primary care can be provided in an efficient and cost-effective manner by the same practitioner who provides more sophisticated, specialized, and up-to-date medical services (18).

MEETING THE POSTREHABILITATION HEALTH-CARE NEEDS OF PEOPLE WITH DISABILITIES

The traditional distinctions between primary care and specialty care become much less clear when we consider the ongoing postrehabilitative health-care needs of people with disabilities (11). Here the boundaries between primary and specialty care overlap considerably. It is not clear where one ends and the other begins. The handoff from rehabilitative care in the rehabilitation center to primary care in the community is not straightforward. This is best understood when we consider the nature of the ongoing health-care needs of people with disabilities and why many primary-care issues have significant rehabilitative or functional content.

It is difficult to generalize about the ongoing health-care needs of people with disabilities, in part because different disabling conditions have widely varying pathophysiologies, comorbidities, and functional consequences. These differences often obscure the fact that people with disabilities experience most of the same health conditions experienced by people without disabilities. However, people with disabilities are at greater risk for certain common health conditions than are those in the general population, often experience these conditions differently, and may require a somewhat different and extended therapeutic regimen that takes into account both their underlying impairment and their functional limitations. However, people with disabilities observe that many health-care providers are often unable to look beyond the disabling condition to address the health problem that precipitated the provider-patient encounter in the first place.

SIX CHARACTERIZATIONS

There are many ways one can characterize the ongoing health-care needs of people with disabilities relative to those without disabilities. At the risk of overgeneralization, we note six ways in which the ongoing health-care needs of people with disabilities are different from those in the general population. These characterizations are limited mainly to people with the types of conditions commonly seen in inpatient rehabilitation settings (19,20).

First, people with disabilities generally have a thinner margin of health that must be carefully guarded if medical problems are to be averted (21). This observation applies to health conditions that people with disabilities share with the nondisabled population (e.g., upper respiratory infection, pneumonia), as well as to conditions more likely to appear among people with disabling conditions (e.g., urinary tract infections, renal failure, pressure sores). It should be emphasized that people with disabilities are not "sick" and that most are generally very healthy. However, their impairments and functional limitations often render them more vulnerable to certain health problems.

Second, people with disabilities often do not have the same opportunities for health maintenance and preventive health as those without disabilities. For example, people with mobility limitations usually have fewer opportunities to participate in aerobic activity needed for good cardiovascular health, and people with paralysis may not be able to detect certain health conditions early because they cannot experience pain in certain body regions (21).

Third, people with disabilities who acquired their impairment early in life may experience onset of chronic health conditions earlier than people in the general population. For example, it is believed that people with long-standing mobility limitations are likely to have an earlier onset of coronary artery disease than the general population. Likewise, people with mobility limitations may experience an earlier onset of adult diabetes because of obesity and may experience an earlier onset of renal disease (e.g., pyelonephritis) because of a neurogenic bladder dysfunction (22).

Fourth, people with disabilities who acquire a new health condition, apart from their original impairment, are likely to experience secondary functional losses. Thus the functional consequences of a new chronic health condition are usually more significant for a person who already has a disabling impairment. The onset of exertional angina, for example, may require that the person upgrade from a manual to an electric wheelchair and from a conventional automobile to an adapted van.

Fifth, people with disabilities may require more complicated and prolonged treatment for a given health problem than do people without disabilities. For example, using a plaster cast for a broken leg may be complicated by the individual's vulnerability to a pressure sore when the individual has no sensation in the lower limbs. Likewise, a person with a disability may require a longer recovery period after an acute episode of illness or injury because of preexisting functional limitations that limit a person's participation in various therapies (e.g., using a treadmill or exercise bicycle after an acute myocardial infarct).

And sixth, people with disabilities may need durable medical equipment and other assistive technologies that require some level of functional assessment. Today these devices are often prescribed by physicians who have only a rudimentary understanding about the fit between various types of equipment and the needs of the individual consumer. A poor fit between the individual and an assistive device can reduce functional capacity and may induce the individual to abandon the device, the combination of which is wasteful for both the individual and for society.

These six characterizations are not exhaustive. A more complete characterization will be important in sorting out the respective roles of traditional primary-care disciplines and the various specialty disciplines in managing the health-care needs of people with disabilities. The six characterizations point out that traditional distinctions lose their meaning when managing the health-care needs of a person with a disabling or chronic health condition.

IMPACT ON HEALTH-CARE UTILIZATION AND EXPENDITURES

These six characterizations are borne out in the higher-than-average rates of health-care utilization and expenditures among people with disabilities. The 1996 Medical Expenditure Panel Survey provides a broad overview of the health-care utilization and expenditure experience of adults with selected functional limitations. Using variables available in the Medical Expenditure Panel Survey, a person is defined as having a disability if they meet any one of the following criteria: (a) use mobility aids or equipment; (b) have difficulty bending, lifting, or stooping; (c) are limited in major activity; or (d) require help or supervision with at least one activity of daily living or instrumental activity of daily living (23).

Using this definition of disability, individuals with disabilities comprise approximately 16% of the adult population (age 18 and older). Yet in 1996, they accounted for about 34% of all physician visits made by adults, 41% of all adult prescriptions (including refills), nearly half of all hospital discharges, 62% of all nights spent in the hospital by adults, and 46% of all adult-related healthcare expenditures (Fig. 69-1).

The disproportions reported above are also reflected in estimates of the utilization and expenditure experience of individ-

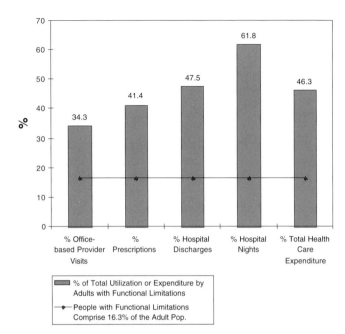

Figure 69-1. Percent of total health-care utilization and expenditures by adults with a functional limitation. United States, 1996. (From NRH Center for Health and Disability Research 1996 Medical Expenditure Panel Survey, with permission.)

ual adults with disabilities. Although only 3% of adults with disabilities had zero health-care expenditures in 1996, 16% of individuals without disabilities had zero health-care expenditures. Of those with at least a $1 expenditure, the median expenditure for people with disabilities was $2,489, compared with $420 for people without disabilities. According to these median figures, adults with disabilities typically pay more out of their own pocket ($427) for health care than the no-disabled expenditure paid from all sources ($420). The median out-of-pocket expenditure for adults without limitations was $1441 (Fig. 69-2). (Median total and out-of-pocket expenditures are calculated only for those who had at least a $1 total, or $1 out-of-pocket expenditure, respectively. Out-of-pocket expenditures do not include health plan premiums.)

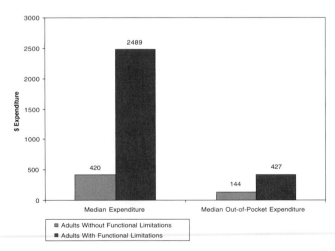

Figure 69-2. Median total and out-of-pocket expenditures for adults by functional limitation, United States, 1996. (From NRH Center for Health and Disability Research 1996 Medical Expenditure Panel Survey, with permission.)

ACCESS TO PRIMARY CARE

Many of the secondary health conditions experienced by people with disabilities are entirely preventable through scrupulous health maintenance strategies and timely interventions by knowledgeable practitioners before new health conditions become emergent or even life-threatening (23–25). People with disabilities often express frustration about their access to primary-care providers who are knowledgeable about the management of secondary health conditions and the impact of these new health conditions on their functional capacities (21,26,27). People with disabilities often remark that they must spend considerable effort educating their primary-care providers about their disability and how it needs to be taken into consideration when new health conditions are addressed (28, 29).

In a survey of 607 respondents with disabilities (e.g., spinal cord injury, multiple sclerosis, cerebral palsy, postpolio syndrome) in the Washington, D.C., area, it was found that many people had difficulty finding a physician who was knowledgeable about their health-care needs (28). Respondents who had a previous rehabilitation experience often indicated that they consulted with their original physiatrist when they were not confident about a therapy recommended by their primary-care physician. Respondents also reported that many physician offices were not fully accessible, as in the case of examining tables that failed to accommodate the transfer requirements of wheelchair users.

In subsequent interviews with primary-care providers in the Washington, D.C., area, it was also found that many preferred to serve only a very limited number of people with disabilities because people with disabilities often took longer to process in the course of an ordinary office visit and slowed down a busy office practice (30). With rapid growth of capitation-based managed care since then, primary-care physicians have even less incentive to serve high-use populations, such as people with disabilities.

These findings are as current today as they were more than a decade ago when this line of research was first initiated. One of the major themes to emerge from several studies conducted in the late 1990s at the National Rehabilitation Hospital in Washington, D.C., is the lack of what researchers call "disability literacy" and "disability competence" on the part of both health plans and providers (31–33). The lack of "disability literacy" and "competence" occurs despite the fact that health plans and providers have considerable contact with individuals with disabilities because of their disproportionate utilization of health-care.

The rise of managed care in the 1990s is commonly thought to be adverse to individuals with disabilities. Researchers report that managed care has made access to downstream services, such as rehabilitation and assistive technology, more difficult than under traditional fee-for-service plans. Yet, they also report that individuals participating in managed health-care plans had a more regular source of primary care than those in fee-for-service plans but also had somewhat less choice as to whom their primary-care provider would be (34,35).

MULTIDIMENSIONAL CHARACTER OF THE ISSUES

This brief review illustrates how the boundary issues between primary and specialty care in the case of people with disabilities need to be addressed at several different levels. First, there is the issue of the functional and rehabilitative implications inherent in many primary-care encounters. Second, there is the issue of knowledge base and whether traditional primary-care providers are adequately equipped to address the needs of people with disabilities. Third, there is the issue of whether primary-care providers have the facilities to accommodate people with disabilities. And fourth, there is the issue of whether our systems of health-care financing discourage providers, primary care or otherwise, from addressing the primary health-care needs of people with disabilities.

PHYSICAL MEDICINE AND REHABILITATION AS A PRIMARY-CARE SPECIALTY

With these issues in mind, the notion of PM&R as a primary-care specialty can now be brought into focus. PM&R is the medical specialty that deals with the needs of severely disabled persons. Primary-care physicians often refer these patients after a catastrophic illness. When these patients require comprehensive inpatient rehabilitation, the physiatrist usually serves as their primary caregiver during their relatively short hospital stay but subsequently sends the patient back to the referring physician for follow-up general medical care. Follow-up visits at the physiatrist's office typically deal with rehabilitation issues (11).

In contrast, patients with spinal cord and brain injuries often present from referring specialists, i.e., neurosurgeons and orthopedic surgeons, with no regular primary-care physician. After hospitalization, their follow-up care and health maintenance to prevent rehospitalization become major issues. Physicians in spinal cord and brain injury centers often choose to become the primary-care physicians for these patients. Because of the specialized and often complex medical needs of the person with severe disability, primary-care physicians in the community often welcome the physiatrist's involvement and encourage their assistance in providing for the primary-care needs of their mutual patients (11).

Primary-care services are often requested, by those persons with severe disability, to be performed at the rehabilitation facility. In a survey (36) of 144 outpatients with spinal cord injury, it was found that 48% considered their rehabilitation physician as their primary-care physician. Fifty-one percent of persons also requested that all of their general medical care be provided by the physicians at the rehabilitation facility. The primary reasons for these requests included maintaining continuity of care with the physician who the patients felt best understood their specialized needs, as well as easier integration with the rehabilitation hospital for other ancillary health needs (e.g., seating clinic, physical and occupational therapy).

Although it appears that many patients would like their primary-care needs met by the physiatrists, there is not a clear consensus of whether this is a practical approach to the issue of providing this care. The problems described in developing PM&R as a primary-care specialty were outlined partially earlier in this chapter. Additional considerations include manpower or work-force issues, the preferences professed by current practitioners in the field as well as those in training, and concerns dealing with PM&R residency curricula and the ability to provide adequate training in primary-care issues based on our present residency requirements.

As previously noted, it is widely believed that there is a shortage of generalists. There are several ways to reach the goals previously set forth by COGME (13,17) and the Association of American Medical Colleges (15). They include having more medical school graduates enter primary-care fields, reducing the number of specialty residency positions, and encouraging current practitioners in subspecialties to broaden the scope of their practice to include a more primary-care role (38). An additional option is to change the current curriculum of some of our residency programs to include more training in primary-care issues.

Even with the proposed paucity of generalist physicians, it was widely held in the 1990s that there would be an oversupply of physicians by the year 2000. In fact, in COGME's fourth report (16) and eighth report (17), it was proposed that the number of federally funded entry-level positions in graduate medical education be restricted to 110% of the number in medical school in 1993 and that 50% of the graduates should be generalist physicians. Since that time, others have made alternative suggestions, including expanding the enrollment of U.S. medical schools to fulfill the shortfall between the supply of graduates of U.S. medical schools and entry-level positions in graduate medical education (39). More recently, a new model for work-force projections has been proposed, with the emphasis now on a future serious shortage of physicians, especially specialists (40). This model emphasizes the U.S. population growth, economic expansion, the decreasing work effort of physicians, and the services provided by nonphysician clinicians (i.e., nurse practitioners and physician assistants), which has been increasing. Paradoxically, most of this growth will be concentrated in primary care; at this juncture, the thought is that we have shown more recent relative stability. A greater demand for physician services is in the non–primary-care specialties, to which the nonphysician clinicians contribute less. This model, however, has not been without controversy (41). Critics of the model argue that too great an emphasis is made on the need for specialty care (secondary to higher cost without higher quality). It is also argued that individual physician productivity remains high and that the work effort remains stable. There is also disbelief that the U.S. spending in health care will continue to grow unabated over the next 20 years (as noted in this model). Finally, it is accepted that nonphysician clinicians can help to extend and support specialty care as well as assist in providing generalist care.

In the late 1990s, a work-force study was performed to determine the current and future manpower needs for the PM&R practitioner (42). The model was based on the assumption that current residency capacity as well as utilization of physiatry skills remains constant at its 1994–1995 level. The results were that the demand for physiatrists will continue to exceed supply, on average, through the year 2000. Excess supply has emerged and will continue to emerge in selected geographic areas in the future. In order to maintain a level of demand, it was recommended that the field should emphasize the role of physiatrists in providing efficacious and cost-effective health care. An additional option would be to further broaden the scope of practice to include primary-care services. An increasing trend of current graduates of PM&R residencies to enter musculoskeletal outpatient practices has also expanded this demand but not in the area of primary care. There is an ongoing effort to reassess the current and future PM&R work-force needs to help us to address our role in the provision of primary-care services.

Unfortunately, there are several issues that will likely dampen the success of this effort. The above work-force projection is based on the premise that managed care will continue to grow at a moderate level. PM&R is not typically designated as a primary-care provider in our current HMO and managed-care systems. In addition, even if PM&R were designated as a primary-care provider for persons with severe disability, it is unlikely that this would have a significant impact on the shortage of generalists. The total percentage of currently practicing physiatrists as compared with the total number of U.S. physicians is less than 1% (11). Based on our current training capacity, it is doubtful that there will ever be the number of physiatrists necessary to provide direct primary care for the large majority of persons with disability (11).

Some of the above assumptions are based on the premise that current practitioners and those in training in PM&R are willing to provide primary-care services. A recent survey (38) of 106 PM&R physicians (55 physiatrists and 51 PM&R residents) showed that only 39% agreed that PM&R should be designated as a primary-care specialty. The majority also felt that these services should be restricted to those with severe disability (e.g., spinal cord and brain injury). Overall, 53% felt that physiatrists are competent in providing general medical care, but only 38% were convinced that the current 4-year PM&R residency sufficiently prepares physiatrists to assume the role of a primary-care provider.

Current PM&R training and residency curricula do not place a great focus on several areas that are essential to providing primary-care services. These include health promotion and education, as well as preventive services (11). Significant changes would need to occur in our current residency requirements to provide the above training. This would likely require extension of our current 4-year training requirement, as well as substantial adjustments to our current residency experiences. A series of recommendations (43) for changes in the current PM&R residency curriculum were proposed to assist PM&R residency programs in providing for education in the provision of primary care. These include applying general preventive care principles and interventions to those with disabilities, expanding the role of "continuity clinics," publishing a "study guide" on the topic of primary care for the disabled similar to the study guides currently published by the American Academy of Physical Medicine and Rehabilitation, and providing continuing education on common medical problems seen in the disabled and nondisabled population. Additional consideration was given to developing special or added qualifications in primary care for the disabled or expanding the availability of double board certification (current primarycare–oriented combined programs involve internal medicine and pediatrics) to include family practice. Proposals such as these would require significant changes in our current training programs that may ultimately result in a negative impact on the continued growth and attractiveness of our field (11). Changes such as increasing the length of residency training and altering "quality of life issues" for residents and practicing physiatrists (the three "Ls" of primary care: low pay, long hours, low prestige) may be viewed as adverse by prospective PM&R residents (11). In fact, this may ultimately lead to further limitation of the accessibility of care to those persons with severe disabilities. Since the publication of the above recommendations, the issue of primary care within PM&R has become less prominent. A primary-care special interest group has been developed within the American Academy of Physical Medicine and Rehabilitation, but there has been little published within our PM&R literature on this topic. There have been no changes or additions in ACGME PM&R residency requirements relating to the primary-care issue, and no additional qualifications have been developed by the American Board of Physical Medicine and Rehabilitation.

Other potential options to ensure provision of primary-care services to those with severe disabilities include collaboration with other medical specialties as well as allied health providers. Several models have been developed that include close working relationships of physiatrists with internal medicine specialists, as well as physician extenders, such as nurse practitioners (27). The nature of this collaboration can be achieved in numerous ways; however, at a minimum, it should include physiatric education of the other primary-care providers and team ventures with them to provide primary care for this population (11). A more detailed description of these types of collaborations is provided later in this chapter.

HEALTH PROMOTION IN PERSONS WITH DISABILITIES

The overall life course health profile of an individual with a disabling condition is the result of interaction among disability management strategies, general health-care practices, biological and socioenvironmental factors, and lifestyle behaviors. Therefore, when physiatrists address the longitudinal health-care needs of those with chronic disabilities, they must view disability-related health management and general health-promoting strategies as equally important components of care. In order to do this, they must enhance their frames of reference and incorporate the concepts of health promotion and secondary condition risk reduction.

Health Promotion and Related Models

Health promotion has several features that overlap with both primary care and medical rehabilitation. Most notable, all three emphasize education and encouragement of self-responsibility, and all address the potential or actual impact of a given physical or cognitive/emotional condition across several dimensions of health. Finally, all address both health maintenance and disease prevention so as to enhance and protect functional capacity over the life span.

As a general concept, health promotion describes all efforts directed toward helping individuals modify their lifestyles and behavior so as to promote a state of optimal health. Health promotion per se is not disease or health problem specific. However, the most important health-promoting behaviors recommended are proper nutrition, weight control, smoking cessation, stress management, physical fitness, elimination of any drug or alcohol misuse, disease and injury prevention, development of social support, and maintenance of a regularly scheduled health surveillance plan to monitor health status (44). The U.S. Department of Health and Human Services' initiative Healthy People 2010 added responsible sexual behavior, environmental quality, immunization, and access to health care to the core list of national health promotion and disease prevention health indicators for the first 10 years of the twenty-first century (45). These behaviors all emphasize enhancement of health status in the absence of a specific health threat. Additionally, Healthy People 2010 includes specific objectives related to the health and well-being of people with disabilities. These goals include reducing the number of people with disabilities who report feelings of sadness, unhappiness, or depression that prevent them from being more active, and increasing the percentage of adults with disabilities who participate in community and social activities.

It is, therefore, clear that although early-twentieth-century definitions of optimal health emphasized freedom from disease and issues related to hygiene, contemporary definitions of health typically reflect its complex multidimensional nature, incorporating themes related to disease, environment, capacity or potential, and effective coping (46). Indeed, the Department of Health and Human Services defined optimal health as having a "full range of functional capacity at each life stage, allowing one the ability to enter into satisfying relationships with others, to work, and to play" (45).

These multidimensional definitions of health continue to find parallels in the revised International Classification of Impairments, Disabilities, and Handicap model of disablement [The International Classification of Functioning, Disability and Health (ICF), referred to as ICIDH-2] (47) and its variations (48–51). These models of the disablement process attempt to describe the "health impact" or disease or injury in three principle domains of the human experience. Specifically, attention is directed to the impact on the organ level (impairment), the impact on the performance of routine tasks, skills, and human behaviors (activity), and the impact on social role performance, community integration, and opportunity (participation and context) (47,49). Several models (48,49) have attempted to incorporate biological, environmental, lifestyle, and behavioral influences on the disabling process and the interaction with quality of life/perceptions of personal well-being. In addition, various investigators (52,53) have proposed that a more complete accounting of the health impact of a given injury or disease also requires inclusion of a fourth domain: subjective well-being, reflecting an individual's own assessment of health, life satisfaction, and other life experiences rather than the objective nature of these experiences. The merging of contemporary definitions of health, the physiatry-oriented models of disablement, and the disabled individual's own perceptions of well-being can provide a conceptual framework on which specific health-promoting and secondary condition risk reduction strategies can be formulated within the context of chronic disability.

Health Protection and Secondary Risk Reduction

Intimately related to health promotion is health protection. Health-protecting behaviors, although overlapping to some degree with health-promoting behaviors, emphasize preventive measures that guard or defend an individual against specific injuries or illnesses (54). Public health interventions designed to protect health have traditionally been conceptualized as primary, secondary, and tertiary preventive measures. Primary prevention refers to those activities undertaken to reduce the circumstances that would result in the subsequent development of a disease process or illness (e.g., addressing risk factors). Attention can be directed to the host (e.g., immunization, counseling on lifestyle behaviors), to the environment (e.g., elimination of physical hazards), or to a specific agent, if one is identified (e.g., contaminated water). Secondary prevention emphasizes the early detection and prompt intervention against asymptomatic disease processes in evolution. Screening efforts characterize this level of prevention. Tertiary prevention attempts to minimize disability from existing disease through medical treatment, education, and rehabilitation. Efforts to prevent the development of secondary conditions (i.e., secondary impairments, disabilities, or handicaps) known to occur in those with specific disabilities incorporate principles from all three of these traditional models of prevention/health protection (48,55). To emphasize the importance of clarifying the nature of health promotion and secondary condition prevention in those with disability, the Center on Health Promotion Research for Persons with Disabilities was established in 1997 with a grant from the Centers for Disease Control and Prevention. Results of their interventions demonstrated that substantial benefits can be attained in core health indicators in targeted populations (45,56).

Expansion of these public health concepts for application among those with disabilities can provide additional conceptual grounding for the development of disability-specific prevention protocols. Specifically, primary prevention for those

TABLE 69-1.   Health Promotion Assessment and Health Maintenance Activities in Those with Physical Disabilities

Physical Health Functions	Assessment
Respiratory	Smoking/exposure to second-hand smoke
	Influenza and pneumococcal vaccine status, particularly in those with advanced age, higher levels of paraplegia/tetraplegia, or neuromuscular compromise that influences muscles of respiration
	Fund of knowledge regarding management of early signs of chest congestion
	Access to assistance with secretion mobilization
	Posture/kyphosis/truncal spasticity/abdominal distention/obesity problems that can have potential impact on chest expansion/respiratory function
	Aspiration risk/gastroesophageal reflux
	Forced vital capacity and forced expiratory volume in 1 second
	Aging-related phenomena
Cardiovascular	Risk factors: family history, physical inactivity/decreased exercise capacity, dyslipidemia, abnormal carbohydrate metabolism, obesity, smoking, impaired peripheral circulation, hypertension
	Exercise practices in individuals capable of exercise/adapted exercise
	Fund of knowledge regarding diet, weight control, physical activity options, and smoking cessation resource options
Skin	Fund of knowledge on risk factors for skin breakdown and how to resolve early problems
	Frequency of visual skin inspections
	Frequency of pressure reliefs
	Evolving latex sensitivity/allergic reactions
	Moisture issues/fecal or urinary incontinence/friction
	Age and condition of wheelchair cushion/seating system
	Posture/pelvic obliquity/spasticity-induced shearing and pressure issues
	Weight/nutritional status and impact on skin vulnerability
	Transfer skills
	Pedal edema/shoe or orthotic trim lines and fit
	Palmar skin protection
	Cigarette smoking
	Sunscreen utilization
	Aging-related changes
Neuromusculoskeletal	Upper-extremity neuromusculoskeletal pain issues with or without current functional impact rotator cuff pathology; shoulder, elbow, wrist, or phalangeal joint contractures; ulnar and median nerve entrapment syndromes
	Lower extremity/axial skeleton degenerative changes with impact on ambulation skills
	Osteoporosis/fractures
	Spasticity/tone-related impact on transfer safety, posture, or shearing phenomenon on skin
	Stability of sensory/motor profile
	Charcot joint arthropathy and impact on trunk stability/dysreflexia patterns/pain issues
	Neuropathic pain phenomena (new onset versus stable pattern; functional impact)
	Motor coordination
	Activities to enhance strength, endurance, and flexibility
Genitourinary	Bladder hygiene/bladder management technique and equipment/supplies/adjunct therapies
	Infection/incontinence rates
	Urinary tract stone formation (upper and lower tracts)
	Genitourinary system surveillance history to date
	Gynecologic history: including access to Papanicolaou smear/bimanual examination/amenorrhea/breast examination habits/postmenopausal hormone replacement
	Prostate health assessment
	Fertility and sexuality concerns
Gastrointestinal	Bowel evacuation technique/duration/predictability
	Early identification of hypomobility patterns
	Latex allergy or evolving sensitivity
	Nutrition and hydration
	Anticholinergic use for detrusor hyperreflexia
	Gallstone disease
	Colon cancer (age specific)
	Symptomatic hemorrhoids (bleeding: dysreflexia-inducing)
Functional status	Interval changes in function secondary to changes in strength; endurance, balance, vision, hearing, hypotension, fatigue levels, pain status, cognition, polypharmacy, access to personal care assistance/transportation/health-care resources in community, or lifestressors
	Mobility
	Cognitive intellectual
	Communication
	Social attitudinal
	Depression
	Knowledge base regarding physical activity/exercise options appropriate for the nature of their disability
	Family and social support systems
	Support systems for primary care providers/family

(continued)

TABLE 69-1. (continued)

Physical Health Functions	Assessment
Nutritional assessment	History and physical examination
	Body weight
	High-density lipoprotein and low-density lipoprotein cholesterol, fasting serum glucose
	Swallowing difficulties
	Functional, economic, or environmental influences on dietary habits/adequacy of nutrient intake
	Medication effect on appetite/bowels
	Nutrition intake/diet composition
Tobacco, alcohol, and	Smoking/second-hand smoke exposure
substance use evaluation	CAGE screening questionnaire/brief MAST screening tool
	Adult immunizations
	Dental health
	Ocular health

Adapted with permission from Lanig IS. *A practical guide to health promotion after spinal cord injury.* Gaithersburg, MD: Aspen, 1996:55.

with an existing disability should include appropriately tailored measures to eliminate risk factors for chronic conditions not necessarily directly related to their primary disability. Interventions may include protocols for health-promoting activities such as smoking cessation, weight control, reduction of substance abuse, increasing physical activity, and screening for age- and sex-specific carcinoma (53). Tailoring of these measures includes deliberate attention to the economic, logistic, architectural, and attitudinal obstacles to primary health care often encountered by persons with disabilities.

Secondary prevention measures in those with chronic disability should focus on ongoing anticipatory strategies to minimize the adverse health impact over time of the primary disability, superimposed aging issues, or new injuries. Emphasis is placed on early detection of secondary conditions that, if left unaddressed, can have deleterious effects on organ systems, performance of activities of daily living, and community reintegration over time (48,49,57–59). Tertiary prevention measures are then activated when appropriate.

Tertiary prevention incorporates ongoing interval efforts to maximize and maintain functional capacity over the life course. Education in new skills and equipment is pursued as functional abilities change. Strategies to combat secondary handicaps are pursued with attention directed to stabilizing or improving access to comprehensive specialized care and stabilizing access to personal care assistance/support services. Additional attention may be given to ongoing vocational rehabilitation and problem solving, the socioeconomic disincentives and obstacles often experienced by disabled individuals seeking a place in the work force.

Building a Knowledge Base

Thoughtful advice and counsel (i.e., patient education) about behaviors, lifestyle, and self-care practices that influence overall health can have far greater impact on health and longevity than specific screening tests or procedures (60). It is for this reason that emphasis on awareness and education is at the crux of health-promotion activities. However, the success of health-promotion education efforts depends on a variety of issues that can be grouped into three categories: (a) issues related to health-care professionals themselves; (b) issues related to the patient; and (c) issues related to clinical/environmental circumstances (55). Comments here are limited to the first category. Rehabilitation professionals may lack self-efficacy regarding their knowledge base and skills necessary for education and motivating individuals in health-promoting behaviors. Additionally, their own personal health enhancement beliefs and practices, inability to overcome the inertia of previous practice, time limitations, lack of a reminder system, underestimation of patient interest or motivation, or lack of outcome expectancy will also influence the nature of clinical encounters and related patterns of education or referral (55,61,62). Continuing education activities, collaboration with primary-care providers in the community, hands-on skills training, small group discussion, and case studies can be useful to physiatrists interested in building their knowledge base over time (62,63).

In order to facilitate effective patient education and behavioral change, the rehabilitation professional must have a clear understanding of available epidemiology assessment and intervention information related to commonly encountered disability-related and general health-related issues. Upon establishing this knowledge base, the physiatrist who so chooses can than routinely pose and answer the following questions during routine medical encounters:

1. What are potential disability-related or general health-related problems of which the patient should be aware?
2. What steps are necessary to clarify if the patient is at risk for specific conditions?
3. Is the problem present?
4. If present, what should be done?

Questions 1 and 2 require knowledge of (a) available epidemiologic data and risk-factor information and (b) specialty-specific technical assessment skills. Question 3 requires skills in interpretation of the data secured, and question 4 requires knowledge in appropriate education and therapeutic intervention options (45,64,65).

The Interdisciplinary Assessment of Health

A systematic health assessment is necessary to establish and document an individual's current health status, lifestyle practices, and psychosocial variables that can influence health. Thereafter, goals can be established and pursued in a manner appropriate to the individual's unique circumstances, resources, and personal desires (64). Particular attention must be directed to the social and environmental aspects of disability that are typically of a magnitude sufficiently significant to greatly influence health-promoting activities (57,63,66,67).

Health-risk appraisal or health-status assessment instruments are often used in the general population in risk-factor assessment, education, and behavioral change programs. However, there are no such validated instruments for use in the disabled populations. Additionally, concerns have been raised regarding the validity and reliability of the data yielded by some of these instruments, even in the nondisabled population (68). Nonetheless, simple icebreaker-type health-status assessments designed for use in the general population can be used to stimulate interest and initiate health-promotion discussions between disabled individuals and rehabilitation professionals. Additionally, despite the current lack of valid and reliable health-risk appraisal instruments for those with disabilities, the adoption of certain general health-risk assessment principles related to smoking, weight control, nutrition, physical activity, cancer screening, and family history risk factors for disease seems appropriate for those with chronic disabilities (55). In addition, there is a fair degree of consensus in the medical rehabilitation literature on the core concepts that should be incorporated into disability-specific health-status assessments (63,68). Table 69-1 provides a partial list of health-assessment questions appropriate for individuals with physical disabilities. The following section reviews general health-promoting activities that should be addressed and encouraged during physiatric encounters wherein the physiatrist is the functional primary provider.

GENERAL HEALTH-PROMOTING ACTIVITIES

Smoking Cessation

Smoking only further compromises a disabled person's already impaired physiologic reserves for good health. Therefore, it is vitally important for physiatrists to encourage and help every patient they encounter who smokes to quit. Cigarette smoking is the single most preventable cause of death and disability in the United States (69,71). It is known to cause heart disease, stroke, and chronic obstructive pulmonary disease. More than 400,000 Americans die from tobacco use each year—more than the number of individuals who die from acquired immunodeficiency syndrome, cocaine use, heroin use, gang violence, alcohol use, fires, automobile accidents, driving under the influence, suicide, and homicide combined (71–73). One in every five deaths in the United States is smoking related (70,71). Numerous studies have demonstrated that physicians' advice is a strong motivator and that their efforts to encourage patients to quit do make a difference (70–72). Unfortunately, only half of smokers report that their primary-care physicians in the previous year have even asked about their smoking status during the past year (74).

This lack of physician attention to smoking status and smoking cessation recommendations is particularly disturbing in light of the fact that options for office practice-based smoking cessation strategies are readily available from a variety of sources (75,76). Most notably, in 1996, the Centers for Disease Control and Prevention and the Agency for Health Care Policy and Research produced clinical practice guidelines on smoking cessation (77). Emphasis was placed on assessment and intervention strategies designed to be brief, requiring 3 minutes or less of direct clinician time. Physicians were encouraged to include smoking status (current, former, never) on the vital signs stamp at every clinic/office visit. Nicotine replacement therapy (patch or gum) was recommended for smoking cessation unless special circumstances were present, such as pregnancy, the early post–myocardial infarction period, serious arrhythmias,

or severe angina pectoris. The practice guidelines recommend that clinicians acknowledge that the majority of smokers who quit smoking will gain weight. Patients should be told that most individuals will gain less than 10 pounds, although a small minority may gain substantially more (73,78). Follow-up for positive reinforcement for behavioral change over time is encouraged. The physiatrist and interdisciplinary team, in particular, are often in a relationship with patients wherein cross-discipline reinforcement and follow-through can be instituted during routinely scheduled inpatient or outpatient clinical encounters.

Nutrition and Weight Control

For many individuals with chronic disability, the promotion and protection of their nutritional health can be compromised by a variety of physical and socioeconomic difficulties. Bulbar signs/swallowing difficulties, limitations in upper-extremity function, income restrictions, and food procurement and preparation difficulties are several confounding variables that can adversely impact food selection and consumption.

Mounting scientific evidence, however, has underscored the direct relationship between diet and health (79). Poor diet has been implicated or identified as a risk factor in several chronic diseases that have become the leading causes of death in the United States: heart disease, diabetes, stroke, and some forms of cancer. In response to these, numerous health agencies—most notably the U.S. Department of Health and Human Services, American Heart Association, and National Cancer Institute—have proposed dietary guidelines for the American population (73,80,81).

For those with disabilities, nutritional health-related secondary conditions can manifest themselves in the form of compromised skin integrity, increased skin vulnerability from cachexia, suboptimal wound-healing capacity, adult-onset glucose intolerance and dyslipidemias (82), bowel evacuation problems, fluid intake-related genitourinary tract difficulties, and functional compromise associated with weight gain. Identifying and reducing environmental, socioeconomic, and disability-related physiologic or functional skills risk factors for poor nutritional health often require a team approach (83).

Physiologic and body composition differences in many individuals with chronic disability influence the reliability and utility of standard nutritional assessment tools. Basic biochemical and clinical assessment can be pursued based on principles described elsewhere in this text. Data relating to dietary history, social situation history, and functional status components of the nutritional health assessment can be obtained through the interdisciplinary treating team's collaborative efforts. Action plans can be proposed based on the assembled data.

Physical Fitness

The cycle of disability has been characterized as a vicious cycle, wherein physical disability and dysfunction through physical inactivity and deconditioning leads to additional/perpetuated physical disability and dysfunction (84) (Fig. 69-3). Health promotion and related educational efforts for those with disabilities would therefore be incomplete without the provision of a physical fitness component. Exercise regimens adapted to the characteristic limitation or physiologic vulnerabilities created by their specific impairments/disabilities are a must.

Physical fitness encompasses the physiologic attributes of (a) cardiopulmonary fitness, (b) muscular strength, (c) muscular endurance, (d) flexibility, and (e) body composition. Training principles and programs for those with disabilities have

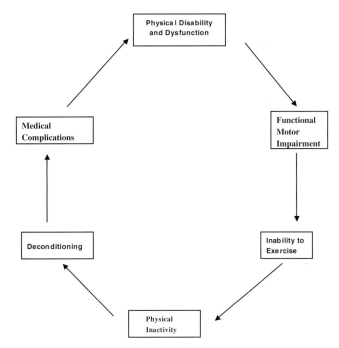

Figure 69-3. The cycle of disability.

steadily been investigated and developed in recent years (85–93).

In 1996, the Surgeon General's Report on Physical Activity and Health included an unprecedented section specifically directed to persons with disabilities (90). Benefits of physical activity—including improvements in stamina, muscle strength, promotion of general feelings of well-being, and modulation of joint swelling and pain associated with arthritis—were cited. The importance and positive correlation of social support and regular physical activity in those with disabilities was noted.

However, for many with disabilities, physical fitness cannot be defined in terms of the traditional concepts of fitness in the general population. Rather, it must be defined in a broader sense that encompasses not only appropriately modified descriptions of endurance, strength, and flexibility, but also (a) conscientious nutritional health practices to nourish the body, (b) health practices and medical follow-up to minimize the risk of secondary impairments and disabilities, and (c) a balanced commitment to maximizing functional capabilities in both necessary and discretionary activities of daily living (91).

Well-planned, clinically sound physical exercise can improve cardiovascular and peripheral muscle endurance, enhance strength and coordination, and improve flexibility in many individuals with chronic disabilities. Therefore, despite a variety of practical challenges often articulated, the interdisciplinary team should systematically evaluate and recommend physical exercise activities for most individuals with chronic disability. In those with neuromuscular disease, there is a common concern that strength and endurance exercises have the potential to create exercise-induced weakness. This concern can be tempered through specific recommendations for nonfatiguing intensity and duration of exercise activities and with monitoring of functional capacity after introduction of regular exercise activities (94,95). For those with arthritis, isometric exercise programs can often maintain strength if pain and inflammation with movement is particularly problematic. However, attention must be directed to maintaining functional range of motion. Overall, strength and endurance programs for individuals with arthritis have been shown to result in better disease

outcomes (96,97). Exercise programs to reverse deconditioning associated with multiple sclerosis can be beneficial to those with stable or mild to moderately impaired neurologic profiles. Attention should be directed to balancing frequency, duration, and time of day so that the exercise activity does not compromise the individual's ability to perform activities of daily living (98). For those with spinal cord injury, the level of injury will influence the cardiovascular response to exercise. Generally speaking, the higher the level of injury, the more likely a significant reduction in cardiopulmonary capacity and fitness as compared with those of the nondisabled population (99). However, the gains in peripheral muscle strength and endurance often enhance functional capacity and should therefore be encouraged. Recommendations for adaptation of exercise equipment and regimens to accommodate weakness, sensory deficits, and orthopedic limitations created by various disabilities are increasingly more available through a variety of resources.

Screening for Substance Abuse

The importance of screening for drug and alcohol abuse in the disabled population is necessitated by both the impact of these substances on bodily functions and by the behavioral aberrations associated with excessive use (100). The prevalence of hazardous or frankly abusive alcohol use patterns in the general population varies from 7.5% to 19.7%, depending on the limits selected (101). When limits recommended by the National Institute on Alcohol Abuse and Alcoholism (102) are used (14 drinks/week for men, more than 7 drinks/week for women, or binge drinking), findings have suggested that one in five adults in the general outpatient population will screen positive for at-risk alcohol use. World Health Organization criteria focus on persons at highest risk for alcohol-related events and therefore focus attention on screening for those who consume more than 21 drinks per week or engage in binge drinking (101–104). A large percentage of individuals admitted to rehabilitation services with neurotrauma were intoxicated at the time of injury and often had preinjury histories of hazardous ethanol consumption patterns (105–107). Additionally, for some individuals with chronic disabilities, maladaptive coping may include hazardous or frankly abusive alcohol consumption. For others, excessive alcohol consumption may be a form of maladaptive self-medication for chronic pain phenomena. Finally, given the high prevalence of alcoholism found in the community-based general population studies and the morbidity and mortality associated with alcohol abuse and dependency, public health agencies recommend that screening for alcoholism should be a routine part of every medical evaluation (60). One first seeks to help the problem drinker acknowledge the problem, understand its consequences, and recognize the need for treatment. Thereafter, attention shifts to negotiating and carrying out an acceptable, customized treatment plan (108).

The U.S. Preventive Services Task Force recommends screening all adolescents and adult patients for potential harmful and hazardous use of alcohol, rather than just for frank abuse and dependence (109). Many screening instruments are widely used in medical practice, but their performance is known to vary according to the age, sex, ethnicity, and other characteristics of the population being screened, including the prevalence of cases in the population. As such, it may be unreasonable to assume that the same screen will be effective for all individuals in any given setting (101). The CAGE questionnaire was designed as an easy, expedient instrument to evaluate a patient's alcohol usage and to determine if further assessment

TABLE 69-2.   The CAGE/CAGE-AID Questions

The original CAGE questions appear in plain type. The adaptations to include drugs (CAGE-AID) are indicated in *italics*. The CAGE or CAGE-AID should be preceded by these two questions:

1. Do you drink alcohol? If yes, how much? How Often?
2. Have you ever experimented with drugs? Which ones?

If the person has experimented with drugs, ask the CAGE-AID questions. If the patient only drinks alcohol, ask the CAGE questions.

CAGE and CAGE-AID questions

1. In the last 3 months, have you felt you should cut down or stop drinking or *using drugs*?
   Yes   No
2. In the last 3 months, has anyone annoyed you or gotten on your nerves by telling you to cut down or stop drinking or *using drugs*?
   Yes   No
3. In the last 3 months, have you felt guilty or bad about how much you drink or *use drugs*?
   Yes   No
4. In the last 3 months, have you been waking up wanting to have an alcoholic drink or *use drugs* (eye-opener)?
   Yes   No

Each affirmative response earns one point. One point indicates a possible problem. Two points indicate a probable problem.

is necessary (110). Although a limitation of this instrument is that it relies on self-report, it appears that those who drink intemperately are more inclined to give accurate responses to CAGE questions when they are part of a series of lifestyle questions that include diet, exercise habits, smoking, and safe sex practices (111). The CAGE interview questions are shown in Table 69-2. The *italicized* words in the CAGE interview questions reflect adaptations made to include drug-use screening questions. The CAGE adapted to include drugs is called the CAGE-AID. Other screening tools that have been shown to be useful in health screening activities include the 25-question Michigan Alcoholism Screening Test (MAST) (112), the 10-question brief MAST (113), and the World Health Organization Alcohol Use Disorders Identification Test (AUDIT) (103,104). The AUDIT attempts to identify drinkers whose consumption patterns place them at risk for direct or indirect medical problems and alcohol dependency before frank dependency has developed. Because the majority of alcohol-related problems occur in at-risk nondependent drinkers (114), public health officials and alcohol epidemiologists have often encouraged use of the AUDIT or other consumption pattern questionnaires to screen for this subpopulation (101).

Formal diagnosis of alcohol dependence or abuse involves tracking the quantity and duration of consumption and identifying physiologic manifestation of ethanol addiction, loss of control over drinking, and damage to physical health and social functioning (108). Routine screening may facilitate early detection of hazardous consumption patterns before frank dependency or abuse develops. Hazardous consumption has been defined by alcohol epidemiologists as five or more drinks per day in men and two or more drinks per day in nonpregnant women (115). A "drink" is defined as approximately 12 ounces of beer, 5 ounces of wine, or 1.5 ounces of distilled liquor—the equivalent of 0.6 ounces of ethanol.

Once a problem is identified, a multifaceted, personalized, long-term management plan operationalized in collaboration with available community resources and family should be pursued. Transportation issues, architectural and attitudinal barri-

ers within community-based resource facilities, and sometimes united social support are specific challenges to systematic management in those individuals with both chronic disability and substance abuse problems.

PRIMARY MEDICAL CARE IN THE GENERAL POPULATION

Earlier in this chapter, several definitions of primary care were reviewed. The definitions were notable for the broad spectrum of services a primary-care physician must address, including disease prevention, health education, and risk reduction. Additionally, this chapter presented differences regarding the ongoing health-care needs of people with disabilities relative to those without disabilities. Several of those differences—such as people with disabilities having an increased vulnerability to certain health problems, an increased risk that a new health problem may impose significant secondary functional losses, and concerns that a given health condition may result in unusually complicated and prolonged treatment—make the attention to health prevention and risk-factor modification in people with disabilities of paramount importance. Arguably, primary care for people with disabilities takes on a more critical role than for people without disabilities.

The United States Preventive Services Task Force

The United States Preventive Services Task Force (USPSTF) was convened by the United States Public Health Service in 1984. The USPSTF consists of 15 experts from the specialties of family medicine, pediatrics, internal medicine, obstetrics and gynecology, preventive medicine, public health, behavioral medicine, and nursing. Its mission is to systematically review the evidence of effectiveness of clinical preventive services and create age-, sex-, and risk-based recommendations about services that should routinely be incorporated into primary medical care (116). The initial efforts culminated in the *Guide to Clinical Preventive Services* in 1989, with a second edition published in 1996. As of spring 2001, the task force has been releasing updated recommendations on selected topics that will ultimately make up the third edition.

In addition to the USPSTF, there are many other major health organizations that propose recommendations. These organizations, which include the American College of Physicians, the American Heart Association, the American Academy of Family Physicians, and the American Cancer Society, oftentimes disagree on recommendations, as the literature available for review may be inconclusive.

Most primary-care organizations comprehensively focus their recommendations on the following services, which will provide an outline for the discussion to follow:

- Immunizations
- Screening tests
- Chemoprevention
- Counseling (discussed earlier in the chapter)

Immunizations

Immunizations are one of the easiest and most effective ways to prevent potentially catastrophic illnesses. Unfortunately, they are often overlooked during patient encounters that are already full of multiple issues, especially in adults. However, it is incumbent on physicians providing primary care to address the need for immunization as one component of preventive

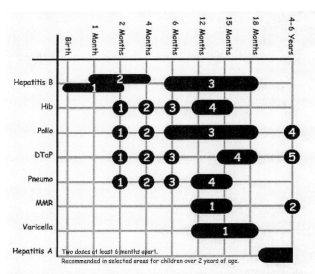

This chart is based on the Immunization schedule recommended by CDC, the American Academy of Pediatrics, and the American Academy of Family Physicians.

Figure 69-4. Childhood immunization schedule.

services. The following is a list of immunizations, and the appropriate dosing schedules, that are recommended by the Centers for Disease Control and Prevention's Advisory Committee on Immunization Practices (117).

CHILDHOOD VACCINES
For a childhood immunization schedule, see Figure 69-4.

Diphtheria, Tetanus, and Pertussis Immunization
A child needs five diphtheria, tetanus, and pertussis immunization (DtaP) shots for maximum protection. The first three shots should be given at 2, 4, and 6 months of age. The fourth (booster) shot is given between 15 and 18 months, and a fifth shot (another booster) is given when the child is about to enter school, at 4 to 6 years of age. When DTaP vaccine is given according to this schedule, it protects most children from all three diseases. If a child does get one of the diseases in spite of the vaccine, it will probably be milder than it would have been otherwise.

Polio Immunization
There are two types of polio vaccine: inactivated (killed) polio vaccine (IPV), which is an injection, and live oral polio vaccine (OPV). The Centers for Disease Control and Prevention recommends only IPV, except in very limited circumstances. Children should get a total of five doses of IPV. The first three doses should be given at 2, 4, and 6 months of age. The fourth dose is given between 6 and 18 months, and a fifth dose (booster) is given when the child is about to enter school, at 4 to 6 years of age.

Measles, Mumps, and Rubella Immunization
Most children get measles, mumps, and rubella vaccines all together in a single injection called MMR. All three of these vaccines work very well and will protect most children for the rest of their life. Children should get two doses of MMR vaccine. The first is given between 12 and 15 months of age. The second may be given at any time, as long as it is at least 28 days after the first. It is usually given at 4 to 6 years of age, before the child enters kindergarten or first grade.

Haemophilus Influenza Type B Immunization
Haemophilus influenza type B immunization (Hib) vaccine has had a dramatic impact on *Haemophilus influenzae* type B. As soon as the first vaccine was introduced in 1985, the disease began to disappear. Several improved vaccines have been licensed since then, and the age for the first shot has been lowered from 24 months to 2 months. There were an estimated 20,000 cases of Hib disease a year in the mid-1980s, but now there are only a few hundred cases a year.

Children should get either three or four doses, depending on which company's vaccine is used. All children should get the vaccine at 2 and 4 months of age, and a booster dose between 12 and 15 months. Some children should get an additional dose at 6 months. Children who have passed their fifth birthday do not need Hib vaccination.

Pneumocococcal Immunization
Until very recently, pneumococcal vaccine was recommended mostly for adults older than 65 years and was not licensed at all for children younger than age 2. The lack of licensing for children was because the only type of vaccine that was available (pneumococcal polysaccharide vaccine) didn't work very well for young children. Now a different type of vaccine (pneumococcal conjugate vaccine) has been licensed that is efficacious for children younger than 2. Thus, it is finally possible to prevent pneumococcal disease in that vulnerable age group.

Children should routinely get four doses of the vaccine, one dose each at 2, 4, 6, and 12–15 months of age. Children who begin the series later may not need as many doses. Children older than 5 years generally will not need the pneumococcal conjugate vaccine.

Hepatitis B Immunization
Children can be protected from hepatitis B via immunization with three doses of hepatitis B vaccine. Babies can get their first injection between birth and 2 months of age, the second at 1 to 4 months of age, and the third at 6 to 18 months of age. After the third injection, most children are protected and will not need booster doses.

Varicella Immunization
Varicella vaccine is a live-virus vaccine. It has been used in some parts of the world, such as Japan, for more than 20 years. It was licensed in the United States in 1995. A single dose of varicella vaccine is recommended for children between 12 and 18 months of age. It is usually given at the same time as the MMR injection. Children who miss this dose can still get a single dose of the vaccine until their 13th birthday. A child who has already had chickenpox disease does not need to get the vaccine. Occasionally, even children who respond to the vaccine get a very mild case of chickenpox (about one to two children out of a hundred).

Hepatitis A Immunization
Hepatitis A vaccine is an inactivated (killed) vaccine. It can be given to children 2 years old or older. Two doses are needed, the second dose given 6 to 18 months after the first. Hepatitis A vaccine is recommended for children in Alaska, Arizona, California, Idaho, Nevada, New Mexico, Oklahoma, Oregon, South Dakota, Utah, and Washington and may also be considered for children in Arkansas, Colorado, Missouri, Montana, Texas, and Wyoming. The vaccine is also recommended for communities with high levels of hepatitis A, including Alaskan native villages, American Indian reservations, some Hispanic communities, and some religious communities. Additionally, it is recom-

mended for others who are at high risk, including people traveling to countries where the disease is common, illegal drug users, homosexuals, people with clotting disorders, and people with liver disease.

ADULT VACCINATIONS

Some adults incorrectly assume that the vaccines they received as children will protect them for the rest of their lives. Generally this is true, except that:

- Some adults were never vaccinated as children.
- Newer vaccines were not available when some adults were children.
- Immunity can begin to fade over time.
- As we age, we become more susceptible to serious disease caused by common infections (e.g., flu, pneumococcus) (118).

The following vaccines are recommended for adults:

- Varicella (chicken pox)
- Hepatitis B (adults at risk)
- Measles-mumps-rubella (MMR)
- Diphtheria-tetanus
- Influenza
- Pneumococcal

Varicella

The varicella vaccine is recommended for persons of any age without a reliable history of varicella disease or vaccination, or who are seronegative for varicella. It is also recommended for persons who live or work in environments in which transmission of varicella is likely, such as teachers of young children, day-care employees, college students, or military personnel. For persons 13 years of age and older, two doses separated by 4 to 8 weeks is the appropriate schedule.

Hepatitis B

Hepatitis B vaccine is recommended for adults with multiple sexual partners, a recent diagnosis of a sexually transmitted disease, occupational risk of exposure to blood or body fluids, household contacts and sexual partners of those with chronic hepatitis B infection, injection drug users, and all unvaccinated adolescents. The schedule is three doses, with the second dose 1 to 2 months after the first, and the third dose 4 to 6 months after the first.

Measles-Mumps-Rubella

MMR is recommended for adults born after 1956 without written documentation of immunization, health-care personnel born after 1956, and adolescents entering college. Women should be asked if they are pregnant before receiving the vaccine. At least one dose should be given. A second dose should be given a month after the first for people entering college or in the health-care profession.

Diphtheria-Tetanus

All adults should maintain their diphtheria-tetanus vaccination by receiving a booster dose at 10-year intervals.

Influenza

Influenza is a viral illness that occurs yearly from November through March. The elderly, infirm, and many people with disabilities are more susceptible to an influenza infection causing serious morbidity and mortality. Therefore, it is recommended that all adults 50 years of age and older; people with chronic medical conditions, including diabetes, asthma, renal insuffi-

ciency, and human immunodeficiency virus (HIV); residents of nursing homes and other chronic-care facilities; and health-care professionals receive a vaccination yearly in the late fall or winter.

Pneumococcal

Pneumococcus is the most common pathogen responsible for pneumonia in adults of all ages. Those people most at risk for serious infection and death include the elderly, chronically ill, and immunosuppressed. Therefore, it is recommended that all adults 65 years of age and older, and people with chronic medical conditions, splenic dysfunction, asplenia, multiple myeloma, or HIV, receive one dose of the pneumococcal vaccine. Those people vaccinated before the age of 65, or who are at high risk of fatal infection, should receive a second vaccination at least 5 years after the first dose.

Screening Tests

The three leading causes of death in the United States, in order of incidence, are coronary artery disease, cancer, and stroke (119). The risk of developing coronary artery disease and stroke can be reduced greatly by the treatment of major risk factors. The major risk factors that are modifiable are hypertension, diabetes mellitus, hyperlipidemia, obesity, and smoking. Early detection of certain cancers has been found to increase survival. The cancers that benefit from early detection are the ones that people commonly are screened for, which include breast, cervical, colon, and prostate cancers.

SCREENING FOR CARDIOVASCULAR RISK

Hypertension

In addition to being a major risk factor for coronary artery disease and cerebrovascular disease, hypertension is also a major risk factor for congestive heart failure, renal disease, abdominal aortic aneurysm rupture, and retinopathy. Multiple studies over the last 30 years have demonstrated that reduction in elevated blood pressure leads to a reduction in risk of these diseases regardless of ethnicity, sex, or age (120). Summarizing the current screening recommendations from all major authorities calls for routine blood pressure measurements at least once every 1 to 2 years in adults beginning at age 18–21 (121). Recently, *The Sixth Report of the Joint National Committee on Detection, Evaluation and Treatment of High Blood Pressure* (JNC VI) redefined high blood pressure to include a high-normal range of 130–139 systolic or 85–89 diastolic (122). It is felt that people at high risk for vascular disease, or with known vascular disease, should have their blood pressure lowered below this high-normal range.

The initial treatment of choice in managing hypertension is lifestyle modification. This includes losing weight, reducing sodium intake, limiting alcohol intake, and increasing aerobic physical activity (30 minutes most days of the week). If this is not effective at achieving the lowering of blood pressure to the desired range, then medication should be started. There are many medications available for the treatment of hypertension. The JNC VI suggests that in uncomplicated hypertension, the agents of choice—based on randomized controlled trials—are diuretics and beta-blockers. However, there are many specific and compelling clinical indications to use other antihypertensive agents, such as angiotensin-converting enzyme inhibitors for patients with diabetes, congestive heart failure, or post–myocardial infarction. A comprehensive list of such indications and medication choices is listed in the JNC VI (123).

Diabetes Mellitus

Diabetes mellitus is an established risk factor for both macrovascular (coronary artery disease, cerebrovascular disease) and microvascular (retinopathy, neuropathy, nephropathy) disease. Careful control of blood sugar has been proven to reduce the development of these diseases (124,125). Despite this information regarding reduced risk of disease in the diabetic population, most major authorities, including the American College of Physicians, the American Academy of Family Physicians, and the American Diabetes Association, recommend against routine screening for diabetes among asymptomatic adults (126). The USPSTF finds insufficient evidence to recommend for or against routine screening (127). However, most authorities agree that selective screening in high-risk individuals is warranted. High-risk people would include those with obesity, a strong family history of diabetes, or women with a history of gestational diabetes.

According to the American Diabetes Association, the best screening test for detecting diabetes is the fasting plasma glucose (FPG). An FPG >125 is an indication for retesting, which should be repeated on a different day to confirm the diagnosis. Individuals with an FPG >110 but <125 are considered to have impaired fasting glucose and be at an increased risk of developing diabetes in the future. Normoglycemia is defined as an FPG <110 (128).

Treatment options for diabetes, both insulin dependent and non–insulin dependent, have expanded significantly over the last 5 years. Oral agents are now available that sensitize cells to the effects of insulin, as well as stimulate insulin secretion. It is now common to use oral agents in conjunction with insulin to decrease the insulin requirement. Additionally, the array of insulin preparations available have increased to include longer-acting agents that provide a more stable basal level, as well as agents that act quickly to provide better postprandial effects. Although a comprehensive review of these medications is beyond the scope of this chapter, the goal of treatment, regardless of the treatment option selected, is to achieve a hemoglobin A1C <7.0% (see chapter 56 for further discussion of the above medications).

Hyperlipidemia

There is a significant body of literature that demonstrates that lowering cholesterol levels results in a reduction in primary cardiovascular events (129–131). As a result, most major authorities agree that routine screening of people for lipid abnormalities at least every 5 years is important. Additionally, these same authorities agree that appropriate screening entails obtaining a nonfasting total cholesterol and high-density lipoprotein (HDL) cholesterol level. However, there is disagreement as to the age to begin the screening process. The USPSTF and the American College of Physicians recommend screening men age 35 years and older and women age 45 years and older (132). For people with other risk factors for coronary artery disease, these organizations recommend beginning the screening process as early as 20 years of age.

The National Cholesterol Education Panel–Adult Treatment Panel III (NCEP-ATP III) recommends that screening begin for all people at the age of 20 by obtaining a fasting lipid profile. The fasting lipid profile should include total cholesterol, low-density lipoprotein (LDL), and HDL levels. Subsequently, a person's cardiovascular risk-factor profile should be determined to help determine their target LDL level. People with known coronary artery disease, peripheral vascular disease, or diabetes mellitus should ideally have an LDL value less than 100. People with two or more cardiovascular risk factors (including hypertension, cigarette smoking, obesity, family history of premature coronary artery disease, an HDL cholesterol level less than 40, a man older than 45 years of age or a woman older than 55 years of age) should ideally have an LDL value less than 130. For people with less than two of the above risk factors, an LDL value less than 160 is desirable (133).

The initial approach to a person with elevated cholesterol is dietary modification. A diet low in fat and cholesterol should be tried for several months in attempts to reach the target LDL. If this is unsuccessful, then pharmacologic therapy is instituted. The most common class of medications to treat an elevated LDL cholesterol is the statin class. It is important to monitor the effects of these drugs on the cholesterol profile 2 months after initiating therapy or increasing the dose of the medication. At the same time, careful monitoring of liver function tests and muscle enzymes (CPK) is strongly recommended.

Obesity

Approximately one-third of adults are overweight, based on data from the third U.S. National Health and Nutrition Examination Survey (NHANES III) (134). Persons who are overweight are more likely to have adult-onset diabetes, hypertension, and risk factors for other diseases (135). Observational studies have established a clear association between being overweight and hypercholesterolemia and suggest a relationship between being overweight and coronary artery disease (136). Obesity has also been associated with an increased risk of certain cancers (including those of the colon, rectum, prostate, gallbladder, biliary tract, breast, cervix, endometrium, and ovary) and with other disorders such as cholelithiasis, obstructive sleep apnea, venous thromboembolism, and osteoarthritis (137). Finally, obesity can affect the quality of life by limiting mobility, physical endurance, and other functional measures, as well as through social, academic, and job discrimination.

As a result of the above information linking obesity to a myriad of diseases, the USPSTF recommends periodic height and weight measurements for all patients (138). The weight and height are then used to calculate a body-mass index (BMI). A normal BMI is 18.5–27. Obesity is defined as a BMI greater than 30.

CANCER SCREENING

Breast Cancer

Breast cancer is the most common malignancy in women in the United States. A woman's lifetime risk of developing breast cancer is approximately one in eight (139). There will be an estimated 203,500 cases of breast cancer in American women in 2002, with an estimated 39,600 deaths (140). Treatment for breast cancer, especially when detected early, is effective at decreasing mortality. As a result, the American Cancer Society, American College of Radiology, American Medical Association, American College of Obstetricians and Gynecologists, and a number of other organizations recommend screening mammography and clinical breast examination every one to two years beginning at the age of 40, and annual mammography and clinical breast examination beginning at age 50 (141).

Cervical Cancer

Approximately 13,000 cases of cervical cancer will occur in the United States in 2002, with 4,100 deaths (142). The disease is usually preceded by an asymptomatic phase that is preinvasive and therefore ideal for early detection and screening. Cervical cancer is caused by human papilloma virus, a sexually trans-mitted disease, in 95% of the cases (143).

A consensus recommendation that all women who are sexually active, or who have reached the age of 18, should have annual Pap smears has been adopted by the American Cancer Society, National Cancer Institute, American College of Obstetricians and Gynecologists, American Medical Association, and the American Academy of Family Physicians. The recommendation permits Pap testing less frequently after three or more annual smears have been normal (144).

Colorectal Cancer

Colorectal cancer is the second leading cause of cancer mortality in the United States, with more than 57,000 deaths in 2001 (145). More than 90% of colorectal cancers begin as an adenomatous polyp that can often be detected through screening procedures. As a result, the need for screening is agreed on by all major authorities, but the mode of screening and age at which to begin vary. The USPSTF recommends that all persons aged 50 and older be screened with annual fecal occult blood testing, flexible sigmoidoscopy every 5 years alone or with fecal occult blood testing, or colonoscopy every 10 years (146). A single optimal strategy cannot be determined at this time from the currently available data. The American Cancer Society recommends annual digital rectal examination for all adults beginning at age 40, annual fecal occult blood testing at age 50, and sigmoidoscopy every 3–5 years beginning at age 50 (147).

Sigmoidoscopy can detect adenomatous polyps within the left side of the colon. If an adenomatous polyp is found, the patient is referred for a colonoscopy to look for proximal polyps. Unfortunately, studies have demonstrated 30% to 50% of patients will only have polyps proximal to the reach of the sigmoidoscope (148,149), thereby negating the benefits of early detection. This fact prompted Medicare, as of July 2001, to reimburse screening colonoscopy every 5 years for their recipients. Increasingly, physicians are recommending this screening approach to Medicare patients.

Prostate Cancer

Prostate cancer is the most common cancer in men and accounts for the second-highest number of cancer deaths in men (150). Public awareness of this disease and the opportunity to be screened with a blood test [prostate-specific antigen (PSA)] has grown tremendously in the last decade. Unfortunately, there has been no research to date demonstrating that systematic early screening for prostate cancer with PSA or digital rectal examination would save lives. As a result, the USPSTF does not recommend screening for prostate cancer. However, the American Cancer Society and American Urological Association do recommend annual digital rectal examination beginning at age 40, with an annual serum PSA beginning at age 50. PSA screening should begin at age 45 for those men at high risk for prostate cancer, including African American men and those with a family history of prostate cancer (151).

Chemoprevention

ASPIRIN THERAPY

Coronary artery disease is associated with well-established risk factors, such as hypertension and smoking. In addition to the commonly discussed risk factors, coronary artery disease has also been linked to platelet activity and inflammation. The fact that aspirin possesses both antiplatelet and antiinflammatory properties has made it an interesting option for coronary artery disease prevention.

There have been five major randomized trials of aspirin therapy for the primary prevention of coronary events (152–156). Four out of the five studies showed a reduction in the rates of cardiovascular events, most notably myocardial infarction. The reduction in relative risks of cardiovascular events ranged from 4% to 44%.

The USPSTF recently published strong recommendations for clinicians to discuss aspirin chemoprevention with adults who are at increased risk for coronary artery disease (157). Increased risk is considered for men older than 40, postmenopausal women, and younger people with risk factors for atherosclerotic disease. Other authorities recommend calculating the risk of coronary artery disease over 5 or 10 years and using aspirin in people who reach a certain threshold of risk.

Unfortunately, the available studies do not provide information regarding the optimal dose of aspirin to recommend. The five primary prevention studies used aspirin doses ranging from 75 to 500 mg. There has been no study to date comparing different doses of aspirin with each other.

POSTMENOPAUSAL HORMONE REPLACEMENT

Hormone replacement therapy (HRT) for postmenopausal women has been a controversial topic over the last 20 years. In the 1980s and early 1990s, observational studies suggested that women who were treated with HRT had a lower risk of developing coronary heart disease, more favorable lipid profiles, and a better quality of life (158). Unfortunately, as with all observational studies, confounding factors were significant, including the facts that women treated with HRT were usually healthier at baseline, more physically active, and of higher socioeconomic status. Given the concerns that HRT is associated with a relative risk of 1.3 of developing breast cancer (determined from metaanalysis) made the limitations of observational studies important to consider.

Over the last four years, randomized double-blind trials have demonstrated that HRT in women with known coronary artery disease does not decrease the risk of secondary cardiac events when followed up to 4 years (159). Angiographic studies also showed no difference in the rate of progression of atherosclerotic plaques in women on HRT for 3 years (160). As a result of this information from randomized trials, the American Heart Association does not recommend HRT in women with known heart disease and recommends discontinuing HRT in women who suffer a cardiovascular event (161).

The Women's Health Initiative is a large, clinical primary prevention trial that is due to be completed in 2005. Initiated in 1998, the study was designed to evaluate the efficacy of HRT in the primary prevention of cardiovascular disease, cancer, and stroke. Women were randomized to receive estrogen plus progestin if they had not had a hysterectomy, estrogen alone if they had a hysterectomy, or placebo (162). In July 2002, the Women's Health Initiative Data and Safety Monitoring Board recommended that women in the study group of estrogen and progestin stop their study pills, as the risks now exceeded the benefits. The decision to prematurely terminate this arm of the study was based on the observation that heart attacks, strokes, blood clots, and breast cancer occurred in more women taking estrogen and progestin than in women taking placebo (163). The study is continuing to further assess the effects of estrogen alone.

The Women's International Study of Long Duration of Oestrogen after Menopause trial is an international study currently enrolling postmenopausal women in a long-term, randomized, placebo-controlled trial of HRT involving 10 years of treatment plus an additional 10 years of follow-up of major health outcomes (164). Preliminary results are not yet available.

OSTEOPOROSIS

Osteoporosis is characterized by low bone mass, leading to bone fragility and an increased susceptibility to fractures (165). One out of every two women and one out of every eight men older than the age of 50 will have an osteoporosis-related bone fracture in their lifetime. The estimated direct expenditures for osteoporosis and related fractures is $14 billion each year (166). There are many risk factors for osteoporosis, including age, female sex, body size (small, thin women having the highest risk), family history, ethnicity (Caucasian and Asian women having a higher risk), cigarette smoking, excessive alcohol consumption, medications such as steroids and anticonvulsants, and extended bed rest or inactivity.

Prevention of osteoporosis is of paramount importance given the tremendous impact that it, and the resulting hip and vertebral fractures, have on subsequent quality of life and duration of life (there is a 15% to 20% 1-year mortality rate following a hip fracture) (167). As many people with disabilities suffer from a loss of mobility, especially weight-bearing activity, osteoporosis can develop at an earlier age than average. Prevention is therefore even more important in this segment of the population.

There are several aspects of prevention that can be addressed during patient encounters. It is important to ensure that people are taking adequate dietary intake of calcium and vitamin D (vitamin D is necessary for the absorption of calcium). For most people, 1,000–1,200 mg of calcium a day and 400–800 LU of vitamin D are recommended (168). Furthermore, counseling regarding smoking cessation and moderation of alcohol consumption is essential. Whenever possible, weight-bearing exercise should be encouraged.

The diagnosis of osteoporosis can only be made definitively by obtaining a bone mineral density examination. The World Health Organization has recommended that osteoporosis be defined as a bone density more than 2.5 standard deviations below the normal bone mass in young women and osteopenia (low bone mass) be defined as bone density 1–2.5 standard deviations below the normal mean (169). Dual energy x-ray absorptiometry is the bone mineral examination that is most reproducible and precise.

There are several medications available to treat osteoporosis. These include biphosphonates, calcitonin, and estrogens. The biphosphonates work by inhibiting osteoclast-mediated bone resorption, whereas calcitonin may affect both the osteoclast resorption and osteoblast formation of bone. Estrogens exert their effects on bone by decreasing the production of interleukin-6 (which increases bone resorption) in the bone microenvironment. Additionally, estrogens increase the production of osteoprotegerin, a protein that decreases bone resorption (170).

Low Back Injuries

A leading cause of missed days in the workplace, acute low back pain has not yet received the scientific inquiry and educational priority that it deserves. A recent report revealed that treatment from family physicians, orthopedists, and chiropractors had equal success in resolving uncomplicated acute low back pain (171). However, ambulatory patients surveyed in the study were significantly more satisfied with the care they received from chiropractors, probably because of the chiropractors' more thorough physical examination and patient education efforts. This study's conclusions should not be surprising because undergraduate and resident medical education programs have not adequately stressed orthopedic examination and patient education techniques. The Agency for Health Care Policy and Research published clinical guidelines for the evaluation and management of acute low back pain (172). Authorities propose that prevention programs emphasizing weight reduction, proper lifting techniques, ergonomic design of the home and workplace, and strengthening and flexibility enhancement will reduce the incidence of this common illness.

Overuse Injuries

Sports-related and work-related overuse injuries present principally in ambulatory medical settings. Therefore, primary medical care providers should be familiar with their evaluation and management.

SPORTS

Exercise is an important risk reducer for the chronic diseases mentioned above. Providers should know how to manage the adverse reactions (overuse injuries) of an exercise prescription, just as they should know how to manage the adverse reactions of medication. Common running and walking overuse injuries include metatarsal and tibial stress fractures, metatarsalgia, Morton neuroma, shin splints, patellofemoral pain syndrome, infrapatellar tendinitis, Achilles tendinitis, pes anserine bursitis, and iliotibial band friction syndrome. Although overuse injuries of the lower extremities are usually precipitated by improper training techniques and excessive exercise duration or intensity, sports medicine practitioners now know that the root cause is often a biomechanical imbalance such as overpronation and inflexibility (173). Thus, a working knowledge of strength and flexibility assessment, biomechanical foot disorders, and proper athletic shoe prescription is an essential requirement of the modern primary-care provider.

REPETITIVE INJURIES IN THE WORKPLACE

Because primary-care providers aim to view patients in the full context of their home and work, occupational medicine issues are an integral component of comprehensive health care. For example, our "keyboard society" has hastened a dramatic increase in the reporting of carpal tunnel syndrome cases. Primary-care providers must become well versed in the assessment, conservative treatment, and knowledgeable referral of patients with carpal tunnel syndrome and other work-related repetitive injuries.

Trauma-Related Injuries

MOTOR VEHICLE INJURIES

In 1998, motor vehicle crash-related injuries were the seventh-leading cause of death in the United States (174). In 2000, the cost of unintentional injuries totaled $512.4 billion, with motor vehicle injuries being responsible for almost half of this cost ($201.5 billion) (174). Motor vehicle fatality rates are highest for young and elderly adults, whereas injury rates peak in young adulthood (174,175). Although alcohol-related traffic fatality rates have declined by more than one-third since 1979 (176), alcohol use remains an important risk factor for motor vehicle injuries. Evidence also indicates that impairment with drugs other than alcohol also may play an important role in traffic injuries and deaths, although the relationship is not as well defined as for alcohol. In addition to driving while impaired by alcohol or drugs, failing to use occupant protection (e.g., safety belts, child safety seats, motorcycle helmets) is also an important risk factor for motor vehicle injury (177). Substance abuse screening and intervention are likely to be efficacious in reducing motor vehicle injuries and fatalities, whereas the use of occupant restraints has been shown to reduce the risk of motor vehicle injury and death (177).

Recommendations (177) from the U.S. Preventive Services Task Force for the prevention of motor vehicle–related injuries are listed as follows:

1. Clinicians should regularly urge their patients to use lap and shoulder belts for themselves and their passengers while riding in automobiles, including automobiles equipped with air bags.
2. Operators of vehicles carrying infants and toddlers should be urged to install and regularly use federally approved child safety seats in accordance with the manufacturer's instructions and the child's size.
3. Those who operate or ride on motorcycles should be counseled to wear approved safety helmets.
4. All patients should be counseled regarding the dangers of operating a motor vehicle while under the influence of alcohol or other drugs, as well as the risks of riding in a vehicle operated by someone who is under the influence of these substances.

HOUSEHOLD AND RECREATIONAL INJURIES

Unintentional injuries accounted for nearly 97,300 deaths in the United States in 2000, more than half of these being related to household, recreational, and other etiologies unrelated to motor vehicles (174). Falls, poisoning, fires and burns, drowning, suffocation and aspiration, firearms, and bicycling cause nearly two-thirds of these deaths (174). Almost 90% of deaths relating to sports and recreation occur during swimming, boating, bicycling, riding off-road vehicles such as all-terrain vehicles, or using firearms (174). All of the above are also common causes of nonfatal injuries, with falls being the most common (177).

Recommendations (177) from the U.S. Preventive Services Task Force for the prevention of household and recreation related injuries are listed as follows:

1. Parents should be counseled on measures to reduce the risk of unintentional injuries to their children from residential fires and hot tap water, drowning, poisoning, bicycling, firearms, and falls.
2. Homeowners should install smoke detectors and carbon monoxide detectors in appropriate locations and test the devices periodically to ensure proper operations. Encourage the use of flame-resistant nightwear during sleep, and reduce or cease smoking in the home.
3. Households are advised to keep a 1-ounce bottle of ipecac, display the telephone number of the local poison control center, and place all medications, toxic substances, and matches in child-resistant containers.
4. Bicyclists and parents of children who ride bicycles should be counseled about the importance of wearing approved safety helmets and avoiding riding bicycles in motor vehicle traffic.
5. Families should be encouraged to install fences with gates around swimming pools.
6. All windows that pose high risk for falls should have window guards.
7. All residents of homes with swimming pools, young children, or elderly persons should be encouraged to learn cardiopulmonary resuscitation and maneuvers to manage choking incidents.
8. All firearms should be removed from the home or at a minimum kept unloaded in a locked compartment separated from the ammunition.
9. Elderly patients should be counseled on measures to reduce the risk of falling, including exercise (particularly training to improve balance), safety-related skills and behaviors, and environmental hazard reduction, along with monitoring and adjusting medications.

Organization of the Medical Care Team

Managed care has dramatically and irrevocably changed the delivery of health care in the United States. Managed-care organizations now carefully define the roles of their primary-care providers and specialty providers. Powerful practice-management computer databases are being developed that track patient populations, case mix and levels of service acuity, resource utilization, prescribing patterns, referral patterns, individual practice profiles, and treatment outcomes. Individual practices, regional health-care systems, and Fortune 500 health-care conglomerates are implementing continuous quality improvement programs.

A concept in managed-care delivery that depends on continuous quality improvement for its success is called disease-state management (178). This health-care organization model targets high-cost and high-volume diagnoses and those conditions that tend to have wide variations in provider practices and resource utilization. The intention of disease-state management is to improve outcomes while maintaining or lowering overall costs. The process of disease-state management must include evidence-based clinical policies, an accurate and complete database that can measure the well-defined outcomes, and a team-oriented, multidisciplinary approach. The multidisciplinary approach will require careful and extensive communication between generalist and specialist members of the team (179). Advocates of this organizational system recognize that its success critically depends on a sophisticated information system and the rapid development of evidence-based clinical policies that focus on patient outcomes. Unfortunately, outcome studies in primary care need further development. Thus, outcome-based studies will be important research objectives for primary care scholarship.

Family and Community Issues

Primary-care providers assess and treat patients within the context of their family and community. Indeed, comprehensive longitudinal care is incomplete and ineffective without addressing the meshwork of stresses and supports that surround individual patients (178). Quality primary care addresses and explores the following family/community issues:

- The family circle
- Patient birth order
- Family genogram
- Childhood traumas, expressed and suppressed
- Family violence
- Marital history and marital stresses
- Chronic illness in other family members
- Family organization and identity (chaotic? crisis-oriented? nurturing? etc.)
- Educational level of the patient
- Educational resources available for the patient and family
- Child day-care services
- Health belief models expressed by the patient and family members
- Timing of illnesses in a patient's life-cycle stage
- Patient's work/employment history
- Co-worker stress/support

- Patient hobbies and stress relievers
- Patient's pets
- Home safety
- Neighborhood safety
- Family and nonfamily members living in the same household
- Transportation availability
- Services and support for persons with disabilities
- Financial resources
- Legal difficulties and legal aid services
- Spiritual support (and stress)
- Recreation resources
- Available community health and counseling agencies
- Self-help and support groups
- Respite care for families of the elderly
- Elderly day-care programs
- Extended care facilities
- Rehabilitative services
- Hospice

Model Programs for Providing Primary Care for Persons with Disabilities

Few models are currently in place in the United States that provide comprehensive primary care for adults with physical disabilities. Many multidisciplinary pediatric programs provide care for children with disabilities, but few of these programs incorporate long-term primary-care management. Many rehabilitation providers are currently exploring the development of primary-care programs as a response to unmet needs in their patient populations.

Barriers

There are multiple barriers to access of appropriate health-care services for adults with disabilities (25). Individuals with physical or cognitive challenges often have complex medical management needs (29). Few clinicians have had experience managing the long-term care needs of this population (21). Little exposure to the specific needs of the person with disability occurs in most primary-care residency programs. This lack of experience may result in attitudinal barriers that can impact the health-care choices primary-care practitioners make for their patients. In addition, there are major financial disincentives for physicians caring for this complex population. Rarely do the care needs of these adults fit the typical time framework allotted for outpatient visits (26,181).

Physical access to health care remains a barrier for the person with a disability. Outpatient offices may not be wheelchair accessible. Examination rooms are frequently too small to accommodate patients, their mobility devices, and their families or caretakers. Many of the staff in community-based outpatient settings are not familiar with transfer techniques, and examination tables often do not adjust to heights that facilitate transfers. This may lead to inadequate physical examinations, with patients being examined in their wheelchairs.

Lack of reliable transportation also can inhibit access to timely primary care (182). Patients without access to transportation often use the emergency room for all outpatient care, which leads to inappropriate and fragmented care as well as increasing the cost of care. This leads to a lack of adequate coordination of care, which as noted previously is an essential factor in promoting wellness and providing for optimal utilization of resources. The following will provide an overview of previously developed models for the provision of primary care to persons with disabilities.

Physiatric Model

Many physiatrists provide primary care to a proportion of their patients with severe disabilities (38). This is especially common among physiatrists who work with large numbers of patients with spinal cord injuries and traumatic brain injuries. Many of these patients are young and did not have consistent primary-care providers before injury. In addition, multiple barriers can limit the ability to establish new primary-care access after injury. Unfortunately, most of the PM&R primary-care providers do not have a structured primary-care programs that can provide a full range of primary-care services. They tend to provide medical management on an as-needed basis with coverage provided by emergency departments when they are not available. Few current PM&R providers have an adequate support system established to facilitate the provision of efficient comprehensive primary-care management.

Home-Care Model

The Wisconsin Partnership Program is a fully capitated dual Medicaid and Medicare program providing collaborative interdisciplinary care for frail elderly and physically disabled patients who are certified at a Medicaid nursing-home level of care. The program integrates health and long-term support services, and includes home- and community-based services, physician services, and all medical care. The care management team consists of a patient, their primary-care physician, a registered nurse, a nurse practitioner, a social worker, and other appropriate team members as needed. The nurse practitioner establishes a collaborative practice alliance with the patient's primary-care physician to coordinate care. The state collaborates with nonprofit community-based organizations to establish care teams and take on risk for a population of patients. Services are provided in the participant's home or a setting of their choice. As of 2002, the program was providing care for 1,280 patients enrolled at four sites (183).

Boston's Community Medical Group (BCMG) was established in 1983 as an outgrowth of the Urban Medical Group (UMG). UMG was established in 1978 by a group of Boston area physicians, nurse practitioners, and physician assistants to provide continuous primary care to inner-city nursing-home residents and frail home-bound older adults (184). In cooperation with a center for independent living, BCMG set forth to provide these same benefits to younger adults living independently with major disabilities, including spinal cord injury, cerebral palsy, traumatic brain injury, and other neurologic diseases. Many of the patients are ventilator dependent. Primary-care services are provided in the patients' homes, ambulatory-care sites, hospitals, and long-term-care facilities. A team approach is used but with heavy reliance on nurse practitioners as the providers of first-contact care and gatekeeper functions. Initially this program functioned on a fee-for-service basis via a unique contract with the Massachusetts Medicaid Program; however, beginning in April 1992, BCMG converted to a prepaid, capitated method of payment (185). The program has been able to maintain its identity as the Community Medical Alliance, serving patients with severe disabilities and acquired immunodeficiency syndrome (AIDS) while becoming a part of the Neighborhood Health Plan, a Massachusetts HMO. A pediatric program for severely disabled children in foster care is being developed.

In 2002, the program was providing primary care for 250 patients with severe physical disabilities. A primary-care physician and nurse practitioner perform an initial comprehensive evaluation of each new patient and develop a plan of medical, nursing, rehabilitation, and social work care that the nurse practitioner implements. The nurse practitioner evaluates all new medical problems and provides regular home visits. The primary-care physician and nurse practitioner collaborate via regular meetings and emergency consultation. Emergency access is available 24 hours per day. The team includes a social worker and a psychologist who provides mental health and substance abuse services. A consulting physiatrist provides rehabilitation evaluations. A physical therapist provides home assessments and equipment evaluations and coordinates therapy services as needed.

Internal Medicine Model

An internal medicine model has been developed at the Anixter Center, a not-for-profit community-based agency in conjunction with Schwab Rehabilitation Hospital. The outpatient health-care center was established on site at the Anixter Center sheltered workshop and provides primary care to adults with mental retardation and childhood-onset disabilities who are living in group homes. On-site services are provided by internal medicine, psychiatry, psychology, and podiatry, with consulting rehabilitation services provided at Schwab Rehabilitation Hospital. The program also specializes in providing substance abuse treatment for persons with disabilities. Health maintenance and preventative services are provided on a regular basis, decreasing costly hospitalizations that may occur after long delays for identification and treatment of medical problems. If inpatient hospitalization is required for their clients, care is coordinated by a physician familiar with their medical and rehabilitative needs. Additional services provided at Anixter Center, adding to its holistic approach to treatment, include vocational evaluations and training, addiction recovery, independent living training, job placement, and residential and in-home support services. The program is fee for service, predominantly funded through Medicaid.

Health-Care Coordination Model

The concept of care coordination is the basis of AXIS Healthcare, a specialty disability care management organization based in St. Paul, Minnesota (186). Through a grant from the Center for Health Care Strategies, AXIS developed a voluntary care-coordination model for Medicaid beneficiaries with physical disabilities. The development of AXIS, founded in 1997, was based on the premise that the traditional managed-care approach was not a practical way to deliver appropriate, cost-effective care for persons with severe disabilities (187). Persons with severe disabilities require ongoing health care, as opposed to short-term crisis management, and usually have well-developed relationships with specialty providers. Managed care was not designed to provide either of the above but instead tends to focus on treatment of short-term illnesses and is designed to manage costs by restricting access to specialty services.

There are several unique aspects to this model, one of which is the utilization of health coordinators. the health coordinators are nurses who serve in the role of a clinical case manager. They perform initial health assessments, develop and implement a consumer-centered plan of care, respond to urgent issues or illness 24 hours a day, triage with the primary-care physician (i.e., generalist), establish a network of specialty providers, and facilitate communication and collaboration among all providers and services. The focus of the model is to provide

services that are integrated and seamless within a system that allows for the consumer to assume optimal independence and responsibility. Health-care utilization and costs within this model are also monitored to allow for comparison to the traditional managed-care approach.

The initial pilot project included 46 adults with complex disabilities and health-care needs. As a result of the success of this pilot project, the Center for Health Care Strategies provided additional funding for a much larger care coordination program for up to 500 voluntary enrollees with physical disabilities. As of 2002, the program is ongoing.

Physiatrist-Internist Collaborative Practice Model

A primary-care program using a physiatrist-internist collaborative practice model was developed at the Rehabilitation Institute of Michigan to provide coordinated comprehensive care for Medicaid patients with physical disabilities. The program focused on addressing key concerns of patient access and care coordination (188). The initial concept for the institute's model was a multispecialty, interdisciplinary model with specialty physicians on site in the clinic on a regularly scheduled basis. As the model evolved with protocol development, it moved toward a collaborative practice model with specialty consultation as needed. Urology evaluations were coordinated on site because of the large population of patients with spinal cord injuries. The program staff were able to facilitate transfers and positioning of patients with tetraplegia, improving efficient delivery of services. The collaborative development of protocols with specialty physicians and surgeons included pathways to facilitate the efficiency of the consultation process, including preconsultation information gathering and testing when appropriate.

The collaborative team included an internist, physiatrist, and a nurse clinician. The program provided 24-hour, 7 days-per-week team access via an answering service. Patients were able to be evaluated in the clinic on an urgent basis during the week. Special arrangements with the emergency department were established to manage urgent needs at night and on weekends. The emergency department would contact the program before providing care, allowing for essential medical history to be communicated and facilitating continuity of care. This type of access was essential to triage care in a population frequently using the emergency department for primary care in the past.

One of the major lessons learned from the initial implementation of the program related to time. The time necessary for initial office visits was greater than initially expected, averaging 2.5 hours. Half of the follow-up visits lasted 15 to 45 minutes. The team clearly felt that the time spent in the initial visit, obtaining as complete a database as possible and initiating patient and family education, was the major factor in improving management of long-term primary-care needs.

The initial outcomes of the program included a focus on prevention and health maintenance, not just crisis intervention. It helped to shift patient management out of the high-cost settings of the emergency department and inpatient hospital bed into the outpatient clinic. Careful evaluation and optimization of the number of medications and frequency of administration improved compliance, especially for patients with cognitive impairments. The collaborative practice model in a rehabilitation setting allowed for the integration of functional goals into the health maintenance paradigm. The program facilitated longer-term follow-up related to achievement of vocational goals, independent driving, community reintegration, and recreation and leisure skills.

Program development was initially supported by a grant from Michigan Medicaid. Patient care was supported through Medicaid on a fee-for-service basis. As Michigan Medicaid shifted patients to capitated HMO programs, the continuation of the program would have required negotiation of a separate enhanced capitation program similar to the Massachusetts and Wisconsin models. Unfortunately, these negotiations did not occur, and the program as described above is no longer in operation. Lessons learned included that primary-care programs for persons with disabilities need to anticipate greater time allocation per patient visit than traditional primary-care models. Inclusion of the patient's support system in the primary-care process is essential to facilitate follow-through in the home and community. Cognitive deficits are a frequent impairment requiring a strong focus on patient and caregiver education.

Lastly, Rancho Los Amigos in Southern California has had a long-standing program providing primary care for spinal cord injury and stroke patients in a very similar physiatrist-internist collaborative practice model. The primary team includes an internist, physiatrist, and nurse practitioner. The physiatrist is the team leader during the acute rehabilitation phase of treatment. Once the patient becomes stable, the nurse practitioner provides first-contact primary care. Protocols have been developed for annual physicals and common complications, including urinary tract infections. The team also includes a urologist, pulmonologist, and pressure-ulcer management team. There is a specialized orthopedic clinic focusing on elective orthopedic surgery to improve function in spinal cord patients.

CONCLUSION

All of us, including persons with disabilities, want the same things for ourselves and our families: a compassionate, knowledgeable, and available physician to help us maintain our health when we are well and to manage our minor illnesses when we are sick, and the best specialists available when we have a major acute or chronic medical problem (11). In this chapter, we have reviewed some of the obstacles that those with disabilities endure to achieve the above ideal. It is not expected that the field of physical medicine and rehabilitation will be declared a primary-care specialty, nor would this be a viable solution to providing primary-care services for all of those with disabilities. However, one of the goals of writing this chapter was to provide those physiatrists who currently perform continuity of care and gatekeeper functions with some guidelines, as well as resources, to continue to provide state-of-the-art primary care. The majority of practicing physiatrists, however, do not fulfill this role.

Our health-care system is changing rapidly, and in order to assist our patients with disabilities to achieve optimal health, we need to frequently reevaluate and modify our methods of health-care delivery. The last section of this chapter provided alternatives and models for the provision of primary-care services in this population. Some of the programs have become very successful within their own health-care systems but may not directly apply to all practitioners interested in providing these services. At a minimum, rehabilitation-care providers should collaborate with existing primary-care providers, including generalist physicians and physician extenders, to achieve the goal of providing adequate, high-quality primary care for persons with disabilities. This collaboration could include educating primary-care providers on physiatric issues

and team ventures with them to provide primary care for this population.

REFERENCES

1. Williamson JW, Walters KW, Cordes DL. Primary care, quality improvement, and health systems change. *Am J Med Qual* 1993;8:37–44.
2. Health Resources and Services Administration. The fiscal year 2002 budget. *Health Resources and Service Administration.* http://newroom.hrsa.gov/factsheet.htm (Feb 2002).
3. Shi L. Balancing primary versus specialty care. *J R Soc Med* 1995;88:428–432.
4. Rosenthal MP, Rabinowitz HK, Diamond JJ, Markham FW. Medical student's specialty choice and the need for primary care: our future. *Prim Care* 1996;23(1):155–167.
5. Lishner DM, Richardson M, Levine P, Patrick D. Access to primary health care among persons with disabilities in rural areas: a summary of the literature. *J Rural Health* 1996;12:45–53.
6. American Academy of Physical Medicine and Rehabilitation. AAPM&R position on physiatrists as primary care providers. In: *AAPM&R handbook.* Chicago: American Academy of Physical Medicine and Rehabilitation, 1993: 1–4.
7. Bockenek WL, Currie DM. Physical medicine and rehabilitation as a primary care specialty? A report from the Association of Academic Physiatrists Academic Affairs committee. *AAP Newsletter* 1993:5–7.
8. *Status and future.* Health Research and Services Administration National Research Service Awards Program, 17 April 1991.
9. Institute of Medicine. *Defining primary care: an interim report.* Washington, DC: National Academy Press, 1994.
10. Hurd WW, Barhan SM, Rogers RE. Obstetrician-gynecologist as a primary care provider. *Am J Manag Care* 2001;7:SP19–SP24.
11. Bockenek WL, Currie DM. Physical medicine and rehabilitation as a primary care specialty: commentary. *Am J Phys Med Rehabil* 1994;73:58–60.
12. Brown CV. Primary care for women: the role of the obstetrician-gynecologist. *Clin Obstet Gynecol* 1999;42:306–313.
13. Rivo ML, Satcher D. Improving access to health care through physician work force reform: direction for the 21st century. Third report of the Council on Graduate Medical Education. *JAMA* 1993;270:1074–1078.
14. Rivo ML, Saultz JW, Wartman SA, Dewitt TG. Defining the generalist physician training. *JAMA* 1994;271:1499–1504.
15. Association of American Medical Colleges. AAMC policy on the generalist physician. *Acad Med* 1993;68:1–6.
16. Council on Graduate Medical Education. *Fourth report: recommendations to improve access to health care through physician workforce reform.* Rockville, MD: U.S. Public Health Service, Health Resources and Services Administration, Bureau of Health Professions, 1993.
17. Council on Graduate Medical Education. *Eighth report: patient care physician supply and requirements.* Rockville, MD: U.S. Public Health Service, Health Resources and Services Administration, Bureau of Health Professions; 1996.
18. Gabriel SE. Primary care: specialists or generalists? *Mayo Clin Proc* 1996;71: 415–419.
19. DeJong G, Brannon RW, Batavia AI. Financing health and personal care. In: Whiteneck GG, Charlifue SW, Gerhart KA, et al., eds. *Aging with spinal cord injury.* New York: Demos Publishers, 1993:275–294.
20. DeJong G. Primary care for persons with disabilities: an overview of the problem. *Am J Phys Med Rehabil* 1997;76[Suppl]:2–8.
21. Institute of Medicine, Committee on a National Agenda for Prevention of Disabilities Disability in America. In: Pope AM, Tarlov AR, eds. *Toward a national agenda for prevention.* Washington, DC: National Academy Press, 1991.
22. Bauman WA. The endocrine system. In: Whiteneck GG, Charlifue MA, Gerhart KA, et al., eds. *Aging with spinal cord injury.* New York: Demos Publications, 1993:275–294.
23. DeJong G, Palsbo S, Beatty P, et al. The organization and financing of health services for individuals with disabilities. *Milbank Q* 2002 (in press).
24. American Congress of Rehabilitation Medicine. Addressing the post-rehabilitation health care needs of persons with disabilities. *Arch Phys Med Rehabil* 1993;74[Suppl]:8–14.
25. DeJong G, Batavia A, Griss R. America's neglected health minority: working age persons with disabilities. *Milbank Q* 1989;67[Suppl 2]:311–351.
26. Burns TJ, Batavia AI, Smith QW, DeJong G. The primary health care needs of persons with physical disabilities: what are the research and service priorities? *Arch Phys Med Rehabil* 1990;71:138–143.
27. Gans BM, Mann NR, Becker BE. Delivery of primary care to the physically challenged. *Arch Phys Med Rehabil* 1993;74[Suppl]:15–19.
28. Batavia AI, DeJong G, Burns TJ, et al. *A managed care program for working-age persons with physical disabilities: a feasibility study.* NRH Research Center. Washington, DC: Robert Wood Johnson Foundation, 1989.
29. Batavia A, DeJong G, Halstead L. Primary medical services for people with disabilities. *Am Rehabil* 1989;14:4, 9–12, 26–27.
30. Brannon R, Naierman N, DeJong G. Unpublished report to the Robert Wood Johnson Foundation. Washington, DC: National Rehabilitation Hospital Research Center, 1990.
31. Palsbo S. A call for disability literacy. *SCI Life* 2002(spring):14–15.

32. DeJong G, Frieden L. It's not just managed care; it's the larger health care system. *Research Update.* Washington, DC: National Rehabilitation Center for Health and Disability Research, spring supplement, 2002.

33. O'Day B, Palsbo S, Dhont K, Sheer J. Health plan selection and assessment criteria by consumers with mobility impairments: implications for report cards and the CARPS project. *Med Care* 2002 (in press).

34. Beatty P, Dhont K. Medicare health maintenance organizations and traditional coverage: perceptions of health care among beneficiaries with disabilities. *Arch Phys Med Rehabil* 2001;82(8):1009–1017.

35. Neri M, Beatty P, Dhont K. Individuals with disabilities are less likely to have the primary care doctor of their choice—especially in managed care. *Health and Disability Data Brief.* Washington DC: National Rehabilitation Hospital Center for Health and Disability Research.

36. Bockenek WL, Blom JM. Health care needs assessment in a population with severe disability. *Am J Phys Med Rehabil* 1994;73:144.

37. Kindig DA, Cultice JM, Mullan F. The elusive generalist physician: can we reach a 50% goal? *JAMA* 1993;270:1069–1073.

38. Francisco GE, Chae JC, DeLisa JA. Physiatry as a primary care specialty. *Am J Phys Med Rehabil* 1995;74:186–192.

39. Mullan F. The case for more U.S. medical students. *N Engl J Med* 2000;343;3: 213–217.

40. Cooper RA, Getzen TE, McKee HJ, et al. Economic and demographic trends signal an impending physician shortage. *Health Affairs* 2002;21(1):140–154.

41. Perspectives. *Health Affairs* 2002;21(1):155–171.

42. Hogan PF, Dobson A, Haynie B, et al. Physical medicine and rehabilitation work force study: the supply of and demand for physiatrists. *Arch Phys Med Rehabil* 1996;77:95–99.

43. Buschbacher RM, DeLisa JA, Kevorkian CG. Commentary: the physiatrist as primary care provider for the disabled. *Am J Phys Med Rehabil* 1997;76:149–153.

44. U.S. Department of Health and Human Services. *Healthy people 2000* (PHS 91, 50212–50213).Washington, DC: Government Publishing Office, 1991.

45. U.S. Department of Health and Human Services. *Healthy people 2010.* U.S. Department of Health and Human Services. http://www.health.gov/healthypeople/(Jan 2000).

46. Noack H. Concepts of health and health promotion. In: Abelin T, Brzezinski ZJ, Carstairs VDL, eds. *Measurement in health promotion and protection.* Copenhagen: World Health Organization Regional Publications European Series, 1987:5–28.

47. World Health Organization. International classification of functioning, disability and health. World Health Organization. http://www.who.int/ (Nov 2001).

48. Pope AM, Tarlov AR, eds. *Disability in America.* Washington, DC: National Academy Press, 1991.

49. Patrick DL, Richardson M, Starks HE, Rose MA. A framework for promoting the health of people with disabilities. In: Lollar DJ, ed. *Preventing secondary conditions associated with spina bifida or cerebral palsy. Proceedings and recommendations of a symposium, February 17–19, 1994, Crystal City, VA.* Washington, DC: Spina Bifida Association of America, 1994.

50. Fuhrer MJ. Subjective well-being: implications for medical rehabilitation outcomes and models of disablement. *Am J Phys Med Rehabil* 1994;73:358–364.

51. National Institutes of Health. *Research plan for the National Center for Medical Rehabilitation Research.* Washington DC: National Institutes of Health, Publication No 93–3509, 1993.

52. Fuhrer MJ. The subjective well-being of people with spinal cord injury: relationships to impairment, disability, and handicap. *Top Spinal Cord Inj Rehabil* 1996;1:56–71.

53. Whiteneck GG. Outcome evaluation and spinal cord injury. *Neuro Rehabil* 1992;2:30–40.

54. Bigbee JL, Jansa N. Strategies for promoting health protection. *Nurs Clin North Am* 1991;26:895–913.

55. Lanig IS. The interdisciplinary assessment of health. In: Lanig IS, Chase TM, Butt LM, et al. *A practical guide to health promotion after spinal cord injury.* Gaithersburg, MD: Aspen, 1996:50–77.

56. National Center of Physical Activity and Disability. Executive summary of the Center on Health Promotion Research for Persons with Disabilities. Rimmer JH, principal investigator.http://www.ncpad.org/whtpprs/ch-pexecsum.htm (2002).

57. Simeonsson RJ, McDevitt LN, eds. *Issues in disability and health: the role of secondary conditions and quality of life.* Chapel Hill, NC: North Carolina Office on Disability and Health, 1999.

58. Ravesloot C, Seekins T, Young Q. Health promotion for people with chronic illness and physical disabilities: The connection between health psychology and disability prevention. *Clin Psychol Psychother* 1998.5:76–85.

59. Rimmer JH. Health promotion for people with disabilities: the emerging paradigm shift from disability prevention to prevention of secondary conditions. *Phys Ther* 1999;79:495–502.

60. Mulley AG Jr. Health maintenance and the role of screening. In: Goroll AH, May LA, Mulley AG Jr, eds. *Primary care medicine: office evaluation of the adult patient,* 3rd ed. Philadelphia: JB Lippincott, 1995:13–16.

61. Green LW, Cargo, M, Ottoson JM. The role of physicians in supporting life style changes. *Med Exerc Nutrition Health* 1994;3:119–130.

62. Cabana MD, Rand CS, Powe NP, et al. Why don't physicians follow clinical practice guidelines? A framework for improvement. *JAMA* 1999;282(15): 1458–1465.

63. Gans KM, Jack B, Lasater TM. Changing physicians' attitudes, knowledge, and self efficacy regarding cholesterol screening and management. *Am J Prev Med* 1993;9:101–106.

64. Lanig IS. Principles of effective patient education. In: Lanig IS, Chase TM, Butt LM, et al. *A practical guide to health promotion after spinal cord injury.* Gaithersburg, MD: Aspen, 1996:34–39.

65. Pololi LH, Coletta EM, Kern DG, et al. Developing a competency based preventive medicine curriculum for medical schools. *Am J Prev Med* 1994;10: 240–244.

66. Institute of Medicine, Committee on a National Agenda for Prevention of Disability in America. *Toward a national agenda for prevention.* In: Pope AM, Tarlov AR, eds.Washington, DC: National Academy Press, 1991.

67. Lollar DJ. *Preventing secondary conditions associated with spina bifida or cerebral palsy. Proceedings and recommendations of a symposium, February 17–19, 1994, Crystal City, VA.* Washington, DC: Spina Bifida Association, 1994.

68. Heim C. Health assessment. In: O'Donnell MP, Harris J, eds. *Health promotion in the workplace,* 2nd ed. Albany, NY: Delmar, 1994:219–239.

69. Centers for Disease Control. Cigarette smoking-attributable mortality and years of potential life lost: United States, 1990. *MMWR* 1993;42:645–649.

70. Centers for Disease Control and Prevention. Cigarette smoking-attributable mortality and years of potential life lost: United States, 1990, MMWR 1993; 42:645–648.

71. Centers for Disease Control. Cigarette smoking among adults: United States, 1993. *MMWR* 1994;43:925–930.

72. National Cancer Institute. Tobacco and the clinician: interventions for medical and dental practice. NIH Publication No. 94–3693. *Monogr Natl Cancer Inst* 1994;5:1–22.

73. National Cancer Institute. http://cancer.gov/cancer_information/prevention (June 2002).

74. Roberson MD, Laurent SL, Little JM Jr. Including smoking status as a new vital sign: it works. *J Fam Pract* 1995;40:556–563.

75. Rigotti NA. Smoking cessation. In: Gorroll AH, May LA, Mulley AG, eds. *Primary care medicine: office evaluation and management of the adult patient,* 3rd ed. Philadelphia: JB Lippincott, 1995:300–308.

76. Glynn TJ, Manley MW. *How to help your patients stop smoking: a National Cancer Institute manual for physicians.* Bethesda, MD: U.S. Department of Health and Human Services, Public Health Service, National Institutes of Health, National Cancer Institute. NIH Publication No. 90–3064, 1990.

77. Fiore MC, Bailey WC, Cohen SJ, et al. *Smoking cessation: clinical practice guideline no. 18.* Rockville, MD: U.S. Department of Health and Human Services, Public Health Service, Agency for Health Care Policy and Research. AHCPR Publication No. 96–0692, April 1996.

78. Williamson DF, Madans J, Anda RF, Ket al. Smoking cessation and the severity of weight gain in a national cohort. *N Engl J Med* 1991;324:739–745.

79. Weinsier RL, Morgan SL, Perrin VG. *Fundamentals of clinical nutrition.* St. Louis: Mosby Year Book, 1993.

80. Department of Health and Human Services and Department of Agriculture. *Report of the dietary guidelines: Advisory Committee on the Guidelines for Americans 2000.* http://www.health.gov/dietaryguidelines/#related (June 2002).

81. Krauss RM, Eckel RH, Howard B, Appel LJ. American Heart Association Dietary Guidelines: Revision 2000: A statement for healthcare professionals from the nutrition committee of the American Heart Association. *Circulation* 2000;102(18):2284–2299.

82. Bauman WA, Spungen AM. Metabolic changes in persons after spinal cord injury. In: Hammond M, ed. *Physical medicine and rehabiliation clinics of North America: topics in spinal cord injury medicine.* Philadelphia: WB Saunders, 2000:109–140.

83. Lanig IS. Promoting nutritional health. In: Lanig IS, Chase TM, Butt LM, et al. *A practical guide to health promotion after spinal cord injury.* Gaithersburg, MD: Aspen, 1996:205–229.

84. Figoni SF. *Cycle of disability: national handicapped sports—adapted fitness instructor handbook.* Rockville, MD:1991:2.

85. The National Center on Physical Activity and Disability. Department of Disability and Human Development; College of Applied Health Sciences, University of Illinois at Chicago. http://www.ncpad.org (2002).

86. Cooper RA, Quatrano LA, Axelson PW, et al. Research on physical activity and health among people with disabilities: a consensus statement. *J Rehabil Res Dev* 1999,36:142–154.

87. Lockette KF, Keyes AM. *Conditioning with physical disabilities.* Champaign, IL: Human Kinetics, 1994.

88. Reynolds JP. Stepping out of the medical model: fitness and physical therapy. *PT Magazine* 1993;May:24–41.

89. Rimmer JH. *Fitness and rehabilitation programs for special populations.* Champaign, IL: Human Kinetics, 1994.

90. U.S. Department of Health and Human Services. *A report of the Surgeon General: physical activity and health—persons with disabilities.* Atlanta, GA: Centers of Disease Control and Prevention, National Center for Chronic Disease Prevention and Health Promotion, the President's Council on Physical Fitness and Sports, 1996.

91. Chase TM. Physical fitness strategies. In: Lanig IS, Chase TM, Butt LM, et al. *A practical guide to health promotion after spinal cord injury.* Gaithersburg, MD: Aspen, 1996:243–306.

92. Turk MA. The impact of disability on fitness in women: musculoskeletal issues. In: Krostoski DM, Nosekl MA, eds. *Women with physical disabilities.* Baltimore: Brookes, 1996:391–405.

93. Heath GW, Fentem PH. Physical activity among persons with disabilities: a public health perspective. In: Hollszy JO, ed. *Exercise and sport sciences review.* Baltimore: Williams & Wilkins, 1997:195–234.
94. Ernstoff B, Wetterquist H, Kvist H, et al. The effects of endurance training on individuals with postpoliomyelitis. *Arch Phys Med Rehabil* 1996;77:843–848.
95. Burk J, Agre J. Characteristics and management of postpolio syndrome. *JAMA* 2000;284(4):412–414.
96. Fisher NM, Pendergast DR, Gresham GE, et al. Muscle rehabilitation: its effect on muscular and functional performance of patients with knee osteoarthritis. *Arch Phys Med Rehabil* 1991;72:367–374.
97. Penninx BW, Messier SP, Rejeski WJ, et al. Physical exercise and the prevention of disability in activities of daily living in older persons with osteoarthritis. *Arch Intern Med* 2001;161(19):2309–2316.
98. Cobb ND, Dietz MA, Grigsby J, Kennedy DM. Rehabilition of the patient with multiple sclerosis. In: DeLisa JA, Gans BM, Currie DM, et al., eds. *Rehabilitation medicine: principles and practice,* 2nd ed. Philadelphia: JB Lippincott, 1993:861–885.
99. Jacobs PL, Nash MS, Rusinowski JW. Circuit training provides cardiorespiratory and strength benefits to persons with paraplegia. *Med Sci Sports Exerc* 2001;33(5):711–717.
100. Rohe DE. Psychological aspects of rehabilitation. In: DeLisa JA, Gans BM, Currie DM, et al., eds. *Rehabilitation medicine: principles and practice,* 2nd ed. Philadelphia: JB Lippincott, 1993:131–150.
101. Fleming MF. At risk drinking in an HMO primary care sample: prevalence and health policy. *Am J Public Health* 1998;88(1):90–93.
102. National Institute on Alcohol Abuse and Alcoholism. *The physicians guide to helping patients with alcohol problems.* Washington, DC: U.S. Department of Health and Human Services, NIH Publication: 95–3769, 1995.
103. Saunders JB, Aasland OG, Amundsen A, Grant M. Alcohol consumption and related problems among primary health care patients: WHO collaborative project on early detection of persons with harmful alcohol consumption, II. *Addiction* 1993;88:791–804.
104. Saunders JB, Aasland OG, Amundsen A, Grant M. Alcohol consumption and related problems among primary health care patients: WHO collaborative project on early detection of persons with harmful alcohol consumption, I. *Addiction* 1993;88:349–362.
105. Heinemann AW, Manott BD, Schnoll S. Substance use by persons with recent spinal cord injuries. *Rehabil Psychology* 1990;35:217–228.
106. McKinley WO, Kolakowsky, Kreutzer JS. Substance abuse, violence and outcome after traumatic spinal cord injury. *Am J Phys Med Rehabil* 1999;78(4):306–312.
107. Wells S, Macdonald S. Relationship between alcohol consumption patterns and car, work, sports and home accidents for different age groups. *Accid Anal Prev* 1999;31(6):663–665.
108. Hanna EZ. Approach to the patient with alcohol abuse. In: Goroll AH, May LA, Mulley AG Jr., eds. *Primary care medicine: office evaluation of the adult patient,* 3rd ed. Philadelphia: JB Lippincott, 1995:1044–1053.
109. Preventive Services Task Force. *Guide to clinical preventive services,* 2nd ed. Baltimore: Williams & Wilkins, 1996.
110. Ewing JA. Detecting alcoholism: the CAGE questionnaire. *JAMA* 1984;252:1905–1907.
111. Kitchens JM. Does this patient have an alcohol problem? *JAMA* 1994;272:1782–1787.
112. Selzer ML. The Michigan Alcoholism Screening Test: the quest for a new diagnostic instrument. *Am J Psychiatry* 1971;127:1653–1658.
113. Porkony AD, Miller BA, Kaplan HB. The brief MAST: a shortened version of the Michigan Alcoholism Screening Test. *Am J Psychiatry* 1972;192:3.
114. Institute of Medicine, Division of Mental Health and Behavioral Medicare. *Broadening the base of treatment for alcohol problems.* Washington, DC: National Academy Press, 1990.
115. Rankin JG, Ashley MH. Alcohol-related problems. In: Last JM, Wallace RB, eds. *Public health and preventive medicine,* 12th ed. East Norwalk, CT: Appleton & Lange, 1992:1039–1975.
116. U.S. Preventive Services Task Force. *Guide to clinical preventive services: an assessment of the effectiveness of 169 interventions. Report of the U.S. Preventive Services Task Force.* Baltimore: Williams & Wilkins, 1995.
117. Center for Disease Control and Prevention. *Advisory committee on immunization practices.* Atlanta, GA: CDC, 2001.
118. Center for Disease Control and Prevention. *Advisory committee on immunization practices.* Atlanta, GA: CDC, 2002.
119. American Stroke Association. What is stroke? http://www.strokeassociation.org/presenter.jhtml?identifier=2528.
120. National Heart, Lung and Blood Institute. Cardiovascular information for health professionals. http://www.nhlbi.nih.gov/health/prof/heart/hbp/hbpstmt/index.htm.
121. U.S. Preventive Services Task Force. *Guide to clinical preventive services,* 2nd ed. Screening for Hypertension, 1996. http://www.ahrq.gov/clinic/uspstf/uspshype.htm.
122. National Institutes of Health: National Heart, Lung and Blood Institute. *The sixth report of the Joint National Committee on Detection, Evaluation and Treatment of High Blood Pressure.* Bethesda, MD: National Institutes of Health, NIH Publications No. 98–4080.
123. NHLBI. *The sixth report of the Joint National Committee on Detection, Evaluation and Treatment of High Blood Pressure.* http://www.nhlbi.nih.gov/guidelines/hypertension/jnc6.pdf.
124. The Diabetes Control and Complications Trial Research Group. The effects of intensive treatment of diabetes on the development and progression of long-term complications in insulin-dependent diabetes mellitus. *N Engl J Med* 1993;329:977–986.
125. Turner RC. The U.K. Prospective Diabetes Study: a review. *Diabetes Care* 1998;21[Suppl 3]:C39–43.
126. U.S. Preventive Services Task Force. *Guide to clinical preventive services,* 2nd ed., 1996. Screening: Metabolic, Nutritional and Environmental Disorders, Diabetes Mellitus. http://www.ahcpr.gov/clinic/cpsix.htm.
127. U.S. Preventive Services Task Force. Guide to clinical preventive services, 2nd ed., 1996. Screening: Metabolic, Nutritional and Environmental Disorders, Diabetes Mellitus. http://www.ahcpr.gov/clinic/cpsix.htm.
128. *Diabetes Care* 2002;25:S21–S24.
129. Marschner IC, Colquhoun D, Simes RJ, et al. Long-term risk stratification for survivors of acute coronary syndromes: results from the Long-term Intervention with Pravastatin in Ischemic Disease (LIPID) Study. *J Am Coll Cardiol* 2001;38(1):56–63.
130. Shepherd J. The West of Scotland Coronary Prevention Study: a trial of cholesterol reduction in Scottish men. *Am J Cardiol* 1995;28;76(9):113C–117C.
131. Downs JR, Clearfield M, Weis S, et al. Primary prevention of acute coronary events with lovastatin in men and women with average cholesterol levels: results of AFCAPS/TexCAPS. Air Force–Texas Coronary Atherosclerosis Prevention Study. *JAMA* 1998;279(20):1615–1622.
132. U.S. Preventive Services Task Force. Guide to clinical preventive services, 2nd ed., 1996. Screening: High Blood Cholesterol and Other Lipid Abnormalities. http://www.ahcpr.gov/clinic/cpsix.htm.
133. National Cholesterol Education Program. *Third report of the Expert Panel on the Detection, Evaluation and Treatment of High Blood Cholesterol in Adults (Adult Panel Treatment Panel III).* http://www.nhbli.nih.gov/guidelines/cholesterol/profmats.htm.
134. Kuczmarski RJ, Carroll MD, Flegal KM, Troiano RP. Varying body mass index cutoff points to describe overweight prevalence among U.S. adults: NHANES III (1988 to 1994). *Obes Res* 1997;5(6):542–548.
135. Pi-Sunyer FX. Medical hazards of obesity. *Ann Intern Med* 1993;119:655–660.
136. Manson JE, Colditz GA, Stampfer MJ, et al. A prospective study of obesity and risk of coronary heart disease in women. *N Engl J Med* 1990;322:882–889.
137. Foster WR, Burton BT, eds. National Institute of Health consensus conference: health implications of obesity. *Ann Intern Med* 1985;103:977–1077.
138. U.S. Preventive Services Task Force. Guide to clinical preventive services, 2nd ed., 1996. Screening for Obesity. http://www.ahrq.gov/clinic/2nd cps/obesity.pdf.
139. National Cancer Institute. *Cancer facts: lifetime probability of breast cancer in American women.* http://cis.nci.nih.gov/fact/5_6.htm
140. American Cancer Society. *Statistics for cancer: cancer facts and figures 2002.* http://cancer.org/downloads/STT/CFF2002.pdf.
141. U.S. Preventive Services Task Force. Guide to clinical preventive services, 2nd ed., 1996. Screening: Neoplastic diseases: Breast Cancer. http://www.ahrq.gov/clinic/cpsix.htm
142. American Cancer Society. Statistics for Cancer. Cancer Facts and Figures 2002. http://cancer.org/downloads/STT/CFF2002.pdf.
143. Primary Care Reports. American Health Consultants. 2002;8:11.
144. U.S. Preventive Services Task Force. *Guide to clinical preventive services,* 2nd ed, 1996. Screening: Neoplastic diseases: Cervical Cancer. http://www.ahrq.gov/clinic/cpsix.htm
145. American Cancer Society. Statistics for Cancer. Cancer Facts and Figures 2002. http://cancer.org/downloads/STT/CFF2002.pdf.
146. Pignone M, Saha S, Hoerger T, Mandelblatt J. Cost-effectiveness analysis of colorectal cancer screening: a systematic review for the U.S. Preventive Services Task Force. *Ann Intern Med* 2002;137:96–104.
147. U.S. Preventive Services Task Force. *Guide to clinical preventive services,* 2nd ed., 1996. Screening: Neoplastic diseases: Colorectal Cancer. http://www.ahrq.gov/clinic/cpsix.htm
148. Lieberman DA, Smith FW. Frequency of isolated proximal colonic polyps among patients referred for colonoscopy. *Arch Intern Med* 1988;148(2):473–475.
149. Okamato M, Shiratori Y, Yamaji Y, et al. Relationship between age and site of colorectal cancer based on colonoscopy findings. *Gastrointest Endosc* 2002;55(4):548–551.
150. American Cancer Society. Statistics for Cancer. Cancer Facts and Figures 2002. http://cancer.org/downloads/STT/CFF2002.pdf.
151. U.S. Preventive Services Task Force. *Guide to clinical preventive services,* 2nd ed., 1996. Screening: Neoplastic diseases: Prostate Cancer. http://www.ahrq.gov/clinic/cpsix.htm
152. Steering Committee of the Physicians' Health Study Research Group. Final report on the aspirin component of the ongoing Physician Health Study. *N Engl J Med* 1989;321:129135.
153. Peto R, Gray R, Collins R, et al. Randomized trial of prophylactic daily aspirin in British male doctors. *Br Med J (Clin Res Ed)* 1988;296:313–316.
154. The Medical Research Council's General Practice Research Framework. Thrombosis Prevention Trial: randomized trial of low-intensity oral anticoagulation with warfarin and low-dose aspirin in the primary prevention of ischaemic heart disease in men at increased risk. *Lancet* 1998;351:233–241.
155. Hansson L, Zanchetti A, Carruthers SG, et al. Effects of intensive blood-pressure lowering and low-dose aspirin in patients with hypertension: principal results of the Hypertension Optimal Treatment (HOT) randomized trial. *Lancet* 1998;351:1755–1762.

156. Collaborative Group of the Primary Prevention Project. Low-dose aspirin and vitamin E in the people at cardiovascular risk: a randomized trial in general practice. *Lancet* 2001;357:89–95.

157. U.S. Preventive Services Task Force. *Chemoprevention: aspirin for the primary prevention of cardiovascular events.* Update, 2002 release. http://www.ahrq.gov/clinic/uspstf/uspsasmi.htm.

158. The Writing Group for the PEPI Trial. Effects of estrogen or estrogen/progestin regimens on heart disease risk factors in postmenopausal women. The Postmenopausal Estrogen/Progestin Interventions (PEPI) Trial. *JAMA* 1995; 273(3):199–208.

159. Hulley S, Grady D, Bush T, et al. Randomized trial of estrogen plus progestin for secondary prevention of heart disease in postmenopausal women. Heart and Estrogen/Progestin Replacement Study (HERS) Research Group. *JAMA* 1998;280(7):605–613.

160. Herrington DM, Reboussin DM, Brousnihan KB, et al. Effects of estrogen replacement of the progression of coronary-artery atherosclerosis. *N Engl J Med* 2000;343(8):522–529.

161. American Heart Association Media Advisory 07/09/2002. http://www.americanheart.org/presenter.jhtml?identifier=3003700.

162. The Women's Health Initiative Study Group. Design of the Women's Health Initiative clinical trial and observational study. *Control Clin Trials* 1998; 19(l):61–109.

163. WHI HRT Update. http://www.nhlbi.nih.gov/whi/hrtupd/upd2002.htm.

164. Murkies A. What is WISDOM and why should Australia participate? *Aust Fam Physician* 2000;29(8):796.

165. National Institutes of Health, Osteoporosis and Related Bone Diseases National Resource Center. *Osteoporosis overview.* http://www.osteo.org/about.html.

166. National Institutes of Health, Osteoporosis and Related Bone Diseases National Resource Center. *Osteoporosis overview.* http://www.osteo.org/newfile.asp?doc=osteo&doctitle=Osteoporosis&doctype=HTML+Fact +Sheet.

167. Kanis JA, Melton LJ, Christiansen C, et al. The diagnosis of osteoporosis. *J Bone Miner Res* 1994;8:1137–1141.

168. National Osteoporosis Foundation. *Prevention.* http://www.nof.org/prevention/index.htm.

169. Kanis JA, Melton LJ, Christiansen C, et al. The diagnosis of osteoporosis. *J Bone Miner Res* 1994;8:1137–1141.

170. Authors. Estrogens, progestins, and other agents to treat gynecologic conditions. In: Editors. *Drug evaluations,* 6th ed. Chicago: American Medical Association, 1989:xx–xx.

171. Carey TS, Garrett J, Jackman A, et al. The outcomes and costs of care for acute low back pain among patients seen by primary care practitioners, chiropractors, and orthopedic surgeons. *N Engl J Med* 1995;333:913–917.

172. Agency for Health Care Policy and Research. *Low back pain problems in adults: assessment and treatment.* Rockville, MD: Agency for Health Care Policy and Research, AHCPR Publication No. 95–0643, 1994.

173. Beatty LA. Plantar fasciitis. In: Rakel RE, ed. *Saunders manual of medical practice.* Philadelphia: WB Saunders, 1996:81.413816.

174. National Safety Council. *Injury facts, 2001 edition.* Itasca, IL: National Safety Council, 2001.

175. National Highway Traffic Safety Administration. *Traffic safety facts 1992: a compilation of motor vehicle crash data from the Fatal Accident Reporting System and the General Estimates System.* Washington, DC: Department of Transportation, 1994.

176. Zobeck TS, Grant BF, Stinson FS, et al. Alcohol involvement in fatal traffic crashes in the United States: 1979–90. *Addiction* 1994;89:227–231.

177. Report of the U.S. Preventive Services Task Force. *Guide to clinical preventive services,* 2nd ed. Alexandria, VA: International Medical Publishing, 1996:643–678.

178. American Academy of Family Physicians. A position paper on disease state management. Compendium of AAFP positions on selected health issues. AAFP, 1996.

179. Lanier DC, Clancy CM. The changing interface of primary and specialty care. *J Fam Pract* 1996; 42:303–305.

180. Benedict S. Role of the community. In: Sloan PD, Slatt LM, Curtis P, ed. *Essentials of family medicine.* Baltimore: Williams & Wilkins, 1993;31–38.

181. DeJong G. Post-rehabilitation health care for people with disabilities: an update on the 1988 white paper of the American Congress of Rehabilitation Medicine. *Arch Phys Med Rehabil* 1993;74[Suppl]:2–7.

182. Batavia Al, DeJong G, Burns TJ, et al. *Physical disabilities: a feasibility study.* Washington, DC: National Rehabilitation Hospital Office of Research, 1989.

183. Wisconsin Partnership program. www.dhfs.state. wi.us/wipartnership

184. Meyers AR, Master RJ. Managed care for high-risk populations. *J Aging Social Policy* 1989;1:197–215.

185. Meyers AR, Glover M, Master RJ. Primary care for persons with disabilities: the Boston, Massachusetts program. *Am J Phys Med Rehabil* 1997;76[Suppl]:37–42.

186. Center for Health Care Strategies, Inc. http://www.chcs.org.

187. AXIS Healthcare. http://www.axishealth.com

188. Mann NR. Primary care for persons with disabilities: rehabilitation of Michigan's model program. *Am J Phys Med Rehabil* 1997;76[Suppl]:47–49.

CHAPTER 70

Children with Disabilities

Martin Diamond and Michael Armento

The rehabilitation of children with physical impairments both resembles and differs from that established for adults. It is a challenging combination of normal child care and the best of rehabilitation intervention strategies. With the understanding that a child is not merely a miniature adult, and that specific physiologic parameters exist that either complicate or allow unique intervention opportunities, successful aid may be offered. This chapter reviews the scope of disabling disorders that occur in childhood, the specific differences between children and adults that relate to their special needs, and the basic principles of management of disabled children. The specific management of various childhood disorders will be found both within this chapter and within relevant sections of other chapters.

The various disabling disorders that occur in childhood may be characterized as congenital if they are acquired before birth and are not due to known external environmental factors during the birth or postbirth period, in which case, they are termed *acquired*. Congenital problems may be further specified by cause as either genetic or influenced by some extrinsic factor, even though the effect was expressed in the prenatal period (e.g., fetal alcohol syndrome).

Acquired disabilities usually are the result of trauma, disease, or its treatment. An estimate of the frequency of disabilities for students 6–21 years of age is presented in Table 70-1.

Developmental disabilities in children not only exert a major impact on the child's ability to function in the family and in society, but also result in 1.5 more doctor visits and 3.5 more hospital days per year than for the nondisabled child. In addition, these children typically lose twice the number of school days annually, and there is a 2.5-fold increase in the likelihood of repeating a grade in school when compared with the general population of children. The extent of this impact is much greater in children with multiple disabilities or with either cerebral palsy, seizures, delays in growth and development, or emotional or behavioral problems (1).

THE PEDIATRIC PATIENT: DIFFERENCES TO CONSIDER

Knowledge of the patterns of growth and development is essential to understanding, anticipating, and managing the difficulties that disabled children experience. In the early years, head circumference, weight, and height are important parameters to monitor. Standard tables of growth and development may be used to record and compare disabled children with the normal population (Table 70-2).

Physiologic Performance

Children vary in accordance with age and size in a number of physiologic parameters. Normal heart rate, respiratory rate, heat transfer behavior, and various chemical assessments all change as a function of age. For example, the serum alkaline phosphatase level may be elevated in an adolescent not because of the presence of an occult heterotopic ossification but rather because of normal accelerated bone growth.

The question of enhanced neural plasticity in youth remains open. Conflicting data appear in the literature to support or reject this concept, but the clinical management implications are generally well accepted: the more treatment that is administered earlier and younger, the better the outcome seems to be.

A number of neurologically mediated reflex behaviors are age and development dependent. For example, the asymmetric tonic neck reflex (Fig. 70-1) is a normal behavior when elicited at 2 to 6 months of age, but may be distinctly abnormal when it is persistent and dominant many months later.

Primitive Reflex Patterns

Because they are commonly observed in children with physical disabilities, the major primitive reflex patterns that may either interfere with or facilitate skilled motor actions should be well understood. The times of appearance and disappearance of these reflexes in the developmental sequence are summarized in Table 70-3.

The most basic proprioceptive patterns are the flexion and extension synergies of the arms and legs. In the upper extremity, the full flexor pattern is more commonly seen in central nervous system (CNS) lesions, whereas in the legs, extensor patterns are usually seen. Upper-extremity flexor patterns show shoulder adduction, flexion, and internal rotation with elbow flexion, wrist pronation and flexion, and finger and thumb flexion (Fig. 70-2). The thumb is frequently tightly adducted and flexed into the palm. The extension posture of the leg includes hip adduction, extension, and internal rotation, along with knee extension, internal tibial rotation, and equinovarus foot posturing (Fig. 70-3). In both of these postures, the fingers and toes appear to be influential in establishing the dominance of one or the other posture. It is frequently noted that forcing the toes into extension will facilitate a full flexor synergy of the

TABLE 70-1.   Number and Percentage of Students 6–21 Years of Age Served under IDEA Part B and Chapter 1 of ESEA (SOP) by Disability: School Year 1991–1992

Disability	IDEA Part B		Chapter 1 (SOP)		Total	
	Number	Percent[a]	Number	Percent[a]	Number	Percent[a]
Specific learning disabilities	2,218,948	98.7	30,047	1.3	2,248,995	100.0
Speech or language impairments	990,016	98.9	10,655	1.1	1,000,671	100.0
Mental retardation	500,986	90.4	53,261	9.6	554,247	100.0
Serious emotional disturbance	363,877	90.8	36,793	9.4	400,670	100.0
Multiple disabilities	80,655	82.0	17,747	18.0	98,402	100.0
Hearing impairments	43,690	71.0	17,073	28.1	60,763	100.0
Orthopedic impairments	46,222	89.4	5,468	10.6	51,690	100.0
Other health impairments	56,401	95.8	2,479	4.2	58,880	100.0
Visual impairments	18,296	75.7	5,873	24.3	24,189	100.0
Deaf-blindness	773	54.3	650	45.1	1,423	100.0
Autism	3,555	68.3	1,653	31.7	5,208	100.0
Traumatic brain injury	285	85.4	45	13.6	330	100.0
All disabilities	4,323,704	96.0	181,744	4.0	4,505,448	100.0

[a]Percentages sum across rows.
Reprinted with permission from Ing CD. *Summary of data on children and youth with disabilities.* Washington, D.C.: U.S. Department of Education, National Insititute on Disability and Rehabilitation Research, Office of Special Education Programs, 1993.

leg. Similarly, placing the flexed thumb in an abducted and extended position will frequently facilitate a full extensor response in the arm.

Lateral rotation of the head on the trunk produces the asymmetric tonic neck reflex (see Fig. 70-1). This is the classical fencer's posture of extension in the upper and lower extremities on the nasal side, and flexion of both limbs on the occipital side. The symmetric tonic neck reflex (Fig. 70-4) describes midline effects of flexing and extending the head on the body. Flexion of the head facilitates flexion in the upper extremities and extension of the lower extremities. Extension produces the opposite pattern.

TABLE 70-2.   Examples of Gross Motor Milestones for Comparing Disabled Children with the Normal Population

Age	Activity
2 months	Head in midline
3 months	Prone prop on extended elbows
4 months	Rolls prone to supine
5 months	Rolls supine to prone
	Infantile "swimming"
	Pivot circles in prone
6 months	Sits with straight back
9 months	Crawls on hands and knees ("creeps")
	Transitions into sit from four-point
10 months	Pulls to stand through half-kneel
	cruises
12 months	Independent ambulation
15 months	Comes to stand independently
18–19 months	Climbs into adult-size chair
21–24 months	Up and down stairs with hands on rail
30 months	Jumps clearing ground and lands on feet together
3 years	Pedals tricycle
	Climbs up stairs alternating feet
	True run
4 years	Hops, gallops (not true skipping)
	Walks down stairs alternating feet
5 years	True skipping

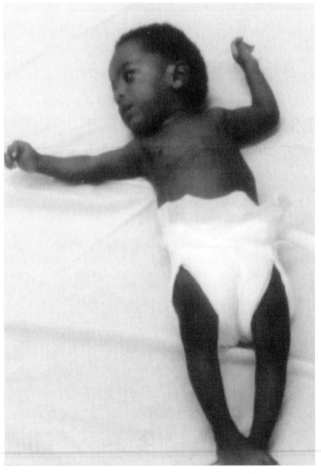

Figure 70-1. The asymmetric tonic neck reflex.

TABLE 70-3.   Normal Acquisition and Regression of Primitive Reflex Behaviors

Reflex	Age of Onset	Age Reflex Disappears
Moro	Birth	6 months
Palmar grasp	Birth	6 months
Plantar grasp	Birth	9–10 months
Adductor spread of patellar reflex	Birth	7 months
Tonic neck	2 months	5 months
Landau	3 months	24 months
Parachute response	8–9 months	Persists

Reprinted with permission from Swaiman KF, Jacobson RI. Developmental abnormalities of the central nervous system. In: Baker AB, Joynl RJ, eds. *Clinical neurology.* Philadelphia: Harper & Row, 1984.

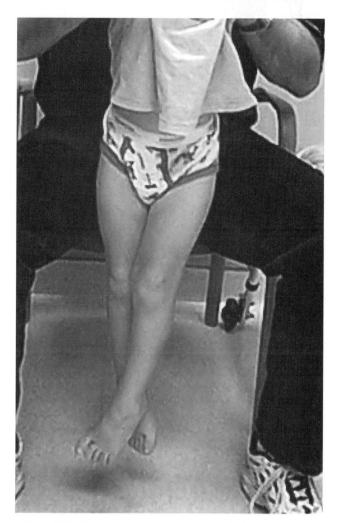

Figure 70-3. The extensor synergy posture in the lower extremity.

The vestibular system mediates static postures and dynamic postural reactions. These are important movement patterns that facilitate the development of mobility skills. The most commonly seen static vestibular pattern is the tonic labyrinthine reflex. This pattern, facilitated by the supine position of the head, demonstrates lower-extremity symmetrical extension with upper-extremity shoulder abduction and external rotation. In the prone position, shoulder adduction and internal rotation are accompanied by lower-extremity flexor posturing.

Cutaneously mediated reflex patterns include palmar and plantar grasp, elicited by tactile pressure over the respective sites.

In young infants, the stepping response is an example of a kinesthetic reflex and will be seen as a result of loading one limb (e.g., by vertical suspension) and stimulating the dorsum of the opposite foot, which is presumably a cutaneous influence as well. The positive supporting reaction occurs pathologically in older children when a loading of the suspended child's plantar surface results in a symmetric extension pattern of the lower extremities.

Child Development

In any assessment of children, one cannot overemphasize the importance of measuring performance against age-expected norms. An understanding of all areas of normal development (see Tables 70-2 and 70-3) is essential if abnormality is to be recognized (2,3).

Psychosocial Development

Frequently, children may be infantilized by family and caretakers as a response to guilt or pity for the child. Conversely, they may be assumed to be more mature than is really the case, particularly if much time has been spent in the company of adults

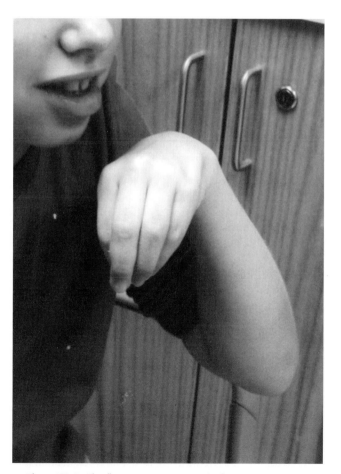

Figure 70-2. The flexor synergy posture in the upper extremity.

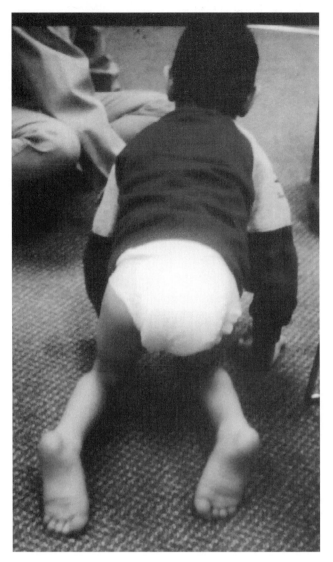

Figure 70-4. The symmetric tonic neck reflex.

in hospitals and other health-care settings and if they are verbal and articulate.

Children who grow up with a physical limitation usually do not have a sense of loss of ability. It is usually around adolescence when social sensitivity and maturity cause adaptation problems to surface. In the early years, it is important to help the child and family identify the child's strengths and abilities so that, despite the disabilities, a sense of confidence and self-worth can be built (4).

COMMON CONCERNS IN TREATING DISABLED CHILDREN

Although the disabling disorders of childhood are widely varied, they share a number of common medical issues and potential as well as active problems. These will be discussed below as well as under specific clinical conditions. Routine well-child care should not be overlooked, with careful attention paid to monitoring of growth parameters (especially weight gain, because obesity is often an added disability), nutrition, and especially immunizations, because the more seriously ill child may slip through the cracks of the well-child system and fall behind

in immunizations. Due to their particular susceptibility to infection, pneumococcal and influenza vaccinations should be given routinely.

Additional areas of medical concern will be discussed as part of specific clinical conditions as they differ somewhat in their presentation and treatment approach. These include spasticity and the various orthopedic conditions of contractures, scoliosis, and hip dysplasias (5), bowel and bladder incontinence, decubitus prevention, and gastroesophageal reflux.

There are also common functional issues. Specific management strategies vary with the particular disease, but the determination of goals and objectives is largely independent of the specific disease.

The desire and ability to communicate is the highest priority in managing a child with a disability. This allows the child to interact with his environment in spite of what may be profound physical impairment. It is also vital to remember that communication need not be vocal in nature to be effective. Gestures and signs may be used if motor control allows. As simple a movement as control of eye gaze may allow use of assistive devices as primitive as object boards or as sophisticated as computer-assisted voice output devices. What is important is not the technology but the identification of the potential for communication and the development of a system that allows a child to live up to his or her potential.

Second to communication in priority is the child's ability to control his or her motion in three-dimensional space. Frequently, children are provided with passive transportation instead of the technical ability to achieve independent mobility. From a developmental perspective, newborns start experiencing self-directed movement in space in their cribs, and a child who is crawling and creeping is acquiring substantial knowledge about the world by navigating within it. It is important not only to provide convenient transportation for parents but also to give the child control over his or her own mobility. As in communication, the devices used are dictated by whatever movement control the child demonstrates. Early prone mobility may be facilitated by wheeled prone boards, whereas once the child can be positioned in sitting, this can be replaced by caster carts and later by appropriately designed wheelchairs. For the child who is unable to propel a manual wheelchair, there are powered vehicles. Limited research has been performed that agrees with clinical observations about the age at which a child can control the powered wheelchair (6). By 18 months, the child may be able to acquire the eye-hand coordination necessary to control a wheelchair with a joystick. More sophisticated steering controls such as wafer, head, or mouth switches require more advanced developmental levels. For the child with ambulation potential, lower-extremity orthotics provide optimum positioning of pivots for safe gait, whereas upper-extremity assistive devices may provide necessary stability.

The more severely impaired children frequently need adapted seating and positioning systems to achieve a number of developmental goals. General goals include normalization of tone, symmetric positioning, and improved trunk alignment. This often facilitates use of the head or upper extremities for communication, self-care, and educational activities. Side-lying devices may facilitate function and maintain trunk flexibility for floor and bed-level activities. Adapted seats are useful for spasticity management and the facilitation of upright activities. Car seating that is safe from both a postural and a crash safety perspective gives secure travel capacity to the child and family. Standing devices allow vertical alignment, weight bearing, and experiences in the upright posture although the effectiveness in reducing osteoporosis has not been shown.

Self-Care Activities

Appropriate goal setting is most important. Infantilization will often limit the achievement of the child's potential. However, unrealistic goal setting should also be avoided. Few methods for the quantified assessment of functional abilities in children exist.

Education

Whereas vocational rehabilitation is an important consideration for the adult with a disability, special education is important to the child with a disability. The laws and services for children with disabilities vary with state and local school systems, but some common features are present. According to federal law (PL 94–142 and PL 99–457), the goals of special education are to provide "free and appropriate public education" in the "least restrictive environment" for a child. Part H of PL 99–457 mandates that participating states also provide early intervention services for children with developmental disabilities from birth to 2 years of age. Services that may variably be included in this type of educational program include special education, physical therapy, occupational therapy, speech and language therapy, adaptive physical education, psychological and social work services, and nursing services. In each case, these services become school system responsibilities in that they are necessary for the child to participate in an individualized education program, a specific educational plan with goals, objectives, definition of services, and time frames.

The role of health professionals in the special education system is an advisory and participatory one. Programs developed within a school setting should be consistent with those established out of school, in both the home and other therapy settings. School programs should not let therapeutic goals obscure their educational objectives. Programs that effectively integrate medical rehabilitation needs with those of education are the most effective (7).

Play

Children with disabilities frequently need special assistance in achieving the ability to play successfully. Recreational therapy, music therapy, art therapy, play therapy, and other interventions may be helpful in allowing a child to find mechanisms to express himself or herself and to experiment with future skills and roles.

Adapted toys and games are useful. Battery adapters that allow external switch control of any electric or electronic device may give the child with a severe disability the option to play with age-appropriate toys while possessing only limited physical skill.

Children also may need special assistance in experiencing group play. Participation in nursery school programs, playgroups, and other endeavors will allow the child to experience play with other children with and without disabilities. Parental counseling and resource identification may be necessary to facilitate these activities.

Social Skills

Children with disabilities are often found to be deficient in adaptive social skills because of a variety of factors, including limited normal childhood experiences and intensive involvement with the health-care community. Efforts may need to be taken to assist a child and family to identify specific behavioral issues and find methods to overcome them. The concept of a child having acquired learned helplessness is useful as a perspective in dealing with these issues.

As these children reach adulthood, they frequently remain in the home setting with their parents long after most young adults have elected to live independently. They also demonstrate a much higher rate of unemployment than their nondisabled counterparts (8).

Parenting Skills

Just as normal child parenting is a challenging experience, so too is parenting a child with a disability. It is further complicated by the challenges of health and social functions experienced by the child and family. Many parents need assistance and guidance in coping with what are really normal parenting issues in their care for the child with a disability.

Common problems include discipline maintenance and difficulty in setting appropriate levels of expectation of responsible behavior, and balancing the schedules of school, work, and other siblings activities. Counseling for the parents on how to distinguish the special limits and expectations that are appropriate for the disability from normal parenting issues, such as control and authority challenging, may be very helpful. Introducing families to parents of other children with disabilities is also a very positive strategy.

Sexuality

Managing the emerging sexuality of a child with a disability requires knowledge, an openness and willingness to discuss, and anticipatory strategies. Many of the early needs of these children are simply for accurate and age-appropriate information about sex and reproduction in general, as well as the child's specific abilities or limitations based on the disability. Frequently, knowledge about the child's sexual and reproductive potential is also needed by the parents.

Education and counseling for the adolescent child are often necessary. Children may express their underlying sexual concerns through other behaviors, including social withdrawal and depression. A high index of suspicion of the need for sexual education and counseling should be maintained by the involved health professional.

Independent Living

A long-term perspective on the child's potential to live independently should be adopted from an early age. Realistic goal setting is the essential first step for any long-term rehabilitation program and for attaining independence. It is frequently possible to distinguish at an early age the child who will need some type of supported living situation in the long term. Helping the family and school system to identify these expectations early on will facilitate appropriate school programming and long-term planning. For the child with a severe physical disability but with cognitive preservation, the possibility of operating an adapted motor vehicle (either car or van) should not be overlooked and appropriate, timely evaluation and training undertaken.

It is unfortunately all too frequent that we encounter a seriously developmentally disabled adult 30 to 40 years of age who lives with his or her parents until the parents become infirm or die. Many times there has been inadequate planning for legal, estate, and practical matters that suddenly become crises. The solution to these types of problems is anticipation and proper planning so that needs can be met during and after the parents' lives.

EVALUATION OF THE CHILD WITH A DISABILITY

There are several objectives to be achieved in the evaluation of a child with a disability. First, determine the type and etiology of the disability. This is based on a careful history and physical examination, including careful assessment of all areas of development from birth to present. Review of previous medical records and evaluations by other members of the rehabilitation team may be helpful to determine where and how severe developmental delays may have been. Next, assess the child's potential to benefit from rehabilitation services. In addition to biological potential, outcome may be affected by the family's adjustment to their child's disability and their ability to support the therapy program.

Evaluation by the Physician

It is essential that the physician establish rapport with the child and family members present. Young children are typically frightened by any encounter with health-care personnel. The most critical factor in obtaining useful data from the initial history and physical examination of a child is the development of a cordial relationship with the child and family as early and rapidly as possible during the interview process. The environment in which the examination is conducted must be as non-threatening as the demeanor of the physician. Toys and children's artwork are useful tools in creating such an atmosphere. The physician should present as much of a friendly image to the child as possible. Attention to seemingly unimportant factors, such as not wearing a white coat in the child's presence and sitting while examining or interviewing the child, can have a major impact on the development of a cordial relationship. Other helpful measures include smiling frequently and assuring the child that he or she is not in your office to receive shots from you. When size permits, use the parent's lap as the "examining table." In the history, a careful review of the pregnancy and birth history as well as the family history is essential. In children with acquired disabilities, detailed information about the illness or injury that produced the disability should be obtained. A detailed developmental history should be elicited. Comparing the development of the child with a disability with other normal children in the family will often facilitate this process. The administration of standard developmental assessment tests will add valuable information in identifying the specific areas of developmental delay in all functional areas.

The initial physical examination should be brief with as much of the examination as possible conducted by observation of the child. Much of this can be accomplished while taking the history. Everything the child does is a hint to their developmental levels in all areas of performance. Actual physical contact can be kept to a minimum. Considerable data regarding basic motor skills such as head and trunk control, reciprocal creeping, standing balance, and gait patterns can be obtained in this manner. Quality of movement can be easily assessed and may actually be more reliable than when performed on request (i.e. the "doctor walk" of the mildly affected child with cerebral palsy). Toy play may allow observation of fine motor skills as well as the ability for imaginative play and social interaction.

Assessment of the developmental reflex profile should be performed. Manual muscle testing is often not possible in a child less than 5 years old at initial evaluation. Observation of an infant's spontaneous movements as well as of the child during play will provide the examiner with information about antigravity muscle strength. Muscle tone should be assessed not only for the degree of tone (i.e., low, normal, or high), but also for the pattern of tone and what activities may trigger abnormal tone. Significant fluctuations in muscle tone should be noted, along with a description of factors that seem to cause the fluctuation. For example, in children with spasticity, a marked increase in tone of a given muscle may be produced by a sudden stretch of that muscle or its tendon. In children with athetoid cerebral palsy, tone fluctuations may be produced by startling the child with an unexpected touch or loud noise.

Deviations from normal range of motion in any of the body parts should be recorded. In cases in which limitation of range of motion exists, the family should be questioned regarding their observations as to whether such tightness is static or progressive and approximately how long it has been present. Monitoring of height, weight, and head circumference is an important routine assessment. Use of the normative charts for comparison purposes is appropriate. Significant deviations in the pattern of growth should be noted and explained. Difficulties in growth may be the result of chronic illness, nutritional deficiency, or chronic gastroesophageal reflux, along with a host of other specific problems.

In children of school age and above, the sensory examination, including vision and hearing, can usually be completed successfully. In younger children and particularly in infants, the sensory examination will primarily consist of the child's response to noxious stimuli such as a pinprick. The response is usually crying and/or withdrawal.

Sensorineural testing in children younger than 4 years of age will usually be limited to simple screening examinations because of the inability of the child to provide consistent responses to testing. The child's ability to follow objects with his or her eyes combined with observation of spontaneous eye movements or their absence will assist the physician in determining whether more definitive testing is needed. The child's ability to respond or localize sounds will help to make similar determinations with regard to hearing. Vision and hearing testing in infants and younger children suspected of abnormality in these functions will require the use of sophisticated measurement devices by physicians specializing in those areas. Auditory and visual brain stem response testing has proved to be very useful in assessing these functions in children too young to respond to standard screening tests. Older children can be screened for visual and auditory function using the same testing techniques used for adults.

Instruments used in the neurologic examination such as reflex hammers and tuning forks should be shown to the child before they are used. It is often helpful to allow the child to play with them before the testing.

The data obtained at the initial evaluation may be synthesized using various tools described below and used as a basis for future comparisons during the treatment process as the child grows. Commonly used screening tests for developmental assessment are the Bailey Scales of Infant Development, designed for children from birth to 30 months, and the Denver Developmental Screening Test. Both are easy to perform but are relatively insensitive to increments of developmental progress that may occur in children with severe disabilities.

Quantitative analysis of motor performance of children is accomplished by several strategies. First is the measurement of physical parameters, such as range of motion and strength, and physiologic parameters, such as heart rate and respiratory rate.

Timed trials of specific activities, such as the Jebson Taylor Hand Function test, may be useful as norm-referenced comparisons or sequential performance reassessments.

Quantitative descriptions of the functional activities of children with disabilities are essential for monitoring and planning rehabilitation programs. The few pediatric tools currently available include the WeeFIM (9), the Gross Motor Functional Measure (10), and the Pediatric Evaluation of Disability Inventory (11). In addition, the analytic tool for children with spina bifida described by Sousa and colleagues and the generally useful Tufts Assessment of Motor Performance may be used. The Tufts Assessment of Motor Performance provides a method for structured quantitative description of developmentally oriented activities that are commonly performed by children with serious disabilities.

The Rehabilitation Plan

Once the initial evaluations are completed, rehabilitation goals and a comprehensive management program should be developed at staffing conferences, involving as many members of the rehab team as possible (physical therapist, occupational therapist, speech therapist, teacher, social worker, psychologist, nutritionist, nurse, etc., and especially the child and family). Often, however, services are delivered at distant sites, and face-to-face conferencing may not be practical. Written, telephone, and even e-mail communication among treating professionals helps coordinate the therapeutic approach and avoids sending "mixed messages." The involvement of the family in daily carryover of treatment strategies is vital.

Prediction of Outcome

One of the major responsibilities of the health professional is the establishment of medical and functional prognoses for a child with a disability. From these estimates of outcome, the specific objectives and plans of management can be drawn that will guide the daily activities of the child and family. It is therefore most important to both accurately predict and be cognizant of the limits of predictability for any individual child. In general, it is important to emphasize the importance of cognition and communication over ambulation. Discussion of the child's strengths as well as weaknesses is vital. Even for the most severely impaired child, comfort and a stimulating environment should be the minimum achievable goals. The correct approach is to admit uncertainty when it exists, make cautiously optimistic predictions, and move forward with goals that at least provide for comfort and care for both the child and family.

SPECIFIC CLINICAL CONDITIONS

Cerebral Palsy

Cerebral palsy is a disorder of movement control and posture resulting from a nonprogressive lesion to an immature brain, occurring in utero, near the time of delivery or within the first 3 years of life. Although 30% to 40% of cases of cerebral palsy have no known etiology, several factors occurring at different points in time are thought to be risk factors for future cerebral palsy.

In the prenatal period, congenital infections (TORCH—toxoplasmosis, rubella, cytomegalovirus, herpes, and others), often clinically unrecognized in the mother, can cause a spectrum of involvement, from severe microcephaly, seizures, and spastic quadriplegia to mild diplegia. Gestational toxins include iodine, which may lead to diplegia, and organic mercury intoxication, which may lead to quadriplegia. Intrauterine subdural hemorrhage may cause hemiplegia (12). During the perinatal period, complications of prematurity include birth weight less than 800 g, grades III and IV intraventricular hemorrhage, prolonged seizures, and an Apgar score of less than 3 at 20 minutes. In full-term gestations, abruptio placenta, placenta previa, nuchal cord, or meconium aspiration can result in neonatal asphyxia, although recent evidence suggests asphyxia may be secondary to underlying prenatal malformations that also result in cerebral palsy. Finally, hyperbilirubinemia secondary to Rh disease, G6PD, or ABO incompatibility may result in kernicterus, with deposition of bilirubin in cranial nerve nuclei and basal ganglia resulting in athetoid (dyskinetic) cerebral palsy.

During the postnatal period, bacterial or viral sepsis or meningitis, especially within the first 6 months, can cause motor residuals. Traumatic brain injury can be due to child abuse ("shaken baby" syndrome with subdural hematoma and retinal hemorrhage), fall from heights, and motor vehicle accidents. Near drowning causes hypoxic ischemic encephalopathy. Stroke syndromes with hemiplegia may be caused by traumatic delivery as well as by cyanotic congenital heart disease (e.g., tetralogy of Fallot), clotting disorders, and ruptured arteriovenous malformations (13). Heavy metal and organophosphate ingestions can cause quadriplegia.

Clinically, gross motor delay is seen in 100%, with lack of sitting after 6 months being the most common initially recognized deficit. Poor head control may be recognized earlier in the more involved child, whereas delayed ambulation to after 16–18 months is seen in the more mildly involved. Motor delay, however, demonstrates poor sensitivity, because the overwhelming majority of children showing isolated gross motor delay will eventually develop normally.

Abnormal motor characteristics (quality of movement) are often mistaken for "early" milestones, but represent influences of abnormal tone on the child's movement capabilities, e.g., "rolling" at 2 months by opisthotonic posturing (Fig. 70-5), "handedness" at less than 1 year in hemiplegics, "walking" at 4 months by reflex steppage. Additional abnormal movement patterns include W-sitting (Fig. 70-6) and sacral sitting with posterior pelvic tilt that is due to hamstring spasticity, bunny

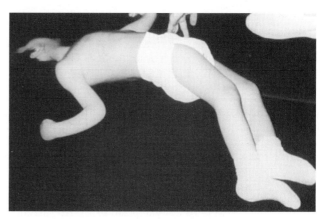

Figure 70-5. Opisthotonic posture in a spastic quadriplegic.

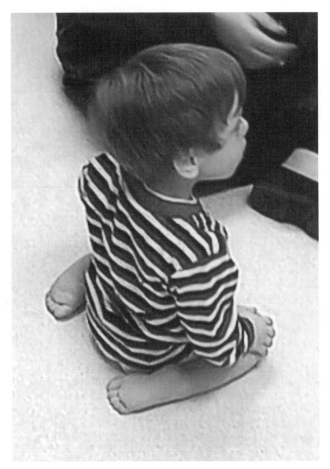

Figure 70-6. W-sitting that is due to hamstring spasticity in a child with spastic diplegia.

hop crawling and coming to stand through symmetric extension of the legs as a result of poor pelvic dissociation in diplegics, and buttock hitching in hemiplegics. As the child achieves ambulation, abnormal gait patterns (crouch gait, "jump" stance, etc.) are seen.

Alterations in tone are seen both chronologically and positionally. Early hypotonia, seen universally, gives way to later hypertonia. Hypotonia or normal tone seen when the child is supine gives way to hypertonia when posturally stressed (ventral or vertical suspension).

Reflex abnormalities include muscle stretch reflexes as well as primitive reflex abnormalities. Infants, however, tend to be relatively hyperreflexic normally, limiting the usefulness of this finding, unless associated with either asymmetry (suggestive of a hemiplegia) or excessive spread of the reflexogenic zone (seen in severe spasticity). Hypo- or areflexia is useful, however, in the differential diagnosis of infantile hypotonia (early cerebral palsy vs. neuromuscular disease).

Primitive reflexes are body postures dictated by head position that are seen at birth, become more elicitable in the first 2 to 3 months of life, and start to fade by 4 to 6 months. Their presence after 6 months is deemed abnormal. However, the ability to obtain the reflex on every attempt or the infant's persistence in the reflex posture for more than 30 seconds is considered abnormal at any age. Commonly elicited reflexes include the asymmetric and symmetric tonic neck reflexes, tonic labyrinthine reflex, and Moro reflex. Abnormal postures at rest are often manifestations of primitive reflex patterns. Examples include

fisting with cortical thumb position, extensor thrusting of the legs with scissoring, and asymmetric tonic neck posturing.

The differential diagnosis of cerebral palsy includes syndromes of early hypotonia (14) and developmental delay but without marked facial dysmorphisms. Two such common examples are the Prader-Willi syndrome of low birth weight, normal neonatal length, hypogonadism, small hands and feet with tapered digits, and a deletion of the long arm of chromosome 15, and Sotos syndrome of large birth weight, macrosomia with megencephaly, large hands and feet, prominent forehead, and advanced bone age. The Rett syndrome of normal early development leading to loss of speech by 9 to 18 months, stereotypic hand movements, sighing respirations, and spasticity is seen in girls only and is associated with a genetic abnormality on the long arm of the X-chromosome (15).

Metabolic disorders include endocrine (thyroid, infant of diabetic mother), amino acid (phenylketonuria), and storage disorders (mucopolysaccharidoses).

Congenital neuromuscular diseases presenting with hypotonia, hypo- or areflexia, and delayed motor development can be confused with the early hypotonic phase of cerebral palsy. Examples include infantile Werdnig-Hoffman disease, congenital muscular dystrophy, congenital myotonic dystrophy, hereditary motor/sensory neuropathies, etc. These will be discussed in greater depth later in this chapter.

Progressive central nervous system diseases may mimic cerebral palsy until the appearance of neurologic deterioration. Examples include metachromatic leukodystrophy, olivopontocerebellar degeneration, Friedrich's ataxia, and ataxia telangiectasia. Human immunodeficiency virus (HIV) encephalopathy, however, is the most common intrauterine acquired neurodegenerative disease.

A thorough history for predisposing factors as well as possible neurologic deterioration should be obtained. Physical examination should stress recognition of dysmorphic features (syndromes), muscle weakness, hypo- or hyperreflexia, joint malalignment, the presence of abnormal movement patterns, and the abnormal retention of primitive reflex postures. Laboratory examination should include blood and/or urine screens for amino acids, organic acids, serum lysosomal hydroxylase enzyme battery, thyroid function, and creatine kinase (CK) as indicated. Cultured skin fibroblasts for metabolic assay may be necessary if serum or white blood cell testing is unrevealing.

Electrodiagnosis allows differentiation of neuropathy from myopathy from normal with 85% to 90% accuracy for neuropathy but with only 40% accuracy for myopathy. Muscle and/or nerve biopsy as well as DNA analysis may be indicated for confirmation. Magnetic resonance imaging (MRI) and cranial ultrasound in the perinatal period demonstrating cystic periventricular leukomalacia as well as ventricular enlargement may be predictive of disabling cerebral palsy (16,17). CNS imaging studies are also useful in ruling out anteriovenous malformation (AVM) or tumor in hemiplegia of unclear etiology.

Classification of cerebral palsy is by tonal type and part of body involved. Spastic cerebral palsy comprises 70% to 85% of cases, with further subdivision based on the topographic distribution of the spasticity. Hemiplegia, diplegia, and quadriplegia account for about 90% of the patients suffering from spastic cerebral palsy with each contributing equally. Triplegia and monoplegia account for the other 10% of the patients suffering from spastic cerebral palsy.

Hemiplegia may result from focal perinatal injury and has the highest incidence of computerized axial tomography (CAT)/MRI abnormalities, usually in the distribution of the middle cerebral artery. The most common presentation is failure to use the involved hand, although hitching on the buttocks rather than crawling on hands and knees is also seen. The arm is invariably more involved than the leg. Sensory deficits are difficult to evaluate in children younger than 4 years and are likely underappreciated (18). Ambulation is usually achieved by 2 years unless severe retardation is an associated finding. Growth retardation of the affected side and an associated parietal lobe syndrome are seen in 50%. Initial seizures may occur as late as 5 years old. Long-term disability is usually more cosmetic than functional.

Diplegia represents the most common type of cerebral palsy seen in preterm babies. There is disproportionate involvement of the legs, although upper-extremity abnormalities, manifested as motor perceptual dysfunction, are very common. Most diplegics eventually ambulate, although both lower-extremity orthoses and upper-extremity devices may be required and distances covered vary.

Triplegia presents with relatively symmetric involvement of the legs and marked asymmetric involvement of the arms.

Quadriplegics, also termed "total body involved," have the highest incidence of significant cognitive disability, with 25% severely involved, 50% moderately involved, and 25% mildly involved. Legs are usually more involved than arms, with asymmetries not unusual. A brief period of hypotonia giving way to early spasticity is usually a poor prognostic sign for independent mobility.

Dyskinetic (athetoid/dystonic) cerebral palsy accounts for 5% to 8% of cases. In the past, most cases were associated with kernicterus that was due to Rh disease. Athetosis, dysarthria, sensorineural deafness, and paralysis of upward gaze were the usual signs; intelligence was often normal, because the cerebral cortex was spared. Today, dyskinetic cerebral palsy is more commonly seen as part of the picture of diffuse hypoxia and may be associated with spasticity, seizures, and retardation (19). The period of hypotonia is usually longer, from 18 to 36 months, before the abnormal movement disorder appears.

Rarer types include atonic (hypotonic) and ataxic cerebral palsy. The latter is usually associated with hypotonia. If spasticity is present, progressive CNS diseases, such as Friedrich's ataxia, must be ruled out.

PROGNOSIS FOR AMBULATION IN CEREBRAL PALSY

"Will my child walk?" is usually the question asked most frequently by parents of a newly diagnosed cerebral palsy child. In the discussion that would follow, one must clarify not only distances involved (household versus community), but also the quality of the gait and need for both orthoses and upper-extremity assistive devices. Several clinical factors are relevant. The clinical type of cerebral palsy is important. All patients with hemiplegic cerebral palsy will walk, as will those with true ataxic cerebral palsy, whereas patients with atonic cerebral palsy usually will not walk. Quadriplegics, diplegics, and dyskinetics vary. Molnar and Gordon have shown that if independent sitting occurs by 2 years, prognosis for ambulation is good (20). Badell felt that ability to crawl on hands and knees by 1.5 to 2.5 years was a good prognostic sign (21). Persistence of three or more primitive reflexes at 18 to 24 months is a poor prognostic sign (22). Recently, the ability to transition from supine to prone by 18 months was shown to be a predictor of independent ambulation in spastic diplegics (23). Marginal ambulators during childhood may lose functional ambulation during or after adolescence as a result of progressive orthopedic deformity, insufficient muscle power, or control to accommodate increased height and weight and social/emotional

problems. Combinations of independent ambulation and use of wheeled mobility for greater distances should be introduced. Power mobility as a means of independent function should not be delayed; children as young as 3 years can learn to "drive" (24). Parental negative feelings are rapidly replaced by positive ones once independent movement and its effect on the child are observed (25).

ASSOCIATED DISABILITIES

Mental retardation of moderate to severe degree is seen in one-third of patients with cerebral palsy, mildly in another one-third, with the remaining one-third showing normal intelligence. In the latter group, fewer than expected fall into the superior range. Pure dyskinetics as a rule are the brightest, whereas atonics and quadriplegics are most involved. Retardation is usually mild in diplegics and hemiplegics and may be confused with learning disabilities. Preservation of receptive language skills is a better indicator of good cognitive function than expressive language. Hearing loss should be ruled out before making judgments regarding receptive skills. Early educational intervention is a reasonable, if unproven, "treatment" and has been mandated by law (PL 99–457, 1986).

Seizures are seen in up to 35% to 40% (26) and are most common in patients with postnatal hemiplegic and quadriplegic cerebral palsy at about 60% to 70%. Seizures are rarer in patients with dyskinetic and diplegic cerebral palsy at 25% to 33%. Imaging may be considered to rule out structural lesions, and electroencephalgram characterization is useful. Anticonvulsant management is similar to those patients with idiopathic epilepsy, although the risk of breakthrough seizures when medications are discontinued after being seizure free for 2 years is higher in children with hemiplegic cerebral palsy (approximately 60%) than in children without cerebral palsy(40%). Children with diplegic cerebral palsy have a low rate of breakthrough (approximately 14%) (27).

Abnormal vision is seen in 50%. Muscle imbalances cause esotropia, exotropia, or hyperopia and are most frequent in children with diplegic and quadriplegic cerebral palsy. Secondary amblyopia can occur. Homonymous hemianopsia can be seen in patients with hemiplegic cerebral palsy. Paralysis of upward gaze is seen in children with pure dyskinetic cerebral palsy. Nystagmus is seen in patients with ataxic cerebral palsy. Defective tracking can be seen in all types. Most importantly, the possibility of refractory errors as a cause of poor vision should not be overlooked. This is twice as common in children with spastic cerebral palsy as in those with dyskinetic cerebral palsy. Surgical correction of muscle imbalances is mostly cosmetic; optometric "exercises" are controversial, with little evidence of lasting improvement.

Hearing loss may be conductive as a result of abnormal eustachian tube function secondary to palatal distortion or sensorineural deafness that is due to aminoglycoside treatment during the neonatorum. Early assessment is possible with brainstem auditory responses, although this modality assesses high frequencies only and is subject to false positives in the first 6 months. Amplification of bilateral loss is justified.

Dental problems include malocclusions and enamel dysplasias secondary to palatal distortions and abnormal oromotor reflexes (suckle/swallow, tonic bite, rooting, etc.). Inappropriate administration of tetracycline in the newborn nursery is an avoidable cause of enamel dysplasia. Children with cerebral palsy are also at increased risk for dental caries because of poor handling of secretions and food and chronic drooling. This can be a source of pain, leading to increased agitation, worsened spasticity, and greater difficulty in parental handling. The adverse social implications for the child are obvious. Early dental treatment before 3 years old is therefore vital. Anticholinergic treatment, including scopolamine patching for drooling, holds promise, with several studies showing consistent long-term decrease. Potential side effects include constipation, urinary retention, and mood changes, all reversible with discontinuing medication. Most recently, botulinum toxin injection into the parotid glands has been tried, with effects lasting up to 4 months reported (28).

Increased risk of respiratory infections is due to both extrinsic (abnormally high tone and poor control over chest muscles, leading to poor sigh and cough mechanisms) and intrinsic (bronchopulmonary dysplasia) reasons. Early antibiotic treatment is justified. Malnutrition is more common in moderately to severely involved children but can also affect the more mildly involved (29). Abnormal oral motor function affects ability to handle food, with a resulting increased risk of aspiration. The effect of poor feeding skills on survival to adulthood is profound (30). Disordered gastrointestinal motility with reflux proximally and poor transit time distally is seen. Video swallow studies with multiple temperatures and textures of food may define abnormal mechanisms, but the question of relevance to everyday feeding situations has been raised. For many children, gastrostomy tube placement not only improves nutrition but resolves the tension associated with feeding, thereby improving social emotional conditions.

A "neurogenic" bladder can occur in the face of normal sensation and takes the form of either a disinhibited bladder or a spastic dyssynergic bladder because of external sphincter spasticity coupled with uncontrolled spastic detrusor contraction. Abnormal urodynamic studies have been seen in more than 85% of symptomatic patients. Similarly, spasticity of the external anal sphincter can lead to difficult initiation of bowel evacuation and secondary constipation. Cutaneous stimulation and sacral cleft massage may be useful. Ditropan for the spastic detrusor may also be helpful (31).

Behavior disorders include true emotional lability as part of an organic pseudobulbar palsy consisting of dysarthria, drooling, and poor chewing. Attention deficit disorder with hyperactivity may be seen. Poor peer acceptance leading to a negative self-image, school phobia, depression, and anger may be exacerbated during normal periods of transition; i.e., preschool to kindergarten and early adolescence. The more mildly physically involved child may actually have more social and peer group difficulties than the severely involved, wheelchair-bound patients with quadriplegic cerebral palsy (e.g., spastic hand posturing, lurching "effeminate" gait, etc.). Limited participation in school results from both physical impairment as well as cognitive-behavioral abnormalities (32). Psychosocial support, including psychotherapy, is indicated as soon as a problem is identified.

THERAPY IN THE MANAGEMENT OF CEREBRAL PALSY
The multidisciplinary management of the motor handicap in children with cerebral palsy maximizes potential but does not "cure" brain damage.

"Physical" therapy consists of a hands-on approach by physical, occupational, and speech therapists to improve gross motor, fine motor and oromotor function. Developed in the early 1960s by the Bobaths, neurodevelopmental therapy (33), the most popular "system" of therapy in use today, emphasizes hands-on facilitation of movement and positioning to "normalize" tone and reduce the influence of abnormal postures (including primitive reflexes). This can be further assisted by the use of positioning aids: side-liers, adaptive seat inserts, prone standers, etc.

Conductive education (34), developed at the Peto Institute in Hungary, has received recent support as a system capable of "treating" many children in a non–staff-intensive setting. "Educators" or "conductors" encourage spontaneous achievement of motor activity without regard for abnormal quality of movement. The end is more important than the means. Additional therapy systems include craniosacral manipulation, hyperbaric oxygen (35), and various electrical stimulation systems, both functional electrical stimulation (36) and threshold electrical stimulation (37,38). No system of therapy has been objectively shown to result in a greater degree of improved motor function than that expected with a program of passive range of motion only (39). The role of progressive resistive exercises for strengthening has been questioned, although increased spasticity has not been seen. Although strength could be increased, the extent of functional improvement was not clear (40).

Bracing goals include reduction of abnormal tone, avoidance of deformity, and facilitation of normal movement patterns. Lightweight plastics are widely used and include aquaplast (low temperature, softer, direct fabrication possible) and polypropylene (high temperature, more rigid, fabricated from cast mold). Where metal components are necessary, lighter weight alloys have replaced steel.

In the lower extremities, inframalleolar and supramalleolar orthoses are used to control primarily foot and talocalcaneal alignment with little direct tibio-talar control (41). Ankle foot orthoses add direct tibio-talar control and indirect control of the knee. Setting the ankle in neutral to slight dorsiflexion promotes heel strike and limits knee recurvatum. Articulated ankle foot orthoses allow setting of a plantar-flexion stop while allowing free dorsiflexion and promote active use of anterior tibialis as well as passive dorsiflexion necessary in stair-climbing, crouching, and half-kneeling. The addition of twisters (either rod or elastic) attached to a pelvic belt adds an element of control over hip internal or external rotation. Floor reaction ankle foot orthoses, with the ankle set at neutral dorsiflexion and molded anteriorly to just below the patella, limit crouch gait secondary to hamstring spasticity. Posterior leaf spring orthoses are solid ankle orthoses, thinned posteriorly to simulate push-off at the end of stance phase, following passive dorsiflexion in early to midstance. Knee-ankle-foot orthoses add direct control over knee flexion and extension as well as varus and valgus, but add bulk and weight. Similarly, hip-knee-ankle-foot orthoses (HKAFOs) add control over hip position. Neither of the latter two braces significantly improves gait capability, but do prevent deformity and may facilitate standing. Use of ratchet joints may allow for gradual reduction of flexion contractures over lengthy time periods.

The primary use of upper extremity orthoses is to prevent fixed deformity. Minimal improvement in hand function is seen. The cortical thumb loop orthosis, a simple fabric loop providing pressure into the thenar eminence, promotes abduction and extension of the thumb and facilitates thumb-opposed grasp. Wrist and/or elbow extension splints can be used during the day to extend reach or at night to prevent flexion deformities. More recently, restrictive casts and slings have been used on the functional upper limbs of hemiplegic patients in constraint-induced therapy or "forced use" programs with early encouraging results (42,43).

MEDICATIONS FOR SPASTICITY
By limiting the effects of spasticity, deformity can be prevented, nursing care improved, bracing better tolerated, and function

enhanced. Most commonly used medications include baclofen (Lioresal), diazepam (Valium), dantrolene sodium (Dantrium), clonidine, and zanaflex (Tizanidine).

Baclofen acts at GABA-B receptors in the spinal cord. Dose starts at 2.5–5 mg twice daily, increasing 2.5 mg per dose every 3 days. Effects can be expected by 1 mg/kg/day, although doses as high as 2 mg/kg/day may be well tolerated. Side effects include confusion, depression, weakness, gastrointestinal upset, and lowered seizure threshold.

Diazepam acts at both the brain stem reticular activating system and spinal cord. Doses start at 1–2 mg twice daily and are titrated up to the desired effect. Side effects of lethargy, urinary retention, and dependence may limit usefulness. Prompt withdrawal may cause seizures.

Dantrium acts at the level of intra- and extrafusal muscle fibers, resulting in decreased release of calcium from sarcoplasmic reticulum. Dose starts at 0.5 mg/kg/day. Weakness, fatigue, lethargy, and diarrhea are potential side effects. Liver functions and blood counts are monitored during use.

Clonidine, an α-agonist originally used to treat hypertension in autonomic dysreflexia, was found serendipitously to reduce spasticity. Dose starts at 0.05 to 0.1 mg twice daily, increasing as needed. Side effects include temporary sedation, as well as hypotension. Delivery by transdermal patches in 0.1-mg, 0.2-mg or 0.3-mg doses, each lasting 7 days, adds a measure of convenience. More recently, zanaflex, starting with 1–2 mg/day, has replaced oral clonidine.

Although medications have been shown to be capable of reducing tone, the doses required may cause significant side effects (most commonly sedative or gastrointestinal) so as to limit the amount of functional improvement realized.

Intrathecal Baclofen Infusion

Intrathecal infusion of baclofen offers the advantage of bypassing the poor solubility of baclofen to cross the blood-brain barrier, leading to cerebrospinal fluid (CSF) concentrations 30 times higher than when given by mouth. Incidence of side effects are also reduced. The intrathecal catheter is inserted by lumbar puncture and positioned at the T-10 level. The dose varies from 30 to 800μg/day and is delivered by a programmable pump implanted in a subcutaneous abdominal pouch. Changes in dose as well as mode of delivery (continuous infusion, bolus, or variable rate) can be made by transcutaneous telemetry. Although tone reduction is most significant in the lower extremities, effects on the upper extremities and trunk are also seen by upward migration of infused baclofen. Functional changes in gait and upper-extremity use can be seen (44). Potential complications are multiple and include CSF seroma, leaks, catheter kinking or dislodging, infection, and pump failure. However, the rate for any single complication is quite low (45–47). Battery life is currently up to 7 years, but replacement requires a surgical procedure. The cost of pump and its placement is approximately $25,000, with refills every 2–3 months costing approximately $750.

Injection Therapy in the Management of Spasticity

Previously used in various movement disorders (blepharospasm, spasmodic torticollis, spasmodic dysphonia), botulinum neurotoxin type A (Btx-A) has recently been used in the treatment of spasticity in children. Btx-A acts by irreversibly blocking presynaptic release of acetylcholine (ACh). Given as an intramuscular injection, the onset of effect is delayed by 24–72 hours because of a complex process of binding to presynaptic receptor sites, neuromotor junction uptake by endocytosis, and interruption of ACh-release mechanisms. Clinical effects peak at 2–6 weeks and last 3–6 months with reinnervation by nerve sprouting. Large muscles may require several injection sites. Common clinical practice allows injection of 12–14 U/kg divided among all injected muscles.

Advantages over nerve block include no need for anesthesia, no sensory side effects, and no apparent tolerance to repeated injections. Loss of effect due as a result of the development of antibodies to Btx-A has been described in adults receiving higher doses (more than 400U) every 2 to three months. In one study of 27 patients, Btx-A significantly improved positioning in severely involved quadriplegics, including those with paraspinal spasticity (48), as well as improving gait function in patients with hemiplegic cerebral palsy and diplegic cerebral palsy with severe gastrocnemius spasticity (49). In another recent study, Btx injected into thenar muscles reduced the cortical thumb and gave significant hand opening for patients with cerebral palsy. Injection of biceps and forearm flexors reduces "flexion synergy" pattern in patients with hemiplegia, but verification of functional improvement still forthcoming. Typical injection patterns and suggested doses for individual muscles are available (50,51).

Local injections of phenol or alcoholnear a peripheral nerve or muscle motor points cause chemical neurolysis, resulting in temporary decrease in tone and strength of the affected muscle. Distal regeneration from the site of injection results in loss of effect after 4 to 6 months (less for motor points). Potential benefits include prevention of deformity and improved function by facilitation of other therapies—physical therapy, tolerance of orthoses or positioning devices, etc.—and, in younger children, may buy time before requiring surgical intervention. Potential negative effects include temporary sensory dysesthesias (nerve blocks only), especially in the main tibial and upper-extremity nerves, and permanent weakness leading to deformity (e.g., tibial block leading to calcaneovalgus foot).

In the lower extremities, obturator nerve blocks (anterior and posterior branches) reduce adductor tone, diminish scissored gait, and promote passive abduction as a means of protecting hip joint integrity. Sciatic branch blocks to the medial hamstrings (semimembranosus and semitendinosus) lessen crouch gait and internal rotation postures (52). Tibial nerve blocks (and more recently, tibial branch blocks to the heads of the gastrocnemius) diminish plantar-flexion tone and allow better tolerance of ankle foot orthosis. Femoral nerve blocks diminish spastic recurvatum. In the upper extremities, musculocutaneous nerve blocks promote elbow extension and facilitate reach. Median and ulnar nerve blocks are generally avoided because of the high risk of sensory dysesthesias. Motor point injections into the forearm, wrist, and finger flexors are preferred. Except for obturator block, Btx-A is the preferred agent of choice for affecting spasticity in the muscles supplied by the above nerves.

SURGERY IN CEREBRAL PALSY

Orthopedic surgical intervention can be classified as either soft tissue or bony. Soft-tissue procedures are done at the muscle or tendon level and consist of either releases, lengthenings, or transfers. Recurrence of abnormalities tend to occur with the former two, especially if done before 4 years old (53). Transfers also tend to weaken the muscle at its new position but may balance forces across a joint; e.g., medial hamstring transfer leading to less knee flexion, split posterior tibialis transfer leading to less ankle inversion, and rectus femoris transfer to sartorius leading to less knee recurvatum (usually done in conjunction with hamstring lengthenings). Bony procedures consist of either fusions (ankle or spine), (de)-rotations (femur or tibia), or

TABLE 70-4. Orthopedic Surgical Procedure by Joint

Foot and ankle
  Tendoachilles lengthening for ankle equinus
  Split anterior tibialis transfer for inversion and dorsiflexion
  Split posterior tibialis transfer for inversion and plantar flexion
  Subtalar arthrodesis for calcaneovalgus. Often combined with
    lateral column (fifth metatarsal ray) lengthening
Knee
  Hamstring lengthening for crouch, internal rotated gait
  Rectus transfer (to sartorius or semitendinosus) to balance hamstring
    weakness and prevent recurvatum
  Tibial derotation osteotomy for internal rotation
Hip
  Psoas lengthening (intramuscular over the pelvic brim) for hip
    flexion
  Adductor tenotomy for scissored gait or early hip subluxation
  Varus derotational osteotomy for hip subluxation
  Pelvic shelf procedures (Salter, Chiari, etc.) for subluxation with
    severe acetabular dysplasia

angulations (femur). A list of specific procedures in presented below (Table 70-4). Current trend is for multilevel soft-tissue surgery (rectus transfer, hamstring lengthening, and tendoachilles lengthening) and bilateral bony surgery (bilateral femoral varus osteotomies) to avoid imbalances and asymmetries. Computerized gait analysis measuring joint kinematics, kinetics, and dynamic electromyography (EMG) is recommended by many before undertaking complex orthopedic surgery (54,55).

Intensive postoperative rehabilitation is required to maximize gains and can be started while the child is still casted. Activities include upper-extremity strengthening, tilt table to decrease postural hypotension and increase trunk control, and wheelchair and scoliosis cart ambulation to maintain cardiovascular conditioning. Once casts are removed, aggressive passive and active assistive range of motion, lower-extremity strengthening, transfer training, and gait training are begun. Generally, for complex procedures, as many as 6 months may be required before the child's preoperative functional status is regained, with further progress made for up to another year.

Selective posterior (or dorsal) rhizotomy involves sectioning a variable percentage of sensory nerve rootlets after L2-S1 laminectomy. Theoretically, this results in a decrease in peripheral excitatory influences on the anterior horn cell in a patient with spastic cerebral palsy. Favorable patient selection criteria include lack of dystonia or athetosis, preservation of functional strength independent of spasticity, presence of selective motor control, younger age (3–8 years), lack of significant joint contracture, and few previous orthopedic procedures. In addition, cognitive preservation, motivation, and positive family supports are important. Selection of "abnormal" rootlets is based on EMG (sustained contraction after a 1-second stimulation train, spatial spread of contraction to different spinal root level muscles) and clinical (briskness and overflow of contraction) criteria at the time of surgery. It is preferable not to section all rootlets at any given level. More recent studies suggest contralateral spread of the EMG response or spread to the upper body may be the most valid abnormal criteria (56). Early postoperative therapy avoids excessive hip flexion (>70 degrees), straight leg raising (>30 degrees) or trunk rotation, and passive flexion or extension in order to avoid stress on the operative site. By 6 weeks, full passive range of motion can be started, as well as functional strengthening and mobility training with or without orthoses. Small but statistically significant improvements in gait function as measured by the Gross Motor Functional Measure have been documented at 1 year after surgery (57). Additional improvement in gait function has been documented for up to 2 years, but may not be significant when compared with physical therapy alone (58).

Negative effects of selective posterior rhizotomy include hypotonia (usually transitory immediately postoperation, but occasionally lasting up to 6 months), weakness (unmasked by reduction of tone), sensory changes and bladder dysfunction (both usually of brief duration), hip dislocation (thought exacerbated by sparing of L-1 root leading to unbalance hip flexor spasticity) (59), and spinal deformity (no significant evidence of scoliosis but possibly lordosis also may be due to sparing of L-1) (60). Some centers now start selective posterior rhizotomy at L-1.

There are recent report of decreased plantar-flexor spasticity by sectioning rootlets at S-2. By doing a "pudendal neurogram" (SSEP technique) and not sectioning rootlets carrying pudendal nerve responses, bladder dysfunction was reduced from 24% to 0% (61). Results of selective posterior rhizotomy have been mixed, and there is still great controversy regarding advantages of selective posterior rhizotomy over orthopedic surgery. Additional unanswered questions regarding selective posterior rhizotomy include the need for EMG monitoring during surgery (62) as well as the role of limited selective posterior rhizotomy, either by level (only L-4 through S-1) or percentage of rootlets cut (only 25% to 35%).

Progressive Neuromuscular Disease

EARLY DIAGNOSTIC FEATURES AND DIFFERENTIAL DIAGNOSIS

With the site of pathology within the motor unit, these disorders can be classified as originating from the anterior horn cell, peripheral nerve (either myelin or axonal), neuromuscular junction, or muscle.

APPROACH TO DIAGNOSIS

In the history and physical exam, look for evidence of hypotonia with weakness, disproportionately delayed motor milestones compared with other developmental areas, and hypo- or areflexia. Laboratory tests include serum CK for primary muscle disease, although consistent elevations are seen in dystrophinopathies and inflammatory muscle disease only. Serum electrolytes (particularly potassium), organic acids (lactate, pyruvate), and amino acids (carnitine) may also be useful. Genetic testing (high-resolution banding and DNA analysis) has allowed diagnosis of many diseases based on abnormal genetic loci (Table 70-5) and may avoid the need for biopsy as well as allow for prenatal diagnosis. Electrodiagnostic studies give about 90% positive correlation with neuropathy but only 44% with myopathy. Biopsy of either muscle or nerve, done as open procedures, confirms diagnosis. H&E stain of muscle shows gross structure—size of cells, uniformity, fatty or fibrous proliferation—and histochemical studies divide cells into subpopulations of type I (light) and type II (dark) cells (APTase), and show abnormal intracellular organelles (NADH-trichrome) or accumulations of storage material (PAS). Electron microscopy gives additional resolution. Fluorescent antibody staining techniques can be used for dystrophin analysis in the dystrophies. Nerve biopsy assesses involvement of large vs. small fibers and myelinated vs. unmyelinated fibers.

TABLE 70-5. Genetic Loci of Select Neuromuscular Diseases	
Locus	**Disorder**
1q21.2-q23	Charcot-Marie-Tooth, type 1B
1q21-q23	Nemaline myopathy, autosomal dominant
4q35	Facioscapulohumeral muscular dystrophy
5q13	Werdnig-Hoffman (infantile) spinal muscle atrophy
5q13	Kugelberg-Welander (juvenile) spinal muscle atrophy
15q	Limb-girdle muscular dystrophy
17p13.1	Charcot-Marie-Tooth, type 1A
17q13.1-q13,5	Paramyotonia congenita
19q13.3	Myotonic muscular dystrophy
19q12-q13.2	Malignant hyperthermia syndrome
19q13.1	Central core disease
Xp21.2	Duchenne muscular dystrophy
Xp21.2	Becker muscular dystrophy
Xq13	Charcot-Marie-Tooth, X-linked
Xq28	Emery-Dreifuss muscular dystrophy
Xq28	Myotubular (centronuclear) myopathy
Mitochondrial	MERRF –(myoclonic seizures, ragged red fibers)
	MELAS –(encephalomyopathy, lactic acidosis, stroke)
	Cytochrome oxidase deficiency
	—Benign infantile myopathy
	—Fatal infantile myopathy

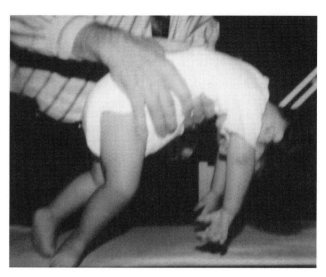

Figure 70-7. Global hypotonia in spinal muscle atrophy (SMA) I.

SPECIFIC DISEASE OF INFANTS AND TODDLERS: THE "FLOPPY BABY"

Although the overwhelming majority of "floppy babies" will eventually show normal motor development (63), nonneuromuscular causes of pathologic hypotonia should be considered (64). Early in children with cerebral palsy, clues in the history (prematurity, asphyxia, etc.) and physical exam (superimposed hypertonicity, hyperreflexia, abnormal primitive reflex profile) should arouse suspicion. Syndromes include the Prader-Willi syndrome of hypotonia, small for gestational age, typical facies, failure to thrive early replaced by hyperphagia and marked obesity after 3–4 years, hypogonadism, small hands and feet, tapered digits, and a deletion at the long arm of chromosome (15q-). At the opposite end of the spectrum is Sotos syndrome or cerebral gigantism. Characteristics include hypotonia with macrosomia, megencephaly, large hands and feet, and typical facies. Both syndromes are easily confused with congenital myopathies that are due to the hypotonia without obviously marked facial dysmorphisms. CNS infections—including bacterial and viral meningitis and sepsis, as well as botulism—cause acute presentations of hypotonia in a child who appears toxic.

Anterior Horn Cell Diseases

Spinal muscle atrophy (SMA) presents in two forms during infancy. Infantile SMA I or Werdnig-Hoffman disease is seen in 1/25,000 live births. Transmission is autosomal recessive. The onset of hypotonia (Fig. 70-7) and global weakness with facial muscle sparing within the first weeks of life is typical. Fasciculations are seen in the tongue only, and there are no joint contractures. Stretch reflexes are absent, but sensation is normal as is the serum CK. Electrodiagnosis reveals normal motor conduction velocities but markedly decreased compound muscle action potential amplitudes. Sensory latencies and amplitudes

are normal. EMG may be "chronic neuropathic," although fibrillations may also be seen. Muscle biopsy shows rounded fibers, with areas of atrophy and compensatory hypertrophy. DNA analysis reveals a deletion on the long arm of the fifth chromosome (5q13) near the area of the survival motor neuron gene (65). DNA testing is 95% reliable for diagnosis and can also be used for prenatal testing. The clinical course is progressively downhill to death in 90% by 2 years, although long-term survival is now possible with the use of home ventilator support (66,67). Rehabilitative efforts should focus on provision of appropriately supportive adaptive seating and assistive technology for mobility and activities of daily living.

Intermediate spinal muscle atrophy (SMA II, also called chronic Werdnig-Hoffman disease) has the onset of progressive weakness and areflexia later in infancy, usually after sitting is achieved. A few patients become limited household ambulators during childhood with the assistance of ankle foot orthosis and walkers. Fasciculations are more common, and minipolymyoclonus is seen. CK may be as much as five times normal and increases with age. In addition to the nerve conduction abnormalities seen in type I spinal muscle atrophy, large amplitude motor units are more frequent on EMG. A tremulous baseline in the electrocardiogram (ECG) represents cardiac muscle fasciculations and is almost pathognomonic. Muscle biopsy shows more angular fibers and type grouping. Genetic findings are similar to spinal muscle atrophy type I. The clinical course is one of gradual progression, with long-term complications of chronic wheelchair existence (scoliosis, contractures, respiratory insufficiency) leading to death in early adulthood (Fig. 70-8). Contracture prevention, early spinal bracing, and surgical correction of scoliosis are necessary to allow optimum respiratory status to be maintained. As weakness progresses, noninvasive assisted ventilation may prolong life.

Diseases at the level of the neuromuscular junction include *transient neonatal myasthenia gravis* and *congenital myasthenic syndromes.* The former is seen in newborns of mothers with autoimmune myasthenia gravis that is due to transplacental transmission of AntiChR antibodies. The onset is usually within the first 24 hours, with feeding disorders, hypotonia, respiratory distress, weak cry, and facial weakness seen in decreasing order of frequency from more than 90% to 50%. Ptosis is seen in only 15%. Diagnosis is by either Tensilon test or electrodiagnosis (see discussion of autoimmune myasthenia gravis

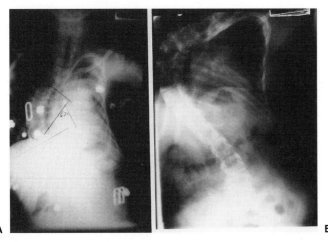

Figure 70-8. Progression of scoliosis (**A**) after 1 year (**B**) in spinal muscle atrophy (SMA) II

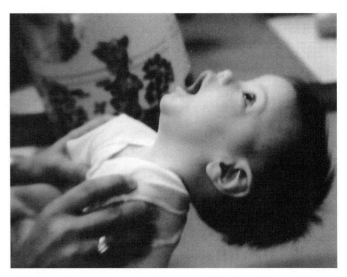

Figure 70-10. Head lag in congenital muscular dystrophy.

in the section "Disease of Older Children," below). Symptoms are self-limiting and nonrecurring. Treatment is primarily supportive, although anticholinesterase drugs (Mestinon) may be required in severe cases. Congenital myasthenic syndromes are an as yet poorly delineated group of neuromuscular junction disorders that usually present at birth, but possibly not until years later. Most are autosomal recessive, but sites of pathology within the neuromuscular junction can be variably presynaptic, post-synaptic, or both. Diagnosis requires sophisticated electrodiagnostic and biopsy techniques and are available in few specialized centers only.

Peripheral nerve disorders include the hereditary motor-sensory neuropathies, which are much more common in older children and will be discussed below.

Congenital Myopathies of Infancy

Congenital myotonic dystrophy is an autosomal dominant disorder transmitted from an affected mother. Typical features include severe hypotonia at birth with respiratory distress often

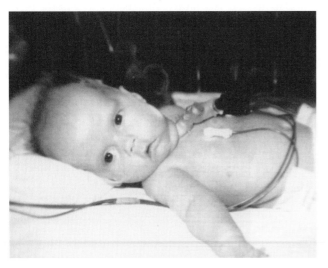

Figure 70-9. Typical facies of congenital myotonic dystrophy.

requiring prolonged ventilator support (68). Facial diplegia with a characteristic triangular-shaped mouth (Fig. 70-9), equinovarus contractures, and mental retardation are also seen. Clinical myotonia may not appear until age 3–4 years, and electrical myotonia is rarely seen at birth and may be absent until age 2–3 years. Clinical diagnosis is confirmed by examining the mother, who invariably has the adult form of the disease. An abnormal genetic locus on the long arm of chromosome 19 (19q13.3) results in a trinucleotide repeating sequence (69). The number of repetitions, normally between 5 and 35, may be as high as 2,000 and is directly correlated with severity of disease, including cardiomyopathy (70). The genetic and clinical abnormalities tend to increase in severity with successive generations (termed *genetic anticipation*). Muscle biopsy is now rarely required. The clinical course is one of gradual improvement, with hypotonia no longer clinically significant by 4 years. All will eventually become at least household ambulators, although soft-tissue surgeries and bracing may be required. Mild to moderate mental retardation, exacerbated by oromotor immobility affecting expressive language skills more than receptive skills, requires special education placement. Multisystem disease consisting of frontal baldness, cataracts, testicular atrophy in boys, smooth muscle and cardiac muscle dysfunction, all typical of the adult form of myotonic dystrophy, is seen in adults with congenital myotonic dystrophy and leads to a typically shortened life span, with death most commonly due to cardiac dysrhythmias.

Congenital muscular dystrophy, a disorder of variable severity, is transmitted as an autosomal recessive disorder. Severe forms present early with hypotonia, proximal weakness with head and neck muscles involved early (Fig. 70-10), and congenital contractures usually seen distally only (ankles, wrists—"arthrogrypotic"). Cognition is usually normal. Patients with milder forms may present with less severe gross motor delays and weak gait. CK is variably increased, and electrodiagnosis may or may not show "myopathic" patterns. Muscle biopsy is similar to that of patients with Duchenne's muscular dystrophy, with variation in fiber size, fiber splitting, central nuclei, and fibrous proliferation. Severity of biopsy abnormalities are not necessarily correlated with clinical abnormalities. The clinical course can be static or slowly progressive, with scoliosis a common complication. *Fukuyama congenital muscular dystrophy,* a more severe form of congenital muscular dystrophy—associated with seizures, mental retardation, and abnormal CNS imaging (71)—is seen primarily but not exclusively in the Japanese population. With the discovery of the dystrophin-glycoprotein complex, specific component deficiencies have been associated with different forms of congenital dystrophy, the most common being merosin (or laminin) deficiency, which may also be associated with a peripheral neuropathy (72).

Other myopathies, once considered questionably distinct clinical entities, are named after histologic changes seen in biopsy specimens treated with special staining techniques. Examples include nemaline (rod-body) myopathy, central core disease, centronuclear (myotubular) myopathy, and fiber-type disproportion (73). In addition, each can demonstrate a broad spectrum of involvement (74). Recent discovery of abnormal genetic loci (see Table 70-5) for many of these histologic myopathies supports the concept that these may indeed be true entities.

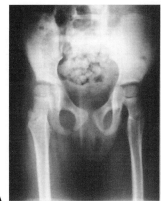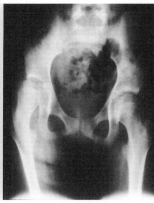

Figure 70-11. Coxa valga **(A)** and mild hip subluxation **(B)** in Charcot-Marie-Tooth

DISEASE OF OLDER CHILDREN

In older children, *spinal muscle atrophy III (Kugelberg-Welander disease)* presents with proximal weakness during early childhood to young adulthood. Ambulation may be maintained into later years. Calf hypertrophy is seen in 25%, fasciculations in 75%. CK may be elevated two to five times normal. EMG shows a chronic neuropathic pattern (minimal fibs/pos sharps with large amplitude polyphasics and diminished recruitment). Biopsy can show a mixed neuropathic/myopathic picture or can be nonspecific in 30%. The abnormal genetic locus on the long arm of chromosome 5 (5q13) is seen.

Several *hereditary motor-sensory neuropathies* (HMSN) exist and have been classified by Dyck and Lambert. Most common are HMSN I (Charcot-Marie-Tooth) and HMSN II (neuronal Charcot-Marie-Tooth). HMSN III (Dejerine-Sotas) presents in early infancy, involves sensory nerves more often than in other types, and has more palpable nerve hypertrophy. Type IV (Refsums disease) is associated with hearing loss and deficiencies in phytanic acid. Type V (familial spastic paraplegia) may have upper motor neuron findings (75). Clinical findings in types I and II are similar. Foot problems (pes cavus, claw toes, intrinsic atrophy) are most common but can be clinically insignificant. In young children, pes planus is the more common presentation. Lower-leg atrophy occurs later. The cavus foot appearance is secondary to progressive denervation leading to atrophy, fibrosis, and contracture in a distal to proximal direction. Type I can be distinguished from type II by electrodiagnosis. Type I gives a demyelinating picture (markedly slowed nerve conduction velocity with few needle EMG abnormalities), whereas type II gives an axonal picture [relatively normal nerve conduction velocity with a more abnormal EMG (76) and nerve biopsy]. Several abnormal genetic loci have been found: the long arm of chromosome 1 (1q), long arm of chromosome 17 (17q) and an X-linked form. Orthopedic complications include hip dysplasia in about 6% to 8%, often asymptomatic (Fig. 70-11), and neuromuscular scoliosis in about 10%. Progressive cavus deformities and scoliosis may lead to the need for orthoses to improve ambulation and slow progression of spinal deformity. Resistant deformities may require surgical intervention (foot reconstructions, spinal fusions). As near normal physical activity as possible should be allowed.

Autoimmune myasthenia gravis occurs with a prevalence of 5–10/100,000 population and is four times as frequent in girls. Clinically, abnormal fatigue occurs after activity and improves with rest. The onset is usually insidious, although it may present precipitously after a febrile illness, allergic reaction, or emotional upset. The most common presenting sign is ptosis (ocular myasthenia gravis), which increases with reading and is accompanied by compensatory forehead wrinkling. Facial weakness (presenting as a slack jaw, slurred speech, or difficulty swallowing) and limb weakness (proximal more than distal with a positive Gower sign and Trendelenburg gait) may also be seen. Tensilon, a short-acting anticholinesterase, given intravenously, reverses weakness within 30–60 seconds and lasts 5–10 minutes. Electrodiagnostic testing reveals a decrement of more than 10% on 2–3 Hz stimulation, and single-fiber electromyography shows abnormal jitter but is difficult to perform in children. Finally, antibodies to ACh receptors (anti-AChR antibodies) can be measured and are elevated in 85% to 90% of patients with generalized myasthenia gravis, but in only 50% in ocular myasthenia gravis. Treatment is based on either improving neuromuscular junction transmission with anticholinesterases (AChEs) or decreasing the lytic effect of Anti-AChR antibodies by steroids, immunosuppressive therapy, or thymectomy. Commonly used AChEs include Prostigmin (neostigmine) or Mestinon (pyridostigmine). Steroids may be given in high doses once daily, low doses every other day, or pulsed, each method having its proponents. Immunosuppression can be achieved by drugs (azathioprine, cyclosporin), intravenous gamma-globulin, or plasma exchange (during crisis). The role of thymectomy is still controversial, with optimal response seen when surgery is done within 5 years of onset and in relatively mild cases. Paradoxically, though, thymectomy is usually performed only after other treatments have failed.

The presentation of *fascioscapulohumeral muscular dystrophy* is often in adolescent or early adult years. Facial weakness often precedes shoulder girdle weakness. In later years, there may be progression to abdominal and pelvic girdle muscles. Associated abnormalities include high- (and rarely, low-) frequency hearing loss and retinal abnormalities (telangiectasia, microaneurysms) in up to 75%. There are no cardiac abnormalities, and cognition is preserved. CK elevation and muscle biopsy changes may be minimal. An abnormal genetic locus has been found at the 4q35 site. Fascioscapulohumeral muscular and *limb girdle dystrophy* have many overlapping features;

prominent facial involvement and autosomal dominant transmission favors fascioscapulohumeral muscular dystrophy; proximal weakness and autosomal recessive transmission favors limb girdle dystrophy. Both show variable severity and in their extremes can be like Duchenne's muscular dystrophy, with scoliosis, respiratory disease, and early death. The abnormal genetic locus is on chromosome 15.

Duchenne muscular dystrophy, a sex-linked recessive disorder, is seen in 1–3/10,000 male births. Gait deviations present in patients after 2 years of age, eventually leading to a Trendelenburg gait, pathognomonic of gluteus medius weakness. Patients come to stand through the Gower maneuver, pathognomonic of proximal pelvic girdle weakness. Gradually a characteristic posture of tight heel cords, calf pseudohypertrophy (deltoid pseudohypertrophy also common but less visually obvious), a widely abducted stance, and hyperlordosis develops. Dull mentation is seen in about one-third. CK is markedly elevated, maximally in the preclinical stage, with values greater than 10,000 not unusual. Values decrease with age as muscle loss progresses, but never approach normal. A "myopathic" EMG (BSAPPs, early recruitment) is seen. ECG shows cardiomyopathy with tall R-waves in the right precordial leads and deep Q-waves in the limb and precordial leads. These abnormalities are seen in 70% to 90% of patients, and cardiomyopathy causes death in about 10% (77). Biopsy shows variation in fiber size, fiber splitting, central nuclei, fibrous/fatty replacement, and absence of type 2B fibers.

The abnormal genetic locus is at the Xp21 site, resulting in deficient or abnormal muscle protein, dystrophin, assayed by immunofluorescent techniques in muscle biopsy specimens. Quantification of dystrophin now allows classification of the dystrophies based on the level of dystrophin deficiency. Less than 3% is characteristic of Duchenne, whereas between 3% and 10% suggests severe Becker muscular dystrophy, and 10% to 20% suggests mild to moderate Becker muscular dystrophy. Levels greater than 20% suggests non–Becker/Duchenne dystrophies. Detailed DNA analysis on blood will soon be available using DNA probes, as will prenatal diagnosis with accuracy approaching 95%. Therapeutically, ongoing drug trials continue. Currently both prednisone as well as androgenic steroids are used (78).

The clinical course is variable but inexorably downhill, with ambulation typically lost by 8–12 years of age. Ambulation can be prolonged by bracing and timely surgical intervention to release contractures (79). Specifically, resection of the iliotibial band, TAL with or without posterior tibialis lengthening or release, can prolong ambulation an average of 2 years if done before initial entry into the wheelchair. Success depends on having a cognitively preserved patient motivated for ambulation with a supportive family. Early remobilization is vital, and only minimal orthotic support is needed. The wheelchair phase is characterized by progressive weakness, scoliosis in 80% (although 15% of these will not show significant progression and do not require surgical correction), and death by late teens to early twenties, usually secondary to respiratory failure on the basis of restrictive lung disease. Prolongation of useful life is possible by early surgical correction of scoliosis suggested once the curve exceeds 20 degrees and before lung vital capacity becomes less than 20%, and appropriate portable ventilator support (Fig. 70-12).

Becker muscular dystrophy occurs with an incidence only one-tenth that of Duchenne. All clinical findings are the same as in Duchenne's muscular dystrophy. Dystrophin deficiency is only partial (between 3% and 20%), rather than complete (<3%) as in Duchenne's. The clinical course is protracted compared with Duchenne, with ambulation maintained into the twenties and

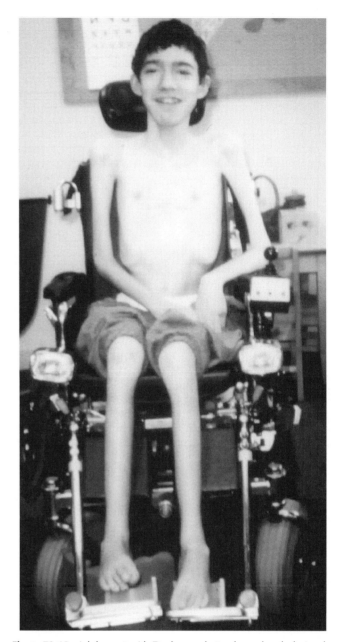

Figure 70-12. Adolescent with Duchenne dystrophy and early fusion for scoliosis.

survival to the forties. Each form of dystrophy is genetically distinct (see Table 70-5).

SPINAL CORD DYSFUNCTION

There are multiple etiologies of pediatric spinal cord dysfunction. These include congenital etiologies, such as spinal dysraphism and ligamentous laxity in children with Down syndrome. They also include acquired etiologies, such as spinal cord injury, either as a complication of birth, later trauma, or vascular events (i.e., a ruptured arteriovenous malformation), and infectious/autoimmune disorders, such as transverse myelitis or tumors. The rehabilitation principles are similar for these disorders regarding bowel and bladder management, skin care, sexuality, and therapeutic intervention. Spinal dys-

TABLE 70-6. Distribution by Level of Traumatic Spinal Cord Injury			
Injury Type	Group 1 (0–8 years)	Group II (9–16 years)	Total
Total cervical	49 (79%)	63 (53%)	112 (62%)
Upper cervical (0 to C3)	33 (53%)	31 (26%)	64 (36%)
Lower cervical (C4 to C7)	16 (26%)	32 (27%)	48 (26%)
Thoracic (T1 to T11)	7 (11%)	16 (14%)	23 (13%)
Thoracolumbar (T12 to L1)	2 (3%)	17 (15%)	19 (11%)
Lumbar (L1to L5)	4 (7%)	21 (18%)	25 (14%)

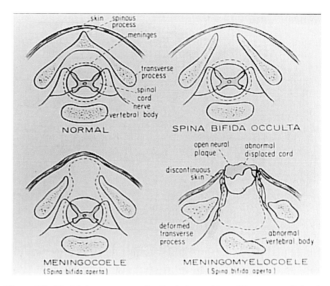

Figure 70-13. Major patterns of spinal dysraphism. The name of the lesion depends on the contents of the abnormal sac.

raphism will be the focus because it represents a significant proportion of children with spinal cord dysfunction. However, key distinctions between pediatric and adult traumatic spinal cord injury will also be discussed.

Traumatic Spinal Cord Injury

Pediatric traumatic spinal cord injury constitutes approximately 3% to 5% of all spinal cord injuries (80–82). There are several key anatomic differences between the child and adult patient that predispose the child to spinal cord injury without radiographic abnormalities (SCI WORA). These differences include wedge-shaped vertebral bodies and horizontally oriented facet joints in the younger child; usually by age 8–10 years, the pediatric vertebral column resembles that of an adult. Paraspinal muscle weakness and ligamentous laxity are present, as they are not fully developed in the younger patients. These factors favor ligamentous injury over bony injury (83,84). Young children also tend to have proportionally large heads compared with their body size. Therefore the fulcrum of injury is higher, resulting in higher cervical injuries (82,85) (Table 70-6). The incidence of patients with spinal cord injury without radiographic abnormalities varies but has been reported to be as high as 60% of pediatric spinal cord injuries in children younger than 8 years of age (82).

It is important to be aware of the presence of spinal cord injury without radiographic abnormalities. For the unconscious pediatric patient in the emergency room, a lateral neck x-ray does not rule out spinal cord injury. Further diagnostic tests, such as cervical MRI and computerized tomography scans may be warranted. Delayed onset of neurologic symptoms has been reported. There are several hypotheses, including compression from an undetected unstable spine, vascular compromise, and inflammation leading to expansion of an injury. Motor vehicle accidents are the most common cause of injury in children. Boys are more commonly injured than girls, but less so in the toddler and younger-child years, with a ratio of approximately 3:2.

The management of the pediatric spinal cord–injured patient is similar to the adult, with a couple of exceptions. The exam of the pediatric patient is usually limited by the child's ability to cooperate. At approximately age 5, accurate manual muscle testing can be performed. It is important to remember that when assessing the pediatric patient, the resistance during manual muscle testing is not the same as required by an adult. Also, in the young patient, especially in infants, the sensory exam should be done caudal to cranial. The child should be calmed, and then pinprick testing can be done, with the onset of a cry as the indication that sensation is present. Grading the sensory exam in infants is nearly impossible.

There is limited data on deep venous thrombosis (DVT) in the pediatric population. A retrospective review by Radecki and Gaebler-Spira found 1 in 20 patients younger than age 13 had a DVT. For the immature adolescent and child, the issue of DVT prophylaxis is not clear-cut, and further investigation is warranted (86). Scoliosis and hip dislocations are encountered more commonly in the pediatric population because of the effects of abnormal tone on a developing neuromuscular system.

Spinal Dysraphism

There are several different forms of spinal dysraphism with several different terminologies used (Fig. 70-13). *Spinal bifida occulta,* a normal variant seen in 5% to 10% of the population, is the failure of fusion of the posterior elements of the spine with an intact thecal sac and normal spinal cord. There is usually no associated neurologic deficit, although it is rarely associated with a sacral lipoma or tethered cord. *Meningocele* is the failure of fusion of the posterior elements with cystic-outpouching of the thecal sac filled with CSF, but with no neural tube disruption. Therefore, there are no neurologic deficits. The skin may or may not be intact. *Meningomyelocele* is the significant disruption of all elements of the bony spine, typically with an open malformed neural tube covered by a membranous sac. There are variable degrees of neurologic deficits. Another term that may be seen is *spina bifida aperta,* which is any lesion that is open to the environment. Some authors also use *spina bifida occulta* as any lesion that is not open to the environment.

Embryology

Normally neural tube closure starts in the third week of gestation from the midcervical level and proceeds in both cephalad and caudad directions. The defect of neural tube closure is thought to occur around day 26 and accounts for most lesions through midlumbar. The most caudal cell mass forms between days 26 and 30, eventually resulting in formation of a central canal in the embryonic tail. Caudal regression with rostral extension resulting in fusion with the neural tube results in the formation of the spinal cord by day 53. Lesions of the lumbrosacral levels occur before day 53.

Demographics

The incidence worldwide is approximately 1–2/1,000 births, depending on the populations studied. U.S. studies showed declining incidence to 0.3/1,000 births (live and stillborn) in 1990 (87). Yen found that the incidence decreased from 1.3/1,000 births in 1970 to 0.6/100 births in 1989 (88). Comparison of two surveillance systems found the birth-prevalence rate for patients with spina bifida in the United States from 1983 to 1990 to be 0.46/1,000 and 0.40/1,000 births (89). Differences have also been noted between races and nationalities. The rates were highest for Hispanics and lowest for Asians/Pacific Islanders (89). African blacks have the lowest incidence of 1/10,000, whereas Celts (Eastern Irish, Western Scots, and Welsh) have a birth incidence reported as high as 1/80 (90). The incidence is decreasing worldwide and is felt to be due to several factors, including better prenatal diagnosis and termination of the pregnancy, better nutritional support, and the use of folic acid.

Prenatal Detection

Early detection can be done via serum alpha-fetoprotein with levels peaking at the sixteenth week of gestation. False positives can be caused by incorrect dates, multiple gestations, maternal cancer, gastrointestinal or renal disease (maternal or fetal). False negatives occur with incorrect dates, intrauterine growth retardation, maternal diabetes, and Down syndrome. Fetal ultrasound can be used to assist with diagnosis. Amniocentesis for alpha-fetoprotein and acetylcholinesterase can be performed to confirm the diagnosis.

Etiology

The specific etiology of neural tube defects has not been elicited. However, the mode of inheritance appears to be multifactorial with genetic and gestational influences, such as folic acid deficiency, fetal exposure to valproic acid (91) or Tegretol (92), and maternal diabetes mellitus. Maternal hyperthermia, such as the use of hot tubs or saunas, during early pregnancy has also been implicated as a risk factor (93). Risk of recurrence is 2% to 4% after the first affected child and as high as 10% after the second. The risk of an affected mother giving birth to an affected child is 4% to 10%.

The risk of recurrence can be reduced by as much as 70% with periconceptual use of folic acid in doses up to 4 mg/day. Multiple studies worldwide using 0.4–5 mg/day, given 1 month preconception through the first trimester, have been done with the majority citing a 60% to 70% reduction in risk of recurrence of neural tube defects. The Centers for Disease Control and Prevention recommends that all women of childbearing years consume 0.4 mg/day of folic acid. Folic acid intake should be kept less than 1 mg/day unless under a physician's care. Some physicians feel that higher doses, such as 4 mg/day, should be used if the woman has already had a child with a neural tube defect (94,95).

Neural Tube Closure

Sac closure is usually performed within the first 24–48 hours to reduce the risk of infection. Microsurgical closure with reapproximation of the neural tube and construction of a fluid-filled pouch to "bathe" the cord reduces the incidence of early tethering of the spinal cord.

Newer neurosurgical techniques now involve repair. Tulipan and Bruner reported three successful cases of *in utero* repair (96). A case study of 29 patients repaired *in utero* suggests that intrauterine repair of meningomyelocele decreases the incidence of hindbrain herniation and shunt-dependent hydrocephalus. However, there was an increase in prematurity (97,98).

Associated Neurologic Abnormalities

The Chiari malformation type II, seen in 90% of patients, is defined as downward displacement of the inferior portion of the cerebellar vermis, medulla, and lower pons, and an elongated fourth ventricle through the foramen magnum. There may be an associated kinking of the medulla.

Hydrocephalus occurs in 80% to 90% of patients. A "cork in the bottle" phenomenon, related to the abnormal placement of the above-mentioned structures through the foramen magnum; aqueductal stenosis; and a defect in CSF uptake are all causative factors (99). More than 80% of children require ventriculoperitoneal shunting.

Symptoms of the Chiari malformation or hydrocephalus include laryngeal and pharyngeal paresis and may be associated with stridor or apnea during infancy and early childhood. Infants may be born with symptoms, but typically develop them within the first 2 months, with the peak mortality between 9–12 weeks. Mild inspiratory stridor with crying is usually the initial symptom because of paresis of the vocal cord abductors. Progressive cardiorespiratory problems, including apnea and bradycardia, may develop, as well as aspiration pneumonia. Approximately one-third of infants develop symptoms, and about one-third of these will die (99).

Tethered spinal cord may be due to a lipoma, scarring at the closure site, or diastematomyelia. Presenting symptoms include deterioration in bladder and bowel function, loss of strength or sensation, spasticity, low back pain, or radicular pain and/or rapidly progressive scoliosis. It is felt that microinfarctions of the spinal cord occur with repetitive flexion and extension. Treatment requires early surgical detethering. Herman and associates reported that 93% of patients that were detethered had improvement or stabilization of presenting symptoms (100). Spontaneous resolution of scoliosis has been reported after detethering. Tethering of the cord is felt to develop in almost all patients with meningomyelocele (101).

Syringomyelia is felt to be due to high CSF pressure within the central canal. Presenting symptoms include deterioration of neurologic function, loss of sensory and motor function in the upper extremities, and spasticity resulting in progressive joint deformity. It may also be present in 25% of asymptomatic patients. Shunting may be necessary.

Orthopedic Issues

Associated musculoskeletal malformations that may cause a structural scoliosis include vertebral body anomalies, such as wedge or hemivertebrae; unilateral bars; or block vertebrae, alone or in combination. Paralytic scoliosis is secondary to loss of truncal support and is seen in most thoracic-level patients. Kyphosis may be structural or paralytic, with the higher levels at greater risk for a paralytic kyphosis. Rib anomalies are also seen, including fused or malformed ribs. Contractures at any joint that are due to muscular imbalance, hip dysplasia, and club feet also occur. Pathologic fractures occur below the level of the neurologic lesion, may be caused by trivial trauma, and present as painless swelling, warmth, or redness. There is no good data to indicate that passive standing alone reduces the risk of pathologic fractures.

Scoliosis is typically treated initially with spinal bracing of curves greater than 20 degrees and regular radiographic monitoring. Curves greater than 40 degrees are considered surgical curves. Rapidly progressive scoliosis should raise suspicion of a tethered cord. A severe kyphosis (gibbus) may be corrected by a kyphectomy. Bilateral hip dislocations without restricted range of motion may be left alone. Unilateral hip dislocation in low level lesions should be corrected, but in high-level lesions, surgery may have no benefit (102). Unilateral hip dislocation may lead to pelvic obliquity. The relationship between pelvic obliquity and scoliosis has been questioned. Serial casting or soft-tissue releases to improve range of motion may be needed to increase mobility and improve positioning for seating and bracing.

After surgical procedures, postoperative immobilization should be limited as much as possible to prevent further osteoporosis and pathologic fractures.

Genitourinary

The majority of patients have a neurogenic bladder, with a flaccid bladder being more common than a spastic bladder. In addition, there are associated genitourinary abnormalities seen in as many as 20% of patients, including horseshoe kidneys, hypoplastic kidneys. or renal agenesis, as well as ureteral duplications and posterior urethral valves.

An ultrasound should be performed early in infancy to define the anatomy. VCUG will define bladder contour and determine the presence of reflux. Renal scan and urodynamics can be performed after 2 weeks of age. Because the physiology can change over the first year of life, serial ultrasounds should be performed every 2 to 3 months to monitor the status of the kidneys and detect any abnormal changes that would necessitate further intervention. Most patients will be managed with clean intermittent catheterization. The age at which this may begin is debatable. Clean intermittent catheterization may be started at birth because the child has a known neurogenic bladder. Alternatively, because infants are normally not continent, if bladder pressures are not elevated, there are no changes on ultrasounds, and the patient is free of urinary tract infections, then clean intermittent catheterization can be started at the age when continence is normally achieved, perhaps 3–4 years old. However, once the first urinary tract infection occurs, then catheterizations must be started. The long-term goals of bladder management are to prevent renal damage by preventing infection and reflux and to prevent wetness between catheterizations.

Pharmacologic intervention with Ditropan, Urecholine, or other medications may be needed based on the results of the urodynamics and the patient's clinical status.

Surgical procedures include bladder augmentation for small capacity bladders, urethral implantation for patients with reflux, and suprapubic vesicostomy to allow for an alternative method of drainage. The Mitrofanoff procedure is used to provide an alternative conduit for urinary catheterization. The artificial sphincter is an implantable device used to help achieve urinary continence. It can be considered in a motivated patient after all other conservative methods have failed. Clean intermittent catheterization is still required. Patients should be free of infection and have normal renal function, adequate bladder capacity, and low-pressure bladders with no uninhibited contractions. Problems include rejection, foreign body reaction, and infection. Neural stimulation involving stimulation of the sacral roots (103) and pudendal nerve stimulation have also been reported. Children with good fine motor skills and good cognition can be taught self-catheterization at approximately age 5 years. Controversial issues include the use of prophylactic medications, such as antibiotics or vitamin C.

Bowel

The management of the bowel program in patients with meningomyelocele is a constant process. Bowel incontinence can cause terrible social stigmatization. Training in timed bowel regulation may be started by 2–3 years of developmental age. Because peristalsis and the gastrocolic reflex are still intact, postmealtime evacuations are usually more successful. Diet is an important component of the bowel program. Adequate fluid intake is important, as well as knowing which foods soften or harden the stools. Bulk additives, stimulant suppositories, and enemas may be needed. For patients with uncontrollable incontinence, the Malone antegrade continence enema provides a surgical alternative, with a conduit using either the cecum or the appendix between the intestine and the abdominal wall. This is a catheterizable conduit that can be used to deliver tap water or saline enemas and allow for evacuation through the rectum.

Sexuality

Women may have relatively normal function in spite of sensory loss. Men have variable ability for erection and ejaculation, but fertility may be compromised by recurrent urinary tract infection, repeated mechanical trauma to the testicles, testicular hypoplasia, and decreased temperature control of the scrotum resulting in decreased sperm count.

Latex

Latex allergy should be considered in every child with meningomyelocele. Numerous different types of allergic reaction have been reported, including anaphylaxis. Protein in the latex is the primary allergen. The Food and Drug Administration estimated that 18% to 40% of children with meningomyelocele and 6% to 7% of surgical personnel are latex sensitive (104), with the prevalence as high as 64.5% (80). Niggemann and associates report that atopic disposition, number of operations, and presence of a shunt all increase the risk of becoming not only sensitized but also allergic to latex. Sensitization may occur at any time, so serum IgE levels may give a false sense of security (105). Therefore, latex should be avoided in all patients with meningomyelocele.

Rehabilitation

The rehabilitation program for children with meningomyelocele begins in the newborn period. A working knowledge of normal development is important. A careful examination in the newborn period, often by observation of the position of the infant, can help discern the functional level of the patient that result from imbalance of muscular forces around major pivots. Thoracic level is most often associated with flaccid lower extremities and with frog-legged positioning. High lumbar (L1–2) levels lay with hips flexed and adducted. The knees are often flexed because of intrauterine positioning. This position predisposes to early hip dislocation. Low lumbar (L3–5) levels lay with the hips flexed and adducted but with the knees in extension and possibly the ankles dorsiflexed. Hip dislocation may be a late complication. Sacral level may assume normal postures, but pes cavus and clawing of the toes may be seen.

Children develop psychosocially by interacting with their environment. If motor limitations exist, adaptive devices will be needed to help facilitate this interaction. Adaptive equipment in infancy is designed to allow attainment of functional milestones at as near to normal time as possible. Proper seating with appropriate relief for deformities allows the infant to sit upright and view the environment. At about 1 year of age, standing devices can be considered. The data are limited in regards to passive standing alone and the prevention of osteoporosis. The devices include a stander or parapodium for thoracic-level patients, although the parapodium is typically not used for mobility until at least 18 months of age. For thoracic-level patients, the parapodium can be replaced by HKAFOs with the use of a walker or Lofstrand crutches, depending on the child's abilities. Ambulation in childhood, even in high-level patients, is a reasonable goal, although by adolescence, wheelchair ambulation may be required as a result of the energy demands of upright ambulation. The reciprocating gait orthosis allows for an upright energy-efficient gait pattern. The isocentric reciprocating gait orthosis is the newest version, using a bar with a central pivot (Fig. 70-14). The quality of gait

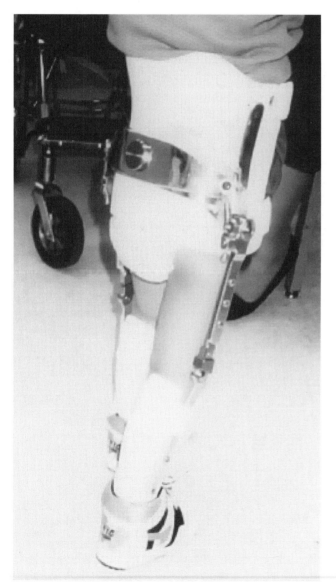

Figure 70-14. Isocentric reciprocating gait orthosis for spinal dysfunction.

is improved if the patient can assist with active hip flexion. The energy consumption of ambulation with reciprocating gait orthosis approaches that of wheelchair mobility (81). In the study by Cuddeford and associates, energy consumption and energy efficiency of HKAFOs and reciprocating gait orthosis were compared. Previous studies had shown less energy consumption with reciprocating gait orthosis than with a swing-through gait. The children who ambulated with HKAFOs had significantly higher energy consumption than those with reciprocating gait orthosis, but they ambulated faster. Therefore, the energy efficiency was less for the HKAFO group. The study felt that further investigation was needed to confirm the importance of energy efficiency during ambulation in considering a mode of locomotion with the child with meningomyelocele (106). High–lumbar-level patients may be able to be braced as early as 10–12 months, usually with HKAFOs. For lower-level patients, the residual motor movements will dictate the type of orthotic needed.

Wheelchair ambulation can be achieved by 18–24 months, and steering a power wheelchair can be achieved before 3 years of age.

There are multiple factors that affect ambulation, including level of paralysis, age when first braced (107), obesity, degree of scoliosis, lower-extremity deformities, weight and efficiency of the orthosis, child's motivation, parental support, cognition, and upper-extremity function. Charney and Melchionni, in a retrospective study, evaluated high-lumbar and thoracic-level patients and found that the significant factors determining ambulation were degree of mental retardation, whether the child received physical therapy for ambulation, and parental involvement (108). Typically, most sacral-level patients will ambulate as adults, and most thoracic-level patients will require wheelchair mobility.

One key aspect of the rehabilitation program that needs to be stressed is parental involvement. The parents must be taught all aspects of care in order for the appropriate carryover at home to occur.

A high proportion of these children will have learning disabilities, and the appropriate supports need to be provided in the school setting. Supportive counseling may be needed to help the child cope and effectively manage his/her disability.

Prognosis

There are several studies regarding follow-up of patients with meningomyelocele.

Worley and associates monitored patients for 5 years: 63 patients were followed from infancy. There were 32 boys and 31 girls. Ninety-eight percent had VP shunts; 23% had symptoms of brain-stem dysfunction, with the median age of 3 months (1–22 months). Eleven of fifteen underwent brain-stem decompression. In four of fifteen, symptoms resolved spontaneously. Mortality rate at 5 years was 14%; five of nine died as a result of brain-stem dysfunction (109). Hunt and Poulton reported a 25-year follow-up of 117 patients born between 1963 and 1970. Fifty-two percent, or 61 patients, were alive in 1992. Seventy-nine percent lived to their first birthday, 63% to their tenth birthday, and 56% to their twentieth birthday. The most severely disabled patients had the highest mortality. Sixteen deaths were due to renal failure. Clean intermittent catheterization was not a standard of care when many of these patients were younger, however. Of the 61 survivors, only 33 were able to live independently (110).

A Team Approach

The rehabilitation of the child with spinal cord dysfunction is multifaceted and requires a team approach. The physiatrist can guide the team, which may include an orthopedic surgeon, neurosurgeon, urologist, psychologist, social worker, physical therapist, occupational therapist, speech therapist, and nutritionist. Finally, it is important to include not only the child as part of the team, but the parents as well.

CONGENITAL BRACHIAL PLEXUS PALSIES

The reported incidence of brachial plexus injuries is 0.6–2.6/1,000 live births The mechanism of injury is by traction to the brachial plexus. Most frequent is a neuropraxic injury, from which more than 90% will recover fully. Axonal damage, rupture of the nerve, or nerve root avulsion result in variable residual damage. Risk factors include primiparous mothers, prolonged labor, birthweight more than 8.5 pounds, shoulder dystocia in more than 50%, traumatic delivery with mid- to high forceps, and breech presentation

Injuries are divided and classified anatomically (111). Erb's palsy, involving the upper plexus (C-5,6,7), accounts for about 80% of injuries. Klumpke's palsy, involving the lower plexus (C-7,8,T-1) exclusively, is now felt to be quite rare, with total plexus injuries accounting for 15%. Bilateral plexus injuries are also quite rare. Associated injuries secondary to the use of forceps include facial palsies, cephalohematomas, and torticollis. Fractures of the clavicle, humerus, and, in worst cases, cervical spine can occur, as can diaphragmatic paralysis. Horner's syndrome (ptosis, miosis, anhydrosis) can be seen with lower plexus injuries and is secondary to stellate ganglion injury.

On initial examination, the position of the arm is related to muscle imbalances around the pivots. Erb's palsies present with the typical "waiters tip" posture of shoulder internal rotation and adduction, elbow extension and pronation, wrist flexion. and thumb in palm (due to loss of extensor pollicis) (Fig. 70-15). Klumpke's palsy is the reverse, with shoulder external rotation (abduction usually not seen due to gravity), elbow flexion and supination, wrist extension, and the intrinsic minus hand deformity because of loss of C-8, T-1 muscles (Fig. 70-16). Muscle stretch reflexes are often lost. Sensory deficits often present may difficult to test for in newborns. MRI has shown pseudomeningoceles in both severe and mildly involved patients and may be unreliable (112). Early electrodiagnostic testing may distinguish neuropraxic from axonal injury and defines severity. Most ominous is the preservation of sensory potentials in the face of clinically absent sensation, suggesting root avulsion. The appearance of small polyphasic potentials, so-called "nascent" potentials, may be an early sign of recovery (113).

Treatment (114) in the first week must take into account the presence of a traumatic neuritis. Gentle range of motion should be done, as well as pinning the end of a long sleeve shirt to the diaper waist to avoid stretching of the shoulder capsule. Later, aggressive range of motion should include shoulder abduction with scapular stabilization to stretch scapulohumeral adhesions, elbow supination as well as extension, and thumb abduction. Splinting of tight pivots may be considered as may functional electrical stimulation to flaccid muscles. Developmental handling encourages activity and provides functional strengthening. Prone propping and wheelbarrow walking strengthens shoulder girdle, and eliciting righting reactions can strengthen deltoid, triceps, and wrist extensors. Active reaching in all di-

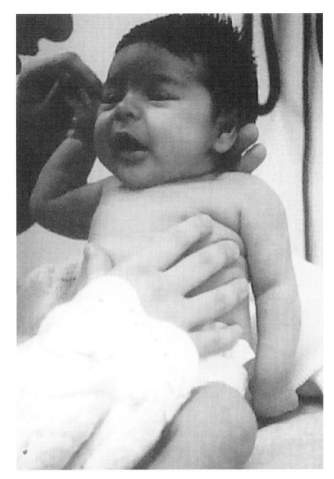

Figure 70-15. "Waiters tip" posture in Erbs Palsy (upper plexus injury).

rections is encouraged. Complete recovery occurs in more than 65%, whereas mild and moderate deficits are seen in 10% each. Fifteen percent will have severe residual deficits. Poor-grade elbow flexion with 0 to trace strength in wrist and finger extensors at 6 months old may be predictive (115).

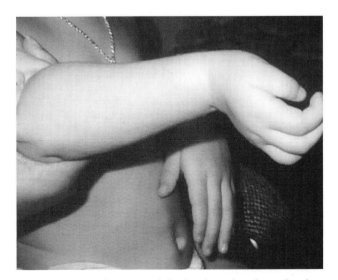

Figure 70-16. Typical posture of the hand in Klumpkes palsy (lower plexus injury).

Since the mid-1990s, early neurosurgical repair of the injured brachial plexus has been advocated by some (116,117). Candidates for surgery have zero to one-fifth strength in the biceps at 3–4 months or have plateaued at two-fifths for 4 months. The optimum age for surgery is younger than 9 months because nerve growth factor is at a maximum before 1 year of age, and there is less nerve scarring and distal muscle atrophy at that age. Procedures done include surgical neurolysis of scars, end-to-end anastomosis with microsurgical fascicular repair, and cable graft of nerve rupture. Intraoperative SSEPs may identify root avulsions not amenable to repair, and motor responses may distinguish neuropraxia from rupture. Postoperatively, as many as 12 months may be needed for return to be seen. In one study, all muscles improved at least one grade by 9 months, with average strength in biceps and deltoids being three-fifths. Surgical neurolysis also resulted in at least one grade improvement, whereas those patients requiring nerve graft showed the most dramatic improvement of between two and three grades. Others have questioned the criteria for early surgical repair, with recovery starting as late as 1 year seen (118). Additionally, soft-tissue procedures may be helpful (119). Subscapularis release improves passive shoulder external rotation, especially if done before 4 years of age. Latissimus dorsi transfers can improve either elbow flexion or extension, and shoulder abduction can be improved if coupled with trapezius transfer. Late deficits are largely cosmetic, with the presence of a high-riding, hypoplastic scapula with winging and loss of scapulohumeral rhythm. An elbow flexion contracture that is due to radial head subluxation and biceps contracture is almost always seen, and there is frequent shortening of the humeral segment. Finally, as with any disfiguring injury, the adverse effect on psychosocial development should not be underestimated, and appropriate counseling services provided.

CHILDHOOD TORTICOLLIS

The incidence of congenital muscular torticollis is about 4/1,000 live births, with 75% involving the right side (related to left occiput anterior presentation). More recent studies have shown more equal presentation of right- and left-sided signs (120). A nontender, soft enlargement in the sternocleidomastoid muscle, the so-called "olive" sign, may be seen within the first 6 weeks. It is mobile within the belly of the muscles, gradually decreases in size, and is usually gone within 4 to 6 months. Between 10% and 20% develop persistent torticollis, and an additional 25% have mild sternocleidomastoid asymmetry. Secondary deformities, including flattening of the ipsilateral face, contralateral occipital flattening, and orbital asymmetry, can be seen (121). Ipsilateral hip dysplasia is seen in up to 12%. Typically, there are no spinal abnormalities or neurologic deficits. The differential diagnosis is quite extensive and is outlined in Table 70-7.

The treatment of torticollis should be based first on correcting identified etiologic factors (122,123). Conservative therapy should include stretching of the tight neck muscles, as well as functional strengthening of contralateral neck muscles by use of lateral and anterior head righting reactions. Directing the gaze toward the ipsilateral superior direction should also be encouraged. The use of skull-shaping orthotics has recently been advocated as an additional cosmetic corrective measure, although much controversy exists (124). Surgical intervention should be considered when there has been no improvement by 18–24 months and consists of resection of a fibrotic sternocleidomastoid muscle. Successful correction can be achieved as late as 12 years old (125).

TABLE 70-7.   Differential Diagnosis of Torticollis

Congenital postural torticollis
  Intrauterine crowding
  No olive seen
  Resolve with conservative treatment
Congenital vertebral anomalies
  Segmentation failures
  Formation failures
  Combinations: Klippel-Feil, Sprengel's
Congenital ocular torticollis
  Strabismus
  Nystagmus: spasmus nutans
Acquired structural torticollis
  Traumatic
    Rotary subluxation
    Fracture/dislocation
    Muscular injury
    Basilar skull fracture
  Infection
    Cervical osteomyelitis
    Tuberculosis
  Ligamentous laxity and synovitis that is due to adjacent
    inflammation:pseudosubluxation, calcified cervical disc
Juvenile rheumatoid arthritis
Tumor of the cervical spine
  Metastatic
  Osteoid osteoma/osteoblastoma
  Eosinophilic granuloma
  Rare primary bone/muscle tumor
Atlantooccipital subluxations
  Associated with Down syndrome
  Mucopolysaccharidoses and other conditions causing ligamentous
    laxity
Ocular strabismus (most commonly CN 4)
Infection
  Retropharyngeal abscess
  Vestibular infection (otitis media)
  Cervical adenitis
Vestibular
  Mastoiditis
  Paroxysmal torticollis of infancy
Tumor
  Midbrain tumors
  Posterior fossa/intracranial tumor
  Cervical cord tumor
  Lymphoma
  Acoustic neuroma
  Orbital tumor (neurofibromatosis)
Miscellaneous
  Migraine headache
  Myasthenia gravis
  Associated with gastroesophageal reflux (Sandifer's syndrome)
  Syringomyelia
  Habitual, hysterical
  Oculogyric crisis (phenothiazine toxicity)

OSTEOGENESIS IMPERFECTA

Clinical Features

These skeletal dysplasias are characterized by the Sillence classification originally described in 1979 (126). As a group, skeletal dysplasias occur in 1 in 15,000 newborns. Type I is most common but may not be recognized in the neonatal period when fractures are not as common as after the first 2 to 3 years, when fractures occur with minimal trauma. Frequency diminishes after adolescence only to increase again in postmenopausal women and in men after age 60. With good orthopedic care, fractures heal rapidly with good callous formation and without deformity. Intense blue sclerae are noted at birth and persist. Conductive hearing loss may be seen in 50% during the second decade, but sensorineural deficits may occur later. Other associated abnormalities include thin, easily bruised skin, hypotonia with ligamentous laxity, and scoliosis (127). Type II, osteogenesis imperfecta congenita, presents in the newborn with multiple fractures and leads to death early. Type III occurs with one-eighth the frequency of type I. Multiple fractures are often present at birth and occur *in utero* as well as during labor and delivery. An undermineralized calvarium with wormian bones and basilar impression is typical. Biconcave vertebral bodies are seen on x-ray, and scoliosis is a common later complication. Bowing of the long bones in both coronal and sagittal planes is seen. The typical body habitus is one of extreme short stature, short trunk, and megaencephaly. Although blue sclerae are seen at birth, they normalize with age. Dentinogenesis imperfecta is also common. Finally, type IV is much less common than type III and is associated with normal sclerae and a milder fracture history (128).

Genetics

Osteogenesis imperfecta is transmitted as an autosomal dominant condition. Eighty percent to 90% of the patients with osteogenesis imperfecta have mutations of one of the two type I collagen genes encoding for the pro-α1 or pro-α2 protein chains, resulting in abnormal collagen formation. However, the severity of symptoms in patients with osteogenesis imperfecta correlates poorly with the type and site of the expressed mutations, and there is often phenotypic variability within members of the same family (129)

Management

Treatment strategies can best be divided into medical, orthopedic, and (re)habilitation measures. Molecular genetic treatment will likely be the most effective treatment in the future, but best current medical management consists of intravenous cyclical administration of pamidronate, a bisphosphonate shown to decrease osteoclastic activity, thereby increasing cancellous bone mineral density and significantly decreasing the frequency of fractures (130). Treatments of 2 mg/kg/cycle are given every 4–6 months (131). Synthetic growth hormone may be appropriate for type IV patients with moderate short stature (132).

In addition to careful immobilization of fractured long bones, orthopedic management consists of appropriately timed intramedullary rodding of long bones. Extensible rods can be used after 4 years of age, and although the complication rate is higher, revisions necessitated by growth are done much less frequently. A recent study has shown a marked decrease in complications with overlapping rods instead of Bailey-Dubow rods (outer sleeve with inner obturator rods) (133). Improved preambulatory skills (standing, transfers, etc.) in types III and IV and improved ambulation in type I has been seen. Loss of knee flexion may be seen in types III and IV but is much less likely in type I. Extensible rods have been used little in upper extremities, especially the forearms.

Surgery for basilar impression is done in the presence of neurologic signs suggestive of brain-stem or cervical-cord compression. Controversy exists regarding the most appropriate decompression technique, either suboccipital craniectomy with C-1 laminectomy or an anterior transoral approach. Similarly, scoliosis surgery may have up to a 50% complication rate. Rodding may fail because of bone fragility. Fusion with Keil grafts without rodding may be a better alternative (134).

(Re)habilitation strategies should address not only impairments (range of motion, poor strength, deformity) but also functional disabilities (diminished mobility, poor self-care skills, and delayed social development). A comprehensive program was first described by Binder et al. in 1984 (135). Beginning early in infancy, careful positioning in best neutral alignment in well-padded frames was done along with instruction in careful handling to avoid fractures. Hydrotherapy was begun early to increase strength, encourage spontaneous movement, and increase aerobic capacity. Developmental exercises to increase strength and advance motor milestones included use of antigravity righting reactions and led to independent sitting. Appropriate "containment" braces (HKAFO with spinal extension) were used by 2 years for standing. As ambulation skills improved, jointed braces were used with "weaning" of proximal components as tolerated. Wheeled mobility was also encouraged where appropriate and transitioned to power mobility when greater speed and distances were required.

When patients were reviewed at 10 years, they could be classified into three functional groups of increasing mobility. Preventable complications impeding function in each group included upper-extremity contracture and weakness in standers only (group A), hip flexion and plantar-flexion contractures along with upper-extremity weakness in household ambulators (group B), and poor lower-extremity alignment, balance, and endurance in community ambulators (group C) (136).

Engelbert et al. have looked at osteogenesis imperfecta children comparing levels of impairment with functional capability over time. Interestingly, they found that although impairment did not often improve, activities of daily living skills did with aggressive training in children younger than 7.5 years. In older children, there was a closer correlation with impairment level and activities of daily living capabilities (137–139).

Finally, when scales of "perceived competence" were applied, osteogenesis imperfecta children scored fairly well for all levels except "athletics" in type I and "romance" in type III, suggesting that perceived self-image could be shaped independently of physical impairment (140).

Overall, these studies support the validity of aggressive rehabilitation strategies for children with osteogenesis imperfecta and incorporation into "normal" society for these children with preserved intelligence.

REFERENCES

1. Boyle CA, Decoufle P, Yeargin-Allsopp M. Prevalence and health impact of developmental disabilities in U.S. children. *Pediatrics* 1994;93:399–403.
2. Illingworth RS. *Development of the infant and young child: normal and abnormal*, 8th ed. New York: Churchill-Livingstone, 1987.
3. Berninger VW, Gans BM. Language profiles in nonspeaking individuals of normal intelligence with severe cerebral palsy. *Augmentative Alternative Communication* 1986;2:56–63.
4. Arnold P, Chapman M. Self-esteem, aspirations and expectations of adolescents with physical disability. *Dev Med Child Neurol* 1992;34:97–102.
5. Tachdjian MO. *Pediatric orthopedics*, 3rd ed. Philadelphia: WB Saunders, 2001.
6. Butler C, Okamoto GA, McKay T. Motorized wheelchair driving by disabled children. *Arch Phys Med Rehabil* 1984;65:95–97.
7. Chess S, Fernandez P. *The handicapped child in school: behavior and management.* New York: Brunner/Mazel, 1981.
8. Kokkonen J, Saukkonen AL, Timonen E, et al. Social outcome of handicapped children as adults. *Dev Med Child Neurol* 1991;33:1095–1100.
9. Granger CV, Hamilton BB, Kayton R. Guide for the use of the functional independence measure (WeeFIM) of the uniform data set for the medical rehabilitation. Buffalo, NY: Research Foundation, State University of New York, 1988.
10. Russell DJ, Rosenbaum PL, Cadman DT, et al. The gross motor function measure: a means to evaluate the effects of physical therapy. *Dev Med Child Neurol* 1989;31:341–352.

11. Feldman AB, Haley SM, Coryell J. Concurrent and construct validity of the Pediatric Evaluation of Disability Inventory. *Phys Ther* 1990;70:602–610.
12. Akman CI, Cracco J. Intrauterine subdural hemorrhage. *Dev Med Child Neurol* 2000;42:843–846.
13. Rivkin MJ, Volpe JJ. Strokes in children. *Pediatr Rev* 1996;17:265–278.
14. Ricker LP, Shevell MI, Miller SP. Diagnostic profile of neonatal hypotonia: an 11-year study. *Pediatr Neurol* 2001;25:32–37.
15. Schanen NC. Molecular approach to the Rett syndrome gene. *J Child Neurol* 1999;14:806–814.
16. Pinto-Martin JA, Riolo S, Cnaan A, et al. Cranial ultrasound prediction of disabling and non-disabling cerebral palsy at age two in a low birth weight population. *Pediatrics* 1995;95:249–254.
17. Olsen P, Paakko E, Vainionpaa L, et al. Magnetic resonance imaging of periventricular leukomalacia and its clinical correlation in children *Ann Neurol* 1997;41:754–761.
18. Cooper J, Majnemer A, Rosenblatt B, et al. The determination of sensory deficits in children with hemiplegic cerebral palsy *J Child Neuro* 1995;10:300–309.
19. Rosenbloom L. Dyskinetic cerebral palsy and birth asphyxia. *Dev Me Child Neurol* 1994;36:285–289.
20. Molnar GE, Gordon SU. Cerebral palsy: predictive value of selected clinical signs of early prognostication of motor function. *Arch Phys Med Rehabil* 1976;57:153.
21. Badell A. Cerebral palsy: postural locomotor prognosis in spastic diplegia. *Arch Physl Med Rehabil* 1985;66:614–619.
22. Bleck EE. Locomotor prognosis in cerebral palsy. *Dev Med Child Neurol* 1975;17:18.
23. Fedrizzi E, Facchin P, Marzaroli M, et al. Predictors of independent walking in children with spastic diplegia. *J Child Neurol* 2000;15:228–234.
24. Bottos M, Bolcati C, Sciuto L, et al. Powered wheelchairs and independence in young children with tetraplegia. *Dev Med Child Neurol* 2001;43:769–777.
25. Berry ET, McLaurin SE, Sparling JW. Parent/caregiver perspectives on the use of power wheelchairs. *Pediatric Physical Therapy* 1996;8:146–150.
26. Zafeiriou DI, Kontopoulos EE, Tsikoulas I. Characteristics and prognosis of epilepsy in children with cerebral palsy. *J Child Neurol* 1999;14:289–294.
27. Delgado MR, Riela AR, Mills J, et al. Discontinuation of antiepileptic drug treatment after two seizure-free years in children with cerebral palsy. *Pediatrics* 1996;97:192–197.
28. Suskind DL, Tilton A. Clinical study of botulinum-a toxin in the treatment of sialorrhea in children with cerebral palsy. *Laryngoscope* 2002;112:73–81.
29. Samson-Fang LJ, Stevenson RD. Identification of malnutrition in children with cerebral palsy: poor performance of weight-for-height centiles. *Dev Med Child Neurol* 2000;42:162–168.
30. Strauss DJ, Shavelle RM, Anderson TW. Life expectancy of children with cerebral palsy. *Pediatr Neurol* 1998;18:143–149.
31. Reid CJD, Borsyzkowski M. Lower urinary tract dysfunction in cerebral palsy. *Arch Dis Child* 1993;68:739–742.
32. Mancini MC, Coster WJ, Trombly CA, et al. Predicting elementary school participation in children with disabilities. *Arch Phys Med Rehabil* 2000;81:339–347.
33. Bobath K. *A neurophysiologic basis for the treatment of cerebral palsy.* Philadelphia: JB Lippincott, 1980.
34. Hari M, Tillemans T. Conductive education. In: Scrutton D. ed. *Management of the motor disorders of children with cerebral palsy.* Philadelphia: JB Lippincott, 1984.
35. Montgomery D, Goldberg J, Amar M, et al. Effects of hyperbaric oxygen therapy on children with spastic diplegic cerebral palsy: a pilot project. *Undersea Hyperbaric Medicine* 1999;26:235–242.
36. Carmick J. Clinical use of neuromuscular electrical stimulation for children with cerebral palsy, part I: lower extremity. *Phys Ther* 1993;73:505–516.
37. Steinbok P, Reiner A, Kestle JRW. Therapeutic electrical stimulation following selective dorsal rhizotomy in children with spastic diplegic cerebral palsy: a randomized clinical trial. *Dev Med Child Neurol* 1997;39:515–520.
38. Sommerfelt K, Markestad T, Berg K, et al. Therapeutic electrical stimulation in cerebral palsy: a randomized, controlled, crossover trial. *Dev Med Child Neurol* 2001;43:609–613.
39. Butler C, Darrah J. Effects of neurodevelopmental treatment (NDT) for cerebral palsy: an AACPDM evidence report. *Dev Med Child Neurol* 2001;43:778–790.
40. Darrah J, Fan JSW, Chen LC, et al. Review of the effects of progressive resisted muscle strengthening in children with cerebral palsy: a clinical consensus exercise. *Pediatric Physical Therapy* 1997;9:12–17.
41. Morris C. A review of the efficacy of lower-limb orthoses used for cerebral palsy. *Dev Med Child Neurol* 2002;44:205–211.
42. Charles J, Lavinder G, Gordon AM. Effects of constraint-induced therapy on hand function in children with hemiplegic cerebral palsy. *Pediatric Physical Therapy* 2001;13:68–79.
43. Willis JK, Morello A, Davie A, et al. Forced use treatment of childhood hemiparesis. *Pediatrics* 2002;110:94–96.
44. Butler C, Campbell S. Evidence of the effects of intrathecal baclofen for spastic and dystonic cerebral palsy. *Dev Med Child Neurol* 2000;42:634–645.
45. Stempien L, Tsai T. Intrathecal Baclofen pump use for spasticity: a clinical survey. *Am J Phys Med Rehabil* 2000;79:536–541.
46. Meythaler JM, Guin-Renfroe S, Law C. Continuously infused intrathecal baclofen over 12 months for spastic hypertonia in adolescents and adults with cerebral palsy. *Arch Phys Med Rehabil* 2001;82:155–161.
47. Gilmartin R, Bruce D, Storrs BB, et al. Intrathecal baclofen for management of spastic cerebral palsy: multicenter trial. *J Child Neurol* 2000;15:71–77.
48. Koman LA, Mooney JF, Smith BP, et al. Management of spasticity in cerebral palsy with botulinum-a toxin: report of a preliminary, randomized, double-blind trial. *J Pediatr Orthop* 1994;14:299–303.
49. Boyd RN, Graham HK. Objective measurement of clinical findings in the use of botulinum toxin type A for the management of children with cerebral palsy. *Eur J Neurol* 1999;6[Suppl 4]:523–535.
50. Graham HK, Aoki KR, Autti-Ramo I, et al. Recommendations for the use of botulinum toxin type A in the management of cerebral palsy. *Gait Posture* 2000;11:67–79.
51. Boyd RN, Damiano DL, Graham HK, eds. Clinical considerations for the therapeutic use of botulinum toxin type a in cerebral palsy: an evidence-based examination. *Eur J Neurol* 2001;8[Supp 5]:1–202.
52. Seidel PMP, Seidel GK, Gans BM, et al. Precise localization of the motor nerve branches to the hamstring muscles: an aid to the conduct of neurolytic procedures. *Arch Phys Med Rehabil* 1996;77:1157–1160.
53. Brunner R, Baumann JU. Long-term effects of intertrochanteric varus-derotation osteotomy on femur and acetabulum in spastic cerebral palsy: an 11 to 18 year follow-up study. *J Pediatr Orthop* 1997;17:585–591.
54. Gage JR, DeLuca PA, Renshaw TS. Gait analysis: principles and applications. *J Bone Joint Surg Am* 1995;77:1607–1623.
55. DeLuca PA, Davis RB, et al. Alterations in surgical decision making in patients with cerebral palsy based on three-dimensional gait analysis. *J Pediatr Orthop* 1997;17:608–614.
56. Steinbok P, Keyes R, Langill L, et al. The validity of electrophysiological criteria used in selective functional posterior rhizotomy for treatment of spastic cerebral palsy. *J Neurosurg* 1994;81:354–361.
57. McLaughlin J, Bjornson K, Temkin N, et al. Selective dorsal rhizotomy: meta-analysis of three randomized controlled trials. *Dev Med Child Neurol* 2002;44:17–25.
58. McLaughlin J, Bjornson K, Astley SJ, et al. Selective dorsal rhizotomy: efficacy and safety in an investigator-masked randomized clinical trial. *Dev Med Child Neurol* 1998;40:220–232.
59. Carroll KL, Moore K, Stevens PM. Orthopedic procedures after rhizotomy. *J Pediatr Orthop* 1996;18:69–74.
60. Crawford K, Karol LA, Herring JA. Severe lumbar lordosis after dorsal rhizotomy. *J Pediatr Orthop* 1996;16:336–339.
61. Lang FF, Deletis V, Cohen HW, et al. Inclusion of the S2 dorsal rootlets in functional posterior rhizotomy for the reduction of spasticity in cerebral palsy. *Neurosurgery* 1994;34:847–853.
62. Hays RM, McLaughlin JF, Stephens K, et al. Electrophysiological Monitoring during selective dorsal rhizotomy, and spasticity and GMFM performance. *Dev Med Child Neurol* 1998;40:233–238.
63. Carboni P, Pisani F, Crescenzi A, et al. Congenital hypotonia with favorable outcome. *Pediatr Neurol* 2002;26:383–386.
64. Richer LP, Shevell MI, Miller SP. Diagnostic profile of neonatal hypotonia: an 11-year study. *Pediatr Neurol* 2001;25:32–37.
65. Devriendt K, Lammens M, Schollen E, et al. Clinical and molecular genetic features of congenital spinal muscular atrophy. *Ann Neurol* 1996;40:731–738.
66. Moyniham Hardart MK, Burns JP, Truog RD. Respiratory support in spinal muscular atrophy type I: a survey of physician practices and attitudes. *Pediatrics* 2002;110:1–5.
67. Bach JR, Baird JS, Plosky D, et al. Spinal muscular atrophy type I: management and outcomes. *Pediatr Pulmonol* 2002;34:16–22.
68. Keller C, Reynolds A, Lee B, et al. Congenital myotonic dystrophy requiring prolonged endotracheal and noninvasive assisted ventilation: not a uniformly fatal condition. *Pediatrics* 1998;101:704–706.
69. Lieberman AP, Fischbeck KH. Triplet repeat expansion in neuromuscular disease. *Muscle Nerve* 2000;23:843–850.
70. Igarashi H, Momoi MY, Yamagata T, et al. Hypertrophic cardiomyopathy in congenital myotonic dystrophy. *Pediatr Neurol* 1998;18:366–369.
71. Itoh M, Houdou S, Kawahara H, et al. Morphological study of the brainstem in Fukuyama type congenital muscular dystrophy. *Pediatr Neurol* 1996;15:327–331.
72. Shorer Z, Philpot J, Muntoni F, et al. Demyelinating peripheral neuropathy in merosin-deficient congenital muscular dystrophy. *J Child Neurol* 1996;10:472–475.
73. Bodensteiner JR. Congenital myopathies. *Muscle Nerve,* 1994;17:131–144.
74. Tsuji M, Higuchi Y, Shiraishi K. Congenital fiber type disproportion: severe form with marked improvement. *Pediatr Neurol* 1999;21:658–660.
75. Coutinho P, Barros J, Zemmouri R, et al. Clinical heterogeneity of autosomal recessive spastic paraplegias. *Arch Neurol* 1999;56:943–949.
76. Emeryk-Szajewska B, Badurska B, Kostera-Pruszczyk A. Electrophysiological findings in hereditary motor and sensory neuropathy type I and II: a conduction velocity study. *Electromyogr Clin Neurophysiol* 1998;38:95–101.
77. Melacini P, Fanin M, Duggan DJ, et al. Heart involvement in muscular dystrophies due to sarcoglycan gene mutations. *Muscle Nerve* 1999;22:473–479.
78. Johnson SD. Prednisone therapy in Beckers muscular dystrophy. *J Child Neurol* 2001;16:870–871.
79. Vignos PJ, Wagner MB, Karlinchak B. Evaluation of a program for long-term treatment of Duchenne muscular dystrophy. *J Bone Joint Surg Am* 1996;78:1844–1852.
80. Vogel LC, Betz RR, Mulcahey MJ. Pediatric spinal cord disorders. In: Kirshblum S, Campagnolo DI, DeLisa JA, eds. *Spinal cord medicine.* Philadelphia: Lippincott Williams & Wilkins, 2002:438–470.

81. Nelson VS. Spinal cord injuries. In: Molnar GE, Alexander MA, eds. *Pediatric rehabilitation*, 3rd ed. Philadelphia: Hanley & Belfus, Inc., 1999:269–288.

82. Massagli TL. Medical and rehabilitation issues in the care of children with spinal cord injury. *Phys Med Rehabil Clin N Am* 2000; 11(1):169–182.

83. Pang D, Wilberger JE. Spinal cord injury without radiographic abnormalities in children. *J Neurosurg* 1982;57:114–129.

84. Reynolds R. Pediatric spinal injury. *Curr Opin Pediatr* 2000;12:67–71.

85. Eleraky MA, Theodore N, Adams M, et al. Pediatric cervical spine injuries: report of 102 cases and review of the literature. *J Neurosurg* 2000;92:12–17.

86. Radecki RT, Gaebler-Spira D. Deep vein thrombosis in the disabled pediatric population. *Arch Phys Med Rehabil* 1994;75:248–250.

87. Centers for Disease Control. Spina bifida incidence at birth: United States, 1983. *MMWR Morb Mortal Wkly Rep* 1992;41:497–500.

88. Yen IH, Khoury MJ, Erickson JD, et al. The changing epidemiology of neural tube defects, United States, 1968–1989. *Am J Dis Child* 1992;146:857–861.

89. Lary JM, Edmonds LD. Prevalence of spina bifida at birth: United States, 1983–1990: a comparison of two surveillance systems. *MMWR Morb Mortal Wkly Rep* 1996;45:15–26.

90. Shurtleff DB, Lemaire RJ. Epidemiolgy, etiologic factors, and prenatal diagnosis of open dysraphism. *Neurosurg Clin N Am* 1995;6:183–193.

91. Omtzigt JG, Los FJ. The risk of spina bifida aperta after first-trimester exposure to valproate in a prenatal cohort. *Neurology* 1992;42[Suppl]:119–125.

92. Rosa FW. Spina bifida in infants and women treated with carbamazepine during pregnancy. *N Engl J Med* 1991; 324:674–677.

93. Milunsky A, Ulcickas M, Rothman K, et al. Maternal heat exposure and neural tube defects. *JAMA* 1992;268:882–885.

94. Centers for Disease Control and Prevention. Use of folic acid for prevention of spina bifida and other neural tube defects: 1983–1991. *MMWR Morb Mortal Wkly Rep* 1991;40:513–516.

95. Centers for Disease Control and Prevention. Recommendations for the use of folic acid to reduce the number of cases of spina bifida and other neural tube defects. *MMWR Morb Mortal Wkly Rep* 1992;41(RR-14):1–7.

96. Tulipan N, Bruner JP. Myelomeningocele repair in utero: a report of three cases. *Pediatr Neurosurg* 1998; 28:177–180.

97. Bruner JP, Tulipan N, Paschall RL. Fetal surgery for myelomeningocele and the incidence of shunt-dependent hydrocephalus. *JAMA* 1999;288:1819–1825.

98. Sutton LN, Adzick NS, Bilaniuk LT. Improvement in hindbrain herniation demonstrated by serial fetal magnetic resonance imaging following fetal surgery for myelomeningocele. *JAMA* 282:1826–1831.

99. Rekate HL, ed. *Comprehensive management of spina bifida*. Boston: CRC Press, 1991.

100. Herman JM, McLone DG, Storrs BB. Analysis of 153 patients with myelomeningocele or spinal lipoma reoperated upon for a tethered cord. *Pediatr Neurosurg* 1993;19:243–249.

101. McEnery G, Borzyskowski M, Cox TC. The spinal cord in neurologically stable spina bifida: a clinical and MRI study. *Dev Med Child Neurol* 1992;34:342–347.

102. Fraser RK, Bourke HM, Broughton NS. Unilateral dislocation of the hip in spina bifida. *J Bone Joint Surg Br* 1995;77:615–619.

103. Schmidt R, Royan BA, Tanayho EA. Neuroprosthesis in the management of incontinence in myelomeningocele patients. *J Urol* 1990;143:779–782.

104. Meeropol E, Frost J, Pugh L, et al. Latex allergy in children with myelodysplasia: a survey of Shriners hospitals. *J Pediatr Orthop* 1993;13:1–4.

105. Niggemann B, Buck D, Michael T, et al. Latex provocation tests in patients with spina bifida: who is at risk of becoming symptomatic? *J Allergy Clin Immunol* 1998;10:665–670.

106. Cuddeford TJ, Freeling RG, Thomas SS, et al. Energy consumption in children with myelomeningocele: a comparison between reciprocating gait orthosis and hip-knee-ankle-foot orthosis ambulators. *Dev Med Child Neurol* 1997;39:239–242.

107. Findley T. Ambulation in the adolescent with myelomeningocele I: early childhood predictors. *Arch Phys Med Rehabil* 1987;68:518–522.

108. Carney E, Melchionni J. Community ambulation by children with myelomeningocele and high level paralysis. *J Pediatr Orthop* 1991;11:579–582.

109. Worley G, Schuster JM, Oates WJ. Survival at 5 years of a cohort of newborn infants with myelomeningocele. *Dev Med Child Neurol* 1996;38:816–822.

110. Hunt GM, Poulton A. Open spina bifida: a complete cohort reviewed 25 years after closure. *Dev Med Child Neurol* 1995;37:19–29.

111. McCann PD, Bindelglass DE. The brachial plexus; clinical anatomy. *Orthopedic Review*, 1991;20:413–419.

112. Yilmaz K, Caliskan M, Oge E, et al. Clinical assessment, MRI and EMG in congenital brachial plexus palsy. *Pediatr Neurol* 1999;21:705–710.

113. Eng GD, Koch B, Smokvina MD. Brachial plexus palsy in neonates and children. *Arch Phys Med Rehabil* 1978;59:458–464.

114. Ramos LE, Zell JP. Rehabilitation program for children with brachial plexus and peripheral nerve injury. *Semin Pediatr Neurol* 2000;7:52–57.

115. Noetzel MJ, Park TS, Robinson S, et al. Prospective study of recovery following neonatal brachial plexus injury. *J Child Neurol* 2001;16:488–492.

116. Laurent JP, Lee R, Shenaw S, et al. Neurosurgical correction of upper brachial plexus birth injuries. *J Neurosurg* 1993;79:197–203.

117. Grossman JAI. Early operative intervention for birth injuries to the brachial plexus. *Semin Pediatr Neurol* 2000;7:36–43.

118. Strombeck C, Krumlinde-Sundholm L, Forssberg H. Functional outcome at 5 years in children with obstetrical brachial plexus palsy with and without microsurgical reconstruction. *Dev Med Child Neurol* 2000;42:148–157.

119. Price A, Tidwell M, Grossman JAI. Improving shoulder and elbow function in children with Erbs palsy. *Semin Pediatr Neurol* 2000;7:44–51.

120. Cheng JCY, Tang SP, Chen TMK, Sternocleidomastoid pseudotumor and congenital muscular torticollis in infants: a prospective study of 510 cases. *J Pediatr* 1999;134:712–716.

121. Golden KA, Beals SP, Littlefield TR. Sternocleidomastoid imbalance versus congenital muscular torticollis: their relationship to positional plagiocephaly. *Cleft Palate Craniofac Jo* 1999;36:256–261.

122. Ballock RT, Song KM. The prevalence of nonmuscular causes of torticollis in children. *J Pediatr Orthop* 1996;16:500–504.

123. Gupta AK, Roy DR, Conlan ES, et al. Torticollis secondary to posterior fossa tumors. *J Pediatr Orthop* 1996;16:505–507.

124. Persing J. Controversies regarding the management of skull abnormalities. *Journal of Craniofacial Surgery* 1997;8:4–5.

125. Minamitani K, Inoue A, Okuno T. Results of surgical treatment of muscular torticollis for patients >6 years of age. *J Pediatr Orthop* 1990;10:754–759.

126. Sillence DO, Senn A, Danks DM. Genetic heterogeneity in osteogenesis imperfecta. *J Med Genet* 1979;16:101–116.

127. McKusick VA. Osteogenesis imperfecta, type I. OMIM Database, #166200, 2002:1–20.

128. McKusick VA, et al. Osteogenesis imperfecta, progressively deforming with normal sclerae. OMIM Database, #259420, 2001:1–5.

129. Cole WG. Advances in osteogenesis imperfecta. *Clin Orthop* 2002;401:6–16.

130. Rauch F, Travers R, Plaotkin H, et al. The effects of intravenous pamidronate on the bone tissue of children and adolescents with osteogenesis imperfecta. *J Clin Invest* 2002;110(9):1293–1299.

131. Giraud F, Meunier PJ. Effect of cyclical intravenous pamidronate therapy in children with osteogenesis imperfecta: open-labeled study in seven patients. *Joint Bone Spine* 2002;69(5):486–490.

132. Marini JC, Gerber NL. Osteogenesis imperfecta: rehabilitation and prospects for gene therapy. *JAMA* 1997;277746–277750.

133. Luhman SJ, Sheridan JJ, Capelli AM, et al. Management of lower extremity deformities in osteogenesis imperfecta with extensible intramedullary rod technique: a 2-year experience. *J Pediatr Orthop* 1998;18:88–94.

134. Engelbert RHH, Pruijs JEH, Beemer FA, et al. Osteogenesis imperfecta in childhood: treatment strategies. *Arch Phys Med Rehabil* 1998;79:1590– 1594.

135. Binder H, Hawks L, Graybill G, et al. Osteogenesis imperfecta: rehabilitation approach with infants and young children. *Arch Phys Med Rehabil* 1984;65:537–541.

136. Binder H, Conway A, Gerber LH. Rehabilitation approaches to children with osteogenesis imperfecta: a ten-year experience. *Arch Phys Med Rehabil* 1993;74:386–390.

137. Engelbert RHH, Custers JWH, van der Net J, et al. Functional outcome in osteogenesis imperfects: disability profiles using the PEDI. *Pediatric Physical Therapy* 1997;9:18–22.

138. Engelbert RHH, van der Graff Y, van Empelen R, et al. Osteogenesis imperfecta in childhood: impairment and disability. *Pediatrics* 1997;99(2):E3.

139. Engelbert RHH, Beemer FA, van der Graff Y, et al. Osteogenesis imperfecta in childhood: impairment and disability—a follow-up study. *Arch Phys Med Rehabil* 1999;80:896–903.

140. Engelbert RHH, Gulmans VA, Uiterwaal CS, et al. Osteogenesis imperfecta in childhood: perceived competence in relation to impairment and disability. *Arch Phys Med Rehabil* 2001;82(7):943–948.

CHAPTER 71

Congenital and Childhood-Onset Disabilities: Age-Related Changes and Secondary Conditions in Mobility Impairments

Margaret A. Turk and Robert J. Weber

The issues of secondary conditions and aging in persons with disabilities have become of considerable interest to researchers and clinicians in recent years. Nevertheless, persons with disabilities have been concerned about these issues throughout their lifetimes and have been questioning healthcare professionals about the expectations for lifelong function. For years, children with disabilities and their families have been told that health and functional status, mobility, and musculoskeletal problems essentially stabilize by early adulthood. However, as more people with lifelong mobility impairments live through their adult years, it is apparent that mobility, functional status, and musculoskeletal changes commonly continue in adulthood. In fact, questions and concerns about mobility, function change, and pain are common among the majority of adults with mobility impairments caused by any etiology (1). These ongoing changes occurring in adulthood may be a part of the dynamic aging process, may be related to personal lifestyle choices, or may be in and of themselves secondary conditions.

There is a growing body of literature about aging issues and secondary conditions among persons with congenital and childhood-onset mobility impairments. Systematic studies of secondary conditions have only recently been initiated. Most scientific information has been published in the last 5 to 10 years, and much of the conventional wisdom in this area has been communicated through the network of persons with disabilities. There is minimal information regarding the impact of commonly practiced interventions over a lifetime. Therefore, health-care providers and consumers have limited knowledge from which to base decisions regarding adult health issues and anticipated changes in function in these individuals with disabilities.

This chapter will define secondary conditions and aging as it relates to congenital and childhood-onset disabilities, identify common lifelong functional status and health issues of adults with congenital and childhood-onset motor impairments, and discuss health promotion strategies in a disability population.

DEFINITIONS

Aging is the conception-to-death series of developmental changes that impact a person's ability to respond to the demands of the environment (2). It encompasses a person's entire lifetime, and not just the later stages of life. Aging is not simply a process of becoming older, less functional, and dying. Growth, development, acquisition of skills, maintenance of skills and functional capabilities, repair and replacement, and decline are all parts of aging. During the early stages of aging (infancy, childhood, adolescence), attainment of skills and capabilities is on the rise; in the middle stages (adulthood), maintaining and retaining function is the focus. All body systems are affected by aging. It is only in the later stages of life that function declines, if disease is not a factor at any of the preceding stages. Aging is also genetically moderated.

The underlying assumption has been that the pattern of aging for all body systems is the same in persons with lifelong disabilities as it is in the general population. Data to substantiate this assumption are not available. To understand the aging process, one must encompass all the changes that occur in a person from conception until death. Regarding motor performance, persons with disabilities follow a course of aging, although likely with a slower and lower attainment of skills, and a smaller capacity to adjust to acute or intercurrent health or medical and surgical interceders (Fig. 71-1).

Secondary conditions are impairments, functional limitations, disabilities, diseases, injuries, or other conditions that occur during the life of a person with a disability, in which the primary disabling condition is a risk factor for that secondary condition or may alter the standard intervention for prevention or treatment of any health condition (Syracuse Conference, 1994).

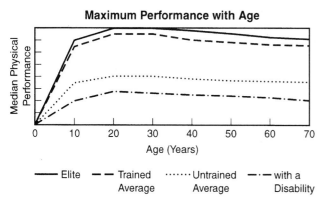

Maximum Performance with Age

Figure 71-1. Aging and performance is explained through this graph. (Adapted from Fries JF. The compression of morbidity. *Milbank Memorial Fund Quarterly/Health and Society* 1983;61(3):397–419.) Maximum performance (an arbitrary quotient) is achieved after a period of skill attainment, followed by maintenance of skills and linear decline. As noted, elite and trained individuals achieve significantly higher performance than an untrained average individual. Persons with childhood onset motor impairments have a slower achievement of optimal performance, lower optimal performance level, and quicker and lower performance with age, showing a smaller reserve for acute, recurrent, or chronic limitations to performance; there is still the capability for improved performance with training as in the nondisabled individual.

This is based on the new paradigm that people with disabilities are healthy; that is, a disabling condition does not imply illness and disease. Secondary conditions may be insidiously progressive or have onset in late adolescence or adulthood. They may include progression of pathology or impairment, either through complications or through the aging process. There may be variable expression, and some may not be preventable. With better supporting information, some of the reported early aging changes experienced by persons with congenital or childhood-onset disabilities may be considered secondary conditions. They may be modified by environmental or adaptive equipment measures. Secondary conditions may be difficult to identify if there is no index of suspicion by the clinician, or if there is an expectation of declining health and function of persons with disabilities as they mature. Commonly reported secondary conditions include pain, contractures, recurrent urinary tract infections, pressure sores, and osteoporosis.

Secondary conditions should not be confused with *associated conditions* or residual impairments. These are terms commonly used to describe conditions that result from the defect, injury, or disease and often may be considered primary impairments depending on their severity. For cerebral palsy or other brain injuries, the list of associated conditions includes seizures, learning disabilities, mental retardation, sensory problems, and oral motor and communication problems. Some conditions associated with the diagnosis of spina bifida include neurogenic bladder, neurogenic bowel, learning disabilities, mental retardation, and seizures. For the rheumatologic disorders, renal, cardiac, or pulmonary conditions may supersede the motor impairments as the primary health concern. Persons with a primary disabling condition may have any combination of associated conditions, all of which will impact on their ultimate functional capabilities.

Secondary conditions also do not include other *comorbidities*, that is, other medical conditions unrelated to the primary disabling condition. As an example, persons with cerebral palsy may also develop hypertension or diabetes mellitus should they have the risk factors or genetic predisposition for these conditions.

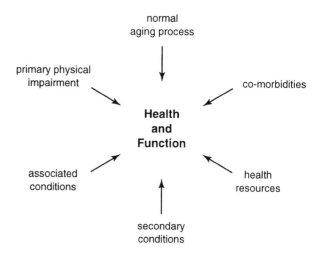

Figure 71-2. The medical paradigm is changing from illness and disease to health and wellness for persons with disabilities. Multiple factors affect function and health, and should be recognized by clinicians who serve persons with disabilities.

Health, then, is the absence of disease or illness beyond the disabling condition. In fact, the World Health Organization defines health as "a state of complete physical, mental, and social well-being and not merely the absence of disease or infirmity" (3). Health perception is an individual determination and is affected by personal expectations, experiences, sense of vulnerability, support, and locale. Often the health of persons with disabilities is perceived as poor by clinicians when the individual has a positive perception of her own health. In general, persons with nonprogressive disabilities should be considered healthy, with a shift of the health-care model from an illness and disability paradigm to one of wellness and prevention or early identification of secondary conditions, aging issues, or comorbidities (Fig. 71-2).

A body of literature has accumulated regarding aging and secondary conditions. Spinal cord injury and aging is the best developed, with information in the areas of quality of life (4), functional changes over time (5,6), premature and interactive effects of disability and aging (7–9), aging and secondary conditions (10), and psychological adjustment (11), among other issues. Other disability groups that have been studied are cerebral palsy (12), spina bifida (13,14), and polio (15).

Identification of age-related changes and secondary conditions with their risk factors has been better explored (1,16–20) than have prevention or intervention strategies. Recent research has been directed toward maintaining function with age and preventing secondary conditions. The person with a disability may have less reserve against the onset of functional or health changes compared with a nondisabled person.

Each factor in the interaction of disability and aging or secondary conditions has the capability to become a "negative feedback loop" (21) that may lead to further disability or a new medical condition. In effect, as a person with a disability ages, a series of new pathologies, impairments, and functional limitations may become superimposed on the previous ones.

HEALTH AND FUNCTIONAL STATUS: SECONDARY CONDITIONS AND AGE-RELATED CHANGES

The majority of information available regarding adults with congenital and childhood-onset motor impairments involves persons with cerebral palsy and spina bifida. This is because of their higher prevalence rates and the many organized pediatric clinics dedicated to these conditions. There is also increasing available information regarding adults with skeletal dysplasias and rheumatologic diseases. The accumulated information is a combination of scientifically observed and anecdotal information. Most reported research information is from cross-sectional or convenience samples and represents patient reports and clinical observations, not longitudinal studies using standardized measures. Although there is also supporting information from studies on cross-disability groups, persons with spinal cord injury, and polio survivors, generalization to other disability groups should be considered with caution.

Most problems of adults with congenital or childhood-onset motor impairments focus on musculoskeletal and physical performance symptoms and changes. This is not surprising for a group of people defined by impaired motor function. Although these groups are not homogeneous (i.e., they vary widely in severity and functional capacity), the prevalence of these symptoms indicates that musculoskeletal issues have a significant impact on the individual. The clinician therefore should anticipate these symptoms and be prepared to identify their cause and manage the problems appropriately.

The personal and social impact of functional changes in performance for adults with congenital and childhood-onset mobility impairments will not be addressed. The transition from childhood to adult management, lifestyles, goals, and issues will also not be highlighted. However, these aspects should not be ignored, nor can they be easily separated from discussions regarding implications for independence and recognition of changes. People with mobility impairments work hard to meet expectations for achieving independence both for themselves and for parents, professionals, and peers. Changes that compromise these hard-earned achievements can cause a significant emotional injury that should be addressed.

The following listing is designed to provide a core of knowledge to increase awareness of clinically important issues and to encourage further investigation. Table 71-1 provides a guide to commonly occurring secondary conditions and age-related changes for persons with disabilities and prevention strategies.

Health Status

Adults with cerebral palsy report that they enjoy generally good health (17,22). In fact, this self-rated health is comparable to that of the community at large (23). Adults with spina bifida report more health-related problems (e.g., pressure sores, burns, urinary tract infections, obesity) than do individuals with cerebral palsy, but general and comparative health data are not available (13,24). A cross-sectional study of adult women with mobility impairments from a variety of causes noted that women with lifelong or early-onset disabilities had a more positive health perception than those with adult-onset disabilities (25). Studies of polio survivors or persons with spinal cord injury report elevated cardiovascular system risk factors, including hypercholesterolemia, inactivity, and smoking; ischemic heart disease is a leading cause of death in spinal cord injury (15,26,27). These factors and an adverse outcome have not yet been found to be prevalent in adults with cerebral palsy or spina bifida.

Mortality statistics are limited. In a retrospective review of a British cerebral palsy registry (28), the most common reported cause of death in children and young adults with cerebral palsy was respiratory. In a retrospective, time-limited, population-based study (29), children with severe or profound mental retardation had an increased risk of dying at a younger age. In a population-based study of adults with cerebral palsy in a mid-sized metropolitan area, persons with cerebral palsy were generally healthy (based on clinical information and self-report), but noted worries and concerns about their health status (17). Spina bifida studies reported in the early 1970s noted survival to adulthood to be 60% to 70% for infants referred to regional centers (30). More recent studies reported a survival rate of 60% (31) and 76% (32) for consecutive cases, treated unselectively, within a 20-year time frame. Shortened life expectancy was reported in a state service registry for persons with developmental disabilities including mental retardation, severe motor impairments, and, in particular, a feeding disability (33).

Recent reports about juvenile rheumatoid arthritis are conflicting. It is reported that only a small percentage of adults with juvenile rheumatoid arthritis have recurrence of the arthritis, yet continued inflammatory activity into adulthood is also recognized (34). A U.S. midwest clinic cohort study reported an increased mortality for adults with juvenile rheumatoid arthritis that was associated with other autoimmune disorders (35). Regarding health perceptions, a clinic study of adults with juvenile rheumatoid arthritis showed poor health perception and continued pain in the face of typical health insurance coverage and income levels for age-matched controls (36).

Age-Related Changes

Information about age-related changes in a nondisabled population is available in the literature. Wide differences exist between individuals in the rate of aging and its effect on their physical function. Different organ systems age at different rates. There is no reason to believe that similar age-related changes will not occur in persons with disabilities. However, the changes related to the musculoskeletal system and performance should be considered more closely, because they may have a more profound expression in persons with long-term motor impairments. There are known aging changes that can be anticipated in the general population. Physical work capacity decreases with age, although muscle strength generally is maintained through the middle adult years. Complex performance activities can show greater change with aging because they require coordination and integration of multiple functions (e.g., endurance, sequence of muscle activity, balance, vision). The risks and causes for arthritic changes are complicated; however, degenerative joint changes in weight-bearing joints are universally noted by age 60 in both sexes and are hypothesized to be due to "wear and tear." Any predisposing factors (e.g., occupational activities, congenital joint malalignment, hereditary trends) may modify their onset or progression. Postmenopausal osteoporosis and aging-associated osteoporosis (senile osteoporosis) are age-related changes and can clinically present as the basis for fractures.

The impact of these general aging factors on a person with a mobility impairment is not well understood. It is, however, known that persons with mobility impairments use more energy to perform mobility activities than their nondisabled peers (37). Skeletal malalignment, deformities, and contractures are well described in persons with mobility impairments, and it is theorized that these contribute to pain and joint changes. It has been suggested through cross-sectional and convenience samples that adults with congenital or childhood-onset disabilities may show musculoskeletal or performance changes typical of advanced aging earlier than their nondisabled peers (22,24,38). In fact, published reports of adults with cerebral palsy show that about one-third of the study populations (cross-sectional or convenient samples) describe a decline in walking ability since early adulthood (25,39–43). Pain is also

TABLE 71-1.   Lifelong Motor Disabilities, Aging, and Secondary Conditions[a]

Body System	Pathology, Impairment, or Other Conditions Leading to Potential Secondary Conditions	Potential Prevention Strategies
Skin and subcutaneous tissues	Insensate skin; increased areas of pressure due to poor positioning, obesity, or limited weight shifts because of cognitive, behavioral, or personal care issues; decreased elasticity or turgor in aging with top layer thinning resulting in increased susceptibility to shearing and tearing; urinary or bowel incontinence.	Regular weight shift routine; appropriate seating systems and surfaces; good nutrition and hygiene habits; social or cognitive support to follow through with prevention.
Musculoskeletal system	Decreased strength and endurance; decreased range of motion; pain; osteoporosis (must recognize hereditary and all acquired forms); asymmetric motor performance; overuse or repetitive activities on unprepared system; aging issues of decreased flexibility, strength, endurance, and balance; risk of falls; obesity.	Maintenance of exercise programs (endurance, strength, flexibility); fall avoidance practices; osteoporosis prevention or management—must determine type of osteoporosis and state of clinical/scientific information; use of proper body mechanics and posture; appropriate assistive devices utilization; environmental accessibility; consideration of ergonomically correct work and activity surroundings; use of energy conservation and joint protection techniques.
Cardiovascular system	Hypertension; atherosclerosis (similar risk factors as in nondisabled individuals); limited activity and exercise; deep venous thrombosis and resulting pulmonary emboli—more often an early complication; obesity; age-related changes of slower responsiveness to position or heart rate change.	Health practices to identify risk factors for atherosclerosis (hypertension, smoking, hypercholesterolemia or hyperlipidemia, diabetes, menopause, etc.) and initiation of prevention or management strategies; good nutrition; maintenance of exercise or activity programs.
Genitourinary system	Urinary retention or incontinence; changes in urinary function from existing underlying condition (expected or unexpected progressive changes); progressive and chronic kidney filtration changes from poor or unchanged bladder management techniques; chronic urinary tract infections; kidney stones; prostate enlargement; urinary continence changes with menstrual cycle; urinary function changes from aging (e.g., reduced bladder capacity, decreased tissue compliance, reduce flow rate).	Monitoring of fluid intake and output; maintaining regular voiding schedule (e.g., intermittent catheter program, use of medication, timed voiding program); achieving acceptable hygiene program; participation in regular evaluation of urinary management (e.g., urodynamics, renal scans, post-void residual checks); reporting of urinary habit changes; consideration surgical opinions when appropriate; education in the consequences of urinary management, pros and cons of suggested interventions.
Respiratory system	Compromised breathing or cough due to underlying weakness; aspiration; existing obstructive or restrictive pulmonary disease or progression; breathing changes associated with aging (e.g., loss of reserve capacity, decreased tissue compliance); obesity; progressive weakness due to underlying condition; recurrent pneumonia.	Monitoring pulmonary function as appropriate and reporting changes; cessation of smoking or contact with secondary smoke; use of assistive coughing; maintaining exercise or activity program and healty diet; education of management strategies in progressive conditions; use of vaccinations when appropriate.
Gastrointestinal system	Decreased bowel motility with increased transit time; esophageal reflux; peptic ulcer disease; constipation or obstipation; megacolon; abnormal swallow function; hemorrhoids or risk for hemorrhoids with bowel program; malabsorption.	Good nutrition with diet modification (e.g., consistencies, textures, tastes); maintaining and monitoring routine bowel evacuation with consideration of fiber, fluid, and medication; review of routine medications which could contribute to decreased bowel motility; avoiding overuse of bowel medications; monitoring diet history and weights; reporting changes in bowel evacuation.

[a]This is not an inclusive table and serves as a practical guide only.
Reprinted with permission from Elrandt EN Jr, Pope AM, eds. *Enabling America: assessing the role of rehabilitation science and engineering.* Washington, D.C.: National Academy Press, 1997.

reported across a variety of disabilities at relatively younger adult ages and may influence performance at these young ages (25,36,42–44). These observations require confirmation through longitudinal controlled studies. Although risk factors may predispose a person to these changes, they are, as yet, unproven. These earlier-than-expected aging changes may be secondary conditions and are awaiting scientific confirmation.

Therefore, we should anticipate that persons with congenital or childhood-onset disabilities will progress over a disability continuum that includes age-related changes. The traditionally held belief that function is static is no more true for persons with disabilities than it is for persons without disabilities. As adolescents and young adults with disabilities transition to more independence, they and their families must be educated about potential age-related changes. While speculative, the use of appropriate adaptive equipment (e.g., power and manual wheelchairs, ergonomically correct work stations) as a potential moderator of chronic wear should be discussed. Health-

care providers should routinely question their adult patients with childhood-onset disabilities about pain and changes in function. Prevention strategies (e.g., energy conservation, joint protection, exercise) must be considered, and reports of change in function must be evaluated and treated appropriately. Exercise (flexibility, strengthening, and conditioning) should be a part of a regular routine and should be initiated and focused in response to complaints of pain or change in function. Exercise and activity programs can be individually modified and can be accomplished at home or through a health club. However, it must be recognized that aging alone does not cause dramatic decline in function and that when dramatic decline occurs, specific causes must be sought.

Musculoskeletal Issues

Decreased independence (increased need for assistance) in mobility and self-care is a common complaint of adults with mobility impairments. The reasons for change are varied and may include those related to age changes (e.g., decreased endurance, flexibility, strength, or balance), progressive pathology or secondary conditions (e.g., pain, contractures, spasticity, osteoporosis and fractures, tethering, stenosis), or personal choices (e.g., use of powered mobility to conserve energy). The change in mobility is often a response to a secondary condition or age-related change. Falls may also be such a response. Significant change in mobility or falls should not automatically be accepted as a part of a congenital or childhood-onset disabling condition in adult years; treatable etiologies should be sought.

Pain is a typical symptom of adults with mobility impairments and is commonly described by adults with spina bifida (24), cerebral palsy (18,22,25,43), juvenile rheumatoid arthritis (36), and osteogenesis imperfecta (44). Pain may be present for a variety of reasons, and it may be acute, recurrent, or chronic. Chronic pain may be present in adults with juvenile rheumatoid arthritis in the face of no active disease (45). Increased spasticity, weakness, falls, or progression of contractures or deformities can result from pain, particularly when pain is not reported because of communication difficulties or severe mental retardation. Symptoms or indications of pain should be noted by the adult with the mobility impairment or their health-care provider, and evaluation, diagnosis, and intervention should ensue. Pain is often the reason for a change in function, living arrangement, or social interaction.

Pain is usually identified with a specific location, most frequently a joint. Most people report arthritis as the etiology; however, these pains may originate from either joints or muscles. A good history and clinical exam will help sort out the issues and direct appropriate treatment. Back and leg pain symptoms are common in persons with cerebral palsy (18,22,23) and spina bifida (24). Adults with osteogenesis imperfecta types I, III, and IV commonly report pain in their lower limbs (44). Various forms of neck pain are frequently reported in any of these conditions. Although shoulder pain is a prominent problem in persons with spinal cord injury (46,47), it is reported less frequently in persons with cerebral palsy and spina bifida. Joint pain is likely to be related to recurring stresses during walking or other joint-loading activities (e.g., propelling a wheelchair) on normally or abnormally aligned joints, which also may have arthritic changes. Degenerative changes may not always be appreciated on x-rays in osteogenesis imperfecta because of the underlying bone density defect. Degenerative changes have been noted radiographically in dislocated and subluxed hips, not always related to weight-bearing activities, in persons with cerebral palsy (48). Femoral head resection as a treatment strategy for control of pain in hip disease for persons with cerebral palsy has been suggested (49); however, pain often persists or recurs postoperatively. Joint fusion has been an accepted intervention, but it may have a negative impact on positioning or on function. Muscle pain or tendonitis may result from functional activities and repetitive motions, and this is often the etiology of pain in young adults with lifelong motor impairments. Muscular pain is often noted by adults with spasticity as they age, and the spasticity often increases in response to pain. It has been reported that fatigue often incites pain, and exercise most commonly relieves pain (43). Appropriate management includes initial identification of the problem and its source (Table 71-2). Common musculoskeletal etiologies include poor er-

TABLE 71-2.   Pain Considerations in Adults with Childhood Onset Disabilities

Etiology	Assessment	Management
Musculoskeletal: • Fracture • Position; deformities or contractures • Ergonomics • Overuse • Weakness • Hypertonia • DJD	Elicit the history identifying areas of pain or function change Complete a clinical examination impairment and function based; compare to previous documentation Determine position or task causing discomfort Determine task requirement Request radiography as needed	Adjust position or task for function within capabilities Assess workplace ergonomically Consider adaptive equipment, temporary and permanent Use standard pain management • NSAIDs • Pain medications as appropriate • Manual medicine • Trigger point injections • Cognitive coping strategies Prescribe an exercise program • Strengthening • Flexibility • Conditioning • Aquatics-based Manage tone Prescribe modalities • Traditional • Nontraditional Consider joint replacement
Neurologic: • Radiculopathy • Peripheral nerve entrapment (CTS, Ulnar at elbow or wrist) • Cervical spine stenosis • Tethered cord/syrinx	Elicit a history characterizing pain, identifying change in function Complete a clinical examination distribution of findings; compare to previous documentation Request radiology, including imaging, as appropriate Consider urodynamics if urinary changes Electrodiagnosis EMG; peripheral and central conductions as appropriate	Standard non-surgical management; modification as needed for disability Surgical management requires planning for post-op capabilities, possible rehabilitation admission post-op

gonomics and biomechanics in tasks (secondary to deformity or limited motor control), underlying weakness and therefore overuse, hypertonia, and degenerative joint disease. Management includes traditional interventions (e.g., analgesics, anti-inflammatories, therapy modalities), more aggressive pain management strategies (e.g., manual medicine, trigger point injection, massage), and reevaluation of functional activities or positioning that may predispose to the pain symptoms. Use of tone management techniques can be helpful, including anti-spasticity medications, use of botulinum toxin injections for focal pain symptoms related to spasticity, or intrathecal baclofen. Any technique used to modify hypertonia requires a directed therapy approach to improve strength, position, and function (e.g., serial casting, orthotic change, strengthening program, neuromuscular electrical stimulation, surface electromyography biofeedback). Total hip replacements as a treatment option for hip pain from severe arthritis in adults with cerebral palsy is now more common, but its lifelong efficacy remains unknown (50); revision may be anticipated with placement at younger ages. Joint replacements are much more common for children and adults with juvenile rheumatoid arthritis and juvenile ankylosing spondylitis, and need for replacement may extend beyond 20 years (34), likely because of more limited or less rigorous activity level. Radiculopathies may also be the cause for painful symptoms, and appropriate evaluation and treatment should ensue. It is most important that treatment strategies are based on the person's history of function, that there is effective input from that person or their care provider, and that practical outcome goals are identified.

Although not as common as a musculoskeletal etiology, nerve entrapment is also a cause of pain. The most common nerves and areas of entrapment as reported by adults with developmental disabilities are those susceptible to compression in the nondisabled population: the median nerve at the carpal tunnel and the ulnar nerve in the hand distally and at the elbow. Compression points are often related to use of crutches, transfer techniques, propelling wheelchairs, or deformity. Work-related or positional activities may also cause entrapments, just as in the nondisabled population. All hand pain or sensation change does not represent nerve entrapment. Often these symptoms are actually problems of repetitive motion or are position related. Although they may be ascribed to carpal tunnel syndrome, they often respond poorly to surgery (22). Appropriate testing (including electrodiagnostic testing) is necessary to determine their etiology. When treatment options are similar for disabled and nondisabled adults, some modification of management will be required if functional independence is changed by or during treatment.

Contractures are a common secondary condition. Their impact on functional status or general health-care needs is variable. Increasing contractures, particularly when associated with pain or increased spasticity, may be an indication of progressing pathology. Aging changes include decreased flexibility, and the clinician must distinguish pathologic causes of increasing contracture through appropriate diagnosis. Charcot joints occur in spina bifida as a result of deformity and impaired sensation. In cerebral palsy, severe motor impairment is associated with scoliosis and other deformities (16). It has been reported in spina bifida that contractures are associated with partial or total dependence (24). Scoliosis in cerebral palsy and spina bifida seldom progresses during adulthood, but it can cause seating and pressure problems, impaired respiratory function, and pain. Adults with osteogenesis imperfecta type I (mild form) may have scoliosis noted in the second or third decade of life (51).

In persons with cerebral palsy, spinal stenosis must be ruled out whenever significant functional change is noted, particularly for change in or loss of walking skills, increased leg spasticity, change in bladder habits, neck pain, vague sensory changes, and (late) change in arm and hand function (52,53). A tethering effect on the spinal cord also may occur, resulting in cranial nerve changes. Some early reports noted a higher risk in those with an athetoid or dyskinetic component (54,55); however, more recent reports show these problems are present in spastic forms of cerebral palsy as well. It is generally held that stenosis is due to early spondylosis and compression, but there may also be a predisposition to it in those with a congenitally narrow canal. Diagnosis is made through imaging studies, and comparative evoked potentials may also be helpful in determining neurologic function. Surgical decompression may prevent further, often catastrophic loss of function, but does not assure complete return of lost function, particularly in cases of long-standing compression with spinal cord atrophy. Postoperative management planning should accommodate change in functional capabilities and care needs. The presence of an athetoid movement component will affect postoperative spine stabilization and possibly head positioning and neck mobility. When no surgical intervention is undertaken, a frank discussion of possible respiratory compromise and the future need for ventilator assistance should be provided.

In persons with spina bifida, the presence of a tethered cord or syringohydromyelia must be ruled out when they experience changes in bladder or bowel habits, increase in leg weakness, change in sensory level, onset of spasticity, report of pain (usually backache), or progression of scoliosis or foot deformities. In adults, an antecedent event such as in direct trauma to the back or buttocks often initiates symptoms. Prominent are diffuse leg pain with referral to the anorectal area, and changes in bladder or bowel habits; there is usually not progressive deformity noted as is reported in children (56). Diagnostic suspicion should be high for tethered cord in all persons who had immediate closure of the defect (57). The diagnosis may be supported through evoked potentials, urodynamic studies, and ultrasound or other imaging modalities, although the diagnosis remains a clinical one. However, recent studies report that a low-lying conus, tethering, cord thinning, lipomas, cavities within the cord, and diastematomyelia are present in some asymptomatic persons with spina bifida so that comparative studies that show internal change are more definitive diagnostically (58). Primary treatment is neurosurgical, but symptomatic management of pain, spasticity, and functional changes may be indicated when surgery is not possible. In particular, tethering associated with lipomeningoceles can be a difficult surgical procedure and has been associated with a higher risk of permanent loss of function.

Osteoporosis is a secondary condition associated with mobility impairments, often referred to as secondary osteoporosis of immobilization. This is not the osteoporosis associated with aging (postmenopausal or senile, both primary causes), but a condition noted much earlier in the lives of persons with mobility impairments. Reductions both in weight bearing and in physical activity with associated changes in muscular contraction forces are believed to play an etiologic role. Other contributing factors for osteoporosis in this population include poor nutrition, medications (e.g., phenytoin, barbiturates), and endocrine-related problems. Secondary osteoporosis is a known problem in persons with spina bifida and in persons with cerebral palsy who are categorized as severe and have no effective independent weight bearing (15,59,60). It has been shown that muscle activity is a more important determinant than weight bearing in persons with spina bifida (61). It has never been proven that passive, supported standing has any positive effect on secondary osteoporosis. Fractures of the extremities (not of the vertebrae as is seen in postmenopausal or senile osteoporosis) often are the first signs of significant secondary osteoporosis. Fractures are reported in adults with cerebral palsy and spina bifida (22,24). Unfortunately, treatment options for fractures are often limited because of the poor healing of severely osteoporotic bones with casting or surgical plating. Adequate pain management is of utmost importance. The impact on the individual of functional changes associated with the fracture needs to be addressed. Early recognition of osteoporosis and heightened efforts to protect against fractures in mobility-impaired individuals (e.g., appropriate transfer techniques, protection of distal limbs, fall prevention) are the initial management approaches. Assuring appropriate calcium and vitamin D intake is also important. There is recent interest in the use of bisphosphonates (62,63) as a treatment strategy in children and adults with disabilities; although studies note an increase in bone mineral densities, there is no information about the influence on rates of fracture. There are no published studies in adults with childhood-onset disabilities, nor on the lifelong positive (or negative) effects of medications used in childhood. The interrelationship of age-related osteoporosis with secondary osteoporosis is unknown.

Adults with spinal dysplasias have lifelong concerns with complicating skeletal changes. Adults with osteogenesis imperfecta (particularly type III) may continue to experience fractures, possibly being at a higher risk of bone loss with aging because of abnormal or diminished amounts of collagen matrix. Management of the fractures must allow continued activity and pain control. The circumstances, individual's function, and fracture characteristics direct the choice of treatment from soft immobilization of the fracture site to intramedullary rodding. There have been reports of improved bone mineral density with bisphosphonates in children with osteogenesis imperfecta noting a decrease in fractures (64), but there are no published studies regarding the maintenance of the changes or use in adults (63). Spinal stenosis at a variety of levels must be considered in adults with achondroplasia, osteogenesis imperfecta, or other dysplasias who note changes in urinary, bowel, sensory, or motor function.

In order to accomplish their daily routines, adults with mobility impairments often find they must conserve energy. The most practical way to do this is usually by making adjustments in the amount of walking or through use of power mobility aides. Although these adaptations are functional changes, they may not represent pathology, but rather normal aging effects. Normal aging and limited activity reduce physical performance reserve. Because mobility in the face of physical impairment requires vigorous effort, it is sometimes assumed that this alone provides conditioning. However, simply maintaining a daily activity will not enhance endurance or strength beyond that required of the activity. For instance, independent transferring maintains shoulder strength at the minimum level for that activity; it does not create endurance capacity in the arm or prepare one to perform weighted activities above the head. Participation in a fitness or exercise program should be considered, particularly when capability is marginal or waning.

Other Body-Systems Issues

Pressure ulcers are a commonly occurring secondary condition in persons with disabilities. In cerebral palsy, they may be seen as a result of poorly fitting orthotics or seating devices and are not common in the juvenile rheumatologic disorders or skeletal dysplasias. However, pressure ulcers are frequent in persons with spina bifida, related to their impaired protective sensation. The incidence and location of the sores is directly related to the functional motor level (24,65). Pressure ulcers are a persistent problem at all ages and do not necessarily decrease with age (13,24). Interestingly, obesity and burns are commonly associated with recurrent and chronic pressure sores (66), and are themselves acknowledged secondary conditions in spina bifida (13). A study conducted of a self-selected population of adults with spina bifida noted that preventive measures were generally not practiced or were ineffectively practiced in this group (24). Osteomyelitis is a complication of recurrent or chronic pressure ulcers and may ultimately require amputation for management (13,66).

Urologic problems are reported in both cerebral palsy and spina bifida. In spina bifida, lifelong issues are similar to those for persons with spinal cord injury: routine follow-up, recurrent urinary tract infections, renal calcifications, and renal failure or impairment (13,24,66). Renal failure is a serious secondary condition, and dialysis is an effective treatment in this group. Urinary diversion is associated with adverse affects on both health and renal function (67). Clean intermittent catheterization is an effective long-term management strategy for properly selected persons with neurogenic bladders from spina bifida (67). Urinary incontinence persists into adulthood, can be a socially limiting condition, and is shown in at least one study to be associated with partial or full unemployment (24). A survey of persons identified in a state registry as having spina bifida reported only a slight majority of the adults had achieved independence in urinary management (13). Neurogenic bladders in adults with cerebral palsy are only infrequently associated with upper tract pathology (68). Some women report that incontinence consistently occurs at a particular point of their menstrual cycle (25,69,70). Urinary incontinence can be effectively addressed through well-established diagnostic and intervention approaches. There are no available data that assess the adverse impact of urinary incontinence on social integration in cerebral palsy, but anecdotal support for this association is abundant. In both cerebral palsy and spina bifida, urinary habit changes may indicate other central or spinal pathology. Cognitive function also can affect urinary continence and should be taken into account. Self-imposed prevention strategies to manage incontinence (e.g., extreme fluid restriction, infrequent voiding) can cause other medical conditions. In older men, high index of suspicion of prostate enlargement as the cause of urinary symptoms should be maintained. In both men and women, urinary incontinence should be identified and addressed regardless of age or other conditions.

Gastrointestinal conditions occur in association with some mobility impairments. Usually they are chronic rather than new or late-onset problems. Changes in oral motor function affecting eating and swallowing may indicate spinal cord or brain-stem pathology. Symptomatic Arnold-Chiari malformation should be considered in spina bifida, and cervical cord stenosis should be ruled out in cerebral palsy and skeletal dysplasias. Dental hygiene and health have been reported as problems for adults with cerebral palsy (12,23,71) and osteogenesis imperfecta types I and IV (51,72). Although children with cerebral palsy are reported to have multiple gastrointestinal problems (73), studies of adults indicate these conditions are not common (17,22), despite anecdotally reported concerns (12). Bowel evacuation problems may be seen across motor impairments and are often related to fluid management (e.g., limited intake, excessive sweating), dietary intake, and limited gastrointestinal motility. Constipation, diarrhea, or incontinence may continue through adulthood; megacolon can develop if management is inadequate. Typical management strategies should be implemented, including use of fiber, osmotic agents, stimulants (oral and rectal), and softeners. In spina bifida, it has been noted that assistance is commonly required for bowel management, even in adulthood (13,74).

Obesity or overweight is a significant problem in the U.S. population overall and has been noted to be problematic for adults with disabilities in general (75). Obesity is a problem in spina bifida in adolescence through adulthood. There are higher levels of body fat in women and those not walking (76), and there is a correlation of increased body fat with previous hydrocephalus (77). Obesity may be less common in adults with cerebral palsy; however, the result of growth retardation (e.g., short stature) seen in children with cerebral palsy persists with age (78). Obesity and overweight may also be a problem in adults with skeletal dysplasia who are sedentary and adults with rheumatologic diseases who are treated with exogenous steroids in adolescence through adulthood. Appropriate nutrition and adequate exercise and activity are lifelong goals in persons with disabilities.

Because obesity and deconditioning may be common in adults with childhood-onset disabilities, screening for type 2 diabetes mellitus, hypercholesterolemia, or hyperlipidemia should be considered. Eliciting a positive family history for cardiac disease or diabetes mellitus would strengthen the need for such screening. Presently, there are no studies that identify these conditions in the cerebral palsy, spina bifida, or spinal dysplasia populations. However, preliminary data from a study investigating type 2 diabetes mellitus in obese children with spina bifida does identify high fasting and 2-hour postprandial insulin levels, indicating that there may in fact be insulin resistance in this population (personal communication, Craig McDonald, MD, 2003).

Adults with juvenile rheumatologic diseases may require vigilance regarding cardiac disease. In particular, atherosclerotic complications of systemic lupus erythematosus, aortitis (rare) in juvenile ankylosing spondylitis, and history of cardiac manifestations in any of the diseases may contribute to later morbidity or mortality even in early adulthood. Steroid use may be a risk factor, but is not substantiated. Comparison with adult-onset diseases notes no correlations to allow predictions of risks for complications in adulthood (34).

In general, pulmonary secondary conditions are not common for adults with congenital or childhood-onset mobility impairments. However, chest expansion restrictions from weakness (e.g., spinal cord dysfunction, muscle diseases, poor central motor control) or skeletal changes (e.g., arthritis, skeletal dysplasia, deformities) should be recognized. Pneumonia, bronchitis, and asthma should be managed in an anticipatory manner and aggressively treated when necessary. Preparation for possible surgeries should include pulmonary hygiene peri- and postoperatively. In osteogenesis imperfecta, particularly type III, there is an increased risk for premature death secondary to pulmonary disease with thoracic scoliosis greater than 60 degrees associated with vital capacities below 50% (79).

The issues of women's health apply for this population as well, with perhaps even greater questions of access and preventive maintenance programs in addition to reproductive health. Generally, women with disabilities have limited participation in typical health maintenance activities, such as routine pelvic examinations, Pap smears, and breast examinations (80). This is documented for women with cerebral palsy (69) and very likely to be true for women with spina bifida. Although

architectural barriers (e.g., inaccessible offices, inaccessible exam tables) may be a part of the problem, attitudinal barriers also contribute. Women with spasticity or contractures may find a pelvic examination to be difficult, painful, and too hurried to allow their effective participation. Health-care providers often consider women with disabilities to be asexual, and, therefore, not in need of routine obstetric or gynecologic care, including provision of information on contraception and protection during sex. However, these women are typically able to conceive and carry pregnancies to term without the expectation of major complications. It has been suggested that women with severe forms of osteogenesis imperfecta consider elective caesarean section for delivery because of the potential for fracture or cephalopelvic disproportion (72). Often women with childhood-onset disabilities report fewer sexual encounters as compared with other women with disabilities (25). Women with early-onset disabilities also experience high levels of sexual desire compared with other women with disabilities, postulated as being related to reduced social opportunities, frustrated satisfaction of sexual urges, discouragement of childhood sexual expression, or perceived social stereotypes (80,81). Although sample sizes are small, studies do indicate there could be associated problems with pregnancies in this group, emphasizing the importance of prenatal care (24,69). In spina bifida, back pain and deterioration in urologic status has been reported to be associated with pregnancy (82).

Men with childhood-onset disabilities also should receive information on sexual functioning, including information on contraception and protection. For men with spina bifida, the level of the neurologic lesion is not predictive of erectile or ejaculation function, but there is greater reproductive potential for those with low spinal cord lesions (82). Serum testosterone levels have been reported as normal (83) and possibly low (84).

Latex sensitivity and allergy occurs in persons with spina bifida, with the incidence of latex antibodies in this group approaching 40% (85). The sensitivity has been noted across disability severity and periodically across disabilities. In children, risk factors for the development of latex sensitization are atopy and atopic dermatitis; risk factors for allergic response are elevated IgE to latex, positive history of allergic response to latex contact, and frequent operations (86). This remarkably high level of sensitivity must be considered across a wide range of management (e.g., catheters, therabands, gloves), which includes discussion of condoms.

Hearing impairment is associated with osteogenesis imperfecta type I and is usually recognized in the second to third decade. The hearing loss is typically conductive and may be amenable to surgical intervention (72). There may also be a sensorineural hearing loss in conjunction with the conductive loss or independently; it occurs much less often and is seen in types III and IV (44). Audiologic assessment is imperative.

Access to Health Care

Access to health care for persons with disabilities has become a more public issue. Access involves environment, attitudes, and systems. Architectural barriers have been addressed through the Americans with Disabilities Act, although accessible health-care providers' offices and accessible examination and procedure tables continue to be available on only a limited basis. Attitudinal barriers involve both consumers and providers. Providers may have a limited knowledge regarding persons with lifelong disabilities. This lack of knowledge or understanding is perceived as a lack of caring and interest and as condescension. Through lack of knowledge, providers may in fact make erroneous assumptions of a consumer's cognitive status or ability to understand and make decisions. A consumer with communication impairment (e.g., hearing impairment, speech production impairment) may need more time to communicate, require an interpreter, or require personal preparation time for the appointment in order to have his/her needs conveyed. A consumer may avoid routine medical appointments because of bad experiences. Consequently, the consumer may seek help only late in the course of an acute medical condition or change and limit the options of care, increasing the risk for serious complications. In particular, consumers report that their routine health-care providers know little about their disability and its impact on health and function (38).

The present managed-care environment may not authorize the increased follow-up care appropriate for persons with disabilities or may limit access to specialists well versed in issues of lifelong disabilities. This is not to suggest that persons with disabilities are ill and require excess medical care. Rather, it is to recognize the need for knowledgeable monitoring and timely intervention to prevent loss of function; to identify secondary conditions, age-related changes, or anticipated health issues; and to implement appropriate intervention and prevention strategies to maintain health and function.

HEALTH AND WELLNESS AGENDA

As a result of the steady improvement in medical care and social support systems during the last 50 years, persons with disabilities are healthy, conducting active and productive lives, and generally living longer. The medical paradigm must now shift from that of illness and disease to one of health and wellness. The health-care delivery system must view persons with disabilities through a typical health maintenance and preventive medicine approach. This requires a change in attitudes and care models. Both prevention and promotion strategies should be employed: prevention of activities that lead to illness and disease (e.g., smoking cessation, dietary discretion, routine laboratory and examinations, protected sexual activity), and promotion of activities that improve general well-being (e.g., stress management, exercise) adapted to meet individual requirements and performance. However, positive health behaviors require social, health, and community resources. The more resources a person has, the more likely that individual will engage in health promotion and protective behaviors (87) (Fig. 71-3). Again, access is an important issue. Availability of information and the education of consumers are important, but not the most effective public health strategy. To participate in positive health behaviors, one must be interested, ready to make changes, and have the needed resources and a supportive environment. Early involvement of adolescents with mobility impairments in health-promotion activities may pave the way for maintaining these behaviors into adulthood.

Because musculoskeletal conditions are the most common age-related changes and secondary conditions that affect performance, it would seem most reasonable to view typical physiatric strategies and interventions as preventive management techniques. Use of adaptive equipment, energy conservation techniques, joint protection, and ergonomic positioning may enhance function, decrease musculoskeletal symptoms, and possibly prevent or delay some functional changes. Personal attitudes (of the person with a mobility impairment or their personal support system) may have to change before a person with impaired mobility will consider such assistance or be supported in considering the value of employing more supported (less independent) techniques.

Exercise is a well-known health-promoting behavior, and its effects are also positively demonstrated in persons with disabilities (88). Benefits of a regular exercise program include improved fitness, weight reduction, improved mood, and im-

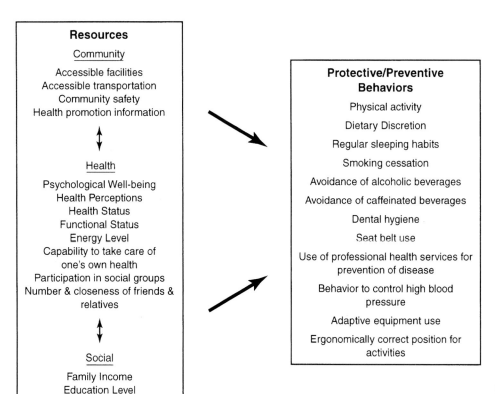

Figure 71-3. The resource model for persons with disabilities.

proved sleep. It is also known that persons must be judicious in participating in exercise programs. Of course, care must be taken in prescribing exercise for persons with impaired mobility; they should participate in an appropriate program of exercise or activity, especially keeping in mind their risk factors for musculoskeletal injury. Regular exercise involving repetitive joint-loaded activities (jogging, running) started by young adults without disabilities more often resulted in discontinuation of exercise because of joint pain than for persons who started an exercise program in their middle years. Aquatics programs can eliminate the wear and tear to joints, and an exercise program can be prescribed for strengthening, flexibility, and conditioning. Adults with cerebral palsy tend to report perceived changes in balance and then fear of falling (34), which usually improved with a general fitness program. Exercises, including strengthening exercises, are not contraindicated for persons with spasticity. Generally, adults and young adults with mobility impairments do not participate in routine fitness or exercise programs. This is as much from limited knowledge in this area as well as attitudes of care providers and persons with disabilities relative to exercise as a self-directed nonmedical activity. Consideration of exercise programs at home, with a health club, or as a part of an individual recreation program (with or without modifications) must be initiated earlier than adulthood to achieve long-term participation. And, just as in the nondisabled population, priorities for persons with a mobility impairment may not include exercise and fitness.

SUMMARY

Adults with congenital and childhood-onset mobility impairments are generally healthy, although the rheumatologic diseases may remain active into adulthood. Not all adults have serious health problems, and many now recognize the aging process as a natural course of events. The most common age-related changes and secondary conditions involve physical performance and the musculoskeletal system. Prevention strategies require knowledge of expected changes and possible risk for changes, recognition of changes that alter function and require intervention, and an understanding of interventions that have an impact on function. This requires that a person with a mobility impairment have access to knowledgeable health care; environmental, communication, attitudinal, and systems barriers must be overcome.

It is time to reconsider the model of illness and disease for persons with lifelong disabilities. Particularly in the realm of mobility, a health and wellness model should be developed. Use of prevention strategies must be considered in childhood and adolescence to address the more frequent secondary conditions. Programs of fitness and exercise have been proven beneficial in nondisabled groups and disability groups alike. Health promotion strategies should be employed for persons with congenital and childhood onset mobility impairments.

REFERENCES

1. Seekins T, Clay J. *Secondary disabilities in a population of adults with physical disabilities served by three independent living centers in a rural state.* Missoula, MT: Research and Training Center on Rural Rehabilitation Services, University of Montana, 1991.
2. Machemer RH. Biology of human aging. In Machemer RH, Overeynder JC, eds. *Aging and developmental disabilities: an in-service curriculum.* Rochester, NY: University of Rochester, 1993:1–23.
3. World Health Organization. *About WHO: mission statement.* http://www.who.int/about who/en/mission/htm (25 Aug 2000).
4. Evans RL, Hendricks RD, Connis RT, et al. Quality of life after spinal cord injury: a literature critique and meta-analysis (1983–1992). *Journal of the American Paraplegia Society* 1994:17:60–66.
5. Gerhart KA, Bergstrom E, Charlifue SW, et al. Long-term spinal cord injury: functional changes over time. *Arch Phys Med Rehabil* 1993;74;1030–1034.
6. Pentland WE, Twomey LT. The weight-bearing upper extremity in women with long term Paraplegia. 1991;29:521–530.
7. Bauman WA, Spungen AM. Disorders of carbohydrate and lipid metabolism in veterans with paraplegia or quadriplegia: a model of premature aging. *Metabolism* 1994;43:749–756.
8. Lammertse DP, Yarkony GM. Rehabilitation in spinal cord disorders: outcomes and issues of aging after spinal cord injury. *Arch Phys Med Rehabil* 1991;72:S309–S311.
9. Ohry A, Shemesh Y, Rozin R. Are chronic spinal cord injured patients (SCIP) prone to premature aging? *Med Hypotheses* 1983;11:467–469.
10. Whiteneck GG, Charlifue SW, Gerhart KA, et al. *Aging with spinal cord injury.* New York: Demos, 1993.
11. Krause JS, Crewe NM. Chronologic age, time since injury, and time of measurement: effect on adjustment after spinal cord injury. *Arch Phys Med Rehabil* 1991;72:91–100.
12. Turk MA, Overeynder JC, Janicki MP, eds. *Uncertain future—aging and cerebral palsy: clinical concerns.* Albany, NY: New York State Developmental Disabilities Planning Council, 1995.
13. Farley T, Vines C, McCluer S, et al. Secondary disabilities in Arkansans with spina bifida (abstract). *Eur J Pediatr Surg* 1994[Suppl I]:39–40(abst).
14. Lollar D. *Preventing secondary conditions associated with spina bifida or cerebral palsy: proceedings and recommendations of a symposium.* Washington, DC: Spina Bifida Association of America, 1994.
15. Maynard FM, Julius M, Kirsch N, et al. *The late effects of polio: a model for identification and assessment of preventable secondary disabilities: final report.* Atlanta: Centers for Disease Control and Prevention, 1991.
16. Turk MA, Weber RJ, Pavin M, et al. Musculoskeletal Problems among adults with cerebral palsy: findings among persons who reside at a developmental center. *Arch Phys Med Rehabil* 1995;1055(abst).
17. Turk MA, Weber RJ, Pavin M., et al. Medical secondary conditions among adults with cerebral palsy. *Arch Phys Med Rehabil* 1995;76:1055.
18. Turk MA, Weber RJ, Geremski CA, et al. Pain complaints in adults with cerebral palsy. *Arch Physl Med Rehabil* 1996;77:940.
19. Turk MA, Weber RJ, Geremski CA, et al. The reproductive functioning of women with cerebral palsy. *Arch Phys Med Rehabil* 1996;77:979.
20. Whiteneck GG, Charlifue SW, Frankel HL, et al. Mortality, morbidity and psychosocial outcomes of persons spinal cord injured more than 20 years ago. *Paraplegia* 1992;30:617–630.21.
21. Guralnik JM. Understanding the relationship between disease and disability. *J Am Geriatr Soc* 1994;42:1128–1129.
22. Murphy KP, Molnar GE, Lankasky K. Medical and functional status of adults with cerebral palsy. *Dev Med Child Neurol* 1995;37:1075–1084(abst).
23. Turk MA, Geremski CA, Rosenbaum PF. Secondary conditions of adults with cerebral palsy: final report. Syracuse, NY: Health Science Center at Syracuse, NY; Centers for Disease Control and Prevention, R04/CCR208516, 1997.
24. Dunne KB, Gingher N, Olsen LM, Shurtleff DB. A survey of the medical and functional status of members of the adult network of the Spina Bifida Association of America. Unpublished, 1984.
25. Turk MA, Scandale J, Rosenbaum PF, Weber RJ. The health of women with cerebral palsy. *Phys Med Rehabil Clin N Am* 2001;12(1):153–168.
26. Ragnarsson KT. The cardiovascular system, aging with spinal cord injury. In: Whiteneck CG, Charlifue SW, Gerhart KA, et al., eds. *Aging with spinal cord injury.* New York: Demos, 1993.
27. Stover SL, Fine PR. *Spinal cord injury: the facts and figures.* Birmingham, AL: University of Alabama, 1986.
28. Evans PM, Alberman E. *Certified cause of death in children and young adults with cerebral palsy.* London: London Hospital Medical College, Department of Clinical Epidemiology, 1990.
29. Kudrjavcev T, Schoenberg BS, Kurland LT, et al. Cerebral palsy: survival rates, associated handicaps, and distribution by clinical subtype (Rochester, MN, 1950–1976). *Neurology* 1985;35:900–903.
30. Shurtleff DB, Hayden PW, Chapman WH, et al. Myelodysplasia: problems of long-term survival and social function. *West J Med* 1975;122:199–205.
31. Hunt GM. Open spina bifida: outcome for a complete cohort treated unselectively and followed into adulthood. *Dev Med Child Neurol* 1990;32:108–118.
32. Bowman RM, McClone DG, Grant JA, et al. Spina bifida outcome: a 25-year prospective. *Pediatr Neurosurg* 2001;34(3):114–120.
33. Eyman RK, Grossman HJ, Chaney RH, et al. The life expectancy of profoundly handicapped people with mental retardation. *N Engl J Med* 1990;323:584–589.
34. Cassidy JT, Petty RE, eds *Textbook of pediatric rheumatology,* 4th ed. Philadelphia: WB Saunders Company, 2001.
35. French AR, Mason T, Nelson AM, et al. Increased mortality in adults with a history of juvenile rheumatoid arthritis: a population based study. *Arthritis Rheum* 2001;44(3):523–527.
36. Peterson LS, Mason T, Nelson AM, et al. Psychosocial outcomes and health status of adults who have had juvenile rheumatoid arthritis: a controlled, population-based study. *Arthritis Rheum* 1997;40:2235–2240.
37. Williams LO, Anderson AD, Campbell J, et al. Energy cost of walking and of wheelchair propulsion by children with myelodysplasia: comparison with normal children. *Developmental Medicine & Child Neurology* 1983;25:617–624.

38. Overeynder JC, Turk MA, Dalton AJ, et al. *I'm worried about the future . . . the aging of adults with cerebral palsy.* Albany, NY: New York State Developmental Disabilities Planning Council, 1992.

39. Andersson C, Mattsson E. Adults with cerebral palsy: a survey describing problems, needs, and resources, with special emphasis on locomotion. *Dev Med Child Neurol* 2001;43:76–82.

40. Ando N, Ueda S. Functional deterioration in adults with cerebral palsy. *Clin Rehabil* 2000;14:300–306.

41. Bottos M, Feliciangeli A, Sciuto L, et al. Functional status of adults with cerebral palsy and implications for treatment of children. *Dev Med Child Neurol* 2001;43:516–528.

42. Murphy K, Molnar G, Lankasky K. Medical and functional status of adults with cerebral palsy. *Dev Med Child Neurol* 1995;37:1075–1084.

43. Schwartz L, Engel J, Jensen M. Pain in persons with cerebral palsy. *Arch Phys Med Rehabil* 1999;80:1243–1246.

44. Wacaster PR, ed. *Managing osteogenesis imperfecta: a medical manual.* Gaithersburg, MD: Osteogenesis Imperfecta Foundation, Inc., 1996.

45. Flato B, Aasland A, Vinje O, et al. Outcome and predictive factors in juvenile rheumatoid arthritis and juvenile spondyloarthropathy. *J Rheumatol* 1998;25: 366–375.

46. Sie IH, Waters RL, Adkins RH, et al. Upper extremity pain in the postrehabilitation spinal cord injured patient. *Arch Phys Med Rehabil* 1992;73:44–48.

47. Subbarao JV, Klopfstein J, Turpin R. Prevalence and impact of wrist and shoulder pain in patients with spinal cord injury. *J Spinal Cord Med* 1994;18: 9–13.

48. Bagg MR, Farber J, Miller F. Long-term follow-up of hip subluxation in cerebral palsy patients. *J Pediatr Orthop* 1993;13(1):32–36.

49. Perlmutter MN, Synder M, Miller F, Bisbal R. Proximal femoral resection for older children with spastic hip disease. *Dev Med Child Neurol* 1993;35:525–531.

50. Buly RL, Huoo M, Root L, et al. Total hip arthroplasty in cerebral palsy: long-term follow-up results. *Clin Orthop* 1993;296:148–153.

51. Carey JC, Bamshad MJ. Constitutional disorders of bone. In: Rudolph CD, Rudolph AM, Hostetter MK, et al. *Rudolph's pediatrics,* 21st ed. New York, McGraw-Hill. 2002;1:713–786.

52. Reese ME, Msall M, Owen S, et al. Case reports: acquired cervical spine impairment in young adults with cerebral palsy. *Dev Med Child Neurol* 1991; 33:153–166.

53. Turk MA, Machener RH. Cerebral palsy in adults who are older. In: Machemer RH, Overeynder JC, eds. *Aging and developmental disabilities: an inservice curriculum.* Rochester, NY: University of Rochester, 1993:111–130.

54. Fuji T, Yonenobu K, Fujiwara K, et al. Cervical radiculopathy or myelopathy secondary to athetoid cerebral palsy. *J Bone Joint Surg Am* 1987;69:815–821.

55. Kidron D, Steiner I, Melamed E. Late onset progressive radiculomyelopathy in patients with cervical athetoid-dystonic cerebral palsy. *Eur J Neurol* 1987;27:164–166.

56. Pang D, Wilberger J. Tethered cord syndrome in adults. *J Neurosurg* 1982;57: 32–46.

57. Venes JL. Surgical considerations in the initial repair of meningomyelocele and the introduction of a technical modification. *Neurosurgery* 1985;17: 111–113.

58. McEnery G, Borzyskowski M, Cox, TCS, Nelville BGR. The spinal cord in neurologically stable spina bifida: a clinical and MRI study. *Dev Med Child Neurol* 1992;34:342–347.

59. Henderson R. Bone density and other possible predictors of fracture risk in children and adolescents with spastic quadriplegia. *Dev Med Child Neurol* 1997;39:224–227.

60. Henderson RC, Lark RK, Gurka MJ, et al. Bone density and metabolism in children and adolescents with moderate to severe cerebral palsy. *Pediatrics* 2002;110:5.

61. Rosenstein BD, Green WB, Herrington RT, Blum AS. Bone density in myelomeningocele: the effects of ambulatory status and other factors. *Dev Med Child Neurol* 1987;29:486–494.

62. Ott SM. Osteoporosis in women with spinal cord injuries. *Phys Med Rehabil Clin N Am* 2001;12:111–131.

63. Apkon SD. Osteoporosis in children who have disabilities., *Phy Med Rehabil Clin N Am* 2002;13:839–855.

64. Chevrel G, Meunier P-J. Osteogenesis imperfecta: lifelong management is imperative and feasible. *Joint Bone Spine* 2001;68:125–129.

65. Harris MB, Banta, JV. Cost of skin care in the myelomeningocele population. *J Pediatr Orthop* 1990;10:355–361.

66. Dorval J: Achieving and maintaining body systems integrity and function: clinical issues. In Lollar DJ ed. *Preventing secondary conditions associated with spina bifida or cerebral palsy.* Washington, DC: Spina Bifida Association of America, 1994:65–77.

67. Koch MO, McDougalWS, Hall MC, et al. Long-term metabolic effects of urinary diversion: a comparison of myelomeningocele patients managed by clean intermittent catheterization and urinary diversion. *J Urol* 1992;147: 1343–1347.

68. Murphy K, Kliever E, Steele BM. Cerebral palsy: neurogenic bladder, treatment and outcomes. *Dev Med Child Neurol* 1996; 38[Suppl 74]:7(abst).

69. Turk MA, Weber RJ, Geremski CA, et al. Health and functional characteristics of women with cerebral palsy. *Dev Med Child Neurol* 1996; 38[Suppl 74]:19.

70. Turk MA, Geremski C, Rosenbaum PF, Weber RJ. The health status of women with cerebral palsy. *Arch Phys Med Rehabil* 1997;78:S10–17.

71. Swedan NG, Gaebler-Spira DJ. Adults with developmental disabilities: cerebral palsy in adults over 40: lifestyle issues related to aging. *Arch Phys Med Rehabil* 1996;77:979(abst).

72. Glauser HC, ed. *Living with osteogenesis imperfecta: a guidebook for families.* Gaithersburg, MD: The Osteogenesis Imperfecta Foundation, Inc., 1994).

73. Pugliese JM, Edwards G. *Secondary and associated conditions of children with cerebral palsy or spina bifida: final report.* Birmingham, AL: United Cerebral Palsy of Greater Birmingham, 1996.

74. Lie HR, Lagergren J, Rasmussen F. Bowel and bladder control of children with myelomeningocele: a Nordic study. *Dev Med Child Neurol* 1991;33: 1053–1061.

75. Centers for Disease Control and Prevention. State-specific prevalence of obesity among adults with disabilities: eight states and the District of Columbia, 1998–1999. *MMWR Morb Mortal Wkly Rep* 2002;51:805–808.

76. Shepherd K, Roberts D, Thomas S, et al. Body composition in myelomeningocele. *Am J Clin Nutr* 1991;53:1–6.

77. Mita K, Akataki K, Itoh K, et al. Assessment of obesity of children with spina bifida. *Dev Med Child Neurol* 1993;35:305–311.

78. Ferrang TM, Johnson RK, Ferrara MS. Dietary and anthropometric assessment of adults with cerebral palsy. *J Am Diet Assoc* 1992;92(9):1083–1086.

79. Widman RF, Bitan FD, Laplaza FJ, et al. Spinal deformity, pulmonary compromise, and quality of life in osteogenesis imperfecta. *Spine* 1999;24(16): 1673–1686.

80. Nosek MA, Rintala DH, Young M, et al. *National study of women with physical disabilities (draft report).* Austin, TX: Baylor College of Medicine, 1996.

81. Nosek M, Rintala D, Young ME, et al. Sexual functioning among women with physical disabilities. *Arch Phys Med Rehabil* 1996;77:107–114.

82. Dunne KB, Arata M, Grover S, Bryan AD. Pregnancy in women with spina bifida: antenatal complications. *Dev Med Child Neurol* 1996;74[Suppl]:7.

83. Deter RM, Furness PD III, Nguyen TA, et al. Reproductive understanding, sexual functioning and testosterone levels in men with spina bifida. *J Urol* 1997;157:1466–1468.

84. Reilly JM, Oates RD. Preliminary investigation of the potential fertility status of postpubertal males with myelodysplasia. *J Urol* 1992;147:251A(abst).

85. Tosi LL, Slater JE, Shaer C. Latex allergy in pediatric spina bifida patients: incidence and implications. *Dev Med Child Neurol* 1993;69:17.

86. Liebke C, Niggemann C, Wahn U. Sensitivity and allergy to latex in atopic and non-atopic children. *Pediatr Allergy Immunol* 1996;7(2):103–107.

87. Kulbok PP. Social resource, health resources, and preventive behaviors: patterns and predictions. *Public Health Nurs* 1985;2:67–81.

88. Turk MA. The impact of disability on fitness in women: musculoskeletal issues. In: Krotoski MA, Nosek M, Turk MA, eds. *Women with physical disabilities: achieving and maintaining health and well-being.* Baltimore: Brookes Publishing, Inc., 1996:387–405.

CHAPTER 72

Geriatric Rehabilitation

Gary S. Clark and Hilary C. Siebens

Aging, an integral part of living, typically is accompanied by gradual but progressive physiologic changes and an increased prevalence of acute and chronic illness. Although neither a disease nor disability per se, aging nonetheless is associated with a higher incidence of physical impairment and functional disability. Many of these functional difficulties occur from the interactions of decreased physiologic reserve with chronic illness. Ongoing research suggests effective interventions to prevent, delay, minimize, or reverse such physiologic declines. Appropriate roles for geriatric rehabilitation accordingly include not only intervening to reverse disability caused by specific disease or injury (e.g., stroke, hip fracture), but also contributing to preventive gerontology by virtue of promoting structured physical fitness (i.e., wellness) programs and early rehabilitation for common musculoskeletal disorders to avoid progression to disability (1,2).

Significant contributions of rehabilitation to care of geriatric patients include functional assessment (including evaluation of underlying impairments contributing to functional loss and disability) with realistic goal setting, interdisciplinary team care, and efficacious adjustment of therapy interventions (e.g., timing, setting, intensity) to prevent, reverse, or minimize disability (3,4). Given the burgeoning number of older persons living longer, Rusk's observation, as modified by Kottke, becomes ever more relevant: "As modern medicine adds years to life, rehabilitation becomes increasingly necessary to add life to these years" (5).

AGING: EPIDEMIOLOGY AND PHYSIOLOGY

Demography and Epidemiology of Aging

DEMOGRAPHIC IMPERATIVE

The context for the increasing interest and concern about health-care needs of older adults is found in demographic projections of an expanding elderly population in the United States and other developed countries. At the turn of the twentieth century, 1 of every 25 Americans (4%) was 65 years of age or older. By 1994, this population had increased to one of every eight Americans (12.6%), or 33.2 million (6,7). Although the elderly population grew 11-fold during this interval, the younger-than-65 population only increased by a factor of three. Current projections indicate that 80 million, or one of every five Americans (21%), will be 65 years of age or older by 2030 (7,8). The peak growth of older persons is predicted to occur between 2010 to 2030, when the majority of baby boomers will turn 65, creating the "elder boom" (6).

Distribution of the elderly is uneven across the United States, with 50% living in just nine states. California has the greatest number of citizens older than the age of 65, but Florida has the highest proportion of elderly (18.6%) (6). There are also ethnic aging trends, with projections that by 2050, the proportion of older white individuals will have decreased to 67% (from 87% in 1990), with corresponding increases of older Hispanic and black American citizens of 16% and 10%, respectively.

This demographic phenomenon is not limited to the United States, as a number of developed countries (including Italy, Japan, Germany, Sweden, and Great Britain) currently show 20% or more of their populations older than age 65 (6). As of 1994, there were 357 million older people worldwide, representing 6% of the total population. Interestingly, the rate of growth of elderly appears to be greatest in developing countries.

There is increasing recognition of differences in health-care needs and issues among subgroups of older people. Of particular significance from a health-care standpoint are the rapidly expanding relative proportions of the population age 65 years and older who are 75 to 85 years of age (old-old) and 85 years of age or older (oldest-old). These groups include many of the so-called "frail elderly," with a disproportionately high prevalence of disabilities and consumption of health services (9). In the United States, as well as many other countries, the 85-or-older group is the fastest growing segment of the population, both proportionately and in actual numbers (8). Making up approximately 1% of the population (3.2 million) in 1994, the number of oldest-old is predicted to more than double (to 7 million) by 2020 and reach 19 million by 2050 (6).

COMPRESSION OF MORBIDITY

Older people also are living longer. 1990 statistics estimate a longevity at 65 years of age of 15.0 years for men and 19.5 years for women; this is projected to increase further to 17.1 and 22.6 years, respectively, by 2040 (8). The increasingly delayed occurrence of death at all ages appears in large part to be due to delays in onset and reduced lethality of such diseases as stroke, cancer, and myocardial infarction, resulting from risk-factor reduction as well as improved health-care interventions (7). Increasingly, people are surviving their initial encounter with these previously fatal diseases, resulting instead in chronic illness. This trend has been termed the fourth stage of epidemiologic transition (i.e., the postponement of death from degenerative diseases) (10). These significant reductions in mortality are associated with an increasing risk for development of various chronic diseases. Certainly the incidence and prevalence of many potentially disabling chronic illnesses increases substantially among older adults, including arthritis, osteoporosis with associated fractures, stroke, amputation, and various neurodegenerative disorders (e.g., Alzheimer's disease, Parkinson's disease) (8,9).

This demographic imperative has far-reaching implications for increasingly limited United States health-care resources and dollars. Current national direct costs of medical services for older individuals with chronic conditions is in excess of $470 billion (in 1990 dollars), with a projected near doubling by 2050 (8). The old-old and oldest-old groups consume the greatest proportion of resources, and a disproportionate amount of these health-care costs represent nursing home and other institutional care (9). While the overall proportion of elderly individuals residing in nursing homes decreased from 6.8% in 1982 to 4.2% in 1999, these rates vary dramatically by age (11). Only 1% of young old (65- to 74-year-olds) reside in nursing homes, contrasted with 20% of the oldest old (85 years of age or older) (7). In fact, the latter group composes 45% of all elderly nursing home residents.

From another perspective, however, the vast majority of the 85-or-older population is not in nursing homes, and half of those in nursing homes do not necessarily need to be there because they have potentially preventable (or reversible) disabilities related to their chronic disorders (12). In fact, it appears that much of the increased health-care costs associated with aging (across all health-care settings) is significantly related to activity limitation, rather than chronic disease (13). Fortunately, there is increasing evidence that disability among older individuals may be decreasing (11,14).

These findings lend credence to the concept advanced by Fries in 1980 of "compression of morbidity", in which he predicted that if the age of onset of disability could be significantly delayed (e.g., with regular exercise, healthier diets, elimination of smoking, and improved health-care interventions) in the context of a relatively "fixed" life span, then terminal predeath disability could be compressed into a shorter interval (15). He postulated that health-care needs for older people would decrease because they would be relatively healthy and functional until shortly before their demise. A related prediction was that this anticipated short duration of predeath morbidity, and accompanying disability, would be expected and accepted with acknowledged futility of medical intervention. Interestingly, although a number of reports have documented dramatically increasing health-care costs near the end of life, it should be noted that these are costs of dying, not of aging per se (16). Further, there is evidence suggesting the incremental costs associated with extending life may actually plateau or even decrease (17). These findings are of critical significance in the context of increasing focus on cost containment and debate over the feasibility and appropriateness of rationing of health care (18). Twenty years after his initial predictions, Fries cites increasing evidence in support of the trend of compression of morbidity, even though the mechanisms are not clear (19). He reiterates the importance of a research agenda focused on delineation of the epidemiology of disability, determination of the fundamental basis of age-associated chronic conditions, and identification of effective interventions for preventing or delaying resulting disability (12).

ACTIVE LIFE EXPECTANCY

A derivative of research into longevity and epidemiology of aging relates to issues of quality of life, given the increased incidence of frequently disabling chronic disorders, such as degenerative neurologic diseases (e.g., Alzheimer's disease, Parkinson's disease), degenerative musculoskeletal conditions (e.g., osteoporosis, osteoarthritis), and multisensory losses (e.g., cataracts, presbycusis). One concept that attempts to delineate quality of life for older individuals has been termed "active life expectancy," referring to the proportion of remaining life span characterized by functional independence (20). This concept has been expanded to consider both physical and cognitive impairments, as well as their interrelationships (21). A significant gender difference in active life expectancy with aging has been identified. As can be seen in Table 72-1, older men have a greater proportionate active life expectancy at all ages. However, because of greater longevity, older women enjoy longer actual durations of active life expectancy than older men, until age 85 (21,22). Although there is no racial difference in longevity, older black people have a shorter active life expectancy than nonblack populations. This is apparently the result of greater and earlier incidence of disabling chronic conditions (22).

Although the increasing incidence and prevalence of (often multiple) chronic diseases with aging is well documented, there is no one-to-one correlation between either disease and illness (23) or disease and disability (14). A significant proportion of older people are limited in the amount or kind of their usual activity or mobility secondary to chronic impairments: more than 60% of adults with functional impairments that are due to chronic health problems are 65 years of age or older (8). Furthermore, there are often fluctuations in levels of disability in older individuals. In a 2-year follow-up study, a number of older persons who were initially disabled had recovered their functional independence, and vice versa (24). Also, the overall health of progressive cohorts of older persons has been changing. Future generations may well be healthier than current generations, partly because of higher levels of education and health awareness (24). However, Kane raises disturbing questions regarding potentially adverse economic, cultural, and individual consequences of successfully overcoming the aging (and dying) process and urges ongoing dialogue to further explore these ethical questions (25).

In summary, an increasingly large number of older people are living longer and are at increased risk of developing varying (and changing) degrees of functional losses and disability. The challenge for health-care providers, accordingly, is to try to prevent, reverse, or at least minimize functional loss resulting from the various chronic illnesses to which the elderly are prone.

Biology of Aging

From a clinical and physiological standpoint, normal aging involves a steady decrease in organ system reserves and homeostatic controls, in conjunction with an increase in prevalence of disease (23). Of increasing interest and focus in aging research is the degree to which these processes influence each other and whether they are indeed interdependent (26).

SUCCESSFUL AGING

Distinctions have been made between aging processes representing "primary aging" (i.e., apparently universal changes that occur with aging, independent of disease and environ-

TABLE 72-1.   Active Life Expectancy (Remaining Years of Functional Independence, Compared to Projected Longevity) by Gender and Age Cohort

Age	Males	Females
65	82% (11.9 of 14.4 years)	73% (13.6 of 18.6 years)
85	50% (2.6 of 5.2 years)	35% (2.3 of 6.4 years)
95	20% (0.6 of 3.2 years)	10% (0.4 of 3.7 years)

Adapted from: Manton KG, Stallard E. Cross-sectional estimates of active life expectancy for the U.S. elderly and oldest-old populations. *J Gerontol* 1991; 46(suppl):170–182.

mental effects) and "secondary aging," which includes lifestyle and environmental consequences and disease as part of the aging syndrome (27,28). A number of tenets associated with aging research are being reexamined, particularly with the observation that a pathologic process may exaggerate an aging process believed to be normal, even before the disease is detected clinically (27). There is increasing speculation that the nonpathologic processes of aging are distinct from, but not necessarily independent of, the pathologic processes of disease (29).

Most studies of normal aging have focused on the physiological and biochemical changes occurring with aging, with explicit exclusion of disease. However, it is increasingly apparent that such factors as personal habits (e.g., diet, exercise, nutrition), environmental exposures, and body composition may have significant impact on observed aging changes (28). Rowe has proposed a conceptual distinction between "successful aging" and "usual aging" (30). He suggests that "successful aging" could be characterized by minimal or no physiologic losses in a particular organ system and would comprise a relatively small subset of the total normal (i.e., nonpathologic) aging population. The remaining majority of normal older adults demonstrate "usual aging," with significant declines in various physiologic functions.

The significance of this concept lies in the implications for modifiability of usual aging by virtue of addressing such variables as level of physical activity, diet and nutrition, and environmental exposures (19,28,29). This principle is demonstrated in studies documenting the effects of exercise, diet, and drugs on the usual aging observations of carbohydrate intolerance. Rowe proposes that geriatric research into health promotion initiatives concentrate on increasing the proportion of older adults who "successfully age" by identifying and modifying extrinsic risk factors contributing to "usual aging" and decreasing the manifestations of "pathologic aging" by preventing or minimizing adverse effects of acquired disease processes (30). This would reinforce the previously described concept of compression of morbidity with greater active life expectancy. Indeed, studies are now beginning to determine which factors distinguish high-functioning older adults from other populations of older adults (28,31).

THEORIES OF AGING

With continuing research, it appears likely that there is no single cause of aging (29). The concept that comes closest to a unifying theory might integrate hypotheses based on passive (i.e., random) or active processes of genetic programming, perhaps with superimposed nongenetic mechanisms (e.g., environment, lifestyle) that could result in varying individual vulnera-

bility (27,29,30,32). Certainly this would help explain the well-documented phenomenon of differential aging, whereby individuals of the same species appear to age at different rates (29,31). Multiple levels of research suggest that rates of aging are affected to varying extents by heredity, lifestyle, environment, occurrence of disease, and psychological coping abilities (12,22,27,31).

Active investigation continues in the areas of neuroendocrine pacemakers, telomere shortening, and attenuation of inducible stress responses (32–34). A number of studies also have focused on the phenomenon of apoptosis—which refers to the gradual and orderly form of cell death—with evidence suggesting that pathologic stimulation of apoptosis may result in a number of degenerative disorders commonly associated with aging, whereas inhibition appears to be associated with a variety of forms of cancer (35).

Physiology of Normal Aging

The normal aging process involves gradual decreases in organ system capabilities and homeostatic controls that are relatively benign (i.e., asymptomatic or subclinical) in the absence of disease or stress (23). Although the older person progressively adapts to these changes without need (or desire) for outside intervention, the steady decreases of physiologic reserves make older adults potentially vulnerable to functional decline as a result of acute or chronic illnesses (27,36).

Characteristics of aging include:

- Decreased reserve capacity of organ systems, which is apparent only during periods of exertion or stress
- Decreased internal homeostatic control (e.g., blunting of the thermoregulatory system, decline in baroreceptor sensitivity)
- Decreased ability to adapt in response to different environments (e.g., vulnerability to hypothermia and hyperthermia with changing temperatures, orthostatic hypotension with change in position)
- Decreased capacity to respond to stress (e.g., exertion, fever, anemia) (23)

The end result of these age-related declines is an increased vulnerability to disease and injury.

PROBLEMS IN STUDY DESIGN

Definition of Normal

A significant concern, in view of the heterogeneity of the aging population, is what is truly normal. As noted, there is great variability in rates of aging among healthy elderly and wide variations in individual performance. Further complicating any analysis is a superimposed dispersion of skills that is due to frequency of significantly impaired function from disease, environment, and lifestyle (22,23). More than 80% of the 65-or-older population has at least one chronic disease, and 50% have two or more disorders (21). Of concern is whether the relative minority of older people who have escaped serious illness should be considered "normal" for the purpose of studies of aging and whether the results of such studies can be generalized to the rest (majority) of the older population.

On the other hand, it is important clinically to be able to differentiate the physiologic consequences of aging (i.e., normal aging) from those of accompanying disease (i.e., pathologic aging) (1). Because detection of disease depends on determination that a patient is other than normal, it is critical to define appropriate age-adjusted criteria for clinically relevant variables in the elderly (37). Although many laboratory values do change gradually with aging, abnormalities should not be a priori attributed to old age. In fact, a number of age-related changes may resemble the changes associated with a specific disease (29). For example, an age-related decline in glucose tolerance is well documented. So dramatic is this change that most people older than 60 years would be diagnosed as diabetic if traditional criteria, based on studies of primarily younger patients, were applied (26).

Methodology Limitations
A number of methodological problems are associated with the study of aging. Well recognized are frequent discrepancies in age reporting, with a tendency to distort upwardly (38). This is coupled with difficulties in verifying reported ages, which is due in part to lost or nonexistent birth records.

A major problem in the design and evaluation of aging studies is the relative validity of both cross-sectional and longitudinal studies. Cross-sectional studies, although easier and less costly in time and money to perform, often overemphasize (but may also underestimate) age changes (39,40). This can result from a cohort bias that is due to significant differences in educational, nutritional, health, and social experiences of people born in different decades. Contributing further to this distortion is the high proportion of elderly in the United States who were foreign born, with relatively less schooling. This has implications in particular for studies of psychological and cognitive changes with aging (14).

On the other hand, longitudinal studies tend to underestimate changes that result from aging, primarily because of withdrawal and survivor biases with high drop-out rates (31,36,39). Some studies have experienced as much as a 50% drop-out rate over just a 10-year period, leading to questions of self-selection for relative preservation of function (and again, the issue of supernormals). Subtle changes in methodology over time may introduce laboratory drifts that are difficult to differentiate from true age-related changes (6). A further concern whenever serial measurements are made is the potential for distortion as a result of learning effects.

Mean Versus Maximal Performance
Another issue in the characterization of aging is that a focus on "average" or "mean" changes in various parameters can hide remarkable individual variation, particularly of peak performance (15). Consider marathon running, which although involving a very select ("supernormal") population, does measure maximal aerobic performance. A 50-year-old male runner with a time of 3.5 hours is in the ninety-ninth percentile for his age group, yet not until 73 years of age would that time set an age-group record. Although there also is a slow linear decline in maximal performance with aging based on world age-group records, this is only on the order of about 1% per year between the ages of 30 and 70 years (15).

EFFECTS OF AGE ON ORGAN SYSTEM PERFORMANCE
There are several general principles regarding aging effects on performance of various organ systems (41).

Wide Individual Differences in Rate of Aging
Variation between healthy people of the same age is far greater than the variation that is due to aging alone, and the range of variability increases with aging (15). Linear regressions show average changes with aging, but variation between subjects is so great that it is not possible to determine accurately if age decrements are linear over the entire age span or whether the rate of decline accelerates in later years (42).

Different Organ Systems Age at Different Rates
There is great variation in the rate of decline for various organ system functions (23). For instance, there is up to a 60% decline in maximal breathing capacity with aging, but only 15% declines in nerve conduction velocity and basal metabolic rate during the same interval. Another demonstration of this principle is the localized cellular growth, aging, and death occurring continually in some tissues and organs (e.g., hematopoietic system, skin, mucosa). Furthermore, significant decline in function of one organ system (e.g., kidney) does not entail a similar decline in other organ systems (41).

Age Changes with Complex Performances
Complex performances (e.g., running) will show greater changes with aging because of the need to coordinate and integrate multiple organ system functions (e.g., rate, degree, and sequence of muscle contraction, balance, proprioception, vision, cardiovascular response), as opposed to simple performances involving a single system (e.g., renal glomerular filtration) (41).

Age Changes in Adaptive Responses
Adaptive responses (e.g., to temperature change or change in position) are most affected by aging owing to a decline in effectiveness of physiologic control mechanisms (e.g., sensory feedback), which is magnified with stress situations (e.g., disease, sudden changes in environment) (23,41).

PREVENTION AND REVERSIBILITY OF PHYSIOLOGIC DECLINE
There is little question that biologic systems, regardless of direct effects of aging, can be profoundly influenced by environment and lifestyle (22,23,28). Obvious examples include effects of smoking and sedentary versus active lifestyles (43).

The modifiability or plasticity of aging is demonstrated by studies in which performance can be improved despite age within relatively broad ranges (15,44). Physical training can improve or even reverse age-related declines in aerobic power and muscle strength (45,46). These gains have been demonstrated to translate to improvements in functional skills (47,48).

FUNCTIONAL IMPLICATIONS OF ORGAN-SYSTEM AGING
The clinician must be aware of specific age-related physiologic changes to properly understand disease in the elderly because these changes significantly influence not only the presentation of disease, but response to treatment and potential complications that may ensue. Such knowledge similarly is essential to understand underlying mechanisms of functional deterioration secondary to disease and to formulate effective rehabilitation approaches (1). The following is a summary of clinically significant physiologic changes that occur with aging.

Hematologic System
Although anemia occurs with increasing prevalence with aging, there is convincing evidence that it is not a normal consequence of aging and should be investigated, especially if hemoglobin is < 10.5 g/dL (49–51). Anemia in older people appears to be due most commonly to iron deficiency (typically from gastrointestinal blood loss) or chronic disease (such as infection, pressure ulcers, polymyalgia rheumatica, or cancer) (50). Other potential causes include hemolysis (e.g., secondary to lymphoma, leukemia, or medication effect), B_{12} deficiency (pernicious anemia, diet), or folate deficiency (diet). Of note, D-dimer levels have been shown to double with aging, with even more dramatic increases among blacks and functionally im-

paired older individuals (52). Increases in the erythrocyte sedimentation rate and C-reactive protein levels also have been noted with aging.

The functional consequences of anemia can be significant because of further reduction of reserve capacity, such that previously subclinical disease states may become symptomatic (e.g., orthostatic blood pressure changes, change in anginal pattern with lower exercise tolerance) (51,53). This has obvious implications with regard to tolerance of relatively intensive and sustained rehabilitation exercise programs. There is also evidence of correlation of even relatively mild anemia with impaired mobility (54). A very anemic older patient may present with nonspecific fatigue and confusion, with the potential for misdiagnosis and mistreatment (49).

There are several related hematologic changes with aging that can affect pharmacokinetics, particularly drug distribution. Decreased drug binding for highly protein-bound drugs (e.g., warfarin, meperidine, tolbutamide) may result in a higher unbound, or free, drug concentration with correspondingly magnified actions (55). This effect is even more significant for patients taking multiple drugs because of competition for fewer binding sites.

There also commonly is an altered volume of distribution, due to reduction in total body water and lean body mass, with a relative increase in body fat. As a result, water-soluble drugs (e.g., digoxin, cimetidine) tend to have a smaller volume of distribution, with higher plasma concentrations and greater pharmacological effect (56). Conversely, fat-soluble drugs (e.g., diazepam, phenobarbital) usually have a larger volume of distribution because of relatively greater storage in fatty tissue. This may result in delayed therapeutic effects, with the potential for unexpected late toxicity. By the same token, prolonged drug effects are seen after dosage change or discontinuation because of the amount of drug stored in adipose tissue (55).

Gastrointestinal System

The term *presbyesophagus* has been used to describe multiple changes in esophageal function commonly observed with aging, such as delayed esophageal emptying, incomplete sphincter relaxation, and decreased amplitude of peristaltic contractions. Only the latter appears to be a direct result of aging, but it is without clinical significance; the other changes, with potentially significant clinical ramifications, are related to associated disease processes (57). There is an increased risk of aspiration with aging because of less coordinated swallowing.

Age-related changes in colon function include slightly decreased force and coordination of smooth muscle contraction resulting in slower transit time, as well as impaired rectal perception of feces (58). The high incidence of constipation in older people accordingly is thought to be related to multiple additional factors, such as low dietary fiber and fluid intake, sedentary habits, and various associated diseases interfering with intrinsic bowel function (e.g., parkinsonism, stroke) (59). A variety of medications are potentially constipating, including minerals (e.g., aluminum antacids, iron, calcium), opiates, nonsteroidal antiinflammatory drugs (NSAIDs), antihypertensives (e.g., calcium channel blockers, clonidine), anticholinergics (e.g., tricyclic antidepressants, neuroleptics, antispasmodics), and sympathomimetics (e.g., pseudoephedrine, isoproterenol, terbutaline) (60). Prolonged use of stimulant laxatives or enemas can also impair bowel contractility and result in constipation or even obstipation (59). Older adults often report straining and hard bowel movements along with their constipation (61). Straining may indicate rectal dyschezia (in which rectal sensation and contractility are impaired).

Fecal incontinence in older people is due most commonly to overflow incontinence secondary to fecal impaction, but can also occur as a result of decreased sphincter tone, cognitive impairments (e.g., from drugs, dementia), diarrhea, or dyschezia (59,61). Diarrhea among elderly patients is most frequently caused by fecal impaction, intestinal infection, or drugs (e.g., broad-spectrum antibiotics, digoxin toxicity), but also can be due to chronic laxative abuse (62). More appropriate interventions for bowel regulation include increasing diet fiber, using bulk agents or stool softeners, and avoiding frequent use of enemas or laxatives.

Despite these physiologic changes with aging, little effect is seen on absorption of most orally administered drugs (56). Drug absorption in general is more significantly affected by concomitant administration of multiple drugs; in particular, antacids and laxatives bind to or reduce dissolution of other medications (55).

Hepatic System

The primary changes in the hepatic system with aging involve progressive decreases in liver size and hepatic blood flow, as well as slowing of hepatic biotransformation, specifically and most consistently microsomal oxidation and hydrolysis (56,58). This can have major implications for circulating concentrations of certain drugs and their metabolites, depending on mode of metabolism and clearance. Drugs with high first-pass clearance (e.g., propranolol, propoxyphene, major tranquilizers, tricyclic antidepressants, antiarrhythmic drugs) are cleared less effectively owing to reduced hepatic blood flow, resulting in greater bioavailability (55). Comorbid processes, such as congestive heart failure, can exacerbate these effects.

Drugs metabolized by means of phase I biotransformation (i.e., oxidation, reduction, hydrolysis) tend to have prolonged elimination in older people (e.g., diazepam, chlordiazepoxide, prazepam), whereas those undergoing phase II metabolism (i.e., glucuronication, acetylation, sulfation) generally are not affected by aging changes (e.g., oxazepam, lorazepam, triazolam) (55,60).

It is important to note that studies of drug elimination with aging demonstrate significant differences between people, contributed to by wide interindividual variability and effects of such factors as smoking, alcohol, caffeine intake, diet, and concurrent use of other medications (56). As a result, caution should be exercised when using age-based guidelines for dosage determination (42).

Renal System

There are a number of age-related anatomic and physiologic changes in the kidney, including decreases in renal mass, number and functioning of glomeruli and tubules, renal blood flow, and glomerular filtration rate (63,64). These reductions in renal function have major implications for drug excretion, with prolonged half-lives for those drugs cleared primarily by glomerular filtration (e.g., cimetidine, aminoglycosides, digoxin, lithium, procainamide, penicillin, chlorpropamide) (55).

Studies show a mean age-related decrease in renal function of about 1% per year, with a decrease in creatinine clearance of 7.5 to 10 mL per decade; however, there is wide variability, with as many as one-third of older individuals showing no significant decline (64). Because of a corresponding decline in daily urinary creatinine excretion (reflecting decreases in muscle mass), there is no significant change in serum creatinine level with aging. As a result, neither serum blood urea nitrogen (which is dependent on dietary intake and metabolic function) or creatinine is valid for accurately gauging renal function in older people (55).

Other common physiologic changes with aging include impaired ability to concentrate or dilute urine, impaired sodium conservation, reduction of urine acidification, and decreased ability to excrete an acid load (63). This erosion of reserve capacity allows maintenance of fluid and electrolyte homeostasis under normal conditions, but not with sudden changes in volume, acid load, or electrolyte balance. As a result, older people are more vulnerable to hyponatremia, hyperkalemia, dehydration, and perhaps most seriously, water intoxication (26,65).

Because of difficulty in concentrating urine in conjunction with a blunted thirst mechanism, a hypernatremic state with attendant mental confusion can result if an elderly person is stressed by higher-than-usual insensible losses (e.g., high or prolonged fever, exercise) with poor fluid intake (65). This is pertinent in a rehabilitation setting because patients often are engaged in vigorous activities and may become dehydrated relatively easily.

Just as older patients are prone to volume depletion when salt deprived, acute volume expansion from an elevated sodium load caused by inappropriate intravenous fluids, dietary indiscretion, or intravenous radiographic contrast dye can result in congestive heart failure, even in elderly patients without preexisting myocardial disease (55,66). A further potential complication of the use of radiocontrast materials in the elderly is the risk of acute renal failure, which is exacerbated by the presence of preprocedure dehydration (63). Because renin and aldosterone plasma concentrations are decreased by 30% to 50% in the elderly, with increased susceptibility to hyperkalemia, potassium-sparing diuretics (e.g., spironolactone, triamterene) should be used with great caution (60).

Hyponatremia that is due to water intoxication may be the most serious electrolyte disorder of geriatric patients (26,65). Most frequently complicating an acute illness, the clinical picture includes nonspecific signs of depression, confusion, lethargy, anorexia, and weakness. Serum sodium concentrations below 110 mEq/L may result in seizures and stupor. The syndrome of inappropriate antidiuretic hormone secretion, with water retention and hyponatremia, can occur with infections (e.g., pneumonia, meningitis), strokes, various drugs including diuretics, or the stress of anesthesia and surgery (64).

Pulmonary System

Although progressive declines in pulmonary function are observed with aging, in the absence of significant pulmonary, cardiovascular, or neuromuscular disease, these declines are reflected primarily as a loss of reserve capacity without major functional limitations at rest (67). However, impaired pulmonary function on spirometric testing does indicate increased risk for several common causes of death in older people, including cardiovascular disease and chronic obstructive pulmonary disease (68). Changes in pulmonary function observed with aging reflect effects of aging per se (in the pulmonary as well as cardiovascular and neuromuscular systems), together with the cumulative effects of inhaled noxious agents (especially cigarette smoke and air pollutants) and infectious processes (67). The latter typically have a far greater impact on pulmonary function.

Progressive decline in a number of pulmonary function tests has been documented with aging, including vital capacity, maximum voluntary ventilation, expiratory flow rate, and forced expiratory ventilation (67). These declines reflect aging changes in the pulmonary system combined with those in related organ systems, which are collectively stressed by the maximum volitional inspiration and expiration required to complete the tests. Examples include stiffening of the rib cage from degenerative calcification of costochondral cartilage (i.e., decreased compliance), weakening of intercostal and abdominal muscles, and increased airflow resistance from small airway narrowing that is due to decreased elasticity (68). Residual volume and functional residual capacity increase, which is related to the loss of elastic recoil (increased compliance), although total lung capacity remains unchanged.

Normal gas exchange requires both uniform ventilation of alveoli and adequate blood flow through the pulmonary capillary bed. With increasing age, there is a progressive ventilation-perfusion imbalance that is due to collapse of small peripheral airways with decreased ventilation of alveoli, resulting in a linear decline in pO_2 with aging [$pO_2 = 110 - (0.4 \times age)$] (67). Because of altered thoracic mechanics, pO2 in older individuals is lower in the supine position than sitting or standing. No changes occur in pCO_2 or pH, and oxygen saturation is typically normal or only slightly reduced.

This reduction in arterial oxygen tension is clinically relevant because it represents a further loss of reserve. Elderly patients are more vulnerable to significant hypoxia from a relatively minor insult (e.g., anemia, congestive heart failure, respiratory infection) or the stress of physical inactivity because they are closer to the steep slope of the oxygen-hemoglobin dissociation curve (67). Blunting of central and peripheral chemoreceptor responsiveness exacerbates this vulnerability further: Both hypercapneic and hypoxic ventilatory responses markedly diminish with aging, independent of lung mechanics. Apparently related to this is the significant increase in sleep-related breathing disorders noted with aging (26).

Maximal oxygen consumption (VO_2max), an overall measure of exercise capacity and cardiopulmonary fitness, depends on pulmonary ventilation, cardiac output, peripheral circulatory control (i.e., ability to shunt blood to exercising muscles), and muscle oxidative capacity. Although a progressive decline in VO_2max is observed with aging, this does not appear to be on a pulmonary basis (68,69). In fact, it appears that decreases in VO_2max in older adults with mild to moderate chronic obstructive pulmonary disease are due primarily to cardiac deconditioning resulting from limited activity levels (68). Regular exercise to maintain or improve fitness is critical with aging because it is possible to improve fitness with training at any age, and this is associated with reduced vulnerability to stress or disease (and thereby increased active life expectancy) (44,47, 70). The tendency of physicians and society to tolerate (or even encourage) decreased activity among older people, in conjunction with trends toward obesity and increased recumbency, probably contributes more to poor pulmonary function than aging alone (68,71).

Although most attention regarding the high incidence of pneumonia in the elderly is focused on immunologic declines, there appear to be contributing factors relating to the pulmonary system directly or indirectly. Because many pneumonias result from aspiration of the infecting organism, impaired mucociliary function and decreased chest wall compliance with weaker cough (resulting in impaired ability to clear aspirated material or secretions) likely play a role (67,68). Other nonimmunologic contributing factors may include dysphagia, disruption of lower esophageal sphincter integrity, various esophageal disorders, and reduced levels of consciousness.

Cardiovascular System

A number of established tenets about the aging cardiovascular system have been revised, based on continuing research using more rigorous methodologies to exclude occult disease and controlling for degree of habitual physical activity. As a result, it now appears that cardiac output at rest and during graded exercise is relatively unaffected by age directly (26,69,72). Although resting heart rate does not change with aging, maximal heart rate with exercise does decrease progressively, related to decreased chronotropic responsiveness to adrenergic stimuli. The clinical formula reflecting this decline in maximal heart rate involves subtracting the age from 220 for men, and subtracting (0.8 × age) from 190 for women (70,72). Decreased inotropic responsiveness to adrenergic stimulus results in decreased myocardial contractility, with decreased ejection fraction and increased risk of congestive heart failure (73). Maintenance of cardiac output at rest and with modest exercise is accomplished by early involvement of the Frank-Starling mechanism, with increased stroke volume via higher left ventricular end-diastolic volumes (26,72).

Another age-associated change is a decrease in the rate of early diastolic filling, with a much greater dependency on late filling through atrial contraction (72). As a result, older people are more vulnerable to deleterious effects of atrial tachycardia or fibrillation, including congestive heart failure (69,73).

Both cross-sectional and longitudinal studies demonstrate decreases in maximal oxygen consumption with aging, regardless of habitual activity level (43,69). However, physically active people retain significantly greater maximal aerobic capacity with aging compared with their sedentary counterparts (44). In fact, trained elderly subjects may have greater maximal oxygen consumption than sedentary subjects who are much younger (45). Furthermore, endurance training, even when begun in old age, can significantly improve exercise capacity (44,70). Of clinical relevance is that the energy of walking represents an increasing percentage of the total aerobic capacity with advancing age, such that walking becomes a very effective physical conditioning activity (74).

A final age-related physiologic change in the cardiovascular system with important clinical applications is decreased baroreceptor sensitivity (74). This results in a diminished reflex tachycardia on rising from a recumbent position and accounts in part (possibly along with blunted plasma renin activity and reduced angiotensin II and vasopressin levels) for the increased incidence of symptomatic orthostatic hypotension in the elderly, as well as cough and micturition syncope syndromes (72,75).

Immunologic System

Significant alterations in immunocompetence occur with aging, involving both cellular and humoral immune functions (76). Although the total number of lymphocytes decreases by about 15% in older adults, this does not appear to contribute significantly to the marked decline in immunocompetence (77). There is a decline in lymphocyte proliferation in response to antigen stimulation in older adults, as well as a higher incidence of anergy (76). Age-related shifts have been observed in the regulatory activities of T cells (i.e., fewer T cells with suppressor or helper activity) and monocytes or macrophages.

Changes in humoral immunity with aging include increases in circulating autoantibodies and immune complexes, with decreased antibody production (76). The latter is characterized by an attenuated response to immunization, with difficulty maintaining specific serum antibody levels.

The increased susceptibility of the elderly to infection is a function of both these age-related changes in immune function and the frequency of concomitant factors that further impair host defenses (e.g., diabetes, malignancy, vascular disease,

malnutrition, and stress) (76). Altered local barriers to infection, such as skin breakdown or an indwelling urinary catheter, often compromise resistance to infection further. Common infectious processes in the elderly include influenza, pneumonia, urinary tract infection, sepsis, herpes zoster, and postoperative wound infections.

Of particular clinical relevance is the fact that older people react differently to infections than do their younger counterparts. There is a less active leukocytosis in response to inflammation, and the total white blood cell count often is not increased (although usually there is still a shift of the differential count to the left) (78). The older patient may have less pain or other symptomatology and frequently absent or only low-grade fever.

Endocrine System

The endocrine system also undergoes significant changes as we grow older. There is a gradual decrease in glucose tolerance with aging, although the fasting blood sugar level remains relatively unchanged (26). Accordingly, age-adjusted criteria for diabetes mellitus have been developed. This age-related decline in glucose tolerance is due to reduced sensitivity of tissues to the metabolic effects of insulin or insulin resistance (79). Compounding these aging changes are secondary conditions that further reduce tissue sensitivity to insulin, including lifestyle changes (e.g., obesity, diet changes, stress, sedentary lifestyle), other diseases (e.g., chronic infections, prolonged immobilization), and effects of medications (30,80).

Of clinical importance is the risk for untreated hyperglycemia, osmotic diuresis, and dehydration, potentially leading to hyperosmolar nonketotic coma or ketoacidosis (80). Certain drugs can cause or potentiate hyperglycemia (e.g., thiazide diuretics, glucocorticoids, tricyclic antidepressants, phenothiazines, phenytoin) (81). Control of serum glucose in older diabetic patients with oral sulfonylureas or insulin can be fragile, with significant risk for hypoglycemia. However, even borderline hyperglycemia appears to result in accelerated atherosclerosis and multiple end-organ involvement (26). Of interest is the contribution of obesity and physical inactivity to increased incidence of diabetes in older adults, and the benefits of weight loss and regular exercise in improving control (30).

There are multiple other endocrine changes associated with aging. The primary clinical impact of altered thyroid physiology with aging is the need to maintain a high index of suspicion for the unusual presentation of thyroid disease. Presenting signs and symptoms of the older thyrotoxic patient may include palpitations, congestive heart failure, angina, atrial fibrillation, major weight loss associated with anorexia, and either diarrhea or constipation (82). Goiter and serious ophthalmopathy frequently are absent. Apathetic hyperthyroidism may not be recognized until late in the course of illness: patients appear depressed and withdrawn, with clinical clues of muscle weakness, dramatic weight loss, and cardiac dysfunction (80). Signs and symptoms of hypothyroidism essentially are unchanged with aging, but the diagnosis still may be delayed because of the many similarities between the stereotype of senescence and the hypothyroid state (e.g., psychomotor retardation, depression, constipation, cold intolerance). In view of the higher incidence of hypothyroidism in older adults, routine periodic screening of thyroid function is warranted (82).

The relationships between the hypothalamus, pituitary, and adrenal cortex remain unchanged with age, with preserved diurnal rhythm and stress response (80). Although cortisol production decreases progressively, basal and adrenocorticotrophic hormone–stimulated serum cortisol levels are unchanged with aging. Primary adrenocortical disease is uncommon in the elderly. Significant hyponatremia or hyperkalemia, suggestive of adrenocortical insufficiency, is not uncommon in the elderly but more often is secondary to drugs (e.g., thiazide diuretics, chlorpropamide, carbamazepine) (60).

Age-related changes in gonadal function are well documented. There are variable and gradual declines in serum testosterone levels in healthy men with aging, likely because of partial testicular failure; however, there is no indication for routine androgen replacement (26). Postmenopausal declines in estrogen levels are well documented, with clinical expression variably including vasomotor instability syndrome (i.e., hot flashes), atrophic vaginitis, and osteoporosis (28). Controversy continues over prophylaxis and treatment of the latter, particularly with regard to potential benefits of dietary supplements and exercise (28,30). The reader is referred to Chapter 30 for further details.

Thermoregulatory System

Older people have impaired temperature regulation because of a combination of diminished sensitivity to temperature change and abnormal autonomic vasomotor control. As a result, they have a reduced ability to maintain body temperature with changes in environmental temperature and are vulnerable to both hypothermia and hyperthermia (26,65). The risk of hypothermia is compounded further by impaired thermogenesis (i.e., inefficient shivering), with potential aggravation by a variety of conditions (e.g., hypothyroidism, hypoglycemia, malnutrition) or medications (e.g., ethanol, barbiturates, phenothiazines, benzodiazepines, narcotics) (65). Conversely, diminished sweating (a result of higher body temperature needed to initiate sweating and decreased sweat production) is a major contributing factor in heat exhaustion and heat stroke in hot conditions. Hypohidrosis is aggravated by anticholinergics, phenothiazines, and antidepressants (60). Two-thirds of deaths from heat stroke occur in people older than 60 years, reflecting this impairment in regulatory systems. This has major implications for rehabilitation exercise programs, particularly when combined with a tendency for dehydration (44).

Sensory System

Deterioration of vision is one of the most recognized sensory changes occurring with aging. The most common visual change with increasing age is a gradual loss of the ability to increase thickness and curvature of the lens to focus on near objects (i.e., presbyopia) and physiologic miosis (26). Cataract formation, with opacification of the lens, occurs to some degree in 95% of the 65-or-older population. The elderly also are at significantly higher risk for further disease-related visual decrements (e.g., glaucoma, macular degeneration, diabetic retinopathy) (83). The result of these various changes is a loss of visual acuity, decrease in lateral fields of vision, decline in both dark adaptation ability and speed of adaptation, and higher minimal threshold for light perception. These changes have obvious implications in relation to the higher incidence of falls in the elderly, particularly at night (84,85).

Gradual decline in hearing acuity (i.e., presbycusis) also is characteristic of aging, although again a number of treatable disorders can cause superimposed damage (e.g., wax occluding the outer canal, cholesteatomas, acoustic neuromas). Older people most commonly manifest a conductive hearing loss, possibly because of increased stiffness of the basilar membrane, or distortion of perceived sound with increase in threshold sensitivity, narrower range of audibility, abnormal loudness, and difficulty discriminating complex sounds (86). Continuing advances in hearing aid technology make remediation of such hearing deficits increasingly feasible (87). Early recognition and treatment of hearing impairments is particularly critical in the presence of cognitive deficits to avoid adverse sequelae of social isolation and development of paranoid ideations or frank psychiatric reactions (84).

Neurologic System

Numerous changes in the functioning of the neurologic system have been noted with aging. Three important areas of dysfunction accompanying normal aging include decreases in short-term memory, loss of speed of motor activities (with slowing in the rate of central information processing), and impairments in stature, proprioception, and gait (26).

The major controversy over neurologic changes with aging concerns cognitive functioning. A significant proportion of the observed decline in fluid intelligence with aging appears to be related to a decrease in the rate of central information processing (88,89). There is progressive deterioration in performance after age 20 on timed motor or cognitive tasks, including abstraction tests (e.g., digit symbol substitution test), reaction time tasks, and other tests requiring speed in processing of new information. Although there are declines with aging in motor and sensory nerve conduction velocities and rate of muscle contraction, they account for only a fraction of these slowed responses (89).

Many aspects of learning and memory remain relatively intact during normal aging, including immediate or primary memory as measured by digit span recall, retrieval from long-term storage, storage and retrieval of overlearned material, and semantic memory (90). However, age-related impairments have been documented consistently in tasks involving episodic short-term memory and incidental learning (91). Examples include difficulties with free recall of long (i.e., supraspan) lists of digits or words and paired associate and serial rate learning, for both visually and verbally presented material. What these investigations indicate is that older adults are capable of new learning, but at a slower rate (90).

Because much of rehabilitation involves learning, these findings have major implications for rehabilitation programming for disabled elderly people. This is particularly true in the context of superimposed cognitive deficits, given that intellectual ability is an important determinant of the effectiveness of a standard geriatric rehabilitation program (2).

A final area of neurologic age-related physiologic changes involves posture, proprioception, and gait. Older people in general are noted to demonstrate progressive declines in coordination and balance, related in part to impaired proprioception (92). This has significant implications for degree of mobility and stability, although there are a number of common, potentially concomitant, pathologic changes that may contribute further to gait problems in the elderly (e.g., vertebral compression fractures with kyphosis, arthritis, degenerative cerebral changes, cerebral infarcts) (85,93).

Musculoskeletal System

There is a well-documented progressive loss of muscle strength with aging, on the order of 14% to 16% per decade (men and women) for lower extremity muscles, and 2% (women) to 12% (men) per decade for upper extremity muscles (40). A major contributing factor to this observed decline in strength appears to be an overall decrease in muscle cross-sectional area and mass with age (94). However, there may be significant contributions of cellular, neural, or metabolic factors to changes in strength, as decline of strength was observed even without loss of muscle mass (40). Further, significant gains in muscle strength, as well as functional mobility, have been demonstrated in older individuals with a structured, high-intensity resistance exercise program, even in frail nursing home residents up to 96 years of age (95).

The high prevalence of both osteoporosis and degenerative joint disease (i.e., osteoarthritis) in the elderly again raises the question about normal physiologic changes versus ubiquitous pathologic processes (30,96). The physiologic changes and sequelae associated with osteoporosis are discussed further in Chapter 30.

Distinction of the "disease" of osteoarthritis from the normal or usual aging changes that occur in weight-bearing joints can be made on a biochemical basis: with osteoarthritis, there are increases in the water content of cartilage and the ratio of chondroitin-4-sulfate to chondroitin-6-sulfate, with decreases in keratin sulfate and hyaluronic acid content (the opposite of what occurs in aging) (96). There is a strong relationship between aging and osteoarthritis: Degenerative joint changes in weight-bearing joints are essentially a universal occurrence in both sexes by 60 years of age (97). These changes include biochemical alteration of cartilage, especially the proteoglycan component, with reduced ability to bear weight without fissuring, focal fibrillation and ulceration of cartilage, and eventual exposure of subchondral bone (96). The wear-and-tear hypothesis of osteoarthritis suggests that this process is the result of the cumulative stresses of a lifetime of joint use. Accordingly, "primary" osteoarthritis results from the stress of repetitive weight loading (e.g., spine, knees) or strain (e.g., distal interphalangeal joints), whereas "secondary" osteoarthritis may be related to occupational factors or congenital factors with unusual patterns of stress (e.g., congenital hip dysplasia). There appear to be other factors operating, however, because there are specific differences in distribution and prevalence between sexes and races (97). Obesity appears to be a risk factor for knee osteoarthritis in particular, although it is not clear whether this is due to a mechanical or a metabolic etiology. Further details regarding arthritis can be found in Chapter 32.

Genitourinary System

Benign prostatic hyperplasia is an almost universal occurrence in men older than 40 years of age and develops under hormonal rather than neoplastic influence (98). Of note is that the median lobe of the prostate, which is not palpable rectally, can cause a ball-valve obstruction during micturition. Accordingly, after ruling out other etiologies (such as anticholinergic medication side effects), cystoscopy should be considered in patients with persisting obstructive symptomatology but minimal prostatic tissue on rectal examination to detect median lobe hypertrophy (99). Usual indications for surgical intervention (e.g., prostatectomy) include increasing obstructive symp-

TABLE 72-2. Common Medical Conditions Associated with Incontinence in the Elderly

Condition	Effect on Continence
Neurologic disease	
Cerebrovascular disease; stroke	DO from damage to upper motor neurons; impaired sensation to void from interruption of subcortical pathways; impaired function and cognition
Delirium	Impaired function and cognition
Dementia	DO from damage to upper motor neurons; impaired function and cognition
Multiple sclerosis	DO, areflexia, or sphincter dyssynergia (dependent on level of synergy)
Multisystem atrophy	Detrusor and sphincter areflexia from damage to spinal intermediolateral tracts
Normal-pressure hydrocephalus	DO from compression of frontal inhibitory centers; impaired function and cognition
Parkinson's disease	DO from loss of inhibitory centers; impaired function and cognition; retention and overflow from constipation
Spinal cord injury	DO, areflexia, or sphincter dyssynergia (dependent on level of injury)
Spinal stenosis	DO from damage to detrusor upper motor neurons (cervical stenosis); DO or areflexia (lumbar stenosis)
Metabolic disease	
Diabetes mellitus	Detrusor underactivity due to neuropathy, DO, osmotic diuresis; altered mental status from hyper- or hypoglycemia; retention and overflow from constipation
Hypercalcemia	Diuresis; altered mental status
Vitamin B12 deficiency	Impaired bladder sensation and detrusor underactivity from peripheral neuropathy
Infectious disease	
Herpes zoster	Urinary retention if sacral dermatomes involved; outlet obstruction from viral prostatitis in men; retention and overflow UI from constipation
Human immunodeficiency virus	DO, areflexia, or sphincter dyssynergia
Neurosyphilis	DO, areflexia, or sphincter dyssynergia
Tuberculosis	Inanition and functional impairments (sterile pyuria found in ≤50% of genitourinary TB cases)
Psychiatric disease	
Affective and anxiety disorders	Decreased motivation
Alcoholism	Functional and cognitive impairment; rapid diuresis and retention in acute intoxication
Psychosis	Functional and cognitive impairment; decreased motivation
Cardiovascular disease	
Arteriovascular disease	Detrusor underactivity or areflexia from ischemic myopathy or neuropathy
Congestive heart failure	Nocturnal diuresis
Other organ system diseases	
Gastrointestinal disease	Retention and overflow UI from constipation
Musculoskeletal disease	Mobility impairment; DO from cervical myelopathy in rheumatoid arthritis and osteoarthritis
Peripheral venous insufficiency	Nocturnal diuresis
Pulmonary disease	Exacerbation of stress UI by chronic cough

DO, detrusor overactivity; TB, tuberculosis; UI, urinary incontinence.
Adapted with permission from DuBeau CE. Interpreting the effect of common medical conditions on voiding dysfunction in the elderly. *Urol Clin North Am* 1996;23(1):11–18.

TABLE 72-3. Precipitating Causes of Transient Incontinence in the Elderly

Cause	Comment
Delirium, confusion state	UI resolves once underlying cause(s) treated
Urinary infection	UI may be only symptom of infection; antibiotic trial warranted in asymptomatic persons only on initial evaluation and with new onset/exacerbation of UI
Atrophic urethritis, vaginitis	Aggravates stress or urge UI; agitation can be presenting symptom in demented patients
Medications	Any agent that impairs cognition, mobility, fluid balance, bladder contractility, or sphincter function; many agents impair several functions
Psychiatric disorders	Severe depression or psychosis
Increased urine output	Frequency or nocturia; causes: excessive fluid intake, diuretics, hyperglycemia, hypercalcemia, volume overload (congestive heart failure, venous insufficiency, hypothyroidism, hypoalbuminemia, and drug-induced peripheral edema)
Restricted mobility	Treat underlying cause; provide a urinal or bedside commode
Stool impaction	Urge or overflow UI; fecal incontinence common

UI, urinary incontinence.
Adapted from Resnick NM. Urinary incontinence in the elderly. *Medical Grand Rounds*. 1984;3:281–290.

toms, recurrent hematuria, bladder calculi, recurrent infections, and postvoid residual volumes greater than 100 mL (98).

Incontinence in the elderly, although increasingly prevalent with advancing age, should be regarded as a symptom of underlying disease; it does not result from the natural aging process (100). Normal aging typically results in decreases in bladder capacity, ability to postpone voiding, detrusor contractility, and urinary flow rate (101). Postvoid residual volumes are typically increased, with a tendency for increased urine output later in the day, as well as propensity for uninhibited detrusor contractions. Each of these changes predispose older adults to incontinence, but none alone precipitates it. Common medical conditions associated with incontinence are listed in Table 72-2, and precipitating (and reversible) causes of transient incontinence are detailed in Table 72-3.

The primary clinical significance of these aging changes is that the new onset or exacerbation of incontinence in an older person is likely due to a precipitating factor outside the urinary tract (100). Usually, remedial intervention can restore continence without necessarily correcting the underlying urologic abnormalities.

Contrary to stereotypes, although there is a decrease in sexual functioning with aging, most older people retain sexual interest and desire, and to a variable extent, capability (102,103). Older men experience a decrease in ability to have psychogenic erections and require more intense physical stimulation for erection; erections may be partial, and orgasm with ejaculation may occur without full engorgement (104). The force of ejaculation is less, along with a less intense sensation of orgasm. Impotence may be caused by a variety of diseases (e.g., diabetes, hypothyroidism) and medications (e.g., antihypertensives, phenytoin, cimetidine). Treatment of erectile dysfunction in older men has been revolutionized with development of the vacuum tumescent device, advances in penile prostheses, and availability of such medications as sildenafil and alprostadil (105,106).

Older women experience postmenopausal changes, including increased fragility of the vaginal wall and attenuation of the excitement phase (e.g., decreased vaginal lubrication) (102). Common sexual difficulties identified included partner's impotence, anorgasmia, decreased libido, and insufficient opportunities for sexual encounters. Despite these changes, most women maintain the ability to engage in sexual intercourse throughout the life cycle (107).

THE ENVIRONMENT OF OLDER PERSONS WITH DISABILITY: PSYCHOLOGICAL AND SOCIAL ISSUES IN AGING

Ageism and Myths of Aging

Butler coined the term *ageism* to describe negatively biased perceptions of older people by the younger population in today's youth-oriented culture, as well as perceptions of old age by elderly individuals themselves (108). There are many adverse sequelae of ageism, including devaluation of older people (by themselves, as well as others both younger and older), diversion of health-care professional focus from the real health problems of older patients, the dearth of physicians interested and trained in geriatric medicine, and lack of curriculum time in medical schools regarding geriatrics (109,110). According to Rowe and Kahn, it is time to "discard the many derogatory myths about older people, who are often seen as sick, senile, silly, sexless, and sedentary, as well as inflexible, irritable, noncontributing, and too old for preventive interventions" (111). Many of today's older adults are survivors of the Depression and the World Wars; they built much of the life and standard of living we now enjoy. The evidence is clear: The majority of elderly are cognitively intact, live independently in the community, and are fully independent in activities of daily living (12,14).

Cumulative Changes

There is increasing awareness of the critical interrelationships, particularly for older people, of physical health, mental health, and life circumstances. The emotional and life stress associated with major losses is well documented, and older people may be exposed progressively to multiple significant losses: job, income, health, functional ability and independence, parents, spouse, siblings, children, friends, social roles and status, and self-esteem (112). There are in fact few norms or defined role expectations regarding appropriate behavior or activities in old age (113,114). Bereavement, isolation, poverty, illness, and physical disability all are associated with a higher incidence of depression in older adults (115), which in turn is associated with decreased physical and cognitive functioning, disability, and increased mortality (116–118).

Social Support Networks

Social support networks include a wide variety of sources that can be categorized as informal (family), semiformal (church, clubs, family doctor, local pharmacist), and formal (health-care system, social service agencies, insurance companies, etc.) (119). Older persons often use supports from a combination of these networks (8).

Elderly people with children usually live near them and visit frequently, or at least maintain regular telephone contact (120). Older people without children tend to maintain closer ties with young relatives or with siblings (121). It is important to consider the extended family, including cousins, in-laws, and others, with regard to support networks, rather than just immediate household members (113,122).

Institutionalization of an impaired older person usually is the last resort for families, used only when all other efforts fail; in fact, 64% of individuals older than the age of 85 who are dependent in self-care or homemaking still live in the community (123). Families, rather than the formal system of government and agencies, provide the bulk (up to 90%) of personalized long-term care for their disabled older relatives (8). This includes home health and nursing care, personal care, household maintenance, transportation, cooking, and shopping. In 1990, 73% of elderly disabled individuals relied exclusively on such informal support and care networks (8).

With advancing age, however, older adults tend to have increasingly limited and relatively fragile support systems. Dependency in aging parents results in significant physical, emotional, and financial stresses on their family network (120). An alternative support system may evolve gradually over a period of time as the older person loses family support (e.g., death of spouse and siblings, children moving away and unable to actively assist). Such a system might include friends and neighbors in an extended network to assist with shopping, cooking, cleaning, and self-care (124).

With whatever combination of support systems, a significant additional insult (e.g., onset of a new disease or complication) may overtax an already marginal arrangement. It is commonly observed that as the patient's dependence on the formal network of the health-care system increases, the informal or family network support decreases (119). Furthermore, if the elderly person is hospitalized for a prolonged period, the network(s) may dissipate and may be difficult or impossible to reassemble (125). The critical importance of maintaining the integrity of support networks is illustrated by the observation that for every aged impaired person in a nursing home there are two equally impaired older people living in the community (1). The difference is the role played by the latter's informal support systems, providing most of their long-term care.

Increasingly, issues concerning family functioning with aging are being studied. Even when family members are seemingly available to assist older relatives, their support cannot always be counted on unless they too receive help. Fortunately, there is evidence that patients' families can benefit from educational interventions to help prevent weakening in this crucial source of patient support. Caregivers of older patients with cancer and chronic pain are often frustrated, fearful, and anxious. Patient care improved when caregivers were provided with guidelines on what they could do within the home to help the patient (119). Similarly, caregivers of stroke survivors had less depression with more formal teaching (126). Nursing home placement has been delayed by specific family interventions for patients with Alzheimer's disease (127).

Caregiver burden is another dynamic receiving increasing attention (128). Increased caregiver burden can be associated with increased mortality after controlling for known risk factors (129). Adding to the physical stress of providing personal care aid may be the unpleasantness of incontinence or exhaustion because of a relative's sleep disorder. Behavioral problems, such as agitation or impulsivity with poor safety awareness, create proportionately greater caregiver burden than the demands of providing physical assistance (128). Physical and emotional health problems among caregivers have been documented, including depression and immunosuppression. Physical aggression on a caregiver by a patient is not uncommon and may lead to reciprocal abuse (130). Potential intervention strategies include encouraging use of other support systems to augment care provided by family members, as well as the use of respite programs (131,132).

Functional Impact

Physically impaired older people tend to become socially isolated, which can result in exacerbation of medical problems, functional deficits, and mental health problems (particularly depression) (117). Other factors contributing to a vicious cycle of depression, withdrawal, and functional decline may include the stress of multiple losses, malnutrition, chronic ill health, pain, and adverse drug effects that aggravate depression (118). Unfortunately, the environment too often fosters dependency. A classic illustration is the acute hospital setting, where the focus is on routinely providing care and assistance, rather than encouraging self-care (133).

Additional psychosocial barriers can interfere with maintaining or improving functional ability in the elderly. Handicapping sequelae of ageism include devaluation of elderly disabled (by themselves as well as others), lack of interest (actual or perceived) among health-care professionals in their problems, and limited opportunity for access to appropriate rehabilitation services (109,111). Further attitudinal obstacles encountered among disabled elderly include the "right of dependency," perceived as earned by virtue of longevity, and the "apathy of fatigue," both physical and emotional, associated with multiple illnesses and hospitalizations (134).

Increasingly physical environments are being recognized as either preventing, or contributing to, disability (135). Although full discussion is beyond the scope of this chapter, the development of a requirement for some housing to meet visitability criteria (one entrance without stairs, bathroom on first floor, and wide bathroom doorway to accommodate a wheelchair) is encouraging. Housing adapted in this manner may more easily accommodate older adults as they age and facilitate social visits to or from friends by minimizing physical barriers.

The obvious conclusion, and why rehabilitation plays a key role in restoring function in disabled older people, is the importance of awareness and intervention regarding significant psychoemotional and social factors affecting their health. Many of these factors can be anticipated and prevented, or at least minimized in terms of their adverse effects. As with any complication, prevention is the best treatment.

TRAJECTORIES OF FUNCTIONAL DECLINE

Cumulative Functional Sequelae of Disease

Older adults can experience acute (sudden) onset of disability (just as in younger people) from such conditions as stroke, amputation, spinal cord injury, and traumatic brain injury. However, many experience a gradual progression of difficulties in function. The effects of multiple and chronic illnesses usually are gradual over time with cumulative erosion of organ reserves, leaving the elderly person reasonably functional with various adaptations, such as walking more slowly or taking more frequent rests (19,23,30). As functional problems develop, it can be hard to determine if the disability can be treated generically, regardless of the contributing diseases and other factors, and when a reversible underlying disease process needs to be treated. Also, an elderly individual may be only marginally functional with little or no reserve capacity, so that even a relatively minor superimposed acute complication or disease process (e.g., influenza) may result in functional decompensation (1). Of even greater concern is that this significant functional decompensation may be difficult to reverse even though the intercurrent acute illness is appropriately treated and resolves (136,137).

Older people as a group are more vulnerable to functional sequelae of diseases for a variety of reasons, including ageism. The latter commonly results in underreporting symptomatology related to illness (23,108). Health-care providers may not be trained adequately to evaluate and treat symptoms and signs of functional disability in older patients, and may as a result not recognize the significance of vague and inconsistent symptoms. Older people themselves may think that such vague symptoms are a natural result of aging (138). As a result, the underlying disease process may become quite advanced before care is sought, making treatment that much more difficult.

From the older person's viewpoint, the available system of care may seem unresponsive (23). Physician offices can be perceived as inconveniently located, with inadequate parking and limited access for the physically impaired. A typically brief physician encounter may not allow for development of rapport and full elaboration of symptoms. Busy office staff may appear to be uninterested or discourteous.

Other issues may contribute further to underreporting of illness. There may be denial of disease coupled with fear of consequences, especially financial (108). Depression is common among older people and may result in the attitude, "What have I got to gain?" (23,117). Increasing isolation, with fewer opportunities for others to observe and react to changes in appearance or behavior, are additional barriers. Finally, older people may not recognize significant symptoms or seek medical attention because of cognitive impairments, which not infrequently may be secondary to or aggravated by an underlying and potentially reversible disease process (89).

There is often an altered response to illness in the elderly, which contributes to delayed or incorrect diagnosis (23). Many specific diseases present with atypical and nonclassic signs and symptoms. For example, the presentation of a myocardial infarction in an elderly person is less likely to include classic retrosternal chest pain; more often it will involve nausea, dizziness, syncope, or congestive heart failure with decreased activity tolerance (53). Furthermore, a wide variety of diseases may present with similar nonspecific symptoms, including confusion, weakness, weight loss, and general "failure to thrive" (23,139). Accordingly, the differential diagnosis of possible disease processes is much broader in elderly patients.

TABLE 72-4. Chronic Conditions Associated with Disability in Older Adults

Characteristics Entered into Each Model	Association with Disability in:			
	A Mobility/Exercise Tolerance Demanding Tasks	B Upper-Extremity Tasks	C Complex Household Management Tasks	D Self-Care Tasks
Age	•		•	
Sex (male)		•		
Angina (nitroglycerine use)	•		•	
Myocardial infarction				•
Congestive heart failure	•			
Stroke	•	•	•	•
Claudication	•		•	
Arthritis	•	•	•	•
Lung disease	•			
Depressive symptomology	•	•		•
Hearing impairment			•	•
Cognitive impairment: digit symbol substitution	•		•	•
Cancer	•			
Weakness	•	•	•	•
Balance problems, last year	•	•		
Dizziness, last 2 weeks				•
Body Mass Index[a]	•			•
Weight[a]	•			

• Indicates significant association (P < .01), adjusting for: clinical sizes, Minimental State Exam Score, hypertension, visual impairment, diabetes, left ventricular systolic dysfunction by echocardiography, carotid stenosis, and grip strength as well as variables in the table.
[a]Increase of 10 lbs.
Reprinted with permission from Fried LP, Guralnik JM. Disability in older adults: evidence regarding significance, etiology, and risk. *J Am Geriatr Soc* 1997;45(1):97.

Further confounding accurate elucidation of the underlying illness are the frequent changes in disease patterns and distribution (23). Abnormalities in one organ system may be accompanied by secondary abnormalities in other organ systems. Traditional medical training focuses on disease recognition and treatment in a relatively young population, with emphasis on synthesizing multiple signs and symptoms into a single unifying diagnosis (23,140). Older people more typically have concurrent symptomatology, relating to multiple diseases. Although accurate diagnosis is important, the functional impact of each disease, particularly the cumulative and additive impact of multiple diseases, must be determined (1).

There is an increased frequency of many chronic diseases in this population, including anemia, osteoarthritis, osteoporosis, cardiovascular disease, malignancy, and malnutrition. Table 72-4 lists types and patterns of disability associated with various chronic conditions. Palliation and prevention of secondary complications frequently is a more appropriate and realistic goal than is cure of the primary condition (23,140). There often are atypical (and potentially confusing) behaviors and responses to treatment, however, because of coexisting diseases and decreased functional reserves of multiple organ systems (e.g., affecting drug metabolism and distribution) (23).

Older people also are more prone to a wide variety of concomitant and complicating diseases, which may further cloud diagnosis and treatment decisions. Examples include thrombophlebitis, dehydration, fluid and electrolyte disturbances, adverse drug interactions or toxicity, decubitus ulcers, pneumonia, and general deleterious effects of deconditioning as a result of inactivity, which occurs earlier and with greater severity in older adults (141,142).

Frailty as a concept refers to more than older individuals who experience functional losses; it represents a state of vulnerability resulting from the balance and interplay of medical and social factors (143). Characteristics of frail older institutionalized persons included female sex, being unmarried, absence of a caregiver, presence of cognitive deficit, functional impairment, and medical condition (e.g., diabetes mellitus, stroke, Parkinson's disease) (144).

"Frailty" is becoming better characterized as a biological syndrome of decreased reserve and resistance to stressors occurring frequently in older adults (145). Contributing are the multiple decrements in physiologic systems, as previously discussed. Clinical characteristics have been defined as unintentional weight loss (10 pounds in prior year), self-reported exhaustion, weakness (grip strength), slow walking speed, and low physical activity.

Given these multiple dynamics, alternative models of disease presentation in older persons may prove useful (140). In one series of proposed models (Table 72-5), the Medical Model, in which the patient's symptoms and signs are fully explained by one disease, is the most basic. The Synergistic Morbidity Model portrays the functional loss that may have suddenly occurred as the result of additive effects of several diseases. In the Attribution Model, a patient might attribute a deterioration in health to an already diagnosed chronic illness when in fact another undiagnosed problem is present (e.g., hypothyroidism superimposed on stroke). In the more complex Causal Chain Model, a medical-psychiatric interaction occurs in which one illness causes another as well as causing functional decrements, with the presenting symptom representing the proverbial last straw of decompensation. Finally, in the Unmasking Event Model, a stressful external event unmasks an underlying, stable, or slowly progressive chronic condition that had previously been well compensated and unrecognized (140). Alternative classification models such as these help organize the

TABLE 72-5. Alternative Models of Illness Presentation

Model of Illness	Characteristics
1. Medical Model	Symptoms and signs correlate directly (and solely) with a specific disease (traditional model of medical diagnostic thinking).
2. Synergistic Morbidity Model	Multiple concurrent chronic diseases, subclinical (or at least not severe enough to seek medical attention) until reaching a threshold of cumulative morbidity and functional decline.
3. Attribution Model	Underlying stable chronic disease(s), with new onset of symptoms attributed by the patient (and possibly, the clinician) to the known chronic disease(s), but in actuality caused by a new, unrecognized condition.
4. Causal Chain Model	Medical-psychiatric interaction involving an underlying disease with multiple secondary conditions/impairments (potentially including mental health problems, such as depression) which aggravate the underlying disease, forming a "vicious cycle."
5. Unmasking Event Model	Underlying stable or slowly progressive chronic disease(s), effectively compensated to minimize functional impact, until the occurrence of a new stressful event (e.g., death of a loved one; relocation) which results in decompensation (and the risk of being misinterpreted as a new condition).

Adapted from Fried LP, Storer DJ, King DE, Lodder F. Diagnosis of illness presentation in the elderly. *J Am Geriatr Soc* 1991;39:117–123.

significant and varying complexity of signs and symptoms to more rapidly and accurately diagnose and treat older persons with multiple interacting problems.

Effects of Acute Hospitalization

There is increasing recognition of the multiple deleterious effects of acute hospitalization on older people separate and distinct from sequelae that are due primarily to their presenting illness (136,146). Disorientation that is due to the foreign hospital environment and relatively infrequent and brief interactions with unfamiliar health-care personnel may contribute to bizarre and inappropriate behavior, including agitation (117, 133). Contributing to this may be relative sensory and social isolation with few familiar environmental cues or social interactions, especially if the patient is confined to a private room or intensive care setting. Moreover, there are atypical routines and schedules (e.g., blood drawing, vital sign checks at odd hours), which, coupled with unusual noises (e.g., overhead paging, machines, other patients), may contribute to insomnia. A patient with insomnia typically is treated with a sedative medication, which may begin a cycle (or cascade) of drug side effects and interactions that may adversely affect the patient's health (136,146).

Increased incidence of medical and iatrogenic complications in older adults is well documented (23,140). Drug side effects, complications, and toxicity, together with adverse interactions related to polypharmacy, make up a large proportion of such morbidity (23,55). There also is a greater frequency of diagnostic and therapeutic misadventures in this age group, related in part to decreased organ reserve with resultant increased vulnerability (146).

There also are a variety of emotional sequelae of hospitalization that may affect health and functional status. Anxiety and confusion relating to the underlying illness and prognosis, or just to hospitalization itself, may interfere with cooperation with medical treatment or therapy programs (147–149). Depression from similar origins may result in dependency and poor motivation to cooperate or improve function (116,117). Functional dependency frequently is reinforced during acute hospitalizations, both by the older people who expect hospital staff to assist and by hospital staff who tend routinely to perform self-care tasks without taking the extra time to supervise the patient in performing his or her own self-care (134,136). Documented functional decline after hospitalization for acute medical illnesses also may result from other, as yet unexplained factors (146). Deconditioning from inadequate activity during the hospital stay may contribute to poorer functional outcomes, and preliminary results suggest exercise can help improve functional outcomes (150).

In addition to significant implications for health care in the hospital setting, these sequelae related to acute hospitalization often affect social support systems and discharge disposition (125,136). The elderly patient may experience loss of confidence or motivation as a result of multiple insults and complications, coupled with erosion of functional abilities from deconditioning (141,142). This in and of itself will put greater stress on often relatively fragile social support systems, making it more difficult for elderly patients to return home to their prior living situation (125).

To try to address these problems, several randomized trials have investigated alternative models attempting to change the organization of care (and outcomes) for older persons during hospitalization. Use of a geriatric consultation team approach did not yield improved outcomes (151). In another randomized clinical trial of 651 patients 70 years of age and older, the experimental patients received care on a special unit, which had the additional components of daily team conferences, active discharge planning, and use of therapy staff for functional training—the core components on typical acute rehabilitation units. Patients in the experimental group were discharged at higher functional levels, and fewer were discharged to skilled nursing facilities (SNFs)(14% versus 22%). Neither cost of hospitalization nor length of stay was increased (152). In a Veterans Administration Study, older patients, after stabilization, were randomized to usual care or to a geriatric unit(153). At hospital discharge, patients receiving the geriatric unit care had greater improvements in scores for four of the eight SF-36 subscales, activities of daily living, and physical performance. These studies suggest potential strategies to improve acute hospital care for older persons, with fewer functional sequelae.

Effects of Deconditioning

Deconditioning can be defined as the multiple changes in physiology and anatomy induced by physical inactivity and reversed through physical activity (142). This topic is covered in detail in Chapter 68 (Immobility and Inactivity), but will be discussed here relative to unique aspects relating to aging.

Older adults' (75 to 120 years old) physical functioning and associated physical activities has been classified by Spirduso into five categories: physically elite, physically fit, physically independent, physically frail, and physically dependent (154) (Fig. 72-1). Deconditioning can be one component, in addition to disease, that may be contributory to a patient's lower level of function.

Reversal of deleterious effects of deconditioning has been amply demonstrated through focused muscle-strengthening programs as well as comprehensive exercise programs in both nursing homes and the community (46,155–157). These programs variably included exercises for flexibility, muscle strength, and aerobic endurance.

The functional consequences of deconditioning in older people may be of major clinical significance and may be confused with changes intrinsic to aging or changes from diseases (142). Deconditioning per se may result in functional losses when certain threshold values for physical performance are crossed (158). Quadriceps weakness may progress to the point of dependency in getting in and out of a car solely from progressive deconditioning, not related to intrinsic aging or new onset of disease (141). Multiple factors associated with falls may originate from deconditioning or be exacerbated by deconditioning (159,160). For people living in the community, factors associated with falls include impairments in static balance, leg strength, and hip and ankle flexibility (161,162). In nursing home patients, falls are associated with decreased muscle strength at the knees and ankles (163,164). Weakened muscles also may contribute to other injuries and pain syndromes by allowing abnormal forces to act on bone, joints, ligaments, and tendons. In addition, lack of exercise is being viewed increasingly as a risk factor not only for functional loss but for onset of various disease processes, including cardiovascular disease and diabetes, among others (165).

Deconditioning affecting older people can be differentiated into acute inactivity secondary to bed rest (such as during acute illness) and chronic inactivity from sedentary lifestyles (often more difficult to reverse) (142). A variety of types and combinations of exercises are available to treat deconditioning in older individuals; a precise prescription of a therapeutic exercise and activity program, including appropriate precautions and instruction, is essential (44,74,166).

Psychological issues in maintaining exercise habits are being studied increasingly (155). Currently health professionals can help older persons increase their physical activity levels by discussing the issue openly and then helping the patient decide what approach may be most appropriate (71). One option may be group classes, which offer the benefits of social interaction and support, and perhaps even friendly competition. Exercising on their own at home may be preferable for some, especially if they are self-conscious about their own abilities (167).

Disability Prevention in Older Adults

The potential future impact of increased disability as populations age is of major concern to clinicians, health-care administrators, insurers, and policy makers. Increasingly, prevention strategies are being proposed both to improve the number of disability-free years of life as well as to contain health-care costs (11,14,21,24). Some of the themes around prevention can be organized according to the concepts of primary, secondary, and tertiary prevention. Primary prevention involves preventing the onset of a disease (e.g., annual influenza vaccine), whereas secondary prevention involves the diagnosis and treatment of asymptomatic diseases to prevent the development of symptoms (e.g., treatment of hypertension to prevent stroke or myocardial infarction). Tertiary prevention involves treatment once a disease becomes symptomatic to avoid complications (e.g., deep venous thrombosis prophylaxis and appropriate mobilization to prevent skin breakdown in poststroke patients). However, what becomes increasingly important in older persons with chronic disease is disability prevention, or avoidance of frailty. A model for risk factors in the development of frailty has been proposed by Buchner and Wagner (168) (Fig. 72-2). In this model, strategies required to prevent

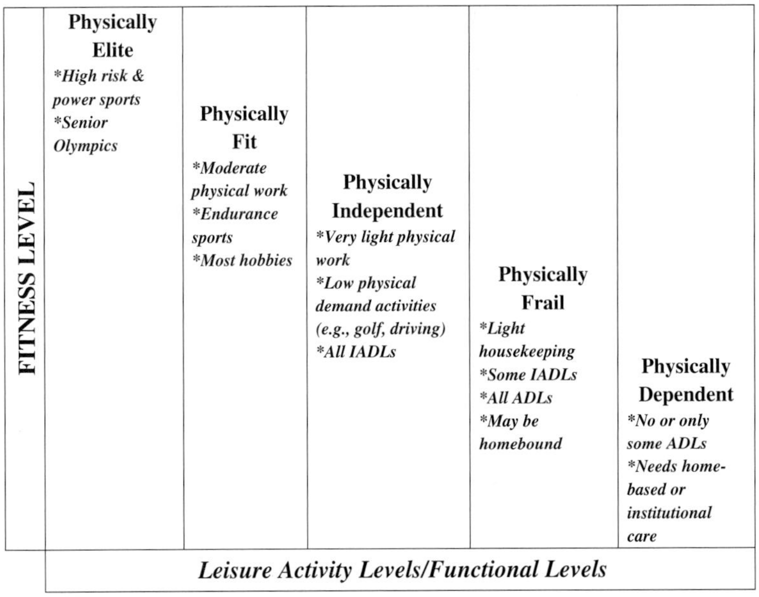

FITNESS LEVEL	Physically Elite *High risk & power sports *Senior Olympics	Physically Fit *Moderate physical work *Endurance sports *Most hobbies	Physically Independent *Very light physical work *Low physical demand activities (e.g., golf, driving) *All IADLs	Physically Frail *Light housekeeping *Some IADLs *All ADLs *May be homebound	Physically Dependent *No or only some ADLs *Needs home-based or institutional care
	Leisure Activity Levels/Functional Levels				

Figure 72-1. Hierarchy of physical function of the old (75–85 years) and oldest-old (86–120 years). (From Spirduso W. *Physical dimensions of aging.* Champaign, IL: Human Kinetics, 1995:339, with permission.)

disability in older age involve multiple interventions on living environment and lifestyle (169).

Another important theoretical model that may help in the development of prevention strategies has been proposed by Lawrence and Jette (170). They have studied the application of a model for the disablement process in 1,048 community-residing adults (mean age 74 years) without functional limitations or disabilities over a 6-year period. The model hypothesized a process in which risk factors (age, sex, education, body mass, and physical activity measured as frequency of walking 1 mile) would lead to functional limitations with or without the presence of pathology or impairments. Over time the functional limitations (e.g., inability to walk well) led to subsequent disability, such as inability to go shopping. Guralnik and colleagues likewise found that among nondisabled persons living in the community, impairments in the lower extremity were highly predictive of later disability (171). Fried and colleagues characterized a functional level of "preclinical disability" (task modification but no difficulty by self-report) in a study of women 70 to 80 years old (172). Measurement of their physical function was intermediate between women with high function

(no modifications) and disability (difficulty with tasks). Such studies support the potential role of interventions with increased physical activity and exercise as types of primary prevention of disability for older persons.

There may in fact be significant overlap of risk factors for multiple problems in older persons. For instance, the risk factors associated with falls, incontinence, and functional dependence are similar—slowed chair stand, decreased arm strength, decreased vision and hearing, and either a high anxiety or depression score (173).

From these types of models, successful prevention strategies are being tested, often entailing multiple interventions covering multiple domains. For instance, incidence of falls can be reduced by a combination of medication adjustments, exercise, safety training, and environmental modifications. A comprehensive nurse-practitioner evaluation program for community-residing seniors resulted in a delay in onset of disability and decreased nursing home admission (174). Another study demonstrated that higher self-efficacy was associated with lesser functional decline in persons with diminished physical capacity (175). Research also suggests that self-efficacy (a person's

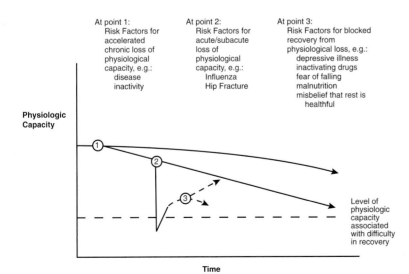

Figure 72-2. Conceptual model of risk factors for frailty. (From Buchner DM, Wagner EH. Preventing frail health. *Clin Geriatr Med* 1992;8:1–17, with permission.)

confidence or belief that he or she can achieve a specific behavior or cognitive state) may be modifiable and therefore may help guide preventive strategies (176). Research continues to identify which targeted intervention for which specific risk factor in which specific patient at what specific point in time will be most efficacious in preventing or minimizing disability.

PRINCIPLES OF ASSESSMENT AND MANAGEMENT OF OLDER ADULTS WITH DISABILITY

Assessment of the Older Patient

There is increasing evidence of the merits of specialized geriatric evaluation clinics or programs to improve early diagnosis of such common health problems as cognitive impairment, depression and anxiety, and incontinence (177–180). When combined with focused geriatric medical management, such clinics proved significantly more effective than traditional primary medical care in improving the quality of health care, decreasing mortality and frequency of acute hospitalization, and increasing patient and caregiver satisfaction (179). Geriatric evaluation and management programs have also demonstrated the ability to delay functional decline and decrease need for home health-care services (180,181).

A standardized framework for assessing older patients can be very useful to busy practitioners. It facilitates efficient use of the clinical time available, helps avoid oversight of a factor that might be important in planning an appropriate rehabilitation approach, and can help with communication among team members caring for the patient (in both inpatient and office settings). Further, because many older patients experience several settings of care sequentially, a standard framework can help in the handoffs between settings of care (182).

Elderly patients often have multiple issues (sometimes 10 or more) being addressed concurrently during their rehabilitation. Because psychological research suggests that the human brain can only deal with three to seven ideas at a time when problem solving, a standard framework may assist with categorization of issues to facilitate clinical care (183).

The Domain Management Model is one approach that operationalizes the biopsychosocial model, a model relevant to the care of older patients (184) (Fig. 72-3). It is consistent with basic rehabilitation concepts and the International Classification of Functioning, Disability, and Health, in which contextual factors like a person's environment need to be considered, in the clinical setting, in order to understand function (135). Four domains cover the spectrum of clinical problems patients and their families face when confronted with disability: domain I—medical/surgical issues, domain II—mental status/emotions/coping, domain III—physical function, and domain IV—living environment (182,185). Although sometimes patients have an isolated problem in one area, often management requires concomitant actions in all four domains. This is especially true for geriatric syndromes like falls.

Domain I (medical/surgical issues) includes the salient disease diagnoses requiring management (e.g., diabetes, hypertension, osteoarthritis, or stroke). For older patients, various clinical syndromes also require explicit identification and management (e.g., incontinence, malnutrition).

Domain II (mental status/emotions/coping) identifies any concerns with patients' mental status or cognitive function, such as attention, memory, and executive function or complex problem solving. Delirium and dementia are especially important to identify, if present, given their major impact on functional status and rehabilitation management. Key emotional problems to identify include depression and anxiety disorders. Coping represents patients' ways of behaving when confronted with stressors of ill health. Many patients cope well, but those who do not require additional assessment and help from the rehabilitation team. Spirituality is another key factor for many older patients confronting disability and can be a source of strength. Although health-care professionals often have to be alert for problems in their patients' function, here a focus can highlight strengths as well (prior coping with difficult situations, etc.).

Assessment of domain II is especially dependent on the ability of clinicians and patients to communicate effectively. Issues affecting communication should also be included in this domain, including visual and hearing problems, as well as aphasia or dysarthria. Advance directives, including health-care proxy and medical directives, are also included in this domain, as they reflect specific patient preferences.

Domain III (physical function) includes the full spectrum of functional activities performed by the patient. These range from basic activities of daily living (dressing, toileting, etc.) to instrumental activities of daily living (shopping, transportation, money management, medication management, etc.) to the advanced activities of daily living (social activities, fulfilling social roles like parenting, vocational and avocational activities). Here interesting patient reports of prior accomplishments and even ongoing unique activities are worth noting.

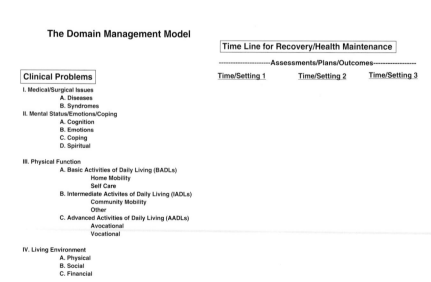

The Domain Management Model

Time Line for Recovery/Health Maintenance

---------------------Assessments/Plans/Outcomes-----------------

Time/Setting 1   Time/Setting 2   Time/Setting 3

Clinical Problems

I. Medical/Surgical Issues
    A. Diseases
    B. Syndromes
II. Mental Status/Emotions/Coping
    A. Cognition
    B. Emotions
    C. Coping
    D. Spiritual

III. Physical Function
    A. Basic Activities of Daily Living (BADLs)
        Home Mobility
        Self Care
    B. Intermediate Activites of Daily Living (IADLs)
        Community Mobility
        Other
    C. Advanced Activities of Daily Living (AADLs)
        Avocational
        Vocational

IV. Living Environment
    A. Physical
    B. Social
    C. Financial

Figure 72-3. The domain management model. The two organizing constructs of the domain management model are the domain classification of patients' problems (vertical, or Y, axis) and time, including identification of process factors (assessments and plans), outcomes, and care setting (horizontal, or X, axis). BADLs = eating, grooming, bathing, dressing, transfers, etc.; IADLs = money and medication management, meal preparation, shopping, etc.; AADLs = hobbies, work, etc. Copyright Siebens 1996. (From: Siebens H. Applying the domain management model in treating patients with chronic diseases. *Jt Comm J Qual Improv* 2001;27(6):304, with permission.)

Domain IV (the living environment) includes three practical components: physical, social, and financial. The patients' physical environment includes man-made structures as well as the natural world (186). Specific details include the type of housing and job site, building access, and proximity of basic necessities like food and banking services. For older persons with progressive disabilities, transitioning to more supportive home environments may be a critical goal in their care.

Patients' social environment is their interface with other people at many levels of association, ranging from social networks to social institutions (186). Relationships with pets as well can be important. These interactions determine whether personal physical help or assistance with instrumental or advanced activities of daily living is available. The psychological and financial burdens families face when patients survive with severe chronic disability are huge. Assessing caregiver burden, and assisting through education and additional supports, is an integral part of rehabilitation management.

Finally, financial resources are critical to determining what medical and rehabilitation services are covered by insurance, as well as what personal financial resources patients and their families may have. This can facilitate determination of what medications, services, or additional equipment are feasible as part of the rehabilitation program if and as needed.

Goal Setting

Increasingly, there is recognition that health-care and rehabilitation goals may not be uniformly shared by patients and their caregivers (187,188). For example, patients may often want to return home after rehabilitation, but rehabilitation staff strongly disagree, at times, out of undue fear of what may occur (189). Our focus as health-care providers is typically on general health and well-being and functional independence. Our tacit assumption is that these goals are necessarily shared by our patients and their caregivers, and perhaps that these are the only goals they value. However, there is evidence of differing goals, and priorities of goals, between health-care providers, case managers, patients, and their caregivers (187, 188, 190). Alternative goals also valued by patients and their caregivers included such areas as education and referrals, social/family relations, emotional issues, and caregiver burden. Of significance is that patients and family caregivers often focused on process goals and shorter time frames, as opposed to typical health-care provider emphasis on specific outcomes and longer-range time frames (188).

Prescription of Rehabilitation Programs

An appropriate therapeutic prescription is critical to the success of rehabilitation program. It must be based on a careful analysis of the patient's current functional limitations, with realistic goal setting in the context of premorbid functioning and anticipated improvement in medical status (191). Specific therapy techniques will be used based on physical status (e.g., neurologic, musculoskeletal, cardiovascular systems) and medical stability. Social and cultural barriers to certain exercises or activities also must be taken into account. The patient should participate in goal setting, such that the rehabilitation plan is relevant to his or her own goals. Without a strong therapeutic alliance between all health professional team members and the patient (and family), progress will be slow and limited.

Functional training approaches usually are well accepted by most older individuals because they can clearly see the relevance and importance. Many therapeutic goals can be achieved by incorporating formal therapy techniques into the context of functional tasks. Examples of this approach include the following techniques:

- Remediate perceptual problems during eating or meal preparation
- Increase range of motion with dressing training
- Strengthen through inclined sanding or woodworking projects
- Aerobically condition through adapted competitive sports

Prescription of the rehabilitation program must be tailored to the person to accommodate limitations imposed by comorbid medical problems (44,70,74). Cardiovascular (e.g., blood pressure/pulse response, cardiac symptomatology) and pulmonary (e.g., use of oxygen) restrictions should be established as appropriate. Weight-bearing limits can be accommodated by means of assistive devices or aquatic therapy. In patients with limited exercise tolerance, it may be necessary to use flexibility with therapy scheduling and duration of treatment, with frequent rest periods. A number of authors have suggested practical rehabilitation guidelines that summarize these recommendations (74,192,193). Resnick proposes a seven-step model to help motivate older individuals to exercise, including education, goal setting, role modeling, and verbal encouragement/rewards (194).

Realistic goal setting is complex in any rehabilitation setting but may be complicated further in older patients in two unique respects. First, older adults frequently have potential caregivers (e.g., spouse, siblings, children) who also are aging and have medical problems of their own; fitness and capability of the proposed caregiver after discharge must be considered in the discharge planning process (121,122,125). The second problem relates to the limited remaining life expectancy of the older disabled patient. For example, diabetic amputees older than 65 years have average survivals of approximately a year (195). In view of the potentially limited longevity, an expedited rehabilitation program to facilitate return home with family would be most appropriate. This would also apply to people with conditions that are progressively disabling and require increasingly frequent episodes of hospitalization or skilled nursing care.

A number of potentially negative or counterproductive team dynamics can develop in rehabilitation settings that may interfere with or limit a patient's progress (196, 197). Patients and families tend to trust their health-care providers as the experts who will know and do what is best for them. It is critical that the rehabilitation team maintain vigilance for and strive to counter such negative attitudes as paternalism (e.g., overriding patient goals judged by the team to be unrealistic or inappropriate), arrogance (e.g., presumptive familiarity by addressing patients by their first name without requesting permission or preference), and self-fulfilling prophecies (e.g., patients judged not to have potential for improvement not receiving as much attention or effort as patients felt to have a good prognosis). Other team issues that can impact effectiveness include relative team member roles (either lack of clarity or excess rigidity), communication barriers, or decision-making conflicts (196). The ongoing challenge for rehabilitation teams is to foster an individual and collective philosophy of respect for and empowerment of the individuals they treat, facilitating functional independence. The latter includes (appropriate) risk-taking (referred to as dignity of risk).

Significance of Functional Status in Placement Issues

Reference already has been made to the critical nature of functional status with regard to ability to live independently in the community. Older people often live alone and must perform their own self-care and other daily activities, including home-making. Issues of safety in this home environment frequently are raised, particularly after an acute adverse event or illness (e.g., a fall with hip fracture). A patient who achieves a level of mobility (i.e., ambulation or transfers) requiring only close supervision or contact guarding because of occasional loss of balance may not be able to safely return home alone. Home-based supervision by an aide, unless paid privately, typically is available only a few hours a day, 5 days a week, for relatively limited intervals. Return to a community setting may be possible if a relative is available to live with this individual. If not, he or she may not even qualify for a boarding home or intermediate-care facility; most intermediate-care facility admission criteria include independent safe locomotion. This patient accordingly may require an SNF (or nursing home) admission as the only source of 24-hour-per-day supervision available. Unfortunately, alternatives are limited for more homelike settings with other residents of similar functional level.

Health-Care Policy Issues

There is increasing evidence that health-care financing can have a significant (if unintended) impact on the structure, delivery, and outcomes of health care. Chan and colleagues have analyzed the effect of changes in the Medicare payment system for rehabilitation hospitals on length of stay and charges, as well as discharge destinations (198,199). Their analysis revealed that lengths of stay and charges dropped significantly the year after implementation of the new Medicare prospective payment system for rehabilitation, compared with the base year, for all diagnostic categories (198). A further dynamic involved an increased likelihood of discharge from a rehabilitation hospital to an SNF, particularly for (often older) patients with longer lengths of stay, under the new prospective payment system with its fixed reimbursement cap (199).

Chan et al. have also documented associations between type of insurance (Medicaid, health maintenance organizations, commercial fee-for-service plans) and relative frequency of postacute hospital discharge settings (SNF versus rehabilitation hospital) for patients with traumatic brain injury (200). Discharges from acute-care hospitals to SNFs were significantly more likely with Medicaid, and to a lesser extent with health maintenance organization (HMO) coverage, than for patients with fee-for-service commercial insurance.

On the other hand, there is also evidence that programs specifically designed to improve quality of care for older patients can effect changes in health-care delivery and outcomes. Coleman and Fox, on behalf of the HMO Care Management Workgroup, describe an evidence-based approach to improving quality of geriatric care within managed care organizations (201). Their premise is that by expanding the managed care organization focus to include older members at risk for functional decline and subsequent frail health (with higher health-care costs), "upstream" approaches to maintain or improve functional reserve will result not only in improved health, but also lower health-care costs.

Jencks et al. cite improvement in care rendered to Medicare patients over a 2-year interval based on tracking of (and possibly related to feedback for) a number of quality of care indicators by the Quality Improvement Organization program of the Centers for Medicare and Medicaid Services (202). The quality indicators included inpatient management of acute myocardial infarction, heart failure, stroke and pneumonia, as well as ambulatory preventive measures for breast cancer, diabetes, and pneumonia. Despite the historical shortcomings of quality improvement efforts on a national level as documented in *Healthy People 2010* (203), Jencks is optimistic that improvement in health-care quality is not only possible but is occurring. He notes this trend should be reinforced by alignment of quality indicator tracking between such national agencies as Centers for Medicare and Medicaid Services, the Joint Commission on Accreditation of Healthcare Organizations, and the National Quality Forum.

Along similar lines, Calkins and colleagues propose changes in components of the health-care system to improve the health of older people, such as more detailed emergency room evaluations and more focused (and sustained) home health-care services (204). What is clear in any case is that health-care policy continues to be in flux, trying to address the challenges of financing and delivering appropriate care to older persons.

MANAGEMENT OF COMORBIDITY AND GERIATRIC SYNDROMES

Medical Issues

REASSESSMENT OF MEDICAL STATUS

Transfer of a patient from an acute medical or surgical service to a rehabilitation unit has been identified as an opportunity for a fresh and objective reassessment of medical status (205). Such an appraisal is even more critical in geriatric rehabilitation and should include confirming the accuracy of referral diagnoses, evaluating for previously unrecognized conditions, and reviewing medications for continuing appropriateness (140). Often an elderly patient's physiologic status has markedly improved or stabilized by the time of transfer, warranting consideration of altering dosage or discontinuing certain medications. Creating and using tools like a patient care notebook with medication lists is one process that can help clarify medication use (206). Patients can be encouraged to take these notebooks to all health-care appointments.

AVOIDING ADVERSE DRUG EFFECTS

The incidence of adverse drug reactions approaches 25% in people older than 80 years (23). Adverse drug reactions account for 11% to 20% of hospitalizations in people older than 65 years and are a frequent cause of mental deterioration (207–209). The reasons for drug problems in older adults revolve around five key interrelated areas:

1. Polypharmacy
2. Medications not taken as prescribed
3. Increased susceptibility to adverse reactions
4. Altered pharmacokinetics
5. Altered receptor sensitivity

Polypharmacy

Polypharmacy is frequent in older people and often compounded by the frequent use of nonprescription drugs, resulting in preventable adverse drug reactions and unnecessary financial costs (210,211). Physicians all too often contribute to this problem, with one in five older patients receiving a prescription for a potentially inappropriate medication in 1996 (212). A compounding factor frequently is not taking known risk factors into account before prescribing a particular medication and dosage (213,214). Medication histories obtained by physicians often are inaccurate in both inpatient and outpatient settings (215,216), related in part to lack of questioning and underreporting of over-the-counter (OTC) medications, which are used almost as much as prescription medications by older adults (217,218). More than 50% of OTC medications are oral analgesics, with the remainder consisting of cough-and-cold preparations, vitamins, antacids, and laxatives (216,218).

The hospital setting is an excellent one in which to discontinue drugs of questionable value because careful monitoring is possible. Accordingly, all medications should be reviewed carefully on admission and regularly thereafter. In addition to OTC medications, special attention should be directed to digitalis preparations, NSAIDs, and psychotropic medications (219).

In addition to unawareness of concurrent medications, other factors have been identified as potentially influencing prescribing habits and contributing to polypharmacy in older people. These include pharmaceutical advertising (particularly involving new drugs inadequately tested in older people) and patient and family expectations (or even demands) for treatment, usually in the form of a prescription (220). In one nursing home study, treatments (i.e., medication prescriptions) occurred more often if a patient's problem produced ongoing discomfort for the staff (e.g., agitation); undertreated were conditions in which symptoms were intermittent or had less impact on staff (e.g., arthritis) (221).

Medications Not Taken as Prescribed

Patients do not take medications as prescribed in one-third to one-half of all cases (222). Patients older than 75 years who live alone are especially likely to not take medications as prescribed (216,218). Reasons given by patients in one study for not taking medications included "feeling the prescribed dosage was too high" and experiencing problematic side effects (223). These patient choices can cause postdischarge deterioration; patient education before discharge is critical to try to avoid such problems. Allowing patients to self-medicate in the hospital with flexible administration times may be a useful way to monitor their understanding and an opportunity to reinforce the need for medications (224). This strategy also may help to decrease the frequency of incorrect drug frequency or dosage, omitted medications, and use of expired medications (225). However, challenges remain in determining the best methods for enhancing patient adherence to medication prescriptions (226).

Drug toxicity can result when a patient is admitted to the hospital and given all the drugs (in the "correct" dosages and frequency) that have been previously prescribed but were not being taken at home. Such a problem should be suspected when a patient shows a decline in cognitive or functional status 5 to 10 days after admission and other medical workup is unrevealing (227).

Increased Susceptibility to Adverse Reactions

Adverse drug reactions appear to be more common in older patients, even when medications are given in the proper dosages (228). This may be related to a relative lack of resiliency in their homeostatic mechanisms (23,219). Although not all adverse drug reactions are avoidable, some investigators suggest that 70% to 90% could be anticipated and prevented (211, 221,222). That some patients choose not to adhere to prescriptions given by physicians may in fact help decrease the frequency of adverse drug reactions (223). Serious side effects can occur secondary to OTC medications, especially from antihistamines with anticholinergic side effects, leading to fatigue and confusion even in middle-aged adults (217).

Altered Pharmacokinetics

There are a number of age-related changes in pharmacokinetics, previously reviewed, with significant implications for drug dosing, timing of dosage changes, and potential for unex-

pected toxicity or interactions. The reader is referred to the previous discussion of organ-system aging for hematologic, gastrointestinal, hepatic, and renal systems.

Altered Receptor Sensitivity

Age-related changes in receptor sensitivity to drug effects are a further reason for untoward drug effects in older people. There is evidence, for example, that benzodiazepines and warfarin have a greater effect at similar concentrations in the young compared with the elderly (220,228). Such changes are difficult to evaluate separately from the pharmacokinetic changes related to aging.

The common philosophy of "go low, go slow" is sound advice when prescribing drugs for older people. Evaluation of response to drug therapy is critical, and elimination of unnecessary medication is essential for improving function. Patient and family education as to the indications, contraindications, and adverse effects of drugs is even more important in older individuals to try to improve adherence and avoid adverse reactions (224,225).

HYPOTENSION

Symptomatic orthostatic hypotension can occur in many older patients after even relatively short periods of bed rest (142). It is accordingly a frequent problem during early remobilization of elderly patients in rehabilitation settings. Symptoms can persist if there are underlying problems with blood pressure maintenance related to drug therapy, salt restriction, or autonomic dysfunction (53). Orthostatic hypotension is defined as a decline of 20 mm Hg or more in systolic blood pressure when rising from supine to standing, usually accompanied by symptoms of dizziness or lightheadedness (229).

Evaluation of the patient should include a review of medications (particularly nitrates, antihypertensives, levodopa, diuretics, phenothiazines, and tricyclic antidepressants), examination for autonomic dysfunction (e.g., pupillary response, abnormal sweating, central nervous system disease, response to Valsalva maneuver) or recent fluid loss, and laboratory tests to rule out abnormalities in aldosterone and cortisol levels (140,229,230). Metanephrines should be evaluated when hypotension occurs with episodic hypertension, a hallmark of pheochromocytoma (230).

Treatment for symptomatic orthostasis includes discontinuing any prescribed or OTC medication that could be contributing to the hypotension. The patient should be instructed to exercise (i.e., ankle dorsiflexion/plantar flexion) before arising, to sit up initially, and then to stand up slowly while holding onto a support. Thigh-high elastic stockings or an abdominal binder may help minimize lower-extremity blood pooling (229). High-sodium diet and fludrocortisone acetate, a synthetic mineralocorticoid, are useful for plasma expansion in the absence of congestive heart failure. Other medications to consider include NSAIDs (which inhibit prostaglandin synthesis), clonidine or midodrine (which are α_2-adrenergic agonists), propranolol (which blocks α_2 vasodilatory receptors), pindolol (which is a α-adrenergic antagonist with intrinsic sympathomimetic activity), or phenylpropanolamine (which is a sympathomimetic) (219,220, 229).

Mental and Emotional Status

DEPRESSION

Depressed mood is a significant problem in older persons and is often missed. Given the importance of improving recognition of depression, several recent reviews have covered the topic in detail (231–233). Rates of major depression vary from

16% to 30% for elderly clinical populations, and prevalence rates in community-dwelling older persons ranges from 2% to 5%. The risk of depression has been estimated to be threefold greater for older persons with disability compared with their functionally independent counterparts (116, 234). Essential is the distinction, sometimes hard to make, between depressed mood that will respond to supportive counseling and more severe depression requiring more aggressive intervention (e.g., psychotherapy, medication, electroconvulsive therapy) (235). The rehabilitation team should maintain a high index of suspicion for the presence of depression that may require aggressive treatment. Vegetative signs suggestive of more severe depression may include the following:

- Sleep disturbance
- Loss of appetite
- Constipation
- Impaired concentration
- Poor memory
- Psychomotor retardation (117)

Symptoms can include depressed mood, poor motivation, fatigue, and suicidal ideation. Other less specific, somatic symptoms include pain and ill-characterized dyspnea (115). Depressed patients may appear as if they have a dementia syndrome (231,232).

In many patients with mild reactive depression, the activity and milieu of the rehabilitation unit will alleviate the depression. Progress in therapy and the support of peers and staff often are therapeutic. When the depression is more profound, antidepressants may prove helpful; however, medical contraindications may limit or preclude their use (231). Newer medications such as trazodone and the selective serotonin reuptake inhibitors have lower anticholinergic activity and should be considered in addition to those tricyclic antidepressants with the fewest anticholinergic side effects (e.g., doxepin, nortriptyline, desipramine) (232). Doses should be started low, usually at night initially, and increased gradually.

Few studies have investigated the role of psychological and social interventions for older persons (231,233). Depressed outpatient volunteers in generally good health have shown benefits with cognitive behavior, interpersonal, and short-term psychodynamic therapies. Clinically, interventions like these are potentially beneficial and require more evaluation, especially because medication alone cannot address such associated issues as altered life role (especially with disabilities), chronic medical illness, and losses of spouses and close friends (117, 233).

ANXIETY

Anxiety syndromes are another frequent problem during rehabilitation (236). Symptoms can manifest in multiple systems, as in depression. Careful differential diagnosis is required to distinguish between primary anxiety disorders and those secondary to medical illness or medication. A detailed interview and chronology of onset is needed, and assistance from psychiatry often is needed. Diagnostic categories include adjustment disorder with anxious mood, generalized anxiety disorder, posttraumatic stress disorder, and panic attacks (237). When feasible, nonpharmacologic interventions should first be used, such as behavioral management techniques, physical therapy for muscle relaxation, or psychotherapy (238). Nonetheless, judicious and appropriate medication use is frequently necessary to control anxiety symptoms and facilitate participation in the rehabilitation process. Commonly used options include lorazepam, buspirone, imipramine, and serotonin selective reuptake inhibitors (238).

A baseline anxiety disorder may be exacerbated by hospitalization, leading to agitation with nonpurposeful excessive motor activity. Depression, as well as preexisting psychoses, can also present with agitation (236). The former usually responds to the more sedating tricyclic antidepressants (e.g., doxepin). Paraphrenia is an example of a psychosis occurring in the elderly that often presents with agitation (238). A paranoid psychosis with onset typically late in life, it is characterized by bizarre paranoid delusions in a socially isolated person. Antipsychotics are critical to the management of this problem, coupled with therapeutic alliance with a physician and an attempt to redevelop social contacts for the patient. A history of preexisting psychiatric disorders always should be sought in the agitated patient. Schizophrenia can continue into old age, although exacerbations respond well to antipsychotics (236).

DELIRIUM

Delirium, a syndrome characterized by the acute onset of fluctuating cognitive deficits in conjunction with attention disorder and disorganized thought, can cause sleep disturbances, hallucinations, and agitation (239). It occurs more often in patients with prior cognitive impairments and can coexist with a dementia, making accurate diagnosis very difficult (240). Any acute medical illness can present in the older person with delirium without the classic signs of the underlying acute illness (140). Infections, dehydration, stroke, hypothermia, uremia, heart or liver failure, and pulmonary emboli are the most common examples of this phenomenon (241). Drug toxicity is another frequent cause of delirium in the elderly, with common offenders including neuroleptics and narcotics (240,241). There are evolving data on factors associated with postoperative delirium states (242). Delirium is still present in 16% of admissions to postacute facilities, presenting diagnostic and management challenges in the SNF setting (243). Delirium represents a medical emergency, with significant independent morbidity (244); identifying the cause is critical to its resolution (140).

DEMENTIA

Severe dementia occurs in about 5% of individuals older than 65 years (with mild to moderate forms in another 10%) and in about 20% of those older than 80 years (245,246). It is found in more than half of nursing home residents and is the most common precipitating cause of admission (245). Women appear to be affected more frequently than men. Insidious onset of memory loss, loss of abstract reasoning and problem-solving ability, impairment of judgment and orientation, and personality changes with relatively intact alertness and awareness are hallmarks of the disease (247). A patient with early dementia, premorbidly not interfering with daily activities, can become severely disoriented during an acute hospitalization (140,248). This agitated confusion may resolve without any specific therapy in 1 to 2 weeks. Appreciation of this possibility is important with regard to evaluating and working with this population in rehabilitation settings.

Fifty to sixty percent of dementias represent dementia of the Alzheimer type, and another 20% are multiinfarct in origin (246). The remaining large number of potentially reversible causes of dementia include the following conditions:

- Subdural hematoma
- Brain tumor
- Occult hydrocephalus
- Syphilis
- Hypothyroidism or hyperthyroidism
- Hypercalcemia
- Vitamin B_{12} deficiency

- Niacin deficiency
- Drug toxicity
- Depression
- Cardiac, renal, or hepatic failure (247)

Diagnostic evaluation always should be performed to rule out these possible causes. Even if one of these potentially treatable etiologies is established, however, reversibility of the dementia may be limited because of permanent damage from the condition (249). Although there are differing guidelines for recommended laboratory tests for evaluating dementia (247), a standard dementia workup, in addition to detailed history and physical examination with cognitive screening, should include at least a complete blood count, blood chemistry profiles (including electrolytes, creatinine, blood urea nitrogen), erythrocyte sedimentation rate, and thyroid function studies.

Other investigative studies, such as serologic test for syphilis, serum folate, serum cobalamin, drug screening, collagen vascular profile, urinalysis for heavy metals, or imaging of the brain (e.g., computed tomography, magnetic resonance imaging) can be undertaken if there is concern that they will clarify the etiology, such as multiinfarct dementia versus Alzheimer's disease (247,250). A trial off all medications probably is warranted in all patients with new onset of dementia. Many clinicians also routinely give a trial of antidepressants to newly identified dementia patients because an occult depression frequently coexists with mild dementia (139,251). Amelioration of the depression may improve overall functioning in this situation.

Patients with moderate or severe dementia can be limited in their new learning in rehabilitation settings because their ability to form new memory is poor. Day-to-day carryover may be limited and makes certain types of therapeutic gains difficult to achieve (252). A rehabilitation trial may still be justified in such situations to clarify learning abilities and to train the family in appropriate care of a patient with a new disability. For instance, the patient may show the ability for procedural learning (learning by performing the activity) even if declarative learning (learning from verbal instruction) is impaired (127,147).

When evaluating the elderly patient for admission to a rehabilitation program, it is critical to determine the mental status before onset of the new disability by talking to family or others who have observed the patient. Too often the mental status as seen in the acute hospital setting underestimates the patient's cognitive function when healthier and in a more supportive and stimulating environment (such as a rehabilitation unit) (253).

Discharge planning for patients with dementia needs to include family education as to the nature of the patient's cognitive strengths and weaknesses and how to handle potential behavioral problems (127). Community resources for adult day-care and respite-care programs may be very helpful for families, as well as educational materials such as the Agency for Health Care Policy and Research's booklet on early Alzheimer's disease (254).

Geriatric Syndromes

INCONTINENCE

An all too common complication, devastating to patient self-esteem and family commitment to patient care, is urinary incontinence. For diagnostic classification and evaluation procedures, the reader is referred to Chapter 76. Several recent reviews cover this topic thoroughly (255,256). Treatment for incontinence in the older patient hinges on proper diagnosis, which usually is possible with a complete history of the problem combined with careful neurologic, pelvic, rectal, and mental status examinations. Laboratory studies should include urinalysis, culture and sensitivity, serum creatinine and blood urea nitrogen, and a postvoid residual urine volume (255,257). A voiding diary often is helpful in determining the nature of the problem, and cystometrics also may be indicated (258).

Treatment is directed at the cause of the incontinence. Unfortunately, many of the etiologies have no uniformly successful therapy, and there may even be multiple causes. A timed voiding program is useful in many patients, offering toileting opportunities at regular intervals to try to maintain continence (255). Initially, the intervals are very short (e.g., every 15 to 20 minutes), with progressive increase as indicated. Modifications of this technique include patterned urge-response toileting (PURT) (259) and functional incidental training (FIT) (260), with reports of excellent success in nursing home settings.

Surgical procedures may be useful in the treatment of prostatic hypertrophy and sphincteric incompetence (256,258). Anticholinergics (e.g., propantheline) frequently are useful in the management of detrusor instability, but with the potential risk of retention (257). Other pharmacologic approaches include direct smooth muscle relaxants (e.g., oxybutynin), calcium channel blockers, and imipramine (255,256). Overflow incontinence that is due to detrusor decompensation (from overstretching) may require long-term indwelling catheterization, although frequent intermittent catheterization and cholinergic drugs to stimulate detrusor contraction may be helpful (261). Excellent patient and health-care professional educational materials are available (262,263).

Bowel incontinence may imply severe bilateral brain disease or loss of sensory input from the rectal ampulla (264). Biofeedback has been shown to be helpful in managing sensory bowel incontinence (265,266), but the management of incontinence secondary to diffuse brain disease usually requires a behavioral approach, with bowel movements induced by suppositories at regular intervals (264).

SLEEP DISORDERS

Sleep disorders and daytime fatigue are related problems common in the hospitalized elderly person as well as those living in the community (141,146,267). The hospital environment alone can disrupt the sleep cycle, an effect further compounded by foreign routines (vital sign checks and medication administration at odd hours), unfamiliar noises (from machines, overhead paging, and neighboring patients), and the depression often associated with the onset of new major chronic illness (146). Sleep deprivation at night leads to fatigue during the day. Napping during the day further disrupts nocturnal sleep patterns, and a vicious cycle can ensue (267).

It is important to document whether insufficient sleep is actually occurring because patients can report sleep difficulties when no problem is documented, and they remain alert throughout the day. Simple reassurance in such cases is warranted. In cases of documented sleep disorder, contributing factors such as delirium, medication toxicities, depression, anxiety, restless leg syndrome, chronic pain syndrome, or nighttime medical problems (e.g., congestive heart failure, angina) should be considered (140,146). It is also important to differentiate acute insomnia from chronic insomnia. Acute insomnia (present for less than 1 month) is often related to a stressor (e.g., bereavement) and is treated with support and short-term, intermittent medication. Chronic insomnia (persisting for more than 1 month) should be viewed more as a symptom of another illness (267). Hypnotics should be used judiciously and only if other interventions, such as improved sleep hygiene and treatment of the underlying illness, are unsuccessful.

After addressing these issues, good sleep hygiene practices may help. These include a regular sleep schedule, keeping the patient out of the bed and bedroom until bedtime, a snack before bedtime, daily exercise, relaxing activities in the evening before bedtime, and instruction in mental imagery or deep breathing relaxation techniques to be used as needed in bed at night (268). In addition, patients should not watch clocks during the night. Naps during the day should be avoided unless absolutely needed briefly after lunch.

Only if these interventions fail should a sleep medication be considered. Selected antidepressants can be used in low doses at night to take advantage of sedative side effects while minimizing anticholinergic activity (e.g., nefazodone, trazodone) (269). If a benzodiazepine-type hypnotic is used, the choice should be one with a very short half-life (e.g., zaleplon, zolpidem) to avoid accumulation with hangover effects (270,271). In general, diphenhydramine should be avoided because of anticholinergic effects (219,220). In the patient who remains persistently fatigued without clear organic cause, occult depression should be suspected (139,230). Additional nonmedication treatments that appear promising in older adults include behavioral treatments (e.g., stimulus control to induce good sleep hygiene behaviors) and increased exposure to light (272,273). Recent research indicates melatonin can be a useful adjunct in the management of sleep disorders in the elderly (274,275).

PAIN

Pain is very common in older people, and studies are increasingly focused on the subject (276–278). Prevalence estimates range from 25% to 50% of community-dwelling elderly people to 45% to 80% of nursing home residents (277,279). The consequences of pain are significant and include depression, decreased socialization, sleep disturbance, impaired ambulation, and increased health-care use and costs (276). The pain experienced and reported by older people is no less threatening than that experienced by younger people and must similarly be addressed promptly (277).

Special considerations in managing pain in older persons include difficulty in assessment secondary to patient fears, the higher incidence of comorbid illnesses compared with younger persons, complications in reporting pain in patients with memory and other cognitive impairments, validity difficulties with proxy reporting, and the importance of assessing functional implications of the pain (277,280). Furthermore, physicians understandably tend to attribute new pain to prior conditions. Cognitive impairment does not mask pain at the time of patient questioning, but accurate reporting of past pain is not necessarily reliable (281). Patients may be able to respond appropriately to pain intensity scales concerning current pain, with visual cueing as needed and taking short attention spans into account (282). Special functional considerations include the recognition that advanced and elective activities of daily living may be more sensitive to changes in pain.

Common etiologies of pain in older people include osteoarthritis, cancer, herpes zoster, temporal arteritis, polymyalgia rheumatica, and atherosclerotic peripheral vascular disease (279). Approaches to pain management are similar across age groups and include use of physical modalities (e.g., heat, cold, massage), transcutaneous electrical nerve stimulation, biofeedback, hypnosis, and distractive techniques (276). Concurrent depression with pain may occur as in younger persons, requiring direct assessment for depression and appropriate intervention (232). Of note, older patients with depression are more likely to report pain as a somatic expression of their mood disturbance (281).

Medications for pain should be prescribed judiciously and in conjunction with nonpharmacologic approaches (276). Acetaminophen remains one of the best initial medications to be used routinely in patients with pain (283,284). Nonsteroidal antiinflammatory medications are problematic in this population, given the limited study of patients older than age 65 (285) and the known fourfold higher risk of peptic ulcer disease (286). Long-term use of opiate analgesics is appropriate for malignant pain and probably in some cases of nonmalignant chronic disabling pain unresponsive to other medications. Tricyclic antidepressants or anticonvulsants may be useful in treating neuropathic pain (276). Physical mobility and activities should be encouraged as much as possible. All these treatments are best administered as part of a multidisciplinary team approach, regardless of the setting (e.g., home, SNF, or outpatient department) (277).

A particularly challenging clinical population includes older adults who experience chronic pain, often with repeated failures to respond to traditional medical or surgical treatments. The cognitive-behavioral model of therapy, developed with younger persons, may prove useful in these patients (277, 278). This therapy is safer, more effective, and probably lower in cost than a long-term analgesic regimen, especially if applied early in the course of an evolving pain syndrome. The model divides contributory factors to the pain experience into biomedical variables, psychological variables (e.g., pain coping strategies, depression, personality), and socioenvironmental variables (e.g., social support, spousal criticism). Behavior therapy encourages wellness behaviors, and cognitive therapy helps patients reassess how they view themselves and their pain experience. This model also highlights the importance of assessing family behaviors in the presence of pain. Specific interventions for family coping can be beneficial (287,288). Family and caregiver training, as well as semiformal social supports in the community, may be especially important in the setting of chronic pain in older persons (277). For example, chronic back pain sufferers (typically with associated depression) tend to exhaust their social support (289). Preventing the resulting social isolation would likely improve efficacy of treatment intervention and avoid a cascade of complications (137).

FALLS

Many of the age-related physiologic declines in multiple organ systems combine to increase dramatically the incidence of falls in the elderly, including visuoperceptual difficulty, postural instability, impaired mobility, orthostatic hypotension, lower-extremity weakness, and vertigo that is due to degenerative or vascular changes in the vestibular apparatus (159,160). Other factors contribute to increase the risk of falling, including environmental hazards, adverse effects of medications, concomitant acute or chronic disease states, depression, apathy, or confusion (246,290–292). A model attempting to identify the degree of risk for recurrent falls stratified patients into high and low risk depending on sitting and standing balance, walking ability, and stair climbing (293). In addition, attitudes toward risk were measured, as were social supports and environmental status. Recurrent falls were associated with impaired mobility, risk-taking behavior, and environmental score.

Prevention of these injurious falls is more problematic. A recent prospective study of 9,516 community-residing white women (average follow-up 4.1 years) found that the likelihood of hip fracture increased in the presence of multiple risk factors and low bone density (294). Suggested possible interventions to decrease risk include maintaining body weight, walking for exercise, avoiding long-acting benzodiazepines, minimizing caffeine intake, and treating impaired visual function. Tai chi reduced risk of multiple falls by 48% in a randomized control trial in community-residing persons 70 years of age and older without chronic illness, many of whom had fallen in the prior year (295).

Whether this intervention would work for older persons with chronic illnesses needs to be assessed. In another study of community-dwelling elderly with at least one risk factor for falls, a multifactorial intervention (medication adjustments, behavioral instruction, and exercise) reduced falls from 47% in the control group to 35% in the intervention group (296). What multiple studies appear to consistently substantiate is that exercise is an important component of any fall prevention strategy (297,298).

Fear of falling resulting in decreased mobility is also a clinical problem in many older adults (299,300). Patient training in fall recovery techniques and education regarding adaptive and preventive strategies are being evaluated as methods to help prevent activity restriction from the fear of falling.

MANAGEMENT OF COMMON DISABLING CONDITIONS

Hip Fracture

Although 95% of falls in older persons fortunately do not result in serious injury (301), hip fractures continue to be one of the most serious sequela (302). Strategies considered for intervention to prevent hip fracture have included both public health initiatives (e.g., emphasizing weight-bearing exercise) and individualized approaches focused on high-risk patients (303, 304). The most effective approaches have yet to be worked out. In situations involving rehabilitation of an elderly patient after repair of hip fracture secondary to fall, it is critical to evaluate and treat the cause of the incident fall to prevent future recurrence.

A number of controversies involve proper care of the elderly patient after hip fracture. The literature is increasingly evaluating factors affecting outcomes from hip fractures and potential cost-effective changes in practice (305,309).

Issues relating to preoperative decisions include how long to wait for medical stabilization. One guideline suggests that hip fracture patients who have two or fewer comorbidities should have the operation within 2 days of admission, but that a longer delay is beneficial for patients with three or more comorbidities (310).

Several factors affect the decision to operate and what type of surgery. A tendency to treat hip fractures conservatively (i.e., nonsurgically) in demented elderly patients is countered by findings of better function with less morbidity and mortality with surgical management (311). For patients with severe cardiovascular disease that contraindicates general anesthesia, percutaneous pinning with Ender rods under local anesthesia can be performed. Femoral neck fractures can be treated either by resection of the femoral head with endoprosthesis with immediate postoperative weight bearing, or by internal fixation with multiple pins with delayed weight bearing. Although intertrochanteric fractures traditionally are managed by internal fixation with nail or compression screw with delayed weight bearing, some studies suggest patients can be mobilized much earlier without complication and with improved morbidity and function (305,308,311).

The postoperative period can be divided into the acute hospital period and posthospital (or postacute) care. The urgency of early mobilization after repair of hip fracture is twofold: the vulnerability to many postoperative complications (e.g., pulmonary problems, thromboembolism, genitourinary sequelae) and the risk of secondary complications from bed rest or relative inactivity (305,306). In one recent study of the acute hospital period after surgical repair of hip fracture, factors associated with discharge directly to home (which occurred in only 17% of 162 hip fracture survivors) included prior community residing status, age younger than 85 years, absence of postoperative complications, achieving independence in bed mobility and ambulation with a walker, and a greater number of physical therapy sessions during hospitalization (308).

By far the majority of hip fracture patients in the United States receive postacute hospital care in other facilities—either acute rehabilitation hospitals/units or SNFs. These settings are increasingly necessary as lengths of hospital stay continue to dramatically decline. Which setting is best for which patients is still not clear. What is necessary during the recuperative phase from hip fracture, regardless of setting, is close attention to multiple medical problems that can arise (306,307). Optimal length of stay in these settings likewise is not yet clear and also continues to decline.

Arthritis and Joint Replacements

Management of arthritic conditions in older people, just as in a younger population, must be individualized with close monitoring of benefits (311,312). Treatment principles are comparable, although the balance between rest and activity is much more delicate because of the adverse sequelae of inactivity in the elderly. There is evidence that older people with arthritis may respond better to therapeutic programs and often are more patient and compliant with long-term exercise and activity programs (313,314). Treatment goals include relief from fear, fatigue, stiffness, and pain; suppression of the inflammatory process; prevention or correction of deformity; and maximizing function (284,313). This is accomplished via a combination of psychological, pharmacologic, physical, and surgical measures.

Important psychological approaches have been developed through the Arthritis Self-Help Course. The multifaceted interventions include education and exercise (315). Part of the benefit may derive from facilitating the patient's ability to manage his or her own chronic condition. Successful exercise interventions include programs of focused muscle strengthening (e.g., quadriceps strengthening for osteoarthritis of the knee), general conditioning, and aerobic activities (316–318).

Patients can be educated about the beneficial results of using various assistive devices to maintain independent community living, such as a firm chair of appropriate height with armrests, utensils with built-up handles, elevated toilet seat with grab bars, or ambulation aids (e.g., cane, walker). As with any patient care equipment, having patients try to use various devices before purchase will help ensure actual functional use (284).

Pharmacologic interventions for pain control should start with acetaminophen (up to 2 to 4 g/day) (283,284). Opiates (codeine or hydrocodone) can provide additional analgesia for breakthrough pain. Topical capsaicin cream may be helpful for persistent knee or finger pain, although usage may be limited by cost, need for frequent application, and initial burning sensation with application. NSAIDs may be needed for control of pain and inflammation, but should be used with great care and close monitoring given the increased risk of acute renal impairments and gastrointestinal bleeding (283). In older patients with a history of gastritis or ulcers who require use of NSAIDs, concurrent administration of misoprostol or other cytoprotective agent should be considered (284,319). The use of the nutraceuticals glucosamine and chondroitin sulfate has been controversial in terms of efficacy, but is currently the focus of a National Institutes of Health multicenter trial (320).

A limited number of intraarticular steroid injections can be considered (generally no more than two to three per year for any joint), but with anticipation of only short-term benefit (284). The Food and Drug Administration has approved another type of intraarticular injection (hyaluronan, a glycosaminoglycan) for patients who have failed other forms of therapy (284).

Age should not be a primary factor in considering potential benefits of surgical intervention in the elderly arthritic patient (283,320). Significant functional gains may be realized with an appropriately timed procedure (e.g., ligament or tendon repair, osteotomy, arthroplasty, prosthetic joint replacement) to improve stability and range or to decrease pain (313). Attention to preoperative and postoperative therapy programs and early mobilization is critical to maximize functional gains and minimize secondary complications from inactivity. Further details of rehabilitation management, including principles for prescription of medication and therapeutic modalities, can be found in Chapters 31, 34, and 36.

Stroke

Appropriateness of intensive rehabilitation for older stroke patients sometimes is questioned, given limited and sometimes conflicting research data. Studies to date suggest that age may have a negative or no effect on functional outcomes, that elderly stroke patients may require longer lengths of stay to achieve the same functional gains as younger patients, and that functional outcomes may be similar in differing rehabilitation settings (321–330). The most significant aspects of rehabilitating elderly stroke patients relate to the severity of their neurologic and functional deficits, medical stability and impact of their frequent multiple comorbid conditions on endurance, and their ability to understand, cooperate, and learn in therapy sessions. Severe language or cognitive deficits, significant neglect or apraxia, poor balance or endurance, or recurrent medical complications/instability may negatively impact the feasibility and goals of a rehabilitation program. The Agency for Health Care Policy and Research has published clinical practice guidelines for stroke rehabilitation which incorporate these and other variables (331).

It is clear that depression, a common complication after stroke at any age, is particularly problematic in older patients as a result of the deleterious effect on cognitive functioning (332). There is evidence of potential to enhance neural plasticity after stroke, even in older individuals, with improved functional recovery (333). Research continues in an effort to clarify the most appropriate (and cost-effective) role, timing, methods, setting, intensity, and duration of rehabilitation services for older people after stroke (334). Chapter 76 reviews concepts of stroke rehabilitation in detail, with reference to older patients.

Amputation

Although a detailed review of rehabilitation of patients with dysvascular amputation can be found in Chapters 32 and 60, several aspects require emphasis here. An ageist bias may result in the belief that a patient's age should be a factor in determining whether to prescribe a prosthesis. Other comorbidities rather than age per se are the relevant determinants for prosthetic fitting (335,336). A number of studies have documented the successful outcomes of rehabilitation programs for older

amputees, including bilateral amputees and amputees with concurrent hemiplegia (336–339). Even in the face of severe medical comorbidity (e.g., cardiovascular disease), a prosthesis still may be both therapeutic and functional, even if only from the standpoint of standing, transfers, or cosmesis (335). For bilateral amputees, although energy costs are significantly higher and ambulation training more difficult, prosthetic fitting still may be useful to allow periodic standing during the day and for walking short distances in the home, which are therapeutic from both an aerobic exercise and psychological standpoint (337). Wheelchair locomotion will usually be a preferable alternative for longer distance travel in view of significantly lower energy costs and ability to stop and rest. The former criterion of successful crutch ambulation to justify prosthetic prescription is no longer justified (335,336).

Spinal Cord Injury

Although spinal cord injury (SCI) usually is considered a disability occurring primarily in the younger population, there is increasing recognition of its significance for older people. Not only is there a significant incidence of SCI in a growing older population (5.4% in the 61- to 90-year-old age group) (340), but increased survival in an aging population injured earlier in their lives (341). The result is a much higher prevalence of older SCI patients, subject to the usual age-related morbidity and mortality. Similarities have been observed between aging morbidity and that of chronic SCI patients who are not old (342).

Epidemiology of SCI with older age at onset differs from that of younger populations. The etiology of injury is much more likely to be falls (60% in the 75-and-older age group), followed by motor vehicle accidents (32% in the 75-and-older group) (340,343). SCI from metastatic disease and cervical myelopathy occurs primarily in older adults. There is a marked increase in proportionate incidence of quadriplegia and quadriparesis in the elderly (67% in the 61- to 75-year-old age group, 88% in the 75-and-older group), as opposed to the more nearly equal distribution between paraplegia and paraparesis and quadriplegia and quadriparesis in younger age groups (340). Elderly SCI patients are much more likely to have quadriparesis as opposed to quadriplegia (343).

There is a progressive disparity in 10-year survival rates between SCI and non-SCI populations with advancing age at injury (340). For those 70 to 98 years of age, the grouped SCI 10-year survival rate is 32%, compared with 48% for their non-SCI counterparts. Life expectancies reported for SCI patients differ depending on whether patients who die before discharge from rehabilitation programs—usually within the first year postinjury—are included in the analysis. If such first-year fatalities are included, life expectancy for SCI patients injured at 60 years of age is 6.5 years for paraparesis, 5.9 years for paraplegia, 4.2 years for quadriparesis, and 1.9 years for quadriplegia, compared with 20.0 years for the non-SCI population (340). Two-year life expectancy is 59% for SCI patients between 61 and 86 years of age, compared with 95% for their younger counterparts (341,344). Older patients with SCI were more likely than their younger counterparts to develop various medical complications, such as pneumonia, gastrointestinal hemorrhage, pulmonary emboli, or renal stones (345). Although overall survival post-SCI is reduced for older adults, with increased morbidity, there does not appear to be a direct relationship between age and functional outcome (346).

These significant life expectancies and potential for functional gains make rehabilitation efforts appropriate for all patients following SCI, regardless of age (346). Rehabilitation goals should be comparable with those for a younger SCI population (see Chapter 79), except as impacted by comorbidity (e.g., arthritis with limitation of hand function, deconditioning, etc.). Personal care assistance becomes more critical with regard to ability to return to the community to live.

Traumatic Brain Injury

Although the concerns regarding falls in older persons are focused primarily on the risk of hip or other skeletal fractures, there is evidence of a significant incidence of traumatic brain injury as well (347). Similarly to older individuals after stroke, the rehabilitation interventions after brain injury must factor in premorbid and current cognitive status, severity of neurologic and functional deficits, and comorbidity issues. Experience with the federally designated Traumatic Brain Injury Model Systems Project reveals that elderly brain-injured patients are capable of significant functional improvement, but more often at a slower pace (with longer lengths of stay and higher costs) (347). A further consideration in the differential diagnosis of an older individual with new onset of cognitive deficits in the context of multiple falls may be the possibility of a postconcussion syndrome rather than a traditional etiology of dementia (348).

THE FUTURE

Role of the Physiatrist in Geriatrics

Physicians from various specialties traditionally have had differing perspectives on their respective roles in geriatrics (349). Physiatrists may serve a variety of roles relating to geriatrics, depending on the practice setting. These contributions range from providing primary care in a rehabilitation inpatient hospital setting or subacute (SNF-based) setting (252,350) to consulting in various health-care settings (such as acute care hospital, SNF, day hospital, or home health care) to outpatient care (252,309,351). In the latter settings, the physiatrist assesses functional and medical status, works closely with therapy staff, helps formulate realistic goals, helps coordinate interdisciplinary team care if needed, and monitors efficacy of therapy.

Hoenig provides an interesting analysis of rehabilitation providers, noting that physicians of whatever specialty typically act at the disease or impairment level (e.g., prescription of medication, surgical procedure, etc.), may function as rehabilitation team leaders, and are often designated as gatekeepers in facilitating access to rehabilitation services (via prescription of therapies, insurance authorization, etc.) (352). She points out that there is a great deal of overlap and variability in the roles played by various rehabilitation providers, with a need to network, communicate, and coordinate to best serve the needs of older patients.

Further progress in this regard is demonstrated by an interdisciplinary interaction and consensus process among 10 medical and surgical specialties, spearheaded and funded by the American Geriatrics Society and John A. Hartford Foundation, respectively (353). As part of this process, Strasser and colleagues articulate the overlapping principles and complementary treatment approaches of geriatrics and physiatry, and the importance of improving the consistency and level of expertise of all physiatrists regarding geriatric rehabilitation, to facilitate improved health care and functional outcomes of our older patients (354).

Geriatric Rehabilitation Settings

Older people with disabling medical conditions may have difficulty tolerating and participating in an intensive comprehen-

sive medical rehabilitation (CMR) hospital-based program, owing to such factors as severity of deficits, medical comorbidity, and deconditioning. Combined with the quest for least costly health-care alternatives, the ideal system of rehabilitative care would provide for varying levels of intensity and settings (191). Indeed, there is evolving interest in the role and effectiveness of subacute rehabilitation, which provides rehabilitation programs of varying intensity in hospital or SNF settings (329,330).

Another nontraditional setting for rehabilitation is the day hospital, which provides comprehensive, relatively intensive and structured rehabilitation therapies designed to reverse disability and train family members to facilitate maintenance of the patient at home (351,355). This provides a greater intensity of therapy with a wider array of equipment and under closer medical supervision than usually is feasible in a home-based treatment program. Day hospitals may allow earlier transition from hospital-based CMR centers to the more familiar and comfortable home setting, with lower health-care costs (351).

There also is increasing interest and program development in augmented home-care services, including rehabilitative care (356,357). New and innovative programs to provide intensive, CMR-level rehabilitation services in the home are being developed and tested (358). A randomized controlled trial of an occupational therapy preventive assessment and treatment program for older people living in the community showed improvements across various health, function, and quality-of-life domains (359). Such community-based programs may prove cost-effective and feasible and help resolve accessibility problems in both urban and rural settings.

These alternative levels and settings of rehabilitation services for older adults provide the potential for a continuum of care, facilitating individually tailored rehabilitative care that can be modified to meet an individual patient's changing needs over time. Further research is required to document the cost-effectiveness and benefits of these varied rehabilitation programs, particularly among subsets of different disability and age groups.

Critical Issues Relating to Outcomes

In summary, the rehabilitation approach to care of older individuals with disability, like geriatric care in general, must be longitudinal in perspective and coordinated with other aspects of the individual's health care, not episodic and in isolation. The teamwork background and training of the physiatrist is an ideal base to accomplish this critical goal of geriatric care.

There are a number of critical issues impacting the quality, cost-effectiveness, and outcomes of rehabilitation interventions. Determining the appropriate treatment setting, timing, and duration of care is of obvious importance. Coupled with this is the need for individualized, realistic, functional, and relevant goal setting, which includes the older person during formulation. Facilitating access to needed services is critical, whether referencing insurance coverage or physical transportation to the care setting. In keeping with the longitudinal perspective, periodic reevaluation is necessary, with review and revision of therapeutic goals as warranted.

Even though "maintenance" treatment or activity is typically unfunded (as opposed to "restorative" care), the concept nonetheless is appropriate. By maintaining an older individual's functional status, he or she can stay in the community at far lower costs than if institutionalized. Waiting for a patient to deteriorate from lack of maintenance care risks initiating a cascade of complications with concomitant decreased prospects of regaining premorbid function. It is also important to remember the potential benefits of group therapy/activities, as opposed to individual treatment (peer support and encouragement, even friendly competition).

The need for patient and family education and training, perhaps on multiple occasions or even continually, should be recognized with respect to compliance and follow-through with health-care recommendations and treatment. Finally, the longitudinal perspective mandates long-term follow-up to monitor (with prompt intervention) for complications, recidivism, or underlying disease progression, as well as to assess counseling or respite needs.

REFERENCES

1. Fried LP, Guralnik JM. Disability in older adults: evidence regarding significance, etiology, and risk. *J Am Geriatr Soc* 1997;45(1):92–100.
2. Hoenig H, Nusbaum N, Brummel-Smith K. Geriatric rehabilitation: state of the art. *J Am Geriatr Soc* 1997;45(11):1371–1381.
3. Hoenig H, Mayer-Oakes SA, Siebens H, et al. Geriatric rehabilitation. what do physicians know about it and how should they use it? *J Am Geriatr Soc* 1994;42:341–345.
4. Strasser DC, Solomon DH, Burton JR. Geriatrics and physical medicine and rehabilitation: common principles, complementary approaches, and 21st century demographics. *Arch Phys Med Rehabil* 2002;83:1323–1324.
5. Kottke FJ. Deterioration of the bedfast patient: causes and effects. *Public Health Rep* 1965;80:437–450.
6. Hobbs FB, Damon BL. *Sixty-five plus in America.* Current Population Reports, Special Studies, P23–P190. Washington, DC: U.S. Department of Commerce, Economics, and Statistics Administration, Bureau of the Census, 1996.
7. National Center for Health Statistics. *Health, United States, 1999 with health and aging chartbook.* Hyattsville, MD: U.S. Department of Health and Human Services, National Center for Health Statistics, 1999; DHHS Pub. No. (PHS) 99–1232.
8. *Chronic care in America: a 21st century challenge.* Princeton, NJ: Robert Wood Johnson Foundation Publications, 1996.
9. Schneider EL, Guralnik JM. The aging of America: impact of health care costs. *JAMA* 1990;263:2335–2340.
10. Olshansky SJ, Ault AB. The fourth stage of the epidemiologic transition: the age of delayed degenerative diseases. *Milbank Q* 1986;64:355–391.
11. Manton KG, Gu X. Changes in the prevalence of chronic disability in the United States black and non-black population above age 65 from 1982 to 1999. *Proc Natl Acad Sci USA* 2001;98:6354–6359.
12. Fries JF. The sunny side of aging. *JAMA* 1990;263:2354–2355.
13. Chan L, Beaver S, MacLehosse R, et al. Disability and health care costs in the Medicare population. *Arch Phys Med Rehabil* 2002;83:1196–1201.
14. Freedman VA, Martin LG, Schoeni RF. Recent trends in disability and functioning among older adults in the United States: a systematic review. *JAMA* 2002;288(24):3137–3146.
15. Fries JF. Aging, natural death, and the compression of morbidity. *N Engl J Med* 1980;303:130–135.
16. Experton B, Ozminkowski RJ, Branch LG, Li Z. A comparison by payor/provider type of the cost of dying among frail older adults. *J Am Geriatr Soc* 1996;44:1098–1107.
17. Lubitz J, Beebe J, Baker C. Longevity and Medicare expenditures. *N Engl J Med* 1995;332:999–1003.
18. Fisher ES, Welch HG, Wennberg JE. Prioritizing Oregon's hospital resources: an example based on variations in discretionary medical utilization. *JAMA* 1992;267:1925–1931.
19. Fries JF. Reducing disability in older age. *JAMA* 2002;288(24):3164–3166.
20. Katz S, Branch LG, Branson MH, et al. Active life expectancy. *N Engl J Med* 1983;309:1218–1224.
21. Manton KG, Stallard E. Cross-sectional estimates of active life expectancy for the U.S. elderly and oldest-old populations. *J Gerontol* 1991;46[Suppl]:170–182.
22. Crimmins EM, Hayward MD, Saito Y. Differentials in active life expectancy in the older population of the United States. *J Gerontol B Psychol Sci Soc Sci* 1996;51(3):S111–S120.
23. Williams ME, Hadler NM. The illness as the focus of geriatric medicine. *N Engl J Med* 1983;308:1357–1360.
24. Manton KG, Stallard E, Liu K. Forecasts of active life expectancy: policy and fiscal implications. *J Gerontol* 1993;48(special issue):11–26.
25. Kane RS. The defeat of aging versus the importance of death. *J Am Geriatr Soc* 1996;44:321–325.
26. Abrass IB. The biology and physiology of aging. *West J Med* 1990;153:641–645.
27. Fozzard JL, Metter EJ, Brant LJ. Next steps in describing aging and disease in longitudinal studies. *J Gerontol* 1990;45:P116–P127.
28. Holloszy JO. The biology of aging. *Mayo Clin Proc* 2000;75[Suppl]:S3–9.
29. Vijg J, Wei JY. Understanding the biology of aging: the key to prevention and therapy. *J Am Geriatr Soc* 1995;43:426–434.
30. Rowe JW. Toward successful aging: limitation of the morbidity associated with "normal aging." In: Hazzard WR, Andres R, Bierman EL, Blass JP, eds. *Principles of geriatric medicine and gerontology,* 2nd ed. New York: McGraw-Hill, 1990:138–141.
31. Seeman TE, Charpentier PA, Berkman LF, et al. Predicting changes in physical performance in a high-functioning elderly cohort: MacArthur studies of successful aging. *J Gerontol* 1994;49:M97–M108.
32. Johnson FB, Sinclari DA, Guarente L. Molecular biology of aging. *Cell* 1999; 96(2):291–302.
33. Lipsitz LA, Goldberger AL. Loss of complexity and aging: potential applications of fractals and chaos theory to senescence. *JAMA* 1992;267:1806–1809.
34. Martin GR, Danner DB, Holbrook NJ. Aging: causes and defenses. *Annu Rev Med* 1993;44:419–429.
35. Thompson CB. Apoptosis in the pathogenesis and treatment of disease. *Science* 1995;267:1456–1462.
36. Manton KG, Vaupel JW. Survival after the age of 80 in the United States, Sweden, France, England, and Japan. *N Engl J Med* 1995;333:1232–1235.
37. Robbins J, Wahl P, Savage P, et al. Hematological and biochemical laboratory values in older Cardiovascular Health Study participants. *J Am Geriatr Soc* 1995;43:855–859.
38. Sorlie PD, Rogot E, Johnson NJ. Validity of demographic characteristics on the death certificate. *Epidemiology* 1992;3(2):181–184.
39. Desrosiers J, Hebert R, Bravo G, et al. A comparison of cross-sectional and longitudinal designs in the study of aging of upper extremity performance. *J Gerontol A Biol Sci Med Sci* 1998;53(5):B362–368.
40. Hughes VA, Frontera WR, Wood M, et al. Longitudinal muscle strength changes in older adults: influence of muscle mass, physical activity, and health. *J Gerontol A Biol Sci Med Sci* 2001;56(5):B209–217.
41. Shock NW. Aging of regulatory systems. In: Cape RDT, Coe RM, Rossman I, eds. *Fundamentals of geriatric medicine.* New York: Raven, 1983:51–62.
42. Rochon PA, Gurwitz JH. Drug therapy. *Lancet* 1995;346(8966):32–36.
43. McGuire DK, Levine BD, Williamson JW, et al. A 30-year follow-up of the Dallas Bed Rest and Training Study: I. Effect of age on the cardiovascular response to exercise. *Circulation* 2001;104:1350–1357.
44. Christmas C, Andersen RA. Exercise and older patients: guidelines for the clinician. *J Am Geriatr Soc* 2000;48(3):318–324.
45. McGuire DK, Levine BD, Williamson JW, et al. A 30-year follow-up of the Dallas Bed Rest and Training Study: II. Effect of age on cardiovascular adaptation to exercise training. *Circulation* 2001;104:1358–1366.
46. Fiatarone MA, Marks EC, Ryan ND, et al. High-intensity strength training in nonagenarians: effects on skeletal muscle. *JAMA* 1990;263:3029–3034.
47. Gill TM, Baker DI, Gottschalk M, et al. A program to prevent functional decline in physically frail, elderly persons who live at home. *N Engl J Med* 2002;347(14):1068–1074.
48. Coleman EA, Fox PD. Translating evidence-based geriatric care into practice: lessons from managed care organizations—Part I: introduction and physical inactivity. *Ann Long Term Care: Clin Care Aging* 2002;10(9):33–38.
49. Aapro MS, Cella D, Zagari M. Age, anemia, and fatigue. *Semin Oncol* 2002; 29(3[Suppl 8]):55–59.
50. Smith DL. Anemia in the elderly. *Am Fam Physician* 2000;62(7):1565–1572.
51. Lipschitz D. Medical and functional consequences of anemia in the elderly. *J Am Geriatr Soc* 2003;51[Suppl 3]:S10–13.
52. Pieper CF, Rao KM, Currie MS, et al. Age, functional status, and racial differences in plasma D-dimer levels in community-dwelling elderly persons. *J Gerontol A Biol Sci Med Sci* 2000;55(11):M649–657.
53. Stern N, Tuck ML. Geriatric cardiology: homeostatic fragility in the elderly. *Cardiol Clin* 1986;4:201–211.
54. Chaves PH, Ashar B, Guralnik JM, Fried LP. Looking at the relationship between hemoglobin concentration and prevalent mobility difficulty in older women: should the criteria currently used to define anemia in older people be reevaluated? *J Am Geriatr Soc* 2002;50(7):1257–1264.
55. Podrazik PM, Schwartz JB. Cardiovascular pharmacology of aging. *Cardiol Clin* 1999;17(1):17–34.
56. Parker BM, Cusack BJ, Vestal RE. Pharmacokinetic optimisation of drug therapy in elderly patients. *Drugs Aging* 1995;7(1):10–18.
57. Altman DF. Changes in gastrointestinal, pancreatic, biliary, and hepatic function with aging. *Gastroenterol Clin North Am* 1990;19:227–234.
58. Shamburek RD, Farrar JT. Disorders of the digestive system in the elderly. *N Engl J Med* 1990;322:438–443.
59. DeLillo AR, Rose S. Functional bowel disorders in the geriatric patient: constipation, fecal impaction, and fecal incontinence. *Am J Gastroenterol* 2000;95 (4):901–905.
60. Beers MH. Explicit criteria for determining potentially inappropriate medication use by the elderly: an update. *Arch Intern Med* 1997;157(14):1531–1536.
61. Harari D, Gurwitz JH, Avorn J, et al. How do older persons define constipation? *J Gen Intern Med* 1997;12:63–66.
62. Holt PR. Diarrhea and malabsorption in the elderly. *Gastroenterol Clin North Am* 1990;19:345–359.
63. Roy AT, Johnson LE, Lee DB, et al. Renal failure in older people. *J Am Geriatr Soc* 1990;38:239–253.
64. Brown W, ed. Aging and the kidney. *Adv Renal Replace Ther* 2000;7(1):1–92.
65. Pandolf KB. Aging and human heat tolerance. *Exp Aging Res* 1997;23(1): 69–105.
66. Luchi RJ, Taffet GE, Teasdale TA. Congestive heart failure in the elderly. *J Am Geriatr Soc* 1991;39:810–825.

67. Chan ED, Welsh CH. Geriatric respiratory medicine. *Chest* 1998;114(6):1704–1733.
68. Enright PL. Aging of the respiratory system. In: Hazzard WR, Blass JP, Ettinger WH Jr, et al., eds. *Principles of geriatric medicine and gerontology*, 4th ed. New York: McGraw-Hill, 1999:721–728.
69. Lakatta EG. The aging heart. *Ann Intern Med* 1990;113:455–466.
70. Evans WJ. Exercise training guidelines for the elderly. *Med Sci Sports Exerc* 1999;31(1):12–17.
71. Damush TM, Stewart AL, Mills KM, et al. Prevalence and correlates of physician recommendations to exercise among older adults. *J Gerontol A Biol Sci Med Sci* 1999;54(8):M423–M427.
72. McLaughlin MA. The aging heart: state-of-the-art prevention and management of cardiac disease. *Geriatrics* 2001;56(6):45–49.
73. Tresch DD, McGough MF. Heart failure with normal systolic function: a common disorder in older people. *J Am Geriatr Soc* 1995;43(9):1035–1042.
74. Heath JM, Stuart MR. Prescribing exercise for frail elders. *J Am Board Fam Pract* 2002;15(3):218–228.
75. Linzer MD, Yang EH, Estes M, et al. Diagnosing syncope: Part 2: unexplained syncope. *Ann Intern Med* 1997;127:76–86.
76. Burns EA, Goodwin JS. Immunology and infectious disease. In: Cassel CK, Reisenberg DE, Sorenson LB, Walsh JR, eds. *Geriatric medicine*, 2nd ed. New York: Springer-Verlag, 1990:312–329.
77. Geokas MC, Lakatta EG, Makinodan T, et al. The aging process. *Ann Intern Med* 1990;113(6):455–466.
78. Makinodan T. Immunologic aspects of aging. *Ann Intern Med* 1990;113:455–466.
79. Halter JB. Diabetes mellitus. In: Hazzard WR, Blass JP, Ettinger WH Jr, et al., eds. *Principles of geriatric medicine and gerontology*, 4th ed. New York: McGraw-Hill, 1999:991–1012.
80. Gruenewald DA, Matsumoto AM. Aging of the endocrine system. In: Hazzard WR, Blass JP, Ettinger WH Jr, et al., eds. *Principles of geriatric medicine and gerontology*, 4th ed. New York: McGraw-Hill, 1999:949–966.
81. Miller M. Fluid and electrolyte homeostasis in the elderly: physiological changes of aging and clinical consequences. *Baillieres Clin Endocrinol Metab* 1997;11:367–387.
82. Chiovato L, Mariotti S, Pinchera A. Thyroid diseases in the elderly. *Baillieres Clin Endocrinol Metab.* 1997; 11:251–270.
83. Fine SL, Berger JW, Maguire MG, et al. Age-related macular degeneration. *N Engl J Med* 2000;342(7):483–492.
84. Keller BK, Morton JL, Thomas VS, et al. The effect of visual and hearing impairments on functional status. *J Am Geriatr Soc* 1999;47(11):1319–1325.
85. American Geriatrics Society, British Geriatrics Society, and American Academy of Orthopaedic Surgeons Panel on Falls Prevention. Guidelines for the prevention of falls in older persons. *J Am Geriatr Soc* 2001;49(5):664–672.
86. Cohn ES. Hearing loss with aging. *Clin Geriatr Med* 1999;15(1):145–161.
87. Mansour-Shouser R, Mansour WN. Nonsurgical management of hearing loss. *Clin Geriatr Med* 1999;15(1):163–177.
88. Rubichi S, Neri M, Nicoletti R. Age-related slowing of control processes: evidence from a response coordination task. *Cortex* 1999;35(4):573–582.
89. Keefover RW. Aging and cognition. *Neurol Clin* 1998;16(3):635–648.
90. Corey-Bloom J, Wiederholt WC, Edelstein S, et al. Cognitive and functional status of the oldest-old. *J Am Geriatr Soc* 1996;44:671–674.
91. Petersen RC, Doody R, Kurz A, et al. Current concepts in mild cognitive impairment. *Arch Neurol* 2001;58(12):1985–1992.
92. Wolfson L, Whipple R, Derby C. Balance and strength training in older adults: intervention gains and Tai Chi maintenance. *J Am Geriatr Soc* 1996;44(5):498–506.
93. Rubinstein TC, Alexander NB, Hausdorff JM. Evaluating fall risk in older adults: steps and missteps. *Clin Geriatr* 2003;11(1):52–60.
94. Frontera WR, Hughes VA, Fielding RA. Aging of skeletal muscle: a 12-yr longitudinal study. *J Appl Physiol* 2000;88(4):1321–1326.
95. Fiatarone MA, Marks EC, Ryan ND, et al. High-intensity strength training in nonagenarians: effects on skeletal muscle. *JAMA* 1990;263:3029–3034.
96. Creamer P, Hochberg MC. Management of osteoarthritis. In: Hazzard WR, Blass JP, Ettinger WH Jr, et al, eds. *Principles of geriatric medicine and gerontology*, 4th ed. New York: McGraw-Hill, 1999:1155–1162.
97. Lawrence RC, Helmick CG, Arnett FC, et al. Estimates of the prevalence of arthritis and selected musculoskeletal disorders in the United States. *Arthritis Rheum* 1998;41(5):778–799.
98. Medina JJ, Parra RO, Moore RG. Benign prostatic hyperplasia (the aging prostate). *Med Clin North Am* 1999;83(5):1213–1229.
99. Krahn MD, Mahoney JE, Eckman MH, et al. Screening for prostate cancer: a decision analytic view. *JAMA* 1994;272:773–780.
100. Fantl JA, Newman DK, Colling J, et al. *Urinary incontinence in adults: acute and chronic management*. Clinical Practice Guideline No. 2, 1996 Update. Rockville, MD: U.S. Department of Health and Human Services, Public Health Service, Agency for Health Care Policy and Research, March 1996; AHCPR Pub. No. 96–0682.
101. Ouslander JG. Aging and the lower urinary tract. *Am J Med Sci* 1997;314 (4):214–218.
102. Meston CM. Aging and sexuality. *West J Med* 1997;167(4):285–290.
103. Duffy LM. Lovers, loners, and lifers: sexuality and the older adult. *Geriatrics* 1998;53[Suppl 1]:S66–69.
104. Kaiser FE. Sexuality in the elderly. *Urol Clin North Am* 1996;23(1):99–109.
105. Kaiser FE. Erectile dysfunction in the aging man. *Med Clin North Am* 1999;83 (5):1267–1278.
106. Montorsi F, Salonia A, Deho F, et al. The aging male and erectile dysfunction. *World J Urol* 2002;20(1):28–35.
107. Roughan PA, Kaiser FE, Morley JE. Sexuality and the older woman. *Clin Geriatr Med* 1993;9(1):87–106.
108. Butler RN. Age-ism: another form of bigotry. *Gerontologist* 1969;9:243–246.
109. Hummert ML. Age and typicality judgments of stereotypes of the elderly: perceptions of elderly vs. young adults. *Int J Aging Hum Dev* 1993;37(3):217–226.
110. Strasser DC, Solomon DH, Burton JR. Geriatrics and physical medicine and rehabilitation: common principles, complementary approaches, and 21st century demographics. *Arch Phys Med Rehabil* 2002;83;1323–1324.
111. Rowe JW, Kahn RL. *Successful aging: the MacArthur Foundation Study*. New York: Pantheon Books, 1998:11–35.
112. Solomon R. Coping with stress: a physician's guide to mental health in aging. *Geriatrics* 1996;51(7):46–48, 50–51.
113. Medalie JH. The elderly and their families. In: Reichel WR, ed. *Clinical aspects of aging*, 3rd ed. Baltimore: Williams & Wilkins, 1989:477–486.
114. Fried LP, Freedman M, Endres TE, Wasik B. Building communities that promote successful aging. *West J Med* 1997;167(4):216–219.
115. Kennedy GJ, Kelman HR, Thomas C, et al. Hierarchy of characteristics associated with depressive symptoms in an urban elderly sample. *Am J Psychiatry* 1989;146:220–225.
116. Harris RE, Mion LC, Patterson MB, Frengley JD. Severe illness in older patients: the association between depressive disorders and functional dependency during the recovery. *J Am Geriatr Soc* 1988;36:890–896.
117. Covinsky KE, Fortinsky RH, Palmer RM, et al. Relation between symptoms of depression and health status outcomes in acutely ill hospitalized older people. *Ann Intern Med* 1997;126:417–425.
118. Penninx BW, Leveille S, Ferrucci, et al. Exploring the effect of depression on physical disability: longitudinal evidence from the established populations for epidemiologic studies of the elderly. *Am J Public Health* 1999;89(9):1346–1352.
119. Roy R, Thomas M, Cook A. Social context of elderly chronic pain patients. In: Ferrell BR, Ferrell BA, eds. *Pain in the elderly*. Seattle: IASP Press, 1996: 111–117.
120. Lang FR, Carstensen LL. Close emotional relationships in late life: further support for proactive aging in the social domain. *Psychol Aging* 1994;9(2):315–324.
121. Connidis IA. Sibling support in older age. *J Gerontol* 1994;49(6):S309–317.
122. Mendes de Leon CF, Gold DT, Glass TA. Disability as a function of social networks and support in elderly African Americans and whites: the Duke EPESE 1986–1992. *J Gerontol B Psychol Sci Soc Sci* 2001;56(3):S179–190.
123. Hing E, Bloom B. Long-term care for the functionally dependent elderly. *National Center for Health Statistics Vital Health Stats* 1990;13:104.
124. Unger JB, McAvay G, Bruce ML, et al. Variation in the impact of social network characteristics on physical functioning in elderly persons: MacArthur Studies of Successful Aging. *J Gerontol B Psychol Sci Soc Sci* 1999;54(5):S245–251.
125. Brody EM. Informal support systems in the rehabilitation of the disabled elderly. In: Brody SJ, Ruff GE, eds. *Aging and rehabilitation: advances in the state of the art*. New York: Springer-Verlag, 1986:87–103.
126. Evans RL, Matlock AL, Biship DS, et al. Family intervention after stroke: does counseling or education help? *Stroke* 1988;19:1234–1239.
127. Mittelman MS, Ferris SH, Shulman E, et al. A family intervention to delay nursing home placement of patients with Alzheimer disease. *JAMA* 1996; 276:1725–1731.
128. Tsuji I, Whalen S, Finucane TE. Predictors of nursing home placement in community-based long-term care. *J Am Geriatr Soc* 1995;43:761–766.
129. Schultz R, Beach S. Caregiving as a risk factor for mortality; the Caregiver Health Effects Study. *JAMA* 1999;282:2215–2219.
130. Lachs MS, Berkman L, Fulmer T, et al. A prospective community-based pilot study of risk factors for the investigation of elder mistreatment. *J Am Geriatr Soc* 1994;42:169–173.
131. Von Korff M, Gruman J, Schaefer J. Collaborative management of chronic illness. *Ann Intern Med* 1997;127(12):1097–1102.
132. Levine C. The loneliness of the long-term care giver. *N Engl J Med* 1999; 340(20):1587–1590.
133. Creditor MC. Hazards of hospitalization of the elderly. *Ann Intern Med* 1993;118(3):219–223.
134. Hesse KA, Campion EW, Karamouz N. Attitudinal stumbling blocks to geriatric rehabilitation. *J Am Geriatr Soc* 1984;32:747–750.
135. World Health Organization. *International classification of functioning, disability, and health*. Geneva: World Health Organization, 2001:1–303.
136. Hirsch CH, Sommers L, Olsen A, et al. The natural history of functional morbidity in hospitalized older patients. *J Am Geriatr Soc* 1990;38:1296–1303.
137. Mold JW, Stein HF. The cascade effect in the clinical care of patients. *N Engl J Med* 1986;314:512–514.
138. Williamson JD, Fried LP. Characterization of older adults who attribute functional decrements to old age. *J Am Geriatr Soc* 1996;44:1429–1434.
139. Sarkisian CA, Lachs MS. Failure to thrive in older adults. *Ann Intern Med* 1996;124:1072–1078.
140. Fried LP, Storer DJ, King DE, Lodder F. Diagnosis of illness presentation in the elderly. *J Am Geriatr Soc* 1991;39:117–123.
141. Hoenig HM, Rubenstein LZ. Hospital-associated deconditioning and dysfunction. *J Am Geriatr Soc* 1991;39:220–222.
142. Siebens H. Deconditioning. In: Kemp B, Brummel-Smith K, Ramsdell JW, eds. *Geriatric rehabilitation*. Boston: Little, Brown, 1990:177–192.

143. Rockwood K, Fox RA, Stolee P, et al. Frailty in elderly people: an evolving concept. *Can Med Assoc J* 1994;150:495–498.

144. Rockwood K, Stolee P, McDowell I. Factors associated with institutionalization of older people in Canada: testing a multifactorial definition of frailty. *J Am Geriatr Soc* 1996;44:578–582.

145. Fried LP, Tangen CM, Walston J et al. Frailty in older adults: evidence for a phenotype. *J Gerontol A Biol Sci Med Sci* 2001;56:M146–M156.

146. Sager JA, Franke TF, Inouye SK, et al. Functional outcomes of acute medical illness and hospitalization in older persons. *Arch Intern Med* 1996;156:645–652.

147. Kemp B. Psychosocial and mental health issues in rehabilitation of older persons. In: Brody SJ, Ruff GE, eds. *Aging and rehabilitation: advances in the state of the art*. New York: Springer-Verlag, 1986:122–158.

148. Inouye SK. Delirium in hospitalized older patients: recognition and risk factors. *J Geriatr Psychiatry Neurol* 1998;11:118–125.

149. Marcantonia ER, Flicker JM, Michaels M, Resnick NM. Delirium is independently associated with poor functional recovery after hip fracture. *J Am Geriatr Soc* 2000;48:618–624.

150. Siebens H, Aronow H, Edwards D, Ghasemi Z. A randomized controlled trial of exercise to improve outcomes of acute hospitalization in older adults. *J Am Geriatr Soc* 2002;48:1545–1552.

151. Reuben DB, Borok GM, Wolde-Tsakid G, et al. A randomized trial of comprehensive geriatric assessment in the care of hospitalized patients. *N Engl J Med* 1995;332:1345–1350.

152. Landefeld CS, Palmer RM, Kresevic DM, et al. A randomized trial of care in a hospital medical unit especially designed to improve the functional outcomes of acutely ill older patients. *N Engl J Med* 1995;332:1338–1344.

153. Cohen HJ, Feussner JR, Weinberger M, et al. A controlled trial of inpatient and outpatient geriatric evaluation and management. *N Engl J Med* 2002;346:905–912.

154. Spirduso W. *Physical dimensions of aging*. Champaign, IL: Human Kinetics, 1995:1–432.

155. American College of Sports Medicine. *ACSM's resource manual for guidelines for exercise testing and prescription*. Philadelphia: Lea & Febiger, 1993.

156. Frontera WR, Meredith CN, O'Reilly KP, et al. Strength conditioning in older men: skeletal muscle hypertrophy and improved function. *J Appl Physiol* 1990;68:329–333.

157. Morey MC, Pieper CF, Sullivan RJ Jr, et al. Five-year performance trends for older exercisers: a hierarchical model of endurance, strength, and flexibility. *J Am Geriatr Soc* 1996;44:1226–1231.

158. Young A. Exercise physiology in geriatric practice. *Acta Med Scand (Suppl)* 1986;711:227–232.

159. Lach HW, Reed AT, Arfken CL, et al. Falls in the elderly: reliability of a classification system. *J Am Geriatr Soc* 1991;39:197–202.

160. Robbins AS, Rubenstein LZ, Josephson KR, et al. Predictors of falls among elderly people: results of two population-based studies. *Arch Intern Med* 1989;149:1628–1633.

161. Gehlsen GM, Whaley MH. Falls in the elderly: Part I. gait. *Arch Phys Med Rehabil* 1990;71:735–738.

162. Gehlsen GM, Whaley MH. Falls in the elderly: Part II. balance, strength and flexibility. *Arch Phys Med Rehabil* 1990;71:739–742.

163. Tinetti ME. Factors associated with serious injury during falls by ambulatory nursing home residents. *J Am Geriatr Soc* 1987;35:644–648.

164. Whipple RH, Wolfson LI, Amerman PM. The relationship of knee and ankle weakness to falls in nursing home residents: an isokinetic study. *J Am Geriatr Soc* 1987;35:13–16.

165. Fentem PH. Exercise in prevention of disease. *Br Med Bull* 1992;48:630–650.

166. Edwards D. *Prime moves: an exercise program for mature adults*. New York: Avery, 1990.

167. Mills KM, Stewart AL, Sepsis PG, King AC. Consideration of older adults preferences for format of physical activity. *J Aging Phys Activity* 1997;5:50–58.

168. Buchner DM, Wagner EH. Preventing frail health. *Clin Geriatr Med* 1992;8:1–17.

169. Wilcox S, King AC. Health behaviors and aging. In: Hazzard WR, Blass JP, Ettinger WH Jr, et al., eds. *Principles of geriatric medicine and gerontology*, 4th ed. New York: McGraw-Hill, 1999:287–302.

170. Lawrence RH, Jette AM. Disentangling the disablement process. *J Gerontol* 1996;51B[Suppl]:173–182.

171. Guralnik JM, Perrucci L, Simonsick EM, et al. Lower-extremity function in persons over the age of 70 years as a predictor of subsequent disability. *N Engl J Med* 1995;332:556–561.

172. Fried LP, Young Y, Rubin G, Bandeen-Roche K. Self-reported preclinical disability identifies older women with early declines in performance and early disease. *J Clin Epidemiol* 2001;54:889–901.

173. Tinetti ME, Inouye SK, Gill T, Doucette JT. Shared risk factors for falls, incontinence, and functional dependence. *JAMA* 1995; 273:1348–1353.

174. Evans LK, Yurkow J, Siegler EL. The CARE program: a nurse-managed collaborative outpatient program to improve function of frail older people. *J Am Geriatr Soc* 1995;43:1155–1160.

175. Mendes de Leon CF, Seeman TE, Baker DI, et al. Self-efficacy, physical decline, and change in functioning in community-living elders: a prospective study. *J Gerontol* 1996;51B[Suppl]:183–190.

176. Tinetti ME, Powell L. Fear of falling and low self-efficacy: a cause of dependence in elderly persons. *J Gerontol* 1993;48(special issue):35–38.

177. Boult C, Boult L, Murphy C, et al. A controlled trial of outpatient geriatric evaluation and management. *J Am Geriatr Soc* 1994;42(5):465–470.

178. Silverman M, Musa D, Martin DC, et al. Evaluation of outpatient geriatric assessment: a randomized multi-site trial. *J Am Geriatr Soc* 1995;43(7):733–740.

179. Toseland RW, O'Donnell JC, Engelhardt JB, et al. Outpatient geriatric evaluation and management: results of a randomized trial. *Med Care* 1996;34(6):624–640.

180. Boult C, Boult LB, Morishita L, et al. A randomized clinical trial of outpatient geriatric evaluation and management. *J Am Geriatr Soc* 2001;49(4):51–359.

181. Cohen HJ, Feussner JR, Weinberger M, et al. A controlled trial of inpatient and outpatient geriatric evaluation and management. *N Engl J Med* 2002;346:905–912.

182. Siebens H. Applying the domain management model in treating patients with chronic diseases. *Jt Comm J Qual Improv* 2001;27(6):302–314.

183. Berwick D, Godfrey D, Roessner J, eds. *Curing health care*. San Francisco: Josey-Bass, 1990.

184. Engel G. The clinical application of the biopsychosocial model. *Am J Psychiatry* 1980;137:535–544.

185. Siebens H. The Domain Management Model: organizing care for stroke survivors and other persons with chronic diseases. *Top Stroke Rehabil* 2002;9:1–25.

186. Germain CB, Gitterman A. The life model approach to social work practice revisited. In: Turner F, ed. *Social work treatment*. New York: Free Press, 1986:618–643.

187. Bogardus ST, Bradley EH, Tinetti ME. A taxonomy for goal setting in the care of persons with dementia. *J Gen Intern Med* 1998;13(10):675–680.

188. Bradley EH, Bogardus ST Jr, van Doorn C, et al. Goals in geriatric assessment: are we measuring the right outcomes? *Gerontologist* 2000;40(2):191–196.

189. Frost FS. Rehabilitation and fear: what happens if the house catches on fire? *Am J Phys Med Rehabil* 2001;80:942–944.

190. Stineman MG, Maislin G, Nosek M, et al. Comparing consumer and clinician values for alternative functional states: application of a new feature trade-off consensus building tool. *Arch Phys Med Rehabil* 1998;79:1522–1529.

191. Clark GS, Bray GP. Development of a rehabilitation plan. In: Williams TF, ed. *Rehabilitation in the aging*. New York: Raven, 1984:125–143.

192. Hunt TE. Homeostatic malfunctions in the aged. *Br Columbia Med J* 1980;22:379–381.

193. Karani R, McLaughlin MA, Cassel CK. Exercise in the healthy older adult. *Am J Geriatr Cardiol* 2001;10(5):269–273.

194. Resnick B. Testing a model of exercise behavior in older adults. *Res Nurs Health* 2001;24:83–92.

195. Bodily KC, Burgess EM. Contralateral limb and patient survival after leg amputation. *Am J Surg* 1983;146:280–282.

196. Clark GS. Rehabilitation team: process and roles. In: Felsenthal G, Garrison SJ, Steinberg FU, eds. *Rehabilitation of the aging and elderly patient*. Baltimore: Williams & Wilkins, 1994:439–448.

197. Strasser DC, Falconer JA. Rehabilitation team process. *Top Stroke Rehabil* 1997;4:34–39.

198. Chan L, Koepsell TD, Deyo RA, et al. The effect of Medicare's payment system for rehabilitation hospitals on length of stay, charges, and total payments. *N Engl J Med* 1997;337(14):978–985.

199. Chan L, Ciol M. Medicare's payment system: its effect on discharges to skilled nursing facilities from rehabilitation hospitals. *Arch Phys Med Rehabil* 2000;81(6):715–719.

200. Chan L, Doctor J, Temkin N, et al. Discharge disposition from acute care after traumatic brain injury: the effect of insurance type. *Arch Phys Med Rehabil* 2001;82(9):1151–1154.

201. Coleman EA, Fox PA. Translating evidence-based geriatric care into practice: lessons from managed care organizations. Part I. introduction and physical inactivity. *Ann Long Term Care* 2002;10(9):33–38.

202. Jencks SF, Huff ED, Cuerdon T. Change in the quality of care delivered to Medicare beneficiaries, 1998–1999 to 2000–2001. *JAMA* 2003;289(3):305–312.

203. U.S. Department of Health and Human Services. *Healthy people 2010: understanding and improving health*. Washington, DC: U.S. Government Printing Office, 2000.

204. Calkins E, Boult C, Wagner EH, Pacala JT. *New ways to care for older people—building systems based on evidence*. Springer Publishing, 1999.

205. Felsenthal G, Cohen BS, Hilton EB, et al. The physiatrist as primary physician for patients on an inpatient rehabilitation unit. *Arch Phys Med Rehabil* 1984;65(7):375–378.

206. Siebens H, Weston H, Parry D, et al. The patient care notebook: quality improvement on a rehabilitation unit. *Jt Comm J Qual Improv* 2001;27:555–567.

207. Beers MH, Dang J, Hashegawa J, Tamai IY. Influence of hospitalization on drug therapy in the elderly. *J Am Geriatr Soc* 1989;39:679–683.

208. Colt HG, Shapiro AP. Drug-induced illness as a cause for admission to a community hospital. *J Am Geriatr Soc* 1989;37:323–326.

209. Sinoff GD, Kohn D. Prevalence of adverse drug reactions. *J Am Geriatr Soc* 1990;38:722–729.

210. Brook RH, Kamberg CJ, Mayer-Oakes A, et al. Appropriateness of acute medical care for the elderly: an analysis of the literature. *Health Policy* 1990;14:225–242.

211. Willcox SM, Himmelstein DU, Woolhandler S. Inappropriate drug prescribing for the community-dwelling elderly. *JAMA* 1994; 272:292–296.

212. Zhan C, Sangl J, Bierman AS, et al. Potentially inappropriate medication use in the community-dwelling elderly: findings from the 1996 Medical Expenditure Panel Survey. *JAMA* 2001;286(22):2823–2829.

213. Doucet J, Jego A, Noel D, et al. Preventable and non-preventable risk factors for adverse drug events related to hospital admission in the elderly. *Clin Drug Invest* 2002;22(6):385–392.

214. Juurlink DN, Mamdani M, Kopp A, et al. Drug-drug interactions among elderly patients hospitalized for drug toxicity. *JAMA* 2003;289(13):1652–1658.

215. Beers MH, Munekata M, Storrie M. The accuracy of medication histories in the hospital medical records of elderly persons. *J Am Geriatr Soc* 1990;38: 1183–1187.

216. Spagnoli A, Ostino G, Borga AD, D'Ambrosio R. Drug compliance and unreported drugs in the elderly. *J Am Geriatr Soc* 1989;37:619–624.

217. Abrams RC, Alexopoulos GS. Substance abuse in the elderly: over-the-counter and illegal drugs. *Hosp Community Psychiatry* 1988;39:822–823.

218. Stoehr GP, Ganguli M, Seaberg EC, et al. Over-the-counter medication use in an older rural community: the MoVIES project. *J Am Geriatr Soc* 1997;45:158–165.

219. Goldberg PB, Roberts J. Pharmacologic basis for developing rational drug regimens for elderly patients. *Med Clin North Am* 1983;67:315–331.

220. Beers MH, Ouslander JG. Risk factors in geriatric drug prescribing: a practical guide to avoiding problems. *Drugs* 1989;37:105–112.

221. Rozzini R, Bianchetti A, Zanett O, Trabucchi M. Are too many drugs prescribed for the elderly after all? *J Am Geriatr Soc* 1989;37:89–90.

222. Morrow D, Leirer V, Sheikh J. Adherence and medication instructions. *J Am Geriatr Soc* 1988;36:1147–1160.

223. Cooper JK, Love DW, Raffoul PR. Intentional prescription non-adherence (non-compliance) by the elderly. *J Am Geriatr Soc* 1982;30:329–332.

224. Pereles L, Romonko L, Murzyn T, et al. Evaluation of a self-medication program. *J Am Geriatr Soc* 1996;44:161–165.

225. Hsia Der E, Rubenstein LZ, Choy GS. The benefits of in-home pharmacy evaluation for older persons. *J Am Geriatr Soc* 1997;45:211–214.

226. McDonald HP, Garg AX, Haynes RB. Interventions to enhance patient adherence to medication prescriptions: scientific review. *JAMA* 2002;288:2868–2879.

227. Larson EB, Kukull WA, Buchner D, Reifler BV. Adverse drug reaction associated with global cognitive impairment in elderly persons. *Ann Intern Med* 1987;107:169–173.

228. Nolan L, O'Malley K. Prescribing for the elderly: Part II. prescribing patterns: differences due to age. *J Am Geriatr Soc* 1988;36:245–254.

229. Lipsitz LA. Orthostatic hypotension in the elderly. *N Engl J Med* 1989;321: 952–957.

230. Samily AH. Clinical manifestations of disease in the elderly. *Med Clin North Am* 1983;67:333–344.

231. NIH Consensus Development Panel on Depression in Late Life. Diagnosis and treatment of depression in late life. *JAMA* 1992;268:1018–1024.

232. Rothschild AJ. The diagnosis and treatment of late-life depression. *J Clin Psychiatry* 1996;57[Suppl 5]:5–11.

233. Hirschfeld RM, Keller MB, Panico S, et al. The National Depressive and Manic-Depressive Association consensus statement on the undertreatment of depression. *JAMA* 1977;277:333–340.

234. Gurland BJ, Wilder DE, Berkman C. Depression and disability in the elderly: reciprocal relations and changes with age. *Int J Geriatr Psychiatry* 1988;3:163–179.

235. Rapp SR, Davis KM. Geriatric depression: physicians' knowledge, perceptions, and diagnostic practices. *Gerontologist* 1989;29:252–257.

236. Flint AJ. Epidemiology and comorbidity of anxiety disorders in the elderly. *Am J Psychiatry* 1994;151:640–649.

237. Brown CS, Rakel RE, Wells BG. A practical update on anxiety disorders and their pharmacologic treatment. *Arch Intern Med* 1991;151:873–884.

238. Martin LM, Fleming KC, Evans JM. Recognition and management of anxiety and depression in elderly patients. *Mayo Clin Proc* 1995;70:999–1006.

239. Francis J, Martin D, Kapoor WN. A prospective study of delirium in hospitalized elderly. *JAMA* 1990;263:1097–1101.

240. Schor JD, Levkoff SE, Lipsitz LA, et al. Risk factors for delirium in hospitalized elderly. *JAMA* 1992;267:827–831.

241. Inouye SK, Charpentier PA. Precipitating factors for delirium in hospitalized elderly persons: predictive model and interrelationship with baseline vulnerability. *JAMA* 1996;275:852–857.

242. Marcantonio ER, Goldman L, Mangione CM, et al. A clinical prediction rule for delirium after elective noncardiac surgery. *JAMA* 1994;271:134–139.

243. Kiely DK, Bergmann MA, Murphy KM, et al. Delirium among newly admitted postacute facility patients: prevalence, symptoms, and severity. *J Gerontol A Biol Sci Med Sci* 2003;58(5):M441–445.

244. O'Keeffe S, Lavan J. The prognostic significance of delirium in older hospital patients. *J Am Geriatr Soc* 1997;45:174–178.

245. Rowe JW. Health care of the elderly. *N Engl J Med* 1985;312:827–835.

246. Wolfson LI, Katzman R. The neurologic consultation at age 80. In: Katzman R, Terry RD, eds. *The neurology of aging*. Philadelphia: FA Davis, 1983;221–244.

247. Fleming KC, Adams AC, Petersen RC. Dementia: diagnosis and evaluation. *Mayo Clin Proc* 1995;70:1093–1107.

248. Warshaw GA, Moore JT, Friedman SW, et al. Functional disability in the hospitalized elderly. *JAMA* 1982;248:847–850.

249. Clarfield AM. The reversible dementias: do they reverse? *Ann Intern Med* 1988;109:476–486.

250. Siu AL. Screening for dementia and investigating its causes. *Ann Intern Med* 1991;115:122–132.

251. McKhann G, Drachman D, Folstein M, et al. Clinical diagnosis of Alzheimer's disease. *Neurology* 1984;34:939–944.

252. Schuman JE, Beattie EJ, Steed DA, et al. Geriatric patients with and without intellectual dysfunction: effectiveness of a standard rehabilitation program. *Arch Phys Med Rehabil* 1981;62:612–618.

253. Beck JC, Benson DF, Scheibel AB, et al. Dementia in the elderly: the silent epidemic. *Ann Intern Med* 1982;97:231–241.

254. *Early Alzheimer's disease: recognition and assessment.* Consumer Version, Clinical Practice Guideline No. 19. Rockville, MD: U.S. Department of Health and Human Services, Public Health Service, Agency for Health Care Policy and Research, 1996; AHCPR Publication No. 96–0704.

255. Resnick NM. An 89-year-old woman with urinary incontinence. *JAMA* 1996; 276:1832–1840.

256. Ham RJ, Lekan-Rutledge DA. Incontinence. In: Ham RJ, Sloane PD, eds. *Primary care geriatrics*. St. Louis: CV Mosby, 1997;321–349.

257. National Institutes of Health Consensus Development Conference. Urinary incontinence in adults. *J Am Geriatr Soc* 1990;38:265–272.

258. Resnick NM, Yalla SV. Management of urinary incontinence in the elderly. *N Engl J Med* 1985;313:800–805.

259. Colling J, Ouslander J, Hadley BJ, et al. The effects of patterned urge-response toileting (PURT) on urinary incontinence among nursing home residents. *J Am Geriatr Soc* 1992;40:135–141.

260. Schnelle JF, MacRae PG, Ouslander JG, et al. Functional incidental training, mobility performance, and incontinence care with nursing home residents. *J Am Geriatr Soc* 1995;43:1356–1362.

261. Williams ME, Pannill FC III. Urinary incontinence in the elderly: physiology, pathophysiology, diagnosis, and treatment. *Ann Intern Med* 1982;97:895–907.

262. Burgio KC, Pearce KL, Lucco AJ. *Staying dry: a practical guide to bladder control.* Baltimore: Johns Hopkins University Press, 1989.

263. Urinary Incontinence Guideline Panel. *Urinary incontinence in adults: clinical practice guideline.* Rockville, MD: Agency for Health Care Policy and Research, Public Health Service, United States Department of Health and Human Services, 1992; AHCPR publication no. 92–0038.

264. Ouslander JG, Schnelle JF. Incontinence in the nursing home. *Ann Intern Med* 1995;122:438–449.

265. Marzuk PM. Biofeedback in gastrointestinal disorders: a review of the literature. *Ann Intern Med* 1985;103:240–244.

266. Wald A. Biofeedback therapy for fecal incontinence. *Ann Intern Med* 1981; 95:146–149.

267. Gottlieb GL. Sleep disorders and their management. *Am J Med* 1990;88: 29S–33S.

268. King AC, Oman RF, Brassington GS, et al. Moderate-intensity exercise and self-rated quality of sleep in older adults: a randomized controlled trial. *JAMA* 1997;277:32–37.

269. Ancoli-Israel S. Insomnia in the elderly: a review for the primary care practitioner. *Sleep* 2000;23[Suppl 1]:S23–S30.

270. Toney G, Ereshefsky L. Sleep disorders: assisting patients to a good night's sleep. *J Am Pharm Assoc (Wash)* 2000;40(5[Suppl 1]):S46–47.

271. Folks DG, Burke WJ. Psychotherapeutic agents in older adults: sedative hypnotics and sleep. *Clin Geriatr Med* 1998;14(1):67–86.

272. Morin CM, Azrin NH. Behavioral and cognitive treatments of geriatric insomnia. *J Consult Clin Psychol* 1988;56:748–753.

273. Campbell SS, Dawson D, Anderson MW. Alleviation of sleep maintenance insomnia with timed exposure to bright light. *J Am Geriatr Soc* 1993;41:829–836.

274. Garfinkel D, Laudon M, Nof D, et al. Improvement of sleep quality in elderly people by controlled-release melatonin. *Lancet* 1995;346:541–544.

275. Olde Rikkert MG, Rigaud AS. Melatonin in elderly patients with insomnia: a systematic review. *Z Gerontol Geriatr* 2001;34(6):491–497.

276. Ferrell BA. Pain management in elderly people. *J Am Geriatr Soc* 1991;39: 64–73.

277. Ferrell BR, Ferrell BA, eds. *Pain in the elderly: a report of the task force on pain in the elderly of the International Association for the Study of Pain.* Seattle: IASP Press, 1996.

278. AGS Panel on Chronic Pain in Older Persons. The management of chronic pain in older persons. *J Am Geriatr Soc* 1998;46:635–651.

279. Ferrell BA, Ferrell BR, Osterweil D. Pain in the nursing home. *J Am Geriatr Soc* 1990;38:409–414.

280. Nishikawa ST, Ferrell BA. Pain assessment in the elderly. *Clin Geriatr Long Term Care* 1993;1:15–28.

281. Parmelee PA, Smith B, Katz IR. Pain complaints and cognitive status among elderly institution residents. *J Am Geriatr Soc* 1993;41:517–522.

282. Ferrell BA, Ferrell BR, Rivera L. Pain in cognitively impaired nursing home patients. *J Pain Symptom Manage* 1995;10:591–595.

283. Michet CJ, Evans JM, Fleming KC, et al. Common rheumatologic diseases in elderly patients. *Mayo Clin Proc* 1995;70:1205–1214.

284. Altman RD, Hochberg MC, Moskowitz RW, et al. Recommendations for the medical management of osteoarthritis of the hip and knee. *Arthritis Rheum* 2000;43(9):1905–1915.

285. Rochon PA, Fortin PR, Dear KB, et al. Reporting of age in data in clinical trials of arthritis. *Arch Intern Med* 1993;153:243–248.

286. Griffin MR, Piper JM, Doughtery JR, et al. Nonsteroidal antiinflammatory drug use and increased risk for peptic ulcer disease in elderly persons. *Ann Intern Med* 1991;114:257–263.

287. Evans RL, Matlock AL, Biship DS, et al. Family intervention after stroke: does counseling or education help? *Stroke* 1988;19:1234–1239.

288. Ferrell B, Rivera L. Cancer pain: impact on elderly patients and their family caregivers. In: Roy R, ed. *Chronic pain in old age: an integrated biopsychosocial perspective.* Toronto: University of Toronto Press, 1995.

289. Billings AG, Moos R. The role of coping responses and social resources in attenuating the stress of life events. *J Behav Med* 1981;4:139–157.

290. Tinetti ME. Performance-oriented assessment of mobility problems in elderly patients. *J Am Geriatr Soc* 1986;34:119–126.

291. King MB, Tinetti ME. Falls in community-dwelling older persons. *J Am Geriatr Soc* 1995;43:1146–1154.

292. Lipsitz L. An 85-year old woman with a history of falls. *JAMA* 1996;276:59–66.

293. Studenski S, Duncan PW, Chandler J, et al. Predicting falls: the role of mobility and nonphysical factors. *J Am Geriatr Soc* 1994;42:297–302.

294. Cummings SR, Nevitt MC, Browner WS, et al. Risk factors for hip fracture in white women. *N Engl J Med* 1995;332:767–773.

295. Wolf SL, Barnhart HX, Kutner NG, et al. Reducing frailty and falls in older persons: an investigation of tai chi and computerized balance training. *J Am Geriatr Soc* 1996;44:489–497.

296. Tinetti ME, Baker DI, McAvay G, et al. A multifactorial intervention to reduce the risk of falling among elderly people living in the community. *N Engl J Med* 1994;331:821–827.

297. Oakley A, Dawson MF, Holland J, et al. Preventing falls and subsequent injury in older people. *Qual Health Care* 1996;5:243–249.

298. Gillespie LD, Gillespie WJ, Cumming R, et al. Interventions for preventing falls in the elderly. *Cochrane Database Syst Rev* 2000; CD000340.

299. Tinetti ME, Richman D, Powell L. Falls efficacy as a measure of fear of falling. *J Gerontol* 1990;45:239–243.

300. Lawrence RH, Tennstedt SL, Kasten LE, et al. Intensity and correlates of fear of falling and hurting oneself in the next year: baseline findings from a Roybal Center fear of falling intervention. *J Aging Health* 1998;10:267–286.

301. Bezon J, Echevarria KH, Smith GB. Nursing outcome indicator: preventing falls for elderly people. *Outcomes Manag Nurs Prac* 1999;3:112–116.

302. Gardner MM, Robertson MC, Campbell AJ. Exercise in preventing falls and fall related injuries in older people: a review of randomised controlled trials. *Br J Sports Med* 2000;34(1):7–17.

303. American Geriatrics Society, British Geriatrics Society, and American Academy of Orthopaedic Surgeons Panel on Falls Prevention. Guidelines for the prevention of falls in older persons. *Ann Long Term Care* 2001;9(11):42–54.

304. Rubinstein TC, Alexander NA, Hausdorff JM. Evaluating fall risk in older adults: steps and missteps. *Clin Geriatrics* 2003;11(1):52–60.

305. Koval KJ, Zuckerman JD. Functional recovery after fracture of the hip. *J Bone Joint Surg Am* 1994;76:751–758.

306. Bernardini B, Neinecke C, Pagani M, et al. Comorbidity and adverse clinical events in the rehabilitation of older adults after hip fracture. *J Am Geriatr Soc* 1995;43:894–898.

307. Kiel DP, Eichorn A, Intrator O, et al. The outcomes of patients newly admitted to nursing homes after hip fracture. *Am J Public Health* 1994;84:1281–1286.

308. Guccione AA, Fagerson RL, Anderson JJ. Regaining functional independence in the acute care setting following hip fracture. *Phys Ther* 1996;76:818–826.

309. Cameron ID, Lyle DM, Quine S. Cost effectiveness of accelerated rehabilitation after proximal femoral fracture. *J Clin Epidemiol* 1994;47:1307–1313.

310. Zuckerman JD; Skovron ML; Koval KJ, et al. Postoperative complications and mortality associated with operative delay in older patients who have a fracture of the hip. *J Bone Joint Surg Am* 1995;77(10):1551–1556.

311. Hochberg MC, Altman RD, Brandt KD, et al. Guidelines for the medical management of osteoarthritis. Part I. osteoarthritis of the hip. *Arthritis Rheum* 1995;38:1535–1540.

312. Hochberg MC, Altman RD, Brandt KD, et al. Guidelines for the medical management of osteoarthritis. Part II. osteoarthritis of the knee. *Arthritis Rheum* 1995;38:1541–1546.

313. Nesher G, Moore TL, Zuckner J. Rheumatoid arthritis in the elderly. *J Am Geriatr Soc* 1991;39:284–294.

314. van Baar ME, Assendelft WJ, Dekker J. Effectiveness of exercise therapy in patients with osteoarthritis of the hip or knee: a systematic review of randomized clinical trials. *Arthritis Rheum* 1999;42(7):1361–1369.

315. Lorig K, Mazonson PD, Holman HR. Evidence suggesting that health education for self-managment in patients with chronic arthritis has sustained health benefits while reducing health care costs. *Arthritis Rheum* 1993;36:439–446.

316. Minor MA. Exercise in the management of osteoarthritis of the knee and hip. *Arthritis Care Res* 1994;7:198–204.

317. Puett DW, Griffin MR. Published trials of nonmedicinal and noninvasive therapies for hip and knee osteoarthritis. *Ann Intern Med* 1994;121:133–140.

318. Ettinger WH, Burns R, Messier SP, et al. A randomized trial comparing aerobic exercise and resistance exercise with a health education program in older adults with knee osteoarthritis. *JAMA* 1997;277:25–31.

319. Silverstein FE, Faich G, Goldstein JL, et al. Gastrointestinal toxicity with celecoxib vs nonsteroidal anti-inflammatory drugs for osteoarthritis and rheumatoid arthritis: the CLASS study: a randomized controlled trial. Celecoxib long-term arthritis safety study. *JAMA* 2000;284(10):1247–1255.

320. Felson DT, Lawrence RC, Hochberg MC, et al. Osteoarthritis: new insights. Part 2. treatment approaches. *Ann Intern Med* 2000;133(9):726–737.

321. Shah S, Vanclay F, Cooper B. Efficiency, effectiveness and duration of stroke rehabilitation. *Stroke* 1990;21:241–246.

322. Schmidt EV, Smirnov VE, Ryabova VS. Results of the seven-year prospective study of stroke patients. *Stroke* 1988;19:942–949.

323. Lindmark B. Evaluation of functional capacity after stroke with special emphasis on motor function and activities of daily living. *Scand J Rehabil Med* 1988;21[Suppl]:1–40.

324. Granger CV, Clark GS. Functional status and outcomes of stroke rehabilitation. *Top Geriatr Rehabil* 1994;9:72–84.

325. Wade DT, Langton-Hewer R, Wood VA. Stroke: the influence of age upon outcome. *Age Ageing* 1984;13:357–362.

326. Granger CV, Hamilton BB, Gresham GE. Stroke rehabilitation outcome study: Part I. general description. *Arch Phys Med Rehabil* 1988;69:506–509.

327. Granger CV, Hamilton BB, Gresham GE, Kramer AA. The stroke rehabilitation outcome study: Part II. relative merits of the total Barthel Index score and a four-item subscore in predicting patient outcomes. *Arch Phys Med Rehabil* 1989;70:100–103.

328. Osberg JS, DeJong G, Haley SM. Predicting long-term outcome among postrehabilitation stroke patients. *Am J Phys Med Rehabil* 1988;68:94–103.

329. Keith RA, Wilson DB, Gutierez P. Acute and subacute rehabilitation for stroke: a comparison. *Arch Phys Med Rehabil* 1995;76:495–500.

330. Kramer AM, Steiner JF, Schlenker RE, et al. Outcomes and costs after hip fracture and stroke: a comparison of rehabilitation settings. *JAMA* 1997;277:396–404.

331. Gresham GE, Duncan PW, Stason WB, et al. Poststroke rehabilitation: assessment, referral and patient management. Clinical Practice Guideline. Quick Reference Guide for Clnicians, No. 16. Rockville, MD: US Department of Health and Human Services, Public Health Service, Agency for Health Care Policy and Research, 1995; AHCPR Publication No. 95–0663.

332. Kimura M, Robinson RG, Kosier JT. Treatment of cognitive impairment after poststroke depression: a double-blind treatment trial. *Stroke* 2000;31(7):1482–1486.

333. Liepert J, Bauder H, Wolfgang HR, et al. Treatment-induced cortical reorganization after stroke in humans. *Stroke* 2000;31(6):1210–1216.

334. Cifu DX, Stewart DG. Factors affecting functional outcome after stroke: a critical review of rehabilitation interventions. *Arch Phys Med Rehabil* 1999;80:S35–S39.

335. Clark GS, Blue B, Bearer JB. Rehabilitation of the elderly amputee. *J Am Geriatr Soc* 1983;31:439–448.

336. Cutson TM, Bongiorni DR. Rehabilitation of the older lower limb amputee: a brief review. *J Am Geriatr Soc* 1996;44:1388–1393.

337. DuBow LL, Witt PL, Kadaba MP, et al. Oxygen consumption of elderly persons with bilateral below knee amputations: ambulation vs. wheelchair propulsion. *Arch Phys Med Rehabil* 1983;64:255–259.

338. Wolf E, Lilling M, Ferber I, Marcus J. Prosthetic rehabilitation of elderly bilateral amputees. *Int J Rehabil Res* 1989;12:271–278.

339. O'Connell PG, Gnatz S. Hemiplegia and amputation: rehabilitation in the dual disability. *Arch Phys Med Rehabil* 1989;70:451–454.

340. Stover SL, Fine PR, eds. *Spinal cord injury: the facts and figures.* Birmingham, AL: University of Alabama, 1986.

341. DeVivo MJ, Fine PR, Maetz HM, Stover SL. Prevalence of spinal cord injury: a reestimation employing life table techniques. *Arch Neurol* 1980;37:707–708.

342. Ohry A, Shemesh Y, Rozin R. Are chronic spinal cord injured patients (SCIP) prone to premature aging? *Med Hypotheses* 1983;11:467–469.

343. Roth EJ, Lovell L, Heinemann AW, et al. The older adult with a spinal cord injury. *Paraplegia* 1992;30(7):520–526.

344. DeVivo MJ, Stover SL, Black KJ. Prognostic factors for 12-year survival after spinal cord injury. *Arch Phys Med Rehabil* 1992;73:156–162.

345. DeVivo MJ, Kartus PL, Rutt RD, et al. The influence of age at time of spinal cord injury on rehabilitation outcome. *Arch Neurol* 1990;47:687–691.

346. Yarkony GM, Roth EJ, Heinemann AW, Lovell LL. Spinal cord injury rehabilitation outcome: impact of age. *J Clin Epidemiol* 1988;41:173–177.

347. Cifu DX, Kreutzer JS, Marwitz JH, et al. Functional outcomes of older adults with traumatic brain injury: a prospective, multicenter analysis. *Arch Phys Med Rehabil* 1996;77(9):883–888.

348. Glenn MB. Post-concussion syndrome. In: Frontera WR, Silver JK, eds. *Essentials of physical medicine and rehabilitation.* Philadelphia: Hanley & Belfus, Inc., 2002:687–693.

349. Kaufman SR, Becker G. Content and boundaries of medicine in long-term care: physicians talk about stroke. *Gerontology* 1991;31:238–245.

350. Felsenthal G, Cohen BS, Hilton EB, et al. The physiatrist as primary physician for patients on an inpatient rehabilitation unit. *Arch Phys Med Rehabil* 1984;65:375–378.

351. Cummings V, Kerner JF, Arones S, Steinbock C. Day hospital service in rehabilitation medicine: an evaluation. *Arch Phys Med Rehabil* 1985;66:86–91.

352. Hoenig HM. Rehabilitation. In: Duthie, ed. *Practice of geriatrics,* 3rd ed. Philadelphia: WB Saunders Co., 1998:159–172.

353. American Geriatrics Society, John A. Hartford Foundation. A statement of principles: toward improved care of older patients in surgical and medical specialties. *Arch Phys Med Rehabil* 2002;83:1317–1319.

354. Strasser DC, Solomon DH, Burton JR. Geriatrics and physical medicine and rehabilitation: common principles, complementary approaches, and 21st century demographics. *Arch Phys Med Rehabil* 2002;83:1323–1324.

355. Fisk AA. Comprehensive health care for the elderly. *JAMA* 1983;249:230–236.

356. Council on Scientific Affairs. Home care in the 1990s. *JAMA* 1990;263:1241–1244.

357. Grieco AJ. Physician's guide to managing home care of older patients. *Geriatrics* 1991;46:49–60.

358. Frank JC, Miller LS. Community-based rehabilitation for the elderly. In: Felsenthal G, Garrison SJ, Steinberg FU, eds. *Rehabilitation of the aging and elderly patient.* Baltimore: Williams & Wilkins, 1994:477–485.

359. Clark F, Azen SP, Zemke R, et al. Occupational therapy for independent-living older adults. *JAMA* 1997;278:1321–1326.

CHAPTER 73

Health Issues for Women with Disabilities

Kristi L. Kirschner, Carol J. Gill, Judy Panko Reis, and Cassing Hammond

BARRIERS: PHYSICAL, ATTITUDINAL, KNOWLEDGE, AND FINANCIAL

People with disabilities are no strangers to barriers. The most overt barriers are physical (e.g., stairs, narrow doorways, curbs, inaccessible bathrooms), communication (e.g., lack of sign language interpreters or materials in Braille), and programmatic (e.g., lack of assistants, flexible scheduling, and transportation). The more insidious barriers are erected by ignorance and negative social attitudes about life with disability. Economic barriers also play a significant role in preventing people with disabilities from accessing community services, such as health care (1–3). Women with disabilities, in particular, are disproportionately affected by discriminatory practices in employment, education, vocational services, economic programs, access to benefits and services, health care, and parenting activities (4,5) (Fig. 73-1). With the passage of civil rights laws such as the Americans with Disabilities Act in 1990, and expanding clinical services targeting the needs of women with disabilities, this situation is beginning to improve (6). Women with disabilities are a long way from full integration, when a woman with a disability can go to a community health center with the expectation that it will be fully accessible with wheelchair-adapted equipment and have knowledgeable staff trained to assist women with a variety of disabilities in a manner respectful of their womanhood.

Recent attention has also focused on the unequal representation of women in health-care research. Historically, women have often been excluded from medical research for a variety of offered reasons ranging from methodological issues about the menstrual cycle to liability concerns related to potential pregnancies (7). As a result, there is little information about the use of medications in women to prevent coronary artery disease, the number-one killer for both sexes (8). Major causes of morbidity and mortality for women, such as osteoporosis and breast cancer, have only recently been receiving priority funding, as the National Institutes of Health has attempted to rectify these neglected areas through the multicenter studies of the Women's Health Initiative. Data is even more limited in guiding the treatments for women with disabilities. For example, what is the best treatment for osteoporosis in a woman with spinal cord injury? Can combined oral contraceptives be used safely in women with mobility impairments?

This chapter provides an overview of disabled women's health issues with particular attention to the psychosocial concerns that dominate this area. Little time is spent in discussing sexuality per se, as another chapter in this book (Chapter 74) is devoted to this topic. The topics in this chapter represent issues that women from the disability community have told the authors are important to them—from their writings, conferences, research, and their collaboration with health-care providers. This chapter is meant to highlight principles and provide a guide for comprehensive care for women with disabilities. A list of resources and model programs is provided in the Appendix for those who wish further information beyond the scope of this chapter.

A few words about language: the terms that persons with disabilities use for self-identification are still evolving. In this chapter, the phrases *women with disabilities* and *disabled women* are used interchangeably. This usage takes into account public statements by prominent disability community leaders (e.g., Judith Heumann, University of Minnesota, Minneapolis, MN, August 1, 1994; Barbara Waxman, Health of Women with Physical Disabilities conference, National Institutes of Health, Bethesda, MD, May 10, 1994), suggesting that an insistence on exclusive "person first" terminology might convey disparagement of the disability experience, whereas the term "disabled person" can convey pride in the disability identity. Consistent with this emphasis on disability as a social minority identity rather than purely medically defined deficiency, we have chosen to use neutral rather than negative terms when possible to describe disabilities, e.g., *extensive disability* rather than *severe disability*.

Although this textbook is primarily directed toward the health-care services of people with physical disabilities, at times examples of women with sensory and developmental disabilities are used to illustrate the principle of inclusiveness that is central to disabled women's health and to reflect the fact that women with physical disabilities can have other disabilities concurrently. Health care needs to embrace issues of men and women; women-s health care needs to embrace nondisabled and disabled; and disabled women's health care needs to embrace physical and nonphysical disabilities.

DEMOGRAPHICS

According to current estimates, there are approximately 28.6 million women and girls with disabilities living in the United States, representing approximately 21.3% of all female citizens (9). Their disabilities range from mild (i.e., they report difficulty with one or more functional activities, such as lifting

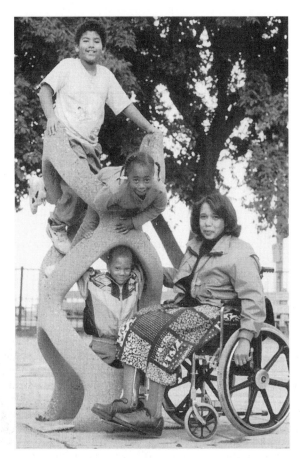

Figure 73-1. Disabled mother and children.

heavy objects) to severe* (i.e., they are unable to manage one or more basic activities of daily living, have one or more specific impairments, or require mobility aids, such as wheelchairs or crutches, to function; *severe* is the descriptor used in many survey instruments). Disability types include mobility, sensory, cognitive, mental illness, and disabilities that are due to various chronic disease conditions. Based on respondents' reports of their primary disabling conditions, the three leading causes of activity limitation in women are, in descending order, back disorders, arthritis, and heart disease (10). Approximately 6.5 million women 15 years and older use a wheelchair, cane, crutches, or walker (11), and 62.4% of people needing assistance with one or more activities of daily living are women (12).

Among women and girls, Native Americans report the highest disability rate (21.8%), followed by black women at 21.7%, white women at 20.3%, and Hispanic women at 16.2%. Asian/Pacific Islander women have the lowest disability rate at 10.7% (9). These ethnic differences may be linked to multiple factors, including income, education, and socioeconomic status (10), as well as possible cultural differences in how disability is experienced and reported. Among working-age women, African Americans and Native Americans have the highest incidence of extensive disability (11).

Women with disabilities have been described as socially isolated and deprived of the social roles and relationships available to most nondisabled women (13). Demographic data support this characterization. Women with activity limitations are less likely to be married compared with other women and men with or without activity limitations. Only 50% of women with activity limitations are currently married compared with 64% of women with no activity limitation. Some of these differences

are probably attributable to women's greater longevity and the positive association between advanced age and disability, especially because the women with activity limitations have higher rates of being widowed. However, there is evidence that having a functional impairment may decrease a woman's likelihood of forming or sustaining a marital relationship. Only 44% of women with extensive activity limitations are married, and these women have higher rates of divorce than women with less extensive limitations (10). As another index of social isolation, only about 11% of the total estimated population of 57.9 million parents in the United States are people with disabilities (9).

In general, women's education level is inversely related to degree of disability. Approximately 20% of all women between 25 and 64 years of age have disabilities. Of all women in that age group who never completed high school, 36.4% have disabilities. Of those who completed 16 or more years of education, 10.6% have disabilities, and only 3.7% are women with extensive disabilities (11).

Poverty is a common experience for women with disabilities. Employment rates for disabled women fall behind those of their nondisabled counterparts. Only 24.7% of women with an extensive disability and 27.8% of men with an extensive disability had a job or business. Nonextensive disability also diminishes the likelihood of working, particularly for women. Among those with a nonextensive disability, 68.4% of women and 85.1% of men were working at a job or business. In comparison, 74.5% of women with no disability and 89.8% of men with no disability were working (12). Furthermore, the earning power of women with disabilities who do find employment falls far below that of nondisabled women and even that of men with disabilities. For every dollar earned by nondisabled men, nondisabled women earn 66 cents, men with disabilities earn 88 cents, and women with disabilities earn only 49 cents. If the male experience is extracted from the calculations and nondisabled women's earnings are used as the standard, women with extensive disabilities earn only 71% of the standard (14). Of women with an extensive work disability, 40.5% are living in poverty, compared with 31.2% of men with an extensive work disability (9). Of all working-age American women receiving means-tested cash assistance, about half are women with disabilities, and 40.5% are women with extensive disabilities (11).

Women with disabilities are as likely as nondisabled women to have health-care coverage. However, the types of coverage differ significantly between the two groups. Women with disabilities are more likely to have publicly funded coverage (as opposed to private insurance) than nondisabled women. Disabled women report approximately twice the number of annual health service visits as nondisabled women, but given the greater likelihood that their disabling conditions demand more medical attention, it is not yet determined whether this greater number of visits provides adequate service (14).

REPRODUCTIVE HEALTH-CARE ISSUES

Women with disabilities have typically not been seen as wives and mothers (15). Dating back to the early 1900s, fears of women with disabilities producing children with disabilities led to some social policies encouraging sterilization and criminalization of marriage (16). Other fears have colored the reproductive history of disabled women, including the perceived inability of women with disabilities to be "good" mothers and exaggerated health risks for women with disabilities who choose to bear children (17,18).

Improved research and education have helped to break down these stereotypes and oppressive policies, though much work remains to be done. Women with disabilities overwhelmingly report difficulties obtaining balanced information about reproductive health-care issues, e.g., techniques for managing menstruation, birth control, risks associated with pregnancy, techniques for labor and delivery, information about sexual functioning, dating, and sexual identity (19–22). This section provides a brief overview of reproductive health-care issues for women with disabilities with an emphasis on further resources for providing more detailed information. Consistent with the rehabilitation model, it is our recommendation that the physiatrist work with a team of health-care professionals—in particular an obstetrician/gynecologist who has an interest in reproductive health-care issues for women with disabilities—to deliver knowledgeable, respectful reproductive health care.

Menstruation and Fertility

MANAGEMENT OF MENSTRUATION

Menarche is a symbolic moment in most women's lives, marking the transition from "girlhood" to "womanhood," with the attendant procreative possibilities. Although management of the menstrual flow is an issue for all women, it can be particularly cumbersome for women with physical impairments. For girls growing up with disabilities, options for managing menstrual flow should be explored, if possible, before the onset of menstruation. Such discussions offer opportunities for girls with disabilities to develop a sense of control over their emerging sexuality and evolving images of themselves as women. For women with acquired disabilities who are still menstruating, management of menstrual flow should be addressed shortly after the onset of disability, preferably as a part of a rehabilitation program.

Some women may be able to work with a nurse or occupational therapist to develop a system for managing menstrual hygiene. Switching from tampons to sanitary pads may be all that is needed. Other women may elect to work with a personal assistant to manage their menstrual hygiene. Some women, particularly those with more extensive physical disabilities, may find these options impractical and choose to look for pharmacological options (i.e., hormonal interventions) to regulate or curtail the menstrual flow (23–27). There are a number of options used by women in general, but there is little data on the safety and usage of these treatments in women with disabilities. Unfortunately, some physical disabilities and chronic disease states are inherently associated with menstrual irregularities, leading exactly to the unpredictable flow that is so unwelcome.

MENSTRUAL IRREGULARITY AND FERTILITY IN WOMEN WITH PHYSICAL DISABILITIES

For most women with physical disabilities, fertility potential is preserved, and menses resemble the patterns of women without disabilities. In some cases, menstrual irregularity and fertility problems can occur. The most common hormonal imbalances found in women in general are disorders of prolactin secretion or thyroid function. Women after traumatic brain injury or spinal cord injury (SCI) occasionally exhibit elevated levels of prolactin, with or without galactorrhea (28,29). This hyperprolactinemia interferes with the normal functioning of the hypothalamic-pituitary-ovarian axis, causing menstrual irregularity. This is usually in the form of oligo- or amenorrhea but can manifest in irregular menses as well. Almost all women after SCI will resume their normal cycle within the first 9 to 12

months postinjury (30). About 25% of one population of women studied report increased autonomic symptoms (sweating, headaches, flushing, and gooseflesh) around the menses (31).

Occasionally medications can also cause menstrual irregularities. Phenytoin (Dilantin) and corticosteroids may affect thyroid function and ovulation; tricyclic antidepressants, antipsychotic medications, and some antihypertensives may also cause menstrual irregularities by affecting prolactin levels (32,33). Treatment of menstrual irregularities varies with age and medical condition. Pregnancy should always be considered in evaluating menstrual irregularity. Thyroid function tests and prolactin levels can be helpful in evaluating women with irregular menstrual periods (34,35). Correcting hormonal causes of menstrual irregularities can often regulate the menstrual cycle successfully and reverse subfertility if desired. Abnormal bleeding can also occur with structural problems, such as uterine or endocervical polyps, fibroids, cervical pathology, and vulvovaginal lesions (36). Menstrual irregularities become more common as women reach the climacteric years. Careful gynecologic evaluation is required to determine an appropriate course of treatment. Again, although an increasing number of hormonal interventions are now available, little data exists to guide their use in women with disabilities (23–27).

Women with disordered menstrual cycles often have fertility difficulties. Although many women with physical disabilities have unaltered fertility potential, some women may have fertility problems related to hormonal irregularities. If these women desire conception, they need to undergo workups identical to those that would be given to nondisabled women, which might include evaluation of fallopian tube pathology with hysterosalpingography, blood work, and biopsies. The male partner needs to be involved in the process by providing a semen specimen for analysis, as almost half of all couples, in general, who present with infertility problems will have a male factor contribution (37).

Contraception

The history of contraception for women with disabilities has at times been coercive and oppressive. Compulsory sterilization, particularly for people with psychiatric and cognitive disabilities, took root in the United States in the early 1900s and in some venues persisted until the 1960s as part of the general eugenics movement (16,18). Concerns about "physician-controlled" contraceptives, such as Depo-Provera (Upjohn, Kalamazoo, MI), still percolate in segments of the disability community as a result of this history and the fear that a woman's reproductive choices might be curtailed by physicians, parents, or guardians who make decisions on her behalf (38).

Sensitivity to this history is essential in establishing patient-centered, trusting relationships between health-care providers and women with disabilities. Women with disabilities have the same right to knowledgeable information about contraception as nondisabled women and should participate in their reproductive health-care decision making to the fullest extent possible. Contraceptive choices may be influenced by the nature of the woman's physical impairment or chronic disease condition (39). For example, a woman with impaired hand function may have difficulty using barrier methods such as the diaphragm, sponge, or spermicidal product without assistance. Problem solving with an occupational therapist, or working with the woman's partner, may result in an adequate solution for the use of barrier methods. Condoms, of course, always remain an effective method, if the male partner is in agreement, and provide the dual benefits of contraception and protection from sexually transmitted diseases (40).

There are a rapidly growing array of hormonal options for contraception that include not only a variety of combination pills, progestin-only minipills, injections [e.g., Depo-Provera—medroxyprogesterone acetate; Lunelle—medroxyprogesterone acetate/estradiol cypionate (Pharmacia, Inc. Peapack, NJ, USA)], the progestin cervical ring [Nuvaring, etonogestrel/ethinyl estradiol vaginal ring (Organon Inc; West Orange, NJ, USA)], the progestin impregnated intrauterine device (IUD) (Mirena Levonorgestrel-releasing intrauterine system; Berlex Laboratories, Inc., USA), and transdermal patches such as OrthoEvra (norelgestromin/ethinyl estradiol transdermal system; Ortho-McNeil Pharmaceutical, USA). For women who desire hormonal methods of contraception, information about the risks and benefits of various hormonal contraceptive options in women with disabilities is limited. For example, some women with mobility limitations (such as women with spina bifida, SCI, and multiple sclerosis) might have an increased risk for developing thrombotic events when using combination oral contraceptives, but definite statistics are not available (41). The progestin-only contraceptive pills are associated with an increased risk of abnormal uterine bleeding and are less effective than the combination pills (42).

Depo-Provera, an injectable form of progesterone that is effective for at least 12 weeks, is highly effective, and patients are often pleased with the decreased menstrual flow or amenorrhea that additionally result from this method if taken long enough (43,44). This method is also efficacious and convenient to use. Unfortunately, many women experience some weight gain and have reduced estrogen levels, which can lead to osteoporosis (45,46). Norplant [subdermal levonorgesterel (Wyeth-Ayerst, Philadelphia, PA)], which was previously available as another option for a progestin-only contraceptive, is no longer on the market. As an implantable contraceptive requiring a minor surgical procedure to place and remove, it was again associated with menstrual irregularities and amenorrhea (44). It is expected that other implantable contraceptives may become available in the future.

The Nuvaring and Ortho Evra are two new options, offering both effective contraception and ease of use. Ortho Evra is a transdermal patch applied weekly on the buttocks, abdomen, upper torso, or outer arm. Nuvaring is a flexible, transparent ring placed in the vagina 3 out of 4 weeks per month. Both Nuvaring and Ortho Evra offer different means of delivering hormonal contraception into the systemic circulation. Indications and contraindications to both devices resemble traditional oral contraception. Patients unable to remember daily pills or unable to swallow pills might find the patch or vaginal ring convenient. Other women with disabilities might find it difficult to check for the ring's presence in the vagina or the patch's adherence to skin without assistance.

IUDs represent the most popular form of reversible contraception throughout much of the world, but remain underutilized within the United States. Despite contraceptive efficacy that approaches that of surgical sterilization, many clinicians still fear infections and other risks previously attributed primarily to shield-type IUDs. Although most of these risks are unsupported by best evidence, American clinicians hesitate to place IUDs in nulliparous patients and patients who are not monogamous (47–52).

No literature specifically evaluates the risk of IUD use among women with disabilities, although physicians should clearly exercise caution in some circumstances. Women with impaired pelvic sensation, for example, might be less able to detect symptoms consistent with pelvic infection as well as

spontaneous expulsion of the IUD. Other women will require assistance in palpating vaginally for the IUD string, one sign that the IUD remains properly placed. Although the Food and Drug Administration has not approved IUDs for noncontraceptive indications, progestin-bearing IUDs offer an opportunity to control menometrorrhagia without resorting to more invasive surgical methods (53). This might offer significant hygienic advantage to women with mobility impairments who experience heavy or irregular menses regardless of their need for contraception.

Pregnancy and Prenatal Preparation

When possible, as with any nondisabled woman, it is best to discuss issues and concerns about pregnancy and motherhood *before* becoming pregnant (54–56). Counseling about health behaviors that can maximize the woman's and fetus's well-being during pregnancy is just one potential benefit. As many women with disabilities are on multiple medications, such as antiepileptics and antispasticity agents, careful consideration of the potential effects of the medications on a developing fetus is warranted (57–61). Information about diet; potential adverse effects on the fetus of smoking, alcohol, and illicit drug use; and the benefits of various vitamin supplementations may maximize the woman's ability to make choices and be an active participant in managing her pregnancy.

For some women, information about their health risks with pregnancy may be useful in facilitating a decision to pursue biological motherhood. A few disabilities may progress with pregnancy, perhaps irreversibly, or require higher-risk interventions and support (62–66). For example, a woman with multiple sclerosis may expect that her multiple sclerosis could worsen postpartum (63,67), or a woman with spinal muscular atrophy may need ventilatory assistance as the gravid uterus pushes on her diaphragm and impedes ventilatory excursion (65).

Other women could expect a temporary decrement in their functional abilities, necessitating more physical assistance as pregnancy progresses (57,68–71). Most women with mobility impairments will be affected to some degree by changes in their center of gravity with the expected weight gain of pregnancy. Women who had previously managed their mobility with braces or assistive devices may find their stamina and balance affected as the pregnancy progresses and elect to temporarily use a manual wheelchair. Women who had previously been independent with manual wheelchairs may notice that they fatigue much more quickly and are unable to navigate the environment independently; these women may choose to use an electric wheelchair in the latter stages of pregnancy. Anticipating these changes will allow the woman and her health-care provider to anticipate needs that might arise during the pregnancy and proactive interventions (such as referrals to physical therapy in the second trimester) that can be instituted to lessen the impact of some of these changes.

Information about other potential risks associated with pregnancy may assist in a plan of care to obviate or lessen these risks (40,71–73). For example, for women who use indwelling catheters and are chronically colonized with bacteria, the risk of recurrent pyelonephritis may be heightened as the growing uterus causes pressure on the ureters (71). Prompt recognition and prevention of urinary tract infections is extremely important in preventing preterm labor (73). Women who have been accustomed to intermittent catheterization may find their bladder capacitance to be significantly decreased and opt to use pads or an indwelling catheter to maintain continence for the latter part of their pregnancies.

Excellent skin care and vigilance are extremely important in preventing decubitus ulcers during pregnancy for any woman with a mobility impairment and areas of insensate skin (71,73). A pressure-relief program that had previously been adequate in preventing decubiti may no longer be adequate with the increasing weight gain of pregnancy, coupled with hormonal changes that may predispose the skin to break down more easily. Counseling about more frequent pressure reliefs, changing wheelchair cushions, and frequent skin checks can go a long way in preventing this complication.

Constipation and hemorrhoids are potential problems in any pregnancy with changes in diet, hormonal influences on the intestinal tract, iron supplementation, and the gravid uterus pushing on pelvic veins, but these potential complications can be particularly difficult for a woman with neurogenic bowel dysfunction (74). Vigilance coupled with modifications in diet and the bowel program can help prevent bowel impaction and hemorrhoidal complications.

Pressure on the pelvic veins, hormonal changes in pregnancy, and immobility may predispose a woman to deep venous thrombosis (DVT), a potential complication of any pregnancy but especially for a woman with paralysis (40,75). Frequent examinations and counseling about signs and symptoms of DVT are extremely important in helping women and care providers quickly recognize and seek assistance in managing this potentially life-threatening complication. Elevation of the legs, restriction of salt, range of motion, and the use of compression stockings may help minimize dependent edema.

For women with respiratory impairments from SCI, neuromuscular disorders such as spinal muscular atrophy, or extensive scoliosis with restrictive lung disease, respiratory function may also be affected with lowering of the functional residual capacity as the uterus grows (40,73,76). Pregnant women frequently hyperventilate and develop a mild degree of respiratory alkalosis, believed to be an effect of progesterone (76). Women with limited respiratory reserve may be particularly affected by these changes and require some modification in their activities, sleeping positions, and occasionally assisted ventilation to manage the latter stages of pregnancy, labor, and delivery.

A few potential complications of pregnancy can be life-threatening for a woman with disability (77). One of the best-recognized and frequently documented complications is autonomic hyperreflexia in a woman with tetraplegia or high paraplegia (usually T-6 or above) (73,78–82). Not only can hyperreflexia signal an issue requiring attention such as bladder distention or infection, bowel impaction, or labor, but the signs and symptoms can be misinterpreted as preeclampsia and lead health-care providers down an incorrect path of diagnosis and treatment, with potentially disastrous results, including intracerebral hemorrhage and even death. For women who are at risk for hyperreflexia, consultation with an anesthesiologist well before delivery may be prudent (77,83–86). A team approach to pregnancy, with a specialist in SCI working closely with the obstetric staff, can facilitate prevention and management of these potential complications (40,71,73,87).

Preventive health care is a major focus for any woman with a disability going through pregnancy, but this period also offers an excellent opportunity to help the woman prepare for her future role as a mother (70,88,89). If a woman has severe mobility impairment, referrals to an experienced occupational therapist and physical therapist may help her to develop a variety of anticipated skills to maximize her ability to parent (90–93). For example, how will she carry the baby? How will she feed the baby? If she plans to breast-feed, what positioning techniques will work best for her? What about diapering, dressing, and bathing? A home visit may be helpful in setting up the environment with adaptive equipment to facilitate her functional abilities (94). If the woman will require or chooses to use assistance in managing some of the care tasks required, working out a plan before the baby is born is important.

Many women with disabilities also yearn to talk to other women with similar disabilities about their experiences as mothers. Peer support and referrals can be extremely helpful in facilitating successful adjustment for both mother and baby and in anticipating the needs of each subsequent developmental stage (95,96). If a woman uses a wheelchair, how will she manage her toddler and maintain safety and discipline? How will she work with her child around the child's growing perception of her disability (97–100)? Women also report that continued contact with child-care specialists from occupational therapy and psychology can be extremely important in adapting to each new developmental stage. More detailed information and resources on mothering with a disability is presented later in the chapter.

Labor and Delivery

Preparation for labor and delivery is an important consideration for the woman with a disability, but depending on her disability, the traditional Lamaze classes (or variations thereof) may not make sense for her and her partner (70). Information to assist the woman in proper recognition of labor involves understanding expected signs and symptoms in the context of her particular disability (57,71). For example, a woman with extensive sensory impairments may not be able to sense pain from uterine contractions but have to rely on manual or electronic detection of the contractions. If she has high paraplegia or tetraplegia, periodic headaches from recurring autonomic hyperreflexia (occurring with each contraction of the uterus) may be the first symptom she recognizes. Recognition of amniotic fluid leakage and knowing when to seek a checkup with her care provider are also important to discuss. Of course, frequent regular checkups with her obstetrician will also be helpful in predicting impending labor.

As previously mentioned, a discussion of anesthesia before labor and delivery is important in establishing a care plan (101). For example, a woman with an SCI who develops autonomic hyperreflexia with labor may do well with epidural anesthesia as a way to block the afferent signal from the uterus to the spinal cord, which triggers the sympathetic response (57,77,79). For a woman with respiratory compromise, a plan for providing ventilatory support should be discussed. If general anesthesia is needed for any reason, pertinent knowledge about disability-related issues that could influence the safety of general anesthesia should be considered. For example, a woman with a SCI should not receive succinylcholine as a depolarizing agent secondary to the risk of hyperkalemia (77,84). If a woman has had a cervical fusion of her neck, intubation may be more difficult with traditional methods.

Working with the labor and delivery staff may also be important in anticipating the needs of a woman with disability. If she is at risk for skin breakdown, proper padding and frequent position changes are important. If she has significant contractures and spasticity, tips for managing these issues with range of motion, positioning, and occasionally medication may be advisable (57,71,101). An increasing number of women are being recognized with latex allergies, in particular a large proportion of women with spina bifida (102), and this should always be mentioned to the staff as well. It is always optimal if the woman (and her partner) has an opportunity to tour the facility where she will deliver and to discuss her wishes for her peripartum care with her obstetrician and the nursing staff.

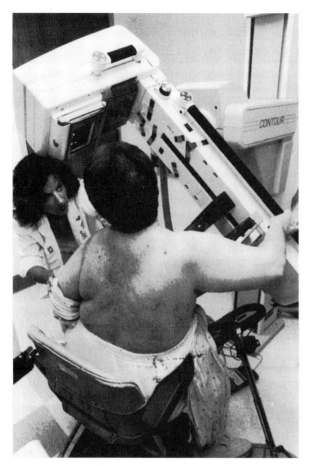

Figure 73-2. Patient who uses a wheelchair receiving a mammogram.

Preventive Health-Care Services

PAP TESTS AND GYNECOLOGIC EXAMINATIONS

Basic preventive health and gynecologic screening for women with disabilities is often overshadowed by more obvious physical or neurologic problems, which may require more immediate focus. Thus, screening for diabetes, hypertension, hyperlipidemia, and thyroid imbalance, all of which are common concerns for women, may be neglected in women with disabilities. Many women avoid gynecologic care because of difficulty in obtaining an accessible, comfortable, and dignified examination (21,22,40). As a consequence, treatable early-stage problems may escalate and become much more difficult to manage. These concerns include Pap test screening as well as breast evaluation.

Performance of the pelvic examination must be tailored to a woman's physical impairments (103–105). An accessible examination table that lowers to wheelchair height and has security features such as hand rails, boots, and straps can be indispensable (104). Leg adjustments should be performed slowly and gradually to minimize pain and spasticity. Liberal application of lidocaine gel to the perineal area can be helpful in minimizing spasticity or in preventing episodes of autonomic hyperreflexia in some spinal-cord-injured women with high lesions (above T-6) (57,106).

BREAST SELF-EXAM AND MAMMOGRAMS

National Cancer Institute statistics report that breast cancer is the most prevalent gynecologic cancer occurring in women, with approximately 1.75 million women affected in 1995 (107) (Fig. 73-2). Currently, it is estimated that one in eight women will develop breast cancer. It is generally recommended that women learn their breast anatomy and examine themselves on a regular basis to detect changes or abnormalities that may signal breast cancer (108,109), although breast self-exam has low sensitivity and specificity, making some question the wisdom or need to focus on breast self-exam as a screening tool (110). If a woman with a disability is unable to perform breast self-exam, she may want to work out a system with her physician, personal care assistant, partner, or other available person to assist in breast exam techniques. Those who endorse manual breast exams usually recommend performing the exam each month 1 week after menses and on a monthly basis in post-menopausal women.

As a screening tool, mammography has much greater sensitivity but it still fails to detect 10% to 15% of all lesions. Although there is general agreement that all women age 50 and older should have yearly screening mammograms, there is still no clear consensus regarding women ages 40 to 49 (110). Women with disabilities should, at the very least, obtain screening mammography at rates comparable to nondisabled peers. Unfortunately, not all facilities have staff and equipment able to accommodate mobility-impaired women. Women with disabilities should ask their health-care provider for the names of facilities in their area best able to accommodate their disability and should contact the center in advance to notify them of any special needs she might have.

MENOPAUSE AND AGING WITH A DISABILITY

More than half of women with disabilities in this country are older than age 50, and this poses unique issues in preventive health-care services (111,112). Menopause is the "permanent cessation of menses that occurs after the cessation of ovarian function" and is frequently preceded by oligoovulatory bleeding (113). Menopause usually occurs in women between 45 and 55 years of age with a mean age of 51 and is suspected after 6 months of amenorrhea (114). Diagnosis can be confirmed by findings of low estradiol and high follicle-stimulating hormone. These tests can be performed if the diagnosis is in question. The age of onset of menopause can occur earlier in women with chronic disease states, such as thyroid disease, diabetes, and multiple sclerosis (115,116). Symptomatology may also vary in its manifestation and effects on women with disabilities. For example, women with neurologic conditions that are particularly heat sensitive, such as multiple sclerosis, may have difficulty distinguishing hot flashes and vasomotor instability of menopause from symptoms commonly attributed to their disability (117).

Women with physical disabilities may be at higher risk than their nondisabled counterparts for the consequences of estrogen deprivation, such as osteoporosis or difficulties with skin integrity. For example, a woman with weakness or paralysis from a neurologic disease or dysfunction may have extensive immobilization osteoporosis that occurred around the onset of the disability (118,119). She is still at risk for age-related and menopause-related bone loss but will be entering these phases with a lower bone mass to begin with. If she is at increased risk for pressure sores from immobility or loss of sensation, she may note increasing difficulty with maintenance of her skin integrity and turgor around menopause with the loss of estrogen.

Although hormone replacement therapy has been believed to be a safe and effective agent for many postmenopausal women and has also been used in the hope of preventing cardiovascular disease, osteoporosis, and even cognitive decline, recent studies have questioned the wisdom of routine use. The Heart and Estrogen/Progestin Replacement Study Follow-up (HERS II) found that hormone replacement therapy was not effective in preventing coronary artery disease and in fact increased the risk of biliary tract disease and venous thromboembolism (120–122). The Women's Health Initiative arm that evaluated estrogen plus progestin was stopped early, as this large randomized controlled trial found an increased incidence of coronary events, strokes, pulmonary emboli, and invasive breast cancer in those receiving the combination hormone replacement therapy versus those receiving placebo. The Women's Health Initiative study did indicate some potential benefit in those receiving combination hormone replacement therapy for a lower risk of colorectal cancer and hip fracture (123). Studies are still pending regarding the estrogen-only group, but the current recommendations are not to use hormone replacement therapy as primary preventive treatment of heart disease or osteoporosis, as many other more effective treatments are available (122). Aspirin, β-blockers, angiotensin-converting enzyme inhibitors, statins, and other lipid-lowering strategies are important agents to consider as preventive strategies for coronary artery disease and cerebral vascular disease (122). A number of agents, including bisphosphonates and selective estrogen receptor modulators such as raloxifene, are useful in preventing fractures in women with low bone mineral density. Patients experiencing acute symptoms related to estrogen deprivation, including vasomotor symptoms, should realize that relative risks of major cardiac events and invasive breast cancer were low and only demonstrable after 4 years of therapy in the Women's Health Initiative trial. Immediately following release of the Women's Health Initiative trial data, the American College of Obstetricians and Gynecologists formed a task force to review and revise previous recommendations regarding hormone replacement therapy. Until final recommendations from the panel become available, the American College of Obstetricians and Gynecologists recommends that short-term use of this therapy be a "personal, individualized decision, made after consultations between a woman and her physician and taking into account a woman's individual benefits and risks of such use" (124)

SEXUALITY

The World Health Organization definition of sexual health (1975) is "the integration of the somatic, emotional, mental, and social aspects of being sexual beings, in ways that are positively enriching and that include personality and love," whereas body image is "an image of self and includes physical appearance, inner feelings, how other people act or react (or one's interpretation of how they react or do not react) and identification" (125).

Sexuality is much more than penile-vaginal intercourse, though prior research has focused heavily on this area to describe sexuality after disability (126–137). People with disabilities have been pioneers of sorts, expanding our concepts of human sexuality to include the quality of relationships, imagery, sensuality, self-image, creativity, and emotional connectedness (138–142).

Access to knowledgeable health-care professionals can be important in facilitating successful sexual adjustment after disability and problem-solving issues that may arise (143–156). For example, sexual desire may be suppressed in women who experience significant fatigue or discomfort from a chronic disease or disability. In such cases, analgesics can be considered and timing centered around peak energy level periods. Current studies are ongoing to assess the efficacy of Viagra in women (157). Communication between members of the sex partner about individual needs can help transcend barriers to desire.

For women with sensory impairments, exploration of nontraditional erogenous zones as well as traditional areas may help her to discover pleasurable touching. Discussions about bowel programs, the management of catheters, spasticity, hyperreflexia, contractures, and positioning may help to alleviate anxiety about resuming intimate relationships. Of course, it is important to remember that not all women with disabilities are heterosexual, and their lives may include lesbian relationships (158). The need to have access to knowledgeable, caring, and open health-care professionals is the same.

SELF-ESTEEM/GENDER

The development of positive identity is a challenge for any member of a socially devalued community. It is especially difficult for an individual to sustain positive identity and self-esteem when surrounded by messages that she/he fails to measure up to culturally prescribed norms. For that reason, scholars specializing in women's issues have denounced the unforgiving standards of physical and functional perfection imposed on all young girls as they mature into womanhood. Heterosexual attractiveness and social success, in particular, are still highly associated with self-esteem in young women (154).

These standards are exceptionally harsh for women with disabilities. Girls who grow up with visible impairments learn early in life that they are not expected to succeed at womanhood, either aesthetically or functionally. In research interviews and their own written accounts of growing up with disabilities (13,159,160), they frequently report that their parents carefully avoided discussions of romance or, worse, explicitly predicted that the daughters would never attract or please a mate. Instead of offering tips on dating, mothers might urge them to hide their limps or cover up disabled body features with clothing to prevent social rejection. Fathers often encouraged them to study hard and prepare for a good job in lieu of a husband. Nondisabled classmates sometimes openly ridiculed their sexual appeal. The consequences for many adolescent girls with disabilities have been alienation and shame.

Some young women with disabilities, however, including those with extensive physical limitations, have demonstrated amazing resilience in the face of invalidating messages. They have developed positive self-concepts as women and have established enduring intimate relationships despite all predictions (161). Many give credit to unusually perceptive family members who affirmed their sex roles and who facilitated their social contacts. Others, surrounded by discouragement, refused to internalize it. Seeking strong disabled women role models for support or simply finding validation from within, they have integrated their disabilities into sound and positive identities as women (154,162). Accepting disability as a familiar and normal part of their lives, they seem to set their own standards for what is valuable, sexually appealing, and womanly.

Women who acquire their disabilities after adolescence may be spared the unique barriers to self-esteem development and sex-role definition experienced by women with early-onset disabilities. However, they frequently report feeling shaken by a change in others' regard for them as women immediately following disability. One author has referred to this phenomenon as "degenderization"—being treated as asexual and as no longer female (163). Divested of the qualities and roles that define women in our society, women with late-onset disabilities may feel a profound loss of identity and meaningful place in their social network (164).

In addition to invalidating messages about their womanliness from family, friends, and greater society, women with disabilities experience degenderization and patronizing attitudes from professionals in medical settings (161). An experience that is so pervasive and distressing to women with disabilities that they have written about it extensively and given it a name is "public stripping" (165). By this term, they refer to the practice of requiring children and adults with disabilities to disrobe for medical educational display and/or clinical photographs, sometimes without adequate preparation or request for permission. Women with disabilities report enduring psychological trauma from their perceived violation of body space and privacy in medical settings, describing such events as assaultive, objectifying or dehumanizing, and dismissive of their sex roles. Many women and girls with disabilities struggle to be respected as valid women with genuine women's health issues, including contraception, fertility, and sexually transmitted disease. When a primary care physician expresses undue curiosity or overriding concern regarding aspects of their disability rather than gynecologic health, they may feel "treated like a disability instead of a woman."

In addition to adopting a responsive and respectful clinical approach that acknowledges women with disabilities as women in every way, physicians can help link their patients to community resources for peer support and opportunities for self-expression. Physicians can acquaint themselves with independent living centers—a national network comprising hundreds of centers run by people with disabilities to provide disability-related information, services, and advocacy to others with disabilities and deafness. Most cities have one or more such centers, and many offer peer support groups and domestic violence programs as well as information on housing, health services, transportation, and in-home personal assistance services (see National Council on Independent Living in the Appendix). Additionally, in many cities, there are disability rights and consumer organizations that can be contacted for resources helpful to women with disabilities. State, county, and municipal government offices routinely have departments addressing the needs of citizens with disabilities. By contacting these organizations and programs, physicians and the women with disabilities they serve can inquire about local recreational, artistic, employment, and peer support programs that welcome women with disabilities and encourage their development of positive identity.

Recently, the national disability community has developed a multitude of projects to celebrate the history, culture, and group identity of people with disabilities. Women with disabilities have figured prominently in this movement. As poets, playwrights, scholars, and performers, they have asserted the importance of disabled women's perspectives on the world. In the past three decades, women with disabilities across the country have established programs to encourage networking for support and mentoring (Fig. 73-3). Health professionals can locate such projects by entering the words *women with disabilities* in their favorite Internet search engine. Historically speaking, the Networking Project for Disabled Women and Girls, established in New York by Harilyn Rousso in 1984, was a model for many current mentoring projects that promote connections between girls with disabilities and disabled women who have achieved career and relationship goals (162). The Project on Women and Disability in Boston led by Marsha Saxton developed a variety of projects in the 1980s and 1990s to encourage women with disabilities to exchange information about their experiences and to learn useful skills, such as assertiveness and strategies for effective communication and partnership-building with health-service providers (166). For example, the pro-

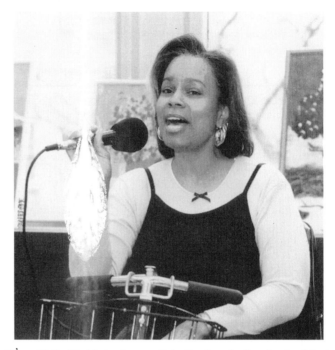

Figure 73-3. Disabled actress participating in a "coffee-shop" celebrating the arts and talents of disabled women.

ject linked with the famous Boston Women's Health Book Collective to ensure that the classic handbook, *Our Bodies, Ourselves*, included issues of importance to women with disabilities (146). The motto of the project—"Female, Disabled, and Proud!"—aptly expresses the philosophy underpinning most of the ongoing efforts by women with disabilities to support each others' empowerment.

ACCESS TO INFORMATION

Lack of access to information can prevent women with disabilities from achieving self-determination in health and other aspects of life. Their exclusion from sources of information about sexuality and reproductive health options has been caused by inadequate disability accommodations, negative disability attitudes, or a combination of both types of barriers.

Many girls with disabilities grow up outside the usual channels for learning about sexuality. For example, they may be denied admission to their neighborhood schools and recreation programs due to access barriers and discriminatory enrollment practices (162). Consequently, they are denied important informal opportunities to exchange information and experiences regarding sexuality with their peers. Instead, they might be placed in a sheltered and closely supervised special education school, where even formal sex education may not be offered. Their parents are less likely to talk to them about sexuality and reproduction than to their nondisabled sisters (154). Girls and young women who are blind are rarely given tactile anatomical models so they can safely explore and understand the form and function of human body parts. Those who are deaf or hard of hearing may miss conversations about "the facts of life" whispered between hearing friends. Girls and women with cognitive disabilities may not fully understand spoken and written information about sexuality and health matters unless it is presented in an illustrated, uncomplicated manner.

In adulthood, information barriers interfere with health maintenance for women with disabilities. Blind women and those with low vision confront clinic signs, instructions, release forms, and educational materials that have not been translated into accessible formats, such as Braille, audiotape, or computer disk versions. Deaf women are not offered interpreters to insure accurate doctor/patient communication. Women with cognitive disabilities are not allowed adequate time and explanation to insure comprehension and informed consent.

Provider attitudes affect the amount and quality of information offered to women patients with disabilities. Negative disability attitudes in physicians have been associated with their lack of complete knowledge about health options for persons with disabilities and even the inclination to withhold options that are known (167). There is some empirical evidence to confirm that disabled women garner negative judgments from health professionals. In one study of allied health professionals' knowledge of men and women with disabilities, for example, the researchers found that men generally were perceived by the professionals as better at coping with their disabilities than women (168). There is also evidence that physicians' perceptions of a woman's disability may result in the withholding of information about her health options. One of the first systematic studies to document disabled women's health-service experiences revealed that physicians' inclination to offer disabled women patients information regarding sexuality and contraception was mediated by such factors as the age of onset or extent of a woman's disability (22).

Some reproductive health agencies, such as Planned Parenthood and Regional Family Planning, have taken important steps to insure that their information and services are accessible to women with disabilities. State or city government offices specializing in disability services can guide physicians in providing accessible information and communication to patients with disabilities. To find out more about health professionals' responsibilities to comply with the Americans with Disabilities Act, call (800) 949–4232 to be connected with the nearest U.S. Department of Education funded Disability and Business Technical Assistance Center. (Further resources available in Appendix). A useful rule of thumb in working clinically with any woman with a disability, particularly early-onset disability, is to ask if she would like information or guidance about sexuality, reproductive health options, or any other aspect of health. Some women with disabilities are extraordinarily sophisticated about their health options and the workings of their bodies; others lack basic information about anatomy and human sexuality. Many are experts regarding their particular disability but have gaps in general health maintenance knowledge because of the information barriers discussed above. It is useful to explore each woman's level of knowledge and desire for more information before concluding any health-service contact.

MOTHERING WITH A DISABILITY

A growing number of women with disabilities have been choosing to become mothers, shattering stereotypes of asexuality and maternal incompetency historically ascribed to them by a society that stigmatizes disability. They and mothers who later acquired disabilities are seeking recognition and support for their capabilities. This surge was generated in the 1970s by the independent living movement and in the 1990s by the passage of the Americans with Disabilities Act and is forcing health-care providers to take a closer look at ways to assist mothers with disabilities to achieve self-determination over their parenting activities. Although mothers with disabilities share the same basic needs and concerns as nondisabled mothers, their capabilities to function aptly in a parenting role are greatly enhanced with the use of adaptive equipment, adequate personal assistance, regular access to peer support, and knowledgeable health-care providers who understand the concept of self-determination, as well as the sociopolitical barriers confronting women with disabilities (169).

Research

Research on disabled parents is still relatively scarce, but some significant strides have been made in the past 5 years that include the following demographics. Of the 6.9 million disabled parents in the United States, approximately 60% are women, and about one-third of these women, compared with 25% of disabled men, have children in the home (170). Findings from a national study of parents with disabilities confirm the prevalence of discrimination that face mothers with disabilities regarding their rights to bear and raise children (170,171). Of the more than 1,000 parents with disabilities surveyed, 15% report attempts to remove their children. As a result of such findings and other literature that demonstrates a pervasive belief among professionals "that disability severely limits parenting ability and often leads to maladjustment in children," there has been more than two decades of disability-friendly research focusing on the capabilities of mothers with disabilities (172–174). Conducted from a disability cultural perspective, this approach is grounded in the view that disability does not reside solely within the mother, but rather is socially constructed in her experiences of discrimination and marginalization. In an attempt to counter the literature that pathologizes mothering with a disability and that perpetuates their marginalization, Through the Looking Glass was founded in 1982 in Berkeley, California. Working in synergy with its provision of disability culture-based clinical services and resources to parents with disabilities, Through the Looking Glass focuses its research on issues that are considered essential for social change to improve the lives of parents with disabilities and their children.

Through the Looking Glass and its National Institute on Disability and Rehabilitation Research–funded Research and Training Center for Parents with Disabilities remain on the forefront of conducting research that documents the capabilities in mothers with disabilities in an effort to combat pervasive stereotypes that emphasize the negative effects of a mother's disability on the well-being of her children. Its early research was driven by data showing that parents with physical, visual, and hearing disabilities were offended that professionals, in questioning their child-care abilities, were also suggesting that the parents had never considered the implications of being disabled and providing child care (172).

From 1985 to 1988, Through the Looking Glass conducted groundbreaking research that established the reciprocal process of adaptation to disability obstacles as it developed between 10 mothers with physical disabilities and their babies (175). In this videotaped project—which explored basic care, including feeding, lifting, bathing, diapering, and dressing—Through the Looking Glass captured the gradual process for mutual adaptation that emerged between mother and baby during their interaction (172). For example, the study documented the process of reciprocal cooperation between a mother with paraplegia and her 1-month-old infant. The infant would help his mother lift him by balling up his legs and head on his mother's lap and remain still until his mother completed the lift. The videotape documented the mother's cueing process that facilitated the infant's adaptation through a series of strategies that included positioning the baby on his back and a variety of tugs on his clothing that signaled her intention to lift him. This study offered practitioners an expanded working sense of a range of acceptable parenting practices that include issues of physical difference in mothers (172). The findings demonstrated that mothers with physical disabilities were naturally resourceful in creating their own adaptations to baby care and that adaptation in infants was easily facilitated by their disabled mothers.

Consistent with these findings is anecdotal evidence that suggests that adaptations can continue as the child develops. For example, mothers with hemiplegia report that their children knew at an early age to approach the mother on her stronger side and to refrain from extending arms to be picked up when their mother was standing as opposed to the more stable, seated position (175,176). Through the Looking Glass's videotape evaluation and analysis methods documenting the mutual adaptation process between children and their disabled moms can be an invaluable tool for clinicians and health providers called upon to assist parents with disabilities involved with child protective services (172). In one renowned incident, Tiffaney Callo, a mother with cerebral palsy, lost her two sons to foster care. Through the Looking Glass discredited presumptions of her incompetency by demonstrating with video documentation and analysis that Callo's diapering skills were within the range of "good enough" (172). Furthermore, when Callo's lack of a mutual gaze with her infant was interpreted by social service professionals to be pathological, Through the Looking Glass researchers directly challenged this assessment with the introduction of a lap tray and well-positioned pillows that allowed Callo to establish a mutual gaze with her infant. Through the Looking Glass determined that this experience, and that of many others, underscored the necessity for ensuring the provision of adaptive baby equipment when attempting an accurate assessment of a disabled woman's full range of mothering abilities. This is especially important in situations that involve a disabled woman's legal rights as a parent or in custody decisions.

Against a background of scant high-quality research on mothering with a disability and prevalence of literature condemning the activity of parenting with a disability as a source of potential damage to the children, Through the Looking Glass continues to spearhead research that helps improve the quality of family life for individuals parenting with a disability (172). Through the Looking Glass has focused on three research initiatives conducted over the past decade involving (1) the development and evaluation of baby care equipment, (2) a national survey of parents with disabilities, and (3) a study examining the effects that mothers with disabilities have on their children.

BABY-CARE EQUIPMENT

Through the Looking Glass has undertaken some pioneering work in baby-care equipment, including three projects that included the design and evaluation of lifting harnesses for use by mothers with physical disabilities to lift their children (177–181). The studies found that this equipment can have a beneficial effect on mother/infant interaction. By lessening the disabled mother's level of physical stress and fatigue, these studies demonstrated that the provision of adaptive equipment can help prevent the need for additional rehabilitation services caused by secondary disabilities, such as back or repetitive stress injuries. Another significant finding was that use of the equipment played a role in "alleviating depression associated

with post-natal exacerbations of disability such as in multiple sclerosis" (172).

NATIONAL PARENTING SURVEY

In the largest national study of its kind, 1,175 parents with disabilities were surveyed on their needs and experiences encountered in their role as parents (170). Noteworthy are findings that reveal that parents with disabilities face significant social barriers that impede their parenting activities, such as the lack of accessible transportation (87%) and lack of accessible housing (69%). Also of interest are the problems they report in accessing adaptive parenting equipment despite a predominance of respondents who indicated that equipment could improve their lives by increasing their independence, maximizing their time, and alleviating their stress and fatigue. Of the sample answering questions on equipment, 50% indicated that they were unable to locate such equipment, and 48% reported that they were unable to pay for it.

IMPACT OF A MOTHER'S DISABILITY ON HER FAMILY

Another study examined mothers with physical or visual impairments with latency-age children (from about 5 years of age to puberty) and found an absence of ill effects of a mother's disability on her family. In fact, the predictors of problem parenting were more likely linked to a history of abuse in the mother's family of origin—e.g., physical, sexual, or substance abuse—and not to the disability per se (182). This research is important in the challenge it poses to the common stereotype that children of mothers with disabilities will be "parentified" or obliged to care for the emotional or physical needs of their disabled mothers at too early of an age (172). In fact, contrary to being "parentified," this study found that children of disabled mothers were often spared the responsibilities of common family chores, such as taking out the garbage, when the mothers felt that the request was "necessitated" by their disabilities (172). Another study looking at mothers with SCI found that there were no significant differences between children raised by mothers with SCI and children raised by mothers without disabilities in regard to individual adjustment, atti-

TABLE 73-1. The Blessings/Positive Aspects of Parenting with a Disability

	# of Responses
Child learns compassion	70
Child has open attitude toward others	40
More time with kids	36
My child's love	35
Child more resourceful	29
No difference	24
Can be a good role model for my kids	23
High value on having kids	17
Being a mom or dad	16
Life is more precious	15
Understanding of children's needs	15
None/There is no blessing	15
Makes family pull together	14
Focused on important issues	11
Physical closeness	11
Can advocate for children's needs	4

N=296

tudes toward their parents, self-esteem, sex roles, and family functioning (100). It is commonly reported that among the multitude of positives that disabled parents offer their children are the ability to learn compassion and an openness toward others (Table 73-1).

Facilitating Self-Determination

Although the introduction of adaptive equipment and parenting resources early in the mothering experience can minimize problems and significantly improve a disabled mother's capacity to provide independent care for her baby, this is not feasible for all mothers. Financial constraints, scarcity of customized equipment, and physical limitations may still prevent many women from becoming fully self-sufficient in managing the

care of a child. In fact, more than half (57%) of disabled parents report that they need help with parenting tasks (170). It is thus essential for mothers and health-care providers alike to recognize that a disabled woman's lack of independence does not diminish her mothering skill. Rather, it shifts the focus to the value of facilitating self-determination instead of self-sufficiency in the parenting role. This distinction is a crucial one. It suggests that parents with disabilities should be (a) the primary decision makers in the care of their children, (b) encouraged to personally perform as many parenting tasks as they can carry out safely, and (c) supported with a caregiver when they cannot or choose not to perform an activity independently. A caregiver can be a family member, spouse, friend, or hired personal assistant. Caregivers are most beneficial when they enhance the special bond between a parent and child

Item Name: Care of Others (Child Care)

Definitions:

a. **Physical daily care**--Selects proper equipment, uses correct positioning, and performs the following:

- Feeding--breastfeeding, bottle feeding (includes set-up and clean-up), spoon feeding (includes opening jars)
- Changing a diaper--donning and removal (specify type: cloth with pins or diaper cover or plastic with tape) and managing hygiene
- Dressing/undressing--Donning and removal (specify type: one-piece jumpsuit, t-shirt, plastic pants, dress with snaps or buttons, socks, shoes, booties)
- Bathing--Holding, washing, drying off (indicate location: tub, sink, positioning device)
- Preparing for bed--Changing clothes, lifting and lowering side of crib, moving child from crib to lap or wheelchair, covering child with blanket
- Carrying/lifting--Lifting to and from floor and transporting 50 feet

b. **Playing/nurturing**--Selects appropriate toys/activities, uses age-appropriate interaction, and is aware of various intervention strategies for behavior management and facilitation emotional growth

c. **Illness/first aid**--Takes temperature, uses nasal aspirator, manages suppositories, and gives medication. Is aware of symptoms and is able to perform minor emergency procedures (cuts choking, CPR, poisoning), "baby-proofing" of home, and seeking assist in an emergency

d. **Community access/resourcing**--is able to select and access day care/preschool, child supplies, physician, babysitter. Is able to instruct babysitter. Is able to manage stroller and car seat (includes placement and removal from car, placing child in/out of devices), diaper bag, back pack.

Note: Select and note activities appropriate to the patient's lifestyle/abilities.

SCALE POINTS

NO CAREGIVER REQUIREMENT:
7. Complete independence: Patient can perform task safely and consistently within a functional amount of time in any environment without specialized equipment, modifications, or verbal/physical assist.
6. Modified independence: Patient can perform task safely and consistently without caregiver assistance but requires specialized equipment, an adapted environment, and/or excessive time to complete task.
REQUIRES CAREGIVER ASSISTANCE
5. Set-up/infrequent assistance: Patient consistently requires caregiver presence to initiate and/or complete task (e.g., with set-up and/or clean-up), but patient safely and consistently completes interim components independently, *or* patient requires caregiver's assistance for unpredictable occurrences only.
4. Minimal assistance: Patient performs more than three quarters of the task safely and consistently. Because of physical or cognitive impairment, patient requires caregiver to provide physical or verbal assist to complete one quarter of the task.
3. Moderate assistance: Patient performs half to three quarters of the task safely and consistently. Because of physical or cognitive impairment, patient requires caregiver to provide physical or verbal assist to complete on quarter to half the task.
2. Maximal assistance: Patient performs one quarter to half of the task safely and consistently, or may be physically unable to perform any part of the activity but can accurately direct the caregiver. Patient requires caregiver to provide physical or verbal assist to complete the remainder of the task.
1. Dependent: Patient performs less than one quarter of the task consistently. Patient is unable to direct the caregiver and is dependent of the caregiver's physical or verbal assistance for completing more than three quarters of the task.

Figure 73-4. Rehabilitation Institute of Chicago Functional Assessment Scale. The occupational therapy department would like to recognize the contribution made by Sharon Gartland, OTR/L, and Sheila Gupta, OTR/L, in the development of the definition for child care. (Used by permission of the Rehabilitation Institute of Chicago.)

(183). Health professionals and occupational therapists can help maximize the value of hired caregivers by training the caregiver how to assist the disabled mother "without taking over the role of the parent" (93).

Although efforts are under way to develop comprehensive assessment tools to evaluate a disabled mother's full range of parenting capabilities, many clinicians and therapists are continuing to rely on a protocol and activity analysis to assess child-care and parenting skills that facilitate self-determination in mothers with cognitive as well as physical disabilities (93) (Figs. 73-4 and 73-5). This approach. developed by occupational therapists at the Rehabilitation Institute of Chicago, identifies a disabled mother's abilities regarding selective child-care tasks and gives her final say in parenting decisions. On the basis of the assessment, therapist, mother, and spouse or caregiver collaborate to determine the tasks the disabled mother needs simplified, is comfortable performing independently, or will delegate to helpers.

Despite the growing numbers of mothers with disabilities and the positive impact of support resources, the lack of disability-aware social institutions and services can pose real threats to their self-determination. A profound problem related to personal assistance stems from the fact that some states exclude child care as an activity of daily living for which a disabled person can get personal assistant support. Tasks involving dinner preparation for a child or assistance in positioning for breast-feeding or bathing are not considered viable activities for state-funded assistance. Note that this issue is relevant only in cases when the parents are disabled and have nondis-

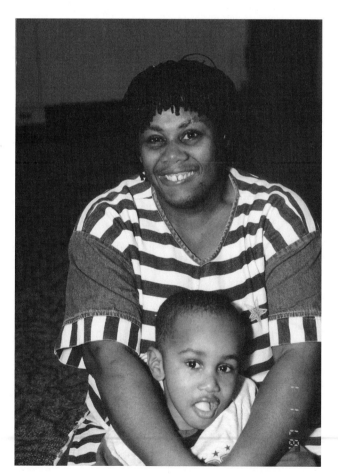

Figure 73-5. Disabled mother.

abled children. When the child is also disabled, funds for personal assistance are common (184).

Unfortunately, women with disabilities who have a low income and are unable to afford private child care have lost custody of their children because the state refused to provide assistant services and then deemed them incompetent in parental functioning (184,185). Full knowledge of state policies on the provisions of personal assistants will create realistic expectations on the part of prospective parents and assist practitioners in educating their clients.

Adoption

Stereotypes depicting women with disabilities as having to be "cared for" rather than as caregivers presents ongoing challenges to those women wishing to adopt children. Other barriers to adoptive services include the lack of universal definitions for good parenting and permitting agency staff to impose arbitrary standards onto disabled individuals applying for adoptive services (186–188). Despite these disincentives, many disabled men and women are taking advantage of the advocacy services of disability service groups and the supports of knowledgeable physicians and health providers to successfully negotiate the social and attitudinal obstacles to become adoptive parents. When screening for the parenting capabilities of a prospective parent, it is common for an adoption agency to require a physician's certification documenting the individual's good health and ability to raise a child (189). Before rendering a determination, rehabilitation and medical practitioners should carefully consider the prospective parent's support network and full spectrum of parenting abilities. To focus on the disability as a negative to the exclusion of a woman's full range of beneficial attributes may result in the denial of a child's placement with a caring and competent parent. Disabled women report that an unfavorable medical determination adds to the frustrations of an already stressful adoption process and can reinforce a host of self-doubts and low self-esteem (190). In one case, a physician (familiar to a disabled couple) arbitrarily determined that their cerebral palsy represented a potential hazard to raising a child. The mother subsequently documented the couples' challenges and successes in becoming adoptive parents by engaging in a national writing and speaking campaign to enlighten disabled women and their service providers about strategies for maximizing adoption options. Among the suggestions that she offers to medical professionals are the following:

- Read the literature on adoption for people with disabilities available via the Through the Looking Glass Web site, www.lookingglass.org.
- Remember that the same screening standards should be applied in adoption screening for all potential parents, whether they have a disability or not.
- Learn about the disabled parent's support system—what resources are available to them (e.g., family, friends neighbors, child-care assistance)?
- Examine your own concerns and be honest about your discomfort—you may not be the best person to handle this issue (191).

Rehabilitation clinicians can also be of service to prospective disabled mothers by encouraging them to become aware of their rights as they proceed with the adoption process (189).

Increasingly, a growing number of women with disabilities are publishing accounts of how they have come to remove the effects of stereotypes and discrimination by developing innovative adoption resources and methods. This includes the narra-

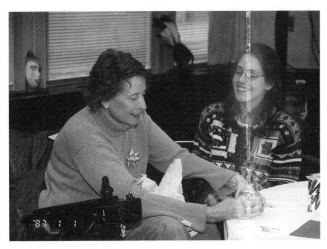

Figure 73-6. Peer support.

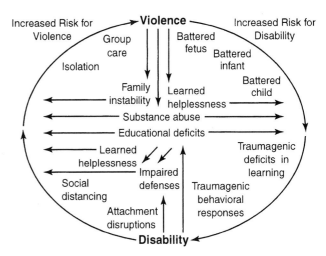

Figure 73-7. Mechanisms that contribute to the abuse and disability cycle. (From Sobsey D. *Violence and abuse in the lives of people with disabilities: the end of silent acceptance?* Baltimore: Paul H. Brookes, 1994:47, with permission.)

tives of disabled women who are lesbians and have chosen to adopt and raise a disabled child (192). Health providers are recommended to direct women with similar interests to literature that documents the expertise and adaptations derived from these personal experiences.

Peer Support

Facing the onslaught of negative messages concerning one's reproductive and parenting capacities can reinforce self-doubts in even the most confident of disabled women (Fig. 73-6). Advocates and experts around the world are finding that a disability consciousness and culture emerging from the power of peer-to-peer contact is the tried-and-true remedy for counteracting the isolation and devaluation women experience when parenting with a disability (169,193). From each other, many women are hearing for the first time that their decision to become mothers is a valid one—a cause for celebration. They rely on one another for a wholeness and strength that come not from independence and self-sufficiency, but from interdependence and self-determination. As disabled mothers increase in number, so are the national and international parenting networks for people with disabilities, many of them online (see Appendix). Most independent living centers can assist health providers in identifying the peer-support groups and networks for disabled mothers and women in their area.

VIOLENCE AND ABUSE

Unlike many traditional health concerns, domestic violence is a complex social problem rather than a biomedical one (194). It is a crime of power that utilizes fear to control a victim and is an everyday reality in the United States. Above all, domestic violence is an insidious process frequently invisible to the public and many health practitioners. Moreover, ground-breaking work by Dick Sobsey has established that disability is intrinsically linked to violence (195). This association creates a cycle of disability and violence, begetting more disability and violence, which easily entraps and proves difficult for a woman to escape (195) (Fig. 73-7). Growing evidence suggests that women with disabilities are victims of violence and abuse at rates that are similar to or higher than nondisabled women (195–199). When it comes to experiencing violence in relationships with intimate partners, this form of violence can be the same

for women with disabilities as compared with nondisabled women, but often more complex (197). This is evidenced by forms of neglect and abuse that the Center for Research on Women with Disabilities at Baylor College of Medicine (CROWD) defines as the following:

Emotional abuse can manifest in "behaviors such as emotional abandonment and rejection, or denial of disability."

Physical abuse "includes physical restraint or confinement; withholding orthotic equipment, medications, transportation; or refusing to provide assistance with essential daily living needs such as dressing or getting out of bed."

Sexual abuse "includes demanding or expecting sexual activity in return for help or taking advantage of a physical weakness and inaccessible environment to force sexual activity" (199).

Although there are no known rigorous studies that have empirically explored risk factors for abuse among women with disabilities, CROWD analyzed data from a sample of 415 women with disabilities and discovered that "women with disabilities who are younger, more educated, less mobile, more socially isolated and who have higher levels of depression are more likely to have experienced abuse within the past year" (200,201). Other factors that may elevate the susceptibility of women with disabilities to abuse include their reliance on others for personal assistance, their inability to escape, their lack of adaptive equipment, increased risk in institutional settings, stereotypes of vulnerability, and dependence on perpetrators for survival activities (198,202).

It is incumbent on health-care providers who work with women with disabilities to grasp the multiplicity of contexts in which disability factors can define the experience of violence and abuse. In a recent study, researchers from CROWD identified two findings specific to women with disabilities. First, it was established that women with disabilities were more likely than their nondisabled peers to experience abuse from a significantly greater number of perpetrators, such as attendants and disability service/health providers. Other offenders included spouses, ex-spouses, family members, strangers, and dates. Second, the study found that women with disabilities were more likely to experience abuse for longer periods of time (203). Environmental and attitudinal barriers may play a critical role in accounting for significantly longer periods of abuse

(200). The shortage of disability friendly resources, such as accessible housing, battered women's shelters, transportation, personal-care attendants, disability-aware law enforcement officers, and accessible courtrooms can cause women with disabilities who are victims of partner or caregiver abuse to feel revictimized and frustrated when they attempt to obtain help (198,204).

Another factor that may contribute to the likelihood of women with disabilities to experience sustained abuse is the lack of abuse screening administered to disabled women by disability-related service providers (200). A survey conducted by CROWD found that less than 20% of rehabilitation providers screen for abuse and violence (200). Despite this low percentage, there is evidence revealing that disabled women would welcome providers asking these questions and that asking abuse screening questions can increase the detection of violence and abuse from 0.8% to 7% (198,205). Routine abuse screening is likely to substantially increase detection of abuse among women with disabilities and to decrease their tendency to experience longer periods of abuse compared with nondisabled women.

Given that women with disabilities are at high risk for experiencing abuse from attendants and disability health/service providers, it is important to use disability specific screening tools. Asking questions that screen solely for intimate partner or spousal abuse may miss the wide range of abuse that women with disabilities can experience from caregivers or service providers. The Abuse Assessment Screen-Disability screening tool developed by researchers at CROWD (Fig. 73-8) exemplifies a tool that can be used to screen women with disabilities for general and disability-specific abuse.

The DisAbled Women's Network Canada were among the first to determine that the abuse experiences of women with disabilities are often not reported to law officers because of their fear of and dependency on the offender (206). Anecdotal evidence suggests that like other abused women, those who are disabled tend to resist reporting their experiences because of denial, guilt, self-contempt, and fear of loss of financial security. However, some experts believe that disabled women are often discouraged from disclosure because they are commonly regarded as less credible and easily discredited as witnesses by virtue of having a disability (207). Threats from abusers to withdraw assistive devices, such as wheelchairs and ventilators, as well as personal assistant services, add to the fears of disabled women and further inhibit their disclosure of violent

incidents. These threats and fears also serve as disincentives to leave abusive relationships with caregivers and family members, and reinforce the cycle of violence.

In studies investigating abuse among women with disabilities from personal assistance services, a variety of forms were identified, "including physical and sexual abuse, medication manipulation, equipment disablement or abuse" (198). Women revealed that they often refused to confront abusive personal assistance services providers because of fear of retribution and to avoid having to find a new provider (208). In in-depth studies on personal assistance services abuse conducted by the Center for Self-Determination at Oregon Health and Science University, participants described several barriers to addressing abuse: "(a) difficulty recognizing it and having their experiences validated; (b) feelings of shame or embarrassment; (c) lack of [personal assistance services] providers and emergency backup services; (d) fear of institutionalization or loss of their children if they reported the abuse; (f) lack of access to abuse services such as crisis, services, support groups and domestic violence shelters" (198). Findings from this study also indicated that women found professionals of little help in helping them to identify or to address abuse from a personal assistance service provider, but indicated they would welcome being asked about these experiences and being assisted to discover management options (198). Clinicians working with women with disabilities who are experiencing abuse from personal assistance service providers are urged to assist women in connecting with disability support groups and resource centers that can support them in developing strategies for effectively managing personal assistance service providers, e.g., learning how to draw clear boundaries and how to recognize qualified safe providers.

Sexual abuse among women with physical disabilities is commonly perpetrated by male strangers rather than acquaintances or family members (as is often the case with women with developmental disabilities) (198,209). Health-care providers are cautioned to discriminate between the signs of sexual abuse and those of disability. Frequently, symptoms of abuse are confused with the sequelae of a woman's disability, or they may be overlooked completely. Common symptoms of sexual abuse include pain, bruises, and bleeding in the genital area, behavioral disturbances, loss of weight, fear of sexual intimacy, and fear of intervention (209,210).

Practitioners are also urged to be mindful in recognizing and treating the symptoms of posttraumatic stress disorder, which can manifest in survivors of violence. When she has had previous brain trauma or injuries acquired through violence, the compounded effects may overwhelm the woman and require physicians to invoke the expertise of mental health workers familiar with such cases. Moreover, physicians must take a supportive and facilitative role in identifying and treating violence and abuse. Many states have mandatory reporting laws that require health providers to report incidents of abuse detected in their disabled patients or clients. Because the specifics of these laws can vary from state to state, it is essential that health providers educate themselves about their responsibilities.

Domestic violence requires practitioners to move beyond the biomedical model and collaborate with advocacy groups committed to ending violence against women (194). They can assist by working to facilitate access to high-quality personal assistants and to increase living options beyond nursing homes and other institutional facilities (210). Health-care providers can help prevent sexual abuse in women with disabilities by collaborating with other social services to develop comprehensive outreach strategies that are accessible to women with

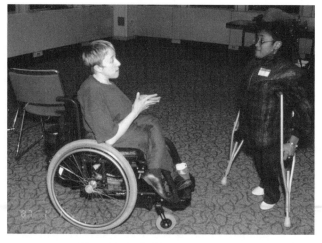

Figure 73-8. Girls' mentoring group.

physical, cognitive, sensory, and communication disabilities, including those living in institutions.

Offering high-quality health services to disabled women obliges providers to make their services available with accessible equipment, signers, and TTYs (teletype writers). It also dictates that they become knowledgeable about local accessible shelters and their policies regarding personal assistants and children. Shelters and support services are accessible only if they can be accessed by a woman at any time regardless of her disabilities. Physicians should be aware of their role in breaking the cycle of violence and disability. They are encouraged to work with disabled women's centers and social services to prevent isolation by involving the expertise of disabled women in the design and execution of outreach and education strategies. For example, transportation is a key component in any emergency. It should be factored into any protocol developed in response to abuse encounters. Most important, health providers can assist in breaking the cycle of violence and disability by implementing a system of detection, reporting, and prosecution for cases of assault. Assaults will continue unless practitioners are willing and able to implement a comprehensive protocol (211).

MENTAL HEALTH

It has been well established that women are troubled by significant depression at a rate approximately twice that of men (212–214). Among the causes hypothesized to explain this disparity have been physiology, particularly hormones; social oppression, including restricted choices and narrow standards for appearance and behavior; and socially imposed powerlessness. Although research has insufficiently addressed depression in women with disabilities, there is no reason to believe this population would be immune from the dynamics of depression affecting all women.

Women with disabilities are often members of multiple minority groups, leading to marginalization and increased risk for stress and mental health problems (215). The complexities and pressures of living with a disability command a balancing act of finding transportation, making appointments, filling out forms, negotiating with service agencies, managing personal assistants, worrying about equipment breakdowns, and coping with discrimination. For women, who are more likely than men with disabilities to confront poverty and social isolation, the lack of adequate resources can compound the routine pressures of disability, leading to depression and feelings of hopelessness. A study of women with SCIs found that these women reported significantly higher levels of perceived stress and scored higher in depression than both men with the same disability and women in the general population (216).

A survey study of women with disabilities in Canada found a significant association between suicide, depression, and abuse (217). Of 371 women with a variety of disabilities, more than 60% had contemplated suicide, of which 45% had attempted suicide at least once. Approximately half had experienced physical abuse or sexual abuse, and two-thirds had experienced emotional abuse. The more abuse a woman had experienced, the more likely she was to have considered suicide. Aside from abuse, the two factors mentioned most by the women as contributing to their suicidality were poverty and isolation.

The social role loss that all too often accompanies disablement in our society may be a significant risk factor for depression and suicide in elderly women. One study has found that women who enter nursing homes because of age-related disability often respond to their powerlessness, loss of control over life, and cessation of meaningful social involvement by passively foregoing life-sustaining behaviors, e.g., taking medications. The authors refer to this phenomenon as "acquiescent suicide" (218). In contrast, another researcher found that many older women with disabilities maintain a high level of psychological well-being as they age, a quality they authors refer to as "emotional vitality" (219). Along with such variables as income and cognitive functioning, aspects of the social environment were correlated strongly with emotional vitality. The researchers found that the critical element of social relationships was not frequency of contacts but the availability of "enough warmth and understanding to meet an individual's needs."

Treatable depression in disabled women remains undiagnosed when health-service providers incorrectly assume that depression is a natural concomitant of disability. Although depression is an expected feature of the initial disability adjustment process, it should be noted and addressed with support, counseling, and other interventions appropriate to situational distress. Beyond the adjustment phase, depression in women with disabilities calls for a thorough exploration of specific causes (whether directly related to the woman's disability or not) and a review of potentially effective interventions by professionals knowledgeable about disability issues. Peer support can be a powerful adjunct to professional treatment.

Unfortunately, many women's clinics and community mental health centers are inaccessible to women with disabilities. Residential treatment programs for substance abuse and psychiatric disorders commonly refuse to admit women who use equipment or need physical assistance with activities of daily living. Sexual counseling, psychotherapy, and suicide intervention are rarely available from therapists who are adequately informed about the stressors and options resulting from the interaction of being a woman and being disabled. A concerned physician can be an important ally in a disabled woman's journey through depression, from identification of the problem to support in surmounting the barriers to adequate mental health services. The management of depression is a critical facet of disabled women's health care, and the consequences of failing to address it can be grave, as evidenced by the disproportionate number of women with disabilities who have requested assisted suicide (220).

HEALTH CONSIDERATIONS FOR GIRLS WITH DISABILITIES

It is estimated that girls with disabilities comprise somewhere between 5% and 8% of female youth. This includes girls with physical, cognitive, emotional, and learning disabilities (221). Research also suggests that compared with their nondisabled female and disabled male counterparts, girls with disabilities "experience higher rates of physical and sexual abuse, higher rates of adolescent pregnancy, and lower employment rates and income levels upon leaving school. They may also have more limited access to quality health care and sexuality education"(221).

Although girls and young women with disabilities share similar health-care issues with their nondisabled peers, their health encounters are likely to be more frequent, intense, and complex. In addition to routine adolescent health needs, disabled girls may encounter a regime of repeated disability-specific hospitalizations, health visits, and medication schedules that can intrude into their family, school, and social lives (222).

Sensitivity to the medicalization of these girls' lives is important and should be demonstrated by actively engaging the girls in the decision-making process as it affects their health issues. This can be accomplished in partnership with a parent or caregiver as long as the girl is not coerced into unwanted decisions, and is supported with information in a user-friendly format that allows her to be self-determining. The promotion of self-determination in girls and young women with disabilities serves to decrease the incidence of negative health encounters while optimizing the likelihood of compliance with healthy life choices.

Given that disabled girls frequently do not have access to accurate formal sexuality education and that their access to informal information on the subject acquired through friends, family, and the media is often limited or inaccurate, the role of the health-care provider as educator is critical (222). This is especially important when it comes to issues of management of menses, contraception, pregnancy, sexually transmitted diseases, breast health, and how these reproductive or gynecologic issues may interact with their disabilities. It is also likely that, as is the case with many girls in general, disabled girls may also want to talk to their doctors and clinicians about drugs, smoking, alcohol, sexual abuse, and emotional concerns, such as anger and sadness (222).

Given the higher rates of pregnancy and single parenthood for adolescent women than for nondisabled peers or disabled young men (222), it is essential that health providers offer disability-friendly contraception options or connect disabled young women with pregnancy prevention services, as well as teen parenting programs. These programs need to be accessible and take into consideration strategies to minimize the risks of pregnancy for disabled young women and the harmful secondary social consequences (e.g., school dropout, limited employment), and to "expand their options . . . should they become pregnant" (222).

Recent surveys polling disabled teens on their health care indicate that the teens were "eager to take charge of their own health care and that they need more information and support to address the formidable barriers they face" (222). Among the barriers they identified were parental overprotection and their own fears. In addition to expressing an interest for more information about their disability and medical issues from their health providers and clinicians, disabled teens also indicated an interest in having contact with an adult with a disability who can serve as a mentor to discuss health promotion, risk behaviors, and concerns, including sexuality and family planning (222).

TABLE 73-2.   Abuse Assessment Screening Measure

Abuse Assessment Screen-Disability (AAS-D) (Circle YES or NO)

1. *Within the last year,* have you been hit, slapped, kicked, pushed, shoved, or otherwise physically hurt by someone?   YES ____   NO ____

   If YES, who? (Circle all that apply)

   Intimate partner   Care provider   Health professional   Family member   Other

   Please describe: _____

2. *Within the last year,* has anyone forced you to have sexual activities?   YES ____   NO ____

   If YES, who? (Circle all that apply)

   Intimate partner   Care provider   Health professional   Family member   Other

   Please describe: _____

3. *Within the last year,* has anyone prevented you from using a wheelchair, cane, respirator, or other assistive devices?   YES ____   NO ____

   If YES, who? (Circle all that apply)

   Intimate partner   Care provider   Health professional   Family member   Other

   Please describe: _____

4. *Within the last year,* has anyone you depend on refused to help you with an important personal need, such as taking your medicine, getting to the bathroom, getting out of bed, bathing, getting dressed, or getting food or drink?   YES ____   NO ____

   If YES, who? (Circle all that apply)

   Intimate partner   Care provider   Health professional   Family member   Other

   Please describe: _____

From McFarlane J, Hughes RB, Nosek MA, et al. Abuse Assessment Screen-Disability (AAS-D): measuring frequency, type and perpetrator of abuse toward women with physical disabilities. *Journal Womens Health Gend Based Med* 2001;10(9):861–866.

Among the cluster of programs serving youth with disabilities (see Appendix) is a gender-specific mentoring program in Chicago that has experienced success in tackling many of the issues identified by the teens above. The Mentee/Mentor Roll Model Program sponsored by the Health Resource Center for Women with Disabilities at the Rehabilitation Institute of Chicago is a community based program that pairs disabled teen girls between the ages of 13 and 19 with disabled women mentors, and aims to break down social isolation and promote self-determination skills to achieve emotional and physical wellness among the girls (Table 73-2). Mentoring pairs are required to have three contacts per month and to attend monthly meetings with the entire mentoring group to enhance a sense of disability pride and membership in the disabled women's community. Under the supervision of disabled women professionals who work closely with staff from the rehabilitation hospital, the girls themselves developed the program format as well as its activities and topics for group discussion. Dating, sexuality, sexual abuse and violence, career planning, higher education, self-advocacy, and visits to an accessible gynecologic clinic, accompanied by a discussion with a knowledgeable health-care professional on reproductive health issues, have routinely been included in this model program.

MODEL HEALTH SERVICES: THE ROLE OF COMMUNITY

A list of health-service organizations focused on disabled women's issues is given in the Appendix.

In 1988, Aimee Jackson, M.D., Director of the Spain Rehabilitation Center at the University of Alabama in Birmingham, inaugurated the first clinic in the United States offering reproductive health services specifically for women with disabilities (the Women's Clinic for the Disabled). The treatment center is fully wheelchair accessible and has a flexible examining table that facilitates unassisted transfers and eases the examination process. Working closely with an obstetrician/gynecologist, Dr. Jackson offers disabled women the benefit of "combined expertise" (223).

After a long history of neglect by both the medical and women's communities, disabled women are currently finding a voice in both planned and existing health services. Gaining increased respect as the experts in their own lives, they are acquiring decision-making authority and local ownership in programs designed to serve their needs. Although the manifestations of these efforts are varied in health-service delivery throughout North America, the community-driven perspective emerges as a common theme in several prominent programs addressing disabled women's health concerns. This is illustrated in three programs that developed their community orientation in different ways in Los Angeles, Chicago, and Houston.

The California Family Planning Council initiated a federally funded Americans with Disabilities Act and Reproductive Health Project in 1993 under the direction of Barbara Fiduccia Waxman, a disabled woman and certified sex educator expert in disabled women's reproductive concerns. The project, originating in Los Angeles, aimed to enable federally funded family planning clinics in the United States to provide accessible medical, educational, and counseling services to individuals with a wide variety of disabilities: mobility, hearing, visual, and cognitive. An important goal of this project was to build significant relationships between the council's clinics and women from local disability communities.

Programs like this are predicated on a community organization approach to health that encourages community participation rather than institutional dependency (224). This concept stresses that the role of health clinicians is to facilitate community health programs. Successful implementation of a community empowerment model obliges physicians to work collaboratively with members from the local disabled women's community in shaping the delivery of medical services, conducting research, and developing educational resources.

The Health Resource Center for Women with Disabilities at the Rehabilitation Institute of Chicago brings to life the vision of a balanced partnership between local disabled women activists and the staff of a rehabilitation hospital (see Appendix). The center started in 1991 as a clinic offering accessible, collaborative reproductive health-care services. Its goal is to assist disabled women to become self-determining in achieving physical and emotional wellness.

The backbone of the center from its inception has been a community board of 20 women of diverse backgrounds and disabilities who work with medical and rehabilitation staff to find solutions to the access problems preventing women from obtaining reproductive health-care services. As members of its community board, they have expanded services to include the center's research component and an educational mission emphasizing psychosocial resources, such as parenting, aging, teen mentoring, and antiviolence support. The lifeblood of the center, the community board, sets research and training priorities and provides ongoing feedback to the center's medical director, a woman physiatrist, and the administrative director, a disabled woman professional.

The Health Resource Center for Women with Disabilities is committed to its investment in the leadership abilities of its disabled women professionals who conduct research, ongoing peer support groups, and periodic conferences, seminars, and in-services targeting physicians, clinicians, and consumers. They have also created a resource library that handles information and referrals and collaborates in producing educational videos and an international newsletter published once a year. Hospital medical and administrative staff assist with fund-raising and program development as needed.

CROWD was founded in 1993 by Margaret Nosek, Ph.D. When Nosek, a researcher with a disability, received a grant from the National Institutes of Health to study the psychosocial concerns of women with disabilities, including sexuality, domestic violence, and self-esteem, she was besieged with nationwide requests from disabled women asking to participate in the study. The grant and ensuing outcry from community women moved Nosek to start the center. In contrast to other community health initiatives, the center offers no treatment services. Instead, Nosek, as the center's director, works with a team of other researchers with disabilities toward the end of improving reproductive health services for disabled women. Nosek supports mainstreaming services for disabled women into community health centers as opposed to offering services solely in specialty clinics (223). To meet this goal, Nosek and her team are committed to dismantling attitudinal and knowledge barriers preventing disabled women from receiving quality care by developing research and training materials for primary care physicians and ob/gyn providers.

This raises a crucial question: Are reproductive health services for disabled women more viable when they reside in specialty clinics or when they are mainstreamed into community health settings? Advocates favoring equal access to neighborhood health centers caution that taken to the extreme, specialty clinics reinforce negative stereotypes, emphasizing the disability over the woman and suggesting that the disabled woman is without legitimate women's concerns. But others, preferring treatments from physicians who understand their disabilities, warn that traditional community clinics are often staffed with disability-unaware physicians whose practices can unwittingly cause them harm or humiliation. This structure also guarantees outreach to larger numbers of disabled women using the rehabilitation center for other services. Mindful of the merits inherent in each model, many professionals and advocates agree that creating a full spectrum of health services available to disabled women is an ideal worth striving for and one that gives women the choices they need to become truly self-determining.

ACKNOWLEDGMENTS AND DEDICATION

We would like to thank Virginia Dare White for her invaluable assistance and support, and Dr. Raymond Curry and Dr. Eileen Murphy for their critical review of the manuscript.

We would like to dedicate this chapter to Dr. Sandra Welner and Ms. Barbara Fiduccia Waxman, whose untimely deaths have left a significant void. Dr. Welner, a disabled ob/gyn, was a coauthor on the original version of this chapter and a pioneer in disabled women's health-care services. Ms. Waxman was a disability activist and feminist who led the way in integrating federally funded family planning clinics and victim service centers for individuals with disabilities.

APPENDIX: SELECTED MODEL PROGRAMS AND RESOURCES FOR WOMEN WITH DISABILITIES

National Council on Independent Living (NCIL)
(877) 525–3400 (toll-free)
www.ncil.org.

Domestic Violence Initiative for Women with Disabilities
P.O. Box 300535
Denver, CO 80203
(303) 839–5510 (V)
E-mail: dvidenver@aol.com
Director: Sharon Hickman

This is a nationally respected center of information and support for women with disabilities experiencing domestic violence and for their allies and health professionals.

National Clearinghouse for Women and Girls with Disabilities
Educational Equity Concepts, Inc.
114 East 32nd Street
New York, NY 10016
(212) 725–1803 (V)
www.calcna.ab.ca/actlibrary/contents.html

This is a national repository of information on organizations and services for women with disabilities that publishes and disseminates the publication, Bridging the Gap: A Directory of Services for Women and Girls with Disabilities.

Berkeley Policy Associates (BPA)
440 Grand Avenue, Suite 500
Oakland, CA 94610
(510) 465–7884 (V)
(510) 465–4493 (TTY)
E-mail: info@bpacal.com
www.bpacal.com
Director: Linda Toms Barker

Researching and identifying access barriers to mainstream services for women with disabilities nationally.

Americans with Disabilities Act and Reproductive Health Project
Los Angeles Family Planning Council
Satellite Office
19907 Beekman Place
Cupertino, CA 94014–2452
(408) 996–9005

Project works to enable federally funded family planning clinics and victim services centers in United States to provide accessible medical, educational, and counseling services to individuals with a wide variety of disabilities.

Center on Research on Women with Disabilities
Department of Physical Medicine and Rehabilitation
Baylor Medical College
3440 Richmond, Suite B
Houston, TX 77046
(713) 960–0505 (V and TTY)
(713) 961–3555 (fax)
E-mail: crowd@bcm.tmc.edu
www.bcm.tmc.edu/crowd
Director: Margaret Nosek

The center works to develop research and training materials for primary care physicians and ob/gyn providers.

Disability, Pregnancy, and Parenthood International
National Centre for Disabled Parents
Unit F9, 89–93 Fronthill Road
London, N4 3JH
England
www.dppi.org.uk

Periodic newsletter by subscription for professionals and parents to exchange information and experience. A forum in the United Kingdom for professionals and parents to exchange information and experience

The Women's Center at Premier Healthcare
175 Remsen Street
Brooklyn, NY 11201
(212) 273–6100, ext 2132 (V)
(212) 273–6458 (fax)
E-mail: thewomenscenter@yai.org
www.yai.org
Chief of Staff: Dr. Debra Shabas

The Women's Center provides high-quality, coordinated health care for women with disabilities. Their practice includes primary and specialty care, dentistry, rehabilitation and mental health services

The Center for Women with Physical Disabilities
Magee-Women's Hospital of UPMC Health Systems
300 Halket Street
Pittsburgh, PA 15213
(412) 647–4747, (800) 804–7750 (toll-free) (V)
E-mail: www.pd@mail.magee.edu
Director: Jaye E. Hefner, MD

Comprehensive health-care center for women with physical disabilities dedicated to meeting the unique needs of these women by significantly reducing social and physical barriers to the access and application of comprehensive health services and preventive care.

Center on Self-Determination Oregon Health and Science University
3608 S.E. Powell Boulevard
Portland, OR 97202
(503) 232–9154
www.ohsu.edu
Director: Dr. Laurie Powers

The center is dedicated to identifying, developing, validating, and communicating policies and practices that promote the self-determination of people with and without disabilities. Projects include domestic violence program and youth program.

Breast Health Access for Women with Disabilities (BHAWD)
Alta Bates Comprehensive Breast Center—Herrick Campus
2001 Dwight Way
Berkeley, CA 94704
(510) 204–4866
www.bhawd.org

Clinic devoted to breaking barriers for breast health access for women with disabilities. The clinic is equipped with Bennett's Contour Mammography System and trains disabled women in breast self-examination.

Health Resource Center for Women with Disabilities (HRCWD)
Rehabilitation Institute of Chicago
345 East Superior, #106
Chicago, IL 60611
(312) 238–8003 (V)
(312(238–1205 (fax)
E-mail: HRCWD@RIC.ORG
Director: Judy Panko Reis, MA, MS
Medical Director: Kristi L. Kirschner, MD

Newsletter Resourceful Woman *written by, about, and for women with disabilities is published three times a year, available at no charge. Includes a parenting peer advice column for disabled mothers and mothers-to-be written by professionals with personal parenting with a disability experience.*

M&M Roll Model Program—Health Resource Center for Women with Disabilities at the Rehabilitation Institute of Chicago fosters new and ongoing mentoring relationships between teen girls with disabilities between 13 and 19 and women with disabilities. This disabled teen girl-centered mentoring program is an opportunity for girls with disabilities to:

- *Develop self-confidence and self-esteem*
- *Increase leadership and advocacy skills*
- *Explore different ways to integrate their disability with their self-identity*

Partners for Youth with Disabilities, Inc.
95 Berkeley Street, #407
Boston, MA 02116
(617) 556–4075 (V and TDD)
E-mail: holt_ty@hotmail.com
http://www.pyd.org/home.html
Program Coordinator: Ty Holt

Mentoring program for youth with disabilities in Boston area.

Through the Looking Glass
P.O. Box 8226
Berkeley, CA 94707–8138
(510) 525–8138 (V)

(800) 644–2666 (toll-free)
(510) 527–8137 (TTY)
www.lookingglass.org
Director: Megan Kirshbaum

National research and training center on families of adults with disabilities offering free periodic publication, Parent with a Disability. *If you are caring for a child and you have a physical disability, you should look at the wonderful ideas from Through the Looking Glass at* http://www.ncddr.org/rr/parent/result.html

Want to know more about parenting with a disability? Go to this comprehensive Web site: www.disabledparents.net. There you will find books, medical information, adaptive parenting products, and toy ideas, as well as stories from other disabled parents. This is a great, one-of-a-kind resource.

The National Parent-To-Parent Network connects parents with disabilities who want to share their experiences and learn from each other. To learn more about this network, or to join it, please call or write to:

Nikki Brown-Booker, MFTI
Through the Looking Glass
2198 Sixth Street, Suite 100
Berkeley, CA 94710
Local and international calls: (510) 848–1112, ext 101
Toll-free TTY: (800) 804–1616
www.lookingglass.org

Disabled Women's Health Center
Spain Rehabilitation Hospital
1717 6th Avenue South
Birmingham, AL 35233
(205) 934–3330 (V)
Director: Aimee Jackson, MD

First collaborative clinic designed to meet the reproductive health-care issues of women with disabilities.

Access WOW (Women's Outpatient Wellness)
SSM Rehabilitation
6420 Clayton Road
St. Louis, MO 63117
Voice: (314) 768–5200 (press "1")
Toll-free TTY: (800) 735–2966
Medical Director: Thy Huskey, MD
Manager of Women's Services: Angela Allen, (312) 768–5321

Opened in summer 2002, this disabled women's health clinic was designed to provide comprehensive health care in the St. Louis region, including gynecologic exams and mammograms, in close collaboration with Paraquad Inc., the local independent living center.

REFERENCES

1. Gill CJ, Kirschner KL, Panko Reis J. Women with disabilities: barriers and portals. In: Dan A, ed. *Reframing women's health.* San Francisco: Sage Publications, 1994:257–266.
2. Nosek MA, Young ME, Rintala DH. Barriers to reproductive health maintenance among women with physical disabilities. *J Womens Health* 1995;4 (5):505.
3. health care professionals. Educational video produced by the Health Resource Center for Women with Disabilities at the Rehabilitation Institute of Chicago (2002), 345 East Superior Street, Chicago, IL 60611.
4. Tate DG, Roller S, Riley B. Quality of life for women with physical disabilities. In Cardenas D, ed. *Women's issues, physical medicine and rehabilitation clinics of North America.* Philadelphia: WB Saunders, 2001;12:1, 23–37.
5. Perlman L, Arneson D. *Women and rehabilitation of disabled persons: a report of the sixth annual Mary E. Switzer Memorial Seminar.* Washington, D.C.: National Rehabilitation Association, 1982.

6. Grabois E. Guide to getting reproductive health care services for women with disabilities under the Americans with Disabilities Act of 1990. *Sexuality and Disability* 2001;19(3):191–208.
7. Bulger RE. Special reports: inclusion of women in clinical trials—policies for population subgroups. *N Engl J Med* 1993;329:288–296.
8. Wenger NK, Speroff L, Packard B. Cardiovascular health and disease in women. *N Engl J Med* 1993;329:247–272.
9. Jans L, Stoddard S. *Chartbook on Women and Disability in the United States.* An InfoUse Report. Washington, DC: U.S. Department of Education, National Institute on Disability and Rehabilitation Research, 1999.
10. LaPlante MP, Carlson D. *Disability in the United States: prevalence and causes, 1992.* Disability Statistics Report (7). Washington, DC: National Institute on Disability and Rehabilitation Research, 1996.
11. McNeil JM. *Americans with disabilities: 1991–1992.* U.S. Bureau of the Census. Current Population Reports, P70–33. Washington, DC: U.S. Government Printing Office, 1993.
12. McNeil JM. *Americans with disabilities: 1994–95.* U.S. Bureau of the Census, Current Population Reports, P70–61. Washington, DC: U.S. Department of Commerce, 1997.
13. Fine M, Asch A. Introduction: Beyond pedestals. In Fine M,. Asch A, eds. *Women with disabilities: essays in psychology, culture, and politics.* Philadelphia: Temple University Press, 1988.
14. Altman BM. Causes, risks, and consequences of disability among women with physical disabilities. In: Krotoski DM, Nosek MA, Turk MA, eds. *Achieving and maintaining health and well-being.* Baltimore: Paul H. Brookes, 1996:35–56.
15. Tilley CM. Sexuality in women with physical disabilities: a social justice or health issue? *Sexuality and Disability* 1996;14:139–151.
16. Larson EJ. *Sex, race, and science: eugenics in the deep south.* Baltimore: John Hopkins University Press, 1995.
17. Mathews J. *A mother's touch: the Tiffany Callo story.* New York: Henry Holt, 1992.
18. Shapiro JP. *No pity: people with disabilities forging a new civil rights movement.* New York: Times Books, 1993.
19. Jackson AB. Pregnancy and delivery. In: Krotoski DM, Nosek MA, Turk MA, eds. *Women with physical disabilities: achieving and maintaining health and well-being.* Baltimore: Paul H. Brookes, 1996:91–99.
20. Waxman BF. It's time to politicize our sexual oppression. *Disability Rag* 1991;Mar/Apr:23–26.
21. Nosek MA, Rintala DH, Young ME, et al. Sexual functioning among women with physical disabilities. *Arch Phys Med Rehabil* 1996;77:107–115.
22. Beckmann CRB, Gittler M, Barzansky BM, Beckmann CA. Gynecologic health care of women with disabilities. *Obstet Gynecol* 1989;74:75–79.
23. Jensen JT, Speroff L. Health benefits of oral contraceptives. *Obstet Gynecol Clin North Am* 2000;27:705–721.
24. Mishell DR Jr. Noncontraceptive benefits of oral contraceptives. *J Reprod Med* 1993;38[Suppl 12]:1021–1029.
25. Coleman M, McCowan L, Farquhar C. The levonorgestrel releasing intra-uterine device: a wider role than contraception. *Aust N Z J Obstet Gynaecol* 1997;37:195–201.
26. Luukkainen T, Toivonen J. Levonorgestrel-releasing IUD as a method of contraception with therapeutic properties. *Contraception* 1995;52:269–276.
27. Istre O, Trolle B. Treatment of menorrhagia with the levonorgestrel intra-uterine system versus endometrial resection. *Fertil Steril* 2001;76:304–309.
28. Yarkony GM, Novick AK, Roth EJ, et al. Galactorrhea: a complication of spinal cord injury. *Arch Phys Med Rehabil* 1991;73(9):878–880.
29. De Leo R, Petruk KC, Crockford P. Galactorrhea after prolonged traumatic coma: a case report. *Neurosurgery* 1981;9:177–178.
30. Reame NE. A prospective study of the menstrual cycle and spinal cord injury. *Am J Phys Med Rehabil* 1992;71:15–21.
31. Jackson AB, Wadley V. A multicenter study of women's self reported reproductive health after spinal cord injury. *Arch Phys Med Rehabil* 1999;80:1420–1428.
32. Smith PJ, Surks MI. Multiple effects of 5,5N-diphenylhydantonin on the thyroid hormone systems. *Endocr Rev* 1984;5:514–524.
33. Kletzky OA, Davajan V. Hyperprolactinemia. In: Mishell DR, Davajan V, Lobo RA, eds. *Infertility, contraception, and reproductive endocrinology.* Boston: Blackwell Scientific Publications, 1991:809–851.
34. Wathen PI, Hendersen MC, Witz CA. Abnormal uterine bleeding. *Med Clin North Am* 1995;2:329–344.
35. Ratchev E, Dokumov S. Premenopausal bleeding associated with hyperprolactinaemia. *Maturitas* 1995;3:197–200.
36. Severino M. Endocrinology, infertility, and genetics. *Gynecol Obstet* 1995;5:2.
37. Mosher WD, Pratt WF. *Fecundity and infertility in the United States, 1965–1988: advance data from vital and health statistics, no. 192.* Hyattsville, MD: National Center for Health Statistics, 1990.
38. Gill CJ. Cultivating common ground: women with disabilities. *Health/PAC Bull* 1992;22:32–37.
39. Hakim-Elahi E. Contraception for the disabled. *Female Patient* 1991;16:19–27.
40. Welner SL, Hammond C. Gynecologic and obstetric issues facing women with disabilities. In: Sciarra JJ, ed. *Gynecology and obstetrics,* vo. 1, rev. ed. Philadelphia: Lippincott Williams and Wilkins, 1999:xx–xx.
41. World Health Organization. Effect of different progestagens in low estrogen oral contraceptives on venous thromboembolic disease: collaborative study of cardiovascular disease and steroid hormone contraception. *Lancet* 1995;346:1582–1588.
42. Speroff L, Glass RH, Kase NG. *Clinical gynecologic endocrinology and infertility,* 5th ed. Baltimore: Williams & Wilkins, 1994.

43. East Tennessee State University James H Quillen College of Medicine, Johnson City. Depo-Provera: an injectable contraceptive. *Am Fam Physician* 1994;49:891–894, 897–898.
44. Datey S, Gaur LN, Saxena BN. Vaginal bleeding patterns of women using different contraceptive methods (implants, injectables, IUDs, oral pills). *Contraception* 1995;51:155–165.
45. Mainwaring R, Hales HA, Stevenson K, et al. Metabolic parameter, bleeding, and weight changes in U.S. women using progestin only contraceptives. *Contraception* 1995;51:149–153.
46. Cundy T, Evans M, Roberts H, et al. Bone density in women receiving depot medroxyprogesterone acetate for contraception. *BMJ* 1991;303:13–16.
47. Forrest JD. US women's perceptions of and attitudes about the IUD. *Obstet Gynecol Surv* 1996;51[Suppl]:S30–34.
48. Darney PD. Time to pardon the IUD? *N Engl J Med* 2001;345:608–610.
49. Cheng D. The intrauterine device: still misunderstood after all these years. *South Med J* 2000;93 859–864.
50. Fortney JA, Feldblum PJ, Raymond ED. Intrauterine devices: the optimal long-term contraceptive method? *J Reprod Med* 1999;44:269–274.
51. Dardano KL, Burkman RT. The intrauterine contraceptive device: an often forgotten and maligned method of contraception *Am J Obstet Gynecol* 1999;181:1–5.
52. ACOG technical bulletin: the intrauterine device. *Int J Gynaecol Obstet* 1993;41:189–193.
53. Hubacher D, Grimes D. Noncontraceptive health benefits of intrauterine devices: a systemative review. *Obstet Gynecol Surv* 2002;57:120–128.
54. DisAbled Women's Network (DAWN). *I want to be a mother I have a disability: what are my choices?* Available from DAWN, Toronto, Ontario M4A 1Z3, 1993.
55. Pischke ME. Parenting with a disability. Special issue: reproductive issues for persons with physical disabilities. *Sexuality and Disability* 1993;11:3.
56. Asrael W. An approach to motherhood for disabled women. *Rehab Literature* 1982;43:214–218.
57. Baker ER, Cardenas DD. Pregnancy in spinal cord injured women. *Arch Phys Med Rehabil* 1996;77:501–507.
58. Koren G, Pastuszak A, Ito S. Drugs in pregnancy. *N Engl J Med* 1998;338(16):1128–1137.
59. Zahn CA, Morreel MJ, Collins SD, et al. Management issues for women with epilepsy: a review of the literature. *Neurology* 1998;51;949–956.
60. Morrell MJ. Guidelines for the care of women with epilepsy. *Neurology* 1998;51[Suppl 4]:S21–S27.
61. Quality Subcommittee of the American Academy of Neurology. Practice Parameter: Management issues for women with epilepsy (summary statement). 1998;51:944–948.
62. Rudnik-Schoneborn S, Rohrig D, Nicholson G, Zerres K. Pregnancy and delivery in Charcot-Marie-Tooth disease type 1. *Neurology* 1993;43:2011–2016.
63. Abramsky O. Pregnancy and multiple sclerosis. *Ann Neurol* 1994[Suppl];36:S38–S41.
64. Birk K, Ford C, Smeltzer S, et al. The clinical course of multiple sclerosis during pregnancy and the puerperium. *Arch Neurol* 1990;47:738–742.
65. Carter GT, Bonekat HW, Milio L. Successful pregnancies in the presence of spinal muscular atrophy: two case reports. *Arch Phys Med Rehabil* 1994;75:229–231.
66. Sadovnick AD, Eisen K, Hashimoto SA, et al. Pregnancy and multiple sclerosis: a prospective study. *Arch Neurol* 1994;51:1120–1124.
67. Damek DM, Shuster EA. Pregnancy and multiple sclerosis. *Mayo Clin Proc* 1997;72:977–989.
68. Asrael W. The rehabilitation team's role during the childbearing years for disabled women. *Sexuality and Disability* 1987;8:47–62.
69. Guthrie M. Bringing up baby: products for parents with disabilities. *Team Rehab Report* 1997;June:17–19.
70. Rogers J, Matsumura M. *Mother to be: a guide to pregnancy and birth for women with disabilities.* New York: Demos Publications, 1991.
71. Yarkony GM. Spinal cord injured women: sexuality, fertility and pregnancy. In: Goldstein PJ, Stern BJ, eds. *Neurologic disorders of pregnancy.* Mt. Kisco, NY: Futura, 1992:203–222.
72. Cohen BS, Hilton EB. Spinal cord disorders and pregnancy. In: Goldstein PJ, ed. *Neurological disorders of pregnancy.* Mt. Kisco, NY: Futura, 1986:139–152.
73. Baker ER, Cardenas DD. Pregnancy in spinal cord injured women. *Arch Phys Med Rehabil* 1996;77:501–507.
74. Craig DI. The adaptation to pregnancy of spinal cord injured women. *Rehabil Nurs* 1990;15:6–9.
75. Cunningham FG, MacDonald PC, Gant NF, et al., eds. *Williams obstetrics,* 20th ed. New York, NY:Appleton and Lange, 1997.
76. Ling FW, Duff P. *Obstetrics and gynecology: principles for practice.* New York: McGraw-Hill Medical Publishing Division, 2001.
77. Santos AC, Petrikovsky BM, Kaplan GP. Neurologic and muscular disease. In:Datta S, ed. *Anesthetic and obstetric management of high risk pregnancy.* St. Louis: Mosby, 1991:135–168.
78. Greenspoon JS, Paul RH. Paraplegia and quadriplegia: special considerations during pregnancy and labor and delivery. *Am J Obstet Gynecol* 1986;155:738–741.
79. American College of Obstetricians and Gynecologists. Committee on Obstetrics, Maternal-Fetal Medicine. *Committee Opinion 121: Management of labor and delivery for patients with spinal cord injury.* Washington, DC: ACOG, 1993:1–2.
80. McGregor JA, Meeuwsen J. Autonomic hyperreflexia: a mortal danger for spinal cord-damaged women in labor. *Am J Obstet Gynecol* 1985;151:330–333.

81. Verduyn WH. Spinal cord injured women, pregnancy and delivery. *Paraplegia* 1986;24:231–240.
82. Wanner MB, Rageth CJ, Zach GA. Pregnancy and autonomic hyperreflexia in patients with spinal cord lesions. *Paraplegia* 1987;25:482–490.
83. Creasy RK. Medical complications of labor and delivery. In: *Management of labor and delivery*. Malden, MA: Blackwell Science, 1997:506–526.
84. Brooke MM, Dononvon WH, Stolov WC. Paraplegia: succinylcholine-induced hyperkalemia and cardiac arrest. *Arch Phys Med Rehabil* 1978;59:306–308.
85. Schonwald G, Fish KJ, Perkash I. Cardiovascular complications during anesthesia in chronic spinal cord injured patients. *Anesthesiology* 1981;55:550–558.
86. Tabsh KMA, Brinkman CR III, Reff RA. Autonomic dysreflexia in pregnancy. *Obstet Gynecol* 1982;60:119–121.
87. Letcher JC, Goldfine LJ. Management of a pregnant paraplegic patient in a rehabilitation center. *Arch Phys Med Rehabil* 1986;67:477–478.
88. Saxton M, ed. Special issue: Women with disabilities: reproduction and motherhood. *Sexuality and Disability* 1994;12.
89. Westgren N, Levi R. Motherhood after traumatic spinal cord injury. *Paraplegia* 1994;32:517–523.
90. Campion MJ, ed. Who's carrying the baby? *Dis Pregnancy Parent Int* 1993;3.
91. Freda M, Cioschi HM, Nilson C. Childbearing issues for women with physical disabilities. *Am Occup Ther Assoc* 1989;12:1–4.
92. Stewart C. Raising children from a wheelchair. *Am Occup Ther Assoc Spec Int Sect Newslett* 1989;12:5–8. .
93. Culler KH, Jasch C, Scanlon S. Childcare and parenting issues for the young stroke survivor. *Top Stroke Rehabil* 1994;1:48–64.
94. Kirshbaum M. Mothers with physical disabilities. In: Kratoski DM, Nosek MA, Turk MA, eds. *Women with physical disabilities: achieving and maintaining health and well-being*. Baltimore: Paul H. Brookes, 1996:125–133.
95. Hughes HE, ed. *The creative woman, swimming upstream: managing disabilities*. University Park, IL: Governors State University, 1991.
96. Finger A. *Past due: a story of disability, pregnancy and birth*. Seattle: Seal Press, 1990.
97. Beck V, Beck K. Who'll teach Michael to play baseball? *Spinal Network Extra* 1991;spring:26–28.
98. Buck FM, Hohmann GW. Parental disability and children's adjustment. *Annu Rev Rehabil* 1983;3:203–241.
99. Crown-Fletcher J. *Mama zooms*. New York: Scholastic, 1993.
100. Alexander CJ, Hwang K, Sipski ML. Mothers with spinal cord injuries: impact on marital, family, and children's adjustment. *Arch Phys Med Rehabil* 2002;83:24–30.
101. Delhaas EM, Verhagen J. Pregnancy in a quadriplegic patient treated with continuous intrathecal baclofen infusion to manage her severe spasticity: case report. *Paraplegia* 1992;30:527–528.
102. Posch A, Chen Z, Raulg-Heimsoth M, Baur X. Latex allergens: review of current knowledge. *Pneumologie* 1997;51:1058.
103. Welner SL. Compassion and comprehension key to care of the disabled woman. *Focus* 1992;5:1–6.
104. Waller L, Reader G, Etingen O, et al., eds. *Textbook of women's health: caring for the woman with a disability*. Boston: Little, Brown, 1998.
105. Ferreyra S, Hughes K. *Table manners: a guide to the pelvic examination for disabled women and health care providers*. San Francisco: Planned Parenthood Alameda/San Francisco, 1984.
106. Colachis SC III. Autonomic hyperreflexia with spinal cord injury. *J Am Paraplegia Soc* 1992;15:171–186.
107. National Cancer Institute. *National Cancer Institute fact book*. Bethesda: National Cancer Institute, 1992.
108. American College of Obstetrics and Gynecology. *Committee Opinion 140: Role of ob-gyns in diagnosis and treatment of breast disease*. Washington, DC: ACOG, 1994.
109. American College of Obstetrics and Gynecology. *Patient Education Pamphlet AP026: Detecting and treating breast disease*. Washington, DC: ACOG, 1993.
110. Recommendations of the U.S. Preventive Services Task Force 2002. www.hhs.gov/news/press/2002pres/20020221.html.
111. Vandenakker CB, Glass DD. Menopause and aging with a disability. In: Cardenas D, ed. *Women's issues, physical medicine and rehabilitation clinics of North America* 2001;12:1, 133–151.
112. Welner SL, Simon JA, Welner B. Maximizing health in women with disabilities. *Menopause* 2002;9:208–219.
113. Hurd WW. Menopause. In: Berek JS, Adashi EY, Hillard PA, eds., *Novak's gynecology*, 12th ed. Baltimore: Williams & Wilkins, 1988:981–988.
114. Coney P, Cefalo RC. Menopause: acceptance and understanding of its impact. *Women's primary health care: office practice and procedures*. New York: McGraw-Hill, 1995.
115. Grinsted L, Heltberg A, Hagen C, Djursing H. Serum sex hormone and gonadotropin concentrations in premenopausal women with multiple sclerosis. *Intern Med* 1989;226:241–244.
116. Hoek A, Van Kasteren Y, De Haan-Meulman M, et al. Dysfunction of monocytes and dendritic cells in patients with premature ovarian failure. *Am J Reprod Immunol* 1993;30:207–217.
117. Smith R, Studd JWW. A pilot study of the effect upon multiple sclerosis of the menopause, hormone replacement therapy, and the menstrual cycle. *J R Soc Med* 1992;85:612–613.
118. Ott SM. Osteoporosis in women with spinal cord injuries. In: Cardenas D, ed. *Women's issues, physical medicine and rehabilitation clinics of North America* 2001;12(1)111–113.
119. McIlree N, Kirschner KL. Osteoporosis in women with disabilities: a view of the past, present, and future. *Sexuality and Disability* 1999;17(3):237–253.
120. Grady D, Herrington D, Bittner V, et al. Cardiovascular disease outcomes during the 6.8 years of hormone therapy: Heart and Estrogen/Progestin replacement study follow-up (HERS II). *JAMA* 2002;288:49–57.
121. Hulley S, Furber C, Barret-Connor E, et al. Noncardiovascular disease outcomes during 6.8 years of hormone therapy: Heart and Estrogen/Progestin replacement study follow-up (HERS II). *JAMA* 2002;288:58–66.
122. Petitti DB. Hormone replacement therapy for prevention: more evidence, more pessimism. *JAMA* 2002;288:99–101.
123. Writing Group for the Women's Health Initiative Investigators. Risks and benefits of estrogen plus progestin in healthy postmenopausal women: principal results from the Women's Health Initiative randomized clinical trial. *JAMA*. 2002;288:321–333.
124. American College of Obstetricians and Gynecologists. Policy Statement, July 2002. www.acog.org.
125. Griggs W. Sexuality. In: Martin N, Holt NB, Hick D, eds. *Comprehensive rehabilitation nursing*. New York: McGraw-Hill, 1980.
126. Aloni R, Schwartz J, Ring H. Sexual function in post-stroke female patients. *Sexuality and Disability* 1994;12:191–199.
127. Sipski ML, Alexander CJ. *Sexual function in people with disabilities and chronic illness: a health professionals guide*. Gaithersburg, MD: Aspen, 1997.
128. Boldrini P, Basaglia N, Calanca MC. Sexual changes in hemiparetic patients. *Arch Phys Med Rehabil* 1991;72:202–207.
129. Charlifue SW, Gerhart KA, Menter RR, et al. Sexual issues of women with spinal cord injuries. *Paraplegia* 1992;30:192–199.
130. Donohue J, Gebhard P, eds. Special issue: The Kinsey/Indiana University report on sexuality and spinal cord injury. *Sexuality and Disability* 1995;13:7–85.
131. Finger WW. Prevention, assessment and treatment of sexual dysfunction following stroke. *Sexuality and Disability* 1995;11:39–56.
132. Freda M, Rubinsky H. Sexual function in the stroke survivor. *Phys Med Rehabil Clin North Am* 1991;2:643–658.
133. Garden FH, Bontke CF, Hoffman M. Sexual functioning and marital adjustment after traumatic brain injury. *J Head Trauma Rehabil* 1990;5:52–55.
134. Kreuter M, Sullivan M, Siosteen A. Sexual adjustment and quality of relationships in spinal paraplegia: a controlled study. *Arch Phys Med Rehabil* 1996;77:541–547.
135. Lundberg PO, Hulter B. Female sexual dysfunction in multiple sclerosis: a review. *Sexuality and Disability* 1996;14:65–72.
136. Monga TN. Sexuality post stroke. *Phys Med Rehabil State Art Rev* 1993;7:225–236.
137. Hulter BM, Lundberg PO. Sexual function in women with advanced multiple sclerosis. *J Neurol Neurosurg Psychiatry* 1995;59:83–86.
138. Badeau D. Illness, disability and sex in aging. *Sexuality and Disability* 1995;13:219–237.
139. Anderson BL, Cyranowski JM. Women's sexuality: behaviors, responses, and individual differences. *J Consult Clin Psychol* 1995;63:891–906.
140. Cole SS, Cole TM. Sexuality, disability, and reproductive issues through the lifespan. *Sexuality and Disability* 1993;11:189–205.
141. Holland NJ, Cavallo PF. Sexuality and multiple sclerosis. *Neurorehabilitation* 1993;3:48–56.
142. Kroll K, Klein EL. *Enabling romance*. New York: Harmony Books, 1992.
143. Bullard DG, Knight SE, eds. *Sexuality and physical disability: personal perspectives*. St Louis: CV Mosby, 1981.
144. Leyson JFJ, ed. *Sexual rehabilitation of the spinal cord injured patient*. Clifton, NJ: Humana Press, 1991.
145. O'Carroll RE, Woodrow J, Maroun F. Psychosexual and psychosocial sequelae of closed head injury. *Brain Inj* 1991;5:303–313.
146. The Boston Women's Health Book Collective. *Our bodies, ourselves for the new century: a book by and for women*. New York: Simon and Schuster, Touchstone, 1998.
147. Medlar TM. Sexual counseling and traumatic brain injury. *Sexuality and Disability* 1993;11:57–71.
148. McCormick GP, Riffer DJ, Thompson McDougall M. Coital positioning for stroke afflicted couples. *Rehabil Nurs* 1986;11:17–19.
149. Perduta-Fulginiti PS. Sexual functioning of women with complete spinal cord injury: nursing implications. *Sexuality and Disability* 1992;10:115–118.
150. Rousso H. Special considerations in counseling clients with cerebral palsy. *Sexuality and Disability* 1993;11:99–108.
151. Vermote R, Peuskens J. Sexual and micturition problems in multiple sclerosis patients: psychological issues. *Sexuality and Disability* 1996;14:73–82.
152. Hatzichristou DG. Preface to the special issue: management of voiding, bowel and sexual dysfunction in multiple sclerosis: towards a holistic approach. *Sexuality and Disability* 1996;14:3–6.
153. Finger WW, ed. Special issue: Sexual counseling for people with disabilities. *Sexuality and Disability* 1993;11:1.
154. Rousso H. Sexuality and a positive sense of self. In: Krotoski DM, Nosek MA, Turk MA, eds. *Women with physical disabilities: achieving and maintaining health and well-being*. Baltimore: Paul H. Brookes, 1996:109–116.
155. Haseltine F, Cole S, Gray D, eds. *Reproductive issues for persons with physical disabilities*. Baltimore: Paul H. Brookes, 1993.
156. Lemon MA. Sexual counseling and spinal cord injury. *Sexuality and Disability* 1993;11:73–97.
157. Sipski ML. Sexual function in women with neurologic disorders. In: Cardenas D, ed. *Women's issues, physical medicine and rehabilitation clinics of North America* 2001;12:1, 79–90.

158. Corbett O'Toole J. Disabled lesbians: challenging monocultural constructs. In: Krotoski DM, Nosek MA, Turk MA, eds. *Women with physical disabilities: achieving and maintaining health and well-being.* Baltimore: Paul H. Brookes, 1996:135–152.

159. Gill CJ, Voss LA. *Inclusion beyond the classroom: asking persons with disabilities about education.* Paper presented at the annual meeting of the Society for Disability Studies, Rockville, MD, June 1994.

160. Rousso H. Daughters with disabilities: defective women or minority women? In: Fine M, Asch A, eds. *Women with disabilities: essays in psychology, culture, and politics.* Philadelphia: Temple University Press, 1988:139–171.

161. Nosek MA, Howland C, Rintala DH, et al. National Study of Women with Physical Disabilities: final report. *Sexuality and Disability* 2001;19(1):5–39.

162. Rousso H Wehmeyer ML. *Double Jeopardy: Addressing Gender Equity in Special Education Supports and Services.* New York: State University of New York Press, 2001.

163. Hannaford S. *Living outside inside.* Berkeley, CA: Canterbury Press, 1985.

164. Klein BS. We are who you are: feminism and disability. *Ms* 1992;70–74.

165. Blumberg L. Public stripping. *Disability Rag* 1990;11:18–20.

166. Saxton M. Teaching providers to become our allies. In: Krotoski DM, Nosek MA, Turk MA, eds. *Women with physical disabilities: achieving and maintaining health and well-being.* Baltimore: Paul H. Brookes, 1996:175–178.

167. Paris MJ. Attitudes of medical students and health-care professionals toward people with disabilities. *Arch Phys Med Rehabil* 1993;74:818–825.

168. Westbrook MT, Adamson BJ. Gender differences in allied health students' knowledge of disabled women and men. *Women Health* 1989;15:93–110.

169. Loyola University of Chicago. *Mothers with disabilities: an introduction to the issues (video).* Chicago: Loyola University of Chicago, 1992.

170. Toms Barker LT, Maralani V. *Challenges and strategies of disabled parents: findings from a national survey of parents with disabilities.* Oakland, CA: Berkeley Planning Associates, 1997.

171. Kirshbaum M. Disability cultural perspective on early intervention with parents with physical or cognitive disabilities and their infants. *Infants and Young Children* 2000;23(2):9–20.

172. Kirshbaum M, Olkin R. Parents with physical systemic or visual disabilities. *Sexuality and Disability* 2002;20(1)65–80.

173. Buck F, Hohmann G. Personality behavior, values and family relations of children of fathers with spinal cord injury. *Arch Phys Med Rehabil* 1981;62:432–438.

174. Greene BF, Norman R, Searle M, et al. Child abuse and neglect by parents with disabilities: a tale of two families. *J Appl Behav Anal* 1995;28(4):417–434.

175. Kirshbaum M. Parents with physical disabilities and their babies. *Zero to Three* 1988;8(5)8–15.

176. Brentan A. *Acts of creativity, acts of love: mothering with disabilities.* University Park, IL: Governors State University, 1991.

177. Tulja C, DeMoss A. Babycare assistive technology. *Technology and Disability* 1999;11(1,2);71–78.

178. Through the Looking Glass. *Adaptive equipment and adaptive techniques for physically disabled parents and their babies within the context of psychosocial services.* Berkeley, CA: Through the Looking Glass, 1995.

179. Tulja C, Rogers J, Vens and K, DeMoss A. Continuation of adaptive parenting equipment development. Berkeley, CA: Through the Looking Glass, 1998.

180. DeMoss A .Jans L. Kirshbaum M. Assistive technology and parenting: teamwork component—the parenting with a disabilities survey Berkeley, CA. Through the Looking Glass,1998.

181. DeMoss A, Kirshbaum M, Tuleja C, et al.. Adaptive parenting equipment: evaluation development, dissemination and marketing. Berkeley, CA: Through the Looking Glass, 2000.

182. Cohen L. *Mothers' perception of their influence of their physical disabilities on the developmental tasks of children.* Unpublished doctoral dissertation, California School of Professional Psychology, Alemeda, CA, 1998.

183. Panko Reis J. Parenting with a disability: how different is it really? *Resourceful Woman* 1992;1:1–4.

184. Gill CJ. A grieving mother shares her story. *Resourceful Woman* 1992;1:2.

185. Mathews J. *A mother's touch: the Tiffany Callo story.* New York: Henry Holt, 1992.

186. Angelis T. Custody battles challenging parents with disabilities. *APA Monitor* 1995;26–39.

187. Cupolo A, Srong M, Barker LT, Haight S. *Meeting the needs of women with disabilities: a blueprint for change. Preliminary summary of key issues.* Berkeley, CA.: Berkeley Planning Associates, 1995.

188. Starkloff C. The adoption option. In: Haseltine FH, Cole SS, Gray DB, eds. *Reproductive issues for persons with disabilities.* Baltimore: Paul H. Brookes, 1993:103–105.

189. Toms Barker L, Kirshbaum M. You may be able to adopt: a guide to the adoption option for prospective mothers with disabilities and their partners. Oakland, CA: Berkeley Planning Associates, 1997.

190. Jacobson D. *The question of David: a disabled mother's journey through adoption, family, and life.* Berkeley, CA: Creative Arts Book Company, 1999:88.

191. Panko Reis J. Author provides answers to the adoption with disability question. *Resourceful Woman* 1997:1:1—5, 193.

192. O'Toole C, Doe T. Sexuality and disabled parents with disabled children. *Sexuality and Disability* 2002;2(1):89–100.

193. Kirshbaum M. Family context and disability culture reframing: Through the Looking Glass. *Family Psychologist* 1994;10:8–12.

194. Warshaw C. *Violence against women with disabilities: responding to partner abuse.* April 23, 1996, monograph of conference proceedings, "We've come a long way but can we survive managed care?" Chicago, IL: Rehabilitation Institute of Chicago, 1996:39–42.

195. Sobsey D. *Violence and abuse in the lives of people with disabilities: the end of silence and acceptance?* Baltimore: Paul H. Brookes, 1994.

196. Gill C. Becoming visible: personal health experiences of women with disabilities. In: Krotoski DM, Nosek MA, Turk M, eds. *Women with physical disabilities: achieving and maintaining health and well-being.* Baltimore: Paul H. Brookes, 1996:5–16.

197. Nosek MA, Howland C, Rintala DH, et al. *National study of women with physical disabilities: final report.* Houston: Center for Research on Women with Disabilities, 1997.

198. Saxton M, Curry MA, Powers L, et al. "Bring my scooter so I can leave you": A study of disabled women handling abuse by personal assistance providers. *Violence Against Women* 2001;7(4):393–417.

199. Nosek MA, Hughes RB. *Violence against women with physical disabilities: findings from studies conducted by the Center for Research on Women with Disabilities at Baylor College of Medicine 1992–2002.* Fact Sheet. Houston: Center for Research on Women with Disabilities at Baylor College of Medicine, 2002:3–4.

200. Nosek MA, Hughes RB, Taylor HB, Howland C. *Violence against women with disabilities.* Commissioned paper for national conference on preventing and intervening with violence against children and adults with disabilities, Washington, DC, May 6–7, 2002;12.

201. Nosek MA, Taylor HB, Hughes RB, et al. Demographic disability and psychosocial characteristics of abused women with disabilities, (in preparation). 2004.

202. Nosek MA, Foley CC, Hughes RB, Howland CA. Vulnerabilities for abuse among women with disabilities. *Sexuality and Disability* 2001;19:177–189.

203. Nosek M.A, Howland C, Young MEp Abuse of women with disabilities: Policy implications. *J Dis Policy Studies* 1997;8:157–176.

204. Panko Reis J. When violence meets disability. *Advance for Directors in Rehabilitation* 1995;4(9):6.

205. McFarlane J, Hughes R, Nosek M, et al. Abuse assessment screen—disability (AAS-D): measuring frequency , type and perpetrator of abuse toward women with physical disabilities. *J Womens Health* 2001;10(9):862.

206. Dington J. Beating the odds: violence and women with disabilities (Position paper 2). Vancouver, BC: DisAbled Women's Network Canada, 1987.

207. Cusitar L. Strengthening the links—stopping violence. Toronto: DisAbled Women's Network, 1989.

208. Ulincy GR, White GW, Bradford B, Matthews RM. Consumer exploitation by attendants: how often does it happen and can anything be done by it? *Rehabilitation Counseling Bulletin* 1990;33:240–246.

209. Nosek MA. Sexual abuse of women with disabilities. In: Krotoski DM, Nosek MA, Turk MA, eds. *Women with physical disabilities: achieving and maintaining health and well-being.* Baltimore: Paul H. Brookes, 1996:153–173.

210. Cole S. Facing the challenges of sexual abuse in persons with disabilities. *Sexuality and Disability* 1984–1986;7:71–88.

211. Bacon J. *Violence against women with disabilities: practical considerations for health care professionals.* Toronto: DisAbled Women's Network, 1994.

212. Burt VK, Stein K. Epidemiology of depression throughout the female life cycle. *J Clin Psychiatry* 2002:63,9–15.

213. Nolen-Hoeksema S, Grayson C, Larson J. Explaining the gender difference in depressive symptoms. *Personality and Social Psychology* 1999;77(5):1061–1072.

214. Seeman MV. Psychopathology in women and men: focus on female hormones. *Am J Psychiatry* 1997;154(12):1641–1647.

215. Krause JS, Kemp B, Coker J. Depression after spinal cord injury: relation to gender, ethnicity, aging, and socioeconomic indicators. *Arch Phys Med Rehabil* 2000;81(8):1099–1109.

216. Rintala DH, Hart KA, Fuhrer MJ. Perceived stress in individuals with spinal cord injury. In: Krotoski DM, Nosek MA, Turk MA, eds. *Women with physical disabilities: achieving and maintaining health and well-being.* Baltimore: Paul H. Brookes, 1996.

217. Masuda S. *Research summary. SAFETY NET/WORK Community kit: from abuse to suicide prevention and women with disabilities.* Toronto: DisAbled Women's Network of Canada, 1996

218. Osgood NJ, Eisenhandler SA. Gender and assisted and acquiescent suicide: a suicidologist's perspective. *Issues Law Med* 1994;9:361–374.

219. Penninx B, Guralnik JM, Simonsick EM, et al. Emotional vitality among disabled older women: the women's health and aging study. *J Am Geriatr Soc* 1998;46(7):807–815.

220. Canetto SS, Hollenshead JD. Gender and physician-assisted suicide: analysis of the Kevorkian cases, 1990–97. *Omega—Journal of Death and Dying* 1999;40(1):165–208.

221. Rousso H. A call to action for girls. *Resourceful Woman* 2001(fall):xx.

222. Rousso H. *Strong proud sisters: girls and young women with disabilities.* Barbara Waxman Fiduccia Papers on Women and Girls with Disabilities Center for Women Policies Studies, 2001.

223. Reichley M. Women with disabilities resource centers. *Adv Phys Ther* 1995; May 8:8–10.

224. McKnight JL. Services are bad for people. *Organizing* 1991;Spring/Summer:41–44.

CHAPTER 74

Sexuality and Disability

Marca L. Sipski, Craig Alexander, and Andrew Sherman

Sexuality is an important part of life. It is both a means of expressing one's feelings toward self or others and the means of procreation of the species. Unfortunately, during medical crises and serious chronic illness, health-care professionals often ignore issues pertaining to sexuality and sexual functioning. Furthermore, some physicians are uncomfortable speaking about their patients' sexual concerns, and the patient perceives this discomfort. Hence, the patient or his or her partner may have a concern about sexuality or sexual functioning that is overlooked. This is unfortunate, because sexuality can be a source of great comfort for many individuals and couples.

It is the goal of this chapter to provide the reader with an up-to-date understanding of sexual functioning in the able-bodied individual and how that can be affected by aging or medications. The general impact of disability on sexual functioning is then discussed, as is the method of performing a sexual history and physical examination. Specific disorders and their impact on sexual functioning are then reviewed, and wherever possible, specific research results are addressed. Finally, classification and treatment of sexual dysfunction is addressed.

THE SEXUAL RESPONSE CYCLE

Probably the most widely accepted model of sexual response is the four-stage model of Masters and Johnson (1). The four phases of the Masters and Johnson model for sexual response include excitement, plateau, orgasm, and resolution. These phases were chosen on the basis of laboratory-based analysis of the sexual responses of more than 600 able-bodied men and women. Male and female pathways were overall similar; however, men would have only one orgasm with each cycle, whereas women could achieve one or multiple orgasms. Moreover, it was noted that women could become "stalled" at the plateau phase of sexual response and go straight down to a resolution period.

During the excitement phase, men demonstrate engorgement of the corpora cavernosa of the penis, beginning testicular elevation, and scrotal skin flattening. In women, there is clitoral enlargement in diameter, vaginal lubrication, constriction of the lower third of the vagina coupled with dilation of the upper two-thirds, and beginning uterine elevation out of the deep pelvis. Two-thirds of men and women develop nipple

erection, and in women there is associated areolar enlargement and deepening in color. Myotonia also becomes obvious in both men and women late in the excitement phase.

The plateau phase of men is characterized by an increase in the diameter and color of the glans penis, an increase in testicular size of 50% to 100% over baseline, and the potential for a drop of secretion from the Cowper's gland to appear at the urethral meatus. In women, as a result of continued vasocongestion, the orgasmic platform develops in the vagina with further ballooning out of the upper two-thirds while the clitoral shaft and glans retract. Furthermore, female breast size can increase up to 50%. In both sexes, increased muscle tone, heart rate, and respiratory rate are expected. Moreover, the sex flush, a measles-like rash over the chest, neck, and face, may occur.

Orgasm is characterized by further increases in heart rate, blood pressure, and respiratory rate. Furthermore, involuntary rhythmic contractions occur in the perineal musculature. In men, contraction of the seminal vesicles, vas deferens, and prostate occur, resulting in pooling of seminal fluid, which is followed by ejaculation. Concomitant closure of the bladder neck also occurs. In women, there is contraction of the uterus and fallopian tubes; moreover, one or more orgasms may occur.

The resolution phase is marked by general perspiration in conjunction with gradual reversal of the above-described anatomic and physical changes. Furthermore, in men there is a postejaculation refractory period for repeated ejaculation.

Critics of the Masters and Johnson four-stage model have indicated that there is an unnecessary separation of the plateau and orgasm phases of sexual response (2). Furthermore, the model does not consider factors associated with subjective arousal and does not offer an explanation for the pattern of neurologic components of sexual response (3). Kaplan's model of sexual response, which was incorporated into the third edition of the Diagnostic and Statistical Manual of Mental Disorders (DSM-III), involves the phases of desire, excitement, and orgasm (4,5). By desire, Kaplan means "the experience of specific sensations that motivate the individual to initiate or become responsive to sexual stimulation" (3, p. 42), a process that is said to be under central neurophysiologic control. According to Kaplan, the excitement phase is simply characterized by genital vasocongestion, and the orgasm phase consists of reflex muscle contractions in the pelvis. Furthermore, Kaplan indicates that these other two phases are associated with stimulation of peripheral reflex pathways of the spinal cord. Critics point out that Kaplan's model does not always hold true; for instance, desire is not always a necessary precursor to arousal or orgasm (3).

THE NEUROLOGIC PATHWAYS INVOLVED IN SEXUAL RESPONSE

The predominant model of the neurophysiology of male sexual arousal predicts a dual innervation, which in large part was derived from the studies of men with spinal cord injury (SCI) (6). Innervation for reflex erectile function includes excitation of the dorsal penile nerve with resultant transmission of the impulse to the sacral cord via the pudendal nerve. Sacral parasympathetic excitation of the pelvic nerve is later followed by cavernosal nerve stimulation and resultant engorgement (7). Evidence for brain control of erectile function has been noted at the level of the medial amygdala, the hypothalamus (8), and specifically the medial preoptic area (9,10). Within this area, α_2-adrenergic receptor-mediated inhibitory pathways and dopaminergic-mediated facilitory pathways appear to regulate erectile function. Thus, apomorphine, a dopaminergic agonist, and yohimbine, an α_2-adrenergic receptor-mediated antagonist, have been studied for the treatment of erectile dysfunction (ED) (11). It is further thought that the neurologic pathways travel down the lateral columns of the spinal cord near the pyramidal tracts and then connect to thoracolumbar sympathetic and sacral parasympathetic pathways to produce erection (12). Studies of spinal cord injured men support the hypothesis that the presence of intact sympathetic innervation to the genitals in the absence of parasympathetic supply is sufficient to produce psychogenic erection (13–15). However, the relative role of the sympathetic and parasympathetic pathways in producing able-bodied men's psychogenic erection is as of yet uncertain, and other evidence indicates that the sympathetic pathways may also be inhibitory to erectile function (16).

Ejaculation involves two processes: emission and ejaculation. Emission is produced via thoracolumbar sympathetic stimulation, which results in prostatic, seminal vesicle, and vas deferens contractions. Ejaculation involves the forceful propulsion of semen from the urethra and relies on sacral parasympathetic and somatic efferent stimulation in addition to sympathetic stimulation to close the bladder neck (17).

Recent research has increased our awareness of the neurologic pathways for vaginal lubrication. It is likely that these pathways are at least somewhat similar between men and women. Human and animal studies have provided evidence that reflex lubrication is regulated via the sacral cord (18–20), and psychogenic lubrication is regulated via the thoracolumbar cord and sympathetic nervous system (20–23).

SEXUALITY AND AGING

Any discussion regarding sexuality must take into account the effects of age on sexual functioning. Age results in predictable changes in sexual response and psychological functioning, which must be considered in evaluating sexual functioning. Previously, it was thought that aging itself resulted in a great decrease in frequency of sexual activity (24). However, other surveys have not revealed a significant change in the frequency of sexual activity for elderly persons as compared with their youth (25,26).

With aging, there are predictable changes in the sexual organs and sexual response. In women, menopause leads to a decrease in estrogen levels and resultant loss of labial fullness, thinning of pubic hair, and dryness, thinning, and increased friability of the vaginal mucosa (27). With regard to sexual response, Masters and Johnson (1) found that elderly women had less vaginal lubrication, and it took longer to develop, than in younger women. Other changes during the excitement phase included smaller increases in breast size and a loss of the flattening, separation, and elevation of the major labia along with a decrease in the vasocongestive thickening of the genital organs during advanced excitement. During the plateau phase, there was a decrease in the intensity of areolar engorgement, loss of the preorgasmic color change of the minor labia, and a decrease in the vasocongestion in the outer one-third of the vagina. Orgasm was characterized by an overall decrease in myotonia with less muscular tension during both voluntary and involuntary contractions. Rectal contractions also occurred less frequently, as did contractions of the orgasmic platform. It was further noted, however, that those women who were more sexually active did not have changes in their muscular contractions.

Elderly men were also studied (1). The time it takes to achieve an erection was increased by two- to threefold. Furthermore, the older a man was, the longer it would take to achieve an erection, and if the erection was lost without ejaculation, it would take even longer to regain it. Scrotal vasocongestion was also markedly reduced in older men. During the plateau phase, myotonia is diminished except in more sexually active men. Nipple rigidity is decreased, and the sex flush is lost. Testicular elevation occurs later and is decreased. Full erection may not occur, and erection may be maintained a long time without ejaculation. The decrease in myotonia continues during orgasm, along with less frequent contractions of the penis and rectal sphincter. Ejaculatory fluid is decreased and travels less than in the young. Resolution is remarkable for more rapid reversal of genital changes; however, there is an extended refractory period, which may last for days.

In addition to the physical changes associated with aging, there are psychological changes that occur. As people age, their bodies are less physically taut, and weight gain is common. Hair may gray or else be lost. These physical changes may contribute to a decrease in self-esteem, which can contribute to sexual problems. Moreover, changes in sexual responsiveness can cause further insecurities and sexual difficulties. The classic story is of the man who becomes emotionally disturbed about his declining erectile function (all normal and physically based) and therefore develops psychogenic ED. Through adequate education regarding normal physical changes, it is hoped psychogenic sexual dysfunction can be avoided.

Other emotional changes that occur with aging include fears about illness and death, which can preclude an individual's interest in sex. Depression, which is more common in the elderly, may also decrease interest in sex. Moreover, elderly people may have lost their partners through death or divorce and may not feel that pursuing a new relationship is something they should do. Some aging individuals may also feel that sex is for procreation and the young, and therefore, it is something they should not be concerned about.

In addition to the expected physical and emotional changes accompanying aging, the elderly are also more prone to having medical problems that can affect sexual functioning. Diabetes, cardiac, and pulmonary disease each can produce its own effects on sexual functioning and must be taken into account in evaluating the sexual functioning of the elderly person. Moreover, the elderly can suffer from myriad other diseases and disabilities that can affect their sexual functioning by increasing

TABLE 74-1.   Medications and Sexual Functioning

Drug Class	Impact on Sexual Function
Antihypertensives	Diminished sex drive, erectile ability, ejaculatory function
Anticholesterolemics	Erectile dysfunction, low sexual desire
Digoxin	Decreased testosterone and luteinizing hormone in conjunction with increased estrogen; decreased desire, arousal, and erectile function
Antiarrhythmics	Erectile dysfunction
Antidepressants	Erectile and ejaculatory dysfunction, anorgasmia, spontaneous orgasms and ejaculation, decreased sexual desire
Benzodiazepines	Delayed orgasm or anorgasmia in women, delayed ejaculation in men, decreased sexual desire and arousal
Anticonvulsants	Erectile dysfunction, diminished sexual desire
H₂ blockers	Decreased libido, erectile dysfunction, decreased sperm count

methyldopa. A recent metaanalysis of the effects of β-blockers on sexual function has, however, questioned their effects on sexual function, reporting there is a small but significant annual increase in risk of reported sexual dysfunction (5 per 1,000 patients; 95% CI, 2–8) (32). Thiazide diuretics were studied in a randomized, placebo-controlled study of 176 men (33). Sex drive, erectile ability, and ejaculatory function were all adversely affected in the men on thiazides.

Other medications taken by patients with cardiac disease have been associated with sexual dysfunction in men. The antihypercholesterol agent clofibrate has been associated with ED and low sexual desire (34–36). In contrast, pravastatin and lovastatin may result in slight improvements in sexual functioning (29). Digoxin has been shown to cause sexual dysfunction, including decreased testosterone and luteinizing hormone in male patients in conjunction with increased estrogen (37). Moreover, another study found that men treated with digoxin for 2 years had diminished desire, arousal, and erectile functioning as compared with those receiving other treatments (38). The antiarrhythmic disopyramide has also been associated with ED (39,40).

their overall level of fatigue, thereby decreasing their interest in sexual activity. Furthermore, elderly patients may need to take medications, many of which may have a negative impact on sexual functioning.

One must not underestimate the impact medications can have on a person's sexual desire or response. Open communication can allow these problems to be uncovered, and a change in medication may be all that is necessary to regain the lost or altered function. Alternatively, the use of sildenafil is often a viable means to treat drug-induced sexual dysfunction. For instance, in the male patient with an SCI, high doses of baclofen will cause a decrease in the ability to attain an erection. In this case, a modification in the drugs used to treat spasticity may help with the problem, or the intermittent use of sildenafil may be beneficial.

Many types of medications can have an impact on sexuality and sexual functioning, and a complete discussion of this topic is beyond the scope of this chapter; therefore, we limit our discussion here to those medications most likely to be seen in a physiatric practice. These include antihypertensives, anticholesterolemics, antidepressants, and antianxiety medications. Anticonvulsants, antiulcer medications, anticancer drugs, and medications used to treat prostate problems can also be problematic. Unfortunately, most research that has assessed the impact of medications on sexual functioning has relied on self-report information rather than laboratory-based analysis, and data are thus subject to bias. Moreover, the study of sexual functioning in men is far advanced over that in women (Table 74-1).

Antihypertensive drugs are some of the most commonly prescribed medications, and sexual side effects are one of the main reasons for noncompliance with these drugs (28). Of the antihypertensives, two major classes have been strongly associated with adverse effects on sexual function. These include the sympatholytic or adrenergic-inhibiting drugs and the diuretics (29). Hogan and associates (30) noted that of 861 hypertensive men, 23% of those treated with propranolol and diuretics reported sexual dysfunction, compared with 15% taking clonidine and 13% taking methyldopa. Furthermore, they noted only 4% of untreated controls had sexual dysfunction. Croog et al. (31) also found a greater incidence of sexual dysfunction in patients on propranolol as compared with captopril and

PSYCHOTROPIC DRUGS

Many of the psychotropic drugs can cause sexual side effects; however, it is difficult to differentiate these from the effects of the disorder itself. For instance, the tricyclic antidepressants can have a negative impact on sexual functioning, but depression in and of itself will also cause a decline in sexual functioning. Therefore, the clinician must carefully perform the history in an attempt to determine which problem came first.

Among the antidepressants, imipramine has been shown to cause erectile or ejaculatory problems in about one-third of men (41). In contrast, clomipramine has been associated with high rates of anorgasmia in both men and women (42), and other reports claim spontaneous orgasms and ejaculation have occurred in relation to clomipramine administration (43). Orgasmic problems have also been noted in both men and women taking imipramine, amoxapine, and monoamine oxidase inhibitors (44–46).

Selective serotonin-specific reuptake inhibitors (SSRIs) are also known to cause sexual dysfunction. In a recent retrospective review of 596 men and women taking fluoxetine, sertraline, paroxetine, or venlafaxine, 16.3% of cases had sexual dysfunction. Anorgasmia and decreased sexual desire were most common and generally occurred within 1 to 2 months of taking the medications. Men (23.4%) were more likely than women (13.8%) to have sexual dysfunction (33). Antidotes for this SSRI sexual dysfunction have been tried, and sildenafil has been shown to be quite effective in ameliorating this dysfunction (47). Another report revealed that 81% of patients responded positively to yohimbine. Other, newer antidepressant drugs may have fewer sexual side effects. These include bupropion, trazodone, and nefazodone (29).

The benzodiazepines diazepam, alprazolam, and clonazepam have been noted to cause sexual dysfunction, including delayed orgasm or anorgasmia in women (48–51) and delayed ejaculation in men (52,53). Decreased sexual desire and arousal have also been reported (48,54). In contrast, buspirone has not been associated with negative sexual side effects.

Other commonly used drugs can cause sexual side effects. The anticonvulsants primidone and phenobarbital have been associated with ED and diminished sexual desire (55). In another study, 85 epileptic patients receiving carbamazepine, valproate, or phenytoin had a prevalence of sexual dysfunction similar to that in controls (56). Cimetidine, a histamine antagonist used to treat ulcer disease, has been shown to cause low libido and ED (57,58). Decreased sperm count has also been noted in men taking 1,200 mg/day of cimetidine (59). Ranitidine, another commonly used antiulcer drug, has not been shown to have sexual side effects, and switching to ranitidine can resolve the symptoms caused by cimetidine (60–61). The use of high-dose narcotics to treat chronic pain is also a likely source of decreased sexual desire and arousal.

PERFORMANCE OF THE SEXUAL HISTORY AND PHYSICAL EXAMINATION

Sexuality issues may be approached as primary or secondary concerns. In the former case, it is appropriate to begin the discussion with sexual concerns, whereas in the latter, questions about sexual functioning may accompany questions of bladder and bowel function.

Once the chief sexual symptom is obtained, the examiner should assess duration of the dysfunction, its relationship to the overall disability or illness, what the predisability sexual functioning was, and how it differs from that at present.

A listing of the person's other medical problems and treatments must be obtained. Any history of sexually transmitted diseases should be elicited, as well as prior radiation therapy or surgical procedures. Finally, any history of alcohol or illicit drug use should be determined.

For women, the presence and quality of their menstrual cycles should be elicited; furthermore, in those women who are peri- or postmenopausal, the circumstances surrounding these events should be ascertained. Method of birth control, if any, should be noted. A full obstetric history should also be obtained determining the number of pregnancies, miscarriages, abortions, and live births. With regard to sexual response, women should be queried about their ability to be sexually aroused and whether they are able to lubricate. Moreover, an attempt should be made to distinguish reflex from psychogenic lubrication. Adequacy of lubrication should be noted, as should the ability to achieve orgasm. Situational factors associated with arousal and orgasm should be sought, and any history of and timing of change in function should be elicited.

Men should be queried about the quality of their erections, both reflex and psychogenic. Their ability to sustain the erection should be noted, as should their ability to ejaculate in an anterograde fashion and achieve orgasm. Situational difficulties should be elicited, and any history of change in pattern of response should be noted. Furthermore, if there was a change in their response pattern, when it occurred and any associated events should be noted. Whether birth control is used and what type should be determined.

Finally, the person's psychosocial history should be taken. Sexual orientation, relationship, and family status should be noted. Any history of current or former psychiatric illness must be noted. Occupational status, ability to care for oneself, and living status should be discussed. Furthermore, any transportation difficulties should be addressed.

The sexual physical examination of the person with a disability is similar to the general physiatric examination. However, special attention must be paid to range of motion at the hips, arms, and hands, the presence of neurologic deficits and altered tone, and the presence of dryness in the mouth or genital area. These areas can all affect a person's ability to engage in sexual activity.

UNIVERSAL PSYCHOLOGICAL ISSUES

Trieschmann (62) has described a model of assessment of sexual functioning following disability that emphasizes the psychological along with the physical components affecting the desire for sex, the sexual act itself, and the broader concept of sexuality. Sexuality involves interplay between the psychological and the physical. In fact, most sexual dysfunctions originate in reaction to psychological processes or are compounded by psychological reaction to organic pathology (63). Thus, in discussing sexuality, we must examine the emotional and physical elements involved.

The rate and manner in which a person adjusts to disability will affect his or her sense of sexuality. Emotional adjustment to disability, however, will vary. Although some theorists have advanced defined stages of adjustment, including depression as a necessary component, each person tends to adjust in his or her own way and own time. Disability is an insult to our innate sense of narcissism, resulting in a blow to self-esteem. The issue of self—how we think of ourselves, feel about ourselves, and perceive our ability to act and influence the world—must be addressed following disability. Failure to resolve these issues can result in emotional consequences affecting one's adjustment and sense of sexuality. As Taylor (64) points out, there are at least three issues that one must address following disability. First is the universal question, "Why did this happen to me?" Individuals wrestle with this question until it is somehow put to rest. Of course, there is no correct answer to this question. It is through the process of attempting to answer the question that the issue can become resolved. Second, one must attempt to regain a sense of control in life. This can be accomplished in a variety of ways, from immersing oneself in the physical therapy process to practicing self-regulation techniques such as relaxation or meditation. Last but not least is the long-term process of self-enhancement, the feeling that one is a "survivor" and is a "better" person for what he or she has experienced.

Failure to adequately resolve or develop a functional method for addressing these issues can result in mood disorders such as depression or anxiety. On the other hand, for some people mood depression and anxiety may be normal parts of the adjustment process and may not necessarily signal an abnormal reaction. These reactions, whether considered normal or abnormal, are painful. The individual must do the work necessary to resolve his or her depression in order to successfully resolve the issue and become functional and achieve satisfaction. At times, however, the pain becomes too much, and the person is unable to persist in completing the work necessary for healing. Regardless, this process will likely interfere with one's energy level and sense of self, temporarily affecting one's sexual life.

The age at which one acquires a disability can significantly affect one's adjustment to the condition. Developmental psychologists have theorized various models involving critical stages of both psychological and sexual development. Typically, these theories hold that individuals progress through a prescribed sequence of stages of development. In each stage, critical issues are addressed as the individual matures and develops. When traumatic events occur that interfere with the smooth progression through these developmental stages, emotional problems can ensue. Take, for example, the instance of a catastrophic injury leading to a disability. If a teenage boy sustains an SCI, its impact will be quite different than the same injury experienced by an elderly man. Because of the nature of SCIs, they often occur in more youthful and active individuals. It is understandable then that a high incidence of SCIs occurs in young active men, usually in their late teens or early adulthood. According to the late psychologist Erik Erikson, late adolescence and early adulthood is the critical time for one to resolve the developmental conflicts of "identity versus role confusion" as well as "intimacy versus isolation" (65). It is during this critical period of life that one struggles with answering the question "Who am I?," gains comfort with his or her physical and sexual development, achieves a sense of independence from family, and develops the skills necessary for sexual intimacy. We all can think back and relate to that time in our lives as teenagers when we looked forward to, with enthusiasm and excitement in search of our freedom and independence, the very aspects interfered with by the paralyzing effects of an SCI. The young victim of an SCI may struggle more than his ablebodied counterpart at developing a sense of self and identity and, along with them, a sense of self-esteem, self-image, and sense of intimacy acquired through productive relationships with peers of the same and opposite sex. Presumably, the elderly man will have already experienced and resolved these psychosocial developmental crises and will have moved on to other age-appropriate issues. Thus, the age of onset of a disability or chronic illness predicts the issues one must confront. Certainly, these psychological issues are closely linked to one's sense of sexuality.

Disability and illness affect both the patient and his or her partner. Thus, when we evaluate the patient's sexuality, we must assess the factors affecting the couple. Some of these issues may have existed before the onset of disability and illness and have become exacerbated, but in other instances, the illness may have brought on an issue that did not previously exist. There is no question that disability and illness create stress, which can lead to increased conflict in a relationship. One must determine the degree of conflict that presently exists between the partners and to what extent it is related to the illness. Similarly, the amount of hostility in both the patient and partner must be assessed. Following illness or disability, there is the inevitable question of "Why did this happen to me?" Of course, there is usually no good answer to this question, which often leads to frustration and more anger on the patient's part. The partner too has similar questions and can be left feeling cheated and hostile about the changes in his or her life situation. Moreover, disability can disrupt the usual balance of power that exists within any relationship, leading to struggles to regain the homeostasis that is comfortable for both partners. The disabled person may feel particularly vulnerable and replete with fears. These fears may be rational or irrational but exist nonetheless. The disabled partner might harbor feelings of inadequacy both as a person and as a sexual partner. These feelings can lead to an intense fear of disappointing his or her partner sexually or even a broader fear of abandonment, that the partner will leave him or her for a more "adequate," "healthy," and "worthy" person. Disability and illness may have changed the couple's lives significantly to the point that their life goals, which were once compatible, may no longer be compatible.

Situational and cultural factors can also interfere with the couple's sexual relationship. Disability and illness can highlight some issues that existed previously but posed few problems. Differing attitudes and values regarding intimacy, reli-

gion, and roles within the family system can lead to conflict both within the individual and between the partners. A common scenario occurs when the traditional role played by the man (e.g., masculine, wage earner) is disrupted by disability, forcing a reversal of roles with his wife. Some cultures place a premium on maintaining the traditional masculine role, and any deviation from this can be a blow to the self-esteem, leading to a variety of insecurities and conflict. The economic impact of disability often is substantial, may have significant impact on self-esteem, and may be associated with role reversal within the family.

All of these issues underscore the need for healthy communication, mutual trust and openness, and a strong sense of commitment on the part of each partner. Of course, these issues are not unique to the disabled. However, because of the magnitude of the potential problems that may exist, these qualities are even more important for the satisfaction of the couple's relationship and sexual lives. It has been said that there is no greater test of love than disability. It is easy to see why this might be the case. However, with these problems and obstacles comes the opportunity through resolution for an even greater degree of intimacy and satisfaction for the couple.

DISABILITY-SPECIFIC ISSUES PERTAINING TO SEXUAL FUNCTIONING

Little is known about the impact of many specific disabilities on sexual functioning. Most research that has examined this has relied on self-report methodology. Most studies lack control groups, and very few reports include any type of psychophysiological measures. In addition, there is a disproportionate amount of information examining the issues of men as compared with those of women. For this reason, it may be helpful to consider specific groups of disabilities with similar pathology together in order to better understand their effects on sexual function. For instance, the individual with hemiparesis from a traumatic brain injury will have some similarities to an individual with hemiparesis from a cerebrovascular accident. Moreover, the individual with paraplegia related to multiple sclerosis will have some similarities to an individual with the same level and degree of paraplegia related to an SCI. Although all aspects of these disabilities will not be the same, their similarities can be equal to if not more important than their differences in determining their impact on sexual function.

Spinal Cord Injury

With regard to sexual function, we probably understand more about SCI than any other disability. However, to understand its impact, we must first understand the natural history of sexual response after SCI. Furthermore, the best way to do this is to determine what the impact of the injury is, based on its level and severity.

In men with upper motor neuron complete spinal injuries affecting the sacral spinal segments, based on the neurologic pathways involved, we would anticipate that all would be able to achieve reflex erections; however, none would be able to have psychogenic erections. The literature reports that as many as 93% (15) to as few as 70% (66) of men with this pattern of injury have reflex erections, although none are reported to have psychogenic erections. With consideration for the neurologic pathways involved in the production of anterograde ejaculation, we would anticipate this to be unlikely. Bors and Comarr (15) noted that 4% of patients with this type of injury reported they could achieve anterograde ejaculation.

In men with upper motor neuron incomplete spinal injuries, one would anticipate that reflex erection should remain intact and that psychogenic erection should be possible depending on where the neurologic damage occurred. Furthermore, it has been postulated that whether or not psychogenic erections will occur may be dependent on the integrity of the lateral columns of the spinal cord (8,9). Via self-report studies, Bors and Comarr (15) noted that 80% of men with this injury pattern should have an isolated reflex erection, whereas 19% of these men should have combined reflex and psychogenic erections. Comarr and Vigue (67) noted that 100% of these men would have some type of nonspecified erection. Because of the need to coordinate various neurologic impulses, one would anticipate the ability to achieve anterograde ejaculation to be diminished. This is consistent with the findings of Bors and Comarr (15), who reported that 32% of these patients were able to experience ejaculation, 72% following reflex erection and 26% following psychogenic erections.

With complete lower motor neuron injury affecting the sacral spinal segments, it follows that the ability to achieve psychogenic erection should persist based on the integrity of the thoracolumbar part of the spinal cord and sympathetic genital input. Bors and Comarr (15) noted that 26% of patients with complete lower motor neuron injuries affecting the sacral segments could achieve psychogenic erection; however, none of these patients could achieve reflex erections. In contrast, Comarr and Vigue (67) reported that 50% of these patients could achieve psychogenic erections. Perhaps the discrepancy in these figures arose in part from the fact that attention was not paid to the degree of remaining function these patients had in the thoracolumbar region. With regard to ejaculatory function, 18% of the men in Bors and Comarr's study had anterograde ejaculations, and it was noted that these occurred in conjunction with psychogenic erections.

With regard to incomplete lower motor neuron injuries, the ability to achieve psychogenic erections should theoretically be based on the integrity of the thoracolumbar cord, and the ability to achieve reflex erections should be diminished in varying degrees. The ability to achieve these functions has not been examined through research studies; however, reports have noted that between 67% (67) and 95% (68) of these patients will have some type of erectile function remaining. Bors and Comarr (15) noted that 70% of these patients were able to ejaculate.

The impact of SCI on female sexual response has recently been systematically studied in a laboratory-based controlled setting. In women with documented complete upper motor neuron injuries affecting the sacral spinal segments, reflex genital arousal, but not psychogenic, was found to remain (19). Regardless of the degree of incompleteness or level of SCI, the combined ability to perceive light touch and pinprick sensation in the T11–L2 dermatomes was noted to be predictive of women's ability for psychogenic genital vasocongestion (20). These findings are believed to be indicative of sympathetic control of psychogenic sexual arousal and of reflex control of arousal through the sacral cord.

Based on self-report studies, orgasm is known to occur in men with SCI. Recent reports revealed that 42% (69) to 47% (70) of men with SCI reported the capacity to achieve orgasm. Similarly, recent questionnaire studies revealed that 44% (70) to 50% of women with SCI (71) reported the ability to achieve orgasm. Self-report studies, however, are unable to allow characterization of the physiological responses accompanying orgasm. A laboratory-based assessment of the orgasmic potential of women with SCI has recently been conducted. In the larger series, 69 women with SCI were included along with 21 able-bodied, age-matched controls (20). Women with complete lower motor neuron injuries affecting their S3–S5 spinal segments were noted to be significantly less likely to achieve orgasm than women with all other levels and degrees of SCI. Women with SCI were significantly less likely to be orgasmic and took significantly longer to achieve orgasm than able-bodied women. However, in a blinded assessment, the descriptions of the orgasms of able-bodied and spinal-cord injured women were indistinguishable. The authors felt these findings support the belief that orgasm is a reflex response of the autonomic nervous system. Animal studies of the urethrogenital reflex, which is known to occur in spinal-injured rats, also provide evidence for this hypothesis (72). Based on these results, the development of therapeutic programs to improve the capacity of women with SCI to achieve orgasm should be explored.

Frequency of sexual activity, satisfaction, and which activities people participate in after SCI have been studied in both men and women. These concepts, however, are largely subjective and difficult to measure (73), which may be why there are many inconsistencies in the literature. Frequency of sexual activity has been reported to decrease in men and women after SCI (7,70,71,74); however, level or severity of injury has not been related to frequency (58). Satisfaction has also been shown to decrease in men (70,74–76) and women (76,77) after SCI. Except for a lower frequency of intercourse, the types of activities men engaged in were similar pre- and postinjury. Moreover, women did not demonstrate a significant difference in the types of activities they participated in post-SCI (70). The issue of when interest in sexual activities resumes post-SCI was recently studied in a prospective longitudinal fashion (76). According to these investigators, "The first 6 months after discharge . . . were found to be a point in the adjustment process when persons with recent SCI are more amenable to sexual education and counseling." These findings underscore the need for timely, proactive interventions from health-care professionals caring for persons with recent SCIs.

REPRODUCTIVE CONCERNS IN MEN

Fertility has been shown to be impaired in men with SCI. One reason for infertility is the inability of most men with SCI to achieve an anterograde ejaculation (78). Furthermore, decreased number and motility of sperm are present, and sperm motility is compromised (78). Possible reasons include recurrent urinary tract infections, stasis of fluid, prolonged sitting in a wheelchair, long-term use of medications, and retrograde ejaculation causing sperm to come in contact with urine (78). Previously it was thought that semen quality was affected by lack of scrotal temperature control, however, this theory has recently been disproven (79). The seminal plasma of men with SCI has been shown, however, to inhibit the sperm motility of men without SCI (80); moreover, the level of reactive oxygen species in the semen of men with SCI correlates negatively with sperm motility (81). Timing of SCI has also been studied in an animal model, and testicular function and sperm were noted to degenerate in the first few weeks after injury with partial recovery delayed until 4 to 6 months postinjury (82). Yet another group evaluated 638 ejaculatory specimens from 125 men with SCI, finding an initial decline in semen quality, which probably occurs in the first few weeks after injury; however, they did not find evidence of a progressive decline in semen quality in the years postinjury (83). Based on these results, it is thought that a combination of factors results in the decline in semen quality after SCI (84).

Remediation of male infertility after SCI has been possible through the development of electroejaculation and electrovibration, which are often successfully used in conjunction with assisted reproductive technologies. The technique of electroejaculation was first used in men with SCI in 1948 (85). It was not until 1975, however, that a live birth was reported (86).

Performance of an electroejaculation procedure begins with preparation. The urine is cultured and treated if infection is present; moreover, prophylactic antibiotics may be administered if the urine is clear. The evening before the procedure, the patient performs his bowel program. The bladder is drained of urine just before the procedure and rinsed with a physiological solution in case of retrograde ejaculation. Prophylaxis for autonomic dysreflexia is then provided, followed by digital rectal examination and anoscopy to rule out any preexisting rectal lesions. Electrical stimulation is then performed via a rectal probe with the electrodes placed on the prostate until an ejaculate is obtained or the blood pressure elevation is too high. If unable to stimulate an ejaculate after 15 times, the procedure is aborted. Any ejaculate that is produced is collected for insemination. In addition, postprocedure the individual should be catheterized to obtain any retrograde ejaculate. The rectum is examined to rule out any damage, and the semen is processed for insemination (84).

The penile vibratory stimulation (PVS) procedure is similar pre- and postejaculation to electroejaculation; however, there is no need to examine the rectum. The vibrator is applied on the underside of the penis near the glans, and vibration is applied until an ejaculate occurs or for up to 5 minutes. Autonomic dysreflexia is also a risk with this procedure in patients with levels of injury at T-6 and above; therefore, blood pressure monitoring and potentially prophylaxis are necessary (84).

Recent research pertaining to electroejaculation and PVS has targeted determination of success rates and ways to improve the procedures. For PVS, optimum stimulation parameters of 100-Hz frequency and 2.5-mm amplitude have been defined (87). Utilizing these parameters, Ohl and colleagues (88) found that of 34 men with SCI undergoing PVS, 65% had anterograde ejaculation. Furthermore, sperm averaged 26% motility with counts of 968 million. Bracket et al. (89) noted the percentage of motile sperm and the percentage of sperm with rapid linear motion were significantly higher when obtained with PVS than electroejaculation. Differences were present when both the total ejaculate and the antegrade fraction of the ejaculate were studied. No differences were noted in the sperm quality between vibrator responders and nonresponders. Ohl et al. (90) also compared the semen of 11 subjects obtained via electroejaculation and PVS, and noted that there was no difference between the two groups in the antegrade sperm counts; however, the antegrade PVS specimens had greater motility, viability, total motile sperm count, and hamster egg penetration than the electroejaculation specimens. Based on these studies, it appears that PVS results in better overall sperm quality than electroejaculation. Another issue that should be compared is what associated considerations also affect sperm quality. Ohl noted that using electroejaculation (91), 44% of men with SCI using intermittent catheterization achieved pregnancy as compared with 7% of men using other bladder management techniques. Furthermore, the presence of sterile male urine improved the pregnancy rates from 10% to 30%.

REPRODUCTIVE CONCERNS IN WOMEN
In the woman with SCI, although the outlook for successful childbirth is much more positive, other issues related to gynecologic health are altered by SCI and warrant consideration. In the largest series to date, Jackson studied 472 women from the

model SCI systems (92) who were at least one year posttraumatic SCI. In general, with the exception of cramping, which occurred in 42% of women preinjury and only 27% postinjury, menstrual cycles were similar postinjury. These findings were generally similar to a previous study of 38 women with SCI (93) where temporary amenorrhea of an average of 5 months' duration was found in about 58%; however, in this report, menstrual pain was stable pre- and post-SCI, occurring in 56% of women.

With resumption of a regular ovulatory menstrual cycle, there should be no decrease in the potential for women with SCI to be able to conceive. However, of 231 women with SCI who were studied, the pregnancy rate postinjury was only 0.34 per person as compared with a preinjury rate of 1.3 per person (71). Furthermore, there was a lower pregnancy rate for those women with more significant impairments.

When a woman with an SCI does become pregnant, there can be unique problems because of her injury. Urinary tract infections, increased spasticity, and decubitus ulcers have all been noted (92, 94–96). Whereas anemia has also been noted as a problem (97), Baker and Cardenas point out that anemia is also common in the able-bodied pregnant woman, and the outcomes of anemic women with SCI should be correlated with specific blood levels (94). Other issues that must be monitored in the pregnant woman with SCI include declining pulmonary function as the growing fetus takes up more room. Frequent autonomic dysreflexia has also been reported (91). Care must be taken to differentiate autonomic dysreflexia from preeclampsia. Although various methods have been described for treating dysreflexia, continuous epidural anesthesia has been most commonly recommended (94).

Management of pregnancy in the woman with SCI must take into account the poor sensation that these women have. Labor is often perceived through nontraditional symptoms postinjury. These can include spasms, pain in the back or above the level of injury, ruptured membranes, difficulty breathing, or symptoms of autonomic dysreflexia (92,98). Preterm labor may occur slightly more commonly than the 5% to 10% rate in the general population; however, although the incidence was greater, differences in the frequency of preterm labor and delivery failed to reach statistical significance in Jackson and Wadley's sample (92). Baker and Cardenas recommend that women with paraplegia be instructed in uterine palpation to detect preterm labor, and patients with sensation should have symptom-generated examinations in addition to routine pregnancy visits (94). Furthermore, consideration should be given to home uterine contraction monitoring in women who are unable to detect any symptoms of preterm labor (94). Of note, postinjury pregnancies were significantly more likely to produce low-birth-weight infants (92).

Menopause was also recently studied (92). Whereas the average age of women who went through menopause before injury was 45.5, postinjury the average age was 43.3. Menopausal symptoms were generally similar in women pre- and post-SCI. Further research is needed in this area.

Multiple Sclerosis

The impact of multiple sclerosis (MS) on a person's sexuality and sexual functioning varies tremendously, just as the extent of the neurologic compromise can vary. Despite this, the incidence of sexual dysfunction associated with MS is generally considered high. In fact, more than 50% of women with MS and 75% of men are thought to experience some type of sexual dysfunction at some point in time (99,100). A decrease in libido has been documented in 28% (101) to 60% of women. Because of the changing nature of MS, the sexual symptomatology associated with it can fluctuate. Moreover, the affective and biological impacts of MS are highly interdependent and can influence sexual function separately or in concert.

For patients with some patterns of MS, such as transverse myelitis with associated bladder and bowel incontinence and paraplegia, the changes that occur in sexual functioning may be similar to those occurring in men and women with SCI. Sexual response changes have been noted in both the arousal and orgasm phases of response. In a group of 47 women with advanced MS, 36% of women reported difficulties with lubrication (102), 38% reported decreased orgasmic capacity, and 28% noted anorgasmia. Another study of 149 women with MS reported a 74% incidence of orgasmic dysfunction (99). Another report correlated the presence of orgasmic difficulties in MS with significant abnormalities or the absence of one or both pudendal somatosensory evoked potentials (103); pelvic floor weakness and bladder and bowel dysfunction have also been correlated with changes in lubrication and orgasm (102).

Alternatively, other people with MS may have neurologic deficits resembling those of a stroke or brain injury, and their sexual difficulties may approach those of persons with similar dysfunctions. Other issues associated with sexual dysfunction in persons with MS can include loss of the ability to achieve orgasm, fatigue, tremor, muscle weakness, and spasticity (104). Moreover, the cognitive changes and psychological impact of the disorder can result in anxiety, depression, poor self-image, and lack of interest in sex in both patient and partner.

Modifications of sexual activity may be useful to preserve the sexual relationships of persons with MS. Timing of activity so as to diminish the impact of fatigue may be helpful. Furthermore, assurance that sexual activity will not cause disease progression may help some couples adjust to the disorder. Appropriate education about management of bladder and bowel incontinence can make sexual activity more desirable. Finally, special attention to treating spasticity in the adductor muscles, both through range of motion and medical management, can help maintain the capacity for active participation in sexual activities.

Based on what is known about MS, it follows that some men will be unable to achieve erections or will have difficulty maintaining them. Moreover, other men will be unable to have anterograde ejaculations. If erectile or ejaculatory dysfunction is present in the man with MS, these can be treated in a similar fashion to men with SCI or other disabilities (see SCI section for discussion of treatment of infertility). Sexual dysfunction in women with MS should be treated similarly to that in other disabilities.

Fertility is generally unimpaired in the woman with MS. Birth control should be used for those women not wishing to conceive. There are no contraindications associated with pregnancy for those women who become pregnant.. It has been noted that there is a decrease in exacerbations during pregnancy (105); however, the risk of aggravation of MS increases with childbirth. Three extensive studies have, however, found that pregnancy does not affect the long-term prognosis for women with MS (106–108). Therefore, women with MS should be appropriately counseled regarding their potential for childbirth, and consideration should be given to obtaining extra help at home during the postpartum period.

Stroke

Despite the high incidence and prevalence of stroke, surprisingly little is known about its effects on sexual functioning. Furthermore, most reports that have examined the impact of stroke on sexual functioning have relied on small numbers of subjects and have focused on the presence or absence of libido and patient's frequency of intercourse (109). Our understanding of the effect of stroke on sexuality is also clouded by the fact that most patients with stroke are elderly, suffer from concomitant medical problems that can impact their sexuality, and may take many medications.

Men and women who sustain strokes have been noted to have a decrease in libido (110–112). Multiple reports have also found there is a decrease in the frequency of sexual activity poststroke in men and women (110,113,114).

With regard to sexual response, one prospective study recently evaluated the sexual responses of 38 male and 12 female stroke patients, free from concomitant neurologic dysfunction, severe aphasia, psychiatric, or medical disorders. At 6 months postinjury, 57% of men reported decreased or absent erectile function, and 64% of men reported decreased or absent ejaculation. Of 10 female subjects, 6 noted a negative change in their ability to lubricate poststroke (115). Of 117 male stroke patients, only 22% retrospectively reported normal erectile capability poststroke as compared with prestroke (116). In women, of 75 patients studied retrospectively, 57% reported normal lubrication preinjury, whereas only 24% reported normal lubrication poststroke. Forty-eight percent reported normal orgasm prestroke compared with only 16% poststroke. The findings are similar to another older retrospective study in which 29% of 35 women reported normal lubrication poststroke as compared with 63% prestroke. Orgasm has also been noted to be less frequent in women who sustain strokes (110,113,117), and ED (113,117) and premature ejaculation (110) are more common poststroke.

Traumatic Brain Injury

The effect of traumatic brain injury (TBI) on sexual functioning is also minimally studied. Furthermore, because of the profound interpersonal and cognitive effects of TBI, research should take into account the distinct effects of the psychological and physiological effects of the injury. This is especially unfortunate because brain injuries occur most frequently between the ages of 15 and 24 (118), at a time when people are often just beginning to explore their sexual potential and develop sexual relationships.

The reported incidence of ED in men with TBI varies from 71% to 10% (119–121). In women, difficulty with lubrication after TBI has also been documented, occurring in 18% of 129 post-TBI as compared with 7% of 112 nondisabled control subjects (120). Ability to achieve orgasm was also significantly decreased in this population of women with TBI, with 16% of subjects reporting orgasmic difficulties compared with only 2% of controls (120). Statistically significant decreases in energy for sex, sex drive, and ability to initiate sexual activities were also noted. Moreover, statistically significant differences in sexual difficulties were reported with regards to positioning, body movement, attractiveness, and comfort with having partner view body during sexual activities when TBI survivors were compared with nondisabled control subjects.

The effects of various brain lesions on sexual responsiveness have been studied primarily in animals. Injury to the brain stem may decrease the general level of arousal, thereby impairing sexual functioning (122). Stimulation of the thalamus has been noted to cause erection in animals (123). Because the hypothalamus secretes gonadotropin-releasing hormone, it is involved in regulation of the menstrual cycle in female subjects and testosterone secretion in male animals. Hypothalamic injury during childhood can therefore result in precocious puberty (124), whereas injury as an adult can lead to amenorrhea or sexual dysfunction. Lesions in the medial preoptic area of the hypothalamus result in reduced or absent copulatory behavior. Stimulation of the dorsomedial nucleus of the hypothalamus results in ejaculation in animals, whereas stimulation of the ventromedial nucleus is thought to play a role in female sexual behaviors (125). Damage to the limbic and paralimbic systems can cause hypersexual behaviors. Damage to the dorsolateral frontal lobes can cause impairments in libido and sexual assertiveness (125); furthermore, frontal lobe damage can result in an inability to fantasize (126). Erections have been produced via stimulation of the hippocampus, septal complex, and amygdala (127). The Kluver-Bucy syndrome results from lesions in the anterior temporal poles and leads to hypersexual and exploratory behaviors with hyperorality (128–130). Temporal lobe seizures can result in genital sensations and either hypo- or hypersexual behavior (125). Finally, stimulation of the hippocampus results in erection in animals, and damage may result in sexual dysfunction (123).

Research in 100 male TBI survivors has indicated that location and severity of injury are related to erectile functioning (119). Miller et al. (131) also studied eight TBI patients and noted that medial basal–frontal injury or diencephalic injury would result in hypersexuality and that limbic injury could result in changes in sexual preference. Sandel et al. (132) noted in 52 persons with TBI that those with frontal lobe lesions reported higher levels of sexual satisfaction and functioning and more sexual cognitions and fantasies than persons with brain injuries in other locations. Furthermore, persons with right hemisphere injuries had higher sexual arousal and more sexual experiences than did other brain injury survivors.

When working with couples or persons with TBI, it is important to take into account the effects of the brain injury on the person's cognitive status and personality. These psychological factors may impact significantly on the quality of their relationships. With regard to physical factors, the impact of paralysis, loss of sensation, altered mental status, and potential bladder and bowel dysfunction on sexual functioning must be taken into account. Spasticity, hypersensitivity, and the inability to transfer also may affect the ability to engage in sexual activities.

Education is important in working with couples affected by TBI. The general effects of the injury should be discussed in addition to the potential impact on sexual functioning. Issues surrounding positioning and problems with sexual functioning should be addressed. Most importantly, if necessary, appropriate psychological and sexual counseling should be pursued.

Neuromuscular Diseases

As a whole, the impact of neuromuscular diseases on sexuality and sexual functioning is primarily related to peripheral rather than genital dysfunction. These disorders have a wide span in the degree of illness and disability they cause, ranging from significant paralysis—including loss of pulmonary capacity, which can result in as serious a consequence as death—to as small a consequence as moderate degrees of loss of stamina and strength in peripheral musculature. These disorders also vary significantly in the times they manifest themselves, which can range from birth to the elderly. Because of these factors, the effects of neuromuscular diseases on sexual functioning can vary greatly.

Treatment of sexual dysfunction in the person with a neuromuscular disease begins with education regarding the impact of the disability on sexual functioning. Specific problems such as difficulties with positioning or difficulty achieving orgasm

should be elicited and specific suggestions provided to remediate the patient's concerns. These may include showing the patient pictures demonstrating positioning with their degree of paralysis or recommending the use of a vibrator for persons with limited mobility in order to allow more effective genital stimulation. Psychological counseling or sex therapy may be necessary if significant depression or anxiety are detected or for couples issues.

Arthritis and Connective Tissue Diseases

The impact of arthritis on sexual functioning is primarily related to the associated pain, joint stiffness, and fatigue (133). Other factors can also cause sexual dysfunction, however, including loss of mobility, altered body image (134), and depression (135). Medications can also cause sexual dysfunctions, such as corticosteroids, which can cause a decrease in libido, and those used to decrease pain and improve sleep (136).

Rheumatoid arthritis (RA) is known to cause sexual dysfunction in both men and women. Of 31 men with RA, 33% reported episodes of ED, and 50% reported decreased libido during active inflammatory periods (137). In another study of 91 married women with RA, more than 50% noted a decrease in their desire for sex since their disease onset, and 50% noted arthralgia associated with intercourse. Furthermore, 22% of women noted their arthritis symptoms were worse the day after intercourse (138). Seventeen women with RA were grouped with six women with systemic lupus erythematosus (SLE) (139), and significant decreases were noted in sexual satisfaction, frequency of sexual intercourse, and desire for sexual intercourse 1 year after disease onset. The majority of women considered joint pain and fatigue as factors affecting their sexual performance. In another report, 100 women with SLE were noted to more frequently abstain from sex and have less frequent sex, poorer sexual adjustment, and diminished vaginal lubrication as compared with a group of 71 controls (140).

Progressive systemic sclerosis (PSS) has also been noted to impact sexual functioning in both men and women. Sixty women with PSS were compared with an age- and disease-matched control group of women with RA and SLE (139). Decreased desire, sexual satisfaction, and frequency of sexual intercourse were noted with PSS. A greater frequency of vaginal dryness, dyspareunia, and perineal fissures and ulcerations were also noted since the onset of PSS; furthermore, these women reported a decrease in the number and intensity of their orgasms. One-third to one-half of men with PSS have been noted to have erectile problems (141,142), which are thought to result from vascular changes limiting penile blood flow (143).

Treatment of sexual dysfunction in the patient with arthritis or other connective tissue disorders begins with assuring maximal overall physical functioning. Educating the patient and his or her partner about the impact of the disease on sexual functioning is also important. Pamphlets demonstrating proper positioning, such as those available through the Arthritis Foundation, may be useful aids. During sexual activity, prolonged pressure on painful joints must be avoided. Premedication or the use of heat before sexual activity may also be useful (144). Lubricants may be useful, as may the use of adapted erotic aids such as vibrators for people with poor hand functioning. As with all disabilities, counseling should be used when appropriate.

Total Joint Replacement

Joint disease can have a significant effect on sexual functioning. Consequently, total hip replacement can substantially improve sexual functioning. In one survey (145), 57% of 121 patients who underwent total hip replacement reported some relief of sexual difficulties after surgery, and 34% had complete or considerable improvement. Another report noted that 65% of patients were free from sexual difficulties after hip replacement. Nevertheless, one study reported that 81% of surgeons did not discuss with their patients when to resume sexual activity (146).

Sexual intercourse can typically be resumed within 1 to 2 months after total hip surgery. By this time significant healing should have taken place, reducing the risk of dislocation. Preferred positions include the missionary for men, as excess motion is eliminated at the hip joint, and side lying with the nonoperative side down and the operative side supported by pillows for women (147). Other joint replacements generally cause less impact on sexual activity; however, proper positioning to decrease stress across the operated joint should be practiced.

Diabetes

Approximately 16 million Americans have diabetes (148). Many of these patients develop secondary complications such as amputation or stroke, which a physiatrist may treat. Therefore, it is important to be aware of the sexual consequences of diabetes, and the subject deserves special mention.

The impact of diabetes on male sexual functioning has been extensively studied. ED is known to occur in 50% of men with diabetes and is at least three to five times more prevalent among men with diabetes than in the general population. Timing is an important factor in determining the reversibility of ED in the diabetic population. ED can occur when poor glycemic control results in temporary chemical changes in the autonomic nerves and resolves when the metabolic derangements are corrected. Alternatively, ED that develops more slowly is most likely related to permanent changes in the autonomic nerve fibers of the corpora cavernosa (149). Furthermore, ED has been shown to occur whenever there are other signs and symptoms of diabetic autonomic neuropathy (150–153). The effect of microangiopathy is less clear on sexual functioning. One histopathologic autopsy study of diabetic men found no correlation between ED and diabetic microangiopathy (154). In contrast, two larger studies of diabetic men noted a positive association between ED and microangiopathic changes (151,155).

There is less impact of diabetes on ejaculation and orgasm than on ED. One study of 80 diabetic men revealed that 27 had ED, whereas only 5 had any orgasmic dysfunction, and of these, 3 had premature ejaculation and 2 had delayed ejaculation (156). Retrograde ejaculation can also be a problem for diabetic men whose internal vesical sphincter does not close properly during ejaculation as a result of autonomic neuropathy (150).

The impact of diabetes on female sexual functioning has been studied much less than that in men. Conflicting reports have arisen as to whether there is an impact of diabetes on lubrication (156–159); however, the majority of reports were based on questionnaire studies, which are notoriously inaccurate in assessing lubrication. One laboratory-based study included 10 women and used vaginal photoplethysmography to compare able-bodied and diabetic subjects' responses to erotic videos (160). Women with autonomic neuropathy were not excluded, and decreased vaginal responsiveness in diabetic women was demonstrated. In contrast, another study used labia minora temperatures to compare the responses of women with insulin-dependent diabetes mellitus and able-bodied age-matched controls to erotic videos and revealed no significant differences. Studies of orgasm in diabetic women have also been inconclusive as to whether there is (161–163) or is not (156,157,164) a decrease in their ability to achieve orgasm.

Fertility is affected in men and women with diabetes. There is a lower than expected rate of pregnancy in the partners of diabetic men. Proposed reasons include ED, retrograde ejaculation, and endocrine abnormalities (126). Whereas the ability of a dihabetic woman to conceive is only slightly decreased, the likelihood of a live birth is decreased (165). Furthermore, preexisting and gestational diabetes can result in macrosomia and birth defects, including congenital heart disease, kidney disease, poorly developed colon and central nervous system, and spinal deformities (166).

Amputation

The effect of amputation on sexual functioning is primarily related to peripheral rather than genital causes. The loss of a limb and loss of range of motion may result in difficulties with positioning in sexual activity and require the individual to alter patterns of sexual behavior. Preservation of the knee joint is helpful to maintain balance during coitus; however, for transfemoral amputees, positioning with pillows can help maintain stability (144). Those individuals with upper limb amputations may benefit from a side-lying position for intercourse, thereby permitting free movement of the intact arm.

Psychological issues are also important in the sexuality of persons with amputations. Depression in adults with amputation may persist for years (167). Amputees need to adjust to their altered body image. Furthermore, anxiety about disease progression can be a problem for nontraumatic amputees.

Cardiac Disease

A large body of literature exists concerning the impact of cardiac disease on sexual functioning. Although cardiac disease does not have a direct impact on genital sexual functioning, the psychological and peripheral effects on physical functioning are great. As with most other studies examining sexual functioning, there is a great imbalance in the attention paid to male as opposed to female sexual response.

Frequency of sexual activity has been shown to decrease in 40% to 70% of men after myocardial infarction (MI) (168). Of 130 women who sustained an MI (169), 44% reported decreased frequency of intercourse, and another 27% became completely abstinent. In another report of 100 male veterans surveyed 6 months after MI (170), common reasons for not resuming intercourse included ED (39%), chest pain (28%), deconditioning (28%), decreased libido (19%), anxiety about recurrence of MI (16%), boredom (15%), and depression (14%).

Denial, anxiety, and depression have been noted as the psychological disturbances most common after MI (171). Denial is usually the first response and does not affect sexual functioning. Anxiety, however, can become chronic after MI and can result in ED. What's more, anxiety is often inappropriately focused on the occurrence of MI during sexual activity. Of 858 patients with acute MIs who were sexually active in the previous year, only 3% reported sexual activity in the 2 hours preceding their MI; moreover, the risk of MI during sexual activity was no different in patients with or without a preexisting history of MI, and sexual activity was thought to contribute to the etiology of MI in only 0.9% of cases (172). Of the psychological impacts of MI, depression is felt to be the most clearly established cause for sexual dysfunction (173) and can result in decreased libido and erectile and orgasmic dysfunctions.

Physical consequences of cardiac disease on sexual functioning include diminished cardiac reserve, which can make the patient less physically able to perform (174), and angina (175). Notably, angina after MI is more frequent during the resolution phase of sexual response than during orgasm (176). Sternal incisional pain is common in the first 6 to 8 weeks after coronary artery bypass grafting (168) and can infrequently persist, causing long-term sexual difficulties. Most patients with cardiac disease are also on multiple medications, many of which can cause sexual dysfunction.

Energy requirements during sexual activity have been studied. Orgasm requires 4 to 6 metabolic equivalents (METs) for 10 to 15 seconds, whereas the other phases of sexual response require 3 to 4 METs (177). Furthermore, in a study of middle-aged married men, requirements generally did not exceed 4 METs (178). Walking on a treadmill at 3 miles/hour at a 5% grade and climbing two flights of stairs at a rate of 20 steps in 10 seconds (179) are felt to require equivalent amounts of energy as sexual intercourse. Furthermore, the energy requirements for sexual intercourse are thought to be less for familiar positions than unfamiliar positions, regardless of what they may be (180).

The two-flight test has been used to determine safe return to sexual activity after MI; however, it has been noted that the test can be used only to make a rough estimate (181), and the test is unable to detect silent ischemia. One study of 88 men (182) undergoing ambulatory electrocardiogram monitoring revealed that one-third of patients had ischemia during sexual activity, and silent ischemia was more common than symptomatic. Furthermore, they noted that a positive exercise stress test was noted in all patients with ischemia. Therefore, a true exercise stress test may be the best mechanism to determine safe return to sexual activity post-MI.

Treatment of the patient with cardiac disease and sexual difficulties begins with education and reassurance of the patient about the effects of cardiac disease on sexual functioning. The importance of a general conditioning program should also be emphasized, as one report noted that heart rate reduction and increased exercise tolerance should theoretically decrease ischemic episodes during sex (182). Timing of sexual activity when not fatigued (183,184), and possibly in the morning with rest periods before and after, is important for patients with cardiac disease (185,186). Foreplay has also been noted to be particularly important in order to allow a gradual increase in heart rate (176). Sexual intercourse should be avoided after a heavy meal and for at least 3 hours after drinking alcohol (183–187). Sex should also be avoided during emotional stress or in association with anxiety-producing conditions (185,186,188). Positioning during sexual activity should stress comfort, ease, and familiarity.

Patients should also be counseled about what symptoms should be reported to their physicians (183). These include a rapid heart rate or breathing pattern persisting for 7 to 10 minutes after orgasm, angina, extreme fatigue after orgasm, or the development of other sexual difficulties. For those persons with angina, prophylactic nitroglycerin may be useful during sexual activity (187–192). With the availability of sildenafil to treat ED, however, one must be cautious not to prescribe this to any patients with access to nitrates and to make certain that nitrates are not given to any patients that may have take sildenafil in the last 24 hours. The treatment of ED in this population is discussed later on in this chapter, particularly the use of sildenafil.

Pulmonary Disease

Patients with chronic pulmonary disease are likely to experience sexual dysfunction, although little research has been done on this topic (193). Dyspnea leading to decreased activity tolerance can cause sexual difficulties in patients with chronic obstructive pulmonary disease (COPD) (194). Because respiratory rates of 40 to 60 per minute may be reached during sexual activity, the ability to achieve full exhalation may be diminished in COPD patients. Furthermore, if the patient is underneath his or her partner, dyspnea can be exacerbated through the pressure of the partner on the chest (195). This can lead to anxiety and fear, beginning a vicious cycle that makes the sexual act even more difficult. Bronchospasm with resultant coughing can also diminish an erection (194), leading to further psychological and sexual difficulties.

An association has been demonstrated between COPD and ED (196). Other potential causes of sexual dysfunction in the individual with pulmonary disease include side effects of medications such as corticosteroids, antihypertensives, digoxin, and antidepressants. Deconditioning can impair one's ability to participate in sexual activity. In addition, altered body image, depression, and general anxiety can cause sexual difficulties.

Patients with cystic fibrosis deserve special mention with regard to the impact of their disease on sexual functioning. Of 30 married male and female cystic fibrosis patients (197), 57% reported no or only occasional problems in sexual functioning; however, 30% reported serious sexual problems. Men with cystic fibrosis are also noted routinely to have bilateral absence or atrophy of the vas deferens (198), and azoospermia is universal (199). Despite these abnormalities, successful pregnancies have resulted from microsurgical epididymal sperm aspiration followed by intracytoplasmic sperm injection (200).

Treatment of patients with pulmonary disease involves education about the impact of their pulmonary dysfunction on sexual activity. Patients should be encouraged to talk about anxieties associated with sexual functioning and may benefit from trying mutual masturbation rather than oral sex or intercourse as a form of sexual activity (195).

Patients should be instructed to plan their sexual activity (194). This includes getting a good night's rest before sex but avoiding sex on awakening because of accumulated secretions (195,201). One should wait 2 to 3 hours after meals before having sex (201) and avoid physical activity right before sex (194,195). A familiar, relaxing atmosphere should help reduce anxiety (202,203). Furthermore, some persons with pulmonary dysfunction may feel it is easier to have sex on firm surfaces, whereas other persons may feel that a waterbed is useful (194). The use of an inhaler or cough drop just before sex can help prevent bronchospasm and coughing (194). Oxygen should also be used if helpful, but with adequate length and positioning of tubing. Restrictive clothing should be removed before sexual activity, and having a box of tissues nearby can help prevent interruptions during sexual activity. Avoiding prolonged kissing and oral sex before intercourse should be considered if they result in dyspnea. Finally, patients should adjust the rate and intensity of intercourse to their breathing needs (194), and positions for intercourse should avoid putting pressure on the chest (195). The side-lying position and seated positions make breathing easier (202).

Cancer

The emotional impact of a diagnosis of cancer cannot be overestimated. Nevertheless, advances in treatment of persons with cancer have made extended survival and cure a realistic possibility in many cases, and issues pertaining to sexuality and sexual functioning are important. The physical impact of cancer on sexual functioning is in a large part determined by the location of the primary tumor. Furthermore, various treatments for cancer can often cause iatrogenically induced sexual dysfunction.

Prostate cancer is the most common form in men, with an incidence of approximately 244,000 in l995 (203). All treatment options can cause sexual changes (204). Radical prostatectomy, an option for early-stage cancer that includes removal of the entire prostate, seminal vesicles, and vas deferens, results in permanent ED in 85% to 90% of men. Fortunately, nerve-sparing surgery will result in a 76% return of erectile ability if both neurovascular bundles are preserved and a 60% return of erectile capacity if only one neurovascular bundle is preserved (205). With radiation therapy, sexual dysfunction is influenced by the size of the radiation field and whether there is damage to the pelvic vascular bed, sympathetic nerves, or testicles with resultant decreased testosterone levels (206). ED and ejaculatory pain from a reduction in semen flow (207) can both result from radiation. With internal beam radiation therapy, 15% of men report subsequent ED (208). Hormonal manipulation is aimed at decreasing androgen availability to prevent tumor growth. Testosterone levels decrease 90% to 95%, with associated side effects including decreased libido, hot flashes, and ED. Furthermore, it is felt that the effect of hormonal therapy on sexual functioning may be greatest through its effect on the brain in decreasing desire and arousability (209).

Testicular cancer is the most common form of cancer in men between the ages of 15 and 35 (203). Retroperitoneal lymphadenectomy may be undertaken, resulting in severance of paraaortic sympathetic nerves necessary for ejaculation. Retrograde ejaculation along with decreased semen volume occurs almost universally (210); therefore, nerve-sparing procedures are advocated when possible. Although desire, erection, and orgasm are usually unchanged physiologically, the psychological impact of testicular cancer may decrease a person's desire for sexual activity. Fertility will be impaired through both direct damage to the sperm and altered ejaculation, and sperm banking and assisted ejaculation procedures may be considered.

Penile carcinoma makes up only 1% of male cancers, generally occurring after the age of 50 (211). Treatment can range from partial penectomy, radiation therapy, or topical chemotherapy for small lesions to total penectomy with perineal urethrostomy for more advanced disease (204). Despite changes in erectile functioning, the capacity for arousal of other erotically sensitive areas including the mons, scrotum, perineum, and anus, and capacity for ejaculation and orgasm persist. For those individuals with complete penectomy, penile implants have been reported to result in satisfaction with function and appearance in 89% of patients and their mates (210).

Breast cancer is diagnosed in approximately 182,000 women in the United States annually (203). Administration of antiestrogens can result in temporary or permanent menopause, as can chemotherapy. Soreness, dryness, vaginal atrophy, hot flashes, and decreased sexual desire can result (212). Local estrogen cream may alleviate some of these symptoms. In addition to the physical changes associated with treatment, the profound psychological impact of breast cancer results in orgasmic difficulties and reduced frequency of intercourse in up to 39% of women (213). These effects have been noted despite the attempts to preserve women's breasts through breast-saving surgery or reconstruction.

Ovarian cancer is the third most frequently diagnosed gynecologic malignancy (203). Sexual dysfunction, including postcoital bleeding or pelvic pain, can be the presenting symptom (213). Surgical removal of the ovaries results in the onset of menopause with the symptomatology mentioned above. In addition, the resultant infertility can be psychologically devastating. For advanced cancers, total pelvic exenteration including surgical removal of the bladder, vagina, uterus, rectum, and associated structures may be necessary, after which most women cease all sexual activity (214,215).

Women with cervical cancer may experience sexual dysfunction related to fibrosis, pain with penetration, decreased lubrication, and vaginal stenosis associated with radiation therapy (204). Vaginal dilators and lubricants may be useful to minimize these side effects, and alternative positioning during intercourse may minimize discomfort.

Other gynecologic cancers are rare. Cancer of the vulva most often occurs in postmenopausal women (203). Treatment can include simple vulvectomy, after which sexual functioning and the capacity for orgasm may be preserved. However, removal of the clitoris results in more substantial impairment. Despite this, because adrenal androgens and ovarian hormone function are unaffected, some women retain the capacity for desire, arousal, and orgasm after radical vulvectomy. Additionally, it is thought that psychological distress may be a factor in those women with an inability to achieve orgasm (204). Cancer of the vagina and associated treatments may result in shortening and narrowing of the vagina, dryness, and dyspareunia. For those women who undergo total vaginectomy, however, 30% to 70% of patients will have a return of orgasm provided the clitoris is left intact (216).

Colorectal cancer is the third most common cause of cancer in both sexes. Abdominoperineal resection can result in ED in 50% to 100% of patients (217) and ejaculatory dysfunction in 50% to 75% of patients. What's more, both sexes experience changes in self-image and sexuality as a result of colostomy.

Bladder cancer is usually treated by surgery followed by radiation. Radical cystectomy results in ED in nearly 100% of cases, and ejaculation is retrograde. However, orgasm and sexual desire remain unaffected. In women, total abdominal hysterectomy, bilateral oophorectomy, and removal of the anterior vaginal wall can result in numbness in the perineum and decreased estrogens with resultant decreases in vaginal size and lubrication and dyspareunia. The ability to achieve orgasm, however, should remain in women who successfully resume sexual activity (213). The use of an ileal conduit can also result in changes in self-image and resultant sexual dysfunction similar to those resulting from colostomy.

Other cancers, though primarily nongenital, can also have enormous impact on sexual functioning. Head and neck cancers and their associated treatments can result in profound disfigurement and change in self-image. Metastatic tumors to the brain or spinal cord can result in changes in sexual functioning from neurologic dysfunction. Depression and anxiety will be associated with a diagnosis of cancer no matter where the primary tumor is, and weakness and fatigue will occur regardless of the location of the primary tumor. Additionally, treatments prescribed for cancer, including chemotherapeutic agents, radiation therapy, and hormonal manipulation, can cause general side effects of fatigue and other medical problems in addition to specific sexual side effects regardless of the types of tumors they are treating.

Treatment of sexual dysfunction in the person with cancer should begin with giving them permission to talk about their concerns regarding sexuality and then providing them with basic information, tailored to their particular problem. Recommendations regarding timing for sexual activity when free from fatigue and about positioning to decrease energy requirements may be useful. Treatment of specific dysfunctions is warranted, as is referral for further psychological and sexual counseling, if appropriate.

Chronic Pain and Sexual Dysfunction

Physicians treating patients with chronic painful conditions have more recently begun to characterize the pain separate from the underlying cause in terms of a disease itself rather than a symptom. Persons with the condition of chronic daily pain often suffer from not just the pain, but from multiple disabilities related to their pain. Depression, weight loss or gain, physical deconditioning, and loss of self-image all often accompany chronic pain (218). The underlying medical conditions causing chronic pain range from benign lower back or neck injuries to terminal malignant cancers.

Each of these conditions that cause chronic pain can limit that person's ability to function mentally and physically. For many reasons, chronic pain sufferers are left vulnerable to disruption of sexual functioning. The complex nature of chronic pain and its underlying causes often makes it difficult to pinpoint a single cause of such disruption and thus makes it difficult to treat.

There are few published studies on chronic pain and its effect on sexual function. It is often difficult to tease out the specific effect of pain on sexual interest and function from the other medical and psychological conditions that may be present. As stated above, many persons with pain also suffer from psychological or organic illness. Additionally, they may be on psychotropic drugs, muscle relaxants, or narcotic pain medications, many of which cause sexual dysfunction (218). Finally, in certain types of chronic pain, such as pelvic pain, sexual abuse is identified as a contributing cause more often than in "no-pain" control subjects (219).

A few studies have been published despite the difficulties. Ambler et al. (218) surveyed 237 patients with chronic pain; 73% had difficulty with sexual function that the patient felt was directly related to their pain. These problems included difficulties with arousal, position, low confidence, performance worries, and pain exacerbation. Most responders reported a combination of the above factors. There was no statistically significant difference between men and women. Responders were younger and less depressed than those who did not respond to the survey. No attempt was made to correlate drug use to sexual dysfunction. Smaller studies (219,220) have found similar percentages. Monga et al. (221) found that in 70 patients (62 men) attending a chronic pain program, 53% were sexually active less than once per month, and 73% suffered from some type of sexual dysfunction. Despite the limitations inherent in these studies, the percentage of patients with chronic pain who suffer from sexual dysfunction seems to be relatively consistent.

Ambler et al. (218) also surveyed a subset of 68 patients concerning their preferences for help. In that group, 47% wanted written information only, 26.5% wanted discussion, and 20% wanted both discussion and information. There was no gender difference in these preferences. In a survey by Dunn et al. (222), only one-tenth of the respondents who wished for professional help had previously received such help.

It is evident from these studies that a problem exists on many levels. First, there is a clear disruption of sexual function in patients suffering from chronic pain (223). Second, the causes of this disruption are many and complex. Comprehensive multidisciplinary medical and psychological treatment will therefore be required if these patients' needs are to be met and their function improved. Finally, it seems that their needs are not currently being met by their pain-management physicians, despite the wish to have their sexual dysfunction treated along with their pain. Therefore, it is important for all physicians regularly treating patients with chronic pain to have an avenue where patients can discuss their sexual problems related to their condition and then seek treatment in the most appropriate manner.

Other Disorders

Discussion of the sexual problems associated with all potential physical disorders is beyond the scope of this chapter. However, the basic principles discussed here should be used when working with persons with other diagnoses. Determination of premorbid sexual dysfunction is important, and the impact of medication use and other concomitant medical problems must be addressed. The psychological status of the patient, including evidence of depression and anxiety, must be considered. Physical examination should look for signs previously discussed associated with changes in sexual functioning. For those disorders similar to another for which we do have some understanding of sexuality, it may be useful to discuss the effects of the other disorder with the patient. Basic education should be provided regarding sexuality, supplemented by referral for further psychological and sexual counseling and treatment if appropriate.

TREATMENT STRATEGIES

Sexuality Counseling

Sexuality is a sensitive topic and one that many of us feel uncomfortable addressing with our patients. The reasons for this are at least twofold. First, few of us have received professional training in the area of sexuality. Second, the subject of sexuality is replete with our own personal values and biases based on our own upbringing and life experiences. For many, it is difficult to separate our own values and attitudes to address the issue objectively. It is not therefore surprising that the subject is not approached with our patients, or raised inappropriately, or simply dismissed when the patient raises the topic. Annon (224) has proposed a multilayered framework for sexual counseling incorporating all health-care personnel working with the patient. The so-called *PLISSIT* model is an acronym for *p*ermission, *l*imited *i*nformation, *s*pecific *s*uggestions, and *i*ntensive *t*herapy. According to this model, all personnel working with the patient should feel comfortable enough with their own sexuality and knowledgeable enough to engage in the first two levels of this model. That is, professionals should feel comfortable raising the issue with the patient to "permit" discussion of the topic. In addition, practitioners should possess enough knowledge about sexuality and the specific disability/illness to impart limited information. Moreover, they should possess enough information to know their limits or to "know what they do not know." In this case, they would move up to the next level of the model, which involves referring the patient to a more knowledgeable professional for specific suggestions or intensive therapy. Successful implementation of this model would require an ongoing institutional commitment to train all staff having contact with patients on basic sexuality issues. This model also argues for the existence of a standing multidisciplinary hospitalwide committee addressing sexuality issues, including education of patients and staff, along with ongoing ethical issues.

The need for sexual counseling has been reported differently depending on the population. Pauly and Goldstein (225) reported that 10% of the general population is in need of some sort of sexual counseling. Burnap and Golden (226) reported that 15% of their general medical practice needed sexual therapy, whereas Stuntz (227) stated that 50% of his gynecologic patients were in need of sexual counseling services. More recently, Fisher et al. (76) reported that between 60% and 70% of SCI inpatients acknowledged a request for sexual information and counseling as inpatients, more than 40% noted this need at 6 months postinjury, and at 12–18 months postinjury, more than 30% still acknowledged this need.

Schover (228) described a model for brief, problem-focused sexual counseling following chronic illness. According to her model, there are at least five criteria for counseling: (a) a sexual dysfunction that predated the illness or disability, (b) a relationship that is conflicted by the illness, (c) sexual dysfunction as a result of poor coping, (d) difficulty coping because of severe changes in sexual self-image, and (e) adjustment to medical or surgical procedures. The model calls for practical, realistic, and humane interventions with clear goals. When referring someone for sexual counseling, one must be sensitive to the emotional concerns of patients. The patient referred for sexual counseling may react with disapproval because of fear that the problem is interpreted as emotional. However, a patient referred to the urologist with ED following illness or disability will probably be quite receptive to help. This situation, viewed as clearly medical, is less threatening and therefore more acceptable to the individual. Thus, one must use sensitivity in educating a patient to the emotional and physical roles involved in sexual problems.

Schover (228) delineates five aspects to her model of brief sexual counseling: (a) sexual education, (b) changing maladaptive sexual attitudes, (c) helping couples resume sex, (d) overcoming the physical handicaps, and (e) decreasing any marital conflict. The issue of sexual education cannot be overstated. Couples must be educated about the normal sexual response cycle and the impact of their specific disability on it. Couples must also be knowledgeable about the impact of medications, lifestyle changes, and the aging process on their sexuality. Chronic illness and disability often result in maladaptive attitudes (e.g., sex is unhealthy, sex must be spontaneous, intercourse is the only worthwhile form of sexual expression) that must be challenged and corrected (228). Not infrequently, couples will need assistance resuming their sexual activity. This can be accomplished through improving communication and self-esteem, along with educating the couple on alternative methods of sexual expression and caring. This will help decrease any performance anxiety. Disability will usually present physical barriers that must be successfully hurdled. Issues such as diminished movement and sensation, bowel and bladder programs, and chronic pain must be addressed. Last, when marital conflict exists because of changes in roles, changes in the homeostasis of power in the relationship, or fear that the able-bodied partner will leave, it must be confronted and corrected. An all too common conflict arises when the spouse ends up serving in the dual role of lover as well as caretaker. This situation should be actively avoided whenever possible.

Sexuality involves interplay between physiological and psychological components, and disability and illness impact each of these areas. As Trieschmann (62) has noted, the physiological and psychological contributions to the sexual act, the desire for sex, and the broader concept of sexuality must be assessed. All too often, when discussing sexuality, we only focus on the narrow aspect of the sexual act and forget the more important global aspects of sexuality. The late and noted social worker

Mary Romano (229) eloquently described female sexuality as the following: "Sexuality is more than the act of sexual intercourse. It involves for most women the whole business of relating to another person; the tenderness, the desire to give as well as take, the compliments, casual caresses, reciprocal concerns, tolerance, the forms of communication that both include and go beyond words. For women, sexuality includes a range of behaviors from smiling through orgasm; it is not just what happens between two people in bed" (p. 28). The goal with couples in sexual counseling is to help them expand their personal definition of sexuality. To the extent that their personal definition is narrow, they will have more difficulties adjusting to disability. On the other hand, when their definition of sexuality is broad and encompassing, they will likely adjust more smoothly to the physical challenges in their lives.

What is Sexual Dysfunction?

WOMEN

The effects of disability on sexual function must also be considered in light of the question of whether the individual experiences sexual dysfunction. Previously, the DSM-IV (230) was the "gold standard" for diagnosis of sexual dysfunctions, which were considered mainly psychological; however, with the advent of sildenafil, the preponderance of medical causes of sexual problems has recently been acknowledged. In fact, this resulted in a new classification of female sexual dysfunction based on a multidisciplinary international consensus development panel that included representation from physical medicine and rehabilitation (231).

Based on this new classification, there are four categories of female sexual dysfunction: sexual desire disorders, sexual arousal disorder, orgasmic disorder, and sexual pain disorders. Each of these diagnoses should then be subtyped as lifelong versus acquired, generalized versus situational, and by etiologic origin (organic, psychogenic, mixed, unknown). Moreover, a common requirement among these is that each must cause personal distress.

From a practical physiatric standpoint, this last issue bears further discussion. It follows that if an individual has decreased interest in sex directly as a cause of a TBI, there may be a sexual problem that goes undiagnosed by virtue of its effects. Furthermore, a woman with an SCI could have a physiologic change in her ability to achieve lubrication; however, it would only be considered a sexual dysfunction if this change causes her personal distress (232). Describing the expected physiologic effect of an individual's neurologic dysfunction, such as an SCI, on their sexual function, along with whether there is accompanying sexual dysfunction, then becomes a challenge. Also, the development of more detailed classification systems for sexual dysfunction, such as the Spinal Sexual Function Scale (233) recently proposed for classifying female sexual function potential post-SCI, may be warranted for other diagnoses in the future.

MEN

In the DSM-IV-TR (234), the male sexual dysfunctions are characterized by a disturbance in the psychophysiological changes that characterize the sexual response cycle. These changes cause marked distress and interpersonal difficulty. The sexual dysfunctions include sexual desire disorders, sexual arousal disorders, orgasmic disorders, sexual pain disorders, sexual dysfunction due to a general medical condition, substance induced sexual dysfunction, and sexual dysfunction not otherwise specified. Subtypes are provided to indicate the onset, context, and etiological factors associated with the sexual dysfunctions. These include lifelong or acquired, generalized or situational, and due to psychological or combined factors.

Management of Erectile Dysfunction

Since the advent of sildenafil, the management of ED has changed dramatically. Previously a topic that was almost taboo, it is now common to see television and magazine advertisements for various treatments. Ideally, despite the "quick fix" available through the use of sildenafil, management of the patient with ED should still begin with a thorough history and physical examination designed to elicit the cause. For instance, you may find that the patient is on medications that cause ED but which may be substituted by other, less disruptive drugs. If appropriate, a comprehensive evaluation should also include a psychological evaluation or determination of serum testosterone level, electrodiagnostic studies, penile Doppler, and nocturnal penile tumescence monitoring via Rigiscan (Dacomed, Minneapolis, MN). However, in many cases of disability, such as a young man with decreased ability to sustain a reflex erection following SCI, comprehensive testing may result in unnecessary cost without resultant change in treatment.

SILDENAFIL

Since the Food and Drug Administration (FDA) approved it for the treatment of ED, sildenafil has been prescribed to more than 10 million people (235). It is a selective inhibitor of cyclic guanosine monophosphate (cGMP)-specific phosphodiesterase type 5 (PDE5). By inhibiting PDE5, the enzyme responsible for cGMP catabolism, sildenafil causes nitric oxide–induced cGMP concentrations to stay elevated in penile corporeal smooth muscle. This results in increased smooth muscle relaxation with vasodilatation and penile erection (235). The most common adverse events associated with sildenafil are headache, flushing, dyspepsia, nasal congestion, and transient vi-

sual symptoms (236). The main absolute contraindication to the use of sildenafil is the use of nitroglycerin or other nitrate medications, which could result in significant reductions in blood pressure (237). Since the widespread use of the drug, cardiovascular safety has been studied extensively, without finding any adverse effects. In an analysis of 5,601 men treated for an average of 4.9 months with sildenafil in the United Kingdom, no evidence was found that age-standardized mortality for MI, MI death, or ischemic heart disease death or morbidity for MI or ischemic heart disease were higher in sildenafil-treated patients than the normal population (238). Based on the risks of sexual activity with cardiac disease, a consensus panel has recently published an algorithm for management of ED according to graded cardiovascular risk (239) (Table 74-2).

The use of sildenafil has been extensively studied in patients with ED secondary to medical and psychological causes. Efficacy of sildenafil has been demonstrated in patients with diabetes (240,241) and cardiovascular disease (242). In patients with cancer and radical prostatectomy (235,243,244), men with nerve-sparing procedures have been shown to have better responses. Men with ED subsequent to radiation therapy have also been shown to improve erectile function with the use of sildenafil (245,246), as have those treated with androgen deprivation for early prostate cancer (247). Patients with end-stage renal disease have been shown to benefit from the use of sildenafil (248), as have transplant recipients (249,250). In a study of subjects with ED and untreated depression, 83% of responders had received sildenafil (251). Moreover, sildenafil has been effectively used in men with clinically controlled major depression and subsequent SSRI-associated sexual dysfunction (47).

Patients with neurologic disorders have been especially helped with sildenafil. Men with SCI have been shown to be safely and effectively treated with sildenafil for ED (252–254). However, the drug does generally not help those with baseline complete absence of both reflex and psychogenic function (13). Efficacy has also been demonstrated in Parkinson's disease (74) and spina bifida (77).

TABLE 74-2. Erectile Dysfunction Management Algorithm According to Graded Cardiovascular Risk

Grading of Risk	Cardiovascular Status	ED Management Recommendations
Low risk	Controlled hypertension Asymptomatic, <3 risk factors for CAD	Manage within the primary care setting
	Uncomplicated past MI (>6 weeks) Mild valvular disease Mild stable angina	Review treatment options with patient and partner (whenever possible)
	Postsuccessful revascularization LVD/CHF (NYHA class I)	Reassess at regular intervals (6–12 months)
Intermediate risk	Recent MI or CVA (<6 weeks)	Specialized evaluation recommended (e.g., exercise test for angina, echocardiogram for murmur)
	≥3 risk factors for CAD, excluding age and sex LVD/CHF (NYHA class II) Moderate stable angina CVA or peripheral vascular disease	Patient to be placed in high- or low-risk category, pending outcome of testing
High risk	Unstable or refractory angina Uncontrolled hypertension (SBP > 180 mmHg) LVD/CHF (NYHA class III, IV)	Refer for specialized cardiac evaluation
		Treatment for ED to be deferred until cardiac condition stabilized and then at specialist's recommendation
	Recent MI or CVA (<14 days) High-risk arrhythmias Hypertrophic cardiomyopathy Moderate/severe valvular disease	

CAD, coronary artery disease; CHF, congestive heart failure; CVA, cerebral vascular accident; ED, erectile dysfunction; LVD, MI, myocardial infarction; NYHA, New York Heart Association; SBP, systolic blood pressure.

OTHER ORAL MEDICATIONS

Multiple oral medications have been tried to improve erectile functioning, with mixed results. Yohimbine, an alkaloid agent that blocks presynaptic α_2-adrenergic receptors, is thought to augment the physiological shunting of blood to the corporal bodies. Although some researchers (255) note there is inadequate evidence to support the use of yohimbine in persons whose ED is a result of altered shunting mechanisms or other etiologies, it was found to be useful in treating ED associated with SSRIs (256). Oral phentolamine was noted to produce erection adequate for vaginal penetration in 42% of 100 men with ED (257). Effectiveness was greatest in men with nonspecific, psychogenic, or mild vascular impotence; however, side effects included dizziness, palpitations, and nasal congestion. Apomorphine is known to produce selective activation in the nucleus paraventricularis leading to proerectile signals (258) and is marketed in a sublingual format in Europe under the name Uprima. Another PDE5 inhibitor BAY 38–9456 (vardenafil) is in clinical trials (259). With so much interest in the field of sexual dysfunction, we can anticipate more medication approvals from the FDA and new drug developments over the next few years.

TOPICAL AND INTRAURETHRAL THERAPIES

Several different medications have been applied to the penis with the goal of improving erectile functioning, including topical nitroglycerin and minoxidil, with limited clinical efficacy. Intraurethral application of prostaglandin E_1 is also available. The overall efficacy of these drugs is much less than sildenafil. Further studies are examining the use of other topical and intraurethral medications to treat ED.

VACUUM-ASSISTED ERECTIONS

One of the least invasive means of achieving penile rigidity involves the use of a vacuum erection device. These devices generally consist of a hard plastic cylindrical tube, at the end of which is a smaller, soft plastic tube leading to the pump. A manual or electrically powered pump is used to generate a vacuum, which results in engorgement of both corporeal and extracorporeal tissues. Once the erection is attained, a constricting ring is placed on the base of the penis to maintain the erection.

Vacuum-assisted erections are less esthetically pleasing than those achieved through the use of medications. Because of the engorgement of the extracorporeal tissues, there will be superficial dilation of veins, and the penis will be wider than its usual diameter. Furthermore, there is an abrupt lack of erection proximal to the constricting band. Although less invasive, vacuum erections are not without potential complications and must not be used in persons on anticoagulants because of the potential risk of hematoma. Most importantly, the maximum time the constricting band may remain in place is 30 minutes because of the potential development of necrosis of the penile skin and injury to the corporeal tissues, resulting in permanent penile deformity (260). For those men who are able to achieve an erection but unable to sustain it, the use of constricting bands may be adequate to remediate their ED; however, similar time precautions should be adhered to.

INJECTION ERECTIONS

Intracavernosal injection therapy is useful to treat most types of ED, although it is less successful in men with impaired penile arterial blood flow. Relaxation of the sinusoidal smooth muscle by the medications enhances corporeal filling, with the duration of the erection being directly related to the dose of medication administered (261). Various medications, including papaverine and Regitine, have been used for intracavernosal injections. However, prostaglandin E_1 (PGE$_1$), is most commonly used and is available in a convenient package, and intracavernosal PGE$_1$ has been demonstrated to be efficacious (262). Potential complications include penile pain, prolonged erections, priapism, penile fibrosis, and ecchymosis or hematoma (262).

Chronic administration of intracorporeal mediations can result in scarring of the tunica albuginea with resultant permanent curvature in the erect penis (263). Priapism must be treated as a medical emergency. Blood is aspirated from each corporeal body, and an α-adrenergic agonist should be injected to promote contraction of the smooth muscle and restore venous drainage to the system (264).

THE PENILE PROSTHESIS

Historically, the penile prosthesis was the mainstay of treatment for ED. Unfortunately, it is the most invasive therapy available and often results in complications in persons with impaired genital sensation. These can include mechanical failures of the devices, infections, and extrusion of the devices.

Prostheses include the malleable, which results in permanent erection, although the penis can be manipulated in order to hide it, and the inflatable. Two erectile cylinders containing fluid reservoirs at the base, an inflation pump at the tip, and an expansile chamber in the middle are surgically implanted into the corporeal bodies. Manual pumping of the device results in an erection without great increase in the diameter of the penis. Postcoitus, pressure on a relief valve causes detumescence (260).

Satisfaction rates approximate 75% with an implantable inflatable prosthesis. Complaints include altered orgasm and ejaculation, and persistence of inadequate erection to enjoy intercourse (265). Potential complications include internal scar formation resulting in device dysfunction, mechanical failure resulting in penile deformity, and extravasation of the internal fluid of the device. The rate of prosthesis infection can be as high as 16.5% (266) in patients with SCI, and infection coupled with the risk of extrusion led to a 25% explantation rate in another study of men with SCI (267). Currently, this should be considered a treatment of last resort.

Management of Hypoactive Sexual Desire

Hypoactive sexual desire disorder is a persistent or recurrent lack of sexual fantasies and desire for sexual activity that causes the individual marked personal or interpersonal distress (DSM-IV-TR). Hypoactive sexual desire is one of the most common problems addressed in general sex therapy, occurring in 15% to 34% of the able-bodied population (268). In addition to being primary and premorbid, decreased desire associated with disability or illness can also be related to depression or other psychological distress related to disability or illness, or related to the use of medications or to the illness. Treatment involves discontinuing any medications that could be responsible for the dysfunction and referral for counseling.

Management of Premature Ejaculation

Premature ejaculation is one of the most common male sexual dysfunctions (269). Although that name persists in the DSM-IV-TR, practitioners have been notoriously unable to come to a consistent definition, and the term *early ejaculation* has been recommended to be less pejorative and more accurate (270). Masters and Johnson's (63) definition for early ejaculation was that the male ejaculated before the female was orgasmic at least 50% of the time. However, because some women are unable to experience orgasm through genital intercourse, this definition has pitfalls. Other researchers have utilized time, such as 1 or 2 minutes of intercourse thrusting, whereas others have noted the inability to maintain control with more than 20 seconds of rapid thrusting (270). The DSM-IV-TR defines premature ejaculation as "persistent or recurrent ejaculation with minimal sexual stimulation before, on, or shortly after penetration and before the person wishes it. The clinician must take into account factors that affect duration of the excitement phase . . . " (230). Furthermore, the disturbance must cause marked distress.

In men with disabilities, premature ejaculation is usually present premorbidly (271). New diagnoses should prompt a workup for prostate or urinary infection (272) and may be easily treatable with antibiotics. For other cases, a cognitive-behavioral treatment model is used. New attitudes and skills are taught to increase the man's pleasure and decrease the pressure to perform for the woman. Ejaculatory control is then relearned as a couple, through progressively increasing stimulation and identifying the point of ejaculatory inevitability, at which point stimulation is stopped and then resumed. Furthermore, alternative intercourse positions and movements are added as control is achieved (270).

Recent research has also demonstrated that medical treatment may be appropriate to treat problems with early ejaculation. For those couples who have failed behavioral interventions, medical treatment with SSRIs may help improve ejaculatory latency. Fluoxetine and clomipramine have both been shown to have beneficial effects in this regard (269).

Management of Inhibited Ejaculation

Inhibited ejaculation is rare in the nondisabled population but extremely common in men with some neurologic disorders, particularly SCI. In this population, inhibited ejaculation may or may not be accompanied by anorgasmia. To date, treatments have relied on the restoration of ejaculatory function, solely for fertility purposes. However, some of these procedures may be accompanied by pleasant sexual sensations including orgasm. As some men with complete SCI still retain the ability to achieve orgasm, future research should include a focus on what can be done to improve orgasmic capabilities in men with SCI and other neurologic disabilities.

Management of Female Sexual Arousal Disorder

The International Female Sexual Dysfunction Classification defines female sexual arousal disorder as the persistent or recurrent inability to attain or maintain sufficient sexual excitement, causing personal distress, which may be expressed as a lack of subjective excitement, or genital or other somatic responses. Subtypes of dysfunction were previously described. Treatment should include assessment of whether the condition was premorbid, along with removal of any potential causative agents. The use of water-based lubricants is appropriate, as is education about the impact of the particular disability on sexual functioning. The use of sildenafil was shown to be potentially beneficial in a small double-masked placebo-controlled study of women with SCI (273). Furthermore, the use of vibratory stimulation may increase arousal (274). Cognitive therapies may also be beneficial in subgroups. False-positive feedback was shown to be beneficial in women with SCI (275). Sexual counseling is appropriate in cases of premorbid disorders.

Orgasmic Disorder

Orgasmic disorder is the persistent or recurrent difficulty, delay in, or absence of attaining orgasm following sufficient sexual stimulation and arousal, which causes personal distress. As with all sexual dysfunctions when working with women with disabilities, it is important to determine if the dysfunction was premorbid, as treatments may differ. For those women with primary anorgasmia, learning about their bodies through masturbation with gradual increasing stimulation until they reach orgasm is one treatment method. Sex therapy may also be beneficial. For those women with disabilities, only those with complete disruption of their sacral reflex arc appear to have anorgasmia based solely on their neurologic dysfunction (20). Therefore, we recommend that the liberal use of vibrators and other sexual aids to augment sexual response be tried in women with disabilities, and women should be taught to masturbate to learn what now feels good to them. The use of the EROS therapy should also be considered (276). Future research should focus on improving the capabilities of women with disabilities to achieve orgasm.

Sexual Pain Disorders

Dyspareunia is recurrent or persistent genital pain associated with intercourse. Vaginismus is the recurrent or persistent involuntary spasm of the musculature of the outer third of the vagina that interferes with vaginal penetration and that causes personal distress. Noncoital sexual pain disorder is recurrent or persistent genital pain induced by noncoital sexual stimulation. Treatment should include a search for comorbidities, such as neuropathic pain. It also includes assurance of adequate vaginal lubrication and relaxation training, as well as physical and sex therapy. Increasing sizes of well-lubricated dilators may be used by the patient to practice stimulation. Above all, it is important that the woman always be in charge of when and how penetration takes place (277).

REFERENCES

1. Masters WH, Johnson VE. *Human sexual response*. Boston: Little, Brown, 1966.
2. Robinson P. *The modernization of sex*. New York: Harper & Row, 1976.
3. Rosen RC, Beck JG. *Patterns of sexual arousal: psychophysiological processes and clinical applications*. New York: Guilford Press, 1988.
4. Kaplan HS. Hypoactive sexual desire. *J Sex Marital Ther* 1977;3:3–9.
5. Kaplan HS. *Disorders of sexual desire*. New York: Simon and Schuster, 1979.
6. Weiss HD. The physiology of human penile erection. *Ann Intern Med* 1972;76:793.
7. Sipski ML, Alexander CJ. Sexual function and dysfunction after spinal cord injury. *Phys Med Rehab Clin N Am* 1992;3:811–828.
8. McKenna KE. Some proposals regarding the organization of the central nervous system control of penile erection. *Neurosci Biobehav Rev* 2000;24:535–540.
9. Andersson K-E, Wagner G. Physiology of penile erection. *Physiol Rev* 1995;75:191–236.
10. Nehra A. Treatment of male erectile dysfunction: past, present and future. *Sex Dysfunction Med* 2001;2:66–71.
11. Traish A, Kim NN, Moreland RB, et al. Role of alpha adrenergic receptors in erectile function. *Int J Impot Res* 2000;23[Suppl 1]:S48–S63.
12. Bennett CJ, Seager SW, Vasher EA, McGuire EJ. Sexual dysfunction and electroejaculation in men with spinal cord injury: review. *J Urol* 1988;139:453–457.
13. Schmid DM, Schurch B, Hauri D. Sildenafil in the treatment of sexual dysfunction in spinal cord-injured male patients. *Eur Urol* 2000;38:184–193.
14. Courtois FJ, Goulet MC, Charvier KR, et al. Post-traumatic erectile potential of spinal cord injured men: how physiologic recordings supplement subjective reports. *Arch Phys Med Rehabil* 1999;80:1268–1272.
15. Bors E, Comarr AE. Neurological disturbances of sexual function with special reference to 529 patients with spinal cord injury. *Urol Surv* 1960;110:191.
16. De Groat WC, Booth AM. Neural control of penile erection. In: Maggi CA, Harwood J, eds. *The autonomic nervous system*. London: Academic Publishers, 1993:467–524.

17. Sipski ML. Spinal cord injury: what is the effect on sexual response? *J Am Paraplegia Soc* 1991;14:40–43.
18. Giuliano F, Allard J, Compagnie S, et al. Vaginal physiological changes in a model of sexual arousal in anesthetized rats. *Am J Physiol Regul Integr Comp Physiol* 2001;281:R140–R149.
19. Sipski ML, Alexander CJ, Rosen RC. Physiological parameters associated with psychogenic sexual arousal in women with complete spinal cord injuries. *Arch Phys Med Rehabil* 1995;76: 811–818.
20. Sipski ML, Alexander CJ, Rosen RC. Sexual arousal and orgasm in women: effects of spinal cord injury. *Ann Neurol* 2001;49:35–44.
21. Meston CM, Gorzalka BB. The effects of sympathetic activation following acute exercise on physiological and subjective sexual arousal in women. *Behav Res Ther* 1995;33:651–664.
22. Meston CM, Heiman JR. Ephedrine-activated sexual arousal in women. *Arch Gen Psychiatry* 1998;55:652–656.
23. Meston CM. Sympathetic nervous system activity and female sexual arousal. *Am J Cardiol* 2000;86:2[Suppl 1]:30–34.
24. Kleitsch EC, O'Donnell PD. Sex and aging. *Phys Med Rehabil State Art Rev* 1990;4:121–134.
25. Starr BD, Weiner MB. *The Starr-Weiner report on sex and sexuality in the mature years.* New York: McGraw-Hill, 1981.
26. Whitten P, Whiteside EJ. Can exercise make you sexier? *Psychology Today* 1989;April:42–44.
27. Sipski ML, Alexander CJ, eds. *Sexual function in people with disability and chronic illness: a health professional's guide.* Gaithersburg, MD: Aspen Publishers, 1997.
28. Breckenridge A. Angiotensin converting enzyme inhibitors and quality of life. *Am J Hypertens* 1991;4:79S–82S.
29. Weiner DN, Rosen RC. Medications and their impact. In: Sipski ML, Alexander CJ, eds. *Sexual function in people with disability and chronic illness: a health professional's guide.* Gaithersburg, MD: Aspen Publishers, 1997:85–118.
30. Hogan MJ, Wallin JD, Baer RM. Antihypertensive therapy and male sexual dysfunction. *Psychosomatics* 1980;21:235–237.
31. Croog SH, Levine S, Sudilovsky A, et al. Sexual symptoms in hypertensive patients: a clinical trial of antihypertensive medications. *Arch Intern Med* 1988;148:788–794.
32. Ko DT, Hebert PR, Coffey CS, et al. β-Blocker therapy and symptoms of depression, fatigue, and sexual dysfunction. *JAMA* 2002;288:351–357.
33. Chang SW, Fine R, Siegel D, et al. The impact of diuretic therapy on reported sexual function. *Arch Intern Med* 1991;151:2402–2408.
34. Blane GF. Comparative toxicity and safety profile of fenofibrate and other fibric acid derivatives. *Am J Med* 1987;83:26–36.
35. Coronary Drug Research Group. Clofibrate and niacin in coronary heart disease. *JAMA* 1975;231:360–388.
36. Schneider J, Kaffarnik H. Impotence in patients treated with clofibrate. *Atherosclerosis* 1975;21:455–475.
37. Stoffer SS, Hynes KM, Jiang NS, Ryan RJ. Digoxin and abnormal serum hormone levels. *JAMA* 1973;225:1643–1644.
38. Neri A, Aygen M, Zuckerman Z, Bahary C. Subjective assessment of sexual dysfunction of patients on long-term administration of digoxin. *Arch Sex Behav* 1980;9:343–347.
39. Amahd S. Disopyramide and impotence [Letter to the editor]. *South Med J* 1980;73:958.
40. McHaffie DJ, Guz A, Johnston A. Impotence in a patient on disopyramide. *Lancet* 1977;1:859.
41. Couper-Smartt JD, Rodham R. A technique for surveying side effects of tricyclic drugs with reference to reported side effects. *J Intern Med Res* 1973;1: 473–476.
42. Monteiro WO, Noshirvani HF, Marks IM, Lelliott PT. Anorgasmia from clomipramine in obsessive-compulsive disorder: a controlled trial. *Br J Psychiatry* 1987;151:107–112.
43. McLean JD, Forsyth RG, Kapkin IA. Unusual side effects of clomipramine associated with yawning. *Can J Psychiatry* 1983:28:569–570.
44. Sovner R. Anorgasmia associated with imipramine but not desipramine: case report. *J Clin Psychiatry* 1983;44:345–346.
45. Shen WW. Female orgasmic inhibition by amoxapine. *Am J Psychiatry* 1982; 139:1220–1221.
46. Nurnberg HG, Levine PE. Spontaneous remission of MAOI-induced anorgasmia. *Am J Psychiatry* 1987;144:805–807.
47. Nurnberg HG, Gelenberg AJ, Fava M et al. Sildenafil for serotonin reuptake inhibitor-associated sexual dysfunction: a 3-center, 6-week, double-blind, placebo-controlled study in 90 men. *American Psychiatric Association abstract book 2000.* Arlington, VA: APA, 2000.
48. Ashton AK, Hamer R, Rosen RC. SSRI-induced sexual dysfunction and its treatment: a large-scale retrospective study of 596 psychiatric outpatients. *J Sex Marital Ther* 1997;23(3):165–175.
49. Nutt D, Hackman A, Hawton K. Increased sexual function in benzodiazepine withdrawal. *Lancet* 1986;2:1101–1102.
50. Riley AJ, Riley EJ. Cyproheptadine and antidepressant-induced anorgasmia. *Br J Psychiatry* 1986;148:217–218.
51. Sangal R. Inhibited female orgasm as a side effect of alprazolam. *Am J Psychiatry* 1985;142:1223–1224.
52. Uhde TW, Tancer ME, Shea CA. Sexual dysfunction related to alprazolam treatment of social phobia [Letter to the editor]. *Am J Psychiatry* 1988;145: 531– 532.
53. Hughs JM. Failure to ejaculate with chlordiazepoxide. *Am J Psychiatry* 1964; 121:610–611.
54. Segraves RT. Treatment of premature ejaculation with lorazepam. *Am J Psychiatry* 1987;144:1240.
55. Balon R, Ramesh C, Pohl R. Sexual dysfunction associated with diazepam but not clonazepam. *Can J Psychiatry* 1989;34:947–948.
56. Mattson RH, Cramer JA, Collines JF, et al. Comparison of carbamazepine, phenobarbital, phenytoin, primidone in partial and secondary generalized tonic-clonic seizures. *N Engl J Med* 1985;313:145–151.
57. Jensen P, Jensen SB, Sorensen PS, et al. Sexual dysfunction in male and female patients with epilepsy: a study of 86 outpatients. *Arch Sex Behav* 1990; 19:1–14.
58. Niv Y. Male sexual dysfunction due to cimetidine. *Ir Med J* 1986;79:352.
59. Wolfe MM. Impotence of cimetidine therapy. *N Engl J Med* 1979;300:94.
60. Van Thiel PH, Gavaler BS, Smith WI, Paul G. Hypothalamic-pituitary-gonadal dysfunction in men using cimetidine. *N Engl J Med* 1979;300:1012– 1015.
61. Peden NR, Wormsley KG. Effect of cimetidine on gonadal function in man [Letter to the editor]. *Br J Clin Pharmacol* 1982;14:565.
62. Trieschmann RB. *Spinal cord injuries: psychological, social and vocational adjustment,* 2nd ed. New York: Pergamon, 1988.
63. Masters WH, Johnson VE. *Human sexual inadequacy.* Boston: Little, Brown, 1970.
64. Taylor SE. Adjustment to threatening events: a theory of cognitive adaptation. *Am Psychol* 1983;38(11):1161–1173.
65. Erikson EH. *Identity: youth and crisis.* New York: Norton, 1968.
66. Talbot HS. The sexual function in paraplegia. *J Urol* 1955;73:91.
67. Comarr AE, Vigue M. Sexual counseling among male and female patients with spinal cord injury and/or cauda equina injury. *Am J Phys Med* 1978;57: 107–122, 216–227.
68. Geiger RC. Neurophysiology of sexual response in spinal cord injury. *Sexuality and Disability* 1979;2(4):257–266.
69. Phelps G, Brown M, Chen J, et al. Sexual experience and plasma testosterone levels in male veterans after spinal cord injury. *Arch Phys Med Rehabil* 1983; 64:47–52.
70. Alexander CJ, Sipski ML, Findley TW. Sexual activities, desire, and satisfaction in males pre- and post-spinal cord injury. *Arch Sex Behav* 1993;22(3): 217–228.
71. Charlifue SW, Gerhart KA, Menter RR, et al. Sexual issues of women with spinal cord injuries. *Paraplegia* 1992;30:192–199.
72. McKenna KE, Chung SK, McVary KT. A model for the study of sexual function in anesthetized male and female rats. *Am J Physiol* 1991;30:R1276– R1285.
73. Willmuth ME. Sexuality after spinal cord injury: a critical review. *Clin Psychol Rev* 1987;7:389–412.
74. Sjogren K, Egberg K. The sexual experience in younger males with complete spinal cord injury. *Scand J Rehabil Med Suppl* 1983;9:189–194.
75. Berkman AH, Weissman R, Frielich MH. Sexual adjustment of spinal cord injured veterans living in the community. *Arch Phys Med Rehabil* 1978;59: 29–33.
76. Fisher TL, Laud PW, Byfield MG, et al. Sexual health after spinal cord injury: a longitudinal study. *Arch Phys Med Rehabil* 2002;83:1043–1051.
77. Sipski ML, Alexander CJ. Sexual activities, response and satisfaction in women pre- and post-spinal cord injury. *Arch Phys Med Rehabil* 1993;74: 1025–1029.
78. Linsenmeyer TA, Perkash I. Infertility in men with spinal cord injury. *Arch Phys Med Rehabil* 1991;72:747–754.
79. Brackett NL, Lynne CM, Weizman MS, et al. Scrotal and oral temperatures are not related to semen quality or serum gonadotropin levels in spinal cord-injured men. *J Androl* 1994;15:614–619.
80. Brackett NL, Davi RC, Padron OF, Lynne CM. Seminal plasma of spinal cord injured men inhibits sperm motility of normal men. *J Urol* 1996;155:1632–1635.
81. Padron OF, Brackett NL, Sharma RK, et al. Seminal reactive oxygen species and sperm motility and morphology in men with spinal cord injury. *Fertil Steril* 1997;67:1115–1120.
82. Linsenmeyer TA, Pogach LM, Ottenweller JE, Huang HFS. Spermatogenesis and the pituitary-testicular hormone axis in rats during the acute phase of spinal cord injury. *J Urol* 1994;152:1302–1307.
83. Brackett NL, Ferrell SM, Aballa TC, et al. Semen quality in spinal cord injured men: does it progressively decline postinjury? *Arch Phys Med Rehabil* 1998;79:625–628.
84. Linsenmeyer TA. Management of male infertility. In: Sipski ML, Alexander CJ, eds. *Sexual function in people with disability and chronic illness: a health professional's guide.* Gaithersburg, MD: Aspen Publishers, 1997:487–509.
85. Horne HW, Paul DA, Munro D. Fertility studies in the human male with traumatic injuries of the spinal cord and cauda equina. *N Engl J Med* 1948; 239:959–951.
86. Thomas RJS, McLeish G, McDonald IA. Electroejaculation of the paraplegic male followed by pregnancy. *Med J Aust* 1975;2:798–799.
87. Sonksen J, Biering-Sorensen F, Kristensen JK. Ejaculation induced by penile vibratory stimulation in men with spinal cord injuries: the importance of the vibratory amplitude. *Paraplegia* 1994;32:651–660.
88. Ohl DA, Menge AC, Sonksen J. Penile vibratory stimulation in spinal cord injured men: optimized vibration parameters and prognostic factors. *Arch Phys Med Rehabil* 1996;77:903–905.
89. Brackett NL, Padron OF, Lynne CM. Semen quality of spinal cord injured men is better when obtained by vibratory stimulation versus electroejaculation. *J Urol* 1997;157:151–157.

90. Ohl DA, Sonksen J, Menge AC, et al. Electroejaculation versus vibratory stimulation in spinal cord injured men: sperm quality and patient preference. *J Urol* 1997;157;2147–2149.

91. Ohl DA, Denil J, Fitzgerald-Shelton K, et al. Fertility of spinal cord injured males: effect of genitourinary infection and bladder management on results of electroejaculation. *J Am Paraplegia Soc* 1992;15(2):53–59.

92. Jackson AB, Wadley V. A multicenter study of women's self-reported reproductive health after spinal cord injury. *Arch Phys Med Rehabil* 1999;80;1420–1428.

93. Axel SJ. Spinal cord injured women's concerns: menstruation and pregnancy. *Rehabil Nurs* 1982;7(5):10–15.

94. Baker ER, Cardenas DD. Pregnancy in spinal cord injured women. *Arch Phys Med Rehabil* 1996;77:501–507.

95. Feyi-Waboso PA. An audit of five years experience of pregnancy in spinal cord damaged women: a regional unit's experience and a review of the literature. *Paraplegia* 1992;30:631–635.

96. Westgren N, Hultling C, Levi R, Westgren M. Pregnancy and delivery in women with a traumatic spinal cord injury in Sweden, 1980–1991. *Obstet Gynecol* 1993;81:926–930.

97. Robertson DNS, Guttman L. The paraplegic patient in pregnancy and labour. *Proc R Soc Med* 1963;56:381–387.

98. Wanner MB, Rageth CJ, Zach GA. Pregnancy and autonomic hyperreflexia in patients with spinal cord lesions. *Paraplegia* 1987;25:482–490.

99. Valleroy ML, Kraft G. Sexual dysfunction in multiple sclerosis. *Arch Phys Med Rehabil* 1984;65:125–128.

100. Mattson DH, Petrie M, Srivastava DK, McDermott M. Multiple sclerosis—sexual dysfunction and its response to medications. *Arch Neurol* 1995;52: 862–868.

101. Barak Y, Achiron A, Elizur A, et al. Sexual dysfunction in relapsing-remitting multiple sclerosis: magnetic resonance imaging, clinical, and psychological correlates. *J Psychiatry Neurosci* 1996;21:255–258.

102. Hulter BM, Lundberg PO. Sexual function in women with advanced multiple sclerosis. *J Neurol Neurosurg Psychiatry* 1995;59:83–86.

103. Yang CC, Bowen JR, Kraft GH, et al. Cortical evoked potentials of the dorsal nerve of the clitoris and female sexual dysfunction in multiple sclerosis. *J Urol* 2000;164:2010–2013.

104. Smeltzer SC, Kelley LC. Multiple sclerosis. In: Sipski ML, Alexander CJ, eds. *Sexual function in people with disability and chronic illness: a health professional's guide.* Gaithersburg, MD: Aspen Publishers, 1997: 177–188.

105. Birk K, Rudick R. Pregnancy and multiple sclerosis. *Arch Neurol* 1986;43: 719–726.

106. Korn-Lubetzki I, Kahana E, Cooper G. Activity of multiple sclerosis during pregnancy and puerperium. *Ann Neurol* l984;16:229–231.

107. Thompson DS, Nelson LM, Burns A, et al. The effect of pregnancy in multiple sclerosis: a retrospective study. *Neurology* l986;36:1097–1099.

108. Weinshenker BG, Hader W, Carriere W, et al. The influence of pregnancy on disability from multiple sclerosis: a population-based study in Middlesex County, Ontario. *Neurology* 1989;39:1438–1440.

109. Monga TN, Kerrigan AJ. Cerebrovascular accidents. In: Sipski ML, Alexander CJ, eds. *Sexual function in people with disability and chronic illness: a health professional's guide.* Gaithersburg, MD: Aspen Publishers, 1997:189–219.

110. Monga TN, Lawson JS, Inglis J. Sexual dysfunction in stroke patients. *Arch Phys Med Rehabil* 1986;67(1):19–22.

111. Aloni R, Ring H, Rozenthul N, Schwart J. Sexual function in male patients after stroke: a follow-up study. *Sexuality and Disability* 1993;11(2):121–128.

112. Kinsella GH, Duffy FD. Psychosocial readjustment in the spouses of aphasic patients: a comparative survey of 79 subjects. *Scand J Rehabil Med* 1979;11 (3):129–132.

113. Sjogren K, Damber JE, Liliequist B. Sexuality after stroke with hemiplegia. 1. Aspects of sexual function. *Scand J Rehabil Med* 1983;15:55–61.

114. Boldrini P, Basaglia N, Calanca MC. Sexual changes in hemiparetic patients. *Arch Phys Med Rehabil* 1991;72:202–207.

115. Korpelainen JT, Kauhanen M-L, Kemola H, et al. Sexual dysfunction in stroke patients. *Acta Neurol Scand* 1998;98:400–405.

116. Korpelainen JT, Nieminen P, Myllyla VV. Sexual functioning among stroke patients and their spouses. *Stroke* 1999;30:715–719.

117. Bray GP, DeFrank RS, Wolfe TL. Sexual functioning in stroke patients. *Arch Phys Med Rehabil* 1981;62(6):286–288.

118. Elovic E, Antoinette T. Epidemiology and primary prevention of traumatic brain injury. In: Horn LJ, Zasler ND, eds. *Medical rehabilitation of traumatic brain injury.* Philadelphia: Hanley and Belfus, 1996:1–28.

119. Meyer JE. Die sexuellen storungen der hirnverletzten. *Arch Psychiatr Z Neurol* 1955;193:449–469.

120. Hibbard MR, Gordon WA, Flanagan S, et al. Sexual dysfunction after traumatic brain injury. *NeuroRehabilitation* 2000:15:107–120.

121. Walker AE, Jablon S. *A follow-up study of head wounds in World War II.* Washington, DC: Veterans Administration Medical Monograph, 1961.

122. Boller F, Frank E. *Sexual dysfunction in neurologic disorders: diagnosis, management and rehabilitation.* New York: Raven Press, 1982.

123. MacLean O. Brain mechanisms of primal sexual functions and related behavior. In: Sandler M, Gessa G, eds. *Sexual behavior: pharmacology and biochemistry.* New York: Raven Press, 1975.

124. Blendonohy P, Philip P. Precocious puberty in children after traumatic brain injury. *Brain Inj* l991;5:63–68.

125. Sandel ME. Traumatic brain injury. In: Sipski ML, Alexander CJ, eds. *Sexual function in people with disability and chronic illness: a health professional's guide.* Gaithersburg, MD: Aspen Publishers, 1997:221–245.

126. Horn LJ, Zasler ND. Neuroanatomy and neurophysiology of sexual dysfunction. *J Head Trauma Rehabil* 1990;5:1–13.

127. Heath RG. Pleasure response of human subjects to direct stimulation of the brain: physiologic and psycho-dynamic considerations. In: Heath RG, ed. *The role of pleasure in behavior.* New York: Harper & Row, 1964.

128. Kluver H, Bucy PC. Preliminary analysis of functions of temporal lobes in monkeys. *Arch Neurol Psychiatry* 1939;42:979–1000.

129. Lilly R. The human Kluver-Bucy syndrome. *Neurology* 1983;33:1141.

130. Mesulum M. *Principles of behavioral neurology.* Philadelphia: FA Davis, 1985.

131. Miller B, Cummings J, McIntyre H, et al. Hypersexuality or altered sexual preference following brain injury. *J Neurol Neurosurg Psychiatry* 1986;49:867–873.

132. Sandel ME, Williams KS, DellaPietra L, Derogatis LR. Sexual functioning following traumatic brain injury. *Brain Inj* 1996;10:719–728.

133. Blake DJ, Maisiak R, Alarcon GS, Brown S. Sexual quality of life of patients with arthritis compared to arthritis-free controls. *J Rheumatol* 1987;14:570–576.

134. Pigg JS, Schroeder PM. Frequently occurring problems of patients with rheumatic disease: the ANA outcome standards for rheumatology nursing practice. *Nurs Clin North Am* 1984;19(4):697–708.

135. Lipe H, Longstreth WT, Bird TD, Linde M. Sexual function in married men with Parkinson's disease compared to married men with arthritis. *Neurology* 1990;40:1347–1349.

136. Conine TA, Evans JH. Sexual reactivation of chronically ill and disabled adults. *J Allied Health* 1982;11:261–270.

137. Gordon D, Beastall GH, Thomson JA, Sturrock RD. Androgenic status and sexual function in males with rheumatoid arthritis and ankylosing spondylitis. *QJM* 1986;231:671–679.

138. Yoshino S, Uchida S. Sexual problems of women with rheumatoid arthritis. *Arch Phys Med Rehabil* 1981;62:122–123.

139. Bhadauria S, Moser DK, Clements PJ, et al. Genital tract abnormalities and female sexual function impairment in systemic sclerosis. *Am J Obstet Gynecol* 1995;172:580–587.

140. Curry SL, Levine SB, Conty E, et al. The impact of systemic lupus erythematosus on women's sexual functioning. *J Rheumatol* 1994;21:2254–2260.

141. Lally EV, Jimenez SA. Erectile failure in systemic sclerosis. *N Engl J Med* 1990;322:1398.

142. Simeon CP, Fonollosa V, Vilardell M, et al. Impotence and Peyronie's disease in systemic sclerosis. *Clin Exp Rheumatol* 1994;12:464.

143. Saad CS, Behrendt AE. Scleroderma and sexuality. *J Sex Res* 1996;33:215–220.

144. Buckwalter KC, Wernimont T, Buckwalter JA. Musculoskeletal conditions and sexuality (Part I). *Sexuality and Disability* 1982;4(3):131–142.

145. Currey HLF. Osteoarthritis of the hip joint and sexual activity. *Ann Rheum Dis* 1970;29:488–493.

146. Stern SH, Fuchs MD, Ganz SB, et al. Sexual function after total hip arthroplasty. *Clin Orthop Rel Res* 1991;269:228–235.

147. Nadler SN. Arthritis and other connective tissue diseases. In: Sipski ML, Alexander CJ, eds. *Sexual function in people with disability and chronic illness: a health professional's guide.* Gaithersburg, MD: Aspen Publishers, 1997;:261–278.

148. Karan JH, Forsham PH. Pancreatic hormones and diabetes mellitus. In: Greenspan FS, Baxter JD, eds. *Basic and clinical endocrinology.* Norwalk, CT: Appleton & Lange, 1994:50.

149. Tilton MC. Diabetes and amputation. In: Sipski ML, Alexander CJ, eds. *Sexual function in people with disability and chronic illness: a health professional's guide.* Gaithersburg, MD: Aspen Publishers, 1997:279–302.

150. Faerman I, Jadzinsky M, Podolsky S. Diabetic neuropathy and sexual dysfunction. In: Podolsky S, ed. *Clinical diabetes: modern management.* New York: Appleton-Century-Crofts, 1980:306–316.

151. McCulloch DK, Young RJ, Prescott RJ, et al. The natural history of impotence in diabetic men. *Diabetologia* 1984;26:437–440.

152. Melman A, Henry DP, Felten DL, O'Connor B. Effect of diabetes upon penile sympathetic nerves in impotent man. *South Med J* 1980;73(3):307–317.

153. Baum N, Neiman M, Lewis R. Evaluation and treatment of organic impotence in the male with diabetes mellitus. *Diabetes Educ* 1988;14(2):123–129.

154. Faerman I, Glocer L, Fox D, et al. Impotence and diabetes: histological studies of the autonomic nervous fibers of the corpora cavernosa in impotent diabetic males. *Diabetes* 1974;23(12):971–976.

155. Buvat J, Lemaire A, Buvat-Herbaut M, et al. Comparative investigations in 26 impotent and 26 nonimpotent diabetic patients. *J Urol* 1985;133:34–38.

156. Jensen SB. Diabetic sexual dysfunction: a comparative study of 160 insulin treated diabetic men and women and an age-matched control group. *Arch Sex Behav* 1981;10(6):493–504.

157. Tyrer G, Steel JM, Ewing DJ, et al. Sexual responsiveness in diabetic women. *Diabetologia* 1983;24:166–171.

158. Whitley M, Berke P. Sexuality and diabetes. In: Woods NF, ed. *Human sexuality in health and illness.* St Louis: CV Mosby, 1984;328–340.

159. Leedom L, Feldman M, Procci W, Zeidler A. Symptoms of sexual dysfunction and depression in diabetic women. *J Diabetes Complications* 1991;5(1): 38–41.

160. Albert A, Wincze JP. *Sexual arousal in diabetic females: a psychophysiological investigation.* Unpublished manuscript, Brown University, 1990.

161. Campbell LV, Redelman MJ, Borkman M, et al. Factors in sexual dysfunction in diabetic female volunteer subjects. *Med J Aust* 1989;151:550–552.

162. Kolodny RC. Sexual dysfunction in diabetic females. *Diabetes* 1971;20:557–559.

163. Zrustova M, Rostlaplil J, Kabrhelova A. Sexual disorders in diabetic women. *Csek Gynekol* 1978;43:277–281.

164. Ellenberg M. Sexual aspects of the female diabetic. *Mt Sinai J Med* 1977;44:495–499.

165. Williams RH. The endocrine pancreas and diabetes mellitus. In: Williams RH, ed. *Textbook of endocrinology.* Philadelphia: WB Saunders, 1981:831.

166. Hare JW. Diabetes and pregnancy. In: Kahn CR, Weir GC, eds. *Joslin's diabetes mellitus.* Philadelphia: Lea & Febiger, 1994:889–899.

167. Rybarczyk B, Nyenhuis DL, Nicholas JJ, et al. Body image, perceived social stigma, the prediction of psychosocial adjustment to leg amputation. *Rehabil Psychol* 1995;40(2):95–110.

168. Blocker WP Jr. Coronary heart disease and sexuality. In: *Physical medicine and rehabilitation: state of the art reviews,* vol 9. Philadelphia: Hanley and Belfus, 1995:387.

169. Papadopoulos C, Beaumont C, Shelley SI, Larrimore P. Myocardial infarction and sexual activity of the female patient. *Arch Intern Med* 1983;143:1528–1530.

170. Mehta J, Krop H. The effect of myocardial infarction on sexual functioning. *Sexuality and Disability* 1979; 2:115–121.

171. Blocker WP. Cardiac rehabilitation. In: Halstead L, Grabois M, eds. *Medical rehabilitation.* New York: Raven Press, 1985:181–192.

172. Muller JE, Mittleman MA, Maclure M, et al. Triggering myocardial infarction by sexual activity: low absolute risk and prevention by regular physical exertion. *JAMA* 1996;275:1405–1409.

173. Cassem NH, Hackett TP. Physiological rehabilitation of myocardial infarction patients in the acute phase. *Heart Lung* 1973;2:382–388.

174. Stitik TP, Benevento BT. Cardiac and pulmonary disease. In: Sipski ML, Alexander CJ, eds. *Sexual function in people with disability and chronic illness: a health professional's guide.* Gaithersburg, MD: Aspen Publishers, 1997:303–335.

175. Hamilton GA, Seidman RN. A comparison of the recovery period for women and men after an acute myocardial infarction. *Heart Lung* 1993;22:308–315.

176. Conine TA, Evans JH. Sexual reactivation of chronically ill and disabled adults. *J Allied Health* 1982;264:261–270.

177. Cohen JA. Sexual counseling of the patient following myocardial infarction. *Crit Care Nurs* 1986;6(6):18–29.

178. Skinner JB. Sexual relations and the cardiac patient. In: Pollock ML, Schmat DH, eds. *Heart disease and rehabilitation.* New York: John Wiley & Sons, 1986:583–589.

179. Hellerstein HK, Friedman EH. Sexual activity and the postcoronary patient. *Med Aspects Hum Sexuality* 1969;3(3):70–96.

180. Bohlen JG, Held JP, Sanderson MO, Patterson RP. Heart rate, rate pressure product and oxygen uptake during four sexual activities. *Arch Intern Med* 1984;144:1745–1748.

181. Elster SE, Mansfield LW. Stair climbing as a test of readiness for resumption of sexual activity after a heart attack (abstracted). *Circulation* 1977;55–56 [Suppl III]:102.

182. Drory Y, Shapira I, Fisman E, Pines A. Myocardial ischemia during sexual activity in patients with coronary artery disease. *Am J Cardiol* 1995;75:835–837.

183. Scalzi CC. Sexual counseling and sexual therapy for patients after myocardial infarction. *Cardiovasc Nurs* 1982;18:13–17.

184. McCauley K, Choromanski JD, Wallinger C, Liu K. Learning to live with controlled ventricular tachycardia: utilizing the Johnson model. *Heart Lung* 1984;13(6):637.

185. Griffith GC. Sexuality and the cardiac patient. *Heart Lung* 1973;2:70–73.

186. Masur FT. Resumption of sexual activity following myocardial infarction. *Sexuality and Disability* 1979;2:98–114.

187. Abbott MA, McWhirter DP. Resuming sexual activity after myocardial infarction. *Med Aspects Hum Sexuality* 1978;12(6):18–28.

188. Semmler C, Semmler M. Counseling the coronary patient. *Am J Occup Ther* 1974;28:609–614.

189. Eliot RS, Miles RR. Advising the cardiac patient about sexual intercourse. *Med Aspects Hum Sexuality* 1975;9(6):49–50.

190. Friedman JM. Sexual adjustment of the postcoronary male. In: LoPicolo J, LoPicolo L, eds. *Handbook of sex therapy.* New York: Plenum Press, 1978.

191. Koller R, Kennedy KW, Butler JC, Wagner NN. Counseling the coronary patient on sexual activity. *Postgrad Med* 1972;51(4):133–136.

192. Wagner NN. Sexual activity and the cardiac patient. In: Green R, ed. *Human sexuality: a health practitioner's text.* Baltimore: Williams & Wilkins, 1975:173–179.

193. Plummer JK. Psychosocial factors in pulmonary rehabilitation. In: O'Ryan, Burns, eds. *Pulmonary rehabilitation from hospital to home.* Chicago: Year Book Medical Publishers, 1984:162–165.

194. Hahn K. Sexuality and COPD. *Rehabil Nurs* 1989;14(4):191–195.

195. Rabinowitz B, Florian V. Chronic obstructive pulmonary disease—psychosocial issues and treatment goals. *Soc Work Health Care* 1992;16(4):60–86.

196. Fletcher EC, Martin R. Sexual dysfunction and erectile impotence in chronic obstructive pulmonary disease. *Chest* 1982;81:4.

197. Levine SB, Stern RC. Sexual function in cystic fibrosis: relationship to overall health status and pulmonary disease severity in 30 married patients. *Chest* 1982;81(4):422–428.

198. Kaplan E, Shwachman H, Perlmuter AD, et al. Reproductive failure in males with cystic fibrosis. *N Engl J Med* 1968;279:65–69.

199. Stern RC, Boat TF. Doershuk cystic fibrosis: obstructive azoospermia as a diagnostic criterion for cystic fibrosis syndrome. *Lancet* 1983;1:1401–1404.

200. Fogdestam I, Hamberger L, Ludin K, et al. Successful pregnancies after in vitro fertilization with sperm from men with cystic fibrosis. Paper presented at 19th European Cystic Fibrosis Conference, 1994.

201. Campbell M. Sexual dysfunction in the COPD patient. *Dimensions Crit Care Nurs* 1987;6(2):70–74.

202. Thompson WL. Sexual problems in chronic respiratory disease: achieving and maintaining intimacy. *Postgrad Med* 1986;79:41–52.

203. American Cancer Society. *Cancer facts & figures—1995.* New York: American Cancer Society, 1995.

204. Waldman TL, Eliasof B. Cancer. In: Sipski ML, Alexander CJ, eds. *Sexual function in people with disability and chronic illness: a health professional's guide.* Gaithersburg, MD: Aspen Publishers, 1997:337–354.

205. Brender C, Walsh P. Prostate cancer: evaluation and radiotherapeutic management. *CA Cancer J Clin* 1992;42:223–240.

206. Perez CA, Fair WR, Ihde DC. Carcinoma of the prostate. In: DeVita VT, Hellman S, Rosenberg S, eds. *Cancer principles and practice of oncology,* 3rd ed. Boston: Jones & Bartlett, 1989:1023–1058.

207. Heinrich-Rynning T. Prostatic cancer treatments and their effects on sexual function. *Oncol Nurs Forum* 1987;14(6):37–41.

208. Porter A, Forman J. Prostate brachytherapy: an overview. *Cancer* 1993;71 [Suppl 3]:953–958.

209. Taylor R. Endocrine therapy for advanced stage D prostate cancer. *Urol Nurs* 1991;11(3):22–26.

210. Krebs LU. Sexual and reproductive dysfunction. In: Groenwald SL, Goodman M, Frogge MH, Yarbro CH, eds. *Cancer nursing: principles and practice.* Boston: Jones & Bartlett, 1993:697–719.

211. Anderson BL, Lamb MA. Sexuality and cancer. In: Lanhard R, Lawrence W, Murphy G, eds. *Textbook of clinical oncology.* New York: American Cancer Society, 1995:700–711.

212. Kaplan HS. A neglected issue: the sexual side effects of current treatments for breast cancer. *J Sex Marital Ther* 1992;18(1):3–19.

213. Lamb M. Alterations in sexuality and sexual functioning. In: Baird SB, McCorkle R, Grant M, eds. *Cancer nursing: a comprehensive textbook.* Philadelphia: WB Saunders, 1991:831–849.

214. Vera MI. Quality of life following pelvic exenteration. *Gynecol Oncol* 1981;12:355–366.

215. Auchincloss SS. Sexual dysfunction in cancer patients: issues in evaluation and treatment. In: Holland JC, Rowland JH, eds. *Handbook of psychooncology: psychological care of the patient with cancer.* New York: Oxford University Press, 1989:383–413.

216. Hubbard JL, Shingleton HM. Sexual function of patients after cancer of the cervix treatment. *Clin Obstet Gynecol* 1985;12:247–264.

217. Grunberg KJ. Sexual rehabilitation of the cancer patient undergoing ostomy surgery. *J Enterostom Ther* 1986;13:148–152.

218. Ambler N, Williams AC, Hill P, et al. Sexual difficulties of chronic pain patients. *Clin J Pain* 2001;17:138–145.

219. Maruta T, Osborne D, Swanson DW. Chronic pain patients and spouses: marital and sexual adjustment. *Mayo Clinic Proc* 1981;56:307–310.

220. Flor H, Turk DC, Scholz OB. Impact of chronic pain on the spouse: marital, emotional and physical consequences. *J Psychosom Res* 1987;31:63–71.

221. Monga TN, Tan G, Ostermann JH. Sexuality and sexual adjustment of patients with chronic pain. *Disabil Rehabil* 1998;20:317–329.

222. Dunn KM, Croft PR, Hackett GI. Sexual problems: a study of the prevalence and need for health care in the general population. *Fam Pract* 1998;15:519–524.

223. Ritchie MH, Daines B. Sexuality and low back pain: a response to patients needs.

224. Annon J. *The behavioral treatment of sexual problems: brief therapy.* New York: Harper & Row, 1976.

225. Pauly IH, Goldstein SG. Prevalence of sexual dysfunction. *Med Aspects Hum Sexuality* 1970;4:48–52.

226. Burnap DW, Golden JS. Sexual problems in medical practice. *J Med Educ* 1967;42:673–680.

227. Stuntz RC. Assessment of organic factors in sexual dysfunctions. In Brown RA, Field JR, eds. *Treatment of sexual problems in individual and couples therapy.* Columbia, MD: PMA, 1988:187–207.

228. Schover LR. Sexual problems in chronic illness. In Leiblum SR, Rosen RC, eds. *Principles and practice of sex therapy: update for the 1990s,* 2nd ed. New York: Guilford Press, 1989:319–351.

229. Romano M. Sexuality and the disabled female. *Accent on Living* 1973;winter:27–34.

230. American Psychiatric Association. *Diagnostic and statistical manual of mental disorders,* 4th ed. Washington, DC: American Psychiatric Association, 1994.

231. Basson R, Berman J, Burnett A, et al. Report of the international consensus development conference on female sexual dysfunction: definitions and classifications. *J Urol* 2000;163:888–893.

232. Sipski ML. A physiatrist's view regarding the report of the International Consensus Conference on Female Sexual Dysfunction: definitions and classification. *J Urol* 2000;163:888–893.

233. Sipski ML, Alexander CJ. Documentation of the impact of spinal cord injury on female sexual function: the female spinal sexual function classification. *Top Spinal Cord Inj Rehabil* 2002;8(1):63–73.

234. American Psychiatric Association. *Diagnostic and statistical manual of mental disorders,* 4th ed., Text Revision. Washington, DC: American Psychiatric Association, 2000.

235. Sadovsky R, Miller R, Moskowitz M, et al. Three-year update of Sildenafil citrate (Viagra®) efficacy and safety. *Int J Clin Pract* 2001;55 (2):115–128.

236. Morales A, Gingell C, Collins M, et al. Clinical safety of oral sildenafil citrate (Viagra™) in the treatment of erectile dysfunction. *Int J Impot Res* 1998;10: 69–74.

237. Webb DJ, Freestone S, Allen MJ, et al. Sildenafil citrate potentiates the hypotensive effects of nitric oxide donor drugs in male patients with stable angina. *Am J Cardiol* 1999;83[Suppl 5A]:21C–28C.

238. Shakir S, Wilton L, Pearce F. IHD morbidity and mortality in a community-based cohort of sildenafil users: phase I results from prescription event monitoring (PEM) in England. Presented at the 8th European Society of Pharmacovigilance Annual Meeting; September 21–23, Verona, Italy.

239. DeBusk R, Drory Y, Goldstein I, et al. Management of sexual dysfunction in patients with cardiovascular disease; recommendations of the Princeton Consensus Panel. *Am J Cardiol* 2000;86:175–181.

240. Rendell MS, Rajfer J, Wicker P. Sildenafil for the treatment of erectile dysfunction in men with diabetes. *JAMA* 1999;281:421–426.

241. Blonde L, Feiner C, Siegel R. Partner's evaluation of the efficacy of Viagra (sildenafil citrate) for the treatment of erectile dysfunction in men with diabetes. *Diabetes* 1999;48[Suppl]:A89.

242. Olsson AM, Persson CA, for the Swedish sildenafil investigators group. Efficacy and safety of Viagra ® (sildenafil citrate) for the treatment of erectile dysfunction in men with cardiovascular disease and erectile dysfunction. *J Am Coll Cardiol* 2000;35[Suppl A]:329.

243. Zippe CD, Jhaveri FM, Klein EA. et al. Role of Viagra after radical prostatectomy. *Urology* 1998;52:963–966.

244. Zippe CD, Jhaveri FM, Klein EA, et al. Role of Viagra after radical prostatectomy. *Urology* 2000;55:241–245.

245. Kedia S, Sippe CD, Agarwal A, et al. Treatment of erectile dysfunction with sildenafil citrate (Viagra) after radiation therapy for prostate cancer. *Urology* 1999;54:308–312.

246. Zelefsky MJ, McKee AB, Lee H, et al. Efficacy of oral sildenafil in patients with erectile dysfunction after radiotherapy for carcinoma of the prostate. *Urology* 1999;53:775–778.

247. Scholz M, Strum S. Recovery of spontaneous erectile function after nerve-sparing radical retropubic prostatectomy with and without early intracavernous injections of alprostadil: results of a prospective, randomized trial. *J Urol* 1999;262:1914–1915.

248. Paul HR, McLeish D, Rao TKS, et al. Initial experience with sildenafil for erectile dysfunction in maintenance dialysis (MD) patients. *J Am Soc Nephrol* 1998;9:222A.

249. Wagoner LE, Giesting RM, Bell BJ, et al. Is Viagra (sildenafil citrate) safe and effective in cardiac transplant recipients? *Transplantation* 1999;67:S102.

250. Chait J, Kobashigawa J, Chuang J, et al. Efficacy and safety of sildenafil citrate (Viagra) in male heart transplant patients. *J Heart Lung Transplant* 1999;18:58.

251. Menza M, Roose S, Seigman S, et al. Effect of sildenafil citrate on depression scores in men with erectile dysfunction and comorbid depression. *J Gen Intern Med* 1999;[Suppl 2]:55.

252. Derry FA, Dinsmore WW, Fraser M, et al. Efficacy and safety of oral sildenafil (Viagra) in men with erectile dysfunction caused by spinal cord injury. *Neurology* 1998:51:1629–1633.

253. Maytom MC, Derry FA, Dinsmore WW, et al. A two-part pilot study of sildenafil (Viagra™) in men with erectile dysfunction caused by spinal cord injury. *Spinal Cord* 1999;37:110–116.

254. Green BG, Martin S. Clinical assessment of sildenafil in the treatment of neurogenic male sexual dysfunction: after the hype. *NeuroRehabilitation* 2000:15:101–105.

255. Gousse AE, Lambert M-M, Kester RR. Oral pharmacotherapy to manage erectile dysfunction in spinal cord-injured men. *Top Spinal Cord Inj Rehabil* 2002;8(1) 51–62.

256. Ashton AK, Hamer R, Rosen RC. SSRI-induced sexual dysfunction and its treatment: a large-scale retrospective study of 596 psychiatric outpatients. *J Sex Marital Ther* 1997;23(3):165–175.

257. Zorgniotti AW, Lizza AF. On demand oral drugs for erection on impotent men. *J Urol* 1993;147:308A.

258. Altwein JE, Keuler FU. Oral treatment of erectile dysfunction with apomorphine SL. *Urol Int* 2001;67:257–263.

259. Stark S, Sachse R, Liedl T, et al. Vardenafil increases penile rigidity and tumescence in men with erectile dysfunction after a single oral dose. *Eur Urol* 2001;40:181–188.

260. Rivas DA, Chancellor MB. Management of erective dysfunction. In: Sipski ML, Alexander CJ, eds. *Sexual function in people with disability and chronic illness: a health professional's guide.* Gaithersburg, MD: Aspen Publishers, 1997: 429–464.

261. Wein AJ, Malloy TR, Hanno PM. Intracavernosal injection programs—their place in management of erectile dysfunction. *Prob Urol* 1987;1:496–506.

262. Linet OI, Ogrinc FG. Efficacy and safety of intracavernosal alprostadil in men with erectile dysfunction. *N Engl J Med* 1996;334:873–877.

263. Lakin MM, Montague DR, Vanderbrug MS, et al. Intracavernous injection therapy: analysis of results and complications. *J Urol* 1990;143:1138–1141.

264. Lue TF, Tanagho EA. Physiology of erection and pharmacological management of impotence. *J Urol* 1987;137:829–836.

265. Lewis RW. Long-term results of penile prosthetic implants. *Urol Clin North Am* 1995;22:847–855.

266. Rossier AB, Fam BA. Indication and results of semirigid penile prostheses in spinal cord injury patients: long-term follow-up. *J Urol* 1984;131:59–62.

267. Kabalin JN, Kessler R. Infectious complications of penile prosthesis surgery. *J Urol* 1988;139:953–955.

268. Spector I, Carey M. Incidence and prevalence of the sexual dysfunctions: a critical review of the empirical literature. *Arch Sex Behav* 1990;19:389–408.

269. Rosen RC, Leiblum SR. Treatment of sexual disorders in the 1990s: an integrated approach. *J Consult Clin Psychol* 1995;63(6):877–890.

270. McCarthy BW. Cognitive-behavioral strategies and techniques in the treatment of early ejaculation. In: Leiblum SR, Rosen RC, eds. *Principles and practice of sex therapy.* New York: Guilford Press, 1989:141–167.

271. Ducharme S, Gill K. Management of other male sexual dysfunctions. In: Sipski ML, Alexander CJ, eds. *Sexual function in people with disability and chronic illness: a health professional's guide.* Gaithersburg, MD: Aspen Publishers, 1997:465–485.

272. Tordjman G. A new therapeutic perspective for premature ejaculation disorder. *Cah Sexol Clin* 1993;10:5–6.

273. Sipski ML, Rosen RC, Alexander CJ, Hamer RM. Sildenafil effects on sexual and cardiovascular responses in women with spinal cord injury. *Urology* 2000;55: 812–815.

274. Sipski ML. Future options for improving sexual satisfaction in persons with spinal cord injuries. *Top Spinal Cord Inj Rehabil* 2000;6[Suppl]:148–154.

275. Sipski ML, Rosen R, Alexander CJ, Hamer R. A controlled trial of positive feedback to increase sexual arousal in women with spinal cord injuries. *NeuroRehabilitation* 2000;15:145–153.

276. Billups KL, Berman L, Berman J, et al. A new non-pharmacological vacuum therapy for female sexual dysfunction. *J Sex Marital Ther* 2001;27:1435–1441.

277. Whipple B, McGreer KB. Management of female sexual dysfunction. In: Sipski ML, Alexander CJ, eds. *Sexual function in people with disability and chronic illness: a health professional's guide.* Gaithersburg, MD: Aspen Publishers, 1997:511–536.

CHAPTER 75

Pressure Ulcers

Kevin O'Connor

Pressure ulcers have been challenging societies for centuries. Despite new understanding of wound causation and management, pressure ulcers continue to be a significant health-care concern. The number of persons affected and costs in terms of dollars, productivity, and life is enormous. Failure to maintain skin integrity will extend length of stay in a health-care facility, increase health costs, increase nosocomial infections, and increase comorbidities and other complications (1). As our health-care system becomes more cost conscious and result oriented, pressure ulcers must be viewed as preventable and not merely as a complication of illness and immobility (2).

The purpose of this chapter is to review pressure ulceration and to explore advances in the prevention and treatment of this clinically significant problem. More advancement has been made in the area of tissue biomechanics, and there has been extensive effort toward producing surfaces and products that prevent and help heal pressure ulceration.

SCOPE OF THE PROBLEM

Definition

The National Pressure Ulcer Advisory Panel (NPUAP) defines a pressure ulcer as an area of unrelieved pressure over a defined area, usually over a bony prominence, resulting in ischemia, cell death, and tissue necrosis (3). Although in the past the terms *decubitus ulcers* and *bedsores* originated from the observation that sores or ulcers occurred frequently in people who were bedridden, the term *pressure ulcer* is more accurate and useful as it includes the etiology rather than specific body position. The term *pressure ulcer* reflects our current belief that the etiology is excessive pressure, which causes ischemia and necrosis, eventually leading to tissue ulceration (4).

Economic Implications

The Agency for Healthcare Research and Quality clinical practice guideline on prevention of pressure ulcers notes that the national total cost of pressure-ulcer treatment exceeded $1.3 billion (5,6), an estimated $2,000 to $30,000 per pressure ulcer. More recent estimates of the national economic burden are $3 to $6 billion each year (7). Pressure ulcers are responsible for physical, social, and vocational costs, as well as the economic cost of treating the ulcer, so the actual total costs are likely far greater. This economic impetus has created innumerable industries ranging from wound-care products and specialists to outpatient treatment centers (7).

Incidence and Prevalence

It is estimated that more than 1 million persons in acute and chronic facilities have pressure ulcers (8). The incidence and prevalence of pressure ulcers vary widely by population and setting. The incidence of pressure ulcers in acute-care hospitals ranges from 3% (9) to 29% (10), with a prevalence as high as 69% (11). In critical care settings, the incidence can increase to 33% (12), with a prevalence of 41% (13). Age is a definite factor with incidence rates of 23% to 37% in hospitalized elderly patients (14). In a large-scale, longitudinal multisite study of elderly persons, 83% who developed pressure ulcers had been treated in the hospital (15). Unfortunately, each year approximately 60,000 people die of pressure ulcer–related complications (16), and pressure-ulcer development has been associated with a 4.5 times greater risk of death than for persons with the same risk factors but without pressure ulcers (17).

Long-term-care facilities have an incidence that ranges from 10.8% to 38.5%, with prevalence ranges from 1.2% to 11.2% (18). About 25% of residents admitted from an acute-care hospitalization have pressure ulcers (19), but long-term follow up demonstrates that the majority of ulcers healed within a year (17,20). The wide variation of prevalence of pressure ulcers in long-term-care facilities may be a reflection of implementation of care practices. Accordingly, because the prevalence of pressure ulcers is an indicator of overall quality of care, it is monitored by both state and federal governments in the Minimum Data Set. The incidence of pressure ulcers in persons cared for in the home with professional supervision ranges from 4.3% to 20% (21).

ANATOMY AND PATHOPHYSIOLOGY: NORMAL SKIN

Skin is the largest organ in the human body, and its functions include thermoregulation of body temperature, protection from injury, sensation, and metabolism. The outermost layer, the epidermis, shields the underlying tissues from water and electrolyte loss, mechanical injury, harmful chemicals, and microorganisms. The dermis supports the epidermis and contains fibroblasts that synthesize and secrete collagen and elastin. Collagen gives skin its tone and tensile strength, and elastin provides for stretch and elastic recoil.

The blood supply to the skin serves to provide oxygen and nutrients to the skin as well as thermoregulation for the body. The avascular epidermis is nourished by the microcirculation of the dermal and hypodermal layers (22). Thermoregulation is accomplished by circulation and sweating. Vasodilation dissipates body heat; vasoconstriction maintains it. Sweat glands under control of the nervous system respond to temperature changes and emotional stimulation while evaporation of sweat on the skin lowers body temperature. Vitamin D is synthesized in the skin with exposure to sunlight and is important in calcium and phosphate metabolism.

Many changes occur in the skin throughout our life span that increase the susceptibility to injury and extend the time for wound healing. With aging, the epidermal turnover rate decreases, epithelialization slows, and vitamin D production and inflammatory response slow. There is a decrease in subcutaneous fat, reduced numbers of sweat glands, and diminished vascularity, which affects thermoregulation. Skin becomes thinner and less elastic and consequently more susceptible to forces of pressure and shear.

Many nutrients, including protein, carbohydrates, fats, minerals, and vitamins, are essential to healthy skin, and inadequate intake of calories, protein, and iron is a causative factor in pressure-ulcer development (5,23). Many other factors can influence aging and healing of skin, ranging from ultraviolet rays to skin-cleansing products.

PRESSURE-ULCER PATHOPHYSIOLOGY

Although pressure ulcers develop in response to a number of factors, the most important external ones are pressure and shear. In addition, risk factors can include intrinsic factors such as mobility status, sensory-motor function, nutrition, age, hemopoietic changes, incontinence, and psychosocial issues, and external factors such as long times without movement (24).

Pressure

Unrelieved static pressure applied directly to the skin is a critical factor in the development of pressure ulcers. External pressure applied in excess of capillary closure pressure for pro-

longed or unrelieved periods will produce ischemia in underlying tissue. The pressure that exceeds tissue capillary closure pressure was first quantified by Landis to be 32 mmHg (25). Pressure-reducing and -relieving products use 32 mm Hg as the standard for judging efficacy; however, more recent studies have shown that much lower pressures are needed to occlude capillaries in elderly and debilitated individuals, and the actual capillary closure pressures can vary widely over different sites of the body (26–28).

There are three important aspects of pressure in ulcer development: intensity, duration, and tissue tolerance. There is an inverse relationship between pressure and the duration of the pressure necessary to cause ulceration. Intense pressure applied for a short duration can be as damaging as lower-intensity pressure for extended periods (29,30). In order to prevent pressure ulcers, pressure must be relieved frequently as well as reduced at the surface-skin interface. It is on these studies that the clinical practice of weight shifting while sitting and the use of 2-hour bed-turning regimen to provide pressure relief are based (5,31,32). If pressure is relieved by shifting the body's weight, blood flows back into the tissue again, and the area becomes hyperemic. This phenomenon is called reactive hyperemia, because a bright red flush appears as the body attempts to flood the starved tissue with oxygen. This protective mechanism of local vasodilatation is a naturally occurring compensatory response to temporary ischemia. If the pressure-time threshold has been exceeded, damage continues to occur even after relief of the pressure (33).

The concept of tissue tolerance was initially described by Husain (34) and further studied by Daniel and colleagues (35), who found that muscle tissue is much more sensitive to the effects of pressure than is skin. When pressure is placed on a body surface, the greatest pressure is to the tissues overlying the bone. The pressure is distributed in a conelike fashion, with the base of the cone on the underlying body surface. This is why the greatest damage is often seen at the muscle layer, rather than on the skin. Ulcer presentations often reflect this concept when they appear with a small skin defect and a larger area at the base of a deep ulcer. When muscle is damaged without skin breakdown, a second application of less pressure and less time is needed to result in an ulcer. Clinically, at the first sign of skin impairment or blanchable hyperemia, pressure must be relieved to allow for tissue recovery.

Shear

Shear, as an opposing force to friction, is the application of force tangential to the skin surface and occurs when the skin remains stationary and the underlying tissue shifts (5) (Fig. 75-1). Shear, combined with pressure, can lower the threshold for skin ulceration sixfold (36). Reichel (37) found that shearing forces cause the perforating arteries to become angulated, disrupting the supply of blood.

In its mildest form, shear causes skin tears, abrasions limited to the epidermal and dermal layers. Skin tears can result from varied activities, including grasping an extremity, transferring, bathing, and dressing (38). Epidemiological studies suggest that at least 1.5 million skin tears occur each year in institutionalized adults (39). Common other causes of shearing include sitting in the semirecumbent position, spasticity, and sliding rather than lifting during transfers.

Immobility

The inability or decreased ability to change or control body position is the most frequently cited factor in the risk of pressure

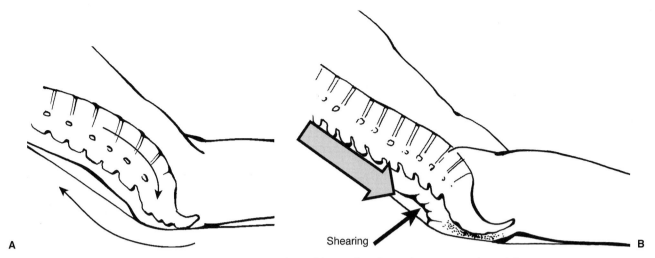

Figure 75-1. Shear forces are biomechanical factors that play a role in pressure ulcer etiology.

ulceration (40). Impaired mobility often follows spinal cord injury (SCI), traumatic brain injury, stroke, multiple sclerosis, arthritis, depression, weakness, and confusion.

Nutrition

Low serum albumin levels are highly associated with pressure-ulcer development (41,42), and several studies have shown that a poor diet is a causative factor in pressure-ulcer development and delayed healing. Lean mass is a good measure of adequate nutrition, whereas weight and total mass are not. Adipose tissue, which is poorly vascularized, should not be equated with adequate nutrition (43). Balanced diets are recommended to provide a positive nitrogen balance to meet the metabolic and nutritional requirements crucial to pressure-ulcer prevention.

Moisture and Incontinence

Moisture alone can make the skin more susceptible to injury (5) by weakening the connective tissue of the skin. Excessive moisture may result from perspiration, wound drainage, and fecal or urinary incontinence. Incontinence is the most reliable predictor of pressure-ulcer formation, especially fecal incontinence (41) or urinary incontinence occurring with both friction and neurologic disorders (44). Bowel incontinence may be a more important risk factor than urinary incontinence; the exposure of the skin to the bacteria and toxins in stool may be important in the pathogenesis of pressure ulcers (45).

Smoking

In individuals with SCI, there is a positive correlation with smoking and pressure-ulcer development: the more persons smoked, the greater the incidence of pressure ulcers (46).

Spinal Cord Injury

Individuals with SCI are the most studied population for pressure-ulcer formation. Factors that are associated with the development of pressure ulcers in SCI are the higher level and completeness of the SCI, longer duration of the SCI, a decreased level of activity (47), and those who have had previous ulcers (48). Psychosocial factors that have *not* been found to be associated with pressure ulcers in SCI include age at onset (49),

quality of life (50), depression (51), satisfaction with social support (52), and social integration (49).

Temperature

Researchers correlated increases in body temperature with increased risk of pressure ulceration. Elevated temperature may place increased metabolic demands on an already compromised area. It is estimated that an increase of 1°C causes a 10% increase in tissue metabolism and oxygen demand (53). If temperature is a factor in a patient's care, attention should be given to clothing and support surfaces that either insulate or conduct heat away from the individual's skin.

Psychosocial Factors

Psychosocial factors influence pressure ulcer formation and healing. Anderson and Andberg (54) found life satisfaction, self-esteem, and practice of responsibility to be important factors in both initial development and recurrence of pressure ulcers. An elevated cortisol level, which affects wound healing and immune function, places the person at risk for pressure ulcer development (55).

WOUND HEALING

Classification

The Wound Healing Society defines healing as complete closure of the integument. Wound healing has three levels, or intentions: primary, secondary, and tertiary or delayed primary closure. Wounds that close with primary intention have no tissue loss and take 3 to 14 days to complete. Examples include surgical incisions with closure. Wounds with tissue loss that requires connective tissue to fill the defect may close by secondary intention. Closure by secondary or spontaneous intention involves no active intent to seal the wound, and the wound is allowed to close by reepithelialization and contraction. Healing time depends on the extent of the tissue loss, and examples include pressure ulcers and wound dehiscence (56). Tertiary intention wounds are wounds in which primary closure has been delayed or are left open and subsequently closed (57). The chronic wound, for some reason, does not proceed to restoration of functional integrity. It is stalled in the inflammatory phase of wound healing and does not proceed to closure.

Phases of Wound Healing

There are three major phases of wound healing: inflammatory phase, proliferative phase, and maturational or remodeling phase. All three phases may occur simultaneously, and the phases within their individual processes may overlap.

In the immediate reaction of the tissue to injury, hemostasis and inflammation occur. The body's defenses are aimed at limiting the amount of damage and preventing further injury by stopping the bleeding, sealing the surface of the wound, and removing any necrotic tissue, foreign debris, or bacteria. Key to wound healing is the subsequent breakdown of platelets releasing growth factors that attract the cells needed to begin healing. In the inflammation phase, vasodilation leads to increased blood vessel permeability, vasocongestion, and leakage of serous fluid into the surrounding tissue. As the acute responses of hemostasis and inflammation begin to resolve, the foundation is made for wound repair.

During the proliferative phase, the repair processes are angiogenesis, fibroplasias, and epithelialization. This stage is characterized by the formation of granulation tissue, consisting of a capillary bed, fibroblasts, macrophages, and a loose arrangement of collagen, fibronectin, hyaluronic acid, and bacteria. The desired outcome of the proliferative phase is to fill the wound defect with connective tissue and cover it with epithelium. In the process of granulation, neoangiogenesis and collagen synthesis provide a new capillary network to provide nutrients to the collagen bed. Collagen synthesis is performed by the fibroblasts, which also synthesize other connective tissue. The collagen fibers thicken and assume parallel orientation, which provides the tensile strength of the wound. The granulation tissue itself appears red and is fragile, bleeding easily.

In the maturational phase, the wound contracts. Contraction is the reduction of the size of the wound by the inward movement of the tissue and the surrounding skin. Wound contraction occurs by a complex interaction of extracellular materials and the fibroblasts. Once the wound is healed, it will remodel and mature. Wound strength increases rapidly within 1 to 6 weeks and then levels off as a sigmoid curve up to 1 year after injury. Compared with unwounded skin, the tensile strength is only 30% in scar, mostly because of cross-linked collagen (58).

ASSESSMENT OF PRESSURE ULCERS

Staging

The most frequently used staging system is that recommended by the NPUAP and the Agency for Health Care Policy and Research (AHCPR) (Fig. 75-2). The descriptions allow for recording only visually observed changes in the skin (59) (Table 75-1).

Staging can only be used when the wound bed can be visualized. If it is not able to be visualized, such as when it is secondary to necrotic tissue, then the wound is unable to be staged. Healing wounds can be difficult to classify and thus cannot be staged with this scale (60). Numerical progression of stages does not necessarily imply progression in ulcer severity. Likewise, when a wound is healing, it does not become a lower-stage wound. For example, a stage II wound does not become a stage I—it is a healing stage II wound.

Measurement

Wounds are monitored at least weekly on a regular schedule to provide consistent and timely evaluation in the treatment plan.

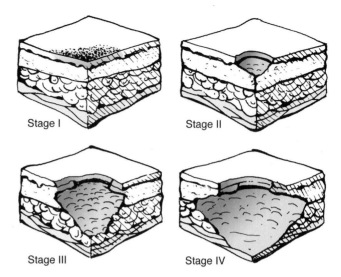

Figure 75-2. The depth of tissue for each grade of pressure ulcer.

Both the wound bed and surrounding tissues are examined and characterized, including granulation tissue, necrotic tissue, erythema, maceration, induration, and other wound characteristics. In addition, accurate notation of location can assist in determining pathophysiologic factors that need to be resolved before healing (61).

Rulers, tracing, and photography are the most commonly used methods of wound measurement. Rulers are a simple and accurate way to measure wounds that have a clean wound bed, but are less helpful with necrotic tissue: As the necrotic tissue is removed, the wound will increase in measurement size. Nevertheless, repeated measurements over time will depict a trend of the wound repair process.

Tracing using concentric circles or rulers can also be useful to describe the wound's progress; however, they are more advantageous for lower-extremity ulcers rather than buttock wounds, as these pressure ulcers often undermine, so that the wound outline can underestimate volume (62).

Color photography accurately captures color of tissues, but depth of the wound can be difficult. Nevertheless, the presence of exudates, or necrotic tissue in the wound, as well as the condition of the surrounding skin, can be accurately detailed with a picture.

Stage	Description
I	Nonblanchable erythema of intact skin not resolved within 30 minutes; epidermis intact
II	Partial-thickness loss of skin involving epidermis, possibly into dermis; may appear as blisters with erythema
III	Full-thickness destruction through dermis into subcutaneous tissue
IV	Deep-tissue destruction through subcutaneous tissue to fascia, muscle, bone, or joint

TABLE 75-1.   Staging of Pressure Ulcers

Data from Panel for Prediction and Prevention of Pressure Ulcers in Adults. *Prediction and prevention.* Clinical Practice Guideline No. 3, AHCPR publication No. 92–0047. Rockville, MD: Agency for Health Care Policy and Research, Public Health Service, U.S. Department of Health and Human Services, 1994.

		TABLE 75-2.	**Braden Risk Assessment Scale**		
Subscale	**1**	**2**	**3**	**4**	**Score**
Sensory perception	Completely limited	Very limited	Slightly limited	No impairment	
Moisture	Constantly moist	Very moist	Occasionally moist	Rarely moist	
Activity	Bedfast	Chairfast	Walks occasionally	Walks frequently	
Mobility	Completely immobile	Very limited	Slightly limited	No limitation	
Nutrition	Very poor	Probably inadequate	Adequate	Excellent	
Friction and shear	Requires moderate to maximum assistance in moving	Moves freely or requires minimum assistance	Moves independently		

Adapted from Braden B, Bergstrom N. A conceptual schema for the study of the etiology of pressure sores. *Rehabilitation Nursing* 1988;12:8–16.

Risk-Assessment Scales

The goal of risk assessment is to identify at-risk individuals needing preventive methods, as well as the specific factors placing them at risk, so that resources can be allocated toward appropriate situations (63). Risk-assessment scales include factors of immobility, incontinence, nutritional factors, and altered levels of consciousness. Patients are assessed at admission as well as during follow-up (64). The Braden Scale and the Norton Scale are the two most commonly used assessment tools for assessing pressure-ulcer risk.

The Braden Scale consists of six factors: mobility, activity, moisture, sensory perception, nutrition, and friction and shear. The subscales are rated 1 to 4, except for friction and shear, which is rated 1 to 3. Scores range between 4 and 23, with 16 or below considered at risk (65). The Braden Scale has been tested and validated in both acute- and long-term-care settings and has a high interrater validity (66) (Table 75-2).

The Norton Scale consists of five factors: physical condition, mental condition, activity, mobility, and incontinence. Each factor is rated 1 to 4, with total scores ranging from 5 to 20 (Table 75-3). A combined score of 14 indicated onset of risk, whereas a score of 12 or less indicated a high risk of pressure-ulcer formation (67).

SITES OF PRESSURE ULCERS

Pressure ulcers occur most frequently over bony prominences. The most common sites for pressure ulcers are the ischium, sacrum, greater trochanter of the femur, and the heel (Table 75-4). Pressure ulcers will occur anywhere on the body where there is compression of soft tissue, including compression from splints, orthoses, and orthopedic immobilizers. In studies of

the SCI population, the sacrum was found to be the most common site of severe pressure ulcers. As more time is spent in the wheelchair, the pressure ulcer incidence is reflected in increased frequency at the ischial tuberosities and feet. Forty-seven percent of all ulcers discovered during follow-up were on the foot (68). In a study of children aged 10 weeks to 13 years, the occiput was the site of greatest pressure, changing to the sacrum as the child aged. This is not surprising given the percentage of body weight a child's head represents, and the child's positioning needs must be considered separately from the adult's (69).

PRINCIPLES OF TREATMENT

Prevention

Prevention is the most cost-effective management of pressure ulcers. Prevention of pressure ulcers is based on an understanding of the etiology of ulcers as well as associated risk factors. The AHCPR (6) recommends four target goals:

1. Identify at-risk individuals who need prevention and the specific factors placing them at risk.
2. Maintain and improve tissue tolerance to pressure to prevent injury.
3. Protect against the adverse effects of pressure and shear.
4. Utilize educational programs to reduce pressure-ulcer incidence.

Further recommendations for skin care include:

1. Inspect the skin of at-risk individuals at least twice daily.
2. Cleanse the skin at the time of soiling and at routine intervals.

		TABLE 75-3.	**Norton Scale**		
Subscale	**1**	**2**	**3**	**4**	**Score**
Physical condition	Very bad	Poor	Fair	Good	
Mental condition	Stupor	Confused	Apathetic	Alert	
Activity	Bed	Chairbound	Walk/help	Ambulant	
Mobility	Immobile	Very limited	Slightly limited	Full	
Incontinent	Doubly	Usually/urine	Occasional	Not	

From Norton D, McLaren R, Exton-Smith AN. *An investigation of geriatric nursing problems in hospitals.* London: Churchill Livingstone, 1975.

TABLE 75-4. Common Sites for Pressure Ulcers

Body Position	Wound Sites
Prone	Knee (6%)
	Pretibial crest (2%)
Supine	Sacrum (23%)
	Heel (8%)
	Elbow (3%)
	Occiput (1%)
Sitting	Ischium (24%)
Side-lying	Greater trochanter (15%)
	Lateral malleolus (7%)

Data from Panel for Prediction and Prevention of Pressure Ulcers in Adults. *Prediction and prevention.* Clinical Practice Guideline No. 3, AHCPR publication No. 92–0047. Rockville, MD: Agency for Health Care Policy and Research, Public Health Service, U.S. Department of Health and Human Services, 1994.

3. Use mild cleansing agents to reduce dryness and skin irritation.
4. Minimize environmental factors leading to skin drying.
5. Minimize skin exposure to moisture.
6. Use proper positioning, equipment, and transferring techniques to minimize shear forces.
7. Provide nutritional support, including nutritional supplements to maintain adequate intake of protein and calories.
8. Reposition individuals at risk every 2 hours while in bed and weight shifts every 20 minutes while in a wheelchair.
9. Use pillows or foam wedges while in bed to protect bony prominences.
10. Maintain the head of the bed at the lowest degree of elevation possible.
11. Use lifting devices to transfer and position rather than dragging.
12. Use pressure-relieving cushions and bed support surfaces to lessen risk of pressure-ulcer development; do not use doughnut-shaped devices.

Education

A comprehensive educational program for patients and their family/caregivers should begin throughout the continuum of care to include new self-care techniques and technology. Information should be presented at an appropriate level for the target audience (70); include principles of adult learning, including explanation, demonstration, group discussion, and drills; and designed to meet the listener's needs, interests, and background (71). The educational program should include information on etiology and pathology, risk factors, comorbid conditions, proper positioning, equipment, complications, and the principles of wound prevention, skin care, and wound treatment (72). The educational program can be modified to include additional specific information regarding a particular treatment for those patients who have developed an ulcer. Studies have shown that compliance is greater and the treatment more successful when the patient actively participates in the learning process (73,74). In addition, it is important that family/caregiver education is also comprehensive, as this may help decrease the incidence of new pressure ulcers (75).

Nutrition

Normal tissue and skin integrity depend upon adequate calorie, protein, and vitamin intake (76). Individuals who develop pressure ulcers often have significantly lower calorie and protein intake than those who do not develop pressure ulcers (10). For the purposes of assessing nutritional status, several blood chemistry tests are available and have been associated with the presence or development of pressure ulcers. For example, prealbumin is the most sensitive indicator for monitoring nutritional status because of its short half-life (2–3 days) and has been found to be significantly lower in patients with pressure ulcers compared with those without pressure ulcers (77). In addition, decreases in total protein (< 6.4 g/dL) and albumin (< 3.5 g/dL) (78) have similarly been found to be associated with pressure-ulcer development. Factors associated with hypoalbuminemia include losses of protein and albumin in pressure ulcer exudates (1) and the presence of a chronic inflammatory state (79).

Consequently, nutritional intake should be adequate to help prevent pressure ulcers as well as heal those that develop. Equations, such as the Harris-Benedict Equation, have been used to estimate the patients' recommended caloric need, both with and without pressure ulcers (80). In addition, the AHCPR Guidelines recommend that an individual without a pressure ulcer should intake 1.0–1.25g/kg of body weight/day of protein; with a pressure ulcer, this should increase to 1.25–1.5 g/kg/day. However, indirect calorimetry is the best method of determining the energy expenditures (81–83).

Other nutritional factors studied for wound healing include vitamins and minerals such as vitamins C and E and zinc. Vitamin C is an antioxidant and also necessary for the hydroxylation of proline and lysine during collagen formation and there-

TABLE 75-5. Support Surface Characteristics

Performance Characteristics	Air Fluidized	Low Air Loss	Alternating Air	Static Flotation	Foam	Standard Mattress
Increased support area	Yes	Yes	Yes	Yes	Yes	No
Low moisture retention	Yes	Yes	No	No	No	No
Reduced heat accumulation	Yes	Yes	No	No	No	No
Shear reduction	Yes	?	Yes	Yes	No	No
Pressure reduction	Yes	Yes	Yes	Yes	Yes	No
Dynamic	Yes	Yes	Yes	No	No	No
Cost per day	High	High	Moderate	Low	Low	Low

Data from Panel for Prediction and Prevention of Pressure Ulcers in Adults. *Prediction and prevention.* Clinical Practice Guideline No. 3, AHCPR publication No. 92–0047. Rockville, MD: Agency for Health Care Policy and Research, Public Health Service, U.S. Department of Health and Human Services, 1994.

TABLE 75-6. Examples of Static Support Surfaces

Foam	Air	Gel/Water
Eggcrate	Roho™ (Roho)	Rik® Fluid
Geo-Matt®	Sof-Care®	Overlay (KCI)
(Span America)	(Gaymar Industries)	
Comfortline™	First Step®	
(Hill-Rom)	(Kinetic Concepts)	

TABLE 75-8. Examples of Wheelchair Cushions

Foam	Gel	Air	Alternating Air
Stimulite™	The Cloud™	Roho®	Altern8®
(Sepracor)	(Otto Bock)	(Roho)	(Pegasus)
Combi® Jay	Jay® (Jay	Nexus®	ErgoDynamic™
Medical)	Medical)	(Roho)	(ErgoAir)
Varilite™			
(Cascade			
Designs)			

fore may help with wound healing. However, supplementation of vitamin C has not been shown to accelerate healing of pressure ulcers (84), nor does intake of vitamin C predict pressure ulcer development (85). Vitamin E is also an antioxidant and although reported to improve the healing of pressure ulcers, there is limited scientific evidence of this (86). Zinc is involved in the structural integrity of collagen and, like vitamin E, there are anecdotal reports of improved healing with supplementation, but scientific evidence is limited (87).

Because catabolism, or loss of body protein, occurs with any open wound as a result of inflammation or infection, it is important to maintain adequate nutrition to prevent further loss of protein stores (88). With injury or chronic debilitation, there are decreased levels of the normal anabolic hormones human growth and testosterone (89,90). Because of this, several investigators have used the anabolic agent oxandrolone, combined with good nutrition, to restore weight and accomplish a significant increase in the healing rate of wounds (91,92). The use of these hormones for wound healing continues under investigation (93).

Although inadequate nutritional intake has been found to correlate with the development of new pressure ulcers, in the patient who requires surgery, neither serum albumin nor total protein has been found to correlate with postsurgical wound outcomes. Moreover, although wound closure is not advised in nutritionally depleted individuals, a particular serum albumin or total protein level has not been identified that would avert surgical intervention.

Finally, weight control is important for preventing pressure ulcers. Increases or decreases in weight may alter contributing factors to pressure-ulcer development. For example, if an individual gains weight, he or she may become more susceptible to developing an ulcer from shear, especially if his or her own strength or that of the caregiver is insufficient to transfer without sliding along the surface. Additionally, weight gain may lead to a piece of equipment no longer fitting properly, such as a wheelchair, so that the device itself can create a pressure risk. Given the limitations of most exercise facilities to adapt to the wheelchair user, weight control may become a challenge to SCI patients with compromised energy expenditure.

TABLE 75-7. Examples of Dynamic Support Surfaces

Low-Air-Loss Overlays	Low-Air-Loss Beds	Air-Fluidized Beds
Micro Air®	Flexicair® (Support	Clinitron®
(Invacare)	Systems International)	(Support Systems
Clini-Care®	Kinair®	International)
(Gaymar)	Kinetic (Concepts)	Skyton® (Skytron)
First Step	Mediscus®	FluidAir®
Select® (KCI)	(Mediscus Group)	(Kinetic Concepts)

Support Surfaces

Because of advances in technologies and difficulties that have arisen in the acute-care setting, including staffing and medical conditions that prevent or limit turning, numerous beds and overlays have been developed to help prevent pressure ulcers. Although there is a large body of literature available on support surfaces, there is insufficient evidence to recommend one support surface over another for cost-effectiveness and appropriate patient characteristics of a specific mattress (Table 75-5). Static support surfaces, which can be filled with foam, air, or gel, can be chosen for an individual without an ulcer, without bottoming out on the support surface, or for an individual with a pressure ulcer who can be positioned without weight bearing on the ulcer (94,95). Examples of static support surfaces are in Table 75-6.

Dynamic support surfaces should be used if the individual cannot be positioned without pressure on the ulcer, if there is no evidence of ulcer healing, or if a new ulcer develops (96). Dynamic support surfaces include low-air-loss beds and overlays and air-fluidized beds. Examples of dynamic support surfaces are seen in Table 75-7.

Low-air-loss and air-fluidized beds should be used if there are multiple pressure ulcers, with large stage III or IV pressure ulcers, or after myocutaneous flap surgery. In comparison with air-fluidized beds, in general, low-air-loss beds and overlays are lighter, and patient transfers are more easily managed. Air-fluidized beds are advantageous for excessive moisture, whether from the wound, perspiration, or incontinence, and the ceramic fluidized beads have a bactericidal effect that is due to the sequestration and desiccation of microorganisms (97,98).

Wheelchair cushions complement bed support surfaces in the prevention of pressure ulcers. Clinically useful computerized systems have been developed to evaluate the pressure exerted on various cushions, although they are limited in their ability to measure shear (99). The same materials are now available in wheelchair cushions as for support surfaces, including foam, air, and gel static cushions as well as low-air-loss cushions, which can allow ischial wound healing even with sitting because of the alternating air function. As with bed supports, the use of donut-shaped ring cushions should be avoided, as the ring will prevent perfusion of the central area (100). Examples of the different types of cushions are in Table 75-8.

Age-associated changes in the patient's skin and mobility mean that the support surface, wheelchair, and wheelchair cushion initially prescribed may not be the most appropriate across the life span. It is therefore recommended that routine and regular assessment of each patient occurs to determine if a change in equipment or additional equipment is needed before development of a pressure ulcer.

WOUND CARE

Débridement and Cleansing

Optimal wound healing can only occur in a clean wound. Cleaning the wound of inflammatory stimuli, such as devitalized tissue and reactive chemicals, involves débridement and cleansing. In addition, effective wound cleansing and débridement can reduce the bio-burden and minimize colonization in pressure ulcers. Evidence is accumulating that effective débridement and cleansing improves wound healing. Chronic wounds may persist because of chronic inflammation secondary to devitalized tissue, wound exudate, and bacteria (101, 102). Débridement can be accomplished in a variety of ways. The most common methods include chemical, mechanical, autolytic, or surgical débridement. Cleansing uses specific types of fluid, usually saline based, to remove loosely adherent foreign material so as to facilitate wound healing (103).

Sharp débridement uses a scalpel or scissors to remove the devitalized tissue and is the quickest way to remove devitalized tissue (104). In a multicenter study, Steed and colleagues (101) reported a lower rate of healing in those centers that performed less frequent débridement, independent of treatment. These findings suggest a correlation between aggressive wound débridement and improved wound healing. Mechanical débridement uses woven cotton gauze in a wet-to-dry technique, wound irrigation, or dextranomers. Although a variety of gauzes are available, the most effective gauzes for mechanical débridement are coarse and have large pores (105). Mechanical débridement can also be accomplished through hydrotherapy, such as with a whirlpool. Feedar and Kloth (106) recommend twice-daily whirlpool cleansing to remove debris and residue.

Whirlpool should be discontinued when the ulcer is clean, because the potential benefits of wound cleansing are outweighed by the potential trauma to fragile regenerating tissue as a result of the agitated water. Autolytic débridement is the process of keeping devitalized tissue hydrated and allowing reactive enzymes within the wound to digest the denatured tissues (107,108). This can be accomplished using moisture-retentive dressings or the use of hydrogels to moisturize the devitalized tissue. *In vivo* enzymes self-digest devitalized tissue. Mulder and colleagues (109) reported that when compared with a wet-to-dry gauze, a hypertonic gel was more effective in both tissue removal and overall costs (110). When clinicians use autolytic débridement, the wound must frequently be cleansed to wash out partially degraded tissue fragments. Overall, autolytic débridement can be more selective and less traumatic to the surrounding tissue and healthy wound tissue than mechanical débridement. Autolytic débridement is contraindicated for infected wounds.

Enzymatic débridement uses commercially prepared enzymes such as Collagenase® (Medical Services Group, Inc., Wayne, PA) and Accuzyme® (Healthpoint, Fort Worth, TX), similar to autolytic débridement, to degrade devitalized tissue. However, although the commercial enzymes are expected to work faster, one study indicates that similar results can be achieved with hydrogel alone, which is much less expensive (111).

Wounds should be cleansed at each dressing change using a technique and solution that minimizes trauma to healthy wound tissue (112). Most wounds can be cleansed with normal saline and for clean, granulating wounds, a gentle flushing with isotonic saline will cleanse the wound. For dirty wounds, stronger cleansing solution may be required, and clinicians can

TABLE 75-9. Relative Toxicity Indexes of Nonantimicrobial and Antimicrobial Wound Cleansers

Product	Manufacturer	Toxicity Index
Nonantimicrobials		
Dermagran®	Derma Sciences, Inc.	10
Shur-Clens® Wound Cleanser	Convatec®	10
Biolex™	Bard Medical Division, CR Bard, Inc.	100
Cara-Klenz™ Wound and Skin Cleanser	Carrington Laboratories, Inc.	100
Saf-Clens®Chronic Wound Cleanser	Convatec®	100
Clinswound™	Sage Laboratories, Inc.	1,000
Constant-Clens™ Dermal Wound Cleanser	Sherwood Medical-Davis and Geck	1,000
Curaklense™ Wound Cleanser	Kendall Healthcare Products Co.	1,000
Curasol™	Healthpoint Medical	1,000
Gentell Wound Cleanser™	Gentell	1,000
Sea-Clens® Wound Cleanser	Coloplast Sween Corp	1,000
Ultra-Klenz™ Wound Cleanseer	Carrington Laboratories, Inc.	1,000
Antimicrobials		
Clinical Care® Dermal Wound Cleanser	Care-Tech® Laboratories, Inc.	1,000
Dermal Wound Cleanser	Smith and Nephew United, Inc.	10,000
MicroKlenz™ Antimicrobial Wound Cleanser	Carrington Laboratories, Inc.	10,000
Puri-Clens™ Wound Deodorizer and Cleanser	Coloplast Sween Corp.	10,000
Restore™	Hollister, Inc.	10,000
Royl-Derm™	Acme United Corp.	10,000
SeptiCare™ Antimicrobial Wound Cleanser	Sage Laboratories, Inc.	10,000

Data from Panel for Prediction and Prevention of Pressure Ulcers in Adults. *Prediction and prevention.* Clinical Practice Guideline No. 3, AHCPR publication No. 92–0047. Rockville, MD: Agency for Health Care Policy and Research, Public Health Service, U.S. Department of Health and Human Services, 1994.

TABLE 75-10.   Irrigation Pressures by Various Devices

Device	Irrigation Impact Pressure (PSI)
Bulb syringe	2.0
Piston irrigation syringe (60 mL) with catheter tip	4.2
Saline squeeze bottle (250 mL) with irrigation cap	4.5
Water-Pik at lowest setting (#1)	6.0
35-mL syringe with 19-gauge needle or angiocatheter	8.0
Water-Pik at middle setting (#3)	42
Water-Pik at highest setting (#5)	>50

Data from Panel for Prediction and Prevention of Pressure Ulcers in Adults. *Prediction and prevention.* Clinical Practice Guideline No. 3, AHCPR publication No. 92–0047. Rockville, MD: Agency for Health Care Policy and Research, Public Health Service, U.S. Department of Health and Human Services, 1994.

use commercial cleansing agents containing surfactants, such as Dermagran® (Derma Sciences, Inc.), Biolex™ (Bard Medical Division, CR Bard, Inc), and Ultra-Klenz™ Wound Cleanser (Carrington Laboratories, Inc.) (Table 75-9). As the wound becomes cleaner, because surfactants are harmful to wound cells, the strength of the cleansing solution should be decreased (6). Although their benefit in addition to cleansing solutions has not been documented, antiseptic agents can be added to the cleanser, such as Dermal Wound Cleanser (Smith and Nephew United, Inc.) and MicroKlenz™ Antimicrobial Wound Cleanser (Carrington Laboratories, Inc.), which will dramatically increase the toxicity index of the solution (113).

Cleansers must be applied gently so as to minimize trauma to healthy tissue. Irrigation streams must keep the impact force below 15 psi. Wound irrigation pressures of 10–15 psi were superior to those of 1 or 5 psi, and direct application should only be with the smoothest and softest device available (6). As seen in Table 75-10, irrigation with a 35-mL syringe and a 19-gauge needle or angiocatheter meets these requirements.

Infected Wounds

Several bacteriologic studies found a direct correlation between high levels of bacteria in pressure ulcers and failure to heal. Wound cleansing and débridement can enhance healing. It is not recommended to use swab cultures to diagnose wound infection as all pressure ulcers are colonized (114). Documenting a wound infection requires culture of needle aspiration fluid or biopsy of ulcer tissue (115).

If the pressure ulcer is clean and either continues to produce exudate or is not healing after 2 to 4 weeks of optimal care, a 2-week trial of topical antibiotics is recommended that is effective against gram-negative and gram-positive organisms as well as anaerobic organisms (e.g., sulfadiazine, triple antibiotic ointment) (6). Approximately 25% of nonhealing pressure ulcers have underlying osteomyelitis (116). The standard for diagnosing osteomyelitis is bone biopsy, although noninvasive strategies may include magnetic resonance imaging (MRI), bone scans, and plain x-ray. Plain films, although inexpensive, have a sensitivity of 78%, but a specificity of just 50% (117). Conventional bone scans, although more sensitive than plain films, also have a specificity of only 50% (118). Because of their false-positive rate, bone scans are rarely useful in clinical practice (119). MRI is an effective tool for the diagnosis of os-

teomyelitis and has been shown to have sensitivity of 95% with a specificity of 88% (120). In addition, in contrast to plain films and bone scan, MRI reveals anatomic detail of the wound as well as spatial resolution (121).

GENERAL DRESSING GUIDELINES

In general, wounds should be assessed at a minimum of weekly intervals, and more frequent assessment is warranted if the wound is rapidly changing or deteriorating (Table 75-11). With each dressing change, the wound should be gently irrigated. If no improvement is seen in approximately 3 weeks, consideration should be given to changing the management or reassessment of risk factors for the pressure ulcer (122). To decrease wound maceration, management techniques include application of zinc oxide or Vaseline to wound edges, or a stomal adhesive wafer around the wound. In choosing a dressing, exudates should be controlled without desiccating the ulcer while also optimizing caregiver time. To prevent abscess formation, all cavities should be loosely filled with dressing material without overpacking, which can lead to worsening the wound.

Dressings Based on Exudate Amounts

For wounds with minimal to mild exudates, dressing choices can include a hydrocolloid, polyurethane foam, or a saline gauze dressing. With moderate to heavy exudates, a calcium alginate dressing or even a hypertonic saline dressing can be used, although the hypertonic dressing may cause tissue destruction.

Dressings Based on Wound Tissue Color

For a wound with thick necrotic eschar, it will first need to be débrided. After débridement or on a wound with yellow slough, wound management should absorb excess exudate and débride any nonviable tissue. For these wounds, a saline gauze can be used, or, alternatively a hydrocolloid or calcium alginate, depending on the amount of exudate. With a red, healthy-appearing wound, the wound should be kept clean and slightly moist to maximize wound healing. Dressing choices include a moist saline dressing or a film dressing.

Dressings for Wound Cavities

For wound cavities, it is important that the wound be loosely filled to avoid excessive pressure on the fragile tissues, but packed sufficiently to avoid abscess formation. Dressings used for packing include calcium alginate packing, hydrocolloid pastes, polyurethane foam fillers, and expandable dressings. Although iodine-impregnated gauze can be used, it should be used only briefly as it may cause tissue destruction (123,124). Table 75-12 lists some suggested wound dressings based on ulcer stage.

Wound-Care Modalities

Adjunctive therapies have long been described in the pressure-ulcer literature. The AHCPR recommendations critically evaluated the strength of the literature on adjunctive therapies. Based on the clinical evidence available, only electrical stimulation merited recommendation and is to be considered for stage III and IV pressure ulcers that have proved unresponsive to conventional therapy, and also for recalcitrant stage II ulcers (6). Hydrotherapy should be considered for pressure ulcers containing large amounts of exudate and necrotic tissue, where

TABLE 75-11. Wound Dressings

Type	Description	Functions	Examples
Semiocclusive films	Semiocclusive/ semipermeable polyurethane film	Mimic skin performance Water vapor permeable Water/bacterial impermeable Provides moist environment for epithelialization	Tegaderm™ (3M) Op-Site® (Smith and Nephew) Bioclusive™ (Johnson and Johnson)
Impregnated gauze	Mesh or gauze impregnated with antibacterial, moisturizing compounds; nonadherent	Promotes epithelialization	Adaptic™(Johnson & Johnson) Xeroform™ (Kendall) Mesalt® (hypertonic saline) (Tendra) Iodoform™ (iodine) (Johnson & Johnson)
Hydrocolloid films	Colloid particles in an adhesive	Absorb fluid Autolytic débridement Encourages granulation Protects from trauma	Duoderm® (Convatec) Restore™ (Hollister) Comfeel®(Coloplast) Ultec™(Kendall)
Hydrogels	Cross-linked polymer with 90% water	Provides moist environment for epithelialization Minimal débridement Low absorbency	Carrington gel™ (Carrington Labs) Vigilon® (Bard)
Polyurethane foam	Hydrophilic or hydrophobic polyurethane foam	High absorbency	Allevyn™ (Smith & Nephew) Polymem® (Ferris Polymem) Lyofoam® (activated charcoal) (Convatec)
Absorptive powders	Starch, copolymers, colloidal particles	High absorbency Débridement	Duoderm granules Bard absorptive dressing
Calcium alginate	Calcium alginate (seaweed) fibers	Highly absorbent With exudate, becomes a gel to create moist environment	Sorbsan® (Bertek) Kaltostat® (Convatec)
Gauze	Cotton or rayon/polyester blend, woven	Highly absorbent Débridement Packing Prepping	Versalon™ (Kendall) Nu Gauze® (Johnson & Johnson)

it can assist in débridement. However, once the wound is clean and has healthy granulation tissue, the agitating water may cause damage to the delicate new tissue and should be discontinued. The therapeutic efficacy of hyperbaric oxygen, infrared, ultraviolet, and low-energy laser irradiation, and ultrasonography have not been sufficiently established for recommendation in the treatment of pressure ulcers (6). Currently, the Health Care Financing Administration uses a case-by-case evaluation of electrical stimulation for wound management for Medicare reimbursement (125).

Since the AHCPR recommendations were published, the strength of the scientific evidence for the use of electrical stimu-

TABLE 75-12. Wound Dressings for Ulcer Stages

Stage	Suggested Dressing
I	Polyurethane or hydrocolloid dressing
II or III Clean	Wet to moist saline dressing Hydrogel dressing Polyurethane foam dressing Hydrocolloid dressing
II or III Infected	Topical antiseptic Wet-to-dry saline dressing
IV Clean	Wet to moist saline dressing Hydrogel dressing Hydrocolloid dressing
IV Infected	Topical antiseptic Wet-to-dry saline dressing

From Bello YM, Phillips JT. Recent advances in wound healing. *JAMA* 2000;
283:716–718.

lation has advanced (126,127), and there is evidence that growth factors may be efficacious in the treatment of pressure ulcers (128–131). Since the publication of the AHCPR guidelines, there are three new adjunctive therapies for the healing of pressure ulcers that have had initial evidence of efficacy: vacuum-assisted therapy (subatmospheric pressure therapy) (132,133), normothermia (134), and constant tension approximation (135). Vacuum assisted therapy or subatmospheric pressure therapy entails placing an open-cell foam into the wound, sealing the site with an adhesive drape, and applying subatmospheric pressure (125 mm Hg below ambient) that is transmitted to the wound in a controlled manner. This will increase blood flow in the wound and adjacent tissue, thereby increasing oxygen and nutrient delivery, and increase clearance of bacteria from infected wounds, resulting in an environment that promotes wound healing (136,137). It has been shown to be cost-effective in the home care of chronic wounds (138). Normothermia employs the use of a radiant-heat dressing to hasten wound healing. Normothermia has been shown in one small study with stage III and IV pressure ulcers to decrease the mean wound surface area by 61% over a 4-week period (139). Constant tension approximation has been reported in one study on ulcers on patients with a variety of comorbidities to increase the rate of healing through use of a device for wound approximation.

SURGICAL TREATMENT

In general, stage I and II pressure ulcers can be treated nonsurgically. Stage III and IV pressure ulcers, because of their high rate of recurrence as well as the long duration necessary for wound closure, often require surgical intervention. In general,

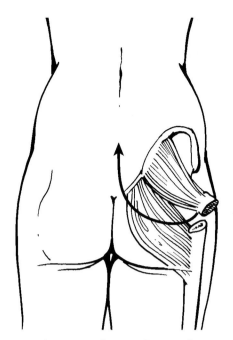

Figure 75-3. Musculocutaneous flaps, used to cover large extensive pressure ulcers.

the goals of surgical wound closure can include reduction in the time to healing, lower costs, improved patient hygiene and appearance, decreased amount of care needed, and prevention of secondary complications, including renal amyloidosis and Marjolin's ulcer (140). Proper selection of the surgical candidate is important because of the cost and postoperative recovery time, both of which can be extensive. In addition, if musculocutaneous flaps are performed (Fig. 75-3), there are only a limited number that can be performed, which may be of consequence if the individual has repeated pressure ulcers or additional risk factors are added with aging.

Operative procedures to repair pressure ulcers include direct closure, skin grafting, skin flaps, musculocutaneous flaps, fasciocutaneous flaps, and free flaps. The simplest type of repair that can adequately close the wound with a reasonable success rate should be chosen (140,141). Free flaps, skin flaps, and skin grafts are rarely used for pressure ulcers in SCI, as they are poorly able to tolerate any future pressure or shear. Direct closure is rarely of benefit unless the source of the pressure has been eradicated and the wound is small (142). Musculocutaneous and fasciocutaneous flaps have become the coverage of choice for SCI patients who require surgical closure of the pressure ulcer. Because of their blood supply, these flaps are better able to withstand pressure and shear and can be particularly useful in osteomyelitis by bringing highly vascularized muscle tissue into the area of infection (143,144).

Factors that impair postoperative healing include smoking, spasticity, nutritional concerns, and bacterial colonization. Smoking is one of the strongest inhibitors of wound healing as a result of carbon monoxide and nicotine, both of which are potent vasoconstrictors. In addition to compromises in arterial blood flow and oxygen delivery, smoking increases blood viscosity (145) and increases oxidase release by neutrophils (146), all of which impair wound healing. Nicotine patches should not be used, as they provide the same drug as cigarettes. Spasticity can also impair postoperative healing through repeated contraction of muscles, causing joint movement during the period of postoperative immobilization (147,148). In addition, significant contractures may impair pressure-relief efforts

(149). Adequate nutrition must be maintained during the postoperative period to allow for wound healing, although serum albumin and total protein levels have not been found to correlate with postoperative wound outcome (150). Finally, exposure to bacterial contamination, particularly of urine and feces, increases colonization of wounds and is associated with slower rates of healing (95).

At the sacral area, the gluteus maximus muscle may be used in its entirety or in portions. At the ischium, a posterior thigh fasciocutaneous flap, inferior gluteus maximus myocutaneous flap, hamstring V-Y advancement flap, and tensor fascia lata fasciocutaneous flap can all be used to cover defects in this region. Prophylactic unilateral or bilateral ischiectomy is not recommended. Unilateral ischiectomy, because weight is diverted to the contralateral ischium, is associated with occurrence of a contralateral ischial ulcer (151). Bilateral ischiectomy will transfer weight bearing to the anterior pelvis and perineum, causing perineal ulcers and urethral fistulae (152,153). At the greater trochanter, the tensor fascia lata fasciocutaneous flap is considered the flap of choice in this area, although alternatives include use of the vastus lateralis, inferior gluteus maximus, and rectus femoris muscles. Girdlestone arthroplasty for ulcers that communicate with the hip joint may be necessary, although patients may experience a pistoning of the distal femur after this procedure, which may be detrimental to the flap (154).

Postoperatively, strict bed rest is prescribed with immobilization and pressure relief. Usually, a low-air-loss mattress or an air-fluidized bed is prescribed. The head of the bed should not be elevated greater that 15 degrees to avoid risk of shear. Bed rest should be maintained postoperatively to allow sufficient time for the surgical site to heal. There is no consensus in the literature on the necessary length of immobilization, ranging from 2 to 6 weeks (155). A progressive sitting program is initiated after the period of immobilization, although there is no consensus regarding rate of progression in the sitting schedule. Overall, a 13% to 56% recurrence rate has been reported following surgical repair of pressure ulcers (156).

COMPLICATIONS OF PRESSURE ULCERS

Pressure ulcers have been associated with many complications, including endocarditis (157), heterotopic bone formation, maggot infestation (158), perineal urethral fistula, septic arthritis (159), sinus tract or abscess (160), squamous cell carcinoma in the ulcer (161), systemic complications of the treatment (162, 163), and, specifically in SCI, contractures (164).

In addition, once a pressure ulcer has occurred, there is the risk of recurrence. Niazi and associates (46) found a 35% recurrence rate of pressure ulcers regardless of whether the treatment was medical or surgical; however, Disa and colleagues (165) found that in 69% of patients and 61% of sores, a recurrent ulceration can occur. Smoking, diabetes mellitus, and cardiovascular disease were associated with the highest rates of recurrence in these studies. Patients often have misconceptions about pressure ulcers: one study found that 82% of people with SCI who had an ulcer did not believe that they were at risk for the development of a future ulcer (166). Other factors, including age, employment status, and psychological well-being, are less well defined in their association with pressure ulcer recurrence (167).

Long-standing ulcers (20 years or more) can rarely (<0.5%) develop Marjolin's ulcers, a type of squamous cell carcinoma. Biopsy can identify the carcinoma that is suspected clinically with pain, increasing discharge, verrucous hyperplasia, and bleeding (168,169).

SUMMARY

Pressure ulcers remain a significant source of morbidity and cost, despite advances in our understanding of their pathophysiology and risk factors. Education of these risk factors, as well as interventions to prevent ulcers from occurring, can help maintain skin integrity as well as assist in the treatment of pressure ulcers. Treatment options—aimed at wound care, minimizing risk factors, mobilization, and surgery—require careful management and follow-up.

REFERENCES

1. Allman RM, Goode PS, Burst N, et al. Pressure ulcers, hospital complications, and disease severity: impact on hospital costs and length of stay. *Advances in Wound Care* 1999;12:22–30.
2. Copeland-Fields LD, Hoshiko BR. Clinical validation of Braden and Bergstrom's conceptual schema of pressure sore risk factors. *Rehabilitation Nursing* 1987;14:257–260.
3. National Pressure Ulcer Advisory Panel. Pressure ulcers prevalence, cost and risk assessment: consensus development conference statement. *Decubitus* 1989;2:24–28.
4. Maklebust J. Pressure ulcers: etiology and prevention. *Nurs Clin North Am* 1987;22:359–377.
5. Panel for Prediction and Prevention of Pressure Ulcers in Adults. *Prediction and prevention.* Clinical Practice Guideline No. 3, AHCPR publication No. 92–0047. Rockville, MD: Agency for Health Care Policy and Research, Public Health Service, U.S. Department of Health and Human Services, 1992.
6. Panel for Prediction and Prevention of Pressure Ulcers in Adults. *Prediction and prevention.* Clinical Practice Guideline No. 3, AHCPR publication No. 92–0047. Rockville, MD: Agency for Health Care Policy and Research, Public Health Service, U.S. Department of Health and Human Services, 1994.
7. Glover D. Let's own up to the real cost of pressure ulcers. *Journal of Wound Care* 2003;12:43.
8. Kynes PM. A new perspective on pressure sore prevention. *Journal of Enterostomal Therapy* 1986;13:42–43.
9. Staas WJ, Lamantia J. Decubitus ulcers and rehabilitation medicine. *Int J Dermatol* 1982;21:437–444.
10. Tourtual DM, Riesenberg LA, Korutz CJ, et al. Predictors of hospital acquired heel pressure ulcers. *Ostomy/Wound Management* 1997;43(9):24–34.
11. Gerson L. The incidence of pressure sores in active treatment hospitals. *Int J Nurs Stud* 1975;12:201–204.
12. Clarke M, Kahdom H. The nursing prevention of pressure sores in hospital and community patients. *J Adv Nurs* 1988;13:365–373.
13. Meehan M. Multisite pressure ulcer prevalence survey. *Decubitus* 1990;3:14–17.
14. Bergstrom N, Braden B, Laguzza A, et al. The Braden scale for predicting pressure sore risk. *Nurs Res* 1987;36:205–210.
15. Robnett M. The incidence of skin breakdown in a surgical intensive care unit. *Journal of Nursing Quality Assurance* 1986;1:77–81.
16. Allman RM, Laprade CA, Noel LB, et al. Pressure sores among hospitalized patients. *Ann Intern Med* 1986;105:337–342.
17. Brandeis GH, Morris JN, Nash DJ, et al. The epidemiology and natural history of pressure ulcers in elderly nursing home residents. *JAMA* 1990;264:2905–2909.
18. Berlowitz DR, Bezerra HQ, Brandeis GH, et al. Are we improving the quality of nursing home care: the case of pressure ulcers. *J Am Geriatr Soc* 2000;48:59–62.
19. Reed J. Pressure ulcers in the elderly: prevention and treatment utilizing the team approach. *Maryland State Medical Journal* 1981;30:45–50.
20. Berlowitz D, Wilking S. Risk factors for pressure sores: a comparison of cross-sectional and cohort-derived data. *J Am Geriatr So* 1989;37:1043–1050.
21. Hentziem B, Bergstrom N, Poxehl B. Prevalence and incidence of pressure sores and associated risk factors in a rural-based home health population. Poster presented at 17th Annual Midwest Nursing Research Society, Cleveland, Ohio, March 28–30, 1993.
22. Bates-Jensen B. *Wound care: a collaborative manual for physical therapists and nurses.* Gaithersburg, MD: Aspen, 1998.
23. Bergstrom N, Braden B. A prospective study of pressure sore risk among the institutionalized elderly. *J Am Geriatr Soc* 1992;40:747–758.
24. Russel L. Physiology of the skin and prevention of pressure sores. *British Journal of Nursing* 1998;7:1088–1092.
25. Landis EM. Micro-injection: studies of capillary blood pressure in human skin. *Heart* 1930;15:209–228.
26. Bryant R, Shannon ML, Pieper B, et al. Pressure ulcers. In: Bryant R, ed. *Acute and chronic wounds: nursing management.* St. Louis: Mosby Year Book, 1992.

27. Garber SL, Krouskop TA. Body build and its relationship to pressure distribution in the seated wheelchair patient. *Arch Phys Med Rehabil* 1982;63:17–20.
28. Seiler WO, Allen S, Stahelin HB. Influence of the 30 degrees laterally included position and the "super-soft" 3-piece mattress on skin oxygen tension on areas of maximum pressure—implications for pressure sores prevention. *Gerontology* 1986;32:158–166.
29. Kosiak M, Kubicek WG, Olso M, et al. Evaluation of pressure as a factor in the production of ischial ulcers. *Arch Phys Med Rehabil* 1958;39:623–629.
30. Koziak M. Etiology and pathology of ischemic ulcers. *Arch Phys Med Rehabil* 1959;40:62–69.
31. Staas WE Jr, Cioschi HM. Pressure sores: a multifaceted approach to prevention and treatment. *West J Med* 1991;154:539–544.
32. Reswick JB, Rogers JE. Experience at Rancho Los Amigos Hospital with devices and techniques to prevent pressure ulcers. In: Kenedi R, Cowden J, Scales J, eds. *Bedsore biomechanics.* London: University Park Press, 1976:300.
33. Daniel RK, Hall EJ, MacLeod MK. Pressure sores: a reappraisal. *Ann Plast Surg* 1979;3:53–63.
34. Husain T. An experimental study of some pressure effects on tissues with reference to the bedsore problems. *Journal of Pathology and Bacteriology* 1953;66:347–382.
35. Daniel RK, Priest DL, Wheatley DC. Etiologic factors in pressure sores: an experimental model. *Arch Phys Med Rehabil* 1981;62:492–498.
36. Dinsdale S. Decubitus ulcers: role of pressure and friction in causation. *Arch Phys Med Rehabil* 1974;55:147–152.
37. Reichel S. Shearing force as a factor in decubitus ulcers in paraplegics. *JAMA* 1958;166:762–763.
38. Bryant R. Skin pathology and types of damage. In: R. Bryant, ed. *Acute and chronic wounds: nursing management.* St. Louis: Mosby, 2000.
39. Thomas DR, Goode PS, LaMaster K, et al. A comparison of an opaque foam dressing versus a transparent film dressing in the management of skin tears in institutionalized subjects. *Ostomy/Wound Management* 1999;45:22–24, 27–28.
40. Yarkony GM. Pressure ulcers: a review. *Arch Phys Med Rehabil* 1994;75:908–917.
41. Allman RM. Epidemiology of pressure sores in different populations. *Decubitus* 1989;2:24–48.
42. Pinchocofsky-Devin G. Nutritional assessment and intervention. In: Krasner D, ed. *Chronic wound care.* King of Prussia, PA: Health Management Publications, 1990.
43. Natow AB. Nutrition I. prevention and treatment of decubitus ulcers. *Topics in Clinical Nursing* 1983;5:32–44.
44. Haalboom JR, den Boer J, Buskens E. Risk-assessment tool in the prevention of pressure ulcers. *Ostomy/Wound Management* 1999;45:20–26.
45. Bates-Jensen BM, Alessi CA, Al-Samarrai NR, et al. The effects of an exercise and incontinence intervention on skin health outcomes in nursing home residents. *J Am Geriatr Soc* 2003;51;348–355.
46. Niazi ZBM, Salzberg CA, Byrne DW, et al. Recurrence of initial pressure ulcers in persons with spinal cord injuries. *Advances in Wound Care* 1997;10:38–42.
47. Salzberg CA, Byrne DW, Cayten CG, et al. Predicting and preventing pressure ulcers in adults with paralysis. *Advances in Wound Care* 1998;11:237–246.
48. Lehman CA. Risk factors for pressure ulcers in the spinal cord injured in the community. *Sci Nurs* 1995;12:110–114.
49. McKinley WO, Jackson AB, Cardenas DD, et al. Long-term medical complications after traumatic spinal cord injury: a regional model systems analysis. *Arch Phys Med Rehabil* 1999;80:1402–1410.
50. Carlson CE, Matthews-Kirk P, Stevens K, et al. Psychosocial factors associated with pressure sores after spinal cord injury. *Arch Phys Med Rehabil* 1990;71:788(abst).
51. Fuhrer MJ, Rintala DH, Hart KA, et al. Depressive symptomatology in persons with spinal cord injury who reside in the community. *Arch Phys Med Rehabil* 1993;74:255–260.
52. Rintala DH, Young ME, Hart KA, et al. Social support and the well-being of persons with spinal cord injury living in the community. *Rehabil Psychol* 1992;37:155–163.
53. Fisher BH. Topical hyperbaric oxygen treatment of pressure sores and skin ulcers. *Lancet* 1969;2:405–409.
54. Anderson T, Andberg M. Psychological factors associated with pressure sores. *Arch Phys Med Rehabil* 1979;60:341–346.
55. Braden BJ. The relationship between serum cortisol and pressure sore formation among the elderly recently relocated to a nursing home. *Reflections* 1988;14:182–186.
56. Kravitz M. Outpatient wound care. *Critical Care Nursing Clinics of North America* 1996;8:217–233.
57. Carlson CE, King RB, Kirk PM, et al. Incidence and correlates of pressure ulcer development after spinal cord injury. *Rehabilitation Nursing Research* 1992;1:34–40.
58. Witte M, Barbul A. General principles of wound healing. *Surg Clin North Am* 1997;77:509–528.
59. Bethell E. Controversies in classifying and assessing grade I pressure ulcers. *Journal of Wound Care* 2003;12:33–36.
60. Stotts NA, Rodeheaver GT, Thomas DR, et al. An instrument to measure healing in pressure ulcers: development and validation of the pressure ulcer scale for healing (PUSH). *J Gerontol A Biol Sci Med Sci* 2001;56:M795–799.
61. Lyder CH. Pressure ulcer prevention and management. *JAMA* 2003;289:223–226.
62. Motta G. *Skin and wound care: dressing for success.* Providence, RI: Workshop American Healthcare Institute, April 1993.

63. Pieper B, Weiland M. Pressure ulcer prevention within 72 hours of admission in a rehabilitation setting. *Ostomy/Wound Management* 1997;43:14–22.

64. Ayello EA. Predicting pressure ulcer sore risk. *MEDSURG Nursing* 2003;12:130–131.

65. Curley MA, Razmus IS, Roberts KE, et al. Predicting pressure ulcer risk in pediatric patients: the Braden Q Scale. *Nurs Res* 2003;52:22–33.

66. Bergquist S. Subscales, subscores, or summative score: evaluating the contribution of Braden Scale items for predicting pressure ulcer risk in older adults receiving home health care. *Journal of Wound, Ostomy, and Continence Nursing* 2001;28:279–289.

67. Norton D. Calculating the risk: reflections on the Norton Scale. *Decubitus* 1989;2:24–31.

68. Yetzer EA, Sullivan RL. The foot at risk: identification and prevention of skin breakdown. *Rehabilitation Nursing* 1992;17:247–251.

69. Baldwin KM. Incidence and prevalence of pressure ulcers in children. *Advances in Skin and Wound Care* 2002;15:121–124.

70. Maklebust J, Magnan MA. Approaches to patient and family education for pressure ulcer management. *Decubitus* 1992;5:18–20, 24, 26.

71. Warren VB, ed. *A treasury of techniques for teaching adults.* Washington, DC: National Association for Public Continuing and Adult Education, 1977.

72. Gray D. Deep cell prime: preventing and healing pressure ulcers. *British Journal of Nursing* 2002;11:S44, S46–S48.

73. Engstrand JL. A nursing challenge: effective patient education. *AORN J* 1979;4:15–18.

74. Barnes SH. Patient/family education for the patient with a pressure necrosis. *Nurs Clin North Am* 1987;22:463–474.

75. Krouskop TA, Noble PC, Garber SL, Spencer WA. The effectiveness of preventative management in reducing the occurrence of pressure sores. *J Rehabil Res Dev* 1983;20:74–83.

76. Collins N. Vegetarian diets and wound healing. *Advances in Skin and Wound Care* 2003;16:65–66.

77. Bonnefoy M, Coulon L, Bienvenu J, et al. Implication of cytokines in the aggravation of malnutrition and hypercatabolism in elderly patients with severe pressure sores. *Age Ageing* 1995;24:37–42.

78. Blaylock B. A study of risk factors in patients placed on specialty beds. *JWOCN* 1995;22:263–266.

79. Segal JL, Gonzales E, Yousefi S, et al. Circulating levels of IL-2R, ICAM-1, and IL-6 in spinal cord injuries. *Arch Phys Med Rehabil* 1997;78:44–47.

80. Chin D, Kearns P. Nutrition in the spinal-injured patient. *Nutr Clin Pract* 1997;6:213–222.

81. Alexander LR, Spungen AM, Liu MH, et al. Resting metabolic rate in subjects with paraplegia: the effect of pressure sores. *Arch Phys Med Rehabil* 1995;76:819–822.

82. Liu MH, Spungen AM, Fink L, et al. Increased energy needs in patients with quadriplegia and pressure ulcers. *Advances in Wound Care* 1996;9:41–45.

83. Saltzman E. Nutrition in disease prevention and treatment. *Caring* 2002;21:22–24.

84. terRiet G, Kessels A, Knipschild P. Randomized clinical trial of ascorbic acid in the treatment of pressure ulcers. *J Clin Epidemiol* 1995;48:1453–1460.

85. Collins N. Vitamin C and pressure ulcers. *Advances in Skin and Wound Care* 2002;15:186–188.

86. Houwing R, Overgoor M, Kon M, et al. Pressure-induced skin lesions in pigs: reperfusion injury and the effects of vitamin E. *Journal of Wound Care* 2000;9:36–40.

87. Kohn S, Kohn D, Schiller D. Effect of zinc supplementation on epidermal Langerhans' cells of elderly patients with decubitus ulcers. *J Dermatol* 2000;27:258–263.

88. Lawrence W. Clinical management of non-healing wounds. In: Cohen C, ed. *Wound healing.* Philadelphia, PA: WB Saunders, 1992:541.

89. Jeevendra M, Ramos L, Shamos R, et al. Decreased growth hormone levels in the catabolic phase of severe injury. *Surgery* 1992;111:495–502.

90. Demling R, DeSanti L. Oxandrolone, an anabolic steroid significantly increases weight gain in the recovery phase after major burns. *J Trauma* 1997;43:47–51.

91. Demling R, DeSanti L. Closure of the "non-healing wound" corresponds with correction of weight loss using the anabolic agent oxandrolone. *Ostomy/Wound Management* 1998;44:58–68.

92. Fox M, Minor A. Oxandrolone: a potent anabolic steroid. *J Clin Endocrinol Metab* 1962;22:921–923.

93. Lyder CH. Pressure ulcer prevention and management. *Annual Review of Nursing Research* 2002;20:35–61.

94. Charles MA, Oldenbrook J, Catton C. Evaluation of a low-air-loss mattress system in the treatment of patients with pressure ulcers. *Ostomy/Wound Management* 1995;41:46–52.

95. Ferrell BA, Osterweil D, Christenson P. A randomized trial of low-air-loss beds for treatment of pressure ulcers. *JAMA* 1993;269:494–497.

96. Day A, Leonard F. Seeking quality care for patients with pressure ulcers. *Decubitus* 1993;6:32–43.

97. Sharbaugh RJ, Hargest TS, Wright FA. Further studies on the bactericidal effect of the air-fluidized bed. *Ame Surg* 1973;39:253–256.

98. Sharbaugh RJ, Hargest TS. Bactericidal effect of the air-fluidized bed. *Am Surg* 1971;37:583–586.

99. Barr CA. Evaluation of cushions using dynamic pressure measurement. *Prosthet Orthot Int* 1991;15:232–240.

100. Crewe RA. Problems of rubbering nursing cushions and a clinical survey of alternative cushions for ill patients. *Case SCI Pract* 1987;5:9–11.

101. Steed DL, Donohoe D, Webster MW, et al. Diabetic Ulcer Study Group. Effect of extensive débridement and treatment on the healing of diabetic foot ulcers. *J Am Coll Surg* 1996;183:61–64.

102. Burke DT, Ho CH, Saucier MA. Hydrotherapy effects on pressure ulcer healing. *Arch Phys Med Rehabil* 1997;78:1053.

103. Rodeheaver GT. Pressure ulcer débridement and cleansing:a review of current literature. *Ostomy/Wound Management* 1999;45[Suppl 1A]: 80S–85S.

104. Witkowski JA, Parish LC. Débridement of cutaneous ulcers: medical and surgical aspects. *Clin Dermatol* 1992;9:585–591.

105. Mulder GD. Evaluation of three nonwoven sponges in the débridement of chronic wounds. *Ostomy/Wound Management* 1995;41:62–67.

106. Feedar JA, Kloth LC. Conservative management of chronic wounds. In: Kloth LC, McCulloch JM, Feedar JA, eds. *Wound healing: alternatives in management.* Philadelphia: FA Davis, 1990.

107. Flanagan M. The efficacy of a hydrogel in the treatment of wounds with non-viable tissue. *Journal of Wound Care* 1995;4:264–267.

108. Bale S, Banks V, Haglestein S, et al. A comparison of two amorphous hydrogels in the débridement of pressure sores. *Journal of Wound Care* 1998;7:65–68.

109. Mulder GD, Romanko KP, Sealey J, et al. Controlled randomized study of a hypertonic gel for the débridement of dry eschar in chronic wounds. *Wounds* 1993;5:112–115.

110. Mulder GD. Cost-effective managed care: gel versus wet-to-dry for débridement. *Ostomy/Wound Management* 1995;41:68–76.

111. Martin SJ, Corrado OJ, Kay EA. Enzymatic débridement for necrotic wounds. *Journal of Wound Care* 1996;5:310–311.

112. Lyder CH. Pressure ulcer prevention and management. *JAMA* 2003;289:223–226.

113. Hellewell TB, Major DA, Foresman PA, et al. A cytotoxicity evaluation of antimicrobial and non-antimicrobial wound cleansers. *Wounds* 1997;9:15–20.

114. Heggers JP. Assessing and controlling wound infection. *Clin Plast Surg* 2003;30:25–35.

115. Thomas DR. Prevention and treatment of pressure ulcers: what works? What doesn't? *Cleve Clin J Med* 2001;68:704–707, 710–714, 717–722.

116. Black JM, Black SB. Surgical management of pressure ulcers. *Nurs Clin North Am* 1987;22:229–232.

117. Deloach E, Christy R, Ruf L. Osteomyelitis underlying severe pressure ulcers. *Contemporary Surgery* 1992;40:25–32.

118. Han H. Lewis VL Jr., Wiedrich TA, et al. The value of Jamshidi core needle bone biopsy in predicting postoperative osteomyelitis in grade IV pressure ulcer patients. *Plast Reconstr Surg* 2002;110:118–122.

119. Lewis VL Jr., Bailey MH, Pulawski G, et al. The diagnosis of osteomyelitis in patients with pressure sores. *Plast Reconstr Surg* 1988;81:229–232.

120. Santiago Restrepo C, Gimenez CR, McCarthy K. Imaging of osteomyelitis and musculoskeletal soft tissue infections: current concepts. *Rheum Dis Clin North Am* 2003;29:89–109.

121. Ruan CM, Escobedo E, Harrison S, et al. Magnetic resonance imaging of nonhealing pressure ulcers and myocutaneous flaps. *Arch Phys Med Rehabil* 1998;79:1080–1088.

122. Hess CT. When to use gauze dressings. *Advances in Skin and Wound Care* 2000;13:266–268.

123. Belmin J, Meaume S, Rabus MT, et al. Sequential treatment with calcium alginate dressings and hydrocolloid dressings accelerates pressure ulcer healing in older subjects: a multicenter randomized trial of sequential versus nonsequential treatment with hydrocolloid dressings alone. *J Am Geriatr Soc* 2002;50:269–274.

124. Bello YM, Phillips JT. Recent advances in wound healing. *JAMA* 2000283:716–718.

125. Ovington LG. Dressings and adjunctive therapies: AHCPR guidelines revisited. *Ostomy/Wound Management* 1999;45:94S–106S.

126. Wood JM, Evans PE III, Schallreuter KU, et al. A multicenter study on the use of pulsed low-intensity direct current for healing chronic stage II and stage III decubitus. *Arch Dermatol* 1993;129:999–1009.

127. Gardner SE, Frantz RA, Schmidt FL. Effect of electrical stimulation on chronic wound healing. *Wound Repair Regeneration* 1999;7:495–503.

128. Robson MC, Phillips LG, Lawrence WT, et al. The safety and effect of topically applied recombinant basic fibroblast growth factor on the healing of chronic pressure sores. *Ann Surg* 1992;216:401–406.

129. Robson MC, Phillips LG, Thomason A, et al. Recombinant human platelet-derived growth factor-BB for the treatment of chronic pressure ulcers. *Ann Plast Surg* 1992;29:193–201.

130. Robson MC, Phillips LG, Thomason A, et al. Platelet-derived growth factor BB for the treatment of chronic pressure ulcers. *Lancet* 1992;339:23–25.

131. Rees RS, Robson MC, Smiell JN, et al. Becaplermin gel in the treatment of pressure ulcers: a phase II randomized, double-blind, placebo-controlled study. *Wound Repair Regeneration* 1999;7:141–147.

132. Mullner T, Mrkonjic L, Kwasny O, et al. The use of negative pressure to promote healing of tissue defects: a clinical trial using the vacuum sealing technique. *Br J Plast Surg* 1997;50:194–199.

133. Argenta LC, Morykwas MJ. Vacuum-assisted closure: a new method for wound control and treatment: clinical experience. *Ann Plast Surg* 1997;38:563–576.

134. Kloth LC, Berman JE, Dumit-Minkel S, et al. Effects of a normothermic dressing on pressure ulcer healing. *Advances in Skin and Wound Care* 2000;13(2):69–74.

135. Ger R. Wound management by constant tension approximation. *Ostomy/Wound Management* 1996;42:40–46.

136. Morykwas MJ, Argenta LC, Shelton-Brown EI, et al. Vacuum-assisted closure: a new method for wound control and treatment: animal studies and basic foundation. *Ann Plast Surg* 1997;38(6):553–562.

137. Wanner MB, Schwarzl F, Strub B, et al. Vacuum-assisted wound closure for cheaper and more comfortable healing of pressure sores: a prospective study. *Scand J Plast Reconstr Surg Hand Surg* 2003;37:28–33.

138. Hartnett JM. Use of vacuum-assisted wound closure in three chronic wounds. *Journal of Wound, Ostomy and Continence Nursing* 1998;25:281–290.

139. Peirce B, Gray M. Radiant heat dressings for chronic wounds. *Journal of Wound, Ostomy, and Continence Nursing* 2001;28:263–266.

140. Daniel RK, Faibusoff B. Muscle coverage of pressure points: the role of myocutaneous flaps. *Ann Plast Surg* 1982;8:446–452.

141. Fulda GJ, Khan SU, Zabel DD. Special issues in plastic and reconstructive surgery. *Crit Care Clin* 2003;19:91–108.

142. Anthony JP, Huntsman WT, Mathes SJ. Changing trends in the management of pelvic pressure ulcers: a 12-year review. *Decubitus* 1992;5:44–51.

143. Daniel RK, Hall EJ, Macleod MK. Pressure sores: a reappraisal. *Ann Plast Surg* 1979;2:53–63.

144. Mathes SJ, Feng LJ, Hunt TK. Coverage of the infected wound. *Ann Surg* 1983;198:420–429.

145. Read RC. Presidential address: systemic effects of smoking. *Am J Surg* 1984;148:706–711.

146. Fincham JE. Smoking cessation: treatment options and the pharmacist's role. *Ann Pharmacother* 1992;32:62–70.

147. Ger R, Levine SA. The management of decubitus ulcers by muscle transposition: an 8-year review. *Plast Reconstr Surg* 1976;58:419–428.

148. Herceg SJ, Harding RL. Surgical treatment of pressure sores. *Arch Phys Med Rehabil* 1978;59:193–200.

149. Haher JN, Haher TR, Devlin VJ, et al. The release of flexion contractures as a prerequisite for the treatment of pressure sores in multiple sclerosis: a report of ten cases. *Ann Plast Surg* 1983;11:246–249.

150. Goodman CM, Cohen V, Armenta A, et al. Evaluation of results and treatment variables for pressure ulcers in 48 veteran spinal cord injured patients. *Ann Plast Surg* 1999;43:572–574.

151. Arregui J, Canon B, Murray JE. Long-term evaluation of ischiectomy in the treatment of pressure ulcers. *Plast Reconstr Surg* 1965;36:583–590.

152. Hackler RH, Zampieri TA. Urethral complications following ischiectomy in spinal cord injury patients: a urethral pressure study. *J Urol* 1987;137:253–255.

153. Karaca AR, Binns JH, Blumenthal FS. Complications of total ischiectomy for the treatment of ischial pressure sores. *Plast Reconstr Surg* 1978;62:96–99.

154. Evans GR, Lewis VL Jr., Manson PN, et al. Hip joint communication with pressure sore: the refractory wound and the role of Girdlestone arthroplasty. *Plast Reconstr Surg* 1993;91:288–294.

155. Stal S, Serure A, Donovan W, et al. The perioperative management of the patient with pressure sores. *Ann Plast Surg* 1983;11:347–356.

156. Tavakoli K, Rutkowski S, Cope C, et al. Recurrence rates of ischial sores in para- and tetraplegics treated with hamstring flaps: an 8-year study. *Br J Plast Surg* 1999;52:476–479.

157. Schwartz IS, Pervez N. Bacterial endocarditis associated with permanent transvenous cardiac pacemaker. *JAMA* 1971;218:736–737.

158. Roche S, Cross S, Burgess I, et al. Cutaneous myiasis in an elderly debilitated patient. *Postgrad Med J* 1990;66:776–777.

159. Klein NE, Moore T, Capen D, et al. Sepsis of the hip in paraplegic patients. *J Bone Joint Surg* 1988;70:839–843.

160. Putnam T, Calenoff L, Betts HB, et al. Sinography in management of decubitus ulcers. *Arch Phys Med Rehabil* 1978;59:243–245.

161. Berkwits L, Yarkony GM, Lewis V. Marjolin's ulcer complicating a pressure ulcer: case report and literature review. *Arch Phys Med Rehabil* 1986;67:831–833.

162. Johnson CA. Hearing loss following the application of topical neomycin. *J Burn Care Rehabil* 1988;9:162–164.

163. Shetty KR, Duthie EH Jr. Thyrotoxicosis induced by topical iodine application. *Arch Intern Med* 1990;150:2400–2401.

164. Dalyan M, Sherman A, Cardenas DD. Factors associated with contractures in acute spinal cord injury. *Spinal Cord* 1998;36:405–408.

165. Disa JJ, Carlton JM, Goldberg NH. Efficacy of operative cure in pressure sore patients. *Plast Reconstr Surg* 1992;89:272–278.

166. Gibson L. Perceptions of pressure ulcers among young men with a spinal injury. *British Journal of Community Nursing* 2002;7:451–460.

167. Heilporn A. Psychological factors in the causation of pressure sores: case reports. *Paraplegia* 1991;29:137–139.

168. Dumurgier C, Pujol G, Chevalley J, et al. Pressure sore carcinoma: a late but fulminant complication of pressure sores in spinal cord injury patients: case reports. *Paraplegia* 1991;29:390–395.

169. Ratliff CR. Two case studies of Marjolin's ulcers in patients referred for management of chronic pressure ulcers. *Journal of Wound, Ostomy, and Continence Nursing* 2002;29:266–268.

CHAPTER 76

Neurogenic Bladder and Bowel Dysfunction

Todd A. Linsenmeyer, James M. Stone, and Steven A. Steins

Voiding dysfunctions are commonly encountered in patients who are referred for rehabilitation. These voiding problems may result from medications, cognitive changes, physical impairments, or neurologic etiologies. Timely identification of voiding dysfunctions, treatment, and follow-up are important. This is particularly true in the rehabilitation setting, where voiding dysfunctions may cause patient embarrassment, interruption of therapy, and increased morbidity, and ultimately may make the difference between reintegration into the community and being confined to a home or nursing home.

ANATOMY AND PHYSIOLOGY OF THE UPPER AND LOWER URINARY TRACTS

Upper Urinary Tracts

The kidney can be thought of as two parts: the renal parenchyma, which secretes, concentrates, and excretes urine, and the collecting system, which drains urine from multiple renal calyces into a renal pelvis. The renal pelvis then narrows to become the ureter; this is known as the ureteropelvic junction (1).

The ureter is approximately 30 cm in length in the adult. It has three areas of physiologic narrowing that take on clinical significance with respect to possible obstruction from stones. These areas are the ureteropelvic junction, the crossing over of the iliac artery, and the ureterovesical junction (2,3).

The ureterovesical junction is the place where the ureteral orifice opens up into the bladder. Its function is to allow urine to flow into the bladder but prevent reflux into the ureter. This can be accomplished because the ureters traverse obliquely between the muscular and submucosal layers of the bladder wall for a distance of 1 to 2 cm before opening into the bladder (Fig. 76-1). Any increase in intravesical pressure simultaneously compresses the submucosal ureter and effectively creates a one-way valve (4). Presence of ureteral muscle in the submucosal segment also has been shown to be important in preventing reflux (5).

Normal Urine Transport from the Kidneys to the Bladder

Urine transport is the result of both passive and active forces. Passive forces are created by the filtration pressure of the kidneys. The normal proximal tubular pressure is 14 mm Hg, and the renal pelvis pressure is 6.5 mm Hg, which slightly exceeds resting ureteral and bladder pressures. Active forces are the result of peristalsis of the calyces, renal pelvis, and ureter. Peristalsis begins with the electrical activity of pacemaker cells at the proximal portion of the urinary collecting tract (6).

For the ureter to propel the bolus of urine efficiently, the contraction wave must completely coapt the ureteral walls (7). Ureteral dilation for any reason results in inefficient propulsion of the urine bolus, and this can delay drainage proximal to that point. This can result in further dilation and, over time, lead to hydronephrosis.

Lower Urinary Tracts

Anatomically, the bladder is divided into the detrusor and the trigone. The detrusor is composed of smooth muscle bundles that freely crisscross and interlace with each other. Near the bladder neck, the muscle fibers assume three distinct layers. The circular arrangement of the smooth muscles at the bladder neck allows them to act as a functional sphincter. The trigone is located at the inferior base of the bladder. It extends from the ureteral orifices to the bladder neck. The deep trigone is continuous with the detrusor smooth muscle; the superficial trigone is an extension of the ureteral musculature (see Fig. 76-1) (4).

There is no clear demarcation of the musculature of the bladder neck and the beginning of the urethra in the man or woman. In the woman, the urethra contains an inner longitudinal and outer semicircular layer of smooth muscle. The circular muscle layer exerts a sphincteric effect along the entire length of the urethra, which is approximately 4 cm long.

In the man, the urethra runs the length of the penis. It begins at the meatus and is surrounded by the spongy tissue of the corpora cavernosus. In addition to the corpora cavernosus, which runs on the underside of the penis, the penis is made up of two corpora cavernosa that contain the spongy erectile tissue. The urethra is divided into the posterior or prostatic urethra, extending from the bladder neck to the urogenital diaphragm, and the anterior urethra, which extends to the meatus. The junction between the anterior and posterior urethra is known as the membranous urethra.

Urinary Urethral Sphincters

Traditionally the urethra has been thought to have two distinct sphincters, the internal and the external or rhabdosphincter. The internal sphincter is not a true anatomic sphincter. Instead, in both men and women, the term refers to the junction of the

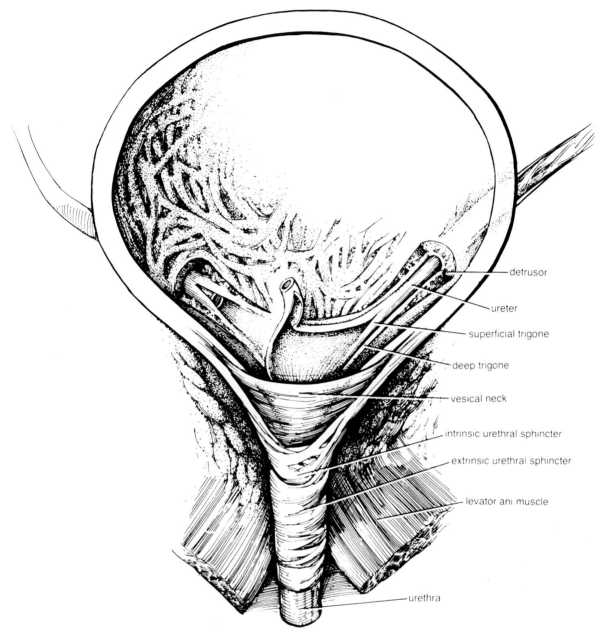

Figure 76-1. Anatomy of the bladder and related structures in a woman. Note how the ureter tunnels for a distance through the bladder wall, helping to prevent vesicoureteral reflux. Also note that there is not a clear demarcation between the bladder neck and sphincter mechanism. (From Hinman F Jr. Bladder repair. In: Hinman F Jr., ed. *Urological surgery.* Philadelphia: WB Saunders, 1989:433.)

bladder neck and proximal urethra, formed from the circular arrangement of connective tissue and smooth muscle fibers that extend from the bladder. This area is considered a functional sphincter because there is a progressive increase in tone with bladder filling so that the urethral pressure is greater than the intravesical pressure. These smooth muscle fibers also extend submucosally down the urethra and lie above the external rhabdosphincter (8).

In the man, the external or urethral rhabdosphincter often is diagrammatically illustrated as a thin circular band of striated muscle forming a diaphragm just distal to the prostatic urethra (i.e., membranous urethra). In an anatomic study, however, Myers and associates reconfirmed earlier studies showing that the urethral external striated sphincter does not form a circular band but has fibers that run up to the base of

the bladder (8). The bulk of the fibers are found at the membranous urethra (9). This sphincter is under voluntary control. The striated muscular fibers in both the man and woman are thought to have a significant proportion of slow-twitch fibers with the capacity for steady tonic compression of the urethra. In the woman, striated skeletal muscle fibers circle the upper two-thirds of the urethra (9).

STRUCTURE AND FUNCTION OF THE MALE AND FEMALE CONTINENCE MECHANISM

In the man, the structures responsible for continence at the level of the membranous urethra include the mucosa, longitudinal smooth muscle of the urethra, striated sphincter, and levator ani musculature. Traditionally, the striated sphincter has been considered responsible for maintaining continence. However, experimental paralysis of the striated sphincter and levator ani following surgery for prostate outlet obstruction did not result in incontinence. This demonstrated the important role of the smooth muscle fibroelastic component of the membranous urethra. The increased tone at the bladder outlet (i.e., internal sphincter) also helps maintain continence (10).

In the woman, there are three important factors in maintaining continence:

1. Adequate pelvic floor support from the endopelvic fascia and anterior vagina.
2. Good sphincter function.
3. Maintenance of the intraabdominal position of the proximal urethra.

During an increase in intraabdominal pressure, continence is maintained by the downward-moving pelvic viscera compressing the urethra against the layer of endopelvic fascia and distribution of the increase of intraabdominal pressure to the proximal intraabdominal urethra. The urethral epithelium, which is sensitive to estrogen, is believed to help maintain continence by forming a mucosal seal (9).

NEUROANATOMY OF THE LOWER URINARY TRACT

Urine storage and emptying is a function of interactions among the peripheral parasympathetic, sympathetic, and somatic innervation of the lower urinary tract. Additionally, there is modulation from the central nervous system (CNS).

Bladder Neuroanatomy

EFFERENT SYSTEM
The parasympathetic efferent supply originates from a distinct detrusor nucleus located in the intermediolateral gray matter of the sacral cord at S-2 to S-4. Sacral efferents emerge as preganglionic fibers in the ventral roots and travel through the pelvic nerves to ganglia immediately adjacent to or within the detrusor muscle to provide excitatory input to the bladder. After impulses arrive at the parasympathetic ganglia, they travel through short postganglionics to the smooth muscle cholinergic receptors. These receptors, called cholinergic because the primary postganglionic neurotransmitter is acetylcholine, are distributed through the bladder. Stimulation causes a bladder contraction (11,12).

The sympathetic efferent nerve supply to the bladder and urethra begins in the intermediolateral gray column from T-11 through L-2 and provides inhibitory input to the bladder. Sympathetic impulses travel a relatively short distance to the lumbar sympathetic paravertebral ganglia. From here, the sympathetic impulses travel along long postganglionic nerves in the hypogastric nerves to synapse at α- and β-adrenergic receptors within the bladder and urethra. Variations in this anatomic arrangement do occur; sympathetic ganglia sometimes also are located near the bladder, and sympathetic efferent fibers may travel along the pelvic as well as the hypogastric nerves (Fig. 76-2) (11,12).

Sympathetic stimulation facilitates bladder storage because of the strategic location of the adrenergic receptors. Beta-adrenergic receptors predominate in the superior portion (i.e., body) of the bladder. Stimulation of β-receptors causes smooth muscle relaxation. Alpha receptors have a higher density near the base of the bladder and prostatic urethra; stimulation of these receptors causes smooth muscle contractions and therefore increases the outlet resistance of the bladder and prostatic urethra (Fig. 76-3) (11–13).

After spinal cord injury (SCI), several changes occur to the bladder receptors that alter bladder function. There is evidence that when smooth muscle is denervated, its sensitivity to a given amount of neurotransmitter increases (i.e., denervation supersensitivity). Therefore, smaller doses of various pharmacologic agents would be expected to have a much more pronounced effect in those with SCI as compared with those with nonneurogenic bladders (14).

A change in receptor location and density may also occur. Norlen and colleagues found that after complete denervation there was a change from a β-receptor predominance to an α-receptor predominance (15). Because α-receptors cause contraction of smooth muscle, a change in receptors may be one reason for some individuals to have poor compliance of the bladder after SCI.

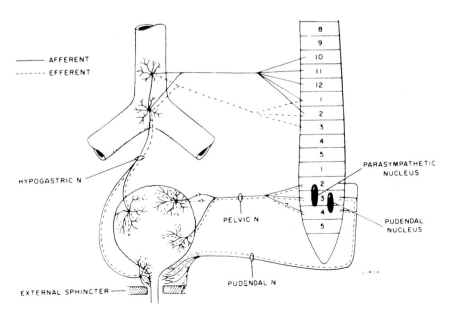

AFFERENT
EFFERENT

8
9
10
11
12
1
2
3
4
5
1
2
3
4
5

HYPOGASTRIC N

PARASYMPATHETIC NUCLEUS

PELVIC N

PUDENDAL NUCLEUS

PUDENDAL N

EXTERNAL SPHINCTER

Figure 76-2. Peripheral innervation of the bladder and urethra. Sympathetic stimulation responsible for storage travels through the hypogastric plexus. Parasympathetic stimulation causing bladder contractions travels through the pelvic nerve. (From Blaivas JG. Management of bladder dysfunction in multiple sclerosis. *Neurology* 1980;30:73.)

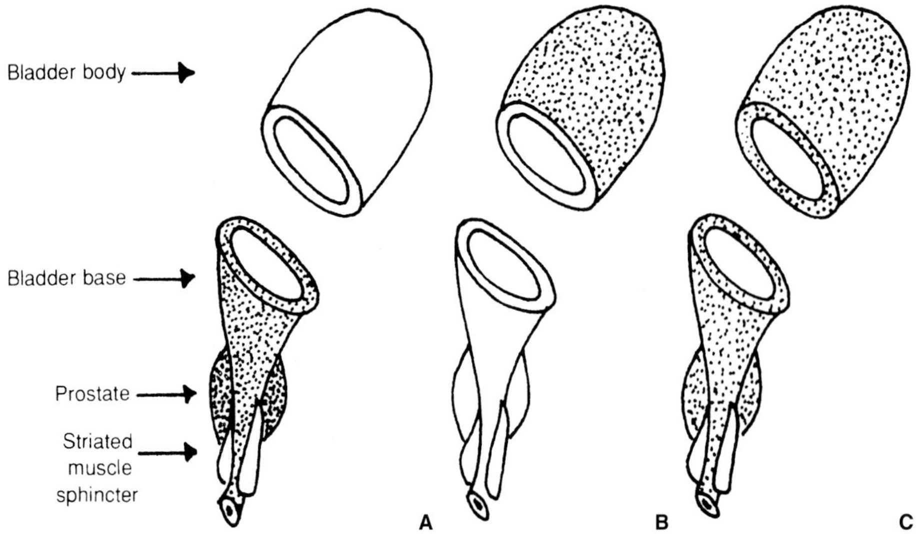

Figure 76-3. Location of bladder receptors. Bladder storage is maintained by simultaneous sympathetic alpha-adrenergic receptor (contraction) **(A)** and beta-adrenergic receptor (relaxation) stimulation **(B)**. Bladder emptying occurs with parasympathetic cholinergic receptor stimulation **(C)**.

Animal studies have revealed that, although the previously described long postganglionic neurons exist, there are ganglia close to the bladder and urethra in which there are both cholinergic and adrenergic fibers. This has been termed the *urogenital short neuron system*. These ganglia are composed of three cell types, adrenergic neurons, cholinergic neurons, and small intensely fluorescent cells, which are believed to be responsible for this interganglionic modulation of the adrenergic and cholinergic neurons. Further work is needed to define this system in humans (16).

AFFERENT SYSTEM

The bladder afferent system transmits the mechanoreceptive input that is essential for voiding. The most important afferents that stimulate voiding are those that pass to the sacral cord via the pelvic nerves. These afferents include two types of afferents, small myelinated A-delta and unmyelinated (C) fibers.

The small myelinated A-delta fibers respond in a graded fashion to bladder distention and are needed for normal voiding. The unmyelinated (C) fibers have been termed *silent C-fibers* because they do not respond to bladder distention and therefore are not essential for normal voiding. However, these silent C-fibers do exhibit spontaneous firing when they are activated by chemical or cold temperature irritation at the bladder wall. Additionally, the unmyelinated (C) fibers (rather than A-delta afferents) have been found to "wake up" and respond to distention and play an important role in stimulating uninhibited bladder contractions in following suprasacral SCI.

This role of the unmyelinated (C) fibers has been demonstrated in studies using intravesical administration of capsaicin and resiniferatoxin. Both of these agents are potent C-fiber afferent neurotoxins. In non-SCI animals (with A-delta afferents), there was no blockage of bladder contractions with bladder distention. However, in SCI animals (with "awake" C-fiber afferents), capsaicin completely blocked rhythmic bladder contractions induced with bladder distention (16). While intravesical capsaicin and resiniferatoxin are considered investigational drugs, similar results have been found in human studies in those with suprasacral SCI and multiple sclerosis (17). These findings have important potential therapeutic implications. However, further work is needed to determine the optimal dosage and vehicle for intravesical instillation. (See Management of Voiding Dysfunctions: Therapy for Incontinence Caused by the Bladder: Pharmacologic Treatment Options later in this chapter.)

BLADDER NEUROTRANSMITTERS

It is known that there are more transmitters than acetylcholine and norepinephrine, including nitric oxide, vasoactive intestinal polypeptide, endogenous opioid peptides, and neuropeptide Y. These transmitters may work independently or help modulate the classic neurotransmitters. Nitric oxide and vasoactive intestinal polypeptide have smooth muscle relaxant effects. This helps to explain the concept of atropine resistance. It has been found that a single neurotransmitter-blocking agent such as atropine fails to suppress 100% of the bladder or urethral activity (14,18). This explains why a combination of agents may be more effective than a higher dose of a single agent.

URETHRAL SPHINCTER INNERVATION

The external urethral sphincter classically has been described as having somatic innervation, allowing the sphincter to be closed at will. Somatic efferents originate from a pudendal nucleus of sacral segments from S-1 to S-4. Somatic efferents then travel through the pudendal nerve to the neuromuscular junction of the striated muscle fibers in the external urethral sphincter.

The internal urethral sphincter has been described as being under control of the autonomic system. This area has a large number of sympathetic α-receptors, which cause closure when stimulated. Animal studies have revealed that nitric oxide is an important parasympathetic neurotransmitter mediating relaxation of the urethral smooth muscle (8,18).

The distinction between the internal and external sphincter is becoming less clear. Elbadawi and Schenk reported histochemical evidence of a triple innervation pattern of the external sphincter (i.e., rhabdosphincter) in five mammalian species, with dual sympathetic and parasympathetic autonomic components superimposed on the somatic component (19). Sundin and Dahlstrom demonstrated sprouting and increasing adrenergic terminals after parasympathetic denervation in cats (20). Crowe and associates reported a substantial invasion of adrenergic nerve fibers in smooth and striated muscle in the urethra in SCI patients with lower motor neuron lesions (21).

Influences of the Central Nervous System on the Lower Urinary Tract

Facilitation and inhibition of the autonomic nervous system are under control of the CNS. There are several theories of how this occurs. Denny-Brown and Robertson suggested that micturition was primarily mediated by a sacral micturition reflex (22). According to their theory, descending nervous system pathways modulate this micturition reflex (21). Barrington, Bradley, and de Groat thought that facilitative impulses to the bladder originated from a region of the anterior pons termed "Barrington's center" (23).

De Groat and associates additionally stressed the importance of the sympathetic nervous system in facilitating urine storage (24). Carlsson provided evidence that this pontine mesencephalic area also plays a role in coordinating detrusor and sphincter activity. Stimulation of Barrington's center significantly decreased electromyographic (EMG) activity in the periurethral-striated sphincter while causing a bladder contraction (25).

Transection experiments in cats suggest that the net effect of the cerebral cortex on micturition is inhibitory. This also is true for the basal ganglia and corresponds to clinical findings of detrusor hyperreflexia in those with basal ganglia dysfunction (e.g., Parkinson's disease). The cerebellum is thought to maintain tone in the pelvis floor musculature and influence coordination between periurethral striated muscle relaxation and bladder emptying (15,25).

NORMAL VOIDING PHYSIOLOGY

Micturition should be considered as having two phases: the filling (storage) phase and the emptying (voiding) phase. The filling phase occurs when a person is not trying to void. The emptying phase occurs when a person is attempting to void or told to void.

During filling (filling or storage phase), there should be very little rise in bladder pressure. As filling continues, low intravesical pressure is maintained by a progressive increase in sympathetic stimulation of the β-receptors located in the body of the bladder that cause relaxation, and stimulation of the α-receptors located at the base of the bladder and urethra that cause contraction. Sympathetic stimulation also inhibits excitatory parasympathetic ganglionic transmission, which helps suppress bladder contractions. During the filling phase, there is a progressive increase in urethral sphincter EMG activity (26). Increased urethral sphincter activity also reflexly inhibits bladder contractions. When a bladder is full and has normal compliance, intravesical pressures are between 0 and 6 cm H_2O and should not rise above 15 cm H_2O. Filling continued past the limit of the viscoelastic properties of the bladder results in a steady progressive rise in intravesical pressure (27). This part of the filling curve usually is not seen in a person with normal bladder function, because this much distension would cause significant discomfort and not be tolerated.

When a patient is told to void (voiding or emptying phase), there should be cessation of urethral sphincter EMG activity as well as a drop in urethral sphincter pressure and funneling of the bladder neck. There is no longer reflex inhibition to the sacral micturition center from the sphincter mechanism. This is followed by a detrusor contraction. The urethral sphincter should remain open throughout voiding, and there should be no rises in intraabdominal pressure during voiding. In younger individuals, there should be no postvoid residual, although postvoid residuals may increase with aging.

GERIATIC VOIDING PHYSIOLOGY

The aging process often affects voiding physiology. The kidneys undergo an age-related decrease in glomerular blood flow

and renal blood flow (28). The elderly also experience a loss in concentrating ability and often excrete most of their fluid intake at night, even in the absence of medical conditions such as prostate outlet obstruction, diabetes, remobilization of lower-extremity edema, and use of evening diuretics (29).

Detrusor overactivity has been reported as the most common type of voiding dysfunction in incontinent elderly men and women (29). More recently, this has been called an *overactive bladder*. This may be associated with a central nervous lesion (such as a stroke, head injury, cervical disk disease, etc.) and be called *detrusor hyperreflexia*. Alternatively, it may result from local changes in the bladder and be called *detrusor instability*. A replacement of normal muscle cell junctions by novel "protrusion junction cells" and ultraclose abutments, connecting cells into chains, which facilitates and increases spontaneous smooth muscle activity, has been found in incontinent elderly patients (30). There is often a combination of causes that result in an overactive bladder. Detrusor hyperactivity may coexist with impaired contractility of the bladder wall, resulting in both incontinence and retention. This combination was found to be one of the most common urodynamic findings in the elderly incontinent nursing home population (29). A combined pattern may also occur if there are cognitive/mobility issues and a person begins to void (incontinence) and then stops voiding.

Outlet obstruction by prostatic hypertrophy is the second most common cause of incontinence in men, although most men with outlet obstruction do not have incontinence (29). Outlet obstruction results in a significant increase in collagen, leading to bladder trabeculation. This in turn can cause a decrease in the viscoelastic properties for storage as well as the ability to contract and may be one reason for increasing postvoid residuals and decreasing bladder capacity with aging (31). It should be noted that outlet obstruction in women is rare; however, it may occur from various etiologies, such as urethral stenosis or kinking from a large cystocele or a previous bladder neck suspension. A trabeculated bladder appearance in older women without obstruction usually results from a thinning of the bladder wall with more prominent muscle bundles rather than deposition of collagen (31).

Stress incontinence is the second most common cause of incontinence in elderly women (29). In younger women, stress incontinence frequently results from pelvic laxity; however, in elderly women, it is also caused by a decrease in urethral closure pressure. This decrease in urethral pressure has been attributed to a decrease in estrogen, which causes a loss of muscle bulk and atrophic changes of the urethra and vagina. This, in turn, can cause inflammation and friability of these tissues, decreased periurethral blood flow, further laxity of pelvic structures, and possible urethral prolapse (31).

Detrusor underactivity may also occur with aging. At a cellular level, this has been characterized by widespread degenerative changes of both muscle cells and axons without accompanying regenerative changes (32). Ouslander and associates reported that approximately 25% of elderly patients evaluated had postvoid residuals greater than 100 mL (33). Approximately 10% of geriatric incontinence has been attributed to overflow incontinence (29).

PEDIATRIC VOIDING PHYSIOLOGY

Voiding physiology also changes with age in children. In the newborn, the sacral micturition reflex is primarily responsible for voiding. Because the brain stem is intact, there is coordination of the bladder contraction with sphincter relaxation; how-

TABLE 76-1. Urodynamic and Functional Classification

Incontinence
  Caused by the bladder
    Uninhibited contractions
    Decreased capacity
  Low bladder wall compliance
    Normal (cognitive/mobility issue)
  Caused by the outlet
    Decreased bladder neck pressure
    Decreased external sphincter tone
Retention
  Caused by the bladder
    Detrusor areflexia
    Large capacity/high compliance
    Normal (cognitive/mobility issue)
  Caused by the outlet
    High voiding pressure with low flow rate
    Internal sphincter dyssynergia
    External sphincter dyssynergia
    Overactive sphincter mechanism (i.e., sphincter or
      pseudosphincter dyssynergia)
Retention and Incontinence
  Caused by the bladder
    Uninhibited contractions with underactive detrusor
  Normal (cognitive/mobility issue)

ever, there is little inhibition of the micturition reflex from the cerebral cortex. As the child grows, the voided volume increases, and voiding frequency decreases. By 3 years of age, most children have some voluntary control of voiding. This control usually is complete by the age of 4 years. There are some neurologically intact children, however, for whom complete control of voiding may take 5 or 6 years (34).

CLASSIFICATION OF VOIDING DYSFUNCTION

There are a wide variety of classifications to describe voiding dysfunctions. Ideally, the system should describe the type of neurologic lesion, clinical symptoms, urodynamic data, and treatment options. A single classification focusing on all of these factors does not exist. Current classifications have been based on neurologic lesion (e.g., Bors–Comarr, Bradley), urodynamic findings (e.g., Lapides, Krane–Siroky), functional classification (e.g., Wein), and combination of bladder and urethral function based on urodynamics (e.g., International Continence Society) (35–40).

Table 76-1 shows a combination of Wein's classification and possible urodynamic findings. This classification is helpful at directing treatment because it is based on, then can be directed at the specific urodynamic findings.

VOIDING DYSFUNCTIONS FOUND IN COMMON NEUROLOGIC DISORDERS

Suprapontine Lesions

Any suprapontine lesion may affect voiding. Lesions may result from cerebrovascular disease, hydrocephalus, intracranial neoplasms, traumatic head injury, Parkinson's disease, and multiple sclerosis. It should be noted that multiple sclerosis is unique among the suprapontine lesions because it also affects the white matter of the spinal cord and often has a relapsing and remitting nature. The expected urodynamic finding following a suprapontine lesion is detrusor hyperreflexia without detrusor sphincter dyssynergia. Because of various factors

such as medications, prostate obstruction, and possible normal bladder function but poor cognition, however, the voiding dysfunctions may be very different from expectations. Voiding dysfunction following cerebrovascular accident (CVA), Parkinson's disease, and multiple sclerosis has been studied more extensively than those associated with other suprapontine lesions and is reviewed in the following discussion.

Cerebrovascular Accidents

After a CVA, some patients initially have acute urinary retention. The reason for this detrusor areflexia is unknown. Urinary incontinence, however, is the most common urologic problem following an acute CVA. Various series have reported that 40% to 60% of patients are incontinent 1 week post-CVA (41–43). In the inpatient rehabilitation setting, a 33% incidence of incontinence during the first 3 months post-CVA has been reported (44). It also has been well documented that this problem significantly improves or resolves in the majority of patients. At 1 month, the percentage of incontinent patients dropped to between 29% and 42%. By 6 months to 1 year post-CVA, 14% to 15% of patients still were incontinent, which is similar to the 15% to 30% incidence in the general geriatric population (41–43). Risks for incontinence poststroke include age greater than 75 years, dysphagia, motor weakness, and visual field defects. At 2 years poststroke, incontinent patients versus continent patients had higher case fatality rates (67% versus 20%), higher institutional rates (39% versus 16%), and grater disability (39% versus 5%) (43).

Detrusor hyperreflexia with uninhibited bladder contractions is the most common urodynamic finding following a stroke. It has been reported to occur 70% to 90% of the time (42,45,46). One hypothesis for this finding is the release of the spinal micturition reflexes from the inhibitory higher centers. Symptoms, however, often do not correlate with urodynamic findings. Linsenmeyer and Zorowitz evaluated 33 consecutive incontinent patients who were 1 to 3 months post-CVA. They found that whereas 82% of men had uninhibited contractions, 43% also had urodynamic evidence of outlet obstruction. Six percent of the incontinent group had no bladder contractions, and 12% had normal urodynamic findings (46). Voluntary sphincter contractions (i.e., pseudodyssynergia) to keep from voiding should not be misinterpreted as true detrusor sphincter dyssynergia. In a review of 550 patients, Blaivas reported that patients with CVAs do not develop true detrusor sphincter dyssynergia (47). EMG studies by Siroky and Krane gave similar results (48).

Parkinson's Disease

Symptoms of bladder dysfunction have been reported in 37% to 72% of patients with Parkinson's disease. These symptoms may be frequency or urgency (57%), obstruction (23%), or a combination of the two (20%). Detrusor hyperreflexia with uninhibited bladder contractions has been the most common urodynamic finding (72% to 100%) (49–51). Detrusor hyperreflexia is thought to occur because of loss of the inhibitory input from the basal ganglia on the micturition reflexes; however, detrusor instability also has been associated with benign prostatic obstruction. Detrusor areflexia may result from bladder decompensation through a combination of bladder outlet obstruction and chronic use of anticholinergic and α-adrenergic medications (51).

EMG studies of the external sphincter reveal that patients may have pseudodyssynergia or bradykinesia but not have true detrusor sphincter dyssynergia (49–51). The majority of patients (63% to 75%) have normal sphincter function (49–51).

Multiple Sclerosis

Only 6% of patients with multiple sclerosis first present with urologic symptoms (52). Bemelmans and associates, however, reported that 50% of asymptomatic patients with early multiple sclerosis had urodynamic abnormalities that needed further follow-up, and 50% of these required therapeutic intervention (53). As the disease progresses, urologic symptoms become common, eventually affecting at least 50% of men and 80% of women (54). The type of voiding dysfunction often is difficult to predict because of the diffuse involvement and changing nature of the disease.

Goldstein and colleagues reported that in a series of 86 symptomatic patients, 49% had incontinence, 32% had urgency and frequency, and 19% had obstructive hesitancy and retention. They also documented that patients with similar neurologic findings may have different voiding dysfunctions and that urologic signs and symptoms do not accurately reflect the voiding dysfunction (55). Wheeler and associates found that 55% of patients who were studied had changes in their urodynamic picture. The urodynamic pattern varied from detrusor areflexia to detrusor hyperreflexia and vice versa (56).

Because suprapontine and suprasacral plaques occur most frequently, detrusor hyperreflexia is the most common urodynamic finding; however, as many as 50% of patients have poorly sustained uninhibited bladder contractions with inefficient bladder emptying. Detrusor areflexia is found in approximately 20% of patients with urologic symptoms. This is believed to be a result of sacral plaque involvement (57).

True detrusor sphincter dyssynergia may occur in multiple sclerosis when there is involvement of the suprasacral spinal cord. Approximately 15% to 20% of patients develop detrusor sphincter dyssynergia. Blaivas and Barbalias reported that this was an ominous sign because of the potential for upper-tract damage and development of reflux as a result of the increased intravesical pressures needed to force urine past the dyssynergic sphincter (58). Upper-tract pathologic processes, including pyelonephritis, renal calculi, reflux, and hydronephrosis, have been reported to occur in 10% to 20% of patients with multiple sclerosis (58,59).

Suprasacral Spinal Cord Lesions

Traumatic SCI is the most common suprasacral lesion affecting voiding. Other suprasacral lesions include transverse myelitis, multiple sclerosis, and primary or metastatic spinal cord tumor.

Patients with suprasacral spinal cord lesions would be expected to have detrusor hyperreflexia with detrusor sphincter dyssynergia. However, in cases of partial lesions, occult lesions of the sacral cord, or persistent spinal shock, this is not always the case (60).

Traumatic suprasacral SCI results in an initial period of spinal shock, in which there is hyporeflexia of the somatic system below the level of injury and detrusor areflexia. During this phase, the bladder has no contractions, even with various maneuvers such as water filling, bethanechol supersensitivity testing, or suprapubic tapping. The neurophysiology of spinal shock and its recovery is not known. Recovery of bladder function usually follows recovery of skeletal muscle reflexes. Uninhibited bladder contractions gradually return after 6 to 8 weeks (61).

Clinically, a person with a traumatic suprasacral SCI may begin having episodes of urinary incontinence and various visceral sensations, such as tingling, flushing, increased lower-extremity spasms, or autonomic dysreflexia with the onset of uninhibited contractions. As uninhibited bladder contractions become stronger, the postvoid residuals decrease. Rudy and associates reported that voiding function appears optimal at 12 weeks postinjury (62). However, detrusor hyperreflexia has been reported to have a delayed onset of up to 22 months postinjury. Eventually, all of these patients did develop uninhibited contractions (63). Bors and Comarr considered the bladder "balanced" when postvoid residuals were less than 20% of the total bladder capacity in those with detrusor hyperreflexia (35). Graham reports that 50% to 70% of patients will develop balanced bladders without therapy (64). Unfortunately, high intravesical voiding pressures usually are required for the development of a balanced bladder. These high pressures may cause renal deterioration.

Traditionally, it has been thought that there is decreased activity of the external urethral sphincter during acute spinal shock. However, Downie and Awad noted in dogs that with surgical transection between T-2 and T-8, there was no change in the activity of the periurethral striated musculature despite detrusor areflexia (65). In humans, Nanninga and Meyer found that in 44 patients in spinal shock with suprasacral lesions, all had a positive bulbocavernosus reflex, and 30 of 32 had sphincter activity despite detrusor areflexia within 72 hours of injury (66). Koyanagi and colleagues noted that external sphincter electrical activity was not affected during acute spinal shock but was likely to increase after recovery from spinal shock. This increase was more marked in those with high suprasacral lesions than in those with low suprasacral lesions (67).

Detrusor–external sphincter dyssynergia often occurs following suprasacral lesions. Blaivas and associates noted that it occurred in 96% of patients with suprasacral lesions. They found several different patterns of striated sphincter dyssynergia (68). Rudy and associates proposed that detrusor sphincter dyssynergia is an exaggerated continence reflex. The continence reflex is the normal phenomenon of increasing urethral sphincter activity with bladder filling. They believed that the patterns described by Blaivas and colleagues represented variations of the single continence reflex (62).

In addition to the detrusor external sphincter dyssynergia, internal sphincter dyssynergia also has been reported, often occurring at the same time as detrusor external sphincter dyssynergia.

Sacral Lesions

There are a variety of lesions that may affect the sacral cord or roots. These include spinal trauma, herniated lumbar disk, primary or metastatic tumors, myelodysplasia, arteriovenous malformation, lumbar stenosis, and inflammatory process (e.g., arachnoiditis). In Pavlakis and associates' series, trauma was responsible for conus and cauda equina lesions more than 50% of the time. The next most common cause was L-4/L-5 or L-5/S-1 intervertebral disc protrusion. The incidence of lumbar disc prolapse causing cauda equina syndrome is between 1% and 15% (69). Damage to the sacral cord or roots generally results in a highly compliant acontractile bladder; however, particularly in patients with partial injuries, the areflexia may be accompanied by decreased bladder compliance, resulting in progressive increases in intravesical pressure with filling (70). The exact mechanism by which sacral parasympathetic decentralization of the bladder causes decreased compliance is unknown (70,71).

It has been noted that the external sphincter is not affected to the same extent as the detrusor. This is because the pelvic nerve innervation to the bladder usually arises one segment higher than the pudendal nerve innervation to the sphincter (72). The nuclei also are located in different portions of the sacral cord, with the detrusor nuclei located in the intermediolateral cell column and the pudendal nuclei located in the ventral gray matter. This combination of detrusor areflexia and an intact sphincter helps contribute to bladder over distention and decompensation.

Peripheral Lesions

There are multiple etiologies for peripheral lesions that could affect voiding. The most common lesion is a peripheral neuropathy secondary to diabetes mellitus. Other peripheral neuropathies that have been associated with voiding dysfunction include chronic alcoholism, herpes zoster, Guillain-Barré syndrome, and pelvic surgery (73,74). A sensory neuropathy is the most frequent finding in diabetes. Urodynamic findings, including decreased bladder sensation, chronic bladder over distention, increased postvoid residuals, and possible bladder decompensation, may result from bladder overdistention secondary to decreased sensation of fullness. Andersen and Bradley reported that in their series, mean bladder capacity was 635 mL, with a range of 200 to 1,150 mL (75). An autonomic neuropathy also may be responsible for decreased bladder contractility. Guillain-Barré syndrome and herpes zoster are predominantly motor neuropathies. Transient voiding symptoms, predominantly urinary retention, have been reported to occur in 0% to 40% of patients and are thought to represent involvement of the autonomic sacral parasympathetic nerves. Detrusor hyperreflexia occasionally has been found in those with Guillain-Barré syndrome (76). Voiding dysfunctions resulting from pelvic surgery or pelvic trauma usually involve both motor and sensory innervation of the bladder (75).

COMPREHENSIVE EVALUATION OF VOIDING DYSFUNCTION

Neurourologic History

A thorough patient history is required to identify the neurologic diagnosis, cognitive deficits, and associated medical problems. The urologic history should focus initially on the patient's voiding symptoms. Symptoms related to urinary retention may include a decreased urinary stream, intermittent stream, feeling of the bladder not being empty, or having to strain to void. Symptoms of urinary incontinence may include frequency, urgency, and feeling of wetness. Information can be obtained in those who are poor historians by reviewing the nurses' notes, from family members, and from the patient's intake and output chart. Outpatients should be asked to record their intake and output and incontinent episodes for at least 48 hours. The history should establish whether the onset of the current symptoms is new, has become worse, or has remained unchanged since the neurologic insult. This will allow for more meaningful discussions when patients and family ask about "returning to normal." A preexisting problem such as urinary frequency may cause incontinence from decreased mobility.

Despite the importance of getting a clear understanding of the patient's symptoms, it is important not to initiate treatment based on symptoms. It is well established that symptoms often correlate poorly with the actual voiding problem. Katz and Blaivas, in a prospective study of 425 consecutive patients, found that the clinical assessment based on symptoms did not correlate with the objective urodynamic findings in 45% of patients thought to have storage problems, in 25% believed to have emptying problems, and in 54% of those believed to have storage and emptying problems (77). Ouslander and associates found in the geriatric female population that presenting symptoms were predictive of the urodynamic diagnosis in only 55% of those with pure urge incontinence (78).

Significant past history includes additional medical problems that may contribute to present problems, such as diabetes, previous CVAs, hypertension, and use of diuretics. The past history also needs to focus on surgery that may affect voiding, such as previous transurethral resection of the prostate, surgery for stress incontinence, or pelvic surgery. Questions about past and present bowel and erectile function should be asked. Potentially reversible causes of voiding disorders need to be investigated. A helpful mnemonic coined by Resnick and Yalla to describe the reversible causes of incontinence in the elderly is *DIAPPERS* (79). These same factors also may be responsible for problems with retention. The mnemonic can be broken down as follows:

> Delirium
> Infection
> Atrophic vaginitis, urethritis
> Pharmaceuticals
> Psychological
> Endocrine
> Reduced mobility
> Stool impaction

The physiatric history that has particular significance for voiding dysfunction is hand function, dressing skills, sitting balance, ability to perform transfers, and ability to ambulate. These factors not only play a role in why a person may be incontinent (e.g., not being able to undress, get to the bathroom, or transfer to a commode) but also are important considerations in developing management strategies.

Neurourologic Examination

The neurourologic physical examination should focus on the abdomen, external genitalia, and perineal skin. In performing the rectal examination, it is important to note that it is not the overall size of the prostate but the amount of prostate growing inward that causes obstruction. Therefore, urodynamic study rather than rectal examination is needed to diagnose outflow obstruction objectively.

In the postmenopausal woman, the urethra and vaginal introitus should be examined for atrophic changes suggestive of estrogen deficiency. In women, the examination also should focus on the degree of pelvic support. A determination of masses producing extrinsic compression on the bladder should be made during the vaginal examination.

The mental status portion of the neurourologic examination should, as a minimum, evaluate the patient's level of consciousness, orientation, speech, long- and short-term memory, and comprehension. Voiding disorders may be secondary to or made worse by disorientation, inability to communicate the desire to void, or lack of understanding when the patient is told to void.

The sensory examination should focus on determining the level of injury in those with SCI. Especially important is establishing if the level of injury is above T-6, which would make the patient prone to autonomic dysreflexia. Sacral sensation evaluates the afferent limb (i.e., pudendal nerve) of the sacral micturition center. Loss of pinprick and light touch sensation in the hands and feet is suggestive of a peripheral neuropathy.

The motor examination helps to establish the level of injury and degree of completeness in those with SCI. Hand function should be assessed to determine the ability to undress or possibly perform intermittent catheterization. Upper- and lower-extremity spasticity with sitting, standing, and ambulating need to be evaluated. Anal sphincter tone also should be evaluated. Decreased or absent tone suggests a sacral or peripheral nerve lesion, whereas increased tone suggests a suprasacral lesion. Voluntary contraction of the anal sphincter tests sacral innervation, suprasacral integrity, and the ability to understand commands.

Cutaneous reflexes that are helpful to the neurourologic examination are the cremasteric (L-1 to L-2), bulbocavernosus (S-2 to S-4), and anal reflex (S-2 to S-4). Absence of these cutaneous reflexes suggests pyramidal tract disease or a peripheral lesion. The bulbocavernosus reflex has been reported to be present only 70% to 85% of the time in neurologically intact people (80). A false negative often results from a person being nervous and already having his or her anal sphincter clamped down at the time of the examination. Muscle stretch reflexes also should be evaluated. A sudden increase in spasticity may indicate a urinary tract infection (UTI). In addition, pathologic reflexes (e.g., Babinski reflex) may help localize the neurologic lesion.

UROLOGIC ASSESSMENT OF THE UPPER AND LOWER URINARY TRACT

Indications for Testing

A variety of tests can be performed to evaluate the upper and lower urinary tract. The exact types of tests and follow-up depend on the disease process, the patient's clinical course, and any preexisting urologic problems needing further follow-up.

If the disease process is one that is not known generally to affect the upper tracts, such as a stroke, hip replacement with retention, or peripheral neuropathy, then the evaluation can be directed at the lower urinary tracts. Evaluation of the upper tracts should be undertaken if there is any suggestion of upper-tract involvement ,such as an episode of fever or chills attributed to pyelonephritis or hematuria.

Patients with disease processes that occasionally affect the upper tracts, such as multiple sclerosis, should undergo baseline testing of the upper tracts and then periodic screening. Emphasis otherwise is directed primarily at the lower tract with the use of urine analysis, culture and sensitivity, postvoid residual, and urodynamics. Testing usually is done annually, but may be needed more or less frequently depending on the patient's clinical course.

Spinal-cord-injured patients, particularly those with potential high intravesical voiding pressures, need constant surveillance of the upper tracts as well as lower tracts. Although there is no agreement on exactly which tests and the frequency at which testing should be done, there is agreement that upper- and lower-tract testing is necessary. The American Paraplegia Society has developed recommendations for the urologic evaluations of those with SCI (81).

Institutions often will have SCI patients undergo a yearly evaluation for the first 5 to 10 years, and if their upper tracts are stable, then evaluations every other year. However, there is evidence that bladder function continues to change even after 20 years postinjury, suggesting that yearly evaluations should be considered (82). People with an indwelling suprapubic or Foley catheter, however, often will get yearly cystoscopy to rule out stones and bladder tumors.

Specific Upper- and Lower-Tract Tests

Tests designed to evaluate the upper tracts include an intravenous pyelogram (IVP), renal ultrasound, 24-hour urine creatinine clearance, and quantitative renal scan (83,84). The IVP traditionally has been used to visualize kidneys and ureters but has largely been replaced by ultrasound and renal scan. Reasons for not using IVPs to screen patients include potential allergic reactions, radiation exposure, and patient inconvenience, specifically getting an IVP laxative preparation the night before the test. Because an IVP with tomograms gives good anatomic detail, this test is helpful when there is a concern about possible kidney or ureteral tumors, possible ureteral stones, or equivocal ultrasound or renal scan findings.

The kidney ultrasound is helpful for detecting hydronephrosis and kidney stones (83). The major advantages of ultrasound is that it is noninvasive and does not involve any contrast agents. The major disadvantages of ultrasound are that it is user dependent and does not show renal function. Some institutions use renal ultrasound for initial screening, and many use it as an adjunctive study if there is a possible anatomic abnormality or stone noted on kidney/ureter/bladder scan, IVP, or renal scan. In one study, ultrasound was found to have a 0.96 sensitivity and 0.90 specificity at detecting hydronephrosis. Renal scan had a 0.91 sensitivity and 0.84 sensitivity at detecting hydronephrosis (85).

If further anatomic definition is needed to evaluate for stones or tumors, computerized tomography (CT) should be considered. It has largely replaced IVPs in a number of institutions. In a prospective study of nonenhanced helical CT scans versus IVP, CT correctly identified 36 of 37 ureteral stones with one false positive. CT had a sensitivity 97%, specificity of 96%, and accuracy of 97% at detecting ureteric stones. This was double that of IVP (86). The quantitative renal scan is able to detect hydronephrosis, but its primary purpose is to monitor renal function and drainage. Many institutions use this as the primary modality to evaluate renal function. Attempts should be made to obtain the glomerular filtration rate (GFR) or effective renal plasma flow (ERPF) (84). If the nuclear medicine department does not have the capability to obtain a GFR or ERPF, a renal scan and a 24-hour urine creatinine clearance can be used to follow year-to-year renal function quantitatively. Serum creatinine is not helpful for monitoring yearly kidney function because it may remain normal despite moderate to severe renal deterioration (87).

Tests to evaluate the lower tracts include cystogram, cystoscopy, and urodynamics. Because each of these involves instrumentation, it is best to obtain a urine culture and sensitivity test, and give antibiotics if positive before the testing.

Some indications for cystoscopy in those with voiding disorders include hematuria, recurrent symptomatic UTIs, recurrent asymptomatic bacteriuria with a stone-forming organism (i.e., *Proteus mirabilis*), an episode of genitourinary sepsis, urinary retention or incontinence, pieces of eggshell calculi obtained when irrigating a catheter, and long-term indwelling catheter. Cystoscopy also is indicated when one is removing an indwelling Foley catheter that has been in place 4 to 6 weeks or changing to a different type of management, such as intermittent catheterization or a balanced bladder. Cystoscopy can reveal a pubic hair or eggshell calculus that may be missed on radiography and serve as a nidus for bladder stones. Urodynamics provides objective information on voiding function (Table 76-2).

TABLE 76-2.   Common Tests for Neurourologic Evaluation
Upper Tracts
Intravenous pyelogram
Quantitative renal scan
24-hour urine creatinine clearance
Renal ultrasound
Lower Tracts
Urine culture and sensitivity tests
Cystoscopy
Postvoid residual
Cystogram
Urodynamics

Urodynamics

Urodynamics is defined as the study of normal and abnormal factors in the storage, transport, and emptying of urine from the bladder and urethra by any appropriate method (40). When deciding on an appropriate urodynamic test, one needs to consider whether information is needed about the filling phase, emptying phase, or both phases of micturition.

The following are some of the more common indications for a urodynamics evaluation:

Recurrent UTIs in a patient with neurogenic bladder
Urinary incontinence
Urinary frequency
Large postvoid residuals (i.e., retention)
Deterioration of the upper tracts
Monitoring of voiding pressures
Evaluation and monitoring of pharmacotherapy

The physician's presence is important to help direct the urodynamics study. Typical decisions include how much water to put in the bladder, whether to repeat the study, and whether to have the patient sit or stand to void. Observing the patient during urodynamics also will help in getting an idea of factors that might influence the test, such as patient anxiety or inability to understand when told to void. Blood pressure monitoring is particularly important in SCI patients prone to autonomic dysreflexia. Urodynamics is particularly helpful for detecting autonomic dysreflexia in men with SCI at T-6 and above who reflexly void. Otherwise normal blood pressures are noted to rise during the uninhibited bladder contractions. Moreover, 43% of the men were found to have "silent dysreflexia" during voiding, which would have not been detected without urodynamics (88).

EVALUATION OF BLADDER FILLING (STORAGE PHASE)

The bedside cystometrogram involves filling the bladder with water through a Foley catheter. It is often attached by means of a Y-connector to a manometer, which is used to measure the rise in water pressure. This test can be used to evaluate sensation, stability, and capacity, and as a screening test to determine if an SCI patient has come out of spinal shock. There are several limitations to the bedside cystometrogram, however. It is difficult to determine if small rises in the water column result from intraabdominal pressure (i.e., straining) or a bladder contraction. An iatrogenic bladder contraction can be elicited if the tip of the Foley catheter rubs against the trigone pressure sensors, which can then trigger bladder contractions. Most important, the voiding phase cannot be evaluated.

The carbon dioxide urodynamics apparatus often has an additional channel to measure intraabdominal pressure, making it easier to interpret rises in the intravesical pressure. Although the gas is cleaner and neater to use than water, the major disadvantage is that the voiding phase of micturition cannot be eval-

uated (89). Therefore this test is of little use when evaluating bladder function.

EVALUATION OF BLADDER EMPTYING

One of the easiest screening tests to evaluate bladder emptying is a postvoid residual; however, it should not be used to characterize the specific type of voiding dysfunction. The postvoid residual can be determined with catheterization or bladder ultrasound. A younger person should have no postvoid residual; however, an elderly person with no voiding symptoms may have a postvoid residual or 100 to 150 mL. A normal postvoid residual does not rule out a voiding problem. For example, a postvoid residual may be normal despite significant outflow obstruction (e.g., benign prostate hypertrophy, sphincter–detrusor dyssynergia) as a result of a compensatory increase in the strength of detrusor contractions or of absent bladder contractions in the presence of increasing intraabdominal pressure (e.g., Valsalva maneuver, Crede maneuver). Caution also has to be taken in interpreting a large postvoid residual. It may be abnormal because it was not taken immediately after voiding, because of poor patient understanding, or because of an abnormal voiding situation (e.g., the patient was given a bedpan at 2:00 A.M.).

A multichannel water-fill urodynamic study is the gold standard to evaluate bladder function because it measures both the filling and the emptying phase of micturition. Multichannel refers to the fact that each of the various urodynamics parameters are measured as a separate channel such as detrussor pressure, abdominal pressure, and flow rate. Urodynamic studies also may incorporate urethral pressure recordings, urethral sphincter or anal sphincter EMG, videofluoroscopy, and the use of various pharmacologic agents, such as bethanechol (Fig. 76-4).

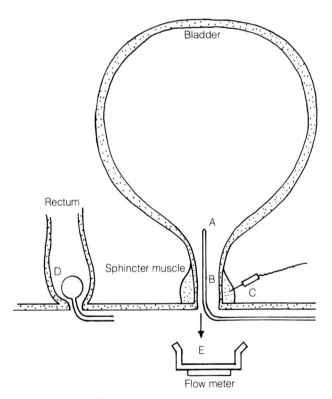

Figure 76-4. Waterfill urodynamics setup. Simultaneous monitoring of various urodynamics parameters are shown. Intravesical pressure minus intraabdominal pressure will produce the detrusor pressure (P_{det}). **A:** Intravesical pressure, P_{ves}. **B:** Urethral sphincter pressure, P_{ur}. **C:** Urethral sphincter electromyography. **D:** Intraabdominal pressure, P_{abd}. **E:** Urine flow rate.

NORMAL WATER-FILL URODYNAMICS STUDY

A water-fill urodynamic study evaluates two distinct phases of bladder function. The first is the filling (storage) phase, during which water is being infused into the bladder. Urodynamic parameters that can be evaluated during this phase include bladder sensation, bladder capacity, bladder wall compliance, and bladder stability (whether or not there are uninhibited contractions). The second portion of the study is the voiding (emptying) phase. The voiding phase is considered to begin when a person is told to void. In those who have neurogenic bladders and reflexly void, the voiding phase is considered to begin when the person has an uninhibited contraction and voiding begins. Urodynamic parameters that can be evaluated during the voiding phase include opening or leak-point pressure (bladder pressure at which voiding begins), maximum voiding pressure, urethral sphincter activity (EMG or actual pressure), flow rate, voided volume, and postvoid residual. In those who have the potential for autonomic dysreflexia, changes in blood pressure before, during, and after voiding can also be evaluated.

With an empty bladder, there should be no sensation of fluid within the bladder. During the filling phase, the first sensation of fullness usually occurs with 100 to 200 mL within the bladder. The sensation of fullness occurs around 300 to 400 mL, and the onset of urgency usually occurs between 400 to 500 mL. There is, however, variability in bladder capacity, which ranges between 400 and 750 mL in adults. There should be little to no rise in the intravesical pressure, which indicates normal bladder wall compliance. Additionally, there should be no involuntary bladder contractions during this part of the study.

During the voiding phase, the detrusor pressures usually are less than 30 cm H_2O in women and between 30 and 50 cm H_2O in men. A normal maximum flow rate is 15 to 20 mL/sec-ond and should not be less than 10 mL/second in any age group. The patient should have at least 150 mL in the bladder because the flow rate depends on the voided volume (44). The flow usually has a bell-shaped curve, progressively increasing to its maximum rate and then decreasing. The urethral sphincter should remain open throughout voiding, and there should be no rises in intraabdominal pressure during voiding. As previously discussed, there should be no postvoid residual, although postvoid residuals increase with age.

A single elevated postvoid residual during urodynamics should be interpreted with caution because the patient may be nervous and voluntarily stop the urine stream. Several catheterized or ultrasound postvoid residual tests should be done to confirm an increased urodynamic postvoid residual (Fig. 76-5). Urodynamics is able to characterize specific types of voiding patterns (Fig. 76-6).

SPECIAL CONSIDERATIONS IN CHILDREN

At one time, urodynamic evaluation was delayed until a child was school aged and definitive corrective surgery was to be

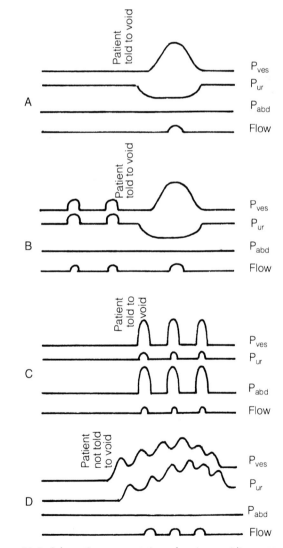

Figure 76-6. Schematic representation of various voiding patterns. **A:** Normal. **B:** Uninhibited contractions occur with filling. The sphincter is attempting to inhibit contractions. Patient has a normal voiding phase. **C:** No bladder contractions. Rises in bladder pressure result from rises in abdominal pressure (i.e., Valsalva voiding). **D:** Uninhibited contractions occur with simultaneous sphincter contractions (i.e., detrusor sphincter dyssynergia). P_{abd}, intraabdominal pressure; P_{ur}, urethral sphincter pressure; P_{ves}, intravesical pressure.

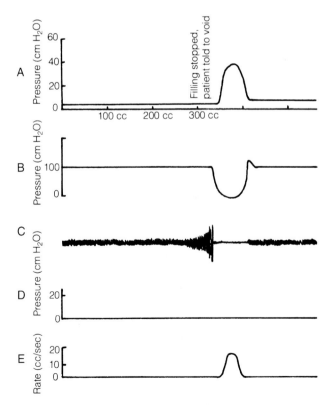

Figure 76-5. Normal urodynamic findings. There is a minimal rise in intravesical pressure during the filling phase. The voiding phase is initiated with quieting of electromyographic activity, and relaxation of the external urethral sphincter is followed by a bladder contraction. **A:** Intravesical pressure (P_{ves}). **B:** Urethral sphincter pressure (P_{ur}). **C:** Urethral sphincter electromyography. **D:** Intraabdominal pressure (P_{abd}). **E:** Urine flow rate.

performed. However, reflux and renal deterioration often occur during the first 3 years of life. McGuire and colleagues reported that there was a high incidence of renal deterioration in patients with urethral leak-point pressures greater than 40 cm H_2O (90). Therefore, it is recommended that all myelodysplastic newborn children be evaluated as soon as possible (91).

It is difficult to obtain high-quality water-fill urodynamic studies on children younger than 4 or 5 years. In younger children, it sometimes is necessary to use sedation or general anesthesia. It is important that children feel comfortable with the physician, nurses, and test. As a general principle, the amount of additional information gained from insertion of EMG needles usually is not enough to warrant the risk of obtaining poor urodynamics results from a crying, fearful child. This is especially true if it is anticipated that the child will come back for follow-up studies.

PHARMACOLOGIC TESTING

Pharmacologic testing sometimes is done in conjunction with this urodynamics test. Lapides and associates popularized the bethanechol supersensitivity test. A 15-cm rise in pressure of subcutaneous bethanechol is considered positive (92). Wheeler and colleagues have pointed out that false-positive tests may be caused by UTIs, psychogenic stress, and azotemia (93). Therefore, when this test is used, it should be interpreted in light of the rest of the neurologic examination.

MANAGEMENT OF VOIDING DYSFUNCTIONS

A useful way to organize management of voiding dysfunctions is to base options on a modification of the Wein classification: incontinence caused by (a) the bladder or (b) the outlet (e.g., bladder neck, sphincter, or prostate) or retention caused by (a) the bladder or (b) the outlet. Management can be categorized as behavioral, pharmacologic, surgical, or supportive. Table 76-3 shows various treatment options. Although each of these modalities is listed separately, it is important to note combinations within the same category (e.g., behavioral—timed voiding, fluid restriction, biofeedback) and separate categories (e.g., behavioral—timed voiding, pharmacologic—anticholinergics). Men undergoing community-based and referral center–based urodynamics have been found to have a variety of urodynamics findings despite having similar symptoms (94).

It is important to characterize the type of voiding dysfunction that a person has with a urodynamics evaluation, particularly when considering pharmacologic and surgical options (see Table 76-3). Empirical pharmacotherapy should be discouraged because there is a risk of potential side effects of drugs that may have no benefit or make the problem worse. In addition to the type of voiding dysfunction, the physician needs to consider the type of disease process (i.e., progressive, stable, or remitting), cognition, mobility, family support, and medical conditions when recommending a bladder-management program.

The following are goals of management in patients with voiding dysfunctions:

Prevent upper-tract complications (e.g., deterioration of renal function, hydronephrosis, renal calculi, pyelonephritis).

Prevent lower-tract complications (e.g., cystitis, bladder stones, vesicoureteral reflux).

Develop a bladder management program that will allow patient to reintegrate most easily back into the community.

TABLE 76-3. Treatment Options for Voiding Disorders

Incontinence Caused by the Bladder
Behavioral: Scheduled (timed) voiding, limited fluid intake, biofeedback
Pharmacologic: oral anticholinergics, antispasmodics, tricyclic antidepressants, DDAVP (vasopressin), intravesical oxybutynin, intravesical c fiber afferent neurotoxins (capsacin, resiniferatoxin),[a] calcium antagonists,[a] prostaglandin inhibitors[a]
Surgical: Augmentation cystoplasty, urinary diversion, interruption of innervation, neurostimulation, botulinum toxin injections into the bladder wall[a]
Supportive: Diapers, external condom catheter, intermittent catheterization, indwelling catheter
Incontinence Caused by the Sphincter
Behavioral: Scheduled voiding, pelvic floor exercises, biofeedback
Pharmacologic: Alpha-adrenergic agonists, estrogen, injectable periurethral bulking agent
Surgical: Artificial sphincter, urethral suspension, neurostimulation[a]
Supportive: Same as with bladder
Retention Caused by the Bladder
Behavioral: Scheduled voiding ($\downarrow$ cognition/mobility), suprapubic tapping (bladder hypocontractility), Valsalva, Credé
Pharmacologic: Cholinergic agonists, intravesical prostaglandin,[a] narcotic antagonists[a]
Surgical: sphincterotomy, neurostimulation (if bladder contraction present)
Supportive: intermittent catheterization, indwelling catheter
Retention Caused by the Sphincter/Outlet
Behavioral: biofeedback, suprapubic tapping, anal stretch/scissoring
Pharmacologic: alpha-adrenergic blockers, baclofen, diazepam, dantrolene
Surgical: sphincterotomy, botulinum toxin injections, pudendal neurectomy, bladder outlet surgery, urethral stents, balloon dilation[a]
Supportive: same as with bladder

[a]Investigational use.

Therapy for Incontinence Caused by the Bladder

BEHAVIORAL TREATMENT OPTIONS

Many patients with incontinence caused by the bladder benefit from a scheduled (timed) voiding regimen. Patients with incontinence resulting from poor cognition, aphasia, or poor mobility but normal bladder function often are helped by being placed on a commode or offered a urinal at set intervals (i.e., timed voiding). Patients who have uninhibited contractions also can have decreased incontinence by voiding by the clock rather than waiting for a sense of fullness. They are taught to void before reaching their full bladder capacity because uninhibited contractions often become more forceful and frequent as the bladder is reaching its full capacity.

Another type of behavioral intervention is bladder training. This is done by progressively increasing the time between voiding by 10 to 15 minutes every 2 to 5 days until a reasonable interval between voidings is obtained (95). Bladder training often is effective for a person who has recovered or is recovering from a neurologic lesion (e.g., head injury, stroke) with improved bladder function but is voiding frequently out of habit or from fear of incontinence based on past experience.

PHARMACOLOGIC TREATMENT OPTIONS

Pharmacologic treatment often is needed in addition to timed voiding in patients with incontinence caused by uninhibited contractions. There are a number of anticholinergic agents whose primary action is to block acetylcholine receptors competitively at the postganglionic autonomic receptor sites. Some agents, such as oxybutynin, also have a localized smooth-muscle antispasmodic effect distal to the cholinergic receptor site and a local anesthetic effect on the bladder wall. It sometimes is helpful to combine an agent such as propantheline, with primarily anticholinergic effects, with one that also has local effects (96). Potential side effects of anticholinergic medications include dry mouth, pupillary dilatation and blurred vision, tachycardia, drowsiness, and constipation from decreased gastrointestinal motility. Newer anticholinergic agents that are more selective to the bladder, such as terodiline and slower-release oxybutynin, have been developed to lessen anticholinergic side effects, particularly dry mouth. It has not been shown whether these agents maintain their effectiveness for an entire 24-hour period. Twenty-four-hour effectiveness is important in those with SCI who have the potential to develop autonomic dysreflexia if their medications "wear off" and they begin to develop uninhibited contractions.

Tricyclic antidepressants sometimes are used alone or in combination with anticholinergic agents. These medications, of which imipramine has been used most extensively, are thought to have a peripheral anticholinergic effect and a central effect. They have been found to suppress uninhibited bladder contractions, increase bladder capacity, and increase urethral resistance (97). There have been several reports of severe autonomic dysreflexia in SCI patients secondary to overdistention of the bladder with urine (98). Therefore, caution should be taken in giving these medications that depend on uninhibited contractions to void (reflex voiders).

Intravesical medications are gaining interest because oral anticholinergic medications have a number of side effects. The major advantage of intravesical medications is that there are minimal to no systemic side effects. This is particularly helpful for those with a neurogenic bowel, because anticholinergic medications frequently cause constipation that could lead to fecal impaction. Anticholinergic medications may also cause a dry mouth, which can be particularly difficult to tolerate for those trying to limit their fluids because of being on intermittent catheterization.

Intravesical lidocaine has been shown to be effective at suppressing uninhibited bladder contractions in those with overactive bladders (99). Although it has a rapid onset of action, it does not have a long duration of action. Therefore this medication is best reserved for use in acute problems. For more long-term suppression of uninhibited bladder contractions, oxybutynin is the anticholinergic medication of choice for intravesical instillation (100). It not only has an anticholinergic effect, but also a topical anesthetic effect. This medication is effective at suppressing uninhibited bladder contractions, but it still has the disadvantage of only being effective for 4–6 hours. We have found 5–10 mg dissolved in 30 cc of normal saline instilled into the bladder four times a day to be effective in most individuals. We will also combine intravesical oxybutynin with oral oxybutynin if they are not able to use intravesical oxybutynin throughout the entire day. One study using this dose noted in the seven men studied that there was improvement in body image and enhanced sexuality because of the significant improvement in incontinence (101). Another investigator examined 32 patients, comparing standard dosages of intravesical Ditropan (0.3 mg/kg body weight per day) with increasing dosages in steps of 0.2 mg/kg body weight up to 0.9 mg/kg body weight per day. Twenty-one of 32 (66%) patients became continent with the standard dose. Seven of the 11 failures at the lower dose became continent with a median dose of 0.7 mg/kg body weight for an overall success rate of 28 of 32 (87%). Four of the 11 (12.5%) had no improvement, and 2 of the 11 patients

had side effects with a dosage of 0.9 mg/kg body weight per day (102).

The fact that two patients had side effects at high doses suggests that there is some systemic absorption of intravesical Ditropan. There is no commercial preparation for intravesical oxybutynin instillation. Therefore, a person has to dissolve the medication in sterile saline and instill it at 4- to 6-hour intervals. A large number of individuals abandon this because it is so labor intensive. Intravesical instillations may, however, assume a more important role of helping to control uninhibited contractions with the development of longer-acting agents. Of particular interest is afferent C-fiber neurotoxins. The prototype medication is capsaicin, which is effective at suppressing uninhibited contractions for several months at a time. In a double-blind placebo-controlled study in 20 patient with spinal cord lesions, bladder capacity increased from 169±68 cc to 299±96 cc, and maximum detrusor pressure decreased from 77±24 to 53±27 when given capsaicin (103).

Unfortunately, capsaicin frequently causes discomfort or suprapubic pain, urgency, hematuria, and autonomic dysreflexia, which can last to up to 2 weeks postinstillation.

A newer afferent C-fiber neurotoxin, resiniferatoxin toxin, is being investigated. It is 1,000 times stronger than capsaicin and is long acting. It is has an extremely rapid onset of action at desensitizing the C-fiber afferent neurons, which causes minimal discomfort when it is instilled. In one study, 14 patients with detrusor hyperreflexia were instilled with 100 mL (or the bladder capacity if lower than that volume) of 50 to 100 nm resiniferatoxin instillation in 10% alcohol in saline. Treatment improved or abolished incontinence in 9 of 12 (75%) patients. Mean cystometric capacity increased from 182 cc to 330 cc. Maximal detrusor pressure was not modified by treatment. The effects were long lasting, up to 12 months in 7 patients (104). Other studies to date also appear very promising (17, 105).

A more recent study showed resiniferatoxin to be superior to capsaicin at improving bladder capacity and the uninhibited detrusor contraction threshold, as well as not having the inflammatory side effects of capsaicin (106). It is our understanding that Food and Drug Administration (FDA) multicenter trials evaluating resiniferatoxin in the United States have been stopped due to funding issues.

Desmopressin acetate has been found to decrease the number of episodes of nocturia in patients with multiple sclerosis. However, further studies are needed to determine its usefulness in the elderly because of the high prevalence of contraindications such as renal insufficiency, heart failure, and risks of inducing hyponatremia and fluid retention (29). Potential side effects and contraindications must be weighed against potential benefits when using any pharmacologic agents for treatment of incontinence caused by the bladder (96,97).

SURGICAL TREATMENT OPTIONS

Bladder Augmentation

Surgical treatment is sometimes needed to improve bladder capacity in adult patients who are incontinent and want to perform intermittent catheterization. The indications for surgical intervention include inability to tolerate or not wanting to take pharmacologic agents, severe detrusor hyperreflexia or poor bladder wall compliance, recurrent UTIs, autonomic dysreflexia, or continued upper-tract deterioration despite aggressive pharmacotherapy and other types of management.

Bladder augmentation is a surgical technique that is frequently used to create a large bladder capacity with low intravesical pressures. Because this is a surgical procedure, other alternatives, such as pharmacologic treatment, should first be tried.

An extensive preoperative evaluation is important. The history should include questions about any gastrointestinal problems. Urodynamics should be done to evaluate bladder and sphincter function. Various treatments may be needed to treat the sphincter if there is a low leak point pressure. Laboratory work should include liver and renal function. To help reduce the risk of significant acidosis and metabolic abnormalities, bladder augmentation is best reserved for those with serum creatinine less than 2.0 mg/dL. A cystogram should be done to evaluate for vesicoureteral reflux. Ureteral reimplantation may be considered if there is significant reflux. Upper-tract evaluation is also important, both to rule out any problems and also to serve as a baseline for follow up postaugmentation (107).

There are a number of different techniques of bladder augmentation in which different segments of bowel can be used. The most common type of bladder augmentation is the clam cystoplasty. This procedure involves isolating a piece of intestine, being careful to keep it attached to its mesentery, detubularizing it, and sewing it onto the bladder, which is first partially bivalved. Various bowel segments can be used and depend on the surgeons preference.

There are predictable metabolic abnormalities depending on the segment being used. The stomach mucosa has secretory epithelium with little resorptive function. Gastric mucosa secretes hydrochloric acid in conjunction with systemic bicarbonate release. Therefore, hypochloremic metabolic alkalosis can result if the stomach is being used, particularly if there is poor renal function. However, the stomach has the least absorptive properties and is best if one is concerned about metabolic acidosis from reabsorption of urinary solutes through the bowel wall. However, this is technically more difficult than an intestinal segment closer to the bladder.

The jejunal mucosa is different from the ileum and large intestine in that it secretes sodium and chloride and may result in hyponatremia, hypochloremia, and hyperkalemia. This segment is most likely to result in metabolic abnormalities and rarely used in diversions. The ileum and colon have similar transport mechanisms. Ammonia and chloride are reabsorbed. This can lead to hyperchloremic metabolic acidosis.

The most frequent changes that occur after this are an increase in mucus noted in the urine, possible metabolic changes, abnormal drug absorption (especially those that are absorbed by the gastrointestinal tract and excreted unchanged by the kidneys, such as Dilantin and certain antibiotics), osteomalacia from chronic acidosis, and stones, particularly in those with urea-spitting organisms and hyperchloremic metabolic acidosis. Long-term consequences of bowel attached to bladder are unknown. There have also been case reports of cancer in those with bladder augmentations, ileal conduits, and colon conduits. These have been adenocarcinomas, undifferentiated carcinomas, sarcomas and transitional cell carcinomas (108,114). There have been a few reports of patients who had an augmentation cystoplasty more than 10 years previously developing adenocarcinoma in the bladder (110).

Mast and associates reported a 70% success rate at stopping incontinence (mean length of follow-up 1.5 years), and this was increased to 85% with the addition of an artificial sphincter in those with low sphincter resistance (111).

Complications included recurrent UTI (59%) and stone formation (22%). As a result of complications, however, further surgery was required for 44% of the patients. Another study evaluated clinical outcome and quality of life after enterocystoplasty in 18 patients with neurogenic bladders and 3 with contracted bladders because of radiation cystitis (112). Entero-

cystoplasty was performed using a 40-cm segment of terminal ileum. Mean bladder capacities improved from 165 mL preoperatively to 760 mL posteroperatively. At a mean of 36 months, 90% had acceptable continence rates, and 95% reported improved quality of life (112).

Another method of surgically increasing bladder size without mucus formation and use of a bowel segment is a bladder autoaugmentation. This is also called a also called a detrusor myomectomy. Through an abdominal approach, the bladder muscle is stripped away from the inner mucosal lining. Without this muscle lining, the bladder mucosa gradually stretches to become a large diverticulum, thus increasing bladder capacity. Autoaugmentation has the advantage of not causing metabolic and absorption problems as described previously for bladder augmentation using a bowel segment. However, this procedure is often technically difficult, particularly in those with a neurogenic bladder who frequently have a small, a heavily trabeculated bladder, and it offers only an approximate 25% increase in bladder capacity. The capacity does not immediately increase, but gradually increases over time. One investigator reported on bladder autoaugmentation of 50 men with neurogenic bladders. Bladder capacity increased over a period of 1 to 6 months. One patient had a bladder rupture and two were reported to have "failed" because of psychological reasons (113).

Urinary Diversions

Another method of management is urinary diversion. Although there are many types of diversions, they can be grouped into two types: standard (noncontinent) and continent diversion. Preoperative workup should be the same as that for bladder augmentation.

The most common standard noncontinent diversion is an ileal conduit. Ten to 15 cm of ileum, along with its mesentery, is isolated from the ileum. The isolated segment of ileum is closed off at one end, and the other end is brought out through the abdominal wall and everted as a nipple stoma. The ureters are implanted onto the side of the ureters.

Standard noncontinent diversions are primarily used in those with SCI who need to have the urinary stream diverted from the perineum. Common indications include impaired healing of a decubitus because of urinary incontinence, or a urethral stricture or fistula.

Continent diversions may be used in those who need to have their urinary stream diverted, but are frequently used in those who would like to perform intermittent catheterization but are not able to do this for a variety of reasons, such as a small bladder capacity or severe leg spasticity. Continent diversions are divided into two types. The first are orthotopic diversions, in which the bowel reservoir is anastomosed to the urethra, and the second is a continent catheterizable pouch.

Orthotopic diversions are much like bladder augmentations and used to increase bladder capacity. Because they are attached to the urethra, people can catheterize themselves through their urethra in the same manner that they would if they were catheterizing their bladder. Continent catheterizable pouches have the advantage that the stoma can be placed in a location that makes catheterization easier. For example, the stoma can be created within the umbilicus so that a person does not have to undress to catheterize himself or herself. The most difficult part of the continent diversion is the creation of a continent mechanism. The most commonly used bowel segment for this is the ileocecal valve. The right colon with or without a segment of small bowel to increase volume is used for the pouch, and the terminal ileum is used to create the catheterizable limb (107,108).

Postoperatively patients need to catheterize their pouch frequently to prevent rupture. Because there is an increase in mucus, patients need to be taught how to irrigate their pouch. Irrigations can be decreased over time, but irrigation is recommended at least once a month as there may be malabsorption of bile salts because of the use of the ileal cecal valve. This increase in bile salts in the colon may cause diarrhea. This is best treated with oral administration of cholestyramine (114).

Long-term follow-up of bladder augmentations and urinary diversions includes regular monitoring of the upper tracts and careful monitoring of blood chemistries and renal function. Cystoscopy is used to monitor for stones or tumors (107,108).

Surgical methods also have been designed to interrupt innervation to the bladder. This can be done centrally (e.g., subarachnoid block, cordectomy), peripherally (e.g., anterior or anteroposterior rhizotomy), or perivesically (e.g., extensive mobilization of the bladder) (115–117). Although there usually is a successful short-term outcome, decreased compliance or detrusor hyperreflexia may return. This may result from an increased sensitivity of receptors following decentralization (24). Impotence usually occurs after these procedures.

Neurostimulation is a relatively new area of research. Electrical stimulation has a number of uses in treating those with voiding dysfunction. It has been used both to facilitate storage by decreasing uninhibited bladder contractions and also to improve voiding by helping to trigger uninhibited contractions. Methods to inhibit bladder contractions has had its widest use in able-bodied individuals with overactive bladders. Ohlsson and Frankenberg-Sommar reported an average 49% increase in bladder capacity by stimulation of the pudendal nerve with anal and vaginal electrode plugs (118). Tanago has reported success at selective sacral root stimulation to increase sphincter tone, which in turn suppresses detrusor activity (119).

In those with neurogenic bladders, investigators continue to try to improve voiding through the use of neurostimulation. Techniques include placing electrodes on the bladder itself, the pelvic nerves, conus medullaris, sacral nerves, and the sacral anterior roots. Of these, sacral anterior root stimulation has been most successful.

Brindley and colleagues developed an anterior root stimulator that produces micturition by stimulating the sacral nerve roots (120). The largest experience is with surgically implanted Finetech-Brindley sacral afferent stimulator, in which there have been an estimated 800 implants over 15 years.

Prerequisites for successful neurostimulation include an intact sacral reflex arc and a detrusor capable of contracting. Stimulation of the sacral afferent nerves causes reflex activation of the efferent nerves to the sphincter. However, this reflex accommodates so that fatigue of the sphincter occurs and the pressure generated in the urethra is overcome by the bladder contraction. A posterior rhizotomy is often performed at the same time as the sacral implant to abolish uninhibited bladder contractions, abolish contractions of the sphincter, and improve bladder wall compliance. The disadvantage of the posterior rhizotomy is the loss of reflex erections and reflex ejaculations, loss of perineal sensation, and loss of reflex bladder contractions (121). Van-Kerrebroeck reviewed the worldwide experience with the Finetech-Brindley sacral stimulator. In 184 cases, of which 170 were using the stimulator, 95% had postvoid residuals less than 60 cc. There was no deterioration of the upper tracts. Two-thirds of men reported stimulated erections, but only one-third used these for coitus (122). The FDA recently approved the extradural version of this device. It was developed by NeuroControl Corporation and known as the Vocare Bladder System. Individuals must have a suprasacral injury with an intact sacral reflex arc so that the stimulator can trigger uninhibited bladder contractions.

SUPPORTIVE TREATMENT OPTIONS

Diapers often are helpful either as primary management or as backup to management for timed voiding. Custom-fit diapers are much more cosmetic than in the past. Major drawbacks include expense, patient embarrassment, difficulty getting them on and off, and potential skin breakdowns if they are not changed within 2 to 4 hours after getting wet.

External condom catheters often are a good option for men with detrusor hyperreflexia or normal bladder function with incontinence secondary to mobility or cognitive factors. An advantage over diapers is that the condom catheter needs to be changed only once a day. Major drawbacks include wearing of a leg bag, potential for penile skin breakdown, condom catheter falling off, and slight increase in bladder infections.

Intermittent catheterization, usually combined with anticholinergics, is another effective way to manage patients with detrusor hyperreflexia and incontinence. Guttman and Frankel popularized sterile intermittent catheterization for SCI patients in the 1960s. They reported that in 476 SCI patients monitored over 11 years on sterile intermittent catheterization, only 7.4% developed hydronephrosis, 4.4% had vesicoureteral reflux, 1.7% developed kidney stones, and 0.6% developed bladder stones (123). In the mid-1970s, Lapides and colleagues reported on the effectiveness of intermittent catheterization. They attributed the success of intermittent catheterization to the ease of performing intermittent catheterization compared with sterile technique so that patients were more likely to catheterize themselves and prevent bladder overdistention than with sterile technique (124). Maynard and Glass reported that 80% of patients on intermittent catheterization monitored for 60 months continued on intermittent catheterization, suggesting low morbidity and high patient acceptance (125). Although clean technique works well in the outpatient setting, Anderson reported that there was a high rate of significant bacteriuria despite antibiotic prophylaxis in the hospital setting and suggested that sterile technique may be preferred in the acute spinal cord center (126).

The important principles of intermittent catheterization are to restrict fluids to 2 liters a day and to catheterize frequently enough to keep the bladder from becoming overdistended (<400 mL). Use of prophylactic antibiotics is controversial (125, 126). Relative contraindications to intermittent catheterization are women with significant adductor leg spasticity, patients with history of a urethral false passage, or those with poor hand–eye coordination, poor cognition, or poor motivation.

Because there is no satisfactory external collecting device for women, an indwelling catheter may be needed if diapers cannot be changed regularly and the patient is unable to perform intermittent catheterization. With shorter lengths of stay, patients are often discharged from the hospital while their bladder is still is in spinal shock. Both men and woman with cervical injuries and poor hand function have much more independence as outpatients with an indwelling catheter than depending on others for intermittent catheterization. Indwelling catheters are particularly helpful at preventing bladder distention, which can provoke autonomic dysreflexia.

An indwelling catheter also may be an option for men who are unable to wear a condom catheter or have contraindications to performing intermittent catheterization such as a urethral diverticulum. If an indwelling catheter is going to be used as a long-term bladder management option, some men prefer to switch to a suprapubic catheter so that it is easier to have intercourse. An indwelling catheter is used more often in women than men with suprasacral injuries and poor hand function. This is because there is no satisfactory external collecting device for women.

Once out of spinal shock, an indwelling catheter can irritate the bladder and provoke uninhibited contractions in those with suprasacral injuries. This in turn can cause high intravesical pressure resulting in a functional obstruction at the ureteral orifices that in turn may cause decreased drainage from the upper tracts. Therefore, use of an anticholinergic also should be strongly considered in men and women alike who have an indwelling catheter in place, particularly if there is urodynamic evidence of detrusor hyperreflexia.

Principles of management include an oral fluid intake of at least 2 liters a day, keeping the catheter taped up to the abdomen of men when they are laying down to decrease the risk of a penile scrotal fistula, cleaning the urethral meatus of incrustations with soap and water twice a day, preventing reflux of urine into the bladder by never raising the drainage bag above the level of the bladder, and changing the Foley catheter every 2 to 4 weeks. Before removing an indwelling Foley catheter, we believe it is important to obtain urine culture and sensitivity tests, and to treat the patient with an appropriate antibiotic for several days before and after catheter removal. This is to decrease the risk of bacteremia if the patient is unable to void and gets a distended bladder. If a Foley catheter has been in place for 4 to 6 weeks before switching a patient over to intermittent catheterization, cystoscopy is recommended to remove eggshell calculi and debris that may have collected in the bladder and have the potential of becoming a nidus for large bladder stones. Prophylactic antibiotics are not recommended for a patient with an indwelling catheter because of the risk of developing resistant organisms.

Although there is a lack of prospective studies, risks are generally felt to be higher with an indwelling Foley catheter compared with intermittent catheterization. The most common complications of indwelling catheter include the development of bladder stones; hematuria; bacteremia, especially if the catheter becomes obstructed; meatal erosions; penile scrotal fistulas; and epididymitis. Perhaps the highest risk with any type of indwelling catheter compared with other types of management are bladder stones. A suprapubic catheter has been found to be safer than an indwelling Foley catheter because it decreases the risk of epididymitis, urethral stricture disease, and urethral irritation (127,128). Another study reported a significant increase in febrile UTIs, dysreflexia, and bladder stones, and a 54% incidence of urethral erosions in women with indwelling Foley catheters compared with intermittent catheterization (129). Care in using a small-caliber (16 French) catheter and keeping the leg bag from getting overfilled and pulling down on the catheter will decrease the frequency of urethral erosions.

It has also been noted that the risk of bladder cancer in those with SCI is increased by 15 times. The risk of bladder cancer was noted to be 4.9 times greater in those using indwelling catheters compared with those who were not. One study showed no cancer in those with a Foley in place for less than 10 years. However, the risk increased after that time (130).

Many criticize the use of suprapubic catheters, but one group of investigators evaluated complications in 44 individuals with SCI who had been treated with an indwelling suprapubic catheter. They found no renal deterioration and a low incidence of incontinence, UTI, and calculi (131). Another study retrospectively evaluated 32 patients with SCI with an indwelling catheter and 25 with SCI without a catheter. There was a statistically higher incidence of bladder stones, but no

overall statistically significant difference in upper-tract or lower-tract complications between the two groups. The authors suggested that the decision to manage a person with quadriplegia should not be based on relative risks of complications of renal deterioration. Rather, the decision to avoid an indwelling catheter should reflect patient comfort, convenience, and quality of life (132).

A controlled prospective study would be helpful to confirm their observations. As with any type of bladder management, one needs to monitor carefully for potential problems of the upper and lower urinary tracts.

Reflex Voiding

Another method of management that can be used in men with an intact sacral micturition reflex is reflex (spontaneous) voiding. This type of voiding involves having the person wear a condom catheter attached to a leg bag. The bladder has a spontaneous uninhibited contraction when it reaches a certain bladder volume. However, the volume that "triggers" the uninhibited bladder contraction is different for each person. One advantage to an external condom catheter and a leg bag is that is does not require good hand function. A caregiver can place on the condom catheter in the morning and not have to be change it until the next day. Some assistance is needed, however, because the leg bag is 1,000 cc and should be emptied when it is half full. Similar to an indwelling catheter, another advantage is that there is no limit on fluid intake like there is with those who use intermittent catheterization as their method of bladder management. Major disadvantages are potential penile skin breakdown and having to wear an external condom catheter and leg bag and possibly a slightly increased risk of bladder infections compared with intermittent catheterization.

Because men who reflexly void usually have detrusor sphincter dyssynergia, their upper tracts and lower tracts have to be monitored. Although there is agreement that elevated voiding pressures cause upper-tract problems, there is no consensus as to what voiding pressure will cause this damage (133–135).

A recent study revealed that the most important voiding parameter causing upper-tract stasis in those who reflexly void was the duration of the bladder contraction (136). Until we have a better understanding of what is causing upper-tract and lower-tract problems, and until treatments are not without complications, it is best to treat a person if they are having or are beginning to have problems. Problems may include autonomic dysreflexia, recurrent bladder infections, vesicoureteral reflux, kidney or bladder stones, kidney infection, or deterioration in bladder function (progressively higher postvoid residuals) or renal function (137).

There are a variety of treatment options for those who reflexly void and are having problems. Various methods to improve voiding secondary to outlet obstruction without the presence of detrusor sphincter dyssynergia is discussed later in the chapter.

Suprasacral Incontinence That Is Due to the Sphincter

It would be extremely unusual for a person with a suprasacral injury to have urinary incontinence solely because of the sphincter. It is possible that this may occur if the person's bladder is still in spinal shock and urinary incontinence occurs as a result of overflow from an overdistended bladder. However, if urinary incontinence were found because of the sphincter in the absence of uninhibited bladder contractions, one should suspect a secondary sacral injury. Because detrusor sphincter dyssynergia is common following suprasacral SCI, treatment of the sphincter should not be undertaken because of the risk of making the dyssynergia worse.

Therapy for Incontinence Caused by the Outlet or Sphincter

BEHAVIORAL TREATMENT OPTIONS

Timed voiding sometimes is helpful in patients with mild incontinence who have normal bladder function but an underactive urethral sphincter mechanism. The object is to have the patient void before the bladder reaches full capacity. At full capacity, intravesical pressure is more likely to overcome the urethral pressure, resulting in leakage.

Pelvic floor (i.e., Kegel) exercises also may be tried in neurologically intact patients with mild to moderate stress incontinence caused by the sphincter (138). There is a great variation in the number of sets and repetitions described by various authors, with the total number of exercise contractions varying from eight to 160 per day (139). Exercises sometimes are combined with commercial biofeedback units (140). Patients have to be highly motivated, and effects may not be seen for 4 to 8 weeks.

PHARMACOLOGIC TREATMENT OPTIONS

Alpha-adrenergic agonists may be useful at improving minimal to moderate stress incontinence caused by the sphincter. Wyndaele has reported success at decreasing urinary leakage around the Foley catheter in incomplete SCI women with patulous urethras (98). Ephedrine and phenylpropanolamine are two commonly used agents. Ephedrine causes a release of norepinephrine as well as directly stimulating α- and β-receptors. Phenylpropanolamine is pharmacologically similar to ephedrine but provides less CNS stimulation (141). Recently, phenylpropanolamine has been reported to increase the risk of hemorrhagic stroke (142).

Before these medications are used, it is essential that detrusor hyperreflexia or poor bladder compliance be ruled out with urodynamics; otherwise, increasing the urethral sphincter tone may increase intravesical pressures, which could result in poor drainage from the upper tracts.

A 4- to 6-week course of estrogen supplementation may be helpful in postmenopausal women with atrophy of the urethral epithelium or irritative symptoms from atrophic urethritis (143). Its beneficial effect may result from improving the local mucosal seal effect or increasing sensitivity or improving the number of α-adrenergic receptors (144). The risks of endometrial cancer, thrombosis, or withdrawal bleeding are negligible when estrogen supplementation is used topically for this short duration. Potential side effects and contraindications need to be weighed against potential benefits of using any agents to treat incontinence caused by the sphincter (141).

Periurethral collagen injection therapy has recently received FDA approval for those with intrinsic urethral sphincter deficiency. Although clinical trials have focused primarily on non-SCI individuals, this therapy appears to be a promising method to increase urethral resistance to the flow of urine. Appell reported that 80% of female patients treated by this method were continent after two treatments. The major contraindication in properly selected patients is an allergy to bovine collagen (145). This should also not be used in a person with forceful uninhibited bladder contractions or poor bladder wall compliance, because obstructing the urethra could cause back pressure into the kidneys.

SURGICAL TREATMENT OPTIONS

In patients with a selective injury affecting just the sphincter mechanism, such as postprostatectomy or pelvic fracture, surgical implantation of an artificial urethral sphincter should be strongly considered. Surgery should be delayed at least 6 months to 1 year to make sure there is not going to be a return of sphincter function. Artificial sphincters are used infrequently in the adult SCI population, because they potentially can cause upper-tract damage in those with detrusor hyperreflexia and high intravesical pressure. In addition, there is an increased risk of prosthesis infection or erosion of the cuff in SCI patients because of frequent episodes of bacteriuria. Light and Scott reported that 24% of their SCI patients developed infection requiring removal of the device (146). Artificial sphincters are better tolerated in children with myelodysplasia (147).

For women with stress incontinence caused by the sphincter, or intrinsic sphincter damage, such as from a long-term indwelling catheter, a variety of surgeries have been developed to anatomically improve the urethral support and position. These procedures can be performed transabdominally, transvaginally, and even without surgical incisions. One- to 3-year follow-up success rates have been reported to be 57% to 91% (148). A potential problem is that the operation works too well and causes retention. Patients therefore should be aware of the possibility of needing to perform postoperative intermittent catheterization. Other surgical options for those with intrinsic sphincter damage include surgical closure of the bladder neck followed by urinary diversion with an abdominal stoma that can be catheterized or the insertion of a suprapubic tube.

SUPPORTIVE TREATMENT OPTIONS

Supportive options are similar to those for incontinence caused by the bladder. Specifically, these include diapers, external condom catheters, and indwelling catheters.

Therapy for Retention Caused by the Bladder

BEHAVIORAL TREATMENT OPTIONS

Timed voiding combined with increasing intravesical pressure either manually (i.e., Crede maneuver) or through increased intraabdominal pressure (i.e., Valsalva voiding) may allow bladder emptying. In patients with weak uninhibited bladder contractions, suprapubic bladder tapping may be used to trigger a contraction. The goal for patients who use Crede or Valsalva maneuvers to void should be to become catheter-free. This goal can be reached through an organized program of bladder retraining consisting of fluid restriction and catheterization every 4 to 6 hours to check residual urine volumes. Catheterization is discontinued when the patient is maintaining regular (i.e., every 3 hours) and complete (i.e., < 100 mL residual urine volume) emptying of the bladder (149).

Crede and Valsalva maneuvers may cause exacerbation of hemorrhoids, rectal prolapse, or hernia; they are best reserved for those who are unable to perform intermittent catheterization and have decreased urethral sphincter activity, such as elderly women or SCI men with lower motor lesions and sphincterotomy. Increasing intraabdominal pressure in those with sphincter–detrusor dyssynergia often worsens the dyssynergia (150). Vesicoureteral reflux is a contraindication to this type of voiding.

PHARMACOLOGIC TREATMENT OPTIONS

Bethanechol chloride, which provides relatively selective stimulation of the bladder and bowel and is resistant to rapid hydrolysis by acetylcholinesterase, often is used to augment bladder contractions. A review of the literature shows that bethanechol is most useful in patients with bladder hypocontractility and coordinated sphincter function (151). Light and Scott reported that it failed to induce bladder contractions in SCI patients with detrusor areflexia (152). Sporer and associates found that bethanechol increased external sphincter pressures by 10 to 20 cm H_2O in SCI men (153). Therefore, it should not be used in those with sphincter–detrusor dyssynergia. It also is contraindicated in patients with bladder outlet obstruction. Potential side effects and contraindications must be weighed against potential benefits when pharmacologic agents are used to improve emptying (154).

Two investigational agents to improve bladder emptying are prostaglandins and narcotic antagonists. Intravesical prostaglandin F2a was noted to increase detrusor pressures in SCI patients with suprasacral lesions (155). Narcotic antagonists are thought to block enkephalins, which are believed to inhibit the sacral micturition reflex (156).

SURGICAL TREATMENT OPTIONS

There have been reports of surgically reducing the size of the bladder to decrease the postvoid residual; however, there is no effective way surgically to augment bladder contractions by operating on the bladder itself (157). Sphincterotomy has been reported in SCI men with detrusor areflexia, but this is generally not recommended because there is a high failure rate at decreasing postvoid residuals (158).

Investigators continue to try to improve voiding through the use of neurostimulation. Techniques include placing electrodes on the bladder itself, the pelvic nerves, conus medullaris, sacral nerves, and the sacral anterior roots. The largest experience is with surgically implanted Finetech-Brindley sacral afferent stimulator, in which there have been an estimated 800 implants over 15 years (121,159). Prerequisites for successful neurostimulation include an intact sacral reflex arc and a detrusor capable of contracting. Stimulation of the sacral afferent nerves causes reflex activation of the efferent nerves to the sphincter. However, this reflex accommodates so that fatigue of the sphincter occurs and the pressure generated in the urethra is overcome by the bladder contraction. A posterior rhizotomy is often performed to abolish uninhibited bladder contractions, abolish contractions of the sphincter, and improve bladder-wall compliance. The disadvantage of the posterior rhizotomy is the loss of reflex erections and reflex ejaculations, loss of perineal sensation, and loss of reflex bladder contractions (121). Van Kerrebroeck and colleagues reviewed the worldwide experience with the Finetech-Brindley sacral stimulator. There was no deterioration of the upper tracts. Two-thirds of men reported stimulated erections, however only one-third used these for coitus (122). More recent developments involve research on microstimulation of the spinal cord and a newly proposed closed loop bladder neuroprosthesis (160).

SUPPORTIVE TREATMENT OPTIONS

One of the many important and successful methods for management of failure to empty caused by the bladder is intermittent catheterization. In those unable to tolerate pharmacotherapy and unable to perform intermittent catheterization, an alternative is an indwelling catheter. Principles of management include an oral fluid intake of at least 2 liters a day, keeping the catheter taped up to the abdomen of men when they are lying down to decrease the risk of a penile scrotal fistula, cleaning the urethral meatus of incrustations with soap and water twice a day, preventing reflux of urine into the bladder by never raising the drainage bag above the level of the bladder, and chang-

ing the Foley catheter every 2 to 4 weeks. Before removing an indwelling Foley catheter, we believe it is important to obtain urine culture and sensitivity tests and to treat with an appropriate antibiotic for several days before and after catheter removal. This is to decrease the risk of bacteremia if the patient is unable to void and gets a distended bladder. If a Foley catheter has been in place for 4 to 6 weeks before switching a patient over to intermittent catheterization, cystoscopy is recommended to remove eggshell calculi and debris that may have collected in the bladder and have the potential of becoming a nidus for large bladder stones. Prophylactic antibiotics are not recommended for a patient with an indwelling catheter because of the risk of developing resistant organisms. Complications of indwelling catheter include the development of the following:

Bladder stones
Hematuria
Bacteremia, especially if the catheter becomes obstructed
Meatal erosions
Penile scrotal fistulas
Epididymitis

Therapy for Retention Caused by the Outlet or Sphincter

BEHAVIORAL TREATMENT OPTIONS

Timed voiding and biofeedback methods have not been reported as successful methods of treatment in patients with neurogenic sphincter–detrusor dyssynergia. Biofeedback has been reported to be successful in patients with voluntary pseudo-sphincter–detrusor dyssynergia. These patients, who often are children, voluntarily tighten their sphincters during voiding, resulting in large postvoid residuals and UTIs (161).

In SCI patients with detrusor hyperreflexia and detrusor sphincter dyssynergia, anal stretching or scissoring and suprapubic bladder tapping have been reported as ways temporarily to interrupt the dyssynergia and allow voiding (162).

PHARMACOLOGIC TREATMENT OPTIONS

In those with an intact sacral micturition reflex, reflex voiding into a condom catheter attached to a leg bag is a common method of bladder management in men with SCI. However, upper-tract damage or elevated postvoid residuals can occur secondary to detrusor sphincter dyssynergia. Alpha-adrenergic blocking agents have been shown to be effective at improving bladder emptying in patients with sphincter–detrusor dyssynergia and prostate outlet obstruction (163,164). In those with prostate outlet obstruction, this is because the prostate smooth muscle is mediated by α-adrenergic stimulation. Placebo-controlled studies have shown both a clinical and statistically significant improvement in voiding in subjects taking phenoxybenzamine, prazosin, and more recently, terazosin (165).

Alpha-blocking agents may improve voiding in patients with sphincter dyssynergia secondary to a SCI caused by several factors. After denervation, a supersensitivity of the urethra to α-adrenergic stimulation can occur. In addition, there may be a conversion of the usual β-receptors to α-receptors (24, 26). Scott and Morrow found that phenoxybenzamine worked well at decreasing residual urine volume in patients with suprasacral SCI and autonomic dysreflexia, but had variable effect on those without dysreflexia (166). An added benefit of α-blockers is their ability to blunt autonomic dysreflexia (167). When deciding which α-blocker to use, it is important to know that the manufacturer of phenoxybenzamine has indicated a dose-related incidence of gastrointestinal tumors in rats. There have been no cases of gastrointestinal tumors linked to phenoxybenzamine in humans in more than 30 years of use (168); however, the potential medicolegal issues of long-term use of phenoxybenzamine in young SCI patients should be considered.

Three drugs that have been used for striated external sphincter relaxation are baclofen, diazepam, and dantrolene. In the our experience, these agents are not as effective as α-blocking agents and should not be used as the drugs of choice for external sphincter relaxation. Baclofen functions as an agonist for the inhibitory neurotransmitter gamma-aminobutyric acid (GABA), which blocks excitatory synaptic transmission, resulting in external sphincter relaxation. Diazepam is believed to cause external sphincter relaxation by increasing GABA inhibitory transmission in the spinal cord. Dantrolene acts peripherally by decreasing calcium release from the sarcoplasmic reticulum, thereby inhibiting excitation-contraction of the striated skeletal muscle fibers.

Potential side effects and contraindications must be weighed against potential benefits when using pharmacologic agents to improve emptying (167,169).

SURGICAL TREATMENT OPTIONS

Pudendal block or neurectomy was used in the past in SCI men with sphincter–detrusor dyssynergia (170). This procedure largely has been replaced by sphincterotomy. Pudendal block or neurectomy is being used to relax the sphincter mechanism by some investigators working at perfecting electrical stimulation for voiding (119). A unilateral neurectomy is recommended over a bilateral procedure to help decrease the risk of impotence and fecal incontinence (115).

Transurethral sphincterotomy is a well established treatment for SCI men with sphincter–detrusor dyssynergia. Indications include vesicoureteral reflux, high residuals with severe autonomic dysreflexia or recurrent UTIs, upper-tract changes with sustained high intravesical pressures, and poor compliance or side-effects from medications being used to relax the outlet. Perkash reported a more than 90% success rate at relief of dysreflexic symptoms, decrease in residual urine, decrease in infected urine, and significant radiologic improvement. He stressed the importance of extending the incision to the bladder neck (171).

Longitudinal studies have shown a 25% to 50% sphincterotomy failure rate. This has been attributed to a variety of causes, such as poor patient selection (i.e., those with detrusor areflexia or bladder contractions less than 30 cm H_2O), recurrent detrusor sphincter dyssynergia, failure to recognize the need for a concomitant procedure (such as bladder neck incision or prostate resection), or new onset detrusor hypocontractility (172).

The major concerns of most SCI patients are that the procedure is irreversible, it is a surgical procedure, and they will have to wear a leg bag. The traditional electrocautery method of performing a sphincterotomy has been reported to be at times bloody with hemorrhage requiring blood transfusion varying from 5% to 26%. This risk of bleeding has been largely eliminated with the use of Nd:YAG contact laser sphincterotomy. Perkash reported that in 30 patients undergoing laser sphincterotomy, blood loss was 150 cc in one patient and less than 50 cc in the other 29 patients (173). The major advantages to a sphincterotomy and reflex voiding are that there are no fluid restrictions, the procedure is effective for the previously mentioned problems, and it will decrease attendant care in

those who had previously performed intermittent catheterization (171).

Another method of sphincter dyssynergia treatment is the stainless steel woven mesh stent (e.g., Urolume Endourethral Wallstent, American Medical Systems), which holds the sphincter mechanism open. With an experienced team, this can be done under local anesthesia. Because the sphincter is not cut, the procedure is potentially reversible with removal of the stent. The stent becomes covered by epithelium in 3 to 6 months, preventing calcium encrustations. A multicenter study of 153 men with SCI revealed a significant decrease in voiding pressures and postvoid residual urine volumes up to 2 years. Hydronephrosis resolved in 22 of 28 patients (78.6%). There was no loss or erectile function. Complications included mild postoperative hematuria in 10 patients (7.1%), penile edema in 2 patients, incrustation of the stent in 3 patients, stent removal (usually caused by stent migration) in 10 patients, and subsequent operation for bladder neck obstruction in 13 patients. Long-term follow-up studies are under way. This device has recently been approved by the FDA for the treatment of urethral strictures (174).

Another method under investigation to decrease urethral sphincter pressure is botulism toxin. Dykstra and colleagues reported decreased detrusor dyssynergia in 10 of 11 men with suprasacral SCI with injection of botulism toxin into the sphincter (175).

SUPPORTIVE TREATMENT OPTIONS

Supportive treatment options for the outlet are the same as those for retention caused by the bladder—specifically, intermittent catheterization or indwelling catheters. Occasionally a person has so much sphincter spasticity that it is difficult to pass a catheter. Instillation of lidocaine jelly down the urethra 5 minutes before catheterization, administration of α-adrenergic blockers, or use of a coudé catheter often facilitates catheterization.

Pediatric Considerations

Children with incomplete emptying and sphincter dyssynergia caused by a nonneurogenic learned disorder have been treated successfully with biofeedback. This has involved looking at or listening to their sphincter EMG patterns during voiding. Sugar and Firlit reported that all 10 of their patients aged 6 to 16 years converted to a synergistic voiding pattern within 48 hours of therapy (176).

The same pharmacologic principles discussed under the general management section apply for children. The age of the child and decreased dosages need to be considered.

The same surgical procedures discussed under management can be used in children. In the past, children with vesicoureteral reflux were treated with urinary diversion, but because of long-term complications of urinary diversion and the excellent success of intermittent catheterization and ureteral reimplantation, this rarely if ever is used today. Surgical procedures for children with severe incontinence include an anterior fascial sling around the urethra and artificial urinary sphincter. There have been reports of 90% long-term success rates with the use of the artificial sphincter in children (144). The Kropp procedure, in which a new urethra is formed from a portion of bladder and tunneled submucosally in the trigone, has been described and may be a good alternative to an artificial urinary sphincter (177).

Clean intermittent catheterization has been shown to be effective treatment for children with failure to empty. In those with incontinence caused by the bladder, an anticholinergic medication often is also required (oxybutynin, 1.0 mg/year of age twice daily). Parents often can learn intermittent catheterization in 1 day. It is thought that parents and children adjust to this program if it is started when the child is a newborn. There have been no reported cases of urethral injury, epididymitis, or UTIs requiring hospitalizations caused by this procedure. Children usually can begin performing their own intermittent catheterization at age 5 years (144). A child's bladder capacity can be calculated using the formula: bladder capacity = 2 + (age) (in ounces).

COMPLICATIONS OF VOIDING DYSFUNCTIONS

Urinary Tract Infections

BACTERIURIA

Bacteriuria is a common problem in patients with voiding dysfunctions. Lloyd and associates followed 181 new SCI patients discharged from an acute SCI center initially with sterile urine and on a variety of bladder management programs for 1 year. At 1 year, 66.7% to 100% had at least one episode of bacteriuria, depending on their bladder management program (178). Maynard and Diokno reported on 50 new SCI inpatients on intermittent catheterization and found that 88% had one or more episodes of bacteriuria (i.e., any bacteria present) (179). Elderly patients often compose a large part of the patient population in a rehabilitation hospital. Asymptomatic bacteriuria has been found to be present in 10% to 25% of community-dwelling and 25% to 40% of nursing home patients older than 65 years of age (180). These numbers would be expected to be at least as high, if not higher, in those with a voiding disorder.

Traditionally, a UTI was defined as more than 100,000 organisms in a midstream urine sample (181). The probability increased from 80% to 90% if this was found in two separate specimens. There is increasing controversy, however, as to the true definition of UTI. Studies show that symptomatic patients often have fewer than 100,000 organisms, there is uncertainty about the significance of asymptomatic bacteriuria and the presence or absence of pyuria, and there is the potential impact of other factors, such as high voiding pressures, frequency of voiding, and postvoid residuals. It has been found that 30% of able-bodied women with acute dysuria had less than 10,000 coliforms/mL, and many had less than 200/mL (182,183).

In SCI patients, Rhame and Perkash reported that any specimen with more than 1,000 coliforms/mL was significant (184). Donovan and associates thought that the appearance of any count of the same organism for two consecutive days was significant (185). The National Institute on Disability and Rehabilitation Research UTI consensus conference based the definition of significant bacteria on the method of urine collection and colony count. Significant bacteria did not necessarily mean an infection but, rather, confidence that the bacteria cultured were from the bladder and not contamination. For those on intermittent catheterization, "significant" meant >10^2 colony-forming units (cfu)/mL; for those who did not use catheterization, >10^4 cfu/mL; and for those who used an indwelling catheter, any detectable pathogens (186).

With regard to pyuria, Stamm and colleagues found that 96% of patients with symptomatic infections had > 10 leukocytes/mm³ (183). Deresinski and Perkash reported that 79% of 70 SCI patients with symptoms and bacteriuria also had pyuria; however, 46% of asymptomatic patients also had significant pyuria (187). Anderson and Hsieh-ma also found that gram-negative bacteria caused significant pyuria, but that this

was not true of *Staphylococcus epidermidis* or *Streptococcus faecalis,* even in high numbers (188).

SIGNS AND SYMPTOMS

Signs and symptoms of a UTI involving the lower tract result from tissue invasion of the bladder wall with accompanying inflammation and generation of leukocytes from the bladder mucosal. In general, these may include cloudy urine, dysuria, frequency, urinary incontinence, or hematuria. Unless a person has had acute retention or urologic instrumentation, which can cause a bacteremia, fever is more likely as a result of kidney rather than bladder infections. Because many SCI patients have decreased or no bladder sensation, they may present with less specific signs and symptoms, such as weakness or malaise, increased abdominal or lower-extremity spasticity, new onset of urinary incontinence, occasionally retention from increased sphincter–detrusor dyssynergia, or autonomic dysreflexia in those with a lesion above T-6.

Patients with acute upper-tract involvement may present with any of the above signs and symptoms. They also usually will have fever and chills and an elevated serum white blood cell count. Those with sensation usually report costal vertebral angle tenderness. It should be noted in the elderly that signs and symptoms may be much more subtle and patients may present simply with confusion or lethargy. UTIs also should be considered in the differential diagnosis of new cognitive changes in a head-injured patient.

DEFINITION OF A URINARY TRACT INFECTION

Although there is no agreement on the exact definition of a UTI in a person with a neurogenic bladder, several concepts are important. The first is that bacteria alone in the absence of pyuria and other signs and symptoms should be regarded as bacterial bladder colonization and not a UTI (186). The second is that one has to be very careful that there is not some other cause of a new onset of signs or symptoms if there are no white blood cells in the urine. The third is that because there no single definition, it is important in discussing with patients, families, health-care workers, and research studies what your definition of a UTI is.

Although there are exceptions, we consider a person to have a UTI if the he or she presents with clinically significant bacteriuria; evidence of tissue invasion of the bladder wall, which is exhibited by leukocytes in the urine; and new onset of signs or symptoms.

TREATMENT OF ASYMPTOMATIC URINARY TRACT INFECTION

Guidelines for treatment have been difficult to establish for asymptomatic bacteriuria because of controversy on whether this represents colonization rather than an infection. Ideally, the urine should be sterile; however, the side effects of antibiotics and development of resistant organisms need to be taken into account. Kass and associates followed 225 children on intermittent catheterization for 10 years and reported that in the absence of vesicoureteral reflux, bacteriuria proved innocuous, with only 2.6% of subjects developing fresh renal damage. In high-grade reflux, however, 60% developed pyelonephritis (189).

Lewis and colleagues studied 52 acute SCI patients during their initial hospitalization. Seventy-eight percent of patients had greater than 100,000 organisms, but only 13% had symptoms and required antimicrobial therapy over 6 months. Of interest is that 35% of cultures changed weekly from positive to negative, negative to positive, or one organism to another, necessitating a short course of antibiotics (190).

An accurate characterization of voiding dysfunction—such as voiding pressure, bladder compliance, and postvoid residuals, along with accurate characterization of level and completeness of injury—often is lacking in various studies discussing UTIs in SCI patients. It is hoped that prospective evaluations considering these factors in relation to factors such as bacteriuria, pyuria, upper- and lower-tract anatomy, virulence of organisms, and types of bladder management will allow guidelines to be formulated for the treatment of asymptomatic bacteriuria. There is general agreement that asymptomatic bacteriuria in a patient with an indwelling Foley catheter should not be treated. Attempts should be made to eradicate asymptomatic bacteriuria in those with high-grade reflux, before urologic instrumentation, in hydronephrosis, or in the presence of urea-splitting organisms.

TREATMENT OF SYMPTOMATIC URINARY TRACT INFECTIONS

Once a urine culture has been obtained, empiric oral antibiotic treatment can be started for patients with minimal symptoms while waiting for the culture results. Patients usually do well with a 7-day course of antibiotics. In those with high fevers, dehydration, or autonomic dysreflexia, more aggressive therapy should be instituted. It is our opinion that these patients should be hospitalized, closely monitored, hydrated, and given broad-spectrum antibiotics (e.g., gentamicin and ampicillin) while waiting for the culture results and for defervescence of the fever. It is important to have an indwelling Foley catheter in place during intravenous or oral fluid hydration to keep the bladder decompressed. We believe that it also is beneficial to give an anticholinergic medication while the Foley catheter is in place; this will decrease the intrinsic pressure within the detrusor, allowing relaxation of the ureterovesical junction and improving drainage of the kidneys. Tempkin and associates showed on renal scans that there was improved drainage of the upper tracts in SCI patients given anticholinergics (191). Patients with significant fever should be considered to have upper-tract involvement (i.e., pyelonephritis) and therefore be continued on 2 to 3 weeks of oral antibiotics after the fever has resolved. In addition, these patients should undergo a urologic evaluation for cause of urosepsis. Acutely, this should consist of a plain abdominal radiograph to rule out an obvious stone, followed by a renal ultrasound. If there is a question of a stone, hydronephrosis, or persistent fever, an IVP should be performed. Once the patient has been treated, it is often necessary that he or she undergo a cystogram to evaluate for reflux, a cystoscopy to evaluate the bladder outlet and bladder, and urodynamics to evaluate voiding function.

COMPLICATIONS OF URINARY TRACT INFECTIONS

In addition to acute lower UTIs (i.e., cystitis) and acute upper UTIs (i.e., pyelonephritis), the physician should be aware of other potential problems. Those from lower UTIs include epididymitis, prostatic or scrotal abscess, sepsis, or an ascending infection to the upper tracts. Complications that may occur from upper-tract infections include chronic pyelonephritis, renal scarring, progressive renal deterioration, renal calculi if there is a urea-splitting organism such as proteus, papillary necrosis, renal or retroperitoneal abscess, or bacteremia and sepsis.

ROLE OF PROPHYLACTIC ANTIBIOTICS

There is controversy over the role of prophylactic antibiotics (126,179,192). Anderson reported a statistically significant difference in bacteriuria in SCI inpatients on a combination of oral nitrofurantoin and neomycin/polymyxin B solution compared with controls (126). Merritt and colleagues reported a statistically significant decrease in bacteriuria with methenamine salt or co-trimoxazole compared with controls at 3 to 9 months but not at greater than 15 months (193). Maynard and Diokno reported that antibiotic prophylaxis significantly reduces the probability of a laboratory infection but not the probability of a clinical infection (179). Kuhlemeier and associates evaluated vitamin C and a number of antimicrobial agents as prophylactic agents and found no beneficial effect in SCI patients compared with controls (192). These studies seem to show that prophylactic agents do not have a long-term effect in decreasing bacteriuria compared with controls. The role of prophylactic antibiotics in patients with recurrent clinical infections, anatomic abnormalities such as vesicoureteral reflux, or hydronephrosis is not known. Prophylactic antibiotics should be considered before urologic testing requiring instrumentation, particularly in those with bacteriuria.

Bladder Stones

Bladder calculi are the second most common cause of morbidity (following UTIs) in those with SCI. The reason for this is the common use of indwelling catheters following SCI and the close association of bladder stones and indwelling catheters. In small series, bladder stones have been reported to occur in 5% of those on intermittent catheterization and 22% of those with an indwelling urinary catheter (194). In a large series of 3,670 study participants, 46% of those with an indwelling catheter, versus 10% in the nonindwelling catheter group, developed bladder stones over time (130).

The 1995 National Spinal Cord Injury database found that in women, indwelling catheters are the second most common type of management at discharge (35%) and most common type of management in those at 5 and 10 years out from injury (46.5% and 55.1%, respectively). In men at discharge, indwelling catheters were the third most common type of bladder management (20.5%) and second most common type of management at 5 and 10 years out from injury (27.1% and 36.4%, respectively) (195).

The majority of bladder stones are composed of struvite caused by a urease-producing organism. These organisms lay down a biofilm on the surface of the catheter that then forms into stones. Complications from indwelling catheters include recurrent UTIs, hematuria, and blockage of an indwelling catheter with potential life-threatening autonomic dysreflexia. Prevention of stones is best accomplished by catheter changes on a monthly basis and treatment of stone-forming organisms such as proteus. In those with frequent recurrent bladder stones, daily instillations of Renacidin (3 cc left in the bladder for 5–10 minutes, two to three times a day) may be tried. Weekly catheter changes have also been found to reduce significantly bladder stones in some people (196).

The role of bladder irrigations and high fluid intake at preventing bladder stones is not known. The standard treatment of bladder stones involves cystoscopy and the breaking up and removal of the stones under direct visualization.

Bladder Cancer

As noted in the previous sections on indwelling catheters and bladder augmentations, patients with SCI have been found to have a higher risk for bladder cancer than their able-bodied counterparts (130). These cancers seem to occur after a person has been injured for more than 10 years. Possible causes include chronic irritation from UTIs, stasis of urine, and bladder stones or exposure of the bowel mucosal to urine following a bladder augmentation or urinary diversion. Those with SCI usually get either transitional cell carcinoma (most common in able-bodied individuals) or much more rare squamous cell cancer. Squamous cell carcinoma was more common in patients with SCI and indwelling catheters than those without chronic catheterization (42% versus 19%) (197). There have been a few reports of adenocarcinoma in the bladder in patients who have had an augmentation cystoplasty for more than 10 years (110). Hematuria was frequently a presenting sign in those with bladder cancer (198).

These studies suggest that an evaluation of hematuria is important particularly in the absence of a UTI, and yearly cystoscopy should be performed in people who have had indwelling catheters for more than 10 years. Before 10 years, many centers perform yearly cystoscopy on those with an indwelling catheter, primarily to rule out bladder stones. The role of other screening methods, such as cell cytology, is under investigation.

Vesicoureteral Reflux

Price and Kottke reported in an 8-year study that vesicoureteral reflux was one of the factors frequently associated with renal deterioration after SCI (199). Fellows and Silver found that there was a definite association of the degree of reflux and renal damage (200). Vesicoureteral reflux in children has been associated with a congenital shortening or absence of the submucosal ureter, absence of ureteral muscle in the submucosal segment, or association with a paraureteral diverticulum of the bladder (201). In people with neurogenic voiding dysfunctions, high intravesical pressures are thought to be a major cause of reflux. Recurrent cystitis and anatomic changes in the oblique course of the intravesical ureter caused by bladder thickening and trabeculation are believed to be other causes of reflux. Renal deterioration from reflux is thought to be secondary to recurrent pyelonephritis, resulting in renal scars as well as back-pressure hydronephrosis.

The mainstay of treatment in those with reflux and voiding dysfunction is to lower intravesical pressures and eradicate infections. Ureteral reimplants are technically difficult to perform in a trabeculated bladder and have not been uniformly successful.

Renal Calculi

Approximately 8% of patients with SCI develop renal calculi (i.e., staghorn calculi or struvite stones) (202). Kuhlemeier and associates found that renal calculi were the single most important cause of renal deterioration (203). Without treatment, a patient with a staghorn calculus has a 50% chance of losing the involved kidney (204). DeVivo and Fine evaluated 25 SCI patients who developed calculi compared with 100 SCI patients who did not have calculi and found that those with calculi were more likely to have neurologically complete quadriplegia, have *Klebsiella* or *Serratia* infections, a history of bladder calculi, and high serum calcium values (202). Patients who present with persistent *Proteus* infections also should be monitored for renal calculi. Urea-splitting organisms form alkaline urine that in turn causes supersaturation and crystallization of magnesium ammonium phosphate.

Previously, a surgical pyelolithotomy or nephrolithotomy was performed to remove these stones (Fig. 76-7). Newer techniques, including percutaneous nephrolithotomy and extracorporeal shock wave lithotripsy, have largely replaced open surgical procedures (205). All of these procedures need to be combined with sterilization of the urinary tract of urea-split-

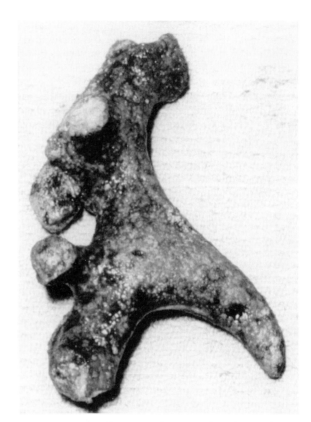

Figure 76-7. Example of a surgically removed staghorn calculus. This calculus completely filled the renal pelvis and calyces and assumed their shape.

ting organisms. DeVivo and Fine reported a 72% recurrence rate within 2 years of the first kidney stone (202). Investigations are under way on the use of acetohydroxamic acid as a prophylactic agent; limitations of this agent are reported side effects and high cost (206).

Hydronephrosis

Ureteral dilation for any reason results in inefficient propulsion of the urine bolus caused by inability of the walls to coapt completely, as well as in decreased intraluminal pressure caused by the increased ureteral diameter. Over time, this may result in further distention of the ureter with eventual hydronephrosis (7,207). There are several causes for ureteral dilation. It can occur transiently from a brisk diuresis effectively overloading the ureters, not allowing enough time for individual boluses to travel down the ureter. Another cause may be a mechanical obstruction, such as a stone or stricture. Those with poor bladder-wall compliance, sphincter–detrusor dyssynergia, or outlet obstruction may develop a functional obstruction caused by high intravesical pressures. The elevated intravesical pressure increases the tension within the bladder wall, which in turn constricts the submucosal ureter as well as increasing the hydrostatic force within the bladder. Ureteral dilation will occur if ureteral peristalsis is unable to overcome these increased pressures (208).

McGuire and colleagues reported that 81% of myelodysplastic children with leak point pressures greater than 40 cm H_2O developed upper urinary tract changes, whereas only 11% with leak point pressures below 40 cm H_2O developed upper-tract changes (91). Hydrostatic forces in the ureter and kidneys also may be increased by vesicoureteral reflux blocking the downward egress of urine (207). Teague and Boyarsky have identified another potential cause of ureteral dilation. They found that *Citrobacter* sp. and *Escherichia coli* from human urine cultures injected into the lumen of dog ureters produced marked suppression of peristalsis and ureteral dilation lasting up to 2 hours (209).

Renal Deterioration

Renal failure previously was the leading cause of death following SCI. The death rate from renal causes was reported in the 1960s at between 37% and 76%. The use of intermittent catheterization and sphincterotomy have markedly reduced death from renal causes. Price and Kottke followed 280 patients for 8 years and reported 78% had good function, 13% mild deterioration, 4% moderate deterioration, and 5% severe deterioration (199). Factors most frequently associated with renal deterioration were vesicoureteral reflux, renal calculi, recurrent pyelonephritis, and recurrent decubitus ulcers. Kuhlemeier and colleagues evaluated 519 SCI patients with renal scans for up to 10 years. They found that factors associated with a statistically significant decreased ERPF were quadriplegia, renal stones, female patients older than 30 years of age, and a history of chills and fever presumably caused by acute UTIs. Renal calculi were the most important cause. Factors not found to be statistically significant included years since injury, presence of severe decubitus, bladder calculi, bacteriuria without reflux, and completeness of injury (203).

Autonomic Dysreflexia

Another potential problem that can occur in those with injuries at thoracic level 6 (T-6) and above from urologic causes is autonomic dysreflexia. Of most concern is a sudden severe elevation in blood pressure that occurs until the cause of the autonomic dysreflexia is removed. Other symptoms may include sweating, flushing, "goose bumps," headache, and bradycardia. "Silent" dysreflexia may also occur, in which there are no symptoms of dysreflexia despite a significant rise in blood pressure (88).

Because autonomic dysreflexia can occur with any noxious stimuli, various urologic problems, such as bladder distention, UTIs, epididymitis, and urologic instrumentation, may provoke its onset. The ejaculation reflex, whether it is induced by vibratory stimulation or electoejaculation, will usually cause autonomic dysreflexia in those with injuries at or above T-6 (210). The onset of uninhibited bladder contractions has been noted on urodynamics studies frequently to cause a rise in the blood pressure (88).

When a person presents with autonomic dysreflexia, one should first sit the person up and loosen any restrictive clothing. It is then important to evaluate for any potential urologic causes, such as a blocked catheter or kinked catheter tubing. If a catheter is blocked and going to be changed, and lidocaine jelly is readily available, consideration should be given to instilling the lidocaine into the urethra before the catheter change. This helps to decrease sensory afferent input that could increase autonomic dysreflexia. A national guideline on the acute management of autonomic dysreflexia for individuals with SCI presenting to health-care facilities has been (210). Lidocaine can also be instilled into the bladder before urologic procedures or during an acute episode of autonomic dysreflexia when a person is felt be having a UTI (99).

THE GASTROINTESTINAL SYSTEM

Traditionally, urinary and gastrointestinal system impairments are grouped together for discussion because of similarities in anatomic location, function, and neurologic innervation. However, there are limits to further extension of this analogy and a few important distinctions. The colon is only the terminal segment of the gastrointestinal tract and is greatly influenced by activity up the alimental pathway. Neurogenic bowel refers primarily to functional changes in the colon and pelvic floor, although a variety of neurologic conditions affect various other gastrointestinal organs as well (211). The sequelae of neurogenic bladder dysfunction can frequently be life-threatening, whereas neurogenic bowel dysfunction is seldom life-threatening but certainly life limiting, affecting quality of life. Neurogenic bowel dysfunction can prevent willful continence, voluntary defecation, and self-management of cleanup; cause dread and fear of incontinence; and constrict full participation in life (212).

SCI is the condition that is most frequently associated with neurogenic bowel dysfunction, although there are many other neurologic conditions contributing to gastrointestinal dysfunction as well. Furthermore, gastrointestinal involvement is not limited to the colon after SCI; all segments are affected (211). Oral hygiene is affected in patients with high tetraplegia. SCI can contribute to dysphagia as a result of local protrusion of osteophytes discs or cervical fixation hardware. Gastric ulcers are more common after SCI and peak during the first few weeks after injury. The prevalence of gallstones after SCI can reach 30%, yet in spite of this high prevalence, acute cholecystitis does not occur with greater frequency or at increased risk for mortality (213,214). Superior mesenteric artery syndrome produces gastric distention, bloating, and vomiting that results from the superior mesenteric artery descending and pinching off the distal duodenum; this is termed the *nutcracker effect*. Nontraumatic pancreatitis occurs infrequently after acute SCI, likely because of sphincter of Oddi spasm, thickening of pancreatic secretions, and vagal dominant innervation (215). Surveillance with stool guaiacs, serum amylase, and calcium levels during the first month after SCI can lead to early identification of complications (211).

Anatomic and Physiological Considerations

COLON

The large intestine serves to desiccate and form fecal matter as it is transported from the ileum to the rectum. There the feces can be willfully evacuated at the right time and place. In addition to its role as a transport and storage organ, the colon functions to absorb water and electrolytes. The colon normally reduces the approximately 1,500 mL of small intestinal content that is introduced into the cecum to about 150 mL per day.

Colonic propulsion of the fecal contents requires motility, a term frequently misused and often misunderstood. Unfortunately, a variety of experimental measurements have been associated with motility and attributed to functional fecal transport (216). Motility and fecal transport are measured differently. For motility, colonic wall contractions can be quantified manometrically (217,218), and electrode placement delivers recordings of the patterns and intensity of smooth muscle activation (219). It is not possible to deduce the movement of material through the colon by the measurement of electrical activity, however. Therefore, unqualified terms such as *increased motility* or *decreased motility* say little about success with fecal transport. Alterations in colonic transport may be caused by events that occur outside of the colon, such as distal obstruction or proximal dilation mediated by the intestinal colic inhibitory reflex. Indices of motility may be abnormal in situations with low transport. Interventions directed solely at correcting the abnormal indices of colonic motility are doomed to failure. The interrelationships of these various inferential measures of motility are yet to be studied and currently of little clinical significance. These local measurements cannot fully account for actual fecal transit through the colon.

The most clinically useful index of overall colonic function is colonic transit time, the amount of time required for contents to pass from the cecum to the outside. Several techniques exist for measuring transit time. A practical economic method uses radiopaque markers that are swallowed and followed through the intestinal tract with serial abdominal radiographs (220,221). Swallowed markers are counted on serial radiographs (220). Although even such objective measures have limitations, as expected, the transit of material through the colon does depend on colonic motility. After SCI, in the absence of regular spontaneous or willful defecation, transit and motility are dependent on regular scheduled bowel care. Rectal distention in itself can reflexively inhibit peristalsis and affect alimentary function as proximal as the stomach, preventing gastric emptying.

ANORECTUM

The anal canal provides the primary mechanism for fecal continence and is the barrier that must be traversed for evacuation to occur. The *internal anal sphincter* (IAS) is the specialized thickening of the circular smooth muscle layer of the rectum that maintains a continuous state of maximal contraction. It is responsible for the majority of resting tone in the anal canal (222).

Normal internal anal canal resting pressures range from 50 to 100 cm H_2O. This resting tone is not altered after SCI (223). The *external anal sphincter* (EAS) is a striated muscle that is continuous with the pelvic floor and is innervated by the pudendal nerves bilaterally. The EAS, along with muscles of the pelvic floor, displays the unusual property of continuous electrical activity in both the waking and sleeping states (224). Presumably, this special property allows the EAS and pelvic floor to maintain continence without conscious will and during sleep. Although the EAS plays a small role in the resting state, contraction of the EAS can double anal canal pressure for short periods of time. External sphincter function is felt to be important during events that are an acute threat to continence, such as coughing, acute rectal contraction, or assuming an upright position.

The puborectalis muscle originates from behind the pubic symphysis and extends posteriorly to loop around the rectum just proximal to the anal canal. The puborectalis tugs the rectum anteriorly and creates an angle between the rectum and anal canal, the *anorectal angle*. This kink in the fecal pathway aids in continence (225,226). Conversely, failure of the puborectalis to relax appropriately, with persistence of an acute anorectal angle, has been associated with inability to defecate (227). The IAS, the EAS, and the puborectalis work together synergistically to maintain continence and are collectively named the *anal sphincter mechanism*.

The mucosa at the proximal end of the rectum and anal canal is rich in sensory receptors. This allows for socially critical judgments about the phases of the matter therein: liquid, solid, and gaseous material. The rectoanal inhibitory or sampling reflex allows a sample of the rectal contents to come into contact with this sensory zone. The *rectoanal inhibitory reflex* consists of a transient relaxation of the IAS stimulated by a rise in rectal pressure. A simultaneous increase in EAS tone, *the guarding reflex*, occurs to preserve continence while sensory receptors of the rectum appraise the contents. The rectoanal inhibitory reflex occurs during sleep and throughout the day, usually at a subconscious level.

Regulation of Gastrointestinal Function

Fortunately, many of the organs, tissues, and cells of the gastrointestinal system operate autonomously. Regulatory influences include the parasympathetic and sympathetic nervous systems, the enteric system within the gut, and endocrine, myogenic, and intraluminal cues. Preliminary knowledge is available but further investigation is required. Rudimentary explanations are offered so that the reader may exploit these systems therapeutically in neurogenic bowel management. The variety of these regulatory influences act in concert and interact in feedback loops. They can be explained from the gut lumen out.

INTRALUMINAL CONTENT

The intraluminal contents can affect gastrointestinal function through alteration of the physical characteristics of stool, bacterial action, and the effects of various substances on mucosal receptors. The physical characteristics of the fecal mass have an important effect on colonic motility and defecation efficiency. The typical Western diet, deficient in fiber, results in small, hard, often scybalous stool that is difficult for the colon to propel and the anorectum to evacuate. The effect of stool consistency on rectal evacuation has been well studied in able-bodied subjects (228,229). Dry, hard stool is not compressible, breaks apart, and contributes to high friction against the colonic wall. These stools produce difficulty with evacuation.

Addition of vegetable fiber to the diet increases stool volume and moisture content, which increases plasticity and decreases transit time (230). With increased dietary fiber, fecal microbial mass also increases (231). Bacterial fermentation of indigestible fiber within the colon generates short-chain fatty acids. These short-chain fatty acids are passively absorbed by colonic mucosa and may be oxidized as an important energy source (232). Bacteria also are important in the metabolism of bile salts. Bile salts stimulate colonic motility and may play a role in the hypermotility of patients with the irritable bowel syndrome (233).

Furthermore, the luminal content also can affect gastrointestinal function by stimulation of specific mucosal receptors. Five types of gastrointestinal sensory receptors are known to exist. These respond to mechanical, chemical, osmotic, thermal, or painful stimuli.

INTRINSIC OR ENTERIC NEURAL REGULATION

The enteric intrinsic nervous system is embedded in the wall of the gut and runs the length of the digestive tube, from pharynx to anus. Meissner's plexus is distributed throughout the submucosa and transmits local sensory and motor signals to Auerbach's plexus, autonomic ganglia, and the spinal cord. This intrinsic nervous system includes Auerbach's plexus (intramuscular myenteric) distributed between the longitudinal and circular muscle layers. The enteric nervous system is organized into three levels:

1. Afferent neurons, which gather sensory information and relay it to an array of interneurons
2. Interneurons, which process information locally, integrate the incoming sensory information, and coordinate local motor and secretory responses
3. Efferent neurons, which exert their influence on target cells, such as secretory, absorptive, or muscle cells

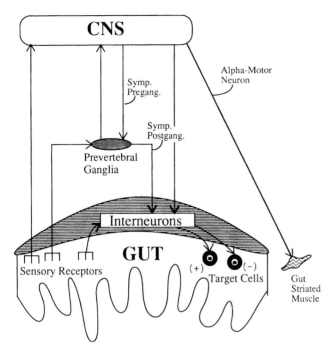

Figure 76-8. General organization of the enteric nervous system. Sensory fibers in the gut send afferents to the central nervous system (CNS) through the vagus nerve (cell bodies in nodose ganglia) or the sympathetic nerves (cell bodies in the dorsal root ganglia); prevertebral ganglia; and interneurons within the gut wall. Input may be processed and efferent fibers sent to effector cells at all three levels. The only efferent neurons that do not involve the enteric nervous system are the alpha-motor neurons that innervate the striated muscle at both ends of the gut (i.e., cricopharyngeus and external anal sphincter).

The enteric nervous system integrates sensory information from the contents and coordinates local and distant secretion and peristalsis. Ablation of all enteric nervous activity by the neurotoxin tetrodotoxin causes the colon to contract, the rectum to undergo tonic and phasic contractions, and the IAS to contract tonically (234). Thus, it appears that the major effect of the enteric nervous system on the lower gastrointestinal tract is to provide an inhibitory influence.

EXTRINSIC OR EXTRAINTESTINAL NEURAL REGULATION
Extrinsic neural influences provide overall coordination of intestinal reflexes as well as integration of the gastrointestinal tract with the whole organism. Sensory receptors in the gut may send afferents directly to the CNS, to prevertebral sympathetic ganglia, or to interneurons within the gut wall. The sensory information may be processed within the CNS, the prevertebral ganglia, or within the enteric nervous system (Fig. 76-8). In fact, the enteric nervous system contains a greater number of neurons than the spinal cord (235). This is no surprise when the complexity and variety of gastrointestinal functions controlled by the enteric nervous system are considered. The important regulatory role of the enteric nervous system also is apparent in the organization of visceral efferents from the CNS. All efferents, except those to striated muscle in the pharynx or EAS (i.e., alpha motor neurons), synapse with enteric interneurons before reaching an effector cell.

The gastrointestinal tract receives both parasympathetic and sympathetic nervous system innervation. The function of the parasympathetic efferents is complex. Separate groups of vagal preganglionic fibers may innervate inhibitory or excitatory neurons in the same organ. Therefore, whole-nerve stimulation may produce excitatory as well as inhibitory effects on

the same organ. For example, transection of the vagus at the level of the lower esophagus (i.e., truncal vagotomy) has been used as treatment for peptic ulcer disease. Gastric acid secretion is diminished to a variable extent, and gastric motility is significantly impaired; however, small bowel and colonic motility are largely unaffected. Injury to the inferior splanchnic nerve (parasympathetic S2–S4) results in impaired defecation and constipation (236). The function of the sympathetic nerves is generally to cause inhibition of motor and secretory activity and contraction of gastrointestinal sphincters. Sympathetic stimulation leads to adynamic ileus and decreased bowel activity. Although surgical sympathectomy has little clinical effect on bowel function in humans, diarrhea has been reported in animal models (237).

The striated muscle of the pharynx and the EAS are innervated by alpha motor neurons directly from the CNS. The cell bodies of the alpha motor neurons to the EAS are located in the anterior horn cells of spinal segments S-2 through S-4. Their axons are carried in the pudendal nerve. Injuries to the pudendal nerves or the sacral cord produce flaccid paralysis of the pelvic floor along with the external sphincter.

As can be inferred from the previous discussion, the regulatory mechanisms for gastrointestinal function are highly interdependent and frequently redundant. Loss of any individual component does not necessarily result in an identifiable syndrome. In fact, the inherent automaticity of the gut often allows it to function quite well in the absence of all extrinsic control. The effects of loss of extrinsic neural control (i.e., neurogenic bowel) are most apparent at the two ends of the gastrointestinal tract, where complex voluntary behaviors occur. The primary function lost with neurogenic bowel is voluntary control over defecation.

GASTROINTESTINAL HORMONES
The gastrointestinal hormones influence activity in three systems throughout the alimentary canal. This influence is communicated by blood-borne chemical messengers (i.e., endocrine action) and secondarily transmitted by locally released messengers that traverse the interstitial space to reach a target cell (i.e., paracrine action). A third chemical messenger system, even more specific in its location of activity, is the neurocrine system. These neuropeptides are active only at the nerve terminals where they are released. The central role of neuropeptides in both neural and endocrine function illustrates the overlap and inseparability of these two systems.

Our understanding of the neuroendocrine potential of the colon has progressed much over the last decade (238). The colon and rectum harbor peptides and amines that come from enterochromaffin cells in rectal crypts and enkephalinergic neurons in the myenteric plexus (238). The colon may be a source of enterogastrone, which is secreted in response to intracolonic nutrients and reduces gastric acid secretion from the stomach. Locally acting neuropeptides, including intestinal peptide, substance P, and GRP/bombesin, stimulate secretion of ions. Conversely, somatostatin, opioid peptide, and neuropeptide stimulate absorption.

Transit and Motility
Studies of colonic transit time in people with SCI generally have shown a prolongation of total colonic transit time that is predominantly caused by slowing through the rectosigmoid segment (239,240). Interpretation of this finding is difficult because transit time studies cannot differentiate slow transit through the rectosigmoid because of altered colonic motility from slow transit because of infrequent or inefficient evacua-

tion of the rectum. In our SCI population, bowel care was performed at a mean interval of approximately 2 days; the interval between bowel movements in a neurologically intact control group was 1 day. Because any movement in the rectosigmoid colon between bowel-care days would not be expected, the difference between SCI and controls may simply be related to the frequency of bowel care and bowel movements. Furthermore, Kellow and associates have demonstrated that distention of the rectum slows intestinal transit in both the fasting and fed states. Inhibition of contraction in one portion of the intestinal tract by distention of another (i.e., intestinointestinal, intestinocolic, and colocolic reflexes) was first reported 50 years ago (241). Interestingly, these reflexes are mediated in the prevertebral ganglia, not the spinal cord, so they likely would be unaffected by SCI (242).

Attempts to describe the effect of SCI on colonic motility by measurement of electrical or pressure events have yielded inconsistent results. Connell and associates, measuring intraluminal pressure waves, concluded that people with injury levels above T-9 had decreased rectosigmoid motor activities, whereas those with lesions below T-9 had increased motor activity (243). However, Aaronson and colleagues found an increase in rectal myoelectric activity in a disparate group of six people with SCI when compared with neurologically intact controls (244). Glick and colleagues found no change in myoelectric activity when nine people with SCI were compared with controls (245). Interpretation of these studies is plagued by many of the previously mentioned methodological problems. The study groups were small and uncontrolled for important variables such as time after injury, age, level and completeness of injury, and presence of gastrointestinal symptoms. Even if a consistent pattern of motility disorder could be found, it could as easily be caused by the inability to evacuate as by a primary motility problem.

Fecal Continence

Fecal continence is achieved with a combination of structures that work together to prevent inadvertent passage of stool. These barriers are removable to allow bowel evacuation to occur. The current state, continence or evacuation, depends on the balance between those forces that favor expulsion of stool and those that resist it (Fig. 76-9). Expulsive forces include intraabdominal pressure, colorectal contraction, elastic forces, and gravity. Resistive forces include the anorectal angle, anal canal tone contributed by the IAS and EAS, and friction. Stool consistency is a pivotal factor that can shift the balance in either direction. Small, hard stool is evacuated less completely and

with more difficulty than soft, bulky stool (228, 229), whereas even subjects with normal continence mechanisms may be incontinent when faced with large volumes of liquid stool as in during an acute diarrheal illness.

CLINICAL EVALUATION

As with any patient, the evaluation begins with a complete history and physical examination. A request for symptoms guides the evaluation. Symptoms typically are vague; clues to their origin may be derived from a careful search for a relationship to exacerbating or remitting factors. The effect of body position, time of day, eating, bowel care, medications, and urinary function should be elicited (246). The presence of associated symptoms, such as autonomic dysreflexia, abdominal wall spasticity, fever, and weight change, should be noted. A gastrointestinal review of symptoms further clarifies function. A careful query of premorbid bowel function should be made, because neurologic lesions may alter the way that preexisting problems are manifest. Recognition of the impact of the symptom on the patient's ability to carry out important life activities is essential; neurogenic bowel dysfunction is notorious for detrimental impact on quality of life (247). Finally, the components of the bowel program should be systematically evaluated. A history of the type of diet–with special emphasis on fluid and fiber intake, use of laxatives, stool softeners, fiber supplements, and medications with anticholinergic properties–should be obtained. The frequency, duration, and technique of bowel care are elicited, as well as problems with stool consistency, lack of stool in the rectum at the time of stimulation, incontinence, and bleeding.

The physical examination is not only an assessment of the colon and pelvic floor but also includes a survey for associated pathology, sensory/motor impairments, and activity limitations that could affect bowel care (211). Abdominal examination allows for motor assessment of the abdominal wall, percussion for tympany, palpation of the colon for impaction, and elicitation of symptoms (246). Pelvic floor innervation and function should be appraised with neurologic and rectal examination. The anocutaneous reflex is recognized with EAS contraction on anal skin contact. The bulbocavernosus reflex is elicited with penile head squeeze or clitoral pressure and the recognition of an increase in anal sphincter tone. Both these reflexes suggest an intact sensory (S3–S4) to motor (S2) reflex arch (212). The rectal examination should assess for sensation, voluntary contraction, puborectalis tone, masses the rectal vault, and stool consistency. The examination is an opportunity for education and explanation of options for various techniques of bowel care.

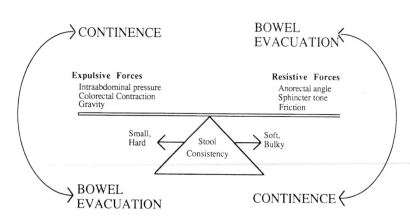

Figure 76-9. Balance of forces favoring continence or bowel evacuation. Physical character of stool is the pivotal variable that can shift the balance in either direction. Small, hard stool shifts the fulcrum to the left, and more force is required to evacuate. Soft, bulky stool causes the fulcrum to shift the opposite way.

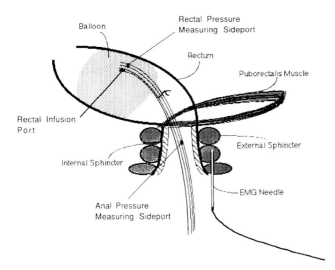

Figure 76-10. Rectodynamics setup. Expulsive forces (e.g., intraabdominal pressure, colorectal contraction, rectal elasticity) are reflected by the pressure in the balloon in the rectum. Resistive forces are measured by the anal sphincter pressure. The contribution of the external sphincter is reflected by the electromyographic activity. Pressures are measured at rest and during stimulation by anal stretch (i.e., digital stimulation); rapid rectal stretch (i.e., rectoanal inhibitory reflex); and continuous infusion of saline into the rectal balloon.

RECTODYNAMICS

To understand the effects of SCI on bowel evacuation, we designed a test to measure the opposing expulsive and resistive forces at work in the anorectum. We call the test *rectodynamics* because of its similarity to urodynamics, the study of bladder emptying (Fig. 76-10). Rectodynamics is performed by placing a triple-lumen catheter through the anus so that one pressure-measuring sideport is in the rectum and another is in the high-pressure zone of the anal canal. The third lumen is used to fill a balloon located in the rectum. A concentric EMG needle is placed in the EAS. Rectal and anal pressures, along with external sphincter EMG, are measured at rest and during stimulation of the anorectum by digital stimulation, the Valsalva maneuver, rapid rectal distention (i.e., air is rapidly injected and removed from rectal balloon to elicit the rectoanal inhibitory reflex), and slow, continuous filling of the rectal balloon with saline.

The typical features of rectodynamic study of an asymptomatic person with upper motor neuron SCI are illustrated in Figure 76-11A. During continuous filling of the rectal balloon, the intermittent rises in rectal pressure (i.e., rectal contractions) are invariably linked with decreases in anal canal pressure. When the rectal threshold pressure is reached (20 to 30 cm H_2O), the external sphincter EMG becomes silent, and anal pressure decreases toward zero. The rectal pressure rises slowly until the rectal reservoir capacity is overcome (usually at 150 to 300 mL) and then rises rapidly until anal pressure is overcome and spontaneous evacuation of the balloon occurs.

BOWEL EVACUATION MECHANICS

In neurologically intact people, the sequence of defecation begins with the perception of rectal fullness. This often occurs in response to a giant migratory contraction that pushes stool into the rectum. Rectal distention may be perceived at volumes as low as 10 mL by stretch receptors in the rectal wall, puborectalis muscle (248), and the pelvic floor. Continued rectal distention triggers rectal contraction and the rectoanal inhibitory reflex (249). Frenckner, while studying a small group of SCI

patients, found that distention of the rectum with small volumes caused increased activity of the EAS (i.e., guarding reflex), whereas distention with large amounts caused the EAS to totally cease its electrical activity (223). This cessation of EAS activity rarely is seen in neurologically intact subjects. We have found that the volume at which the cessation of EAS activity occurs is variable and probably related to rectal capacity but that the intrarectal pressure at which it occurs is quite constant (20 to 30 cm H_2O; see Fig. 76-11A). There is a subgroup of patients with upper motor neuron lesions in whom EAS activity is aberrantly linked to rectal pressure (see Fig. 76-11*B*). In these patients, the spikes in rectal pressure that occur during dynamic rectal filling are met by increases in anal pressure. There is a failure to "turn off" EAS sphincter activity despite the presence of rectal pressures greater than 100 cm H_2O. We call this pattern *anorectal dyssynergia* by analogy with detrusor–sphincter dyssynergia of the bladder. These SCI patients usually have significant difficulty with bowel evacuation.

If the choice is made to defecate, the sitting position is assumed. Sitting makes the angle between the rectum and anal canal less acute (250). In the able-bodied, a rise in intraabdominal and perhaps intrarectal pressure is generated by closing the glottis to retain a full breath in the chest. The abdominal muscles are contracted and the diaphragm is pulled down. Neurologically intact people often are able to increase intrarectal pressure by 100 cm H_2O or more with a Valsalva maneuver. Persons with upper motor neuron SCI often initiate bowel evacuation with digital stimulation. Digital rectal stimulation is done by introducing the entire length of the gloved and lubricated finger into the rectum and dilating the distal rectum by moving in a circular funnel pattern. This key unlocks the sphincter mechanism, stretches the puborectalis, and provides a stimulus for peristalsis (211,246,251). Digital rectal stimulation results in the transient loss of approximately 75% of resting anal tone and presumably further straightens the anorectal angle. Expulsive force is added by performance of a Valsalva maneuver as well as the addition of external abdominal compression. The ability to elevate intraabdominal pressure with the use of these techniques is closely related to the level and completeness of SCI. Patients with C-5 to C-6 level injuries rarely can generate intraabdominal pressures greater than 10 cm H_2O.

The most common rectodynamic finding in patients with symptomatic difficulty with bowel evacuation is a failure to generate expulsive forces that are sufficient to overcome the residual tone of the normal, fully relaxed sphincter mechanism. These patients typically have long-standing cervical cord injuries, often with associated megacolon and megarectum. In these patients, the relationship between rectal pressure and anal relaxation remains intact, although it can take rectal volumes greater than 500 mL to generate enough rectal stretch to trigger anal relaxation. Rectal volumes of 100 to 150 mL usually are sufficient to turn off the anal sphincter mechanism.

Once evacuation is initiated, the entire left colon may empty by mass peristaltic action, or the fecal bolus may be passed bit by bit. The presence of an anocolic reflex (i.e., stool passing through the anus causes colonic contraction) has been postulated but not proven. Stool consistency is probably the major determinant of the pattern of defecation. Stool consistency is of even greater importance in SCI patients, in whom the balance between expulsive and resistive forces is so tenuous.

Neurogenic Bowel Function

Supraspinal bowel dysfunction occurs with lesions rostral to the pons. Voluntary defecation depends on an accurate percep-

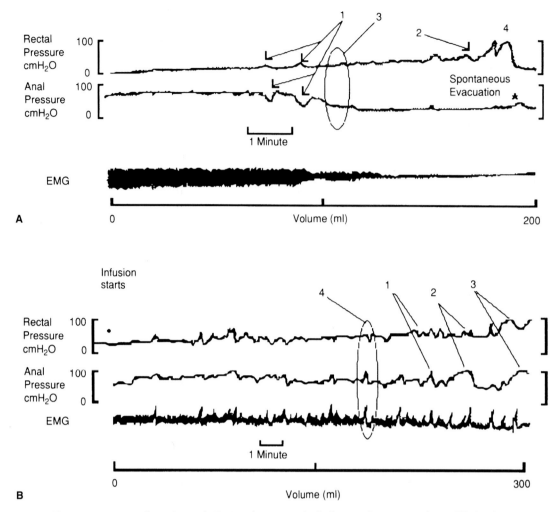

Figure 76-11. Rectodynamics study. During the tracing, the balloon in the rectum is being filled with saline at a constant rate (20 mL/min). **A:** Normal evacuation pattern after spinal cord injury. *(1)* Small rises in rectal pressure (i.e., rectal contractions) are invariably linked to anal pressure relaxation. Later contraction does not show linked relaxation because anal pressure cannot go below zero. *(2)* Gradual rise in rectal pressure becomes rapid when rectal reservoir capacity is overcome (usually 150–300 mlL. *(3)* When rectal threshold pressure (20–30 cm H_2O) is reached, anal pressure goes to zero. *(4)* Spontaneous evacuation of the balloon occurs when expulsive forces exceed resistive forces. **B:** Dyssynergia. *(1)* Loss of normal anal relaxation with rectal contraction. In this patient there is total loss of coordination between the rectum and anus. *(2)* Anal pressure fails to go to zero when the normal threshold (20–30 cm H_2O) of rectal pressure is reached. *(3)* No spontaneous evacuation of the rectal balloon occurs despite rectal pressures of 100 cm H_2O. Anal pressures increase concomitantly. *(4)* Spikes of electromyographic activity reflect contractions of the striated external anal sphincter. These contractions occur inappropriately and cause an elevation in anal pressure.

tion of the need to defecate as well as the necessary motor function to position over a toilet and to initiate the complex motor activity of bowel evacuation. A failure to perceive rectal fullness is common in the elderly and may manifest as overflow incontinence around a fecal impaction (252). Although disorders of continence and bowel evacuation are not uncommon after stroke, few distinct syndromes have been described. One syndrome, frontal lobe incontinence, is caused by lesions involving the anterior cingulate gyri (253). Patients with frontal lobe incontinence are said to have no awareness of bladder or rectal fullness. A pontine defecation center, analogous to the pontine micturition center, has been postulated but not proven (254). Patients with Parkinson's disease and multiple sclerosis often have disordered bowel evacuation; however, it may be difficult to factor out the effects of immobility, diet, and medications in these cases.

Upper motor neuron bowel dysfunction occurs with lesions between the pons and the sacral spinal cord. This is the type of

dysfunction most common in patients with C-1 through T-10 SCI. Associated deficits in function include sensory deficit for perception of fullness, a spastic pelvic floor that retains stool, and less effective peristaltic patterns (212). The gastrocolonic response is preserved after SCI. This is the increase in peristalsis in the large and small intestine in response to a meal. The gastrocolonic response has been demonstrated to be preserved after complete SCI, although it may be somewhat less robust as compared with able-bodied controls (255), A bowel program is a unique plan designed to effectively eliminate stool and prevent incontinence. The components are fluid intake, diet, exercise, medications, and scheduled bowel care (246). Bowel care is the procedure for assisted defection. Through empirical manipulation of diet, hydration, medications, and stimulation techniques, a balance is maintained between continence and evacuation.

Using the rectodynamics technique, we have identified two patterns of bowel evacuation mechanics that are associated with an inability to undergo satisfactory reflex evacuation: anorectal dyssynergia and insufficient expulsive forces. In both situations, spontaneous evacuation of the saline-filled balloon rarely occurs. In asymptomatic patients, spontaneous evacuation at volumes of 150 to 300 mL is the rule. Patients with insufficient expulsive forces tend to be older and to have had their SCI longer than patients with anorectal dyssynergia. It is attractive to postulate that both patterns are different stages of the same process. Chronically obstructed evacuation from dyssynergia may result in an end-stage dilated and decompensated rectum that is unable to generate a sufficient expulsive force. Against this theory is the finding that many patients with the insufficient expulsive force pattern retain a normal linkage between rectal and anal pressures, albeit at much higher volumes. Because patients with insufficient expulsive force all have cervical injuries, it is tempting to implicate a specific neurophysiologic cause, such as an overabundance of sympathetic input, although it is difficult to explain why the majority of patients with complete cervical injuries do not manifest this pattern. A more likely association with cervical injuries is that with denervation of the abdominal wall, only minimal increases in intraabdominal pressure can be generated. Although these studies do not reveal the underlying pathophysiological process of neurogenic bowel, they do provide a practical basis for thinking about the management of patients with neurogenic bowel.

Gastrointestinal Problems after Spinal Cord Injury

It has long been clear to clinicians that gastrointestinal symptoms are very common in the chronic phase after SCI. Colonic and pelvic floor function are entwined in etiquette and governed by social norms. The need for scheduled bowel care and fears of unanticipated evacuation are life limiting (247). Glickman and Kamm evaluated 115 consecutive outpatients with chronic SCI. Eighty-nine were male, the mean duration of injury was 62 months, and the level of injury was categorized as 48% cervical, 47% thoracic, and 5% lumbar. In this group, 95% required at least one therapeutic method to initiate defecation, half were dependent on others for toileting, and 49% took more than 30 minutes to complete bowel care (256). In a prospective study carried out by the Palo Alto Veterans Affairs Medical Center Spinal Cord Injury Service, chronic gastrointestinal problems that were severe enough to alter lifestyle or require chronic treatment occurred in 27% of subjects. The limited way in which people with SCI can manifest symptoms resulted in symptoms that were characteristically nonspecific. The most common problems were difficult bowel evacuation (20%) and poorly localized abdominal pain (14%). The term *pain* was used in its most general sense and was defined as a distressing sensation in a particular part of the body. Presumably, the pain sensation was carried to the brain by means of autonomic afferents (257).

Difficult bowel evacuation was said to be present in patients who required more than 60 minutes per day for their bowel care or needed manual disimpaction more than once a week. When managing persons with SCI, the term *constipation* is avoided because it is and has varied implied meanings. Specific descriptions are preferred, such as prolonged defecation, insufficient results, or abdominal fullness (247). The impact of problems with bowel evacuation on quality of life is formidable. In patients with difficult bowel evacuation, bowel care routinely occupies a significant part of the day, greatly restricted diets are adopted to minimize symptoms, and emergency trips to a physician for disimpaction are common. Episodes of dysreflexia, rectal bleeding, and incontinence from overtreatment with laxatives also occur frequently.

There are a few surgical options to improve success in neurogenic bowel management should conventional bowel care be

ineffective (258). The appendicocecostomy stoma is constructed by bringing the appendix through the abdominal wall. This stoma is irrigated with a 100–500 cc of saline to trigger defecation. This procedure has been used most successfully in patient populations with spina bifida (259). A few carefully selected patients with SCI that have benefited from the catheterizable stoma have been reported (260). Colostomy is an elective procedure that can improve independence in bowel care and enhance quality of life (261–263). The decision for surgical adaptation requires interdisciplinary evaluation (246) to explore implications of surgical risk (261), body image, and functional outcome. Interdisciplinary trials of various appliances and methods for self-management can lead to optimization of stoma location and choice of equipment. Colostomy has been performed with good success in the subgroup of these patients with the most severe disability (261). In patients with severe difficulty with evacuation, unresponsive to alterations in the bowel program colostomy can shorten the time needed for bowel care and enhance self-efficacy and quality of life (264, 265).

Stone and collaborators prospectively reviewed gastrointestinal complications in a cohort of patients with acute and chronic SCI (261). Incontinence is more common in patients with lower motor neuron than upper motor neuron bowel except during diarrheal illness or as a result of overtreatment for difficult bowel evacuation. Autonomic dysreflexia arising from the gastrointestinal tract occurred in almost one-half of the subjects with lesions above T-6 at some time but was rarely a significant problem by itself. Fecal impaction was the most common precipitating cause of autonomic dysreflexia. Other, less common causes were massive abdominal distention and routine digital rectal stimulation. Rectal bleeding during bowel care occurred in 74% of subjects. The majority of these patients were treated with hemorrhoidal bands or expectant management. Twelve percent eventually required operative hemorrhoidectomy. Esophageal reflux symptoms were present in 24% of subjects, and 10% of patients had a proven peptic ulcer. These rates are similar to those seen in the nondisabled population (261).

Gastrointestinal problems have special significance for people with SCI. Some problems, such as autonomic dysreflexia and ventilatory insufficiency caused by massive abdominal distention, are life-threatening problems that are unique to SCI patients. Other problems are shared with the nondisabled population but are associated with disproportionate morbidity when they occur in people with SCI. Twenty-three percent of SCI patients required an admission to the hospital for evaluation or treatment of a chronic gastrointestinal problem. Absence of specific symptoms made emergency operations the rule rather than the exception for problems such as peptic ulcers and gallstones.

Stone and associates further noted that chronic gastrointestinal problems usually do not develop for several years after injury (261). This finding is particularly significant because it suggests that these problems potentially are preventable. The situation may be analogous to that of the urinary tract in years past, when improvement in chronic care protocols has greatly reduced morbidity. For example, if chronic rectal overdistention eventually impairs the ability to evacuate, techniques to reduce rectal distention, such as more frequent bowel care, may be of benefit. In this way, decompensation of the rectum may be analogous to detrusor decompensation from chronic bladder overdistention.

Medical and Rehabilitation Management

The approach of evaluation and intervention to improve gastrointestinal function after SCI should be interdisciplinary and address all domains of disablement (212). The World Health

Organization has recently redefined disablement domains that address the organ (impairment), person (activity limitation), and the person as related to the environment (barriers to participation). A spectrum of inquiry that spans organ function and task capabilities of the person and needs for full community integration will lead to the most effective treatment (212).

Utilization of the entire interdisciplinary team for assessment and goal setting integrates bowel management into the comprehensive rehabilitation plan. Overall bowel management is outlined in the bowel program, which includes the following components: diet, fluid intake, medications, physical activity, and a schedule for bowel care. Bowel care is the procedure for assisted defecation with one or more of the following components: positioning, assistive devices, rectal simulation or trigger for defecation, and assistive maneuvers (abdominal massage) (212,246).

All components of the bowel program should be designed for maximal performance. People with SCI, particularly those with tetraplegia, have very little capability to overcome resistive forces and expel stool with bowel care. Stool consistency should be titrated with diet and medications (see Fig. 76-9). Adjustments in the bowel program that may be trivial in the nondisabled population can shift the balance significantly. Stool consistency is a pivotal variable. A diet containing 15–30 g of dietary fiber per day should be encouraged (212,246,266). Wheat bran and psyllium make the stool more pliable by increasing the fecal water content (266). Other helpful interventions include upright bowel care to utilize gravity, abdominal binders, daily osmotic laxatives, increased frequency of bowel care, more frequent digital stimulation, and stronger triggering medications.

Avoidance of colorectal overdistention is desirable because rectal distention is known to decrease intestinal transit by the colocolic reflex. Frequent bowel care (i.e., every 1 to 2 days) will avoid colonic distention with stool and may also enhance colonic transit by the hypothetical anocolic reflex. A preliminary intervention to promote bowel evacuation is movement of the sigmoid contents into the rectum. This may be accomplished by timing bowel care after a large meal to take advantage of the gastrocolonic response or by giving an oral laxative the day before. SCI persons with upper motor neuron bowel have SCI lesions above the conus and retain bulbocavernosus and anocutaneous reflexes.

The basic bowel care procedure for upper motor neuron neurogenic bowel has been broken down into steps (Table 76-4) and presented in patient education booklets (246) and a film, *Accidents Stink!: Bowel Care 202* (267). Rectal minienemas or suppositories and digital stimulation trigger and facilitate efficient bowel evacuation. A suppository or the contents of a minienema is first inserted as high as possible into the rectal vault and positioned against the mucosal lining. Suppositories containing bisacodyl are frequently used (268,269). They stimulate the sensory nerve endings, resulting in local and conal mediated reflex increases in peristalsis, frequently signaled by flatus. It generally takes 15 to 60 minutes for passage of the first flatus, which is followed shortly thereafter by stool flow (212). A significant reduction in the duration of bowel care can be achieved by using polyethylene glycol-based (PGB) bisacodyl suppositories rather than hydrogenated vegetable oil-based (HVB) bisacodyl (268,269). The average time to first flatus was 10 minutes with the PGB suppository compared with 37 minutes with the HVB suppository. The average total bowel-care time was 46 minutes with the PGB suppository compared with 85 minutes with the HVB suppository (270). Suppositories containing sodium bicarbonate and potassium bitartrate are sometimes used. With this suppository, there is a chemical reaction

---

TABLE 76-4.   Steps of Bowel Care: Reflexic Neurogenic Bowel

1. Getting ready and washing hands: Empty bladder.
2. Setting up and positioning: Transfer to a toilet or commode. If you don't sit up, lie on your left side.
3. Checking for stool: Remove any stool that would interfere with inserting a suppository or minienema.
4. Inserting stimulant medication: Using a gloved and lubricated finger or assistive device, place the medication right next to the rectal wall.
5. Waiting: Wait about 5 to 15 minutes for the stimulant to work.
6. Starting and repeating digital rectal stimulation: To keep stool coming, repeat digital rectal stimulation every 5 to 10 minutes as needed, until all stool has passed.
7. Recognizing when bowel care is completed: You'll know that stool flow has stopped if (a) no stool has come out after two digital stimulations at least 10 minutes apart, (b) mucus is coming out without stool, or (c) the rectum is completely closed around the stimulating finger.
8. Cleaning up – wash and dry the perianal area

---

that releases carbon dioxide. The colonic expansion from this reaction often initiates a rectal-anal reflex. However, use of this type of suppository usually requires significant anal sphincter tone to prevent the carbon dioxide from being expelled before causing expansion within the rectal vault. Glycerine suppositories are often used as a transition from bisacodyl suppositories to no suppositories and digital stimulation. Glycerine draws water into the stool to soften it, provides a mild irritant stimulus to trigger defecation, and lubricates the rectum to reduce resistance for expulsion.

Following an adequate time for the suppository to take effect, digital stimulation is initiated. If a person is having difficulty with autonomic dysreflexia during digital stimulation, pretreatment with topical application of viscous 2% lidocaine may be beneficial. If no stool is present in the rectal vault, stimulation may be repeated a few minutes later. If stool still is not present in the rectal vault, a small-volume saline enema may be given to lubricate the rectum and create acute rectal distention. If this is still unsuccessful, a small-volume bisacodyl enema may be helpful to stimulate colorectal peristalsis.

Patients with lower motor neuron bowel typically have SCI lesions affecting the conus or cauda equina. Anal canal tone is reduced, anocutaneous bulbocavernosus reflexes are absent, and the pelvic floor may passively descend. Bowel care for lower motor neuron SCI typically consists of digital rectal stimulation and manual evacuation after the morning and evening meals. A study of bowel-care patterns of persons with SCI revealed that the average frequency of bowel care in persons with lower motor neuron bowel was twice per day, and the frequency of those with upper motor neuron bowels averaged three times per week (270).

Oral medications may also be used to potentiate the success of bowel care. Oral dioctyl sodium sulfosuccinate functions as a stool softener by having a detergent effect and increasing fluid accumulation in the stool. Oral senna or bisacodyl preparations are sometimes helpful 6 to 12 hours before bowel care. Their action is limited to the colon and felt to stimulate Auerbach's plexus (212,265).

In patients with difficult bowel evacuation, the first step is optimization of stool consistency with fluids, fiber, oral osmotic agents, or glycerin suppositories. If possible, anticholinergic agents such as oxybutynin are discontinued. If rectodynamic studies show anorectal dyssynergia, topical application of viscous 2% lidocaine and providing a prolonged anal stretch occasionally are of benefit. If the rectodynamic study shows that a megarectum already exists, large-volume enemas (300–500 mL) may be necessary to provide the necessary rectal distention to raise rectal pressures and shut down anal sphincter activity. In those prone to autonomic dysreflexia, careful monitoring of blood pressure is necessary.

In patients who have failed all attempts to modify their bowel program, colostomy may provide remarkable relief (212, 246,257,267). We currently reserve colostomy for patients with severe long-term disability, excessively long bowel care with poor results, and exhaustion of all nonsurgical options. Transit time studies are performed before colostomy. If markers accumulate in the rectosigmoid, a sigmoid colostomy is performed. If the entire colon is atonic, an ileostomy is performed.

Traumatic superficial mucosal erosion is by far the most common cause of bright red rectal bleeding after SCI. It usually is manifest as streaks of blood on the glove or stool. This should be distinguished from hemorrhoidal bleeding (i.e., bleeding from high-pressure vessels within hemorrhoids), which usually manifests as blood dripping into the commode or passage of clots. Traumatic erosion usually is treated conservatively. Hemorrhoids need only be treated when they cause a symptom such as bleeding, mucous soilage, or difficulty with anal hygiene. They should be kept clean, wiped with a solution or witch hazel, and supported on an air-filled cushion. A minimal evaluation for bright red rectal bleeding includes digital examination, anoscopy, and proctoscopy or flexible sigmoidoscopy.

Bright red rectal bleeding, when it occurs after SCI, tends to arise from circumferential mucosal excoriation rather than a discrete site on a hemorrhoid. Therefore, treatment of the entire circumference of the anal canal may be necessary to eliminate bleeding. We have had good success with rubber-band ligation of bleeding hemorrhoids. Patients must be aware that the likelihood of recurrent bleeding is high, that multiple applications may be necessary, and that complications, although rare, do occur. Transient episodes of autonomic dysreflexia have occurred at the time of banding, although all have been brief and self-limited (257).

In patients with irreducible hemorrhoidal prolapse, blood loss sufficient to cause anemia, or failure of rubber-band ligation, operative hemorrhoidectomy must be performed. A conventional surgical technique is used. To avoid manipulation of the fresh suture lines, however, we perform a full mechanical bowel preparation before surgery. No bowel care is performed for 4 days after operative hemorrhoidectomy.

The frequency with which rectal bleeding occurs makes screening for colorectal cancer by testing for occult blood of little value. We screen patients older than 45 years old with flexible sigmoidoscopy. If polyps or tumors are seen, a full colonoscopy is performed (257).

REFERENCES

1. Grant JCB. *An atlas of anatomy*, 6th ed. Baltimore: Williams & Wilkins, 1972:181–189.
2. Olsson CA. Anatomy of the upper urinary tract. In: Walsh PC, Gittes RF, Perlmutter AD, Stamey TA, eds. *Campbell's urology*, 5th ed. Philadelphia: WB Saunders, 1986:12–29.
3. Kaye KW, Goldberg ME. Applied anatomy of the kidneys and ureters. *Urol Clin North Am* 1982;9:3–13.
4. Tanago EA. Anatomy of the lower urinary tract. In: Walsh PC, Gittes RF, Perlmutter AD, Stamey TA, eds. *Campbell's urology*, 5th ed. Philadelphia: WB Saunders, 1986:46–61.
5. Stephens FD, Lenaghan D. The anatomical basis and dynamics of vesicoureteral reflux. *J Urol* 1962;87:669–680.
6. Gosling JA, Dixon JS. Species variation in the location of upper urinary tract pacemaker cells. *Investigative Urology* 1974;11:418–423.
7. Griffiths DJ, Notschaele C. Mechanics of urine transport in the upper urinary tract: 1. The dynamics of the isolated bolus. *Neurourol Urodyn* 1983;2:155–166.
8. Myers RP, Goellner JR, Cahill DR. Prostate shape, external striated urethral sphincter and radical prostatectomy: the apical dissection. *J Urol* 1987;138:543–547.
9. Delancey JO. Structure and function of the continence mechanism relative to stress incontinence. In: Leach GE, Paulson DF, eds. *Problems in urology, vol. 1. Female urology.* Philadelphia: JB Lippincott, 1991:1–9.
10. Myers RP. Male urethral sphincteric anatomy and radical prostatectomy. *Urol Clin North Am* 1991;18:211–227.
11. Fletcher TF, Bradley WE. Neuroanatomy of the bladder-urethra. *J Urol* 1978;119:153–160.
12. Benson GS, McConnell JA, Wood JG. Adrenergic innervation of the human bladder body. *J Urol* 1979;122:189–191.
13. Elbadawi A. Autonomic muscular innervation of the vesical outlet and its role in micturition. In: Hinman F Jr, ed. *Benign prostatic hypertrophy.* New York: Springer Verlag, 1983:330–348.
14. Burnstock G. The changing face of autonomic neurotransmission. *Acta Physiol Scand* 1986;126:67–91.
15. Norlen L, Dahlstrom A, Sundin T, Svedmyr N. The adrenergic innervation and adrenergic receptor activity of the feline urinary bladder and urethra in the normal state and after hypogastric and/or parasympathetic denervation. *Scand J Urol Nephrol* 1976;10:177–184.
16. Elbadawi A. Ultrastructure of vesicourethral innervation: III. Axoaxonal synapses between postganglionic cholinergic axons and probably SIF-cell derived processes in feline lissosphincter. *J Urol* 1985;133:524–528.
17. Chancellor MB, De Groat WC. Intravesical capsaicin and resiniferatoxin therapy. *J Urol* 1999;162:3–11.
18. de Groat WC. Mechanism underlying the recovery of lower urinary tract function following spinal cord injury. *Paraplegia* 1995;33:493–505.
19. Elbadawi A, Schenk EA. A new theory of the innervation of bladder musculature: Part 4. Innervation of the vesicourethral junction and external urethral sphincter. *J Urol* 1974;111:613–615.
20. Sundin T, Dahlstrom A. The sympathetic innervation of the urinary bladder and urethra in the normal state and after parasympathetic denervation at the spinal root level. *Scand J Urol Nephrol* 1973;7:131–139.
21. Crowe R, Burnstock G, Light JK. Adrenergic innervation of the striated muscle of the intrinsic external urethral sphincter from patients with lower motor spinal cord lesion. *J Urol* 1989;141:47–49.
22. Denny-Brown D, Robertson EG. On the physiology of micturition. *Brain* 1933;56:149–190.
23. Barrington FJF. The relation of the hindbrain to micturition. *Brain* 1921;44:23–53.
24. de Groat WC. Nervous control of the urinary bladder of the cat. *Brain Res* 1975;87:201.
25. Carlsson CA. The supraspinal control of the urinary bladder. *Acta Pharmacol Toxicol* 1978;43A[Suppl II]:8–12.
26. Bradley WE, Teague CT. Spinal cord organization of micturitional reflex afferents. *Exp Neurol* 1968;22:504–516.
27. Barrett DM, Wein AJ. Voiding dysfunction: diagnosis, classification and management. In: Gillenwater JY, Grayhack JT, Howards SS, Duckett JW, eds. *Adult and pediatric urology*, 2nd ed. St Louis: Mosby Year Book, 1991:1001–1099.
28. Lewis WH Jr, Alving AS. Changes with age in the renal function in adult men. *Am J Physiol* 1938;123:500–515.
29. Resnick NM. Geriatric incontinence. *Urol Clin North Am* 1996;23(1):55–74.
30. Elbadawi A, Yalla SV, Resnick NM. Structural basis of geriatric voiding. III. Detrusor overactivity. *J Urol* 1993;150:1668–1680.
31. Staskin DR. Age-related physiologic and pathologic changes affecting lower urinary tract function. *Clin Geriatr Med* 1986;2:701–710.
32. Elbadawi A, Yalla SV, Resnick NM. Structural basis of geriatric voiding: methods of a correlative study and overview of findings. *J Urol* 1993;150:1650–1656.
33. Ouslander JG, Hepps K, Raz S, Su HL. Genitourinary dysfunction in a geriatric outpatient population. *J Am Geriatr Soc* 1986;34:507–514.
34. Kaplan GW, Brock WA. Voiding dysfunction in children. *Curr Probl Pediatr* 1980;10(8):15–16.
35. Comarr AE. Diagnosis of the traumatic cord bladder. In: Boyarsky S, ed. *The neurogenic bladder.* Baltimore: Williams & Wilkins, 1967:147–152.
36. Bradley WE, Chou S, Markland C. Classifying neurologic dysfunction of the urinary bladder. In: Boyarsky S, ed. *The neurogenic bladder.* Baltimore: Williams & Wilkins, 1967:139–146.
37. Lapides J. Neuromuscular vesical and ureteral dysfunction. In: Campbell MF, Harrison JH, eds. *Urology*, 3rd ed. Philadelphia: WB Saunders, 1970:1343–1379.
38. Krane RJ, Siroky MB. Classification of neuro-urologic disorders. In: Krane RJ, Siroky MB, eds. *Clinical neuro-urology*, 2nd ed. Boston: Little, Brown & Co, 1979:143–158.
39. Wein AJ. Classification of neurogenic voiding dysfunction. *J Urol* 1981;125:605–609.
40. Abrams P, Blaivas JG, Stanton SL, Andersen JT. Standardization of terminology of lower urinary tract function. *Neurourol Urodyn* 1988;7:403–427.
41. Borrie MJ, Campbell AJ, Caradoc-Davies TH, Spears GF. Urinary incontinence after stroke: a prospective study. *Age Ageing* 1986;15:177–181.

42. Brocklehurst JC, Andrews K, Richards B, Laycock PJ. Incidence and correlates of incontinence in stroke patients. *J Am Geriatr Soc* 1985;33:540–542.
43. Patel M, Coshall C, Rudd AG, Wolfe CDA. Natural history and effects on 2-year outcomes of urinary incontinence after stroke. *Stroke* 2001;32:122–125.
44. Linsenmeyer TA. Characterization of voiding dysfunction following recent cerebrovascular accident. *Arch Phys Med Rehabil* 1990;71:778.
45. Tsuchida S, Noto H, Yamaguchi O, Itoh M. Urodynamic studies on hemiplegic patients after cerebrovascular accident. *Urology* 1983;21:315–318.
46. Linsenmeyer TA, Zorowitz RD. Urodynamic findings in patients with urinary incontinence after cerebrovascular accident. *NeuroRehabilitation* 1992;2 (2):23–26.
47. Blaivas JG. The neurophysiology of micturition: a clinical study of 550 patients. *J Urol* 1982;127:958–963.
48. Siroky MB, Krane RJ. Neurologic aspects of detrusor-sphincter dyssynergia with reference to the guarding reflex. *J Urol* 1982;127:953–957.
49. Staskin DR. Intracranial lesions that affect lower urinary tract function. In: Krane RJ, Siroky MB, eds. *Clinical neuro-urology,* 2nd ed. Boston: Little, Brown & Co, 1991:345–451.
50. Pavlakis AJ, Siroky MB, Goldstein I, Krane RJ. Neurourologic findings in Parkinson's disease. *J Urol* 1983;129:80–83.
51. Andersen JT. Detrusor hyperreflexia in benign infravesical obstruction: a cystometric study. *J Urol* 1976;115:532.
52. Ivers RR, Goldstein NP. Multiple sclerosis: a current appraisal of symptoms and signs. *Proceedings Staff Meetings Mayo Clinic* 1963;38:457–466.
53. Bemelmans BL, Hommes OR, Van Kerrebroeck PE, et al. Evidence for early lower urinary tract dysfunction in clinically silent multiple sclerosis. *J Urol* 1991;145:1219–1224.
54. Miller H, Simpson CA, Yeates WK. Bladder dysfunction in multiple sclerosis. *BMJ* 1965;1:1265–1269.
55. Goldstein I, Siroky MB, Sax DS, Krane RJ. Neurourologic abnormalities in multiple sclerosis. *J Urol* 1982;128:541–545.
56. Wheeler JS, Siroky MB, Pavlakis AJ, et al. The changing neurourologic pattern of multiple sclerosis. *J Urol* 1983;130:1123–1126.
57. Gonor SE, Carroll DJ, Metcalfe JB. Vesical dysfunction in multiple sclerosis. *Urology* 1985;25:429–431.
58. Blaivas JG, Barbalias GA. Detrusor-external sphincter dyssynergia in men with multiple sclerosis: an ominous urologic condition. *J Urol* 1984;131:91–94.
59. Wheeler JS. Multiple sclerosis. In: Krane RJ, Siroky MB, eds. *Clinical neuro-urology,* 2nd ed. Boston: Little, Brown & Co, 1991:353–363.
60. Kaplan SA, Chancellor MB, Blaivas JG. Bladder and sphincter behavior in patients with spinal cord lesions. *J Urol* 1991;146:113–117.
61. Yalla SV, Fam BA. Spinal cord injury. In: Krane RJ, Siroky MB, eds. *Clinical neuro-urology,* 2nd ed. Boston: Little, Brown & Co, 1991:319–331.
62. Rudy DC, Awad SA, Downie JW. External sphincter dyssynergia: an abnormal continence reflex. *J Urol* 1988;140:105–110.
63. Light JK, Faganel J, Beric A. Detrusor areflexia in suprasacral spinal cord injuries. *J Urol* 1985;134:295–297.
64. Graham SD. Present urological treatment of spinal cord injury patients. *J Urol* 1981;126:1–4.
65. Downie JW, Awad SA. The state of urethral musculature during the detrusor areflexia after spinal cord transection. *Invest Urol* 1979;17:55–59.
66. Nanninga JB, Meyer P. Urethral sphincter activity following acute spinal cord injury. *J Urol* 1980;123:528–530.
67. Koyanagi T, Arikado K, Takamatsu T, Tsuji I. Experience with electromyography of the external urethral sphincter in spinal cord injury patients. *J Urol* 1982;127:272–276.
68. Blaivas JG, Sinha HP, Zayed AAH, Labib KB. Detrusor-external sphincter dyssynergia. *J Urol* 1981;125:542–544.
69. Pavlakis AJ, Siroky MB, Goldstein I, Krane RJ. Neurourologic findings in conus medullaris and cauda equina injury. *Arch Neurol* 1983;40:570–573.
70. Sharr MM, Carfield JC, Jenkins JD. Lumbar spondylosis and neuropathic bladder investigations of 73 patients with chronic urinary symptoms. *BMJ* 1976;1:645.
71. Hackler RH, Hall MK, Zampieri TA. Bladder hypocompliance in the spinal cord injury population. *J Urol* 1989;141:1390–1393.
72. Sislow JG, Mayo ME. Reduction in human bladder wall compliance following decentralization. *J Urol* 1990;144:945–947.
73. Appell RA, Whiteside HV. Diabetes and other peripheral neuropathies affecting lower urinary tract function. In: Krane RJ, Siroky MG, eds. *Clinical neuro-urology,* 2nd ed. Boston: Little, Brown & Co, 1991:365–373.
74. Bradley WE. Autonomic neuropathy and the genitourinary system. *J Urol* 1978;119:299–302.
75. Andersen JT, Bradley WE. Abnormalities of bladder innervation in diabetes mellitus. *Urology* 1976;7:442–448.
76. Wheeler JS Jr, Siroky MB, Pavlakis A, Krane RJ. The urodynamic aspects of the Guillain-Barré syndrome. *J Urol* 1984;131:917–919.
77. Katz GP, Blaivas JG. A diagnostic dilemma: when urodynamic findings differ from the clinical impression. *J Urol* 1983;129:1170–1174.
78. Ouslander J, Staskin D, Raz S, et al. Clinical versus urodynamic diagnosis in an incontinent geriatric female population. *J Urol* 1987;137:68–71.
79. Resnick NM, Yalla SV. Management of urinary incontinence in the elderly. *N Engl J Med* 1985;313:800–805.
80. Blaivas JG, Zayed AAH, Labib KB. The bulbocavernosus reflex in urology: a prospective study of 299 patients. *J Urol* 1981;126:197–199.
81. Linsenmeyer TA, Culkin D. APS Recommendations for the urological evaluation of patients with spinal cord injury. *J Spinal Cord Med* 1999;22(2):139–142.
82. Linsenmeyer, TA, Chou, F, Millis, S, Ho CH. Long-term change in bladder function following SCI. *J Spinal Cord Med* 2001;24(3):196(abst).
83. Rao KG, Hackler RH, Woodlief RM, et al. Real time renal sonography in spinal cord injury patients: prospective comparison with excretory urography. *J Urol* 1986;135:72–77.
84. Lloyd LK, Dubovsky EV, Bueschen Aj, et al. Comprehensive renal scintillation procedures in spinal cord injury: comparison with excretory urography. *J Urol* 1981;126:10–13.
85. Tsai SJ, Ting H, Ho CC, Bih Li. Use of sonography and radioisotope renography to diagnose hydronephrosis in patients with spinal cord injury. *Arch Phys Med Rehabil* 2001;82(1):103–106.
86. Liu W, Esler SJ, Kenny BJ, et al. Low-dose nonenhanced helical CT of renal colic: assessment of ureteric stone detection and measurement of effective dose equivalent. *Radiology* 2000;215(1):51–54.
87. Kuhlemeier KV, McEachran AB, Lloyd LK, et al. Serum creatinine as an indicator of renal function after spinal cord injury. *Arch Phys Med Rehabil* 1984;65:694–697.
88. Linsenmeyer TA, Campagnolo DI, Chou I. Silent autonomic dysreflexia during voiding in men with SCI. *J Urol* 1996;155: 519–522.
89. Khanna OP. Cystometry: water. In: Barrett DM, Wein AJ, eds. *Controversies in neuro-urology.* New York: Churchill-Livingston, 1984:11–12.
90. McGuire EJ, Woodside JR, Borden TA, Weiss RM. Prognostic value of urodynamic testing in myelodysplastic patients. *Problems in Urology* 1981;126:205–209.
91. Bauer SB. Urologic management of the myelodysplastic child. *Probl Urol* 1989;3:86–101.
92. Lapides J, Friend CR, Ajemian EP, Reus WF. A new test for neurogenic bladder. *J Urol* 1962;88:245–247.
93. Wheeler JS Jr, Culkin DJ, Canning JR. Positive bethanechol supersensitivity test in neurologically normal patients. *Urology* 1988;31:86–89.
94. Fusco F, Groutz A, Blaivas JG, et al. Videourodynamic studies in men with lower urinary tract symptoms: a comparison of community based versus referral urological practices. *J Urol* 2001;166:910–913.
95. Burgio KL, Burgio LD. Behavior therapies for urinary incontinence in the elderly. *Clin Geriatr Med* 1986;2:809–827.
96. Brown JH. Atropine, scopolamine and related antimuscarinic drugs. In: Gilman AG, Rall TW, Nies AS, Taylor P, eds. *Goodman and Gilman's the pharmacologic basis of therapeutics,* 8th ed. New York: Pergamon Press, 1990:150–165.
97. Baldessarini RJ. Drugs and the treatment of psychiatric disorders. In: Gillman AG, Rall TW, Nies AS, Taylor P, eds. *Goodman and Gilman's the pharmacologic basis of therapeutics,* 8th ed. New York: Pergamon Press, 1990:383–435.
98. Wyndaele JJ. Pharmacotherapy for urinary bladder dysfunction in spinal cord injury patients. *Paraplegia* 1990;28:146–150.
99. Yokoyama O, Komatsu K, Kodama K, et al. Diagnostic value of intravesical lidocaine for overactive bladders. *J Urol* 2000;164(2):340–343.
100. Brendler CB, Radebaugh LC, Mohler JL. Topical oxybutynin chloride for relaxation of dysfunctional bladder. *J Urol* 1989;141:1350–1352.
101. Vaidyanathan S, Soni BM, Brown E, et al. Effect of intermittent urethral catheterization and oxybutynin bladder instillation on urinary continence status and quality of life in a selected group of spinal cord injured patients with neuropathic bladder dysfunction. *Spinal Cord* 1998;36:409–414.
102. Haferkamp A, Saehhler G, Gerner HJ, Dorsam. Dosage escalation of intravesical oxybutynin in the treatment of neurogenic bladder patients. *J Spinal Cord* 2000;38:250–254.
103. de Seze M, Wiart L, Joseph PA et al. Capsaicin and neurogenic detrusor hyperreflexia: a double-blind placebo-controlled study in 20 patients with spinal cord lesions. *Neurourol Urodyn* 1998;17:513–523.
104. Silva C, Rio M Cruz F. desensitization of bladder sensory fibers by intravesical resiniferatoxin, a capsaicin analog: long-term results for the treatment of detrusor hyperreflexia. *Eur Urol* 2000;38:444–452.
105. Lazzeri M, Beneforti P, Turini D. Urodynamic effects of intravesical resiniferatoxin in humans: preliminary results in stable and unstable detrusor. *J Urol* 1997;158(6):2093–2096.
106. Giannantoni A, Di Satasi SM, Stephen RL, et al. Intravesical capsaicin versus resiniferatoxin in patients with detrusor hyperreflexia: a prospective randomized study. *J Urol* 2002;167:1710–1714.
107. Gray GJ, Yang C. Surgical procedures of the bladder after spinal cord injuries. *Topics in Spinal Cord Medicine* 2000;11(1):61–69.
108. McDougal WS. Use of intestinal segments and urinary diversion. In Walsh PC, Retik AB, Vaughan ED, Wein AJ, eds. *Cambell's urology,* 7th ed. Philadelphia: WB Saunders Co., 1998:3121–3157.
109. Sakano S, Yoshihiro S, Joko K, Kawano H, Naito K. Adenocarcinoma developing in an ileal conduit. *J Urol* 1995;153:146–148.
110. Golomb J, Klutke CG, Lewin KJ, et al. Bladder neoplasms associated with augmentation cystoplasty: report of 2 cases and literature review. *J Urol* 1989;142:377–380.
111. Mast P, Hoebeke P, Wyndaele JJ, et al. Experience with augmentation cystoplasty: a review. *Paraplegia* 1995;33:560–564.
112. Kuo HC. Clinical outcomes and quality of life after enterocystoplasty for contracted bladders. *Urol Int* 1997;58(3):160–165.
113. Stohrer M, Kramer G, Gopel M, et al. Bladder autoaugmentation in adult patients with neurogenic voiding dysfunction. *Spinal Cord* 1997;35(7):456–462.

114. Anderson B, Mitchell M. Management of electrolyte disturbances following urinary diversion and bladder augmentation. *AUA News* 2000;5(8):1–7.
115. Misak SJ, Bunts RC, Ulmer JL, Eagles WM. Nerve interruption procedures in the urologic management of paraplegic patients. *J Urol* 1962;88:392.
116. Leach GE, Goldman D, Raz S. Surgical treatment of detrusor hyperreflexia. In: Raz S, ed. *Female urology.* Philadelphia: WB Saunders, 1983:326–334.
117. Hodgkinson CP, Drukker BH. Infravesical nerve resection for detrusor dyssynergia: the Ingelman-Sundberg operation. *Acta Obstet Gynecol Scand* 1977;56:401–408.
118. Ohlsson BL, Frankenberg-Sommar S. Effects of external and direct pudendal nerve 110 maximal electrical stimulation in the treatment of the uninhibited overactive bladder. *Br J Urol* 1989;64:374–380.
119. Tanago EA. Concepts of neuromodulation. *Neurourol Urodyn* 1993;12:497–498.
120. Brindley GS, Polkey CE, Rushton DN. Sacral anterior root stimulator for bladder control in paraplegia. *Paraplegia* 1982;20:365–381.
121. Creasey GH, Bodner DR. Review of sacral electrical stimulation in the management of the neurogenic bladder. *NeuroRehabilitation* 1994;4:266–274.
122. Van Kerrebroeck PEV. World wide experience with the Finetech-Brindley sacral anterior root stimulator. *Neurourol Urodyn* 1993;12(5):497–503.
123. Guttmann L, Frankel H. The value of intermittent catheterisation in the early management of traumatic paraplegia and tetraplegia. *Paraplegia* 1966/1967;4:63–84.
124. Lapides J, Diokno AC, Silber SJ, Lowe BS. Clean, intermittent self catheterization in treatment of urinary tract disease. *J Urol* 1972;107:458–461.
125. Maynard FM, Glass J. Management of the neuropathic bladder by clean intermittent catheterisation: 5 year outcomes. *Paraplegia* 1987;25:106–110.
126. Anderson RU. Non sterile intermittent catheterization with antibiotic prophylaxis in the acute spinal cord injured male patient. *J Urol* 1980;124:392–394.
127. Weld KJ, Dmochowski RR. Effect of bladder management on urological complications in spinal cord injured patients. *J Urol* 2000;163:768–772.
128. Donnelan SM, Boulton DM. The impact of contemporary bladder management techniques on struvite calculi associated with spinal cord injury. *Br J Urol Intl* 1999;84:280–285.
129. McGuire EJ, Savastano JA. Comparative urological outcome in woman with spinal cord injury. *J Urol* 1986;135:730–731.
130. Groah SL, Weitzenkamp DA, Lammertse DP, et al. Excess risk of bladder cancer in spinal cord injury: evidence for an association between indwelling catheter use and bladder cancer. *Arch Phys Med Rehabil* 2002;83:346–351.
131. MacDiarmid SA, Arnold EP, Palmer NB, et al. Management of spinal cord patients by indwelling suprapubic catheterization. *J Urol* 1995;154:492.
132. Dewire DM, Owens RS, Anderson GA, et al. A comparison of the urological complications associated with long term management of quadriplegics with and without chronic indwelling urinary catheters. *J Urol* 1992;147:1060–1072.
133. Kim YH, Katten MW, Boone TB. Bladder leak point pressure: the measure for sphincterotomy success in spinal cord injured patients with external detrusor-sphincter dyssynergia. *J Urol* 1998;159:493–497.
134. Killorin W, Gray M, Bennet JK, Green, BG. The value of urodynamics and bladder management in predicting upper urinary tract complications in male spinal cord injury patients. *Paraplegia* 1992;30:437–441.
135. Gerridzen RG, Thijssen AM, Dehoux E. Risk factors for upper tract deterioration in chronic spinal cord injury patients. *J Urol* 1992;147:416–418.
136. Linsenmeyer TA, Bagaria SP, Gendron B. The impact of urodynamic parameters on the upper tracts of spinal cord injured men who void reflexly. *J Spinal Cord Med* 1998;21:15–20.
137. Linsenmeyer TA, Horton J, Benevento J. Impact of alpha-1 blockers in men with spinal cord injury and upper tract stasis. *J Spinal Cord Med* 2002;25(2):124–1–28.
138. Kegel AH. Progressive resistance exercises in the functional restoration of the perineal muscles. *Am J Obstet Gynecol* 1948;56:238–248.
139. Wells TJ, Brink CA, Diokno AC, et al. Pelvic muscle exercise for stress urinary incontinence in elderly women. *J Am Geriatr Soc* 1991;39:785–791.
140. Jeter KF. Pelvic muscle exercises with and without biofeedback for the treatment of urinary incontinence. *Probl Urol* 1991;5:72–84.
141. Hoffman BB, Lefkowitz RJ. Catecholamines and sympathomimetic drugs. In: Gillman AG, Rall TW, Nies AS, Taylor P, eds. *Goodman and Gilman's the pharmacological basis of therapeutics,* 8th ed. New York: Pergamon Press, 1990:187–220.
142. Kernan WN, Viscoli CM, Brass LM, et al. Phenylpropanolamine and the risk of hemorrhagic stroke. *N Engl J Med* 2000;343(25):1826.
143. Walter S, Wolf H, Barlebo H, Jensen HK. Urinary incontinence in post menopausal women treated with estrogens. *Urol Int* 1978;33:135.
144. Hodgson BJ, Dumas S, Bolling DR, Heesch CM. Effect of estrogen on sensitivity of rabbit bladder and urethra to phenylephrine. *Invest Urol* 1978;16:67–69.
145. Appell RA. Periurethral collagen injection for female incontinence. *Probl Urol* 1991;5:134–140.
146. Light JK, Scott FB. Use of the artificial urinary sphincter in spinal cord injury patients. *J Urol* 1983;130:1127–1129.
147. Bosco PJ, Bauer SB, Colodny AH, et al. The long term results of artificial sphincters in children. *J Urol* 1991;146:396–399.
148. Kelly MJ, Leach GE. Long term results of bladder neck suspension procedures. *Probl Urol* 1991;5:94–105.
149. Opitz JL. Treatment of voiding dysfunction in spinal cord injured patients: bladder retraining. In: Barrett DM, Wein AJ, eds. *Controversies in neuro-urology.* New York: Churchill-Livingston, 1984:437–451.
150. Barbalias GA, Klauber GT, Blaivas JG. Critical evaluation of the Crede maneuver: a urodynamic study of 207 patients. *J Urol* 1983;130:720–723.
151. Finkbeiner AE. Is bethanechol chloride clinically effective in promoting bladder emptying? A literature review. *J Urol* 1985;134:443–449.
152. Light KJ, Scott FB. Bethanechol chloride and the traumatic cord bladder. *J Urol* 1982;128:85–87.
153. Sporer A, Leyson JFJ, Martin BF. Effects of bethanechol chloride on the external urethral sphincter in spinal cord injury patients. *J Urol* 1978;120:62–66.
154. Taylor P. Cholinergic agonists. In: Gilman AC, Rall TW, Nies AS, Taylor P, eds. *Goodman and Gilman's the pharmacological basis of therapeutics,* 8th ed. New York: Pergamon Press, 1990:122–130.
155. Vaidyanathan S, Rao MS, Mapa MK, et al. Study of intravesical instillation of 1A(s)-15 methy prostaglandin F_2 in patients with neurogenic bladder dysfunction. *J Urol* 1981;126:81–85.
156. Booth AM, Hisamitsu T, Kawatani M, de Groat WC. Regulation of urinary bladder capacity by endogenous opioid peptides. *J Urol* 1985;133:339–342.
157. Hanna MK. New concept in bladder remodeling. *Urology* 1982;19:6.
158. Lockhart JL, Vorstman B, Weinstein D, Politano V. Sphincterotomy failure in neurogenic bladder disease. *J Urol* 1986;135:86–89.
159. Creasey G. Restoration of bladder, bowel and sexual function. *Topics in spinal cord rehabilitation* 1999;5(1):21–32.
160. Jezernik S, Craggs M, Grill WM, Creasey G, Rijkhoff NJ. Electrical stimulation for the treatment of bladder dysfunction. Current status and future possibilities. *Neurol Res* 2002;24(5):413–430.
161. Maizels M, King LR, Firlit CR. Urodynamic biofeedback: a new approach to treat vesical sphincter dyssynergia. *J Urol* 1979;122:205–209.
162. Kiviat MD, Zimmermann TA, Donovan WH. Sphincter stretch: new technique resulting in continence and complete voiding in paraplegics. *J Urol* 1975;114:895–897.
163. Lepor H. Alpha blockers for the treatment of benign prostatic hypertrophy. *Probl Urol* 1991;5:419–429.
164. Scott MB, Morrow JW. Phenoxybenzamine in neurogenic bladder dysfunction after spinal cord injury: I. Voiding dysfunction. *J Urol* 1978;119:480–482.
165. Lepor H, Gup DI, Baumann M, Shapiro E. Laboratory assessment of terazosin and alpha 1 blockade in prostatic hyperplasia. *Urology* 1988;32[Suppl 6]:21–26.
166. Scott MB, Morrow JW. Phenoxybenzamine in neurogenic bladder dysfunction after spinal cord injury: II. Autonomic dysreflexia. *J Urol* 1978;119:483–484.
167. Hoffman BB, Lefkowitz RJ. Adrenergic receptor antagonists. In: Gilman AG, Rall TW, Nies AS, Taylor J, eds. *Goodman and Gilman's the pharmacological basis of therapeutics,* 8th ed. New York: Pergamon Press, 1990:221–243.
168. Wein AJ. Prazosin in the treatment of prostatic obstruction: a placebo controlled study (editorial comment). *J Urol* 1989;141:693.
169. Cedarbaum JM, Schleifer LS. Drugs for Parkinson's disease, spasticity and acute muscle spasms. In: Gilman AG, Rall TW, Nies AS, Taylor P, eds. *Goodman and Gilman's the pharmacological basis of therapeutics,* 8th ed. New York: Pergamon Press, 1990:463–484.
170. Engel RME, Schirmer HKA. Pudendal neurectomy in neurogenic bladder. *J Urol* 1974;112:57–59.
171. Perkash I. Modified approach to sphincterotomy in spinal cord injury patients. *Paraplegia* 1976;13:247–260.
172. Yang CC, Mayo ME. External sphincterotomy; long term follow up. *Neurourol Urodynam* 1995;14:25–31.
173. Perkash I. Contact laser transurethral external sphincterotomy: a preliminary report. *NeuroRehabilitation* 1994;4(4):249–254.
174. Chancellor MB, Rivas DA, Linsenmeyer T, et al. Multicenter trial in North America of Urolume urinary sphincter prosthesis. *J Urol* 1994;152:924–930.
175. Dykstra DD, Sidi AA, Scott AB, et al. Effects of botulinum A toxin on detrusor sphincter dyssynergia in spinal cord injury patients. *J Urol* 1988;139:919–922.
176. Sugar EC, Firlit CF. Urodynamic biofeedback: a new therapeutic approach for childhood incontinence/infection (vesical voluntary sphincter dyssynergia). *J Urol* 1982;128:1253–1257.
177. Parres JA, Kropp KA. Urodynamic evaluation of the continence mechanism following urethral lengthening: reimplantation and enterocystoplasty. *J Urol* 1991;146:535–538.
178. Lloyd LK, Kuhlemeier KV, Fine PR, Stover SL. Initial bladder management in spinal cord injury: does it make a difference? *J Urol* 1986;135:523–527.
179. Maynard FM, Diokno AC. Urinary infection and complications during clean intermittent catheterization following spinal cord injury. *J Urol* 1984;132:94–946.
180. Romano JM, Kaye D. UTI in the elderly: common yet atypical. *Geriatrics* 1981;36(6):113–120.
181. Kass EH. The role of asymptomatic bacteriuria in the pathogenesis of pyelonephritis. In: Quinn EL, Kass EH, eds. *Biology of pyelonephritis.* Boston: Little, Brown & Co, 1960:399–418.
182. Stamey TA. Recurrent urinary tract infections in female patients: an overview of management and treatment. *Rev Infect Dis* 1987;9[Suppl 2]:S195–S210.
183. Stamm WE, Counts GW, Running KR, et al. Diagnosis of coliform infection in acutely dysuric women. *N Engl J Med* 1982;307:463–468.
184. Rhame FS, Perkash I. Urinary tract infections occurring in recent spinal cord injury patients on intermittent catheterization. *J Urol* 1979;122:669–673.

185. Donovan WH, Stolov WC, Clowers DE, Clowers MR. Bacteriuria during intermittent catheterization following spinal cord injury. *Arch Phys Med Rehabil* 1978;59:351–357.

186. National Institute on Disabilities and Rehabilitation Research. The prevention and management of urinary tract infections among people with spinal cord injuries. National Institute on Disabilities and Rehabilitation Research, Consensus Conference Statement, January 27–29, 1992. *J Am Paraplegia Soc* 1992;15:194–204.

187. Deresinski SC, Perkash I. Urinary tract infections in male spinal cord injured patients: part 2. Diagnostic value of symptoms and of quantitative urinalysis. *J Am Paraplegia Soc* 1985;8:7–10.

188. Anderson RU, Hsieh-ma ST. Association of bacteriuria and pyuria during intermittent catheterization after spinal cord injury. *J Urol* 1983;130:299–301.

189. Kass EJ, Koff SA, Diokno AC, Lapides J. The significance of bacilluria in children on long term intermittent catheterization. *J Urol* 1981;126:223–225.

190. Lewis RI, Carrion HM, Lockhart JL, Politano VA. Significance of asymptomatic bacteriuria in neurogenic bladder disease. *Urology* 1984;23:343–347.

191. Tempkin A, Sullivan G, Paldi J, Perkash I. Radioisotope renography in spinal cord injury. *J Urol* 1985;133:228–230.

192. Kuhlemeier KV, Stover SL, Lloyd LK. Prophylactic antibacterial therapy for preventing urinary tract infections in spinal cord injury patients. *J Urol* 1985;134:514–517.

193. Merritt JLM, Erickson RP, Opitz JL. Bacteriuria during follow up in patients with spinal cord injury: Part II. Efficacy of antimicrobial suppressants. *Arch Phys Med Rehabil* 1982;63:413–415.

194. DeVivo MJ, Fine PR, Cutter GR, Maetz HM. The risk of bladder calculi in patients with spinal cord injuries. *Arch Intern Med* 1985;145:428–430.

195. Cardenas D, Farrell-Roberts L., Sipski M, Rubner D. Management of gastrointestinal, genitourinary and sexual function. In Stover SL, DeLisa JA, Whiteneck GG, eds. *Spinal cord injury clinical outcomes from the model systems.* Gaithersburg, MD: Aspen Publications, 1995:129–130.

196. Park YI, Linsenmeyer TA. A method to minimize catheter calcification and bladder stones in individuals with spinal cord injury. *J Spinal Cord Med* 2001; 24(2):105–108.

197. West DA, Cummings JM, Longo WE, et al. Role of chronic catheterization in the development of bladder cancer in patients with spinal cord injury. *Urology* 1999;53(2); 292–297.

198. Kaufman JM, Fam B, Jacobs SC, et al. Bladder cancer and squamous metaplasia in spinal cord injury patients. *J Urol* 1977;118:967–971.

199. Price M, Kottke FJ. Renal function in patients with spinal cord injury: the eighth year of a ten year continuing study. *Arch Phys Med Rehabil* 1975;56: 76–79.

200. Fellows GJ, Silver JR. Long term follow up of paraplegic patients with vesico-ureteric reflux. *Paraplegia* 1976;14:130–134.

201. Winberg J. Urinary tract infections in infants and children. In: Walsh PC, Gittes RF, Perlmutter AD, Stamey TA, eds. *Campbell's urology,* 5th ed. Philadelphia: WB Saunders, 1986:848–867.

202. DeVivo MJ, Fine PR. Predicting renal calculus occurrence in spinal cord injury patients. *Arch Phys Med Rehabil* 1986;67:722–775.

203. Kuhlemeier KV, Lloyd LK, Stover SL. Long term followup of renal function after spinal cord injury. *J Urol* 1985;134:510–513.

204. Singh M, Chapman R, Tresidder GC, Blandy J. Fate of unoperated staghorn calculus. *Br J Urol* 1973;45:581–585.

205. Irwin PP, Evans C, Chawla JC, Matthews PN. Stone surgery in the spinal patient. *Paraplegia* 1991;29:161–166.

206. Rodman JS, Williams JJ, Peterson CM. Partial dissolution of struvite calculus with oral acetohydroxamic acid. *Urology* 1983;22:410–412.

207. Gillenwater JY. Hydronephrosis. In: Gillenwater JY, Grayhack JT, Howards SS, Duckett JW, eds. *Adult and pediatric urology,* 2nd ed. St. Louis: Mosby Year Book, 1991:789–813.

208. Staskin DR. Hydroureteronephrosis after spinal cord injury. *Urol Clin North Am* 1991;18:309–316.

209. Teague N, Boyarsky S. Further effects of coliform bacteria on ureteral peristalsis. *J Urol* 1968;99:720–724.

210. Spinal Cord Consortium. Acute management of autonomic dysreflexia in individuals with spinal cord injury presenting to health care facilities. *J Spinal Cord Med* 2002;25[Suppl 1]: 67–88.

211. Stiens S, Fajardo N, Korsten M. The gastrointestinal system after spinal cord injury. In: Lin VW, ed. *Spinal cord medicine,* 1st ed. New York: Demos, 2002: 549–570.

212. Stiens SA, Bergman SB, Goetz LL. Neurogenic bowel dysfunction after spinal cord injury: clinical evaluation and rehabilitative management. *Arch Phys Med Rehabil* 1997;78:S86–102.

213. Moonka R, Steins SA, Resnick WJ et al. The prevalence and natural history of gallstones in spinal cord injured patients. *J Am Coll Surg* 1999;189:274–281.

214. Moonka R, Stiens S, Eubank W, Stelzner, M. The presentation of gallstones and results of biliary surgery in a spinal cord injured population. *Am J Surg* 1999;178:246–250.

215. Nobel D, Baumberger M, Eser P, et al. Nontraumatic pancreatitis in spinal cord injury. *Spine* 2002;27(9):E228–232.

216. Wald, A. Colonic and anorectal motility testing in clinical practice. *Am J Gastroenterol* 1994;89:2109–2115.

217. Smout A.J. Manometry of the gastrointestinal tract: toy or tool? *Scand J Gastroenterol Suppl* 2001;234:22–28.

218. Bassotti G, Clementi M, Pelli MA, Tonini M. Low-amplitude propagated contractile waves: a relevant propulsive mechanism of the human colon. *Dig Liver Dis* 2001;33(1):36–40.

219. Fajardo N, Hussain K, Korsten M. Prolonged ambulatory colonic manometric studies using endoclips. *Gastrointestinal Endoscopy* 2000;51:199–201.

220. Arhan P, Devroede G, Jehannin B, et al. Segmental colonic transit time. *Dis Col Rectum* 1981;24:625–629.

221. Harari D, Minaker KL. Megacolon in patients with chronic spinal cord injury. *Spinal Cord* 2000;38:331–339.

222. Duthie HL, Watts JM. Contribution of the external anal sphincter to the pressure zone in the anal canal. *Gut* 1965;6:64–68.

223. Frenckner B. Function of the anal sphincters in spinal man. *Gut* 1975;16:638–644.

224. Parks A, Porter N, Melzack J. Experimental study of the reflex mechanism controlling the muscles of the pelvic floor. *Dis Colon Rectum* 1962;5: 407–414.

225. Madoff R, Williams J, Caushaj P. Fecal incontinence. *N Engl J Med* 1992;326: 1002–1007.

226. Schweiger M. Method for determining individual contributions of voluntary and involuntary anal sphincters to resting tone. *Dis Colon Rectum* 1979; 22:415–416.

227. Wallace W, Madden W. Partial puborectalis resection: a new surgical technique for anorectal dysfunction. *South Med J* 1969;62:1121–1126.

228. Bannister J, Gibbons C, Read N. Preservation of fecal continence during rises in intraabdominal pressure: is there a role for the flap valve? *Gut* 1987; 28:1242–1245.

229. Ambroze W, Bell A, Pemberton J, et al. The effect of stool consistency on rectal and neorectal emptying. *Gastroenterology* 1989;96[Suppl 5]:A11.

230. Findlay J, Smith A, Mitchell W, et al. Effects of unprocessed bran on colon function in normal subjects and in diverticular disease. *Lancet* 1974;1:146.

231. Cummings J. Constipation, dietary fibre and the control of large bowel function. *Postgrad Med J* 1984;60:811–819.

232. Bond J, Currier B, Buchwald H, Levitt M. Colonic conservation of malabsorbed carbohydrate. *J Gastroenterol* 1980;78:444–449.

233. Flynn M, Hammond P, Darby C, et al Faecal bile acids and the irritable colon syndrome. *Digestion* 1981;22:144–149.

234. Goyal R, Crist J. Neurology of the gut. In: Sleisenger MH, Fordtran JS, eds. *Gastrointestinal disease: pathophysiology, diagnosis, management,* 4th ed. Philadelphia: WB Saunders 1989:21–47.

235. Furness J, Costa M. Types of nerves in the enteric nervous system. *Neuroscience* 1980;5:1–20.

236. Devroede G, Arhan P, Duguay C, et al. Traumatic constipation. *Gastroenterology* 1979;77:1258–1267.

237. Graffner H, Ekelund M, Hakanson R, et al. Effects of upper abdominal sympathectomy on gastric acid, serum gastrin, and catecholamines in the rat gut. *Scand J Gastroenterol* 1984;19:711–716.

238. Lluis F, Thompson JC. Neuroendocrine potential of the colon and rectum. *Gastroenterology* 1988;94(3):832–844.

239. Menardo G, Bausano G, Corazziari E, et al. Large-bowel transit in paraplegic patients. *Dis Colon Rectum* 1987;30:924–928.

240. Nino-Murcia M, Stone JM, Chang PJ, Perkash I. Colonic transit in spinal cord-injured patients. *Invest Radiol* 1990;25:109–112.

241. Kellow J, Gill R. Wingate D. Modulation of human upper gastrointestinal motility by rectal distention. *Gut* 1987;28:864–868.

242. Kreulen D, Szurszewski, J. Reflex pathways in the abdominal prevertebral ganglia. evidence for the colo-colonic inhibitory reflex. *J Physiol* 1979;295: 21–32.

243. Connell A, Frankel H, Guttman L. The motility of the pelvic colon following complete lesions of the spinal cord. *Paraplegia* 1963;1:98–115.

244. Aaronson, MJ, Freed MM, Burakoff R. Colonic myoelectric activity in persons with spinal cord injury. *Dig Dis Sci* 1985;30:295–300.

245. Glick ME, Haldeman S, Meshkinpour H. The neurovisceral and electrodiagnostic evaluation of patients with thoracic spinal cord injury. *Paraplegia* 1986;24:129–137.

246. Consortium for Spinal Cord Medicine. Clinical Practice Guideline: Neurogenic bowel management in adults with spinal cord injury. *J Spinal Cord Med* 1998;21:248–293.

247. Roach MJ, Frost FS, Creasey G. Social and personal consequences of acquired bowel 2000;23:263–269.

248. Rasmussen O. Anorectal function . *Dis Colon Rectum* 1994;37 :386–403.

249. Read N, Timms J. Defecation and the pathophysiology of constipation. *Clin Gastroenterol* 1986;15:937–965.

250. Barkel D, Pemberton J, Pezim M, et al. Scintigraphic assessment of the anorectal angle in health and after ileal pouch—anal anastomosis. *Ann Surg* 1988;208:42–49.

251. Sun WM, MacDonagh, R, Forster D, et al. Anorectal unction in patients with complete spinal transection before and after sacral posterior rhizotomy. *Gastroenterology* 1995;108:990–998.

252. Suckling P. The ball-valve rectum due to impacted feces. *Lancet* 1962;2:1147.

253. Adams R, Victor M. Neurologic disorders caused by lesions in particular parts of the cerebrum. *Principles of neurology,* 4th ed. New York: McGraw-Hill 1989:347–376.

254. Weber J, Denis P, Mihout B, et al. Effect of brain-stem lesion on colonic and anorectal motility: study of three patients. *Dig Dis Sci* 1985;30:419–25.

255. Walter A, Morren GL, Ryn AK, Hallbook O. Rectal pressure response to a meal in patients with high spinal cord injury. *Arch Phys Med Rehabil* 2003;84: 108–110.

256. Glickman S, Kamm M. Bowel dysfunction in spinal cord injured patients. *Lancet* 1996;347:1651–1653.

257. Stone J, Nino-Murcia M, Wolfe V, Perkash I. Chronic gastrointestinal problems in spinal cord injury patients: a prospective analysis. *Am J Gastroenterol* 1990;85:1114–1149.

258. Pfeifer J, Agachan F, Wexner S. Surgery for constipation: a review. *Dis Colon Rectum* 1996;39:444–460.

259. Shandling B, Gilmore R. The enema continence catheter in spina bifida: successful bowel management. *J Pediatr Surg* 1987;22:271–273.

260. Yang C, Stiens S. Antegrade continence enema for the treatment of neurogenic constipation and fecal incontinence after spinal cord injury. *Arch Phys Med Rehabil* 2000;81:683–685.

261. Stone JM, Wolfe VA, Nino-Murcia M, Perkash I. Colostomy as treatment for complications of spinal cord injury. *Arch Phys Med Rehabil* 1990;71:514–518.

262. Saltzstein R, Romano J. The efficacy of colostomy as a bowel management alternative in selected spinal cord injured patients. *J Am Paraplegia Society* 1990;13:9–13.

263. Kirk PM, King RB, TEMPLE R. Long term followup of bowel management after spinal cord injury. SCI Nursing 1997;14:556–563.

264. Rosito O, Nino-Murcia M, Wolfe VA, et al. The effects of colostomy on the quality of life in patients with spinal cord injury: a retrospective analysis. *J Spinal Cord Injury Nursing* 2002;25(3):174–183.

265. Saltzstein R, Romano J. The efficacy of colostomy as a bowel management alternative in selected spinal cord injured patients. *J Am Paraplegia Society* 1990;13:9–13.

266. Cameron KJ, Nyulasi IB, Collier GR, Brown DJ. Assessment of the effect of increased dietary fibre intake on bowel function in patients with spinal cord injury. *Spinal Cord* 1996;34:277–283.

267. Stiens SA, Pidde T, Veland B. *Accidents stink!: bowel care 202* (a 50-minute film), PMRSECRETS.com, 2002.

268. Stiens S. Reduction in bowel program duration with polyethylene glycol based bisacodyl suppositories. *Arch Phys Med Rehabil* 1995;76:674–677.

269. House J, Stiens S. Pharmacologically initiated defecation for persons with spinal cord injury: effectiveness of three agents. *Arch Phys Med Rehab* 1997;78:1062–1065.

270. Yim SY, Yoon SH, Lee IY, et al. A comparison of bowel care patterns in patients with spinal cord injury: upper motor neuron bowel vs lower motor neuron bowel. *Spinal Cord* 2001;39(4):204–207.

CHAPTER 77

Stroke Rehabilitation

Murray E. Brandstater

DEFINITION

A stroke is a clinical syndrome characterized by the sudden development of a persisting focal neurologic deficit. *Stroke* is a useful clinical term, its abrupt or rapid onset implying its vascular pathogenesis. A clinical diagnosis of stroke excludes nonvascular causes of focal brain deficits, such as seizure, brain tumor, encephalitis, abscess, trauma, or syncope, all of which represent important differential diagnoses of stroke. The expression *cerebrovascular accident* or *CVA* has been used interchangeably with the term *stroke,* but its use is discouraged. Both terms convey the same information, but CVA is often a source of confusion (does a right CVA describe the lesion location or the clinical deficit?). *Stroke* is a useful term for general description of events secondary to cerebrovascular disease, but, like CVA, it is not specific enough to use as a formal, medical diagnosis. For individual patient description, a pathologic diagnosis should be made, such as cerebral infarction or cerebral hemorrhage.

The focal brain lesions encountered in patients with stroke produce a wide variety of neurologic deficits, such as hemiplegia, hemisensory loss, aphasia, hemianopia, etc., the specific clinical signs in each case reflecting the anatomic site of the lesion. The size and extent of the lesion determine the severity of the deficits, which in rehabilitation medicine are referred to as *impairments.* The objectives of stroke rehabilitation are to achieve a maximum level of functional independence; minimize disability; successfully reintegrate back into home, family, and community; and reestablish a meaningful and gratifying life. These goals are accomplished through therapy to reduce impairments; functional training to compensate for residual impairments; and use of assistive devices, such as braces or wheelchair, to substitute for lost function. Successful rehabilitation also requires resolution of the many psychosocial issues that surround integration of the patient back to home and community.

EPIDEMIOLOGY

Stroke is the most common serious neurologic disorder in the United States, comprising half of all patients admitted to hospital for a neurologic disease. It is the third leading cause of death after heart disease and cancer. The incidence of stroke in the 1960s was reported at around 200 per 100,000 population, or approximately 500,000 to 700,000 new cases per year in the United States. A decline in the overall incidence was noted late in the 1960s and 1970s to levels around 115/100,000, but this decline flattened out in the 1980s. There may have been a small rise in incidence since then. Incidence is age related, being uncommon before age 50 but doubling each decade after age 55. After the age of 80, the incidence of stroke may be as high as 2,500/100,000. The decline in incidence in the 1970s was probably attributable in most part to improved management of hypertension in the general population (1). Stroke is more common in men.

Most patients who die from acute stroke succumb in the first 30 days. The overall 30-day survival following a new stroke is reported to be 70% to 85%, survival being largely dependent on stroke type. The 30-day survival of patients with intracerebral hemorrhage is between 20% and 50%, most of the deaths occurring in the first 3 days. The 30-day survival of patients with cerebral infarction is approximately 85%. Death during the first few days following onset is usually attributed to cerebral causes, especially transtentorial herniation, but pneumonia, pulmonary embolism, and cardiac conditions contribute to the 30-day mortality. After the initial 30 days, the death rate declines. The overall mortality from stroke is declining, reflecting better risk-factor reduction and hence lower incidence and better medical management of patients during the acute phase. It should be noted that long-term survival poststroke is improving, so that despite reduced incidence, prevalence of stroke in the population has stayed the same or has increased.

RISK FACTORS AND PREVENTION

There is only limited potential for successful medical treatment to reverse the neurologic sequelae of a completed stroke; therefore, interventions aimed at stroke prevention are extremely important. The following is a summary of risk factors for stroke and a description of opportunities for stroke prevention. Age, race, sex, and family history are all important biological indicators of enhanced stroke susceptibility, but these are inherent characteristics and cannot be altered. The following discussion focuses on those other risk factors that are modifiable, listed in Table 77-1.

TABLE 77-1. Modifiable Risk Factors for Stroke

Hypertension
Heart disease
    Ischemic/hypertensive
    Valvular
    Arrhythmias
Smoking
Diabetes mellitus
Elevated fibrinogen
Erythrocytosis
Hyperlipidemia

Modifiable Risk Factors in Asymptomatic Patients

Hypertension is the most important risk factor. The degree of risk increases with higher levels of pressure and becomes particularly strong with levels higher than 160/95 mm Hg. Systolic hypertension and high mean arterial pressure represent parallel risks. In the Framingham Study, a sevenfold increased risk of cerebral infarction was observed in patients who were hypertensive (2). Hypertension increases the risk of thrombotic, lacunar, and hemorrhagic stroke and increases the likelihood of subarachnoid hemorrhage. Successful long-term treatment of hypertension greatly reduces the risk of these events. Every effort should be made to diagnose hypertension early and establish adequate blood pressure control before the secondary changes of hypertensive vascular disease develop. Treatment of late hypertension, e.g., after an individual has sustained a stroke, is much less effective in reducing risk of future events.

Heart disease is an important risk factor for stroke. To some degree, this reflects the common underlying precursors of stroke and heart disease: hypertension and atherosclerosis. The risk of stroke is doubled in individuals who have coronary artery disease (3), and coronary artery disease accounts for the majority of subsequent deaths among stroke survivors. Atrial fibrillation and valvular heart disease increase the risk of cerebral infarction because both may cause cerebral emboli. In patients with chronic, stable atrial fibrillation, the risk of stroke is increased fivefold (4). When atrial fibrillation is a manifestation of rheumatic heart disease, the risk of embolic stroke is increased up to 17 times normal (4). Prevention of embolic stroke in these patients is best achieved by long-term anticoagulation with warfarin. Treatment carries the danger of intracranial hemorrhage, especially in elderly individuals and in those with impaired balance and who are likely to fall. When the risk of hemorrhage appears to be high, aspirin in a dose of 325 mg daily may be used as an alternative to warfarin in patients with nonvalvular atrial fibrillation, although aspirin is much less effective than warfarin in preventing embolism.

Diabetes, as an independent risk factor, doubles the risk of stroke. Unfortunately, good blood sugar control does not seem to slow the progression of cerebrovascular disease.

Smoking has been shown to increase the risk of stroke about 1.5 times (1.9 times for cerebral infarction) (5). There is clear evidence that smoking cessation reduces the risk of cerebral infarction in addition to reducing the risk of myocardial infarction and sudden death.

Hyperlipidemia poses only a small additional risk for stroke, mainly for individuals younger than age of 55. Elevated low-density lipoprotein (LDL) cholesterol is an important risk factor for ischemic heart disease, and it is therefore recommended that all patients with cerebrovascular disease and elevated LDL cholesterol should be treated to reduce serum LDL levels.

Elevated fibrinogen levels correlate with higher risk of stroke, and it should be noted that fibrinogen levels are higher in individuals who smoke and have a high-cholesterol diet. A *raised hematocrit* increases the risk of stroke. It is unproven whether reducing the hematocrit lessens the risk for stroke. Elevated serum levels of *homocystine* are associated with premature atherosclerosis, causing stroke, myocardial infarction, and peripheral vascular disease earlier in life. Homocysteinemia can be treated with daily high dose vitamin therapy, including vitamin B_6 (pyridoxine) and folic acid.

Risk Factors in Symptomatic Patients

Transient ischemic attacks (TIAs) and minor stroke are important warning signals of an impending completed stroke. In the first month after onset of TIAs, 4% to 8% of patients will develop a completed stroke, and the risk is 30% in the next 5 years (6,7). Patients with recent onset of TIAs should be treated in an attempt to prevent a stroke. The most widely accepted intervention is prescription of daily antiplatelet drugs, such as aspirin (7). Several clinical trials have reported a reduced incidence of stroke of 20% to 25% using low- and high-dose daily aspirin. There is some controversy about the optimal dose of aspirin, but at present there is no evidence to indicate that a dose higher than 325 mg daily is more efficacious (7).

Ticlopidine is an antiplatelet drug with a different action from aspirin, and it has comparable and perhaps slightly more beneficial effect on stroke risk reduction. However, it is expensive and has side effects (diarrhea, neutropenia), which may diminish its value compared with aspirin (7). Clopidogrel is another antiplatelet agent similar to ticlopidine. In clinical trials, its efficacy in preventing stroke is slightly (7%) better than aspirin. It has few side effects. Another agent, dipyridamole, is about as effective as aspirin when taken alone, but it has an added benefit when taken in combination with aspirin. In a large European trial, there was a 37% reduction in risk of stroke in patients prescribed both aspirin and dipyridamole (8). Anticoagulants have been used to prevent stroke in patients with recent-onset TIAs, but no clinical trial has shown that treatment with warfarin is better than placebo. Warfarin is not recommended unless the patient has a major cardiac source of potential embolism.

Carotid endarterectomy has reduced the risk of stroke in those patients with single or multiple TIAs and with 70% or greater stenosis of the ipsilateral internal carotid artery (9). Patients with stenosis of 50% to 70% do not have a hemodynamically significant lesion but may be considered for surgery if symptomatic, i.e., they are having TIAs ipsilateral to the carotid lesion. Carotid endarterectomy has still not been proven superior to medical treatment in asymptomatic patients (10).

Risk Factors for Recurrent Stroke

The probability of stroke recurrence is highest in the postacute period. For survivors of an initial stroke, the annual risk of a second stroke is approximately 5%, with a 5-year cumulative risk of recurrence around 25% (11,12), although it may be as high as 42% (11). Risk factors for initial stroke also increase the risk of recurrence, especially hypertension, heart disease, and diabetes mellitus (13,14). Heavy alcohol consumption is also a risk factor for recurrent stroke. As a risk factor, hypertension is more important for an initial than a recurrent stroke, probably because stroke occurrence depends more on the duration of elevated hypertension than on the current level of blood pressure. By the time a first stroke occurs, widespread hypertensive vascular damage is already present and will predispose to recurrent stroke even after blood pressure has been controlled. The beneficial effects of therapeutic blood pressure control are seen only after some years through delay or prevention of hypertensive vascular disease. Treatment of severe hypertension in patients who have had a stroke reduces rate of recurrence, but in patients with mild or moderate hypertension, treatment has little effect on rate of recurrent stroke. However, treatment of mild to moderate hypertension is still recommended because successful control reduces the incidence of cardiovascular complications, such as congestive heart failure and myocardial infarction, and therefore prolongs survival.

Many authors have reported on the high mortality of stroke survivors. Reported 5-year cumulative mortality rates depend on the presence of risk factors. Patients with a stroke who have hypertension and cardiac symptoms have only a 25% chance of surviving 5 years. Patients with one of these risk factors have a 50% chance of surviving 5 years, and those without heart disease and without hypertension have a 75% chance of surviving 5 years (12). Leonberg and Elliott (13) were able to achieve 16% reduction in stroke recurrence rate by an energetic and sustained program of control of multiple risk factors. Therefore, efforts should be made to reduce risk of recurrent stroke and mortality through controlling risk factors. The risk of recurrent embolism is reduced by anticoagulation in patients with atrial fibrillation or valvular disease.

CLINICAL PROFILES

Transient Ischemic Attacks

TIAs reflect focal areas of retinal or cerebral ischemia of sufficient duration to cause neurologic symptoms and signs. The ischemia is brief and does not persist long enough to develop a functionally significant cerebral infarction. The symptoms of a TIA begin abruptly, and they may persist for only a few seconds or minutes, finally resolving without any sequelae. By definition, all clinical features of a TIA resolve within 24 hours. A TIA may occur as an isolated event, or it may recur quite frequently, sometimes many times a day. The nature of the symptoms evoked by the TIA usually permits its localization into the distribution of the right or left carotid artery, or the vertebrobasilar system. Recurrent TIAs may be benign, and spontaneously stop, but in as many as 30% of patients, a functionally significant stroke will develop within 5 years (7).

Usually TIAs are caused by microembolism of small platelet aggregates from ulcerated atherosclerotic plaques in large extracranial arteries, or from myocardium or cardiac valves. The small platelet emboli cause symptoms by occluding small blood vessels in the brain or retina before fragmenting enough to allow resumption of blood flow. Alternatively, a TIA may have a hemodynamic basis. Fluctuations in cardiac output or systemic arterial pressure may cause critical hypoperfusion distal to atherosclerotic stenosis of the large extracranial vessels. Cerebral hypoperfusion under these conditions would result in brief and self-limited neurologic symptoms and signs.

Cerebral Thrombosis

Thrombosis of the large extracranial and intracranial vessels occurs on the basis of atherosclerotic cerebrovascular disease and accounts for approximately 30% of all cases of stroke (Table 77-2) (14). Atherosclerotic plaques are particularly prominent in the large vessels of the neck and at the base of the brain. Occlusion of one of these large vessels, in the absence of good collateral channels, usually results in a large brain infarc-

TABLE 77-2. Causes of Stroke

Cause	%
Large vessel occlusion/infarction	32
Embolism	32
Small vessel occlusion, lacunar	18
Intracerebral hemorrhage	11
Subarachnoid hemorrhage	7

tion. Atherosclerosis is accelerated by hypertension, diabetes, and other risk factors. Following arterial thrombosis, the volume of infarcted brain depends on the rate at which the vessel becomes occluded and the adequacy of the collateral circulation. A large vessel such as the internal carotid artery may slowly become stenotic and finally occlude without causing clinical signs or infarction if the slowly progressive stenosis had stimulated the development of sufficient collateral circulation prior to its occlusion.

A thrombotic occlusion occurs most commonly at night during sleep or during periods of inactivity. Often patients only become aware that they have weakness or other impairment when they attempt to get out of bed. The extent of the clinical deficit usually worsens over some hours or several days, then stabilizes, with clinical improvement generally beginning after 7 days postonset. Progression of neurologic deficits in the first several days following a thrombotic stroke is frequently observed and is due to several factors, particularly development of surrounding cerebral edema and alterations in perfusion and metabolism in tissue adjacent to the infarction. With large infarctions, edema may be severe enough to cause brain displacement, herniation, and death.

Cerebral Embolism

Embolism is responsible for about 30% of all cases of stroke. Emboli may arise from thrombi in the heart, or on heart valves or the large extracranial arteries (Table 77-3). Thrombi develop at different sites, such as the endocardium in the region of a recent myocardial infarction, an area of myocardial hypokinesis, the atrium associated with fibrillation, or on diseased or prosthetic values. The clinical neurologic deficit from a cerebral embolus has an abrupt onset that is due to sudden loss of arterial perfusion to a focal area of the brain. The distribution of emboli is not random, being much more common in the middle cerebral artery territory. The embolus is friable and usually undergoes lysis, with fragments lodging in the distal branches of the main vessel. The occlusion of these small cortical vessels results in characteristic, wedge-shaped, superficial cortical in-

TABLE 77-3. Sources of Cerebral Embolism

Cardiac
- Atrial fibrillation, other arrhythmias
- Mural thrombus—recent MI, hypokinesis, cardiomyopathy
- Bacterial endocarditis
- Valve prosthesis
- Nonbacterial valve vegetations
- Atrial myxoma

Large artery
- Atherosclerosis of aorta and carotid arteries

Paradoxical
- Peripheral venous embolism with R-to-L cardiac shunt

farctions seen on brain imaging studies. They are often multiple. However, large vessel occlusions do occur and may involve the carotid or vertebrobasilar circulation.

The initial clinical deficit may change rapidly. With lysis and fragmentation of the embolus, the neurologic signs may fade rapidly. Alternatively, reperfusion of an area of brain infarction may cause arterial bleeding into the lesion. This may, but not always, worsen the neurologic picture. Because of the risk of hemorrhagic transformation of a large embolic infarction, which usually occurs within 48 hours, anticoagulant therapy is usually delayed at least for 2 to 3 days. The risk of hemorrhage from immediate anticoagulation must be weighed against delay in starting therapy. Without anticoagulation, the risk of recurrent embolism is 12% in 2 weeks.

Although emboli commonly affect the elderly, they represent an important cause of stroke in younger adults. It is important for the clinician to recognize that a cerebral infarction is due to embolism because the risk of recurrence can be greatly reduced by long-term anticoagulation. Diagnosis may be difficult in some cases, for example, when all of a mural cardiac thrombus embolizes, leaving no residual thrombus. The echocardiogram in such a case would not show a mural thrombus, although other features suggesting the possibility of thrombus may be present, such as heart dilatation, hypokinetic myocardial segment, acute ischemic electrocardiogram changes, or atrial fibrillation.

Lacunar Stroke

Lacunar lesions constitute approximately 20% of all strokes. They are small, circumscribed lesions, at most 1.5 cm in diameter and frequently much smaller. They represent occlusions in the deep penetrating branches of the large vessels which perfuse the subcortical structures, including internal capsule, basal ganglia, thalamus, and brain stem. Small lacunar infarcts may produce major neurologic deficits if they are strategically located, but in general, the associated deficits are less than those with a large vessel thrombosis, and lacunar infarctions may even occur without overt symptoms. Lacunar lesions are noteworthy because of their earlier, more rapid, and greater degree of neurologic recovery.

The arteries involved in lacunar lesions are small-diameter branches of the middle cerebral artery called lenticulostriate arteries and comparably small penetrating branches of the anterior cerebral, posterior cerebral, and basilar arteries. The disease process affecting these small vessels may involve micro-atheroma, but very commonly the pathology is different, with progressive vessel wall thickening and fibrinoid necrosis, especially in patients with hypertension and diabetes. The clinical features associated with lacunar strokes are often mixed and difficult to distinguish, frequently because the lesions may be multiple. However, several characteristic lesions have been recognized, and these are described below.

Cerebral Hemorrhage

Intracerebral hemorrhage accounts for 11% of all cases of stroke. Spontaneous intracerebral hemorrhage most commonly occurs at the site of small, deep, penetrating arteries, the same vessels responsible for lacunar stroke if they undergo occlusion rather than hemorrhage. It is thought that hemorrhage occurs through rupture of microaneurysms (Charcot–Bouchard aneurysms) that develop in these vessels in hypertensive patients. The majority of lesions occur in the putamen or thalamus, and in about 10% of patients, the spontaneous hemorrhage occurs in the cerebellum.

TABLE 77-4. Causes of Intracranial Hemorrhage
Primary intracerebral hemorrhage
Ruptured saccular aneurysm
Ruptured arteriovenous malformation
Trauma
Cerebral infarction
Brain tumor
Amyloid angiopathy
Hemorrhagic disorders: leukemia, thrombocytopenia, anticoagulant therapy

The clinical onset of the hemorrhage is usually dramatic, with an otherwise fit patient abruptly developing a severe headache and major neurologic deficits within minutes. In many patients, consciousness becomes progressively impaired, with coma developing rapidly. Brain displacement from the hematoma and cerebral edema may give rise to transtentorial herniation and death within the first 2 to 3 days. Mortality rates of patients with this type of clinical presentation are high, more than 80%. The initial deficits may partially be secondary to edema and brain displacement rather than large volumes of tissue disruption from the arterial bleeding, and the degree of functional recovery may be surprisingly good.

Spontaneous intracerebral hemorrhage is a well-recognized complication of anticoagulant therapy, especially when prothrombin times are maintained at the upper level of the therapeutic range or in a patient who falls and sustains a head injury. Other causes of intracerebral hemorrhage include trauma, vasculitis, and bleeding into a tumor (Table 77-4). Patients with a bleeding diathesis—for example, thrombocytopenia or coagulation disorders—may develop an intracranial hemorrhage. Cerebral amyloid angiopathy is an unusual cause of hemorrhage in the elderly. The lesions in this disorder tend to be superficial and recurrent.

Patients with acute hemorrhages in the cerebellum develop a sudden headache and inability to stand, along with nausea, vomiting, and vertigo. With large posterior fossa lesions, the hematoma and edema may occlude cerebrospinal fluid (CSF) flow, causing acute hydrocephalus. Rapid death can be prevented by urgent evacuation of the hematoma in what is a true medical emergency. Patients who survive surgical evacuation of a cerebellar hemorrhage, or who have a less severe lesion, usually make a good functional recovery.

Subarachnoid Hemorrhage

In about 7% of all stroke patients, the lesion is a subarachnoid hemorrhage, usually resulting from rupture of an arterial aneurysm at the base of the brain with bleeding into the subarachnoid space. Aneurysms develop from small defects in the wall of the arteries and slowly increase in size. Eventually they develop a tendency to bleed in midlife. Major rupture of an aneurysm may be preceded by headache from a small bleed or by localized cranial nerve lesions caused by direct pressure by the aneurysm. When rupture occurs, the clinical onset is usually dramatically abrupt. There is severe headache followed by vomiting and signs of meningeal irritation. Focal signs are usually not observed initially but may develop as a result of associated intracerebral bleeding or cerebral infarction occurring as a complication of arterial vasospasm. Coma frequently occurs, and as many as one-third of patients may die acutely. Rebleeding is unfortunately very common, especially in the first 2 to 3 weeks following the initial episode. Within 6 months, 50% of surviving patients will rebleed. The rate of rebleeding in late survivors is 3% per year. Therefore, early surgical intervention has become routine, with the objective of ligation of the aneurysm to prevent recurrent hemorrhage, which is usually fatal. Blood in the subarachnoid space may cause arterial vasospasm, leading to localized areas of cerebral infarction with associated focal neurologic deficits. Hydrocephalus may develop several weeks after the acute event as a result of arachnoiditis from blood in the CSF. Successful surgical clipping of an aneurysm is curative. If the patient has not developed focal deficits or an encephalopathy, there may be total clinical cure.

Subarachnoid hemorrhage may also result from bleeding from an arteriovenous malformation (AVM), which is a tangle of dilated vessels found on the surface of the brain or within the brain parenchyma. These lesions are congenital abnormalities and tend to bleed in childhood or young adulthood. In about half the cases, the hemorrhage is the first clinical indication of the lesion. In approximately one-third of patients, the AVM presents as a seizure disorder or with chronic headaches. In most patients, the lesions eventually bleed. Most patients survive a single hemorrhagic event. The rate of rebleeding is about 6% in the first year and 2% to 3% per year thereafter. The treatment of choice is surgical excision of the AVM or neurovascular ablation through embolization. Irradiation with proton-beam therapy to destroy the lesion has become an attractive alternative to surgery (15).

LESION LOCALIZATION

The pathology of the lesion can be surmised from an analysis of the temporal profile of the clinical presentation, i.e., the history, along with the progression and pattern of recovery of the lesion. Anatomic localization of a lesion can usually be established with reasonable accuracy based on a careful delineation of the neurologic deficits. A complete picture of the neurologic deficits may not be possible initially if the patient is confused and unable to cooperate fully with the examination. Therefore, repeat examinations of the patient in the early recovery phase help to further define the combination of deficits and assist in establishing the precise localization of the lesion. The following discussion describes in some detail the typical features observed in patients with commonly encountered focal stroke syndromes.

Internal Carotid Artery Syndrome

The most minor clinical deficits associated with internal carotid artery ischemia are TIAs caused by microembolic platelet aggregates carried peripherally from atherosclerotic plaques in the internal carotid or other large arteries. Transient occlusion of the retinal branches of an ophthalmic artery produces sudden, transient loss of vision in one eye, the amaurosis fugax syndrome. Cerebral TIAs take the form of brief motor, sensory, or language deficits.

The clinical consequences of complete occlusion of an internal carotid artery vary from no observable clinical deficit if there is good collateral circulation to massive cerebral infarction in the distribution of the anterior and middle cerebral arteries with rapid severe obtundation, with head and eyes turned toward the side of the lesion and dense contralateral motor and sensory deficits. There is often cerebral edema with transtentorial herniation and death. Less extensive infarctions result in partial or total lesions in the distribution of the middle cerebral artery. The anterior cerebral circulation may be preserved through flow from the opposite side via the anterior communicating artery. The first branch of the internal carotid artery is the ophthalmic, and if there is inadequate collateral flow through the orbit from the external carotid artery, there may be ipsilateral blindness from retinal ischemia on the side of the lesion associated with contralateral hemiplegia.

Middle Cerebral Artery Syndromes

The internal carotid artery divides into the middle and anterior cerebral arteries. The middle cerebral artery supplies the lateral aspect of the frontal, parietal, and temporal lobes and the underlying corona radiata, extending as deep as the putamen and the posterior limb of the internal capsule. As the main stem of the middle cerebral artery passes out through the Sylvian fissure, it gives rise to a series of small branches called lenticulostriate arteries, which penetrate deeply into the subcortical portion of the brain and perfuse the basal ganglia and internal capsule. At the lateral surface of the hemisphere, the middle cerebral artery divides into upper and lower divisions, which perfuse the lateral surface of the hemisphere. When the middle cerebral artery is occluded at its origin, a large cerebral infarction develops involving all the structures mentioned above. Because of the cerebral edema that usually accompanies such a large lesion with brain displacement, the patient initially shows depressed consciousness, with head and eyes deviated to the side of the lesion, and there are contralateral hemiplegia, decreased sensation, and homonymous hemianopia. If the dominant hemisphere is involved, a global aphasia is usually present. As the patient's mental status improves, other features become evident, namely dysphagia, contralateral hemianopia, and, in patients with nondominant hemisphere lesions, perceptual deficits and neglect. Patients who survive the acute lesion regain control of head and eye movements, and normal level of consciousness is restored. However, severe deficits involving motor, visuospatial, and language function usually persist with only limited recovery.

Occlusion of the branches of the middle cerebral artery, except for the lenticulostriate, are almost always embolic in origin, and the associated infarctions are correspondingly smaller and more peripherally located. The superior division of the middle cerebral artery supplies the Rolandic and pre-Rolandic areas, and an infarction in this territory will result in a dense sensory-motor deficit on the contralateral face, arm, and leg, with less involvement of the leg. As recovery occurs, the patient is usually able to walk with a spastic, hemiparetic gait. Little recovery occurs in motor function of the arm. If the left hemisphere is involved, there is usually severe aphasia initially with eventual improvement in comprehension, although an expressive aphasia is likely to persist. Small focal infarctions from occlusions of branches of the superior division will produce more limited deficits such as pure motor weakness of the contralateral arm and face, apraxia, or expressive aphasia.

The inferior division of the middle cerebral artery supplies the parietal and temporal lobes, and lesions on the left side result in severe involvement of language comprehension. The optic radiation is usually involved, resulting in partial or complete homonymous hemianopia on the contralateral side. Lesions affecting the right hemisphere often result in neglect of the left side of the body. Initially, the patient may completely ignore the affected side and even assert that the arm on his left side belongs not to him but to somebody else. Such severe neglect seen initially often gradually improves but may be followed by a variety of persisting impairments such as constructional apraxia, dressing apraxia, and perceptual deficits.

The lenticulostriate arteries are branches arising from the main stem of the middle cerebral artery that penetrate into the subcortical region and perfuse the basal ganglia and posterior internal capsule. Several characteristic and rather common isolated syndromes have been described when discrete focal lesions occur. They are frequently referred to as lacunar strokes. The most common is a lesion in the internal capsule causing a pure motor hemiplegia. An anterior lesion in the internal capsule may cause dysarthria with hand clumsiness, and a lesion of the thalamus or adjacent internal capsule causes a contralateral sensory loss with or without weakness. The neurologic deficits in these lesions often show early and progressive recovery with good ultimate outcome.

Patients with hypertension and diabetes are at risk for recurrent lacunar strokes. Pseudobulbar palsy is a syndrome that develops when multiple small lesions affect the anterior limb of both internal capsules, including the corticobulbar pathways. This syndrome consists of excessive emotional lability and spastic bulbar (pseudobulbar) paralysis, i.e., dysarthria, dysphonia, dysphagia, and facial weakness. There are often sudden outbursts of inappropriate and uncontrolled crying and laughter, at times blending into each other, without corresponding emotional stimulus. Drooling is often prominent. The term *pseudobulbar* is applied to this syndrome to distinguish it as an upper motor neuron lesion in contrast to a lower motor neuron lesion in the medulla. More widespread and posterior subcortical lacunar infarctions will often produce a dementia, often called multiinfarct dementia.

Anterior Cerebral Artery Syndromes

Branches of the anterior cerebral arteries supply the median and paramedian regions of the frontal cortex and the strip of the lateral surface of the hemisphere along its upper border. There are deep penetrating branches that supply the head of the caudate nucleus and the anterior limb of the internal capsule. Occlusions of the anterior cerebral artery are not common, but when they occur, there is contralateral hemiparesis with relative sparing of the hand and face and greater weakness of the leg. There is associated sensory loss of the leg and foot. Lesions affecting the left side may produce a transcortical motor aphasia characterized by diminution of spontaneous speech but preserved ability to repeat words. A grasp reflex is often present along with a sucking reflex and paratonic rigidity (gegenhalten). Urinary incontinence is common. Large lesions of the frontal cortex often produce behavioral changes, such as lack of spontaneity, distractibility, and tendency to perseverate. Patients may have diminished reasoning ability.

Vertebrobasilar Syndromes

The two vertebral arteries join at the junction of the medulla and pons to form the basilar artery. Together, the vertebral and basilar arteries supply the brainstem by paramedian and short circumferential branches and supply the cerebellum by long circumferential branches. The basilar artery terminates by bifurcating at the upper midbrain level to form the two posterior cerebral arteries. The posterior communicating arteries connect the middle to the posterior cerebral arteries, completing the circle of Willis.

Some general clinical features of lesions in the vertebrobasilar system should be noted. In contrast to lesions in the hemispheres, which are unilateral, lesions involving the pons and medulla often cross the midline and cause bilateral features. When motor impairments are present, they are often bilateral, with asymmetric corticospinal signs, and they are frequently accompanied by cerebellar signs. Cranial nerve lesions are very frequent and occur ipsilateral to the main lesion, producing contralateral corticospinal signs. There may be dissociated sensory loss (involvement of the spinothalamic pathway with preservation of the dorsal column pathway or vice versa), dysarthria, dysphagia, disequilibrium and vertigo, and Horner syndrome. Of particular note is absence of cortical deficits, such as aphasia and cognitive impairments. Visual field loss and visuospatial deficits may occur if the posterior cerebral artery is involved, but not with brain-stem lesions. Identification of a specific cranial nerve lesion allows precise anatomic localization of the lesion.

Lacunar infarcts are common in the vertebrobasilar distribution, arising from occlusion of small penetrating branches of the basilar artery or posterior cerebral artery. In contrast to cerebral lacunes, most brainstem lacunes produce clinical features. There are a variety of characteristic brainstem syndromes associated with lesions at various levels in the brainstem. The reader is referred to neurologic texts for a comprehensive discussion of these lesions. These brainstem syndromes are not infrequently encountered in patients referred for rehabilitation, and these are described in some detail.

The *lateral medullary syndrome* (Wallenberg syndrome) is produced by an infarction in the lateral wedge of the medulla. It may occur as an occlusion of the vertebral artery or the posterior inferior cerebellar artery. The clinical features of this syndrome, along with the corresponding anatomic structures involved, are impairment of contralateral pain and temperature (spinothalamic tract); ipsilateral Horner syndrome consisting of miosis, ptosis, and decreased facial sweating (descending sympathetic tract); dysphagia, dysarthria, and dysphonia (ipsilateral paralysis of the palate and vocal cords); nystagmus, vertigo, nausea, and vomiting (vestibular nucleus); ipsilateral limb ataxia (spinocerebellar fibers); and ipsilateral impaired sensation of the face (sensory nucleus of the fifth nerve). Patients with this syndrome are frequently quite disabled initially because of vertigo, disequilibrium, and ataxia, but they often make a good functional recovery.

Occlusion of the basilar artery may result in severe deficits with complete motor and sensory loss and cranial nerve signs from which patients do not recover. Patients are often comatose. Less extensive lesions, however, are compatible with life, and a characteristic syndrome observed occasionally is the *locked-in syndrome*. The infarction in such cases affects the upper ventral pons, involving the bilateral corticospinal and corticobulbar pathways but sparing the reticular activating system and ascending sensory pathways. Patients have normal sensation and can see and hear but are unable to move or speak. Blinking and upward gaze are preserved, which provides a very limited but usable means for communication. The patient is alert and fully oriented. Some patients do not survive, and those who do are severely disabled and dependent. Some slow progressive improvement and partial recovery may occur in this group of patients, justifying appropriate levels of rehabilitation intervention.

Focal infarctions may occur in the midbrain and affect the descending corticospinal pathway, sometimes also involving the third cranial nerve nucleus (Weber syndrome), resulting in ipsilateral third nerve palsy and paralysis of the contralateral arm and leg.

The posterior cerebral artery perfuses the thalamus through perforating arteries, as well as the temporal and occipital lobes with their subcortical structures, including the optic radiation. An occipital lobe infarction will cause a partial or complete contralateral hemianopia, and when these visual deficits involve the dominant hemisphere, there may be associated difficulty in reading or in naming objects. When the thalamus is involved, there is contralateral hemisensory loss. A lesion involving the thalamus may cause a syndrome characterized by contralateral hemianesthesia and central pain, although only about 25% of cases of central pain in stroke are caused by lesions of the thalamus. Other lesion sites reported to be associated with central pain are the brainstem and parietal lobe projections from the thalamus. In the thalamic syndrome, patients report unremitting, unpleasant, burning pain affecting the opposite side of the body. The pain usually begins a few weeks after stroke onset and becomes intractable to conventional medication, including narcotics. It may be partly relieved with tricyclic antidepressants. Examination of the patient reveals contralateral impairment of all sensory modalities, often with dysesthesia. There may be involvement of adjacent structures, such as the internal capsule (hemiparesis, ataxia) or basal ganglia (choreoathetosis).

STROKE DIAGNOSIS

The clinical diagnosis of stroke is often self-evident from the dramatic and abrupt onset of the clinical features, but other disorders may cause relatively sudden neurologic deficits and be mistaken for stroke. For example, a patient with hemiparesis and depressed level of consciousness may have a subdural hematoma from a fall, a cerebral abscess, a brain tumor, or be postictal. It is imperative, therefore, that the diagnosis of stroke be firmly established at the beginning of the patient's care. It is the responsibility of the rehabilitation physician to be sure that an adequate diagnostic evaluation has been completed.

Once a firm diagnosis of stroke has been made, the characteristics of the lesion need to be determined. This can be done by answering three questions: What is it (pathologic diagnosis)?, Where is it (anatomic diagnosis)?, and Why did it happen (etiologic diagnosis)? The answers to these questions will influence acute and long-term medical management and will give insights to the rehabilitation team about prognosis and optimum therapeutic procedures.

Pathologic Diagnosis

The pathologic diagnosis—cerebral infarction, intracerebral hemorrhage, or subarachnoid hemorrhage—is suggested by the clinical presentation but is established by imaging studies, which should be done as early as possible. Computed tomography (CT) of the head is performed as soon as possible because hemorrhage can be observed immediately as a hyperdense area, and because CT reveals other structural lesions (subdural hematoma, tumor, abscess) that may require surgical management. CT will often be negative for the first 1 to 2 days in patients with cerebral infarction. The location of a hemorrhage will give clues to its etiology, such as hypertension in lesions involving the basal ganglia or thalamus. A subarachnoid hemorrhage is most likely due to a bleeding aneurysm or AVM. In patients with obvious clinical features of stroke, it is reasonable to conclude that a negative CT scan in the first 48 hours represents an infarction. Magnetic resonance imaging (MRI) shows changes of cerebral infarction as early as a few hours postonset.

In the postacute phase, both CT and MRI show changes of cerebral infarction, but MRI is more sensitive in the first 48 hours. Moreover, MRI is more sensitive in detection of small lacunar strokes because of its greater resolution, and it is more sensitive than CT for detecting lesions in the brainstem and cerebellum. Magnetic resonance angiography is a technique for display of details of cerebrovascular anatomy and pathology without the risks of conventional angiography.

Anatomic Diagnosis

Anatomic localization of the lesion is determined by the neurologic examination, although sometimes the clinical deficits are inconclusive. For example, a patient with a pure motor hemiplegia may have a small embolic infarction involving the motor cortex from occlusion of a branch of the upper division of the middle cerebral artery. Alternatively, a lacunar stroke affecting the internal capsule or brainstem may also result in a pure motor hemiplegia. Imaging studies are therefore very helpful in documenting the location of the structural lesion responsible for the patient's set of neurologic signs.

Etiologic Diagnosis

For many patients, a stroke, either infarction or hemorrhage, is a late event in the natural course of progressive cerebrovascular disease. Such patients will often have risk factors for stroke, such as age, a history of hypertension, diabetes, and smoking, and features of generalized atherosclerosis, especially coronary artery disease and peripheral vascular disease. The etiology of the stroke in these patients is rarely in doubt. But in other patients with thrombotic infarctions, there may be no particular risk factors and no evidence of clinical atherosclerosis. Other less obvious causes of arterial occlusion should then be considered as possible reasons for the stroke. This is particularly important in younger patients who have not had time to develop advanced atherosclerosis. It is a useful strategy for the clinician to always consider the possibility of an alternative cause of arterial occlusion in patients less than 55 years of age when there are no apparent risk factors for atherosclerosis or lipohyalinosis. A list of important causes of arterial thrombosis is noted in Table 77-5. There is a residual group of patients with thrombotic infarction in whom the etiology remains undetermined even after extensive workup. The stroke in these patients may be attributed to a number of uncommon conditions, such as systemic lupus erythematosis, arteritis, dissection, migraine, and a hypercoaguable state. Some may be due to artery to artery embolism.

There should be a thorough search for sources of emboli through careful cardiac examination. Echocardiography is very useful for the detection of a source of cardiac embolism. A transesophageal echogram is superior in evaluation of the left atrium, mitral valve, and the aortic arch.

If CT and MRI are nondiagnostic, angiography may be helpful in revealing conditions such as dissection of extracranial vessels, fibromuscular dysplasia, or cerebral vasculitis. An-

TABLE 77-5.   Causes of Arterial Thrombosis

Atherosclerosis (large vessels)
Lipohyalinosis (small vessels)
Arterial dissection (extracranial trauma)
Fibromuscular dysplasia
Vasculitis
Homocystinuria
Coagulopathy
  Sickle-cell anemia
  Plasma C-protein deficiency
  Antithrombin-3 deficiency

giography is usually not indicated in most cases of cerebral infarction.

STROKE IN CHILDREN AND YOUNG ADULTS

Stroke is a recognized phenomenon in children and is relatively common in young adults. In a significant number of cases, 40% to 50%, no obvious risk factors—such as sources of cardiogenic emboli and atherosclerosis—are found. These patients should be thoroughly investigated for primary etiology of the stroke. A list of possible diagnoses is given in Table 77-6. Coagulation disorders may be inherited or acquired, but they may account for up to 20% of cases with thrombotic infarction in young adults. Deficiencies of antithrombin III, protein C, and protein S are among the most important coagulopathies, as each of these substances is part of the naturally occurring anticoagulant system. Each of these conditions requires long-term treatment with warfarin. There have been many reports of external trauma to the neck in children and adults causing thrombosis or dissection of the carotid artery and corresponding cerebral infarction. There are numerous reports of chiropractic manipulation of the cervical spine causing brain-stem stroke from trauma and subsequent occlusion or dissection of the vertebral arteries.

Vasculitis may exist as a primary disorder or may occur as part of multisystem inflammatory disease, such as juvenile rheumatoid arthritis, systemic lupus erythematosus, polyarteritis nodosa, or Takayasu disease. The pattern of clinical features includes both generalized encephalopathy and focal lesions, such as hemiplegia (16).

The inherited disorder homocysteinuria predisposes individuals to early atherosclerosis, and stroke is a frequent occurrence in young adults with this disorder. Stroke has been reported as an occasional complication occurring during pregnancy or in the postpartum period.

ACUTE INTERVENTION

There has been a dramatic change in the approach to treatment of the acute stroke patient in the last few years. Many centers have established acute stroke units to best implement specific protocols to optimize the neurologic and medical care of these patients. The efficacy of acute stroke units in improving the outcome of patients has been clearly established (17).

Stroke Management

The goals of acute stroke management are: (a) to limit or reverse neurologic damage through thrombolysis or neuroprotection, and (b) to monitor and prevent secondary stroke complications such as raised intracranial pressure.

There is a group of patients with acute infarction who are candidates for intravascular thrombolysis with tissue-type plasminogen activator (18). The treatment must be given within 3 hours of onset of symptoms. This has prompted major centers to develop stroke teams that can respond rapidly 24 hours a day with immediate clinical evaluation, urgent CT scan, and infusion within the therapeutic window. The purpose of thrombolytic therapy is to reestablish arterial circulation and limit or reverse neuronal damage. The use of carotid angioplasty or stenting, or surgical endarterectomy in patients with critical stenosis is controversial because these procedures carry the risk of causing hemorrhage into the infarction when

TABLE 77-6.   Causes of Stroke in Children and Young Adults

Cerebral embolism
Trauma to extracranial arteries
   Thromboembolic occlusion
   Dissection
Subarachnoid hemorrhage
   Aneurysm
   AVM
Sickle-cell anemia
Vasculopathy
   Moya moya disease
   SLE
   Drug induced
   Vasculitis
Coagulopathy
   Deficiency of antithrombin III
   Deficiency of protein C
   Deficiency of protein S
Homocystinuria
Oral contraceptives
Postpartum
Drug-induced

AVM, arteriovenous malformation; SLE, systemic lupus erythematosis.

arterial perfusion is reestablished. They may have a place in patients with ischemia or small infarctions.

The concept of neuroprotection has become important. In the acute phase, brain tissue in the penumbra around an infarction has borderline perfusion and compromised energy metabolism. Cells that have not progressed to structural damage and death have the potential for recovery with early reperfusion, which may occur spontaneously or through thrombolysis. Physiological factors such as arterial perfusion, oxygen tension, intracranial pressure, and serum biochemistry can influence the fate of neurons in the penumbra. Hence monitoring and optimizing all aspects of care may limit the extent of neurologic damage

There is an "excitotoxic theory" that holds that neuronal ischemia in the penumbra around an infarction triggers extracellular accumulation of excitatory amino acids, particularly glutamate, which activate cell membrane channels, allowing toxic levels of calcium to accumulate inside the cells. There may be other sources of excessive intracellular calcium, such as release from storage sites. The high level of intracellular calcium initiates an array of neurochemical changes within the neurons that eventually generate free radicals and progress to cell death. Initial research on the value of glutamate receptor antagonists and free radical scavengers for acute stroke have been disappointing in humans, despite evidence of efficacy in animal models. In the future there is promise that effective treatments will evolve and that medical treatment of cerebral infarction will turn from a realm of fatalism to a field of therapeutic opportunity. For further reading, see reviews by Dobkin (19) and Stein et al. (20).

Patients with cerebral hemorrhage have a high mortality because of the risk of progressive bleeding, raised intracranial pressure, and herniation. In selected patients at risk for brain displacement and herniation, craniotomy and evacuation of the hematoma can be a life-saving procedure. This is particularly the case in patients with cerebellar hemorrhage in whom raised pressure in the posterior fossa can cause acute hydrocephalus and death. With surgical evacuation of the hematoma, these patients will survive and often have very good functional outcome.

General Medical Treatment

Any patients who survive an acute stroke may subsequently die in the acute phase from systemic complications, such as pneumonia or pulmonary embolism. Very careful attention to the general medical management of the patient is therefore important. This involves measures to preserve a good airway, assistance in clearing pulmonary secretions, and prevention of aspiration. Intermittent catheterization is preferable to prolonged indwelling bladder catheterization to minimize the chances of urinary tract infection. The risk of deep venous thrombosis is high, especially in patients with hemiplegia, and many peripheral thrombi appear within the first several days following the stroke. Every patient should therefore have some form of deep vein thrombosis (DVT) prophylaxis, either subcutaneous heparin or external pneumatic compression stockings, or both. There should be adequate hydration and nutrition. Many patients have cardiac arrhythmia, and some have concomitant ischemic heart disease. Appropriate cardiac monitoring and intervention are therefore important.

Rehabilitation during the Acute Phase

Rehabilitation is not a distinctly separate phase of care, beginning after acute medical intervention. Rather, it is an integral part of medical management and continues longitudinally through acute care, postacute care, and community reintegration. Although diagnosis and medical treatment are the principal focus of early treatment, rehabilitation measures should be offered concurrently. Many of these can be considered preventive in nature. For example, patients who are paralyzed, lethargic, and have bladder incontinence are at high risk for developing pressure ulcers. Deliberate strategies should be followed to prevent skin breakdowns, including protection of skin from moisture such as urine, avoidance of undue pressure through use of heel-protecting pads, maintenance of proper position with frequent turning, and daily inspection and routine skin cleansing (21).

Many patients with acute stroke have dysphagia and are at risk for aspiration and pneumonia. Aspiration will usually result in coughing, but in as many as 40% of patients with acute stroke, aspiration is silent, without coughing. Patients who are lethargic or have decreased arousal should not be fed orally. Even in alert patients, the ability to swallow should be assessed carefully before oral intake of fluids or food is begun. This is done with a bedside evaluation, and if any doubt exists about aspiration, a swallowing videofluoroscopy examination is performed. During the acute phase, nasogastric tube feeding is necessary. It should be noted that patients who are lying flat in bed are at significant risk for regurgitation and aspiration (22).

Impairment of bladder control is frequent following a stroke, which initially causes hypotonic bladder with overflow incontinence. If an indwelling catheter is used for drainage, this should be removed as soon as possible because reflex voiding returns quite quickly and retention is rarely a problem. The indwelling catheter may be useful in the first several days to monitor fluid balance, but it carries an increased risk of urinary tract infection. Regular intermittent catheterization is preferable to an indwelling catheter (23).

Hemiplegic patients are at high risk for development of contractures. These are myogenic, induced by prolonged posturing with the muscles in a shortened position. When muscle fibers are unloaded, there is rapid loss of sarcomeres and reduced fiber length, and some accumulation of connective tissue (24). The development of spasticity contributes to development of contractures through sustained posturing of the limbs

TABLE 77-7. Criteria for Admission to a Comprehensive Rehabilitation Program

Stable neurologic status
Significant persisting neurologic deficit
Identified disability affecting at least two of the following: mobility, self-care activities, communication, bowel or bladder control, or swallowing
Sufficient cognitive function to learn
Sufficient communicative ability to engage with the therapists
Physical ability to tolerate the active program
Achievable therapeutic goals

in certain positions. The harmful effects of immobility can be ameliorated by regular passive stretching and moving the joints through a full range of motion, preferably twice daily.

There is a strong belief that early mobilization is beneficial to patient outcome by reducing the risks of DVT, gastroesophageal regurgitation and aspiration pneumonia, contracture formation, skin breakdown, and orthostatic intolerance. Early activation is assumed to have a strong positive psychological benefit for the patient. Mobilization involves a set of physical activities that may be started passively but that quickly progress to active participation by the patient in the activity. Specific tasks include turning from side to side in bed and changing position, sitting up in bed, transferring to a wheelchair, standing, and walking. Mobilization also includes self-care activities such as self-feeding, grooming, and dressing. The timing of patient participation and progression in these activities depends on the patient's condition. The activities would be precluded by progressive neurologic signs, intracranial hemorrhage, coma, or cardiovascular instability. If the patient's condition is stable, however, active mobilization should begin as soon as possible, within 24 to 48 hours of admission (23).

Evaluation for Rehabilitation Program

Within several days of admission, once the patient appears to be neurologically and medically stable, the patient should be evaluated for admission to a comprehensive rehabilitation program. The criteria for admission into a postacute rehabilitation program are listed in Table 77-7. A comprehensive rehabilitation program involving multiple professionals is justified when the patient has identified disability affecting multiple areas of function. A patient with an isolated disability such as a partial aphasia, visual loss, or monoparesis may need rehabilitation, but for these cases, therapy can be provided by a therapist, one discipline only, usually in an outpatient setting. In the very early postonset phase, it may not be possible to judge whether the patient has sufficient cognitive function or communicative ability to engage in the program or sufficient physical tolerance to participate fully. It may be necessary in such cases to offer a short trial of therapy to observe the patient's true capacity and potential before deciding on candidacy.

Evaluation of the acute stroke patient should include information about the patient's general medical status, including the presence of important comorbidities. Equally important, the patient's psychosocial status influences the way the patient copes with the disability, impacts motivation and physical outcome, and forms the basis of discharge planning. It is important to establish at the outset the nature of the patient's family support, living situation, and postdischarge environment. Knowledge of all of these factors will assist the team in counseling the patient and family and in planning for discharge.

Medical stability has traditionally been required for admission of a patient to a specialized rehabilitation unit. However, hospitals are increasingly transferring patients from acute wards to rehabilitation units at earlier stages, often when they still have unresolved medical problems. This practice has forced rehabilitation centers to expand their resources to care for these more complex cases and to provide closer medical and nursing monitoring. Local institutional referral patterns and practices will usually determine the timing of transfer, but if earlier transfer to rehabilitation can be accomplished safely, patient care may be enhanced by earlier active participation of the patient in the rehabilitation program.

The rehabilitation program may be offered in different settings, such as an acute inpatient rehabilitation unit, a subacute rehabilitation inpatient unit, home care, or an outpatient center. The acute rehabilitation setting is appropriate for those patients who meet the admission criteria and are able to tolerate 3 hours or more of active therapy per day. An acute rehabilitation setting is preferred if the patient requires close medical and nursing monitoring of the medical status. If the patient's medical status is stable, but the patient is unable to tolerate more than 1 hour of therapy per day, a subacute rehabilitation setting is more appropriate. Other patients who require only minor degrees of assistance in self-care and mobility would be suitable for outpatient therapy or a home-care program.

PRINCIPLES OF STROKE REHABILITATION

Although rehabilitation intervention is important during the acute phase of care, it is secondary to the activities involved in diagnosis and acute medical treatment. However, when a patient has a persisting major continuing impairment, such as hemiplegia with disabilities, the rehabilitation components of care quickly become the main focus of management. The rehabilitation process for patients with complex problems requires a carefully planned and integrated program. Some general principles have evolved over time to form the basis of stroke rehabilitation. Some of these principles are based on conclusions from clinical trials, but many represent a general consensus based on clinical experience. They are:

1. There is a clear need for committed medical direction. The role of the physician includes provision of medical care. Many patients have ongoing associated medical problems that require appropriate monitoring and therapy. The physician must act as medical counselor, offering reasonable prognostication to patient and family along with guidance in stroke risk-factor reduction and ongoing medical care. The physician must also give leadership to the team and assist in developing treatment protocols and setting treatment expectations.
2. The multiple problems of a patient require the active participation of a team of professionals. The treatment activities of the team members must be coordinated so that detailed evaluations are shared and goals and treatment interventions are agreed on.
3. Each of the professional therapists on the team should be knowledgeable regarding the appropriate interventions within his or her discipline for treating the disabilities of stroke patients.
4. The interventions should be directed at achieving specific therapeutic goals, which may be short term, e.g., week to week, or longer term, e.g., goals to be reached by discharge. Having achieved those goals, the patient moves on to the next phase of rehabilitation or is discharged home to continue treatment as an outpatient.
5. There is evidence from clinical trials that early initiation of therapy favorably influences the outcome. During delays in starting therapy, patients may develop secondary avoidable complications, such as contractures and deconditioning.
6. Therapy should be directed at specific training of skills and functional training. Therapy should be given with sufficient intensity to promote skill acquisition.
7. Planning for discharge from the inpatient rehabilitation program should begin on admission.
8. Psychosocial issues are obviously very important. Numerous studies have reported on the influence of spouse, family, and the patient's own psychological adjustment and coping mechanisms in determining ultimate outcome. Family involvement is essential throughout the treatment program and in discharge planning.
9. There should be an emphasis on patient and family education about stroke, risk-factor reduction, and strategies to maximize functional independence.
10. Rehabilitation requires a functional approach. When impairments cannot be altered, every effort should be made to assist patients to compensate for deficits and adapt with alternative methods to achieve optimal functional independence.
11. Discharge from hospital is often thought of as the end of rehabilitation, with the assumption that a good program prepares the patient for reintegration into home and community. However, hospital discharge should instead be looked on as the end of the beginning of a new life in which the patient faces the challenge of adopting different roles and relationships and a search for new meaning in life. This will involve resuming as much as possible former roles in the family and with friends and finding ways to live a meaningful life in the community.

RECOVERY FROM STROKE

Numerous studies have described the patterns of improvement in neurologic deficits and in recovery of function after stroke. There is marked variation among patients in the time course of recovery and in its degree. An important objective of many of these studies has been identification of specific variables that would predict the course of recovery from neurologic impairments.

Recovery from Impairments

Hemiparesis and motor recovery have been the most studied of all stroke impairments. As many as 88% of patients with an acute stroke have hemiparesis (25). In a classic report, Twitchell (26) described in detail the pattern of motor recovery following stroke. At onset, the arm is more involved than the leg, and eventual motor recovery in the arm is less than in the leg. The severity of arm weakness at onset and the timing of the return of movement in the hand are both important predictors of eventual motor recovery in the arm (27–30). The prognosis for return of useful hand function is poor when there is complete arm paralysis at onset or no measurable grasp strength by 4 weeks. However, even among those patients with severe arm weakness at onset, as many as 11% may gain good recovery of hand function. Some other generalizations can be made. For patients showing some motor recovery in the hand by 4 weeks, as many as 70% will make a full or good recovery. Full recovery, when it occurs, is usually complete within 3 months of onset. Bard and Hirshberg claim that "if no initial motion is noticed during the first 3 weeks, or if motion in one segment is not followed within a week by the appearance of motion in a second segment, the prognosis for recovery of full motion is poor" (28).

The patterns of motor recovery have been described in detail by the authors of the Copenhagen Stroke Study (31). Summary data are shown in Figure 77-1. Ninety-five percent of patients reached their best neurologic level within 11 weeks of onset. Patients with milder stroke recovered more quickly, and those with severe strokes reached their best neurologic level in 15 weeks on average. The course of motor recovery reaches a plateau after an early phase of progressive improvement. Most recovery takes place in the first 3 months, and only minor additional measurable improvement occurs after 6 months postonset (32). However, in some patients who have significant partial return of voluntary movement, recovery may continue over a longer period of time.

About one-third of patients with acute stroke have clinical features of aphasia. Language function in many of these patients improves, and at 6 months or more after stroke, only 12% to 18% have identifiable aphasia (33,34). Skilbeck et al. (34) reported that patients with aphasia continue to show some late improvement in language function, even beyond 1 year after onset. Patients who would be initially classified as having Broca aphasia have a variable outcome. In patients with large hemisphere lesions, Broca aphasia persists with little recovery, but patients with smaller lesions confined to the posterior frontal lobe often show early progressive improvement, the impairment evolving into a milder form of aphasia with anomia and word-finding difficulty. Patients with global aphasia tend to progress slowly, with comprehension often improving more than expressive ability. Communicative ability of patients who initially have global aphasia improves over a longer period of time, up to 1 year or more postonset. Patients with global aphasia associated with large lesions may show only minor recovery, but recovery may be quite good in those patients with smaller lesions. Language recovery in Wernicke's aphasia is variable.

About 20% of patients have a visual field defect. In general, the degree of visual improvement following stroke is not as impressive as recovery of motor and sensory function, and if the field defect persists beyond a few weeks, late recovery is less likely.

Mechanisms of Neurologic Recovery

In the early phase poststroke, there is prompt initial improvement in function as the pathologic processes in the ischemic penumbra–ischemia, metabolic injury, edema, hemorrhage, and pressure resolve. The time frame for recovery of function in these reversibly injured neurons is relatively short and accounts for improvement in the first several weeks. The later, ongoing improvement in neurologic function occurs by a different set of mechanisms that allow structural and functional reorganization within the brain. The processes involved in this reorganization represent neuroplasticity and may continue for many months. There is restitution of partially damaged pathways and expansion of representational brain maps, implying recruitment of neurons not ordinarily involved in an activity. A key aspect of neuroplasticity that has important implications for rehabilitation is that the modifications in neuronal networks are use dependent. Animal experimental studies and clinical trials in humans have shown that forced use and functional training contribute to improved function. On the other hand, techniques that promote nonuse may inhibit recovery. It used to be taught that benefits from rehabilitation are primarily achieved through training patients in new techniques to com-

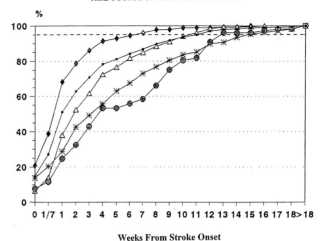

Figure 77-1. The time course of recovery in stroke survivors shown as the cumulated rate of patients having reached their best neurological outcome. The course of recovery is given for patients whose initial stroke severity was mild, ◆; moderate, ▲; severe, *; very severe, ●. All patients are represented by ■.

pensate for impairments, e.g., using the uninvolved hand to achieve self-care independence. This approach avoided intense therapy on the weak upper limb. It is now recognized that repeated participation by patients in active physical therapeutic programs probably directly influences functional reorganization in the brain and enhances neurologic recovery. (See Chapter 78 for more details about neuroplasticity.)

IMPAIRMENT EVALUATION

The focal neurologic lesion that accompanies a stroke confers on the patient a set of neurologic deficits, which in rehabilitation medicine are referred to as impairments. Evaluation of these impairments constitutes an essential first step in rehabilitation management of the patient. When the physician and therapist understand the nature of a patient's impairments, they can provide specific targeted therapy to optimize the rehabilitation program. The relationship between medical diagnosis and rehabilitation diagnosis is described in Table 77-8 (35). The initial clinical examination of a patient with an acute stroke includes a thorough, detailed neurologic examination. The neurologic findings are used by the rehabilitation team for prognostication, development of the specific details of the rehabilitation plan, and selection of the appropriate setting for rehabilitation. Reassessment of the patient during rehabilitation provides a means of monitoring progress and subsequently evaluating outcome. The initial rehabilitation assessment should begin immediately postonset, within 2 to 7 days, and then at repeated subsequent intervals.

The following sections summarize the important details of the neurologic impairments encountered in postacute stroke patients.

TABLE 77-8. Medical Diagnosis versus Rehabilitation Diagnosis
Medical diagnosis
Pathology (e.g., infarction) → Neurologic deficits (e.g., hemiplegia)
Rehabilitation diagnosis
Impairments (e.g., hemiplegia) → Disability (e.g., inability to walk)

TABLE 77-9. Mental Status Examination

Level of consciousness
  Alertness, response to stimulation
Attention
Memory
  Orientation, new learning, remote memory
Cognition
  Fund of knowledge, calculation, problem solving, abstract thinking,
    judgment
Perception, consructional ability, apraxia
Affect and behavior

Higher Mental Function

Focal brain lesions associated with a stroke frequently produce measurable impairments in higher mental function. Even small lesions may significantly impair cognition, particularly when they are multiple. However, interpretation of test information must be made in the context of the clinical situation because other nonstroke factors may contribute to impaired mental status. Many patients are elderly and may have had some premorbid decline in mental status. Further, general medical disorders, such as a fever, electrolyte disturbance, hypothyroidism, congestive heart failure, and reaction to medication, may produce an encephalopathy. Such patients are often confused and may have a diminished level of consciousness; they have a generalized disturbance of mental status with abnormalities in most or all cognitive tests. The encephalopathy associated with these general medical problems is reversible following correction of the complicating disorder. Only when nonstroke factors have been excluded can changes in mental status be attributed to the focal lesion of the brain.

The cognitive impairments observed with focal lesions frequently show specific disturbances, for example, memory loss, neglect, or constructional apraxia. Disturbances such as these can usually be recognized at the bedside. Because cognitive impairments can have a significant influence on the rehabilitation program and on outcome, the bedside mental status examination should be an essential part of the assessment of every stroke patient. The components of the examination are shown in Table 77-9. For a more detailed description of this assessment, see Strub and Black (36). The Mini-Mental State Examination developed by Folstein et al. (37) is a useful bedside tool that screens a variety of mental demands quickly and gives a well-validated measure of overall mental function. It requires less than 10 minutes to administer. Formal psychological tests may be used to establish global intellectual level and to reveal specific areas of diminished performance reflecting focal brain impairment. The Wechsler Adult Intelligence Scale (WAIS) is commonly used in stroke patients.

Perceptual impairments are extremely important in stroke rehabilitation, and their recognition is an essential part of the higher mental function evaluation. A perceptual deficit is an impairment in the recognition and interpretation of sensory information when the sensory input system is intact. Impaired perception is caused by a lesion at the cortical level, almost always in the nondominant parietal lobe. The patient exhibits selective inattention, which can be detected by careful observation of his or her behavior. A patient with hemisensory loss or homonymous hemianopia will also ignore the affected side. However, inattention is only referred to as true neglect when the sensory and visual pathways are intact. Unilateral neglect may be visual, tactile, spatial, or auditory. Visual neglect is demonstrated at the bedside when the patient, on request, attempts to draw numbers on a clock face, draw a stick figure, or bisect a horizontal line on a piece of paper. The patient is inattentive to the affected side. Other bedside tests of perceptual function are failure to recognize palm writing (graphesthesia), inability to identify objects in the hand (astereognosis), and extinction of simultaneous bilateral stimulation.

The term *apraxia* describes the inability of a patient to execute a willed movement when motor and sensory functions are apparently preserved. Apraxia may be detected when a patient is unable to carry out a task on command such as "comb your hair" or "wave goodbye," even though there is no paralysis. Patients with lesions of the nondominant parietal lobe may have apraxia of putting on their clothes and getting dressed.

Communication Disorders

Communication is a complex function involving reception, central processing, and sending of information (see Chapter 45). Communication occurs through the use of language and consists of a system of symbols that are combined to convey ideas, i.e., letters, words, or gestures. Impairment of language is called *aphasia,* and its presence reflects an abnormality in the dominant hemisphere. *Speech,* on the other hand, is a term that refers to the motor mechanism involved in the production of spoken words, namely breathing, phonation, and articulation. Dysphonia and dysarthria are disorders of speech.

Although there are many classifications for aphasia, certain identifiable groups of patients are observed with clinically similar disorders of communication. In the simplest classification, aphasia is divided into two main categories: motor aphasia (sometimes called expressive or anterior aphasia), characterized by nonfluent speech, and sensory aphasia (sometimes called receptive, posterior, or Wernicke's aphasia), characterized by fluent speech. A common system of classification of

TABLE 77-10 Classification of Aphasia

Classification	Fluency	Comprehension	Repetition	Naming
Global	Poor	Poor	Poor	Poor
Broca	Poor	Good	Variable	Poor
Isolation	Poor	Poor	Good	Poor
Transcortical motor	Poor	Good	Good	Poor
Wernicke	Good	Poor	Poor	Poor
Transcortical sensory	Good	Poor	Good	Poor
Conduction	Good	Good	Poor	Poor
Anomic	Good	Good	Good	Poor

TABLE 77-11. The Bedside Test

Questions	Clinical Test
Does the patient understand?	Give verbal commands, ask patient to point to objects.
Is the patient able to talk?	Ask the patient to name objects, describe them, count. Listen for spontaneous speech.
Can the patient repeat?	Ask the patient to repeat words.
Can the patient read?	Give commands in writing.
Can the patient write?	Ask the patient to copy or to write dictated words.

aphasia is listed in Table 77-10 (35). Use of simple bedside tests can allow the clinician to categorize the communication disorder according to this classification. During the evaluation of a patient, the clinician should avoid using nonverbal cues, such as gestures. The questions addressed during the bedside assessment of aphasia are provided in Table 77-11.

Complete evaluations of patients can be performed using formal aphasia tests. Table 77-12 summarizes the more commonly used formal aphasia test instruments.

For assessment of dysarthria, clinicians subjectively rate the degree of impairment as a percentage intelligibility of speech.

Cranial Nerves

In patients with lesions involving the hemispheres, visual field defects may be present. Patients with hemianopia will often fail to detect objects on the affected side of the body, which confers significant disability. The precise nature of the defect can be characterized by confrontation testing. Extraocular palsies involving lesions of the midbrain or pons can produce characteristic dysfunction.

Dysphagia is a frequent impairment with unilateral hemisphere stroke, but it is much more pronounced in bilateral disease and in brain-stem lesions. Other cranial nerve lesions may be identified in lesions involving the brain stem. The reader is referred to standard neurologic texts and to Chapter 45 for detailed descriptions.

TABLE 77-12. Commonly Used Formal Aphasia Test

- The Boston Diagnostic Aphasia Examination (32) produces a classification of the aphasic features observed in a particular patient. Besides classifying the aphasia, it also provides a score of the severity of the aphasia, which can be compared to aphasic patients in general (38).
- The Western Aphasia Battery (39) is somewhat similar to the Boston. It measures various parameters of spontaneous speech and examines comprehension, fluency, object naming, and repetition. It provides a total score called an aphasia quotient, which is a measure of the severity of the aphasia.
- The Porch Index of Communication Ability (PICA) is different from the other tests in that it evaluates verbal, gestural, and graphic responses. It is very structured in its format and must be given by a trained professional. It provides a useful statistical summary of the details of the language impairments and offers outcome prediction.
- The Functional Communication Profile (40) provides an overall rating of functional communication. It is not a diagnostic test. The score indicates severity and can be a useful indicator of recovery.

Motor Impairment

Paralysis is such a common feature among central nervous system impairments with stroke that the terms *hemiplegia* and *stroke* are often used interchangeably. Assessment of motor impairment includes an evaluation of tone, strength, coordination, and balance.

The most widely used scale to assess strength is the Medical Research Council (MRC) six-point scale, 0 to 5, in which 0 represents complete paralysis, 3 is the ability to fully move the joint against gravity, and 5 indicates normal strength. The test is insensitive in its upper range, where the examiner must assess strength by offering manual resistance to maximum muscle activation. The MRC scale is designed to assess the strength of individual muscles, and it is therefore most useful in grading strength in patients with lower motor neuron lesions. There are drawbacks to the use of this scale in patients with upper motor neuron lesions, such as stroke. A patient recovering from hemiplegia may not be able to selectively activate a particular muscle in isolation and hence will be given a 0 grade on the MRC scale. However, the patient may be able to forcefully activate the muscle within a gross motor pattern in which groups of muscles contract together in synergy, for example, a flexor or extensor synergy pattern. Further, as tone increases during recovery, the capacity of the patient to move a joint may be restricted by spasticity in the antagonists. Cocontraction of agonists and antagonists can diminish the force of muscle contraction recorded externally. Despite these shortcomings, the MRC scale may be quite useful in the early phases following a stroke, before significant spasticity develops.

Brunnstrom (41) adopted a different approach for assessment of motor function in hemiplegic patients. She developed a test in which movement patterns are evaluated and motor function is rated according to stages of motor recovery. The clinician assesses the presence of flexor and extensor synergies and the degree of selective muscle activation from the synergy pattern (Table 77-13) (35). The rating can be performed very quickly, and although the scale defines recovery only in broad categories, these categories do correlate with progressive functional recovery (42).

Rather than subjectively assess strength using the MRC scale, Bohannon advocated direct measurement of force with a dynamometer (43). Despite the limitations of assessing and interpreting muscle strength in patients with upper motor neuron lesions, strength does correlate with performance on functional tasks (44). Fugl-Meyer et al. (45) designed a more detailed and comprehensive motor scale in which 50 different

TABLE 77-13. Brunnstrom Stages of Motor Recovery

Stage	Characteristics
Stage 1	No activation of the limb
Stage 2	Spasticity appears, and weak basic flexor and extensor synergies are present
Stage 3	Spasticity is prominent; the patient voluntarily moves the limb, but muscle activation is all within the synergy patterns
Stage 4	The patient begins to activate muscles selectively outside the flexor and extensor synergies
Stage 5	Spasticity decreases; most muscle activation is selective and independent from the limb synergies
Stage 6	Isolated movements are performed in a smooth, phasic, well-coordinated manner

movements and abilities were rated. The test evaluates strength, reflexes, and coordination, and a composite score is derived on a scale of 0 to 100. The Fugl-Meyer Scale is reliable, and repeat scores reflect motor recovery over time. It is quite useful and informative but has not been widely adopted by clinicians because it is time-consuming to complete each evaluation.

Muscle tone refers to the resistance felt when the examiner passively stretches a muscle by moving a joint. The rating is subjective and depends on the judgment of the examiner. Physiological conditions such as position of body segments and body posture strongly influence the level of muscle tone, and these must be controlled as much as possible. For example, tone will be increased if the patient is supine rather than prone or standing rather than sitting. Tone in the leg muscles may be quite modest in a sitting hemiplegic patient but be very severe when the patient is standing. A high level of anxiety will also increase the degree of muscle tone. Quantification of spasticity is difficult. The most widely used scale is the Ashworth Scale (see Chapter 67) (46).

Sensory Impairment

When sensory deficits exist as part of a clinical picture following a stroke, they frequently accompany motor impairment in the same anatomic distribution. Interpretation of sensory testing may be difficult in a confused or cognitively impaired patient. Clinical examination involves testing pain, temperature, touch, joint position, and vibration. Lesions of the thalamus may cause severe contralateral sensory loss. With lesions of the cortex, sensation, although preserved, is qualitatively and quantitatively reduced. Parietal lobe lesions cause perceptual deficits in which primary modalities of sensation may be intact. Typical tests to reveal the presence of perceptual impairment include simultaneous bilateral stimulation for inattention, two-point discrimination, object recognition for stereognosis, and recognition of digits drawn in the palm.

Balance, Coordination, and Posture

Impaired balance may be caused by deficits in motor and sensory function, cerebellar lesions, and vestibular dysfunctions. Clinical testing involves assessing coordination using finger-to-nose pointing and rapid alternating movements. The ability of the patient to sit unsupported or, if able, to stand and walk provides important information. Ataxia caused by sensory impairment can be differentiated from ataxia resulting from cerebellar loss because performance of a motor task with the eyes closed is much poorer in sensory ataxia, when the patient has no vision to compensate for sensory loss.

Evaluation of the neurologic impairments should be made repeatedly during the course of the rehabilitation program. Ideally, evaluation should be made weekly in the early phases of rehabilitation to allow monitoring of the recovery process and to guide the therapeutic intervention.

OUTCOME AND PROGNOSTICATION IN STROKE REHABILITATION

Prognostication regarding outcome for a stroke patient is often expressed in the simple question: "Is this patient a good candidate for rehabilitation?" The benefits of good prognostication are self-evident. Patients and family members need to know the prospects for survival, the degree of recovery that may be expected, and the extent of possible residual disability following rehabilitation. Professionals providing care need information with which to counsel patients and families. Knowledge of prognosis of individual patients can guide physicians and therapists in selection of specific therapies and appropriate intensities of therapies. Finally, good prognostication can help to reduce costs of care through reduction of misdirected therapy and optimal use of facilities and staff.

Accurate prognostication of the ultimate status of patients after recovery from stroke has proven to be elusive because of difficulties encountered in stroke outcome research. Some factors that have made conclusions about prognostication imprecise include the following: The effects of cerebrovascular disease are heterogeneous, and pathologies are different; some patients have only transient symptoms, whereas others have severe and lasting impairment. Many studies are not comparable; for example, it is difficult to compare studies that aggregate all patients regardless of pathology, lesion site, time interval since onset, and degree of impairment with those studies of selected subgroups of patients. A major limitation in interpretation of many early reports on prediction of stroke outcome has been poor definition of prognostic variables and outcome variables. Methodological issues in stroke outcome research were reviewed in a symposium in 1989 (47,48). Important recommendations were made to standardize methodologies in outcome studies in stroke research, and in 1989, the World Health Organization task force issued similar recommendations (49).

It is important to distinguish between prognostic and outcome variables. Prognostic variables influence the survival, recovery, and ultimate outcome of an individual who has sustained an acute stroke (Table 77-14) (50). These variables may be categorized into those that are patient related, those that are lesion related, those that are intervention and therapy related, and those that are psychosocial. Outcome variables, on the other hand, describe different aspects of the status of the patient at a particular end point. Typical outcome variables of interest are listed in Table 77-15 (50).

Predicting Survival

Early death following a stroke is usually related to the underlying pathology and to the severity of the lesion. The 30-day survival for patients with cerebral infarction is 85%, but for patients with intracerebral hemorrhage, survival is reported to be only 20% to 52% (51,52). Better management of cardiac and res-

TABLE 77-14. Classification of Prognostic Variables

Patient demographic variables
General medical characteristics
   Examples: hypertension, heart disease, diabetes
Lesion-related variables
   Pathology
   Lesion site and size
   Impairment characteristics
   Coma at onset
   Bladder and bowel continence
Specific therapy interventions
   Nature of therapy
   Time of initiating therapy
   Intensity of therapy
Psychosocial variables
   Socioeconomic status
   Premorbid personality
   Patient family role

TABLE 77-15.   Outcome Variables
Survival
Impairment: neurologic deficit
Degree of paralysis
Aphasia
Visual field defect, neglect
Disability
Activities of daily living (ADL)
Ambulation
Social variables
Discharge destination
Living arrangements
Social integration

TABLE 77-16.   Factors Predicting Poor ADL Outcome
Advanced age
Comorbidities
Myocardial infarction
Diabetes mellitus
Severity of stroke
Severe weakness
Poor sitting balance
Visuospatial deficits
Mental changes
Incontinence
Low initial ADL scores
Time interval: onset to rehabilitation

ADL, activities of daily living.

piratory disorders has decreased early mortality. Hypertension, heart disease, and diabetes, however, remain as risk factors for recurrence of stroke. Coma following a stroke onset indicates a poor prognosis, presumably because coma occurs frequently in cerebral hemorrhage, and when it occurs in relationship to cerebral infarction, it reflects a large lesion with cerebral edema.

Lacunar lesions are small and affect a very limited amount of tissue. The prognosis for recovery from lacunar lesions is usually excellent, although significant persisting deficits may occur when the lesion is strategically located. Because of their subcortical locations, lacunar lesions rarely if ever affect cortical functions. With large vessel infarctions, due either to thrombosis or embolism, prognosis is related to the volume of the lesion. Outcome is poorest when the lesion involves more than 10% of intracranial volume (53). Large intracerebral hemorrhages can be devastating, with a high mortality because of increased pressure and brain displacement. Small hemorrhages have a good prognosis because the pressure effects are minor.

Predicting Disability and Functional Status

The key outcomes from a rehabilitation perspective are those that describe the disability status of the patient. The central purpose of the rehabilitation program is to lessen ultimate disability; therefore, considerable attention has been directed at the identification of factors that will predict the late functional status of the patient, especially with respect to walking and activities of daily living (ADLs).

Most patients admitted to an inpatient stroke rehabilitation program in the postacute phase have hemiparesis of sufficient severity that walking is impossible. Some recovery of leg function almost always occurs, and improvement in mobility follows. By 3 months postonset, 54% to 80% of patients are independent in walking (54,55). In a retrospective study of 248 patients with stroke treated at a rehabilitation center, Feigenson et al. (56) reported that 85% of patients were ambulatory at discharge. The degree of recovery in walking ability depends on motor recovery (42). As measured on the Brunnstrom Scale for stages of motor recovery, very few patients who remain in stage II (minimal voluntary movement) regain the ability to walk; however, most patients in stage III (active flexion and extension synergy through range of motion) do eventually walk. Data from the Framingham cohort reported by Gresham et al. (57) indicate that long-term survivors of stroke show good recovery of functional mobility, with 80% being independent in mobility.

Most patients with significant neurologic impairment who survive a stroke are dependent in basic ADLs, that is, bathing, dressing, feeding, toileting, grooming, and transfers. The ca-

pacity of individuals to perform these activities is usually scored on disability rating scales, such as the Functional Independent Measure (see Chapter 43). Almost all patients show improved function in ADLs as recovery occurs. Most improvement is noted in the first 6 months (58,59), although as many as 5% of patients show continued measurable improvement to 12 months postonset. Other patients may show some functionally worthwhile improvement beyond 6 months, which the disability scales usually fail to detect because of their limited sensitivity at the upper end of the functional range. The levels of functional independence eventually reached by stroke patients after recovery as reported by different authors are variable. This probably reflects differences between study populations and differences in methods of treatment, follow-up, and data reporting. In most reports, between 47% and 76% of survivors achieve partial or total independence in ADLs (56,58,59).

Most authors who have attempted to determine which factors predict ultimate ADL functional outcome have used multivariate analysis. Of many independent variables tested, those reported to have the most influence on outcome are listed in Table 77-16. Not all of these factors were shown in every study to statistically predict outcome status.

The effect of age on outcome may partly be related to more frequent coimpairments. If elderly patients are less functional prestroke, this alone could explain poorer outcomes following a stroke. Furthermore, elderly patients often do not receive as intensive therapy as younger patients, and they may be discharged from the rehabilitation program sooner. Some studies designed to examine age as an independent prognostic factor have not found a correlation between age and functional ADL outcome in 6 months (60). Coexisting heart disease and diabetes represent comorbidities that are likely to increase the chance of recurrent stroke and may limit a patient's full participation in an intensive program. These comorbidities affect survival, i.e., increase the likelihood of recurrence or death, but it is not known to what degree their presence influences functional recovery from stroke. Such measures of the severity of the stroke as reduced sitting balance, visuospatial impairment, mental changes, and incontinence all influence functional outcome. Intuitively, it would seem reasonable to assume that patients with more severe neurologic deficits would have worse functional outcomes, but this is not necessarily the case when isolated neurologic impairments are considered. For example, analyses of predictive variables have failed to show that patients with sensory deficits have a poorer ultimate outcome (61). The severity of the neurologic deficit is reflected in the overall ADL score, and most authors have reported that the initial ADL score is a good predictor of ultimate ADL function. Patients admitted for rehabilitation with lower ADL scores do not have as good a functional outcome as patients who initially had higher admission ADL scores.

It is generally accepted that early initiation of therapies is desirable. Early rehabilitation minimizes secondary complications, such as contractures and deconditioning, and helps motivation. It is not known whether higher-intensity therapy as an independent variable improves ultimate functional recovery.

Social Variables

The discharge destination of a patient, home or institutional placement, living arrangements, and social integration are all important in reflecting the social status of patients following recovery. Patients most likely to require long-term institutional care are those with severe disabilities who need maximum physical assistance in ADLs and who have bowel or bladder incontinence (56). However, psychosocial variables, especially prestroke family interaction (62) and the presence of an able spouse, also influence whether the patient returns home. A supportive family whose members are willing to provide significant physical care may be able to manage a severely disabled patient at home. By contrast, a patient with much less disability but no family support may require institutional care if not fully independent.

When a clinician is confronted with the challenge of evaluating an individual patient, guidelines for predicting functional outcome are useful but are not precise because multiple variables interact. A patient who might be judged as having a good prognosis for functional outcome may do poorly because of a negative psychosocial factor. The best estimate of prognosis can be made only after a thorough and comprehensive evaluation of the patient's medical, neurologic, functional, and psychosocial status. The clinician at the bedside is in the best position to formulate a prognosis and provide an answer to the question, "Is this patient a good candidate for rehabilitation?"

MEDICAL MANAGEMENT IN THE POSTACUTE PHASE

There is a high incidence of coexisting medical disorders among patients recovering from stroke, reflecting the age of the patient population and the fact that cerebrovascular disease is part of a generalized disease process. If severe, or if poorly managed, these disorders may interfere with the patient's participation in the rehabilitation program and may adversely affect outcome. It is imperative, therefore, that the attending physician assess the patient thoroughly and monitor the medical status closely, being prepared to intervene promptly when required. Some of the important and more frequent disorders are discussed briefly.

Medical Comorbidities

In a large majority of patients, a stroke is an acute event in the course of a systemic disease, e.g., atherosclerosis, hypertensive vascular disease, or cardiac embolism. These patients frequently exhibit other clinical features of the underlying systemic disorder, especially heart disease. As many as 75% of stroke patients may show evidence of coexisting cardiovascular disease, including hypertension (estimates range from 50% to 84%) (63) and coronary artery disease (as many as 65%) (63). Another group of heart diseases cause a stroke through cardiogenic cerebral embolism. These diseases include atrial fibril-

lation and other arrhythmias from multiple causes, valvular disease, cardiomyopathy, endocarditis, recent myocardial infarction, and left atrial myxoma.

Concomitant heart disease has a negative impact on short-term and long-term survival and probably on functional outcome of stroke patients (64,65). Acute exacerbations of heart disease occur frequently during postacute stroke rehabilitation (64). Common problems include angina, uncontrolled hypertension, hypotension, myocardial infarction, congestive heart failure, atrial fibrillation, and ventricular arrhythmias. Development of one of these complications may have minimal or no impact on the patient's progress or outcome if the problem is promptly diagnosed and appropriately treated. However, these complications often do impact the patient's capacity to participate fully in the therapeutic program. Congestive heart failure and angina decrease exercise tolerance and reduce capacity to roll over in bed, transfer, and walk.

All patients should be monitored carefully during postacute rehabilitation for evidence of cardiac disease. The classical features of coronary artery disease and congestive heart failure may be present, but often they are not. Ischemia may be silent. The clinical clues to significant coexisting heart disease may be subtle, e.g., slower than expected progress, excessive fatigue, lethargy, or mental changes. Patients should undergo appropriate cardiac investigation with electrocardiography, Holter monitoring, echocardiography, etc., and should receive optimal therapy. These cardiac complications can be successfully treated and are not contraindications for rehabilitation.

The rehabilitation management of patients with identified cardiac complications should include formal clinical monitoring of pulse and blood pressure during physical activities. Brief electrocardiac monitoring during exercise can add more specific information. A useful set of cardiac precautions in patients undergoing rehabilitation was developed by Fletcher et al. (66) and are listed in Table 77-17. It should be noted that in deconditioned patients, the resting heart rate may be high, and in an elderly patient, the estimated limit for heart rate based on 50% above resting may be too high. For patients on β-blockers, a reasonable limit might be a heart rate at around 20 beats above the resting level.

Medical Complications

Medical complications frequently occur during the postacute phase of rehabilitation, affecting as many as 60% of patients and as many as 94% of patients with severe lesions (67). Common medical and neurologic complications are listed in Table 77-18 (56-59).

PULMONARY ASPIRATION AND PNEUMONIA

Dysphagia is a frequent and serious complication of stroke. It is a usual feature in brain-stem lesions or bilateral hemisphere lesions (68), but it also occurs in patients with unilateral hemisphere lesions (22,69). Difficulty in swallowing may occur in the oral preparatory phase or in the pharyngeal phase. There is usually delay in or absence of the swallowing reflex. Evaluation of a patient includes observation of the muscles of the lips, tongue, cheeks, and jaw and elevation of the larynx during swallowing. Poor muscle control results in trickling of saliva or liquids into the valleculae or inability to handle solids. There is poor protection of the airway, with high risk for aspiration.

Aspiration usually causes coughing, but some studies report a significant number of patients with silent aspiration (70). Careful bedside evaluation should be performed in all patients before oral feeding is started. Muscles of the lips and tongue should be tested, and the patient observed when taking sips of

TABLE 77-17. Cardiac Precautions

Activity should be terminated if any of the following develops:
1. New onset cardiopulmonary symptoms
2. Heart rate decreases >20% of baseline
3. Heart rate increases >50% of baseline
4. Systolic BP increases to 240 mm Hg
5. Systolic BP decreases ≥30 mm Hg from baseline or to <90 mm Hg
6. Diastolic BP increases to 120 mm Hg

BP, blood pressure.
From Fletcher BJ, Dunbar S, Coleman J, Jann B, Fletcher GF. Cardiac precautions for nonacute inpatient settings. *Am J Phys Med Rehabil* 1993;72:140–143.

TABLE 77-18. Medical Complications During Postacute Stroke Rehabilitation

Complication	Frequency (%)
Medical	
Pulmonary aspiration, pneumonia	40
Urinary tract infection	40
Depression	30
Musculoskeletal pain, RSD	30
Falls	25
Malnutrition	16
Venous thromboembolism	6
Pressure ulcer	3
Neurologic	
Toxic or metabolic encephalopathy	10
Stroke progression	5
Seizure	4

RSD, reflex sympathetic dystrophy.
Data are from the following sources: Wade DT, Wood VA, Langton Hewer R. Recovery after stroke—the first 3 months. *J Neurol Neurosurg Psychiatry* 1985; 48:7–13; Feigenson JS, McDowell FH, Meese P, McCarthy ML, Greenberg SD. Factors influencing outcome and length of stay in a stroke rehabilitation unit Part 1. *Stroke* 1977;8:651–656; Gresham GE, Fitzpatrick TE, Wolf PA, MacNamara PM, Kannel WB, Dawber TR. Residual disability in survivors of stroke: The Framingham Study. *N Engl J Med* 1975;293:954–956; Wade DT, Langton Hewer R. Functional abilities after stroke; measurement, natural history and prognosis. *J Neurol Neurosurg Psychiatry* 1987;50:177–182; and Dombovy ML, Basford JR, Whisnut JP, Bergstralh EJ. Disability and use of rehabilitation services following stroke in Rochester Minnesota, 1975–1979. *Stroke* 1987;18: 830–836.

water and during eating. If the patient has a poor cough response, or if there is any question about the safety of swallowing, a videofluoroscopy using a modified barium swallow should be performed to assess swallowing and to detect aspiration. Numerous therapeutic interventions can improve swallowing. Techniques include stimulation to increase arousal, sitting the patient upright in a chair with head forward, close supervision of the patient, modifying the consistency of food to pureed solids and thickened liquids, and exercise. If swallowing is not safe, a nasogastric tube is indicated for enteral feedings. It should be noted that patients fed via a nasogastric tube are still at risk for aspiration because of gastroesophageal reflux, especially when lying flat in bed. Dysphagia rapidly improves in patients with unilateral stroke, and by 1 month postonset, only about 2% of patients still have difficulty (71). Patients with brain-stem lesions or bilateral hemisphere lesions may progress more slowly and hence require gastrostomy.

URINARY TRACT INFECTION

Urinary tract infections are common because of the neurogenic bladder and need for catheterization in the acute phase. Immediately postonset, the sacral reflexes mediating micturition are depressed, and the bladder will overdistend and, if not drained, empty by overflow incontinence. Overdistention is best avoided in the acute stage by intermittent catheterization every 4 or 6 hours, depending on the rate of urine flow. The objective is to prevent the bladder from filling beyond approximately 500 mL and to stimulate physiological emptying. There is a modest risk of urinary tract infection with catheterization, but the risk is greatly increased if an indwelling Foley catheter is used. Intermittent catheterization is preferred, especially as the need for catheter drainage may be very brief, for a few days or less. As soon as spontaneous voiding begins, the intermittent catheterization can be reduced in frequency and may be stopped when postvoid residual bladder volumes are below 100 to 150 mL. The patient can be helped to achieve better bladder control by using a posture that increases intraabdominal pressure, namely, sitting on a commode or toilet or standing to use a urinal.

In the postacute phase of stroke rehabilitation, the problem is not one of bladder overdistention but one of uninhibited bladder with incontinence. The patient has a sense of urgency to micturate and cannot postpone voiding. Bladder volumes and voided volumes are often rather small. At least some improvement in bladder function during the day can be achieved through deliberate training or pharmacologically, using anticholinergics such as oxybutynin chloride (Ditropan) to inhibit bladder contraction. Tricyclic antidepressants, such as imipramine, may also be useful because they exhibit peripheral anticholinergic and α-adrenergic agonist activity, relaxing the bladder and increasing urethral pressure and sphincter tone.

Bladder infections must be promptly recognized and treated. Management of incontinence can be quite difficult and usually involves one or all of the following: intermittent catheterization (self-catheterization whenever possible), medication, fluid restriction, and use of special diapers.

MALNUTRITION

A surprising number of patients admitted for stroke rehabilitation are malnourished, and in one report, 22% of patients showed nutritional deficiencies (72). Elderly patients may be admitted to hospital following a stroke already in a marginal nutritional status, and their condition is exacerbated by the low calorie intake during the initial acute care. If not closely monitored during postacute rehabilitation, a patient's nutritional status may be further compromised because of dysphagia, reliance on others for oral or tube feedings, lack of interest in food, depression, and problems with communication. The risk of malnutrition and dehydration should be recognized, and the intake of fluid, protein, and total calories should be monitored closely in all patients. Oral nutritional supplements may have to be prescribed, and if a patient continues to have inadequate intake, enteral tube feeding may be necessary.

MUSCULOSKELETAL PAIN AND REFLEX SYMPATHETIC DYSTROPHY

Pain in the shoulder and arm is a frequent symptom of patients undergoing postacute stroke rehabilitation. It tends to develop early, several weeks to 6 months postonset, and may affect as many as 72% of individuals, especially those with more severe hemiplegia (73).

Although some patients may have preexisting shoulder problems, such as rotator cuff tendinitis, most hemiplegic patients with shoulder pain have varying combinations of glenohumeral subluxation, spasticity, and contracture. The role of subluxation in generating a painful shoulder has been debated, but it often precedes and then accompanies a painful shoulder.

Subluxation of the glenohumeral joint is a clinical diagnosis that can be quantified by x-ray. It occurs in 30% to 50% of patients and is probably caused by the weight of the arm pulling down the humerus at a stage when the supraspinatus and deltoid muscles are flaccid and weak and by weakness of the scapular muscles, which allow the glenoid cavity to rotate facing downward (74). The shoulder is best managed in the early phases of rehabilitation through proper positioning of the arm and hand and avoidance of pulling on the arm during assisted transfers. Whenever the patient is sitting, the arm should be supported in an arm trough or lapboard. Therapy should be directed at facilitating return of active movement at the shoulder and should include techniques such as stretching to minimize spasticity, especially in shoulder depressors and internal rotators. When spasticity becomes severe and cannot be controlled with stretching, consideration may be given to reducing the tone in the subscapularis muscle with intramuscular phenol neurolysis or with botulinum toxin (75).

The syndrome of reflex sympathetic dystrophy occurs quite commonly in the hemiplegic arm (shoulder–hand syndrome). A clinical diagnosis was made in 12.5% of cases reported by Davis et al. (76) and in 25% of patients studied with a bone scan (77). The clinical features usually develop between 1 and 4 months postonset and, once established, run a rather predictable, protracted course. Pain dominates the clinical picture. The hand is swollen, and contractures develop at the shoulder, wrist, and hand, and these will persist as permanent sequelae unless the syndrome is treated early and aggressively. Treatment is most effective when begun early and consists of medical and physical measures. Some authorities have reported good results with prompt resolution of the clinical features with a short course of relatively high-dose prednisone, tapering and discontinuing the drug over several weeks. A series of stellate ganglion blocks is also advocated in acute cases. The blocks are repeated every few days. Analgesics or nonsteroidal anti-inflammatory drugs are necessary for pain control. The most important intervention is therapy to the limb to maintain range of motion of all joints, reduce swelling, and desensitize the limb through physiological stimulation such as massage and hot and cold contrast baths.

VENOUS THROMBOEMBOLISM

Immediately postonset, stroke patients are at high risk for DVT, the risk being greater when the leg is paralyzed. The risk of DVT may be as high as 75% in untreated hemiplegic patients. The thrombosis begins early, sometimes as soon as the second day and usually within the first week, although some new DVT events are recorded weeks after onset in the postacute rehabilitation phase.

All patients with stroke should receive DVT prophylaxis. Low-dose subcutaneous heparin and low-molecular-weight heparin are effective in reducing the incidence of DVT. External pneumatic compression stockings are an alternative to heparin when the risk of bleeding is high, e.g., in patients with peptic ulcer disease or intracerebral hemorrhage. Prophylaxis should continue well into the postacute phase and preferably until the patient is walking, although there are no studies to indicate the optimal duration of DVT prophylaxis (78).

The clinical signs of DVT are not reliable, being absent in about 50% of cases with proven DVT (78). However, the development of clinical signs suggesting DVT should always prompt laboratory investigation. The test of choice for diagnosis of DVT is venous duplex scanning, which has a high degree of sensitivity and specificity in patients with clinical features suggesting DVT. A positive scan is sufficient to justify treatment for DVT with anticoagulation.

The diagnosis of a new-onset DVT is a medical emergency, and immediate full-dose anticoagulation should be started with heparin infusion or full-dose low-molecular-weight heparin. Warfarin can be started on day 1, and once the prothrombin time is therapeutic, usually within 5 days, the heparin infusion can be stopped. It is advisable to keep a patient with an acute DVT on bed rest for at least 24 hours and until the heparin is therapeutic with a partial thromboplastin time between 55 and 75 seconds. In patients who are at risk of hemorrhage, e.g., those with hemorrhagic stroke, DVT may be treated by installing a vena cava filter to prevent pulmonary embolism. The reader is referred to recent reviews on venous thromboembolism in stroke (78,79).

REHABILITATION MANAGEMENT

Therapy for Hemiplegia

EARLY PHASE

In the early poststroke phase, the hemiplegic limbs are often paralyzed and flaccid. At this stage, which may last for a few hours to days, the limbs and joints are prone to development of contractures. Through poor positioning, a stuporous patient may develop nerve-pressure palsies. If the patient sits up or stands with a flaccid weak arm, the weight of the arm may stretch the capsule of the shoulder joint, leading to development of subluxation and painful shoulder.

Therapy during this early phase should consist of proper positioning of the patient in bed and support of the arm in a wheelchair trough when sitting. Traction on the arm should be avoided when the patient is moved in bed or is transferred to a wheelchair. All joints of the affected limbs should be passively moved through a full range of motion at least once daily to prevent contractures. Within hours or a few days, muscle tone returns to the paralyzed limbs, and spasticity progressively increases. Different approaches are used by therapists during this phase of motor recovery. The most widely accepted method, the neurodevelopmental technique advocated by Bobath (80), stresses exercises that tend to normalize muscle tone and prevent excessive spasticity. This is achieved through the use of special reflex-inhibiting postures and movements. If spasticity becomes severe, tone can be reduced by slow, sustained stretching, which neurophysiologically reduces Ia afferent discharge rate as the muscle spindles accommodate to their elongation. Vibration of an antagonist muscle will also reduce tone in a spastic muscle through reciprocal inhibition, although the effect does not persist after the vibration stops.

DEVELOPMENT OF MOTOR CONTROL

Movements in a hemiparetic limb show typical features of an upper motor neuron lesion. Muscles show increased tone and are weak. Initiation and termination of muscle activation are prolonged, and there is a variable degree of cocontraction of agonists and antagonists, making movements slow and clumsy. Studies of recruitment patterns of individual motor units in affected muscles show slower firing rates and impersistent firing; i.e., there are more gaps in long motor unit firing trains (81–83).

Conventional methods of rehabilitation to regain motor control consist of stretching and strengthening, attempting to retrain weak muscles through reeducation. Use of sensory feedback is often stressed to facilitate muscle activation, e.g., stroking the overlying skin, sudden stretching of the muscle, and vibration of the muscle or its tendon. Some of these latter facilitation techniques are incorporated into well-defined systems of therapy. The system developed by Rood involves superficial cutaneous stimulation using stroking, brushing, tapping, and icing, or muscle stimulation with vibration, to evoke voluntary muscle activation. Brunnstrom emphasized the synergistic patterns of movement that develop during recovery from hemiplegia. She encouraged the development of flexor and extensor synergies during early recovery, hoping that synergistic activation of muscle would, with training, transition into voluntary activation. Proprioceptive neuromuscular facilitation was developed by Kabat and colleagues and relies on quick stretching and manual resistance of muscle activation of the limbs in functional directions, which often are spiral and diagonal. The proprioceptive neuromuscular facilitation methods are more useful when muscle weakness is not due to upper motor neuron lesions. As described above, the neurodevelopmental technique (80) approach aims to inhibit spasticity and synergies, using inhibitory postures and movements, and to facilitate normal automatic responses that are involved in voluntary movement. For a review of these methods, see Lorish et al. (84). As yet, no clinical trial has shown that application of any of these approaches improves patient outcome over conventional therapy.

THERAPY FOR THE HEMIPARETIC ARM

As outlined above, early intervention is important to support the arm, preserve joint range of motion, and maintain shoulder integrity. If the arm becomes quite spastic, frequent slow stretching can help to reduce tone. Spasticity usually dominates in the flexors and may hold the wrist and fingers in a constant position of excessive flexion. A static wrist–hand orthosis is often helpful in maintaining these joints in a functional position.

The challenge of poor function in the hemiparetic hand has prompted therapists to develop new forms of therapy. One approach that has undergone considerable study is focused neuromuscular reeducation supplemented by electromyogram (EMG) biofeedback. Results of trials have been mixed, some showing benefit but others no better results than control therapy. One review of clinical trials of biofeedback did appear to show that biofeedback was an effective treatment method (85). The EMG biofeedback involves recording surface EMG from the test muscle and using auditory or visual display of the EMG signal as feedback to the patient on the ongoing activity status of the muscle. The EMG signal supplements conventional reeducation given by the therapist. Another form of therapy uses functional electrical stimulation (FES) to provide sensory–motor reeducation. The most promising technique for the hemiparetic arm appears to be FES when it is initiated by the EMG signal of the test muscle (86). Recently, EMG-triggered FES has been refined using intramuscular electrodes. The initial case reports appear promising (87). These techniques may be useful in individual patients. They should be viewed as supplemental to all the other forms of therapy given to the patient.

When severe weakness of the hemiparetic arm persists, attention of the therapist and patient is directed toward functional retraining, using the unaffected limb to achieve independence in self-care skills, etc. Several recent reports indicate that some individuals who begin to use the unaffected limb early and ignore the paretic limb succumb to what is called "learned nonuse" of the weak limb. These individuals have latent potential for improved motor function but do not improve because of failure to use the limb (88–90). Forcing patients to use the weak limb by repeated encouragement or even restraint of the unaffected hand produces measurable improvement in function in the weak hand. Trials of constraint-induced movement therapy have shown significant increases in speed and strength

of contraction. These studies appear to confirm the belief that improved function may occur with vigorous and intensive therapy, strong motivation, and good cognition, providing some selective hand movement is present.

THERAPY FOR MOBILITY

An important rehabilitation goal for a hemiplegic patient is to achieve independent ambulation. In the early stages of recovery, or if recovery is limited to weak synergy patterns only, walking will not be possible because of poor upright trunk control, inability to achieve single-limb support during stance, and inability to advance the leg during swing phase. Patients should receive initial therapy to develop gross trunk control and training in pregait activities such as posture, balance, and weight transfer to the hemiparetic leg. As recovery progresses, patients develop better gross motor skills and trunk balance and greater strength in the leg. At Brunnstrom stage III recovery (see above), characterized by strong synergies and spasticity but no selective muscle activation, most patients will walk, although many will require an ankle–foot orthosis and cane and will walk slowly. Ambulation improves as motor recovery provides for selective phasic activation of muscles during the gait cycle. For details on evaluation of hemiplegic gait and therapeutic interventions, see reviews by Perry (91,92).

There have been reports that hemiplegic patients benefit from intensive gait training when therapy consists of walking on a treadmill with body weight partially supported with a harness (93,94). The harness substitutes for poor trunk control, and the motor-driven treadmill forces locomotion. During early training, the patient is assisted by two or three therapists in controlling the trunk, pelvis, and weak leg. Treadmill training with body weight support is superior to conventional therapy. It was found that with treadmill training, some nonambulatory hemiplegic patients learned to walk, and those who were already walking significantly increased their gait speed.

Communication Therapy

Language therapy is based on the detailed evaluation of the patient's cognitive and linguistic capabilities and deficits. Generally, speech pathologists attempt to improve communicative ability by circumventing or deblocking the language deficit or by helping the patient to compensate. In the early stages of rehabilitation, it is important for the therapist to help the patient establish a reliable means for basic yes/no communication. The therapist then progresses to specific techniques based on the patient's deficits. Even though spontaneous recovery is responsible for early improvement, speech therapy plays an extremely important role in minimizing patient isolation and encouraging the patient to actively engage in the program. Although communication may be difficult, simple childish phrases or tasks should be avoided, as patients perceive them as infantile and may withdraw. Specific techniques have been described for improving comprehension, word or phoneme retrieval, and gestures to supplement verbal communication. There have been reports of patients showing continued slow recovery between 6 and 12 months and beyond. It is difficult to predict which patients will show late recovery, but it seems quite justified to continue speech therapy while patients are showing measurable gains in communication.

Disorders of Cognition and Behavior

Cerebrovascular lesions produce a wide spectrum of cognitive and behavioral clinical features. At the extreme end is dementia, which may preclude functional recovery and render efforts at rehabilitation futile. Less severe impairments of higher-level function may be observed frequently in patients undergoing rehabilitation, e.g., poor attention, decreased memory, ignoring the food on one side of a plate, or bumping into one side of a doorway. Other more subtle changes may not be apparent until the patient returns home and family members notice mild behavioral changes, such as decreased judgment or insight. All of these conditions affect performance of functional activities, sometimes profoundly. Therefore, the professional should be able to recognize significant cognitive and behavioral disorders and anticipate how therapeutic strategies may be employed to ameliorate them.

LESION AND COGNITION/BEHAVIOR

In general, the absolute size of a brain lesion determines the severity of behavioral and psychological changes poststroke. For example, large cortical lesions produce more psychological changes than smaller subcortical lesions. Behavioral and organic mental changes occur most often in association with frontal lesions and less often with parietal, temporal, or occipital lesions. Patients with multiple lesions, especially when bilateral, are more likely to show features of dementia (95). Numerous studies have shown that in patients with a history of stroke, those with more extensive white matter changes are at higher risk for dementia.

It has been reported that patients with left hemisphere lesions, especially when they are anterior, are more likely to be depressed, although this has been disputed. Patients with right hemisphere lesions are more likely to be unduly cheerful. Emotional lability occurs in as many as 20% of patients poststroke and is more common in patients with right hemisphere lesions. It is a typical feature of the syndrome of pseudobulbar palsy. The clinical features of emotional lability tend to improve with time and often respond to tricyclic antidepressants (96,97).

UNILATERAL NEGLECT

Many patients with a nondominant parietal lobe lesion have neglect and ignore the opposite side of the body or hemispace. Inattention also occurs with impaired sensation or homonymous hemianopia. Patients with persistent inattention perform functional tasks less well, and various therapies have been tried to remediate the inattention. Therapy is directed at retraining, with repetitive exercises or use of compensatory techniques, to teach new methods of task completion. These therapies include training patients to visually scan from side to side, offering stimuli to draw attention to the left hemispace, and environmental adaptations. An example of environmental adaptation is orientation of the patient's neglected hemispace toward the side most frequently stimulated, e.g., entrance to the room. Specific therapy is usually given to remediate visual neglect and hemianopia, which almost always includes visual scanning. Another strategy for improving vision in patients with complete hemianopia is the use of Fresnel prisms applied to eyeglasses. These devices shift images in the affected hemivisual field toward the center of the retina and hence into the field of view (98).

DEPRESSION

Depression is very common following stroke and, depending on diagnostic criteria, has been reported in as many as 50% of patients (99,100). Although there is some dispute about lesion location and depression, there is apparently a relationship between left frontal lesions and major depression (101), though this relationship may operate only in the early phase poststroke. It has been hypothesized that the depression in these cases may be induced by catecholamine depletion through lesion-induced damage to the frontal noradrenergic, dopaminergic, and serotonergic projections. Many authors have pointed out the important psychological factors that can lead to depression following stroke. These include psychological responses to the physical and personal losses caused by the stroke and the state of helplessness and loss of control that often accompanies severe disability.

The diagnosis of poststroke depression is often difficult because some of the diagnostic criteria used may simply reflect sequelae of the stroke, e.g., vegetative symptoms such as sleep disturbance, fatigue, and psychomotor retardation. Of particular importance in the diagnosis is depressed mood and loss of interest in participating in daily activities, such as the rehabilitation program (102).

Persisting depression correlates with delayed recovery and poorer ultimate outcome. Active treatment should be considered for all patients with significant clinical depression. There is general acceptance of the importance of psychosocial intervention by all professional staff, with individual psychotherapy supplemented by positive reinforcement of the progress being made in rehabilitation. Many patients respond to drug therapy. Antidepressants improve depression in a majority of patients, desipramine or the selective serotonin reuptake inhibitor group being favored because of fewer side effects. Some practitioners prescribe methylphenidate [Ritalin (CibaGeneva, Summit, New Jersey)] with the antidepressant, as this drug will often bring about an abrupt improvement in arousal and motivation to participate in the therapeutic program.

SEXUALITY

It has been well documented that the majority of elderly persons continue to enjoy active and satisfying sexual relationships. By contrast, however, there is considerable sexual dysfunction following stroke (103). Before-and-after studies have reported a marked decline in sexual activity, involving both men and women. There is a marked reduction in libido with a corresponding decrease in coital frequency. In one study (104), male patients reported that before the stroke, 95% had erections, but only 38% reported normal erections poststroke, and 58% believed that after the stroke they had a sexual problem. These and most other poststroke sexual problems are related to emotional factors, such as fear, anxiety, or guilt regarding the stroke itself. Patients have a loss of self-esteem, and they may fear rejection or abandonment by their partner. They are, therefore, reluctant to make emotional demands. Health-care professionals should be sensitive to relationship issues and be prepared to ask questions about intimacy, sexual attitudes, needs, and behavior. Most will require supportive psychotherapy to provide them with better mechanisms to cope with the sequelae of the stroke.

PSYCHOSOCIAL ASPECTS

The psychological, social, and family aspects of stroke rehabilitation are extremely important. The abrupt change in the life situation of the stroke survivor impacts all phases of care. The patient fears loss of independence, and the disabilities reduce self-esteem and self-worth. Patients are often concerned about the capacity of their spouse to sustain them following discharge and whether they will both be able to make the appropriate role adjustments. The response of some patients to the stroke may be catastrophic with subsequent maladaptive behavior. All members of the rehabilitation team should contribute to a positive and supportive milieu to promote appropriate coping strategies on the part of the patient and to assist the patient and family to prepare for discharge and reintegration into the home and community. This will involve early discussions around planning for discharge, education about stroke and its consequences, and detailed discussions about potential problems and opportunities that patient and family will encounter in the future.

Late Rehabilitation Issues

There are important issues that make postdischarge follow-up mandatory. From a medical perspective, the majority of patients have ongoing medical problems requiring monitoring and therapeutic intervention such as hypertension, heart disease, diabetes, etc. Appropriate management will reduce the risk of stroke recurrence and prolong survival. A seizure disorder develops in about 8% of stroke survivors, and this requires conventional monitoring and treatment.

There are also rehabilitation issues that are ongoing. The rehabilitation program does not finish when the patient leaves the hospital, and almost all patients benefit from continued therapy. There are many reports describing continued improvement over many months postdischarge, and many patients require formal therapy to achieve that continued progress. The physician overseeing the rehabilitation program should regularly reevaluate the patient to document physical progress and define ongoing therapeutic goals. Specific problems that may become prominent following discharge from the hospital, during the outpatient therapy phase of care, include psychological maladjustment and depression; reduced sexuality; poor role adjustment in the home and family; equipment needs; transportation and driving; and secondary physical problems, such as excessive spasticity in the arm, reflex sympathetic dystrophy, changing pattern of ambulation, etc. Management of spasticity requires careful evaluation, goal setting, and selection of appropriate therapies (105). Dantrolene (Proctor & Gamble Pharmaceuticals, Cincinnati, OH) has been used for many years for pharmacologic treatment of hemiplegic spasticity caused by stroke (106), but early use of dantrolene did not improve function in a recent double-blind study (107). A small number of patients are bothered by spontaneous spasms occurring mostly at night in bed. These can usually be adequately controlled by small doses of diazepam before bedtime. For localized spasticity, such as biceps, forearm flexors, or calf muscles, intramuscular neurolysis with phenol or chemodenervation with intramuscular botulinum toxin injections can be very effective.

For all of these reasons, the rehabilitation physician should continue to monitor the progress of the patient as long as necessary to be satisfied that the patient has reached a stable, optimal level of function.

REFERENCES

1. Bonita R. Epidemiology of stroke. *Lancet* 1992;339:342–344.
2. Kannel WB, Dawber TR, Sorlie P, Wolf PA. Components of blood pressure and risk of atherothrombotic brain infarction: the Framingham Study. *Stroke* 1976;7:327–331.
3. Wolf PA, Kannel WB, Venter J. Current status of risk factors for stroke. *Neurol Clin* 1983;1:317–343.
4. Wolf PA, Dawber TR, Thomas HE Jr, Kannel WB. Epidemiologic assessment of chronic atrial fibrillation and risk of stroke: the Framingham Study. *Neurology* 1978;23:973–977.
5. Shinton R, Beevers G. Meta-analysis of relation between cigarette smoking and stroke. *BMJ* 1989;298:789–794.
6. Dyken ML, Conneally M, Haener AF, et al. Cooperative study of the hospital frequency and character of transient ischemic attacks. 1. Background, organization and clinical survey. *JAMA* 1997;237:882–886.
7. Feinberg WM, Albers GW, Barnett HJM, et al. Guidelines for the management of transient ischemic attacks. *Stroke* 1994;25:1320–1335.
8. Diener HC, Cunha L, Forbes C, et al. European stroke prevention study. 2. Dipyridamole and acetylsalicylic acid in the secondary prevention of stroke. *J Neurol Sci* 1996;143:1–13.
9. North American Symptomatic Carotid Endarterectomy Trial Collaborators. Beneficial effect of carotid endarterectomy in symptomatic patients with high-grade carotid stenosis. *N Engl J Med* 1991;325:445–453.
10. Barnett HJM, Haines SJ. Carotid endarterectomy for asymptomatic carotid stenosis. *N Engl J Med* 1993;328:276–279.
11. Sacco RL. Risk factors and outcomes for ischemic stroke. *Neurology* 1995;45 [Suppl 1]:S10–S14.
12. Viitanen M, Eriksson S, Asplund K. Risk of recurrent stroke, myocardial infarction and epilepsy. *Eur Neurol* 1988;28:227–231.
13. Leonberg SC, Elliott FA. Prevention of recurrent stroke. *Stroke* 1981;12:731–735.
14. Mohr JP, Caplan LR, Melski JW, et al. The Harvard cooperative stroke registry: a prospective study. *Neurology* 1978;28:754–762.
15. Steinberg GK, Fabrikant JI, Marks MP, et al. Stereotactic heavy-charged-particle Bragg-Peak radiation for intracranial arteriovenous malformations. *N Engl J Med* 1990;323:96–101.
16. Sheets RM, Ashwal S, Szer IS. Neurologic manifestations of rheumatic disorders of childhood. In: Swaiman KF, Ashwal S, eds. *Pediatric neurology: principles and practice*, 3rd ed. St Louis: CV Mosby, 1999.
17. Stroke Unit Trialists' Collaboration. Collaboration SUT: collaborative systematic review of the randomised trials of organized inpatient (stroke unit) care after stroke. *BMJ* 1997;314:1151–1159.
18. The National Institute of Neurological Disorders and Stroke rt-PA Stroke Study Group. Tissue plasminogen activator for acute ischemic stroke. *N Engl J Med* 1995;333:1581–1587.
19. Dobkin BH. *Neurologic rehabilitation*. Philadelphia: FA Davis, 1966.
20. Stein DG, Brailowsky S, Will B. *Brain repair*. New York: Oxford University Press, 1995.
21. Roth EJ. Medical complications encountered in stroke rehabilitation. *Phys Med Rehabil Clin N Am* 1991;2(3):563–578.
22. Horner J, Massey EW, Riski JE, et al. Aspiration following stroke: clinical correlates and outcomes. *Neurology* 1988;38:1359–1362.
23. Gresham GE, Duncan PW, Stason WB, et al. *Post-stroke rehabilitation*. Clinical Practice Guideline No 16. Rockville, MD: U.S. Department of Health and Human Services, Public Health Service, Agency for Health Care Policy and Research. AHCPR Publication No. 95–0662, May 1995.
24. Booth FW. Effect of limb immobilization on skeletal muscle. *J Appl Physiol* 1982;52:1113.
25. Foulkes MA, Wolf PA, Price TR, et al. The Stroke data bank: design, methods and baseline characteristics. *Stroke* 1988;19:547–554.
26. Twitchell TE. The restoration of motor function following hemiplegia in man. *Brain* 1951;74:443–480.
27. Nakayama H, Jorgensen HS, Raaschou HO, Olsen TS. Recovery of upper extremity function in stroke patients: the Copenhagen Stroke Study. *Arch Phys Med Rehabil* 1994;75:394–398.
28. Bard G, Hirshberg CG. Recovery of voluntary motion in upper extremity following hemiplegia. *Arch Phys Med Rehabil* 1965;46:567–572.
29. Gowland C. Management of hemiplegic upper limb. In: Brandstater ME, Basmajian J, eds. *Stroke rehabilitation*. Baltimore: Williams & Wilkins, 1987; 217–245.
30. Wade DT, Langton Hewer R, Wood VA, et al. The hemiplegic arm after stroke: measurement and recovery. *J Neurol Neurosurg Psychiatry* 1983;46: 521–524.
31. Jorgensen HS, Nakayama H, Raaschou HO, et al. Stroke rehabilitation: outcome and speed of recovery. Part II: Speed of recovery: the Copenhagen Stroke Study. *Arch Phys Med Rehabil* 1995;76:406–412.
32. Kelly-Hayes M, Wolf PA, Kase CS, et al. Time course of functional recovery after stroke: the Framingham Study. *J Neurol Rehabil* 1989;3:65–70.
33. Wade DT, Langton Hewer R, David RM, Enderby PM. Aphasia after stroke: natural history and associated deficits. *J Neurol Neurosurg Psychiatry* 1986;49: 11–16.
34. Skilbeck CE, Wade DT, Langton Hewer R, Wood VA. Recovery after stroke. *J Neurol Neurosurg Psychiatry* 1983;46:5–8.
35. Brandstater ME. Basic aspects of impairment evaluation in stroke patients. In: Chino N, Melvin JL, eds. *Functional evaluation of stroke patients*. New York: Springer-Verlag, 1996:9–18.
36. Strub R, Black F. *The mental status examination in neurology*, 2nd ed. Philadelphia: FA Davis, 1995.
37. Folstein MF, Folstein SF, McHugh PR. Mini-Mental State: a practical method for grading the cognitive state for the clinician. *J Psychiatr Res* 1975;12:189–198.
38. Goodglass H, Kaplan E. *The assessment of aphasia and related disorders*. Philadelphia: Lea & Febiger, 1983.
39. Kertesz A. *Western aphasia battery*. New York: Grune & Stratton, 1982.
40. Sarno MT. *The Functional Communication Profile: manual of directions*. Rehabilitation monograph 42. New York: Institute of Rehabilitation Medicine, 1969.
41. Brunnstrom S. *Movement therapy in hemiplegia: a neurophysiological approach*. New York: Harper & Row, 1970.

42. Brandstater ME, deBruin H, Gowland C, Clark B. Hemiplegic gait: analysis of temporal variables. *Arch Phys Med Rehabil* 1983;64:583–587.

43. Bohannon RW. Is the measurement of muscle strength appropriate in patients with brain lesions? *Phys Ther* 1989; 69:225–230.

44. Bohannon RW. Correlation of lower limb strengths and other variables with standing performance in stroke patients. *Physiother Can* 1989;41:198–202.

45. Fugl-Meyer AR, Jaasko L, Leyman I, et al. The post-stroke hemiplegic patient. I: A method for evaluation of physical performance. *Scand J Rehabil Med* 1975;7:13–31.

46. Bohannon RW, Smith MB. Interrater reliability of a modified Ashworth scale of muscle spasticity. *Phys Ther* 1987;67:206–207.

47. Gresham GE. Past achievements and new directions in stroke outcome research. *Stroke* 1990;21[Suppl II]:II-1–II-2.

48. Jongbloed L. Problems of methodological heterogeniety in studies predicting disability after stroke. *Stroke* 1990;21[Suppl II]:II-32–II-34.

49. World Health Organization (WHO). Recommendations on stroke prevention, diagnosis, and therapy: report of WHO Taskforce on Stroke and Other Cerebral Vascular Disorders. *Stroke* 1989;20:1407–1431.

50. Brandstater ME. Prognostication in stroke rehabilitation. In: Chino N, Melvin JL, eds. *Functional evaluation of stroke patients.* New York: Springer-Verlag, 1996: 93–102.

51. Broderick JP, Phillips SJ, Whisnant JP, et al. Incidence rates of stroke in the eighties: the end of the decline in stroke. *Stroke* 1989;20:577–582.

52. Sacco RL, Wolf PA, Kannel WB, MacNamara PM. Survival and recurrence following stroke: the Framingham Study. *Stroke* 1982;13:290–295.

53. Ganesan V, Ng V, Chong WK, et al. Lesion volume, lesion location, and outcome after middle cerebral artery territory stroke. *Arch Dis Child* 1999;81: 295–300.

54. Skilbeck CE, Wade DT, Langton Hewer R, Wood VA. Recovery after stroke. *J Neurol Neurosurg Psychiatry* 1983;46:5–8.

55. Wade DT, Wood VA, Langton Hewer R. Recovery after stroke: the first 3 months. *J Neurol Neurosurg Psychiatry* 1985;48:7–13.

56. Feigenson JS, McDowell FH, Meese P, et al. Factors influencing outcome and length of stay in a stroke rehabilitation unit. Part 1. *Stroke* 1977;8:651–656.

57. Gresham GE, Fitzpatrick TE, Wolf PA, et al. Residual disability in survivors of stroke: the Framingham Study. *N Engl J Med* 1975;293:954–956.

58. Wade DT, Langton Hewer R. Functional abilities after stroke: measurement, natural history and prognosis. *J Neurol Neurosurg Psychiatry* 1987;50:177–182.

59. Dombovy ML, Basford JR, Whisnut JP, Bergstralh EJ. Disability and use of rehabilitation services following stroke in Rochester, Minnesota, 1975–1979. *Stroke* 1987;18:830–836.

60. Wade DT, Langton Hewer R, Wood VA. Stroke: the influence of age on the outcome. *Age Ageing* 1984;13:357–362.

61. Wade DT, Skilbeck CE, Langton Hewer R. Predicting Barthel ADL score at 6 months after an acute stroke. *Arch Phys Med Rehabil* 1983;64:24–28.

62. Evans RL, Bishop DS, Matlock AL, et al. Family interaction and treatment adherence after stroke. *Arch Phys Med Rehabil* 1987;68:513–517.

63. Hertzer NR, Young JR, Beven EG, et al. Coronary angiography in 506 patients with extracranial cerebrovascular disease. *Arch Intern Med* 1985;145: 849–852.

64. Roth EJ, Mueller K, Green D. Stroke rehabilitation outcome: impact of coronary artery disease. *Stroke* 1988;19:42–47.

65. Roth EJ. Heart disease in patients with stroke. Part II: Impact and implications for rehabilitation. *Arch Phys Med Rehabil* 1994;75:94–101.

66. Fletcher BJ, Dunbar S, Coleman J, et al. Cardiac precautions for nonacute inpatient settings. *Am J Phys Med Rehabil* 1993;72:140–143.

67. Kalra L, Yu G, Wilson K, Roots P. Medical complications during stroke rehabilitation. *Stroke* 1995;26:990–994.

68. Horner J, Massey EW, Brazer SR. Aspiration in bilateral stroke patients. *Neurology* 1990;40:1686–1688.

69. Teasell RW, Bach D, MacRae M. Prevalence and recovery of aspiration poststroke: a retrospective analysis. *Dysphagia* 1994;9:35–39.

70. Horner J, Massey EW. Silent aspiration following stroke. *Neurology* 1988; 38:317–319.

71. Blauer D. The natural history and functional consequences of dysphagia after hemispheric stroke. *J Neurol Neurosurg Psychiatry* 1989;52:236–241.

72. Axelsson K, Asplund K, Norberg A, Alafuzoff I. Nutritional status in patients with acute stroke. *Acta Med Scand* 1988;224:217–224.

73. Van Onwenaller C, LaPlace PM, Chartraine A. Painful shoulder in hemiplegia. *Arch Phys Med Rehabil* 1985;67:23–26.

74. Basmajian JV. *Muscles alive: their function revealed by electromyography,* 4th ed. Baltimore: Williams & Wilkins, 1978.

75. Hecht JS. Subscapular nerve block in the painful hemiplegic shoulder. *Arch Phys Med Rehabil* 1992;73:1036–1039.

76. Davis SW, Petrillo CR, Eichberg RD, Chu DS. Shoulder–hand syndrome in a hemiplegic population: 5-year retrospective study. *Arch Phys Med Rehabil* 1977;58:353–356.

77. Tepperman PS, Greyson ND, Hilbert L, et al. Reflex sympathetic dystrophy in hemiplegia. *Arch Phys Med Rehabil* 1984;65:442–447.

78. Brandstater ME, Siebens H, Roth EJ. Venous thromboembolism in stroke: Part I. Literature review and implications for clinical practice. *Arch Phys Med Rehabil* 1992;73:S379–S391.

79. Harvey RL, Green D. Deep venous thrombosis and pulmonary embolism in stroke. *Top Stroke Rehabil* 1996;3(1):54–70.

80. Bobath B. *Adult hemiplegia: evaluation and treatment.* London: Heinemann, 1976.

81. Freund HJ, Hefter H, Homberg V. Motor unit activity in motor disorders. In: Shahani B, ed. *Electromyography in CNS disorders: central EMG.* Boston: Butterworths, 1984:29–44.

82. Kraft GH, Fitts SS, Hammond MC, et al. Motor unit activity in forearm muscles following cerebral vascular accident. *Arch Phys Med Rehabil* 1986;67: 673–674.

83. Hammond MC, Kraft GH, Fitts SS. Recruitment and termination of EMG activity in the hemiparetic forearm. *Arch Phys Med Rehabil* 1988;69:106–110.

84. Lorish TR, Sandin KJ, Roth EJ, Noll SF. Stroke rehabilitation: 3, rehabilitation evaluation and management. *Arch Phys Med Rehabil* 1994;75:S47–S51.

85. Schleenbaker RE, Mainous AG III. Electromyographic biofeedback for neuromuscular reeducation in the hemiplegic stroke patient: a meta-analysis. *Arch Phys Med Rehabil* 1993;74:1301–1304.

86. Kraft GH, Fitts SS, Hammond MC. Techniques to improve function of the arm and hand in chronic hemiplegia. *Arch Phys Med Rehabil* 1992;73:220–227.

87. Chae J, Fang ZP, Walker M, Pourmehdi S. Intramuscular electrically controlled neuromuscular electrical stimulation for upper limb recovery in chronic hemiplegia. *Am J Phys Med* 2001;80:935–941.

88. Wolf SL, Lecraw DE, Barton LA, Jann FF. Forced use of hemiplegic upper extremities to reverse the effect of learned nonuse among chronic stroke and head injured patients. *Exp Neurol* 1989;104:125–132.

89. Taub E, Miller NE, Novack TA, et al. A technique for improving chronic motor deficit after stroke. *Arch Phys Med Rehabil* 1993;74:347–354.

90. Taub E, Wolf SL. Constraint induced movement techniques to facilitate upper extremity use in stroke patients. *Top Stroke Rehabil* 1997;3(4):38–61.

91. Perry J, Montgomery J. Gait of the stroke patient and orthotic indications. In: Brandstater ME, Basmajian JV, eds. *Stroke rehabilitation.* Baltimore: Williams & Wilkins, 1987.

92. Perry J. *Gait analysis: normal and pathological function.* Thorofare, NJ: Slack, 1992.

93. Hesse S, Bertelt C, Jahnke M, et al. Treadmill training with partial body weight support compared to physiotherapy in nonambulatory hemiparetic patients. *Stroke* 1995;26:976–981.

94. Hesse S, Bertelt C, Schaffrin A, et al. Restoration of gait in nonambulatory hemiparetic patients by treadmill training with partial body weight support. *Arch Phys Med Rehabil* 1994;75:1087–1093.

95. Adams RD, Victor M. *Principles of neurology,* 4th ed. New York: McGraw-Hill, 1989.

96. Seliger G, Hornstein A, Flax J, et al. Fluoxetine improves emotional incontinence. *Brain Inj* 1991;5:1–4.

97. Robinson RG, Parikh RM, Lipsey JR, et al. Pathological laughing and crying following stroke: validation of a measurement scale and a double-blind study. *Am J Psychiatry* 1993;150:286–293.

98. Rossi P, Kheyfets S, Reding M. Fresnel prisms improve visual perception in stroke patients with homonymous hemianopia or unilateral visual neglect. *Neurology* 1990;40:1597–1599.

99. Robinson RG, Starr LB, Kubos K. A two-year longitudinal study of poststroke mood disorders: findings during the initial evaluation. *Stroke* 1983;14: 736–741.

100. Coll P, Erickson RJ. Mood disorders associated with stroke. *Phys Med Rehabil State Art Rev* 1989;3:619–628.

101. Robinson RG, Szetela B. Mood change following left hemisphere brain injury. *Ann Neurol* 1981;9:447–453.

102. Lazarus LW, Moberg PJ, Langsley PR, Lingam VR. Methylphenidate and nortiptyline in the treatment of poststroke depression: a retrospective comparison. *Arch Phys Med Rehabil* 1994;75:403–406.

103. Monga TN. Sexuality post stroke. *Phys Med Rehab: State Art Rev* 1993;7:225–236.

104. Monga TN, Lawson JS, Inglis J. Sexual dysfunction in stroke patients. *Arch Phys Med Rehabil* 1986;67:19–22.

105. O'Brien CF, Seeberger LC, Smith DB. Spasticity after stroke: epidemiology and optimal treatment. *Drugs Aging* 1996;9:332–340.

106. Chyatte SB, Bridsong JH, Bergman BA. the effects of dantrolene sodium on spasticity and motor performance in hemiplegia. *South Med* 1971;64:180–185.

107. Katrak PH, Cole AMD, Poulos CM, McCauley JCK. Objective assessment of spasticity, strength, and function with early exhibition of dantrolene sodium after cerebrovascular accident: a randomized double-blind study. *Arch Phys Med Rehabil* 1992;73:4–9.

CHAPTER 78

Rehabilitation Issues in Traumatic Brain Injury

John Whyte, Tessa Hart, Andrea Laborde, and Mitchell Rosenthal

NATURE OF TRAUMATIC BRAIN INJURY

Traumatic brain injury (TBI) is a major health problem in the United States and other countries where vehicular accidents, sporting accidents, and interpersonal violence are commonplace. The systematic study of the residual effects of TBI can be traced to World War II and the work of Alexander Luria, Kurt Goldstein, and others (1,2). In this early work, much was learned about the deficits following penetrating injuries to the brain in soldiers with gunshot wounds. The pattern of residual dysfunction often corresponded to a focal lesion caused by the bullet passing through the brain. These focal deficits were similar to those observed in strokes.

The vast majority of peacetime TBIs seen in hospitals are classified as closed head injuries, wherein the skull is not actually penetrated. The nature of injury sustained in vehicular accidents (e.g., blunt impact, acceleration-deceleration) often results in multifocal lesions and diffuse brain damage with a variety of physical, cognitive, and neurobehavioral impairments that are unique to each person and pose formidable obstacles to community integration.

TBI affects all age groups. However, additional complex issues are posed by children with TBI because the injury interacts with the processes of biological, psychological, and social development. The special problems of children with TBI are not treated in detail here, but there are excellent sources for additional information on this topic (3–5) (See also Traumatic Brain Injury in Children and Adolescents). At the other end of the age spectrum one finds the older adult with brain injury, whose recovery tends to be slower than the younger population and is complicated by preexisting comorbidities and the reduced plasticity of the aged brain (6). Given the increasing percentage of older persons within the general population, it is likely that a growing number of survivors of brain injury will be in this subgroup.

The Range of Outcomes: Death to Complete Recovery

The pattern and severity of injury and resultant outcomes are highly variable. In some injuries, commonly referred to as mild, the person may not suffer any loss of consciousness or only a very brief period of altered consciousness. In these cases, the person may be seen in a hospital emergency room, held for observation, and released several hours later. In the absence of any further medical complications, the person may return to normal activities within a few days. In a minority of cases, somatic, cognitive, and affective symptoms may persist for weeks, months, or longer (see also Mild Traumatic Brain Injury). Mild brain injuries constitute the vast majority of TBIs within the United States, though the rate of hospitalization for mild TBI has declined substantially from 130 per 100,000 population in the 1970s to 51 per 100,000 population in the 1990s (7).

Most rehabilitation efforts are focused on those with severe TBI (i.e., unconsciousness of 6 hours or longer). The Centers for Disease Control and Prevention (CDC) estimates that approximately 80,000 to 90,000 individuals survive each year with disability caused by TBI (7). Within this broad category, a variety of outcomes may be observed. Sosin and colleagues (8) reported a 22% reduction in death rate due to TBI from 1979 to 1992, to an estimated 20.7 per 100,000 population, which they attributed to a decrease in deaths associated with motor vehicle crashes. For the survivors, global outcome usually is defined by the categories of the Glasgow Outcome Scale (GOS) (9). Table 78-1 depicts the percentage of survivors in these categories at various time periods after injury. Even those who achieve a "good recovery" status according to the GOS, however, may have significant psychosocial impairments that preclude a return to premorbid level of function.

Measures of Injury Severity

Both *depth* and *duration* of coma have been considered to be indices of the severity of TBI. Clinical assessment of coma was made more precise and objective with the advent of the Glasgow Coma Scale (GCS) (10), a quantitative measure of the depth of unconsciousness (Table 78-2). Coma is defined as not opening the eyes, not obeying commands, and not uttering understandable words. A GCS score of 8 or less in the acute period is operationally defined as a comatose state (11).

Duration of coma is often defined as the time to follow commands. Both duration of coma and initial GCS score have been reported to predict neurobehavioral outcome from TBI (12,13), varying with the outcome measures selected and the time since

TABLE 78-1.   Outcome in Survivors of Severe Head Injury

Outcome	3 Mos. (n = 534)	6 Mos. (n = 515)	12 Ms. (n = 376)
Vegetative state	7%	5%	3%
Severe disability	29%	19%	16%
Moderate disability	33%	34%	31%
Good recovery	31%	42%	50%
Moderate–good (combined)	64%	76%	81%

n, number of patients.
From Jennett B, Teasdale G. *Management of head injuries*. Philadelphia: FA Davis Co, 1981:309.

injury. Stein and Spettell (14) showed that when the GCS was modified slightly to include complications such as intracranial lesions, its predictive power was improved.

Russell was the first to suggest the duration of *posttraumatic amnesia* (PTA) as a measure of injury severity (15). During PTA, patients are out of coma but remain disoriented and amnesic for day-to-day events. Duration of PTA is measured from the onset of TBI to the resumption of ongoing memory; the duration of coma, if any, is thus included. Researchers have used PTA as an index of injury severity and an important predictor of outcome (16,17). Retrospective measurement of PTA duration from examination of medical records, or by asking the person to estimate the amnestic interval, can be unreliable. The Galveston Orientation and Amnesia Test (GOAT; Table 78-3) has provided an objective, reliable way of measuring PTA prospectively (18). The GOAT has been criticized on the grounds that although it assesses orientation, it fails to capture the amnesia characteristic of PTA. An alternative, the Westmead PTA Scale, includes a measure of day-to-day memory as well as standard orientation questions (19). Duration of PTA, assessed prospectively with the Westmead, is a strong predictor of long-term outcome variables such as future employment status (20). The predictive power of PTA duration is better for patients whose brain damage is caused primarily by diffuse axonal injury than for those with primarily contusions or other focal brain injury (21). Another alternative, known as the Orientation Log (O-Log), has been used increasingly and found to be easier to administer than the GOAT. Unlike the GOAT, the O-Log allows for cueing to assist individuals with language or severe memory impairments, and it does not require the patient to verify information about events relating to the injury (22). The initial O-Log score, combined with measures such as time since injury and number of O-Log administrations, accurately predicted resolution of disorientation in 76% of a sample of 389 individuals between the ages of 10 to 93 years (23).

EPIDEMIOLOGY OF TRAUMATIC BRAIN INJURY

The incidence of TBI requiring hospitalization is estimated to be approximately 95 per 100,000 population in the United States. In all, approximately 230,000 individuals are hospitalized and survive with TBI annually in the United States. This rate of hospitalization represents an approximately 50% decrease from studies conducted 15 to 20 years ago. It is considered to be a reflection of substantially fewer "mild" cases being hospitalized due to managed care practices and changes in admission policies, rather than a drop in incidence of TBI. Precise measures of prevalence within the population are unknown; however, the CDC estimates that approximately 5.3 million Americans are living with a TBI-related disability (24).

The age distribution is bimodal, with young adults (between the ages of 15 to 24 years, 145 per 100,000) and the elderly (75 years and older, 191 per 100,000) showing the highest incidence (24). The elderly population has the highest level of mortality—46 per 100,000 (24). Elderly patients have a much slower and less certain recovery process, compared with the young adult population (25).

In all studies of moderate/severe TBI, men outnumber women by at least two to one. Further, male TBI mortalities are three to four times greater than those in the female population (26). Several studies have noted that TBI tends to occur with slightly greater frequency among minority groups (27).

TABLE 78-2.   Glasgow Coma Scale

Examiner's Test	Patient's Response	Assigned Score
Eye opening		
Spontaneous	Opens eyes on own	4
Speech	Opens eyes when asked in a loud voice	3
Pain	Opens eyes when pinched	2
Pain	Does not open eyes	1
Best motor response		
Commands	Follows simple commands	6
Pain	Pulls examiner's hands away when pinched	5
Pain	Pulls a part of the body away when pinched	4
Pain	Flexes body inappropriately when pinched (decorticate posturing)	3
Pain	Body becomes rigid in an extended position when pinched (decerebrate posturing)	2
Pain	Has no motor response to pinch	1
Verbal response (talking)		
Speech	Carries on a conversation correctly and tells examiner where he or she is, month and year	5
Speech	Seems confused or disoriented	4
Speech	Talks so examiner can understand words being spoken but makes no sense	3
Speech	Makes sounds that examiner cannot understand	2
Speech	Makes no noise	1

From Teasdale G, Jennett B. Assessment of coma and impaired consciousness. *Lancet* 1974;2:81.

TABLE 78-3.   The Galveston Orientation and Amnesia Test

Name _____   Date of test _____

Age _____ Sex M F   Day of the week S M T W T F S

Date of birth _____   Time _____ A.M. P.M.

Diagnosis _____   Date of injury _____

	Error points
1. What is your name? (2) _____	_____
When were you born? (4) _____	_____
Where do you live? (4) _____	_____
2. Where are you now? (5) (City) _____	_____
Hospital (5) (unnecessary to state name of hospital) _____	_____
3. On what date were you admitted to this hospital? (5) _____	_____
How did you get here? (5) _____	_____
4. What is the first event you can remember after the injury? (5) _____	_____
Can you describe in detail (e.g., date, time, companions) the first event you can recall after the injury? (5) _____	_____
5. Can you describe the last event you recall before the accident? (5) _____	_____
Can you describe in detail (e.g., date, time, companions) the first event you can recall before the injury? (5) _____	_____
6. What time is it now? (1 point for each half hour removed from current time to a maximum of 5 points) _____	_____
7. What day of the week is it? (1 point for each day removed from the correct day) _____	_____
8. What day of the month is it? (1 point for each day removed from the correct day to a maximum of 5 points) _____	_____
9. What is the month? (5 for each month removed from the correct month to a maximum of 15 points) _____	_____
10. What is the year? (10 for each year removed from the correct year to a maximum of 30 points) _____	_____
Total error points	_____
Total score (100 minus total error points)	_____

About 50% of all TBIs are transportation related. The other 50% are caused by falls, assaults, and other causes (24). With rising age, increasing numbers of TBIs are caused by falls and suicide attempts, and the increasing mortality is correlated with a rising incidence of subdural hematomas (28,29).

A variety of risk factors have been identified as influential in determining which type of person is likely to sustain a TBI. The most common factor cited is alcohol intake before the TBI (30). In the TBI Model System Database as of 2001, approximately 50% of those screened for blood alcohol level (which includes about 80% of cases) were legally intoxicated at the time of injury (31). Other factors have been noted, such as preinjury personality disturbance, history of attention deficit hypersensitivity disorder (ADHD) (32), family discord, or antisocial behavior, but little systematic research has been done to relate these factors to risk of injury (33). Helmet use by both motorcyclists and bicyclists reduces the severity of injuries that occur (34,35), and both seat belt use and helmet use remain uncommon among those who are seriously hurt, with only 24% using seat belts and 16% wearing helmets (36). Automobile airbags, when used in conjunction with belt restraints, have been shown to reduce fatalities in high-speed crashes (37), and presumably a considerable proportion of the deaths prevented

would have been from TBI. In addition, violence has been rising as an etiology in TBI, especially in the African-American population, where the incidence is two to three times higher than in Caucasians and other racial groups (24). Violence as a cause of TBI has been an increasing focus of research and public health attention.

The economic and social impact of TBI is considered enormous but has not been extensively researched to date. In a study based on 327,907 individuals with TBI, Max and associates estimated that the total lifetime costs for all people who sustained TBI in 1985 in the United States was $37.8 billion (38). Charges simply for acute care and rehabilitation of individuals in the Model Systems Database averaged about $120,000 per patient, excluding physician charges (39). Estimates of return to work vary greatly, from 15% to 100%, depending on selection criteria for the vocational program under study (40,41). In a population-based study, conducted without regard to whether or not individuals received vocational rehabilitation services, 47% of those with severe injuries who were working prior to injury, were working again 1 year later. Comparable figures for those with moderate and mild injuries were 78% and 81%, respectively (42). TBI creates strain in intimate relationships, affects role functioning, fosters economic hardship, and creates a great burden on the family (43). These issues are discussed further later in this chapter.

PATHOPHYSIOLOGY OF TRAUMATIC BRAIN INJURY

Primary Injury

Diffuse axonal injury (DAI) is the distinguishing feature of TBI. Acceleration-deceleration and rotational forces that commonly result from motor vehicle accidents produce diffuse axonal disruption. Depending on the severity of injury, such lesions may be microscopic, or they may coalesce into focal macroscopic lesions, with a preponderance in the midbrain and pons, corpus callosum, and white matter of the cerebral hemispheres (Fig. 78-1) (44–46). DAI is primarily responsible for the initial loss of consciousness (47). The precise mechanism of axonal damage remains controversial but includes disruption of the intraaxonal cytoskeleton which may lead to axonal swelling and disconnection (48). Such injury may be a risk factor for development of Alzheimer's dementia (49). Animal data suggest that some of the loss of axonal integrity may happen after a delay (48), allowing for the possibility that preventive treatments may be developed.

Cerebral contusions are another form of primary injury. These cortical bruises occur at the crests of the gyri and extend to variable depths, depending on severity. Contusions occur primarily on the undersurface of the frontal lobes and at the temporal tips, regardless of the site of impact (Fig. 78-2). The lesions usually are bilateral but may be asymmetric (50). Cerebral contusions may produce focal cognitive and sensory motor deficits and are risk factors for seizure disorders but are not directly responsible for loss of consciousness. In contrast to DAI, contusions may result from relatively low-velocity impact such as blows and falls (51). A given patient's pattern of functional deficits may be more focal (e.g., from contusions) or diffuse (e.g., from DAI) or may include features of both. The balance of these two pathologic features influences the nature of deficits. Deficits related to DAI tend to recover gradually, with the pace of recovery inversely related to the duration of coma, whereas recovery from deficits related to cortical contusions depends more on the size and location of the focal injury rather than coma duration (21).

Secondary Injury and Initial Neurosurgical Management

The initial injury may set in motion a variety of pathologic processes that result in more severe and widespread brain damage. Any factor that leads to increased intracranial pressure (ICP) can decrease cerebral perfusion pressure (CPP) and cause ischemic damage. Expanding extraaxial or intraparenchymal hematomas or acute hydrocephalus can lead to dramatic pressure changes. Impaired autoregulation may lead to disruption of appropriate blood flow to the brain. Low cerebral blood flow may result in abnormalities in cerebral metabolism (52). Cerebral blood flow may be further reduced in tissue near areas of contusion (53). Increased blood volume is a major contributing factor for increasing ICP (54). Intermittent peaks in ICP during the first 24 hours are a risk factor for sustained increases in ICP (55).

In the past, ICP was routinely monitored in severe TBI. More recent guidelines recommend ICP monitoring in patients with severe head injury (GCS of 3 to 8) and an abnormal computed tomography (CT) scan (hematomas, contusions, edema, or compressed basal cisterns); or a normal CT scan and two out of three adverse features (age greater than 40, unilateral or bilateral motor posturing, or systolic blood pressure [BP] less than 90 mm Hg) (56). Increased ICP is no longer treated in an isolated manner but as a determinant of CPP, which is defined as the mean arterial pressure (MAP) minus ICP. Current data suggest CPP should be maintained at 70 mm Hg, or higher (56). Aggressive hyperventilation and the use of barbiturate coma should be reserved for patients refractory to other methods of management (56). Treatment with glucocorticoids, although still common, has been shown to be ineffective (57). Bolus doses of mannitol may be employed for increased ICP secondary to edema, providing MAP is maintained through adequate fluid replacement (58).

The initial DAI may initiate the release of excitatory neurotransmitters, which greatly increases the activity of certain brain regions at a time when their metabolic demand cannot be supported. Use of neuroprotective drugs to prevent excitotoxicity has proved promising in animal models. The efficacy of neurotransmitter blockade in minimizing this type of secondary injury in humans is under investigation (59) (see the following section, "Neuroprotection, Neuronal Recovery, and Functional Recovery").

Systemic factors such as blood loss and hypotension, pulmonary injury, and cardiac or respiratory arrest also may contribute to secondary hypoxic/ischemic brain injury. Brain infection may occur from open skull fractures, cerebrospinal fluid rhinorrhea, or iatrogenically from ICP monitoring (60). Protracted seizures also can lead to deterioration through increased metabolic requirements, disruption of spontaneous respiration, and aspiration.

Neuroprotection, Neuronal Recovery, and Functional Recovery

Recovery from TBI often is incomplete. Reports have identified subtle but persistent deficits after even mild TBI (61,62). Yet many brain-injured people make tremendous gains from coma to the reemergence of a variety of complex skills. This recovery is believed to occur at multiple levels, from alterations in biochemical processes to changes in family structure (63). A better understanding of the pathophysiologic mechanisms involved in secondary injury, as well an improved understanding of the processes that underlie functional recovery may lead to improved treatments to restore functioning in injured individuals.

Secondary neuronal injury is thought to be related to hypoxia, cellular influx of calcium and other ions, release of free radicals and excitotoxic neurotransmitters, and apoptotic cell death (64). Thus, in theory, drugs that block various ion channels, scavenge free radicals, inhibit excitatory neurotransmitters, or block the internal signals for programmed cell death might salvage a greater proportion of neural tissue that is not irreversibly damaged at the time of impact. Despite the theoretical promise, however, the clinical trials that have studied such interventions have been generally disappointing (65). There are many possible reasons for the failure to identify useful neuroprotective treatments (66). In many instances, the therapeutic time windows established in animal models have been exceeded in human trials. Human TBI tends to be considerably more neuropathologically heterogeneous than more controlled animal models, such that treatments that work on a single pathologic process may have insufficient clinical impact in humans (67). In addition, controversy exists about the injury severity levels most appropriate for neuroprotection research, and the outcome measures most likely to demonstrate efficacy of neuroprotective treatments. While no such treatments can

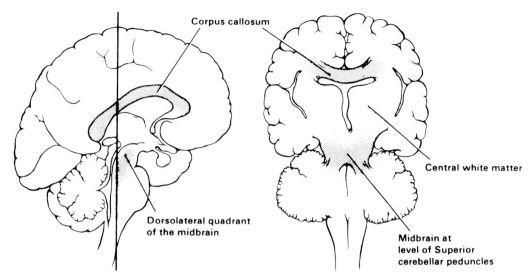

Figure 78-1. Brain regions particularly involved by diffuse axonal injury include the corpus callosum and parasagittal white matter as well as the dorsolateral quadrants of the midbrain. (From Auerbach SH. Neuroanatomical correlates of attention and memory disorders in traumatic brain injury: an application of behavioral subtypes. *J Head Trauma Rehabil* 1986;1:1–12. Reprinted with permission of Aspen Publishers, Inc. © 1986.)

currently be recommended with confidence, it is likely that such treatments will be developed in the future. For example, interest in estrogen and progesterone as neuroprotective agents has recently been spurred by the observation of superior recovery from brain damage in female versus male animals (68,69). Similar patterns have been seen in humans (70), although it is more difficult to ensure that the severity and mechanism are well balanced across genders in human studies.

Once a given degree of brain damage has occurred, a number of processes, overlapping in time, may contribute to functional recovery. Restoration of effective perfusion, resolution of edema, and weaning of sedating drugs can lead to improvements in function in the first days and weeks after injury. Latent neuronal circuitry may be unmasked by injury, to support functions that previously depended on the damaged neural mechanisms (71). Experience, often in the form of intense practice, has been shown to alter sensory-motor cortical representations ("maps") in healthy humans as well as lesioned animals,

suggesting that appropriately structured therapy might directly contribute to improved function after brain damage (72–75). Central nervous system neurons depend on a variety of inputs for their ongoing activity, the sudden loss of which leads to marked depression of undamaged structures (i.e., diaschisis) (76). Over time, alterations can occur in receptor sensitivity to remaining neurotransmitters, such that partially disrupted neural networks develop more normal levels of activity. Along these lines, there is considerable evidence in several animal species and some in humans that certain receptor agonists can hasten functional recovery, whereas doses of antagonists cause regression (77,78). At a more behavioral level, a person with a particular deficit may discover (or be taught) another strategy for accomplishing the task that relies on remaining intact neural systems (79). Finally, as long as individuals remain conscious and retain some learning capacity, it may be possible for them to learn specific tasks and activities, even though their overall capacity may remain fixed.

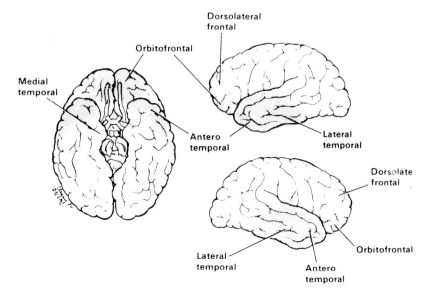

Figure 78-2. Areas predominantly affected by cortical contusions. *Shading* represents more frequently involved areas. Anterotemporal and orbitofrontal regions are particularly involved. Note relative sparing of dorsolateral frontal lobe and medial temporal lobe. (Adapted from Courville CB. *Mythology of the central nervous system.* Mountain View, CA: Pacific Press, 1937; with permission.)

Although there is considerable evidence for all of these recovery mechanisms, particularly in the animal literature, there is as yet limited systematic application of these principles to the design of human rehabilitation efforts. Animal studies of neural transplantation are in progress and human trials in more focal neurologic conditions have already appeared (80). While such trials are promising, TBI is one of the most challenging settings for neural transplantation, given the diffuse neuropathology involving numerous brain systems. Similarly, few controlled pharmacologic trials to enhance neural recovery have been conducted in TBI. With respect to the experiential rehabilitation therapies, their organization and scheduling is dictated by a complex combination of clinical judgment, tradition, and administrative efficiency more than by research on motor or cognitive learning. Nevertheless, the growth of basic science research related to neural recovery is increasingly being translated into clinical research, with the anticipation of more theoretically based rehabilitation efforts in the future.

OUTCOME AFTER TRAUMATIC BRAIN INJURY

Types of Deficits

Most survivors of severe TBI emerge from coma and achieve remarkable progress toward regaining their preinjury functional abilities. A majority, however, are left with a combination of physical and neurobehavioral impairments. These, in turn, interact to produce a broad array of limitations in activity and restrictions in societal participation that may persist for many months or years after the injury. Each individual's specific pattern of deficits is a consequence of the severity of the injury, nature of brain damage, and medical complications, varying greatly from one person to the next. However, deficits in cognition are nearly ubiquitous after moderate or severe TBI.

Changes in behavior, mood, and personality after TBI have been documented by many investigators and are considered by clinicians to be among the most difficult disabilities to manage effectively. Behavior problems range from minor irritability or passivity to labile emotional displays or disinhibited, bizarre, or aggressive behavior. The severely brain-injured person may appear egocentric and childlike, and may display a loss of empathy and concern for others.

Limitations in activities related to self-care, toileting, mobility, basic communication, and feeding commonly occur in severe TBI. In those with less severe injuries, limitations and restrictions may not be revealed until more complex community-oriented skills are attempted, such as time and money management, community mobility, and school or vocational tasks. Restrictions in vocational, educational, and interpersonal domains are widespread. There is frequently loss or diminution of friendships and intimate relationships and a devastating impact on the family system. The psychosocial consequences of TBI, and the cognitive and behavioral impairments that underlie them, are reviewed in greater detail later in this chapter.

Outcomes Measurement

The measurement and prediction of outcomes have taken on increased importance in health care generally and rehabilitation specifically. There are several distinct uses for outcomes measurement, with different implications for the types of outcomes measured and their interpretation. Outcomes data for clinical program evaluation systems in brain injury rehabilitation are required by the Commission for the Accreditation of Rehabilitation Facilities (CARF), with the intent of ensuring that the types of functional outcomes achieved by each program are reasonable and in line with their programmatic missions. However, the quality of functional outcomes can be interpreted only in light of the characteristics of the clients entering the program, and the ability to adjust for the effects of these "case mix" variables (e.g., injury severity, etiology, time postinjury) is still rather primitive.

Outcomes measurement can also be useful in the pilot phases of research: by comparing innovative treatments to the standard system, one can get a sense of whether the new treatment is improving outcomes. Highly accurate outcomes prediction could also, in principle, guide individual treatment decisions. For example, if it could be predicted in the first few days postinjury that a patient would remain permanently vegetative, the physician and family might choose not to pursue aggressive treatment; if independent ambulation were predicted not to be possible, the energies of physical therapy could be redirected to other goals, and a definitive wheelchair could be prescribed earlier. For outcomes prediction to be used in this way, however, it would need to be highly accurate in projecting the specific outcomes of individual patients; unfortunately this goal has not been achieved.

The outcome scale that has been used in most studies of acute TBI is the Glasgow Outcome Scale (GOS). As shown in Table 78-4, the GOS consists of five global categories ranging from good recovery to death. It has been demonstrated to have a high degree of interrater reliability in large, multicenter, international studies (81). It has been used to correlate early injury severity measures (e.g., GCS, length of PTA) and outcome at 6 months postinjury. Several major drawbacks in the use of the scale for rehabilitation purposes have been identified:

- The categories are so broad that it is not a sensitive measure of progress during rehabilitation.
- The global categories do not provide a real indication of functional abilities.
- Cognitive and behavioral dysfunctions are poorly addressed in the outcome categories.

Despite these limitations, the GOS continues to have widespread use for its intended purpose—to provide a quantitative, general way of describing outcome. A recent extension of the GOS, the Glasgow Outcome Scale-Extended (GOS-E) seeks to remedy some of the shortcomings of the GOS by providing a broader range of outcome scores to improve sensitivity, and by incorporating a comparison to preinjury status in both medical and psychosocial domains (82).

Several other outcome measurement scales have been developed to be more sensitive to functional changes that are of interest in rehabilitation. Some of these are brain injury–specific, and others are general rehabilitation scales. The Disability Rating Scale (DRS) was developed specifically for TBI and is intended to assess changes "from coma to community" (83). This scale produces a quantitative index of disability across ten levels of severity, with high interrater reliability. This measure is considerably more sensitive to clinical change than the GOS (84), particularly at the severe end of the spectrum but it has larger scoring gaps between self-care and ability to live independently, and between independent living and employment (85).

The Rancho Los Amigos Levels of Cognitive Function Scale (Table 78-5) focuses on cognitive recovery after TBI and the capacity to interact effectively with the environment. Each level is accompanied by a lengthy description of behaviors that meet the criteria for placement at that level (86). A comparison of this

TABLE 78-4.   Glasgow Outcome Scale

Score	Category	Definition
1	Death	As a direct result of brain trauma. Patient regained consciousness and died thereafter from secondary complications or other causes.
2	Persistent vegetative state	Patient remains unresponsive and speechless for an extended period of time. Patient may open the eyes and show sleep–wake cycles but an absence of function in the cerebral cortex judged behaviorally.
3	Severe disability (conscious but disabled)	Dependent for daily support by reason of mental or physical disability, usually a combination of both. Severe mental disability may occasionally justify this classification in a patient with little or no physical disability.
4	Moderate (disabled but independent)	Can travel by public transport and work in a sheltered environment and can therefore be independent as far as daily life is concerned. The disabilities found include varying degrees of dysphasia, hemiparesis, or ataxia as well as intellectual and memory deficits and personality change. Independence is greater than simple ability to maintain self-care within the patient's home.
5	Good recovery	Resumption of normal life even though there may be minor neurologic and pathologic deficits.

From Jennett B, Bond MR. Assessment of outcome in severe brain damage: a practical scale. *Lancet* 1975;1:480–484.

scale with the DRS revealed that it has slightly lower validity and reliability (87).

The Functional Independence Measure (FIM), an 18-item rating scale, is the most widely used outcome measurement scale in medical rehabilitation. The emphasis of this scale is on physical ability, however, which often is of less interest in TBI. Because of the relative insensitivity of the FIM to cognitive and behavioral deficits, the Functional Assessment Measure (FAM) was developed to supplement it with more cognitively oriented items. Interrater agreement for the FAM is lower (67%) than for the FIM (88%), and although it extends the range of difficulty somewhat compared to the FIM alone, its items are highly redundant with existing FIM items in terms of their scoring (85).

All of the outcome scales discussed herein are well suited to measuring the changes that occur during acute rehabilitation, but none of them adequately addresses higher-level functions for those with mild injuries or for those with severe injuries who have been discharged into the community (88).

Measures of behavioral and social functioning in the community that have been developed specifically for TBI outcome measurement include the Neurobehavioral Functioning Inventory (NFI) (89) and the Mayo-Portland Adaptability Inventory (MPAI) (90). The NFI is a self-report measure of the frequency of neurobehavioral symptoms, completed by either the injured person or a family member, which yields subscale scores in six domains of emotional/behavioral function: depression, somatic, memory/attention, communication, aggression, and

TABLE 78-5.   Rancho Los Amigos Levels of Cognitive Functioning Scale

I. No response
II. Generalized response to stimulation
III. Localized response to stimuli
IV. Confused and agitated behavior
V. Confused with inappropriate behavior (nonagitated)
VI. Confused but appropriate behavior
VII. Automatic and appropriate behavior
VIII. Purposeful and appropriate behavior

From Hagen C, Malkmus D, Durham P. Levels of cognitive functions. In: *Rehabilitation of the head-injured adult: comprehensive physical management.* Downey, CA: Professional Staff Association, Rancho Los Amigos Hospital, 1979.

motor. Both construct validity and criterion-related validity were demonstrated to be at acceptable levels (91). The MPAI was developed to provide an evaluation of progress during postacute brain injury rehabilitation. It is a 30-item rating scale completed by staff or the patient on two fundamental dimensions derived from a principal components analysis: Physical/Cognitive Impairment Scale and Social Participation Scale. Both person reliability (0.82) and item reliability (0.96) were found to be good to excellent (90).

The first outcome measure developed specifically to measure community functioning of persons with brain injury was the Community Integration Questionnaire (CIQ) (92). This 15-item questionnaire has three subscales: Home Integration, Social Integration, and Productivity. It can be completed by the person with brain injury or a significant other. The CIQ has been found useful as a measure of "objective" quality of life and level of productivity, but it has also been subject to criticism for its psychometric properties (93).

Another measure of community functioning, originally developed for persons with spinal cord injury, is the Craig Handicap Assessment and Reporting Technique (CHART) (94). Original subscales included Physical Independence, Mobility, Occupation, Social Integration, and Economic Self-Sufficiency. A revised version of the scale, which included a dimension identified as Cognitive Independence, was developed more recently (95). This additional scale also showed high test–retest reliability (0.87) in a mixed sample of individuals with neurologic illness including TBI, and was also found to be a useful tool in evaluating postacute functioning in persons with TBI (96).

The scales mentioned here, as well as other instruments, are described in more detail on the Center for Outcome Measurement in Brain Injury (COMBI) Web site, located at www.tbims.org/combi.

Prediction of Outcome

The Glasgow Coma Scale (GCS) is the most widely used measure of injury severity and is a primary basis for most predictions of outcome. The total coma score when taken at 2 to 3 or 4 to 7 days postinjury is highly predictive of outcome at 6 months, as measured by the GOS (81). Scores less than 8 are usually predictive of poor outcome. Duration of PTA also is highly correlated with ultimate outcome, with PTA greater than 14 days associated with greater likelihood of moderate or severe disability (81). The rate of early recovery, as reflected in serial DRS scores, is also predictive of final outcome (97).

Multimodality evoked potentials (MEPs) also have been used as an early means of assessing neurologic status and predicting outcome. It appears that MEPs do improve the prognostic value of the GCS and correlate with outcome measures such as the DRS (98). Somatosensory evoked potentials (SEPs), in particular, have been shown to have good sensitivity and specificity (73% to 95%) in grossly predicting outcomes as favorable or unfavorable (99). Greenberg and colleagues found that maximal recovery occurs in approximately 3 months for patients with minimal evoked potential abnormalities (100). Severe evoked potential abnormalities, however, suggest that maximal recovery may extend to 12 months.

Reactive pupils are associated with better outcomes than nonreactive pupils—50% of those with reactive pupils achieve the moderate disability or good recovery range, as opposed to 4% with nonreactive pupils (101). An absent oculovestibular response, elicited by injecting ice water into the ear of a comatose patient, is an indication of severe brain stem dysfunction and poorer outcome (11). The presence of an intracranial hematoma appears to increase the chance of a poor outcome when the patient is under 20 years of age (81). The level of creatine kinase (i.e., BB fraction) measured early after TBI also is a prognostic indicator because it reflects brain tissue destruction (102,103). Hyperglycemia and low levels of thyroid hormones have negative prognostic significance, presumably reflecting the severity of stress response (104,105).

The research from Glasgow and other major TBI centers strongly suggests that the bulk of neurologic recovery from acute brain injury occurs within the first 6 months postinjury. The maximal duration of the recovery period is more controversial. Some researchers affirm that neurologic recovery is virtually complete by 1 year, whereas others assert that recovery can extend 2 years or more postinjury (106). It is clear, however, that certain areas of dysfunction recover more quickly than others. For example, recovery of physical abilities and functional skills such as mobility occurs rapidly, often within 3 months after injury (107). Recovery of more complex mental abilities, as assessed by neuropsychological measures, appears more variable. This aspect of recovery has been studied in large samples in the Traumatic Coma Data Bank study (108) and in the Traumatic Brain Injury Model Systems Project (109,110).

Preinjury medical and psychological factors also may affect the prognosis. For example, the presence of a prior TBI or neurologic deficit is likely to slow the recovery process. Also, if cognitive or behavioral abnormalities existed before the injury, there is a greater likelihood of a slower and less complete recovery. Acquired brain damage is thought to exacerbate preexisting behavior disorders (111).

There probably is no final end point to the recovery process; rather, the pace of recovery slows, and its scope narrows. Even those with permanent cognitive and physical impairments can continue to learn new skills for solving particular functional problems, albeit slowly. Thus, neurologic recovery and cognitive recovery merge imperceptibly into ongoing learning and adaptation.

THE ASSESSMENT AND TREATMENT-PLANNING PROCESS

The rehabilitation needs of the survivor of severe TBI often begin at the roadside or site of emergency care but are not likely to end for many years. Although many medical conditions and physical deficits stabilize within 1 year after injury, the presence of long-term psychosocial disorders often necessitates ongoing intervention (112). Survivors of TBI make indefinite use of the treatment and support services to which they have access, particularly to address psychosocial difficulties (113).

Treatment and Support Options

To help the person with brain injury achieve a reasonable quality of life, a broad spectrum of services may be provided in hospital, community-based, or home settings, depending on the severity of injury and residual sequelae. Changes in private and governmental funding streams stimulated much growth of specialized TBI rehabilitation services in the 1980s and early 1990s, but subsequent funding cutbacks and managed care practices have meant that these services are available to fewer patients and their families.

Initial management takes the form of aggressive neurosurgical intervention to minimize secondary injury. The physiatrist may be called in as a consultant even when the patient is still in the intensive care unit to assist the acute care team in preventing complications such as contractures, pressure ulcers, heterotopic ossification (HO), and bowel and bladder problems that may impede later rehabilitation of surviving patients, and to assist in choosing medications that minimize sedation.

A tremendous variety of treatment programs may be appropriate for a given individual at various points in the recovery process. Acute inpatient rehabilitation is typically provided to individuals who are able to participate actively in treatment, whose array of medical, physical, and cognitive deficits preclude a safe home discharge. Subacute rehabilitation, which is less costly and less intensive, may be given to those who are vegetative, slow to recover, or cannot tolerate intensive therapy. A day treatment program may be provided to individuals who can be managed at home but continue to display a variety of physical or neurobehavioral problems. This type of treatment often combines extensive cognitive rehabilitation, behavior management, daily life skills training, community activities, and prevocational activities (114,115).

Residential programs may be chosen for individuals who display disinhibited, aggressive, or self-abusive behavior that cannot be managed at home. Such programs aim to reduce inappropriate behaviors and teach more effective means of communication and social interaction through contingency management or pharmacologic intervention (116). Transitional living programs assist individuals who have mastered basic activities of daily living (ADLs) and social interaction skills to live increasingly independently in the community. Typically the brain-injured person lives in a supervised group home or apartment setting and is given instruction and increasing responsibility in skills needed to live independently (e.g., cooking, cleaning, money management, community mobility, job seeking), with less supervision required over time. The final goal for many individuals is return to work, most typically through job coaching and supported work, funded by state vocational rehabilitation services. Many clients with TBI have difficulty applying knowledge gained in one setting to related problems or different environments. In such instances, it is particularly important that the independent living and vocational training be given in the actual community or on the actual job that the individual will be attempting.

Telerehabilitation is an emerging facet of service provision that may allow for more accurate assessment and treatment planning in the home-care context, and may allow rural patients to receive services from specialized TBI rehabilitation centers (117,118). During the long rehabilitation process, a case manager may provide crucial coordination and social support. The case manager serves as a liaison among the patient, family, and service providers and gathers medical records, arranges for medical visits, screens programs and facilities, and helps coordinate admission and discharge. With the advent of managed care, intensive case management may be even more crucial although, as previously noted, it is less often provided (119).

The continuum of services discussed herein is not needed by all survivors of TBI, but some individuals are likely to need all of these options and many more. Unfortunately, in many regions, services that are needed by survivors of TBI are either unavailable or difficult to access, due in part to the rapidly evolving changes in health-care financing (120). This calls for creative financing strategies, assisted by case managers or social workers working with the patient, along with advocacy efforts to expand the range of services accessible to individuals with TBI. Some states have developed Medicaid waiver programs that extend the array of available services to TBI survivors through the use of public funds (121,122).

Evidence for the Effectiveness of Traumatic Brain Injury-Specific Services

As in most areas of rehabilitation, there is currently insufficient evidence for the efficacy of the services discussed herein (123,124). However, observational data and randomized pilot studies do provide some evidence to support the impact of comprehensive systems of care for TBI, particularly in the postacute period (115,125,126). One randomized trial comparing an organized program of cognitive rehabilitation to a limited home program failed to find an overall treatment effect, but did find superior outcomes for the cognitive rehabilitation program for the more severely impaired subgroup (127).

Patient Assessment and Treatment Planning

Standards of care and practice for the management of acute and postacute care of persons with TBI have been promulgated by organizations such as the American Association of Neurological Surgeons (56), the Commission on the Accreditation of Rehabilitation Facilities (CARF) (128), and the American Congress of Rehabilitation Medicine (129). Rehabilitation services traditionally are organized on a team model to promote coordination and information sharing across disciplines, since a specific cognitive impairment may interfere with the performance and retention of a mobility, communication, or ADL skill. Similarly, disruptive behaviors and lack of initiation cut across all therapy domains. Each of these problems requires the development of a unified team view of the patient's deficits and needs and the creation of a unified treatment plan.

When a patient enters a rehabilitation service, an initial assessment is needed to guide treatment planning. The goals of this assessment vary with time since injury. A recently injured patient has the potential for considerable recovery. Therefore, assessment usually is aimed at defining broad functional areas in need of treatment (e.g., impaired mobility, memory deficits). As the pace of recovery slows, and discharge to home or another facility approaches, assessment must shift to identification of the specific skills and behaviors that will be prerequisites in the new environment (e.g., toilet transfers, learning a daily schedule). Assessment also depends on injury severity. It is focused more on physical function and basic sensory processing in the severely impaired and on cognitive, social, and vocational function in the mildly impaired.

Discipline-specific assessments must be melded into a patient-oriented assessment for treatment-planning purposes. Typically, severely injured patients have a large number of medical, physical, cognitive, and behavioral problems. Therefore, the team must develop priorities for treatment, framed in terms of long- and short-term goals, based on such factors as estimated length of stay, functional importance of each deficit, age and developmental stage, and prognosis for improvement. As time passes, the goals become more specific and functionally oriented, such that "the patient will have increased range of motion in all joints" becomes "the patient will have adequate hip flexion for erect sitting throughout the day." Identification of the patient's physical and cognitive strengths can also be very helpful in determining the best way to circumvent specific deficits. Goals being addressed by a single discipline must ultimately be shared by the team. For example, a communication strategy designed by a speech pathologist should be carried out by nurses, other therapists, and family to promote generalization of the skill.

Treatment planning also must consider the hierarchy of impairment, activity, and participation and must choose at which of these levels to intervene. For example, it may be concluded that a patient's ambulation *activity limitation* is related to *impairments* in range of motion, tone, strength, balance, proprioception, and attention. Clinicians then must choose whether to try to address each of these impairments to improve ambulation, or whether to assess the patient's mobility skills in a motorized wheelchair instead, which would be an *activity*-level intervention.

A neuropsychological assessment may be important in identifying intact cognitive skills and clarifying cognitive mechanisms responsible for various behavior and skill deficits. In the severely impaired patient, formal testing may be impossible; however, the neuropsychologist's observation of the patient may still be helpful. Higher-level patients should receive formal testing of such core cognitive areas as attention, learning and remembering, language comprehension and production, visual perception, planning, reasoning, and organization. It should be kept in mind that the results of formal neuropsychological testing have limited predictive ability for real-world function (130). Thus, patients' skills also should be assessed in naturalistic settings.

SPECIAL SUBPOPULATIONS

Coma and the Vegetative State

Initial coma is universal in patients with severe TBI. Up to one-half of patients in coma for longer than 6 hours die without ever regaining consciousness (81,99,131). About 10% of the total survivors (20% of survivors) remain unresponsive 1 month after injury, with the remainder emerging from coma and gradually improving in function (132). Patients who remain unresponsive for more than 2 to 4 weeks evolve into the vegetative state, a state of wakeful unresponsiveness that is characterized by the presence of spontaneous sleep–wake cycles but absence of cortical activity as judged behaviorally (133).

Patients who are vegetative 1 month postinjury still may experience substantial recovery, but their chances of doing so diminish over time. Of patients who are vegetative at 1 month, there is approximately a 50% chance of regaining some degree of consciousness within a year and approximately a 28% chance of improving to a level of independence (134).

Patients continue to emerge from the vegetative state following trauma for at least a year and perhaps longer (little research is available for follow-up periods greater than a year), but nearly all are severely disabled if their emergence is this late. Emergence from the vegetative state following nontraumatic injuries (such as cardiac arrest) is far less likely overall, and very few patients emerge beyond 3 months postinjury (134). This suggests that patients with traumatic injuries complicated by substantial secondary anoxic injury are also likely to have a poorer prognosis than those with uncomplicated trauma.

The following factors have positive prognostic significance for emergence from unresponsiveness: young age, reactive pupils and conjugate eye movements, decorticate posturing rather than decerebrate or flaccid states, early spontaneous eye opening, absence of ventilator dependence or hydrocephalus, shorter time between injury and rehabilitation admission, higher scores (within the vegetative range) on the DRS, and more rapid early functional improvement (132,135,136). Unfortunately, no set of prognostic variables is precise enough to guide early clinical decision making (132). The life expectancy of those who remain permanently vegetative is not precisely known, but one study of patients in vegetative states of mixed etiologies revealed that almost 75% had died within 5 years (137). Similarly, TBI survivors with severe mobility impairments (though not necessarily vegetative) have a reduced life expectancy due primarily to cardiovascular disease, respiratory disease, choking, and seizures (138).

The term *persistent vegetative state* has been used extensively in the literature, but without consensus on its definition. Recently, it has been suggested that this term be abandoned because it confuses diagnosis (vegetative) with prognosis (persistent). However, recommendations have been made to add a new term to this topic area: *minimally conscious state (MCS)* (139). This refers to individuals who show some evidence of awareness in the form of visual tracking or motor behavior that is nonreflexive and contingent on environmental events (e.g., intermittent following of simple commands, replicable pulling out of tubes) but who do not consistently follow commands or communicate intelligibly. The MCS, like the vegetative state, can be a transitional state on the way to greater recovery or can be the permanent functional plateau. Misdiagnosing patients who are in the MCS as vegetative may occur more than 40% of the time, highlighting the need for rigorous diagnostic assessment (139,140).

Initial coma in TBI probably reflects disruption of brain stem alerting mechanisms, often with relative preservation of higher brain structures. Brain stem alerting mechanisms tend to recover with time, however, resulting in return of the sleep–wake cycle. Thus, a vegetative state of long duration generally includes extensive damage to subcortical white matter in higher brain regions, including the thalamus (141,142). Akinetic mutism and the locked-in syndrome may be confused with the vegetative state, but akinetic mutism generally involves damage to the medial frontal lobes, and hypertonia and posturing are absent. The locked-in syndrome generally results from a pontine stroke, and there is evidence of preserved consciousness and communication through eye movements (143,144).

Establishing the diagnosis of the vegetative state can be done clinically, by observing for volitional responses to the environment, such as following commands, orienting visually to salient objects, attempting to remove tubes and restraints, and the like. Essentially, any behavior that is nonstereotyped and

that indicates some evaluation of environmental stimuli is evidence of emerging consciousness. A formal and quantitative assessment strategy is an absolute requirement in working with vegetative and minimally conscious patients; without this, staff and family members may disagree about whether or not evidence of consciousness is present and whether improvement is occurring. Several standardized scales are available for objectively grading responsiveness in vegetative and minimally conscious patients (145–148). In addition, the principles of single-subject experimental design can be used to answer important clinical questions in individual patients, such as whether the patient can see (149), follow commands (150), or reliably use a yes/no signaling system; or whether he or she responds to therapeutic medications (151). Assessment should take place repeatedly and at various times of day because patients may respond inconsistently, particularly when they are first emerging from the vegetative state. Individualized staff assessments of relevant behaviors can be conducted when family members report observing volitional behavior that has not been witnessed by others. Although family members may overinterpret reflexive or coincidental behaviors, staff members may fail to elicit the patient's best performance. Definitive assessment of the vegetative state must await withdrawal of potentially sedating drugs and ruling out peripheral sensory deficits (e.g., blindness, deafness) (152).

Many treatments have been attempted in the vegetative state, but none has been subjected to an adequate controlled clinical trial. The pathologic heterogeneity of unresponsive states makes it unlikely that one treatment will help all affected people. Electrical stimulation of the mesencephalic reticular formation or nonspecific thalamic activating system with implanted electrodes has been reported to improve the electroencephalographic (EEG) spectrum and clinical status in some vegetative patients with stroke or TBI (153–156). However, these studies have used small samples of patients with vegetative states of varying intervals and of mixed etiologies. Thus, ruling out spontaneous recovery is difficult. Dopaminergic pharmacologic treatments, including L-dopa, bromocriptine, and amantadine, also have been reported to be of help (157–160). All of these treatments act primarily to augment ascending arousing influences. From a theoretical standpoint, this would seem unlikely to benefit patients with extensive cerebral lesions. Coma stimulation treatment has been used widely in vegetative patients. This involves the systematic and frequent provision of sensory stimulation to all sensory modalities and is based on animal research that shows that enriched environments improve neurologic recovery (63). However, it should be noted that studies that show a role of experience in promoting neurologic recovery have involved active participation of the animal, not merely passive stimulation (161). Several small studies on coma stimulation have been done, but all suffer from serious methodologic flaws, which have been summarized in review articles (162,163). A large, multicenter clinical trial will be needed to settle this issue.

In the absence of definitive treatments to alter the prognosis in the vegetative state, the main goals for rehabilitation are to optimize medical stability, preserve bodily integrity, and objectively define the patient's current sensory and cognitive capacities with measures that can be monitored for change over time (152). This includes screening for adverse medical events such as undiagnosed seizures, hydrocephalus, and endocrine disorders. Attempts to optimize pulmonary hygiene and maintain skin integrity also are essential. Aggressive treatment of hypertonia and contractures is warranted early because they will predispose to skin breakdown and interfere with positioning. Much time, money and pain can be saved for those patients who do recover by preventing the development of severe deformities. Finally, sedating medications should be avoided until the prognosis has declared itself. This includes a variety of antispasticity, anticonvulsant, antihypertensive, anticholinergic, and antihistaminic medications that may have subtle cognitive effects in susceptible patients (164).

Regular evaluation with a quantitative assessment scale should be carried out. This will reveal subtle improvement that should lead to updated treatment plans, deterioration that should lead to further diagnostic evaluation, or no change, which should lead to family counseling about prognosis and planning toward home or chronic care placement. When a patient remains permanently vegetative, or when a patient remains minimally conscious but has left a specific advance directive, the possibility of forgoing further medical treatments and even life-sustaining fluid and nutrition may be discussed with the family after careful review of local legal guidelines relevant to this area and any institutional policies and ethical guidelines relevant to end-of-life determinations. However, a small number of vegetative or minimally conscious patients may continue to improve over several years, making the determination of permanence more difficult (165).

Mild Traumatic Brain Injury

At the other end of the spectrum from unresponsive states is the patient with mild, or minor, traumatic brain injury (MTBI). This is generally defined as a TBI with the following characteristics:

- Loss of consciousness, if any, 30 minutes or less
- PTA 24 hours or less
- Initial GCS 13 to 15
- No focal neurologic deficit
- Negative CT or magnetic resonance imaging (MRI).

The etiology of MTBI involves either direct mechanical trauma or acceleration-deceleration forces only (e.g., whiplash) (166). The initial symptoms of the cerebral injury may be difficult to disentangle from those of the common coincident injuries to the scalp, neck, and peripheral vestibular apparatus (167). Acute complaints after MTBI typically fall into three symptom clusters (168):

1. Cognitive: attention and concentration difficulties, memory impairment
2. Affective: irritability, depression, anxiety
3. Somatic: headache, dizziness, insomnia, fatigue, sensory impairments (169).

These symptoms clear within the first few weeks or months postinjury for the majority of patients. Group studies have generally revealed no decrement, or only modest or transient decrement, on neuropsychological measures for subjects with MTBI compared to uninjured controls (170–172). For some individuals, however, difficulties persist and are associated with social and vocational failure seemingly out of proportion to the severity of the neurologic insult. The etiology of these persistent complaints (often termed *postconcussion syndrome*, or PCS) has been elusive and remains controversial. Premorbid factors such as substance abuse, psychiatric disorder, and age have been implicated but do not explain all cases of persistent disability. Similarly, it has not been confirmed that the idea that pending litigation or financial gain accounts for PCS (168). In a recent single photon emission CT (SPECT) study, MTBI patients with unusually persistent disability showed hypoperfusion in the anterior mesial regions of the temporal lobes (173). There is probably no one cause of PCS; premorbid variables,

idiosyncratic neurologic vulnerability, and psychological reactions to acute symptoms may all be found to play roles.

The treatment of MTBI should include patient and family education about the typical symptoms and their time frame, and guidance on how and when to resume preinjury activities. Patients with persistent symptoms may benefit from psychotherapy (174), pain management protocols (175), or holistic community reentry programs offering these components along with education, vocational counseling, and group support. Many of the somatic symptoms are responsive to interventions that can be provided through an experienced physical therapist in conjunction with judicious use of medications. Therapeutic interventions include vestibular habituation exercises (176), Rocabado exercises (177), myofascial release, trigger point injections, nonsteroidal antiinflammatory medications, and muscle relaxants. For more extensive information, the reader is referred to more detailed publications on this aspect of brain injury (178–180).

Prompt diagnosis and treatment of "concussion" in sports-related injuries has received increased public awareness. Practice parameters have been established by a subcommittee of the American Academy of Neurology (181). A Standardized Assessment of Concussion was developed to provide a sideline evaluation which could be performed by nonphysicians (182). Computerized neuropsychological tests have been developed for more in-depth evaluation (183).

Traumatic Brain Injury in Children and Adolescents

Children and adolescents are a high-risk group for TBI, with etiologies varying by age group. The most common cause of TBI among infants and toddlers is child abuse; in preadolescents the most common causes are accidental injuries and motor vehicle accidents; and among adolescents the most common causes are injuries due to violence and risk-taking behaviors. The management and sequelae of TBI in children and adolescents are very similar to those of adults, but there are a number of issues that are specific to children. Because injured children are in a phase of active development and skill acquisition, it is challenging to disentangle neurologic recovery from normal growth and maturation. On the other hand, young children may appear to have minimal deficits after TBI, since the skills expected of them are minimal, only to reveal increasing developmental lags as they mature. In addition, the appropriate roles of children differ from adults and change during development, and "independence" is not an appropriate goal of pediatric TBI rehabilitation (see Chapter 70 for more discussion of pediatric rehabilitation.) Because of this, many children with TBI are sent home without rehabilitation services, since their parents provide the assistance needed to function safely (184).

It has been estimated that 20,000 children and adolescents reenter school each year with significant disabilities related to TBI. Surveys of special education services in the U.S. however estimate that only about 12,000 of the more than 5 million special education students receive services due to a TBI (185). This discrepancy may have several sources. Children already receiving special education services, particularly those with ADHD, are overrepresented among those injured, and they may retain their original etiology's label; children may "grow into" their educational disability without the educational system recognizing their prior injury; and some school systems keep records by educational needs rather than etiology (184,185). Policy recommendations for improving special education services for this population have been published (185).

Problems with attention and concentration appear to be among the most frequent sequelae of TBI in children, as they are in adults, occurring in up to 50% of survivors, although as many as 19% of those injured carried a premorbid label of ADHD (32,186). Language impairments have also been reported in children injured in the preschool years (187). TBI may also have important effects on emotional adjustment in children and adolescents, with depression, dysthymia, and anxiety disorders among the most common new problems (32). In a study of college students with a history of mild TBI, intellectual impairments were not found, although the students with prior TBI had increased levels of subjective distress in several subscales of the Symptom Checklist-90—Revised (188).

There is also reason to be concerned about the impact of the child's injury on the family. In particular, it has been suggested that siblings of children with TBI-related disability may experience adverse impact themselves. A small study that compared siblings of children with TBI to classmate controls, did not find significantly greater psychopathology, depression, or problems in emotional well-being among the siblings (189). However, there were trends suggesting that such a pattern might be found in a larger study.

The preponderance of data suggests that pediatric TBI is underreported and underrecognized in its importance. A high proportion of children with a history of TBI are likely to present with educational special needs, cognitive problems, and psychological/behavioral problems. This underrecognition may be due to the fact that some of these children had such problems premorbidly, coupled with the delay between injury and appearance of the problems. Thus, it appears crucial that children with significant TBI be identified and tracked so that the relevance of their TBI to future problems and needs does not go unnoticed.

Traumatic Brain Injury in the Elderly

As discussed previously, the incidence of TBI rises again among the older individuals, with up to 86% of TBIs in those over 65 due to falls (190). It has long been known that mortality from TBI at a given level of severity is higher among the older population than among younger individuals. However, considerable controversy exists about the prognosis for functional recovery among older survivors. There are a number of methodologic problems that contribute to this uncertainty. The fact that falls are the predominant etiology among the elderly points to the fact that their premorbid functional status is often already compromised, making a return to "normal functioning" an unrealistic expectation. On the other hand, studies suggesting that elderly patients admitted to acute rehabilitation can achieve functional recovery comparable to their younger counterparts, albeit at a slower pace, are confounded by the bias inherent in the selection process for rehabilitation admission. One recent study that enrolled elderly patients in acute care, thus avoiding this selection bias, found that GOS scores of moderate disability or good recovery never occurred in those with GCS scores less than 11 (191). This was true even among the subgroup with milder original injuries and subsequent deterioration to lower GCS scores. Though it appears likely that the functional prognosis for elderly patients is indeed worse than for younger ones, there is also a concern that this may contribute to a self-fulfilling prophecy in which elderly survivors of TBI are not given the same rehabilitation opportunities as their younger counterparts.

Understanding the rehabilitation problems and needs of the older person presents some of the same challenges as those seen in the pediatric population. In a retired population, what are the appropriate standards for community integration? If the normal developmental sequence is for an increasing prevalence of disability and need for assistance with aging, how does one assess the outcome of the rehabilitation process against this moving functional target? But, unlike children with TBI, whose parents are already in the role of caregiver, elderly survivors of TBI may have few support options. A spouse may already have died or be too frail to provide the necessary care, and adult children, if any, may be occupied providing care for their own dependent children. In the absence of family and community supports, therefore, a nursing home destination may seem to be a foregone conclusion, further eroding optimism about the cost-effectiveness of aggressive rehabilitation interventions.

MEDICAL PROBLEMS AFTER TRAUMATIC BRAIN INJURY

Neurodiagnostic Techniques

Many imaging and neurophysiological technologies are available to assist in TBI management. In the acute postinjury period, CT scanning can detect intracranial hematomas, brain swelling, hydrocephalus, and infarction (192). It is also the neuroimaging technique recommended in the management of brain injury due to penetrating objects (193). However, it is not sensitive in identifying small contusions and white matter injury (194). In the postacute phase, CT scanning is useful in evaluating the progress of hydrocephalus and cortical atrophy.

MRI has advantages over CT, including lack of x-ray exposure, greater resolution in the brain stem, better identification of isodense collections of blood, and detection of small white matter lesions (195).

Even MRI may be normal in patients with mild TBI however, despite a well-documented loss of consciousness (196). Recent advances in MRI have increased the clinically relevant information available. Through the use of quantitative MRI, documentation of where the damage has occurred and how generalized it is can be more clearly defined in areas previously not observable to the trained eye (197). Diffusion-weighted MRI can be helpful in determining the acuity of intracerebral hemorrhage and degree of irreversible damage (198). Functional MRI is presently a tool for research purposes but may prove to be beneficial for evaluating brain reorganization after injury and the efficacy of therapeutic interventions (199).

Like functional MRI, positron emission tomography (PET) can provide information about brain function as well as anatomy. Labeled metabolic substrates or blood components are taken up by brain tissue in proportion to metabolic demand or blood flow. Thus, metabolically hypoactive but anatomically normal tissue may be identified. Studies of motor or cognitive activity can be obtained through the use of a tracer such as oxygen-15 (199).

SPECT scanning is more widely available and shares some of the useful functional features of PET scanning. It has been shown to be more clinically applicable when used in conjunction with neuropsychological testing both in severe and mild TBI (199,200). Its sensitivity may be further enhanced in combination with MRI and quantitative MRI (201).

The standard EEG can provide gross information about the severity, location, and extent of brain damage. In addition, epileptiform activity may suggest seizure risk. Interictal EEGs have low sensitivity for seizure disorders, however, especially in areas distant from the cortical convexities (e.g., medial temporal lobes) (202). Sensitivity can be increased by sleep deprivation or prolonged monitoring with behavioral correlation.

EEG measures may at times be misleading, as in the case of improvement of a patient with an isoelectric EEG (203).

Much research has been done on evoked potentials in brain trauma. SEPs can predict the gross outcome of acutely injured patients (204). While there are those who may advocate the use of evoked potentials to allocate rehabilitation resources to patients with a potential to benefit, studies have shown that evoked potentials should not be the sole basis for prediction of outcome in cerebral injury (205).

Because of the traumatic etiology of the brain injury, peripheral nerves may be stretched or damaged by fractures. Patients who have sustained a TBI and show focal muscle wasting, numbness, unexplained weakness, or flaccid extremities in the context of other upper motor neuron findings should receive electromyelogram (EMG) evaluation.

Fractures

Open reduction and internal fixation are used more aggressively in TBI to promote early mobilization, simplify patient care, and improve predictability of fracture outcome. Early fixation may reduce health-care costs and delay in mobility, but the risks for potential secondary brain injury due to surgery and the effects on ultimate functional recovery need to be further explored (206). Many fractures are diagnosed in the acute injury period, but more subtle ones often are missed until transfer to rehabilitation, when the patient shows increased movement and responsiveness to pain. Any unexplained swelling, deformity, or pain response should prompt evaluation for occult fracture. Fractures in TBI predispose to HO. For example, despite appropriate operative management of 23 acetabular fractures, 61% had poor outcomes because of HO (207).

Seizures

Posttraumatic epilepsy is common after significant TBI. The risk of ongoing seizures is related to injury severity, specifically depressed skull fracture, intracranial hematoma, early seizure, and prolonged disturbance of consciousness (208). The risk of new seizure development is greatest in the first 2 years postinjury and gradually declines. Spontaneous resolution of a seizure disorder also occurs, indicating the need for periodic reevaluation.

Most seizures are diagnosed clinically on the basis of focal or generalized motor activity. Patients with muscle spasms or tremors may present diagnostic dilemmas. In such cases, a routine or sleep-deprived EEG may reveal epileptiform activity. More definitive is a 24-hour EEG correlated with observations of the suspicious activity. Seizures in limbic areas may lead only to altered behavior or states of consciousness, presenting further diagnostic challenges.

Treatment during the first week postinjury with phenytoin and valproic acid can be effective for reducing the incidence of early-onset seizures(209). Long-term seizure prophylaxis is no longer recommended and has not been shown to be beneficial in preventing late-onset posttraumatic seizures (209,210).

Carbamazepine and valproic acid have been found to be more cognitively benign than phenobarbital; their superiority over phenytoin is debated (211),(212). Patients who have difficulties with compliance may benefit from Tegretol-Oros, a slow-release form of carbamazepine. In patients with more refractory seizures, newer agents such as gabapentin, lamotrigine, topiramate, and tiagabine may be employed (213). Fosphenytoin is a water-soluble phenytoin prodrug that can be rapidly infused (either intramuscularly or intravenously) without the side effects of intravenous phenytoin, thus improving the management of status epilepticus and potentially reducing its long-term effects on brain tissue (214).

There are no standard recommendations on duration of treatment. In view of the expense and potential toxicity of anticonvulsants, most clinicians withdraw medications after 1 to 2 seizure-free years. Of patients with previous seizure disorders of mixed etiologies who had been seizure-free for 2 years, 35% relapsed after tapering of their anticonvulsants (215).

Hydrocephalus

Ventricular dilation occurs in up to 40% of patients with severe TBI and usually begins to appear within 2 weeks of injury. In most instances, ventriculomegaly results from diffuse atrophy or focal infarction of brain tissue (i.e., hydrocephalus *ex vacuo*). Flattening of the cortical sulci and periventricular lucency tend to support the diagnosis of clinically important hydrocephalus (216).

Hydrocephalus in TBI is most often of the communicating or normal-pressure type. Unfortunately, the classic diagnostic triad of incontinence, gait disorder, and dementia is of little help in severely disabled patients. Failure to improve or deterioration of cognitive or behavioral function should prompt assessment with a CT scan. If the scan is equivocal, cisternography may be done; however, one study in idiopathic hydrocephalus suggested that the cisternogram does not add to clinical diagnostic accuracy (217). Pressure measurements during fluid infusion into the lumbar space and behavioral changes in response to withdrawal of cerebrospinal fluid via lumbar puncture (the "tap test") also have been reported to be of diagnostic value. Patients with ventricular shunts may experience complications due to shunt failure, infection, or over-/underdrainage.The latter complication has been addressed through use of programmable shunt valves. Though not problem-free, they have improved the ability to make minor changes in cerebrospinal fluid flow noninvasively (218). Even when a patient has definitive hydrocephalus, the prognosis from shunting is uncertain. This may be partly because the patient has other cognitive and motor deficits unrelated to hydrocephalus.

Frequently the patient's therapists and nurses are the best judges of subtle cognitive improvements and deteriorations. Hydrocephalus and shunt failure may not be identified through the standard neurologic examination, especially in a patient with an abnormal baseline examination. Hence, it is critical that consulting neurologists and neurosurgeons incorporate the entire team's assessments of cognitive and behavioral fluctuations into their evaluation.

Hypertension

Hypertension, tachycardia, and increased cardiac output in the acute postinjury period result from the increased release of epinephrine and norepinephrine (219). Therefore, β-blockers represent the most specific intervention in this patient group. Propranolol can cause cognitive impairments in hypertensive patients (220). Consequently, use of highly polar β-blockers such as atenolol or nadolol may be preferable. These agents cross the blood–brain barrier very little in uninjured people (221,222), but this has not been studied in diffuse brain injury, where the blood–brain barrier may be disrupted.

In severe brain injury, hypertension may persist beyond the acute phase. This may be linked to injury to the brain stem, hypothalamus, and orbitofrontal regions, but there may be other contributing factors (223). Evaluation to rule out occult spinal cord injury, increased ICP, renal and adrenal abnormalities, or hypothyroidism should be considered (224).

Sustained hypertension is infrequent after TBI unless there was preexisting hypertension. Where hypertension does exist, angiotensin-converting enzyme (ACE) inhibitors, calcium channel blockers, and diuretics are least likely to cause cognitive impairment. If medication with central nervous system side effects must be used, it is wise to inform therapy staff so that subtle cognitive deterioration is noted and reported to the physician.

Cardiopulmonary Disorders

Severe TBI can produce cardiorespiratory arrest or dysrhythmias. Such disturbances of cardiorespiratory control are indications of severe brain injury and causes of further hypoxic injury. Cardiac injury occurs as a result of blunt trauma to the right ventricle against the sternum. This results in early elevations of cardiac enzymes, cardiac wall motion abnormalities, and decreased cardiac output. Central sympathetic hyperactivity can lead to ongoing myocardial necrosis over the next few days (225). Although these injuries may result in lasting electrocardiogram changes (e.g., Q waves, S-T segment alterations), their relevance to the long-term cardiovascular health of survivors is unknown.

Multiple trauma often causes pneumothorax, pulmonary contusions, and lacerations. In addition, adult respiratory distress syndrome, excessive fluid administration during resuscitation, and intense α-adrenergic outflow may lead to noncardiogenic pulmonary edema (226). These and other problems can further compromise cerebral oxygenation.

Many brain-injured patients require tracheostomies for ventilation and suctioning. Humidified air may be delivered through a tracheostomy collar to maintain moist secretions and prevent tracheitis, and frequent suctioning may be required (227). Patients who initially require supplemental oxygen usually can be weaned from it by assessing pulse oximetry on oxygen and again after it has been stopped. Patients who require long-term tracheostomies but have begun to vocalize may benefit from one of the varieties of tubes that permit vocalization.

Most TBI patients eventually can be decannulated. Indirect laryngoscopy screening can be used to check for adequate vocal cord abduction and to rule out subglottic stenosis (228). In some instances tracheal or subglottic stenosis will prevent decannulation and will require dilation or surgical management. If there is no sign of anatomic obstruction, a small-caliber tracheostomy tube will allow air to bypass the tube while it is plugged for progressive intervals. The patient is checked at the end of each interval or at any sign of distress with pulse oximetry. Once the patient has tolerated 24 hours of plugging without incident, decannulation can take place, and the tracheostomy stoma can be covered by a gauze pad or occlusive dressing until it heals. Some patients will have difficulty with decannulation because of the quantity of secretions and inability to cough them up into the pharynx. Thus, persistent suctioning is required. The tracheostomy tube itself however may be an irritant that evokes secretions. To evaluate this possibility, a tracheal button (i.e., a small plug that keeps the stoma open) can replace the tube temporarily to see if the elimination of the tube allows patients to manage their own secretions; if not, the tube can be replaced (229).

Long-term survivors of severe TBI have been reported to show decreased lung capacity, vital capacity, and forced expiratory volume. The etiology of these abnormalities is not entirely clear but appears to be a combination of muscle weakness and incoordination, decreased compliance, and deconditioning

(230). Parameters regarding cardiopulmonary conditioning specifically for patients with brain injury have not been clearly established.

Hypothalamic and Endocrine Dysfunction

Acute TBI causes numerous endocrine changes, including an outpouring of norepinephrine and epinephrine, a rise in aldosterone, glucose, cortisol, and atrial natriuretic hormone, and a drop in thyroid hormones, all of which are related to injury severity (231–235). Elevation of cortisol is related to increased ICP but only in the presence of an intact brain stem, and is independent of corticotropin secretion (236).

Chronic endocrine alterations also occur after TBI. An autopsy study of 100 brain-injured patients revealed a 62% incidence of pituitary injury (237); hypothalamic injuries coexisted in some patients. In addition, there are prominent axonal connections between orbitofrontal cortex and the hypothalamus, providing a potential mechanism for endocrine derangement without overt damage to the hypothalamus or pituitary (238). The few studies of hormone levels in survivors of TBI have found abnormalities in at least one hormone, ranging from 36% to 69% after severe TBI (239,240). Research to date has used laboratory definitions of endocrine abnormalities. Thus, the actual health impact of these derangements is unclear.

TBI may result in abnormalities in virtually any endocrine system. It may cause either diabetes insipidus or the syndrome of inappropriate antidiuretic hormone secretion (SIADH) (241). Both disorders can be managed acutely by controlling fluid and electrolyte intake and monitoring serum electrolytes and osmolality. Persistent or late appearance of diabetes insipidus usually is permanent and may be managed with a synthetic ADH analogue.

Clinical signs of derangement of anterior pituitary hormones may be subtle and confounded with other causes of cognitive, behavioral, and physiologic abnormalities. Hypotension or hypothermia or cognitive decline may be an indicator of endocrine dysfunction. Secondary amenorrhea in female patients is common and may predispose to osteoporosis. Ironically, precocious puberty after TBI has been reported in children (242).

Gynecomastia and galactorrhea occur from elevations in prolactin. In normal subjects, prolactin secretion is controlled by tonic hypothalamic inhibition. Brain injury frequently disrupts these inhibitory influences (243). Chest trauma and a number of medications also may result in galactorrhea. There is evidence that increased prolactin may be involved in the risk of HO after TBI (244). Sexual dysfunction in brain-injured men is more common than can be accounted for on the basis of endocrine dysfunction but is related to other indices of injury severity, suggesting a psychosocial component (245).

In summary, it appears that endocrine dysfunction is common at least in the severely injured and may remit with neurologic recovery. Clinical evaluation may be difficult because of confounding deficits, so the clinician should have a high index of suspicion. Uncorrected endocrine disorders may limit cognitive and behavioral recovery and lead to serious physical sequelae. The lack of agreement on which endocrine abnormalities are most common unfortunately precludes the development of a simple screening strategy.

Cranial Nerve Dysfunction

Olfactory nerve injuries commonly accompany significant head trauma because of the delicate anatomy of the fibers exiting the cribriform plate; they are particularly likely in association with cerebrospinal fluid rhinorrhea. The diagnosis may be missed by incomplete sensory testing. Objective testing of olfaction using a scratch-and-sniff odor panel is possible (246). Injuries not detected by sensory testing may be revealed through MRI (247). Olfactory deficits may play a role in altered feeding behavior.

Visual impairment may occur as spotty scotomata that differ in the two eyes, as homonymous hemianopsia, or as complete blindness. Optic nerve lesions must be distinguished from hemi-inattention, cortical blindness, and visual agnosia. Early assessment can be done in gross terms through funduscopic examination, visual evoked response studies, and pupillary assessment. Vision and visual attention can be evaluated in severely impaired patients, using repeated presentations of colorful photographs and cards in each hemifield (149). When cooperation allows, more precise visual field and acuity testing should be performed. Neuropsychological assessment may clarify visual perceptual disorders. Information about field cuts and acuity should be shared with all team members to ensure that therapy materials are of appropriate size and placement.

Extraocular movements may be affected by damage to cranial nerves, their brain stem nuclei, or by impairment of coordinative structures in the midbrain and cerebellum (248). In addition, orbital fractures or damage to the extraocular muscles may produce disconjugate gaze. Neuro-ophthalmologic examination may help clarify the pathophysiology of the deficit. Alternating or unilateral eye patching can eliminate diplopia. Prisms and strabismus surgery require that the patient be capable of ocular convergence to maintain binocular vision, but surgery sometimes may be appropriate solely for cosmetic purposes.

Temporal bone fractures may disrupt facial nerve function temporarily or permanently. This must be differentiated from cortical or subcortical central facial weakness. Facial weakness, when combined with corneal insensitivity as a result of trigeminal lesions, can lead to corneal ulceration; corneal lubricants or tarsorrhaphy may be indicated.

Skull fractures also may disrupt the auditory or vestibular pathways (249). Ossicular dislocation can lead to conductive hearing loss. Brain stem auditory evoked responses can be helpful in assessment of auditory function in comatose or uncooperative patients; however, if no response is seen at normal intensity, hearing threshold should be evaluated with increasing intensities. Caloric testing can provide information about vestibular function. Later, standard audiologic evaluation, including speech perception, should be performed. Hearing aids or ossicular repair can be helpful in selected patients. The patient's auditory capabilities should be shared with the entire treatment team so that care can be taken to communicate in the environment and style that optimize comprehension.

Movements of the tongue, pharynx, and larynx often are impaired by severe TBI at various levels in the central nervous system (250). Evaluation of oral motor function including cough and gag reflexes and indirect laryngoscopy may help clarify the location and extent of the problem. Such disturbances will be relevant for safe oral feeding as well as vocal communication.

Sensory Deficits

TBI can produce disturbances of any of the sensory modalities. Depending on the location and severity of the damage, these may be disturbances of basic sensation (e.g., decreased visual acuity) or of perceptual processing of that sensation (e.g., impaired visual spatial perception). Both forms of disturbance can be disabling.

Disorders of somesthetic sensation can result from damage to a variety of brain structures and may distort touch, pain, temperature, and position information. Pain syndromes may result from central injury to the thalamus, other cerebral structures, or from deranged neurotransmission between the thalamus and cerebral cortex (251).

Basic sensation can be assessed in each modality as soon as the patient is able to cooperate. Visual, auditory, and somesthetic sensation can be assessed grossly earlier with evoked potential studies. The presence of normal basic sensation, however, does not ensure that the patient can form the complex perceptions needed to recognize a visually presented object, or identify a letter through stereognosis.

When patients fail at a task for which basic sensory input is intact, other causes of inability to perform can be explored. A patient recovering from cortical blindness, for example, may have full visual fields and functional acuity but may be unable to name visually presented objects. Neuropsychological assessment can help to differentiate among object-naming disorders, visual agnosias, scanning disorders, and disorders of complex visual perception (252).

There is no uniform strategy for coping with sensory deficits. Rather, treatment is planned around the severity of the deficit, strength of remaining sensory capabilities, and cognitive status of the patient. All team members should be involved in this planning because the patient's sensory, motor, and cognitive capacities all are relevant to the process.

Heterotopic Ossification

Clinically significant HO occurs in 11% to 20% of severely injured patients, primarily in proximal joints of the upper and lower extremities (253). The etiology of HO in brain injury is unknown. Risk factors include prolonged coma, increased muscle tone and limited movement in the involved extremity, and associated fractures (254).

HO may present with pain, warmth, swelling, and contracture formation but may be occult. Earliest diagnosis is possible with a bone scan, but ossification subsequently is visible on plain radiographs. Diphosphonates and nonsteroidal antiinflammatory agents, particularly indomethacin, and radiation therapy have been used in an attempt to arrest early HO or to prevent its postoperative recurrence (253). A study of patients with early and intermediate HO found that calcium deposition occurred in the early phase, inflammation in the intermediate phase, and appearance of osteoclasts and osteoblasts in the late phase (255). This suggests that diphosphonates may be beneficial early and antiinflammatories at an intermediate time, but no controlled treatment comparisons have been performed to date. Radiation has been used for prophylaxis, to treat existing HO (256), and after surgery to prevent recurrence (253). Long-term adverse effects have not yet been studied, particularly in young patients. Range-of-motion exercises are indicated to prevent ankylosis. If ankylosis seems inevitable despite exercises, it should be encouraged to occur in the most functional position.

Surgery for removal of ectopic bone should be undertaken only for clear functional goals, such as improved standing posture or ambulation or independent dressing and feeding. In general, surgery is not undertaken earlier than 18 months after injury (257).

Increased Muscle Tone and Contractures

Increased muscle tone following TBI may reflect true spasticity (i.e., increased phasic stretch reflexes). Dystonia, posturing in

TABLE 78-6.   Indications for Treatment of Increased Muscle Tone

Interference with active movement
Contracture formation or progression in a posturing limb
Interference with appropriate positioning or hygiene
Self-inflicted trauma during muscle spasms
Excessive pain on range-of-motion exercises or during muscle
    spasms
Excessive therapy time devoted to contracture prevention rather than
    functional activities

response to head position and cutaneous stimulation, and extrapyramidal syndromes also are common. The mere existence of abnormal tone is not an indication for treatment. Treatment should be based on functional considerations (Table 78-6).

Motor Disturbances

A variety of other motor disturbances result from TBI. The diffuse and multifocal nature of the neuropathologic condition often challenges a precise neurophysiological diagnosis. Deficits may include paralysis or paresis involving isolated muscle groups, combinations of limbs, or the whole body.

Disorders of balance and coordination may result from damage to the cerebellum or its connections. Patients with good muscle strength may be unable to ambulate or even sit independently because of profound ataxia. Similarly, limb ataxia may preclude self-feeding, writing, and independent ADLs. Tremors, bradykinesia, and parkinsonism may accompany basal ganglia and substantia nigra lesions, and it appears that posttraumatic parkinsonism is less likely to respond to dopaminergic or anticholinergic drugs than Parkinson's disease (258).

The patient's movement abilities should be assessed by the physiatrist, physical therapist, and occupational therapist (259). Formal gait analysis may help reveal the specific impairments affecting gait (260). Weakness can be addressed through active assistive range-of-motion and progressive resistive exercises. Ataxia is notoriously difficult to treat. A weighted walker or wrist cuffs may be of modest benefit. If ataxia varies markedly from proximal to distal joints, selective splinting or strategies to stabilize the extremity may be useful.

An attempt should be made to diagnose tremors specifically with reference to their frequency, amplitude, and occurrence during action, rest, and sleep (261). L-Dopa and propranolol both have been used in movement disorders such as tremors and ataxia, but functional tests should be performed on and off medication to assess efficacy in individual patients (262). Some improvement in tremor-related disability may be seen with botulinum toxin injections (263). Stereotactic surgery may be an alternative, but is recommended only for those with severe, disabling tremor (264). Deep brain stimulation has been used to treat patients with movement disorders (265) but its efficacy has not yet been specifically studied following TBI. Orthoses and adaptive devices may assist weak or ataxic patients in performing functional tasks. Dexterity exercises may be used to increase manual speed and coordination.

Slowed motor responses are among the most common deficits associated with TBI and may limit self-care and employment productivity. It appears, however, that much of this motor slowness can be attributed to central processing delays rather than a motor deficit per se (266). There is no consensus on how to treat this generalized slowness.

Dysarthria sometimes is noted after brain injury and may be the result of either peripheral or central nervous system damage affecting motor control of the speech mechanism. The dysarthric patient may receive oral motor strengthening and coordination exercises to improve articulation, a palatal lift for nasality, and breath support training to improve sustained volume. Kinematic articulography may provide more objective data regarding the nature of dysarthria and better target the area of focus for treatment (267).

A number of automated systems for guiding motor-related therapies are in development. These computerized devices deliver movement exercises via various forms of virtual reality, and make use of various kinds of displacement and force sensors to monitor performance. Such devices may prove to be able to enhance the frequency and intensity of movement therapy while reducing personnel costs, and may also allow for remote monitoring of therapy via telerehabilitation (268). However, such devices need to be flexible with respect to a variety of difficulty hierarchies appropriate to different therapeutic goals if they are to allow reduction in direct therapist supervision (269).

Nutrition and Feeding

TBI can produce dramatic increases in basal metabolism, with catabolism, weight loss, and low serum albumin. Thus, the acutely injured patient must have increased caloric and protein intake, but the need for invasive procedures and difficulty in achieving high rates of tube feeding may interfere.

While it is recommended that full nutritional replacement be instituted within the first week of injury (270), there is no consensus on how soon to consider gastrostomy or jejunostomy placement in patients who remain obtunded or lack oral motor capability (271,272). In patients with recurrent pneumonia and possible aspiration, more distal placement of feeding tubes should be considered. This may be done by means of surgical jejunostomy or through fluoroscopic guidance of a tube through the gastrostomy site into the jejunum. The gastric source of the aspiration should be confirmed, however, because some patients may merely be aspirating oral secretions and will not benefit from jejunal tubes. Adding methylene blue or food coloring to gastrostomy tube feedings and suctioning from a tracheostomy or scanning the lungs for radioactive tracers introduced into the stomach are two useful alternatives.

Gastroesophageal reflux is common following brain injury even in those without nasogastric tubes (273). It may lead to aspiration and esophagitis. Antacids and acid suppressants may improve esophagitis. Metoclopramide increases gastroesophageal sphincter tone but it can cause sedation and extrapyramidal side effects (274). Head elevation may reduce aspiration of regurgitated feedings.

Obstacles to oral feeding include both cognitive and oral motor deficits (275). Attempts at oral feeding generally begin with assessment of the reflexive and voluntary components of oral motor function by a speech, occupational, or physical therapist experienced in dysphagia treatment. This is followed, if necessary, by an oral motor facilitation treatment program to decrease the latency of the swallowing reflex and improve oral motor strength and coordination.

When appropriate, small quantities of pureed foods are introduced and increased in amount to build endurance. As performance improves, the variety of thickness and texture is increased until liquids can be handled safely. Failure to become a functional feeder is associated with persistently poor intraoral manipulation or cognitive levels below V on the Ranchos Los Amigos Scale (see Table 78-5).

Patients who appear to be candidates for oral feeding but who have frequent coughing or an episode of clinical aspiration may benefit from a videofluoroscopy performed collaboratively by an experienced feeding therapist and a radiologist (276). By using different food textures and placements, it may be possible to determine a strategy to normalize swallowing. Fiberoptic endoscopy has also been found to be useful in evaluating patients with dysphagia (277).

When the patient has made maximal progress in terms of food quantity and texture, the patient or family and nursing staff should be trained in the optimal oral feeding methods.

Bowel and Bladder Dysfunction

Frontal lobe lesions can impair inhibitory control over bowel and bladder evacuation, leading to urgency and incontinence. Slowed mobility, poor communication, and impaired initiation also contribute indirectly to incontinence, making this issue a significant one in persons with brain injury. For details on management please refer to Chapter XX on bowel and bladder dysfunction.

Pain

Pain is a complex phenomenon that can complicate the rehabilitation process of individuals with both mild and severe injuries, and at any time after injury. In mild TBI (See also Mild Traumatic Brain Injury), pain may be one of the primary complaints, particularly in the form of frequent headaches. In more severe injuries, pain may also be related to hypertonia, contractures, and HO. When TBI occurs in the context of multisystem trauma, fractures and traumatic neuropathies and plexopathies may also contribute to pain. Complex regional pain syndrome is seen relatively frequently in the acute rehabilitation setting (278). Of course individuals with TBI may also have pain in relation to any coexisting painful illness. The most appropriate treatments for pain-producing conditions depend on an assessment of the source and nature of the pain. In patients who are able to describe their symptoms, assessment of pain-producing conditions is similar to such assessment in nonbrain-injured individuals. In minimally conscious patients, however, it may be difficult to distinguish pain syndromes from spontaneous moaning or grimacing that may have no painful etiology. Moreover, more interactive patients with memory problems may have difficulty reporting the frequency, pattern, and precipitating causes of their pain. In such instances it may be helpful to record the behavioral manifestations of pain (e.g., grimacing) and their relationship to potential provoking factors (e.g., ranging of a particular limb). The range of treatment modalities available to able-bodied individuals can also be applied to patients with TBI who are experiencing pain. The possibility of central pain, induced by the patient's primary brain injury, should also be kept in mind, particularly when no physical cause is apparent. Where possible, narcotics or other sedating analgesics should be avoided to optimize cognitive functioning. However, particularly in the case of acute highly painful conditions (e.g., postoperative pain), the patient's participation in therapy will probably be no worse with a short course of regularly scheduled narcotics than if asked to participate with inadequate pain relief.

NEUROCOGNITIVE AND NEUROBEHAVIORAL DEFICITS

TBI is by nature a diffuse and multifocal insult. Partly for this reason, there is great variability in the patterns of cognitive and behavioral impairments seen. Despite this there are certain commonalties across patients, most likely related to the typical areas of injury to the gray matter (i.e., frontal and temporal poles) and white matter (i.e., midbrain and corpus callosum). Thus, difficulty with alertness, memory, and concentration are very common, as are behavioral disturbances related to impulsivity, impaired initiation, and other problems of behavioral control. In the sections that follow, we review some of the most common cognitive and behavioral impairments affecting persons with TBI. Although we discuss problems separately, the reader should keep in mind their interrelatedness. Many difficulties labeled by clinicians and family members as "behavior problems" are highly influenced by cognitive and perceptual disturbances. For example, comprehension deficits or slowed information processing can induce brain-injured persons to act out in frustration when their capacities are overtaxed. Variations in behavioral response may also be related in complex ways to preinjury factors including age, socioeconomic factors, substance use history, and personality differences. The totality of subjective experiences and personal history must be considered when evaluating problems and developing treatments for them.

Neurocognitive and neurobehavioral status may be assessed with standardized tests, as in a neuropsychological evaluation, or by structured observations in real-world situations. The latter are more useful for clarifying the impact of cognitive impairments in persons who are low-functioning or when status is likely to fluctuate (e.g., in the early stages of recovery). Formal neuropsychological assessment is beyond the scope of this chapter but is discussed extensively in the textbook by Lezak (279).

Impairments of Arousal and Attention

Deficits in arousal and attention are among the most widespread (266). The comatose patient suffers from profoundly impaired arousal, and many of the cognitive and emotional complaints in minor TBI are hypothesized to be attentional in nature (266). Arousal may be defined as the general state of responsiveness to environmental stimuli. Normally, arousal undergoes slow fluctuations in relation to diurnal rhythm, food intake, and activity level (i.e., tonic arousal). Arousal also can be modulated over brief intervals by demands in the environment (i.e., phasic arousal) (280). The reticular activating system (RAS) has a primary role in control of arousal, exerting its influence over diffuse cortical regions and receiving cortical inputs in return (281). Damage to the RAS plays a critical part in coma onset (47). In principle, a deficit in tonic arousal could lead to generalized impairments in responsiveness and profound slowing of information processing. Impaired phasic arousal could interfere with the ability to modify arousal to cope with cognitively demanding situations.

Attention may be considered to be the selective channeling of arousal. Attention (associated with conscious awareness) is directed to a particular set of internal or external stimuli out of the infinite set of possible targets of awareness. Attention is not a unitary phenomenon either in psychological or neurophysiological terms, and there is no precise agreement about how to divide up its component processes; at the least, the following phenomena can be distinguished (282,283):

- Arousal: the state of receptivity to sensory information and readiness to respond.
- Selection (sometimes referred to as focused attention): the ability to focus attention on particular stimuli or responses. Selection is often made on spatial grounds (i.e., selecting a stimulus in a certain location), and damage, particularly to right parietal or frontal lobes, can interfere with normal spatial selective attention (hemispatial neglect).
- Strategic control: the ability to sustain attention over time; inhibit disruption by distracting influences; shift attention in line with changing goals and priorities; manipulate information currently held in mind (referred to as working memory); and divide attention between two or more task demands.
- Processing speed: the speed at which information is transmitted within the nervous system to allow cognitive processing to occur.

Numerous brain regions appear to play a role in attentional processes. Research has particularly highlighted the roles of the right hemisphere, bilateral prefrontal and parietal cortices, the anterior cingulate, and portions of the thalamus and basal ganglia in attentional function (284). Disorders of attention may impair learning and performance in several ways. Affected patients may have difficulty focusing on any task, may be easily distracted, or may show hemispatial neglect. Attention deficits can lead to secondary decreases in language comprehension or visuospatial processing because the patient's information processing is interrupted and disorganized. Inability to shift attention might be manifested, for example, in the inability to attend to task instructions and also monitor one's own performance. It has been suggested that PTA is most appropriately considered a confusional state related to attention deficit rather than a true memory disturbance (285). Similarly, frontal lobe disorders such as impulsivity and perseveration may be interpreted in attentional terms. These disorders may reflect a loss of goal-directed control over attention such that it

is easily pulled or dysfunctionally fixed on irrelevant aspects of a task (286).

Exactly which of these aspects of attention are disrupted in TBI remains a subject of some controversy. There is general agreement that processing speed is reduced in TBI, but the location of this slowing in the stream of information processing is still under debate. Recent laboratory research shows that patients with TBI have difficulties with sustained attention (287) but that phasic arousal to auditory stimuli is preserved even in severe injury (280). Tasks requiring divided attention appear to be particularly impaired by TBI, when both tasks require conscious control (288). When performing independent work in distracting environments, individuals with TBI have more off-task behavior than uninjured controls both in the presence of distractions and in their absence (289). On the basis of the many attentional studies in TBI, it appears that, other than slowed processing, most attentional complaints can be linked to strategic control of attention rather than basic arousal or selection. Strategic control, in turn, is believed to be dependent on prefrontal and limbic goals and motivations being linked to basic attentional mechanisms.

Arousal and attention are assessed best by a combination of formal neuropsychological tests and behavioral observation by all disciplines (283). It is critical to arrive at more precise diagnoses than "impaired attention" because impairments of different components of attention may have different therapeutic implications. Unfortunately, there is no consensus on what set of neuropsychological tests are most informative about attention impairments and, in particular, most useful in differential assessment. Digit span forward and backward and other tests of working memory and mental control may be useful (279). In less impaired individuals, tests such as the Paced Auditory Serial Addition Test (PASAT) (290) and Test of Everyday Attention (291) may provide additional insight. In general, treatment of these disorders can be grouped in terms of pharmacologic, behavioral, and compensatory strategies (Table 78-7).

Many medications used for other purposes have negative effects on arousal, attention, and general cognitive function. Anticonvulsants such as phenytoin and phenobarbital, antihypertensives such as methyldopa and propranolol, and antispasticity drugs such as diazepam, baclofen, and dantrolene all

TABLE 78-7. Treatment of Disorders of Arousal and Attention

Component	Pharmacologic[a]	Behavioral[a]	Compensatory Strategy[a]
Tonic arousal	Methylphenidate[b] d-Amphetamine Pemoline Nonsedating tricyclics Amantadine Bromocriptine	Naps Upright position	Engage in tasks when most alert
Phasic arousal		Frequent task changes	Give alerting clues
Selective attention		Reinforce attention	Nondistracting environment
Hemispatial neglect	Bromocriptine	Graded training to attend	Position tasks to the patient's left right
Strategic control		Training in hierarchic attention skills	Simplify decision making, provide supervision, train solutions to specific problems
Processing speed		Reinforce rapid performance	Allow adequate time for responding

[a]Note that most of these treatments are investigational.
[b]All of these medications may have uses beyond regulation of arousal and act on other components of the attentional network. Their respective roles are under investigation.

may impair cognitive performance (221,292–294). Therefore, attempts should be made to withdraw such medications or replace them with less sedating alternatives (e.g., carbamazepine, ACE inhibitors, phenol, or botulinum toxin nerve/muscle blocks) (164,295).

The role of pharmacologic treatment remains controversial. Some studies have suggested attentional benefits from psychostimulants such as methylphenidate but are subject to methodologic criticisms (small numbers of subjects, inadequate control for spontaneous recovery, and failure to specify which attentional components are being assessed) (296). A small randomized controlled pilot study suggested that methylphenidate improves cognitive processing speed, and some aspects of sustained attention, while having little effect on overt orienting to extraneous distracting events (297). Although methylphenidate has been reported to increase seizure risk, this is not well documented, and research suggests that, on the contrary, it may have some anticonvulsant effect (298). Other dopaminergic drugs such as amantadine and bromocriptine have been reported to improve overall attentiveness, increase the ability to divide attention (299), or diminish hemispatial neglect (300,301). Selection of appropriate patients for drug treatment, however, has not been clarified. Therefore, it is recommended that, when a patient is being considered for pharmacologic therapy of attention deficits, individualized measures of the behaviors of interest be assessed both on and off the medication (151).

Behavioral retraining of attention has been advocated but is of uncertain efficacy. Some studies have suggested benefit from retraining of patients with neglect or distractibility (302–304), whereas others have failed to document changes (305–307). Few of the studies that demonstrate improvement have assessed generalization of benefits to the everyday environment. A metaanalysis of behavioral treatments for attention deficits suggests that studies involving a pre–postdesign without an untreated control group show far more improvement than those involving a comparison to a control group, indicating that much of the apparent "benefit" of attention retraining programs results simply from repeated administration of the outcome measures themselves, combined with residual spontaneous recovery. The studies that do demonstrate greater improvement in the treatment than the control group tend to involve attention coaching in complex tasks such as driving and ADLs rather than retraining of specific attentional capacities (308). Together, these results suggest that therapists' energy would be better spent giving feedback about attentiveness in important real-world tasks than supervising repetitive drills of core attentional capacities. In addition, it is important to ensure that strategies learned in a therapy environment are carried over into a variety of functional activities. Therefore, if a team member is training spatial attention in, for example, reading, interdisciplinary plans should be made to transfer the same protocol to other settings such as ambulation and ADL tasks.

In uninjured people, extensive practice of virtually any task leads to the ability to perform it with minimal attention (i.e., automatically). This phenomenon has received little study in brain-damaged patients; however, it would seem possible to deal with some attentional impairments by practicing activities to such a degree that they no longer place much demand on disordered attentional processes.

Impairments of Learning and Memory

Memory impairments are among the most common, persistent, and handicapping of the cognitive complaints after TBI. All patients with moderate to severe injuries and most with mild injuries experience permanent amnesia for the events immediately preceding and following the injury. These intervals are referred to as retrograde and posttraumatic amnesias, respectively. As patients recover from the acute confusional state postinjury, retrograde amnesia typically "shrinks" toward the present (309). The final interval unaccounted for ranges from minutes to weeks or months, depending on the severity of the injury. In severe cases, retrograde amnesias may cover a span of several years and may "eliminate" highly salient preinjury memories, such as the birth of a child or the death of a parent. PTA is the interval of permanently lost memory following the injury; it covers both coma and the acute confusional state and is nearly always longer than retrograde amnesia. As noted earlier, its duration is commonly used as a measure of injury severity.

These permanent gaps in memory are often emotionally disturbing to patients who must reconstruct the missing interval by obtaining reports from others. Retrograde and posttraumatic amnesias also have legal ramifications, particularly when injuries are caused by assaults or reckless driving. Medical professionals may need to intervene with the legal system when persons with TBI are asked to testify about events they are unable to remember.

Most individuals with moderate and severe TBI suffer from ongoing deficits in anterograde memory (i.e., difficulty in storing and retrieving new information), well beyond the resolution of PTA. Because of the diffuse and multifocal nature of TBI, the learning and memory impairments typically affect multiple modalities (e.g., visual/spatial as well as verbal) and have a broad impact on "everyday memory" (310,311). The neural substrate of memory deficits after TBI is not fully understood. However, memory test scores have been shown to correlate with the degree of posttraumatic atrophy of the hippocampus, a limbic structure thought to play an important role in new learning (312). Given the prevalence of attentional deficits in TBI, it is also plausible that some "memory" impairment can be attributed to defective processing of information at the time of presentation (313). One study showed that challenging attentional resources at the time of stimulus encoding did *not* disproportionately affect the later recall of TBI patients (314). However, there is also evidence that when persons with TBI are given extra learning trials, their later retrieval of the learned material can be comparable to that of uninjured controls (315). Other research suggests that even with extra learning experience, persons with TBI fail to take spontaneous advantage of retrieval cues (e.g., categories in a word list) which boost the retrieval scores of control subjects (316). These findings imply that at least some memory deficits may be due to problems with initial acquisition, which might be overcome with extra training or rehearsal of information; and that persons with TBI might need help to notice, and use, aspects of the material that will facilitate later retrieval.

The bulk of the research on memory impairment has concerned memory for past events or past learning (i.e., retrospective memory). However, a very important aspect of real-world function is *prospective* memory, which is the ability to remember to do something in the future. Prospective memory may depend partly on frontal/executive control processes that help to maintain an active goal state over time and provide "triggers" for action at the appropriate moment (317). Prospective memory is significantly impaired in persons with TBI, either when the task is framed as something that must be done at a specific time, or when it is to be performed later in association with another activity or event (318). Real-world prospective memory problems appear as a wide variety of "failures of intention" such as forgetting to run errands or take medications, missing appointments, and neglecting to provide information or messages to others. Of the many commercially available tests and test batteries for the assessment of memory, only a few include a measure of prospective memory (e.g., the Rivermead Behavioural Memory Test) (319).

In the clinical setting, evaluation of memory impairment should not rely exclusively on test results. A functional assessment by the interdisciplinary team and careful interviewing of the family or caretakers will help to identify the environmental situations in which the disorder disrupts function, the frequency with which real-world memory problems occur, and most importantly, the cues or conditions that facilitate memory performance. As noted earlier, it is also important to remember that other cognitive difficulties such as attention, language, or executive function impairments will affect memory performances and may still be interpreted or described by the affected person and family as a "memory" problem. In such cases the memory system may actually be relatively spared, and other difficulties must be sought as the root of poor or inconsistent performance.

An influential model of memory processing which has relevance to TBI rehabilitation highlights the distinction between *implicit* and *explicit* memory. Explicit memory refers to consciously remembered material. For example, remembering yesterday's events, drawing a picture from memory, and recounting a conversation all involve explicit memory. In contrast, implicit learning operates outside of conscious awareness and cannot be precisely verbalized; it is expressed through improved performances (e.g., when new motor skills or other forms of *procedural learning* are acquired) (320). These two memory systems, which interact constantly in normal learning, are thought to be subserved by different neuronal circuitry. Implicit memory may be diffusely represented in cortical networks, making it less vulnerable to cerebral injury than the phylogenetically newer explicit memory system, which is thought to be dependent on focal regions of the hippocampus and medial temporal lobes (321). There is evidence that in TBI as in other organic conditions affecting memory, implicit learning is spared relative to explicit memory (322–324). A training method known as *errorless learning* has been studied in persons with TBI and other forms of organic memory impairment. Errorless learning (in which the trainer minimizes the errors committed by the trainee during the learning process) helps to bypass the need for explicit memory, which is thought to be critical for benefiting from error. Without explicit memory errors may inadvertently be learned by the more intact implicit memory system, interfering with performance. Errorless learning and related methods have been shown to be effective for helping people with TBI to learn new computer tasks, face–name associations, procedures for using memory notebooks, and other materials (325–327). The full range of tasks amenable to errorless learning and its clinical use in rehabilitation environments still need to be explored.

Many other methods have been used in an attempt to remediate the memory problems experienced by persons with TBI. As there is little convincing evidence that memory can be enhanced pharmacologically (300), the most promising methods involve the teaching of compensatory strategies. For example, in a group of people with TBI who were living independently, training in the real-world application of memory enhancement techniques improved memory on objective tests as well as subjective ratings, and the improvement persisted at 4-month follow-up (328). For those with more severe memory deficits, a more commonly used approach is to train the use of reminder systems such as notebooks, planners, and so forth. Electronic organizers and hand-held computers have also been used for this purpose (See also Cognitive Rehabilitation). The success of any reminder system depends partly on an individual's awareness of memory deficits and acceptance of the need to use external strategies, both of which may be problematic. In addition, persons with TBI may have difficulty with the executive demands of these strategies (i.e., knowing *what* to record *when*, remembering to do it consistently, and using recorded information prospectively). Structured training programs in how to use compensatory memory systems however may be worth the effort. In one of the few controlled studies to date, Schmitter-Edgecombe and colleagues used a comprehensive training regimen to teach individuals with TBI how to use memory notebooks, and showed that the training had beneficial effects on measures of everyday memory function (329).

For the rehabilitation setting the following summary points should be considered:

- Many persons with TBI benefit more from hands-on training of procedural skills than from verbally based or didactic instruction, although a combination of modalities may be most effective.
- The learning of persons with TBI may need to be judged by changes in performance in addition to verbal self-report, as much learning can take place of which patients are unaware.
- Errorless learning can be effective for patients with severe explicit memory impairments. It may be necessary to provide cues at each step and hand-over-hand assistance (e.g., during the training of ADLs) to prevent the patient from making errors. This assistance can be gradually faded as the patient begins to initiate more of the actions correctly.
- Persons with TBI may not spontaneously recognize or take advantage of cues or aspects of the material to be remembered that will assist later recall, so therapists may need to provide explicit help in this regard.
- Memory notebooks and other organizing systems are useful for many persons with TBI.

Reminder systems are most effective when the entire rehabilitation team focuses on teaching only one or two applications (e.g., scheduling appointments, recording the contents of phone calls). This allows the team to achieve more consistency in teaching "how and when to record what." New applications can be added as the user achieves mastery of the original functions.

Impairments of Frontal Executive Function

The mark of intelligent behavior is the ability to adapt to change, solve unexpected problems, anticipate outcomes, and otherwise cope with situations that fall outside of one's routine. These abilities in turn require cognitive flexibility, self-monitoring, and self-adjustment of performance as well as simultaneous consideration of multiple alternatives and their probable consequences. From these alternatives an appropriate plan of action must be selected and the intention carried to completion. Complex abilities such as these, which are necessary for adaptive human behavior, have been termed *executive functions*. There is considerable evidence linking these functions to prefrontal cortex (317,330,331). TBI, which often involves damage to the frontal poles and orbitomesial cortex or their connections (332,333), commonly leads to disorders of reasoning, planning, and goal-directed behavior attributable to breakdowns in executive function. Depending on the nature and severity of the injury as well as premorbid factors, these impairments may appear clinically as disorganized or tangential speech and action, a tendency to be "pulled" by irrelevant stimuli, and inappropriate interpersonal behavior (334). Lack of insight into these and other deficits (See also Awareness Deficits) and poor ability to profit from feedback are usually part of the clinical picture.

Most conceptualizations of executive function include the notion of purposeful, controlled deployment of attention and other cognitive/perceptual functions in the service of goal-directed behavior unfolding over time (335). Normal behavior falls under external control at times, as when one attends "involuntarily" to a loud noise or moving object. Behavior must be modulated, however, in the service of one's intentions. For example, if the goal is to get to an appointment in an unfamiliar place on time, one will be more likely to attend to street signs and less likely to attend to shop windows. For such modulation to occur, emotional and motivational states must be linked to perceptual and motor systems so that the appropriate aspects of the environment may be attended to and acted on, and the irrelevant ones screened out. The breakdown of this linkage contributes to the distractibility and aimlessness of many TBI patients. Even when performing so-called overlearned routine actions such as making a sandwich or cup of coffee, persons with TBI omit steps and make errors of planning, sequencing, and object use that can be attributed to failures in this attentional control of action (336). Compared to uninjured control subjects, those with frontal lobe damage due to TBI have difficulty generating "scripts" for action plans for familiar activities such as grocery shopping, and even more difficulty implementing such plans in real time (337). Deficits in planning and goal attainment have been emphasized as central to frontal executive function in the influential research of Duncan, who conceptualizes such impairment as "goal neglect" (338,339).

Another important aspect of executive function is control over one's responses to people and situations, such that some behaviors are inhibited in favor of others that are more appropriate to the context. For example, to meet certain interpersonal needs, one must judge, then select which of many possible behaviors will achieve the goal and fit with the social milieu, and use available social feedback to check the appropriateness of one's behavior. Individuals with TBI often lack these judgments, behaving in ways that appear inappropriate and short-sighted to others, and that seem to entail "personality changes." Thus, a male patient may behave in contradiction to his preinjury interpersonal style by exhibiting a sexually aggressive manner with a female therapist, oblivious both to her reaction and to strong cues and admonitions from members of his own family.

Remaining questions to be addressed about executive function include questions about *what* and *how many* specific cognitive processes underlie these critical functions. For example, working memory (340) and the formation of effective plans (339) have both been proposed as central operations, deficits in which may explain a variety of dysexecutive behaviors. Related lines of research have examined the relationships among seemingly disparate behavioral symptoms often categorized as executive function disorders, such as behavioral dyscontrol, personality change, and various higher cognitive impairments. These symptoms do appear related to one another, and it may turn out that executive functions are comprised of a relatively small number of correlated factors (341,342).

Clinical assessment of executive function deficits is difficult for several reasons. Partly because of the uncertainty in how to conceptualize these functions, there is simply less agreement as to how they should be measured compared to other functions (e.g., learning and memory abilities). In addition, by virtue of late phylogenetic and ontologic development, frontal executive functions may show more interindividual variation than relatively hard-wired functions such as perception and language. Thus, two people could have identical prefrontal injuries yet display different patterns of executive dysfunction (334). Because executive disorders relate to the ability to deal with novelty and change, they are difficult to see within structured tasks but must be looked for in challenging or open-ended situations. Persons with TBI may do fairly well on traditional neuropsychological tests yet show profound life disruption from executive dysfunction (317). Recently developed test procedures now provide standardized analogues to the kinds of tasks that are sensitive to executive dysfunction. For example, the Behavioural Assessment of the Dysexecutive Syndrome (BADS) is a validated battery that includes tests of planning and prioritizing as well as a rating scale to capture personality and behavioral changes affecting daily life (343,344). Schwartz and colleagues have developed the Naturalistic Action Test (NAT), a brief standardized assessment of the ability to plan and carry out everyday actions in real time (345).

Attempts to treat executive impairments have been based on one of three general perspectives (346). At one extreme, the deficits are considered to affect behavior in such a global way that they cannot be remediated. Therefore, the physical and social environment will need to be fully structured to act as "prosthetic frontal lobes" for guiding the person's adaptive behavior. In this view, the treatment consists of determining and implementing the specific environmental conditions that will elicit and support the desired behaviors. An alternative view seeks to retrain or reinforce the separate abilities and tasks that are disrupted by executive dysfunction (e.g., socially acceptable behavior or step-by-step approaches to specific situations). A third approach attempts to remediate one or more cognitive *processes* that are hoped to affect executive function in a variety of contexts. These processes include "metastrategies" such as generic problem-solving approaches (347) or techniques of verbal self-instruction (348). Some of these methods have shown promise. For example, in a study of 30 people with TBI, Levine and colleagues provided empirical support for a strategy training method known as Goal Management Training (349). A short-term trial of this method, which teaches the steps involved in defining goals, breaking them into steps, and checking one's performance, was associated with fewer errors on cognitively demanding tasks compared to a sham training method (practice on cognitive tasks without strategic training). Other methods for addressing executive dysfunction have been discussed in the clinical literature, notably by Mateer (350).

Executive impairments are of profound functional significance for severely brain-injured persons and are major obstacles to independent living, employment, and successful relationships. Until more information is available as to the effectiveness of general strategy training, particularly its impact on real-life problems, it would seem prudent not to focus exclusively on retraining abstract capacities, but to include functional activities such as planning a meal, organizing transportation, and the like.

All team members are likely to be involved in addressing these problems. The neuropsychologist may be able to suggest treatment strategies applicable to all disciplines. In addition, each therapist can assist the patient in solving the specific problems faced within tasks. For example, the physical therapist may help the patient plan how to navigate an unfamiliar route, while the occupational therapist may teach strategies for organizing a menu. Team members should be reminded that executive functions are least challenged in highly structured and routine environments such as hospitals and clinics. Thus, meaningful evaluation and treatment of these difficulties requires clinicians to avoid overstructuring patients and to make use of real-world activities rather than limiting treatment to simulations or paper-and-pencil tasks within the clinical environment.

Impairments of Language and Communication

Because of the diffuse nature of TBI, the classic language disorders found in stroke (i.e., aphasias) are relatively uncommon unless there is a focal dominant hemisphere lesion. More typical problems involving language and communication after TBI are related to the everyday uses of language (i.e., conversation, narrative speech, and "pragmatics") or social rules of communication. Impairments in these areas have an impact on community function, and contribute to social isolation. In research on discourse and conversation, people with TBI have been shown to have difficulty selecting the amount and type of data to provide to others during exchanges of information: they may say too much, not enough, or repeat information unnecessarily (351,352). Ideas may be expressed tangentially, with difficulty staying on topic and reduced coherence in the narrative stream (353). Other social communication problems include overtalkativeness (354), difficulty initiating and taking turns in conversation, and poor use of social cues emitted by the listener. Collectively, these behaviors require others to assume most of the burden of communication during an exchange (353). Impaired conversational skills have been shown to persist for at least several years postinjury (351) and to correlate significantly with limitations in social integration (352).

In the clinical setting, apparent disorders of language and communication may be related to other cognitive impairments. For example, a patient may respond inappropriately to questions asked in a crowded, noisy room because of problems in auditory comprehension, abstract reasoning, or divided attention. For the majority of people with TBI, basic language skills will appear functionally normal to the casual observer. In a more challenging environment such as school or work, however, or in grappling with the demands of intimate relationships, communication difficulties may come to the fore and pose major obstacles to successful community integration. For instance, humor is a critically important mode of communication and social learning in adolescence. Brain-injured adolescents show impairments in interpreting linguistic humor relative to their age-matched peers, even when their scores on standard language tests are within normal limits (355).

The treatment of communication difficulties is frequently coordinated by the speech/language pathologist on the rehabilitation team. It is important that all team members, and especially family members, learn to support and reinforce the same communication methods. Patients with motor speech deficits (dysarthrias) may receive training in the use of augmentative communication devices. These may be low-tech devices such as books of pictures or letters of the alphabet to which the patient points, or computer devices and software for conversion of text to speech and vice versa (356). Pragmatic disorders of communication, such as tangentiality and wordiness, can be treated within structured groups which provide audiotape, videotape, and listener feedback. Persons with TBI can also benefit from modeling of good communication skills by other group members and group leaders. Peer group training for pragmatic communication skills has been validated empirically in a small sample by Wiseman-Hakes and colleagues (357).

Agitated, Aggressive, and Disinhibited Behavior

Problems with behavioral and affective control are common after TBI and present in different forms along the continuum of recovery. In the acute stages of injury, agitation may appear as patients emerge from coma and posttraumatic amnesia. It has been estimated that one-third to one-half of patients display agitation following coma (358). A consecutive series of 100 patients admitted with severe TBI (359) documented restlessness in 35 and agitation (defined as aggressive or threatening behaviors) in 11. The factors that predispose to posttraumatic agitation are not fully understood. One study showed that acutely aggressive patients were likely to be older and more likely to be disoriented to both place and time (360). The possible role of pain (which the patient is unable to verbalize) as well as disturbances in the sleep–wake cycle must be considered. Posttraumatic agitation typically resolves within 2 to 3 weeks of its appearance (361). Its resolution is generally paralleled by improvement in orientation and other cognitive skills as the patient emerges from PTA, lending credence to the clinical view that agitation is a "stage of recovery" for some patients (362). Acute agitation predicts longer hospital stays and lower levels of independence at hospital discharge, although these relationships are confounded to some degree by the fact that agitated patients tend to be more cognitively impaired than those without agitation (363).

Agitation may include a spectrum of behaviors, not all of which occur in all patients. Several quantitative scales have been developed for the objective assessment of these behaviors; probably the most thoroughly studied is the 14-item Agitated Behavior Scale (ABS) developed by Corrigan, Bogner, and colleagues (364). The ABS displays good interrater reliability (365). Rating scale analysis suggests that it measures a unitary construct despite including disparate items pertaining to hyperactivity and repetitive behavior, emotionality, aggression, and cognitive impairment (366). The use of an objective, quantitative scale such as the ABS to track recovery and monitor response to treatment is recommended for several reasons. A single patient may display a variety of behaviors at different times, such that positive or negative changes might be missed if the focus of observation is too narrow. In addition, subjective assessments of behavioral change are unreliable, and may be skewed by a few dramatic incidents or by staff members' own emotional reactions to agitated behavior.

Treatment of acute agitation is a high priority in rehabilitation centers because agitation can place the patient in physical jeopardy, interfere with treatment, and cause general disruption in the therapy environment. Agitation is frequently treated with psychoactive medication. There are few controlled studies of the effectiveness of different medications; one such study showed that propranolol reduced the intensity of acute TBI agitation, although the number of agitated episodes did not change (361). Published recommendations are available based on collations of research and clinical experience (367). A 1997 survey of physicians practicing in TBI rehabilitation facilities (368) listed the medications most commonly prescribed for agitation by "experts" in TBI rehabilitation and contrasted them with medications prescribed by "nonexperts." Experts stated that they prescribed carbamazepine, tricyclic antidepressants, trazodone, amantadine, and β-blockers, in that order. Nonexperts used some of the same medications but also listed neuroleptics (e.g., haloperidol) and benzodiazepines, two classes of drugs that the experts reported avoiding unless other medications had failed. Benzodiazepines and other sedatives have been reported to produce paradoxical agitation (369), perhaps by making the patient less able to process events in the environment and by further impairing inhibitory mechanisms. Neuroleptics may produce akathisia that can mimic agitation (370), and they have been reported to produce paradoxical delusions (371). Much of the published information on the use of drugs for posttraumatic agitation derives from uncontrolled case series or case studies. For example, Rosati (372) described a series of 11 patients who showed rapid recovery from agitation after they were withdrawn from sedating medications and given a specific combination of amantadine, methylphenidate (or dextroamphetamine), and trazodone. Given that acute agitation tends to resolve spontaneously, however, the specific contribution of the drugs to these patients' recovery was not entirely clear. The advantages, disadvantages, and indications of various classes of drugs for acute agitation have been thoroughly reviewed by Mysiw and Sandel (373).

In our experience, optimal treatment of posttraumatic agitation requires a thoughtful combination of repeated observations and assessments of behavior, carefully monitored trials of selected medications (151), and ongoing staff education and support. Since recently injured patients may move rapidly through a stage of combative and agitated behavior (359), therapy and nursing staff may need encouragement to adopt an attitude of "watchful waiting" prior to initiating medications or heavy restraints. Less experienced staff may also need education to realize that there is no medication that specifically targets single, troublesome behaviors (such as screaming), and that drugs effective for such behaviors may also inhibit other, more adaptive behaviors. For patients who may be moving through temporary agitation, treatment may simply consist of providing more intensive staffing in the short term, and removing dangerous objects from the environment. Formal therapies may need to be suspended or moved to environments with low levels of stimulation. The patient may need to be moved to a mattress on the floor to prevent injury. Environmental conditions that promote calm behavior should be observed and implemented as much as possible.

Patients with persistent agitation or ongoing problematic behavior, such as aggression, require more active interventions which may include medications, behavior modification techniques, or both. A behaviorally trained psychologist is often helpful in leading the treatment team in collecting and analyzing behavioral information prior to initiating treatment. Baseline data should be collected by all disciplines using an agreed on operational definition of the problem behavior(s) or a scale such as the ABS or the Overt Aggression Scale (374). Data should document frequency, duration, or intensity of the behavior, possible environmental factors that may have contributed to it (e.g., a difficult task, a late-arriving meal), and the consequences that followed it (e.g., a need was met, the patient was scolded). The team should meet periodically to pool data so they may be analyzed for patterns and factors contributing to the problem. A mood disturbance may be revealed by occurrence of a behavior at times of family contact or by episodes of crying. Cognitive impairments may be implicated if the behavior occurs primarily when the patient is working on one content area or is frustrated by attempts at communication. Such hypotheses generated by the baseline data may be tested by, for example, altering the difficulty of tasks or the method of giving instructions. Generally, in treating persons with acute TBI, working to prevent unwanted behaviors is more effective than trying to design "consequences" that are supposed to affect the occurrence of the behavior in the future. Therapy staff may also experience much success by using redirection techniques that

help the cognitively impaired patient shift his or her attention away from the source of the behavior (375). Whatever approach is taken by the team, it should be consistent across team members until reevaluation of the data can take place. Continued data collection may reveal dramatic improvement, partial response, or no improvement. Reanalysis may clarify the reasons and allow for modification of the treatment plan.

As discussed in earlier sections of this chapter, some patients with TBI do not fully recover control over volatile or disinhibited behavior. The frontal regions so frequently damaged by TBI are believed to play an important role in the inhibition of impulsive and inappropriate responses (376). Thus, in some persons with postacute TBI, a minimal provocation can lead to a dramatic outburst of anger or aggression. In milder form this can present as chronic touchiness or irritability, forcing family members to "walk on eggshells." Typically, the affected person is less aware of problems with irritability and aggression than are family members or caregivers (377). For those who are aware of persistent deficits, the irritability may be part of a reactive depression. A series of 66 consecutive admissions to a trauma center, who were followed for 12 months postinjury (378), found that 18% exhibited "acute" irritability (within 3 months of injury), and 15% showed "delayed" irritability (after 3 months postinjury). The latter group also showed worse functioning and greater dependence at follow-up. In addition to generally increased irritability and decreased inhibitory control, brain injuries can (less commonly) lead to extreme displays of aggressive behavior. For example, focal temporal lobe lesions have been linked to sudden outbursts of rage, which may be associated with partial complex seizure activity. These outbursts may have a stereotyped, undirected quality and may not be remembered clearly by the affected person (379). The role of preinjury behavior patterns also cannot be discounted when dealing with post-TBI anger and aggression, as the TBI population includes disproportionate numbers of persons with other long-standing problems such as personality disorder, impulsive behavior, and substance abuse.

Behavioral and psychotherapeutic interventions may be appropriate, in addition to medication trials, for individuals with postacute behavioral control problems due to TBI. Traditional behavior management techniques may be applied or adapted to this population with success. For instance, Slifer and colleagues (380) reported dramatic increases in prosocial behavior and decreases in uncooperative behavior in acutely brain-injured adolescents using differential reinforcement of appropriate behavior (DRA). In this simple paradigm, social reinforcement (i.e., praise and attention) and other rewards are given for cooperative behaviors, while disruptive behaviors are socially ignored. Another technique, differential reinforcement of low rates of responding (DRL), rewards people for reducing the rates of unwanted behaviors such as shouting or throwing objects (381). Such behavior modification techniques do not appear to require explicit memory and thus can be used effectively with cognitively impaired patients (382,383), although it has been shown that persons with brain injury are less sensitive to response consequences than their uninjured counterparts (384). Rothwell and colleagues (385) and Ducharme (386) provide thoughtful discussions on how to adapt behavioral modification techniques to the particular needs of persons with acquired brain injury. Medd and Tate (387) describe an empirically tested 6-week program for helping people with TBI to learn anger management techniques, following a cognitive-behavioral treatment model.

The literature includes reports of medications that have been used for specific problem behaviors. For example, Emory and colleagues (388) used Depo-Provera (Upjohn, Kalamazoo,

MI) for intractable hypersexuality in eight TBI patients. All problematic sexual behaviors ceased during a 6-month course of medication (combined with psychotherapy), and there were unexpected improvements in concentration and other cognitive functions. When drug therapy was stopped, some patients showed reappearance of the unwanted behaviors, but others remained symptom-free. Kant and colleagues (389) reported on an open trial of sertraline HCl (Zoloft), suggesting that the drug was effective in reducing posttraumatic irritability. Wroblewski and colleagues (390) reported that valproic acid helped to ameliorate persistent aggression after other medications had failed.

When acceptable behavior has been achieved in the controlled clinical environment, it should be generalized into home and community settings. Family members should be taught relevant interventions, including how to deal with behavioral regression when the patient is exposed to new people or environments. Careful attention to generalization of appropriate behavior has been shown to allow transition to less restrictive environments for severely impaired patients (116). With shorter stays in hospital levels of care, there has been more acknowledgment of the critical role played by family members and other caretakers in the long-term maintenance of behavioral gains after severe TBI, and more explicit programming designed to train involved laypersons in basic behavior analysis and modification techniques (391).

Reduced Initiation

Some brain-injured patients simply fail to act without extensive cueing or structure imposed by others. In extreme cases, patients may be able to describe a course of action verbally, and express a sincere intention to carry it out, but still do nothing. The ability to link intention and action, which depends also on the "drive" supplied by limbic circuitry involved in motivational states, may depend on mesial frontal regions (e.g., anterior cingulate cortex) (392). While it is uncommon to see patients with lesions circumscribed to this region, various forms of initiation deficits are not at all uncommon in TBI with diffuse axonal injury (DAI).

Impaired initiation is a difficult rehabilitation problem for a number of reasons. It may be difficult to differentiate from disorders of mood (i.e., depression) or impaired arousal. The construct of *apathy* has been suggested to describe patients with TBI with apparently poor motivation for activity, many of whom are clinically depressed as well (393). While the confluence of symptoms may appear as a problem of differential diagnosis, in fact there could be common neurophysiological mechanisms subserving mood, arousal, and initiation such that they are not completely independent disorders. In fact, we have seen patients demonstrate striking increases in initiation when given psychostimulants, even in the absence of overt signs of depression or lethargy. Noradrenergic agonists such as desipramine and amitriptyline (394) or dopaminergic agonists such as L-dopa, bromocriptine, or pergolide (395) may also be helpful in improving initiation.

Commonly used rehabilitative approaches to impaired initiation include physical, verbal, written, or pictorial cues for the steps involved in a task, with behavioral reinforcement for proceeding from one step to the next rather than for completion of the previous step. Structured time frames for task completion, enforced by timers, may also be of help. We have successfully used tape-recorded step-by-step instructions, in the patient's own voice, to help several patients with large right frontal lobe lesions to initiate and complete the steps of showering, dressing, and grooming without having to rely on a caretaker for

these cues. Recently, alphanumeric pagers, cell phones, and other portable electronic devices that can give automated prompts at specific times have been shown to help people with significant initiation problems to begin their daily tasks and routines in a more timely fashion (396,397). While these emerging technologies show promise in helping people with TBI become more independent in managing their routines, electronic devices are variable in their degree of "user-friendliness," and most are not specifically geared to persons with cognitive impairment. Treatment planning with assistive devices should therefore include careful assessment of the cognitive demands of operating them, as well ongoing staff or family help with training, programming, problem solving, and technical support.

Whatever method is used, generalization across tasks should not be expected without explicit training. That is, the patient may learn to use a specific cueing system to initiate a morning ADL sequence but show no spontaneous improvement in starting homework independently. Development of flexible prompting strategies that can be used across tasks is an ideal goal. For example, if a person learns to use a hand-held computer to prompt a task sequence on the job, it may be possible to use the same device for other tasks with minimal new learning required. However, any application of a common strategy across tasks requires careful interdisciplinary treatment planning to ensure that strategies are trained, supported, and reinforced similarly across domains. Another treatment priority for initiation problems is education for both families and therapy staff. Whereas the need for physical assistance is obvious in patients with severe motor deficits, an ongoing need for cognitive cues and prompts is easily misunderstood and can lead to frustration on the part of the patient who feels "nagged," and on the part of the family or staff who suspect that the patient is "lazy" or simply uncooperative.

Disorders of initiation can have profound effects on independent living and psychosocial function. In some instances, individuals with TBI might be able to live semi-independently with the assistance of someone to check their progress periodically and prompt completion of necessary tasks. However, even if an individual can function with this level of assistance, he or she will probably still have difficulty with initiation beyond the bare necessities (e.g., leisure activities, new friendships, or new ideas for life goals). Initiation problems surely contribute to the social isolation and boredom reported by many survivors of TBI.

Depression

Depression is very common after TBI and has a major impact on functional and psychosocial outcome. A recent multicenter study of 666 patients involved in 17 TBI Model Systems of Care found that 27% of patients, evaluated at 10 to 126 months postinjury, may be considered as clinically depressed (398). A prospective study of 66 unselected, consecutive admissions for acute TBI revealed that 43% met the criteria for major depressive disorder at some time during the first year (399). In most follow-up studies of TBI, depressed mood is reported by both client and family for years after the injury. Posttraumatic depression is often accompanied by other disturbances of emotional function, such as anxiety or lability of mood (400). Concomitant depression and anxiety in patients' spouses is also reported (401).

Depression after TBI probably results from both neurologic and psychosocial factors. The DAI of TBI induces acute disruption of neurotransmitter systems. It is plausible that neurotransmitter depletion, particularly in noradrenergic and serotonergic systems, could contribute to acute depressive symptomatology (400). Interestingly, in the prospective study cited above, Jorge and colleagues (399) found a subgroup of "transiently depressed" patients whose symptoms cleared within 3 months. Transient depression was most often associated with left frontal or subcortical lesions. This is reminiscent of the association between left hemisphere lesions and depression in stroke patients (402). However, other investigators have failed to find correlations between lesion site and depression after TBI, and severity of the injury does not appear to be a good predictor of mood disorder (403).

The development of depression after TBI may be influenced by pre- as well as postinjury psychosocial factors, although these remain poorly understood. Prior psychiatric disorder may predispose to posttraumatic depression (404), although some studies have shown negligible effects of both personal and familial psychiatric history (405).

The diagnosis of TBI-related depression can be complicated. Silver and Yudofsky (367) enumerate the issues that must be considered:

- Medications commonly administered to TBI patients can cause or exacerbate depression. These include anticonvulsants, narcotics, and benzodiazepines.
- Depression may predate the injury even if it has never been diagnosed. Premorbid alcohol abuse and injury circumstances that hint at self-destructive behavior are common indicators.
- The vegetative signs of depression, such as insomnia or hypersomnia, or decreased appetite, may be present for other reasons after TBI in patients who are not depressed. However, one study showed that some vegetative signs do appear more frequently in TBI patients who also complain of depressed mood (406). The usual cognitive signs of depression (e.g., difficulty in concentrating) are useless for making the diagnosis following TBI.
- Self-report measures such as the Beck Depression Inventory (407) and the Neurobehavioral Functioning Inventory (398) may be useful screening tools for assessing the presence of varying levels of depression in persons with TBI.

The incidence of suicide after TBI has not been studied systematically; unfortunately, every experienced clinician can cite at least a few cases. Of 111 patients followed by Klonoff and Lage (408), two committed suicide and another two were hospitalized emergently to prevent self-injury. Interestingly, in a large sample of wartime (mostly penetrating) brain injuries, an almost identical percentage (1.4%) of patients committed suicide (409). In the Klonoff and Lage study, 14 patients reported suicidal ideation; however, half of these had sustained their TBI via self-destructive acts. Simpson and Tate (410) recently completed a study of 172 outpatients with TBI using the Beck Depression Inventory (BDI), the Beck Scale of Suicidal Ideation, and the Beck Hopelessness Scale. Twenty-three percent of their subjects reported suicidal ideation and 18% had made at least one suicide attempt postinjury.

The treatment of depression following TBI usually requires persistent application of more than one therapeutic modality. Medication, psychotherapy, and community reentry programs are all effective, especially in combination. Group and individual psychotherapy can help survivors of TBI reestablish a sense of identity and self-worth. Comprehensive rehabilitation programs help by reestablishing active involvement in work, recreation, and social activities.

Silver and Yudofsky (367) provide guidelines for the use of tricyclic and serotonergic antidepressants in TBI. They point out that although TBI patients are more sensitive to side effects of all medications, antidepressants are worth trying because of studies showing their efficacy in this population. One reason to use caution with tricyclics, however, is their effect on seizure threshold (411). Dopaminergic agonists and other psychostimulants should also be kept in mind for their antidepressant effects, particularly if the clinical picture includes problems with attention and arousal and if the depression is not severe (412).

Awareness Deficits

It has been observed for over 100 years that some persons with acquired brain injury, including TBI, lack insight into deficits that may be obvious to others (413). Persons with TBI frequently seem to be less aware of cognitive and behavioral limitations than they are of physical deficits (377,414,415). Compared with uninjured control subjects, persons with TBI are also less able to detect and correct their errors on everyday tasks (416). For most patients, unawareness of deficit resolves to some degree over time with neurologic recovery and real-world experience of deficit areas (417). Reactive depression has been shown to increase along with awareness of one's limitations, as mentioned previously (418,419).

Unawareness of deficit may be hard to distinguish from psychological denial, which refers to conscious or unconscious refusal to admit to a problem of which one is, at some level, aware. The patient's response to direct feedback may help to sort out relative contributions of neurologic and psychologic aspects (420). Regardless of its root cause, the failure to appreciate deficits creates a significant obstacle to rehabilitation efforts, and predicts poor performance in rehabilitation and poor vocational outcome (415,421). This may be because persons who are unaware of deficits are unmotivated to practice therapy tasks and unwilling to consider changes in employment or educational plans. In extreme cases they may see no purpose in, or need for, the entire rehabilitation effort.

The literature contains several reports of methods used to counteract unawareness of deficit. Treatment strategies may generally be classed as *educational* (based on teaching patients about deficits) (422) or *experiential* (e.g., providing systematic feedback or "planned failure" experiences) (423). Ideally, feedback about deficits should be couched in a "therapeutic milieu" that offers peer and staff support, psychotherapy, family counseling, and an emphasis on the affected person's capabilities as well as limitations (415). In our experience, it is crucial to address awareness issues at all phases of the rehabilitation process in order to avoid patient dropout and frustration on the part of both patients and staff. We begin the education process for patients very early, so that matter-of-fact references to brain injury and accompanying deficits will gradually be accepted as part of everyday parlance. An emphasis on tasks and content areas that are both familiar and important to the patient is also beneficial in promoting recognition of the need for further rehabilitation. Staff should be encouraged to remember that unawareness is often partially an organic deficit and that acceptance of the permanent limitations caused by TBI may take a great deal of time, patience, and support. Therapists should also avoid overemphasizing the negative in their zeal to help patients achieve "insight," as this can sabotage the rapport needed to help the patient develop realistic awareness of deficits and their implications.

Cognitive Rehabilitation

Given that cognitive deficits are among the most common and serious of the effects of TBI, systematic attempts to remediate cognitive functions are included as an essential component in rehabilitation programs in both acute and postacute phases of injury. A task force within the American Congress of Rehabilitation Medicine (ACRM) Brain Injury Special Interest Group defined *cognitive rehabilitation* as "a systematic, functionally oriented service of therapeutic cognitive activities . . . directed to achieve functional changes by . . . reinforcing . . . previously learned patterns of behavior, or . . . establishing new patterns of cognitive activity or compensatory mechanisms for impaired neurological systems" (424). Several important concepts are embedded within this definition, including the idea that cognitive rehabilitation may be conceptualized as *restorative* (i.e., targeted at regaining the previous skill); or *compensatory*, aimed at helping the person to deal with limitations by using new skills (425). Early attempts to develop restorative techniques used repetitive practice, such as memory drills, in the hope that this would improve cognition much as physical repetition can strengthen muscles. Such models have not proved very effective, and most programs now emphasize the development of compensatory strategies that are tailored to the individual and to the situations he or she will face in everyday life (426,427).

With the growing emphasis on evidence-based practice in rehabilitation as in other branches of medicine, several major reviews of the literature have sought to determine whether, and under what circumstances, cognitive rehabilitation is effective (428). Evidence has been sought for both training programs targeted to specific cognitive skills, and more comprehensive or "holistic" programs in which cognitive training is combined with individual, group, and family therapies and vocational counseling/training within a therapeutic milieu (429, 430). However, controlled research on cognitive rehabilitation methods is difficult to achieve for multiple reasons. The bulk of available evidence suggests that, for specific cognitive functions such as attention, training in skill areas that require that function, or training in compensatory strategies as noted earlier, is more effective than training in "generic" cognitive activities (129,308).

Future efforts in cognitive rehabilitation may benefit in several ways from the rapid advances in information technology in the early 21st century. In addition to the potentials for portable "personal reminding technology" mentioned in previous sections, researchers have begun to explore the applications of virtual reality (VR) to cognitive therapies for TBI with promising results (431,432). As technologies for designing and programming virtual environments become more affordable and more accessible, VR could have enormous potential for assisting with the efficient retraining of the cognitive components of complex skills such as route finding and driving. In the future, VR could even be used to create realistic social scenarios, to enable practice of interpersonal and communication skills.

PARTICIPATION IN COMMUNITY LIFE

Concept of Task Analysis

As already discussed, many different impairments may contribute to the defective performance of important skills and, in interaction with the physical and social environment, may limit participation in social and vocational activities. To understand which impairments are responsible for specific limitations in activities and participation, a task analysis must be conducted. This involves considering the physical, cognitive, and social demands that different tasks place on the individual to clarify where task breakdown occurs. Ultimately, a clinician specializing in TBI rehabilitation must be as perceptive and

TABLE 78-8.   Some Component Processes Relevant to Mobility

Component	Role in Mobility
Range of motion	Must allow for required movements
Strength	Necessary for ambulation, wheelchair propulsion, or switch operation
Balance and postural reflexes	Necessary for safe ambulation and transfer and adjustment to sudden perturbations
Muscle tone	Must allow for effective use of strength
Visuospatial perception	Necessary for environmental navigation
Spatial attention	Necessary for awareness of both sides of space
Concentration	Necessary for maintenance of locomotion in presence of distractions
Memory	Necessary for using previous experience of routes and locations
Planning, organization, and reasoning skills	Necessary for mobility in unfamiliar environments and using public transportation
Initiation	Necessary for turning plans into action

knowledgeable about tasks as about patients. In Table 78-8, a simple task analysis has been done for a mobility skill, demonstrating that an ability that is often thought of as physical has important cognitive requirements as well. Once the task demands have been understood, there is a choice about whether to modify the task to be more accommodating to the individual or to try to modify the individual to be more adept at the task. This choice will depend on time since injury, learning ability of the individual, availability of effective treatments, flexibility of the task requirements, and many other factors.

Community Mobility

As shown in Table 78-8, community mobility may be limited by a complex combination of physical, cognitive, and neurobehavioral impairments. These interact with availability of transportation services, where the individual lives, presence of curb cuts, and so forth. Aggressive attempts should be made in the early months postinjury to improve these impairments. Purchase of permanent assistive devices should be postponed until the patient's ultimate level of physical function is relatively certain.

Many survivors of TBI lose the ability to drive because of epilepsy or visual, cognitive, or motor impairments (433). This severely limits community mobility, particularly in rural areas. Some may regain the ability to drive, but the criteria on which to base this judgment are controversial. Certain perceptual and motor tests may reveal impairments that preclude driving, but good performance in basic sensory and motor functions does not guarantee safe driving. Attention-demanding driving simulation tasks (434,435) and virtual reality road tests (436) show promise in helping to evaluate driver safety after TBI, but further validation is necessary before their sensitivity and specificity is known. Actual road tests can also be used, though the range of traffic encounters that will occur during such tests is difficult to control. Preliminary research suggests that some poor drivers may benefit from specific retraining (437).

Self-Care Skills

As with mobility, ADL independence may be limited by a complex combination of physical and cognitive impairments. A similar process of interdisciplinary physical and cognitive assessment may lead to identification of particular component processes that are especially significant. Basic ADL skills such as dressing, bathing, and feeding may be improved with a treatment program aimed at three components:

- Attempts to improve salient physical or cognitive deficits such as serial casting for contractures or stimulant medications for arousal deficits
- Attempts to compensate for salient physical or cognitive deficits through provision of assistive devices for physical deficits, or written or pictorial cue cards for cognitive deficits
- Attempts to retrain a task without specific regard for the contributing deficits using behavioral training methods (e.g., breaking down into small steps, backwards chaining, errorless learning, reinforcement) (438).

Similar treatment principles are involved in addressing instrumental ADLs, which generally place greater demands on executive function. Training provided in a hospital or clinic setting will need to be generalized to the home environment through family training or a process of home visits and home therapy.

Social and Family Impact

Following TBI, the most obvious and disabling impairments are in the sphere of social behavior. The person with brain injury may thus have great difficulty maintaining preinjury relationships or establishing new ones. These behaviors are ultimately attributable to the interplay among neurobehavioral deficits, unique premorbid personalities, and postinjury coping responses. Deficits in frontal executive functions, communication, and behavioral control (described in previous sections of this chapter) may particularly predispose patients to long-standing social problems. Poor performance on tests of cognitive flexibility is predictive of social withdrawal (439), as is impaired initiation (440). Reviewing the literature on social disability after TBI, Morton and Wehman (441) pointed to four recurring themes:

- Decline in friendships and social supports, leading to isolation that does not improve spontaneously (442)
- Lack of opportunity to make new social contacts because of a restricted range of activities (e.g., unemployment, inability to drive)
- Inability to engage in preinjury leisure activities
- Depression, which further reduces social initiative and increases isolation.

Unfortunately, treatment of social behavior problems is seldom completely effective. Group therapy with modeling of appropriate behavior can be beneficial and is part of most comprehensive community reentry programs for TBI. Success has been reported using structured social skills training, with videotaped feedback, in postacute patients (443). Recently, a study of a structured peer support program for persons with brain injury and their families (11 individuals with TBI, 9 family members) indicated that it improved participants' overall quality of life, general outlook, coping skills and knowledge of TBI, but did not enhance level of social support received from family and friends (444). The Internet has also been used as a means of providing information and social support, but its efficacy has not yet been validated (445).

Only a few investigators have systematically examined the effects of TBI on leisure and recreational participation but they concur that TBI significantly disrupts premorbid leisure pursuits, due to residual physical and neurobehavioral impairments (446–448). Because many people with TBI do not return to work, loss of leisure activity may be psychologically devastating. A recreational therapist can be an integral team member, performing leisure skill assessments and developing both individual and group treatments to teach new ways of occupying leisure time or adaptive methods for performing favorite premorbid activities.

In recent years, the Clubhouse Model, an innovative approach to the social isolation of persons with TBI, has emerged (449). Clubhouse programs are organized around a work-ordered day (i.e., up to full-time participation), and are run by clients who have suffered TBI, with staff support. A productive social milieu with peer support and naturalistic learning and opportunities for both recreational and vocational activity are key features of such programs. Client strengths and contributions are stressed, in contrast to the "deficit" emphasis found in many therapy programs.

Numerous studies have attested to the extreme stress placed by TBI on the family system (450,451). An early Israeli investigation of marital adjustment 1 year after war-related brain injury found interpersonal tension within the family; feelings of loneliness, depression, and isolation in the wives; lack of sexual contact with husbands because of loss of feelings of attractiveness and personality changes; and role changes within the family (452). More recent American studies have amply replicated these findings (401,453–456). Furthermore, the stress and family disruption experienced by caretaking spouses may be worse than that experienced by parents in a comparable role (454, 455). Studies of the sources of family stress invariably find greater impact of cognitive and behavioral deficits than physical care needs (446,454,457).

Kosciulek (458) identified five distinct and effective coping strategies used by families after TBI:

- Positive appraisal, which is commitment to seeking the positive while accepting things as they are
- Resource acquisition, or the tendency to seek help and guidance
- Family tension management, which involves open expression of feelings
- Head-injury demand reduction (e.g., seeking support groups or becoming involved in advocacy)
- Acquiring social support from friends and relatives.

Inclusion of the family in rehabilitation programs has become standard practice. Families of TBI patients feel strong needs for regular communication with staff, specific information about the injury, and honest answers to their questions (459). Perhaps in response to this, a great emphasis has been placed on individual or group family education, and, as needed, family counseling, family therapy, and support groups (460). The use of a telephone-based, social work liaison follow-up has been demonstrated to reduce caregiver burden, increase quality of life ratings and enhance feelings of caregiver mastery, compared to an historical control group. Though limitations were cited in the methodology by the investigators, this may be prove to be "a low-cost, nonintensive intervention (which) may offer substantial benefits to families caring for people with brain injury" (461).

Sexual Relationships

Disturbances in sexual function after TBI often have been noted by clinicians but have not been well studied. Sexual dysfunctions may include hypersexuality, hyposexuality, impotence, loss of feelings of attractiveness, inability to find appropriate partners, and incapacity to engage in intimate interpersonal relationships requiring the interpretation and expression of complex emotions (462). Staff members and relatives often are dismayed by the sexual dysfunctions after TBI and have difficulty in managing these problems effectively. Rehabilitation facilities have developed sexual reeducation programs for brain-injured patients where specific information is provided about sexual function and basic social skills in interpersonal intimacy are taught (462).

Sexual behavior most often is perceived by staff as a problem when the patient engages in overtly inappropriate behavior, such as public masturbation or continual advances toward uninterested partners. In these cases, team members often are asked to intervene to help reeducate and redirect the patients toward more appropriate expression of their sexual drives.

Inadequate sexual function too often is neglected because it creates fewer problems for family and staff. Patients may have hormonal or neurologic disorders that interfere with sexual function and may lack the relevant psychosocial skills for forming intimate relationships. As with other patient groups, such information rarely is provided unless it is solicited. Furthermore, patients with memory impairments or lack of awareness of their disabilities may be unable to accurately report presence of erections, lubrication, orgasm, and so forth, or to recognize the interpersonal sources of their lack of intimacy.

It is critical for the physician to provide information regarding safe sex practices and contraception to all patients. These include mutual disease screening if indicated and use of condoms and spermicides. However, education alone is often inadequate for individuals who have difficulties with impulse control and executive function and who may be vulnerable to manipulation by others either through personal contact or through the Internet. Therefore, sexual counseling should occur in the context of a full appreciation of the individual's neuropsychological and emotional status. Communication and intimacy may be enhanced for some patients and their partners through the use of educational materials and individual and couples counseling. Some patients, particularly those with specific sexual disorders, may require the intervention of a sex therapist.

Substance Abuse

Substance abuse is a significant problem in TBI. Even without a TBI, long-term abuse of alcohol and other drugs can affect cognitive function and lead to a host of social problems. Thus, ongoing substance abuse would be expected at the very least to slow or interfere with recovery from TBI. Substance abuse not only complicates the process of recovery and rehabilitation but also has a negative impact on the ultimate outcomes of injury. The relationship between alcohol and TBI is illustrated by the fact that 35% to 50% of persons with TBI are intoxicated at the time of injury (463), and a somewhat higher proportion of individuals have a previous history of alcohol or other drug abuse. While estimates vary, a recent review of published studies reported a substance abuse history in 37% to 64% of persons enrolled in TBI rehabilitation (464). Not surprisingly, studies using more in-depth assessments for substance use, such as focused clinical interviews, have reported more positive histories than studies relying on chart reviews. Quantitative measures of the extent and consequences of substance use are also available, such as the Michigan Alcohol Screening Test (MAST) and

the Quantity-Frequency-Variability Index (465). A composite measure using the short form of the MAST, information on quantity and frequency of consumption, and blood alcohol level at the time of injury has reportedly been useful in identifying problematic drinkers with TBI (466). Other methods to assess intake of alcohol and other drugs include questions developed for national health surveys, such as the National Household Survey on Drug Abuse (467) and the Behavioral Risk Factors Surveillance System (468). Questions from these surveys on what substances are ingested, at what quantities and with what frequency, are now included in the TBI Model System Database. Such questions have the advantage of being referenced to a large population-based sample, which can help in determining whether intake is statistically abnormal. However it is measured, a history of substance abuse predicts poorer TBI outcomes in terms of vocational success and overall quality of life (463,469). After injury, continued substance abuse can exacerbate neurobehavioral deficits, contribute to disruption of family relationships, and further reduce the probability of return to work. Although at least one large-scale study has shown a decline in drinking in the first year or so after TBI (470), it also appears that people tend to return to preinjury drinking patterns by 2 years postinjury (470). There has been less research on the impact of drugs other than alcohol on TBI; there is overlap among samples, as many drug abusers also consume alcohol (464). A history of street drug use was acknowledged by one-third of outpatient TBI participants in one study; marijuana was the most popular, followed by cocaine (471). Substance abuse remains a serious problem for many persons following TBI, and rehabilitation programs must be ready to help patients address the issue either with trained staff or appropriate referral mechanisms.

The implementation and success of treatment approaches commonly used with nondisabled populations, such as the 12-step programs of Alcoholics Anonymous and Narcotics Anonymous, may be complicated by the memory, communication, and reasoning deficits caused by TBI. There are published recommendations for how to adapt these programs for TBI (472), and specialized substance abuse treatment approaches have also been developed for this population. For example, Corrigan and colleagues (464) describe comprehensive models for integrating substance abuse treatment into community-based TBI rehabilitation. These models emphasize patient, family, and staff education, in-depth assessment, careful coordination of services, and specialized therapy techniques such as "motivational interviewing," to help the person internalize the motivation to change substance use habits. Other researchers have emphasized the need to assess each person's receptivity to substance abuse counseling by using questionnaires specialized for this purpose, such as the "Readiness to Change Questionnaire." This brief questionnaire has been validated for use with persons with TBI (473) and may be especially useful for revealing the "windows of opportunity" for drug and alcohol counseling that occur relatively soon after injury (474).

Educational, Prevocational, and Vocational Function

TBI may produce significant educational and vocational handicap. Numerous studies of return to work following TBI suggest that both premorbid and injury-related factors play a strong role in vocational success. Previous education, work history, psychiatric history, and substance abuse are all strong predictors of return to work (475). In addition, injury severity, cognitive impairment, and behavioral disturbances are related to reemployment (475,476). Social isolation after injury has also been negatively associated with return to work (475,477) , but whether this reflects the coexistence of depression, lack of initiation, or poor social skills that interfere with work, or whether the social isolation is the result of loss of work-related social outlets is unclear.

Many of the same factors adversely affect school performance among individuals suffering TBI during their youth. However, since education, unlike employment, is an entitlement, the impact of TBI may be less obvious. Although Public Law 94–142 guarantees educational opportunities for brain-injured children and adolescents, as well as other disability groups, up to the age of 21 years, the implementation of special accommodations for them varies greatly, depending on the local school district's educational philosophy, available resources, and understanding of the nature of the problem. For the elementary and secondary school child, transition back into school can be traumatic. For this reason, it is advisable for school personnel, rehabilitation team members, and the family to help the school develop an individualized education plan.

A growing number of community colleges and universities offer educational programs tailored to individuals with brain injury. At these schools, remedial courses in basic skill areas such as reading or mathematics are provided. In other cases, supplemental tutoring may be made available. To assist with daily living needs, a group-living situation with assistance from a residential counselor sometimes is available. These modifications allow a higher-level brain-injured person to progress at a slower pace with a great deal of support and a far greater likelihood of academic success than in a typical college environment.

Vocational goals are important to many brain-injured people once they complete their acute rehabilitation. The major problem is that vocational goals may be based on premorbid abilities or vocation and may be unrealistic. Some comprehensive rehabilitation programs include prevocational assessment and vocational training (478). After the patient completes a period of extensive cognitive rehabilitation, a vocational counselor designs a vocational program that usually involves work trials within the rehabilitation setting. Another model of vocational rehabilitation after brain injury has been the supported employment approach (479–481). In this approach, the client may be placed directly into a competitive employment situation. A job coach provides daily on-the-job instruction and guidance, advises the employer as to potential job modifications needed to maximize the client's performance, and assists with other job-related issues such as transportation, housing, financial management, and substance abuse. The supported work model has been viewed as the most effective in returning brain-injured people to competitive employment, although there have been very few rigorous studies of efficacy. The conclusion of efficacy is based mainly on successful return to work among individuals who have been previously unsuccessful after participation in such programs (90,482).

Every state has a Department of Vocational Rehabilitation, providing many of a wide variety of services, including prevocational assessment, vocational assessment, work adjustment training, sheltered workshop training, or a supported work program. The neuropsychological assessment usually is requested by vocational counselors as an essential component on which to base the vocational plan. However, it is generally agreed that direct observation of clients in work settings or simulations is a more useful guide to vocational success and appropriate vocational goals than standardized neuropsychological testing (483).

MEDICOLEGAL AND ETHICAL ISSUES

A variety of medicolegal and ethical issues can complicate the rehabilitation process. There is frequently the need to determine the competency of the brain-injured person to manage financial affairs, engage in vocational pursuits, make medical decisions, or provide informed consent for research participation. Obtaining informed consent in the rehabilitation setting for people with TBI poses its own unique difficulties (484,485) related to the use of behavioral or psychopharmacologic restrictive procedures (486), decision making about surgical interventions or transfer to a different type of treatment program, and rights to privacy (487). Competency assessments after TBI can be complex, involving the contributions of many disciplines (488). If the court deems a brain-injured person to be incompetent, a conservator may need to be appointed to manage financial affairs or a guardian appointed to make decisions for the TBI person. To complicate matters, family members are often reluctant to move toward guardianship early, in hopes that the individual will recover sufficiently to remain in charge of his or her own affairs. This often leaves an ethical gray area when clinicians understand that an individual's ability to make decisions is compromised, but there has been no official determination of incompetence or appointment of a guardian. Most often, clinicians seek to involve the individual and their caregivers in such decisions, thus minimizing the importance of the exact decision-making status. However, when the individual with TBI and his or her caregivers disagree about important decisions, or when there is disagreement within a group of caregivers, formal determination may become more necessary.

Another issue for many is personal injury litigation, which often results for persons who sustained a TBI in an accident. In this circumstance, the person with brain injury tries to recoup financially for past medical expenses, pain and suffering, and past and future lost wages. Although a large settlement can be very beneficial to the individual, it often takes 5 years or longer for a case to be settled in the courts. This produces a severe stress on the person with a TBI and their family. Furthermore, individuals with brain injury can be their own worst witnesses because of their memory impairments and normal physical appearance, and many achieve only minimal financial gain (489).

Perhaps the most dramatic ethical issues in brain injury have been raised about the treatment of patients in the vegetative or minimally conscious state. Clinicians, lawyers, and theologians have debated the rights of family members to withdraw life-sustaining nutrition for people in the vegetative state (490,491). Although ethical viewpoints vary, terminating artificial hydration and nutrition for an individual judged to be permanently in the vegetative state is legal in most jurisdictions. Matters are much more complex in the minimally conscious state since such individuals are, by definition, incompetent to make their own decisions about continuing treatments and nutrition. In principle, all individuals can avoid this situation by completing an advance directive that specifies what treatments they would want should they find themselves in such a state. In practice, however, many individuals are injured with no advance directive in place, and those who have one have rarely included enough specifics that are applicable to the minimally conscious state for the courts to be convinced of their prior wishes. Though not legally binding, there have been attempts to assess the perspectives of individuals in this state on life and death issues, using repeated, structured yes/no questions (492). In one case, a minimally conscious patient appeared to indicate her desire to continue to live (165). She made modest further recovery over the next several years, and as her assessments produced more clear-cut responses, these supported the validity of her earliest statement of preference.

Members of the rehabilitation team and outside consultants may help navigate through these complex issues. Many healthcare facilities have ethics committees or consultation teams, which may assist in the evaluation of difficult treatment decisions. A lawyer frequently is hired to represent the brain-injured person in various types of litigation. Unfortunately, most attorneys are not knowledgeable about TBI and must be educated by health professionals. All of the members of the rehabilitation team may be asked to assist in medicolegal cases, although typically the physician specialists (e.g., physiatrist, neurosurgeon, neurologist) and psychologist (e.g., neuropsychologist or rehabilitation psychologist) are those who are asked to provide detailed records and to testify in court.

SUMMARY

Increased interest has been focused on TBI in recent years as more patients survive severe injury and as the long-term sequelae of all grades of injury become clearer. During this time, TBI rehabilitation has emerged as a subspecialty of interest to physiatrists, nurses, psychologists, and therapists.

The focused interest in TBI has led to a number of important advances in knowledge. The epidemiology, pathophysiology, and course of recovery have been substantially defined. Our ability to estimate prognosis has improved. The medical, physical, cognitive, and behavioral sequelae of TBI have been more clearly identified and classified.

Treatment advances also have occurred. The acute management of patients with TBI has benefited from advances in neurosurgical intensive care. Medical management of the complications of TBI also has improved. The physical sequelae of TBI such as paralysis, contractures, and heterotopic ossification have been lessened by the same treatments used in the rehabilitation of other physical and neurologic disabilities. Yet the neurobehavioral deficits of many brain-injured patients represent their most significant obstacles to community reintegration. It is in these cognitive and behavioral realms that our ability to improve function is least clearly defined.

Much research is in progress to refine our classification of these deficits, to clarify the extent to which they are remediable, and to identify the most effective remediation strategies. Because each brain-injured patient's pattern of deficits is unique, however, it will always remain a challenge to apply the knowledge gathered from group studies to the management of the individual patient. For this reason, a thoughtful interdisciplinary treatment-planning process that considers the complex interactions of the many physical, cognitive, and behavioral deficits is essential.

ACKNOWLEDGMENTS

Many thanks are due to Mary Czerniak for preparation of the manuscript.

REFERENCES

1. Goldstein K. *After effects of brain injury in war.* New York: Grune & Stratton, 1942.
2. Luria AR. *Higher cortical functions in man.* New York: Basic Books, 1966.
3. Rosenthal M, Griffith ER, Kreutzer JS, et al. *Rehabilitation of the adult and child with traumatic brain injury,* 3rd. ed. In: Rosenthal M, ed. Philadelphia: FA Davis Co, 1999.
4. Michaud L. Pediatric brain injury. *J Head Trauma Rehabil* 1995;10(5).
5. Massagli TL, Jaffe KM, Fay GC, et al. Neurobehavioral sequelae of pediatric traumatic brain injury: a cohort study. *Arch Phys Med Rehabil* 1996;77(3): 223–231.
6. Englander J, Cifu D. The older adult with traumatic brain injury. In: Rosenthal M, Griffith E, Kreutzer J, et al., eds. *Rehabilitation of the adult and child with traumatic brain injury,* 3rd ed. Philadelphia: FA Davis Co., 1999:453–470.
7. Thurman DJ, Guerrerro J. Trends in hospitalization associated with traumatic brain injury. *JAMA* 1999;282(10):954–957.
8. Sosin D, Sniezek J, Waxweiler R. Trends in death associated with traumatic brain injury. *JAMA* 1995;273:1778.
9. Jennett B, Bond MR. Assessment of outcome after severe brain damage: a practical scale. *Lancet* 1975;1:480–484.
10. Teasdale G, Jennett B. Assessment of coma and impaired consciousness. *Lancet* 1974;2:81–84.
11. Miller JD. The neurologic evaluation. In: Rosenthal M, Griffith ER, Bond MR, et al., eds. *Rehabilitation of the child and adult with traumatic brain injury,* 2nd ed. Philadelphia: FA Davis Co, 1990:52–58.
12. Dikmen S, Ross B, Machamer J, et al. One year psychosocial outcome in head injury. *J Int Neuropsychol Soc* 1995:67–77.
13. Dikmen S, Machamer JE. Neurobehavioral outcomes and their determinants. *J Head Trauma Rehabil* 1995;10:74–86.
14. Stein SC, Spettell C. The Head Injury Severity Scale (HISS): a practical classification of closed-head injury. *Brain Inj* 1995;9:437–444.
15. Russell WR. Cerebral involvement in head injury. *Brain* 1932;35:549–603.
16. Brooks N, Campsie L, Symington C, et al. The effects of severe head injury on patient and relative within seven years post injury. *J Head Trauma Rehabil* 1987;2:1–13.
17. Bishara SN, Partridge FM, Godfrey HPD, et al. Posttraumatic amnesia and Glasgow Coma Scale related to outcome in survivors in a consecutive series of patients with severe closed-head injury. *Brain Inj* 1992;6:373–380.
18. Levin H, O'Donnell V, Grossman R. The Galveston Orientation and Amnesia Test: a practical scale to assess cognition after head injury. *J Nerv Ment Dis* 1979;167(11):675–684.
19. Shores EA, Marosszeky JE, Sandanam J, et al. Preliminary validation of a clinical scale for measuring the duration of posttraumatic amnesia. *Med J Aust* 1986;144:569–572.
20. Ponsford J, Oliver J, Curran C, et al. Prediction of employment status 2 years after traumatic brain injury. *Brain Inj* 1995;9:11–20.
21. Katz D, Alexander M. Traumatic brain injury: predicting course of recovery and outcome for patients admitted to rehabilitation. *Arch Neurol* 1994;51: 661–670.
22. Jackson W, Novack T, Dowler R. Effective serial measurement of cognitive orientation in rehabilitation. The Orientation Log. *Arch Phys Med Rehabil* 1998;79:718–720.
23. Alderson AL, Novack TA. Measuring recovery of orientation during acute rehabilitation for traumatic brain injury: value and expectations of recovery. *J Head Trauma Rehabil* 2002;17(3):210–219.
24. Thurman D, Alverson C, Dunn KA, et al. Traumatic brain injury in the United States: a public health perspective. *J Head Trauma Rehabil* 1999;14(6): 602–615.
25. Cifu DX, Kreutzer JS, Marwitz JH, et al. Functional outcomes of older adults with traumatic brain injury: a prospective, multicenter analysis. *Arch Phys Med Rehabil* 1996;77(9):883–888.
26. Frankowski R. The demography of head injury in the United States. In: Miner M, Wagner KA, eds. *Neurotrauma.* Boston: Butterworths, 1986:1–17.
27. Whitman S, Coonley-Hoganson R, Desai BT. Comparative head trauma experience in two socioeconomically different Chicago-area communities: a population study. *Am J Epidemiol* 1984;4:570–580.
28. Annegers J, Grabow J, Kurland L. The incidence, causes and secular trends of head trauma in Olmstead County, Minnesota. *Neurology* 1980;30:912–919.
29. Goldstein F, Levin H. Neurobehavioral outcome of traumatic brain injury in older adults: initial findings. *J Head Trauma Rehabil* 1995;10(1):57–73.
30. Levin H, Benton A, Grossman R. *Neurobehavioral consequences of closed head injury.* New York: Oxford University Press, 1982.
31. Traumatic brain injury. Facts and figures. *United States Department of Education. National Institute on Disability and Rehabilitation Research. The Traumatic Brain Injury Model Systems National Data Center,* 2001;7(1).
32. Bloom DR, Levin HS, Ewing-Cobbs L, et al. Lifetime and novel psychiatric disorders after pediatric traumatic brain injury. *J Am Acad Child Adolesc Psychiatry* 2001;40(5):572–579.
33. Brown G, Chadwick O, Shaffer D, et al. A prospective study of children with head injuries: III. Psychiatric sequelae. *Psychosom Med* 1981;11:63–78.
34. Sosin DM, Sacks JJ, Holmgreen P. Head injury-associated deaths from motorcycle crashes. Relationship to helmet use laws. *JAMA* 1990;264:2395–2399.
35. Wasserman RC, Buccini RV. Helmet protection from head injuries among recreational bicyclists. *Am J Sports Med* 1990;18:96–97.
36. Gordon W, Mann N, Wilier B. Demographic and social characteristics of the traumatic brain injury model system database. *J Head Trauma Rehabil* 1993;8 (2):26–33.
37. Zador PL, Ciccone ME. Automobile driver fatalities in frontal impacts: airbags compared with manual belts. *Am J Public Health* 1993;83(5):661–666.

38. Max W, MacKenzie EJ, Rice DP. Head injuries: costs and consequences. *J Head Trauma Rehabil* 1991;6(2):76–91.
39. Lehmkuhl LD, Hall KM, Mann N, et al. Factors that influence costs and length of stay with traumatic brain injury in acute care and inpatient rehabilitation. *J Head Trauma Rehabil* 1993;8:88–100.
40. Ben-Yishay Y, Silver SM, Piasetsky E, et al. Relationship between employability and vocational outcome after intensive holistic cognitive rehabilitation. *J Head Trauma Rehabil* 1987;2(1):35–48.
41. Haffey W, Abrams D. Employment outcomes for participants in a brain injury work reentry program: preliminary findings. *J Head Trauma Rehabil* 1991;6(3):24–34.
42. Whiteneck G, Mellick D, Harrison-Felix C, et al. *Colorado traumatic brain injury and follow up system databook.* Englewood, CO: Craig Hospital, 2001.
43. McKinlay W, Brooks D, Bond M, et al. The short term outcome of severe blunt head injury as reported by relatives of the injured persons. *J Neurol Neurosurg Psychiatry* 1981;44:527.
44. Adams JH, Doyle D, Ford I, et al. Diffuse axonal injury in head injury: definition, diagnosis and grading. *Histopathology* 1989;15:49–59.
45. Blumbergs PC, Scott G, Manavis J, et al. Topography of axonal injury as defined by amyloid precursor protein and the sector scoring method in mild and severe closed head injury. *J Neurotrauma* 1995;12:565–572.
46. Sahuquillo J, Vilalta J, Lamarca J. Diffuse axonal injury after severe head trauma. *Acta Neurochir Suppl* 1989;101:149–158.
47. Denny-Brown D, Russell WR. Experimental cerebral concussion. *Brain* 1941;64:93–164.
48. Povlishock JT. Pathophysiology of neural injury: therapeutic opportunities and challenges. *Clin Neurosurg* 2000;46:113–126.
49. Lye TC. Traumatic brain injury as a risk factor for Alzheimer's disease: a review. *Neuropsychol Rev* 2000;10:115–129.
50. Clifton GL, Grossman RG, Makela ME, et al. Neurological course and correlated computerized tomography findings after severe closed head injury. *J Neurosurg* 1980;52:611–624.
51. Auerbach SH. Neuroanatomical correlates of attention and memory disorders in traumatic brain injury: an application of behavioral subtypes. *J Head Trauma Rehabil* 1986;1(3):1–12.
52. Weber M, Grolimund P, Seiler RW. Evaluation of post-traumatic cerebral blood flow velocities by transcranial Doppler ultrasonography. *Neurosurgery* 1990;27:106–112.
53. Garnett M, Blamire A, Corkill R, et al. Abnormal cerebral blood volume in regions of contused and normal appearing brain following traumatic brain injury using perfusion magnetic resonance imaging. *J Neurotrauma* 2001;18 (6):585–593.
54. Marmarou A. Pathophysiology of intracranial pressure. In: Narayan RK, Wilberger JE, Povlishock JT, eds. *Neurotrauma.* New York: McGraw-Hill, 1996:413–429.
55. Klauber M, Toutant S, Marshall L. A model for predicting delayed intracranial hypertension following severe head injury. *J Neurosurg* 1984;61:695–699.
56. Brain Trauma Foundation. The American Association of Neurological Surgeons. The Joint Section on Neurotrauma and Critical Care. Guidelines for intracranial pressure monitoring. *J Neurotrauma* 2000;17:479–491.
57. Brain Trauma Foundation. The American Association of Neurological Surgeons. The Joint Section on Neurotrauma and Critical Care. Use of barbiturates in the control of intracranial hypertension. *J Neurotrauma* 2000;17:527–530.
58. Brain Trauma Foundation. The American Association of Neurological Surgeons. The Joint Section on Neurotrauma and Critical Care. Use of mannitol. *J Neurotrauma* 2000;17:521–525.
59. Clausen T, Bullock R. Medical treatment and neuroprotection in traumatic brain injury. *Curr Pharmacol Res* 2001;7:1517–1532.
60. Kaufmann B, Tunkel A, Pryor J, et al. Meningitis in the neurosurgical patient. *Infect Dis Clin North Am* 1990;4:677–701.
61. Barth J, Macciocchi S, Giordani B, et al. Neuropsychological sequelae after minor head injury. *Neurosurgery* 1983;13:529–533.
62. McLean AJ, Temkin N, Dikmen S, et al. The behavioral sequelae of head injury. *J Clin Neuropsychol* 1983;5:361–376.
63. Whyte J. Mechanisms of recovery of function following CNS damage. In: Rosenthal M, et al., eds. *Rehabilitation of the child and adult with traumatic brain injury,* 2nd ed. Philadelphia: FA Davis Co, 1989:679–688.
64. Verma A. Opportunities for neuroprotection in traumatic brain injury. *J Head Trauma Rehabil* 2000;15(5):1149–1161.
65. Faden A. Neuroprotection and traumatic brain injury. *Arch Neurol* 2001;58: 1553–1555.
66. Narayan RK, Michel ME, et al. Clinical trials in head injury. *J Neurotrauma* 2002;19(5):503–557.
67. Maas AL. Neuroprotective agents in traumatic brain injury. *Expert Opin Investig Drugs* 2001;10(4):753–767.
68. Roof RL, Hall ED. Gender differences in acute CNS trauma and stroke: neuroprotective effects of estrogen and progesterone. *J Neurotrauma* 2000;17(5): 367–388.
69. Stein DG. Brain damage, sex hormones and recovery: a new role for progesterone and estrogen? *Trends Neurosci* 2001;24(7):386–391.
70. Groswasser Z, Cohen M, Keren O. Female TBI patients recover better than males. *Brain Inj* 1998;12(9):805–808.
71. Kaas J. Plasticity of sensory and motor maps in adult mammals. *Ann Rev Neurosci* 1991;14:137–167.
72. Recanzone GH, Schreiner CE, Merzenich MM. Plasticity in the frequency representation of primary auditory cortex following discrimination training in adult owl monkeys. *J Neurosci* 1993;13:87–103.
73. Nudo R, Wise B, SiFuentes F, et al. Neural substrates for the effects of rehabilitative training on motor recovery after ischemic infarct. *Science* 1996;272: 1791–1794.
74. Karni A, Meyer G, Jezzard P, et al. Functional MRI evidence for adult motor cortex plasticity during motor skill learning. *Nature* 1995;377:155–158.
75. Nudo RJ, Plautz EJ, Frost SB. Role of adaptive plasticity in recovery of function after damage to motor cortex. *Muscle Nerve* 2001;2001(24):8.
76. Dail WG, Feeney DM, Murray HM, et al. Responses to cortical injury: II. Widespread depression of the activity of an enzyme in cortex remote from a focal injury. *Brain Res* 1981;211:79–89.
77. Feeney D, Gonzalez A, Law W. Amphetamine, haloperidol, and experience interact to affect the rate of recovery after motor cortex injury. *Science* 1982;217:855–857.
78. Boyeson MG, Harmon RL. Acute and postacute drug-induced effects on rate of behavioral recovery after brain injury. *J Head Trauma Rehabil* 1994;9(3):78–90.
79. Sperry RW. Effect of crossing nerves to antagonistic limb muscles in the monkey. *Arch Neurol Psychiatry* 1947;58(452–473).
80. Kanelos S, McDeavitt J. Neural transplantation: potential role in traumatic brain injury. *J Head Trauma Rehabil* 1998;13(6):1–9.
81. Jennett B, Snoek J, Bond M, et al. Disability after severe head injury: observations on the use of the Glasgow Outcome Scale. *J Neurol Neurosurg Psychiatry* 1981;44:285–293.
82. Wilson JTL, Pettigrew LEL, Teasdale GM. Structured interviews for the Glasgow Outcome Scale and the Extended Glasgow Outcome Scale: guidelines for their use. *J Neurotrauma* 1998;15(8):573–585.
83. Rappaport M, Hall KM, Hopkins K, et al. Disability rating scale for severe head trauma: coma to community. *Arch Phys Med Rehabil* 1982;63:118–123.
84. Hall K, Cope D, Rappaport M. Glasgow Outcome Scale and Disability Rating Scale: comparative usefulness in following recovery in traumatic brain injury. *Arch Phys Med Rehabil* 1985;66:35–37.
85. Hall K, Hamilton B, Gordon W, et al. Characteristics and comparisons of functional assessment indices: Disability Rating Scale, Functional Independence Measure, and Functional Assessment Measure. *J Head Trauma Rehabil* 1993;8(2):60–74.
86. Hagen C, Malkmus D, Durham P. *Levels of cognitive functioning.* Downey, CA: Rancho Los Amigos Hospital, 1972.
87. Gouvier W, Blanton P, LaPorte K, et al. Reliability and validity of the Disability Rating Scale and the Levels of Cognitive Functioning Scale in monitoring recovery from severe head injury. *Arch Phys Med Rehabil* 1987;68:94–97.
88. Hall K, Johnston M. Outcomes evaluation in TBI rehabilitation. Part II: measurement tools for a nationwide data system. *Arch Phys Med Rehabil* 1994: 75SC10–SC18.
89. Kreutzer J, Marwitz J, Seel R, et al. Validation of a neurobehavioral functioning inventory for adults with traumatic brain injury. *Arch Phys Med Rehabil* 1996;77:116–124.
90. Malec J, Moessner A, Kragness M, et al. Refining a measure of brain injury sequelae to predict postacute rehabilitation outcome: rating scale analysis of the Mayo-Portland inventory. *J Head Trauma Rehabil* 2000;15(1):670–682.
91. Kreutzer J, Seel R, Marwitz J. *Neurobehavioral functioning inventory.* San Antonio: Harcourt Brace & Company, 1999.
92. Willer B, Linn R, Allen K. Community integration and barriers to integration for individuals with brain injury. In: Finlayson MAJ, Garner S, eds. *Brain injury rehabilitation: clinical considerations.* Baltimore: Williams & Wilkins, 1993.
93. Dijkers M. Measuring the long-term outcomes of traumatic brain injury. A review of the community integration questionnaire. *J Head Trauma Rehabil* 1997;12(6):74–91.
94. Whiteneck GG, Charlifue SW, Gerhart KA, et al. Quantifying handicap: a new measure of long-term rehabilitation outcomes. *Arch Phys Med Rehabil* 1992;73:519–526.
95. Mellick D, Walker N, Brooks CA, et al. Incorporating cognitive independence into the CHART. *J Rehabil Outcomes Meas* 1999;3(3):12–21.
96. Hall K, Bushnik T, Lakisic-Kazazic B, et al. Assessing traumatic brain injury outcome measures for long-term follow-up of community-based individuals. *Arch Phys Med Rehabil* 2001;82:367–374.
97. Fleming J, Thy B, Maas F. Prognosis of rehabilitation outcome in head injury using the Disability Rating Scale. *Arch Phys Med Rehabil* 1994;75:156–163.
98. Rappaport M. Evoked potential and head injury in a rehabilitation setting. In: Miner M, Wagner K, eds. *Neurotrauma: treatment, rehabilitation and related issues.* Boston: Butterworths, 1986.
99. Judson J, Cant B, Shaw N. Early prediction of outcome from cerebral trauma by somatosensory evoked potentials. *Crit Care Med* 1990;18:363–368.
100. Greenberg R, Becker D, Miller J, et al. Evaluation of brain function in severe head trauma with multimodality evoked potentials: Part 2. Localization of brain dysfunction and correlation with posttraumatic neurological conditions. *J Neurosurg* 1977;47:163–177.
101. Jennett B, Teasdale G, Braakman R, et al. Prognosis in series of patients with severe head injury. *Neurosurgery* 1979;4:283–289.
102. Hans P, Albert A, Franssen C, et al. Improved outcome prediction based on CSF extrapolated creatine kinase BB isoenzyme activity and other risk factors in severe head injury. *J Neurosurg* 1989;71:54–58.
103. Nordby HK, Urdal P. The diagnostic value of measuring creatine kinase BB activity in cerebrospinal fluid following acute head injury. *Acta Neurochir Suppl* 1982;65:93–101.

104. Woolf P, Lee L, Hamill R, et al. Thyroid test abnormalities in traumatic brain injury: correlation with neurologic impairment and sympathetic nervous system activation. *Am J Med* 1988;84:201–208.

105. Young B, Ott L, Dempsey R, et al. Relationship between admission hyperglycemia and neurologic outcomes of severely brain-injured patients. *Ann Surg* 1989;210:466–473.

106. Najenson T, Mendelson L, Schechter I, et al. Rehabilitation after severe head injury. *Scand J Rehabil Med* 1974;6:5–14.

107. Head Injury Rehabilitation Project. Final report: severe head trauma—comprehensive medical approach. San Jose, CA: Santa Clara Valley Medical Center, 1982; Project 13-P-59156/9.

108. Levin H, Gary HJ, Eisenberg H, et al. Neurobehavioral outcome one year after severe head injury: experience of the traumatic coma data bank. *J Neurosurg* 1990;73:699–709.

109. Kreutzer J, Devany C, Myers S, et al. Neurobehavioral outcome following traumatic brain injury: review, methodology, and implications for cognitive rehabilitation. In: Kreutzer J, Wehman P, eds. *Cognitive rehabilitation for persons with traumatic brain injury*. Baltimore: Paul H. Brookes, 1991:55–73.

110. Millis SR, Rosenthal M, Novack TA, et al. Long-term neuropsychological outcome after traumatic brain injury. *J Head Trauma Rehabil* 2001;16(4):343–355.

111. Bond M. The psychiatry of closed head injury. In: Brooks N, ed. *Closed head injury: psychological, social and family consequences*. Oxford, UK: Oxford University Press, 1984:148–178.

112. Brooks N. *Closed head injury: psychological, social and family consequences*. Oxford, UK: Oxford University Press, 1984.

113. Hodgkinson A, Veerabangsa A, Drane D, et al. Service utilization following traumatic brain injury. *J Head Trauma Rehabil* 2000;15(6):1208–1226.

114. Prigatano G. *Neuropsychological rehabilitation after brain injury*. Baltimore: Johns Hopkins Press, 1986.

115. Malec J. Impact of comprehensive day treatment on societal participation for persons with acquired brain injury. *Arch Phys Med Rehabil* 2001;82:885–895.

116. Eames P, Wood R. Rehabilitation after severe brain injury: a follow-up study of a behaviour modification approach. *J Neurol Neurosurg Psychiatry* 1985;48:613–619.

117. Grimes G, Dubois H, Grimes S, et al. Telerehabilitation services using web-based telecommunication. *Study of Health Technology Information* 2000;70:113–118.

118. Kinsella A. Disabled populations & telerehabilitation—new approaches. *Caring* 1999;18(8):20–22, 24, 26–27.

119. Bryant ET, Sundance P, Hobbs A, et al. Managing costs and outcome of patients with traumatic brain injury in an HMO setting. *J Head Trauma Rehabil* 1993;8(4):15–29.

120. Corrigan J. Conducting statewide needs assessments for persons with traumatic brain injury. *J Head Trauma Rehabil* 2001;16(1):1–19.

121. Reynolds WE, Page SJ, Johnston MV. Coordinated and adequately funded state streams for rehabilitation of newly injured persons with TBI. *J Head Trauma Rehabil* 2001;16(1):34–46.

122. Spearman RC, Stamm BH, Rosen BH, et al. The use of Medicaid waivers and their impact on services. *J Head Trauma Rehabil* 2001;16(1):47–60.

123. Chestnut RM, Carney N, Maynard H, et al. Summary report: evidence for the effectiveness of rehabilitation for persons with traumatic brain injury. *J Head Trauma Rehabil* 1999;14(2):176–188.

124. Rehabilitation of persons with traumatic brain injury. *NIH Consensus Statement*, 1998;16(1):1–41.

125. Powell J, Heslin J, Greenwood R. Community based rehabilitation after severe traumatic brain injury: a randomised controlled trial. *J Neurol Neurosurg Psychiatry* 2002;72:193–202.

126. Zhu XL, Poon WS, Chan CH, et al. Does intensive rehabilitation improve the functional outcome of patients with traumatic brain injury? Interim result of a randomized controlled trial. *Br J Neurosurg* 2001;15:464–473.

127. Salazar AM, Warden DL, Schwab K, et al. Cognitive rehabilitation for traumatic brain injury: a randomized trial. *JAMA* 2000;283:3075–3081.

128. CARF (Committee on the Accreditation of Rehabilitation Facilities) guidelines. Tucson: The Rehabilitation Accreditation Commission, 2000.

129. Cicerone K, Dahlberg C, Kalmar K, et al. Evidence-based cognitive rehabilitation: recommendations for clinical practice. *Arch Phys Med Rehabil* 2000; 81:1596–1615.

130. Hart T, Hayden M. The ecological validity of neuropsychological assessment and remediation. In: Uzzell B, Gross Y, eds. *Clinical neuropsychology of intervention*. Boston: Martinus Nijhoff, 1986:21–50.

131. Born JD, Albert A, Hans P, et al. Relative prognostic value of best motor response and brain stem reflexes in patients with severe head injury. *Neurosurgery* 1985;16:595–600.

132. Braakman R, Jennett WB, Minderhoud JM. Prognosis of the posttraumatic vegetative state. *Acta Neurochir Suppl* 1988;95:49–52.

133. Jennett B, Plum F. Persistent vegetative state after brain damage: a syndrome in search of a name. *Lancet* 1972;1:734–737.

134. The Multi-Society Task Force on PVS. Medical aspects of the persistent vegetative state (part 2). *N Engl J Med* 1994;330(22):1572–1579.

135. Sazbon L, Fuchs C, Costeff H. Prognosis for recovery from prolonged posttraumatic unawareness: logistic analysis. *J Neurol Neurosurg Psychiatry* 1991; 54:49–52.

136. Whyte J, DiPasquale M, Childs N, et al. Recovery from the vegetative and minimally conscious states: preparation for a multicenter clinical trial. *Am J Phys Med Rehabil* 1999;78(2):181.

137. Higashi K, Hatano M, Abiko S, et al. Five-year follow-up study of patients with persistent vegetative state. *J Neurol Neurosurg Psychiatry* 1981;44:552–554.

138. Shavelle RM, Strauss D, Whyte J, et al. Long-term causes of death after traumatic brain injury. *Am J Phys Med Rehabil* 2001;80:510–516.

139. Giacino J, Ashwal S, Childs N, et al. The minimally conscious state: definition and diagnostic criteria. *Neurology* 2002;58:349–353.

140. Andrews K, Murphy L, Munday R, et al. Misdiagnosis of the vegetative state: retrospective study in a rehabilitation unit. *Br Med J* 1996;313(7048):13–16.

141. Danze F, Brule JF, Haddad K. Chronic vegetative state after severe head injury: clinical study: electrophysiological investigations and CT scan in 15 cases. *Neurosurg Rev* 1989;12[Suppl 1]:477–499.

142. Kinney H, Korein J, Panigrahy A, et al. Neuropathological findings in the brain of Karen Ann Quinlan—the role of the thalamus in the persistent vegetative state. *N Engl J Med* 1994;330:1469–1475.

143. Nordgren RE, Markesbery WR, Fukunda K, et al. Seven cases of cerebromedullospinal disconnection: the "locked-in" syndrome. *Neurology* 1971; 21(1140–1148).

144. Giacino J, Zasler N, Whyte J, et al. Recommendations for use of uniform nomenclature pertinent to patients with severe alterations in consciousness. *Arch Phys Med Rehabil* 1995;76(2):205–209.

145. Ansell BJ, Keenan JE. The Western Neuro Sensory Stimulation Profile: a tool for assessing slow-to-recover head-injured patients. *Arch Phys Med Rehabil* 1989;70:104–108.

146. Giacino J, Kezmarsky M, DeLuca J, et al. Monitoring rate of recovery to predict outcome in minimally-responsive patients. *Arch Phys Med Rehabil* 1991; 72(897–901).

147. Rader MA, Alston JB, Ellis DW. Sensory stimulation of severely brain injured patients. *Brain Inj* 1989;3:141–147.

148. Rappaport M, Dougherty AM, Kelting DL. Evaluation of coma and vegetative states. *Arch Phys Med Rehabil* 1992;73:628–634.

149. Whyte J, DiPasquale M. Assessment of vision and visual attention in minimally responsive brain injured patients. *Arch Phys Med Rehabil* 1995;76(9):804–810.

150. Whyte J, DiPasquale M, Vaccaro M. Assessment of command-following in minimally conscious brain injured patients. *Arch Phys Med Rehabil* 1999;80:1–8.

151. Whyte J. Toward rational psychopharmacological treatment: integrating research and clinical practice. *J Head Trauma Rehabil* 1994;9(3):91–103.

152. Whyte J, Laborde A, DiPasquale MC. Assessment and treatment of the vegetative and minimally conscious patient. In: Rosenthal M, Griffith ER, Kreutzer JS, et al., eds. *Rehabilitation of the adult and child with traumatic brain injury*, 3rd ed. Philadelphia: FA Davis Co, 1999:435–452.

153. Kanno T, Kamei Y, Yokoyama T, et al. Neurostimulation for patients in vegetative status. *PACE* 1987;10:207–208.

154. Katayama Y, Tsubokawa T, Yamamoto T, et al. Characterization and modification of brain activity with deep brain stimulation in patients in a persistent vegetative state: pain-related late positive component of cerebral evoked potential. *PACE* 1991;14:116–121.

155. Sturm V, Kuhner A, Schmitt HP, et al. Chronic electrical stimulation of the thalamic unspecific activating system in a patient with coma due to midbrain and upper brain stem infarction. *Acta Neurochir Suppl* 1979;47:235–244.

156. Tsubokawa T, Yamamoto T, Katayama Y, et al. Deep-brain stimulation in a persistent vegetative state: follow-up results and criteria for selection of candidates. *Brain Inj* 1990;4:315–327.

157. Di Rocco C, Maira G, Meglio M, et al. L-Dopa treatment of comatose states due to cerebral lesions. *JNeurosurg Sci* 1974;18(3):169–176.

158. Horiguchi J, Inami Y, Shoda T. Effects of long-term amantadine treatment on clinical symptoms and EEG of a patient in a vegetative state. *Clin Neuropharmacol* 1990;13:84–88.

159. Ross ED, Stewart RM. Akinetic mutism from hypothalamic damage: successful treatment with dopamine agonists. *Neurology* 1981;31:1435–1439.

160. Passler MA, Riggs RV. Positive outcomes in traumatic brain injury-vegetative state: patients treated with bromocriptine. *Arch Phys Med Rehabil* 2001; 82(3):311–315.

161. Recanzone GH, Merzenich MM. Changes in the distributed temporal response properties of SI cortical neurons reflect improvements in performance on a temporally based tactile discrimination task. *J Neurophysiol* 1992; 67(5):1071–1091.

162. Zasler ND, Kreutzer JS, Taylor D. Coma stimulation and coma recovery: a critical review. *Neurorehabilitation* 1991;1(3):33–40.

163. Wilson SL, McMillan TM. A review of the evidence for the effectiveness of sensory stimulation treatment for coma and vegetative states. *Neuropsychol Rehabil* 1993;3(2):149–160.

164. Whyte J, Glenn MB. The care and rehabilitation of the patient in a persistent vegetative state. *J Head Trauma Rehabil* 1986;1(1):39–53.

165. McMillan TM, Herbert CM. Neuropsychological assessment of a potential "euthanasia" case: a 5 year follow up. *Brain Inj* 2000;14(2):197–203.

166. Ettlin T, Kischka U, Reichmann S, et al. Cerebral symptoms after whiplash injury of the neck: a prospective clinical and neuropsychological study of whiplash injury. *J Neurol Neurosurg Psychiatry* 1992;55:943–948.

167. Alexander MP. Mild traumatic brain injury: pathophysiology, natural history, and clinical management. *Neurology* 1995;45:1253–1260.

168. McAllister TW. Mild traumatic brain injury and the postconcussive syndrome. In: Silver JM, Yudofsky SC, Hales RE, eds. *Neuropsychiatry of traumatic brain injury*. Washington, DC: American Psychiatric Press, 1994:357–392.

169. Zasler N. Neuromedical diagnosis and management of postconcussive disorders. In: Horn L, Zasler N, eds. *Medical rehabilitation of traumatic brain injury*. Philadelphia: Hanley & Belfus, 1996:133–170.

170. Levin H, Mattis S, Ruff R, et al. Neurobehavioral outcome following minor head injury: a three-center study. *J Neurosurgery* 1987;66:234–243.

171. Newcombe F, Rabbitt P, Briggs M. Minor head injury: pathophysiological or iatrogenic sequelae? *J Neurol Neurosurg Psychiatry* 1994;57:709–716.

172. Dikmen S, McLean A, Temkin N. Neuropsychological and psychosocial consequences of minor head injury. *J Neurol Neurosurg Psychiatry* 1986;49:1227–1232.

173. Varney NR, Bushnell DL, Nathan M, et al. NeuroSPECT correlates of disabling mild head injury: preliminary findings. *J Head Trauma* 1995;10:18–28.

174. Cicerone KD. Psychotherapy after mild traumatic brain injury: relation to the nature and severity of subjective complaints. *J Head Trauma Rehabil* 1991;6:30–43.

175. Richter KJ, Cowan DM, Kaschalk SM. A protocol for managing pain, sleep disorders, and associated psychological sequelae of presumed mild head injury. *J Head Trauma Rehabil* 1995;10:7–15.

176. Schumway-Cook A, Horak FB. Rehabilitation strategies for patients with vestibular deficits. *Neurol Clin* 1990;8:441–457.

177. Rocabado M, Johnson B, Blakney M. Physical therapy and dentistry: an overview. *J Cranio-Mandibular Pract* 1983;1:46.

178. Barth JT, Macciocchi N. Mild traumatic brain injury. *J Head Trauma Rehabil* 1993;8(3).

179. Horn L, Zasler N, eds. Rehabilitation of post-concussive disorders. *Phys Med Rehabil Clin North Am* 1992;6(1).

180. Rizzo M, Tranel D. *Head injury and post-concussive syndrome*. New York: Churchill-Livingstone, 1995.

181. Kelly J, Rosenberg J. American Academy of Neurology Report of Quality Stands Subcommittee. Practice parameter: the management of concussion in sports (summary statement). *Neurology* 1992;48:581–585.

182. McCrea M, Kelly JP, Randolph C, et al. Standardized assessment of concussion (SAC): onsite mental status evaluation of the athlete. *J Head Trauma Rehabil* 1998;13:27–35.

183. Collie A, Darby D, Maruff P. Computerised cognitive assessment of athletes with sports related head injury. *Br J Sports Med* 2001;35:297–302.

184. Cronin AF. Traumatic brain injury in children: issues in community function. *Am J Occup Ther* 2001;55(4):377–384.

185. Ylvisaker M, Todis B, Glang A, et al. Educating students with TBI: themes and recommendations. *J Head Trauma Rehabil* 2001;16(1):76–93.

186. Bakker K, Anderson V. Assessment of attention following pre-school traumatic brain injury: a behavioural attention measure. *Pediatr Rehabil* 1999;3 (4):149–157.

187. Morse S, Haritou F, Ong K, et al. Early effects of traumatic brain injury on young children's language performance; a preliminary linguistic analysis. *Pediatr Rehabil* 1999;3(4):139–148.

188. Marschark M, Richtsmeier LM, Richardson JT, et al. Intellectual and emotional functioning in college students following mild traumatic brain injury in childhood and adolescence. *J Head Trauma Rehabil* 2000;15(6):1227–1245.

189. McMahon MA, Noll RB, Michaud LJ, et al. Sibling adjustment after pediatric traumatic brain injury: a case-controlled pilot study. *J Head Trauma Rehabil* 2001;16(6):587–594.

190. Rapoport MJ, Feinstein A. Outcome following traumatic brain injury in the elderly: a critical review. *Brain Inj* 2000;14(8):749–761.

191. Ritchie PD, Cameron PA, Ugoni AM, et al. A study of the functional outcome and mortality in elderly patients with head injuries. *J Clin Neurosci* 2000;7(4):301–304.

192. The Brain Trauma Foundation. The American Association of Neurological Surgeons. The Joint Section on Neurotrauma and Critical Care. Computed tomography scan features. *J Neurotrauma* 2000;17(6–7):597–627.

193. Neuroimaging in the management of penetrating brain injury. *J Trauma* 2001:S7–S11.

194. Teasdale G, Mendelow D. Pathophysiology of head injuries. In: Brooks N, ed. *Closed head injury: psychological, social, and family consequences*. Oxford, UK: Oxford University Press, 1984:4–36.

195. Levin H, Kalisky Z, Handel SF, et al. Magnetic resonance imaging in relation to the sequelae and rehabilitation of diffuse closed head injury: preliminary findings. *Semin Neurol* 1985;5:221–232.

196. Jordan B, Zimmerman R. Magnetic resonance imaging in amateur boxers. *Arch Neurol* 1988;45:1207–1208.

197. Bigler ED. Quantitative magnetic resonance imaging in traumatic brain injury. *J Head Trauma Rehabil* 2001;16(2):117–134.

198. Schaefer PW, Grant PE, Gonzalez RG. Diffusion-weighted MR imaging of the brain. *Radiology* 2000;217;((2):):331–345.

199. Ricker JH, Hillary FG, Deluca J. Functionally activated brain imaging (O-15 PET and fMRI) in the study of learning and memory after traumatic brain injury. *J Head Trauma Rehabil* 2001;16:191–205.

200. Umile EM, Plotkin RC, Sandel ME. Functional assessment of mild traumatic brain injury using SPECT and neuropsychological testing. *Brain Inj* 1998; 12:577–594.

201. Kesler S, Adams H, Bigler E. SPECT, MR and quantitative MR imaging: correlates with neuropsychological and psychological outcome in traumatic brain injury. *Brain Inj* 2000;14(10):851–857.

202. Riley TI. Electroencephalography in the management of epilepsy. In: Browne T, Feldman R, eds. *Epilepsy: diagnosis and management*. Boston: Little, Brown & Co, 1983.

203. Askenazy JJ, Sazbon L, Hackett P, et al. The value of electroencephalography in prolonged coma: a comparative EEG-computed axial tomography study of two patients one year after trauma. *Resuscitation* 1980;8:181–194.

204. Sleigh JW, Havill JH, Frith R, et al. Somatosensory evoked potentials in severe traumatic brain injury: a blinded study. *J Neurosurg* 1999;91:577–580.

205. Theilen HJ, Ragaller M, von Kummer R, et al. Functional recovery despite prolonged bilateral loss of somatosensory evoked potentials: report on two patients. *J Neurol Neurosurg Psychiatry* 2000;68:657–660.

206. Giannoudid P, Veysi V, Pape H. When should we operate on major fractures in patients with severe head injuries? *Am J Surg* 2002;183:261–267.

207. Poole GV, Miller JD, Agnew SG, et al. Lower extremity fracture fixation in head-injured patients. *J Trauma* 1992;32(5):654–659.

208. Frankowski F, Annegers J, Whitman S. Epidemiological and descriptive studies. Part I. The descriptive epidemiology of head trauma in the United States. In: Becker DP, Prulishock, TT, eds. *Central nervous system trauma status report 1985*. Bethesda, MD: 1986.

209. Temkin NR, Dikmen SS, Anderson GD, et al. Valproate therapy for prevention of posttraumatic seizures: a randomized trial. *J Neurosurg* 1999;91(4): 593–600.

210. The Brain Trauma Foundation. The American Association of Neurological Surgeons. The Joint Section on Neurotrauma and Critical Care. Role of antiseizure prophylaxis following head injury. *J Neurotrauma* 2000;17(6–7):549–543.

211. Dikmen SS, Temkin NR, Miller B, et al. Neurobehavioral effects of phenytoin prophylaxis of posttraumatic seizures. *JAMA* 1991;265:1271–1278.

212. Meador KJ, Loring DW, Huh K, et al. Comparative cognitive effects of anticonvulsants. *Neurology* 1990;40:391–394.

213. Meythaler J, Yablon S. Antiepileptic drugs. *Rehabil Pharmacother* 1999;10: 275–300.

214. Allen FH, Runge JW, Legarda S, et al. Multi-center, open label study on safety, tolerance and pharmacokinetics of intravenous fosphenytoin in status epilepticus. *Epilepsia* 1994;35[Suppl 118]:93.

215. Callaghan N, Garrett A, Goggin T. Withdrawal of anticonvulsant drugs in patients free of seizures for two years. *N Engl J Med* 1988;319:942–946.

216. Guyot L, Michael D. Post-traumatic hydrocephalus. *Neurol Res* 2000;22(1): 25–28.

217. Benzel EC, Pelletier AL, Levy PG. Communicating hydrocephalus in adults: prediction of outcome after ventricular shunting procedures. *Neurosurgery* 1990;26:655–660.

218. Bergsneider M. Management of hydrocephalus with programmable valves after traumatic brain injury and subarachnoid hemorrhage. *Curr Opin Neurol* 2000;13(6):661–664.

219. Clifton G, Robertson C, Grossman R. Cardiovascular and metabolic responses to severe head injury. *Neurosurg Rev* 1989;12[Suppl 1]:465–473.

220. Solomon S, Hotchkiss E, Saravay SM, et al. Impairment of memory function by antihypertensive medication. *Arch Gen Psychiatry* 1983;40:1109–1112.

221. Cruikshank JM, Neil-Dwyer G. Beta-blocker brain concentrations in man. *Eur J Clin Pharmacol* 1985;28[Suppl]:21–23.

222. Nadolol (Corgard)—a new beta-blocker. *Med Lett Drugs Ther* 1980;22 (8):33–34.

223. Sandel ME, Abrams PL, Horn LJ. Hypertension after brain injury: case report. *Arch Phys Med Rehabil* 1986;67:469–472.

224. Manhem P, Hallengren B, Hansson BG. Plasma noradrenaline and blood pressure in hypothyroid patients, effect of gradual thyroxine treatment. *Clin Endocrinol* 1984;20:701–707.

225. Hackenberry L, Miner M, Rea G, et al. Biochemical evidence of myocardial injury after severe head trauma. *Crit Care Med* 1982;10:641–644.

226. Marion DW. Complications of head injury and their therapy. *Neurosurg Clin North Am* 1991;2:411–424.

227. Wiercisiewski DR. Pulmonary complications in traumatic brain injury. *J Head Trauma* 1998;13:28–35.

228. Law J, Barnhart K, Rowlett W, et al. Increased frequency of obstructive airway abnormalities with long-term tracheostomy. *Chest* 1993;104:136–138.

229. Akers SM, Bartter TC, Pratter MR. Respiratory care. *State of the Art Rev/Phys Med Rehabil* 1990;4:527–542.

230. McHenry MA. Vital capacity following traumatic brain injury. *Brain Inj* 2001;15:741–745.

231. Node Y, Nakazawa S, Tusuji Y, et al. A study of changes in plasma aldosterone in patients with acute head injury. *Neurosurg Rev* 1989;12[Suppl 1]: 389–392.

232. Woolf PD, Cox C, Kelly M, et al. The adrenocortical response to brain injury: correlation with the severity of neurologic dysfunction, effects of intoxication, and patient outcome. *Alcoholism* 1990;14:917–921.

233. Ziegler MG, Morrissey EC, Marshall LF. Catecholamine and thyroid hormones in traumatic injury. *Crit Care Med* 1990;18:253–258.

234. Tenedieva VC, Potapov AA, Gaitur EL, et al. Thyroid hormones in comatose patients with traumatic brain injury. *Acta Neurochir Suppl* 2000;76:385–391.

235. Donati-Genet PC, Dubuis JM, Girardin E, et al. Acute symptomatic hyponatremia and cerebral salt wasting after head injury: an important clinical entity. *J Pediatr Surg* 2001;36(7):1094–1097.

236. Feibel J, Kelly M, Lee L, et al. Loss of adrenocortical suppression after acute brain injury: role of increased intracranial pressure and brainstem function. *J Clin Endocrinol Metab* 1983;57:1245–1250.

237. Kornblum R, Fisher R. Pituitary lesions in craniocerebral injuries. *Arch Pathol* 1969;88:242–248.
238. L'vovich AI. Descending pathways of the frontal lobe cortex to nuclei of the hypothalamic mamillary bodies in craniocerebral trauma in humans. *Neurosci Behav Physiol* 2001;31(4):371–374.
239. Kelly D, Gonzalo I, Cohan P, et al. Hypopituitarism following traumatic brain injury and aneurysmal subarachnoid hemorrhage: a preliminary report. *J Neurosurg* 2000;93(5):743–752.
240. Lieberman SA, Oberoi AL, Gilkison CR, et al. Prevalence of neuroendocrine dysfunction in patients recovering from traumatic brain injury. *J Clin Endocrinol Metab* 2001;86(6):2752–2756.
241. Hansen J, Cook J. Posttraumatic neuroendocrine disorders. *Phys Med Rehabil Clin North Am* 1993;7:569–580.
242. Sockalosky JJ, Kriel RL, Krach LE, et al. Precocious puberty after traumatic brain injury. *J Neurotrauma* 1987;110:373–377.
243. de Leo R, Petruk KC, Crockford P. Galactorrhea after prolonged traumatic coma: a case report. *Neurosurg* 1981;9:177–178.
244. Wildburger R, Zarkovic N, Tonkovic G, et al. Post-traumatic hormonal disturbances: prolactin as a link between head injury and enhanced osteogenesis. *J Endrocrinol Investig* 1998;21(2):78–86.
245. Kosteljanetz M, Jensen T, Norgard B, et al. Sexual and hypothalamic dysfunction in postconcussional syndrome. *Acta Neurolog Scand* 1981;63:169–180.
246. Doty RL, Shaman P, Dann M. Development of the University of Pennsylvania Smell Identification Test: a standardized microencapsulated test of olfactory function. *Physiol Behav* 1984;32:498–502.
247. Yosem DM, Geckle RJ, Bilker WB, et al. Posttraumatic olfactory dysfunction: MR and clinical evaluation. *AJNR* 1996;17:1171–1179.
248. Lagreze W. Neuro-ophthalmology of trauma. *Curr Opin Ophthalmol* 1998;9:33–39.
249. Kruse J, Awasthi D. Skull-base trauma: neurosurgical perspective. *J Craniomaxillofac Trauma* 1998;4:8–14.
250. Hammer A. Lower cranial nerve palsies: potentially lethal in association with upper cervical fracture-dislocations. *Clin Orthoped Rel Res* 1991;266:64–69.
251. Canevero S, Bonicalzi V. The neurochemistry of central pain: evidence from clinical studies, hypothesis and therapeutic implications. *Pain* 1998;74:109–114.
252. Gouvier W, Cubic B. Behavioral assessment and treatment of acquired visuoperceptual disorders. *Neuropsychol Rev* 1991;2:3–28.
253. Garland D. A clinical perspective on common forms of acquired heterotopic ossification. *Clin Orthoped Rel Res* 1991;263:13–29.
254. Tsur A. Relationship between muscular tone, movement and periarticular new bone formation in postcoma-unaware (PC-U) patients. *Brain Inj* 1996;10:259–262.
255. Keenan M, Haider T. The formation of heterotopic ossification after traumatic brain injury: a biopsy study with ultrastructural analysis. *J Head Trauma Rehabil* 1996;11(4):8–22.
256. Schaeffer MA, Sosner J. Heterotopic ossification: treatment of established bone with radiation therapy. *Arch Phys Med Rehabil* 1995;76:284–286.
257. Moore TJ. Functional outcome following surgical excision of heterotopic ossification in patients with traumatic brain injury. *J Orthoped Trauma* 1993;7:11–14.
258. Doder M, Jahanshahi N, Turjanski N, et al. Parkinson's syndrome after closed head injury: a single case report. *J Neurol Neurosurg Psychiatry* 1999;66:380–385.
259. Geurts A, Ribber G, Knoop J, et al. Identification of static and dynamic postural instability following traumatic brain injury. *Arch Phys Med Rehabil* 1996;77(7):639–644.
260. Kerrigan D, Bank M, Burke D. An algorithm to assess stiff-legged gait in traumatic brain injury. *J Head Trauma Rehabil* 1999;14(2):136–145.
261. Hallet M. Classification and treatment of tremor. *JAMA* 1991;266:1115–1117.
262. Ellison P. Propranolol for severe head injury action tremor. *Neurology* 1978;28:197–199.
263. Jankovic J. Botulinum toxin treatment of tremors. *Neurology* 1991;41:1185–1188.
264. Krauss J, Jankovic J. Head injury and posttraumatic movement disorders. *Neurosurgery* 2002;50(5):927–939.
265. Volkmann J, Benecke R. Deep brain stimulation for dystonia: patient selection and evaluation. *Mov Dis* 2002;17(3):S112–S115.
266. van Zomeren A, Brower W, Deelman B. Attention deficits: the riddles of selectivity, speed, and alertness. In: Brooks N, ed. *Closed head injury: psychological, social, and family consequences.* Oxford, UK: Oxford University Press, 1984:74–107.
267. Goozee J, Murdoch B, Theodoros D, et al. Kinematic analysis of tongue movements in dysarthria following traumatic brain injury using electromagnetic articulography. *Brain Inj* 2000;14(2):153–174.
268. Popescu VG, Burdea GC, Bouzit M, et al. A virtual-reality-based telerehabilitation system with force feedback. *IEEE Trans Inf Technol Biomed* 2000;4(1):45–51.
269. McGhee-Pierce S, Mayer NH, Whyte J. Computer-assisted exercise systems in traumatic brain injury: cases and commentary. *J Head Trauma Rehabil* 2001;16(4):406–413.
270. The Brain Trauma Foundation. The American Association of Neurological Surgeons. The Joint Section on Neurotrauma and Critical Care. Nutrition. *J Neurotrauma* 2000;17(6–7):539–547.

271. Grahm T, Zadrozny D, Harrington T. The benefits of early jejunal hyperalimentation in the head-injured patient. *Neurosurgery* 1989;25:729–735.
272. Kirby D, Clifton G, Turner H, et al. Early enteral nutrition after brain injury by percutaneous endoscopic gastrojejunostomy. *JPEN* 1991;15:298–302.
273. Vane DW, Shiffler M, Grosfeld JL, et al. Reduced lower esophageal sphincter (LES) pressure after acute and chronic brain injury. *J Pediatr Surg* 1982;17:960–964.
274. Metoclopramide (Reglan) for gastroesophageal reflux. *Med Lett Drugs Ther* 1985;27:21–22.
275. Morgan AS, Mackay LE. Causes and complications associated with swallowing disorders in traumatic brain injury. *J Head Trauma Rehabil* 1999;14:454–461.
276. Logemann J. *Evaluation and treatment of swallowing disorders.* San Diego, CA: College Hill Press, 1983.
277. Spiegel JR, Selber JC, Creed J. A functional diagnosis of dysphagia using videoendoscopy. *Ear Nose Throat J* 1998;77:628–632.
278. Gellman H, Keenan M, Stone L, et al. Reflex sympathetic dystrophy in brain-injured patients. *Pain* 1992;51(3):307–311.
279. Lezak M. *Neuropsychological assessment,* 3rd ed. New York: Oxford University Press, 1995.
280. Whyte J, Fleming M, Polansky M, et al. Phasic arousal in response to auditory warnings after traumatic brain injury. *Neuropsychologia* 1997;35(3):313–324.
281. Plum F, Posner JB. *The diagnosis of stupor and coma,* 2nd ed. Philadelphia: FA Davis Co, 1972.
282. Whyte J. Attention and arousal: basic science aspects. *Arch Phys Med Rehabil* 1992;73:940–949.
283. Whyte J. Neurologic disorders of attention and arousal: assessment and treatment. *Arch Phys Med Rehabil* 1992;73:1094–1103.
284. Fernandez-Duque D, Posner M. Brain imaging of attentional networks in normal and pathological states. *J Clin Exp Neuropsychol* 2001;23(1):74–93.
285. Stuss DT, Binns MA, Carruth FG, et al. The acute period of recovery from traumatic brain injury: posttraumatic amnesia or posttraumatic confusional state? *Neurosurgery* 1999;90(4):635–643.
286. Damasio A. The frontal lobes. In: Heilman K, Valenstein E, eds. *Clinical neuropsychology,* 2nd ed. New York: Oxford University Press, 1985:339–375.
287. Whyte J, Polansky M, Fleming M, et al. Sustained arousal and attention after traumatic brain injury. *Neuropsychologia* 1995;33(7):797–813.
288. Park N, Moscovitch M, Robertson I. Divided attention impairments after traumatic brain injury. *Neuropsychologia* 1999;37:1119–1133.
289. Whyte J, Schuster K, Polansky M, et al. Frequency and duration of inattentive behavior after traumatic brain injury: effects of distraction, task, and practice. *J Int Neuropsychol Soc* 2000;6:1–11.
290. Gronwall D. Paced auditory serial addition task: a measure of recovery from concussion. *Percept Motor Skills* 1977;44:367–373.
291. Robertson IH, Ward T, Ridgeway V, et al. The structure of normal human attention: the test of everyday attention. *J Int Neuropsychol Soc* 1996;2:525–534.
292. Kendall P. The use of diazepam in hemiplegia. *Ann Phys Med* 1964;7(6):225–228.
293. Glenn M. Nerve blocks. In: Glenn M, Whyte J, eds. *The practical management of spasticity in children and adults.* Philadelphia: Lea & Febiger, 1990.
294. Thompson PJ, Trimble MR. Anticonvulsant drugs and cognitive functions. *Epilepsia* 1982;23:531–544.
295. Easton JKM, Ozel T, Halpern D. Intramuscular neurolysis for spasticity in children. *Arch Phys Med Rehabil* 1979;60:155–158.
296. Whyte J. Pharmacologic treatment of cognitive impairments: Conceptual and methodological considerations. In: Eslinger P, ed. *Neuropsychological interventions.* New York: Guilford Publications, 2002.
297. Whyte J, Hart T, Schuster K, et al. The effects of methylphenidate on attentional function after traumatic brain injury. A randomized, placebo-controlled trial. *Am J Phys Med Rehabil* 1997;76(6):440–450.
298. Wroblewski B, Leary J, Phelan A, et al. Methylphenidate and seizure frequency in brain injured patients with seizure disorders. *J Clin Psychiatry* 1992;53(3):86–89.
299. McDowell S, Whyte J, D'Esposito M. Differential effect of a dopaminergic agonist on prefrontal function in traumatic brain injury patients. *Brain* 1998;121:1155–1164.
300. Wroblewski BA, Glenn MB. Pharmacologic treatment of arousal and cognitive deficits. *J Head Trauma Rehabil* 1994;9(3):19–42.
301. Pierce S, Buxbaum LJ. Treatments of unilateral neglect: a review. *Arch Phys Med Rehabil* 2002;83:256–268.
302. Gray J, Robertson I. Remediation of attentional difficulties following brain injury: three experimental single case studies. *Brain Inj* 1989;3:163–170.
303. Sohlberg MM, Mateer CA. Effectiveness of an attention-training program. *J Clin Exp Neuropsychol* 1987;9:117–130.
304. Weinberg J, Diller L, Gordon W, et al. Visual scanning training effect on reading-related tasks in acquired brain damage. *Arch Phys Med Rehabil* 1977;58:479–486.
305. Malec J, Jones R, Rao N, et al. Video game practice effects on sustained attention in patients with craniocerebral trauma. *Cogn Rehabil* 1984;2(4):18–24.
306. Ponsford JL, Kinsella G. Evaluation of a remedial programme for attentional deficits following closed-head injury. *J Clin Exp Neuropsychol* 1988;10:693–708.
307. Robertson IH, Gray JM, Pentland B, et al. Microcomputer-based rehabilitation for unilateral visual neglect: a randomized controlled trial. *Arch Phys Med Rehabil* 1990;71:663–668.

308. Park NW, Ingles JL. Effectiveness of attention rehabilitation after an acquired brain injury: a meta-analysis. *Neuropsychology* 2001;15(2):199–210.

309. Russell WR, Nathan PW. Traumatic amnesia. *Brain* 1946;69:183–187.

310. Kinsella G, Murtagh D, Landry A. Everyday memory following traumatic brain injury. *Brain Inj* 1996;10:499–507.

311. Levin HS. Memory dysfunction after head injury. In: Feinberg T, Farah MJ, eds. *Behavioral neurology and neuropsychology*. New York: The McGraw-Hill, 1997:479–489.

312. Bigler E, Blatter D, Gale S, et al. Traumatic brain injury and memory: the role of hippocampal atrophy. *Neuropsychology* 1996;10:333–342.

313. Nissen MJ. Neuropsychology of attention and memory. *J Head Trauma Rehabil* 1986;1:13–21.

314. Schmitter-Edgecombe M. Effects of divided attention on implicit and explicit memory performance following severe closed head injury. *Neuropsychology* 1996;10:155–167.

315. DeLuca J, Schultheis MT, Madigan NK, et al. Acquisition versus retrieval deficits in traumatic brain injury: implications for memory rehabilitation. *Arch Phys Med Rehabil* 2000;81:1327–1333.

316. Carlesimo GA, Sabbadini M, Loasses A, et al. Forgetting from long-term memory in severe closed-head injury patients: effect of retrieval conditions and semantic organization. *Cortex* 1997;33:131–142.

317. Shallice T, Burgess PW. Deficits in strategy application following frontal lobe damage in man. *Brain* 1991;114:727–741.

318. Shum D, Valentine M, Cutmore T. Performance of individuals with severe long-term traumatic brain injury on time-, event-, and activity-based prospective memory tasks. *J Clin Exp Neuropsychol* 1999;21(1):49–58.

319. Wilson B, Cockburn J, Baddeley A. The Rivermead Behavioral Memory Test. Reading, England: Thames Valley Test Co, 1985.

320. Hartman M, Knopman D, Nissen M. Implicit learning of new verbal associations. *J Exp Psychol Learn Mem Cogn* 1989;15(6):1070–1082.

321. Murre JMJ. Implicit and explicit memory in amnesia: some explanations and predictions by the tracelink model. *Memory* 1997;5(1/2):213–232.

322. Ewert J, Levin H, Watson M, et al. Procedural memory during posttraumatic amnesia in survivors of severe closed head injury: implications for rehabilitation. *Arch Neurol* 1989;46:911–916.

323. Ptak R, Gurbrod K, Schnider A. Association learning in the acute confusional state. *J Neurol Neurosurg Psychiatry* 1998;65:390–392.

324. Nissley HM, Schmiter-Edgecombe M. Perceptually based implicit learning in severe closed-head injury patients. *Neuropsychology* 2002;16(1):111–122.

325. Thoene AIT, Glisky EL. Learning of name-face associations in memory impaired patients: a comparison of different training procedures. *J Int Neuropsycholl Soc* 1995;1:29–38.

326. Wilson B, Evans J. Error-free learning in the rehabilitation of people with memory impairments. *J Head Trauma Rehabil* 1996;11:54–64.

327. Squires EJ, Hunkin NM, Parkin AJ. Memory notebook training in a case of severe amnesia: generalising from paired associate learning to real life. *Neuropsychol Rehabil* 1996;6(1):55–65.

328. Berg I, Konning-Haanstra M, Deelman B. Long term effects of memory rehabilitation. A controlled study. *Neuropsychol Rehabil* 1991;1:97–111.

329. Schmitter-Edgecombe M, Fahy JF, Whelan JP, et al. Memory remediation after severe closed head injury: notebook training versus supportive therapy. *J Consult Clin Psychol*, 1995;63(3):484–489.

330. Mesulam MM. Frontal cortex and behavior. *Ann Neurol* 1986;19:320–324.

331. Goldman-Rakic P. Architecture of the prefrontal cortex and the central executive. In: Grafman J, Holyoak K, Boller F, eds. *Structure and functions of the human prefrontal cortex*. New York: New York Academy of Sciences, 1995:71–83.

332. Mattson AJ, Levin HS. Frontal lobe dysfunction following closed head injury: a review of the literature. *J Nerv Ment Dis* 1990;178:282–291.

333. Levin H, Kraus M. The frontal lobes and traumatic brain injury. *J Neuropsychiatr Clin Sci* 1994;6:443–454.

334. Hart T, Jacobs H. Rehabilitation and management of behavioral disturbances following frontal lobe injury. *J Head Trauma* 1993;8(1):1–12.

335. Hart T, Schwartz M, Mayer N. Executive function: some current theories and their applications. In: Varney N, Roberts R, eds. *The evaluation and treatment of mild traumatic brain injury*. Mahwah, NJ: Lawrence Erlbaum Associates, 1999:133–148.

336. Schwartz MF, Montgomery MW, Buxbaum LJ, et al. Naturalistic action impairment in closed head injury. *Neuropsychology* 1998;12:13–28.

337. Chevignard M, Pillon B, Pradat-Diehl P, et al. An ecological approach to planning dysfunction: script execution. *Cortex* 2000;36:649–669.

338. Duncan J. Disorganisation of behaviour after frontal lobe damage. *Cogn Neuropsychol* 1986;3:271–290.

339. Duncan J, Johnson R, Swales M, et al. Frontal lobe deficits after head injury: unity and diversity of function. *Cogn Neuropsychol* 1997;14(5):713–741.

340. Kimberg D, Farah M. A unified account of cognitive impairments following frontal lobe damage: the role of working memory in complex, organized behavior. *J Exp Psychol:(Gen)* 1993;122:411–428.

341. Burgess PW, Alderman N, Evans J, et al. The ecological validity of tests of executive function. *J Int Neuropsychol Soc* 1998;4:547–558.

342. Tate R. Executive dysfunction and characterological changes after traumatic brain injury: two sides of the same coin? *Cortex* 1999;35:39–55.

343. Alderman N, Ward A. Behavioural treatment of the dysexecutive syndrome: reduction of repetitive speech using response cost and cognitive overlearning. *Neuropsychol Rehabil* 1991;1(1):65–80.

344. Norris G, Tate RL. The behavioural assessment of the dysexecutive syndrome (BADS): ecological, concurrent and construct validity. *Neuropsychol Rehabil* 2000;10(1):33–45.

345. Schwartz MF, Segal M, Veramonti T, et al. The naturalistic action test: a standardized assessment for everyday-action impairment. *Neuropsychol Rehabil(in press)*.

346. Sohlberg M, Mateer C, Stuss D. Contemporary approaches to the management of executive control dysfunction. *J Head Trauma Rehabil* 1993;8:45–58.

347. von Cramon DY, Matthes-von Cramon G. Frontal lobe dysfunctions in patients—therapeutical approaches. In: Wood RL, Fussey I, eds. *Cognitive rehabilitation in perspective*. New York: Taylor and Francis, 1990:164–179.

348. Cicerone K, Giacino J. Remediation of executive function deficits after traumatic brain injury. *Neurorehabilitation* 1992;2:12–22.

349. Levine B, Robertson IH, Clare L, et al. Rehabilitation of executive functioning: an experimental-clinical validation of Goal Management Training. *J Int Neuropsychol Soc* 2000;6:299–312.

350. Mateer CA. Executive function disorders: rehabilitation challenges and strategies. *Semin Clin Neuropsychiatry* 1999;4(1):50–59.

351. Snow P, Douglas J, Ponsford J. Conversational discourse abilities following severe traumatic brain injury: a follow-up study. *Brain Inj* 1998;12(11):911–935.

352. Galski T, Tompkins C, Johnston M. Competence in discourse as a measure of social integration and quality of life in persons with traumatic brain injury. *Brain Inj* 1998;12(9):769–782.

353. Coelho CA. Discourse production deficits following traumatic brain injury: a critical review of the recent literature. *Aphasiology* 1995;9:409–429.

354. Prigatano G, Fordyce D, Zeiner H, et al. Neuropsychological rehabilitation after closed head injury in young adults. *J Neurol Neurosurg Psychiatry* 1984;47:505–513.

355. Docking K, Murdoch BE, Jordan F. Interpretation and comprehension of linguistic humour by adolescents with head injury: a group analysis. *Brain Inj* 2000;14(1):89–108.

356. Manasse NJ, Hux K, Rankin-Erickson JL. Speech recognition training for enhancing written language generation by a traumatic brain injury survivor. *Brain Inj* 2000;14(11):1015–1034.

357. Wiseman-Hakes C, Stewart ML, Wasserman R, et al. Peer group training of pragmatic skills in adolescents in acquired brain injury. *J Head Trauma Rehabil* 1998;13(6):23–38.

358. Sandel M, Mysiw W. The agitated brain injured patient. Part 1: definitions, differential, diagnosis, and assessment. *Arch Phys Med Rehabil* 1996;77:617–623.

359. Brooke M, Questad K, Patterson D, et al. Agitation and restlessness after closed head injury: a prospective study of 100 consecutive admissions. *Arch Phys Med Rehabil* 1992;73:320–323.

360. Galski T, Palasz J, Bruno R, et al. Predicting physical and verbal aggression on a brain trauma unit. *Arch Phys Med Rehabil* 1994;75:380–383.

361. Brooke MM, Patterson DR, Questad KA, et al. The treatment of agitation during initial hospitalization after traumatic brain injury. *Arch Phys Med Rehabil* 1992;73:917–921.

362. Corrigan J, Mysiw W. Agitation following traumatic brain injury: equivocal evidence for a discrete stage of cognitive recovery. *Arch Phys Med Rehabil* 1988;69:487–492.

363. Bogner J, Corrigan J, Fugate L, et al. Role of agitation in prediction of outcomes after traumatic brain injury. *Am J Phys Med Rehabil* 2001;(80):636–644.

364. Corrigan JD. Development of a scale for assessment of agitation following traumatic brain injury. *J Clin Exp Neuropsychol* 1989;11:261–277.

365. Bogner J, Corrigan J, Stange M, et al. Reliability of the agitated behavior scale. *J Head Trauma Rehabil* 1999;14(1):91–96.

366. Bogner JA, Corrigan JD, Bode RK, et al. Rating scale analysis of the agitated behavior scale. *J Head Trauma Rehabil* 2000;15(1):656–669.

367. Silver JM, Yudofsky SC. Psychopharmacological approaches to the patient with affective and psychotic features. *J Head Trauma Rehabil* 1994;9:61–77.

368. Fugate L, Spacek L, Kresty L, et al. Measurement and treatment of agitation following traumatic brain injury: II. A survey of the brain injury special interest group of the American Academy of Physical Medicine and Rehabilitation. *Arch Phys Med Rehabil* 1997;78:924–928.

369. Rall TW. Hypnotics and sedatives: ethanol. In: Gilman A, Rall T, Nies A, et al, eds. *Goodman and Gilman's the pharmacological basis of therapeutics*, 8th ed. New York: Pergamon Press, 1990:345–382.

370. Baldessarini RJ. Drugs and the treatment of psychiatric disorders. In: Gilman AG, Rall TW, Nies AS, et al. eds. *Goodman and Gilman's the pharmacological basic of therapeutics*, 8th ed. New York: Pergamon Press, 1990:383–435.

371. Sandel ME, Olive DA, Rader MA. Chlorpromazine-induced psychosis after brain injury. *Brain Inj* 1993;7:77–83.

372. Rosati DL. Early Polyneuropharmacologic intervention in brain injury agitation. *Am J Phys Med Rehabil* 2002;81(2):90–93.

373. Mysiw J, Sandel E. The agitated brain injured patient. Part 2: pathophysiology and treatment. *Arch Phys Med Rehabil* 1997;78:213–220.

374. Yudovsky SC, Silver JM, Jackson W. The Overt Aggression Scale for the objective rating of verbal and physical aggression. *Am J Psychiatry* 1986;143:35–39.

375. Yuen HK, Benzing P. Guiding of behavior through redirection in brain injury rehabilitation. *Brain Inj* 1996;10:229–238.

376. Bond M. The psychiatry of closed head injury. In: Brooks N, ed. *Closed head injury: psychological, social and family consequences*. Oxford, UK: Oxford University Press, 1984:148–178.

377. Hart T, Hawkey K, Whyte J. Use of a portable voice organizer to remember therapy goals in TBI rehabilitation: a within-subjects trial. *J Head Trauma Rehabil* 2002;17(6):556–570.

378. Kim S, Manes F, Kosier T, et al. Irritability following traumatic brain injury. *J Nerv Ment Dis* 1999;187(6):327–335.

379. Silver J, Yudovsky S. Aggressive disorders. In: Silver J, Yudovsky S, Hales R, eds. *Neuropsychiatry of traumatic brain injury.* Washington, DC: American Psychiatric Press, 1994:313–353.

380. Slifer KJ, Cataldo MD, Babbit RL, et al. Behavior analysis and intervention during hospitalization for brain trauma rehabilitation. *Arch Phys Med Rehabil* 1993;74:810–817.

381. Alderman N, Knight C. The effectiveness of DRL in the management and treatment of severe behaviour disorders following brain injury. *Brain Inj* 1997;11(2):79–101.

382. Lloyd LF, Cuvo AJ. Maintenance and generalization of behaviors after treatment of persons with traumatic brain injury. *Brain Inj* 1994;8:529–540.

383. Wood RLI. Conditioning procedures in brain injury rehabilitation. In: Wood R, ed. *Neuro-behavioural sequelae of traumatic brain injury.* New York: Taylor & Francis, 1990:153–174.

384. Schlund M, Pace G. The effects of traumatic brain injury on reporting and responding to causal relations: an investigation of sensitivity to reinforcement contingencies. *Brain Inj* 2000;14(6):573–583.

385. Rothwell NA, LaVigna GW, Willis TJ. A non-aversive rehabilitation approach for people with severe behavioural problems resulting from brain injury. *Brain Inj* 1999;13(7):521–533.

386. Ducharme JM. A conceptual model for treatment of externalizing behaviour in acquired brain injury. *Brain Inj* 1999;13(9):645–668.

387. Medd J, Tate RL. Evaluation of an anger management therapy programme following acquired brain injury: a preliminary study. *Neuropsychol Rehabil* 2000;10(2):185–201.

388. Emory L, Cole C, Meyer W. Use of Depo-Provera to control sexual aggression in persons with traumatic brain injury. *J Head Trauma Rehabil* 1995;10: 47–58.

389. Kant R, Smith-Seemiller L, Zeiler D. Treatment of aggression and irritability after head injury. *Brain Inj* 1998;12(8):661–666.

390. Wroblewski AB, Kupfer JJ, Kalliel K. Effectiveness of valproic acid on destructive and aggressive behaviours in patients with acquired brain injury. *Brain Inj* 1997;11(1):37–47.

391. Carnevale GJ. Natural-setting behavior management for individuals with traumatic brain injury: results of a three-year caregiver training program. *J Head Trauma Rehabil* 1996;11:27–38.

392. Paus T. Primate anterior cingulate cortex: where motor control, drive and cognition interface. *Nat Rev Neurosci* 2001;2:417–424.

393. Kant R, Duffy J, Pivovarnik A. Prevalence of apathy following head injury. *Brain Inj* 1998;12(1):87–92.

394. Reinhard DL, Whyte J, Sandel ME. Improved arousal and initiation following tricyclic antidepressant use in severe brain injury. *Arch Phys Med Rehabil* 1996;77:80–83.

395. Marin RS, Fogel BS, Hawkins J, et al. Apathy: a treatable syndrome. *J Neuropsychiatry* 1995;7:23–30.

396. Wilson B, Emslie H, Quirk K, et al. Reducing everyday memory and planning problems by means of a paging system: a randomised control crossover study. *J Neurol Neurosurg Psychiatry* 2001;70(4):477–482.

397. Wade TK, Troy JC. Mobile phones as a new memory aid: a preliminary investigation using case studies. *Brain Inj* 2001;15(4):305–320.

398. Seel RT, Kreutzer JS, Rosenthal M, et al. Prevalence, symptom rates and factors associated with depression after TBI: a NIDRR Model Systems multicenter investigation. *Arch Phys Med Rehabil* 2003;84(2):177–184.

399. Jorge R, Robinson R, Arndt S, et al. Depression following traumatic brain injury: a 1 year longitudinal study. *J Affect Dis* 1993;27:233–243.

400. Silver JM, Yudofsky SC, Hales RE, eds. *Neuropsychiatry of traumatic brain injury.* Washington, DC: American Psychiatric Press, 1994.

401. Linn RT, Allen K, Wilier BS. Affective symptoms in the chronic stage of traumatic brain injury: a study of married couples. *Brain Inj* 1994;8:135–148.

402. Robinson RG, Kubos KL, Starr LB. Mood disorders in stroke patients: importance of lesion location. *Brain* 1984;107:81–93.

403. Prigatano GP. Psychotherapy after brain injury. In: Prigatano GP, ed. *Neuropsychological rehabilitation after brain injury.* Baltimore: John Hopkins University Press, 1986:67–95.

404. Fedoroff J, Starkstein S, Forrester A, et al. Depression in patients with acute traumatic brain injury. *Am J Psychiatry* 1992:918–923.

405. Fann J, Katon W, Uomoto J, et al. Psychiatric disorders and functional disability in outpatients with traumatic brain injuries. *Am J Psychiatry* 1995;152: 1493–1499.

406. Jorge R, Robinson R, Arndt S. Are there symptoms that are specific for depressed mood in patients with traumatic brain injury? *J Nerv Ment Dis* 1993; 181:91–99.

407. Green A, Felmingham K, Baguley I, et al. The clinical utility of the Beck Depression Inventory after traumatic brain injury. *Brain Inj* 2001;15(12):1021–1028.

408. Klonoff P, Lage G. Suicide in patients with traumatic brain injury: risk and prevention. *J Head Trauma Rehabil* 1995;10:16–24.

409. Hilbom E. After effects of brain injuries. *Acta Psychiatry Neurol Scand* 1960; 142:107.

410. Simpson G, Tate R. Suicidality after traumatic brain injury: demographic, injury and clinical correlates. *Psychol Med* 2002;32(4):687–697.

411. Wroblewski B, McColgan K, Smith K, et al. The incidence of seizures during tricyclic antidepressant drug treatment in a brain-injured population. *J Clin Psychopharmacol* 1990;10:124–128.

412. Joseph A, Wroblewski B. Depression, antidepressants, and traumatic brain injury. *J Head Trauma Rehabil* 1995;10:90–95.

413. Prigatano G, Schacter D. *Awareness of deficit after brain injury: clinical and theoretical issues.* New York: Oxford University Press, 1991.

414. Prigatano G, Altman I. Impaired awareness of behavioral limitations after traumatic brain injury. *Arch Phys Med Rehabil* 1990;71:1058–1064.

415. Sherer M, Boake C, Levin E, et al. Characteristics of impaired awareness after traumatic brain injury. *J Int Neuropsychol Soc* 1998;4:380–387.

416. Hart T, Giovanenetti T, Montgomery M, et al. Awareness of errors in naturalistic action after traumatic brain injury. *J Head Trauma Rehabil* 1998;13: 16–28.

417. Fleming J, Strong J. A longitudinal study of self-awareness: functional deficits underestimated by persons with brain injury. *Occup Ther J Res* 1999; 19:3–17.

418. Godfrey H, Partridge F, Knight R, et al. Course of insight disorder and emotional dysfunction following closed head injury: a controlled cross-sectional follow-up study. *J Clin Exp Neuropsychol* 1993;15:503–515.

419. Gasquoine P. Affective state and awareness of sensory and cognitive effects after closed head injury. *Neuropsychologia* 1992;6(187–196).

420. Prigatano G, Bruna O, Mataro M, et al. Initial disturbances of consciousness and resultant impaired awareness in Spanish patients with traumatic brain injury. *J Head Trauma Rehabil* 1998;13:29–38.

421. Lam C, McMahon B, Priddy D, et al. Deficit awareness and treatment performance among traumatic head injury adults. *Brain Inj* 1988;2:235–242.

422. Zhou J, Chittum R, Johnson K, et al. The utilization of a game format to increase knowledge of residuals among people with acquired brain injury. *J Head Trauma Rehabil* 1996;11(1):51–61.

423. Rebmann MJ, Hannon R. Treatment of unawareness of memory deficits in adults with brain injury: three case studies. *Rehabil Psychol* 1995;40(4): 279–287.

424. Head Injury Interdisciplinary Special Interest Group of the ACRM. Guidelines for cognitive rehabilitation. *Neurorehabilitation* 1992;2:62–67.

425. Ben-Yishay Y, Diller L. Cognitive remediation in traumatic brain injury: update and issues. *Arch Phys Med Rehabil* 1993;74:204–213.

426. Wilson B. Compensating for cognitive deficits following brain injury. *Neuropsychol Rev* 2000;10(4):233–243.

427. Sohlberg M, Mateer C. *Cognitive rehabilitation.* New York: Guilford Press, 2001.

428. Carney N, Chestnut RM, Maynard H, et al. Effect of cognitive rehabilitation on outcomes for persons with traumatic brain injury: a systematic review. *J Head Trauma Rehabil* 1999;14(3):277–307.

429. Prigatano G, Klonoff P, O'Brien K, et al. Productivity after neuropsychologically oriented milieu rehabilitation. *J Head Trauma Rehabil* 1994;9:91–102.

430. Malec J, Basford J. Postacute brain injury rehabilitation. *Arch Phys Med Rehabil* 1996;77:198–207.

431. Christiansen C, Abreu B, Ottenbacher KJ, et al. Task performance in virtual environments used for cognitive rehabilitation after traumatic brain injury. *Arch Phys Med Rehabil* 1998;79:888–892.

432. Grealy M, Johnson D, Rushton S. Improving cognitive function after brain injury: the use of exercise and virtual reality. *Arch Phys Med Rehabil* 1999; 80:661–667.

433. Hopewell C. Driving assessment issues for practicing clinicians. *J Head Trauma Rehabil* 2002;17(1):48–61.

434. Brouwer WH, Witbaar FK, Tant MLM, et al. Attention and driving in traumatic brain injury: a question of coping with time-pressure. *J Head Trauma Rehabil* 2002;17(1):1–15.

435. Fisk G, Novack T, Mennemeier M, et al. Useful field of view after traumatic brain injury. *J Head Trauma Rehabil* 2002;17(1):16–25.

436. Lengenfelder J, Schultheis MT, Al-Shihabi T, et al. Divided attention and driving: a pilot study using virtual reality technology. *J Head Trauma Rehabil* 2002;17(1):26–37.

437. Kewman D, Seigerman C, Kintner H, et al. Simulation training of psychomotor skills: teaching the brain-injured to drive. *Rehabil Psychol* 1985; 1:11–27.

438. Giles G, Shore M. A rapid method for teaching severely brain injured adults how to wash and dress. *Arch Phys Med Rehabil* 1989;70:156–158.

439. Vilkki J, Ahola K, Hoist P, et al. Prediction of psychosocial recovery after head injury with cognitive tests and neurobehavioral ratings. *J Clin Exp Neuropsychol* 1994;16:325–338.

440. Finset A, Dyrnes S, Krogstad J, et al. Self-reported social networks and interpersonal support 2 years after severe traumatic brain injury. *Brain Inj* 1995;9:141–150.

441. Morton MV, Wehman P. Psychosocial and emotional sequelae of individuals with traumatic brain injury: a literature review and recommendations. *Brain Inj* 1995;9:81–92.

442. Thomsen I. Late psychosocial outcome in severe traumatic brain injury. *Scand J Rehabil Med Suppl* 1992;26:142–152.

443. Brotherton F, Thomas L, Wisotzek I, et al. Social skills training in the rehabilitation of patients with traumatic closed head injury. *Arch Phys Med Rehabil* 1988;69:827–832.

444. Hibbard M, Cantor J, Charatz J, et al. Peer support in the community: initial findings of a mentoring program for individuals with traumatic brain injury and their families. *J Head Trauma Rehabil* 2002;17(2):112–131.

445. Vaccaro MJ, Hart T, Whyte J. Internet resources for traumatic brain injury: a selective review of websites for consumers. *Neurorehabilitation* 2002;17(2):169–174.

446. Bond MR. Assessment of the psychosocial outcome of severe head injury. *Acta Neurochir Suppl* 1976;34:57–70.

447. Oddy M, Humphrey M, Uttley D. Subjective impairment and social recovery after closed head injury. *J Neurol Neurosurg Psychiatry* 1978.

448. Schalen W, Hansson L, Nordstrom G, et al. Psychosocial outcome 5–8 years after severe traumatic brain lesions and the impact of rehabilitation services. *Brain Inj* 1994;8(1):49–64.

449. Jacobs H. The Clubhouse: addressing work-related behavioral challenges through a supportive social community. *J Head Trauma Rehabil* 1997;12(5):14–27.

450. Perlesz A, Kinsella G, Crowe S. Impact of traumatic brain injury on the family: a critical review. *Rehabil Psychol* 1999.

451. Kreutzer J, Marwitz J, Kepler K. Traumatic brain injury: family response and outcome. *Arch Phys Med Rehabil* 1992;73:771–778.

452. Rosenbaum M, Najenson T. Changes in life patterns and symptoms of low mood as reported by wives of severely brain injured soldiers. *J Consult Clin Psychol* 1976;44:681–688.

453. Chwalisz K, Stark-Wroblewski K. The subjective experiences of spouse caregivers of persons with brain injuries: a qualitative analysis. *Appl Neuropsychol* 1996;3:28–40.

454. Leathem J, Heath G, Woolley C. Relatives' perceptions of role change, social support and stress after traumatic brain injury. *Brain Inj* 1996;10:27–38.

455. Hall K, Karzmark P, Stevens M, et al. Family stressors in traumatic brain injury: a two-year follow-up. *Arch Phys Med Rehabil* 1994;75:876–884.

456. Kreutzer J, Gervasio A, Camplair P. Primary caregiver's psychological status and family functioning after traumatic brain injury. *Brain Inj* 1994;8(3):197–210.

457. Williams J, Kay T. *Head injury: a family matter.* Baltimore: Paul Brookes, 1991.

458. Kosciulek J. Relationship of family coping with head injury to family adaptation. *Rehabil Psychol* 1994;39(4):215–230.

459. Kreutzer J, Gervasio A, Camplair P. Patient correlates of caregivers' distress and family functioning after traumatic brain injury. *Brain Inj* 1994;8(3):211–230.

460. Rosenthal M, Geckler CL. The neuropsychology handbook. Vol 2. In: Horton AM Jr, Wedding D, et al, eds. *Treatment issues and special populations,* 2nd ed. New York: Springer, 1997:47–72.

461. Albert SM, Im A, Brenner L, et al. Effect of a social work liaison program on family caregivers to people with brain injury. *J Head Trauma Rehabil* 2002;17(2):175–189.

462. Elliot M, Biever L. Head injury and sexual dysfunction. *Brain Inj* 1996;10:703–717.

463. Corrigan J. Substance abuse as a mediating factor in outcome from traumatic brain injury. *Arch Phys Med Rehabil* 1995;76:302–309.

464. Corrigan J, Bogner J, Lamb-Hart G. Substance abuse and brain injury. In: Rosenthal M, Griffith E, Kreutzer J, et al, eds. *Rehabilitation of the adult and child with traumatic brain injury,* 3rd ed. Philadelphia: FA Davis, 1999:556–571.

465. Kreutzer J, Doherty K, Harris J, et al. Alcohol use among persons with traumatic brain injury. *J Head Trauma Rehabil* 1990;5(3):9–20.

466. Cherner M, Temkin NR, Machamer JE, et al. Utility of composite measure to detect problematic alcohol use in persons with traumatic brain injury. *Arch Phys Med Rehabil* 2001;82:780–786.

467. Substance Abuse and Mental Health Services Administration. National Household Survey on Drug Abuse: Population Estimates. Rockville, MD: Substance Abuse and Mental Health Services Administration, Office of Applied Studies; US Dept of Health and Human Services; 1998.

468. Centers for Disease Control and Prevention. Behavioral risk factor surveillance system user's guide. Rockville, MD: US Dept of Health and Human Services and Atlanta: Centers for Disease Control and Prevention, 1998.

469. Bogner J, Corrigan J, Mysiw J, et al. A comparison of substance abuse and violence in the prediction of long-term rehabilitation outcomes after traumatic brain injury. *Arch Phys Med Rehabil* 2001;82:571–577.

470. Kreutzer J, Witol A, Marwitz J. Alcohol and drug use among young persons with traumatic brain injury. *J Learn Disabil* 1995;29:643.

471. Kreutzer J, Wehman P, Harris J. Substance abuse and crime patterns among persons with traumatic brain injury. *Brain Inj* 1991;5:177–187.

472. Kramer T, Hoisington D. Use of AA and NA in the treatment of chemical dependencies of traumatic brain injury survivors. *Brain Inj* 1992;6:81–88.

473. Bombardier C, Heinemann A. The construct validity of the readiness to change questionnaire for persons with TBI. *J Head Trauma Rehabil* 2000;15(1):696–709.

474. Bombardier CH, Ehde D, Kilmer J. Readiness to change alcohol drinking habits after traumatic brain injury. *Arch Phys Med Rehabil* 1997;78:592–596.

475. Wagner AK, Hammond FM, Sasser HC, et al. Return to productive activity after traumatic brain injury: relationship with measures of disability, handicap, and community integration. *Arch Phys Med Rehabil* 2002;83:107–114.

476. Sherer M, Sander AM, Nick TG, et al. Early cognitive status and productivity outcome after traumatic brain injury: findings from the TBI Model Systems. *Arch Phys Med Rehabil* 2002;83:183–192.

477. Ruffolo CF, Friedland JF, Dawson DR, et al. Mild traumatic brain injury from motor vehicle accidents: factors associated with return to work. *Arch Phys Med Rehabil* 1999;80:392–398.

478. Ben-Yishay Y. Neuropsychological rehabilitation: quest for a holistic approach. *Semin Neurol* 1985;5:252–259.

479. Wehman P, Kreutzer J, West M, et al. Employment outcomes of persons following traumatic brain injury: preinjury, post injury and supported employment. *Brain Inj* 1989;3:397–412.

480. Wehman PH, Kreutzer JS, West MD, et al. Return to work for persons with traumatic brain injury: supported employment approach. *Arch Phys Med Rehabil* 1990;71:1047–1052.

481. Wehman P, West M, Kregel J, et al. Return to work for persons with severe traumatic brain injury: a data-based approach to program development. *J Head Trauma Rehabil* 1995;10:27–39.

482. Yasuda S, Wehman P, Targett P, et al. Return to work for persons with traumatic brain injury. *Am J Phys Med Rehabil* 2001;80:852–864.

483. LeBlanc J, Hayden M, Paulman R. A comparison of neuropsychological and situational assessment for predicting employability after closed head injury. *J Head Trauma Rehabil* 2000;15(4):1022–1040.

484. Caplan A. Informed consent and provider–patient relationships in rehabilitation medicine. *Arch Phys Med Rehabil* 1988;69:312–317.

485. Haffey W. The assessment of clinical competency to consent to medical rehabilitative interventions. *J Head Trauma Rehabil* 1989;4(1):43–56.

486. Cope DN. Legal and ethical issues in the psychopharmacologic treatment of traumatic brain injury. *J Head Trauma Rehabil* 1989;4(1):13–21.

487. Banja JD, Higgins P. Videotaping therapeutic sessions and the right of privacy. *J Head Trauma Rehabil* 1989;4(1):65–74.

488. Hart T, Nagele D. The assessment of competency in traumatic brain injury. *Neurorehabilitation* 1996;7:27–38.

489. Rosenthal M, Kolpan K. Head injury rehabilitation: psycholegal issues and roles for the rehabilitation psychologist. *Rehabil Psychol* 1986;31:37–46.

490. Berrol S. Considerations for management of the persistent vegetative state. *Arch Phys Med Rehabil* 1986;67:283–285.

491. Bontke CF, Dolan JM, Ivanhoe CB. Should we withhold food from persons in a persistent vegetative state? *J Head Trauma Rehabil* 1994;9:62–69.

492. Phipps E, Whyte J. Medical decision-making with persons who are minimally conscious. *Am J Phys Med Rehabil* 1999;78(1):77–82.

CHAPTER 79

Rehabilitation of Spinal Cord Injury

Steven Kirshblum

The earliest reference to spinal cord injury (SCI) is found in the Edwin Smith Surgical Papyrus, written between 2500 and 3000 B.C., where it is described as "an ailment not to be treated" (1). Much has changed in spinal cord care over the centuries, particularly in the last 50 years as it relates to increasing survival, life expectancy, community reintegration, and quality of life. Major advances include the specialized spinal cord centers of care, model SCI centers funded by the National Institute on Disability and Rehabilitation Research (NIDRR) in the United States Department of Education, establishment and growth of organizations and journals dedicated to SCI care, and the development of the subspecialty of SCI medicine in 1998. This subspecialty addresses the prevention, diagnosis, treatment, and management of traumatic and nontraumatic etiologies of spinal cord dysfunction (2). The advances of the last 20 years alone have been dramatic in terms of the understanding of the pathology of the initial and secondary aspects of the injury, and the barriers that must be overcome to enhance recovery. Newer techniques to improve function and intervene at the cellular level for possible cure are being developed. These will further allow individuals who sustain an SCI to be more independent in the future.

EPIDEMIOLOGY OF TRAUMATIC SPINAL CORD INJURY

Incidence and Prevalence

The National Spinal Cord Injury Statistical Center (NSCISC) database consists of data contributed by model SCI systems (3). This database captures approximately 15% of all new traumatic SCIs that occur in the United States each year, and has been used to develop an epidemiological profile (4–6). When compared to population-based studies, persons in this database are representative of all SCIs except that more severe injuries, persons of color, and injuries due to acts of violence are slightly overrepresented (4).

The overall incidence of traumatic SCI in the U.S. has remained relatively constant, at approximately 40 new cases per million population, or just over 11,000 cases per year. The incidence of SCI in the rest of the world is consistently lower than in the U.S. (7). The prevalence of SCI is estimated to be approximately 250,00 persons by 2004, with the growth resulting from improved life expectancy rather than any increase in incidence.

Age, Gender, Race, Marital, and Occupational Status

The mean age at injury is 32.1 years, with the most common age at injury being 19 years (Table 79-1). Approximately 60% of all persons enrolled in the NSCISC database are 30 years of age or younger at the time of injury. The percentage of new persons injured who are older than 60 has increased to over 10% in the last decade. Men suffer traumatic SCI much more commonly than women, at a 4:1 ratio. State registries and NSCISC data reveal higher incidence rates of SCI for African Americans than whites, which is predominantly due to injuries that result from acts of violence.

Approximately 50% of persons enrolled in the NSCISC database have never been married at the time of their injury. Approximately 60% of persons enrolled between the ages of 16 and 59 are employed at the time of injury.

Etiology and Time of Injury

Motor vehicle crashes (MVCs) rank first (accounting for 38.5% of cases since 1990), followed by acts of violence (primarily gunshot wounds, or GSWs), falls, and recreational sporting activities. MVCs cause a lower percentage of cases among men than women while men have a higher percentage of SCI due to GSW, diving mishaps, and motorcycle crashes. MVCs have decreased, while SCI caused by GSWs almost doubled (from 12.7% to 24.1%) among men from the mid 1970s to the early 1990s, before declining slightly in subsequent years. Diving mishaps account for the majority of SCIs due to recreational sports, followed by snow skiing, surfing, wrestling, and football.

MVC is the leading cause of SCI until age 45; however, beginning with the 46- to 60-year-old age group, falls represent the leading cause of SCI. Recreational sports and acts of violence decrease with advancing age as a cause of injury.

Traumatic SCI occurs with greater frequency on weekends, with the greatest incidence on Saturday. Seasonal variation exists, with peak incidence occurring in July followed closely by August and June. The seasonal pattern in incidence is more pronounced in the northern part of the U.S. where seasonal variation in climate is greatest.

TABLE 79-1.   Epidemiology of Traumatic Spinal Cord Injury (Since 1990)

Incidence: Approximately 11,000/y
Prevalence: 200,000–250,000
Average age: 32.1
Gender: 80.5% male
Etiology: Motor vehicle accidents (38.5%); followed by violence (primarily GSW); falls; and recreational sports

Current Percentage of Injuries by ASIA Classification

1. Incomplete tetraplegia (29.6%)
2. Complete paraplegia (27.3%)
3. Incomplete paraplegia (20.6%)
4. Complete tetraplegia (18.6%)

ASIA, American Spinal Injury Association; GSW, gun shot wounds.
From Facts and figures: National Spinal Cord Injury Statistical Center. *J Spinal Cord Med* 2002;25:139–140.

Associated Injuries

SCIs are often accompanied by other significant injuries. The most common include broken bones (29.3%), loss of consciousness (28.2%), traumatic pneumothorax (17.8%), and head injury sufficient to affect cognitive or emotional functioning (11.5%) (4). The nature and frequency of these injuries is significantly associated with the etiology of the SCI. For example, pneumothorax occurs more frequently with GSWs as compared with other causes of SCI.

Neurological Level and Extent of Lesion

Traumatic SCI most commonly causes cervical lesions (approximately 50%) followed by thoracic and then lumbosacral lesions. The C5 segment is the most common lesion level, followed by C4, C6, T12, C7, and L1 at the time of discharge from inpatient rehabilitation programs (7). At time of discharge from inpatient rehabilitation, 48.6% of persons have neurologically complete injuries [American Spinal Injury Association (ASIA) A classification], followed by incomplete injuries of ASIA D, C, B, and E classifications (7).

The etiology of injury is strongly associated with level and severity of the injury. Most recreational sports-related injuries, falls, and approximately 50% of MVCs result in tetraplegia, whereas acts of violence usually result in paraplegia. Neurologically complete injuries are more likely to occur as a result of acts of violence and among younger age groups. Thoracic injuries are the most likely to be neurologically complete while most lower level lesions are incomplete injuries. Cervical injuries are most commonly classified as either ASIA A or ASIA D. There has been a trend toward increased likelihood of cervical injury since 1994 (5).

Marital and Occupational Status after Spinal Cord Injury

The annual marriage rate after SCI is below average for the general population and the annual divorce rate is higher (8,9). Approximately 25% of persons with SCI are employed, but the percentage varies substantially by neurological level and extent of injury (10). The higher the level of and the more severe the injury, the less chance one has of returning to gainful employment. Most employed individuals with SCI have full-time rather than part-time jobs. Predictors of returning to work include being of younger age, male, white, with a greater formal education and being employed at the time of injury; having greater motivation to return to work; having a nonviolent injury etiology; being able to drive; and greater time postinjury (11–13). Persons who return to work within the first year of injury usually return to the same job with the same employer, while those who return to work after more than 1 year has elapsed usually acquire a different job with a different employer, often after retraining. Professional/technical and clerical/sales jobs are the most common.

Discharge Placement

Model SCI systems have a higher percentage of persons discharged to the community relative to nonmodel system centers (6–14). Approximately 90% of persons discharged from a model system are discharged to a private residence within the community; 5% being discharged to a nursing home, and 3% dying during hospitalization. Predictors of nursing home placement include ventilator dependence, older age, cervical level of injury with non-useful motor recovery, being unmarried and unemployed, and having either Medicaid or health maintenance organization (HMO) insurance (15). There has been a significant trend toward an increasing percentage of persons being discharged to nursing homes since 1995 with the advent of shorter inpatient rehabilitation lengths of stay (15,16).

Life Expectancy

Life expectancy of persons with SCI has improved significantly over the past few decades but remains below normal. Predictors of mortality after injury include male gender, advanced age, ventilator dependence, injury sustained by an act of violence, high injury level (particularly C4 or above), neurologically complete injury, poor self-rated adjustment to disability, and having either Medicare or Medicaid third-party sponsorship of care (17,18). Life expectancy estimates are typically based on neurological level of injury, degree of injury completeness, age at injury, and ventilator dependence. Estimates from the NSCISC database appear in Table 79-2.

Causes of Death

Diseases of the respiratory system are the leading cause of death following SCI, with pneumonia being the most common. Heart disease ranks second, followed by septicemia (usually associated with pressure ulcers, urinary tract, or respiratory infections) and cancer. The most common location of cancer is the lung, followed by bladder, prostate, and colon/rectum.

Pneumonia is by far the leading cause of death for persons with tetraplegia while heart disease, septicemia, and suicide are more common among persons with paraplegia (19). Among persons with incomplete motor-function (ASIA D) injuries at any neurological level, heart disease again ranks as the leading cause of death (24.1%), followed by pneumonia (11.0%). While genitourinary disease (i.e., renal failure) was the leading cause of death 30 years ago, this has declined dramatically, most likely due to improved care.

TABLE 79-2.   Life Expectancy (Years) for Postinjury by Severity of Injury and Age at Injury (for Persons Surviving at Least 1-Year Postinjury)

Age at Injury	No SCI	Motor Functional at Any Level	Para	Low Tetra (C5-C8)	High Tetra (C1-C4)	Ventilator-Dependent at Any Level
20	57.2	52.5	46.2	41.2	37.1	26.8
40	38.4	34.3	28.7	24.5	21.2	13.7
60	21.2	18.1	13.7	10.6	8.4	4.0

SCI, spinal cord injury.
From Facts and figures: National Spinal Cord Injury Statistical Center. *J Spinal Cord Med* 2002;25:139–140.

Lifetime Costs

Data are available from the model system that include only the direct costs of the SCI, with the indirect costs (i.e., lost wages, fringe benefits) not included in these estimates (6). Costs vary by year postinjury (first year versus subsequent years), by the level of injury, and severity of injury. Estimates of the total annual costs of SCI are $9.73 billion (12). This includes first-year direct costs estimated at $2.58 billion (based on 10,600 new cases), recurring direct costs of $4.55 billion, and $2.59 billion in lost productivity.

ACUTE MEDICAL AND SURGICAL MANAGEMENT OF SPINAL CORD INJURY

After injury prompt resuscitation, stabilization of the injury, and avoidance of additional neurological injury and medical complications are of greatest importance. During the first seconds after SCI there is release of catecholamines with an initial hypertensive phase. This is rapidly followed by a state of spinal shock, defined as flaccid paralysis and extinction of muscle stretch reflexes below the injury level (20), although this may not occur in all patients. The cardiovascular manifestation of spinal shock is neurogenic shock, consisting of hypotension, bradycardia, and hypothermia. Hypotension is especially common in persons with a neurological level of injury (NLI) at or above T6. The parasympathetic influences on the heart rate are unopposed in persons with a level of injury above T1; thus heart rates are typically less than 60 per minute. Treatment of hypotension involves fluid resuscitation to produce adequate urine output of more than 30 cc/hour, however, in neurogenic shock further fluid administration must proceed cautiously, as the patient is at risk for neurogenic pulmonary edema. The use of vasopressors is preferred in order to maintain a mean arterial blood pressure above 85 mm Hg, as this has been associated with enhanced neurological outcome (21).

Bradycardia is common in the acute period in cervical spinal injury and may be treated, if symptomatic, with intravenous atropine, or prevented with atropine given prior to any maneuver that may cause further vagal stimulation (such as nasotracheal suctioning). In cases of severe bradycardia that may lead to cardiac arrest; temporary cardiac pacing, as well as permanent pacemakers, may be required (22,23). While most pronounced in the first few weeks after injury, by 6 weeks the rhythm usually returns to normal.

Respiratory assessment is critical for acute SCI patients and should include arterial blood gases and measurement of forced vital capacity (VC) as an assessment of respiratory muscle strength. A VC of less than 1 L indicates ventilatory compromise, and the patient usually requires assisted ventilation. Close serial assessments should be obtained for those with borderline values. A nasogastric tube should be inserted during the initial assessment period to prevent emesis and potential aspiration. Aspiration occurs in approximately 5% of all SCI individuals, with a higher risk in patients over the age of 60, those who have undergone anterior approach spine surgery, or in the presence of a tracheostomy (24,25). A Foley catheter should be inserted for urinary drainage and will allow for an accurate assessment of output.

Once the initial resuscitative measures have been taken, attention is turned to spinal realignment. A full initial neurological assessment should be documented, and provides a baseline on which changes in neurological status can be gauged. A standard trauma series includes cross-table laterals and anteroposterior views of the cervical and thoracolumbar spine. There is a 12% incidence of noncontiguous fractures, therefore once one fracture is identified careful inspection of the rest of the spine is imperative (26). Forty-seven percent of patients with spine trauma and 64% of patients with SCI have concomitant injuries, including head, chest, and long bone fractures (27).

Computerized tomography (CT scanning) can help evaluate for the presence of cervical fractures most often at the C1 or C7 levels, provide information for surgical stabilization or decompression, and facilitate selection of appropriately sized hardware for operative stabilization. Magnetic resonance imaging (MRI) is helpful in cases in which a ruptured disc or epidural hematoma is suspected. In addition, an MRI is usually recommended prior to attempting closed reduction after cervical spine injury to identify disc herniation and its potential for neurological worsening with manipulation.

Closed cervical reduction is accomplished with traction. The patient is placed in either a Stryker frame (Stryker Corp., Kalamazoo, MI) or a RotoRest bed (Kinetic Concepts Inc., San Antonio, TX). Gardner-Wells tongs or a Halo ring are applied. Once reduction is confirmed, 10 to 15 pounds of weight is used to maintain reduction. The patient can later be brought to the operating room for open stabilization. The indications for and types of spinal orthotic devices are discussed in Chapter 62.

Stab wounds and GSWs generally do not produce spinal instability and therefore may not require surgical stabilization or orthotic immobilization. Plain films and CT are used not only to assess the extent of bony injury, but to provide information regarding the location and path of the bullet and bone fragments, and the extent of soft-tissue/vascular damage, in which case angiography would also be required. Objects that are embedded around the spinal canal (i.e., knife) should be left in place with removal performed in the operating room under direct visualization of the spinal canal. Bullets that pass through the abdominal viscera are treated with broad-spectrum antibiotics and tetanus prophylaxis (28,29). Bullets do not have to be removed, however, they can be removed if accessible while performing another surgical procedure.

In most trauma centers methylprednisolone (MP) is given after an acute SCI. Mechanisms of action for MP include improving blood flow to the spinal cord, preventing lipid peroxidation, being a free radical scavenger, and having antiinflammatory function. The National Acute Spinal Cord Injury Study (NASCIS) 2 demonstrated that MP given within 8 hours of injury (30 mg/kg bolus and 5.4 mg/kg/hour for 23 hours) marginally improves neurological recovery at 6 weeks, 6 months, and 1 year, although functional recovery was not clearly studied (30). The NASCIS 3 reported that if MP is initiated within 3 hours of SCI, it should be continued for 24 hours, whereas if MP is initiated 3 to 8 hours after SCI it should be continued for 48 hours (31). The administration of MP is not given beyond 8 hours from SCI or to those with SCI due to penetrating injuries as they have shown no benefit and their use is associated with a higher incidence of spinal and extraspinal infections (32,33). Because of some limitations of the NASCIS studies and that these findings have not been consistently replicated, these specific recommendations have not been universally adopted (34–36).

Sygen (GM-1) is a ganglioside that is present in high concentrations in the central nervous system (CNS) and forms the major component of cell membranes. An initial small study treating patients within 48 hours of injury for an average of 26 days found greater mean recovery at 1 year including some improved recovery in muscles with no strength at entry of the study (37). A subsequent large multicenter study reported a trend toward improvement in neurological recovery in ASIA B individuals at 26 weeks after being treated for 8 weeks. No significant effect however was noted at the principal endpoint—26 weeks—in the total group of patients studied (38).

Role of Surgery

Animal model evidence suggests that early decompressive surgery leads to improved neurological recovery after SCI (39). However, the role and timing of cervical decompression has not been substantiated in patients with SCI since most studies have failed to demonstrate any significant neurological recovery among patients with complete or incomplete deficits (40). While there is no conclusive evidence in humans with SCI supporting the benefit of "early" versus "late" surgery (40–42), select patients with incomplete SCI, such as those with cervical facet fracture dislocations, may experience improved neurological recovery if early decompression is performed within 8 hours (43).

In the thoracic and thoracolumbar spine, surgery for patients with complete injuries has not been shown to have significantly improved neurological function after decompression, while those with incomplete injuries do benefit from surgical intervention (44). The indication for emergent surgical treatment is progressive neurological deterioration, due to compression or an expanding epidural hematoma. Despite uncertainty regarding the appropriate timing of surgery, the safety of early surgery after SCI has been validated, and is not

TABLE 79-3. Glossary of Key Terms

Key muscle groups: Ten muscle groups that are tested as part of the standardized spinal cord examination.

Root Level	Muscle Group	Root Level	Muscle Group
C5	Elbow flexors	L2	Hip flexors
C6	Wrist extensors	L3	Knee extensors
C7	Elbow extensors	L4	Ankle dorsiflexors
C8	Long finger flexors	L5	Long toe extensor
T1	Small finger abductors	S1	Ankle plantarflexors

Motor level: The most caudal key muscle group that is graded 3/5 or greater with the segments cephalad graded normal (5/5) strength.
Motor index score: Calculated by adding the muscle scores of each key muscle group; a total score of 100 is possible.
Sensory level: The most caudal dermatome to have normal sensation for both pinprick/dull and light touch on both sides.
Sensory index score: Calculated by adding the scores for each dermatome; a total score of 112 is possible for each pinprick and light touch.
Neurological level of injury (NLI): The most caudal level at which both motor and sensory modalities are intact.
Complete injury: The absence of sensory and motor function in the lowest sacral segments.
Incomplete injury: Preservation of motor or sensory function below the neurological level that includes the lowest sacral segments.
Skeletal level: The level at which, by radiological examination, the greatest vertebral damage is found.
Zone of partial preservation (ZPP): Used only with complete injuries, refers to the dermatomes and myotomes caudal to the neurological level that remain partially innervated. The most caudal segment with some sensory or motor function defines the extent of the ZPP.

From Kirshblum SC, O'Connor K. Levels of injury and outcome in traumatic spinal cord injury. *Phys Med Rehabil Clin North Am* 2000;11:1–27.

associated with greater than expected complications (40,45). Early surgery may contribute to a shorter rehabilitation length of stay and a similar frequency of medical complications than those undergoing surgery beyond 24 hours from injury (46).

NEUROLOGICAL ASSESSMENT

The most accurate way to document impairments in a person with a new SCI is by performing a standardized neurological examination as endorsed by the International Standards for Neurological Classification of Spinal Cord Injury Patients (47). These standards provide basic definitions of the most common terms used by clinicians in the assessment of SCI and describe the neurological examination. Key terms are defined in Table 79-3. The examination has two main components, sensory and motor. The information from this neurological examination is recorded on a standardized flow sheet (Fig. 79-1), and helps determine the sensory and motor index scores; the sensory, motor, and NLI; the completeness of the injury; and to classify the impairment.

For the sensory examination, there are 28 key dermatomes, each tested for pinprick and light touch on each side of the body. A 3-point scale (range 0 to 2) is used, with the face as the normal control point. Absent pinprick, a score of zero, is the inability to distinguish between the sharp and dull edge of the pin. Impaired pin sensation, a score of 1, is assigned when the patient can distinguish between the sharp and dull edge of the pin, but the pin is not felt as sharp as on the face. Normal or intact sensation, a score of 2, is assigned only if the pin is felt as sharp in the tested dermatome as when tested on the face. For light touch, a cotton tip applicator is used, and scored as follows: intact, same sensation as on the face; impaired, less than on the face; and absent, no sensation. To test for deep anal sensation, a rectal digital examination is performed. The patient is asked to report any sensory awareness, touch, or pressure, with firm pressure of the examiner's digit on the rectal wall. Deep anal sensation is recorded as either present or absent.

The required elements of the motor examination consist of strength grading of ten key muscles bilaterally: five in the upper limb (C5-T1 myotomes) and five in the lower limb (L2-S1) on each side of the body (see Table 79-3). Testing is performed with the patient in the supine position, and is graded on a 6-point scale (range 0 to 5). Voluntary anal contraction is tested by sensing contraction of the external anal sphincter around the examiner's finger and graded as either present or absent.

STANDARD NEUROLOGICAL CLASSIFICATION OF SPINAL CORD INJURY

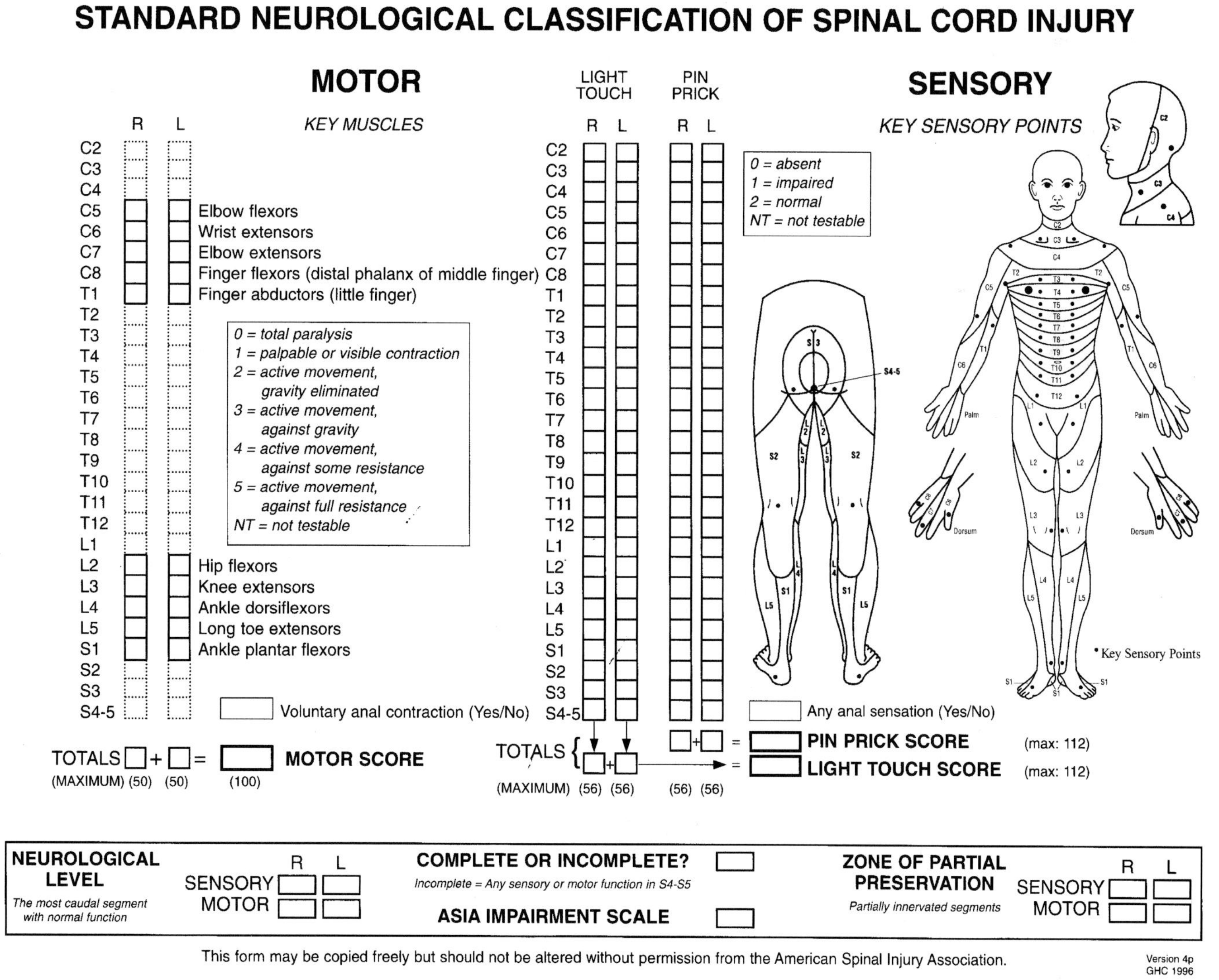

Figure 79-1. American Spinal Injury Association (ASIA) neurological flow sheet.

The NLI is the most caudal level at which both motor and sensory modalities are intact on both sides of the body. The motor and sensory levels are the same in less than 50% of complete injuries, and the motor level may be multiple levels below the sensory level at 1-year postinjury (48). In cases where there is no key muscle available (i.e., cervical levels at and above C4; T2-L1; and sacral levels S2–5), the neurological level is that which corresponds to the sensory level. The motor level and upper extremity motor index score better reflect the degree of function as well as the severity of impairment and disability, relative to the NLI, after motor complete tetraplegia (48). Table 79-4 lists a summary of the steps to be followed in classifying an individual with an SCI (49).

In 1982, the American Spinal Injury Association (ASIA) first published *Standards for Neurological Classification of SCI*, adopting the Frankel Scale (50). These standards were refined with the Frankel Scale being replaced in 1992 by the ASIA Impairment Scale (51), revised in 1996 (52), and again in 2000 (53), with reprinting in 2002 (47). The ASIA Impairment Scale describes five categories of SCI (Table 79-5).

A *complete* injury is defined as the absence of sensory or motor function in the lowest sacral segments, and *incomplete* injury defined as preservation of motor function or sensation below the NLI that includes the lowest sacral segments (termed *sacral sparing*). Sacral sparing is tested by light touch and pin sensation at the anal mucocutaneous junction (S4/5 dermatome), on both sides, as well as testing voluntary anal contraction and deep anal sensation as part of the rectal examination. If any of these are present, whether intact or impaired, the individual has sacral sparing and therefore an incomplete injury.

There were three main revisions to the standards in 2000 (53). First there was clarification that for an individual to receive an ASIA classification of "motor incomplete" (ASIA C or D), the patient must have either (a) voluntary anal sphincter contraction or (b) have sensory sacral sparing with sparing of motor function more than three levels below the motor level. Previously, an individual only needed to have sparing more than two levels below the motor level. Secondly, the *zone of partial preservation* (ZPP) should only be recorded as the most caudal segment with some sensory or motor function bilaterally, rather than all areas spared. Lastly, in the 2000 revision, the Functional Independence Measure (FIM) was eliminated from the standards.

Incomplete Spinal Cord Injury Syndromes

Incomplete SCI syndromes include central cord, Brown-Sequard, anterior cord, conus medullaris, and cauda equina syndromes. The most common of the incomplete syndromes is central cord syndrome (CCS), which applies almost exclusively to cervical injuries and is characterized by motor weakness in the upper extremities greater than the lower extremities, in association with sacral sparing (54). Bladder dysfunction and varying sensory loss below the level of the lesion may also be present. CCS most frequently occurs in older persons with cervical spondylosis who suffer a hyperextension injury, but may occur in persons of any age and is associated with other etiologies, predisposing factors, and injury mechanisms. The postulated mechanism of injury involves compression of the cord both anteriorly and posteriorly by degenerative changes of the bony structures, with inward bulging of the ligamentum flavum during hyperextension in an already narrowed spinal canal (55).

CCS usually has a favorable prognosis. Recovery occurs earliest and to the greatest extent in the lower extremities, followed by bowel and bladder function, proximal upper extremity, and then distal hand function. Prognosis for functional recovery of ambulation, activities of daily living (ADLs), and bowel and bladder function is dependent upon the patient's age (less than or greater than 50 years of age), with a less optimistic prognosis in older patients relative to younger patients (56–58). Older, newly injured individuals however, with a classification of ASIA D tetraplegia, have a good prognosis for recovery of independent ambulation (58).

Brown-Sequard syndrome (BSS) involves a hemisection of the spinal cord, consisting of asymmetric paresis with hypalgesia more marked on the less paretic side and accounts for 2% to 4% of all traumatic SCIs (59–61). In the classic presentation of BSS, there is (a) ipsilateral loss of all sensory modalities at the level of the lesion; (b) ipsilateral flaccid paralysis at the level of the lesion; (c) ipsilateral loss of position sense and vibration below the lesion; (d) contralateral loss of pain and temperature below the lesion; and (e) ipsilateral motor loss below the level of the lesion. This is due to the crossing of the spinothalamic tracts in the spinal cord, as opposed to the corticospinal and dorsal columns that cross in the brainstem. The pure form of BSS is rare; Brown-Sequard plus syndrome (BSPS) is much more common (62) and refers to a relative ipsilateral hemiplegia with a relative contralateral hemianalgesia. Although BSS has traditionally been associated with knife injuries, a variety of etiologies, including those that result in closed spinal injuries with or without vertebral fractures may be the cause (62,63).

Recovery usually takes place in the ipsilateral proximal extensors and then the distal flexors (64,65). Motor recovery of any extremity having a pain/temperature sensory deficit occurs before the opposite extremity and these patients may expect functional gait recovery by 6 months. Overall, patients with BSS have the greatest prognosis for functional outcome and potential for ambulation of the incomplete syndromes, as 75% to 90% of patients ambulate independently at discharge from rehabilitation and nearly 70% perform functional skills and ADLs independently (60,62). Recovery of bowel and bladder function is also favorable.

The *anterior cord syndrome* involves a lesion affecting the anterior two-thirds of the spinal cord while preserving the posterior columns. It may occur with retropulsed disc or bone fragments (66), direct injury to the anterior spinal cord, or with lesions of the anterior spinal artery which provides the blood supply to the anterior spinal cord (67). There is a variable loss of motor as well as pinprick sensation with a relative preservation of light touch, proprioception, and deep-pressure sensation. Patients usually have a 10% to 20% chance of muscle recovery (68).

CONUS MEDULLARIS AND CAUDA EQUINA INJURIES

The conus medullaris, which is the terminal segment of the adult spinal cord, lies at the inferior aspect of the L1 vertebrae. The segment above the conus medullaris is termed the *epiconus*, consisting of spinal cord segments L4-S1. Lesions of the epiconus will affect the lower lumbar roots supplying muscles of the lower part of the leg and foot, with sparing of reflex function of sacral segments. The bulbocavernosus reflex and micturition reflexes are preserved, representing an upper motor neuron (UMN) or suprasacral lesion. Spasticity will most likely develop in sacral innervated segments (toe flexors, ankle plantarflexors, and hamstring muscles). Recovery is similar to other UMN SCIs.

Conus medullaris lesions affecting neural segments S2 and below will present with lower motor neuron (LMN) deficits of the anal sphincter and bladder due to damage of the anterior horn cells of S2-S4. Bladder and rectal reflexes are diminished or absent, depending on the exact level and extent of the lesion. Motor strength in the legs and feet may remain intact if the nerve roots (L3-S2) are not affected (i.e., "root escape").

Injuries below the L1 vertebral level usually affect the cauda equina or nerve rootlets supplying the lumbar and sacral segments producing motor weakness and atrophy of the lower extremities (L2-S2) with bowel and bladder involvement (S2-S4), and areflexia of the ankle and plantar reflexes. Often the patient may have spared sensation in the perineum or lower extremities, but still have paralysis. In cauda equina injuries there is loss of anal and bulbovernosus reflexes, as well as impotence. Cauda equina injuries have a better prognosis for recovery most likely due to the fact that the nerve roots are more resilient to injury. Cauda equina injuries may represent a neuropraxia or axonotmesis and demonstrate progressive recovery over a course of weeks and months. As the cauda equina rootlets are histologically peripheral nerves, regeneration can occur.

Separation of cauda equina and conus lesions in clinical practice is difficult, because some of the clinical features of these lesions overlap. Pain is uncommon in conus lesions but is frequently a complaint in cauda equina lesions. Sensory abnormalities occur in a saddle distribution in conus lesions and, if there is sparing, there is usually dissociated loss with a greater loss of pain and temperature while sparing touch sensation. In cauda equina lesions, sensory loss occurs more in a root distribution and is not dissociated.

THE FUNCTIONAL EVALUATION

Numerous attempts have been made to correlate impairment with disability in SCI. The most commonly used disability measures in SCI are the Functional Independence Measure (FIM), the Modified Barthel Index (MBI), and the Quadriplegia Index of Function (QIF) (69–71). A review of the scales and their reliability and validity have been covered elsewhere (49, 72). The Craig Handicap and Reporting Technique (CHART) is an excellent measure of handicap (limitation of activity) for individuals with SCI (73,74).

The FIM is highly predictive of hours of assistance received by individuals after discharge from inpatient rehabilitation, but the cognitive domain may be inappropriate for use in SCI (75,76). While the FIM was added to the *Standards* in 1992, it was removed in the 2000 revisions (53). There is good correlation between a seven-item short version and the total motor FIM for persons with SCI (77). The QIF is more sensitive and a better indicator of motor recovery as compared to the FIM, since it can reflect small gains in function that parallel small strength gains (78). Another scale described is the Capabilities of Upper Extremity instrument (CUE) that measures upper extremity functional limitations in individuals with tetraplegia (79).

To more precisely measure physical assistance and devices required for walking after SCI, the Walking Index for Spinal Cord Injury (WISCI) has been developed and has shown good validity and reliability (80,81). This is currently being used in research studies.

PROGNOSTICATING RECOVERY AFTER TRAUMATIC SPINAL CORD INJURY

Fundamental to predicting outcome is the knowledge and skill of performing an accurate examination based on the International Standards. The use of radiological and neurophysiological tests can aid and supplement in the diagnosis and prognosis for recovery (82–84). The keys to prognosticating recovery from traumatic SCI depend on the initial level of injury, the initial strength of the muscles, and most importantly, whether the injury is complete or incomplete as determined by physical examination. While the initial examination establishes a baseline, testing over a period of days and at 72 hours is superior to a single early examination (85). Vertebral displacement of less than 30% and age under 30 years at the time of injury is associated with improved recovery (86). No correlation has been found between other variables such as the degree of vertebral wedging or type of fracture. The etiology of the injury only plays a role in determining whether the injury is more likely to be neurologically complete or not (87). The types of injuries that are more likely to cause a complete injury include bilateral cervical facet dislocation, thoracolumbar flexion/rotation injuries, and transcanal bullet locations.

TABLE 79-6.   Summary of Recovery in Complete Tetraplegia

A. Patients (30%–80%) regain one motor level from 1 wk to 1 y.
B. At 72 h to 1 wk, recovery of the next motor level to at least 3/5 at 1 y depends on the motor level and initial strength:
   Approximately 30%–40% of first 0/5 muscles
   70%–90% of muscles 1 or 2/5
   Presence of sensation at that level increases chances of recovery
C. At 1 mo . . . recovery at 1 y:
   Greater than 95% of 1 or 2/5 muscles recover to 3/5
   50%–60% of first 0/5 muscles recover to 1/5
   Approximately 25% of first 0/5 muscles recover to 3/5
   Less than 10% of second 0/5 muscles recover to 1/5
   Approximately 1% of second 0/5 muscles recovers to 3/5
D. The initial strength of the muscle is a significant predictor of achieving antigravity strength and its rate of recovery.
E. The faster an initial 0/5 muscle starts to recover some strength, the better the prognosis for recovery.
F. Most upper extremity recovery occurs during the first 6 mos, with the greatest rate of change during the first 3 mos.
G. Most patients with some initial power plateau at an earlier time and at a higher level than patients with no motor power. Motor recovery can continue, with lesser gains seen in the second year, especially for patients with initially 0/5 strength.

From Ditunno J, Flanders A, Kirshblum SC, et al. Predicting outcome in traumatic spinal cord injury. In: Kirshblum SC, Campagnolo D, DeLisa JE, eds. *Spinal cord medicine.* Philadelphia: Lippincott Williams & Wilkins, 2002:108–122.

Complete Tetraplegia

It has frequently been stated that patients with complete cervical lesions recover one root level of function (88). Table 79-6 lists certain generalizations regarding recovery patterns in patients with complete tetraplegia. The initial strength of a muscle is a significant predictor of achieving antigravity strength at the level caudal to the NLI, as well as the rate of recovering antigravity strength (89,90). The faster recovery begins the greater the chance of recovering antigravity strength (91). Recovery at the C4 level to the C5 level, both motor and sensory, may be less and slower than at the lower cervical segments, especially if there is initially no strength at the C5 myotome (76,92).

Most upper extremity (UE) motor recovery occurs during the first 6 months after injury, with the greatest rate of change during the initial 3 months. Overall, the mean total motor score improvement for persons with complete tetraplegia between 1 and 6 months postinjury is 6.6 ± 4.7; between 1 month and 1 year, 8.6 ± 4.7; and during the second year, 1.7 ± 1.9 (90). In patients with no motor strength at the first caudal level, recovery may continue for up to 2 years after injury (92). Only a small percentage of subjects have motor recovery below the first caudal level from the NLI (90).

Incomplete Tetraplegia

Persons with incomplete tetraplegia have a better prognosis for recovery. UE motor recovery is approximately twice as great as in complete tetraplegia, with the potential for varying degrees of lower extremity (LE) motor recovery and functional ambulation. For patients who are sensory incomplete initially, the prognosis for motor recovery is more favorable in those with sparing of pin sensation rather than light touch sensation alone. Studies using the Frankel Scale found that for Frankel B patients with pin sensation initially intact, the prognosis for

ambulation is 66% to 89%, while for those with only light touch intact it was 11% to 14% (93–95). The basis of a more favorable outcome for pinprick sparing in the initially sensory incomplete patient may be explained by the close anatomical relationship of the motor tracts (mediated through the lateral corticospinal tract), which are just dorsal to the sensory tracts (lateral spinothalamic tract) carrying pain and temperature fibers. A sensory incomplete motor complete patient (ASIA B) at 1 month may still regain LE muscle recovery if bilateral sacral pin sensation is present, although the prognosis for community ambulation is poor (96). Functional and neurological recovery is more favorable for patients with an initial motor incomplete injury (93–98).

For UE motor recovery, the total motor score improvement from 1 month to 1 year is 10.6 ± 6.9, with improvement in the second year of 1.1 ± 2.3 (96). The majority of functional recovery is within the first 6 months after injury and the early appearance of motor function suggests a better functional outcome (85,94,96,98). A greater percentage of key muscles recover antigravity strength or better, as well as earlier, distal to the NLI in individuals with motor incomplete tetraplegia than in those with motor complete injuries (99,100). The mean LE motor recovery in incomplete tetraplegics is 13.5 ± 7 from 1 month to 1 year and 1.8 ± 3.1 in the second year (96). Motor recovery in the UE and LE occur concurrently, rather than sequentially.

Complete Paraplegia

Recovery from injuries resulting in paraplegia has not been studied to the same degree of tetraplegia. For persons with a complete injury with a NLI at T8 or above, Waters and colleagues found that none regained any LE motor function. The potential for LE motor recovery improves with lower initial neurological levels of injury; 15% of patients with an NLI between T9-T11 and 55% of those with an initial NLI below T12 gain some recovery. Most movement gained is in the proximal LE musculature (101). This improvement may represent recovery of partially injured lumbar roots or "root escape" (102).

Incomplete Paraplegia

Individuals with incomplete paraplegia have the best prognosis for LE motor recovery and ambulation (103,104). Eighty percent of individuals with incomplete paraplegia regain antigravity hip flexors and knee extensors at 1 year. Individuals with no LE strength at 1 month may still show significant return by 1 year.

Conversion from Complete to Incomplete Status

While it has been reported that up to 10% of patients with an initial Frankel A classification can progress to Frankel D or E, Maynard and associates prospectively demonstrated that subjects with this degree of change had sustained closed head injuries with cognitive impairment and were incorrectly initially diagnosed as Frankel A (105). Model systems data report that up to 16% of initially neurological complete (Frankel or ASIA A) patients improve at least one classification grade, from initial early examination to the 1-year follow-up, but only up to 5.8% improve to grade C and 3% improve to grade D (76,106). Marino and colleagues reported a small difference when using the Frankel and the ASIA Impairment scales (106).

Between 4% to 10% of patients may undergo late conversion (after 30 days) from complete to incomplete status which has been reported to occur years after injury (90,107,108). Motor recovery seems to be slightly improved and some, usually nonfunctional LE recovery, may take place.

The Effect of Reflexes

The presence of spinal shock may play a role in prognosis; for the same degree of SCI the presence of spinal shock implies a more rapid evolution of injury and a worse prognosis (109). In individual lesions, especially in high level cervical SCI, the most distal sacral reflexes, including the bulbocavernosus (BC) and anal wink, may remain intact.

The order that reflexes return in the postinjury period may help prognosticate outcome (110). The lack of the BC reflex (S3–4 roots) or the anal reflex (S2–4 roots) after the acute period (24 to 72 hours) suggests injury to the conus medullaris or cauda equina (i.e., LMN injury). As such, prognosis regarding recovery and also the potential use of rehabilitation intervention (e.g., electrical stimulation) can be determined. The delayed plantar response, which may be the first of all reflexes to return, occurs within hours or days following SCI, and shows a high correlation with complete injuries and a poor prognosis for LE motor recovery and function (ambulation) (110,111).

Magnetic Resonance Imaging in Predicting Outcome

Numerous studies have shown a direct correlation between the appearance of the spinal cord on MRI and the degree of functional deficit at the time of injury and the capacity for neurological recovery. Overall, the findings on MRI that correspond to a more severe initial injury and have a poor prognosis for neurological recovery include the presence and length of hemorrhage, the length of spinal cord edema, and spinal cord compression. An intramedullary hemorrhage equates with a severe initial neurological deficit, most commonly ASIA A (complete) injury on clinical examination, and carries a poor prognosis (83,112–114). The location of the hemorrhage corresponds anatomically to the level of the neurological injury. If no hemorrhage is seen on initial MRI, these individuals usually have an incomplete lesion by clinical exam and have a better prognosis for motor and functional recovery. Cord edema alone is associated with mild to moderate initial deficits. Cord edema that extends for more than the span of one vertebral segment is associated with a more severe initial injury than smaller areas of edema (114,115).

In the chronic stage after SCI, persons with persistent signal changes in their spinal cord on follow-up MRI exams demonstrate little improvement in ASIA grades relative to the improvements of patients with resolution of signal abnormalities.

Electrophysiological Tests

A number of electrophysiological tests have been used in the acute period after SCI to assess the level and severity of the SCI, as well as to prognosticate neurological and functional outcome. Techniques include nerve conduction studies, late responses (H-reflex and F-wave), somatosensory evoked potentials (SSEPs), motor evoked potentials (MEPs), and sympathetic skin responses (SSRs), all of which can supplement clinical and neuroradiological examinations (83). These tests, however, are most useful in differentiating lesions of the central and peripheral nervous systems and in uncooperative or unconscious patients, since they do not require the cooperation

of the patient. They are not recommended as a routine part of the acute workup of a newly injured individual to offer prognosis for neurological or functional outcome.

Recordings of lower extremity SSEPs enable differentiation between complete and incomplete lesions (116). SSEP recordings are not influenced by spinal shock or by the patient's level of consciousness (117). A return of the early SSEP components in the initial stage after SCI can proceed to clinically detectable improvements of motor or sensory function (118). The presence of an SSEP recording is not always associated with motor recovery since the SSEP represents spared sensory fibers of the posterior columns, while motor activity depends on the functioning of the anterior and anterolateral spinal cord. While many studies have found that SSEPs are no more effective for prognosticating outcome than a proper examination, others report prognostication benefits in terms of gait and hand function (119,120). SSEPs may be especially helpful in an unresponsive or uncooperative patient to determine if they have an SCI, and in the differentiation between SCI and conversion reaction (121,122).

Cortical stimulation examines the corticospinal tract by recording from different peripheral muscles. In neurological complete injuries, MEPs are absent in muscles below the level of injury, whereas in incomplete injuries MEPs can usually be elicited but may be delayed (123,124). MEPs can be used to document the level of injury in the UEs and help predict mobility and ADL function.

Violence-Related Spinal Cord Injury

Individuals with violence-related SCI are typically younger, more likely to be a non–high school graduate from a lower socioeconomic status, and have a higher unemployment rate than other SCI patients at the time of injury (125). GSWs typically result in paraplegia (75%) with an almost equal incidence of complete versus incomplete injuries (which is a higher percentage than from other causes), with most injuries occurring in the thoracic region (125,126). There is increased initial morbidity and mortality associated with GSWs (127). Based on the initial level and severity of the injury, patients with violence-related injuries have a shorter length of hospital stay, with higher admission and discharge FIM scores, but do not have a significant difference in outcome or in discharge to home rates relative to nonviolence-related injuries (90,127–129).

Nontraumatic Spinal Cord Injury

Nontraumatic SCI (NT/SCI) includes such etiologies as spinal stenosis with myelopathy, spinal cord compression from a neoplasm, multiple sclerosis (MS), transverse myelitis, infection (viral, bacterial, fungal, parasitic), vascular ischemia, radiation myelopathy, motor neuron diseases, syringomyelia, vitamin B_{12} deficiency, and others. A significant proportion of SCI rehabilitation admissions are of nontraumatic etiology, primarily due to myelopathy resulting from spinal stenosis and neoplastic spinal cord compression (SCC) (130).

As opposed to those with traumatic-related SCI, individuals with NT/SCI are more likely to be older, female, married, and retired. While traumatic causes are more common in patients under 40 years of age, NT/SCI is more common than trauma in persons over 40. Persons with NT/SCI usually have a less severe neurological impairment as compared with traumatic SCI, as they more often present with paraplegia (73% versus 27% tetraplegia) and with motor incomplete (90% versus 10% complete) lesions (131). This is related to the location of spinal involvement, as tumors tend to involve the thoracic and lumbar regions more than the cervical region.

A comparison of secondary medical complications reveals a significantly lower incidence of spasticity, orthostasis, deep vein thrombosis (DVT), pressure ulcers, autonomic dysreflexia, and wound infections during rehabilitation in patients with NT/SCI (132). However, because cervical stenosis and neoplastic SCC has a peak incidence between the ages of 50 to 70 years, these individuals may have other premorbid medical issues that may impact their rehabilitation. No difference was seen for depression, urinary tract infections, heterotopic ossification, pain, and gastrointestinal bleeds (132).

Comprehensive rehabilitation is justified for persons with NT/SCI with definable goals. Studies report a shorter rehabilitation length of stay (LOS) and lower discharge FIM scores, FIM change, and rehabilitation charges. No statistical differences were found in acute care LOS, admission FIM scores, FIM efficiency, and community discharge rates (131,133–136).

ACUTE MEDICAL ISSUES AFTER SPINAL CORD INJURY

Orthostatic Hypotension

Orthostatic hypotension commonly occurs when the individual with an acute SCI is mobilized from bed. It is defined as a sudden drop in systolic blood pressure (BP) of at least 20 mm Hg or diastolic BP by at least 10 mm Hg within 3 minutes of standing upright or 60 degrees on a tilt table (137). Associated symptoms include lightheadedness, dizziness, ringing of the ears, fatigue, tachycardia, and sometimes syncope, all of which can last for several weeks to months, delaying the rehabilitative process as the patient is given time to acclimate to the upright position. Orthostatic hypotension occurs more frequently in persons with cervical level or neurologically complete injuries. When bedrest is prolonged, the degree of orthostasis tends to be more severe (138). Orthostatic hypotension intensifies after eating, exposure to hot environments, defecation, and rapid bladder emptying (139).

Orthostasis is caused by pooling of venous blood in the LEs and splanchnic vessels in the abdomen after positional changes (140). Carotid and aortic baroreceptors perceive the fall in BP and reduce tonic impulses that travel via the vagus and glossopharyngeal nerves to the medulla. The medullary vasomotor control center stimulates the sympathetic nervous system to release norepinephrine and epinephrine which causes vasoconstriction of the vessels to compensate for the venous pooling. In individuals with a lesion above T6, the efferent pathways to the splanchnic vessels and LEs are interrupted and the sympathetic response is diminished. In addition, plasma catecholamine release is significantly diminished in persons with tetraplegia, with changes in position (138).

Habituation to the symptoms of orthostatic hypotension occurs slowly, although the BP rarely returns to preinjury values. The exact mechanism is unknown, but theories include increased sensitivity of baroreceptors and catecholamine receptors in the vessel walls, development of spasticity, improved autoregulation of cerebral vascular perfusion, and adaptations of the renin-angiotensin system (141).

Physical methods, including compression wraps to the legs and an abdominal binder donned prior to sitting up help to prevent venous distension, should be tried first to mitigate orthostatic hypotension. Repeated postural changes on a tilt table or a high back reclining wheelchair also lessens the drop in BP. However, repeated postural changes are often insufficient by themselves, making pharmacological treatment necessary. Sodium chloride, 1 g qid, can be started to increase intravascular volume. Midodrine hydrochloride, a sympathomimetic agent that acts at the α_1-receptor of arterioles and veins to raise BP, can be given and reaches peak plasma concentrations levels in 1 hour. The initial dose of 2.5 mg is given tid and titrated as needed with avoidance of nighttime dosing because of the risk of supine hypertension (142). Ephedrine, an α- and β-agonist, is not as effective as midodrine in maintaining BP after autonomic failure (143). Fludrocortisone is a mineralocorticoid that promotes sodium and fluid retention in the renal distal tubule. The starting dose is 0.05 to 0.1 mg daily but can be increased to 0.4 mg. Several authors have also noted a rise in BP with functional electrical stimulation (144,145).

Autonomic Dysreflexia

Autonomic dysreflexia (AD), also known as autonomic hyperreflexia, paroxysmal hypertension, and hypertensive autonomic crisis, is a composite of symptoms, most notably a sudden rise in BP, seen in those with SCI due to autonomic dysfunction. It is restricted to those with injuries at or above T6, although patients with injuries down to T8 have been reported. Individuals who are neurologically complete and at higher levels of injury are apt to have more severe symptoms (146). The incidence in susceptible patients varies between 48% to 90%, but rarely presents within the first month after injury, and nearly all patients who will develop AD will do so within the first year (146–148).

AD is caused by a noxious stimulus below the level of injury. The most common source is from the bladder, either from overdistension or infection, followed by fecal impaction. These account for over 80% of all cases. Other causes include pressure ulcers, ingrown toenails, abdominal emergencies, fractures, and body positioning. In females, AD can occur during labor and delivery (149,150). The stimulus travels via the peripheral nerves to the spinal cord and as it ascends in the spinothalamic tracts and dorsal columns, sympathetic neurons in the intermediolateral cell columns are stimulated. Splanchnic vessels, which are innervated by nerves originating from T5-L2, constrict in response to the release of norepinephrine, dopamine, and dopamine-β-hydroxylase and raise the BP. The hypertension from AD is defined as a rise of 20 to 40 mm Hg above baseline (149,151). Symptoms include a headache that is pounding in nature and found in the frontal and occipital areas, sweating, and flushing above level of lesion.

Baroreceptors from the carotid sinus and aortic arch detect the elevated BP and relay impulses to the vasomotor center in the brain stem, which in turn tries to compensate by slowing the heart rate via impulses through the vagus nerve. Signals meant to inhibit the sympathetic system are blocked at the spinal cord lesion.

Since AD does not occur immediately after SCI, loss of supraspinal inhibition alone cannot be the sole mechanism. Resting catecholamine levels are lower in tetraplegics, but there is an exaggerated BP response when challenged with exogenous catecholamine administration (152). Dopamine hydroxylase, an enzyme that converts dopamine to norepinephrine, also is low in nerve terminals in tetraplegics. This suggests that denervation hypersensitivity of the sympathetic receptors occur after SCI (153).

Signs and symptoms reflect sympathetic overflow and the consequent compensatory reaction mediated by the parasympathetic nervous system. The sympathetic discharge causes hypertension and piloerection. The parasympathetic response causes headache, pupillary constriction, sinus congestion, profuse perspiration above the injury level, and bradycardia. More serious and even life-threatening symptoms may occur including cardiac arrhythmias, seizures, intracranial hemorrhage, pulmonary edema, and myocardial infarction (154).

AD requires immediate attention, with the goal to remove the inciting stimulus and reduce the BP. In 2000, the second edition of the clinical practice guideline on the management of AD was published (151). The BP and pulse should be monitored every 2 to 5 minutes until stabilized. A rapid survey of the patient for the causes should be initiated. The patient should sit upright with loosening of all tight fitting clothes. The bladder should be checked for overdistension by flushing an indwelling catheter if one is present or catheterizing those without one. If the catheter is blocked, gentle irrigation with a small amount of fluid at body temperature is used. If available, Xylocaine gel (2%) should be used prior to catheterization. If the bladder was the source, the BP should quickly return to baseline. If the pressure remains elevated (i.e., systolic BP greater than 150 mm Hg), pharmacological management should be considered prior to checking for fecal impaction. Again, Xylocaine gel within the anorectal area should be placed prior to this. If impaction is not present, other possible sources should then be sought, including pressure ulcers, ingrown toenails, infections, fractures, DVT, and heterotopic ossification.

Pharmacological agents that have been used for AD include nitrate gels, nifedipine, clonidine, terazosin, β-blockers, phenoxybenzamine, hydralazine, and chlorpromazine. The use of nitrates is beneficial as they can be easily applied, titrated, and removed immediately if a source is later found. The BP should be monitored frequently because application of too much paste can cause severe hypotension. The individual should be monitored for recurrent symptoms for at least 2 hours after resolution of the AD episode to ensure that it does not recur (151).

Respiratory

Respiratory complications are the leading cause of death for patients with traumatic SCI (24,155,156). The major respiratory problems after acute SCI include secretion management, atelectasis, and hypoventilation. These are due to deficits in both inspiration and the ability to produce an effective cough. Management therefore is related directly to these problems—assisting the patient to mobilize their secretions, stabilizing the alveoli, and inflating and increasing the compliance of the lungs and chest wall.

The three main sets of muscles involved in inspiration include the diaphragm, external intercostals (thoracic innervation), and accessory muscles including the scalenes, sternocleidomastoid, trapezius and pectoralis muscles. The diaphragm, the major muscle of inspiration, is innervated by the phrenic nerve (C3-C5 root levels), and contributes to 65% of the vital capacity (VC) in able-bodied individuals (157). The muscles of expiration include mainly the abdominal muscles (innervated segmentally from T6-L1 root levels), the recti, obliques, and the transversus abdominis. These muscles increase intraabdominal pressure that moves the diaphragm superiorly during high effort expirations and cough.

Patients with an NLI above T12 are at risk for some degree of respiratory dysfunction; the higher the level of injury, the greater the potential deficits. Patients with a complete NLI of C2 and above will have no function of the diaphragm, and will need some type of ventilatory assistance immediately. Those with a C3 or C4 NLI have a good potential to wean from the ventilator if initially required (158). Individuals with an NLI at or below C5 are usually able to breathe without assistance, but may develop difficulty soon after injury due to secretions, at-

electasis, infection, or pulmonary trauma. Vigorous preventive measures with close monitoring are extremely important for these patients.

Persons with SCI typically have a restrictive pulmonary syndrome, with a decrease in all lung volumes except the residual volume (RV), which increases. The VC in the newly injured individual with tetraplegia is reduced between 24% to 31% of predicted normal (159,160) but improves due to increased strength and the development of intercostal and abdominal tone that stabilizes the rib cage and enhances the mechanical effect of the diaphragm (160,161). The typical functional loss of VC in persons with a complete motor lesion at C5 and above who are not ventilator-dependent, is roughly one-half; for C6-C8, approximately one-third; T1-T7, only slightly below the lower limits of normal; and for low paraplegia, only slightly below predicted norms (162–164).

A retrospective review reported that 67% of acute injured individuals experienced some respiratory complication during the initial hospitalization that included atelectasis (36%), pneumonia (31%), and respiratory failure (22.6%) (165). All levels of injury were at risk; 84% of patients with an NLI between C1-C4; 60% of patients between C5-C8; and 65% of those with thoracic level injuries. There is a greater incidence of acute complications with increasing age, higher level of injury, and complete tetraplegia (24,166). Respiratory complications during the acute and initial rehabilitation hospitalizations are associated with increased likelihood of requiring mechanical ventilation, which in turn are associated with lower functional status, greater probability of nursing home placement, greater medical costs, and the potential for decrements in survival and perceived quality of life (167,168).

The VC is the most useful parameter to monitor and should be closely followed over the first few days in persons with high-level cervical injuries, at least every 4 to 8 hours, as immobilization of the patient may predispose to atelectasis and difficulty in clearing secretions. For patients requiring assisted ventilation, arterial blood gases are needed acutely, and then when making changes to the ventilator settings or if there is a change in the medical status of the individual.

Chest physiotherapy, if the stability of the spine is not in question, should be used, as well as a method of secretion management (i.e., suctioning and assisted cough techniques). The "quad cough", is a type of assisted cough technique; a forceful push on the upper abdomen at the end of a deep inspiration. Due to possible displacement of an inferior vena cava (IVC) filter, it is best to not use "quad coughing" in patients who have had a new IVC filter placed (169,170). Mechanical insufflation-exsufflation (MI-E) is the delivery of a deep insufflation (positive pressure) to the airway that is immediately followed by an exsufflation (negative pressure), producing a high expiratory flow rate from the lungs, simulating a cough. This can be used either via tracheostomy, face mask, or mouthpiece. Patients with SCI reported that the MI-E was significantly less irritating, painful, tiring, and uncomfortable than endotracheal suctioning, and overwhelmingly preferred MI-E to suctioning (171). The advantages of MI-E over suctioning in addition to the comfort is that it can better clear secretions from the left side and larger mucous plugs can be removed. The left main stem bronchus branches off at an angle, and the suction catheter has difficulty clearing secretions from this side. This may account for the high frequency of pneumonia in the left lower lobe.

Bronchoscopy may initially be needed to help in removing secretions; however, it should be performed in association with attempts to inflate the lung. Without inflating the lungs, secretions will reaccumulate. If repeated bronchoscopies are required, the patient may require assisted ventilation or some other method to expand the lungs. Interventions that can be used include intermittent positive pressure breathing (IPPB) with or without nebulizer treatments, intrapulmonary percussive ventilation (IPV), or use of a flutter valve.

In contrast to non-SCI patients, those with cervical and high thoracic level injuries have a reduction in VC of about half in the sitting position as compared to the supine position (164, 172,173). This reduction is clinically useful as weaning should be initiated in the supine position, and allowed in the sitting position only after the patient is able to tolerate 1 hour off of the ventilator. The loss in VC in the upright position may be partially corrected by the use of an abdominal binder or corset (173,174).

The use of inspiratory resistance muscle training, abdominal weights, and incentive spirometry (175–179) can improve pulmonary function. Glossopharyngeal breathing (GPB) is a technique that involves rapidly taking small gulps, 6 to 9 gulps of 60 to 200 cc each, and using the tongue and pharyngeal muscles to project the air past the glottis into the lungs. Many patients can use this technique to augment VC to assist with coughing or prolong ventilator-free time (180).

Medications and respiratory treatments are often used after SCI. Because mobilizing secretions is a problem, *mucolytics* are frequently indicated. *Theophylline* medications relax smooth muscle, stimulate the medullary respiratory centers, help stimulate the release of surfactant, may improve diaphragmatic contractility and reduce diaphragmatic fatigue. Patients with tetraplegia have unopposed parasympathetic innervation, and therefore may benefit from the administration of both short-acting and long-acting β-agonist inhaled medications. The use of β-agonists act to offset the unopposed parasympathetic stimulation found in patients with cervical injuries, reduce inflammation, and stimulate the secretion of surfactant.

Criteria for intubation include intractable atelectasis, hypoxemia, or hypercapnia not responsive to noninvasive efforts including continuous positive airway pressure (CPAP) or bilevel positive airway pressure (BIPAP), and rapid shallow breathing with persistent tachycardia or fever related to pneumonia. If the patient requires prolonged ventilation it is best to proceed with a tracheostomy if noninvasive means of ventilation are not an option. Advantages of the tracheostomy tube over the endotracheal tube include less chance of damage to the vocal cords; easier to clear secretions; ability to deflate the tracheostomy tube cuff to allow speech; and ability of the patient to eat. Noninvasive positive pressure ventilation (NIPPV) is an alternative to intubation at centers with experience in these techniques and can be delivered via oral, nasal, or oronasal interfaces (181,182). The benefits of noninvasive ventilation include a decreased risk of infection and tracheomalacia, and greater discharge to home (183). Persons who are not alert, are not medically stable, or have brain stem injury are not candidates for NIPPV.

Persons requiring mechanical ventilation have a high mortality rate, although greater numbers are surviving the initial injury and have greater life spans than in years past. The 1-year survival for initially ventilated patients was approximately half of the 1-year survival for the total admissions to the model systems facilities. For patients who survive the first year on the ventilator, the 15-year survival rate was reported to be 61.4% (167).

Ventilation should be given initially at a tidal volume from 8 to 10 m/kg of ideal body weight and some suggest the volumes to be adjusted upward, while closely monitoring the patient pressures. Higher tidal volumes will result in faster clearing of atelectasis and a better result in weaning off the ventilator (184). Oxygen should only be used as a temporary measure, as most patients have healthy lungs. If the oxygen saturation is low, the patient is usually not being ventilated at a high enough volume, or the patient has secretions that need to be cleared.

Weaning is usually attempted when the patient has a VC approximating 10 mL/kg body weight (185). A weaning protocol has been outlined elsewhere (158,186,187). It is recommended to wean patients using the progressive free breathing technique (PFB), as in comparison to synchronized intermittent mandatory ventilation (SIMV) (158). Advantages include the ability for the patient to rest in between trials, to gradually build up strength, and to maintain expansion of the lungs in between the weaning trials. Another approach to weaning is using noninvasive means of ventilation after extubating or decanulating the patient. This can be performed by having patients wean themselves off the ventilator by taking fewer assisted breaths as the need is felt (188).

Only a few studies report on phrenic nerve pacing in SCI. Full-time use of pacing is seen in approximately 33% of patients who undergo the procedure (188–190). Criteria for use include an injury at or above C2 with intact phrenic nerves as tested by percutaneous stimulation. Other procedures are available for persons with partial damage to the phrenic nerve. Newer less invasive techniques are being developed (191).

Immobilization Hypercalcemia

After acute immobilization, calciuria increases within 2 weeks, reaching a maximum between 1 to 6 months after injury. Hypercalcemia can occur after SCI when bone resorption is increased in association with an impaired fractional excretion of calcium by the kidney. Risk factors for the development of hypercalcemia include multiple fractures, age under 18 because of high rate of bone turnover, male gender, high level lesion, complete neurological injury, prolonged immobilization, and dehydration (192). Ingesting a high-calcium diet does not increase either urinary or serum calcium concentration (193).

Symptoms of immobilization hypercalcemia usually present between 1 to 2 months postinjury but may occur up to 6 months later. These usually include acute onset of nausea, vomiting, anorexia, lethargy, polydipsia, polyuria, or dehydration. For diagnosis, a serum calcium level should be evaluated, with correction for a low serum albumin if present. Ionized calcium can also be measured.

Treatment consists of intravenous fluid (normal saline at 100 to 150 cc/hour), as tolerated to increase calcium excretion. A Foley catheter is recommended due to the volume of fluid being administered. Once the patient is hydrated, furosemide may be given to enhance calcium secretion, but its use is controversial. Other medications that have been used include calcitonin, etidronate, and glucocorticoids (192,194). Pamidronate (30 to 90 mg i.v.) has been reported to be effective, with advantages of only requiring one dose, and has a rapid onset (195, 196). A repeat dose may be required. Standing has been reported to decrease hypercalciuria (197,198).

Heterotopic Ossification

Heterotopic ossification (HO) is the formation of lamellar bone within the soft tissue surrounding a joint. Incidence ranges between 13% and 57%, and is usually found in the first 6 months after injury (199,200). Cases can occur beyond 1 year and are usually associated with a newly developed pressure ulcer, DVT, or fracture. Children and adolescents are less susceptible to its formation with an incidence between 3% and 10% (201).

Although the majority of the cases will have only radiological findings and are not clinically significant, approximately 20% will present with a clinical limitation of the range of motion (ROM), with up to 8% progressing to ankylosis. Only joints below the NLI will develop heterotopic bone, with the most common location being the hips (anteromedial aspect), followed by the knees and shoulders. Besides an initial reduction in the ROM, the joint may appear warm and swollen and must therefore be differentiated from a septic joint, cellulitis, DVT, fractures, and inflammatory arthritis. The patient may also experience pain, malaise, low-grade fever, and an increase in spasticity. In severe cases, adjacent neurovascular structures may be compromised leading to distal extremity swelling and nerve entrapment (202).

Laboratory tests are sensitive but are not specific markers for HO. Serum alkaline phosphatase levels start to increase prior to clinical and radiographic presentation, but may not exceed normal levels for several weeks. Because levels do not correlate with the amount or degree of ossification activity, they should not be used to judge maturity of the new bone or predict its recurrence. Urinary excretion of hydroxyproline and collagen metabolites correlates with alkaline phosphatase levels and can also serve as indirect markers for the presence of HO.

Triple-phase technetium-99m bone scans detect HO within 2 weeks of injury. The first two phases of the bone scan measure the increase in blood flow to a joint during the early inflammatory period. The third phase, or static bone phase, is more specific since it measures the incorporation of the radionuclide into the bony matrix but may take another 3 weeks before it is positive (203). Bone scans are also the most useful technique to assess maturity of the heterotopic bone. Plain x-rays become positive approximately 2 to 6 weeks after a triple-phase bone scan first reveals HO or 1 to 10 weeks after clinical presentation (201). Initially there is a white, smoky appearance that later solidifies as the bone matures. Ultrasonography may be positive early and has the advantage of being a relatively inexpensive examination without requiring radiation (204). Finerman and Stover, Brooker, and Garland have proposed different grading systems for HO (205–207).

The mechanism of formation is unknown but involves change of soft-tissue mesenchymal cells to osteogenic precursor cells by humeral, neural, and local factors. Studies conducted *in vitro* have identified a factor called *bone morphogenic protein* that induces bone formation (208). It is also hypothesized that damage to the sympathetic tracts in the spinal cord may promote HO by increasing the local vascularity and blood perfusion around the joint. When passive ROM is delayed more than 1 week after injury, patients are more likely to develop HO (209). It is also possible that forced ROM of contracted limbs may cause microtrauma and bleeding, which ultimately leads to HO (210). Other risk factors for its development include older age, complete lesions, spasticity, DVT, and pressure sores. These risk factors may be cumulative (199,211).

Treatments for HO include passive- and active-assisted ROM with gentle stretching after the acute inflammatory period is over (1 to 2 weeks), nonsteroidal antiinflammatory drugs (NSAIDs) (e.g., indomethacin), bisphosphonates, radiation therapy, and surgical excision. Disodium etidronate inhibits osteoclastic activity and conversion of calcium phosphate to hydroxyapatite. Although the standard treatment is 20 mg/kg/day for 2 weeks and then 10 mg/kg/day for 10 weeks, a higher dose and longer duration of treatment is more beneficial (212). Banovac and colleagues recommend etidronate 300 mg/day i.v. for 3 days followed by oral administration of 20 mg/kg/day for 6 months, and found quicker resolution of edema with less rebound formation after the medication was discontinued (200,213). While 6-month treatment is currently recommended, it is not concluded that higher dosages are beneficial (201). Surgical excision should be reserved for patients with severely limited ROM that causes functional limitations, and most clinicians recommend waiting until after the ectopic bone has been verified to be mature by bone scan. This may take at least 12 to 18 months to occur (201). Complications of surgery include a great deal of blood loss, infection, and recurrent HO. Postoperative treatment includes NSAIDs for at least 6 weeks, bisphosphonates for 3 to 12 months, or radiation. While radiation is frequently used and decreases the degree of recurrence of HO, complications include delayed wound healing, osteonecrosis, and the risk of developing sarcoma (201, 214).

Prophylaxis of HO in SCI patients has been studied using several agents including etidronate and indomethacin, with less HO formation as compared with placebo (215,216). Warfarin may also be an effective agent by inhibiting the formation of osteocalcin (217). Despite the available therapeutic options, prophylaxis is still not routinely used (201,211,218).

Thromboembolic Disorders

Thromboembolic disorders, which include DVT and pulmonary embolism (PE), are common medical complications after SCI, as well as an important cause of morbidity and mortality. The exact incidence after acute SCI unknown, but has been reported to be 47% to 100% (219–224). Unfortunately these prospective studies did not all use similar diagnostic tests, and the subjects had variable degrees of neurological deficits. The development of DVT is low in the first 72 hours, and occurs most frequently during the first 2 weeks (approximately 80% of cases) following injury (219,225). PE has been reported to occur in approximately 5% of patients, and is the third leading cause of death in all SCI patients in the first-year postinjury. Recent reports have found the incidence to be decreasing, possibly secondary to more effective prophylaxis as well as more accurate diagnostic techniques. Model system data reported an incidence of 9.8% for DVT and 2.6% for PE during acute rehabilitation and an incidence of 2.1% and 1% at 1-year and 2-year follow-up (226).

The high incidence of DVT/PE in individuals with SCI is related to Virchow's triad that includes stasis, intimal injury, and hypercoagulability; which are all sequelae of acute neurological injury (227–230). There is a greater risk of DVT in males, in persons with motor complete injuries, and in those with paraplegia relative to tetraplegia (24). The degree or level of injury does not influence the risk of developing a PE. This is important to recognize, as clinicians often choose not to administer prophylaxis to patients with less severe injuries. Older age is a factor in the development of PE, but not for DVT.

Clinical diagnosis (physical examination) of a DVT in individuals with SCI is difficult and unreliable because edema may be present secondary to immobilization and the patient may have loss of sensation. Suspicion should be high, and diagnostic testing ordered to make the proper diagnosis if suspected. Clinical signs of a DVT may include unilateral edema, low-grade fever, and pain in a patient with an incomplete injury. The most common diagnostic procedure is a duplex ultrasound with vein compression, although this is less sensitive in asymptomatic patients (231). The duplex scan is limited due to poor visualization of the veins proximal to the femoral veins, and in diagnosing calf clots. Contrast venography is the gold standard to diagnose a DVT, but is often not used because of the complications of dye allergy, invasiveness, and the possibility of causing phlebitis (232). If a duplex scan is negative, but there remains high suspicion, further radiological testing (e.g., MRI, venogram) should be performed. Clinical signs of a PE may include fever, tachypnea, dyspnea, tachycardia, chest pain, or hypotension. If suspected, a full workup should be initiated and may include a ventilation/perfusion scan, spiral CT, or pulmonary angiogram.

A consortium for the prevention of thromboembolism in SCI recommends that patients receive both a method of mechanical prophylaxis of DVT as well as anticoagulant prophylaxis (233). Pneumatic compressive devices are recommended during the first 2 weeks following injury. If this measure is delayed for more than 72 hours after injury, a duplex scan to exclude the presence of lower limb clots should be performed. The mechanism of action of the pneumatic compression devices is hypothesized to be due to direct expulsion of blood from the LEs but also enhancement of fibrinolytic activity (234). While electrical stimulation has been shown to be effective (235), this is rarely used.

The consortium guidelines recommend anticoagulant prophylaxis should be initiated within 72 hours following SCI provided that there is no active bleeding, evidence of head injury, or coagulopathy. While these guidelines recommend the use of unfractionated heparin (5,000 units s.c. every 8 or 12 hours) or low-molecular-weight heparin (LMWH) used along with compressive devices for motor-incomplete patients, and dose-adjusted unfractionated heparin to keep a high-normal aPTT, or LMWH for motor-complete patients or those with high-risk factors for DVT(233), current recommendations by specialists in SCI are for the use of LMWH, and this is the current practice by most SCI centers in the U.S. While none of the LMWH products are currently approved by the Food and Drug Administration (FDA) for use in SCI, many reports have shown improved effectiveness over standard unfractionated heparin prophylaxis (236–240). Prophylaxis for those with a motor incomplete injury (ASIA C or D) should continue for at least the time they are in the hospital; for those with a motor complete injury (ASIA A or B) they should be continued for 8 to 12 weeks postinjury depending on other risk factors (233). If the patient is discharged before 8 weeks, many clinicians will continue to administer prophylaxis for the full 8- week period. The consortium guidelines also recommend prophylaxis in chronic individuals with SCI who are admitted to the hospital and require immobilization for medical illness or surgical procedures (233).

Vena cava filter placement is recommended in patients who have failed anticoagulant prophylaxis, or who have a contraindication to anticoagulation. Filters should also be considered in individuals with high-level motor complete tetraplegia with poor cardiopulmonary reserve or with thrombosis of the IVC despite anticoagulant prophylaxis. Filter placement is not a substitute for thromboprophylaxis, and may even be a risk factor for the development of a DVT. The prophylactic insertion of filters is increasingly common in high-risk patients with reported low insertion complication rates (241), and lower incidences of PE as compared to historical controls (242,243). Complications of vena cava filters include cava thrombosis, filter migration, perforation of the vena cava, and complications at the skin insertion site (244,245). A prospective study showed that the initial benefits of vena caval filters were counterbalanced by an excess of recurrent DVT, with no difference in mortality (241).

Once the diagnosis of a DVT is confirmed, pharmacological treatment is by either bolus administration of unfractionated heparin followed by continuous infusion or with LMWH; both are equally effective (246,247). In the rehabilitation facility the use of LMWH in treatment doses is an easier approach (248). Once initiated, oral warfarin follows and the heparin is contin-

ued until the International Normalized Ratio (INR) is therapeutic for at least 24 hours. The proper length of treatment should be at least 3 months for a DVT and 6 months for PE, although some prefer longer treatment in the SCI population. With a documented clot, mobilization and exercise of the LEs is usually withheld for 48 to 72 hours while appropriate pharmacological therapy is implemented; however, there is no recent literature to support this degree of immobilization, especially with the rapid anticoagulation with LMWH.

Thermoregulation

When the body core temperature is cool and requires an adjustment, the hypothalamus, which regulates body temperature, employs shivering and vasoconstriction to increase temperature. Similarly, sweating and vasodilation decreases temperature through increased heat loss. After an SCI above the T6 level, the ability of the hypothalamus to direct the periphery is impaired due to interruption of efferent pathways, and they are partially poikilothermic, in that they may have difficulty maintaining a normal core temperature in response to environmental change in temperature (249,250). This is an important factor to keep in mind when a person with SCI has a high temperature while in a warm environment.

Anemia

Anemia is a common finding following acute SCI and is usually normochromic and normocytic (251–253). Serum iron, total iron binding capacity (TIBC), and transferrin are usually low. Although the exact cause is not known, bleeding may be a factor in some cases. By 1 year postinjury anemia improves in the majority of patients, and if it persists it is usually associated with chronic inflammatory complications such as pressure ulcers or frequent urinary tract infections (253).

Pressure Ulcers

Pressure ulcers are one of the most common and potentially serious complications of SCI. If they develop, they may interfere with the initial rehabilitation and reintegration into the community, as well as being a source of morbidity and mortality.

Model system data report that approximately one-third of patients develop pressure ulcers during their initial rehabilitation and up to 80% of persons with SCI develop a pressure ulcer at some point in their lifetime (226,254–258). Associated risk factors include level and severity of the injury, gender, ethnicity, marital status, employment status, educational achievement, tobacco and alcohol use, nutritional status, and possibly depression. The longer the time a person has been injured the greater the risk of developing an ulcer. Having a previous ulcer is a risk factor as well.

Pressure ulcers can be classified using the National Pressure Ulcer Advisory Panel (NPUAP) staging system (259) (Table 79-7). The costs of a pressure ulcer in SCI are difficult to estimate but range from $20,000 to $30,000 for less serious ulcers and up to $70,000 to heal a full thickness ulcer (258).

Pressure ulcers develop over bony prominences. The most common location in persons with SCI within the first 2 years is the sacrum, followed by the ischium, heel, and trochanter. After 2 years, the ischial tuberosities are the most common site of development (260).

Prevention is the most important aspect, and should begin as early as possible after injury. This includes the proper turning frequency in bed, weight shifting while in the wheelchair, and proper mattress, cushion, and commode chair. In addition,

TABLE 79-7. National Pressure Ulcer Advisory Panel (NPUAP) Stages of Pressure Ulcers

Stage I: Nonblanchable erythema not resolved in 30 min; epidermis intact; reversible with intervention. (Not detectable in persons with darkly pigmented skin.)
Stage II: Partial-thickness loss of skin involving epidermis, possibly into dermis; may appear as blisters with erythema, abrasion, or shallow crater.
Stage III: Full-thickness destruction through dermis into subcutaneous tissue that may extend down to, but not through, the underlying fascia. The ulcer presents clinically as a deep crater with or without undermining of adjacent tissue.
Stage IV: Full-thickness skin loss with deep-tissue destruction through subcutaneous tissue to fascia, muscle, bone, joint, or supporting structures. Undermining and sinus tracts may also be associated with stage IV pressure ulcers.

From National Pressure Ulcer Advisory Panel (NPUAP) Consensus Development Conference, 1989.

maintaining proper nutrition and not smoking are recommendations that will help prevent as well as heal ulcers if they develop. An education program for patients and their caretakers is of utmost importance. See Chapter 75 for further details of pressure ulcer management.

Bowel Management after Spinal Cord Injury

An effective bowel management program is important to prevent potential gastrointestinal (GI) complications and can have a significant influence on successful reintegration of the individual with SCI. More than one-third of persons with paraplegia ranked the loss of bowel and bladder control as the most significant functional loss associated with injury (261). The goal of a "bowel program" is the complete evacuation of the bowel at a specified time, in a short time period, so as to prevent incontinence. The bowel program should be individualized for every patient. The level of injury, previous bowel habits, lifestyle of the patient, and availability of caregivers should be taken into account when planning a bowel program (262). Full details regarding bowel management are detailed in Chapter 76.

The bowel program will vary depending on the type of neurogenic bowel dysfunction (i.e., UMN versus LMN bowel). In LMN lesions, continence is often lost due to weakness of the pelvic floor muscles with a flaccid external anal sphincter. Because spinal-mediated reflexes are absent, digital stimulation and contact irritant suppositories are largely ineffective, necessitating manual disimpaction. The stool is kept firm by use of bulking agents to aid manual disimpaction; performing the disimpaction more than once per day may be required to maintain continence. Assistive techniques such as Valsalva maneuver, abdominal massage in a clockwise direction, increase in physical activity, standing, and completing the bowel program in a commode chair rather than in bed can also greatly facilitate the process.

For persons with UMN bowel, the use of medications (stool softeners with oral stimulants) along with digital stimulation and suppositories on a daily basis are usually required when initiating the bowel program (see Chapter 76). As time goes on, however, the medications may be slowly tapered. In the chronic stage (after 1 year), the following habits have been reported. Alternate-day programs were most common, and most subjects performed their programs more commonly in the morning. Persons with tetraplegia performed their programs less often, used suppositories more often, required greater assistance, and took a longer period of time to complete their programs (263).

Surgical treatments should be considered if diet modifications, medications, and physical techniques have been attempted but fail to produce a consistent bowel movement. Colostomies and ileostomies decrease the time required for bowel management, increase independence, and simplify the overall process. Many patients have reported that they retrospectively wished that these alternatives were offered earlier (264,265). An anterograde continence enema procedure may be an option for adult patients with neurogenic bowel recalcitrant to a bowel program. Originally designed for children with myelomeningocele, it also significantly decreases toileting time and improves quality of life (266,267). Patients also find it more cosmetically acceptable than a colostomy.

Gastrointestinal Complications

Immediately after an SCI, an adynamic ileus is usually present because of spinal shock and typically resolves within a week. In cases where the ileus lasts longer, erythromycin and metoclopramide can be used to stimulate peristalsis (268). Neostigmine has also been effective in refractory cases of pseudo-obstruction (269). Gastric decompression via nasogastric tube with intermittent suction may be necessary for persistent abdominal distention. Parental nutrition should also be considered when the ileus lasts longer than 3 days.

Individuals with cervical cord injuries have a higher risk of developing peptic ulcers compared with the general trauma population (270). The incidence is approximately 5% to 7%, although an incidence as high as 24% has been reported (271, 272). Most ulcers occur acutely, within a few days following injury. Higher-level and more severe injuries (complete versus incomplete) have the greatest risk (273). Although vagal hyperactivity due to loss of sympathetic control after SCI is an attractive hypothesis, animal studies have not reported an increase in gastrin or polypeptide levels after cervical transection (274). The use of ulcer prophylaxis is recommended for the acute person with SCI.

Individuals with SCI above the T10 level have a higher risk (approximately 30%) of developing biliary stasis and gallstone disease compared to able-bodied persons (275,276). Impaired gallbladder motility has been implicated as the cause. The sympathetic nervous system, from T7-T10, innervates the gallbladder via the splanchnic nerve and is responsible for gallbladder relaxation. Patients with lesions above T10 have impaired filling of the gallbladder and lower fasting volumes, which may make the bile more lithogenic.

Although altered sensation after SCI can make the diagnosis more challenging, the majority of patients present with traditional symptoms such as right upper quadrant abdominal pain and tenderness (276,277). A high index of suspicion and radiographic tests are essential in making a timely diagnosis.

Superior mesenteric artery (SMA) syndrome is a condition where the third segment of the duodenum is compressed between the SMA and the aorta. It occurs rarely, more commonly in persons with tetraplegia, with an incidence of less than 0.33%. The patient experiences nausea, vomiting, abdominal tightness, and bloating made worse after a meal or laying supine. The diagnosis is made definitively with an upper GI series. Risk factors that may predispose patients to this condition include weight loss, use of a spinal orthotic, and immobilization in the supine position. Patients may gain some relief by lying on the left side and by taking metoclopramide (278).

Acute abdominal emergencies are often a challenge to diagnose because of the absence of the usual signs and symptoms of abdominal pathology. It is important to have a high suspicion in evaluating patients with SCI presenting with fever, abdominal pain, or pain radiating to the shoulders, and elevated white blood cell count. Performing specialized lab tests, abdominal ultrasonography, or CT scan early is often helpful to confirm the diagnosis.

Spasticity

Spasticity is a common medical complication of UMN SCI. The incidence is approximately 70%, with roughly half the patients requiring pharmacological intervention. (279,280). While spasticity may contribute to improved function (i.e., transfers, standing, ambulation, and assisting in ADLs), it may often lead to various complications including contractures, pain, impaired function, and decreased quality of life. See Chapter 67 for details regarding the basic definitions of spasticity, diagnostic procedures, and treatment options. Spasticity occurs more frequently in persons with cervical and upper thoracic SCI than in those with lower thoracic and lumbosacral SCI, and is usually more significant in persons with partial incomplete injuries, ASIA grades B and C, than persons with grades A or D. The presence of spasticity in persons with SCI may be evidence of some preserved connections, or altered motor control caused by a new spinal cord anatomy after injury.

Clinical evaluation is important, however, the degree of spasticity may vary during the course of the day. Therefore, the patient's description of secondary problems from spasticity becomes extremely important in determining whether to treat. The most common clinical scales used to assess spasticity in SCI include the Ashworth Scale (281), Modified Ashworth (282), and the Penn Spasm Frequency Scale (283), although there is little correlation found between the Ashworth Scale and the Penn Spasm Frequency Scale (284).

Before initiating treatment, potential, nociceptive sources should be evaluated and, if present, treated. Common causes include urinary tract infections, bladder calculi, pressure ulcers, abdominal pathology, ingrown toenails, hemorrhoids, and bowel impaction. Selective serotonin reuptake inhibitors have been reported to increase spasticity (285). Changes in spasticity in an otherwise stable patient may also be an important presenting sign in syringomyelia (286).

Stretching is a mainstay of treatment for spasticity as well as prevention of joint contractures (287), and should be completed twice a day or more. Standing activities, including use of tilt table or standing frame, provide prolonged stretch to joints and may reduce spasticity as well (288,289). Modalities have been used including cold and electrical stimulation (ES), usually with short-term benefits(287). Spinal cord ES has not shown consistent long-term benefits (290). Posture and positioning is extremely important for tone reduction. Adequate low back support to maintain lumbar lordosis and a positive seat plane angle or "dump," with a reduction in seat-to-back angle, encourages proper upright posture and may reduce extensor tone. Inhibitive casting, splinting, and orthotic management of muscles and joints at risk for contracture may be helpful in reducing tone (291).

Numerous pharmacological options are available for persons with SCI-related spasticity (see Chapter 67 and Table 79-8). No medication is universally beneficial to all patients and therefore some amount of trial-and-error may be required. Most medications share common side effects of sedation and asthenia. The person's age, comorbidities, and cognitive status

TABLE 79-8.   Most Common Oral and Transdermal Medications for Spasticity in Spinal Cord Injury

Medication	Dosage
Baclofen	5 mg t.i.d.–40 mg q.i.d.
Diazepam	5 mg q d–15 mg q.i.d.
Klonopin	0.25 mg q.h.s.–1 mg t.i.d.
Dantrolene	25 mg q d–100 mg q.i.d.
Tizanidine	2 mg q d–36 mg/d in divided doses
Catapres	0.1–0.3 TTS patch q wk
Gabapentin	100 mg t.i.d.–1,200 mg q.i.d.
Periactin	4 mg q d–8 mg q.i.d.

should be carefully considered when choosing a medication for spasticity.

Baclofen exerts gamma-aminobutyric acid (GABA) agonist activity by binding presynaptically at the $GABA_b$ receptor and exerts inhibitory activity on monosynaptic and polysynaptic reflexes. If baclofen is to be discontinued it must be tapered, as abrupt discontinuation can result in seizures, visual disturbances, and hallucinations (292). Benzodiazepines may affect cognitive performance measures such as attention, concentration and memory, and are generally not used in persons with concomitant brain injury. A single nighttime dose of diazepam or clonazepam is often used to treat nocturnal spasms that interfere with sleep. Alpha-2-adrenergic agonists, including clonidine and tizanidine, bind to presynaptic α_2-receptors on interneurons in the dorsal horn of the spinal cord, resulting in depression of polysynaptic reflexes. Clonidine can be delivered either orally, via transdermal patch, or intrathecally (293,294). Tizanidine has a shorter half-life and lower incidence of hypotension than clonidine, and has been shown to be effective in patients with SCI and MS (295,296).

Gabapentin, an anticonvulsant, has antispasticity benefits in persons with SCI, especially at higher doses (more than 1,800 mg/day) (297,298). Dantrolene sodium prevents the release of calcium ions from the sarcoplasmic reticulum along muscle fibers, and acts on normal as well as spastic muscle, potentially resulting in weakness (299). Dantrolene may be better at reducing tone rather than spontaneous spasms, but may be of special benefit in persons with concurrent SCI and traumatic brain injury (TBI), since its effects are peripheral rather than in the CNS (299,300). The most worrisome side effect is hepatotoxicity, which occurs in approximately 1.8% of patients.

Cyproheptadine is a nonselective serotonergic (5-HT) antagonist, which has antihistamine activity and reduces clonus and spontaneous spasms in patients with SCI either alone (301–303) or in combination with clonidine (304). Most common side effects include fatigue and excessive weight gain. Opiates exhibit potent antispasticity activity (305,306) by suppressing polysynaptic reflexes to a greater extent than monosynaptic reflexes, but are not considered a primary treatment option for SCI-related spasticity. 4-Aminopyridine (4-AP), a potassium channel-blocking agent has shown some effect on decreasing spasticity and improving function in persons with incomplete SCI (307,308). Although not approved for clinical use, cannabis has shown benefit for persons with SCI-related spasticity (309,310).

Intrathecal baclofen (IT-B) has been shown to be of benefit for persons with SCI, with effective control of spasticity in the lower limbs greater than in the trunk and upper limbs (311, 312). Intrathecal clonidine may also be effective either alone (313) or in combination with baclofen (314), although this is not

FDA-approved. Careful patient selection is critical with close monitoring for pump failure or other complications.

Peripheral nerve blocks, as well as motor point blocks with alcohol or phenol, allow for a focused delivery of drug to manage focal areas of spasticity. These may be particularly effective for the upper limb or in persons with an incomplete injury who may achieve functional goals beyond that achieved by systemic treatment measures alone. These drugs can have effects of up to 1 year or longer by causing destruction of the axons (315). Botulinum toxin can be injected into the affected muscle and blocks neuromuscular transmission by inhibiting the release of acetylcholine into the synapse. It has an onset of action of 4 to 10 days and length of effect lasts on average 3 to 6 months; it has shown effect for improving UE and LE function (316,317). Follow-up stretching, which may include dynamic splinting or serial casting, is recommended to optimize function.

Surgical interventions, including cordectomy and myelotomy, have been performed to reduce spasticity, but with limited long-term success (318). More selective procedures, dorsal rhizotomy, and dorsal root entry zone procedures have been proposed to control spasticity by decreasing the afferent component of spasticity. This treatment is most commonly used for the treatment of pain, and may not result in decreased spasticity.

REHABILITATION OF SPINAL CORD INJURY

"Rehabilitation" begins in the ICU setting and includes meeting the SCI-specific medical and rehabilitative needs to help the individual who suffered the injury meet their potential in terms of physical, social, emotional, recreational, vocational, and functional recovery. If early medical complications can be prevented, the inpatient rehabilitation course is facilitated and the total cost of care is lessened, as is the degree of human suffering (319). The amount of complications appears to be inversely related to the quality of care available at the hospitals that provide early care (320).

The medical aspects of the SCI specialist's acute recommendations are covered earlier in this chapter and can be formulated into a problem list (Table 79-9). The most important aspects include bowel, bladder and pulmonary management, DVT and GI prophylaxis, and proper positioning in bed with the proper turning frequency (at least every 2 hours). Once the spine is stabilized by surgery or orthoses, therapy and nursing will incorporate ROM that will help prevent contractures. The shoulder, elbow, hip flexors, and heel cords are most important to range because they are the most frequently observed contractures on presentation to the acute rehabilitation unit and can potentially serve as a source of pain and functional limitation. Resting splints for paralyzed UEs help prevent contractures and increase comfort. Functional UE splints may also be useful for feeding and other self-care skills in the early period. For persons with high- level tetraplegia, who have undergone tracheostomy, early introduction of communication aids is important. Once medically stable, the patient should be transferred to a specialized spinal cord rehabilitation unit. A specialized SCI center is most beneficial as it offers access to psychology, vocational and SCI educational services, an active peer support program, and the opportunity to undergo rehabilitation with other patients who have similar impairments. Additional opportunities available at larger SCI centers include availability to trial equipment for mobility and accessibility to high-level assistive technology (e.g., environmental control units, or ECU).

The interdisciplinary approach of the rehabilitation team is important for the optimal care of the individual with SCI. As the length of stay shortens in acute rehabilitation, coordination and communication with the entire team is needed to allow for a timely and safe discharge. Frequent team conferences with an early home evaluation should be performed.

Functional Goals

Once the patient's motor level of injury and ASIA Impairment Scale is determined, short- and long-term functional goals are

TABLE 79-9. Sample Medical Problem List in Acute Spinal Cord Injury	
Medical Problem List	**Interventions**
Respiratory	Monitor vital capacity and O_2 saturation. Perform incentive spirometry, assisted cough, deep breathing techniques, chest PT, and respiratory treatments.
Gastrointestinal	Stress ulcer prophylaxis.
Nutrition	Perform calorie count. Monitor weekly weights.
Neurogenic bowel	Initiate bowel program.
Neurogenic bladder	Proper intake and output. Discuss bladder options.
DVT prophylaxis	Adequate pharmacological prophylaxis. Monitor LE circumference.
Skin	Proper mattress. Turn q 2 hours initially. Heel protectors. Frequent weight shifts. Proper cushion.
Orthostasis	Change positions slowly. Ace wrap or LE stockings and abdominal binder. Use tilt table. Pharmacological intervention if needed.
Swallowing	Swallow study if suspect complications, especially in presence of tracheostomy or after anterior approach surgery.
Spine	Precautions based on surgery or orthosis.
Cognition	Screen for dual diagnosis
Heterotopic ossification	Monitor hip and knee range of motion. X-rays and bone scan if suspect.
Contractures	Range of motion.
Autonomic dysreflexia	Monitor vital signs closely.
Hypercalcemia	Monitor for symptoms. Provide fluids; medications as needed.

DVT, deep vein thrombosis; LE, lower extremity; PT, physiotherapy.
From Kirshblum SC, Ho C, Druin E, et al. Rehabilitation after spinal cord injury. In: Kirshblum SC, Campagnolo D, DeLisa JE, eds. *Spinal cord medicine.* Philadelphia: Lippincott Williams & Wilkins, 2002:275–298.

TABLE 79-10.   Projected Functional Outcomes at 1-Year Postinjury by Level

	C1-C4	C5	C6	C7	C8-T1
Feeding	Dependent	Independent with adaptive equipment after set up	Independent with or w/o adaptive equipment	Independent	Independent
Grooming	Dependent	Minimal assistance with equipment after setup	Some assistance to independent with adaptive equipment	Independent with adaptive equipment	Independent
Upper Extremity Dressing	Dependent	Requires assistance	Independent	Independent	Independent
Lower Extremity Dressing	Dependent	Dependent	Requires assistance	Some assistance to independent with adaptive equipment	Usually independent
Bathing	Dependent	Dependent	Some assistance to independent with equipment	Some assistance to independent with equipment	Independent with equipment
Bed Mobility	Dependent	Assistance	Assistance	Independent to some assistance	Independent
Weight Shifts	Independent in power; dependent in manual wheelchair	Assistance unless in power wheelchair	Independent	Independent	Independent
Transfers	Dependent	Maximum assistance	Some assistance to independence on level surfaces	Independence with or without board for level surfaces	Independent
Wheelchair Propulsion	Independent with power Dependent in manual	Independent in power; independent to some assistance in manual with adaptations on level surfaces	Independent—manual with coated rims on level surfaces	Independent—except curbs and uneven terrain	Independent
Driving	Unable	Independent with adaptations	Independent with adaptations	Car with hand controls or adapted van	Car with hand or control adapted van

	T2-T9	T10-L2	L3-S5
ADLs (Grooming, feeding, dressing, bathing)	Independent	Independent	Independent
Bowel/Bladder	Independent	Independent	Independent
Transfers	Independent	Independent	Independent
Ambulation	Standing in frame, tilt table or standing wheelchair. Exercise only	Household ambulation with orthoses. Can trial ambulation outdoors	Community ambulation is possible
Braces	Bilateral KAFO forearm crutches or walker	KAFOs, with forearm crutches	Possibly KAFO or AFOs, with canes/crutches

ADLs, activities of daily living; AFO, ankle-foot orthosis; KAFO, knee-ankle-foot orthosis.
From Kirshblum SC, Ho C, Druin E, et al. Rehabilitation after spinal cord injury. In: Kirshblum SC, Campagnolo D, DeLisa JE, eds. *Spinal cord medicine*. Philadelphia: Lippincott Williams & Wilkins, 2002:275–298.

formulated and a therapy prescription is established. Table 79-10 lists the functional goals expected for a person with a motor complete injury to be achieved at 1 year, and Table 79-11 lists equipment usually prescribed for persons for each level of injury. The ideal outcome may not always be achieved for each patient, as there is a significant amount of variability in individual outcomes despite similar levels of injury. The extent to which an individual can achieve goals from a functional standpoint is dependent on the age of the individual and coexistent conditions.

The projected long-term goals are a starting point for the rehabilitation prescription. The rehabilitation program should be individualized to meet each person's strengths, weaknesses, and particular circumstances. Short-term goals are progressive steps that should be attained to achieve the long-term goals. Monitoring progress at the team conference helps to identify limiting factors along with patients additional needs. Patients

should understand the goals projected to become active participants in their program. Discharge planning should be discussed as early as the first team conference, assuring a timely, but most importantly, a safe discharge.

C1–4 LEVEL

Persons with motor levels at or above C3 will usually require long-term ventilator assistance, whereas most individuals with lesions at C4 will be able to wean off the ventilator. Respiratory equipment including a ventilator, a method for secretion management (i.e., suction machine, mechanical insufflator/exsufflator), backup ventilator batteries, and a generator in case of power failure, should be obtained. One should be in touch with the local power company and emergency services to alert them of the patient's status and condition prior to discharge.

Individuals with these high cervical levels of injury, should be independent in instructing others in providing their care in-

TABLE 79-11. Suggested Equipment for Complete Tetraplegic					
	C1-C4	**C5**	**C6**	**C7**	**C8-T1**
Orthotics					
BFO (mobile arm support)	X	?	—	—	—
Resting hand splint	X	X	X	—	—
Long opponens splint	X	X	—	—	—
Spiral splint	—	X	X	—	—
Powered tenodesis splint	—	X	—	—	—
Wrist-driven tenodesis splint	—	—	X	—	—
Rachet tenodesis splint	—	X	—	—	—
Short opponens splint	—	—	X	X	—
Universal cuff	—	X	X	X	—
Lumbrical bar	—	—	—	—	X
Mouthstick	X	?	—	—	—
Transfers/Mobility					
Power/mechanical lift	X	X	X	—	—
Transfer board	X	X	X	X	X
Power w/c with tilt/recline	X	X	?	—	—
Power w/c	—	—	X	?	—
Manual w/c	X	X	X	X	X
Feeding					
Adapted equipment (plate, etc.)	X	X	—	—	—
Utensils with built-up handles	—	X	X	—	—
Grooming & Dressing					
ADL splints (wash mitt, razor holders)	—	X	X	—	—
Dressing equipment (pant loops, sock aide, dressing stick, long shoe horn, etc.)	—	—	X	X	—
Gooseneck mirror	X	X	X	X	X
Communication					
Environmental control unit	X	X	?	—	—
Computer	X	X	X	X	—
Book holder	X	X	X	X	—
Bathing					
Grab bars	—	—	X	X	X
Reclining shower/commode chair	X	—	—	—	—
Tub seat/shower chair (padded)	—	X	X	X	X
Hand-held spray attachment	X	X	X	X	X
Beds					
Full electric hospital bed	X	X	X	—	—
Full specialized mattress	X	X	?	?	—
Overlay mattress	—	—	X	X	?

ADL, activities of daily living; BFO, balanced forearm orthosis; w/c, wheelchair.
From Kirshblum SC, Ho C, Druin E, et al. Rehabilitation after spinal cord injury. In: Kirshblum SC, Campagnolo D, DeLisa JE, eds. *Spinal cord medicine*. Philadelphia: Lippincott Williams & Wilkins, 2002:275–298.

cluding performing weight shifts, ROM, positioning in bed, donning orthoses, transfers, and in setting up their ECU. These individuals should be independent in power wheelchair mobility, using breath control, mouth stick, head array, and tongue or chin control mechanisms. If the patient can control a power chair, then both a power chair (power recline or tilt wheelchair) and a manual positional wheelchair should be prescribed (321). The manual wheelchair is used when accessibility for a power wheelchair is not available, or in case the power wheelchair fails. Once properly set up, persons at these levels of injury should be independent in their ECU control.

Persons with an NLI at C4 who have some elbow flexion and deltoid strength may be able to use a mobile arm support (MAS) or balanced forearm orthosis (BFO) to assist with feeding, grooming, and hygiene. Once the elbow flexors have antigravity strength with adequate endurance, the MAS is no longer needed. A long straw or a bottle that the person can easily access to drink fluids should be obtained as early as possible.

The benefit of specialized acute rehabilitation for persons with such high levels of injury is justifiable despite their inabil-ity to initially tolerate 3 hours a day of therapy and having what may seem as limited goals. The SCI medical and nursing care during the first few months after injury are crucial for monitoring, treating, and preventing medical complications that can lead to future morbidity and mortality. Patient and family education, emotional and social support, and exposure to advanced technology that may allow independence in the proper environment (i.e., power mobility, ECU) may be the difference for the person between returning to their family/community versus spending a lifetime dependent in a nursing home.

C5 LEVEL
The C5 motor level adds the key muscle group of the elbow flexors (biceps), as well as the deltoids, rhomboids and partial innervation of the brachialis, brachioradialis, supraspinatus, infraspinatus, and serratus anterior. It is important during the acute period after SCI to prevent elbow flexion and forearm supination contractures caused by unopposed biceps activity. Continued stretching should be performed acutely and in the

chronic phase after rehabilitation. An MAS may initially be needed, however, the individual should regain adequate strength to perform these activities without the device.

The addition of the elbow flexors should allow for use of a joystick for a power wheelchair and can allow manual wheelchair propulsion on level surfaces with either rim projections (lugs) or plastic coated hand rims with a protective glove. A power wheelchair, with a power recline or tilt mechanism, is usually still required in addition to the manual wheelchair. A power or manual-assist wheelchair may also be advantageous to improve the distance one can propel the wheelchair.

A long opponens splint, with a pocket for inserting different utensils, is important to assist with many tasks including feeding, hygiene, grooming, and writing. Most functional activities will require the use of assistive devices, and therefore tendon transfers may be considered after neurological recovery is complete. Implanted electrical stimulation units may also be beneficial. (This is discussed in more detail later in the chapter.)

Persons with this level of injury will require almost total assistance for their bowel program. A padded commode/shower chair is recommended as the gravity from the upright position assists with the program and the padding helps to prevent skin breakdown. Bladder management is a decision based on discussion with the SCI specialist and urologist, urodynamic results, amount of assistance available, and lifestyle circumstances. IC usually cannot be performed independently, and will initially require sterile technique to be performed by another person. If using a leg drainage bag, electronic devices to help empty the bag are available. Driving a specially modified van is possible at this level, with a lift for access allowing the patient to be fully independent.

C6 LEVEL

The C6 level adds the key muscle group that performs wrist extension (extensor carpi radialis), as well as partially innervating the supinator, pronator teres, and latissimus dorsi. Active wrist extension can allow for tenodesis, the opposition of the thumb and index finger with flexion as the tendons are stretched with wrist extension. One should avoid overly stretching the finger flexors initially after injury in C5 and C6 motor level patients to avoid potentially losing the tenodesis action. Tenodesis splints can be fabricated but are frequently discarded by patients.

Feeding, grooming, and UE hygiene are usually independent after assistance with setting up the appropriate utensils, however, clothing modifications such as Velcro closures on shoes, loops on zippers, and pullover garments are recommended. Assistance for meal preparation is still required as well as for other homemaking tasks. Transfers may be possible using a transfer board and with loops for LE management, but most often requires assistance. Although persons with a C6 motor level can propel a manual wheelchair with plastic-coated rims, a power wheelchair is often required for long distances, especially if the individual will be returning to the workplace. A power-assist wheelchair may be of benefit as well.

IC is possible for males after assistance for setup with assistive devices, including the HouseHold device (Flexlife Medical, Kingwood, TX) (322). While the use of adaptive equipment may enhance independence for males, this technique is more difficult for females.

C7, C8 LEVELS

The C7 motor level adds the elbow extensors (triceps) as the key muscle group; C8 the long finger flexors. The C7 level is considered the key level for becoming independent in most activities at the wheelchair level, including weight shifts, trans-

fers between level surfaces, feeding, grooming, upper body dressing, and light meal preparation (323). Uneven surface transfers, lower body dressing, and house cleaning may require some assistance. The independent use of a car is possible if the individual can transfer and load/unload the wheelchair.

IC in males can be performed although it is more difficult for females, especially if LE spasticity is present. Bowel care on a padded commode seat, especially suppository insertion, may still require assistance or the use of adaptive devices (i.e., suppository inserter).

T1-T12 THORACIC LEVELS

Individuals with all levels of paraplegia should be independent with basic ADLs, including LE dressing, and mobility skills at the wheelchair level on even and uneven surfaces. This includes advanced wheelchair techniques such as curbs, ramps, wheelies, and floor to wheelchair transfers. Bowel and bladder management should be independent.

For most individuals with higher levels of thoracic injury, community ambulation is not a functional long-term goal. The lower the level of injury, the greater the trunk control due to abdominal and paraspinal muscle innervation. Although individuals with high and midthoracic-level injuries may be interested in gait training, and should undergo this if there are no medical contraindications, it is usually not an inpatient goal. For lower levels of thoracic injuries, there is improved trunk control to allow for ambulation training with bilateral LE orthoses, as an exercise and short distance household ambulation, once the individual has mastered basic wheelchair skills.

L1-L2 LEVELS

Muscles gained at these levels include the hip flexors and part of the quadriceps. While the person may be able to ambulate for short distances, a wheelchair will still be required for functional mobility needs. Bladder care is usually by IC. Individuals with these levels of injury can drive a car with hand controls.

L3-L4 LEVELS

The knee extensors are fully innervated with some strength of ankle dorsiflexion. Ambulation usually requires ankle-foot orthoses (AFOs) with canes and crutches. Bowel and bladder management should be independent. This is typically a LMN injury, and bowel management is usually by contraction of abdominal muscles and manual disimpaction. Suppositories will not be effective because of the loss of reflexes. Bladder management is usually performed via IC or Valsalva maneuver if postvoid residuals are within normal limits and urological workup reveals no contraindication to this method. Absorbent pads can be used.

L5 AND BELOW

Individuals with these injuries should be independent in all activities unless there are associated problems (i.e., severe pain, cardiac conditions, etc.).

Specific Activities in Therapy

RANGE OF MOTION

Shoulder ROM is important to prevent pain in persons with all levels of injury. In persons with C5 and C6 motor levels, ROM should be especially addressed to diminish the development of elbow flexion and supination contractures. For those individuals with active wrist extension and weak or no finger function, the finger flexors should not be fully stretched, but instead allowed to tighten somewhat and naturally curl to improve grip strength and function using a "tenodesis" action. Lying prone when medically able is helpful in preventing and stretching the hip flexors. Prevention of heel cord tightness and contracture is important for proper positioning of the feet on the wheelchair footplate. Stretching of the lumbar spine is initiated when tightness or spasticity interferes with function, but is often avoided to provide the patient with increased postural stability and balance in the short and long sitting positions.

MODALITIES

Modalities such as heat, cold, and ultrasound, can be used above the level of the sensory loss, but in areas with diminished or no sensation, one must be cautious because the risk of causing a burn is high.

PRESSURE RELIEFS

Pressure reliefs are essential to prevent the occurrence of pressure ulcers. When supine, turning for pressure relief is initially performed every 2 hours and progressively extended with close monitoring for signs of erythema that do not quickly dissipate. The use of a mirror will greatly enhance the ability to monitor the sacral area and ischial tuberosities. The method of pressure relief in the sitting position will vary depending on the level of injury and strength of the individual. Persons with high-level injuries (at C5 and above) will usually require a wheelchair with a tilt or recline mechanism. Some individuals with a C5 motor level can perform an anterior weight shift, or a lateral weight shift can be performed. These weight shifts are more effective in pressure relief than tipping the wheelchair backward to 35–65 degrees (324). Individuals with an injury at C7 or below are usually able to perform an independent push-up pressure relief. A pressure relief should be performed for at least 1 minute every 30 minutes while in the wheelchair. Computerized pressure mapping can be used to locate areas of high pressure in the patient's current wheelchair cushion and serve as a teaching tool to demonstrate the pressure relief technique that provides the best results (325).

STANDING

Standing with the use of a tilt-table or standing-frame, after an acute SCI, decreases hypercalciuria and may retard or lessen bone loss (205,206); however it has not been shown to reverse osteoporosis after it has occurred in chronic SCI (326–328). Patients with chronic SCI should undertake the standing procedure with caution, since bone mineral density is often at or below fracture threshold (329).An increase in physical self-concept scores and a decrease in depression scores have been reported with standing after SCI (330). Physiological benefits of standing include a decrease in spasticity, enhancing bowel and bladder programs secondary to the effect of gravity, and preventing pressure ulcers by allowing pressure relief on normally weight-bearing areas (289). Tilt tables can be used early in the rehabilitation process by gradually increasing the degree of vertical positioning in the treatment of orthostatic hypotension.

AMBULATION

Ambulation after SCI is often one of the first goals that many persons with SCI set for themselves. It is important that patients with SCI understand their prognosis in terms of achieving this goal and when it should be worked on. There are four general levels of ambulation: community ambulation, household ambulation, ambulation for exercise, and a nonambulatory period (331). Community ambulation requires independence in performing transfers, capability of going from the sit to stand position, and ambulating reasonable distances unas-

sisted in and outside the home (greater than 150 feet) with or without braces and assistive devices. Household ambulation is the ability to ambulate only within the home with relative independence, but may require assistance for transfers. Ambulation for exercise is for a person who requires significant assistance for ambulation.

Physiological benefits of walking include potentially decreasing the progression of osteoporosis, reduced urinary calcinosis, reduced spasticity, improved digestion and bowel program because of the effect of gravity, and prevention of pressure ulcers (as with standing) (332,333). In addition, it enables reaching objects not obtainable from the wheelchair level and affords access to areas that are not wheelchair-accessible, such as through narrow doorways. While ambulation following SCI has physiological and psychological benefits, it also has significant drawbacks including increased energy consumption, with decreased speed of ambulation when compared to the relatively normal energy expenditure and velocity of wheelchair use; weight-bearing through the UEs that may predispose an individual to shoulder, elbow and wrist problems; and poor long-term follow-through (334–336).

While there is no one definite level at which patients should not perform training with braces, there are factors that will contribute to difficulty in ambulation, including older age, greater weight, lack of motivation, inherent poor agility and coordination, and greater spasticity (337). All patients with the potential for ambulation should be given a trial if they want to pursue this, but for persons with thoracic-level injuries, training should not be initiated until transfer training and wheelchair activities are mastered.

Community ambulation requires bilateral hip flexors greater than 3/5, and one knee extensor to be at least 3/5, with a maximum amount of bracing of one long leg brace and one short leg brace (338). Prognosis for ambulation can be determined early after injury and is determined by the initial level of the injury and the ASIA impairment classification. Waters and colleagues correlated the 1-month lower extremity motor strength (LEMS) in patients with complete and incomplete injuries with the chances for ambulation; the greater the score the greater the chances of ambulation at 1 year (103,107,109,110). Forty-six percent of persons with incomplete tetraplegia advance to community ambulation at 1 year with an additional 14% performing household ambulation. This is compared to 5% of complete paraplegics and 76% of incomplete paraplegics regaining community ambulation. The percentage of persons with incomplete tetraplegia able to achieve community ambulation is lower than for incomplete paraplegia with equivalent LEMS, because the UE strength may be compromised and insufficient to enable assistive-device ambulation if required. (Table 79-12)

A number of orthotic options exist to assist in ambulation, including mechanical orthoses, functional electrical stimulation (FES), and hybrid orthoses—a combination of a mechanical orthosis and FES (319,339). The knee-ankle-foot orthoses (KAFOs) are most frequently prescribed for ambulation. Other devices used occasionally include the Vannini-Rizzoli orthoses, the Parawalker, the reciprocal gait orthosis (RGO), and the advanced RGO (ARGO), and hip-knee-ankle-foot orthoses (HKAFOs), including the hip guidance orthosis (HGO), and may enable persons with thoracic-level paraplegia to ambulate (340,341). The Parastep system is the simplest example of a FES system for walking (342–344). Newer FES systems are being developed for both standing and walking (see Chapter 66).

The Craig Scott orthosis (CSO) is the most commonly prescribed KAFO for individuals with SCI. Advantages of the CSO relative to the conventional or plastic KAFO is that they are

TABLE 79-12.   Estimated Recovery of Community Ambulation at 1-Year Postinjury

1-Mo. LEMS	Incomplete Tetra	Complete Para	Incomplete Para
1–9	21%	45%	70%
10–19	63%	—	100%
≥20	100%	100%	100%

LEMS, lower extremity motor score.
From Waters RL, et al. Motor and sensory recovery following incomplete tetraplegia. *Arch Phys Med Rehabil* 1994;75:306–311; Waters RL, et al. Recovery following complete paraplegia. *Arch Phys Med Rehabil* 1992;73:784–789; Waters RL, et al. Functional and neurologic recovery following spinal cord injury. *J Spinal Cord Med* 1998;21:195–199; and Waters RL, et al. Motor and sensory recovery following incomplete paraplegia. *Arch Phys Med Rehabil* 1994;75:67–72.

more energy efficient; provide more stability so that the patient may be able to balance without using crutches; are easier to unlock; and, because of the cushioned heel, provide a softer landing and improved roll-over.

The use of weight supported ambulation as a rehabilitation intervention has gained a lot of recent attention. Animal models as well as preliminary studies in persons with incomplete SCI have shown improvement in acute and chronically injured individuals in their ability to learn to walk (345,346). Clinical trials are currently underway to better determine its role in SCI rehabilitation.

ASSISTED TECHNOLOGY DEVICES

Assisted technology devices (ATDs) include equipment that is used to increase, maintain, or improve functional capabilities of an individual and may be the key to independence for persons with SCI. Prior to prescription, it is important to identify the patient's capabilities and needed tasks, the patient's goals, and any environmental barriers that may be present (see Chapter 60).

Table 79-11 lists some suggested equipment for each level of motor injury. Telephone access is an important basic skill to allow for socialization as well as in case of medical emergencies. A speakerphone or a headset phone can be used with these devices.

The ECU serves as the control center so that the patient can control electrical appliances in the home, including the radio, television and VCR, DVD, bed, computer, lights, fan, thermostat controls, and so on. The correct ECU can enhance a person's life by giving them a sense of control, security, and independence. A person can essentially use any body part to activate a switch as long as he or she can perform the activity consistently with accuracy. A reliable site can include the head, chin, mouth, shoulder, arm, or hand. Voice activation is also an option. The patient's overall capability (i.e., cognitive status and functional movements) as well as the environment should be evaluated prior to choosing the appropriate switch (347).

Home Modifications for People with Spinal Cord Injury

A number of general guidelines and recommendations for making the home accessible are listed in Table 79-13. A home evaluation, or a floor plan of the residence should be completed early as an important aspect of the rehabilitation process

to allow the injured individual to return home. The main areas to be evaluated include the entrances, bedroom, bathroom, kitchen, and general safety issues. The key pieces of information to know when performing the home evaluation are the patient's level of injury and mobility status, prognosis for functional recovery, social situation for return to home, and financial considerations.

Psychological Adaptation to Spinal Cord Injury

A person who sustains an SCI is at risk for the "four D syndrome": dependency, depression, drug addiction, and, if married, divorce (348). Depressive disorders are the most common form of psychological distress after SCI, estimated to affect 20% to 45% of those injured, and usually occur within the first month postinjury (349–351). When depression occurs, it should be viewed as a complication that is amenable to treatment, rather than a stage that the patient must pass through. A clinical depression is often assessed by a semi-structured interview or a self-report measure such as the Beck Depression Inventory (BDI) (352), although results need to be interpreted carefully. Accurate diagnosis of depressive disorders uses established diagnostic criteria for which clinicians are referred to the *Diagnostic and Statistical Manual of Mental Disorders, Fourth Edition (DSM-IV)* (353).

Risk factors for depression include genetic, psychological, social, and environmental. They include a prior history of or family history of depression, chronic pain, female gender, lack of social support, multiplicity of life stresses, concurrent med-

TABLE 79-13.   General Recommendations for Accessibility in the Home

- The minimum space for turning around is 5' × 5' for a manual wheelchair, and 6' × 6' for a power wheelchair.
- Doorway widths that require a "straight shot" are 32" for a manual chair and 34" for a power wheelchair. This space increases to 36" if there is a turn involved.
- Door handles should be the lever type, which are easier to handle for people with limited hand function. Doors should be hung on offset hinges, which allow the door to swing clear of the doorway.
- Ramps must recognize a 12" length for every 1" in rise.
- All thresholds should be no greater than 1" to allow the person in the wheelchair to maneuver.
- Low-pile carpeting or hard surface flooring is recommended for wheelchair maneuvering.
- Eliminate throw rugs.
- Notify police/fire departments that an individual with a disability resides in the home and provide the bedroom location.
- Backup power should be provided if the person with a spinal cord injury is dependent on equipment for life support, such as a ventilator or stair glide.
- Light switches should be at a height of no more than 36".
- Fireplace/heater cautions: Care should be taken to cover the metal parts of the wheelchair that may contact the person's skin.
- Bathroom sinks should be wall-mounted without a cabinet underneath for knee clearance with pipes insulated to prevent burns.
- Kitchen appliances should be on a surface where the individual can reach inside.
- Power door openers can be installed for people in wheelchairs where a remote can be used, or install a push plate on the wall.

From Kirshblum SC, Ho C, Druin E, et al. Rehabilitation after spinal cord injury. In: Kirshblum SC, Campagnolo D, DeLisa JE, eds. *Spinal cord medicine.* Philadelphia: Lippincott Williams & Wilkins, 2002:275–298.

ical illness, and alcohol or substance abuse. Additional factors include having a complete neurological injury and medical comorbidity with TBI, a poor social network, few financial resources, vocational difficulties, and need for personal and transportation assistance.

Thirty percent of persons with SCI have been found to have raised levels of anxiety and depression up to 2 years postinjury (354). Those who recover from depression have more social supports than those who remain depressed (355). The presence of severe medical complications, a low level of autonomy, poor education, unemployment, insufficient family support, and architectural barriers increases psychological distress postinjury.

The suicide rate following SCI is two to six times greater when compared to the able-bodied population. It is the leading cause of death in individuals with SCI younger than 55 years of age, with 75% of the suicides occurring within 5 years of injury (356–359). The suicide rate is higher for those "marginally" injured (incomplete classification D or E) who have a near complete recovery (359).

The treatment for psychological disturbances after SCI includes counseling and pharmacological intervention. Medications should be considered for patients whose mood disturbance is severe enough to interfere with their ability to perform in activities. It should continue for at least 4 months (360,361) and be tapered slowly as early discontinuation is associated with a high rate of relapse (362,363). Following this, medication may need to be continued to prevent recurrence of symptoms. The patient's presenting signs and symptoms, as well as the potential side-effect profile of each medication, should guide selection of a particular medication. A psychiatrist should be consulted if the patient has suicidal ideation or presents with psychotic features or if the patient does not respond to one or two of the trials of antidepressant medications. Recurrence rates for depression are common.

Acute stress disorder and posttraumatic stress disorder (PTSD) are anxiety diagnoses that may limit adaptation to disability. The prevalence of PTSD following SCI is estimated to range from 12% to 17% (364). To meet the diagnosis these symptoms must be present for 1 month and cause marked distress or impairment in functioning (353).

Most patients are satisfied with their quality of life after a SCI. The level of participation, particularly mobility and social integration, and perceived health status are predictive of quality of life (QOL) (365). An individual's perceived health status seems to be more important to adaptation to the SCI and perceived QOL than direct injury-related deficits. Persons who required initial mechanical ventilation have reported that they are glad to be alive and are satisfied with their lives (366–368). Interestingly, the QOL for persons with high-level injury have been underestimated by health care professionals (367).

Variables affecting successful adjustment include age and time since injury. Individuals injured at a younger age tend to experience successful adjustment and a better QOL than older individuals (369). This may be due to their flexible use of coping strategies and the development of a self-concept that includes the knowledge of future limitations (370).

SCI affects whole families contending with their role changes. Psychological support and support groups with others in similar situations may prove helpful. The rehabilitation team plays an active role in promoting mental health following SCI through active listening, empathy, support, and encouragement. Staff can help to reduce depression, anxiety, and self-neglect behaviors through promoting self-directed behavior and engaging patients in problem-solving to find personally acceptable solutions (351,371).

Substance Abuse

Substance abuse is frequently encountered, even in SCI rehabilitation settings. The CAGE, a four-question screening device for alcoholism, has been found to be a reliable instrument with the SCI population (372). Those with higher CAGE scores have a higher incidence of medical complications (373). Alcohol and drug misuse contributes to SCI by increasing risk taking while intoxicated, and hampers learning and rehabilitation gains, interferes with self-care, places persons at risk for complications, contributes to depression, mortality and morbidity, and limits long-term outcomes and capacity for independent living (356,373,374). Heavy drinkers prior to injury spend less time in educational and vocational activities while in a rehabilitation hospital and alcohol users are less motivated to participate in their rehabilitation than nondrinkers (375). Prevention and treatment programs should be included as part of SCI rehabilitation.

Sexual Function and Fertility

Sexuality issues should be discussed with the individual soon after the injury and in many centers is part of the SCI education classes during inpatient rehabilitation. Chapter 74 discusses this topic in detail. Key aspects for discussion for men include the options for erectile function and capability to father children. For women, SCI does not affect female fertility once menses return. Immediately following SCI, amenorrhea occurs in 85% of premenopausal women with cervical and high thoracic injuries and 50% to 60% of premenopausal women overall. Within 6 months and 1-year postinjury, 50% and 90% of premenopausal women, respectively, have return of menstruation. By 1-year postinjury, 90% of premenopausal women have return of normal menstrual cycles. The level and completeness of injury do not appear to influence the menstrual cycle. During pregnancy, there are a number of potential prenatal, perinatal, and postnatal issues that one needs to be aware of (376), and therefore the patient should be followed closely by the SCI physician in cooperation with the obstetrician.

Driving after Spinal Cord Injury

Driving assessments for the person with an SCI is an essential component of a comprehensive rehabilitation program and for the person to fully return to community activities. Most individuals with a motor level at and below C5 have the potential to return to independent driving with the appropriate adaptive equipment. The timing for a return to driving varies by the level and type of injury. The driver rehabilitation specialist evaluates patients and assists in choosing the proper vehicle and determining the modifications that will be required including the proper controls, lifts, and lock-down and tie-down devices.

A person with a complete paraplegic injury and no additional complications will probably require mechanical hand controls and a few additional minor pieces of equipment to operate a car with an automatic transmission. The evaluation and training for such individuals can usually occur within 3 months of the injury. Individuals with tetraplegia or incomplete motor injuries at any level are usually evaluated at a later time postinjury to allow for neurological recovery to plateau, since any gain in motor function can mean a difference in equipment required. In all cases, the person should be medically stable and be psychologically ready to return to the road.

A pre-driver assessment should be performed on all patients and includes a current and past medical and driving history, current medications, a vision screen, physical skills testing (including ROM and strength of the upper and lower extremities, balance, spasticity, transfer skills, and wheelchair loading skills), wheelchair or mobility equipment required, and reaction time (377,378). The amount of strength as well as the degree of sensation, particularly proprioception, will help determine the proper equipment required. If the individual has a history of brain trauma, cognitive and perceptual screens should also be included.

The behind the wheel assessment involves vehicle entry and exit and operation of primary and secondary controls (377). Evaluation in the vehicle, is important before finalizing the prescription. Training time can range from a few hours for mechanical hand controls and standard steering to over 40 hours for joystick drivers.

For most persons with paraplegia a car with an automatic transmission is an option if there are no problems with transfers. Sport utility vehicles are a possibility but these are more difficult to transfer into as they sit higher from the ground. There are transfer aides available that can raise the person up to the level of a full-size truck seat, but these are costly. If transfers or chair loading become more difficult due to shoulder pain, weight gain, medical complications, or age-related factors then vans should be considered. Loading devices can assist the client in loading the wheelchair. Options include car top devices that fold the manual wheelchair and stow it in a rooftop carrier, or a lift that can stow the folding chair behind the driver's seat in an extended cab three-door pickup truck.

Most persons with tetraplegia choose a modified van. Persons with an NLI above C5, will require a van to accommodate their transportation needs, but will not be able to drive independently. It is usually easier to transport a person while seated in the wheelchair, which is already set up to provide the proper support. A structurally modified full-size van or lowered-floor minivan will usually be required. For dependent passengers, the lowered floor drops eye height to a point where they may be able to see out the side windows.

CHRONIC SPINAL CORD INJURY-SPECIFIC MEDICAL COMPLICATIONS

Upper Extremity Neuromusculoskeletal Pain

Musculoskeletal complications are extremely common after SCI. The upper limbs are primarily designed for prehensile activities, but in persons with SCI they are used for weight-bearing activities including weight shifts, transfers, and wheelchair propulsion as well as for ADLs, thereby increasing the chances of overuse syndromes. Shoulder pain is the most commonly reported painful joint after SCI. Approximately 30% to 50% of patients complain of shoulder pain severe enough to interfere with function, with the prevalence increasing with time from injury (379–382). Pain during the first year after injury is more common in tetraplegics; in later years it is more common in paraplegics. Since the person with SCI relies extensively on the upper limbs, any further loss of upper limb function because of pain may have adverse effects on functional independence (383,384).

It is estimated that two-thirds of shoulder pain is due to chronic impingement syndrome and approximately half involves rotator cuff pathology (380,385). Bicipital tendonitis, subacromial bursitis, adhesive capsulitis, acromioclavicular osteoarthritis, and cervical radiculopathy are other common causes of shoulder pain in chronic SCI (386–388). Other causes that are specific in the SCI population include muscle imbal-

TABLE 79-14. Wheelchair User's Shoulder Pain Index (WUSPI)[a]
1. Pushing wheelchair ≥10 min
2. Pushing wheelchair up ramps/inclines
3. Sleeping
4. Loading wheelchair into car
5. Lifting object from overhead
6. Daily activities at work/school
7. Household chores
8. Wheelchair-car transfer
9. Wheelchair-tub transfer
10. Driving
11. Washing back
12. Bed-wheelchair transfer
13. Putting on t-shirt/pullover
14. Putting on pants
15. Putting on button-down shirt

[a]Listed in order of more to less pain for paraplegic individuals.
From Curtis KA, Roach KE, Applegate EB, et al. Development of the Wheelchair User's Shoulder Pain Index (WUSPI). Paraplegia 1995;33:290–293.

ance, spasticity, contractures, heterotopic ossification, and the presence of a syrinx.

The approach to shoulder pain in the chronic SCI patient is similar to that of the able-bodied, keeping in mind the specific potential causes in SCI. If pain develops acutely, then referred pain should be excluded, including urinary tract infection, peptic ulcer disease, angina, and an acute abdominal problem. Pain associated with neurological changes (i.e., weakness, sensory loss or reflex changes) may be due to peripheral nerve entrapment, radiculopathy, or a posttraumatic syrinx.

ROM, strength and sensory testing, provocative tests for specific abnormalities, as well as a functional assessment should be performed including an evaluation of the patient's posture, function (i.e., pressure reliefs, wheelchair mobility, transfers), and home/work environment. Diagnostic tests are ordered as needed. The Wheelchair User's Shoulder Pain Index (WUSPI) is a 15-item self-report instrument, with a range of 0 to 15, that measures shoulder pain intensity during various ADLs using a visual analogue scale (384,388) (Table 79-14).

Relief of acute pain includes pharmacological intervention (NSAIDs, acetaminophen, muscle relaxants), rest, injections, and modalities. Acupuncture may be helpful (389,390). Complete rest of a painful shoulder is difficult but decreasing stress on the joints should be encouraged by using compensatory techniques (e.g., using a transfer board rather than performing lateral transfers). After the pain has subsided, emphasis should be focused toward preventing further injury by obtaining a balance in strength and flexibility of the musculature surrounding the shoulder (391,392). A proper wheelchair and back support will also play a role in preventing shoulder pain. Surgery can be considered in those who fail conservative management (393).

Overuse injuries may also affect the elbow, wrist, and hand, including the development of carpal tunnel syndrome (CTS), ulnar nerve entrapment at the elbow and wrist, de Quervain's syndrome or other tenosynovitis, osteoarthritis, and stress fractures. Electrodiagnostic criteria for CTS are noted in about half of chronic SCI patients, with a higher incidence at longer times postinjury (379,394–396). This is due to recurrent stress from transfers, wheelchair propulsion, and pressure reliefs. Treatment for CTS includes analgesics, NSAIDs, splinting (especially at night), injections (anesthetic or corticosteroid), physical modalities (ultrasound, friction massage, etc.), and education regarding transfers to avoid end-range stress. Surgical release may be required, with the postoperative recovery time being weighed against the long-term benefits of the procedure.

Since much of the chronic upper limb neuromusculoskeletal problems are due to the overuse from functional activities, it is vital that proper exercise techniques and shoulder protection and conservation be learned early, during acute rehabilitation, and reinforced frequently. Often one hears the phrase "no pain, no gain"; rather the SCI team should teach their patients to "conserve it, to preserve it" (397).

Pain after Spinal Cord Injury

Pain is a major and common problem after SCI. In the acute phase, pain is usually related to damage to the soft tissue and skeletal system from the initial trauma. After the injuries are appropriately treated, this type of pain usually subsides. However, 47% to 96% of the SCI population will develop neuropathic pain several weeks later that is severe enough to hinder rehabilitation and reduce quality of life (398). The pain is often described as burning, tingling, cramping, shocklike, or a sensation of intolerable coldness.

Although the reasons are unknown, several studies have identified cord injuries to the cervical, thoracic, and lumbosacral regions, GSWs, and incomplete injuries as predisposing factors that increase the risk of developing neuropathic pain (399–403), although other studies have not confirmed such an association (404,405). Instead of physical factors, psychosocial deficiencies may better predict subjective pain complaints. Individuals who are depressed, anxious, or experience severe stress are more likely to have pain (404), while those who are active and working are less prone to complain of pain.

No single widely accepted classification scheme for SCI pain has been outlined, which has hindered research and communication among clinicians. To clarify matters, the International Association for the Study of Pain (IASP) proposes to divide SCI-related pain into a multi-tier classification scheme (406). SCI pain is first divided into two broad categories, nociceptive and neuropathic. Nociceptive pain is then divided into musculoskeletal and visceral pain. Neuropathic pain is further described by its relation to the trauma site—either above, at, or below the level of injury. Finally, the anatomic structure that generates the pain is named.

There are several proposed mechanisms for the origin of neuropathic pain after SCI. Deafferentation causes an imbalance of afferent input from the spinothalamic tract and dorsal columns, hyperexcitability of the neurons within the dorsal horn, and loss of inhibition from more rostral structures. Electrophysiological studies have recorded greater spontaneous discharges, reduced thresholds, and protracted firing by wide dynamic range (WDR) neurons in the thalamus and spinal cord. Excitatory amino acids such as glutamate are released at the time of injury and activate N-methyl-D-aspartate (NMDA) receptors (407). The blockade of NMDA receptors with intrathecal administration of ketamine has been shown to reduce continuous and evoked pain (408). The loss of inhibition by GABA-mediated signals is associated with hypersensitivity of WDR neurons. Ischemic models of SCI in animals show reversal of hypersensitivity when the GABA$_B$ agonist baclofen is administered (409). Pain signals are modified in the spinal cord by the release of monoamines such as serotonin and noradrenaline from descending tracts that originated in the brain stem. These nerve fibers synapse with interneurons that release endorphins, which then down-regulate nociceptive input. When the spinal cord is disrupted, this inhibitory system is lost.

Unfortunately, although many treatments have been tried, few have been found to be effective in controlling SCI neuropathic pain. Several studies have not found any advantage to spinal cord stimulation (410–412). Transcutaneous nerve stimulation appears to alleviate neuropathic pain originating at the level of injury but not below (413). Neuroablative procedures are also largely ineffective. Although half of the patients who underwent a dorsal root entry zone procedure reported good pain relief, most of them had either caudal or unilateral pain. The majority of those with below level neuropathic pain had poor results (414). Randomized controlled studies involving amitriptyline, trazodone, mexiletine, and valproate have not shown a consistent benefit. An exception is gabapentin, a synthetic structural analogue of GABA, which increases GABA levels and decreases glutamate levels within the spinal cord (415,416). There are no published studies examining the use of oral opioids in the spinal cord population. However, opioids are gaining acceptance as a therapeutic option in nonmalignant pain syndromes and are rated by SCI patients as one of the more effective treatments (417).

Bone Loss

After SCI, bone loss occurs in the LEs at a rate of 1% to 2% per month, with a more rapid loss in the distal femur and proximal tibia as compared with the proximal and midshaft femur. There is a greater loss of trabecular bone as opposed to cortical bone. Bone loss is most active in the first year postinjury, with a slower loss over the next few years, with resolve by the fourth year postinjury (329). Dual energy x-ray absorptometry (DEXA) scan testing in persons with chronic SCI reveals a loss of 26% of bone mass of the UEs in persons with tetraplegia, approximately 25% in the proximal femur and femoral shaft, 40% in the distal femur, and a slightly higher loss in the proximal and distal tibia. There is an increase in bone mass in the lumbar spine of all patients, possibly due to constant loading while sitting in the wheelchair, and in the forearm of athletes. There is no difference in bone loss in the LEs between persons with paraplegia or tetraplegia (327,329,418–420).

Treatments for bone loss have included weight bearing, FES, and pharmacological intervention. Weight-bearing activities, standing, and ambulation, have not consistently shown an increase in bone mineral density (BMD) (421). Most trials of FES have been in persons with chronic SCI without much benefit. In acute studies, there may be some preventive benefits (422, 423). The use of FES in a person with chronic SCI and low BMD may lead to fracture (424), and caution should be taken. Pharmacological interventions have been trialed. Recent reports of treatment with intravenous pamidronate (425) and oral alendronate (426) have shown some benefits. Many centers are now treating chronic SCI patients with bisphosphonates to improve BMD.

Fracture

As a general guideline, fractures that occur at the time of the acute injury should be treated as usual (i.e., open reduction internal fixation, or ORIF). Fractures that occur in chronic patients with SCI who do not use their lower limbs for functional mobility should be treated conservatively, unless there are mitigating circumstances that require surgical intervention.

The cumulative incidence of chronic long-bone fractures is approximately 2.5% over 20 years after SCI (226); however, the true incidence is probably higher because not all fractures are recognized, nor do these patients all present to SCI centers. Fractures are more common in complete versus incomplete SCI, in women versus men, and in persons with paraplegia versus tetraplegia (427). Most fractures are due to falls during transfers, but fractures can result from minor stresses (e.g., long-sitting or range-of-motion exercises) or without any known etiology. Supracondylar and peritrochanteric femur fractures are most common, followed by femoral shaft, tibial, and humeral fractures (428,429).

The patient may present with a low-grade fever, swollen limb, and malaise. A plain x-ray will usually give a definitive diagnosis. Hospitalization is not always required and should be reserved for those who have severe swelling or who require surgery. The main goals of treatment are to minimize complications, allow for healing with satisfactory alignment and to preserve prefracture function. Most fractures are treated nonoperatively with soft-padded splints (427,430). A well-padded knee-immobilizer is useful for femoral supracondylar, femoral shaft, and proximal tibial fractures; a well-padded ankle immobilizer can be used for distal tibial fractures. In nonambulatory patients, some degree of shortening and angulation are acceptable (430). Rotational deformity, however, is usually less acceptable. Circumferential casts should be avoided; if they are used, they must be well-padded and bivalved for skin inspection at least twice-daily. The patient should be allowed to sit within a few days. Callus formation is usually evident in 3 to 4 weeks, however, ROM is initiated at 6 to 8 weeks, with weight-bearing (tilt table, standing, and stand-pivot transfers) delayed for a longer period. While nonunion of fractures occur (2% to 10%), these are not clinically significant in those who do not weight-bear through their lower limbs.

Surgery, circumferential casting, and external fixation are usually not indicated in the SCI population because of potential complications due to low bone mass, risk of osteomyelitis, recurrent bacteremia, and skin breakdown. Surgery may be indicated when conservative methods will not control rotational deformity, for proximal femur fractures, in patients with severe muscle spasm, if vascular supply is in danger, and in whom shortening and angulation will result in unacceptable function or cosmesis. Femoral neck and subtrochanteric fractures are probably the most difficult to manage and internal fixation may be considered if a minimal device such as an intramedullary rod can be used (430).

Posttraumatic Syringomyelia

The most common cause of progressive myelopathy after an SCI is posttraumatic syringomyelia (PTS). PTS, also called ascending cystic degeneration or progressive posttraumatic cystic myelopathy, may develop at any time, from 2 months to decades postinjury. PTS presents as neurological decline in 3% to 8% of SCI patients, as an elongated cavity by MRI in 12% to 28% of patients, and as an elongated cavity at autopsy in 17% to 20% of patients (286,431–434). A syrinx should be differentiated from posttraumatic cysts, which are small cystic structures that occur in 39% to 59% of SCI patients at the zone of cord injury but do not extend longitudinally and do not cause neurological decline (435).

The pathogenesis is unknown, but the cavity begins at the level of the cord injury in the gray matter between the dorsal horns and posterior columns (436). Initiating factors include cord hematoma, residual spinal canal stenosis, and residual spinal kyphotic deformity. The cyst may extend rostrally or caudally, compressing the cord, by dissecting through intermediate gray matter, and may result from increases in subarachnoid fluid pressure due to intraabdominal or intrathoracic pressure increases (i.e., cough, sneeze, straining or Valsalva, weight lifting, forward-lean pressure release, and quad coughing).

Early symptoms and signs of PTS are often nonspecific and variable; some patients with markedly elongated syrinxes that dilate the spinal cord may have minimal symptoms. The signs and symptoms often present unilaterally early in the evolution of PTS, later becoming bilateral. The most common presenting symptom is pain, usually located at the site of the original injury or may radiate to the neck or upper limbs. The pain is described as aching or burning, often worse with coughing, sneezing, straining, and in the sitting rather than in the supine position. The earliest sign is an ascending loss of deep tendon reflexes. An ascending sensory level is common, typically with a dissociated sensory loss with impaired pain and temperature sensation but intact touch, position, and vibration sense. Loss of pain sensation can lead to a Charcot joint. Weakness occurs, but rarely in isolation. Additional findings may include increased or decreased spasticity, hyperhidrosis, autonomic dysreflexia, neck muscle fatigue with prolonged sitting, loss of reflex bladder emptying, worsening orthostatic hypotension, scoliosis, central or obstructive sleep apnea, new Horner's syndrome, reduced respiratory drive, diaphragmatic paralysis, cranial nerve dysfunction, impaired vagal cardiovascular reflexes, and sudden death (286,431,437).

MRI with gadolinium is the gold standard for diagnosing PTS. MRI characteristics often associated with neurological decline include those that are longer and wider, those with poorly demarcated T2-weighted signal hyperintensity at the rostral extent, those associated with spinal stenosis, or a flow void sign on T2-weighted images suggesting high pressure. (432–434,438). A large syrinx however may be seen without any symptoms noted. Electrodiagnostic findings are occasionally used to aid in the diagnosis (431,439,440).

Both conservative and surgical treatments have been advocated for posttraumatic syringomyelia. A syrinx may spontaneously resolve, progress, then plateau or progress continuously. Neurological monitoring is essential, and includes clinical examination, serial electrodiagnostic tests, or serial MRI. Conservative treatment includes close monitoring, activity restrictions, and providing rehabilitation interventions as needed (i.e., functional training and adaptive equipment). Activity restrictions include avoiding maneuvers that increase intrathoracic/abdominal pressure (i.e., high-force exercise; Valsalva, Credé, and quad coughing with direct compression over the IVC; and avoiding anterior weight reliefs).

Surgical treatment is usually indicated if there is ongoing neurological decline or severe intractable pain. Surgical treatments include shunting (syringo-subarachnoid, syringo-pleural, or syringo-peritoneal); reconstructing the subarachnoid space with dissection of arachnoiditis/meningeal scarring and duraplasty; and cordectomy (441–444). Surgery yields improved strength and improved pain control in some but not all, whereas sensory recovery is not usually as favorable. Reduction of syrinx size on postoperative MRI usually predicts a good surgical result (445); however, complete resolution of the syrinx is not necessary for a good clinical outcome. Recurrence of neurological symptoms is common.

Surgical Interventions of Upper Extremity in Tetraplegia

Reconstructive surgery following tetraplegia can often improve the patient's motor function by one level (446). The most common procedures include tendon transfers where a functioning proximal muscle is used to control distal parts, and arthrodesis of the interphalangeal (IP) joint of the thumb that is often performed with tendon transfer procedures to restore active lateral thumb opposition.

The key components when evaluating potential candidates for UE surgery include the proper timing after injury, and the

**TABLE 79-15. Modified International Classification
for Individuals with Tetraplegia**

Motor Group	Functional Muscles[a]
0	Weak or absent BR (grade 3 or less)
1	BR
2	BR, ECRL
3	BR, ECRL, ECRB
4	BR, ECRL, ECRB, PT
5	BR, ECRL, ECRB, PT, FCR
6	BR, ECRL, ECRB, PT, FCR, finger extensors
7	BR, ECRL, ECRB, PT, FCR, finger extensors, thumb extensors
8	BR, ECRL, ECRB, PT, FCR, finger extensors, thumb extensors, finger flexors
9	Lacks intrinsics only

Sensory	
O:	Two-point discrimination in thumb ≥10 mm
Cu:	Two-point discrimination in thumb ≤10 mm

[a]Functional muscle: grade 4 or 5.
BR, brachioradialis; ECRL, extensor carpi radialis longus; ECRB, extensor carpi radialis brevis; PT, pronator teres; FCR, flexor carpi radialis.

proper physical and behavioral assessments. Most agree that UE surgery should not be performed until the patient has demonstrated neurological stability for a minimum of a few months. The physical assessment includes evaluating occupational performance, UE muscle strength, sensation, ROM, and the presence of spasticity. Occupational performance areas include ADLs, work/productive activities, and play/leisure activities (447). The functional goals and their impact on occupational performance should be discussed with the patient prior to surgical intervention.

To facilitate communication among professionals, the International Classification of the Upper Limb in Quadriplegia is used (448) (Table 79-15). The shoulder muscles should also be evaluated since successful hand function depends on precise placement of the hand. As opposed to the ASIA classification system, a muscle should have 4/5 strength rather than 3/5 to be considered functional, as an initial grade of 3/5 after transfer will most likely not be strong enough to perform the needed tasks (449). Spasticity in the transferred muscle should be absent or minimal.

Sensory testing is performed by using the Weber two-point discrimination test (450). If there is 2-point discrimination of greater than 10 mm at the pulp of the thumb, the patient is classified in the "O" or Ocular group. Subjects who have both visual clues and cutaneous afferents present (2-point discrimination less than 10 mm) are classified as "O-Cu" or Ocular-Cutaneous. ROM of the wrist and fingers should be full for all procedures involving the hand, and for the posterior deltoid or biceps to triceps transfer there should be functional ROM at the shoulder and no more than a 30-degree elbow flexion contracture.

The behavioral assessment includes the motivation and history of compliance of the individual; understanding expected surgical/functional outcome; commitment to postoperative rehabilitation; and psychological status and social support. Candidates should be aware of the time of immobilization, restrictions, and extent of the postoperative rehabilitation program, and how these will affect the patient's lifestyle. Additional assistance or equipment is also necessary during recovery for

many ADLs such as weight shifts, transfers, toileting, and so forth. During the postoperative period, patients who use manual wheelchairs will need to rely on power wheelchairs or assistance from others.

There are a few generalizations regarding tendon transfers that should be remembered.

1. It is generally not possible to simultaneously perform tendon transfers to restore both active opening and closing in one surgical procedure; usually two separate procedures are required.
2. If surgical intervention of both extremities is indicated, the stronger extremity is usually operated on first. If both extremities are of equal strength, the dominant one is reconstructed first.
3. If only visual afferents are present in an individual with bilateral C5 motor level and no digital sensation, surgery should be limited to one extremity. If cutaneous afferents are also present, both extremities may undergo surgical reconstruction, but only one extremity at a time.

At the C5 level, the muscles generally available for transfer are the deltoid and brachioradialis (BR). The most common procedures include the transfer of the BR to the extensor carpi radialis brevis (ECRB) to restore wrist extension and deltoid to triceps to provide elbow extension. For the BR to ECRB transfer, improvement in wrist extensor strength and functional improvement are noted including lifting objects, feeding, grooming, and hygiene (451,452). The posterior deltoid to triceps transfer procedure allows for active elbow extension, enabling patients to stabilize themselves for sitting and transferring and to reach overhead against gravity, with functional improvements in the areas of grooming and personal hygiene, pressure relief, writing speed and clarity, and self-feeding (453). The goal, however, is not to improve the ability to perform a transfer, since the latissimus dorsi, the prime shoulder depressor muscle, is lacking. A biceps to triceps transfer can also be performed (454,455).

At the C6 functional level, the Moberg "key grip" procedure may be performed to restore the lateral or "key" grip in patients without a natural tenodesis (456,457). Improvements in functional activities include grooming, eating, writing, and desktop skills, and these benefits are maintained over time (458). Transfer of an active muscle, like the BR or others to the flexor pollicus longus (FPL) to provide lateral pinch and to the finger flexors to provide grasp, provides better function and is preferable to Moberg's simple FPL tenodesis (459–462).

Posterior deltoid to triceps transfer may also be performed in C6 patients. This procedure is recommended prior to hand reconstruction, or simultaneously without diminishing outcomes (456–463). A supination contracture of the forearm that may occur in individuals with C5 and C6 motor injuries can be corrected by rerouting of the biceps brachii around the radial neck (464).

At the C7 level the goal is to restore active grasp and improve hand control. Transfer of the BR to FPL can achieve restoration of thumb flexion. Restoration of finger flexion is achieved through transfer of ECRL, flexor carpi ulnaris, or physical therapy to the flexor digitorum profundus (FDP). At the C8 level, an intrinsic minus or "claw hand" posture results. A lumbrical bar that prevents hyperextension of the metacarpal phalangeal (MPs) may improve a patient's function, and surgery is rarely indicated.

Immobilization postoperatively of the extremity in a cast is the first step and varies depending on the surgery, but is usually between 1 to 3 months. The patient should be instructed in proper elevation techniques to control edema. Once the patient is cleared for motion, a removable thermoplastic splint is fabricated to protect the transfers from over-stretching. Scar management may include breaking down adhesions, and desensitization techniques. Success following tendon transfer depends on reeducating the pattern of motor recruitment so that the muscle of the transferred tendon fires appropriately to its new function. Biofeedback and therapeutic electrical stimulation can help reeducate muscles following tendon transfers (465, 466). Activities are graded progressively by performance time and resistance applied, eliminating any that create heavy resistance to the tendons until after 3 months.

The Freehand system is a neuroprosthesis that can be implanted in patients with C5 or C6 tetraplegia. Movement of the one shoulder will control the ability to control the opposite hand to allow for grasp. The procedure can be performed in association with tendon transfers. Studies have shown, that the neuroprosthesis is safe, offers improved pinch force and grasp-release abilities, with the ability to be more independent in performing ADLs. Home use of the device for regular function and satisfaction with the neuroprosthesis are high (467–469). For further detail see Chapter 66. Newer techniques of surgery with FES include advanced controls to allow individuals with C4 and higher lesions or C7 lesions to take better advantage of the neuroprosthesis (470), and nerve grafting for persons with C4-C5 level of injury with LMN injuries. The nerve graft is attempted to restore volitional control or to reverse flaccid paralysis into spastic paralysis for application of FES (471).

DUAL DIAGNOSIS: TRAUMATIC BRAIN INJURY IN A PERSON WITH SPINAL CORD INJURY

An impact severe enough to cause an SCI may cause varying degrees of TBI; thus the person sustains a dual disability (dual diagnosis). Prior studies have demonstrated a rate of TBI between 24% and 59% when SCI is the primary injury (5,472,473). Data from the model SCI systems report that 28.2% of SCI patients have at least a minor brain injury with loss of consciousness, while 11.5% have a TBI severe enough to demonstrate cognitive or behavioral changes (5). The higher the level of the SCI the greater are the chances of sustaining a concomitant TBI. When the primary diagnosis is TBI, the incidence of SCI is lower.

In many instances this problem is undiagnosed, especially if the brain injury is mild. Evaluation includes preinjury factors such as substance abuse, premorbid brain injury, and learning disability. Some clinical features include the best and worst Glasgow Coma Scale (474) scores within 24 hours of injury, the duration of coma, and the length of posttraumatic amnesia (PTA) (475,476). This parameter may be challenging to measure retrospectively, and the Galveston Orientation and Amnesia Test (GOAT) is a valuable tool (477). There are a number of scales available to assess the extent of the TBI but all have limitations, and formal neuropsychological testing may be of value. The Halstead-Reitan neuropsychological test battery is widely used, but often not given in its full form.

The individual with a dual diagnosis presents a tremendous challenge to the rehabilitation team. Deficits may be seen in attention, concentration, and memory, as well as interfere with new learning and problem solving. The patient may exhibit agitation, aggression, and disinhibition, as well as depression. This is problematic as SCI rehabilitation requires intensive new learning, with the ability to master new skills in terms of mobility and self-care and adapt to a new lifestyle to be able to integrate into the community. Recognizing that the TBI exists and then developing a comprehensive treatment program to deal with the dual injury is necessary in order for individuals to

meet their maximum potential. Finding the proper setting for therapy should be determined (i.e., whether the patient can tolerate therapy in an active gym, or requires a quiet setting to learn new tasks). Individualized therapy may be more appropriate. Before a patient is diagnosed as having a dual disability based on some behavioral issues, the clinician should seek other causes for such behavior including the possibility of seizures, posttraumatic hydrocephalus, intracranial pathology, neuroendocrine disturbance, metabolic disturbance, side effects of centrally acting medications, hypoxemia, and infectious issues (478).

Treatment of the posttraumatic agitation in a person with dual diagnoses is a coordinated effort from a behavioral and pharmacotherapeutic intervention point-of-view. Patients often require a limitation of distracting environmental tasks and quiet environments (479,480). The most commonly used medications include carbamazepine, valproic acid, amantadine, and β-blockers. Trazodone and nefazodone have been used, especially to enhance sleep. Benzodiazepines and tricyclic antidepressants may be used, but there are potential side effects regarding their effect on cognitive recovery and new learning.

Some of the most frequently prescribed medications in the treatment of medical issues in SCI may cause sedation or impair cognition and should be used with caution in the dual-diagnosis patient. These include medications frequently used in the treatment of spasticity including clonidine, baclofen, tizanidine and diazepam, and GI agents such as histamine-blocking agents and metoclopramide that may produce deleterious cognitive responses as well as extrapyramidal side effects.

DVT prophylaxis in the person who has a dual diagnosis presents a serious dilemma. No clear data exist regarding safety for prophylaxis among those with a traumatic intracranial lesion. It is currently thought that anticoagulation may be safely initiated 10 to 14 days after craniotomy (481), however individualization of each case is important. Those with a high risk of thromboembolic disorders should be considered early for an IVC filter.

The physician caring for patients with a dual diagnosis should be familiar with some of the late complications of TBI. Hydrocephalus is the most common treatable CNS condition after TBI. The symptoms of normal pressure hydrocephalus may be difficult to diagnose in individuals with the impairments related to their SCI and a CT scan can help with the diagnosis. Neuroendocrine complications including pituitary and hypothalamic disorders may present with malaise, hyponatremia, hypothermia, and bradycardia as well as sleep and appetite dysfunction. Sodium metabolism problems include syndrome of inappropriate antidiuretic hormone secretion (SIADH), cerebral salt wasting, and central diabetes insipidus. Central dysautonomia can produce findings of marked temperature dysregulation. The overall incidence of posttraumatic epilepsy has been reported to be 5% and routine use of prophylaxis beyond 1 week is not warranted (482). Risk factors for posttraumatic seizures include depressed skull fracture, early posttraumatic seizure, presence of foreign body, dural tear, cerebral contusions, and posttraumatic amnesia greater than 24 hours.

While few studies have examined the actual effects of TBI on outcome among individuals with SCI, greater adjustment difficulties and unmet needs were noted among persons with dual diagnosis (483–485). Intuitively it seems that the presence of dual diagnoses would have a negative impact on all aspects of care. This would include an increase in the length of stay in acute rehabilitation, a decreased rate of discharge to home, and increased rate of medical complications thus increasing rehospitalization. Medical issues may include pressure ulcers due to the inability to remember to perform a pressure relief, and bladder and bowel difficulties due to the inability to perform these programs adequately.

LONG-TERM FOLLOW-UP

Outpatient programs have recently taken on an even more important role than in previous decades because of the shortened inpatient length of stay. This includes close monitoring of the medical status (i.e., bowel, bladder, skin, and respiratory management), and a comprehensive therapy program that includes not only physical and occupational therapies, but also psychology and vocational counseling. With the shorter length of stay there is less time to help the patient and family adjust to the disability, and to address all of the obstacles present that may interfere with social, vocational, and recreational reintegration.

Long-term follow-up with the SCI specialist is extremely important. Initially visits should occur on a monthly basis, especially while the person is on outpatient therapy. This allows for monitoring of medical issues, reevaluation of the therapy program and updating goals, and equipment prescription. As patients go home from inpatient hospitalization earlier, medical issues that previously were experienced in the hospital now develop while at home. This includes bowel, bladder and spasticity changes, and the development of heterotopic ossification and autonomic dysreflexia. After these issues are stabilized and outpatient therapy has switched to a maintenance-type program, visits to the SCI specialist should be every 3 to 6 months through the second year. For those patients who are medically stable, yearly visits are then recommended. The importance of these visits is to review any medical changes, monitor the neurological examination to make sure that there is no deterioration, ensure that the equipment is being maintained, and prescribe any additional equipment that may be needed. Deterioration of the neurological status may be secondary to a tethered cord, syringomyelia, or peripheral problems such as median or ulnar nerve entrapment or musculoskeletal complications. As a greater amount of persons with SCI are surviving longer after their injury, the importance of their follow-up visits to maintain their quality of life cannot be overemphasized.

At times, readmission to the rehabilitation hospital for medical (i.e., pressure ulcer, autonomic dysreflexia) or rehabilitation issues may be needed. For medical issues the SCI physician is able to care for the patient with consultation as required and the entire rehabilitation staff is most keenly aware of other issues that can occur in the SCI patient. This includes the importance of maintaining the proper bowel and bladder programs, skin issues, and awareness of the signs and symptoms as well as the proper treatment for autonomic dysreflexia. In addition, many times the person with SCI may require a "refresher course" in rehabilitation techniques that can best be taught in an intensive inpatient setting.

Chronic Respiratory Care

The goals of long-term pulmonary care are similar to those acutely: to stabilize the alveoli, clear secretions, and keep the patient free of atelectasis. As pneumonia is the most common cause of death among those with an SCI, patients should periodically have their forced vital capacity (VC) measured, as well as their degree of oxygenation, and they should be questioned as to whether they have symptoms of sleep-disordered breathing, including sleep apnea. Individuals with SCI with a history

of ventilator use at disease onset, a history of repeated atelectasis or pneumonia, a VC of less than 2 L, nocturnal hypercapnia, and a mean SaO_2 of less than 95% are at risk to develop late-onset respiratory insufficiency (186). Patients with a VC below 2 L are at risk for respiratory failure during upper respiratory infections or after surgical anesthesia. These individuals can be taught to monitor their oxygen saturation with a pulse oximeter and use assisted cough techniques (manual or mechanical) or assisted ventilation via NIPPV or BIPAP until they improve.

Individuals with tetraplegia should receive a yearly influenza vaccine. If having undergone a splenectomy, the individual with an SCI should also receive immunization for pneumococcus.

Sleep Apnea

Sleep-disordered breathing occurs in approximately 15% to 60% of patients with SCI (486–489). It is unclear if there is a relationship between sleep apnea and obesity and neck circumference, higher level of injury, VC, the effect of certain medications (i.e., antispasticity medications), and length of time from the original injury. In SCI patients, sleep apnea is primarily obstructive, with a small percentage of patients demonstrating central sleep apnea. Complications include hypertension, pulmonary hypertension and cor pulmonale, congestive heart failure, deterioration in mental function, daytime sleepiness, impotence, and cognitive changes including poor judgment.

It is advisable to review questions about sleep disturbance, snoring, daytime somnolence, and nasal symptoms with SCI outpatients. Optimal workup would include an overnight oximetry recording, followed by a formal sleep study if the oximetry recording is abnormal. Treatment includes CPAP or BIPAP, depending on the situation, as well as possible use of tricyclic antidepressants, theophylline preparations, and medications directed toward relief of upper airway symptoms.

THE FUTURE

The quest for cure is as strong as ever, with many new advances constantly being made. Over the last decade there is increased knowledge regarding the basic pathophysiology of SCI as well as new pharmacological strategies in the acute and chronic treatment to enhance neurological and functional recovery (490). In animal models, scientists have successfully used antibodies to block growth inhibitors, applied growth factors, implanted cells and peripheral nerve bridges, and used gene therapies to stimulate spinal cord regeneration. Some advances are nearly ready for application in the clinical setting. The key factors for cure include: minimizing secondary effects of injury; neutralizing the effects of substrates that inhibit CNS regeneration; delivery of regenerating-promoting substances to the injured spinal cord; allowing a bridge to which the spinal cord axons can attach and grow along after injury; and determining the genes that may allow for "turning on" axonal growth after injury.

For acute SCI, the effect of hyperbaric oxygen treatment may be helpful (491). Further study is needed. A Phase I trial of activated macrophage transplants in patients with complete SCI has been completed in Israel (Proneuron Biotechnology, USA; Weizmann Institute of Science, Rehovot, Israel) and a Phase II trial has been initiated and is expected to begin in the U.S. in 2003.

Currently the only medication being studied for chronic SCI patients is 4-aminopyridine (4-AP). 4-AP is a potassium (K+) channel blocker that blocks fast internodal axonal K+, which blocks conduction of the nerve action potential. It restores conduction in demyelinated nerve fibers and multiple studies in MS and some studies in SCI have shown a trend toward increased bowel and motor function in incomplete injuries, and decreased pain and spasticity (492–495). Newer studies are currently underway. Phase I clinical trials to treat SCI with porcine fetal stem cells have been initiated.

In terms of rehabilitation, body weight support with treadmill training has been discussed earlier, theorizing that upregulation of neurotransmitters due to sensory input and training of a central pattern generator may be the mechanisms responsible for the improved function when using this training method (496–498). The effect of drugs as it relates to enhancing or impeding ambulation has been proposed (499). The combination of rehabilitation techniques and spinal electrical stimulation has been trialed in persons with chronic SCI (500).

While the basic science research continues to make progress, with the ultimate goal of a cure for SCI, what we currently have available is rehabilitation to help maximize functional potential. For individuals who suffer an SCI, the best way for them to be able to take advantage of future research is to be as medically and physically healthy as possible. This includes being active in all areas including social, recreational, and vocational activities. This is what rehabilitation is all about.

REFERENCES

1. Elsberg LA. The Edwin Smith Surgical Papyrus and the diagnosis and treatment of injuries of the skull and spine 5000 years ago. *Ann Med Hist* 1931;3:271.
2. DeLisa JA, Hammond MC. The history of the subspecialty of spinal cord injury medicine. In: Kirshblum SC, Campagnolo D, DeLisa JE, eds. *Spinal cord medicine*. Philadelphia: Lippincott Williams & Wilkins, 2002:1–4.
3. Stover SL, DeVivo MJ, Go BK. History, implementation, and current status of the national spinal cord injury database. *Arch Phys Med Rehabil* 1999;80:1365–1371.
4. Go BK, DeVivo MJ, Richards JS. The epidemiology of spinal cord injury. In: Stover SL, DeLisa JA, Whiteneck GG, eds. *Spinal cord injury: clinical outcomes from the model systems*. Gaithersburg, MD: Aspen, 1995:21–55.
5. Nobunaga AI, Go BK, Karunas RB. Recent demographic and injury trends in people served by the model spinal cord injury care systems. *Arch Phys Med Rehabil* 1999;80:1372–1382.
6. Facts and figures: National Spinal Cord Injury Statistical Center. *J Spinal Cord Med* 2002;25:139–140.
7. Devivo M. Epidemiology of traumatic spinal cord injury. In: Kirshblum SC, Campagnolo D, DeLisa JE, eds. *Spinal cord medicine*. Philadelphia: Lippincott Williams & Wilkins, 2002:69–81.
8. DeVivo MJ, Richards JS. Marriage rates among persons with spinal cord injury. *Rehabil Psych* 1996;41:321–339.
9. DeVivo MJ, Hawkins LN, Richards JS, et al. Outcomes of post-spinal cord injury marriages [published erratum appears in *Arch Phys Med Rehabil* 1995;76:397]. *Arch Phys Med Rehabil* 1995;76:130–138.
10. Krause JS, Kewman D, DeVivo MJ, et al. Employment after spinal cord injury: an analysis of cases from the model spinal cord injury systems. *Arch Phys Med Rehabil* 1999;80:1492–1500.
11. DeVivo MJ, Rutt RD, Stover SL, et al. Employment after spinal cord injury. *Arch Phys Med Rehabil* 1987;68:494–498.
12. Berkowitz M, O'Leary PK, Kruse DL, et al. Spinal cord injury: an analysis of medical and social costs. New York: Demos, 1998.
13. Hess DW, Ripley DL, McKinley WO, et al. Predictors for return to work after spinal cord injury: a 3-year multicenter analysis. *Arch Phys Med Rehabil* 2000;81:359–363.
14. Fiedler RC, Granger CV. Uniform data system for medical rehabilitation: report of first admissions for 1996. *Am J Phys Med Rehabil* 1998;77:69–75.
15. DeVivo MJ. Discharge disposition from model spinal cord injury care system rehabilitation programs. *Arch Phys Med Rehabil* 1999;80:785–790.
16. Fiedler IG, Laud PW, Maiman DJ, et al. Economics of managed care in spinal cord injury. *Arch Phys Med Rehabil* 1999;80:1441–1449.
17. DeVivo MJ, Krause JS, Lammertse DP. Recent trends in mortality and causes of death among persons with spinal cord injury. *Arch Phys Med Rehabil* 1999;80:1411–1419.
18. Krause JS, Sternberg M, Lottes S, et al. Mortality after spinal cord injury: an 11-year prospective study. *Arch Phys Med Rehabil* 1997;78:815–821.
19. DeVivo MJ, Stover SL. Long-term survival and causes of death. In: Stover SL, DeLisa JA, Whiteneck GG, eds. *Spinal cord injury: clinical outcomes from the model systems*. Gaithersburg, MD: Aspen, 1995:289–316.
20. Atkinson PP, Atkinson JL. Spinal shock. *Mayo Clin Proc* 1996;71:384–389.
21. Vale FL, Burns J, Jackson AB, et al. Combined medical and surgical treatment after acute spinal cord injury: results of a prospective pilot study to assess the merits of aggressive medical resuscitation and blood pressure management. *J Neurosurg* 1997;87:239–246.
22. Kay MM. Krana JM. External transcutaneous pacemaker for profound bradycardia associated with spinal cord trauma. *Surg Neurol* 1984;22:344–346.
23. Gilgoff IS, Ward SLD, Holn AR. Cardiac pacemaker in high spinal cord injury. *Arch Phys Med Rehabil* 1991;72:601–603.
24. Ragnarsson KT, Hall KM, Wilmot CB, et al. Management of pulmonary, cardiovascular and metabolic conditions after spinal cord injury. In: Stover SL, DeLisa JA, Whiteneck GG, eds. *Spinal cord injury: clinical outcomes for the model systems*. Gaithersburg, MD: Aspen Publishers, 1995:79–99.
25. Kirshblum S. Johnston MV, Brown J, et al. Predictors of dysphagia after spinal cord injury. *Arch Phys Med Rehabil* 1999;80:1101–1106.
26. Vaccaro AR, An HS, Betz RR, et al. The management of acute spinal trauma: prehospital and in-hospital emergency care. *Instr Course Lect* 1997;46:113–125.
27. Savitsky E, Votey S. Emergency department approach to acute thoracolumbar spine trauma. *J Emerg Med* 1997;15:49–60.
28. Chiles BW III, Cooper PR. Acute spinal injury. *N Engl J Med* 1996;334:514–520.
29. Heary RF, Vaccaro AR, Mesa JJ, et al. Thoracolumbar infections in penetrating injuries to the spine. *Orthop Clin North Am* 1996;27:69–81.
30. Bracken M, Holford T. Effects of timing of methylprednisolone or naloxone administration on recovery of segmental and long-tract neurological function in NASCIS 2. *J Neurosurg* 1993;80:954–955.
31. Bracken NO, Shepard MJ, Holford TR, et al. Administration of methylprednisolone for 24 or 48 hours or tirilazad mesylate for 48 hours in the treatment of acute spinal cord injury. Results of the Third National Acute Spinal Cord Injury Randomized Controlled Trial. National Acute Spinal Cord Injury Study. *JAMA* 1997;277:1597–1604.
32. Heary RF, Vaccaro AR, Mesa JJ, et al. Steroids and gunshot wounds to the spine. *Neurosurgery* 1997;41:576–583.
33. Levy ML, Gans W, Wijesinghe HS, et al. Use of methylprednisolone as an adjunct in the management of patients with penetrating spinal cord injury: outcome analysis. *Neurosurgery* 1996;39:1141–1148.
34. Short DJ, El Amsry WS, Jones PW. High dose methylprednisolone in the management of acute spinal cord injury—a systematic review from a clinical perspective. *Spinal Cord* 2000;38:273–286.
35. Hurlbert RJ. The role of steroids in acute spinal cord injury: an evidence-based analysis. *Spine* 2001;26[24 Suppl]:S39–S46.
36. Nesathurai S. Steroids and spinal cord injury: revisiting the NASCIS 2 and 3 trials. *J Trauma* 1998;45:1088–1093.
37. Geisler FH, Dorsey FC, Coleman WP. Recovery of motor function after spinal cord injury—a randomized, placebo controlled trial with GM-1 ganglioside. *N Engl J Med* 1991;324:1829–1838.
38. Fehlings MG, Bracken MB. Summary statement: the Sygen (GM-I ganglioside) clinical trial in acute spinal cord injury. *Spine* 2001;26[24 Suppl]:S99–S100.
39. Fehlings M, Tator C. An evidence-based review of decompressive surgery in acute spinal cord injury: rationale, indications, and timing based on experimental and clinical studies. *J Neurosurg (Spine 1)* 1999;91:1–11.
40. Vaccaro A, Daugherty R, Sheehan T, et al. Neurologic outcome of early versus late surgery for cervical spinal cord injury. *Spine* 1997;22:2609–2613.
41. Vale F, Burns J, Jackson A, et al. Combined medical and surgical treatment after acute spinal cord injury: results of a prospective pilot study to assess the merits of aggressive medical resuscitation and blood pressure management. *J Neurosurg* 1997;87:239–246.
42. Waters R, Adkins R, Yakura J. Effect of surgery on motor recovery following traumatic spinal cord injury. *Spinal Cord* 1996;34:188–192.
43. Hadley M, Fitzpatrick B, Sonntag V, et al. Facet fracture-dislocation injuries of the cervical spine. *Neurosurgery* 1992;30:661–666.
44. Fessler R, Masson R. Management of thoracic fractures. In: Menezes All, Sonntag VKH, eds. *Principles of spinal surgery*. New York: McGraw-Hill, 1996:899–918.
45. Waters RL, Meyer PR, Adkins RH, et al. Emergency, acute, and surgical management of spine trauma. *Arch Phys Med Rehabil* 1999;80:1383–1390.
46. Campagnolo DI, Esquieres RE, Kopacz KJ. Effect of timing of stabilization on length of stay and medical complications following spinal cord injury. *J Spinal Cord Med* 1997;20:3314.
47. American Spinal Injury Association. *International standards for neurological classification of spinal cord injury*. Chicago: ASIA, 2002.
48. Marino RJ, Rider-Foster D, Maissel G, et al. Superiority of motor level over single neurological level in categorizing tetraplegia. *Paraplegia* 1995;33:510–513.
49. Kirshblum SC, Donovan WH. Neurologic assessment and classification of traumatic spinal cord injury. In: Kirshblum SC, Campagnolo D, DeLisa JE, eds. *Spinal cord medicine*. Philadelphia: Lippincott Williams & Wilkins, 2002:82–95.
50. Frankel HL, Hancock DO, Hyslop G, et al. The value of postural reduction in initial management of closed injuries of the spine with paraplegia and tetraplegia. I. *Paraplegia* 1969;7:179–192.
51. American Spinal Injury Association. *International standards for neurological classification of spinal cord injury*. Chicago: ASIA, 1992.
52. American Spinal Injury Association. *International standards for neurological classification of spinal cord injury*. Chicago: ASIA, 1996.

53. American Spinal Injury Association. *International standards for neurological classification of spinal cord injury.* Chicago: ASIA, 2000.

54. Schneider RC, Cherry OR, Patek H. Syndrome of acute central cervical spinal cord injury with special reference to mechanisms involved in hyperextension injuries of cervical spine. *J Neurosurg* 1954;11:546–577.

55. Taylor AR. The mechanism of injury to the spinal cord in the neck without damage to the vertebral column. *J Bone Joint Surg* 1951;33B:543–547.

56. Penrod LE, Hegde SK, Ditunno JF. Age effect on prognosis for functional recovery in acute, traumatic central cord syndrome. *Arch Phys Med Rehabil* 1990;71:963–968.

57. Roth EJ, Lawler NM, Yarkony GM. Traumatic central cord syndrome: clinical features and functional outcomes. *Arch Phys Med Rehabil* 1990;71:18–23.

58. Burns SP, Golding DO, Rolle WA, et al. Recovery of ambulation in motor incomplete tetraplegia. *Arch Phys Med Rehabil* 1997;78:1169–1172.

59. Bohlman HH. Acute fractures and dislocations of the cervical spine. An analysis of three hundred hospitalized patients and review of the literature. *J Bone Joint Surg* 1979;61A:1119–1142.

60. Bosch A, Stauffer ES, Nickel VL. Incomplete traumatic quadriplegia—a ten year review. *JAMA* 1971;216:473–478.

61. Brown-Sequard CE. Lectures on the physiology and pathology of the central nervous system and the treatment of organic nervous affections. *Lancet* 1868;2:593–595,659–662,755–757,821–823.

62. Roth EJ, Park T, Pang T, et al. Traumatic cervical Brown-Sequard and Brown-Sequard plus syndromes: the spectrum of presentations and outcomes. *Paraplegia* 1991;29:582–589.

63. Tersall R, Turner B. Brown-Sequard and his syndrome. *Lancet* 2000;356:61–63.

64. Graziani V, Tessler A, Ditunno JF. Incomplete tetraplegia: sequence of lower extremity motor recovery. *J Neurotrauma* 1995;12:121.

65. Little JW, Halar E. Temporal course of motor recovery after Brown-Sequard spinal cord injuries. *Paraplegia* 1985;23:39–46.

66. Bauer RD, Errico TJ. Cervical spine injuries. In: Errico TJ, Bauer RD, Waugh T (eds), *Spinal trauma.* Philadelphia: JB Lippincott, 1991:71–121.

67. Cheshire WP, Santos CC, Massey EW, et al. Spinal cord infarction: etiology and outcome. *Neurology* 1996;47:321–330.

68. Bohiman HH, Ducker TB. Spine and spinal cord injuries. In: Rothman RH, ed. *The spine,* 3rd ed. Philadelphia: WB Saunders, 1992:973–1011.

69. Hamilton BB, Granger CV, Sherwin FS. A uniform national data system for medical rehabilitation. In: Fuhrer MJ, ed. *Rehabilitation outcomes: analysis and measurement.* Baltimore: Brooks, 1987:137–147.

70. Granger CV, Albrecht GL, Hamilton BB. Outcomes of comprehensive medical rehabilitation: measurement by PULSES profile and the Barthel Index. *Arch Phys Med Rehabil* 1979;60:145–154.

71. Gresham GE, Labi MLC, Dittmar SS, et al. The quadriplegia index of function (QIF): sensitivity and reliability demonstrated in a study of thirty quadriplegic patients. *Paraplegia* 1986;24:38–44.

72. Marino RJ, Stineman MG. Functional assessment in spinal cord injury. *Top Spinal Cord Inj Rehabil* 1996;14:32–45.

73. Whiteneck GG, Charlifue SW, Gerhart KA, et al. Quantifying handicap: a new measure of long-term rehabilitation outcomes. *Arch Phys Med Rehabil* 1992;73:519–526.

74. Tate D, Forchheimer M, Maynard F, et al. Predicting depression and psychological distress in persons with spinal cord injury based on indicators of handicap. *Am J Phys Med Rehabil* 1994;73:175–183.

75. Hall KM, Werner P. Characteristics of the functional independence measure in traumatic spinal cord injury. *Arch Phys Med Rehabil* 1999;80:1471–1476.

76. Ditunno JF, Cohen ME, Formal CS, et al. Functional outcomes in spinal cord injury. In: Stover SL, DeLisa J, Whiteneck GO, eds. *Spinal cord injury: clinical outcomes from the model system.* Gaithersburg, MD: Aspen, 1995:170–184.

77. Dijkers MP, Yavuzer G. Short version of the telephone motor functional independence measure for use with persons with spinal cord injury. *Arch Phys Med Rehabil* 1999;80:1477–1484.

78. Yavus N, Tezyurck M, Akyuz M. A comparison of the functional tests in quadriplegia: the quadriplegia index of function and the functional independence measure. *Spinal Cord* 1998;36:832–837.

79. Marino RJ, Shea JA, Steinman MG. The capabilities of upper extremity instrument: reliability and validity of a measure of functional limitation in tetraplegia. *Arch Phys Med Rehabil* 1998;79:1512–1521.

80. Ditunno JF, Ditumio PL, Graziani V, et al. Walking Index for Spinal Cord Injury (WISCI): an international multicenter validity and reliability study. *Spinal Cord* 2000;38:234–243.

81. Ditunno PL, Ditunno JF. Walking Index for Spinal Cord Injury (WISCI II): scale revision. *Spinal Cord* 2001;39:654–656.

82. Kirshblum SC, O'Connor K. Levels of injury and outcome in traumatic spinal cord injury. *Phys Med Rehabil Clin North Am* 2000;11:1–27.

83. Ditunno J, Flanders A, Kirshblum SC, et al. Predicting outcome in traumatic spinal cord injury. In: Kirshblum SC, Campagnolo D, DeLisa JE, eds. *Spinal cord medicine.* Philadelphia: Lippincott Williams & Wilkins, 2002:108–122.

84. Kirshblum SC, O'Connor KC. Predicting neurological recovery in traumatic spinal cord injury. *Arch Phys Med Rehabil* 1998;79:1456–1466.

85. Brown PJ, Marino U, Herbison GJ, et al. The 72 hour examination as a predictor of recovery in motor complete quadriplegia. *Arch Phys Med Rehabil* 1991;72:546–

86. Bravo P, Labarta C, Alcarez MA, et al. An assessment of factors affecting neurological recovery after spinal cord injury with vertebral fractures. *Paraplegia* 1996;34:164–166.

87. Waters RL, Sic I, Adkins RH, et al. Injury pattern affect on motor recovery after traumatic spinal cord injury. *Arch Phys Med Rehabil* 1995;76:440–443.

88. Stauffer ES. Neurologic recovery following injuries to the cervical spinal cord and nerve roots. *Spine* 1984;9:532–534.

89. Mange KC, Marino RD, Gregory PC, et al. The course of motor recovery at the zone of injury in complete spinal cord injury. *Arch Phys Med Rehabil* 1992;73:437–441.

90. Waters RL, Adkins, RH, Yakura JS, et al. Motor and sensory recovery following complete tetraplegia. *Arch Phys Med Rehabil* 1993;74:242–247.

91. Wu L, Marino RI, Herbison GJ, et al. Recovery of zero grade muscles in the zone of partial preservation in motor complete quadriplegia. *Arch Phys Med Rehabil* 1992;73;40–43.

92. Ditunno JF, Stover SL, Freed MM, et al. Motor recovery of the upper extremities in traumatic quadriplegia: a multicenter study. *Arch Phys Med Rehabil* 1992;73:431–436.

93. Crozier KS, Graziam V, Ditunno JF, et al. Spinal cord injury: prognosis for ambulation based on sensory examination in patients who are initially motor complete. *Arch Phys Med Rehabil* 1991;72:119–121.

94. Folman Y, Masn WE. Spinal cord injury: prognostic indicators. *Injury* 1989;20:92–93.

95. Foo D, Subrahamyan TS, Rossier AS. Post-traumatic acute anterior spinal cord syndrome. *Paraplegia* 1981;19:201–205.

96. Waters RL, Adkins RH, Yakura JS, et al. Motor and sensory recovery following incomplete tetraplegia. *Arch Phys Med Rehabil* 1994;75:306–311.

97. Stauffer ES. Rehabilitation of post-traumatic cervical spinal cord quadriplegia and pentaplegia. In: *Cervical spine research: cervical spine.* Philadelphia: JB Lippincott Co, 1983:317–322.

98. Crozier KS, Cheng LL, Graziam V, et al. Spinal cord injury: prognosis for ambulation based on recovery of quadriceps function. *Paraplegia* 1992;30:762–767.

99. Ditunno JF, Cohen ME, Belikoff MM, et al. Recovery of upper extremity muscles following cervical spinal cord injury. *J Spinal Cord Med* 1997;20:144.

100. Mange KC, Ditunno JF, Herbison GJ, et al. Recovery of strength at the zone of injury in motor complete and motor incomplete cervical spinal cord injured patients. *Arch Phys Med Rehabil* 1990;71:562–565.

101. Waters RL, Yakura Joy S, et al. Recovery following complete paraplegia. *Arch Phys Med Rehabil* 1992;73:784–789.

102. Holdsworth F. Fractures, dislocations, and fracture-dislocations of the spine. *J Bone Joint Surg Am* 1970;52:1534–1551.

103. Waters RL, Adkins R, Yakura J, et al. Functional and neurologic recovery following spinal cord injury. *J Spinal Cord Med* 1998;21:195–199.

104. Waters RL, Adkins RH, Yakura JS, et al. Motor and sensory recovery following incomplete paraplegia. *Arch Phys Med Rehabil* 1994;75:67–72.

105. Maynard FM, Glen GR, Fountain S, et al. Neurological prognosis after traumatic quadriplegia. *J Neurosurg* 1979;50:611–616.

106. Marino RI, Ditunno JF, Donovan WH, et al. Neurologic recovery after traumatic spinal cord injury: data from the Model Spinal Cord Injury Systems. *Arch Phys Med Rehabil* 1999;80:1391–1396.

107. Waters RL, Adkins RH, Yakura JS. Definition of complete spinal cord injury. *Paraplegia* 1991;29:573–581.

108. McDonald JW, Becker D, Sadowsky CL, et al. Late recovery following spinal cord injury: case report and review of the literature. *J Neurosurg: Spine* 2002;97:252–265.

109. Guttmann L. *Spinal cord injuries. Comprehensive management and research.* Oxford, England: Blackwell Scientific Publications, 1973.

110. Ko HY, Graziam V, Herbison GI, et al. The pattern of reflex recovery during spinal shock. *J Spinal Cord Med* 1997;20:143.

111. Weinstein DE, Ko HY, Graziani V, et al. Prognostic significance of the delayed plantar reflex following spinal cord injury. *J Spinal Cord Med* 1997;20:207–211.

112. Ramon S, et al. Clinical and magnetic resonance imaging correlation in acute spinal cord injury. *Spinal Cord* 1997;35(10):664–673.

113. Marciello M, Flanders AE, Herbison GJ, et al. Magnetic resonance imaging related to neurologic outcome in cervical spinal cord injury. *Arch Phys Med Rehabil* 1993;74:940–946.

114. Flanders AE, Spettell CM, Friedman DP, et al. The relationship between the functional abilities of patients with cervical spinal cord injury and the severity of damage revealed by MR imaging. *AJNR* 1999;20:926–934.

115. Selden NR, Quint DJ, Patel N, et al. Emergency magnetic resonance imaging of cervical spinal cord injuries: clinical correlation and prognosis. *Neurosurgery* 1999;44:785–792.

116. Cheliout-Heraut F, Loubert G, Mastri-Zada T, et al. Evaluation of early motor and sensory evoked potentials in cervical spinal cord injury. *Neurophysiol China* 1998;28:39–55.

117. Grundy BL, Friedman W. Electrical physiological evaluation of the patient with acute spinal cord injury. *Crit Care Clin* 1987;3:519–548.

118. Li C, Houlden DA, Rowed DQ. Somatosensory evoked potentials and neurological grades as predictors of outcome in acute spinal cord injury. *J Neurosurg* 1990;72:600–609.

119. Curt A, Dicta V. Traumatic cervical spinal cord injury: relation between somatosensory evoked potentials, neurologic deficit, and hand function. *Arch Phys Med Rehabil* 1996;77:48–53.

120. Curt A, Dicta V. Ambulatory capacity in spinal cord injury: significance of somatosensory evoked potentials and ASIA protocol in predicting outcome. *Arch Phys Med Rehabil* 1997;78:39–43.

121. Dickson H, Cole A, Engle S, et al. Conversion reaction presenting as acute spinal cord injury. *Med J Aust* 1984;141:427–429.

122. Kaplan BJ, Friedman WA, Gavenstein D. Somatosensory evoked potential in hysterical paraplegia. *Surg Neurol* 1985;23:502–506.

123. Bondurant CP, Haghighi SS. Experience with transcranial magnetic stimulation in evaluation of spinal cord injury. *Neurol Res* 1997;19:497–500.

124. Curt A, Keck ME, Dicta V. Functional outcome following spinal cord injury: significance of motor evoked potentials and ASIA scores. *Arch Phys Med Rehabil* 1998;79:81–86.

125. Waters RL, Adkins RH, Yakura J. Profiles of spinal cord injury after gunshot injury. *Chin Orthop* 1991;267:14–21.

126. Kane T, Capen DA, Waters R, et al. Spinal cord injury from civilian gunshot wounds: the Rancho experience 1980–1988. *J Spinal Cord Disord* 1991;4:306–311.

127. McKinley WO, Johns JS, Musgrove JJ. Clinical presentations, medical complications and functional outcomes of individuals with gunshot wound induced spinal cord injury. *Am J Phys Med Rehabil* 1999;78:102–107.

128. McKinley WO, Cifu D, Keyser-Marcus L, et al. Comparison of rehabilitation outcomes in violent versus non-violent traumatic spinal cord injury. *J Spinal Cord Med* 1998;21:32–36.

129. Waters RL, Adkins RH. Firearm versus motor vehicle related spinal cord injury: predisposing factors, injury characteristics, and initial outcome comparisons among ethnically diverse groups. *Arch Phys Med Rehabil* 1997;78:150–155.

130. McKinley WO, Conti-Wyneken AR, Vokac CN, et al. Rehabilitative functional outcome of patients with neoplastic spinal cord compression. *Arch Phys Med Rehabil* 1996;77:892–895.

131. McKinley WO, Tellis AA, Cifu DX, et al. Rehabilitation outcome of individuals with nontraumatic myelopathy resulting from spinal stenosis. *J Spinal Cord Med* 1998;21:131–136.

132. McKinley WO, Teskbury M, Godbout CJ. Comparison of medical complications following non-traumatic spinal cord injury. *J Spinal Cord Med* 2002;25:88–93.

133. McKinley WO, Conti-Wyneken AR, Vokac CN, et al. Rehabilitative functional outcome of patients with neoplastic spinal cord compression. *Arch Phys Med Rehabil* 1996;77:892–895.

134. McKinley WO, Huang ME, Tewksbury MA. Neoplastic vs. traumatic spinal cord injury: an inpatient rehabilitation comparison. *Am J Phys Med Rehabil* 2000;79:138–144.

135. McKinley WO, Seel RT, Hardman JT. Nontraumatic spinal cord injury: incidence, epidemiology, and functional outcome. *Arch Phys Med Rehabil* 1999;80:619–623.

136. McKinley WO, Seel RT, Gardi RK, et al. Nontraumatic vs. traumatic spinal cord injury: a rehabilitation outcome comparison. *Am J Phys Med Rehabil* 2001;80:693–699.

137. American Autonomic Society and American Academy of Neurology. Consensus statement on the definition of orthostatic hypotension, pure autonomic failure and multiple system atrophy. *Neurology* 1996:46;1470.

138. Mathias CJ, Christensen NJ, Corbett JL, et al. Plasma catecholamines, plasma renin activity and plasma aldosterone in tetraplegics man, horizontal and tilted. *Clin Sci Mol Med* 1975;49:291–299.

139. Maury M. About orthostatic hypotension in tetraplegic individuals: reflections and experience. *Spinal Cord* 1998;36:87–90.

140. Kamelhar DL, Steele JM, Schacht RG, et al. Plasma renin and serum dopamine-beta-hydroxylase during orthostatic hypotension in quadriplegic men. *Arch Phys Med Rehabil* 1978;59:212–216.

141. Teasell RW, Arnold MO, Krassioukov A, et al. Cardiovascular consequences of loss of supraspinal control of the sympathetic nervous system after spinal cord injury. *Arch Phys Med Rehabil* 2000;81:506–516.

142. Mukand J, Karlin L, Barrs K, et al. Midodrine for the management of orthostatic hypotension in patients with spinal cord injury: a case report. *Arch Phys Med Rehabil* 2001;82:694–696.

143. Fouad-Tarazi FM, Okabe M, Goren H. Alpha sympathomimetic treatment of autonomic insufficiency with orthostatic hypotension. *Am J Med* 1995;99:604–610.

144. Ashley EA, Laskin JJ, Olenik LM, et al. Evidence of autonomic dysreflexia during functional electrical stimulation in individuals with spinal cord injuries. *Paraplegia* 1993;31:593–605.

145. Sampson EE, Burnham RS, Andrews BJ. Functional electrical stimulation effect on orthostatic hypotension after spinal cord injury. *Arch Phys Med Rehabil* 2000;81:139–143.

146. Erickson RP. Autonomic hyperreflexia: pathophysiology and medical management. *Arch Phys Med Rehabil* 1980;70:234–241.

147. Campagnolo DI, Merli GJ. Autonomic and cardiovascular complications of spinal cord injury. In: Kirshblum S, ed. *Spinal cord medicine*. Philadelphia: Lippincott Williams & Wilkins, 2002:126.

148. Lindan R, Joiner E, Freehafer AA, et al. Incidence and clinical features of autonomic dysreflexia in patients with spinal cord injury. *Paraplegia* 1980;18:285–292.

149. Guttman, FL, Frankel HL, Paeslack V. Cardiac irregularities during labor in paraplegic women. *Paraplegia* 1965;3:144–151.

150. McGregor JA, Meeuwsen J. Autonomic hyperreflexia: a mortal danger for spinal cord-damaged women in labor. *Am J Obstet Gynecol* 1985;151:330–333.

151. Clinical practice guidelines: acute management of autonomic dysreflexia, 2nd ed. *J Spinal Cord Med* 2002;25[Suppl 1:]S67–S88.

152. Mathias CJ, Frankel HL, Christensen NJ, et al. Enhanced pressor response to noradrenaline inpatients with cervical spinal cord transection. *Brain* 1976:99:757–770.

153. Teasell RW, Arnold MO, Krassioukov A, et al. Cardiovascular consequences of loss of supraspinal control of the sympathetic nervous system after spinal cord injury. *Arch Phys Med Rehabil* 2000:81:506–516.

154. Kiker JD, Woodside JR, Jelinek GE. Neurogenic pulmonary edema associated with autonomic dysreflexia. *J Urol* 1982;128:1038–1039.

155. DeVivo MJ, Black KJ, Stover SL. Causes of death during the first 12 years after spinal cord injury. *Arch Phys Med Rehabil* 1993;74:248–254.

156. Reines HD, Harris RC. Pulmonary complications of acute spinal cord injuries. *Neurosurgery* 1987;21(2):193–196.

157. Sharp JT. Respiratory muscles: a review of older and newer concepts. *Lung* 1980;157:185–199.

158. Peterson W, Charlifue W, Gerhart A, et al. Two methods of weaning persons with quadriplegia from mechanical ventilators. *Paraplegia* 1994;32:98–103.

159. Mansel JK, Norman JR. Respiratory complications and management of spinal cord injuries. *Chest* 1990;97:1446–1452.

160. Ledsome JR, Sharp JM. Pulmonary function in acute cervical cord injury. *Am Rev Respir Dis* 1981;124:41–44.

161. Morgan MD, Gourly AR, Silver JR, et al. The contribution of the rib cage to breathing in tetraplegia. *Thorax* 1985;40:613–617.

162. Roth EJ, Nussbaum SB, Berkowitz M, et al. Pulmonary function testing in spinal cord injury: correlation with vital capacity. *Paraplegia* 1995;33:454–457.

163. Almenoff PL, Spungen AM, Lesser M, et al. Pulmonary function survey in spinal cord injury: influence of smoking and level and completeness of injury. *Lung* 1995;173:297–306.

164. Limi WS, Adkins RH, Gong H Jr, et al. Pulmonary function in chronic spinal cord injury: a cross-sectional survey of 222 southern California adult outpatients. *Arch Phys Med Rehabil* 2000;81:757–763.

165. Jackson AB, Groomes TE. Incidence of respiratory complications following spinal cord injury. *Arch Phys Med Rehabil* 1994;75(3):270–275.

166. Chen D, Apple DF, Hudson LM, et al. Medical complications during acute rehabilitation following spinal cord injury—current experience of the Model Systems. *Arch Phys Med Rehabil* 1999;80:1397–1401.

167. DeVivo MJ, Ivie CS. Life expectancy of ventilator-dependent persons with spinal cord injuries. *Chest* 1995;108:226–232.

168. Fuhrer MJ, Carter RE, Donovan WH, et al. Postdischarge outcomes for ventilator dependent quadriplegics. *Arch Phys Med Rehabil* 1987;68:353–356.

169. Kinney TB, Rose SC, Vaiji K, et al. Does cervical spinal cord injury induce a higher incidence of complications after prophylactic Greenfield filter usage? *J Vasc Interv Radiol* 1996;7:907–915.

170. Balshi ID, Cantelmo NL, Menzoian JO. Complications of caval interruption by Greenfield filter in quadriplegics. *J Vasc Surg* 1989;9:558–562.

171. Garstang SV, Kirshblum SC, Wood KE. Patient preference for in-exsufflation for secretion management in spinal cord injury. *J Spinal Cord Med* 2000;23:80–85.

172. Fugl-Myer AR. Effects of respiratory muscle paralysis in tetraplegic and paraplegic patients. *Scand J Rehabil Med* 1971;3(4):141–150.

173. Estenne M, DeTroyer A. Mechanism of the postural dependence of vital capacity in tetraplegic subjects. *Am Rev Respir Dis* 1987;135(2):367–371.

174. Maloney FP. Pulmonary function in quadriplegia: effects of a corset. *Arch Phys Med Rehabil* 1979;60:261–265.

175. Derrickson J, Ciesla N, Simpson N, et al. A comparison of two breathing exercise programs for patients with quadriplegia. *Phys Ther* 1992;72(11):763–769.

176. Loveridge B, Badour M, Dubo H. Ventilatory muscle endurance training in quadriplegia: effects on breathing pattern. *Paraplegia* 1989;27(5):329–339.

177. Liaw MY, Lin MC, Cheng PT, et al. Resistive inspiratory muscle training: its effectiveness in patients with acute complete cervical cord injury. *Arch Phys Med Rehabil* 2000;81:752–756.

178. Rutchik A, Weissman AR, Almenoff PL, et al. Resistive inspiratory muscle training in subjects with chronic cervical spinal cord injury. *Arch Phys Med Rehabil* 1998;79:29–37.

179. Lin KW, Chuang CC, Wu HD, et al. Abdominal weight and inspiratory resistance: their immediate effects on inspiratory muscle functions during maximal voluntary breathing in chronic tetraplegic patients. *Arch Phys Med Rehabil* 1999;80:741–745.

180. Bach JR, Alba AS. Non-invasive options for ventilatory support of the traumatic high level quadriplegic. *Chest* 1990;98:613–619.

181. Bach JR, Alba AS. Tracheostomy ventilation. A study of efficacy with deflated cuffs and cuffless tubes. *Chest* 1990;97(3):679–683.

182. Bach JR. Non-invasive alternatives to tracheostomy for managing respiratory muscle dysfunction in spinal cord injury. *Top Spinal Cord Inj Rehabil* 1997;2:49–58.

183. Bach JR, Rajarman R, Ballanger F, et al. Neuromuscular ventilatory insufficiency: effect of home mechanical ventilator use v oxygen therapy on pneumonia and hospitalization rates. *Am J Phys Med Rehabil* 1998;77(1):8–19.

184. Peterson WP, Barbalata L, Brooks CA, et al. The effect of tidal volumes on the time to wean persons with high tetraplegia from ventilators. *Spinal Cord* 1999;37:284–288.

185. Garthier BP, Watt JW, Krishnan KR. The artificial ventilation of acute spinal cord damaged patients: a retrospective study of forty-four patients. *Paraplegia* 1986;24:208–220.

186. Peterson P, Kirshblum SC. Respiratory management in spinal cord injury. In: Kirshblum SC, Campagnolo D, DeLisa JE, eds. *Spinal cord medicine*. Philadelphia: Lippincott Williams & Wilkins, 2002:135–154.

187. Peterson P, Brooks CA, Mellick D, et al. Protocol for ventilator management in high tetraplegia. *Top Spinal Cord Injury Rehabil* 1997;2:101–106.

188. Bach JR, Saporito LR. Criteria for extubation and tracheostomy tube removal for patients with ventilatory failure: a different approach to weaning. *Chest* 1996;110:1566–1571.

189. McCrory DC, Samsa GP, Hamilton, BP, et al. Draft evidence report: treatment of pulmonary disease following spinal cord injury. Duke Evidence-based Practice Center, Center for Clinical Health Policy Research. Prepared for the Agency for Healthcare Research and Quality. Durham, NC, February 14, 2000.

190. Weese-Mayer DE, Silvestri JM, Kenny AS, et al. Diaphragm pacing with a quadripolar phrenic nerve electrode: an international study. *Pacing Chin Electrophysiol* 1996;19(9):1311–1319.

191. DiMarco AF, Onders RP, Mortimer JI, et al. Long-term diaphragm pacing via intramuscular diaphragm electrodes. *J Spinal Cord Med.* 2002;25:224–225.

192. Maynard FM. Immobilization hypercalcemia following spinal cord injury. *Arch Phys Med Rehabil* 1986;67:41–44.

193. Stewart AF, Adler M, Byers CM, et al. Calcium homeostasis in immobilization: an example of resorptive hypercalciuria. *N Engl J Med* 1982;306:1136–1140.

194. Meythaler JM, Inch SM, Cross LL. Successful treatment of immobilization hypercalcemia using calcitonin and etidronate. *Arch Phys Med Rehabil* 1993;74:316–319.

195. Massagli TL, Cardenas DD. Immobilization hypercalcemia treatment with pamidronate disodium after spinal cord injury. *Arch Phys Med Rehabil* 1999; 80:998–1000.

196. Kedlaya D, Brandstater ME, Lee JK. Immobilization hypercalcemia in incomplete paraplegia: successful treatment with pamidronate. *Arch Phys Med Rehabil* 1998;79:222–225.

197. de Bruin ED, Frey-Rindova P, Herzog RE, et al. Changes of tibia bone properties after spinal cord injury: effects of early intervention. *Arch Phys Med Rehabil* 1999 Feb;80(2):214–220.

198. Kaplan PE, Roden W, Gilbert E, et al. Reduction of hypercalciuria in tetraplegia after weight-bearing and strengthening exercises. *Paraplegia* 1981; 19:289–293.

199. Lal S, Hamilton BB, Heinemann A, et al. Risk factors of heterotopic ossification in spinal cord injury. *Arch Phys Med Rehabil* 1989;70:387–390.

200. Banovac K, Gonzalez F. Evaluation and management of heterotopic ossification in patients with spinal cord injury. *Spinal Cord* 1997;35:158–162.

201. van Kujik AA, Ceurts A, Kuppevelt H. Neurogenic heterotopic ossification in spinal cord injury. *Spinal Cord* 2002;40:3113–3326.

202. Colachis III SC, Chinchot DM, Venesy D. Neurovascular complications of heterotopic ossification following spinal cord injury. *Paraplegia* 1993;31:51–57.

203. Freed JH, Hahn H, Menter R, et al. Use of the three phase bone scan in the early diagnosis of heterotopic ossification and in the evaluation of didronel therapy. *Paraplegia* 1982;20:208–216.

204. Cassar-Puhicino VN, McCleland M, Badwan DAH, et al. Sonographic diagnosis of heterotopic bone formation in spinal cord patients. *Paraplegia* 1993;31:40–50.

205. Finerman GA, Stover SL. Heterotopic ossification following hip replacement or spinal cord injury. Two clinical studies with EHDP. *Metab Bone Dis Rel Res* 1981;3:337–342.

206. Garland DE, Orwin JF. Resection of heterotopic ossification in patients with spinal cord injuries. *Chin Orthop Related Res* 1989;242:169–176.

207. Brooker AF, Bowerman JW, Robinson RA, et al. Ectopic ossification following total hip replacement. *J Bone Joint Surg* 1973;53A:1629–1632.

208. Gonda K, Nakaoka I, Yoshimura K, et al. Heterotopic ossification of degenerating rat skeletal muscle induced by adenovirus-mediated transfer of bone morphogenic protein-2 gene. *J Bone Miner Res* 2000;15:1056–1065.

209. Daud O, Sett P, Burr RG, et al. Relationship of heterotopic ossification to passive movements in paraplegic patients. *Disabil Rehabil* 1993;15:114–118.

210. Michelsson JE, Rauschning W. Pathogenesis of experimental heterotopic bone formation following temporary forceful exercising of immobilized limbs. *Clin Orthop Rel Res* 1983;176:265–275.

211. Subbarao JV, Garrison SJ. Heterotopic ossification: diagnosis and management, current concepts and controversies. *J Spinal Cord Med* 1999;22:273–283.

212. Garland DE, Alday B, Venos KG, et al. Diphosphonate treatment for heterotopic ossification in spinal cord injury patients. *Clin Orthop* 1983;176:197–200.

213. Banovac K, Gonzalez F, Wade N, et al. Intravenous disodium etidronate therapy in spinal cord injury patients with heterotopic ossification. *Paraplegia* 1993;31:660–666.

214. Kujik AA, Kuppevelt HJM, Schaal DB. Osteonecrosis after treatment for heterotopic ossification in spinal cord injury with the combination of surgery, irradiation and an NSAID. *Spinal Cord* 2000;38:319–324.

215. Stover SL, Hahn HR, Miller JM 3d. Disodium etidronate in the prevention of heterotopic ossification following spinal cord injury (preliminary report). *Paraplegia* 1976;14(2):146–156.

216. Banovac K, Williams JM, Patrick LD, et al. Prevention of heterotopic bone after spinal cord injury with indomethacin. *Spinal Cord* 2001;39:370–374.

217. Buschbacher R, McKinley W, Buschbacher L, et al. Wafarin in prevention of heterotopic ossification. *Am J Phys Med Rehabil* 1992;71:86–91.

218. Jamil F, Subbarao JV, Banovac K, et al. Management of immature heterotopic ossification of the hip. *Spinal Cord* 2002;40:388–395.

219. Merli G, Herbison G, Ditunno J, et al. Deep vein thrombosis: prophylaxis in acute spinal cord injured subjects. *Arch Phys Med Rehab* 1988;69:661–664.

220. Myllynen P, Kammonen M, Rokkanen P, et al. Deep vein thrombosis and pulmonary embolism in patients with acute spinal cord injury: a comparison with nonparalyzed patients immobilized due to spinal fractures. *J Trauma* 1985;25:541–543.

221. Todd J, Frisbie J, Rossier A, et al. Deep venous thrombosis in acute spinal cord injury: a comparison of 125 I fibrinogen leg scanning, impedance plethysmography, and venography. *Paraplegia* 1976;14:50–57.

222. Bors E, Conrad C, Massell T. Venous occlusion of the lower extremities in paraplegic patients. *Surg Gynecol Obstet* 1954;49:451–454.

223. Brach B, Moser K, Cedar L, et al. Venous thrombosis in acute spinal cord paralysis. *J Trauma* 1977;17:289–292.

224. Philipps R. The incidence of deep venous thrombosis in paraplegics. *Paraplegia* 1963;1:116–130.

225. Rossi E, Green D, Rosen J, et al. Sequential changes in factor VIII and platelets preceding deep vein thrombosis in patients with spinal cord injury. *Br J Hematol* 1980;45:143–151.

226. McKinley WO, Jackson AB, Cardenas DD, et al. Long-term medical complications after traumatic spinal cord injury: a regional model systems analysis. *Arch Phys Med Rehabil* 1999;80:1402–1410.

227. Myllynen P, Kammonen M, Rokkanen P, et al. The blood FVIII:Ag/FVIII:C ratio as an early indicator of DVT during post-traumatic immobilization. *J Trauma* 1987;27:287–290.

228. Seifert J, Stoephasius E, Probst J, et al. Blood flow in muscles of paraplegic patients under various conditions measured by a double isotope technique. *Paraplegia* 1972;10:185–191.

229. Ersoz G, Ficicilar H, Pasin M, et al. Platelet aggregation in traumatic spinal cord injury. *Spinal Cord* 1999;37:644–647.

230. Boudaoud L, Roussi J, Lortat-Jacob S, et al. Endothelial fibrinolytic reactivity and the risk of deep venous thrombosis after spinal cord injury. *Spinal Cord* 1997;35:15l–157.

231. Davidson BL, Elliot CG, Lensing AWA, et al. Low accuracy of color Doppler ultrasound in the detection of proximal leg thrombosis in asymptomatic high-risk patients. *Ann Intern Med* 1992;117:735–738.

232. Hall R. Hirsch J, Sackett DL, et al. Combined use of leg scanning and impedance plethysmography in suspected deep venous thrombosis: an alternative to venography. *N Engl J Med* 1977;296:1497–1500.

233. Clinical practice guidelines: prevention of thromboembolism in spinal cord injury. *J Spinal Cord Med* 1997;20:259–283.

234. Salzman EW, McManama GP, Shapiro AH , et al. Effect of optimization of hemodynamics on fibrinolytic activity and antithrombotic efficacy of external pneumatic calf compression. *Ann Surg* 1987;206:636–641.

235. Merli G, Herbison G, Ditunno J. Deep vein thrombosis: prophylaxis in acute spinal cord injured patients. *Arch Phys Med Rehabil* 1988;661–664.

236. Green D, Lee MY, Lim AC. Prevention of thromboembolism in spinal cord injury using low molecular weight heparin. *Ann Intern Med* 1990;113:571–574.

237. Green D, Chen D, Chmiel JS, et al. Prevention of thromboembolism in spinal cord injury: role of low molecular weight heparin. *Arch Phys Med Rehabil* 1994;75:290–292.

238. Geerts WH, Jay RM, Code KL, et al. A comparison of low dose heparin with low molecular weight heparin as prophylaxis against thromboembolism after major trauma. *N Engl J Med* 1996;335:701–707.

239. Harris S, Chen D, Green D. Enoxaparin for thromboembolism prophylaxis in spinal injury. *Am J Phys Med Rehabil* 1996;75:326–327.

240. Shen H, Ho C, Frost FS. Evaluation of the management for prevention and diagnosis of thromboembolic disease in spinal cord injury. *Arch Phys Med Rehabil* 2002;83:1686.

241. Decousus H, Leizorovicz A, Parent F, et al. A clinical trial of vena caval filters in the prevention of pulmonary embolism in patients with proximal deep-vein thrombosis. *N Engl J Med* 1998;338:409–415.

242. Rogers FB, Shackford SR, Ricci MA, et al. Routine prophylactic vena cava filter insertion in severely injured trauma patients decreases the incidence of pulmonary embolism. *J Am Coll Surg* 1995;180:641–647.

243. Wilson JT, Rogers FB, Wald SL et al. Prophylactic vena cava filter insertion in patients with traumatic spinal cord injury: preliminary results. *Neurosurgery* 1994;35:234–239.

244. Balshi JD, Cantelmo NL, Menzoian JO. Complications of caval interruption by Greenfield filter in quadriplegics. *J Vasc Surg* 1989;9:558–562.

245. Kinney TB, Rose SC, Valji K, et al. Does cervical spinal cord injury induce a higher incidence of complications after prophylactic Greenfield inferior vena cava filter use? *J Vasc Interv Radiol* 1996;7:907–915.

246. The Columbus Investigators. Low molecular weight heparin in the treatment of patients with venous thromboembolism. *N Engl J Med* 1997;337:657–662.

247. Simonneau G, Sors H, Charbonnier B, et al. A comparison of low molecular weight heparin and unfractionated heparin for acute pulmonary embolism. *N Engl J Med* 1997;337:663–669.

248. Tomaio A, Kirshblum S, O'Connor K, et al. Enoxaparin for treatment of deep venous thrombosis in spinal cord injury: a cost analysis. *J Spinal Cord Med* 1998;21:205–210.

249. Schniidt KD, Chan CW. Thermoregulation and fever in normal persons and in those with spinal cord injuries. *Mayo Clin Proc* 1992;67:469–475.

250. Menard MR, Hahn G. Acute and chronic hypothermia in a man with spinal cord injury: environmental and pharmacologic causes. *Arch Phys Med Rehabil* 1991;72:421–424.

251. Huang CT, DeVivo MJ, Stover SL. Anemia in acute phase of spinal cord injury. *Arch Phys Med Rehabil* 1990;71:3–7.

252. Hirsch GH, Menard MR, Anton HA. Anemia after traumatic spinal cord injury. *Arch Phys Med Rehabil* 1991;72:195–201.

253. Lipetz JS, Kirshblum SC, O'Connor KC et al. Anemia and serum protein deficiencies in patients with traumatic spinal cord injury. *J Spinal Cord Med* 1997;20:335–340.

254. Rodriguez GP, Garber SL. Prospective study of pressure ulcer risk in spinal cord injury patients. *Paraplegia* 1981;19:235–247.

255. Yarkony GM, Heinemann AW. Pressure ulcers. In Stover SL, DeLisa JA, Whiteneck GG, eds. *Spinal cord injury; clinical outcomes from the model systems.* Gaithersburg, MD: Aspen Publishing, 1995.

256. Pressure ulcer prevention and treatment following spinal cord injury: a clinical practice guideline for health-care professionals. Consortium for Spinal Cord Medicine. 2000. Paralyzed Veterans of America.

257. Salzberg CA, Byrne DW, Cayten CG, et al. Predicting and preventing pressure ulcers in adults with paralysis. *Adv Wound Care* 1998;11:237–246.

258. Young ME, Rintala DH, Rossi CD, et al. Alcohol and marijuana use in a community based sample of persons with spinal cord injury. *Arch Phys Med Rehabil* 1995;76:525–532.

259. National Pressure Ulcer Advisory Panel (NPAUP). Pressure ulcers prevalence, costs, and risk assessment; consensus development conference statement. *Decubitus* 1989;2:24–28.

260. O'Connor KC, Salcido R. Pressure ulcers in spinal cord injury. In: Kirshblum SC, Campagnolo D, DeLisa JE, eds. *Spinal cord medicine.* Philadelphia: Lippincott Williams & Wilkins, 2002:207–220.

261. Hanson RW, Franklin MR. Sexual loss in relation to other functional losses for spinal cord injured males. *Arch Phys Med Rehabil* 1976;57:291–293.

262. Steins SA, Bergman SB, Goetz LL. Neurogenic bowel dysfunction after spinal cord injury: clinical correlation and rehabilitative management. *Arch Phys Med Rehabil* 1997;78:S86–S102.

263. Kirshblum S, Gulati M, O'Connor K, et al. Bowel function in spinal cord injured patients. *Arch Phys Med Rehabil* 1998;79:20–23.

264. Rosito O, Nino-Murcia M, Wolfe VA, et al. Effects of colostomy on the quality of life in patients with spinal cord injury: a retrospective analysis. *J Spinal Cord Med* 2002;25:174–183.

265. Kelly SR, Shashidharan M, Borwell B, et al. *Spinal Cord* 1999;37:211–214.

266. Yang CC, Stems SA. Anterograde continence enema for the treatment of neurogenic constipation and fecal incontinence after spinal cord injury. *Arch Phys Med Rehabil* 2000;81:683–685.

267. Teichnian J, Harris JM, Currie DM, et al. Malone antegrade continence enema for adults with neurogenic bowel disease. *J Urol* 1998;160:1278–1281.

268. Clanton U Jr, Bender J. Refractory spinal cord injury induced gastroparesis: resolution with erythromycin lactobionate, a case report. *J Spinal Cord Med* 1999;22:236–238.

269. Althausen PL, Gupta MC, Benson DR, et al. The use of neostigmine to treat postoperative ileus in orthopedic spinal patients. *J Spinal Disord* 2001;14:541–545.

270. Soderstrom CA, Ducker TB. Increased susceptibility of patients with cervical cord lesions to peptic gastrointestinal complications. *J Trauma* 1985;25:1030–1038.

271. Kiwerski J. Bleeding from the alimentary canal during the management of spinal cord injury patients. *Paraplegia* 1986;24:92–96.

272. Peret G, Solomon A. Gastrointestinal hemorrhage and cervical cord injuries. Proceedings from the 17th Veterans Administration Spinal Cord Injury Conference 1969;17:106–110.

273. Gore RM, Minzter RA, Calenoff L. Gastrointestinal complications of spinal cord injury. *Spine* 1981;6:538–544.

274. MacLellan DG, Shulkes A, Yao CZ, et al. Role of vagal hyperactivity in gastric stress ulceration after acute injury to the cervical cord. *Surg Gynecol Obstet* 1988;166:441–446.

275. Apstein MD, Dalecki-Chipperfield K. Spinal cord injury is a risk factor for gallstones. *Gastroenterology* 1987;92:966–968.

276. Moonka R, Stiens SA, Resnick WJ, et al. Prevalence and natural history of gallstones in spinal cord injured persons. *J Am Coll Surg* 1999;189:274–281.

277. Tola VB, Chamberlain S, Kostyk SK, et al. Symptomatic gallstones in patients with spinal cord injury. *J Gastrointest Surg* 2000;4:642–647.

278. Roth EJ, Fenton LI, Gaebler-Spira DJ, et al. Superior mesenteric artery syndrome in acute traumatic quadriplegia: care reports and literature review. *Arch Phys Med Rehabil* 1991;72:417–420.

279. Maynard FM, Karunas R, Waring WW. Epidemiology of spasticity following traumatic spinal cord injury. *Arch Phys Med Rehabil* 1990;71:566–569.

280. Levi R, Hultling C, Seiger A. The Stockholm Spinal Cord Injury Study: 2. Associations between clinical patient characteristics and post-acute medical problems. *Paraplegia* 1995;33:585–594.

281. Ashworth B. Preliminary trial of carisoprodol in multiple sclerosis. *Practitioner* 1964;192:540–542.

282. Bohannon RW, Smith MB. Interrater reliability of a modified Ashworth scale of muscle spasticity. *Phys Ther* 1987;67:206–207.

283. Pemi RD. Intrathecal baclofen for severe spasticity. *Ann NY Acad Sci* 1988;531:157–166.

284. Priebe MM, Sherwood AM, Thornby JI, et al. Clinical assessment of spasticity in spinal cord injury: a multidimensional problem. *Arch Phys Med Rehabil* 1996;77:713–716.

285. Stolp-Smith KA, Wainberg MC. Antidepressant exacerbation of spasticity. *Arch Phys Med Rehabil* 1999;80:339–342.

286. Schurch B, Wichmann W, Rossier AB. Post traumatic syringomyelia (cystic myelopathy): a prospective study of 449 patients with spinal cord injury. *J Neurol Neurosurg Psychiatry* 1996;60(1)61–67.

287. Kirshblum S. Treatment alternatives for spinal cord injury related spasticity. *J Spinal Cord Med* 1999;22(3)199–217.

288. Bohannon RW. Tilt table standing for reducing spasticity after spinal cord injury. *Arch Phys Med Rehabil* 1993;74:1121–1122.

289. Kunkel CF, Scremin AME, Eisenberg B, et al. Effect of "standing" on spasticity, contracture and osteoporosis in paralyzed males. *Arch Phys Med Rehabil* 1993;74:73–78.

290. Midha M, Schmitt JK. Epidural spinal cord stimulation for the control of spasticity in spinal cord injury patients lacks long term efficacy and is not cost-effective. *Spinal Cord* 1998;36:190–192.

291. Carlson SJ. A neurophysiologic analysis of inhibitive casting. *Phys Occup Ther Pediatr* 1985;4:31–42.

292. Rivas DA, Chancellor MB, Hill K, et al. Neurological manifestations of baclofen withdrawal. *J Urol* 1993;150:1903–1905.

293. Donovan WH, Carter RE, Rossi CD, et al. Clonidine effect on spasticity: a clinical trial. *Arch Phys Med Rehabil* 1988;69:193–194.

294. Weingarden SI, Belen JG. Clonidine transdermal system for treatment of spasticity in spinal cord injury. *Arch Phys Med Rehabil* 1992;73:876–877.

295. Nance P, Bugaresti J Shellenberger K, et al. Efficacy and safety of tizamdine in the treatment of spasticity in patients with spinal cord injury. *Neurology* 1994;44[Suppl 9]:S44–S52.

296. Nance PW, Sheremata WA, Lynch SG, et al. Relationship of the antispasticity effect of tizanidine to plasma concentration in patients with multiple sclerosis. *Arch Neurol* 1997;54(6):731–736.

297. Gruenthal M, Mueller M, Olson W, et al. Gabapentin for the treatment of spasticity in patients with spinal cord injury. *Spinal Cord* 1997;35:686–689.

298. Cutter N, Scott D, Johnson J, et al. Gabapentin effect on spasticity in multiple sclerosis: a placebo-controlled, randomized trial. *Arch Phys Med Rehabil* 2000;81:164–169.

299. Herman R, Mayer N, Mecomber SA. The pharmacophysiology of dantrolene sodium. *Am J Phys Med* 1972;51:296–311.

300. Mayer N, Necomber SA, Herman R. Treatment of spasticity with dantrolene sodium. *Am J Phys Med* 1973;52:18–29.

301. Barbeau H, Richards CL, Bedard PJ. Action of cyproheptadine in spastic paraparetic patients. *J Neurol Neurosurg Psychiatry* 1982;45:923–926.

302. Wainberg M, Barbeau H, Gauthier S. The effects of cyproheptadine on locomotion and on spasticity in patients with spinal cord injuries. *J Neurol Neurosurg Psychiatry* 1990;53:754–763.

303. Norman KE, et al. Effect of drugs in walking after spinal cord injury. *Spinal Cord* 1998;36:699–715.

304. Fung J, Stewart JE, Barbeau H. The combined effects of clonidine and cyproheptadine with interactive training on the modulation of locomotion in spinal cord injured subjects. *J Neurol Sci* 1990;100:85–93.

305. Herman J, D'Luzansky S. Pharmacologic management of spinal spasticity. *J Neurol Rehabil* 1991;5:S15–S20.

306. Advokat C, Moser H, Hutchinson K. Morphine and dextromorphan lose antinociceptive activity but exhibit an antispastic action in chronic spinal rats. *Physiol Behav* 1997;62(4):799–804.

307. Potter PJ, Hayes KC, Segal JL, et al. Randomized double-blind crossover trial of fampridine-SR (sustained release 4-aminopyridine) in patients with incomplete spinal cord injury. *J Neurotrauma* 1998;15(10):837–849.

308. Hansebout RR, Blight AR, Fawcett S, et al. 4-Aniinopyridine in chronic spinal cord injury: a controlled, double-blind, crossover study in eight patients. *J Neurotrauma* 1993;10:1–18.

309. Dunn M, Davis R. The perceived effects of marijuana on spinal cord injured males. *Paraplegia* 1974;12:175.

310. Malec J, Harvey RF, Cayner JJ. Cannabis effect on spasticity in spinal cord injury. *Arch Phys Med Rehabil* 1982;63:116–118.

311. Kroin JS, Ali A, York M, et al. The distribution of medication along the spinal canal after chronic intrathecal administration. *Neurosurgery* 1993;33:226–230.

312. Pemi RI. Intrathecal baclofen for spasticity of spinal origin: seven years of experience. *J Neurosurg* 1992;77:236–240.

313. Remy-Neris O, Barbeau H, Daniel O, et al. Effects of intrathecal clonidine injection on spinal reflexes and human locomotion in incomplete paraplegic subjects. *Exp Brain Res* 1999;129:433–440.

314. Middleton JW, Siddall PJ, Walker S, et al. Intrathecal clonidine and baclofen in the management of spasticity and neuropathic pain following spinal cord injury: a case study. *Arch Phys Med Rehabil* 1996;77:824–826.

315. Botte MJ, Abranis RA, Bodine-Fowler SC. Treatment of acquired muscle spasticity using phenol peripheral nerve blocks. *Orthopedics* 1995;18:151–159.

316. Richardson D, Edwards S, Sheean GL, et al. The effect of botulinum toxin on hand function after incomplete spinal cord injury at the level of C5/6: a case report. *Chin Rehabil* 1997;11:288–292.

317. Sisto SA, Bond Q, Wilen J, et al. Effect of Botox on gait in incomplete spinal cord injury. *J Spinal Cord Med*, 2001:24:199.

318. Smyth M, Peacock W. The surgical treatment of spasticity. *Muscle Nerve* 2000:23:153–163.

319. Kirshblum SC, Ho C, Drum E, et al. Rehabilitation after spinal cord injury. In: Kirshblum SC, Campagnolo D, DeLisa JE, eds. *Spinal cord medicine.* Philadelphia: Lippincott Williams & Wilkins, 2002:275–298.

320. Ragnarsson KT, Stein AB, Kirshblum S. Rehabilitation and comprehensive care of the person with spinal cord injury. In: Capen DA, Haye W, eds. *Comprehensive management of spine trauma.* St. Louis: Mosby, 1998.

321. Outcomes following traumatic spinal cord injury: clinical practice guidelines for health-care professionals. Consortium for Spinal Cord Medicine. 1999. Paralyzed Veterans of America.

322. Adler US, Kirshblum SC. Assistive device for intermittent self-catheterization in men with tetraplegia. *J Spinal Cord Med* 2003;26:155–158.

323. Long C, Lawton EB. Functional significance of spinal cord lesion level. *Arch Phys Med* 1955;36:249–255.

324. Henderson JL, Price SH, et al. Efficacy of three measures to relieve pressure in seated persons with spinal cord injury. *Arch Phys Med Rehabil* 1994;75(5): 535–539.

325. Burns P, Betz K. Seating pressures with conventional and dynamic wheelchair cushions in tetraplegia. *Arch Phys Med Rehabil* 1999;80:566–571.

326. Hangartner T, Rodgers MM, Glaser RM, et al. Tibial bone density loss in spinal cord injury patients: effects of FES exercise. *J Rehabil Res Dev* 1994; 31:50–61.

327. BeDell KK, Scremin AME, Perell KL, et al. Effects of functional electrical stimulation-induced lower extremity cycling on bone density of spinal cord-injured patient. *Am J Phys Med Rehabil* 1996;75:29–34.

328. Leeds EM, Klose KJ, Ganz W, et al. Bone mineral density after bicycle ergometry training. *Arch Phys Med Rehabil* 1990;71:207–279.

329. Szollar SM, et al. Bone mineral density and indexes of bone metabolism in spinal cord injury. *Am J Phys Med Rehabil* 1998;77:28–35.

330. Guest RS, Klose KJ, Needham-Shropshire BM, et al. Evaluation of a training program for persons with SCI paraplegia using the Parastep 1 ambulation system: part 4. Effect on physical self-concept and depression. *Arch Phys Med Rehabil* 1997;78:804–807.

331. Hussey RW, Stauffer ES. Spinal cord injury: requirements for ambulation. *Arch Phys MedRehabil* 1973;54:544–547.

332. Rosenstein BD, Greene WB, Herrington RT, et al. Bone density in myelomeningocele: the effects of ambulatory status and other factors. *Dev Med Child Neurol* 1987;29:486–494.

333. Ogilvie C, Bowker P, Rowley DI. The physiological benefits of paraplegic orthotically aided walking. *Paraplegia* 1993;31:111–115.

334. Waters RL, Lunsford BR. Energy cost of paraplegic locomotion. *J Bone Joint Surg* 1985;67A:1245–1250.

335. Waters RL, Mulroy S. The energy expenditure of normal and pathologic gait. *Gait Posture* 1999;9:207–231.

336. Huang CT, Kuhlemeier KV, Moore NB, et al. Energy cost of ambulation in paraplegic patients using Craig-Scott braces. *Arch Phys Med Rehabil* 1979;60: 595–600.

337. Gordon EE, Vanderwalde H. Energy requirements in paraplegic ambulation. *Arch Phys Med* 1956;36:276–285.

338. Stauffer ES, Hoffer MM, Nickel VL. Ambulation in thoracic paraplegia. *J Bone Joint Surg* 1978;60A:823–824.

339. Nene AV, Hermens HJ, Zilvold G. Paraplegic locomotion: a review. *Spinal Cord* 1996;34:507–524.

340. Lyles M, Munday J. Report on the evaluation of the Vannini-Rizzoli stabilizing limb orthosis. *J Rehabil Res Dev* 1992;29:77–104.

341. Douglas R, Larson PF, D'Ambrosia R, et al. The LSU reciprocating gait orthosis. *Orthopedics* 1983;6:834–839.

342. Chaplin E. Functional neuromuscular stimulation for mobility in people with spinal cord injuries. The Parastep I system. *J Spinal Cord Med* 1996; 19:99–105.

343. Klose KJ, Jacobs PL, Broton JG, et al. Evaluation of a training program for persons with SCI paraplegia using the Parastep 1 ambulation system: part I. Ambulation performance and anthropometric measures. *Arch Phys Med Rehabil* 1997;78:789–793.

344. Nash MS, Jacobs PL, Montalvo BM, et al. Evaluation of a training program for persons with SCI paraplegia using the Parastep 1 ambulation system: part 5. Lower extremity blood flow and hyperemic responses to occlusion augmented by ambulation training. *Arch Phys Med Rehabil* 1997;78:808–814.

345. Protas EJ, Holmes SA, Qureshy H, et al. Supported treadmill ambulation training after spinal cord injury: a pilot study. *Arch Phys Med Rehabil* 2001; 82:825–831.

346. Wernig A, Nanassy A, Muller S. Maintenance of locomotor abilities following Laufband (treadmill) therapy in para- and tetraplegic persons: follow-up studies. *Spinal Cord* 1998;36:744–749.

347. Graf M, Holle A. Environmental control unit considerations for the person with high level tetraplegia. *Top Spinal Cord Inj Rehabil* 1997;2:30–40.

348. Gill M. Psychosocial implications of spinal cord injury. *Crit Care Nurs Q* 1999;22:1–7.

349. Krause JS, Kemo B, Coker J. Depression after spinal cord injury: relation to gender, ethnicity, aging and socioeconomic indicators. *Arch Phys Med Rehabil* 2000;81:1099–1109.

350. Consortium for Spinal Cord Medicine. Depression following spinal cord injury: a clinical practice guideline for primary care physicians; 1998; New York.

351. Fichtenbaum J, Kirshblum SC. Psychological adaptations after spinal cord injury. In: Kirshblum SC, Campagnolo D, DeLisa JE, eds. *Spinal cord medicine*. Philadelphia: Lippincott Williams & Wilkins, 2002:299–311.

352. Beck AT, Ward CH, Mendelson M, et al. An inventory for measuring depression. *Arch Gen Psychiatry* 1967;4:351–363.

353. American Psychiatric Association. *Diagnostic and statistical manual of mental disorders*,4th ed. Washington, DC: APA, 1994.

354. Craig AR, Hancock KM, Dickson, HG. A longitudinal investigation into anxiety and depression in the first two years following a spinal cord injury. *Paraplegia* 1994;32:675–679.

355. Kishi Y, Robinson RG, Forrester AW. Prospective longitudinal study of depression following spinal cord injury. *J Neuropsychiatry* 1994;6:237–244.

356. Heinemann AW. Spinal cord injury. In: Goreczny AJ, ed. *Handbook of health and rehabilitation psychology*. New York: Plenum Press, 1995:341–360.

357. Charlifue SW, Gerhart K. Behavioral and demographic predictors of suicide following traumatic spinal cord injury. *Arch Phys Med Rehabil* 1991;72:448–492.

358. DeVivo MJ, Black BS, Richards JS, et al. Suicide following spinal cord injury. *Paraplegia* 1991;29:620–627.

359. Hartkopp A, Bronnum-Hansen H, Seidenschnur A, et al. Suicide in a spinal cord injured population: its relation to functional status. *Arch Phys Med Rehabil* 1998;79:1356–1361.

360. Altamura AC, Percudam M. The use of antidepressants for long term treatment of recurrent depression: rationale, current methodologies, and future directions. *J Clin Psychiatry* 1993;54:29.

361. Kupfer DJ, Frank E, Perel IM. Five year outcome for maintenance therapies in recurrent depression. *Arch Gen Psychiatry* 1992;49:769–773.

362. Kupfer DJ. Long-term treatment of depression. *J Clin Psychiatry* 1991;52: 28–34.

363. Pnen RF, Kupfer DJ. Continuation therapy for major depressive episodes: how long should it be maintained? *Am J Psychiatry* 1986;143:18–23.

364. Radnitz CL, Tirch D. Substance misuse in individuals with spinal cord injury. *IntJ Addict* 1995;30:1117–1140.

365. Pierce CA, Richards S, Gordon W, et al. Life satisfaction following spinal cord injury and the WHO model of functioning and disability. *SCI Psychosocial Process*. 1999;12.

366. Hall KM, Knudsen ST, Wright J, et al. Follow-up study of individuals with high tetraplegia (C1-C4) 14 to 24 years postinjury. *Arch Phys Med Rehabil* 1999;80:1507–1513.

367. Bach JR, Tilton MC. Life satisfaction and well-being measures in ventilator assisted individuals with traumatic tetraplegia. *Arch Phys Med Rehabil* 1994; 75:626–632.

368. Glass CA. The impact of home based ventilator dependence on family life. *Paraplegia* 1993;31:93–101.

369. Kennedy P, Lowe R, Grey N, et al. Traumatic spinal cord injury and psychological impact: a cross-sectional analysis of coping strategies. *Br J Clin Psychology* 1995;34:627–639.

370. Kennedy P, Gorsuch N, Marsh N. Childhood onset of spinal cord injury: self-esteem and self-perception. *Br J Clin Psychology* 1995;34:581–588.

371. Stems SA, Bergman SB, Formal CS. Spinal cord injury rehabilitation. Individual experience, personal adaptation, and social perspectives. *Arch Phys Med Rehabil* 1997;78:65–72.

372. Tate DG. Alcohol use among spinal cord-injured patients. *Am J Phys Med Rehabil* 1993;72:192–195.

373. Heinemann AW, Hawkins D. Substance abuse and medical complications following spinal cord injury. *Rehabil Psychology* 1995;40:125–140.

374. Young ME, Rintala DH, Rossi D, et al. Alcohol and marijuana use in a community-based sample of persons with spinal cord injury. *Arch Phys Med Rehabil* 1995;76:525–532.

375. Heinemann AW, Goranson N, Ginsburg K, et al. Alcohol use and activity patterns following spinal cord injury. *Rehabil Psychology* 1989;34:191–205.

376. Linenmeyer TA. Sexual function and fertility following spinal cord injury. In: Kirshblum SC, Campagnolo D, DeLisa JE, eds. *Spinal cord medicine*. Philadelphia: Lippincott Williams & Wilkins, 2002:322–330.

377. Anderson BE. Driving assessment in spinal cord injury. In Kirshblum SC, Campagnolo D, DeLisa JE, eds. *Spinal cord medicine*. Philadelphia: Lippincott Williams & Wilkins, 2002: 348–360.

378. Monga TN, Ostermann, HJ, Kerrigan, AJ. Driving: a clinical perspective on rehabilitation technology. *Phys Med Rehabil: State of the Art Rev*. Philadelphia: Hanley & Belfus, 1997;11(1):69–92.

379. Sie IH, Waters RL, Adkins RH, et al. Upper extremity pain in post-rehabilitation spinal cord injured patient. *Arch Phys Med Rehabil* 1992;73:44–48.

380. Bayley JC, Cochran TP, Sledge CB. The weight-bearing shoulder. The impingement syndrome in paraplegics. *J Bone Joint Surg* 1987;69A:676–678.

381. Gellman H, et al. Late complications of the weight-bearing upper extremity in the paraplegic patient. *Chin Orthop* 1988;223:132–135.

382. Curtis KA, Drysdale GA, Lanza RD, et al. Shoulder pain in wheelchair users with tetraplegia and paraplegia. *Arch Phys Med Rehabil* 1999;80:453–457.

383. Goldstein B. Musculoskeletal complications after spinal cord injury. In: Hammond MC, ed. *Topics in spinal cord medicine.Phys Med Rehabil Clin North Am* 2000;11:91–108.

384. Curtis KA, Roach KE, Applegate EB, et al. Development of the Wheelchair User's Shoulder Pain Index (WUSPI). *Paraplegia* 1995;33:290–293.

385. Escobedo EM, Hunter J, Hollister M, et al. Prevalence of rotator cuff tears by MRI in individuals with paraplegia. *Am J Radiol* 1997;168:919–923.

386. Campbell C, Koris M. Etiologies of shoulder pain in cervical spinal cord injury. *Clin Orthop* 1996;322:1405.

387. Lal S. Premature degenerative shoulder changes in spinal cord injury patients. *Spinal Cord* 1998;36:186–189.

388. Curtis KA, Roach KE, Applegate EB, et al. Reliability and validity of the Wheelchair User's Shoulder Pain Index (WUSPI). *Paraplegia* 1995;33:595–601.

389. Dyson-Hudson TA, Shiflett SC, Kirshblum SC, et al. Acupuncture and Trager®. Psychophysical integration in the treatment of shoulder pain in spinal cord injuries. *Arch Phys Med Rehabil* 2001;82:1038–1046.

390. Nayak S, Shiflett SC, Schoenberger NE, et al. Chronic pain following spinal cord injury: the efficacy of acupuncture in pain management. *Arch Phys Med Rehabil* 1999;80:1166.

391. Olenik LM, Laskin JJ, Burnham R, et al. Efficacy of rowing, backward wheeling and isolated scapular retractor exercise as remedial strength activities

for wheelchair users: application of electromyography. *Paraplegia* 1995;33: 148–152.

392. Curtis KA, Tyner TM, Zachary L, et al. Effect of a standard exercise protocol on shoulder pain in long-term wheelchair users. *Spinal Cord* 1999;37:421–429.

393. Robinson MD, Hussey RW, Ha CY. Surgical decompression of impingement in the weight bearing shoulder. *Arch Phys Med Rehabil* 1993;74:324–327.

394. Gellman H, Chandler D, Petrasek J, et al. Carpal tunnel syndrome in paraplegic patients. *J Bone Jt Surg (Am)* 1988;70:517–519.

395. Davidoff G, Werner R, Waring W. Compressive mononeuropathies of the upper extremity in chronic paraplegia. *Paraplegia* 1991;29:17–24.

396. Nemchausky BA, Ubilluz RM. Upper extremity neuropathies in patients with spinal cord injuries. *J Spinal Cord Med* 1995;18:95–97.

397. Kirshblum S, Druin E, Planten K. Musculoskeletal conditions in chronic spinal cord injury. *Top Spinal Cord Inj Rehabil* 1997;2:23–35.

398. Yerzierski RP. Pain following spinal cord injury: the clinical problem and experimental studies. *Pain* 1996;68:185–194.

399. Siddahl PJ, Taylor DA, McClelland JM, et al. Pain report and the relationship of pain to physical factors in the first 6 months following spinal cord injury. *Pain* 1999;81:187–199.

400. Demirel G, Ylhnaz H, Gencosmanoglu B, et al. Pain following spinal cord injury. *Spinal Cord* 1998;36:25–28.

401. Davidoff G, Guarracini M, Roth E, et al. Trazodone hydrochloride in the treatment of dysesthetic pain in traumatic myelopathy: a randomized, double-blind placebo-controlled study. *Pain* 1987;2:151–161.

402. Putzke ID, Richard JS, DeVivo MJ. Preceptors of pain 1 year post-spinal cord injury. *J Spinal Cord Med* 2001;24(l):47–53.

403. Siddall PJ, Loeser JD. Pain following spinal cord injury. *Spinal Cord* 2001; 39:63–73.

404. Stormer S, Gerner HJ, Gruninger W, et al. Chrome pain/dysaethesiae in spinal cord injury patients: results of a multicentre study. *Spinal Cord* 1997; 35:446–455.

405. Turner JA, Cardenas DD, Warms CA, et al. Chronic pain associated with spinal cord injuries: a community survey. *Arch Phys Med Rehab* 2001 82(4): 501–509.

406. Siddall PJ, Yezierski RP, Loeser JD. Pain following spinal cord injury: clinical features, prevalence, and taxonomy. *IASP Newslett* 2000;3–7.

407. McAdoo DJ, Xu GY, Roback G, et al. Changes in amino acid concentrations over time and space around an impact injury and their diffusion through the rat spinal cord. *Exp Neurol* 1999;159:538–544.

408. Eide PK, Stubhaug A, Stenehjem AE. Central dysesthesia pain after traumatic spinal cord injury is dependent on N-methyl-D-aspartate receptor activation. *Neurosurgery* 1995;37(6):1080–1087.

409. Hao JX, et al. Baclofen reverses the hypersensitivity of dorsal horn wide dynamic ranged neurons to mechanical stimulation after transient spinal cord ischemia: implications for a tonic GABAergic inhibitory control of myelinated fiber input. *J Neurophysiol* 1992;68:392–396.

410. Ciom B, Meglio M, Pentimalli L, et al. Spinal cord stimulation in the treatment of paraplegic pain. *J Neurosurg* 1995;82:35–39.

411. Cole J, Illis L, Sedgwick E. Intractable pain in spinal cord injury is not relieved by spinal cord stimulation. *Paraplegia* 1991;20:167–172.

412. Vaarwerk I, Staal M. Spinal cord stimulation in chronic pain syndromes. *Spinal Cord* 1998;36:671–682.

413. Davis R, Lentini R. Transcutaneous nerve stimulation for treatment of pain in patients with spinal cord injury. *Surg Neurol* 1975;4:100–101.

414. Friedman AH, Nashold BS Jr. DREZ lesions for relief of pain related to spinal cord injury. *J Neurosurg* 1986;65(4):465–469.

415. To TP, Lim TC, Hill ST, et al. Gabapentin for neuropathic pain following spinal cord injury. *Spinal Cord* 2002;40(6):282–285.

416. Tai Q, Kirshblum S, Tai Q, Kirshblum SC, Chen B, Millis S, et al. Treatment of neuropathic pain with gabapentin in spinal cord injury. *J Spinal Cord Med* 2002;25:100–105.

417. Warms CA, Turner JA, Marshall HM, et al. Treatments for chronic pain associated with spinal cord injuries: many are tried, few are helpful. *Clin J Pain* 2002;18(3):154–163.

418. Biering-Sorensen F, Bohr H. Bone mineral content of the lumbar spine and lower extremities years after spinal cord lesion. *Paraplegia* 1988;26:293–301.

419. Kiralti B, Smith A, Nauenberg T, et al. Bone mineral and geometric changes through the femur with immobilization due to spinal cord injury. *J Rehabil Res Dev* 2000;37:225–233.

420. Chow Y, Imnan C, Pollintine P, et al. Ultrasound bone densitometry and dual energy x-ray absorptiometry in patients with spinal cord injury: a cross sectional study. *Spinal Cord* 1996;34:736–74l.

421. Needham-Shropshire B, Broton J, Klose K, et al. Evaluation of a training program for persons with SCI paraplegia using the Parastep 1 ambulation system: Part 3. Lack of effect on bone mineral density. *Arch Phys Med Rehabil* 1997;78:799–803.

422. Belanger M, Stein R, Wheeler G, et al. Electrical stimulation: can it increase muscle strength and reverse osteoporosis in spinal cord injured individuals. *Arch Phys Med Rehabil* 2000;81:1090–1098.

423. Mohr T, Podenphant J, Biering-Sorensen F, et al. Increased bone mineral density after prolonged electrically induced cycle training of paralyzed limbs in spinal cord injured man. *Calcif TissInt*1997;61:22–25.

424. Harktopp A, Murphy R, Mohr T, et al. Bone fracture during electrical stimulation of the quadriceps in a spinal cord injured subject. *Arch Phys Med Rehabil* 1998;79:1133–1136.

425. Nance P, Schryvers O, Leslie W, et al. Intravenous pamidronate attenuates bone density loss after acute spinal cord injury. *Arch Phys Med Rehabil* 1999;80:243–251.

426. Luethi M, Zehnder Y, Michel D, et al. Alendronate in the treatment of bone loss after spinal cord injury: preliminary data of a 2 year randomized controlled trial in 60 paraplegic men. *J Bone Min Res* 2001;16[Suppl 1]:S219 (abst).

427. Ragnarsson KT, Sell GH. Lower extremity fractures after spinal cord injury: a retrospective study. *Arch Phys Med Rehabil* 1981;62:418–423.

428. Frisbie JH. Fractures after myelopathy. *J Spinal Cord Med* l997;20:66–69.

429. Garland DE. Pathologic fractures and bone mineral density at the knee. *J Spinal Cord Med* 1999;22:335.

430. Freehafer AA. Limb fractures in spinal cord injury. *Arch Phys Med Rehabil* 1995;76:823–827.

431. Rossier AB, Foo D, Shillito J, et al. Post-traumatic syringomyelia: incidence, clinical presentation, electrophysiological studies, syrinx protein and results of conservative and operative treatment. *Brain* 1985;108:439–461.

432. El Masry W, Biyani A. Incidence, management, and outcome of post-traumatic syringomyelia. *J Neurol Neurosurg Psychiatry* 1996;60:141–146.

433. Perrouin-Verbe B, Lenne-Aurier K, Robert R, et al. Post-traumatic syringomyelia and post-traumatic spinal canal stenosis: a direct relationship: review of 75 patients with a spinal cord injury. *Spinal Cord* 1998;36:137–143.

434. Sett P, Crockard H. The value of magnetic resonance imaging (MRI) in the follow-up management of spinal injury. *Paraplegia* 1991;29:396–410.

435. Backe HA, Beta RR, Mesgarzadeh M, et al. Post-traumatic spinal cord cysts evaluated by magnetic resonance imaging. *Paraplegia* 1991;29:607–612.

436. Abel R, Gerner HJ, Smit C, et al. Residual deformity of the spinal canal in patients with traumatic paraplegia and secondary changes of the spinal cord. *Spinal Cord* 1999;37:14–19.

437. Nogues MA, Gene R, Encabo H. Risk of sudden death during sleep in syringomyelia and syringobulbia. *J Neurol Neurosurg Psychiatry* 1992;55:585–589.

438. Wang D, Bodley R, Sett P, et al. A clinical magnetic resonance imaging study of the traumatised spinal cord more than 20 years following injury. *Paraplegia* 1996;34:65–81.

439. Little JW, Robinson LR, Goldstein B, et al. Electrophysiologic findings in posttraumatic syringomyelia: implications for clinical management. *J Am Para Soc* 1992;15:44–52.

440. Nogues MA, Stalberg E. Electrodiagnostic findings in syringomyelia. *Muscle Nerve* 1999;22:1653–1659.

441. Sgouros S, Williams B. Management and outcome of posttraumatic syringomyelia. *J Neurosurg* 1996;85:197–205.

442. Dautheribes LW, Pointillart V, Gaujard E, et al. Mean term follow-up of a series of posttraumatic syringomyelia patients after syringo-peritoneal shunting. *Paraplegia* 1995;33:241–245.

443. Levi ADO, Sonntag VKH. Management of posttraumatic syringomyelia using expansile duraplasty. *Spine* 1998;23:128–132.

444. Batzdorf U, Klekamp J, Johnson JP. A critical appraisal of syrinx cavity shunting procedures. *J Neurosurg* 1998;89:382–388.

445. Grant R, Handley DM, Lang D, et al. MRI measurement of the syrinx size before and after operation. *J Neurol Neurosurg Psychiatry* 1987;50:1685–1687.

446. Waters RL, Muccitelli LM. Tendon transfers to improve function of patients with tetraplegia. In Kirshblum SC, Campagnolo D, DeLisa JE, eds. *Spinal cord medicine*. Philadelphia: Lippincott Williams & Wilkins, 2002;121 138.

447. Pedretti LW. Occupational performance: a model for practice in physical dysfunction. In: Pedretti LW, ed. *Occupational therapy practice skills for physical dysfunction*, 4th ed. St. Louis: Mosby, 1996;3–12.

448. Mc Dowell CL, Moberg EA, House JH. The Second International Conference on Surgical Rehabilitation of the Upper Limb in Traumatic Quadriplegia. *J Hand Surg* 1986;11A:604–608.

449. Moberg E, Freehafer AA, Lamb DK, et al. International federation of societies for surgery of the hand. A report from the committee on spinal injuries 1980. *Scand J Rehabil Med* 1982;14:3–5.

450. Moberg E. Surgical rehabilitation of the upper limb in tetraplegia. *Paraplegia* 1990;28:330–334.

451. Freehafer AA. Tendon transfers in patients with cervical spinal cord injury. *J Hand Surg* 1991;16A:804–809.

452. Johnson DL, Gellman H, Waters RL, et al. Brachioradialis transfer for wrist extension in tetraplegic patients who have fifth-cervical-level neurological function. *J Bone Joint Surg* 1996;78A:1063–1067.

453. Raczka R, Braun R, Waters RL. Posterior deltoid-to-triceps transfer in quadriplegia. *Chin Orthop* 1984;187:163–167.

454. Revol M, Briand E, Servant JM. Biceps-to-triceps transfer in tetraplegia. The medial route. *J Hand Surg (Br)* 1999;24(2):235–237.

455. Kuz JE, Van Heest AE, House JH. Biceps-to-triceps transfer in tetraplegic patients: report of the medial routing technique and follow-up of three cases. *J Hand Surg (Am)* 1999;24(l):161–172.

456. Moberg E. *The upper limb in tetraplegia, a "new approach" to surgical rehabilitation*. Stuttgart: George Thieme, 1978.

457. Moberg EA. The present state of surgical rehabilitation for the upper limb in tetraplegia. *Paraplegia* 1987;25:351–356.

458. Reiser TV, Waters RL. Long term follow up of the Moberg key grip procedure. *J Hand Surg* 1986;11A:724–728.

459. Water R, Moore K, Graboff S, et al. Brachioradialis to flexor pollicis longus tendon transfer for active lateral pinch in the tetraplegic. *J Hand Surg* 1985;10A(3):385–391.

460. House JH, Shannon M. Restoration of strong grasp and lateral pinch in tetraplegia: a comparison of two methods of thumb control in each patient. *J Hand Surg* 1985;10A(1):22–29.
461. Gansel J, Waters RL, Geilman H. Pronator teres to flexor digitorum profundus transfer in quadriplegia. *J Bone Joint Surg* 1990;72A(3):427–432.
462. Lo IK, Turner R, Connolly S, et al. The outcome of tendon transfers for C6-spared quadriplegics. *J Hand Surg* 1998;23:156–161.
463. Paul SD, Gellman H, Waters R, et al. Single-stage reconstruction of key pinch and extension of the elbow in tetraplegic patients. *J Bone Jt Surg* 1994;76(A):1451–1456.
464. Gellman H, Kan D, Waters RL, et al. Rerouting of the biceps brachii for paralytic supination contracture of the forearm in tetraplegia due to trauma. *J Bone Jt Surg* 1994;76A:398–402.
465. Gellman H. The hand and upper limb in tetraplegia. *Curr Orthop* 1991;5:233–238.
466. Waters RL, Stark LZ, Gubernick I, et al. Electromyographic analysis of brachioradialis to flexor pollicis longus tendon transfer in quadriplegia. *J Hand Surg* 1990;15A:335–339.
467. Peckham PH, Keith MW, Kilgore KL, et al. Implantable Neuroprosthesis Research Group. Efficacy of an implanted neuroprosthesis for restoring hand grasp in tetraplegia: a multicenter study. *Arch Phys Med Rehabil* 2001;82:1380–1388.
468. Mulcahay MJ, Beta RR, Smith BT, et al. Implanted functional electrical stimulation hand system in adolescents with spinal injuries: an evaluation. *Arch Phys Med Rehabil* 1997;78:597–607.
469. Hobby J, Taylor PN, Esnouf J. Restoration of tetraplegic hand function by use of the neurocontrol freehand system. *J Hand Surg (Br)* 2001;26:459–464.
470. Kilgore KL, Pecitham PH, Keith MW, et al. Advanced control alternatives for upper extremity neuroprosthetic systems. *J Spinal Cord Med* 2002;25:228–229(abst).
471. Hutchinson D, Mulcahey MJ, Beta RR, et al. Heterotopic nerve transfer for adolescents with tetraplegia. *J Spinal Cord Med* 2002;25:228(abst).
472. Zafonte RD, Elovic E. Dual diagnosis: traumatic brain injury in a patient with spinal cord injury. In Kirshblum SC, Campagnolo D, DeLisa JE, eds. *Spinal cord medicine.* Philadelphia: Lippincott Williams & Wilkins, 2002:261–274.
473. Davidoff G, Thomas P, Johnson M, et al. Closed head injury in acute traumatic spinal cord injury: incidence and risk factors. *Arch Phys Med Rehabil* 1988;69:869–872.
474. Teasdale G, Jennett B. Assessment of coma and impaired consciousness. A practical scale. *Lancet* 1974;2:81–84.
475. Katz DI, Alexander MP. Traumatic brain injury. Predicting course of recovery and outcome for patients admitted to rehabilitation. *Arch Neurol* 1994;51:661–670.
476. Zafonte RD, Mann NR, Millis SR, et al. Hammond posttraumatic amnesia: its relation to functional outcome. *Arch Phys Med Rehabil* 1997;78:1103–1106.
477. Levin HS, O'Donnell VM, Grossman RG. The Galveston Orientation and Amnesia Test. A practical scale to assess cognition after head injury. *J Nerv Ment Dis* 1979;167:675–684.
478. Mysiw WJ, Sandel ME. The agitated brain injured patient. Part 2: Pathophysiology and treatment. *Arch Phys Med Rehabil* 1997;78:213–220.
479. Uomoto J, Brockway J. Anger management training for brain injury patients and their families. *Arch Phys Med Rehabil* 1992;73:674–679.
480. Crane A, Joyce B. Cool down a procedure for decreasing aggression in adults with traumatic brain head injury. *Behav Res Treat* 1991;6;65–69.

481. Schaible KL, Smith U, Fessler RG, et al. Evaluation of the risks of anticoagulation therapy following experimental craniotomy in the rat. *J Neurosurg* 1985;63:959–962.
482. Tempkin N. A randomized double blind trial of phenytoin following severe head injury. *N Engl J Med* 1990;323;497–502.
483. Richards J, Brown L, Hagglund K, et al. Spinal cord injury and concomitant traumatic brain injury. *Am J Phys Med Rehabil* 1988;67;211–216.
484. Brown M, Vandergoot D. Quality of life for individuals with traumatic brain injury: comparison with others living in the community. *J Head Trauma Rehabil* 1998;13;1–23.
485. Kreuter M, Sullivan M, Dahlof A, et al. Partner relationships, functioning, mood and global quality of life in person with spinal cord injury and traumatic brain injury. *Spinal Cord* 1998;36:252–261.
486. Bach JR, Wang TG. Pulmonary function and sleep disordered breathing in patients with traumatic tetraplegia: a longitudinal study. *Arch Phys Med Rehabil* 1994;75:279–284.
487. Short DJ, Stradling JR, Williams SJ. Prevalence of sleep apnoea in patients over 40 years of age with spinal cord lesions. *J Neurol Neurosurg Psychiatry* 1992;55:1032–1036.
488. Burns SP, Little JW, Hussey JD, et al. Sleep apnea syndrome in chronic spinal cord injury: associated factors and treatment. *Arch Phys Med Rehabil* 2000;81:1334–1339.
489. Klefbeck B, Sternhag M, Weinberg, et al. Obstructive sleep apneas in relation to severity of spinal cord injury. *Spinal Cord* 1998;36:621–628.
490. Young W. Cure research in spinal cord injury. In: Kirshblum SC, Campagnolo D, DeLisa JE, eds. *Spinal cord medicine.* Philadelphia: Lippincott Williams & Wilkins, 2002:600–620.
491. Asamoto S, Sugiyama H, Doi H, et al. Hyperbaric oxygen (HBO) therapy for acute traumatic cervical spinal cord injury. *Spinal Cord* 2000;38:538–540.
492. Segal JL, Brunnemann SR. 4-Aminopyridine alters gait characteristics and enhances locomotion in spinal cord injured humans. *J Spinal Cord Med* 1998;21:200–204.
493. Davis FA, Stefoski D, Rush J. Orally administered 4-AP improves clinical signs in multiple sclerosis. *Ann Neurol* 1990;27:186–192.
494. Segal JL, Brunnemann SR. 4-Aminopyridine improves pulmonary function in quadriplegic humans with longstanding spinal cord injury. *Pharmacotherapy* 1997;17:415–423.
495. Lammerte DP, Graziam V, Katz MA, et al. Evaluation of fampridine-SR in patients with chronic spinal cord injury. *J Spinal Cord Med* 2002;25:239.
496. Dobkin BH, Harkema S, Requejo P, et al. Modulation of locomotor-like EMG activity in subjects with complete and incomplete spinal cord injury. *J Neurol Rehabil* 1995;9:183–190.
497. Wernig A, Nanassy A, Muller S. Laufband (treadmill) therapy in incomplete paraplegia and tetraplegia. *J Neurotrauma* 1999;16:719–726.
498. Wernig A, Nanassy A, Muller S. Maintenance of locomotor abilities following Laufband (treadmill) therapy in para- and tetraplegic persons: follow-up studies. *Spinal Cord* 1998;36:744&#64979;749.
499. Norman KE, Pepin A, Barbeau H. Effects of drugs on walking after spinal cord injury. *Spinal Cord* 1998;36:699–715.
500. Herman R, He J, D'Luzansky S, Willis W, et al. Spinal cord stimulation facilitates functional walking in a chronic, incomplete spinal cord injured. *Spinal Cord* 2002;40:65–68.

CHAPTER 80

Multiple Sclerosis

George H. Kraft and Jimmy Y. Cui

Since publication of the chapter on multiple sclerosis (MS) in the first edition of this text in 1988 (1), there has been an explosion in the understanding of the cause and methods to treat this disease. Prior to 1993, no medication was available that would alter the course of the disease. In late 1993, interferon (IFN) β1b (Betaseron®) was approved by the Food and Drug Administration (FDA) in the United States and a small amount became available to treat patients (2). This medication—a biological product produced by using recombinant technology—was in such short supply that a lottery was held to determine those patients who would receive it. (The situation is much different now; today, three IFN-β products are available in the U.S. and intercorporate competition among manufacturers is strong.) In addition to the IFN-β products, two other medications—glatiramer acetate (Copaxone®) and mitoxantrone (Novantrone®)—have been approved in the U.S. for treatment of MS. Thus, at the present time, five disease-altering immunomodulating medications are available in the U.S. market.

However, none of these medications improve patient function. They all are effective in reducing relapses or slowing down progression in certain stages of the disease, but they do not improve the patient. The only way to improve function in MS is rehabilitation (3).

MS is the most common cause of nontraumatic disability affecting young adults in the Northern Hemisphere (4). In its most common forms—relapsing-remitting (R-R) and secondary progressive (SP)—it is gender-dependent, with more than twice as many females as males developing the disease (5). The mean age of onset is the late 20s, and the typical patient is one of Northern European ancestry living in a temperate latitude (6). Although MS is not a hereditary disease (as defined by Mendelian genetics), there is a familial tendency that increases the likelihood of it occurring in other family members severalfold (7).

Although it is now possible to reduce the frequency of exacerbations and slow the progression of the disease, rehabilitation is still the only way to improve function in patients with MS. Therefore, it is important that physicians be familiar with rehabilitative techniques.

DEMOGRAPHICS AND EPIDEMIOLOGY

Approximately 85% of persons with MS have either relapsing-remitting (R-R) or secondary progressive (SP) disease—the form into which most R-R patients eventually convert (4). These display an approximately 2.5:1 female preponderance (5). A small number of patients —10% to 15%—have progres-

sion of disease from the outset and are considered to have the primary progressive (PP) form of MS. This group tends to be older at onset, and is divided evenly between females and males (8). These differences between the R-R/SP form and the PP form of MS have led some investigators to consider these as two different disorders. Supporting this is the PP form's failure to respond to some immunomodulating therapy in recent clinical trials.

Prevalence in the United States is thought to range from approximately 40 to 220 per 100,000. For some time, it had been noted that MS occurred more frequently in the northern part of the Northern Hemisphere than toward the equator. Although there is less landmass in the Southern Hemisphere, a similar distribution also occurred there: MS was more common toward the South Pole than near the equator (6). This latitudinal discrepancy was investigated further in the early 1970s when MS in Seattle and Los Angeles, as well as migration patterns of patients between the two cities, was investigated (9). This study demonstrated that where a person spent the first 15 years of life predicted her or his likelihood of getting the disease. For example, even though MS is one-third to one-half as common in Los Angeles as in Seattle, a person born in Seattle, then migrating to Los Angeles after age 15, carried the same two to three times greater chance of developing MS as if she or he had stayed in Seattle. These findings have been substantiated by other migration studies in the Southern Hemisphere (10) and throughout the world (11).

Although MS can occur in anyone in any country on the globe, it is preponderantly a disease of persons of Northern European ancestry (11). It also has occurred in patterns suggestive of the presence of an infectious agent. For example, prior to 1943 the Faroe Islands, between Norway and Iceland, was virtually free of MS. However, in 1943, 3 years after British soldiers entered these islands for their defense during World War II, MS started to occur (12). Some associated this with dogs the soldiers brought with them and a subsequent outbreak of distemper, but viral studies failed to support this particular link (13). Yet, these and other observations suggest that some type of infectious agent is active in the etiology of this disease, and that a delay mechanism of some type is operating (14).

ETIOLOGY

MS is considered to be one of a number of "autoimmune" diseases. Like all of these disorders (e.g., rheumatoid arthritis, Sjögren's syndrome, Hashimoto's thyroiditis, Graves' disease, primary biliary cirrhosis, chronic active hepatitis, and lupus erythematosus), it is more common in women than in men. In addition, MS also appears to involve both genetic and latitudinal factors (see section on "Demographics and Epidemiology"). Persons of Northern European ancestry—especially those with HLA–DR2 in DR-positive families—have a greater chance of developing the disease (15). From the standpoint of the latitudinal difference, something during development appears to either cause the disease in the temperate latitudes or protect against the disease in the warmer latitudes—or both (9). This unknown latitudinal factor occurs during the period in which the human immune system initially develops antibodies to environmental antigens (16).

The blood/immune system is a tissue, hence controlled by human leukocyte antigens. An attractive hypothesis of the etiology of MS is that in genetically susceptible individuals, persons with susceptible HLA systems may have an aberration in their antibody-forming systems, allowing environmental stimuli to cause the formations of antibodies to outside agents, cross-reacting to their own cells. When such antigens are later encountered in adulthood, they might set off an attack against components of the person's own central nervous system (CNS) tissue. This concept of "molecular mimicry" might later develop into a self-perpetuating degenerative loop through the concept of "epitope spreading." Other theories are extant (17).

PATHOLOGY, PATHOGENESIS, AND PATHOPHYSIOLOGY

The hallmark of the pathological findings in MS is the presence of multifocal plaques (lesions) of demyelination in the cerebral hemispheres, optic nerves, brain stem, and spinal cord. Microscopically, the typical early plaque has a demarcated area of demyelination with relative axon sparing, inflammatory infiltrates composed of lymphocytes and macrophages, and evidence of astrocytic proliferation and gliosis. In later stages of disease, axon damage is also present (18).

In acute active lesions marked edema due to blood–brain barrier (BBB) interruption accompanies the inflammatory response. Perivenular lymphocytic infiltrates are evident in areas of demyelination. Macrophages are numerically the most prominent inflammatory cells in the lesion and many of them are filled with myelin debris. Proinflammatory CD4+ T cells appear to be critical components in the demyelinating process in active lesions. Proinflammatory cytokines produced in CD4+ T cells are thought to be responsible for direct damage to CNS myelin. B cells from peripheral blood are recruited to the active plaque and differentiate into plasma cells that synthesize and release immunoglobulin. This can be identified as the presence of oligoclonal bands and immunoglobulin G (IgG) index elevation, which can be seen in the cerebrospinal fluid (CSF) of MS patients. However, plasma cells are not universally present. They are more commonly encountered in chronic lesions. New gadolinium-enhancing lesions on magnetic resonance imaging (MRI) in MS represent the breakdown of the BBB that is associated with an acute plaque, which is believed to be the earliest recognizable pathological change in MS.

With progression of the pathological process, chronic inactive lesions are less inflammatory and become hypocellular. Degeneration occurs as oligodendrocytes are destroyed and astrocytes proliferate. As demyelination occurs, there can also be some degree of remyelination in the lesion (19). However, as the disease progresses, demyelination at the plaque margin taking place over the newly remyelinated areas leads to expansion of the lesion, eventually resulting in scarring in the region and loss of the capability of remyelination and reconstruction.

Blood–Brain Barrier

Disruption of the blood–brain barrier (BBB)—the first stage of the MS process—results in an increased permeability across this "wall" which is associated with acute inflammation that allows the entry of a variety of active immune cells and serum proteins into the CNS. Also, tissue culture data indicate that serum from MS patients contains neuroelectric blocking factors that inhibit synaptic transmission. Entry of neuroelectric blocking factors into active plaques near neurons may thus cause synaptic blockade. The BBB is now the targeted site of some currently used and experimental disease-modifying agents (20–22).

The cause of the BBB breakdown has not been well elucidated. Changes of adhesion molecule expression on active immune cells and vascular endothelial cells at the BBB have been reported (23–26). Recent studies have further found the involvement of interendothelial tight junctions (TJ) in BBB breakdown. TJ abnormalities seen in MS were manifested as beading, interruption, absence or diffuse cytoplasmic localization of fluorescence, or separation of junction. Abnormal or open TJ associated with inflammation may contribute to BBB leakage in enhancing MRI lesions (27). Extracellular matrix (ECM) alteration is suggested as a result of BBB breakdown, release, and activation of proteases and synthesis of ECM components. It has been noted that changes such as proteoglycans in white matter ECM may play critical roles in lesion pathogenesis and CNS dysfunction of MS, although further investigation is warranted to fully define its precise role (28).

Demyelination

CNS demyelination probably results from immune-mediated inflammation, but dysfunction of oligodendrocytes has also been suggested (29). Demyelination has important clinical consequences (30). Nerve fibers undergoing demyelination demonstrate suboptimal conduction and poor ability to conduct trains of impulses, due in part to an increased refractory period. Conduction failure is common during the process of demyelination. Although details of conduction failure during demyelination are not fully established, several major components have been described: (a) increased membrane capacitance in the demyelinated region, (b) damage to the nodal sodium channels, and (c) absence of sodium channels from the internodal membrane (30,31). Consequently, secondary to increased intracellular sodium, current leaks through the demyelinated segment resulting in reduced amplitude current prevent the buildup of electrical potential sufficient to cause depolarization at the adjacent internode.

Demyelinated fibers also demonstrate temperature sensitivity. Rasminsky showed a rise in temperature as little as 0.5°C above normal could cause conduction failure in some fibers (32). Transient loss of function in MS patients with fever and Uhthoff's phenomenon (transient scotoma during exercise) are examples of conduction delay/failure and signal dispersion of central demyelinated fibers with increase in temperature. Additional symptoms due to demyelination may relate to increased nerve excitability (transient or sustained paresthesia), the inability to sustain high-frequency transmission (muscle weakness and fatigability), or ephaptic cross-activation (paroxysmal symptoms).

Axonal Damage

Permanent axonal damage with axonal transection and spheroid formation in MS lesions has been described (18). Severing of axons may even occur in acute plaques and is believed to be more common than previously appreciated (33). Clinical and magnetic resonance imaging (MRI) studies show cortical dysfunction and brain atrophy in MS patients, further indicating progressive damage to neurons during the course of MS (34,35). Recent investigation of brain atrophy provides intriguing findings (36); contrary to former belief, significant atrophy, affecting both white and gray matter, occurs early in the clinical course of MS.

Axonal damage in MS is not a new finding (37). In fact, for over a century, neuropathologists have recognized that MS lesions, particularly in old plaques, possess a decreased number of axons (38). Axon loss may be secondary to long-term demyelination, or may be an independent degenerative process. MS may consist of two pathogenic processes:

1. An inflammatory component, associated with BBB breakdown and enhancing lesions on MRI, which predominates in the early stages of R-R MS
2. A progressive, degenerative disease of axons, which is more prominent in later stages of the disease (S-P MS) and in PP MS.

It is unclear to what extent the processes are related or separate. However, it appears that all immunomodulating treatments discovered to date primarily impact the inflammatory, rather than degenerative, process. Axonal damage is considered a determinant of irreversible neurological impairment and long-term disability in MS patients. It is therefore becoming an important focus of investigation.

Restoration, Remyelination, and Neuroprotection

Recovery of function (remission) may be due to resolution of inflammation or the pressure of edema, removal of humoral factors, reattachment of paranodal myelin, or rerouting of nerve transmission through alternative pathways (brain plasticity). Remyelination is a key component in the restoration phase; this usually requires days to weeks. There is abundant evidence of remyelination in MS lesions. Early studies of spinal cord MS lesions suggested that regeneration of central myelin is accompanied by Schwann cell invasion of the CNS and the presence of peripheral myelin within the demyelinated region (19).

One of the classic neuropathological findings in MS with remyelination is "shadow plaques." They are areas of partial reduction of myelin staining, as remyelinated axons have thinner myelin sheaths. They may be seen on MRI as intermediate lesions on T1 images; they will be less dark than the more hypodense "black holes" (which represent significant axon damage). Functionally, the conduction which is restored is not normal. Velocities are slow (2.5% to 5% of normal), high-frequency impulse transmission cannot be maintained, and an estimated 50 to 200 times more energy is required for nerve transmission (39–41).

Recent attention has been shifted to the mechanism of minimizing and preventing axonal damage in the CNS since it is known to be the principal cause of disability. It has been well documented that immune cells are capable of producing a number of potentially neuroprotective factors and neurotrophic mediators, such as NT-3, nerve growth factor (NGF), transforming growth factor-β, and platelet-derived growth fac-

tor. It has been reported that brain-derived neurotrophic factor (BDNF), which can prevent neuronal damage, is expressed in immune cells including T cells, macrophages, and microglia in MS lesions. Furthermore, BDNF receptors are found in neurons in the immediate vicinity of MS lesions, and are likely to be responsive to neuroprotective effects (42).

These findings are in support of a new concept that active immune cells produce not only damaging but also protective factors in MS lesions. As our knowledge is expected to grow in this exciting field, novel therapeutic strategies could possibly be developed based on enhancing neuroprotective effects to preserve axons (43).

TYPES OF MULTIPLE SCLEROSIS

Current terminology separates MS into four subtypes: relapsing-remitting (R-R), secondary progressive (SP), primary progressive (PP), and progressive-relapsing (P-R) (Fig. 80-1). R-R and SP MS are at two ends of the same spectrum. Patients start with relapses which then remit for progressively shorter periods of time; remissions eventually do not return to normal baseline and progression eventually takes over with fewer and

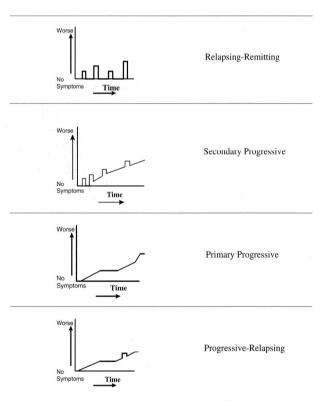

Figure 80-1. Types of multiple sclerosis (MS). The course of the four types of MS, with the horizontal axis designating increasing time and the vertical axis depicting worsening of symptoms. The top two types—relapsing-remitting (R-R) and secondary progressive (SP)—account for 85% of cases. In the R-R type, exacerbations are sudden, relatively brief, and result in return to baseline or slightly worse than baseline. Over time, this form converts to the SP type in which the baseline status worsens between exacerbations, which become less frequent and less severe over time. The primary progressive (PP) form accounts for 10% to 15% of cases. In this type, there is gradual worsening from onset with occasional periods of plateauing. The fourth type, progressive-relapsing (P-R), is very rare, occurring in no more than a few percent of MS patients. This type starts out like the P-P type, but has superimposed relapses and remissions.

less distinct relapses. Eventually the patient develops a progressive disease without relapses. PP disease starts in a progressive manner from the outset, continuing in that mode throughout the duration of the disease. No relapses or remissions occur. The P-R form has short relapses superimposed on a progressive course from the outset.

Relapsing-Remitting Multiple Sclerosis

This is the most common form of MS, with 85% of MS patients initially manifesting this pattern. R-R MS frequently begins with optic neuritis (ON)—transient unilateral visual impairment lasting days to weeks, which may be associated with retrobulbar pain (44). Although ON can occur as a separate disease (see later in the chapter under "Variants of Multiple Sclerosis"), over 50% of persons who have ON eventually develop MS (45). Other patients with R-R MS may initially have tingling or weakness of a limb. Patients initially presenting with afferent or sensory symptoms typically have a better prognosis than those who initially present with motor symptoms (46). In general, patients whose symptoms fully remit after early exacerbations demonstrate a better long-term prognosis (46). It is widely accepted that it is in this early stage of R-R disease that the immunomodulating agents have the most beneficial effect (44,47).

Secondary Progressive Multiple Sclerosis

Secondary progressive (SP) MS is defined as that stage when the baseline to which a patient returns following a relapse gets progressively worse. Approximately 50% of untreated patients with R-R MS convert to this form of disease within 10 years (4). IFN-β1b and mitoxantrone slow the progression of SP MS if given in the early part of this stage (48–50). However, in the late stage, the beneficial effect appears less pronounced. This is the type of MS (along with PP MS) where rehabilitation techniques are the most useful.

Recent autopsy data (51) in SP MS patients have demonstrated that low-grade active demyelination is found to be ongoing in periplaque white matter with deposits of C3d, an opsonin formed during complement activation. C3d coupling is known to be able to markedly promote the immunogenicity of potential antigens, suggesting that disrupted myelin close to plaque provides a possible source of the putative MS antigen ("epitope spreading;" see previous section on "Etiology"). Consequently, ongoing myelin breakdown in periplaque regions, in the absence of perivascular cell cuffing or other signs of acute inflammation, appears to contribute to disease progression in SP-MS (51).

Primary Progressive Multiple Sclerosis

Interestingly, while the R-R/SP form of MS is a 2.5:1 female disease, primary progressive (PP) MS affects both sexes equally (8). It also has an older age of onset. PP MS more often starts with motor symptoms and tends to progress more rapidly, validating observations that patients starting with motor symptoms fare less well than those starting with sensory symptoms, regardless of the type of disease (46).

PP MS is characterized by predominant loss of myelin and axon with only mild inflammatory components (52). There is often a relative paucity of conventional MRI-detectable activity (53). A large cohort study on the pathology of PP MS using MRI and magnetization transfer imaging (MTI) techniques has demonstrated the presence of diffuse tissue damage in the CNS, which is undetectable by conventional MRI. Moreover,

there is prevalent involvement of the cervical cord in PP MS patients, which contributes to the neurological impairment and disease severity in this clinical subtype (54).

There are no FDA-approved immunomodulating agents for PP MS. Although some have been tried, none has shown sufficient statistical benefit for regulatory approval. However, chemotherapeutic agents are often used "off label" to treat this form of disease. Some efficacy has been reported for methotrexate (55). The most important treatment, however, is rehabilitation, as rehabilitative techniques are the only treatments demonstrated to produce functional improvement (3). Since patients with PP MS are more likely to be older men, they also demonstrate many other unique clinical needs (8).

Progressive-Relapsing Multiple Sclerosis

Progressive-relapsing (P-R) MS represents the smallest subtype. Probably no more than 5% of MS patients have this form (4). It is often difficult to distinguish P-R from PP disease, and effective medical treatment for this subtype is unclear. As in the PP form, rehabilitative techniques remain the mainstay of management (3).

VARIANTS OF MULTIPLE SCLEROSIS

Optic Neuritis

Many patients with MS will present with ON, a sudden unilateral loss of vision, which can vary from a slight central scotoma to complete loss of light perception (44). In a long study following ON patients for 11.6 years, 57% eventually developed MS (45). Determining which patients with ON will eventually develop MS is impossible at the onset, but both ON and ON/MS patients respond favorably to intravenous methylprednisolone (44). Because those patients with ON who will eventually develop MS cannot be determined, and because early treatment appears to reduce the percentage of ON patients converting to MS, treatment with IFN-β1a has been recommended (56).

Transverse Myelitis

This variant consists of acute, nontraumatic myelopathy. Similar to ON, some patients with transverse myelitis (TM) will develop MS (57). TM patients who eventually develop MS typically present with asymmetric motor or sensory symptoms, whereas those with pure TM not converting to MS generally have symmetric findings (58).

Devic's Disease (Neuromyelitis Optica)

Devic's disease consists of ON plus TM. The optic nerves and spinal cord are affected; the brain is not involved (59). A large cohort of 71 patients seen over 47 years suggests that this disease has two forms: a monophasic form, which has a good prognosis, and a relapsing form, which develops severe disability in a stepwise manner (59). Neuromyelitis optica does not appear to respond to the usual immunomodulating agents used in R-R MS, but rather should be treated with a combination of azathioprine plus corticosteroids (60).

Other Variants of Multiple Sclerosis

There are several other very rare CNS demyelinating diseases considered variants of MS. The reader interested in learning more about these disorders is advised to consult a recent textbook of neurology.

DIAGNOSIS OF MULTIPLE SCLEROSIS

A clinical course consistent with MS consists of two or more occurrences of CNS symptoms separated in time and space. Common symptoms include fatigue, ataxia, weakness, numbness and tingling, bladder dysfunction, spasticity, cognitive problems, depression, ON, and pain. The diagnosis of MS requires the presence of signs and symptoms separated in space and time.

Diagnostic Criteria

Over the years, several sets of diagnostic criteria have been developed. In the 1960s, Schumacher and colleagues based the diagnosis of MS entirely on clinical findings (61). In the early 1980s, these were modified by Poser and colleagues to allow laboratory tests to substitute for some clinical criteria (62). Much more recently, as laboratory testing—especially MRI—has improved, laboratory results have been allowed to substitute for even more clinical findings (McDonald criteria) (63). Improvements in MRI techniques have diminished the importance of CSF evaluation, but identification of conduction slowing or conduction block with evoked potentials still may be useful. Of these, visual evoked potentials (VEPs) and somatosensory evoked potentials (SEPs) coursing through the longest portion of the neuraxis (i.e., tibial SEPs) are most useful (64). Since immunomodulating drugs appear to be most effective in the earliest stage of R-R MS, it is desirable to diagnose MS at the earliest stage possible.

Magnetic Resonance Imaging

With ever-improved radiologic technology, MRI scans are able to see ever-smaller lesions. Some research MRIs (e.g., 5 Tesla or greater) are able to detect almost microscopic abnormalities in the CNS. T2 scans identify MS lesions as hyperintense areas typically seen as periventricular lesions or subcortical ovoid lesions. Commonly, the periventricular lesions are arranged perpendicular to the roofs of the lateral ventricles, producing what are known as "Dawson's fingers" (65). With disease progression, these opaque white areas coalesce and more subcortical lesions develop. With more chronic and severe disease, brain atrophy becomes apparent. FLAIR (fluid-attenuated inversion recovery) modifications of T2-weighted images darken the CSF and allow the periventricular MS lesions to be more visible. Saggital views demonstrate these pathognomonic features well (Fig. 80-2).

T1-weighted images are useful to document other disorders, and have recently become of interest for the assessment of "black holes" —dark areas on T1 scans indicating severe neural and matrix loss. Also, "shadow plaques" (see previous section "Restoration, Remyelination, and Neuroprotection")—areas of density somewhere between normal brain and black holes—can be identified, suggesting areas of partial remyelination.

For several weeks after the occurrence of the breakdown in the BBB, the affected region will be permeable to gadolinium. Consequently, MRIs taken shortly after the intravenous (i.v.) injection of gadolinium will show "enhancement" or opaque regions on T1-weighted images. Such techniques can identify acute lesions, and can be used to identify a new lesion in time. Double- and triple-dose gadolinium injections are able to show even more subtle disease activity (35).

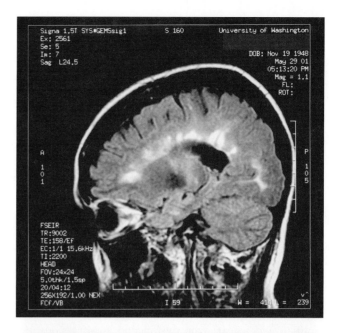

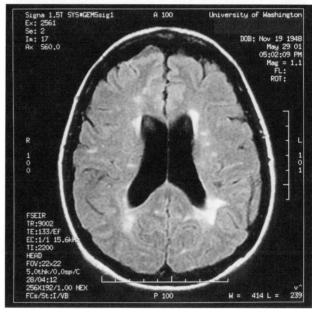

Figure 80-2. Fluid-attenuated inversion recovery-magnetic resonance imaging (FLAIR- MRI) of the brain of a patient with moderately severe multiple sclerosis (MS). **Top:** Sagittal MRI demonstrating the pathognomonic Dawson's fingers, useful in confirming the diagnosis of MS. These "fingers" show up as hyperintense linear areas of disease perpendicular to the roof of the ventricle. **Bottom:** Axial FLAIR-MRI demonstrates the periventricular predilection for disease as well as the subcortical ovoid areas of demyelination characteristic of MS. In addition, this view demonstrates the cortical atrophy (note: enlarged ventricles), which occurs in late-stage disease as axons are destroyed.

Magnetization transfer ratio is a newer imaging approach for the identification of MS lesions. Although not widely available, studies have demonstrated its efficacy in both research and clinical settings (66).

Magnetic Resonance Spectroscopy

Another technique that is primarily available in research laboratories is that of magnetic resonance spectroscopy (MRS). Proton MRS can be used to monitor metabolites such as choline,

TABLE 80-1.   Magnetic Resonance Spectroscopy

Substance Measured	Change	MS Lesions
Free lipids	Increase	Demyelination
N-acetyl-aspartate	Decrease	Axon loss
Lactate	Increase	Acute lesions
Choline/creatine ratio	Increase	MS plaque

MS, multiple sclerosis.

creatine + phosphocreatine, glutamate + glutamine, myo-inositol, N-acetyl-aspartate (NAA), mobile lipids + proteins, and lactic acid (67). Several of these metabolites have been shown to change in MS patients. Lipid metabolism is altered in demyelination, and NAA is a marker of axons. Consequently, a decrease in NAA indicates axon loss and an increase in free lipids indicates demyelination (Table 80-1). MRS studies have identified widespread axon dysfunction in MS lesions, even outside of areas identified as hyper-dense on T2-weighted MRI, suggesting that disease activity may involve a larger area of the CNS than appreciated using MRI alone (67).

Evoked Potentials

Early studies comparing visual evoked potentials (VEPs), brainstem-evoked responses (BAERs), and SEPs reported that VEPs were the most sensitive in demonstrating CNS conduction abnormalities in MS (68,69). However, these generally evaluated the short cord SEP pathway available to median nerve testing; SEPs from the lower limbs were not evaluated. Since MS lesions may occur throughout the spinal cord, brain stem and brain, SEP techniques using the entire central neuraxis are more likely to demonstrate conduction abnormalities. We have found that lower limb SEP testing increases the yield of abnormalities when compared with upper limb testing, and is comparable to the yield of VEPs (64). Consequently, tibial nerve SEPs are excellent tests to perform in both the diagnostic and monitoring stages of the disease.

Although the classic role of evoked potentials is to identify additional "hidden" lesions, conduction slowing also demonstrates a pathological state of myelin. Altered or absent myelin causes conduction slowing or conduction block. If conduction slowing through portions of the central neuraxis is found, the diagnosis of a demyelinating disease is strongly supported (see earlier section on "Demyelination"). Other pathological conditions that might be mistaken clinically for a demyelinating disease (e.g., vascular lesions or tumor) will produce conduction block with attenuation or absence of a response—not significant conduction slowing (70). SEPs assess afferent conduction from a limb and can be a valuable adjunct in planning a rehabilitation program for a patient with MS. Recent recommendations for the use of SEPs in MS can be found in practice topics published by the American Association of Electrodiagnostic Medicine (71).

VEPs are frequently ordered in the diagnostic stage to assess the presence of subclinical ON (or to confirm that a visual deficit was due to ON) in the attempt to confirm the presence of a second site of disease. The technique for these is well established (72). We have documented a correlation between abnormal conduction in the visual pathway and NAA levels (73).

Spinal Fluid Analysis

Lumbar puncture and CSF analysis are less often done today, as improvements in imaging have generally replaced this invasive procedure. However, when done, identification of oligoclonal bands and increased IgG synthesis are associated with a positive diagnosis of MS (74). In the future, it may be possible to obtain similar information about the immune function less invasively from the electrophoresis of tears (75).

Electrodiagnostic Testing

The question frequently arises as to the value of classic electrodiagnostic [electromyogram (electromyography (EMG/nerve conduction studies (NCS)] testing in patients with MS. Because nerve conduction studies are normal in patients with MS, they can be used to differentiate diseases of peripheral nerves from those involving the CNS (76). About one-third of MS patients will demonstrate abnormal late responses with increased amplitude and chronodispersion of F waves, consistent with a myelopathy. Consistent with reduction of central motor drive, abnormal recruitment patterns with slow and incomplete firing of motor unit action potentials having normal configuration will generally be seen. Approximately 20% of patients will demonstrate some positivesharp waves or fibrillation potentials. These will be present diffusely, with no specific myotomal or peripheral nerve distribution, and should therefore not be attributed to a neuropathy or radiculopathy (76).

Because they evaluate brain stem pathways, blink response testing has been shown to be positive in many MS patients, and has been suggested as a laboratory surrogate if MRI is not available (77).

IMPAIRMENT AND DISABILITY RATINGS

MS is a progressive disease. Unfortunately, in spite of current immunomodulating medications, most patients are not totally stabilized. Their relapses will likely be fewer in number, and hopefully their disease courses will be slowed, but over time their diseases are still likely to progress.

In order to assess the effect of treatment, some method of quantifying neurological deterioration is needed. Although MS affects a variety of neurological functions, some unifying assessment is needed. Considerable effort and angst have been expended to achieve this goal (78). MS clinicians and researchers have settled on a widely used scoring system: the Kurtzke Expanded Disability Status Scale (EDSS) (79). Although imperfect, it appears to be the best single measure of an MS patient's neurological changes. Originally designed to be administered by a health-care professional, it is now available in a patient-administered version (80). The EDSS is a 20-step scale ranging from 0 to 10 (using half-steps) where the higher the number, the more serious the impairment/disability (Table 80-2).

MEDICAL MANAGEMENT

Immunosuppressive (Chemotherapeutic) Agents

Because it has been recognized for some time that MS disease activity is related to the immune system (an immune-mediated disease), medications used to suppress the proliferation of cells and cell products (antibodies) have been used to try to sup-

TABLE 80-2.   The Expanded Disability Status Scale (EDSS)[a]

Score	Status	Score	Status	Score	Status
0	Normal neurologic exam	4.0	Fully ambulatory without aid, self-sufficient, active 12 hours a day despite relatively severe disability. Able to walk without aid or rest for about 500 m.	7.5	Unable to take more than a few steps; restricted to wheelchair; may need aid in transfer, wheels self but cannot carry on in standard wheelchair in a full day; may require motorized wheelchair.
1.0	Fully ambulatory	4.5	Fully ambulatory without aid, active much of the day, able to work a full day, may otherwise have some limitation of full activity or require minimal assistance; characterized by relatively severe disability. Able to walk without aid or rest for about 300 m.	8.0	Essentially restricted to bed or chair or perambulated in wheelchair, but may be out of bed much of the day; retains many self-care functions; generally has effective use of arms.
1.5	No disability	5.0	Ambulatory without aid or rest for about 200 m; disability severe enough to impair full daily activities (e.g., working full day without special provisions).	8.5	Essentially restricted to bed much of the day; has some effective use of arm(s); retains some self-care functions.
2.0	Minimal disability in one of seven Functional Systems (FS)[a]	5.5	Ambulatory without aid or rest for about 100 m; disability severe enough to limit full daily activities.	9.0	Helpless bed patient; can communicate and eat.
2.5	Minimal disability in two FS[a]	6.0	Intermittent or unilateral constant assistance (cane, crutch, or brace) required to walk about 100 m with or without resting.	9.5	Totally helpless bed patient; unable to communicate effectively or eat/swallow.
3.0	Moderate disability in one FS[a] or mild disability in three or four FS[a], though fully ambulatory	6.5	Constant bilateral assistance (canes, crutches, or braces) required to walk about 20 m without resting.	10	Death due to MS.
3.5	Moderate disability in one FS[a] and mild disability in one or two FS[a] or moderate disability in two FS[a] or mild disability in five FS[a]	7.0	Unable to walk beyond about 5 m even with aid, essentially restricted to wheelchair, wheels self in standard wheelchair and transfers alone; active in wheelchair about 12 hours a day.		

[a]Functional Systems are defined as pyramidal; cerebellar; brain stem; sensory; bowel and bladder; visual or optic; cerebral or mental functions.
From Kurtzke JF. Rating neurologic impairment in multiple sclerosis: an expanded disability status scale (EDSS). *Neurology* 1983;33(11):1444–1452.

press the disease (81). Immunosuppressive drugs such as methotrexate, azathioprine, and cyclophosphamide are some of the oldest treatments for MS. In general, most have had the same results: there was some beneficial effect, but side effects were too great. The one exception is recent: mitoxantrone (Novantrone®) (50). This agent is a potent immunosuppressive medication effective in R-R and SP MS. However, it has a number of side effects including cardiotoxicity and generally cannot be used longer than a cumulative 2 to 2½ lifetime years (82).

Because MS is considered to be an autoimmune disease and partial immune suppression appears to have value, we hypothesized that more complete immunosuppression might be even more effective or even curative. If the toxicity of complete bone marrow suppression could be prevented by a postsuppression bone marrow transplant, complete immunosuppression might be an effective treatment for severe MS.

The development of the technique to separate autologous peripheral CD34+ blood stem cells from peripheral blood and transplant them back to the immunosuppressed patient seemed a possible solution to the problem of toxicity (83). Thus, complete T-cell suppression using high-dose cyclophosphamide chemotherapy, total body irradiation, and antithymo-

cytic globulin with autologous stem cell transplant "rescue" was carried out in 26 MS patients. To be eligible for the study, patients had to have failed conventional treatment and had progression of disease at least 1.0 EDSS point over the previous year. We found that this treatment appeared to be effective in 77% of patients when analyzed a mean of 15.1 months after transplant (84). These benefits have persisted for a 2-year follow-up (85).

Corticosteroids

Corticosteroids are an old class of medications used for MS (86). They can reduce the severity and duration of exacerbations, but until recently were not thought to have any effect on the long-term course of the disease. As with chemotherapeutic agents, the toxicity profile of oral steroids was considered too great to use on an ongoing basis. In the 1970s, enthusiasm developed over the use of adrenocorticotropic hormone (ACTH) as a means of raising the level of endogenous corticosteroids (87), but at present this treatment is rarely employed. Contrary to previous opinions, a careful recent study suggests that intravenous methylprednisolone (IVMP) may actually have some long-term benefit. Pulsed IVMP given several times a year was shown to slow the development of T1 black holes, delay brain atrophy, and slow progression (88).

In the well-known clinical trial of prednisone versus IVMP for ON, subjects receiving prednisone did worse in the long run than subjects receiving placebo, whereas those getting IVMP did better than the placebo group (44). Therefore, oral corticosteroids are now only rarely used for exacerbations. The current standard of care in the treatment of acute MS exacerbations is 1 g of IVMP for 3 consecutive days. The sooner it can be given—we recommend within 4 days—the more effective it will be. Higher doses for a longer period may be even more beneficial (89).

Interferons

Interferons (IFNs) are large proteins consisting of many amino acids, having a high molecular weight. Theorizing that MS might be related to a viral infection, a clinical trial was carried out with IFN-γ. However, patients receiving this had increased numbers of exacerbations and the trial was stopped. Realizing that IFN-γ can be suppressed by IFN-β, this was studied next. IFN-β showed a remarkable ability to suppress disease activity as monitored by clinical exacerbations and MRI evaluation (2,90). IFN-β1b (Betaseron) was approved by the FDA for use in R-R MS and became available in limited quantities in the United States in late 1993. IFN-β1b was tested in patients with up to a moderate degree of disease severity (EDSS ≤ 5.5). The three-armed Phase III trial clearly demonstrated a dose effect curve. On the high dose [8 million international units (MIU) subcutaneous (s.c.), every other day] which was approved by the FDA, a 34% reduction in exacerbations and an 83% reduction in active MRI lesions was noted.

Three years later, a slightly different IFN-β [IFN-β1a, (Avonex®)] became FDA-approved for R-R MS, based upon a Phase III trial demonstrating 18% reduction in exacerbations and a 33% reduction in MRI activity (56). This once-weekly intramuscularly (i.m.) injected IFN-β was studied in less severely affected patients, with an EDSS ranging up to 3.5.

Recently, a third IFN-β has been approved for the U.S. market: IFN-β1a, s.c., three times a week (Rebif®) (91). This demonstrated efficacy approximately the same as IFN-β1b.

There has been considerable controversy regarding whether there is a dose-effect curve, and whether the route of injection matters. Comparative studies between Betaseron and Avonex and between Rebif and Avonex have shown that higher dose, more frequently administered, s.c. injected IFNs appear to be superior (92,93). This conclusion was also reached by a committee of the American Academy of Neurology, as was the conclusion that the difference in efficacy of the s.c. versus i.m. routes of injection was unknown (94).

Glatiramer Acetate

Glatiramer acetate (GA) (Copaxone) consists of four randomly ordered amino acids. It was tested in R-R MS patients with an EDSS of up to 5.0 and demonstrated a 29% reduction in exacerbations (95). A subsequent study has shown GA to reduce active lesions on MRI by 35% (96). This discrepancy between a good clinical and only modest MRI effect may be explained on a mechanism of activity different from IFNs. Whereas IFN-β is a potent stabilizer of the BBB, GA works as a competitor to attract activated T cells. Copaxone is given s.c. every day; results do not appear dose- or frequency-dependent (97). Efficacy ap-

pears to lie between high dose, frequently administered and low dose, less frequently administered IFN-β (97) (Table 80-3).

All persons with MS may not respond equally well to IFNs and GA. The field of MS care is just beginning to be able to sort out "responders" from "nonresponders" (98,99). Previously, it had been thought that nonresponse to IFN was due to the development of "blocking antibodies." However, that explanation now looks less likely (94).

Other Medications

No other medications have been FDA-approved for MS. The three IFNs, one immunosuppressive agent, and GA remain the only five drugs approved for this disease in the United States. However, research is currently very active, especially with emphasis on finding medications to reduce the breakdown of the BBB, which precedes the MS attack.

Combination Therapy

Perhaps the most promising new area of medical management of MS is combination therapy using one of the IFNs or GA plus another agent—typically a chemotherapeutic drug. Most studies have added azathioprine, methotrexate, or mitoxantrone to one of the IFNs, and results appear promising (100). Early studies are underway to determine if a combination of IFN and GA is efficacious, or whether one interfered with the other's mechanism of action, as has been suspected and suggested by earlier studies on experimental allergic encephalomyelitis.

Treatment of Other Forms of Multiple Sclerosis

All three IFNs and GA are only FDA-approved for R-R MS. Although a European trial of IFN-β1b demonstrated efficacy in early S-P MS (a North American trial in more advanced S-P MS was negative), it is not approved for S-P MS in the United States (101). The only U.S.-approved drug for this stage of this disease is mitoxantrone. No treatment has been approved for PP MS, although one study indicates that methotrexate is slightly effective (55).

SYMPTOM MANAGEMENT

It is only by effectively treating symptoms (e.g., paresis) that individuals with MS can be improved. For example, rehabilitation strategies such as the use of a wheelchair will allow a patient with an EDSS of 8.0 (restricted to bed) to be improved to a 7.0 (wheelchair-reliant). The fitting of braces or the use of a walker might further improve such a patient's function to 6.5 (walking with an ambulation aid). Consequently, rehabilitation is the only way to *improve* function in MS (3).

Fatigue

Although relatively ignored in early research, we identified in the mid-1980s that fatigue was the most common self-identified symptom of MS (102,103). This appeared to be most pronounced in the afternoon, and was perceived by 77% of patients surveyed (102).

Treatment of fatigue has now assumed a much more prominent place in the management of MS, and it can be treated with

TABLE 80-3. Disease Modifying Agents

	Mitoxantrone[a] (Novantrone)	Interferon beta-1b (Betaseron)	Interferon beta-1a (Rebif)	Glatiramer acetate (Copaxone)	Interferon beta-1a (Avonex)
Relative efficacy	1	2[b]	2[b]	3	4
Indications	R-R MS, PP MS, or P-R MS	R-R MS or early PP MS	R-R MS or early PP MS	R-R MS	R-R MS or 1st demyelinating event
Subjects tested (EDSS)[c]	≤6.0[d]	i.v. ≤5.5	≤5.0	≤5.0	≤3.5
Dose	12 mg/M²/q 3 mo (8–10 lifetime doses)	250 mcg (8 million international units (MIU)) S. C. o d	44 mcg (12 million international units (MIU)) S. C. trw.	20 mg S. C. o d	30 mcg (6 million international units (MIU)) I.M. q wk
Relapse rate reduction (compared with placebo)	69%[d]	34%[e]	32%[e]	29%[e]	18%[e]
Effect on MRI (reduction in new lesions)	100%[d]	83%[e]	78%[e]	35%[e]	33%[e]
Advantages	Only 4 times/y treatment	• Autoinjector • Does not need refrigeration	• Autoinjector • Premixed	• No flulike symptoms • Autoinjector • Premixed	Only weekly injection
Side effects	• Menstrual disorders • Cardiotoxicity • Leukemia	Flulike symptoms	• Flulike symptoms • Stings	Transient chest pain	Flulike symptoms
Laboratory monitoring	Initial ECHO LVEF >50% then CBC and liver enzymes before each dose.	CBC and liver enzymes q 3 mo	CBC and liver enzymes q 3 mo	None	CBC and liver enzymes q 3 mo

[a]Although an effective agent, it is limited to 2–2½ years' use, and has the most serious side effects.
[b]Probably comparable effectiveness, although the more frequent dosing of Betaserone may be an advantage.
[c]See Table 80.2.
[d]Hartung HP, Gonsette R, Kopig N, et al. Mitoxantrone in progressive multiple sclerosis: a placebo-controlled, double-blind, randomised, multicentre trial. *Lancet* 2002;360(9350):2018–2025.
[e]Data from Goodin DS, Frohman EM, Germany GP, Jr., et al. Disease modifying therapies in multiple sclerosis: report of the Therapeutics and Technology Assessment Subcommittee of the American Academy of Neurology and the MS Council for Clinical Practice Guidelines. *Neurology* 2002;58(2):169–178.
R-R MS, relapsing-remitting multiple sclerosis; PP MS, primary progressive multiple sclerosis; P-R MS, progressive-relapsing multiple sclerosis; EDSS, Expanded Disability Status Scale; MRI, magnetic resonance imaging; ECHO LVEF, ECHO left ventricular ejection fraction (LVEF); CBC, complete blood count.

a variety of medications or physical agents. Medicines used are amantadine (Symmetrel®), modafinil, (Provigil®), and pemoline (Cylert®) (Table 80-4).

Nonmedical treatments of fatigue include techniques to extract heat from the body or by surface cooling. The most effective method appears to be heat extraction using a vest with a circulating coolant flowing through a radiating system. More widely used, and much less expensive, are cooling vests. It has been demonstrated that core body cooling using heat extraction can improve function in repetitive activities that produce fatigue (104). However, the exact mechanism for this is unclear (105).

Other excellent ways to reduce fatigue are by pacing, taking rests in the afternoon, and using occupational therapy techniques to conserve energy.

Spasticity and Muscle Spasms

Spasticity is common in MS and may go unrecognized by many patients (102). Management of spasticity can be accomplished through frequent (every few hours) stretching of spastic muscles so that agonist muscle groups do not have to "fight" the spastic antagonist muscles. Such stretching should be the fundamental underpinning of all spasticity management (106).

In conjunction with stretching, spasmolytic medications are also generally used. They must be monitored carefully; too little medication will inadequately suppress spasticity and too much may cause the "spaghetti leg" syndrome—limb tone less than adequate for optimal function (107). Muscle stretch reflexes are not the best test to determine the optimal amount of medication; clonus is. Three to five beats of clonus appear to be optimal. Since MS fluctuates, it may be necessary to evaluate a patient at 3-month intervals (an interval recommended to monitor blood and liver function for those patients on IFN-β) to adjust medication dose. Typically, lower limbs are much more spastic than upper limbs.

Baclofen (Lioresal®), tizanidine (Zanaflex®), and dantrolene sodium (Dantrium®) are commonly used, with the majority of patients being managed on Baclofen. (See Table 80-5 for indications and dose ranges of spasmolytic agents.)

One of the difficulties of spasticity management with medications in individuals with MS is that the commonly used spasmolytic agents may make patients fatigued, somnolent, weaker, and slower cognitively. Although this can be minimized by slowly titrating the dose, it may still worsen many MS patients' troublesome symptoms. Consequently, nonsystemic techniques to manage spasticity have an important role in MS. Botulinum toxin (Botox®) injections in spastic muscles and phenol nerve blocks may be used in especially spastic muscles to minimize the dose of oral spasmolytic medication required. Patients with severe lower limb spasticity may be candidates for an implantable baclofen pump—especially since

TABLE 80-4.   Medications for Fatigue

	Generic/Trade Name		
	Amantadine (Symmetryl)	Modafinil (Provigil)	Pemoline (Cylert)
Dose	100 mg b.i.d.	100–600 mg q A.M.	37.5 mg q d or b.i.d.
Action	Unknown	Activator	Stimulant
Advantages	• Also antiviral • Low cost	Very effective	• Effective • Inexpensive
Disadvantages	May be less effective	High cost	May cause liver damage
Laboratory monitoring	None	None	Liver enzymes q 2 wk

the high levels of oral spasmolytics required to control severe spasticity may cause further cognitive impairment.

Nocturnal muscle "spasms" are a subset of problems which may occur in the absence of an increased stretch reflex (spasticity). Tizanidine (Zanaflex) appears to be especially useful to manage these, and produces an additionally beneficial soporific effect.

Weakness

Progressive resistance exercises (PREs) are most effective in persons with normal central and peripheral nervous systems. However, they can also produce some increase in muscle strength in patients with reduced central motor drive (108). Studies have shown that PREs are effective in even profoundly paretic muscles of patients with severe MS, and can also improve function (109).

Since the distal lower limb is the most common site of weakness, severe ankle weakness is best treated with a plastic ankle-foot orthosis (AFO). This is especially true if stretching and exercise have not been adequate to correct the problem and plantarflexion spasticity is also present.

Two conditions may mimic weakness in MS patients when true weakness is not present. In the first, a muscle may appear weak because it is required to "fight" a spastic antagonist. Examples of this are apparent dorsiflexion weakness (foot drop) in patients who have spastic gastrocsoleus mechanisms with tight "heel cords." When such a patient's "heel cords" are stretched and an optimal level of spasmolytic medication is used, adequate dorsiflexion may be possible.

A second example is a uniquely MS phenomenon: progressive weakness with activity. A typical example of this is a patient who complains of foot drop, but who, on examination, has essentially normal tibialis anterior (TA) muscle strength. If

this patient's ambulation is observed, it will be noted that gait is adequate for a short distance, but then shows progressive dorsiflexion weakness. This is a clinical manifestation of conduction impairment associated with partially demyelinated pathways (see earlier section "Pathology, Pathogenesis, and Pathophysiology"). Such a case can be difficult to manage, since use of an AFO would unnecessarily restrict ankle movement during most periods of the day, as well as reduce normal resistance given to the TA at every heel strike, ultimately resulting in disuse atrophy. Yet without ankle support, especially on rough land, such a patient is subject to catching the toe and falling. The clinician's judgment must come into play in such a situation. Perhaps the best solution is to provide the patient with a cane or an AFO to be used only during periods of long-distance ambulation.

Ultimately, however, it may be possible to harness the motor units in the dorsiflexion muscles with heel strike-triggered peroneal nerve stimulation. Preliminary testing has demonstrated that foot dorsiflexion, produced by peroneal nerve stimulation when weight is taken off of a heel switch during the gait cycle, allows for a more natural gait and is favored by subjects with mild MS who experience this type of dorsiflexion fatigue (110).

Another, but presently experimental, approach to weakness and fatigue is the use of 4-aminopyridine or related compounds (111). At present, these are not commercially available in the United States because the window of efficacy is narrow, with heart block an undesired complication. The problem of erratic absorption from the gastrointestinal (GI) tract has not been solved, but pharmaceutical companies are currently working on ways to deliver a more regular and safer dose.

Heat extraction (which enhances the ability to do repetitive activities) (104) would logically appear to be an effective adjunct to resistive exercises to allow a greater amount of work to be done. Preliminary studies appear to support this hypothe-

TABLE 80-5.   Oral Spasmolytic Agents

	Generic/Trade Name		
	Baclofen (Lioresal)	Tizanidine (Zanaflex)	Dantrolene Sodium (Dantrium)
Dose	Up to 30 mg q.i.d.	Up to 24 mg q d in divided doses	Up to 100 mg t.i.d.
Advantages	Inexpensive	Does not cause muscle weakness	Does not cause somnolence
Disadvantages	Causes mild somnolence	Causes marked somnolence	Causes weakness
Laboratory monitoring	None	None	Periodic liver function tests

sis; exercise preceded by heat extraction improves function (112).

In more severely involved patients in whom stretching exercises, spasmolytic medications, and resistive exercises with cooling are not sufficient to provide adequate strength, ambulation aids such as AFOs, canes, crutches, walkers, and wheelchairs may be needed (113). A walker—either rolling or conventional—is an excellent device for individuals with MS as such people often have combinations of fatigue, weakness, sensory deficit, and ataxia. The added stability provided by a walker can provide significant functional improvement. Because fatigue plays such a large part in MS disability, three-wheeled electric "scooters" can be especially helpful to allow long-distance ambulation.

Bladder Dysfunction

Bladder dysfunction is one of the most disturbing symptoms of MS (114). It is the presenting symptom in approximately 5%, and the incidence increases as the disease progresses. It is estimated that 90% of MS patients experience bladder dysfunction at some time (115). The effect of bladder disturbance on MS patients is generally severe; it may even be devastating. Bladder dysfunction is disruptive to social, vocational, and sexual activities.

The most common urinary symptom in MS is urgency, followed by frequency, urge incontinence, hesitancy, and interrupted stream (116). Urological complications in patients with neurogenic bladder have been well-documented, and consist of infections, hydronephrosis, stone formation, vesicoureteral reflux, renal failure, and bladder malignancy. The clinician should be aware of three important factors predisposing to these urological complications: (a) an established diagnosis of detrusor sphincter dyssynergia, (b) elevated detrusor pressure greater than 40 cm H_2O during the filling phase, and (c) use of indwelling catheter for bladder management. Causes of symptoms are related to the stage of the disease, location of the MS lesions, and medications the patient is taking.

There are three types of bladder dysfunction commonly encountered in MS patients: detrusor hyperreflexia, detrusor sphincter dyssynergia, and detrusor areflexia. Treatment depends on the different causes and severity, and in general may include fluid intake adjustment, medications, pelvic muscle exercise, intermittent catheterization (ICP), indwelling catheter, and, rarely, surgical intervention. A specific treatment plan for an MS patient with bladder dysfunction should be individually formulated.

For detrusor hyperreflexia, a simple postvoid residual (PVR) must be obtained before administration of medication. If PVR is less than 100 mL, oxybutynin (Ditropan®) is usually the first drug to be prescribed (5 mg q.h.s., b.i.d. or t.i.d.). Ditropan XL® is a sustained-release preparation given once a day for a patient's convenience, and is also commonly used in MS patients. The newer agent tolterodine (Detrol®) is usually given at 2 mg b.i.d. to those who do not respond to oxybutynin. The advantage of tolterodine is that there is less of a chance to develop an adverse anticholinergic effect: dry mouth. Patients on this type of drug should be advised to watch out for urinary retention due to overdosing.

Our experience with desmopressin acetate (DDAVP) nasal spray indicates that it is a well-tolerated medication for intermittent, short-term use. By reducing the rate of urine production by the kidneys, patients may be able to go for longer periods without visiting toilet facilities. It is also beneficial for those with nocturia, a very disturbing symptom in an individual with MS who is unresponsive to fluid restriction. However,

for safety reasons, it should only be used intermittently. Surgical options include augmentation cystoplasty, denervation procedure (e.g., Ingelman-Sundberg procedure), and selective sacral rhizotomy.

Detrusor-sphincter dyssynergia occurs when detrusor muscle hyperreflexia coincides with outlet obstruction secondary to the sphincter contraction. This condition could be further complicated by coincidentally impaired or ineffective detrusor contractility. If the PVR is more than 150 mL, patients will generally respond to a combination of ICP and anticholinergic agent. Surgical intervention with external sphincterotomy, indwelling urethral stent, and urinary diversion should be considered only in those advanced patients who have failed a nonoperative approach. Patient education is pivotal by informing these patients that Credé and suprapubic tapping maneuvers are contraindicated in this situation.

Detrusor areflexia can cause retention and lead to bladder infection, ureteral reflux, and bladder stone formation. Hydronephrosis and renal failure may eventually occur if unrecognized or treated inappropriately. ICP is the treatment of choice in this condition. Unlike patients with other CNS disorders, MS patients usually respond poorly to cholinergicomimetic agents such as Urecholine®. It is therefore not recommended. Surgical referral for urinary diversion is occasionally made in selected cases.

Tremor and Ataxia

Tremor and ataxia are among the most difficult MS symptoms to treat. Fortunately, they are relatively rare, but can be severe in advanced stages of the disease. Propranolol and isoniazid have been reported to help. However, in our experience they are rarely successful. In mild ataxia, a cane can be used to broaden the base of support. The most practical treatment in most patients with severe tremor and ataxia is the use of a walker or wheelchair (see section on "Weakness") (113).

Although upper limb dysmetria/intention tremor rarely shows any improvement with medication, it may be tried. The most practical physical approach is to apply a several-pound weight to the upper limb, increasing the mass which consequently decreases the excursion produced by any given force applied (117). Fortunately, patients with severe tremor are generally strong and the increased weight does not impair function; it actually increases function as the tremor is reduced. Benefits are small, but may produce some functional improvement.

Severe upper-limb intention tremor can be extremely debilitating. MS patients suffering this complication may be unable to engage in any self-care activities. They cannot eat or perform other activities of daily living without assistance. In cases of severe tremor, the worse side might be treated surgically with a unilateral ventrolateral thalamotomy (118). However, the procedure cannot be performed bilaterally, as potential complications, such as stroke, are too great. Unfortunately, benefit may be only temporary if the disease progresses.

Newer treatments such as deep brain stimulation are still experimental, but might be useful in the future. Similarly, orthotic management may hold promise, but is not currently employed.

Pain

Pain is now recognized as a common symptom in MS patients. It can often be severe, and contributes to disability and reduced quality of life. Nearly 50% of patients with MS experience clinically significant pain at some time during the course of the disease, although pain is the presenting symptom in only about 20% (119,120).

There are multiple potential causes of pain. Treatment should be directed to the particular etiology of the pain problem. Often the pain problem is complex and despite treatment, many MS patients have ongoing pain or develop a chronic-refractory pain syndrome. The pain symptoms in MS patients can be divided into the following categories: (a) pain due to inflammation, (b) neuropathic pain, (c) pain secondary to upper motor neuron damage, and (d) musculoskeletal pain.

PAIN DUE TO INFLAMMATION

A typical example of acute pain due to the inflammatory process is ON. In this condition, inflammation and demyelination occur in or around pain-sensitive structures surrounding the optic nerve. The pain is often triggered or aggravated by eye movement. As discussed later in the "Visual Impairment" section, corticosteroid treatment is generally effective.

Headache in MS is a controversial topic because of its common occurrence in the general population. It is often difficult to prove that the headache is due to MS. The prevalence of headache in MS patients, however, appears to be higher. It is reported that 52% of MS patients have headache as compared with 18% in the general population (121). Evidence suggests that demyelination and inflammation in pain-sensitive structures or around cerebral blood vessels could be an important pathophysiological mechanism.

NEUROPATHIC PAIN

Neuropathic pain is seen in many MS patients. Trigeminal neuralgia, chronic dysesthetic pain, painful Lhermitte's phenomenon, radicular pain, and pain associated with transverse myelitis are all included in this category. Trigeminal neuralgia is a well-known paroxysmal pain syndrome in MS, and has a tendency to affect MS patients at a younger age than in the general population. It occurs in 9% of MS patients during the course of the disease, and is usually located in the second and third divisions of trigeminal distribution (119). This syndrome is believed to arise from ephaptic transmission of nerve conduction, which occurs with demyelination in the area around the trigeminal nerve entry zone. It commonly responds well to pharmacological intervention with anticonvulsants such as carbamazepine (Tegretol®) and gabapentin (Neurontin®). Glycerol, radiofrequency thermal or surgical rhizotomy is reserved for refractory cases.

In contrast to trigeminal neuralgia, dysesthetic extremity pain is a chronic, continuous pain syndrome which is commonly seen in MS. Patients usually describe a burning type of pain. Lower limbs are most frequently involved, followed by the trunk and upper limbs, and it occurs with insidious onset. The underlying mechanism is a central neuropathic pain; these patients have impairment of the posterior column, and nearly half of them have dysfunction of the spinothalamic tract in the spinal cord (119,122). Treatment includes tricyclic antidepressants and anticonvulsants, but it is often difficult to achieve complete relief of symptoms (Table 80-6).

PAIN SECONDARY TO UPPER MOTOR NEURON DAMAGE

The pain related to upper motor neuron damage has variable presentations. Muscle spasm and cramps are reported by many MS patients. Some pain is simply secondary to spasticity, and management is to address the problem with spasmolytic agents. Another type of "muscle spasm" referred to as tonic spinal cord seizure is encountered in less than 10% of MS pa-

TABLE 80-6.   Medications for Neuropathic Pain

	Generic/Trade Name	
	Carbamazepine (Tegretol)	Gabapentin (Neurontin)
Dose	Up to 400 mg t.i.d.	Up to 3,600 mg q d in divided doses
Advantages	More effective	Safer
Disadvantages	Can cause aplastic anemia	Less effective for severe pain
Laboratory monitoring	CBC and platelets	None

CBC, complete blood count.

tients. It is a condition more likely representing neuropathic pain and can therefore be treated by carbamazepine and other anticonvulsants. Others believe that tizanidine (Zanaflex) is helpful, especially for the nocturnal variety.

Medical application of cannabinoids in managing muscle spasm recently has been brought to the attention of the MS field. They appear to have some success in relieving symptoms of muscle pain/spasm and spasticity in some patients with MS (123). For those having both severe spasticity and pain, intrathecal baclofen with morphine or clonidine has been tried in a small group of patients with good results (124).

MUSCULOSKELETAL PAIN

Back pain is a common problem in the general population, and can also occur in MS patients. When occurring in MS it is a complicated issue, as many potential pain structures may be involved. Acute back pain may result from a herniated disc, for which patients with MS are at greater risk (due to muscle weakness), or it may result from a compression fracture in those individuals with osteoporosis from corticosteroid overuse. To complicate matters, radicular pain in MS patients can be caused by an MS lesion in the spinal cord or demyelination in the dorsal root entry zone, a condition more consistent with neuropathic pain. Exclusion of a structural abnormality should be considered first before simply concluding the radicular symptom is due to MS.

Mechanical back pain, posterior element pain (facet syndrome), and myofascial pain may also occur. These result from an increased mechanical stressor and imbalanced muscle force because of weakness or spasticity.

The treatment plan should be formulated according to the cause. In general, MS patients are responsive to corseting, nonsteroidal antiinflammatory agents, analgesics, physical therapy with stretching exercises, and trigger point injections. If related to upper motor neuron symptoms such as spasticity, spasmolytic agents should be used. If neuropathic radicular pain is suspected, a trial of anticonvulsant is worthwhile as well.

Hypesthesia

Numbness and tingling are very common symptoms in MS (102). Numbness, however, rarely creates any type of functional problem. This is good news for those patients with numbness, as there is essentially nothing that can be done to improve sensation.

Visual Impairment

Partial blindness or diplopia occurs in a little over one-fourth of all MS patients. Unfortunately, there is no treatment for the visual loss of ON. However, patients with less incomplete ON are often photophobic and will benefit from the use of sunglasses. The pain of ON is covered in the section on "Pain."

The diplopia associated with MS is not stable; with disease progression it may fluctuate. Therefore, ophthalmologists are rarely enthusiastic about corrective surgery. Diplopia can be a very disturbing symptom and is probably best treated with an eye patch over the less dominant eye.

Sexual Dysfunction

Sexual difficulty is common in MS patients. Men usually report decreased libido, difficulty in achieving or maintaining erection, delayed ejaculation, and impaired genital sensation. Common problems for women are fatigue, decreased vaginal lubrication, anorgasmia, and decreased vaginal sensation. A study of our MS population revealed that 91% of men and 88% of women with MS had some degree of sexual dysfunction (125). A regional survey identified that the single most common female complaint was fatigue-produced anorgasmia (68%), and the most common male complaint was erectile dysfunction (63%) (126).

Research has shown that in both men and women, anorgasmia has been correlated with brain stem pyramidal abnormalities and total lesion volume observed on MRI. Weakness of the pelvic floor and bladder and bowel dysfunctions in females are correlated with changes in lubrication and orgasmic capacity (127). Electrodiagnostic studies demonstrate that the complaints of sexual dysfunction are correlated with abnormalities of pudendal (the dorsal nerve of the penis or clitoris) evoked potentials (128,129).

For better understanding and management of sexual dysfunction in MS, a model has been developed consisting of primary, secondary, and tertiary sexual dysfunction (130–132).

Primary sexual dysfunction is defined as a result of MS-related organic CNS lesions that directly impair sexual feelings and response. Secondary sexual dysfunction occurs as a result of MS-related physical changes or medical and pharmacological treatments that indirectly affect sexual feelings and response—fatigue, bowel and bladder dysfunction, nongenital paresthesias, spasticity, tremor, pain, cognitive impairment, or drug side effects. Tertiary sexual dysfunction refers to the psychological, social, and cultural issues that interfere with sexual feelings and response, such as depression, performance anxiety, changes in body self-image, and role conflict due to family and social role changes.

Therefore, amelioration of sexual dysfunction in MS must be multidisciplinary, starting with a comprehensive assessment of these three areas (132). An appropriate treatment plan should try to address all areas in an attempt to achieve the best possible outcome. Management options usually include counseling, educational, pharmacological, and other medical interventions. Experience indicates that sildenafil citrate (Viagra®) is the most effective medication for erectile dysfunction in men with MS. Other options which may be considered in males include vacuum pumps, papaverine injection, and an implanted prosthesis. For female MS patients, sildenafil may have potential benefit for improving sexual arousal or responsiveness, as a recent study in a small group of women with spinal cord injury has suggested (133).

Bowel Dysfunction

Bowel dysfunction (BD) is less prevalent than bladder dysfunction in MS, but still affects 52% to 68% of patients (134,135). Because BD can affect the integrity of GI function, it can have a major negative impact on critical physiological processes in terms of supplying the water, electrolytes, and nutrients to the body through digestion and absorption.

The most common symptoms of BD are constipation (seen in approximately 50% of patients) and fecal incontinence (30% of patients). The cause of BD is multifactorial, usually resulting from diet, fluid restriction, use of multiple drugs (especially anticholinergics), physical immobility, and neurogenic causes (decreased parasympathetic input in constipation and diminished sphincter control or rectal overloading in incontinence).

The goal of treatment is to enhance GI transit, reduce constipation, and prevent fecal incontinence. Monitoring dietary intake, timed evacuation, adequate hydration, physical exercise, avoiding chronic use of laxatives, and a good bowel program are the keys to minimizing the negative impact of BD. Administration of fiber supplements (e.g., Metamucil®, Perdiem®), bulk forming agents (psyllium), and stool softeners (e.g., docusate sodium, docusate/casanthranol) are often helpful. The addition of a glycerin or Dulcolax® suppository to the bowel program every 2 to 3 days may be of benefit in some patients with more severe conditions. The principles for management of bowel incontinence are similar, with a scheduled defecation program used in conjunction with an appropriate anticholinergic medication such as imipramine.

Heat Intolerance

This section on Symptom Management started with "Fatigue," and ends with "Heat Intolerance." Both of these may seem like minor problems, but for a person with MS, both can be very disabling. Heat intolerance is a very common symptom. It is so characteristic of the disease that before the availability of MRI, one of the best tests for the disease was the confirmation of worsening of neurological signs or development of new ones by body heating (136). The mechanism is still unclear (105); however, heat extraction (see section on "Fatigue") is an effective way to manage patients with severe manifestations of this symptom (104). Although long-term heat extraction may not be a practical solution for most MS patients with symptoms of heat intolerance, avoiding a hot environment is an important rehabilitative strategy. Cooling vests or heat extraction units may be prescribed for patients with heat intolerance. A physician's "prescription" for environmental air conditioning is another practical and valid management tool for heat-sensitive MS patients.

PSYCHOLOGICAL AND COMMUNICATION MANAGEMENT

Depression

Depression is a common problem in MS. We recently conducted a large population survey of 739 MS patients in King County, Washington, and found the point prevalence of significant depressive symptoms [Center for Epidemiologic Studies Depression Scale (CES-D) >16] to be 41.8% (137). Our study indicated that persons with advanced MS are more likely to be depressed than more mildly affected persons. In addition, there also appeared to be a spike in the incidence of depression shortly after diagnosis. Thus, depression in MS may have both organic and situational causes. Treatments to consider include antidepressant medications and behavioral intervention such as counseling.

No large double-blind placebo-controlled study of the selective serotonin reuptake inhibitor (SSRI) antidepressants in depression has been carried out, although one is underway (138). As discussed previously, fatigue is among the most common symptoms of MS. Patients experiencing fatigue may actually be depressed and patients with this symptom should be screened for depression. Energizing antidepressants [e.g., paroxetine (Paxil®)] are reasonable to try in the subset of fatigued patients who also endorse depression. Because of the frequent coexisting fatigue, nonenergizing antidepressants should not be used.

Cognitive Impairment

Cognitive impairment, including memory deficits, represents a significant problem in persons with MS. Comprehensive neuropsychological testing suggests that over 40% of a broad spectrum of MS patients show cognitive impairment of at least some degree of significance (139).

It is easy to miss cognitive impairment among patients with MS. Typically, verbal skills remain relatively intact and a patient with fluent speech and good vocabulary usually gives the initial impression of being cognitively intact. Neuropsychological testing of patients with MS will usually indicate memory to be the most significant area of impairment. However, standard office memory testing may not demonstrate this deficit, as the patient does not forget information immediately. Thus, when asked to recall three items after five minutes during a mental status examination, many MS patients who have serious memory deficits may pass this test (140).

The typical psychological impairment includes loss of higher-level functions such as the ability to multitask. Often, MS patients are able to perform complex activities, but use so much "mental energy" to do so that these activities consume all of their available resources. Consequently, if these tasks are part of their vocational pursuits, these MS patients are exhausted by them, and have little energy remaining for other parts of their daily activities.

Treatment of this problem consists of first identifying the specific deficit, then use of pacing, memory books, and restructuring the environment to assist in maintaining function. In addition, meticulous attention must be paid to treating depression, fatigue, and heat intolerance, as all of these may contribute to cognitive impairment. No drugs have been FDA-approved for improving memory in MS, but medications used to treat Alzheimer's disease [e.g., donepezil (Aricept®)] are used and may be helpful.

Communication Problems

More than one in five MS patients reports problems with speech or communication (141). Because cognition and speech are so intertwined—and because no fully effective medications or surgical treatments are available for amelioration of these problems—therapeutic intervention from speech pathologists or psychologists represent the most effective therapy (140,142).

Dysarthria or faint vocalizations may be a problem in a subset of MS patients with advanced disease (141). Treatments for this include various types of voice amplification technology, breathing exercises, pacing, and behavior modification.

SOCIAL, VOCATIONAL, AND FINANCIAL MANAGEMENT

MS does not just affect the person suffering from the disease; it also involves the family, friends, fellow employees, and all of those interacting socially with the patient (143). Patients are frequently depressed (see section on "Depression") and the relationship with a spouse and children is permanently altered (143). Because of the energy required to fulfill vocational and fiscal obligations (see section on "Cognitive Impairment"), the person with MS may maintain a job but have little energy left over for family, home, and avocational pursuits (144). A patient with such impairment deserves serious consideration for disability retirement (145).

In summary, having significant MS, the patient's entire world has changed. Furthermore, the change represents a future of uncertain progression, disability, and financial loss. In addition to organic brain dysfunction, the uncertainty of the disease can play havoc with a patient's coping mechanisms (140).

Besides the problem with the patient's vocation and family income, there can be difficulty in securing adequate health insurance (146). As health-care costs reach 14% of the gross domestic product (GDP), they come under closer scrutiny. Health care tends to become "rationed," in that health insurance coverage becomes more difficult to get, more expensive, and consists of more limitations of coverage (147). These progressive limitations at a time when an MS patient needs more and more health care services present a problem for both the patient and society as a whole (148).

WELLNESS

Patients with MS are also subject to the complete array of disorders affecting persons without MS. All too frequently, however, MS patients assume that any symptom which may occur is related to MS and not some other disorder. Diabetes mellitus can occur and requires treatment. Heart disease may develop and needs to be managed. Hormonal disorders do not spare persons with MS. And, cancer may develop as MS patients get older. Hypertension, gastrointestinal disorders, and vascular disorders are among the other diseases that can occur in this population as they can occur in those without MS. Thus, it is of primary importance that persons with MS take exquisite care of their health and do not assume that all of their symptoms are related to MS and therefore "untreatable" (we have seen in this chapter that even MS symptoms can be managed).

In addition—and specific to MS—is the fact that infections can increase MS symptoms. Patients with MS often have neurogenic bladders which are subject to repeated infections. These infections can cause an increase in the body temperature which can worsen function (see sections on "Fatigue" and "Heat Intolerance") (149).

Meticulous attention must be paid to patients who appear to have "exacerbations" to be sure that they do not have a fever producing a "pseudoexacerbation." If they do have a fever, the source—most likely bladder, but also possibly pulmonary or sinus—must be identified and treated. Patients with fever should not be given corticosteroids. However, patients who have true exacerbations (not pseudoexacerbations) should be promptly treated with i.v. corticosteroids (see section on "Corticosteroids").

Lastly—and perhaps the most important concept—patients with MS live with MS for the rest of their lives. The better they keep their general health, the better they will do (150). MS is a lifetime disease. Lifetime management and rehabilitation must be employed (151).

CONCLUSION

MS is a lifetime disease. Even though there has been progress in disease course management (no disease-modifying medications were available before 1993), no medication has yet been found to improve function. Only rehabilitative techniques can achieve that. Using techniques reviewed in this chapter can actually improve MS patients by as much as 1.5 EDSS points. By providing bed-bound patients with walkers and giving them physical therapy to learn how to use them, individuals with MS may be freed from their beds and allowed to ambulate (3). MS may be the most difficult neurological disease to manage—far more difficult than spinal cord injury or stroke. MS can produce more disability (cognitive deficits, weakness, spasticity, ataxia, incontinence, pain, dysarthria, and depression) and it progresses with an uncertain course. Such patients require the most comprehensive team of management experts available and should be given frequent reevaluations as the disease progresses.

Such is the complex nature of the disease. And such is the need for its comprehensive management.

REFERENCES

1. Cobble N, Wangaard C, Kraft GH, et al. Rehabilitation of the patient with multiple sclerosis. In: DeLisa J, ed. *Principles and practice of rehabilitation medicine*. Philadelphia: Lippincott Williams & Wilkins, 1988:612–634.
2. Duquette P, Girard M, Knobler RL, et al. Interferon beta-1b is effective in relapsing-remitting multiple sclerosis. I. Clinical results of a multicenter, randomized, double-blind, placebo-controlled trial. *Neurology* 1993;43:655–661.
3. Kraft G. Rehabilitation: Still the only way to improve function in multiple sclerosis. *Lancet* 1999;354(9195):2015–2017.
4. Goodkin D. Treatment of progressive forms of multiple sclerosis. In: Burks J, Johnson KP, eds. *Multiple sclerosis: diagnosis, medical management, and rehabilitation*. New York: Demos Medical Publishing, 2000:177–192.
5. Murray TJ. The history of multiple sclerosis. In: Burks J, Johnson KP, eds. *Multiple sclerosis: diagnosis, medical management, and rehabilitation*. New York: Demos Medical Publishing, 2000: 1–32.
6. Kurtzke JF, Wallin M. Epidemiology. In: Burks J, Johnson KP, eds. *Multiple sclerosis: diagnosis, medical management, and rehabilitation*. New York: Demos Medical Publishing, 2000: 49–71.
7. Baranzini SE, Oksenberg JR, Hauser SL. New insights into the genetics of multiple sclerosis. *J Rehabil Res Dev* 2002;39(2):201–209.
8. Yorkston K, Johnson K, Kuehn C, et al. Age and gender issues related to MS: a survey study . *Int J MS Care* 2002;4(2):94(abst).
9. Detels R, Visscher BR, Haile RW, et al. Multiple sclerosis and age at migration. *Am J Epidemiol* 1978;108(5):386–393.
10. Dean G, Kurtzke JF. On the risk of multiple sclerosis according to age at immigration to South Africa. *Br Med J* 1971;3(777):725–729.
11. Kurtzke JF, Kurland LT, Goldberg ID. Mortality and migration in multiple sclerosis. *Neurology* 1971;21(12):1186–1197.
12. Kurtzke JF, Hyllested K. Multiple sclerosis in the Faroes: 1. Clinical and epidemiologic features. *Trans Am Neurol Assoc* 1978;103:201–205.
13. Krakowka S, Miele JA, Mathes LE, et al. Antibody responses to measles virus and canine distemper virus in multiple sclerosis. *Ann Neurol* 1983;14 (5):533–538.
14. Kurtzke JF, Gudmundsson KR, Bergmann S. Multiple sclerosis in Iceland: 1. Evidence of a postwar epidemic. *Neurology* 1982;32(2):143–150.
15. Barcellos LF, Oksenberg JR, Green AJ, et al. Genetic basis for clinical expression in multiple sclerosis. *Brain* 2002;125(Pt 1):150–158.
16. Bach JF. The effect of infections on susceptibility to autoimmune and allergic diseases. *N Engl J Med* 2002;347(12):911–920.
17. Noseworthy JH, Lucchinetti C, Rodriguez M, et al. Multiple sclerosis. *N Engl J Med* 2000;343(13):938–952.
18. Trapp BD, Peterson J, Ransohoff RM, et al. Axonal transection in the lesions of multiple sclerosis. *N Engl J Med* 1998;338(5):278–285.
19. Hommes OR. Remyelination in human CNS lesions. *Prog Brain Res* 1980; 53:39–63.
20. Waxman SG. Clinical course and electrophysiology of multiple sclerosis. *Adv Neurol* 1988;47:157–184.
21. Waxman SG. Demyelinating diseases–new pathological insights, new therapeutic targets. *N Engl J Med* 1998;338(5):323–325.
22. Miller DH, Khan OA, Sheremata WA, et al. A controlled trial of natalizumab for relapsing multiple sclerosis. *N Engl J Med* 2003;348(1):15–23.
23. Prat A, Al-Asmi A, Duquette P, et al. Lymphocyte migration and multiple sclerosis: relation with disease course and therapy. *Ann Neurol* 1999;46(2): 253–256.
24. Prat A, Biernacki K, Lavoie JF, et al. Migration of multiple sclerosis lymphocytes through brain endothelium. *Arch Neurol* 2002;59(3):391–397.
25. Uhm JH, Dooley NP, Stuve O, et al. Migratory behavior of lymphocytes isolated from multiple sclerosis patients: effects of interferon beta-1b therapy. *Ann Neurol* 1999;46(3):319–324.
26. Stuber A, Martin R, Stone LA, et al. Expression pattern of activation and adhesion molecules on peripheral blood CD4+ T-lymphocytes in relapsing-remitting multiple sclerosis patients: a serial analysis. *J Neuroimmunol* 1996; 66(1–2):147–151.
27. Plumb J, McQuaid S, Mirakhur M, et al. Abnormal endothelial tight junctions in active lesions and normal-appearing white matter in multiple sclerosis. *Brain Pathol* 2002;12(2):154–169.
28. Sobel RA, Ahmed AS. White matter extracellular matrix chondroitin sulfate/dermatan sulfate proteoglycans in multiple sclerosis. *J Neuropathol Exp Neurol* 2001;60(12):1198–1207.
29. Kivisakk P, Trebst C, Eckstein DJ, et al. Chemokine-based therapies for MS: how do we get there from here? *Trends Immunol* 2001;22(11):591–593.
30. Waxman SG. Conduction in myelinated, unmyelinated, and demyelinated fibers. *Arch Neurol* 1977;34(10):585–589.
31. Herndon RM. Pathology and pathophysiology. In: Burks J, Johnson KP, eds. *Multiple sclerosis: diagnosis, medical management, and rehabilitation*. New York: Demos Medical Publishing, 2000:35–45.
32. Rasminsky M. The effects of temperature on conduction in demyelinated single nerve fibers. *Arch Neurol* 1973;28(5):287–292.
33. Ferguson B, Matyszak MK, Esiri MM, et al. Axonal damage in acute multiple sclerosis lesions. *Brain* 1997;120 (Pt 3):393–399.
34. Jeffery DR, Absher J, Pfeiffer FE, et al. Cortical deficits in multiple sclerosis on the basis of subcortical lesions. *Mult Scler* 2000;6(1):50–55.
35. Rovaris M, Filippi M. Contrast enhancement and the acute lesion in multiple sclerosis. *Neuroimaging Clin N Am* 2000;10(4):705–16; viii–ix.
36. Chard DT, Griffin CM, Parker GJ, et al. Brain atrophy in clinically early relapsing-remitting multiple sclerosis. *Brain* 2002;125(Pt 2):327–337.
37. Charcot JM. Histologie de la sclerose en plaques. *Gaz Hosp (Paris)* 1868;140: 554–555.
38. Kornek B, Lassmann H. Axonal pathology in multiple sclerosis. A historical note. *Brain Pathol* 1999;9(4):651–656.
39. Kocsis JD, Waxman SG. Demyelination: causes and mechanisms of clinical abnormality and functional recovery. In: Vilnken PJ, Bruyn GW, Klawans HL, et al, eds. *Demyelinating diseases. handbook of clinical neurology*. Amsterdam: Elsevier Science Publishers, 1985:29–47.
40. McDonald WI. The pathophysiology of multiple sclerosis. In: McDonald WI, Silberberg DH, eds. *Multiple sclerosis*. London: Butterworths, 1986:112–133.
41. Rasminsky M. Pathophysiology of demyelination. *Ann N Y Acad Sci* 1984; 436:68–85.
42. Stadelmann C, Kerschensteiner M, Misgeld T, et al. BDNF and gp145trkB in multiple sclerosis brain lesions: neuroprotective interactions between immune and neuronal cells? *Brain* 2002;125(Pt 1):75–85.
43. Hohlfeld R, Kerschensteiner M, Stadelmann C, et al. The neuroprotective effect of inflammation: implications for the therapy of multiple sclerosis. *J Neuroimmunol* 2000;107(2):161–166.
44. Beck R, Cleary P, Anderson MJ, et al. A randomized, controlled trial of corticosteroids in the treatment of acute optic neuritis. *N Engl J Med* 1992;326 (9):581–598.
45. Francis DA, Compston DA, Batchelor JR, et al. A reassessment of the risk of multiple sclerosis developing in patients with optic neuritis after extended follow-up. *J Neurol Neurosurg Psychiatry* 1987;50(6):758–765.
46. Kraft GH, Freal JE, Coryell JK, et al. Multiple sclerosis: early prognostic guidelines. *Arch Phys Med Rehabil* 1981;62:54–58.
47. Jacobs LD, Beck RW, Simon JH, et al. Intramuscular interferon beta-1a therapy initiated during a first demyelinating event in multiple sclerosis. CHAMPS Study Group. *N Engl J Med* 2000;343(13):898–904.
48. Kappos L, Polman C, Pozzilli C, et al. Final analysis of the European multicenter trial on IFNbeta-1b in secondary-progressive MS. *Neurology* 2001;57(11):1969–1975.
49. Edan G, Miller D, Clanet M, et al. Therapeutic effect of mitoxantrone combined with methylprednisolone in multiple sclerosis: a randomised multicentre study of active disease using MRI and clinical criteria. *J Neurol Neurosurg Psychiatry* 1997;62(2):112–128.
50. Hartung HP, Gonsette R, Konig N, et al. Mitoxantrone in progressive multiple sclerosis: a placebo-controlled, double-blind, randomised, multicentre trial. *Lancet* 2002;360(9350):2018–2025.
51. Prineas JW, Kwon EE, Cho ES, et al. Immunopathology of secondary-progressive multiple sclerosis. *Ann Neurol* 2001;50(5):646–657.
52. Revesz T, Kidd D, Thompson AJ, et al. A comparison of the pathology of primary and secondary progressive multiple sclerosis. *Brain* 1994;117 (Pt 4): 759–765.
53. Kidd D, Thorpe JW, Kendall BE, et al. MRI dynamics of brain and spinal cord in progressive multiple sclerosis. *J Neurol Neurosurg Psychiatry* 1996;60 (1):15–19.

54. Rovaris M, Bozzali M, Santuccio G, et al. In vivo assessment of the brain and cervical cord pathology of patients with primary progressive multiple sclerosis. *Brain* 2001;124(Pt 12):2540–2549.

55. Goodkin DE, Rudick RA, VanderBrug Medendorp S, et al. Low-dose (7.5 mg) oral methotrexate reduces the rate of progression in chronic progressive multiple sclerosis. *Ann Neurol* 1995;37(1):30–40.

56. Jacobs LD, Cookfair DL, Rudick RA, et al. Intramuscular interferon beta-1a for disease progression in relapsing multiple sclerosis. The Multiple Sclerosis Collaborative Research Group (MSCRG). *Ann Neurol* 1996;39(3):285–294.

57. Simnad VI, Pisani DE, Rose JW. Multiple sclerosis presenting as transverse myelopathy: clinical and MRI features. *Neurology* 1997;48(1):65–73.

58. Scott TF, Bhagavatula K, Snyder PJ, et al. Transverse myelitis. Comparison with spinal cord presentations of multiple sclerosis. *Neurology* 1998;50(2):429–433.

59. Filippi M, Rocca MA, Moiola L, et al. MRI and magnetization transfer imaging changes in the brain and cervical cord of patients with Devic's neuromyelitis optica. *Neurology* 1999;53(8):1705–1710.

60. Mandler RN, Ahmed W, Dencoff JE. Devic's neuromyelitis optica: a prospective study of seven patients treated with prednisone and azathioprine. *Neurology* 1998;51(4):1219–1220.

61. Schumacher G, Beebe G, Kibler R. Problems of experimental trials of therapy in multiple sclerosis: report by the panel on the evaluation of experimental trials of therapy in multiple sclerosis. *Ann N Y Acad Sci* 1965;122:552–568.

62. Poser CM, Paty DW, Scheinberg L, et al. New diagnostic criteria for multiple sclerosis: guidelines for research protocols. *Ann Neurol* 1983;13(3):227–131.

63. McDonald WI, Compston A, Edan G, et al. Recommended diagnostic criteria for multiple sclerosis: guidelines from the International Panel on the Diagnosis of Multiple Sclerosis. *Ann Neurol* 2001;50(1):121–127.

64. Slimp JC, Janczakowski J, Seed LJ, et al. Comparison of median and posterior tibial nerve somatosensory evoked potentials in ambulatory patients with definite multiple sclerosis. *Am J Phys Med Rehabil* 1990;69(6):293–296.

65. Fazekas F, Barkhof F, Filippi M, et al. The contribution of magnetic resonance imaging to the diagnosis of multiple sclerosis. *Neurology* 1999;53(3):448–456.

66. Grossman RI. Magnetization transfer in multiple sclerosis. *Ann Neurol* 1994;36[Suppl]:S97–S99.

67. Kraft GH, Richards TL, Heide AC. Correlations of evoked potentials with MR imaging and MR spectroscopy in multiple sclerosis. *Phys Med Rehabil Clin N Am* 1998;9(3):561–567, vi.

68. Trojaborg W, Petersen E. Visual and somatosensory evoked cortical potentials in multiple sclerosis. *J Neurol Neurosurg Psychiatry* 1979;42(4):323–330.

69. Purves SJ, Low MD, Galloway J, et al. A comparison of visual, brainstem auditory, and somatosensory evoked potentials in multiple sclerosis. *Can J Neurol Sci* 1981;8(1):15–19.

70. Kraft G, Janczakowski J, Slimp J. Comparison of MRI and SEP in patients with MS and stroke. *J Clin Neurophysiol* 1993;10(April):243(abst).

71. Kraft GH, Aminoff MJ, Baran EM, et al. Somatosensory evoked potentials: clinical uses. AAEM Somatosensory Evoked Potentials Subcommittee. American Association of Electrodiagnostic Medicine. *Muscle Nerve* 1998;21(2):252–258.

72. Chiappa KH. Pattern-shift visual evoked potentials: Methodology. In: Chiappa KH, ed. *Evoked potentials in clinical medicine*, 2nd ed. New York: Raven Press, 1990:37–109.

73. Heide AC, Kraft GH, Slimp JC, et al. Cerebral N-acetylaspartate is low in patients with multiple sclerosis and abnormal visual evoked potentials. *AJNR Am J Neuroradiol* 1998;19(6):1047–1054.

74. Massaro AR, Tonali P. Cerebrospinal fluid markers in multiple sclerosis: an overview. *Mult Scler* 1998;4(1):1–4.

75. Devos D, Forzy G, de Seze J, et al. Silver stained isoelectrophoresis of tears and cerebrospinal fluid in multiple sclerosis. *J Neurol* 2001;248(8):672–675.

76. Grana EA, Kraft GH. Electrodiagnostic abnormalities in patients with multiple sclerosis. *Arch Phys Med Rehabil* 1994;75(7):778–782.

77. Nazliel B, Irkec C, Kocer B. The roles of blink reflex and sympathetic skin response in multiple sclerosis diagnosis. *Mult Scler* 2002;8(6):500–504.

78. LaRocca NG, Scheinberg LC, Slater RJ, et al. Field testing of a minimal record of disability in multiple sclerosis: the United States and Canada. *Acta Neurol Scand Suppl* 1984;101:126–138.

79. Kurtzke JF. Rating neurologic impairment in multiple sclerosis: an expanded disability status scale (EDSS). *Neurology* 1983;33(11):1444–1452.

80. Bowen J, Gibbons L, Gianas A, et al. Self-administered expanded disability status scale with functional system scores correlates well with a physician-administered test. *Mult Scler* 2001;7(3):201–206.

81. Weiner HL, Hafler DA. Immunotherapy of multiple sclerosis. *Ann Neurol* 1988;23(3):211–222.

82. Ghalie RG, Edan G, Laurent M, et al. Cardiac adverse effects associated with mitoxantrone (Novantrone) therapy in patients with MS. *Neurology* 2002;59(6):909–913.

83. Korbling M. Peripheral blood stem cells for allogeneic transplantation. In: Thomas ED, Blume KG, Forman SJ, eds. *Hematopoietic cell transplantation*, 2nd ed. Malden, MA: Blackwell Science, 1999:469–480.

84. Kraft G, Bowen J, Cui J, et al. Clinical application of autologous stem cell transplantation in severe multiple sclerosis treated with high-dose immunosuppressive therapy. *Neurology* 2002;58[Suppl 3]:A166(abst).

85. Kraft GH, Bowen J, Nash R. Functional stabilization of worsening multiple sclerosis patients treated with high-dose immunosuppression and stem cell rescue. *Arch Phys Med Rehabil* 2002;83:1682(abst).

86. Poser CM. Diseases of the myelin sheath. In: Merritt H, ed. *A Textbook of neurology*, 5th ed. Philadelphia: Lea & Febiger, 1973:683–727.

87. Rose A, Kuzma J, Kurtzke JF, et al. Cooperative study in the evaluation of therapy in multiple sclerosis: ACTH vs. placebo. Final report. *Neurology* 1970;20(5):1–59.

88. Zivadinov R, Rudick RA, De Masi R, et al. Effects of IV methylprednisolone on brain atrophy in relapsing-remitting MS. *Neurology* 2001;57(7):1239–1247.

89. Oliveri RL, Valentino P, Russo C, et al. Randomized trial comparing two different high doses of methylprednisolone in MS: a clinical and MRI study. *Neurology* 1998;50(6):1833–1836.

90. Paty DW, Li DK. Interferon beta-1b is effective in relapsing-remitting multiple sclerosis. II. MRI analysis results of a multicenter, randomized, double-blind, placebo-controlled trial. UBC MS/MRI Study Group and the IFNB Multiple Sclerosis Study Group. *Neurology* 1993;43(4):662–667.

91. PRISMS. Randomised double-blind placebo-controlled study of interferon beta-1a in relapsing/remitting multiple sclerosis. PRISMS (Prevention of Relapses and Disability by Interferon beta-1a Subcutaneously in Multiple Sclerosis) Study Group. *Lancet* 1998;352(9139):1498–1504.

92. Durelli L, Verdun E, Barbero P, et al. Every-other-day interferon beta-1b versus once-weekly interferon beta-1a for multiple sclerosis: results of a 2-year prospective randomised multicentre study (INCOMIN). *Lancet* 2002;359(9316):1453–1460.

93. Panitch H, Goodin DS, Francis G, et al. Randomized, comparative study of interferon beta-1a treatment regimens in MS: The EVIDENCE Trial. *Neurology* 2002;59(10):1496–1506.

94. Goodin DS, Frohman EM, Garmany GP, Jr., et al. Disease modifying therapies in multiple sclerosis: report of the Therapeutics and Technology Assessment Subcommittee of the American Academy of Neurology and the MS Council for Clinical Practice Guidelines. *Neurology* 2002;58(2):169–178.

95. Johnson KP, Brooks BR, Cohen JA, et al. Copolymer 1 reduces relapse rate and improves disability in relapsing-remitting multiple sclerosis: results of a phase III multicenter, double-blind placebo-controlled trial. The Copolymer 1 Multiple Sclerosis Study Group. *Neurology* 1995;45(7):1268–1276.

96. Comi G, Filippi M, Wolinsky JS. European/Canadian multicenter, double-blind, randomized, placebo-controlled study of the effects of glatiramer acetate on magnetic resonance imaging—measured disease activity and burden in patients with relapsing multiple sclerosis. European/Canadian Glatiramer Acetate Study Group. *Ann Neurol* 2001;49(3):290–297.

97. Flechter S, Vardi J, Pollak L, et al. Comparison of glatiramer acetate (Copaxone) and interferon beta-1b (Betaseron) in multiple sclerosis patients: an open-label 2-year follow-up. *J Neurol Sci* 2002;197(1–2):51–55.

98. Petereit HF, Nolden S, Schoppe S, et al. Low interferon gamma producers are better treatment responders: a two-year follow-up of interferon beta-treated multiple sclerosis patients. *Mult Scler* 2002;8(6):492–494.

99. Farina C, Wagenpfeil S, Hohlfeld R. Immunological assay for assessing the efficacy of glatiramer acetate (Copaxone) in multiple sclerosis. A pilot study. *J Neurol* 2002;249(11):1587–1592.

100. Fernandez O, Guerrero M, Mayorga C, et al. Combination therapy with interferon beta-1b and azathioprine in secondary progressive multiple sclerosis A two-year pilot study. *J Neurol* 2002;249(8):1058–1062.

101. Kappos L. Placebo-controlled multicentre randomised trial of interferon beta-1b in treatment of secondary progressive multiple sclerosis. European Study Group on interferon beta-1b in secondary progressive MS. *Lancet* 1998;352(9139):1491–1497.

102. Kraft GH, Freal JE, Coryell JK. Disability, disease duration, and rehabilitation service needs in multiple sclerosis: patient perspectives. *Arch Phys Med Rehabil* 1986;67(3):164–168.

103. Freal JE, Kraft GH, Coryell JK. Symptomatic fatigue in multiple sclerosis. *Arch Phys Med Rehabil* 1984;65(3):135–138.

104. Kraft GH, Alquist AD. Effect of microclimate cooling on physical function in multiple sclerosis. *Mult Scler ClinLab Res* 1996;2(2):114–115.

105. Robinson LR, Kraft GH, Fitts SS, et al. Body cooling may not improve somatosensory pathway function in multiple sclerosis. *Am J Phys Med Rehabil* 1997;76(3):191–196.

106. Arndt J, Bhasin C, Brar SP, et al. Physical therapy. In: Schapiro RT, ed. *Multiple sclerosis: a rehabilitation approach to management*. New York: Demos Medical Publishing, 1991:17–66.

107. Kraft G. Foreword. In: Kraft G, Taylor, RS, ed. Multiple sclerosis: a rehabilitative approach. *Phys Med Rehabil Clin North Am*. Philadelphia: Saunders, 1998:xi–xiii.

108. Kraft GH, Alquist AD, de Lateur B. Effect of resistive exercise on strength in patients with multiple sclerosis. *Veterans Aff Rehabil Res Dev Prog Rep* 1996;33(June):329–330(abst).

109. Kraft GH, Alquist AD, de Lateur B. Effect of resistive exercise on physical function in multiple sclerosis (MS). *Veterans Aff Rehabil Res Dev Prog Rep* 1996;33(June):328–329(abst).

110. Kraft G, Fitts S. Electrical stimulation AFO for MS footdrop. *J Clin Neurophys* 1992;9:301(abst).

111. Rossini PM, Pasqualetti P, Pozzilli C, et al. Fatigue in progressive multiple sclerosis: results of a randomized, double-blind, placebo-controlled, cross-over trial of oral 4-aminopyridine. *Mult Scler* 2001;7(6):354–358.

112. Alquist AD, Kraft G. Optimization of the exercise stimulus by pre-cooling in multiple sclerosis. *Int J MS Care* 2002;4(2):82–83.

113. Kraft GH. Rehabilitation principles for patients with multiple sclerosis. *J Spinal Cord Med* 1998;21(2):117–120.

114. Rothwell PM, McDowell Z, Wong CK, et al. Doctors and patients don't agree: cross sectional study of patients' and doctors' perceptions and assessments of disability in multiple sclerosis. *BMJ* 1997;314(7094):1580–1583.

115. Joy JE, Johnson RB, eds. *Multiple sclerosis: current status and strategies for the future.* Washington, DC: National Academy Press, 2001.

116. Betts CD, D'Mellow MT, Fowler CJ. Urinary symptoms and the neurological features of bladder dysfunction in multiple sclerosis. *J Neurol Neurosurg Psychiatry* 1993;56(3):245–250.

117. Kraft GH. Movement disorders. In: Basmajian J, Kirby L, eds. *Medical rehabilitation.* Baltimore: Williams & Wilkins, 1984:162–165.

118. Cooper IS. Relief of intention tremor of multiple sclerosis by thalamic surgery. *JAMA* 1967;199(10):689–694.

119. Moulin DE, Foley KM, Ebers GC. Pain syndromes in multiple sclerosis. *Neurology* 1988;38(12):1830–1834.

120. Stenager E, Knudsen L, Jensen K. Acute and chronic pain syndromes in multiple sclerosis. *Acta Neurol Scand* 1991;84(3):197–200.

121. Rolak LA, Brown S. Headaches and multiple sclerosis: a clinical study and review of the literature. *J Neurol* 1990;237(5):300–302.

122. Vermote R, Ketelaer P, Carton H. Pain in multiple sclerosis patients. A prospective study using the McGill Pain Questionnaire. *Clin Neurol Neurosurg* 1986;88(2):87–93.

123. Consroe P, Musty R, Rein J, et al. The perceived effects of smoked cannabis on patients with multiple sclerosis. *Eur Neurol* 1997;38(1):44–48.

124. Klein M, Delehanty L, Saidiq S. Use of combination intrathecal medications for spasticity and pain in patients with MS. *Int J MS Care.* 2002;4(2):73(abst).

125. Yang CC. Sexual dysfunction in MS: common electrodiagnostic findings. *Int J MS Care* 2002;4(2):79–80(abst).

126. Valleroy ML, Kraft GH. Sexual dysfunction in multiple sclerosis. *Arch Phys Med Rehabil* 1984;65(3):125–128.

127. Hulter BM, Lundberg PO. Sexual function in women with advanced multiple sclerosis. *J Neurol Neurosurg Psychiatry* 1995;59(1):83–86.

128. Yang C, Bowen J, Kraft G, et al. Cortical evoked potentials of the dorsal nerve of the clitoris and female sexual dysfunction in multiple sclerosis. *J Urol* 2000;164:2010–2013.

129. Yang C, Bowen J, Kraft GH, et al. Physiologic studies of male sexual dysfunction in multiple sclerosis. *Mult Scler* 2001;7(4):249–254.

130. Saunders A, Aisen M. Sexual dysfunction. In: Burks J, Johnson K, eds. *Multiple sclerosis: diagnosis, medical management, and rehabilitation.* New York: Demos Medical Publishing, 2000:461–470.

131. Foley F, Sanders A. Sexuality, multiple sclerosis, and women. *MS Manage* 1997;4(1):1–10.

132. Foley F, Luoto E. Workshop on Sexuality in MS. Consortium of MS Centers (CMSC) Annual Meeting; 2002; Chicago.

133. Sipski ML, Rosen RC, Alexander CJ, et al. Sildenafil effects on sexual and cardiovascular responses in women with spinal cord injury. *Urology* 2000; 55(6):812–815.

134. Chia YW, Fowler CJ, Kamm MA, et al. Prevalence of bowel dysfunction in patients with multiple sclerosis and bladder dysfunction. *J Neurol* 1995;242(2):105–108.

135. Hinds JP, Wald A. Colonic and anorectal dysfunction associated with multiple sclerosis. *Am J Gastroenterol* 1989;84(6):587–595.

136. Berger JR, Sheremata WA. Persistent neurological deficit precipitated by hot bath test in multiple sclerosis. *JAMA* 1983;249(13):1751–1753.

137. Chwastiak L, Ehde D, Gibbons L, et al. Depression and severity of illness in multiple sclerosis: epidemiologic study of a large community sample. *Am J Psychiatry* 2002;159(11):1862–1868.

138. Mohr DC, Boudewyn AC, Goodkin DE, et al. Comparative outcomes for individual cognitive-behavior therapy, supportive-expressive group psychotherapy, and sertraline for the treatment of depression in multiple sclerosis. *J Consult Clin Psychol* 2001;69(6):942–949.

139. Rao S, Leo G, Bernardin L, et al. Cognitive dysfunction in multiple sclerosis: I. Frequency, patterns and prediction. *Neurology* 1991;41:685–691.

140. White DM, Catanzaro ML, Kraft GH. An approach to the psychological aspects of multiple sclerosis: a coping guide for health care providers and families. *J Neurol Rehabil* 1993;7(2):43–52.

141. Beukelman DR, Kraft GH, Freal J. Expressive communication disorders in persons with multiple sclerosis: a survey. *Arch Phys Med Rehabil* 1985;66(10): 675–677.

142. Yorkston K, Klasner E, Swanson K. Communication in context: a qualitative study of the experiences of individuals with multiple sclerosis. *Am J Speech-Lang Path* 2001;10(2):126–137.

143. Schwartz L, Kraft GH. The role of spouse responses to disability and family environment in multiple sclerosis. *Am J Phys Med Rehabil* 1999;78(6):525–532.

144. Fraser R, Clemmons D, Bennett F. *Multiple sclerosis: psychosocial and vocational interventions.* New York: Demos, 2002.

145. Fraser R, Johnson EK, Clemmons D, et al. Vocational rehabilitation in multiple sclerosis: a profile of clients seeking services. *Work* 2003;21(1):69–76.

146. Kraft G. Improving health care delivery for persons with multiple sclerosis. In: Kraft G, Taylor, RS, ed. Multiple sclerosis: a rehabilitative approach. *Phys Med Rehabil Clin North Am.* Philadelphia: Saunders, 1998:703–715.

147. Kraft GH. The 24th Walter J. Zeiter Lecture. Variations on a theme: in defense of health care. *Arch Phys Med Rehabil* 1992;73(3):211–219.

148. Kraft GH. In defense of health care: preserving the capacity for excellence. In: Greenberg HM, Raymond SU, eds. *Beyond the crisis: preserving the capacity for excellence in health care and medical science.* New York: Annals of the New York Academy of Sciences, 1994:39–55.

149. Hillman L, Burns S, Kraft GH. Neurological worsening due to infection from renal stones in a multiple sclerosis patient. *Mult Scler* 2000;6(6): 403–406.

150. Kraft G, Catanzaro M. *Living with MS: a wellness approach,* 2nd ed. New York: Demos Medical Publishing, 2000.

151. Kraft GH. Multiple sclerosis: future directions in the care and the cure. *J Neurologic Rehabilitation* 1989;3(2):61–64.

CHAPTER 81

Rehabilitation for Patients with Cancer Diagnoses

Mary M. Vargo and Lynn H. Gerber

GENERAL ASPECTS OF REHABILITATION FOR CANCER PATIENTS

Historical Background

Patients with cancer diagnoses are living longer because of a combination of early detection, a broader selection of cancer treatment options, and better general medical management. However, cancer and its treatment have long been recognized to have disabling complications. One seminal study of the rehabilitation needs of individuals with cancer assessed 805 hospitalized cancer patients and identified that 54% had physical medicine problems (1). These problems occurred with all tumor types; for those with central nervous system (CNS), breast, lung, or head and neck tumors, rehabilitation needs were present in more than 70%. Psychological problems were found in 42% of patients. There was a large gap between the identified rehabilitation needs and the services actually delivered to this population, which improved dramatically after initiating a program for patient education, automatic screening of patients for their rehabilitation needs, and introducing a physiatrist into the clinical oncology team.

Rehabilitation Expectations in the Cancer Population

This chapter will outline the contributions that rehabilitation can make to meet the needs of cancer patients. There is consensus that cancer patients frequently require treatment for the following general problems: pain, problems of mobility and self-care, fatigue, and weakness. Problems more specific to tumor types include dysphagia, cognitive impairment, lymphedema, neuropathy, and soft-tissue or bony excision. These are situations in which the rehabilitation professions are able to make significant contributions.

Not only can supportive or maintenance care be provided, but prevention of disability and restoration of function have become expectations for the cancer population. Rehabilitation professionals are often introduced into staging and treatment decision making, especially when this involves the musculoskeletal system and when limb surgeries are involved. The rehabilitation team is well organized to evaluate functional needs and deliver functionally based care. Several functional outcome measures developed for cancer patients (2–4) have demonstrated clinical efficacy of these interventions (4–6) (Table 81-1). These indices have helped demonstrate that treatments associated with less morbidity are associated with a more desired outcome and better quality of life, even if life is not prolonged (4). As a result, primary treatment of cancer, including development of surgical procedures, have evolved toward less invasive and more preservation-oriented techniques. Data suggest that the biopsychosocial aspects of cancer are important to survival and tumor recurrence. Higher levels of coping and enhancement of active participation in care over time are predictive of lower rates of recurrence and death (7). Good symptom management is associated with good physical and mental functioning (8).

Options for effective rehabilitation have broadened with the introduction of newer lightweight orthotics and prosthetics. There is better understanding of the mechanisms by which tissue is injured by radiation and chemotherapy. Treatments are often customized to individuals to minimize long-term side effects. Rehabilitation technology advances have produced gains for individuals with communication or mobility problems that are due to cancer.

Demographics of Cancer and Its Relevance to Rehabilitation

Cancer remains the second leading cause of death in the United States and is associated with significant morbidity and disability. The 5-year relative survival rates for a variety of tumors are presented in Table 81-2 (9). The lifetime risk of being diagnosed with cancer is 44% for men and 38% for women (9). The incidence of cancer has increased during the interval 1950–1999 in all tumors except cervix, ovary, oral cavity and pharynx, stomach, and colon. In recent years, however, death rates (per 100,000 population) have been decreasing for younger age groups, especially children and increasing for those older than 65 years of age (9). For the period 1992–1999, incidence and death rates of many tumor types have remained stable or declined, but exceptions include liver malignancies, melanoma, lung cancer (in women), and breast cancer (increased incidence but decreased death rate). The 5-year relative survival rate has increased for most tumors, with overall 5-year survival of 35% in the early 1950s and 64% for the period 1992–1998 (9). No-

TABLE 81-1. Karnofsky Scale

Able to carry on normal activity; no special care is needed.
10 Normal; no complaints, no evidence of disease
9 Able to carry on normal activity; minor signs or symptoms of disease
8 Normal activity with effort; some signs or symptoms of disease
Unable to work; able to live at home; cares for most personal needs; varying amounts of assistance is needed.
7 Cares for self; unable to carry on normal activity or do active work
6 Requires occasional assistance, but is able to care for most of own needs
5 Requires considerable assistance and frequent medical care
Unable to care for self; requires equivalent of institutional or hospital care; disease may be progressing rapidly.
4 Disabled; requires special care and assistance
3 Severely disabled; hospitalization is indicated, although death is not imminent
2 Very sick; hospitalization necessary; active supportive treatment necessary
1 Moribund, fatal process progressing rapidly
0 Dead

tably, however, 5-year survival for individuals with cancers of the stomach, esophagus, liver, pancreas, and lung and bronchus remains less than 30%. Others—e.g., breast, larynx, prostate, and kidney—have a much better prognosis.

When survival statistics are considered by racial background, 5-year survival is improving for both white and black patients, but there remains for most tumor types a discrepancy, with whites living longer after diagnosis (exceptions include ovarian cancer and pancreatic cancer, in which survival is similar, and brain cancer and multiple myeloma, in which survival is more extended among blacks) (9). Knowledge of survival statistics can be important for rehabilitation decision making, because aggressive restorative services may not be appropriate for those with a markedly reduced life expectancy. Expected survival often varies markedly within a given tumor type because of factors such as stage of disease and histology, however, so each case must be approached individually. It is extremely likely that the physiatrist will be consulted in the care of the cancer patient and that this patient is likely to be older and may have comorbidities and reduced tolerance to cancer treatment.

SETTINGS FOR DELIVERY OF REHABILITATION SERVICES FOR CANCER PATIENTS

Cancer rehabilitation care can be provided under various models, including acute inpatient rehabilitation, consultative care, and outpatient care (including home care). The physiatrist is in a strong position to provide concrete strategies that will improve functional status and overall quality of life, often anticipating needs through many stages of cancer. Thus, strong doctor-patient relationships are forged. Individuals with cancer are, as a whole, a highly receptive, motivated, and grateful population.

TABLE 81-2. Summary of Changes in Cancer Incidence and Mortality, 1950–99 and 5-Year Relative Survival Rates, 1950–98. Males and Females. By Primary Cancer Site

	All Races		Whites					
			Percent Change 1950–95				5-Year Relative Survival Rates (Percent)	
	Estimated Cancer Cases in 1999	Actual Cancer Deaths in 1999	Incidence		U.S. Mortality			
Primary Site			Total	EAPC	Total	EAPC	1950–54	1992–98
Oral cavity and Pharynx	29,800	7,486	−44.6	−0.7	−46.9	−1.0	46	58.8
Esophagus	12,500	11,917	0.7	0.3	26.8	0.6	4	14.7
Stomach	21,900	12,711	−77.8	−2.5	−83.0	−3.6	12	20.9
Colon and Rectum	129,400	57,155	−2.1	−0.2	−39.7	−1.0	37	62.6
Colon	94,700	48,433	11.2	0.1	−26.6	−0.5	41	62.7
Rectum	34,700	8,722	−23.9	−0.7	−68.8	−2.7	40	62.4
Liver and Intrahep	14,500	15,972	206.7	1.9	21.5	0.5	1	6.5
Pancreas	28,600	29,081	3.7	0.0	19.3	0.1	1	4.3
Larynx	10,600	3,815	28.6	0.1	−21.0	−0.4	52	65.9
Lung and Bronchus	171,600	152,480	227.9	2.1	248.2	2.3	6	15.0
Males	94,000	89,707	149.0	1.1	180.5	1.6	5	13.3
Females	77,600	62,773	571.5	4.2	600.6	4.6	9	17.0
Melanomas of skin	44,200	7,215	506.7	4.1	161.8	1.9	49	89.3
Breast (females)	175,000	41,144	62.9	1.3	−19.8	−0.2	60	87.6
Cervix uteri	12,800	4,204	−80.4	−2.7	−78.4	−3.5	59	72.1
Corpus and Uterus, NOS	37,400	6,468	1.8	−0.5	−68.9	−2.2	72	86.0
Ovary	25,200	14,035	−1.2	0.2	−2.2	−0.3	30	52.5
Prostate	179,399	31,728	206.1	3.2	−8.2	0.3	43	97.8
Testis	7,400	378	144.6	1.9	−68.3	−3.0	57	95.7
Urinary bladder	54,200	12,205	54.7	0.9	−34.8	−1.1	53	82.3
Kidney and Renal pelvis	30,000	11,461	128.3	1.9	29.0	0.6	34	62.4
Brain and Other nervous	16,800	12,765	112.9	1.1	49.3	0.6	21	31.5
Thyroid	18,100	1,241	169.2	1.9	−49.1	−1.7	80	96.0
Hodgkin's disease	7,200	1,403	2.1	0.1	−73.6	−3.3	30	84.7
Non-Hodgkin's lymphomas	56,800	22,612	189.8	2.8	128.1	1.6	33	56.1
Multiple myeloma	13,700	10,565	183.2	1.6	211.4	1.8	6	29.5
Leukemias	30,200	21,014	2.0	0.2	−3.9	−0.4	10	47.3
Childhood (0–14 yrs)	8,400	1,498	44.3	0.8	−69.0	−2.7	20	78.6
All Sites	1,221,800	549,829	58.7	1.0	0.2	0.1	35	63.9

Close communication with other physicians and care providers is essential. Cancer has become a chronic illness, and for those patients who have sustained a long-term disabling effect from their malignancy or its treatment, the physiatrist may in fact be the primary provider for care over the long term. Patients in whom the cancer progresses may need different interventions. The rehabilitation interventions from which the patient initially benefited may no longer be appropriate. The terminal stage may present a significant challenge to the physician because one must avoid abandoning the patient while at the same time not offering false hope.

The ability to provide support and treatments throughout the various stages of cancer management can be shared, for the physiatrist rarely works alone and is frequently responsible for coordinating interventions from a group of professionals, including occupational therapists (OTs), physical therapists (PTs), recreation therapists (RTs), and speech language pathologists (SLPs). Vocational counselors are consulted, as needed. Each one has unique contributions to offer the cancer patient. Typically, the OT is responsible for those activities that pertain to self-care, adaptive equipment, and bathroom safety. The PT is usually concerned with issues of mobility (including protection of limb/vertebral column stability when appropriate) and trains patients in the use of orthotics and gait aids. The PT is also frequently involved with management of pain and edema. The RT provides support and guidance for leisure-time activity and while in the hospital helps patients develop positive attitudes by producing products (e.g., crafts) and constructively participating in social activities. The SLP helps in the diagnosis and treatment of dysphagia and provides speech therapy for the cognitively impaired. SLPs are highly integrated into programs in which head and neck tumors are frequently seen. They also provide substantial support in the provision of communication strategies.

Inpatient Rehabilitation

In recent years, there has been a growing body of evidence that patients with cancer improve in function during acute rehabilitation comparably to noncancer patients having similar impairments, as measured by the Functional Independence Measure (FIM). Malignancy patients tend to have shorter rehabilitation length of stay and comparable discharge to home rates as controls in studies examining neoplastic spinal cord injury (SCI) (10) and brain tumor (11,12). Functional improvements made during acute rehabilitation are maintained at 3 months postdischarge (13,14). The incidence of transfer back to acute care from rehabilitation may be higher in cancer patients compared to noncancer patients: 33% versus 12% in Marciniak and associates' series (15) and 24% in O'Toole and Golden's series (16), however, only 15/302 (5%) in a more recent series (17). Therefore, communication with referring services must be maintained to promote optimal patient care in the appropriate setting. Chemotherapy and specific tumor type have not been shown to adversely affect rehabilitation outcome (15,17). Brain tumor patients show similar gains between those with primary brain tumor and metastatic disease (18,19); functional gains are better during the initial presentation to rehabilitation than with recurrence (19). Among brain tumor patients, findings regarding radiation therapy have been mixed, with one study finding better functional gains in patients not receiving radiation (12) and another finding better motor efficiency score in the radiation group (19). One study examining brain tumor patients found better outcomes in meningioma patients than in those with other diagnoses and in those with left brain lesions (12). In neoplastic SCI, survival and functional outcome is best in those with less severe neurologic injuries. Neurologically incomplete patients

with primary CNS tumors or radiation myelitis have better outcomes than those with lymphoma or solid tumors (20).

It should be noted that these studies have been performed on a preselected population largely meeting standard acute rehabilitation criteria. Prognosis and the patient's general tolerance of rehabilitation therapies must be weighed in the decision for inpatient rehabilitation, although poor expected long-term survival might not preclude inpatient rehabilitation if substantial functional gains are likely to be made in the short or intermediate term.

Coordinated therapy programs can offer some benefit even for the terminally ill in a hospice setting, where improved mobility scores were demonstrated after 1 month of an individualized physical therapy program (21).

In approaching patients undergoing cancer treatment, it is particularly important to be alert for intercurrent medical problems, which are often related to the treatment regimen. These include infection as a result of myelosuppression, neurologic complications of chemotherapy, and inanition, which may necessitate transfer from rehabilitation back to acute care. Chemotherapy side effects are outlined in Table 81-3 (22).

The physiatrist should routinely check for the following conditions, which when present can have a substantial impact on the ability of the patient to safely tolerate some rehabilitation services, such as exercise or therapeutic heat (23). There is a lack of evidence-based data about these precautions, however, with the best-studied area being metastatic bone disease and the other items largely empiric.

1. Hematologic profile: hemoglobin <7.5 g, platelets <20,000, white blood cell count <3,000 (see "Cancer-Related Fatigue" and "Exercise for the Cancer Patient: General Aspects" sections)
2. Metastatic bone disease with involvement of long bones (femur, tibia, humerus) such that there is more than 50% of the cortex involved, intramedullary lesions more than 50% to 60% cross-sectional diameter, or more than 2.5 cm diameter lesion in the femur (see "Bony Metastatic Disease" section)
3. Compression of a hollow viscus (bowel, bladder, or ureter), vessel, or spinal cord
4. Fluid accumulation in the pleura, pericardium, abdomen, or retroperitoneum associated with persistent pain, dyspnea, or problems with mobility
5. CNS depression or coma, or increased intracranial pressure
6. Hypo/hyperkalemia, hyponatremia, or hypo-/hypercalcemia
7. Orthostatic hypotension, blood pressure in excess of 160/100 mm Hg
8. Heart rate in excess of 110 beats/min or ventricular arrhythmia
9. Fever greater than 101 degrees Fahrenheit

Outpatient Rehabilitation

Outpatient care most commonly addresses specific musculoskeletal or soft-tissue problems, such as lymphedema, contracture, mobility, self-care, and pain. Patients must be mobile enough to be easily transported and should be medically stable. Pain syndromes most amenable to physiatric intervention in outpatient settings include those that are due to bony metastatic disease and to peripheral polyneuropathy, when pharmacologic strategies will intersect with nonpharmacologic treatments. Treatment that is likely to be ongoing, such as supervised exercise, mobility training, proper use of orthotic devices, and other adaptive and ambulatory aides, are best provided in the outpatient setting so that staff can determine how the patient is doing in his or her home environment. The ulti-

TABLE 81-3. Cancer Chemotherapy Agents and Side Effects

Agent	Major Toxicity
Polyfunctional Alkylating Agents	
Mechlorethamine	Therapeutic doses—moderate depression of peripheral blood cell counts
Chlorambucil	Excessive doses—severe bone marrow depression
Melphalan	Maximum toxicity may occur 2–3 weeks after the last dose
Thiotepa	Hemorrhagic cystitis occurs with cyclophosphamide and ifosfamide
Busulfan	Alopecia
Cyclophosphamide; ifosfamide	Nausea and vomiting
Antimetabolites	
Methotrexate; 5-fluorouracil	Oral and digestive tract ulcerations
6-Mercaptopurine; 6-thioguanine	Bone marrow depression
5-Fluorodeoxyuridine	Toxicity enhanced by impaired kidney function
Cytarabine; fludarabine	Alopecia
2-chlorodeoxyadenosine	
2-Deoxycoformycin; gemcitabine	
Antibiotics	
Doxorubicin; daunorubicin	Stomatitis, hypocalcemia, nausea and vomiting, alopecia
Bleomycin	Gastrointestinal injury
Dactinomycin	Bone marrow depression
Plicamycin	Cardiac toxicity at cumulative doses >500mg/m^2 (doxorubicin and daunorubicin)
Mitomycin C	Pneumonitis and pulmonary fibrosis at cumulative doses >400U (bleomycin)
Mitoxantrone	Hepatic toxicity (plicamycin)
Hormonally active compounds	
Androgen (fluoxymesterone)	Fluid retention
Antiandrogen (flutamide)	Masculinization/feminization
Estrogens	Hot flashes (sex hormones)
Antiestrogens (tamoxifen)	Hypertension, diabetes, adrenal insufficiency
Progestin (megestrol acetate)	
Luteinizing hormone-releasing hormone agonist (leuprolide)	
Aminoglutethimide	
Dexamethasone	
Miscellaneous drugs	
Asparaginase	Anorexia, weight loss, somnolence, lethargy, confusion; hypoproteinemia (albumin, fibrinogen) Hyperlipidemia, abnormal liver function tests, fatty liver changes; pancreatis (rare); azotemia Granulocytopenia, lymphopenia, and thrombocytopenia (usually mild, transient)
Altretamine	Bone marrow depression, peripheral neuropathy
AMSA	Bone marrow depression, stomatitis, hepatic dysfunction, nausea and vomiting
Carmustine; lomustine	Bone marrow depression, thrombocytopenia, nausea and vomiting
Streptozotocin	Hypoglycemia, nausea and vomiting
Mitotane	Skin eruptions, diarrhea, mental depression, muscle tremors, adrenal insufficiency, nausea and vomiting
Dacarbazine; hydroxyurea; carboplatin	Bone marrow depression, nausea and vomiting
Etoposide	Alopecia, nausea and vomiting
Cisplatin	Bone marrow depression, renal tubular damage, deafness, nausea and vomiting
Procarbazine	Bone marrow depression, mental depression, nausea and vomiting
Vinblastine	Alopecia, areflexia, bone marrow depression
Vincristine	Areflexia, peripheral neuropathy, paralytic ileus, mild bone marrow depression
Levamisole	None
Cis-retinoic acid	Cheilitis, stomatitis, conjunctivitis
Paclitaxel, docetaxel	Leukopenia, peripheral neuropathy

Adapted from Krakoff IH, Systemic treatment of cancer *CA Cancer J Clin* 1996;46:134–141.

mate goal of the treatments is improved performance. Monitoring how and what the patient is actually doing is best done over time in the outpatient setting. Home health care may need to be prescribed if mobility is a significant obstacle to treatment.

Consultation during Acute Care

Patients in the acute-care setting—being staged for their tumors, receiving definitive oncologic treatment, or admitted for complications of tumor or its treatment—are often in need of rehabilitation services. The problems may be tumor specific or general. Consultative services that are most frequently requested include evaluation and treatment of mobility and self-care needs, as well as assessment of cognitive status, communication, and swallowing skills. Consultative services that

address issues of pain control and the provision of orthotic/prosthetic devices are also requested. The physiatrist will be asked to participate in decision making about the setting for future rehabilitation efforts.

PHYSICAL MEDICINE PRACTICE FOR CANCER PATIENTS

Pain Assessment and Its Treatment

GENERAL APPROACH TO CANCER-RELATED PAIN

It is estimated that 70% of patients with cancer have cancer-related pain that will need treatment during the course of their illness (24). This encompasses about 30% to 50% of ambulatory cancer patients, to more than 90% of those with advanced disease (25). Distinguishing between acute pain and chronic pain syndromes is important for proper selection of pharmacologic and nonmedicinal treatment. Evaluation should include location, severity, and quality of pain; a determination of its impact on sleep; and the ability to perform usual daily routines. Direct tumor spread accounts for most cancer pain (65%–75%), with the remainder related to cancer therapy (15%–25%) or unrelated causes (24,26). In cases of pain that is due to direct tumor spread, antitumor therapy is often highly effective in controlling the pain (25). Treatment guidelines for the management of acute pain have been published by the Agency for Health Care Policy and Research (27), which builds on the World Health Organization (WHO) analgesic ladder (28), matching the intensity of pain to the treatment recommended. The first line of treatment is the nonopioid analgesics (aspirin, acetaminophen, and nonsteroidal antiinflammatories, etc.). Should these fail to control the pain, then an opioid (propoxyphene, codeine, oxycodone, morphine, fentanyl, methadone, etc.) should be added. Dosing depends on the severity of symptoms. The prescribed route of administration depends on whether the patient can consume medication by mouth and whether the severity of the pain can be adequately controlled using oral medication, as well as on the ease of administration. Adjuvant pain medication may be added, if needed, for better control and includes the addition of antidepressants, benzodiazepines, psychostimulants, corticosteroids, and clonidine. Nerve blocks, epidural injections, and surgical ablation also may be useful in the treatment of refractory cancer pain. Modalities of heat, cold, electricity, and nontraditional therapy (such as acupuncture) all have been shown to be helpful in relieving acute pain in patients with cancer diagnoses (29).

The likelihood of cancer pain being chronic is high (30). WHO has strongly urged use of pain management strategies that are designed to totally relieve symptoms. The efficacy of the analgesic ladder described above has been demonstrated to control more than 70% of pain in patients with advanced cancer, with the remainder requiring procedures such as neurolysis for pain control (31). Detailed and systematic assessment of pain must be performed both initially and at regular intervals. Chronic pain in this population is either visceral (poorly localized, cramping, or deep aching), somatic (well localized to discrete anatomic areas, often sharp or stabbing), or neuropathic (burning, tingling, throbbing in the peripheral or central nervous system).

PHARMACOLOGIC MANAGEMENT OF CANCER PAIN

There are four key principles to effective pharmacologic pain management (see also Chapter 15). These include choosing a medication, selecting a route for administration, picking the proper dosage, and recognizing and mitigating side effects or toxicities (Table 81-4). In general, dosing is advanced to the level at which pain is controlled or at which toxicities preclude higher dosing (25). With opioids, the daily effective dose should be established with immediate-release preparations, then converted to a longer-acting preparation. There should also be rescue dosing of an immediate-release preparation available for breakthrough pain, composing about 5% to 15% of the total daily opioid dose (25). Incident pain is discomfort occurring intermittently as a result of usually predictable factors, such as physical activity or time of day. The standing dose of pain medication should be increased surrounding these factors, rather than increasing the around-the-clock dose (32). Adjuvant pain medications are useful for those patients in whom control with opioids alone is inadequate. Nociceptive pain typ-

ically responds well to opioids, but neuropathic pain is often more refractory and benefits from adjuvant medication (25), as does musculoskeletal pain (Table 81-5). Myoclonus may occur with opioid use and responds to clonazepam (32). Stimulants such as methylphenidate can be useful to counteract opioid-related sedation.

OTHER PAIN CONTROL STRATEGIES

In refractory cases, opioids can be administered parenterally via patient-controlled analgesia or spinal analgesia techniques. Long-term catheter systems can be implanted for the latter, with opioids sometimes combined with local anesthetics (33). Other techniques range from local measures, such as joint or trigger-point injections and nerve blocks (sympathetic or somatic), to neurosurgical procedures, such as implantation of dorsal column stimulators and neuroablative procedures (neurectomy, rhizotomy, cordotomy) (33). Comprehensive pain treatment centers offer cognitive and behavioral management strategies as adjuvant treatment for cancer-related pain. These techniques include relaxation training, hypnotherapy, and biofeedback. Controlled trials demonstrating efficacy in treating this population have not been undertaken.

Assessment and Treatment of Mobility Problems in the Cancer Patient

BONY METASTATIC DISEASE

Bony metastatic disease can occur with most types of malignancies but is especially common in tumors involving the prostate, breast, lung, kidney, and thyroid (34–35). Additionally, hematologic malignancies such as multiple myeloma, the lymphomas, and leukemia are often associated with widespread bony infiltration by tumor. Bone is the third most common site for metastases, and the vertebrae, pelvis, femur, ribs, and skull are most frequently involved (36). Bony metastatic lesions usually affect multiple sites and in 20% of cases affect the upper limbs (37).

Bony metastatic disease can produce pain, instability with risk of pathologic fracture, and, in the case of spine or skull metastasis, compromise of adjacent neurologic structures. About 10% of patients with known bone metastases will sustain a fracture (38). One must suspect bony metastatic disease when bone pain is present. Most patients with high-risk conditions for bone metastasis are also followed serially with bone scans to detect occult metastasis because not all lesions are painful. It remains controversial as to whether most large lesions with impending pathologic fracture are painful. Other potential effects of metastatic bone disease include hematopoietic suppression and hypercalcemia (39).

Assessing Bone Stability in the Cancer Patient

Factors such as lesion size, location, and type of metastasis (lytic versus blastic) must be considered (40). When a patient presents with a symptomatic bony lesion, one must investigate whether lesions are present at other sites because more widespread lesions may further impact weight-bearing recommendations.

In evaluating bony stability, plain x-rays are the most useful tool. In the spine, flexion-extension views also should be obtained. Lesions measuring less than 1 cm are not reliably seen on plain films. Total body bone scan is indicated to define the range of bony neoplastic involvement. It is highly sensitive (95% to 97%) but not highly specific for tumor (41). False-negative results can occur in the setting of bone destruction without significant ongoing repair, as can occur in multiple myeloma,

TABLE 81-4. Pharmacologic Management of Pain

Analgesic	Route	Duration of Analgesic	Dosage	Side Effects
Aspirin	Oral	4–6 hr	650 mg every 4 hr	Gastritis, tinnitus
Acetaminophen	Oral	4–6 hr	650 mg every 4 hr	Hepatotoxicity
NSAIDs[a]	Oral	Varies by agent	Varies by agent	Gastritis
Tramadol	Oral	6–8 hr	50–100 mg every 6 hr	Sedation, nausea, constipation
Morphine[b]	Intravenous	1.5–2 hr	2 mg–10 mg	Sedation, respiratory depression, constipation, confusion, pruritus
	epidural/intrathecal	Up to 24 hr	5 mg	
	Oral	2–4 hr	30–60 mg	
Delayed release MS Contin, Roxanol	Oral	8–12 hr	30–60 mg	Sedation, respiratory depression, constipation, confusion, pruritus
Methadone	Oral	8–12 hr	20 mg	Sedation, respiratory depression, constipation, confusion; variable dosing efficacy
Oxycodone	Oral	3–6 hr (standard) 12 hr (sustained release)	30 mg	Sedation, respiratory depression, constipation, confusion
Hydromorphone	Oral	2–4 hr	7.5 mg	Sedation, respiratory depression, constipation, confusion
	Parenteral	2–4 hr	1.5 mg	
	Rectal	6–8 hr	3 mg	
	Oral	3–5 hr	30 mg	
Hydrocodone	Oral	3–5 hr	30 mg	Sedation, respiratory depression, constipation (often more severe than with other opioids), confusion
Fentanyl	Transdermal	48–72 hr	50 µg/hr	Sedation, respiratory depression, constipation, confusion. Use transmucosal form (Actiq opioid-tolerant individuals only, for break pain; per label, transmucosal form is intended for cancer patients only, and not indicated in c
	Transmucosal (buccal)	4 hr (variable)	200 µg	

[a]NSAIDs, nonsteroidal antiinflammatory drugs. Numerous options, including COX-2 inhibitors (rofecoxib, celecoxib) with reduced incidence of gastritis.
[b]Dosing of this agent and other opioids will be highly variable, depending on degree of opioid tolerance. Dosing can be advanced.
[c]Use in opioid–tolerant patients only.

the leukemias, and lymphomas. In the spine, those patients in whom there are neurologic abnormalities or abnormal bone scan findings should be assessed via magnetic resonance imaging (MRI) or computed tomography (CT). This will quantify the extent of tumor infiltration, including any extension to the spinal cord (42). MRI is especially useful in this regard. CT is better for bony detail and is useful in elucidating subtle cortical erosions or fractures. Both studies are useful in distinguishing osteoporotic vertebral collapse from pathologic fracture.

Size criteria for pathologic fracture risk in long bone include lesions measuring more than 2.5 cm in lower-limb long bones (more than 3.0 cm in upper-limb lesions) (43–45), involvement of more than 50% of the bony cortex, intramedullary lesions with greater than 50% to 60% (46,47) cross-sectional diameter,

involvement of a length of cortex equal to or greater than the cross-sectional diameter of the bone, or, in the femoral neck, cortical destruction greater than 1.3 cm in axial length (Table 81-6). Another method of assessing fracture risk involves multiplying the quotient of the diameter of the lesion and the bone diameter at that level by 100 to obtain the percentage probability of fracture (48) (e.g., lesion diameter 2 cm/bone width 5 cm × 100 = 40% chance of fracture). Unfortunately, in practice it is often difficult to gauge the size of bony lesions, especially lytic ones, which may be irregular, permeative, and difficult to distinguish from surrounding osteopenia (49).

Location of a metastatic lesion is also important in assessing stability. One must consider whether weight-bearing bone is involved. In the case of the spine, thoracic lesions are afforded some inherent stability because of the rib cage, whereas lesions

TABLE 81-5. Adjuvants Used in Cancer Pain Management

Type of Pain	Anticonvulsant	Adjuvant Antidepressant	Antispasticity	Steroids	Local Anesthetics[a]	Other
Neuropathic (continuous)	++	+++	0	+	++	Clonidine
Neuropathic (lancinating, stabbing)	++	+	+	0	++	Clonazepam (Carbamazepine) (Baclofen)
Bone	0	+	0	++	+	NSAIDs[b] Bisphosphonates Calcitonin
Soft tissue	0	++	0	++	++	NSAIDs

[a]Includes topical or injected applications, and oral preparations (mexiletine). [b]NSAIDs, nonsteroidal anti-inflammatory drugs.

TABLE 81-6.   Fracture Risk

	Points Assigned		
	1	**2**	**3**
Anatomic site	Upper extremity	Lower extremity	Trochanter
Lesion type	Blastic	Blastic/lytic	Lytic
Lesion size	<1/3 diameter of femur	>1/3, <2/3	>2/3
Intensity of pain	Mild	Moderate	Severe

in the more flexible cervical and lumbar spine are more prone to instability.

In general, lytic lesions are considered more prone to fracture than blastic ones, although blastic lesions are not immune to fracture. Lytic lesions typically occur in tumors of the breast, lung, kidney, thyroid, gastrointestinal tumors, neuroblastoma, lymphoma, and melanoma. Breast cancer is responsible for 30% to 50% of all long-bone pathologic fractures, more than half of those in the proximal femur (49). Renal cell tumors produce large lytic lesions and are at especially high risk for fracture.

In the spine, there are not validated criteria for assessing fracture risk. The three-column model of Denis (50) is often used, with the spine considered to have anterior, middle, and posterior columns. The anterior column includes the anterior longitudinal ligament and anterior wall of the vertebral body, disk, and annulus; the middle column the posterior wall of those structures and the posterior longitudinal ligament; and the posterior column the posterior elements and associated ligaments and facet capsules. If two or more of these columns are involved, or the middle column alone is involved, the lesion is considered unstable. A refinement of this model, described for spine tumors, divides the spine into six columns: anterior, middle, and posterior as per the Denis model, with left and right components. The spine is considered stable if fewer than three columns are destroyed, unstable if three or four columns are destroyed, and markedly unstable if five or six columns are destroyed (Fig. 81-1). The spine is also considered unstable if

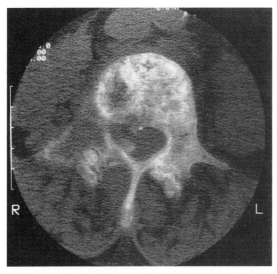

Figure 81-1. Extensive lumbar spinal metastasis, mixed lytic and blastic lesions.

greater than 20 degrees of angulation is present (42). The criteria of Harrington (51) also incorporate neurologic compromise, graded as follows:

I.   No significant neurologic involvement
II. Bone involvement without instability/collapse
III. Major neurologic involvement without bone involvement
IV. Bony collapse without neurologic compromise
V.   Major neurologic compromise and vertebral collapse

Those in categories I–III can benefit from rehabilitation treatment designed to relieve pain and promote function, as well as antitumor therapies (chemotherapy, radiation), and in Stage III cortico-steroids. These patients benefit from lightweight, easily donned corsets, which offer pain relief, as does the use of superficial heat and transcutaneous electrical nerve stimulation (TENS) units. Patients who have stage IV and V involvement, should be considered for surgical stabilization.

Management of Bony Metastatic Lesions

When an unstable lesion is suspected, surgical referral should be placed and the patient made non–weight bearing to the affected structure. Surgical procedures should include the use of methylmethacrylate (38). Often surgical stabilization is followed by radiation therapy to reduce tumor mass, thereby facilitating pain control and eventual regrowth of normal bone. In borderline cases, radiation therapy alone may be applied, especially for radiosensitive tumors such as breast cancer, lung cancer, or multiple myeloma (37). Hormonal treatment in responsive tumor types, such as breast or prostate, may reduce bone pain, as can chemotherapy; and radiation therapy alone is often highly effective in controlling pain. Fracture risk may actually increase over the first 6 to 8 weeks as a result of tumor necrosis and softening of bone (52).

It is important to remember that although bony metastatic disease is a finding of progressive malignancy usually without hope of cure, survival often can be expected for a period of years, especially in breast, prostate, and thyroid malignancies (37).

Depending on the severity of the lesion, mobility recommendations may range from complete non–weight bearing of an affected limb to no precautions whatsoever. Bed rest should be avoided because additional functional loss will occur, and hypercalcemia and thromboembolic disease may complicate the course (38). A walker or crutches will be needed for complete non–weight bearing of a lower limb (40). A single cane can be used in cases of smaller, but painful lesions, or, for somewhat larger or more symptomatic lesions, a forearm crutch that permits about 25% more force transmission than a conventional cane (53). In the spine, Jewett bracing can be used in cases of anterior or middle column involvement, preventing spine flexion, or a custom-molded thoracolumbar orthosis in a two-piece clam shell design (Fig. 81-2) will afford stability in all directions. Bracing alone will not be sufficient in the case of cord compression. Often patients are resistant to the use of spine orthotics because of poor skin tolerance, perceived discomfort, and lack of a clear end point. In such cases, a thoracolumbar corset can provide limited support and pain relief. Use in combination with gait aids such as a walker will minimize torque across the spine.

For the cervical spine, a Philadelphia collar, sternal occipital mandibular immobilizer (SOMI), or even a halo orthotic can be used depending on the severity of the findings (i.e., whether mechanical excursion is seen on plain films or progressing neurologic deficits are present). For cervicothoracic junction lesions, a thoracic extension can be added to a SOMI or Philadel-

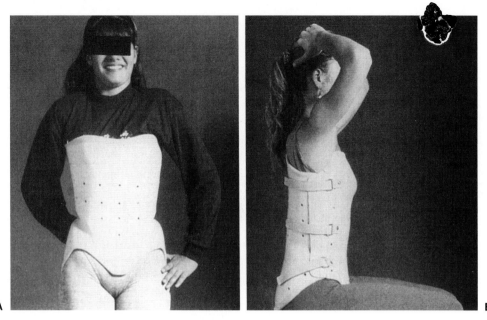

Figure 81-2. Custom-molded body jacket. Front **(A)** and side **(B)** views.

phia collar. One should wear the neck orthosis at all times, especially in the car.

Activity recommendations should focus on exercise that promotes strength and *endurance* but minimizes bony impact, such as isometric strengthening, and *low-impact aerobic activities,* such as swimming, riding a stationary bike, or walking. Climbing steps using a step-to pattern rather than a step-over-step pattern will minimize the period of single limb support (54). Further guidance should focus on attention to proper body mechanics (in particular avoiding sudden spine or limb torsions) and on fall prevention strategies (including environmental modifications) and should address possible influence of medication on balance and orthostatic hypotension. Before prescribing a cane or walker to unload the lower limbs, it becomes quite important to assess the status of the upper limbs, which may also be involved. Those with upper-limb lesions should be treated with a sling or a lightweight humeral cuff and instructed in activities to reduce loads and torsion.

Studies have shown efficacy of bisphosphonates, such as pamidronate and clodronate, in preventing or delaying complications of bony metastatic disease, such as pain and pathologic fractures, as a result of inhibition of osteolysis (55). One recent position paper recommends intravenous pamidronate for breast cancer patients with bone pain caused by osteolytic metastasis, concurrently with chemotherapy or hormonal therapy (56).

CANCER-RELATED FATIGUE

Fatigue is the most common symptom among newly diagnosed cancer patients, reported by 66% (57), and affects 70% to 100% of all cancer patients undergoing treatment (58). Pathophysiologic changes contributing to fatigue include anemia, cachexia, infection, paraneoplastic syndromes, metabolic disorders, psychologic stress, and side effects of cancer treatment (59). The latter includes antitumor therapy, pain medication, and endocrine effects of treatment. Cytokines implicated in cancer-related fatigue include interferon, interleukins 1, 2, 6, 10, and 12, and tumor necrosis factor. Cytokines are proteins produced by cells that mediate cell-to-cell communication, and when physiologic homeostasis breaks down, cytokines appear to mediate such *effects* as anemia, weight loss, fever, infection,

and depression (60). Major depression may be difficult to diagnose, as many of the same somatic symptoms may be attributable to the cancer and its care. For depressed patients with significant fatigue, activating antidepressants such as bupropion or selective serotonin releasing inhibitors may be best (61), although sedating agents such as tricyclic antidepressants or mirtazapine may be preferable if sleep disturbance is contributing to fatigue (61).

In one study, the most common influences contributing to fatigue were pain, sleep disturbance and depression. Five of 40 subjects were also found to be hypothyroid (62). Seventy-five percent of fatigued subjects were prescribed medication, and in 13 of 40 cases, physical medicine and rehabilitation referral was made. (62). Table 81-7 outlines fatigue interventions (63–66).

EXERCISE FOR THE CANCER PATIENT: GENERAL ASPECTS

Moderate exercise is thought to be beneficial for individuals with cancer. Physical activity is encouraged to prevent further muscle wasting or loss of cardiorespiratory fitness (67) and improve efficiency of energy metabolism at the cellular level (68). There may also be benefits of exercise on immune function, such as effects on macrophages, natural killer cells, neutrophils, and regulating cytokines; however, the implications of these effects are not well delineated on a clinical level (69). Exercise studies performed in the cancer population have substantiated gains in functional capacity, decrease in fatigue, and improvements in other parameters examined (67). Aerobic training has been better studied than resistance training.

In establishing exercise precautions, one needs to consider hematologic, cardiac, pulmonary, and skeletal factors. Depression and fatigue may limit exercise participation, and fever will reduce exercise tolerance.

Most hematologic parameters for exercise are empiric. In a study of acute leukemia patients (70), grossly visible hemorrhage was rare with a platelet count greater than 20,000, and no intracranial hemorrhage occurred with a platelet count greater than 10,000. The risk of hemorrhage correlates with the platelet count but is mitigated by other systemic factors, such that a safe threshold level cannot be ascertained. The concern with exercise in the thrombocytopenic state lies in the potential for increased blood pressure, which occurs most dramatically with

TABLE 81-7.   Interventions for Fatigue

Strategy	Examples

Restore energy balance	Correct anemia
	Nutritional and vitamin
	  supplementation
	Correct endocrine dysfunction
	  (thyroid)

Medications	Stimulants (methylphenidate,
	  d-amphetamine)
	Analgesics
	Antidepressants (bupropion, SSRIs,
	  TCAs)
	Regulate sleep/wake
	Glucocorticoids
	Investigational—cytokine-targeted
	  therapy (including NSAIDs)

Exercise	Aerobic exercise is best-studied form. Individualized Attention to precautions Cachectic patients may not tolerate.
Energy conservation	Education Adaptive equipment
Psychologic/coping	Recreational activities Relaxation techniques Support groups Spiritual supports, participation

SSRIs, selective serotonin reuptake inhibitors; TCAs, tricyclic antidepressant agents.
NSAIDs, nonsteroidal anti-inflammatory drugs

isometric exercise, to result in intracranial hemorrhage, and high-impact activities to result in muscular or intraarticular hemorrhage. In general, unrestricted exercise can be pursued with platelet counts greater than about 30,000 to 50,000. Aerobic, but not resistive, activities can be considered with platelet counts greater than 10,000 to 20,000. Active therapy is not advocated with platelet counts less than 10,000 (71). Exercise is also not recommended with fever greater than 40°C (104°F) because of poor tolerance, increased respiratory and heart rates, and increased platelet consumption (72). No specific precautions exist regarding white blood cell count, but exercise can produce transient increases in the white blood cell count, so that patients might be counseled to avoid intense exercise before routine laboratory monitoring (73).

Exercise for Patients Undergoing Bone Marrow Transplantation

Exercise programs have been developed for bone marrow transplant recipients to counteract the debility occurring with medical morbidity and prolonged hospitalization, as well as to counteract other factors such as depression and social isolation (71). Supine or sitting exercise is generally well tolerated, but standing exercise should be attempted at least for brief periods to minimize gastroc-soleus tightness. Supine exercise may be most comfortably performed with the head of the bed slightly elevated. Exercise programs emphasize range of motion; aerobic activity, such as use of a bedside stationary bicycle or walking; light resistive activities, such as bridging and use of light weights; and deep breathing to prevent atelectasis and pneumonia (74). If patients develop hepatic venoocclusive disease, supine exercise or abdominal exercises should be avoided because they may aggravate abdominal pain. In those with graft-versus-host disease, skin erythema and rash may occur, and

protective padding will prevent pain and skin irritation during exercise, especially over the soles of the feet (71). Active assisted range of motion should be performed to prevent contractures in this setting, as well as nighttime orthotic devices to preserve functional positioning of the hands and feet. One study of graft-versus-host disease in children found soft-tissue contractures, mobility deficits, cramping, and self-care impairments in the majority of cases. Improvement was found with medications including quinine, carbamazepine, or baclofen for the cramping, and with stretches along with etretinate for the contractures (75). Often patients will need encouragement to engage in the exercise regimen, but even limited treatment, such as passive range of motion or massage, can build patients' trust and future compliance (72). One study of treadmill training (interval pattern) 30 minutes daily for 6 weeks, with exercise intensity titrated to 80% of calculated maximum heart rate or lactate concentration 3 mmol/L in capillary blood, in bone marrow transplant recipients with stabilized platelet counts and clinical condition resulted in improved physical performance, measured by distance of treadmill walking (76).

Exercise for Patients Undergoing Chemotherapy or Postchemotherapy

Cancer patients treated with cardiotoxic agents such as anthracyclines can sustain permanent cardiac damage that affectsphysical performance. Patients treated with significant doses of these agents (greater than 100 mg/m^2) can have reduced exercise time, reduced maximal oxygen uptake, abnormal heart rate response, ST- and T-wave changes, and exercise-induced hypotension (77). However, a study of children and young adults treated with anthracyclines for childhood cancers found that a 12-week, two-times-per-week hospital-based aerobic conditioning program, supplemented starting at week 7 with one home-based session per week, can improve exercise time (by about 10%), peak oxygen uptake, and ventilatory anaerobic threshold, despite the fact that cardiac parameters, such as exercise heart rate and stroke volume, do not increase (77). A controlled study of patients undergoing aerobic exercise (supervised daily supine bicycle ergometry, to heart rate of 50% of calculated cardiac reserve, for fifteen 1-minute intervals over a 30-minute period) while receiving high-dose chemotherapy (nonanthracycline) followed by autologous peripheral blood stem cell transplantation for solid tumors found multiple benefits in the exercise group, including less decrement in performance per treadmill testing, less pain, decreased duration of neutropenia, and shorter hospitalization (78). A 10-week, three-times-per-week aerobic training program in women undergoing a noncardiotoxic chemotherapy regimen for breast cancer found 40% improvement in functional capacity, improved heart rate, longer work periods, and higher-intensity workload attainable than in controls. This study also had a placebo group doing stretching exercises, and the aerobic training group performed better in the above parameters except heart rate (79). Another study of breast cancer patients receiving adjuvant therapy, stratified by chemotherapy (about two-thirds receiving anthracyclines) or no chemotherapy (radiation or hormonal treatment), found gains in patient-reported physical function whether the exercise program is self-directed (with instruction to exercise five times per week for 26 weeks, including warm-up and cool-down, progressive walking to 50% to 60% maximum oxygen update, and provision of an exercise diary) or supervised (similar program, three times per week supervised and twice weekly at home), and may be greater with the self-directed approach (80). However, measured gains in functional capacity were significant only in the supervised exercised group patients that were not receiving chemotherapy (80). Group exercise therapy, consisting of four sessions of strength training, water exercise, and conditioning, combined with additional sessions for education and training in coping strategies, has also been reported to result in improved self-report of physical strength in a group of primarily breast cancer patients postradiation or postchemotherapy (81). Muscle strength was not actually measured in this study, however. Low- to moderate-intensity home-based aerobic exercise is associated with reduced fatigue in women receiving chemotherapy for breast cancer, although the effect of exercise on fatigue appears to be more immediate (same-day) than long lasting (82).

CACHEXIA

Endogenous tumor necrosis factor, or that administered exogenously as antineoplastic therapy, can reduce skeletal muscle protein stores. The resulting muscle wasting can predispose to fatigue with exercise because the reduced cross-sectional area of muscle results in less force production. Increased effort will be needed by the patient to do the same work. A moderate intensity of exercise (reducing activity at the onset of fatigue), which relies mainly on type I muscle fibers, which are fatigue resistant, should be encouraged (73). Exercise that produces marked fatigue is probably too intense. Patients receiving tumor necrosis factor as therapy might delay exercise a few days to allow muscle regeneration. Those with marked cachexia, possibly tumor necrosis factor alpha-mediated, might not tolerate exercise at all, and rehabilitation efforts should focus on routes other than aerobic conditioning to achieve functional goals (73).

NEUROLOGIC COMPLICATIONS OF CANCER

Brain Metastasis

Brain metastasis occurs in about 20% of patients with cancer and may be intracerebral (77% of cases) or leptomeningeal (40% of cases) (83). The most common primary tumors that metastasize to the brain are lung, breast, and melanoma (84). Tumors of hematologic origin and some genitourinary tract sites also metastasize to the brain. Uterine, cervical, and prostatic carcinoma rarely spread to the brain (83). Eighty percent of brain metastatic lesions are in the cerebrum, and only 20% in the posterior fossa (84).

The clinical presentation may be insidious or sudden in onset. Headache is often present, followed by focal neurologic signs, especially hemiparesis (85). Seizure may also be a presenting feature. Contrast-enhanced MRI or CT is the best diagnostic test. Treatment for the acute condition includes corticosteroids and radiation therapy. Whole-brain irradiation is standard treatment, 2,000 to 4,000 rad given over 5 days to 4 weeks. Radiosensitive tumors such as lymphoma, testicular cancer, and breast cancer respond especially well, but even radioresistant tumors often show some response (84). Corticosteroids will be needed to control edema and should be continued until the completion of radiation therapy (85). Brain irradiation is frequently completed during inpatient rehabilitation, and it is important to remember not to taper the steroids too soon, or neurologic decline can result. Occasionally, chemotherapeutic agents are used concomitantly. Excision of brain metastasis may be indicated, especially if the metastasis is single, the cancer otherwise well controlled, and the brain metastasis appears to be the major factor limiting survival (85).

Relatively favorable prognostic factors are solitary brain lesion and ambulatory status. Presence of headache, visual dis-turbance, or impaired consciousness at presentation are poor prognostic factors (86).

Leptomeningeal involvement is most common at the base of the brain, the major brain fissures, and the cauda equina. Lymphomas, leukemias (especially acute), lung (especially small cell), breast, melanoma, and gastric carcinoma most commonly metastasize to the leptomeninges. Clinically, these patients present with deficits of cranial nerves (in about 50% of cases) (84) and spinal nerve roots (87). Treatment consists of radiation therapy and intrathecal chemotherapy, but prognosis is poor (84,87).

Spinal Cord Involvement

Cancer-related spinal cord involvement may be due to compression by tumor or to bony instability in patients with metastatic bone disease (both oncologic emergencies) or to radiation fibrosis. Spinal metastatic involvement can affect the thoracic spine (70%), lumbosacral spine (20%), and cervical spine (10%) (88).

The most commonly seen primary tumors that cause spinal cord compression are lung (15%), breast (10%), prostate (10%), unknown primary (10%), lymphomas (10%), and myeloma (10%) (88,89). Ninety-five percent of cases are due to epidural extension of tumor (88). Infarction of vertebral blood supply may occur in hematologic malignancies.

Pain is the first symptom of cord compression in 95% of cases, which persists for an average of 6 weeks before irreversible neurologic changes develop (84). Pain can either be local, radicular, or referred. The quality of the pain can vary in each case. Local pain is usually aching and constant. Referred pain may be aching or sharp and is remote from the site involved. Radicular pain is usually sharp, shooting pain. Local vertebral tenderness is present in about one-third of cases (90). Once neurologic abnormalities develop, progression is often rapid. Epidural metastases characteristically are associated with pain when supine, exacerbated by coughing or the Valsalva maneuver (90). Stretching, such as neck and back flexion, is usually poorly tolerated.

In addition to pain, myelopathy is common at the time of diagnosis of spine metastases. Seventy-six percent report weakness, 87% are weak on examination, 57% have autonomic dysfunction, and 78% have sensory deficits (90). Motor abnormalities usually precede sensory abnormalities as a result of epidural extension, preferentially affecting the anterior spinal cord, and recovery occurs in the reverse order. Perineal hypesthesia may be the first sign of a cauda equina syndrome. Sphincter incontinence is a very poor prognostic sign, as is rapid (less than 72 hours) evolution of symptoms (fewer than 5% recover). Complete paraplegia is not reversible (89). Because of the above patterns of involvement, compared with the traumatic SCI population, there is more paraplegia than tetraplegia, and more incomplete lesions in the cancer group (91). Because 1-year survival rates are better in those who remain ambulatory (66% versus 10%) (92), early intervention is appropriate (see Chapter 79, "Rehabilitation of Spinal Cord Injury," for discussion of SCI rehabilitation principles).

Oncologic treatment includes dexamethasone tapered over 2 to 3 weeks (higher dosing with cord compression than with radiculopathy) (89), laminectomy (surgical results best with tumors located posterior or lateral) in selected cases, and radiation therapy (in virtually all cases). A dosage of 3,000 to 4,000 rad over 2 to 4 weeks is typically given. Adjuvant chemotherapy may be considered in certain cases. (See previous section, "Bony Metastatic Disease," for discussion of spine imaging.) Favorable prognostic factors are primary diagnosis of lymphoma, myeloma, or breast cancer; early or slowly progressing neurologic signs; and ambulatory status at time of diagnosis of cord compression (90).

Paraneoplastic Neuromuscular Syndromes

Paraneoplastic syndromes, or remote effects of malignancy that are expressed distant from the primary tumor or metastatic lesions, are often neurologic in nature and include subacute cerebellar degeneration, myopathies, neuromuscular junction disorders, and peripheral neuropathies. Organic dementias may occur (89), as well as metabolic encephalopathy (most often because of electrolyte disturbance including hypercalcemia, hyponatremia, hypoglycemia, and vitamin deficiencies) and sagittal sinus thrombosis (84). Reflex sympathetic dystrophy has been described with local or recurrent tumor (93). Many combinations of motor and sensory neuropathies may occur (see discussion in the next section, "Peripheral Neuropathy").

The ataxia associated with cerebellar degeneration may antedate the diagnosis of tumor, as seen with lung, breast, and ovarian carcinomas (94). The syndrome may be associated with organic dementia. Ataxia also may be induced by cytotoxic drugs, such as fluorouracil, procarbazine, and nitrosureas, as well as by brain metastases. Treatment of the underlying disease may halt the progression, but neurologic improvement of paraneoplastic cerebellar degeneration is rare. However, sustained functional benefit has been reported after comprehensive inpatient rehabilitation (95).

Shy-Drager syndrome may occur as a paraneoplastic syndrome in small-cell lung cancer. Treatment is administered in the form of indomethacin, salt loading, fludrocortisone, and compressive stockings. Proximal myopathies that may occur include inflammatory myopathies, carcinoid myopathy, steroid myopathy, and weakness from cachexia. Treatment of tumor may result in improvement of the myopathy, especially carcinoid and, less consistently, inflammatory forms (96). Isometric exercises in combination with stretching, mobility aides, and adaptive devices to maintain functional independence are indicated for myopathic conditions.

Myasthenia gravis may occur in association with thymoma, and antibodies to thymus are usually present. Myasthenic syndrome occurs in association with small-cell lung cancer. The condition may improve with treatment of the underlying cancer and with guanidine hydrochloride (96).

Devastating paraneoplastic neurologic complications include acute necrotizing myopathy and ascending hemorrhagic myelonecrosis. It is unclear whether amyotrophic lateral sclerosis occurs as a paraneoplastic syndrome.

Peripheral Polyneuropathy

Peripheral neuropathy can occur as a remote effect of tumor. Carcinomatous neuromyopathy, occurring most notably in lung cancer, is a distal peripheral polyneuropathy with associated proximal muscle weakness (97), type II fiber atrophy (98), weight loss, and variable electromyographic changes of proximal myopathy (99). The myopathic changes may be attributable to abnormalities in the intramuscular segments of axons, seen on electron microscopy (99).

Peripheral polyneuropathy has been described in various types of lung cancer (small cell, adenocarcinoma, undifferentiated) (97), as well as in multiple myeloma, breast, and colon malignancies (97). Subacute sensory neuropathy has been reported with carcinoma of the lung, breast, ovary, esophagus, and uterus, and with Hodgkin's disease and sarcoma (100,101). Sensory neuropathy has been associated with pathologic findings of widespread degeneration of the dorsal root ganglia with inflammatory cell infiltrate. Pain, paresthesias, and numb-

ness predominate, with unsteady gait. Face, bowel, and bladder are usually spared. Hematogenous metastases to the dorsal root ganglia also can occur, described with small cell carcinoma and poorly differentiated colon cancer (102). Subacute motor neuropathy occurs with lymphomas, especially Hodgkin's disease. Anterior horn cells degenerate, resulting in progressive weakness, followed by stabilization and subsequent improvement (96). Direct infiltration of roots and peripheral nerves is more likely to occur with lymphomas than with carcinoma.

Paraproteinemic neuropathies with monoclonal serum protein occur in association with multiple myeloma, osteosclerotic myeloma, Waldenström's macroglobulinemia, amyloidosis, gamma heavy-chain disease, and, most commonly, idiopathic cause. Typically the neuropathy is distal, mixed sensory and motor, with axonal loss and segmental demyelination. Amyloidosis often is characterized by autonomic involvement, infiltrative myopathy, and superimposed carpal tunnel syndrome. Compared with other paraproteinemic neuropathies, the neuropathy of osteosclerotic myeloma is most likely to respond to treatment of the underlying condition.

One of the most frequently causes of peripheral neuropathy in the cancer population is chemotherapy. Many agents have impact on the peripheral nervous system, which already may be vulnerable risk because of poor nutrition or prior radiation therapy. A description of the peripheral neuropathies, as well as the tumors or chemotherapies causing them, are presented in Table 81-8.

Treatment includes therapy for the underlying malignancy, and medication to treat pain or cramping includes carbamazepine, gabapentin quinidine, or tricyclic agents (98). Attention should be directed to appropriate nonconstrictive footwear to minimize the likelihood of ulceration resulting from poor sensory feedback. Other measures include exercise to maintain strength and range of motion, appropriate prescription of orthotics, assistive and adaptive devices, and energy conservation strategies.

Radiation-Induced Tissue Damage

Radiation therapy can be applied for curative or palliative intent. Used alone, it can be curative for certain carcinomas of the face, scalp, head and neck, upper esophagus, breast, genitourinary system, nervous system, or hematologic system. It is often used in combination with surgery (head and neck, breast, lung, gastrointestinal, genitourinary, nervous system, and sarcomas) or chemotherapy (small-cell carcinoma, Ewing's sarcoma, hematologic malignancies), or both (Wilms's tumor, rhabdomyosarcoma, and neuroblastoma) for curative intent (89). Use for palliation is indicated for symptom control or prevention, as in the case of pain, brain metastasis, or to prevent complications, such as pathologic fracture or superior vena cava syndrome (89).

Acute adverse effects of radiation therapy include fatigue, desquamation, oral cavity changes (decreased salivation, mucositis, dysphagia loss of taste), nausea, vomiting, anorexia, esophagitis, proctitis, urinary cystitis, decreased libido, sterility, amenorrhea, leukopenia, and thrombocytopenia. Subacute or late effects can include soft-tissue fibrosis with contracture, skin atrophy or ulceration, xerostomia, auditory or visual changes, Meniere's syndrome, osteonecrosis (with more than 6,000 rad), pulmonary fibrosis, gastrointestinal strictures, chronic cystitis or nephritis, impotence, sterility, endocrine insufficiency, brain necrosis, transverse myelitis, lymphedema, and late malignancies including sarcoma, skin cancers, and leukemia (89). Patients receiving combined chemotherapy and

TABLE 81-8. Peripheral Neuropathy in Cancer

Type of Neuropathy	Tumor	Chemotherapy
Distal sensorimotor axonal	Lung (all histologies)	Taxol
	Multiple myeloma (with or without amyloidosis)	Hexamethylmelamine (HMM)
	Leukemia, lymphoma (infiltrative)	Procarbazine
	Prostate, testis, kidney (vasculitic)	Etoposide
Sensory predominant	Lung, breast, ovary, Hodgkin's disease, gastrointestinal sites, kidney, testis, penis	Cisplatin, cytarabine (ARA-C) Platinum (DDP)
Motor predominant	Lung, leukemia (CML), penis	Vincristine (may progress to tetraparesis, involve cranial nerves, produce dysautonomia) Vinblastine
Subacute or chronic demyelinating	Lymphoma (especially Hodgkin's disease) Osteosclerotic myeloma Small cell	Suramin
Mononeuropathy multiplex (vasculitic)	Small cell, lymphoma	
Mononeuropathies	Small cell, multiple myeloma with amyloidosis Lymphoma or leukemia (especially cranial nerve involvement)	Platinum (DDP) hearing loss

radiation therapy are at risk for additive toxicities. Virtually all patients with head and neck cancer receiving radiation therapy develop oral complications.

After radiation therapy of 3,000 to 5,000 rad to bony metastatic lesions, remineralization is noted within 2 months and maximal at 3 months, and remodeling is completed at 6 months to 1 year (103). If the epiphysis is irradiated, growth will be arrested.

Brain effects can include acute changes, which are usually transient and more common with single doses greater than 300 rads; early delayed encephalopathy, presenting within several months due to demyelination; and late delayed encephalopathy (104). Early delayed encephalopathy, with incidence of about 5%, may be distinguished from tumor by its response to steroids (105), with improvement persisting after steroids are discontinued when radiation is the cause. Chronic delayed radiation encephalopathy (rare with a total dose of less than 5,600 rad) begins a year or two after treatment and causes coagulative necrosis of white matter, sparing the cortex. Response to corticosteroids is unpredictable. This chronic irreversible radionecrosis is rare compared with earlier-occurring syndromes (84). Memory loss or cognitive dysfunction may result from brain atrophy after whole-brain irradiation (104).

Radiation to the spinal cord can produce Lhermitte's syndrome (onset 1 to 4 months, lasting weeks to months), which can be seen in patients undergoing radiation for head and neck tumors. Transverse myelitis or delayed radiation myelopathy usually has its onset at 9 to 18 months, typically after more than 5,000 rad, often presenting as a Brown-Sequard syndrome or with radicular pain. For the latter, deficits usually progress slowly, then stabilize without improvement (104). Radiation-induced plexopathies occur and are late findings, seen months to years after completion of treatment (89), typically when more than 6000 rads have been given. (104)

Patients with radiation-induced skin damage should avoid sun exposure, rubbing (such as straps, belts, or collars), tape, or chemical irritants (such a perfumes or deodorants) to the affected site (89,106). For mild cases, improvement may be obtained with lotions such as baby oil or topical "vitamin A&D" ointment, or cornstarch in intertriginous areas. For more severe cases, options can include a topical corticosteroid (1% hydro-cortisone), cleansing with half-strength peroxide, or application of specialized wound care preparations (106).

Nutrition

IMPACT OF CANCER AND CANCER TREATMENTS ON NUTRITION

Cancer and its treatment can impede optimal nutrition. The malignancy itself can lead to cachexia. Weight loss may result from an increase in energy requirements. An increase in cytokines, such as tumor necrosis factor (also known as cachectin), may induce anaerobic glycolysis, fever, amino acid release from muscle, hepatic lipid secretion, and reduced albumin synthesis (107,108). Abnormalities in the regulation of anabolic hormones, such as insulin, growth hormone, and somatostatin, also may contribute to cachexia (108). Dysphagia is a common accompaniment of gastrointestinal and head and neck tumors.

Surgical therapies can interfere with the ability to eat (especially in patients with head and neck tumors) or in those with stomach or bowel tumors, producing malabsorption states with resulting nutritional depletion. Megaloblastic anemia can result from gastric resection that is due to loss of intrinsic factor for binding vitamin B_{12}. Bowel resection can produce deficiencies of vitamins B_{12}, D, B, and A, as well as water and electrolyte imbalance (107). Increased nutrition is needed to allow healing after major surgical procedures.

Radiation to the head and neck can alter taste and salivation and can interfere with swallowing (109). Radiation to the stomach or small intestine may produce nausea, vomiting, and the sensation of fullness. Over the long term, intestinal obstruction, perforation, bleeding, malabsorption, or fistulas may occur. Bowel rest and total parenteral nutrition may be needed in cases of severe radiation enteritis.

Chemotherapy commonly produces nausea, vomiting, and anorexia, as well as oral problems such as stomatitis, glossitis, pharyngitis, and mucosal ulceration. Prolonged vomiting can cause vitamin B_1 deficiency. Folic acid deficiency, common with methotrexate, can produce stomatitis, pharyngitis, gastroenteritis, and proctitis with malabsorption (107). Antimetabolites, such as 5-fluorouracil and 6-mercaptopurine, result in thymine deficiency, producing lip and oral cavity changes. Other common deficiencies are of vitamins B_2 and K. Edema may result from hypoproteinemia (107).

STRATEGIES TO OPTIMIZE NUTRITION

Measures should be taken to maximize intake by the oral route. Often antiemetics such as prochlorperazine, trimethobenzamide, or ondansetron are needed. Prokinetic agents, such as metoclopramide, can be employed to ease early satiety that is due to gastric stasis (110). Oral supplements may be more easily ingested or tolerated than solid foods. Learned food aversions are common, a conditioned response from associating consumption of a food with subsequent gastrointestinal symptoms. To avoid developing aversion to familiar or preferred food items, one might avoid consuming those in the 24 hours before receiving the therapy that produces nausea. Meats, vegetables, and caffeinated beverages in particular often produce food aversions. In patients with dumping syndrome after gastric surgery, small frequent meals should be taken. Medications used as appetite stimulants have included progesterone agents, cxprophetadine, glucocorticoids, and cannabinoids, although side effects can be significant (110). In recent years, there has also been attention to anabolic steroids, especially oxandrolone, and to cytokine inhibitors such as thalidomide; the latter is only available in clinical trials (110). For hyposalivation, dry-mouth products are available in many forms: gum, toothpaste, rinses, etc. Pilocarpine can promote increased salivary flow (107). Medications with anticholinergic side effects should be avoided. Nutritional counseling is often of benefit to advise about strategies for maximizing oral intake. Patients need to be counselled not to rely on appetite alone, because this will be insufficient. Patients may have strong opinions—often complete misconceptions or based on no factual data—about the role of specific foods in being causative or curative of their malignancy. They may be taking toxic doses of nutritional supplements such as fat-soluble vitamins (107). Attention should be paid to adequate fluid intake as well as adequate calories.

Numerous studies have examined parenteral nutrition in the cancer population; findings regarding efficacy have been mixed, and complications such as infection related to the central line can occur. Parenteral nutrition does appear to be of benefit perioperatively in patients who are severely malnourished, and in bone marrow transplant recipients (111).

Cancer-Related Sexual Dysfunction and Its Management

Sexual dysfunction may occur as a primary effect of malignancy but more commonly occurs as a side effect of treatment. Sexual function can be affected by disturbance at many levels, including psychologic, central or peripheral nervous system, endocrine, pelvic vascular, and local effects on gonadal structures. Physical changes may interfere with the patient's concept of his or her sexual attractiveness. Depression may result in low sexual drive. Psychologic distress with impact on sexual function may be more common in younger adults with cancer than in older individuals (112). Sexual dysfunction in cancer patients may persist long after treatment is completed, and thus it is important for the practitioner to inquire about it (113).

Endocrine effects occur in men with prostate cancer treated with orchiectomy or with hormonal regimens to reduce serum testosterone. Sexual desire and function is reduced, but is preserved in a minority of cases.

In men, chemotherapy can have adverse effects on spermatogenesis and testosterone production. Neuropathies, including dysautonomia, can impact sexual function, including the emission phase of male orgasm. Common complications of chemotherapy in men include low sexual desire, erectile dysfunction, dry orgasm, and reduced pleasure with orgasm (112). Less is known about the effects of chemotherapy on female sexual function, but alkylating agents have the most gonadal toxicity. Permanent menopause may occur with combination chemotherapy, accompanied by menopausal symptoms, such as hot flashes. Vaginal mucosal changes can lead to dyspareunia (112).

Radiation therapy to the prostate or testicles can produce erectile dysfunction, possibly as a result of acceleration of pre-existing atherosclerosis from postradiation fibrotic changes. In women, radiation therapy to the pelvis produces premature menopause, with a dose of as low as 600 to 1,000 rad permanently destroying ovarian function. Radiation also produces damage to the vaginal epithelium, and the fibrotic process can continue over years. The result can be dyspareunia, postcoital bleeding, even vaginal ulcers. After local radiation therapy for cervical cancer, stenosis of the upper vagina can occur. Vaginal dilators can preserve the integrity of the vagina. Estrogen therapy also may be of some benefit, as well as vaginal lubricants (112).

Radical prostatectomy has a high rate of erectile dysfunction, although newer surgical procedures sparing the neurovascular bundles permits gradual (up to 1 year) recovery of erectile function (114). More rarely, urinary incontinence occurs. Similar problems may occur after radical cystectomy and abdominoperineal resection of gastrointestinal tumors (115) (lesser incidence of erectile dysfunction after low anterior resection) (114). Sperm banking before surgery should be considered because of incidence of reduced emission secondary to sympathetic plexus dissection. Generally one waits about 6 months after treatment before considering surgery for a penile prosthesis because erectile dysfunction may gradually improve on its own. Medications that may be of benefit for erectile dysfunction include sildenafil (especially with mild erectile dysfunction), bupropion, and, when appropriate, testosterone replacement (113). Vacuum devices and penile injection with papaverine are also options, but have high dropout rates (113).

For women that have undergone resection of pelvic tumors, specific surgical reconstructive measures may be indicated, such as reconstruction of the vagina or labia via myocutaneous flap or split-thickness skin grafting to repair stenosis of the vaginal introitus (112). Among women with history of early-stage cervical cancer, about one-fourth report significant vaginal changes, regardless of the treatment method (116). Vaginal relaxation exercises, vaginal dilators, and water-based lubricants also may be helpful (113,114,117). In general, greasy lubricants, such as petroleum jelly, should be avoided because they may block the urethral opening (115).

Counseling is an important technique in treating sexual disorders in cancer patients because despite the sometimes profound physiologic or anatomic changes, psychologic adjustment has been found to be a more important determinant of sexual satisfaction (117). Counseling is usually short term and optimally includes both partners. Disease or treatment-specific effects on sexual function should be discussed with the patient, including the use of drawings or diagrams when appropriate (115).

Timing of resumption of sexual activity can be an important factor for patients with fatigue, ostomies, or significant psychological trauma associated with their cancer diagnosis. Peer support through ostomy groups can be of benefit (115). Patients should be encouraged to maintain a healthy body through fitness and other strategies, as well as a good personal image. The American Cancer Society's *Look Good, Feel Better and Reach to Recovery* programs can be very helpful (117). Regardless of whether formal counseling is pursued, patients should be encouraged to pursue and not avoid physical closeness and intimacy. The varied aspects of an intimate relationship should be encouraged (117).

SPECIFIC TUMORS AND THEIR REHABILITATION NEEDS

Breast Cancer

The rehabilitation for women with breast cancer should be divided into two groups: those with local disease and disability and those with systemic illness and disability. The general goal for both groups is to help the patient reach her desired level of function when possible. This process is accomplished via education and building a therapeutic alliance that addresses the problems and complications the patient may face. Patients with primary breast cancer are likely to experience limitation of shoulder motion postoperatively and incisional pain of the chest wall (and axillary region for those undergoing mastectomy), and up to 20% may develop lymphedema (118,119). Patients with recurrent regional disease are likely to have shoulder and arm symptoms, not unlike the primary breast cancer patients, and development of lymphedema is likely. Those with distant and metastatic disease are likely to have spread to bone, lung, and liver. Numerous studies of exercise have examined the breast cancer population and found benefits (see previous sections, "Cancer-Related Fatigue" and "Exercise for the Cancer Patient: General Aspects").

POSTSURGICAL ISSUES

Definitive surgical treatment for breast cancer depends on the classification of the tumor and the preference of the patient for breast-conserving therapy or not. The modified radical mastectomy removes all breast tissue and a sampling of axillary nodes. Usually, the pectoralis minor is preserved. In the lumpectomy treatment, only tumor and a margin of breast tissue is removed, and an axillary sampling is taken. The chest is subsequently radiated, as is the axilla when more than three nodes are positive for tumor. The decision to irradiate the supraclavicular region is dependent on the extent of the surgery. Complications of mastectomy include wound complications, axillary web syndrome (120), phantom breast sensations, and arm edema; those that occur after radiation include chest wall pain, shoulder stiffness, and arm edema. Sentinel lymph node dissection shows promise in reducing the morbidity of axillary dissection (121,122). Patients undergoing immediate reconstruction with transverse rectus abdominis myocutaneous (TRAM) flap make similar gains in range of motion as non-TRAM patients (123).

Shoulder mobility and strength are negatively influenced by the extent of surgery, radiation dose and schedule of delivery, and amount of postoperative pain (124,125). Pain should be treated with adequate analgesia, use of heat or cold, and early, but not immediate, mobilization (126). Active motion only should be performed until the drains are out. Includes internal/external rotation to tolerance should be performed from the first postoperative day onward. Until day 4, 40 to 45 degrees of flexion and abduction are permitted. From days 4 to 6, flexion should be advanced from 45 degrees to 90 degrees, but abduction should remain at 45 degrees. Thereafter, flexion, abduction, and rotation should be performed to tolerance. Imme-

diate mobilization through range has been associated with more lymph drainage and wound complications (127,128). Once healing has occurred, there is no need to restrict functional and customary activity.

The use of the overhead pulley helps restore range of motion. However, performing exercises in recumbency is also useful to provide scapular support, especially if there has been damage to the serratus anterior. Transient muscle weakness of the shoulder girdle muscles also may occur (126). Isometric exercise, using resistive elastic bands and gradually progressing to isotonic exercise, is recommended. Recovery of range of motion and strength is usually complete.

LYMPHEDEMA

Lymphedema or a sense of fullness in the arm even without circumferential changes of more than 2 cm are frequently reported by patients undergoing mastectomy or lumpectomy. It tends to develop over a protracted period of time, and the median interval between treatment and presentation is 39 months (119). Risk factors for lymphedema include extent of surgery, receipt of axillary radiation, obesity, and possibly surgical technique (119,125). Comorbid impairments, including range-of-motion deficits, reduced strength, neurologic deficits, pain, and impaired self-care are common (129). Needlesticks should be avoided in the affected limb, but if considered necessary, as for diagnostic or therapeutic procedures for comorbid conditions, should be kept to a minimum, performed with strict aseptic technique, and a stepping-up of the patient's usual lymphedema control regimen (130). Prevention of lymphedema depends on two factors: (a) not interfering with lymph outflow, hence not constricting the arm, and protecting from infection, scarring, and burns; and (b) limiting lymph production by using compression garments when exercising and avoiding vasodilation through heat exposure (sun, sauna, and steam). Raising the arm against gravity is useful. Use of a compression garment that uses 30 to 40 mm Hg (rarely 50 mm Hg) also is effective. There is controversy about the usefulness of compression pumps, either single- or multichannel machines. Some efficacy has been shown to be for this approach (131,132), and it is often advocated, especially in severe cases or when other measures have had only limited success. Manual lymph drainage has been shown effective. The technique requires training in a delicate massage technique, compression bandaging, and a series of exercises (Fig. 81-3) (133). Several reports have surfaced indicating efficacy of the use of benzopyrones, which stimulate macrophage-induced protein breakdown, in the treatment of chronic lymphedema (134); however, one recent study did not show benefit (135). Efficacy of surgical treatments for this problem is not proven. Lymph-edema management entails a daily lifelong regimen, and thus obtaining adequate control represents a significant commitment for the affected person. The

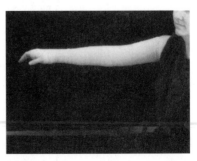

Figure 81-3. Compressive bandage for lymphedema.

TABLE 81-9. Management of Lymphedema in Breast Cancer Patients

	Strategy	Examples
Standard	Education in prevention and precautions	Maintain skin integrity, avoid unaccustomed exertion of the limb; avoid constricting straps or garments
	Attention to comorbidities	Infection; pain syndromes, contracture; self-care impairment; nerve injury or entrapment (including carpal tunnel syndrome); skin ulceration or serous drainage
	Limb elevation	
	Wraps	Short stretch bandaging
	Gradient compression garments	Sleeve; glove; gauntlet
	Exercise	Active exercises; stretches; deep breathing
	Massage	
Controversial; for refractory cases	Compression pumping (attention to precautions, which empirically include local infection, presence of tumor, and, in severe cases, potential for poor cardiac tolerance of fluid shifts; anticoagulation a relative contraindication)	Three-chamber models; (various systems); (multichamber overlapping air chambers clyonphapress)
Unproven	Surgery	
	Medications	Benzopyrones (conflicting data) Diuretics (temporary effect only)

right measures for a particular patient will be determined by the severity and location of the edema, by presence of complications or comorbidities (infections; recurrent or residual tumor), and patient preference, which optimizes compliance with the regimen (Table 81-9).

SYSTEMIC COMPLICATIONS
Involvement of the skeleton, lungs or pleura, and CNS in patients with breast cancer presents a significant problem to the rehabilitation team. Metastatic disease is often accompanied by significant pain, fatigue, mobility, and self-care deficits, as well as depression. It is also a period of resumption of treatment, often including radiation, surgery, and chemotherapies. For some patients, newer experimental treatments are also used. It is a period of great uncertainty, and anxiety and sleep disruption are common. The major goals for the rehabilitation professionals at this stage of the disease are (a) to achieve good pain relief and comfort, (b) to enable self-care and as near normal social and vocational activities as possible, (c) to assure bony stability of the skeleton and long bones, (d) to maintain stamina and strength, and (e) to provide education and support while being realistically hopeful.

The sites for bone metastases in breast cancer are those bones rich in marrow: vertebrae, pelvis, ribs, and proximal long bones. The medical consequences of this involvement include fracture, neurologic compromise (spinal cord or peripheral motor/neuropathy), or metabolic complications. Often the patient presents with dull pain that is nocturnal and often not relieved with rest. Lytic changes with some sclerotic foci are the most characteristic radiographic findings of metastatic breast cancer (see previous section, "Bony Metastatic Disease," for further discussion of long bone and spine metastasis).

Plexopathy that is due to tumor invasion is reported in 4% to 5% of patients attending a cancer pain center (136). The most frequent presenting symptom is pain, which is usually antecedent to paresthesias or focal weakness (137). Pain is usually moderately severe and originates in the shoulder girdle with radiation to the elbow, medial forearm, and fingers. Because 75% of patients have sensory involvement of the lower plexus (138) and 25% have involvement of the entire plexus, sensation in the fourth and fifth fingers is more commonly affected (C7–C8, T1) than thumb and index (C5–C6).

Differentiation between tumor infiltration and radiation-induced plexopathy is often difficult. Spread of tumor through lymphatics will cause lower-trunk involvement because of the proximity of the lymph nodes to the lower trunk. Few nodes are adjacent to the upper trunk. Radiation-induced plexopathy occurs, on average, 5.5 years from therapy (137). Paresthesias occur most commonly, and pain is less common and less severe than in tumor-induced plexopathy. The upper trunk is more frequently involved.

The diagnosis of tumor or radiation-induced plexopathy may require MRI or positron-emission tomography scan to distinguish soft-tissue changes. Electromyography will show fibrillation potentials and positive waves. The presence of myokymic discharges suggest radiation-induced changes (139).

Head and Neck Cancer

Head and neck cancer and its treatment can result in major effects on communication, nutrition, swallowing, dental health, and musculoskeletal function (Table 81-10). Most head and neck malignancies are squamous cell carcinomas. Lesions usually arise at the surface but may invade muscle and spread along muscle or fascial planes. Bone or cartilage invasion usually does not occur until later in the disease process. Perineural

TABLE 81-10. Head and Neck Cancer

Intervention[a]	Impairment
Glossectomy	Communication; dysphagia
Mandibulectomy	Chewing
Radical neck dissection	Shoulder depression and protraction, facial lymphedema; neck asymmetry
Radiation therapy	Contracture (neck, jaw); osteonecrosis; dental changes; decreased salivary flow; dysphagia (usually mild); trismus; central nervous system complications
Partial laryngectomy	Dysphagia; communication
Total laryngectomy	Communication (severe); dysphagia (mild)
Soft palate resection	Communication; dysphagia
Nasopharyngeal tumors/treatment	Cranial nerve abnormalities
Salivary gland tumors/ resection	Facial nerve palsy

[a]See text for treatment strategies

spread may track to the base of the skull, or less commonly, peripherally (140). Lymphatic spread commonly occurs; however, distant metastasis is much less common, and therefore staging workup for distant metastasis is not performed unless the patient is symptomatic (141). Surgery and radiation therapy are the only curative treatment options. Depending on the location, size, and extention of the lesion, either radiation or surgery may be used as the initial option and may or may not need to be followed by the other. Preliminary data in one study found patient report of quality of life to be lower in the group receiving combination treatment than surgery alone. There were no significant differences in swallowing status or speech intelligibility between the groups (142). Comorbid factors, such as alcohol and tobacco abuse, poor nutritional state, diabetes, and pulmonary and cardiovascular disease are common.

RADICAL NECK DISSECTION

Radical neck dissection is performed in cases of locally extensive disease or recurrence (141) and involves removal of the sternocleidomastoid muscle, internal and external jugular veins, spinal accessory nerve, and submandibular gland as a single unit. Deep to the dissection in the posterior triangle lie the nerves to the rhomboids, the long thoracic nerve, brachial plexus (trunk level), subclavian vessels, and phrenic nerve. This area has been referred to as the danger zone and is not routinely included in the dissection. When the spinal accessory nerve is not involved, a modified radical neck dissection can be performed, sparing shoulder function. In some cases, more limited dissection of regional lymph nodes may be appropriate (141).

Complications of radical neck dissection include lymphedema, wound infection and dehiscence, injury to cranial nerves VII, X, and XII, and carotid injury. Asymmetric neck motion results from removal of the sternocleidomastoid, platysma, and other muscles, and shoulder dysfunction from sacrifice of the spinal accessory nerve (143). Loss of trapezius function results in shoulder depression and protraction, and this malalignment produces incomplete and painful active excursion of the shoulder, often with range of abduction of less than 90 degrees. The rhomboids and levator scapula become overstretched and the pectoralis major shortened (143). The sternoclavicular joint bears increased weight from the arm, leading to clavicle subluxation and arthritic changes (144).

Rehabilitation treatment is directed toward preventing or correcting the above deformities. Passive neck range of motion, emphasizing flexion and rotation, is begun when sutures are removed, to the limits of graft or suture line stretch, progressing to active range of motion and isometric strengthening by week 4 (143). Neck exercise is contraindicated if there is felt to be significant risk of carotid rupture, and prolonged coughing also should be discouraged in this setting to avoid increased intrathoracic pressure (145). Some patients with chronic obstructive pulmonary disease may use the sternocleidomastoid and platysma for accessory respiration and may become transiently more dyspneic after this muscle function is lost. Energy conservation measures and breathing exercises can be taught (145). In the setting of radiation therapy, which produces soft-tissue fibrosis and contracture, especially in higher doses, the patient should receive instruction in neck range of motion pretreatment and perform the exercises throughout the radiation course and for an indefinite period thereafter.

The shoulder program includes strengthening, especially of scapular stabilizers such as the serratus anterior, rhomboids, and levator scapula, and stretching of the protractors (144). Internal rotation, which results in protraction, should be avoided. The patient should not do strenuous activities, such as lifting heavy objects with the affected side (143). Spinal accessory nerve grafting may be an option. In the case of neurapraxic lesions, functional electrical stimulation can be considered to maintain the contractile elements as recovery occurs (143).

ORAL MALIGNANCIES AND TREATMENT EFFECTS

In addition to soft-tissue fibrosis in the neck, radiation therapy may induce dental and salivary abnormalities, limited jaw motion, and laryngeal edema with voice changes. The voice changes, such as change in quality or reduced volume, may be most prominent at the end of the day.

Radiation-induced dental disease is due largely to decreased salivary flow (146) and to a lesser extent to a direct effect on the teeth and surrounding soft tissues. Saliva becomes sticky (143), and the patient may convert to a soft, high-carbohydrate diet that further promotes dental caries and plaque. Routine dental hygiene also becomes more painful. Diligent dental follow-up is important to minimize extent of dental caries. Artificial saliva products are recommended (143). Mechanical débridement of the tongue with a soft toothbrush and use of a spray mister before meals maximizes taste-bud access, facilitating the psychic stimulation component of salivary gland secretion (146). A sodium fluoride gel should be used daily, and diluted peroxide, saline rinses, or salt and baking soda (1 teaspoon of each in 1 quart of water) (106) can be used during the course of treatment to cleanse the mouth. Sugarless gum or lozenges may stimulate salivation (143). Pilocarpine has been shown to stimulate saliva production (146). Diet should emphasize fluids, moist foods, and high-calorie supplements. For edentulous patients, one should wait 6 months after radiation therapy before replacing dentures secondary to gingival shrinking and remodeling (143).

Techniques for improving jaw motion include active stretching exercises, mechanical stretching progressively with tongue blades or other devices (such as Therabite, Therabite Corp, Newton Square, PA), and continuous passive motion devices (147).

Drooling or microstomia may result after excision of lip lesions. Mandibulectomy can affect cosmesis and the ability to chew, especially anterior mandible (arch) resections (141). Reconstructive procedures may be considered (141). After unilateral mandibular resections, strengthening of masticatory muscles is needed to prevent drift to the nonsurgical side (143).

Tongue lesions will affect speech and swallowing, especially if extensive muscle infiltration has occurred. Palsy of the hypoglossal nerve rarely occurs from direct invasion in posterior tongue lesions, or postirradiation or surgery (140). Glossectomy is performed initially if the lesion is deeply infiltrative at presentation. Typically, if more than 50% of the tongue is resected, significant speech and swallowing impairments result (148). Enunciation difficulties result if the tongue is bound down by scarring. Radiation therapy produces tongue sensitivity, which is temporary, reduced taste sensation, which usually improves over time, and dry mouth. Fibrosis of the base of the tongue postradiation therapy produces dysphagia, but aspiration is rare (140). Local and systemic pain management strategies for painful soft-tissue necrosis may be needed (140). After glossectomy, the patient should be instructed in strengthening and range of motion of residual tongue tissue, especially if radiation therapy is to follow. The program usually begins 10 to 14 days after surgery. If the residual tongue tissue is unable to contact the hard palate, a palate-lowering prosthesis can be offered (148). Compensatory strategies, such as forward or backward head tilts and strengthening of buccal musculature, may facilitate deglutition. Oral transit can be achieved with use of a syringe or pusher spoon (143).

Buccal mucosa and tonsillar lesions often refer pain to the ear. Trismus may result from posterior extension to the buccinator, pterygoid, or masseter muscles or from high radiation doses to these muscles (149). Soft-palate lesions, when advanced, can cause dysphagia and voice change. If soft-tissue destruction occurs, material may be regurgitated into the nasopharynx. After soft-palate resection, a prosthesis is needed to restore velopharyngeal competence.

Salivary gland tumors often result in facial nerve impairment, either from the tumor itself or after surgery. Facial nerve palsy often recovers over a few months; nerve grafting techniques have also been employed (150).

Strategies for improved communication include use of good eye contact and appropriate gestures, and oral exercises for articulation, and any necessary modification of pitch, loudness, and voice quality (151).

LARYNGEAL AND PHARYNGEAL MALIGNANCIES

Laryngeal lesions are divided into supraglottic, glottic, and subglottic sites. Glottic tumors usually present early with hoarseness, and lymphatic spread is rare because of a sparse lymphatic network. True vocal cord tumors are considered among the most treatable of head and neck tumors, with cure rate of more than 80% (141). Supraglottic lesions most commonly involve the epiglottis but may affect the aryepiglottic fold and false vocal cord and are more likely to undergo regional lymphatic spread (152,153). The subglottic area extends from about 5 mm below the vocal cords to the inferior border of the cricoid cartilage. Lesions in this area are uncommon (153).

Surgical options include vocal cord stripping, hemilaryngectomy and supraglottic laryngectomy (which preserve the voice), and total laryngectomy. With the latter, a permanent tracheostomy is placed, and the pharynx is sutured to the base of the tongue (152). Patients may learn esophageal speech or may use electronic devices for speech. Tracheoesophageal puncture, in which exhaled air is channeled through a voice prosthesis into the esophagus, can result in a more natural-sounding voice than with other communication methods (Fig. 81-4). During speech, the tracheostomy is occluded with a finger or one-way valve (154).

Patients with preexisting pulmonary impairment, specifically low forced expiratory volume in 1 second/forced vital capacity (FEV_1/FVC) ratio are more likely to have intractable aspiration after supraglottic laryngectomy (155). Other risk factors for long-term dysphagia include bilateral supraglottic laryngectomy, bilateral superior laryngeal nerve excision (156), sacrifice of the tongue base (140), and possibly combined treatment with radiation therapy (156). Many patients experience postoperative dysphagia that is transient, with as many as 85% of supraglottic laryngectomy patients attaining a functional swallow (improved from only 39% in the early postoperative period) (155). Techniques such as breath holding during the swallow and throat clear afterward may prevent or minimize aspiration (143). When feasible, occluding the tracheostomy decreases frequency and amount of aspiration (157). In our experience, delayed onset of dysphagia even after many years can rarely occur.

Pharyngeal tumors often involve the pyriform sinus. The recurrent laryngeal nerve may be involved. Extensive regional infiltration is common. Initial symptoms are often unilateral. Partial or total laryngopharyngectomy may be indicated. Total laryngopharyngectomy may be combined with reconstruction from a myocutaneous flap. Either of these procedures may be complicated by fistula, and in the case of the partial laryngopharyngectomy, by dysphagia and aspiration (152). Those

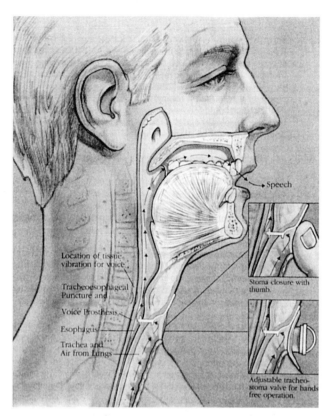

Figure 81-4. Tracheoesophageal fistula for speech production in the laryngectomy patient. Diagram courtesy of InHealth Corporation.

with hypopharyngeal tumors are at greatest risk of severe and permanent dysphagia (148). In some cases, conversion to total laryngectomy has been done to allow eating, but not with consistent success, as this procedure makes it even more difficult to generate enough pressure to drive the bolus through the pharynx (148).

Nasopharyngeal tumors have a high incidence, about 25%, of associated cranial nerve symptoms. Cavernous sinus invasion affects cranial nerves II through VI, and extension from the lateral pharyngeal space laterally can involve nerves IX through XII and the sympathetic chain. Facial neuralgia may result from trigeminal nerve involvement (140). Surgical resection is often not feasible. Radiation therapy complications can include radiation encephalopathy, especially involving the hypothalamus, pituitary, and frontal and temporal lobes; recovery usually occurs (140). Radiation myelitis of the cervical cord or brain stem can be more severe. Radiation fibrosis involving the pterygoid muscles causes trismus, and involvement of the lateral pharyngeal space can cause palsy of cranial nerves IX through XII as a delayed complication (140). Treatment of nasal cavity and paranasal sinus tumors can produce CNS complications, including radiation-induced CNS disease, cerebrospinal fluid leak, meningitis, brain abscess, and a delayed, transient vertiginous syndrome (140).

Hematologic Malignancies

Hematologic malignancies include tumors involving the lymphatics and hematopoietic system. They can result in fatigue as well as more localized disabling effects. Lymphomas include Hodgkin's disease and non-Hodgkin's lymphomas. Non-Hodgkin's lymphomas are seen with increased frequency in patients with acquired immunodeficiency syndrome (AIDS) and in individuals who are immunosuppressed after transplant surgery (158). Many of these cases are primary CNS lymphomas, up to 50% of lymphomas occurring in transplant patients (89). Bone marrow disorders include acute and chronic leukemias and myeloproliferative disorders, such as polycythemia vera, myelofibrosis, and primary thrombocytopenia. Immunoproliferative diseases include multiple myeloma and Waldenström's macroglobulinemia (89).

LYMPHOMAS

Lymphomas characteristically invade lymphatics but can readily invade any tissue. Non-Hodgkin's lymphoma has a greater propensity to invade extranodal sites than Hodgkin's disease (159). Lymphomas are frequently associated with bone pain as a result of tumor invasion. Neuritic pain may result from nerve root infiltration, spinal cord compression, or herpes zoster. Lymphomas have been associated with acute inflammatory demyelinating polyneuropathy. Lymphedema can result from lymphatic obstruction, and thrombophlebitis from extrinsic compression on adjacent veins. Depressed cell-mediated immunity in Hodgkin's disease results in increased risk of opportunistic infection. Herpes zoster is common and may assume a disseminated form (89). Standard chemotherapy with MOPP (mechlorethamine, vincristine, prednisone, and procarbazine) or other vincristine-containing regimens may result in peripheral polyneuropathy (89). Thoracic (mantle) radiation therapy may be complicated by radiation pneumonitis, cardiac abnormalities (constrictive pericarditis, cardiomyopathy), and hypothyroidism (89). Aseptic necrosis of the femoral heads is described in 10% of long-term survivors of inverted y-field (abdominopelvic) irradiation and MOPP (89,160).

Non-Hodgkin's lymphoma is often widely disseminated at the time of presentation. Depending of the aggressiveness of the tumor, treatment of advanced disease may range from a "watch and wait" approach to single- or multiple-agent chemotherapy regimens, to bone marrow transplantation (159). In recent years, newer techniques, such as monoclonal antibody therapy (rituximab) and radioactive monoclonal antibodies, show promise of effectiveness, with a minimum of side effects (89). Aggressive lymphomas, such as Burkitt's lymphoma, which typically presents in childhood, and lymphoblastic lymphoma, which presents in young adulthood, can progress and disseminate rapidly. CNS, skin, and bone marrow involvement are common (159).

Mycosis fungoides is a cutaneous T-cell lymphoma involving helper T-lymphocytes. Patients have significant itching and skin management problems with this lymphoma. Whirlpool treatment may be of benefit for the intractable pruritus and widespread skin scaling that can occur.

IMMUNOPROLIFERATIVE DISORDERS

Immunoproliferative diseases, such as multiple myeloma and Waldenström's macroglobulinemia, occur in older individuals (average age 60 years at diagnosis). With multiple myeloma, multiple lytic lesions are seen in about 70% of patients, single osteolytic lesions or diffuse osteoporosis in 15%, and normal x-rays in 15% (89). The skull, vertebrae, ribs, pelvis, and proximal long bones are the most common sites of involvement (89). Bone scans are of limited usefulness and are only positive in areas of fracture or arthritis, or areas of perilesional osteoblastic activity. Osteoblastic lesions are rare (incidence of less than 2%) and often occur with neuropathy (89). Painful pathologic fractures are common. Neurologic dysfunction is common, including spinal cord or nerve root compression from epidural plasmacytoma, amyloidosis, or vertebral body collapse. Cranial

nerve palsies occur from tumor occluding calvarial foramina, and focal peripheral neuropathies, such as carpal tunnel syndrome, from soft-tissue amyloid infiltration (89). Fatigue, weakness, and weight loss are common. Bone lesions are responsive to radiation therapy, which can be used for pain control and to shrink a bone mass before fracture occurs. Alkylating agents with or without prednisone are also used. Ambulation should be encouraged, with bracing or assistive devices as needed to control pain. Waldenström's macroglobulinemia may produce neurologic symptoms on the basis of hyperviscosity, such as malaise, stroke, and even coma (89).

LEUKEMIA

The leukemias produce fatigue. Bone pain may result from leukemic masses in the bone marrow (89). Leukostasis can produce severe CNS abnormalities when the white blood count is more than 100,000, especially in the later acute stage of chronic myelogenous leukemia. Cerebrospinal fluid involvement may occur, producing leukemic meningitis with associated cranial nerve palsy and mental status changes (160). In children, the skeleton is often the first body system to manifest abnormality, and acute leukemia must be included in the differential diagnosis of unexplained musculoskeletal pain or bony pathology (161).

REHABILITATION INTERVENTIONS FOR PATIENTS WITH HEMATOPOIETIC MALIGNANCIES

Rehabilitation intervention for leukemias and lymphomas involves active exercise, including walking, to maintain endurance (stamina) during the treatment course, which is often protracted. Precautions surround the risk of bleeding in thrombocytopenic patients (see "Exercise for the Cancer Patient: General Aspects," previous section); pressure palsies, especially in patients receiving neurotoxic drugs or with severe immobilization; and orthostasis, especially in those on fluid restriction or with poor nutritional state (160). Restricted weight bearing is advised for bony extensive infiltration or aseptic necrosis.

Bone marrow transplant recipients have additional needs. High-dose steroids are needed to counteract graft-versus-host disease, with potential complications including steroid myopathy, aseptic necrosis, and osteoporosis. The exercise program should include proximal muscle strengthening, back extension, and upper-extremity weight bearing (160). (See previous section, "Exercise for the Cancer Patient: General Aspects," for further discussion of exercise for bone marrow transplant recipients.)

Lung Cancer

Lung malignancies remain very common and are challenging for the physiatrist. Cure is possible in some cases, especially when the disease is detected early and in an operable location, but generally the prognosis remains poor. This often poses a dilemma for the physiatrist because lung cancer produces the fatigue and deconditioning that occur with virtually any chronic illness (plus the fatigue of pulmonary disease), as well as myriad potential neurologic complications. These include peripheral polyneuropathy, mixed sensory-motor axonal in type, and, more rarely, a sensory polyneuropathy that is due to dorsal root ganglionitis. Myasthenic syndrome is linked to small-cell carcinoma and may or may not respond to treatment of the underlying malignancy. Nerve root infiltration may occur, producing pain and weakness. Vertebral bony involvement can produce extradural spinal cord compression, and brain metastasis is common, resulting in severe neurologic impairment. Apical lung tumors, such as Pancoast tumor, can invade the brachial plexus or lower cervical nerve roots by direct extension, producing pain as an early symptom that is often referred to the shoulder; appropriate diagnosis may be delayed while the patient is treated for a nonexistent musculoskeletal shoulder problem. Eventually a full-blown brachial plexopathy occurs, with paresthesias, weakness, and numbness, characteristically involving the lower fibers more than upper fibers.

The neurologic complications often occur early in the clinical course and may even be the presenting feature. Thus, the patient and family are coping with the new diagnosis and with the functional impact of the neurologic complications simultaneously. Often the family is willing but ill equipped to care for the patient at home. In selected cases, a short rehabilitation admission may be appropriate to train the patient and family in safe mobility strategies and to assess for appropriate adaptive equipment. Caution is advised, however, as a traditional rehabilitation admission may not be the best way for the patient to spend his or her remaining days.

Strategies for pain management (see previous section, "General Approach to Cancer-Related Pain"), as well as education about pulmonary hygiene and breathing techniques, may be useful. Patients treated with surgical resection (either lobectomy or pneumonectomy) should be instructed in techniques to promote maximal chest expansion, including coughing, pursed-lip breathing (inhalation through the nose, exhalation through pursed lips), diaphragmatic breathing (patient places hands over the abdomen to consciously promote expansion with inspiration), and segmental (hand over upper or lower portion of the rib cage during inhalation) breathing exercises. Postoperatively, cough may be best tolerated with the knees flexed, and the incision splinted by firm pressure from a pillow or towel roll. Trunk posture and mobility exercise, lower-extremity exercise, and early progressive ambulation are recommended (164).

Gastrointestinal Malignancies

Colorectal cancer is the fourth most prevalent carcinoma in the United States, the second leading cause of cancer death, and the only major malignancy that affects men and women almost equally (163). Efforts in recent years have focused on screening for early detection, as Dukes' disease (tumor limited to the mucosa) is 85% to 95% curable (163). Five-year survival with colon cancer (all stages) has improved somewhat, but is only 62% overall. Surgery is considered the only curative treatment, at times combined with adjuvant chemotherapy or radiation. Pancreatic cancer remains among the most refractory to cure of all malignancies, and favorable prognostic indicators have not been delineated (164). Esophageal, liver, and stomach malignancies also carry a poor prognosis. In general, when liver metastasis occurs, the clinical state deteriorates rapidly (this is also true for nongastrointestinal malignancies).

Gastrointestinal malignancies are low to intermediate in risk for metastasis to bone and neurologic structures. Most often, rehabilitation is indicated for deconditioning, often occurring after extensive abdominal surgical procedures. In selected cases, a short rehabilitation course before return home is beneficial. Tolerance to active therapy and overall medical stability will determine whether this is done on an acute or subacute level. In postsurgical cases, close communication with the referring surgeon is important for management of drains and potential complications.

Brain Tumors

BRAIN TUMOR TYPES: CHARACTERISTICS AND PROGNOSTIC IMPLICATIONS

Brain tumors vary widely in aggressiveness and in prognosis. However, unlike most other regions in the body, even a benign or relatively low-grade lesion may have severe functional consequences, depending on location and the extent to which excision is feasible. Brain-stem lesions in particular can have a profound impact on motor function, cranial nerves, swallowing, and coordination. In patients who have undergone resection, communication with the referring surgeon as to which structures have been sacrificed will be important in advising the patient about recovery of neurologic function.

In adults, meningiomas are the most common benign brain tumor, comprising about 15% of all primary brain tumors. Their growth may have a hormonal component, and increased incidence is seen in breast cancer patients (87). Other benign tumors include pituitary adenomas, acoustic neuromas, craniopharyngiomas, epidermoid tumors, colloid cysts of the third ventricle, and hemangioblastomas associated with Von-Hippel-Lindau disease. Pituitary adenomas present with features of hormonal hypersecretion, bitemporal visual field loss, or headache (87). Variants include prolactinomas, growth hormone producing adenomas causing acromegaly, and corticotrophin-secreting adenomas producing Cushing's disease. Most are resectable. Acoustic neuromas grow on the nerve sheath of the vestibular nerve and may occur sporadically or with neurofibromatosis. Patients can develop hearing loss, vertigo, facial palsy, dysphagia, facial numbness, and even hydrocephalus. Results of microsurgery are generally good, especially with tumors measuring less than 2 cm (87). Craniopharyngiomas arise from pharyngeal epithelium, presenting with growth failure in children and sexual dysfunction or visual loss in adults. After treatment, deficits in memory, behavior, appetite, and endocrine function are common. Adjunctive radiation therapy is often used, with great improvement in the 10-year survival rate (87).

More than 90% of primary brain malignancies are malignant gliomas (165), subdivided into astrocytoma, anaplastic astrocytoma, and glioblastoma multiforme, each carrying a progressively poorer prognosis (87). Low-grade astrocytomas of the cerebral hemispheres may be resectable, but deeper lesions are more difficult to resect, and radiation therapy may be used. With the higher-grade lesions, aggressive surgical excision is performed, except for diffuse pontine, hypothalamic, and deep frontal lesions. Adjunctive radiation therapy prolongs survival, either external beam irradiation or interstitial radiation with iodine 125 or iridium 192. External beam radiation typically consists of 5,000 to 6,000 rad and may be delivered to a limited field rather than the whole brain. Chemotherapy also shows promise in prolonging survival, and trials of immunotherapy are under way (87). Favorable prognostic features are younger age (166), high performance rating at diagnosis (6), and favorable histology (87).

Medulloblastomas compose only about 5% of adult brain tumors, usually presenting in the cerebellar hemispheres, as opposed to the cerebral vermis in children. Primary cerebral lymphomas are increasing in incidence as a result of their association with the human immunodeficiency virus (HIV). Multiple tumor deposits are often present (167), and median survival is less than 1 year (87). Surgical removal does not improve outcome (168).

In children, brain malignancies are the most common type of solid tumor, comprising about one-fourth of all childhood malignancies (89) and of all childhood cancer deaths (165). The most frequent tumors are of glial origin (including astrocytomas, oligodendroglioma, and ependymoma). However, the most common malignant tumor is medulloblastoma, which produces parenchymal invasion and leptomeningeal dissemination (169). Primitive neuroectodermal tumors are highly malignant and may seed the neuraxis (87). Tumors may be associated with underlying diseases such as neurofibromatosis, tuberous sclerosis, and Von Hippel-Lindau disease. Germinomas typically present during the first two decades of life and have a relatively favorable prognosis. Typically, they extend from the suprasellar or pineal region, producing endocrine, visual field, autonomic, cognitive, and behavioral disturbance (170). The lesions are highly radiosensitive. Stereotactic surgery also may be of benefit (170).

In patients 2 to 12 years of age, the majority of tumors are infratentorial (169), and the most common age of presentation is 4 to 8 years (171). Low-grade astrocytomas have a more than 90% 5-year survival rate if they can be surgically excised (89). Surgically accessible low-grade tumors include cerebellar astrocytoma, choroid plexus papilloma, and meningioma (169). In general, more superficial tumors are less likely to be malignant (171). Surgery is also a component of treatment for or anatomically unresectable masses, augmented by radiation therapy. Chemotherapy can be life prolonging but seldom curative (169). It may be considered for very young children (younger than 3 years of age) for whom radiation therapy has the most complications.

REHABILITATION PRINCIPLES FOR BRAIN TUMOR PATIENTS

The most common neurologic deficits in brain tumor patients undergoing acute rehabilitation include impaired cognition (80%), weakness (78%), and visual-perceptual impairment (53%). Most patients have multiple impairments (18). Rehabilitation disposition decisions are guided by the patient's neurologic status and clinical course. A patient whose neurologic status is actively worsening will likely not benefit from intensive rehabilitation. Specific rehabilitation interventions will depend on the combination of deficits and are generally comparable to measures employed for patients with other etiologies of brain disorders, such as traumatic brain injury or stroke (see the chapters addressing those disorders for details of rehabilitation strategies). As noted earlier, brain tumor patients often have a shorter length of stay than other patients in acute rehabilitation for brain disorders. Although this may be related to higher initial FIM score (seen in some studies), it has been speculated that other reasons include fewer behavioral sequelae, better social supports, and expedited discharge planning that is due to prognostic factors (91). One study examining response of 10 brain tumor patients to acute rehabilitation found improved functional status at time of discharge; however, a quality-of-life measure did not improve until after discharge. The FIM and the disability rating scale were found to be more sensitive than the Karnofsky Performance Status Scale in detecting change in functional status (172). See the previous section, "Inpatient Rehabilitation" for further information on outcome studies related to brain tumor patients.

Often, brain tumor patients are undergoing radiation therapy concurrent with the rehabilitation. Because the radiation treatments may produce fatigue, sessions should be scheduled for late in the day, after the rehabilitation therapies have been completed (91). Also, corticosteroids should not be fully tapered while the patient is undergoing radiation treatment, as edema resulting from the radiation can result in mental status changes. Anticonvulsant therapy appears justified in patients with history of seizure and possibly for short-term use perioperatively, but efficacy of long-term prophylaxis for brain tumor patients without history of seizure has not been established (173). Incidence of deep vein thrombosis in brain tumor patients is high, and prophylaxis, such as intermittent pneumatic compression with or without low-dose heparin, is warranted. Incidence of postoperative deep vein thrombosis may be highest in meningioma patients (72%) and lower in brain metastasis (20%) (173).

Sarcomas of Bone and Soft Tissue

Sarcoma represents 1% of the total adult malignancies in the United States (9). These include osteosarcoma, Ewing's sarcoma, chondrosarcoma, giant-cell sarcoma of bone, and soft-tissue sarcoma (muscle, fat, fibrous tissue, neuroectoderm). There is a 1.5:1 male to female ratio, and 45% of the tumors involve the lower extremity; 40% the head, neck, or trunk; and 15% the upper extremity (174). Management of sarcoma of the soft tissue or bone presents a substantial challenge to rehabilitation specialists. The key to successful oncologic management and ultimate functional outcome is good local control. This implies that the initial biopsy was performed carefully, tissue planes were not violated, and adequate margins of uninvolved tissue were obtained. Early detection and treatment are essential if individuals are to have a limb-sparing option. Most patients with soft-tissue sarcoma undergo pretreatment staging, surgery that may consist of wide local excision, and chemotherapy. Many have additional radiation to the primary tumor site. Limb-salvage surgery is possible for those who can achieve good local control without amputation. These patients must have a neurovascular bundle that is not compromised by tumor, have no pathologic fracture, have little extraosseous extension of tumor (for osteosarcoma group), have no distant spread of tumor, and have a high probability for good cosmetic and functional outcome. Patients must be informed of the possibility of subsequent need for amputation in the face of infection, fracture, or continued prosthetic loosening especially in athletic individuals. The conversion rate approaches 15% to 20% in some series (175,176).

For lower-limb procedures, energy expenditure data tend to favor the limb-sparing option over amputation (177), and the advantage in cosmetic outcome of limb-sparing intervention is generally considered self-evident. Comparison of quality-of-life variables between the two groups, however, has not shown a conclusive advantage to either approach (178). Quality-of-life for limb-sparing patients appears to vary with the success of the procedure; those with problematic results often report relief after the late amputation is performed (177).

AMPUTATION

The pretreatment phase of sarcoma provides the rehabilitation team an opportunity to educate family and patient about what to expect, begin a program aimed at strength and stamina, and introduce the patient to the use of ambulation devices and bathroom safety. The amputee is treated similarly to patient undergoing amputation for any reason. The cancer amputee, however, is likely to have relatively shorter residual limb because of the need to achieve adequate tumor-free margins. The primary pathology is often located at a more proximal site in cancer patients than in other amputee populations, resulting in very proximal amputations, such as forequarter or shoulder disarticulation in the upper limb and hemipelvectomy or hip disarticulation in the lower limb (179). The concomitant use of chemotherapy or radiation may prolong the interval between surgery and delivery of a definitive prosthesis. Wound healing may be delayed, and residual limb volume shifts may interfere with weight stabilization. Socket adaptations can be made by adding and subtracting stump socks, using a series of flexible sockets, or padding the lining to adapt the fit. Meticulous wound care is needed, especially for those who have had irradiation to the residual limb. On the positive side, the individuals with amputation that is due to cancer tend to be young (peak incidence in the 10–20-year age group) (179) and without comorbid medical problems, and thus often make excellent prosthetic users. Details of postamputation management and prosthetic fitting are presented in Chapter 60, "Assistive Technology."

LIMB-SPARING PROCEDURES

Rehabilitation after limb-sparing surgery depends on the extent of soft-tissue and bony structural excision. Patients with proximal tibia or distal femur lesions may be eligible for en bloc resection and use of a prosthetic knee (180). An internal hemipelvectomy may be possible for those with proximal femur lesions. After limb-sparing surgery, 1 to 2 weeks (and occasionally longer) of bed rest is needed to promote wound healing, reduce edema, and maintain alignment. Barring complications, quadriceps and gluteal sets, active assisted straight-leg raises, and ankle pumps may be started 1 to 2 weeks postoperatively. Upright activity progresses from non–weight bearing to partial and full weight bearing based on muscle strength and wound healing (180). Rotationplasty may be performed as an alternative to amputation for distal femur lesions. The ankle joint is rotated 180 degrees and substitutes for the absent knee joint, gaining the functional equivalent of a below-knee amputation. Because of poor cosmesis, however, this procedure is done less frequently than in the past (178).

Other limb-sparing procedures that are frequently undertaken in this population include the removal of portions of muscle. Muscles typically removed include the hip adductors, quadriceps, hamstrings, and gastrocnemius. Patients undergoing these procedures will need a period of bed rest until wound drainage stops. Leg elevation, compression garments, and active range of motion should be instituted as part of the rehabilitation process. Patients with quadriceps excision will need a knee immobilizer postoperatively and will need to ambulate with an ankle-foot orthosis (AFO) that keeps the foot plantar-flexed and blocks dorsiflexion to create an extension moment at the knee. Some patients are able to develop a gait pattern substituting hip flexors, such that they have a stable knee and will not require an orthotic device (181). Adductor muscle group and hamstring excision rarely require assistive aides or orthotic device use. However, if there is sciatic nerve excision, an AFO will be needed to provide toe clearance. When the gastrocnemius is excised, a rocker sole needs to be added to the sole of the shoe to promote push-off. Achilles tendon stretching should be performed regularly to maintain ankle range of motion (182).

Prostate Cancer

Prostate cancer is the most common cancer in men and the second leading cause of cancer deaths in men (9). The rehabilitation problems of this population include bone pain (for those who have metastatic lesions), fracture, and impaired mobility (see previous section, "Bony Metastatic Disease"). Survival may be quite prolonged, even after onset of bony metastatic disease. Metastatic lesions are typically blastic, and although it has been stated in the literature that blastic metastasis produces less risk of fracture than lytic lesions, in our experience, pathologic fracture in prostate cancer is quite common. Often there is surrounding or generalized osteopenia, and this may

be the basis or at least contributory to the fracture risk. Men who have undergone radical prostatectomy or radiation therapy are prone to incontinence and impotence (see previous section, "Cancer-Related Sexual Dysfunction and Its Management"). In addition, antiandrogen therapy is often associated with loss of muscle mass, strength, and endurance. These patients are frequently fatigued. Early intervention with strengthening and aerobic conditioning exercise may help mitigate the impact of this treatment. Inguinal or pelvic lymphadenopathy can result in lymphedema or deep vein thrombosis. Studies show that pain, fatigue, and urinary dysfunction are most likely to negatively impact quality of life in prostate cancer patients (183).

CONCLUSION

The focus of rehabilitation interventions for this population is on pain relief, preservation or restoration of function, and education about planning and prioritizing life activities to assure quality. The rehabilitation team is in the unique position of being able to recommend practical suggestions to improve function and preserve independence throughout the course of their illness.

REFERENCES

1. Lehmann J, DeLisa JA, Waarren CG, et al. Cancer rehabilitation assessment of need development and education of a model of care. *Arch Phys Med Rehabil* 1978;59:410.
2. DeRogatis L, Abeloff M, Melisaratos N. Psychological coping mechanisms and survival time in metastatic breast cancer. *JAMA* 1979;242:1504.
3. Bergner M, Bobbitt R, Carter W, et al. The sickness impact profile: development and final revision of a health status measure. *Med Care* 1981;19:787.
4. Ganz PA. Long range effect of clinical trial interventions on quality of life. *Cancer* 1994;74[Suppl 9]:2620–2624.
5. Osoba D. Lessons learned from measuring health-related quality of life in oncology. *J Clin Oncol* 1994;12:608–616.
6. Karnofsky DA, Abelmann WH, Craver LF, et al. The use of the nitrogen mustards in palliative treatment of carcinoma. *Cancer* 1948;1:634–656.
7. Fawzy FI, Fawzy NW, Hyun CS, et al. Malignant melanoma: effects of an early structured psychiatric intervention, coping and affective state on recurrence and survival 6 years later. *Arch Gen Psychiatry* 1993;50:681–689.
8. Given CW, Given BA, Stommel M. The impact of age, treatment and symptoms on the physical and mental health of cancer patients: a longitudinal perspective. *Cancer* 1994;74[Suppl 7]:2128–2138.
9. Ries LAG, Eisner MP, Kosary CL, et al. SEER cancer statistics review 1973–1999. Bethesda, MD: National Cancer Institute,http://seer.cancer.gov/csr/1973 1999/,2002.
10. McKinley WO, Huang ME, Brunsvold KT. Neoplastic versus traumatic spinal cord injury: an outcome comparison after inpatient rehabilitation. *Arch Phys Med Rehabil* 1999;80:1253–1257.
11. Huang ME, Cifu DX, Keyser-Marcus L. Functional outcome after brain tumor and acute stroke: a comparative analysis. *Arch Phys Med Rehabil* 1998; 79:1386–1390.
12. O'Dell MW, Barr K, Spanier D, et al. Functional outcome of inpatient rehabilitation in persons with brain tumors. *Arch Phys Med Rehabil* 1998;79:1530–1534.
13. McKinley WO, Conti-Wyneken AR, Vokac CW, et al. Rehabilitative functional outcome of patients with neoplastic spinal cord compression. *Arch Phys Med Rehabil* 1996;77:892–895.
14. Garstang SV, Gillis TA, Graves DE. Maintenance of functional gains after inpatient cancer rehabilitation. *Arch Phys Med Rehabil* 1998;79:1146–1147(abst).
15. Marciniak CM, Sliwa JA, Spill G, et al. Functional outcome following rehabilitation of the cancer patient. *Arch Phys Med Rehabil* 1996;77:54–57.
16. O'Toole DM, Golden AM. Evaluating cancer patients for rehabilitation potential. *West J Med* 1991;155:384–387.
17. Cole RP, Scialla SJ, Bednarz L. Functional recovery in cancer rehabilitation. *Arch Phys Med Rehabil* 2000;81:623–627.
18. Mukand JA, Blackinton DD, Crincoli MG, et al. Incidence of neurologic deficits and rehabilitation of patients with brain tumors. *Am J Phys Med Rehabil* 2001;80:346–350.
19. Marciniak CM, Sliwa JA, Heinemann AW. Functional outcomes of persons with brain tumors after inpatient rehabilitation. *Arch Phys Med Rehabil* 2001; 82:457–463.
20. Murray PK. Functional outcome and survival in spinal cord injury secondary to neoplasia. *Cancer* 1985;55:197–201.

21. Yoshioka H. Rehabilitation for the terminal cancer patient. *Am J Phys Med Rehabil* 1994;73:199–206.
22. Krakoff IH. Systemic treatment of cancer. *CA Cancer J Clin* 1996;46:134–141.
23. Mellette SJ. The evolving role of cancer rehabilitation in cancer care. *Rehabil Oncol* 1995;13:25.
24. Portenoy RK. Cancer pain pathophysiology and syndromes. *Lancet* 1992; 339:1026.
25. Cheville AL. Pain management in cancer rehabilitation. *Arch Phys Med Rehabil* 2001;82[Suppl 1]:S84–87.
26. Elliott K, Foley KM. Neurologic pain syndromes in patients with cancer. *Neurol Clin* 1989;7:333–360.
27. Acute Pain Management Guideline Panel. *Acute pain management: operative or medical procedures and trauma.* Clinical Practice Guideline, AHCPR Publication No. 92–0032. Rockville, MD: AHCPR, PHS, U.S. Department of Health and Human Services, 1992:145.
28. World Health Organization. *Cancer pain and relief and palliative care.* Geneva: World Health Organization, 1990:75.
29. Management of Cancer Pain Guideline Panel. *Management of cancer pain.* Clinical Practice Guideline No. 9. AHCPR Pub. No. 94–0592. Rockville, MD: U.S. Department of Health and Human Services, PHS, Agency for Health Care Policy and Research, 1994:75–84.
30. Cherry NI, Portenoy RK. Cancer pain: principles of assessment and syndromes. In: Wall PO, Melzack R, eds. *Textbook of pain,* 3rd ed. London: Churchill-Livingstone, 1994:782.
31. Ventafridda V, Tamburini M, Caraceni A, et al. A validation study of the WHO method for cancer pain relief. *Cancer* 1987;59:850–856.
32. Walsh D. Pharmacological management of cancer pain. *Semin Oncol* 2000; 27:45–63.
33. Lamer TJ. Treatment of cancer-related pain: when orally administered medications fail. *Mayo Clin Proc* 1994;69:473–480.
34. Abrams HL, Spiro R, Goldstein N. Metastases in carcinoma: analysis of 1,000 autopsied cases. *Cancer* 1950;Jan:74–85.
35. Tubiana-Hulin M. Incidence, prevalence and distribution of bone metastases. *Bone* 1991;12[Suppl 1]:9–10.
36. Bhalla SK. Metastatic disease of the spine. *Clin Orthop* 1970;73:52–60.
37. Brage ME, Simon MA. Evaluation, prognosis and medical treatment considerations of metastatic bone tumors. *Orthopedics* 1992;15:589–595.
38. Boland PJ, Billings J, Healey JH. The management of pathologic fractures. *J Back Musculoskel Rehabil* 1993;3:27–34.
39. Sim FH. Metastatic bone disease: philosophy of treatment. *Orthopedics* 1992;15:541–544.
40. Vargo MM. Orthopedic management of malignant bone lesions. *PM&R State Art Rev* 1994;8:363–391.
41. Citrin DL, Bessent RG, Greig WR. A comparison of the sensitivity and accuracy of the phosphate bone scan and skeletal radiograph in the diagnosis of bone metastases. *Clin Radiol* 1977;28:107–117.
42. O'Connor MI, Currier BL. Metastatic disease of the spine. *Orthopedics* 1992; 15:611–620.
43. Beals R, Lawton GD, Snell W. Prophylactic internal fixation of the femur in metastatic breast cancer. *Cancer* 1971;28:1350–1354.
44. Behr JT, Dobozi WR, Badrinath K. The treatment of pathologic and impending pathologic fractures of the proximal femur in the elderly. *Clin Orthop Rel Res* 1985;198:173–178.
45. Thompson RC. Impending fracture associated with bone destruction. *Orthopedics* 1992;15:547–550.
46. Habermann ET, Sachs R, Stem RE, et al. The pathology and treatment of metastatic disease of the femur. *Clin Orthop* 1982;169:70–82.
47. Menck H, Schulze S, Larsen E. Metastasis size in pathologic femoral fractures. *Acta Orthop Scand* 1988;59:151–154.
48. Mandi A, Szepesi K, Morocz I. Surgical treatment of pathologic fractures from metastatic tumors of long bones. *Orthopedics* 1991;14:43–49.
49. Keene JS, Sellinger DS, McBeath AA, et al. Metastatic breast cancer in the femur: a search for the lesions at risk of fracture. *Clin Orthop* 1986;203: 282–288.
50. Denis F. Spinal instability as defined by the three-column spine concept in acute spinal trauma. *Clin Orthop* 1984;189:65–76.
51. Harrington KD. Metastatic disease of the spine. *J Bone Joint Surg Am* 1986; 68:1110.
52. Blake DD. Radiation treatment of metastatic bone disease. *Clin Orthop* 1970;73:89–100.
53. Robinson HS. Cane for measurement and recording of stress. *Arch Phys Med Rehabil* 1969;50:457–459.
54. McDonnell ME, Shea BD. The role of physical therapy in patients with metastatic disease to bone. *J Back Musculoskel Rehabil* 1993;3:78–84.
55. Theriault RL, Hortobagyi GN. The evolving role of bisphosphonates. *Semin Oncol* 2001;28:284–290.
56. Hillner BE, Ingle JN, Berenson JR. American Society of Clinical Oncology guideline on the role of bisphosphonates in breast cancer. *J Clin Oncol* 2000; 18:1378–1391.
57. Whelan TJ, Mohide EA, Willan AR, et al. The supportive care needs of newly diagnosed cancer patients attending a regional cancer center. *Cancer* 1997;80:1518–1524.
58. Mock V. Fatigue management: evidence and guidelines for practice. *Cancer* 2001;92[Suppl]:1699–1707.
59. Gutstein HB. The biologic basis of fatigue. *Cancer* 2001;92[Suppl]:1678–1683.
60. Kurzrock R. The role of cytokines in cancer-related fatigue. *Cancer* 2001; 92[Suppl]:1684–1688.
61. Valentine AD, Meyers CA. Cognitive and mood disturbance as causes and symptoms of fatigue in cancer patients. *Cancer* 2001;92[Suppl]:1694–1698.
62. Escalante CP, Grover T, Johnson BA, et al. A fatigue clinic in a comprehensive cancer center. *Cancer* 2001;92[Suppl]:1708–1713.
63. Burks TF. New agents for the treatment of cancer-related fatigue. *Cancer* 2001;92[Suppl]:1714–1718.
64. Homsi J, Walsh D, Nelson K. Psychostimulants in supportive care. *Support Care Cancer* 2000;8:385–397.
65. Sarhill N, Walsh D, Nelson KA. Methylphenidate for fatigue in advanced cancer: a prospective open-label pilot study. *Am J Hospice Palliative Care* 2001;18(3):187–192.
66. Woolridge JE, Anderson CM, Perry MC. Corticosteroids in advanced cancer. *Oncology* 2001;15(2):225–236.
67. Winningham ML. Strategies for managing cancer-related fatigue syndrome. *Cancer* 2001;92[Suppl]:988–997.
68. Dimeo FC. Effects of exercise on cancer-related fatigue. *Cancer* 2001;92 [Suppl]:1689–1693.
69. Shephard RJ, Shek PN. Cancer, immune function, and physical activity. *Can J Appl Physiol* 1995;20(1):1–25.
70. Gaydos LA, Freireich EJ, Mantel N. The quantitative relation between platelet count and hemorrhage in patients with acute leukemia. *N Engl J Med* 1962;226:905–909.
71. Smelz JK, Schlicht LA. Rehabilitation of the cancer patient after bone marrow transplantation *P&R State Art Rev* 1994;8:321–323.
72. James MC. Physical therapy for patients after bone marrow transplantation. *Phys Ther* 1987;67:946–952.
73. St. Pierre BA, Kasper CE, Lindsey AM. Fatigue mechanisms in patients with cancer: effects of tumor necrosis factor and exercise on skeletal muscle. *Oncol Nurs Forum* 1991;19:419–425.
74. Gillis TA, Donovan ES. Rehabilitation following bone marrow transplantation. *Cancer* 2001;92[Suppl]:998–1007.
75. Trovato MK, Pidcock FS, Christensen JR, et al. Chronic graft versus host disease in children: a review of function and rehabilitative needs. *Arch Phys Med Rehabil* 1998;79:1157(abst).
76. Dimeo F, Bertz H, Finke J, et al. An aerobic exercise program for patients with haematological malignancies after bone marrow transplantation. *Bone Marrow Transplant* 1996;18:1157–1160.
77. Sharkey AM, Carey AB, Heise CT, et al. Cardiac rehabilitation after cancer therapy in children and young adults. *Am J Cardiol* 1993;71:1488–1490.
78. Dimeo F, Fetscher S, Lange W, et al. Effects of aerobic exercise on the physical performance and incidence of treatment-related complications after high-dose chemotherapy. *Blood* 1997;90:3390–3394.
79. MacVicar MG, Winningham ML, Nickel JL. Effects of aerobic interval training on cancer patients functional capacity. *Nurs Res* 1989;38:348–351.
80. Segal R, Evans W, Johnson D, et al. Structured exercise improves physical functioning in women with stages I and II breast cancer: results of a randomized controlled trial. *J Clin Oncol* 2001;19(3):657–665.
81. Berglund G, Bolund C, Gustavsson U-L. Starting again—a comparison study of a group rehabilitation program for cancer patients. *Acta Oncol* 1993; 32:15–21.
82. Schwartz AL, Mori M, Gao R, et al. Exercise reduces daily fatigue in women with breast cancer receiving chemotherapy. *Med Sci Sports Exerc* 2001;33: 718–723.
83. Posner JB, Chernik NL. Intracranial metastases from systemic cancer. *Adv Neurol* 1978;19:579–592.
84. Cascino TL. Neurologic complications of systemic cancer. *Med Clin North Am* 1993;77(1):265–278.
85. Patchell RA. Brain metastases: neurologic complications of systemic cancer. *Neurol Clin* 1991;9:817–824.
86. Zimm S, Wampler GL, Stablein D, et al. Intracerebral metastases in solid tumor patient: natural history and results of treatment. *Cancer* 1981;48:384–394.
87. Black P. Medical progress: brain tumors. *N Engl J Med* 1991;324:1471–1476; 1555–1564.
88. Schlicht LA, Smelz JK. Metastatic spinal cord compression. *PM&R State Art Rev* 1994;8:345–361.
89. Casciato DA, Lowitz BB. *Manual of clinical oncology,* 4th ed. Philadelphia: Little, Lippincott Williams and Wilkins, 2000.
90. Gilbert RW, Kim JH, Posner JB. Epidural spinal cord compression from metastatic tumor: diagnosis and treatment. *Ann Neurol* 1978;3:40–51.
91. Kirshblum S, O'Dell MW, Ho C, et al. Rehabilitation of persons with central nervous system tumors. *Cancer* 2001;92[Suppl]:1029–1038.
92. Hill ME, Richards MA, Gregory WM, et al. Spinal cord compression in breast cancer: a review of 70 cases. *Br J Cancer* 1993;68:969.
93. Ku A, Lachmann E, Tunkel R, Nagler W. Upper limb reflex sympathetic dystrophy associated with occult malignancy. *Arch Phys Med Rehabil* 1996;77: 726–728.
94. Hammack JE, Kimmel DW, O'Neill BP, et al. Paraneoplastic cerebellar degeneration: a clinical comparison of patients with and without Purkinje cell cytoplasmic antibodies. *Mayo Clin Proc* 1990;65:1423–1431.
95. Sliwa JA, Thatcher S, Jet J. Paraneoplastic subacute cerebellar degeneration: functional improvement and the role of rehabilitation. *Arch Phys Med Rehabil* 1994;75:355–357.
96. Stubgen JP. Neuromuscular disorders in systemic malignancy and its treatment. *Muscle Nerve* 1995;18:636–648.
97. Campbell MJ, Paty DW. Carcinomatous neuromyopathy: electrophysiological studies. X. An electrophysiological and immunological study of patients with carcinoma of the lung. *J Neurol Neurosurg Psychiatry* 1974;37:131–141.

98. Forman A. Peripheral neuropathy in cancer patients: incidence, features, and pathophysiology. Part 1. *Oncology* 1990;4:57–62.

99. Baryon SA, Heffer RR. Weakness in malignancy: evidence for a remote effect of tumor on distal axons. *Ann Neurol* 1978;4:268–274.

100. Horwich MS, Cho L, Porro RS, et al. Subacute sensory neuropathy a remote effect of carcinoma. *Ann Neurol* 1977;2:7–19.

101. Pourmand R, Maybury BG. AAEM case report #31: paraneoplastic sensory neuronopathy. *Muscle Nerve* 1996;19:1517–1522.

102. Johnson PC. Hematogenous metastases of carcinoma to dorsal root ganglia. *Acta Neuropathol* 1977;38:171–172.

103. Matsubayashi T, Koga H, Nishiyama Y, et al. The reparative process of metastatic bone lesions after radiotherapy. *Jpn J Clin Oncol Suppl* 1981; 11:253–264.

104. DeLattre JY, Posner JB. Neurological complications of chemotherapy and radiation therapy. In: Aminoff MJ, ed. *Neurology and general medicine*. New York: Churchill-Livingstone, 1989:365–387.

105. Watne K, Hager B, Heier M, et al. Reversible edema and necrosis after irradiation of the brain. *Acta Oncol* 1990;29:891–895.

106. Shank B. Radiotherapy: implications for general patient care. In Wittes RE, ed. *Manual of oncologic therapeutics*. Philadelphia: JB Lippincott 1991: 60–61.

107. Spence R. Nutritional concerns in cancer patients. *PM&R State Art Rev* 1994; 8:404.

108. Souba WW. Nutritional support. In: DeVita VT, Hellman S, Rosenberg SA, eds. *Cancer: principles and practice of oncology*, 5th ed. Philadelphia: JB Lippincott, 1997:2841–2857.

109. Berger AM, Kilroy TJ. Oral complications. In: DeVita VT, Hellman S, Rosenberg SA, eds. *Cancer: principles and practice of oncology*, 5th ed. Philadelphia: JB Lippincott, 1997:2714–2725.

110. Nelson KA. The cancer anorexia-cachexia syndrome. *Semin Oncol* 2000;27: 64–68.

111. Rivadeneira DE, Evoy D, Fahey TJ, et al. Nutritional support of the cancer patient. *CA Cancer J Clin* 1998;48:69–80.

112. Schover LR, Montague DK, Lakin MM. Sexual problems. In: DeVita VT, Hellhnan S, Rosenberg SA, eds. *Cancer: principles and practice of oncology*, 5th ed. Philadelphia: JB Lippincott, 1997:2857–2872.

113. McKee AL, Schover LR. Sexuality rehabilitation. *Cancer* 2001;92[Suppl]: 1008–1012.

114. Schover LR. Sexual rehabilitation after treatment for prostrate cancer. *Cancer* 1993;71[Suppl]:1024–1030.

115. Glasgow M, Halfin V, Althausen AF. Sexual response and cancer. *CA Cancer J Clin* 1987;37:322–333.

116. Bergmark K, Avall-Lundqvist E, Dickman PW. Vaginal changes and sexuality in women with a history of cervical cancer. *N Engl J Med* 1999;340: 1383–1389.

117. Gerraughty SM. Sexual function in cancer patients. *P&R State Art Rev* 1994;8:251–260.

118. Kissin MW, dellaRovere QG, Easton D, et al. Risk of lymphedema following the treatment of breast cancer. *Br J Surg* 1986;7:580.

119. Werner RS, McCormick B, Petrek JA, et al. Arm edema in conservatively managed breast cancer: obesity is a major predictive factor. *Radiology* 1991; 180:177.

120. Moskovitz AH, Anderson BO, Yeung RS. Axillary web syndrome after axillary dissection. *Am J Surg* 2001;181:434–439.

121. Woolam GL. What's new in breast cancer surgery? *CA Cancer J Clin* 2000; 50:276–278.

122. Petrick JA, Pressman PI, Smith RA. Lymphedema: current issues in research and management. *CA Cancer J Clin* 2000;50:292–307.

123. Guo Y, Truong AN. Functional outcome after physical therapy of breast cancer patients status post modified radical mastectomy versus mastectomy and transverse rectus abdominis myocutaneous flap. *Arch Phys Med Rehabil* 1998;79:1157(abst).

124. Atkins H, Hayward JL, Klugman DJ, et al. Treatment of early breast cancer: a report after 10 years of a clinical trial. *BMJ* 1972;2:423.

125. Aitken RJ, Gaze MN, Rodger A, et al. Arm morbidity within a trial of mastectomy and either nodal sample with selective radiotherapy or axillary clearance. *Br J Surg* 1989;76:568–589.

126. Gerber LH. Rehabilitation management for women with breast cancer: maximizing functional outcomes. In: Harris JR, Lippman MG, Morrow M, Hellman S, eds. *Diseases of the breast*. Philadelphia: Lippincott-Raven, 1996; 939– 947.

127. Jansen RF, van Geel AN, de Groot HG, et al. Immediate versus delayed shoulder exercises after axillary lymph node dissection. *Am J Surg* 1990; 160:481.

128. Dawson I, Stan K, Heslinga JM, et al. Effect of shoulder immobilization on wound seroma and shoulder dysfunction following modified radical mastectomy: a randomized prospective clinical trial. *Br J Surg* 1989;76:311.

129. Carson CJ, Coverly K, Lasker-Hertz S, et al. The incidence of co-morbidities in the treatment of lymphedema. *J Oncology Management* 1999;8:13–17.

130. Armstrong M, Vargo MM. Safety of diagnostic or therapeutic needle interventions in lymphedema patients. *Arch Phys Med Rehabil* 2001;82:1305 (abst).

131. Zelikovski A, Deutsch A, Reiss R. The sequential pneumatic compression device in surgery for lymphedema of the limbs. *J Cardiovasc Surg* 1983;24:18.

132. Bastien MR, Goldstein BG, Lesher JL Jr, et al. Treatment of lymphedema with a multicompartmental pneumatic compression device. *J Am Acad Dermatol* 1989;20:853.

133. Foldi E, Foeldi M, Weissleder H. Conservative treatment of lymphedema of the limbs. *Angiol J Vasc Dis* 1985;36:171.

134. Casley-Smith JR, Morgan RG, Piller NB. Treatment of lymphedema of the arms and legs with 5,6-benzo-[alpha]-pyrone. *N Engl J Med* 1993;16:329.

135. Loprinzi CL, Kugler JW, Sloan JA, et al. Lack of effect of Coumarin in women with lymphedema after treatment for breast cancer. *N Engl J Med* 1999;340:346–350.

136. Gonzales GR, Elliiot KJ, Portenoy RK, et al. The impact of a comprehensive evaluation in the management of cancer pain. *Pain* 1991;47:141.

137. Kori SH, Foley KM, Posner JB, et al. Brachial plexus lesions in patients with cancer: 100 cases. *Neurology* 1981;31:45.

138. Bagley FH, Walsh JW, Cady B, et al. Carcinomatous versus radiation induced brachial plexus neuropathy in breast cancer. *Cancer* 1978;41:2154.

139. Lederman RJ, Wilbourn AJ. Brachial plexopathy, recurrent cancer or radiation? *Neurology* 1984;34:1331.

140. Million RR, Cassisi NJ, Clark JR. Cancer of the head and neck. In: DeVita VT, Hellman S, Rosenberg SA, eds. *Cancer: principles and practice of oncology*, 3rd ed. Philadelphia: JB Lippincott, 1989:488–590.

141. Shah JP, Lydiatt W. Treatment of cancer of the head and neck. *CA Cancer J Clin* 1995;45:352–368.

142. Perry AR, Shaw MA. Evaluation of functional outcomes (speech, swallowing and voice) in patients attending speech pathology after head and neck cancer treatment(s); development of a multi-centre database. *J Laryngol Otol* 2000;114: 605–615.

143. Dudgeon BJ, DeLisa JA, Miller RM. Head and neck cancer: rehabilitation approach. *Am J Occup Ther* 1980;34:243–251.

144. Saunders WH, Johnson EW. Rehabilitation of the shoulder after radical neck dissection. *Ann Otol* 1975;84:812–816.

145. Roberts WL. Rehabilitation of the head and neck cancers patient. In: McGarvey CL, ed. *Physical therapy for the cancer patient*. New York: Churchill-Livingstone, 1990.

146. Berger AM, Kilroy TJ. Oral complications. In: DeVita VT, Hellman S, Rosenberg SA, eds. *Cancer: principles and practice of oncology*, 5th ed. Philadelphia: JB Lippincott, 1997:2714–2725.

147. Buchbinder D, Currivan RB, Kaplan AJ, et al. Mobilization regimens for the prevention of jaw hypomobility in the radiated patient. *J Oral Maxillofac Surg* 1993;51:863–867.

148. Logemann JA. Rehabilitation of head and neck cancer patients. *Cancer Treat Res* 1999;100:91–105.

149. Schantz S, Harrison L, Lorastiere A. Tumors of the nasal cavity and paranasal sinuses, nasopharynx, oral cavity and oropharynx. In: DeVita VT, Hellman S, Rosenberg SA, eds. *Cancer: principles and practice of oncology*, 5th ed. Philadelphia: JB Lippincott, 1997:741–801.

150. Sessions RB, Harrison LB, Forastiere AA. Tumors of the salivary glands and paragliomas. In: DeVita VT, Hellman S, Rosenberg SA, eds. *Cancer: principles and practice of oncology*, 5th ed. Philadelphia: JB Lippincott, 1997:830–847.

151. LaBlance GR, Kraus K, Karen FS. Rehabilitation of swallowing and communication following glossectomy. *Rehabil Nurs* 1991;16:266–269.

152. Sessions RB, Harrison LB, Forastiere AA. Tumors of the larynx and hypopharynx. In: DeVita VT, Hellman S, Rosenberg SA, eds. *Cancer: principles and practice of oncology*, 5th ed. Philadelphia: JB Lippincott, 1997:802–829.

153. Carew JF, Shah JP. Advances in multimodality therapy for laryngeal cancer. *CA Cancer J Clin* 1998;48:211–228.

154. Lockhart JS, Bryce J. Restoring speech and tracheoesophageal puncture. *Nursing* 1993;23:59–61.

155. Beckhardt RN, Murray JG, Ford CH, et al. Factors influencing functional outcome in supraglottic laryngectomy. *Head Neck* 1994;16:232–239.

156. Weaver AW, Fleming SM. Partial laryngectomy: analysis of associated swallowing disorders. *Am J Surg* 1978;136:486–489.

157. Muz J, Hamlet S, Mathog R, et al. Scintigraphic assessment of aspiration in head and neck cancer patients with tracheostomy. *Head Neck* 1994;16: 17–20.

158. Eyre HJ, Farver ML. Hodgkin's disease and non-Hodgkin's lymphomas. In Holleb AI, Fink DJ, Murphy GP, eds. *American Cancer Society textbook of clinical oncology*. Atlanta: American Cancer Society, Inc., 1991:377–396.

159. Skarin AT, Dorfinan DM. Non-Hodgkin's lymphomas: current classification and management. *CA Cancer J Clin* 1997;47:351–372.

160. Holtzman L, Chesey K. Rehabilitation of the leukemia/lymphoma patient. In: McGarvey CL, ed. *Physical therapy for the cancer patient*. New York: Churchill-Livingstone, 1990:85–110.

161. Gallagher D, Heinrich SD, Craver R, et al. Skeletal manifestations of acute leukemia in childhood. *Orthopedics* 1991; 14:485–492.

162. Shea BD, Vlad G. Rehabilitation of the lung cancer patient. In: McGarvey CL, ed. *Physical therapy for the cancer patient*. New York: Churchill-Livingstone, 1990:29–45.

163. Bond JH. Colorectal cancer update: prevention, screening, treatment and surveillance for high-risk groups. *Advances in Gastroenterology* 2000;84(5): 1163–1182.

164. Gudjonsson B. Cancer of the pancreas: 50 years of surgery. *Cancer* 1987; 60:2284–2303.

165. Bondy ML, Wrensch M. Perspective in 77 prevention: update on brain cancer epidemiology. *Cancer Bull* 1993;45:365–369.

166. Silverstein MD, Cascino TL, Harmsen WS, et al. High grade astrocytomas: resource use, clinical outcomes and cost care. *Mayo Clin Proc* 1996;71:936–944.

167. Remick SC, Diamond C, Migliozzi JA, et al. Primary central nervous system lymphoma in patients with and without the acquired immune deficiency syndrome. *Medicine* 1990;69:345–360.

168. O'Neill BP, Illig JJ. Primary central nervous system lymphoma. *Mayo Clin Proc* 1989;64:1005–1020.

169. Friedman HS, Horowitz M, Oakes WJ. Tumors of the central nervous system: improvement in outcome through a multimodality approach. *Pediatr Clin North Am* 1991;38:381–391.

170. Horowitz MB, Hall WA. Central nervous system germinomas. *Arch Neurol* 1991;48:652–657.

171. Hardwood-Nash DC. Primary neoplasms of the central nervous system in children. *Cancer* 1991;67:1223–1228.

172. Huang ME, Wartella JE, Kreutzer JS. Functional outcomes and quality of life in patients with brain tumors: a preliminary report. *Arch Phys Med Rehabil* 2001;82:1540–1546.

173. Bell K, O'Dell MW, Barr K, et al. Rehabilitation of the patient with brain tumor. *Arch Phys Med Rehabil* 1998;79[Suppl]:S37–S46.

174. Sondak V, Economow J, Eilber F. Soft tissue sarcoma of the extremity and retroperitoneum: advances in management. *Adv Surg* 1991;24:241.

175. Quill G, Gitelis S, Morton T. Complications associated with limb salvage for extremity sarcomas and their management. *Clin Orthop Rel Res* 1990;260:242.

176. Murray JA, Jessup K, Romsdahl M, et al. Limb salvage study in osteosarcoma: early experience at M.D. Anderson Hospital and Tumor Institute. *Cancer Treat Symp* 1985;3:131.

177. Lane JM, Christ GH, Khan S, et al. Rehabilitation for limb salvage patients: kinesiologic parameters and psychologic assessment. *Cancer* 2001;92(4) [Suppl]:1013–1019.

178. Yasko AW, Reece GP, Gillis TA, et al. Limb-salvage strategies to optimize quality of life: the M.D. Anderson Cancer Center experience. *CACancer J Clin* 1997;47:226–238.

179. King JC, Williams RP, McAnelly RD, et al. Rehabilitation of tumor amputees and limb salvage patients. In: *Physical Medicine and Rehabilitation: State of the Art Reviews: Cancer Rehabilitation* 1994;8(2):297–319.

180. Meyer WH, Malawer MM. Osteosarcoma clinical features and evolving surgical and chemotherapeutic strategies. *Pediatr Clin North Am* 1991;38: 317–341.

181. Siegel KL, Stanhope SJ, Caldwell GE. Kinematic and kinetic adaptations in the lower limb during stance in gait of unilateral femoral neuropathy patients. *Clin Biomech* 1993;8:147–155.

182. Lampert M, Gahagen C. Rehabilitation of the sarcoma patient. In: McGarvey CL, ed. *Physical therapy for the cancer patient.* New York: Churchill-Livingstone, 1990:111–135.

183. Herr HW. Quality of life in prostate cancer patients. *CA Cancer J Clin* 1997;47:207–217.

CHAPTER 82

Rehabilitation of the Individual with HIV

Stephen F. Levinson and Steven M. Fine

The quest for effective treatment, prevention, and cure of the acquired immunodeficiency syndrome (AIDS) has resulted in one of the most concentrated research efforts in the history of medicine. Since its discovery in the early 1980s, the human immunodeficiency virus (HIV) has become one of the most studied of human pathogens. Although an outright cure for AIDS still seems to be a distant dream, developments in recent years have been breathtaking, and as of the time of this writing, the possibility of controlling the progression of HIV infection, preventing the decline in immune function that leads to AIDS, and enabling the reconstitution of the immune system destroyed by the virus is within grasp. An effective vaccine, however, remains elusive. Although much is known about the pathogenesis of HIV type I (HIV-I), the most prevalent form of the virus, and about the mechanisms leading to immune dysfunction, the prevalence of disability is far less well known.

HIV is important to the field of rehabilitation for two reasons: because of its occurrence in traditional rehabilitation patients and because it can, in and of itself, cause disability. If nothing else, all rehabilitation professionals should recognize the potential for any of their patients to carry HIV and other blood-borne pathogens and should stringently apply universal precautions. Equally important, however, is the need to recognize that HIV is among the differential diagnoses of many disorders commonly seen in rehabilitation settings. In patients with known HIV infection, rehabilitation professionals need to be familiar with the many chemotherapeutic agents commonly used for treatment and with their side effects and drug interactions. This last task is particularly daunting given the accelerated process for U.S. Food and Drug Administration (FDA) review and approval of new treatments.

This chapter emphasizes the nature of HIV and the many ways that it can cause disability. Current medical treatment strategies are also discussed. However, the discussion is not intended to be comprehensive, and interested readers are urged to follow the literature closely and keep up to date in this rapidly evolving field. The medical management of HIV disease and its complications should be left to experts. Rehabilitation strategies used to manage functional impairments typical of those found in association with HIV, such as spinal cord injury, brain injury, neuropathies, and rheumatologic disorders, however, are similar to those used in disability resulting from other causes, as discussed elsewhere in this book.

HIV-RELATED DISABILITY

The full extent of disability resulting from HIV is unknown. One of the earliest studies attempting to evaluate this, the National Institutes of Health retrospective study, looked only at individuals with AIDS who were involved in research protocols and were referred for various rehabilitation interventions (1). A more comprehensive prospective study of disability in a population of men with HIV was obtained as part of the AIDS Time-Oriented Health Outcome Study (2,3). Of those individuals with AIDS, more than 50% reported difficulty with one or more instrumental activities of daily living (ADLs), such as grasping or driving; nearly 30% with basic ADLs, such as bathing and dressing; and more than 40% with basic mobility. Even among symptomatic seropositive individuals without AIDS, nearly 30% reported difficulties with instrumental ADLs, more than 10% with basic ADLs and 15% with basic mobility. With the introduction of highly active antiretroviral therapy (HAART), it has become possible to control and even reverse the progression of HIV. Although functional abilities generally improve with treatment, some degree of functional impairment often remains, and continued functional decline has been reported (4–8). Quality-of-life issues have also become more significant as survival improves (9–11).

NATURAL HISTORY OF HIV

Pathogenesis

HIV-1 infection results in the destruction of CD4-positive lymphocytes, leading to a decline in their numbers. In acute primary infection, HIV-1 replicates briskly and viral titer rises rapidly (12–14). Within 1 week of onset, 10^5–10^7 infectious particles per microliter of plasma can be measured (15,16). Fifty to 70% of patients experience a clinical syndrome that may include fever, rash, sore throat, lymphadenopathy, splenomegaly, myalgias, arthritis, and, rarely, meningitis.

Within a few weeks to months, seroconversion occurs, and HIV-1 antibodies can be measured by the enzyme-linked immunosorbent assay (ELISA) or Western blot tests. Rapid viral replication persists, however, in the bloodstream, lymphoid tissue, and central nervous system (CNS), leading to a high turnover of infected cells (13,17). A steady state of plasma HIV ribonucleic acid (RNA) level is established within 6 to 12

TABLE 82-1. Classification of HIV			
CD4 Cell Count	Group A: Asymptomatic, Acute HIV or Generalized Lymphadenopathy	Group B: Symptomatic, not A or C	Group C: Indicator Conditions Present
$\geq 500/mm^3$	A1	B1	C1[a]
$200–499/mm^3$	A2	B2	C2[a]
$<200/mm^3$	A3[a]	B3[a]	C3[a]

[a]Indicates the presence of acquired immunodeficiency syndrome (AIDS). HIV, human immunodeficiency virus.

months of seroconversion, and measurements of the viral load are prognostic (18,19). Levels of 10^6 HIV-1 RNA copies per microliter of blood or greater correlate with rapid progression over a few years, 10^3 to 10^5 with progression in 8 to 10 years, and less than 10^3 with long-term nonprogression (20). Unfortunately, rapid viral turnover and mutation leads to the appearance of resistant strains if viral suppression is not complete (21–23).

Classification

The Centers for Disease Control and Prevention (CDC) developed a revised classification scheme in 1993 based on the development of signs and symptoms and the CD4 lymphocyte count (24). This scheme is summarized in Table 82-1. Group A patients are seropositive but essentially symptom free. Group C patients have one or more AIDS-indicator illnesses. A comprehensive list of AIDS-indicator conditions is beyond the scope of this chapter, but suffice it to say that they include most opportunistic infections and malignancies, HIV dementia, and the AIDS wasting syndrome. Group B patients have early symptoms of immune deficiency in the absence of an AIDS-indicator condition. Patients are further subdivided into categories 1, 2, and 3, corresponding to CD4 counts of $500/mm^3$ or above, 200–499, and less than 200, respectively. Patients falling into either group C or category 3 are classified as having AIDS.

Demographics

The World Health Organization estimates that as of December 2001, 40 million adults and 2.7 million children worldwide have been infected with HIV-1 (www.unaids.org) (25). About 850,000 to 950,000 people are infected with HIV in the United States. There are now approximately 15,000 deaths annually, down dramatically from more than 40,000 just a few years ago. In 1999 in the United States, HIV patients were 20% female, 39% white, 40% African American, and 20% Hispanic, reflecting a continuation of the significant shift to minority populations in recent years (www.cdc.gov/hiv/stats/hasr1301.htm) (26).

Documented Routes of Transmission

Documented routes of transmission include sexual contact with infected individuals, percutaneous or mucous membrane exposure to infected blood or body fluids, or transplacental, perinatal, or breast-milk transmission from mother to infant. In 2001, intravenous drug use was the most frequently reported risk behavior in the United States (26). HIV-1 is not transmitted by casual skin contact, airborne routes, or contact with saliva or sweat.

Occupational Exposure

Occupational exposure to HIV-1 among health-care workers has been extensively studied, and an excess number of cases beyond that found in the general population has not been found (27). The risk of HIV-1 infection is estimated to be 0.3% after percutaneous injury involving infected blood (28) and 0.1% after mucous membrane exposure (29). Universal precautions should be used at all times that contact with blood or body fluids may be anticipated. These include the use of gloves to prevent potential exposure to infectious body fluids or broken skin during procedures such as wound care and electromyography (EMG), and the use of a gown, goggles, and a mask during procedures in which spattering of blood is possible.

Postexposure prophylaxis is recommended for percutaneous or mucous membrane exposure to blood or visibly bloody fluid, semen, vaginal secretions, cerebrospinal, synovial, pleural, pericardial, and amniotic fluids. In a case control study, postexposure zidovudine (AZT) decreased HIV-1 infection by 81% (30). Recently updated guidelines by the New York State department of health recommend initiating postexposure prophylaxis as soon as possible after it has been determined that an exposure has occurred, ideally within 2 hours and not later than 36 hours. HAART should be recommended (33). The combination of Combivir with nelfinavir remains the preferred regimen, but consultation with an HIV specialist is highly recommended in order to choose a regimen based on the source patient's HIV strain and antiretroviral resistance, if known. Nevirapine is not recommended for postexposure prophylaxis because of the incidence of severe hepatitis (31). A medical evaluation, counseling, and follow-up by an experienced physician should be provided promptly, but initiation of postexposure prophylaxis should not be delayed (32) (www.hiv guidelines.org, www.hivatis.org). Recommendations for pregnant health care workers are similar except that efavirenz and amprenavir should be avoided (33,34).

Prevention of Transmission among the Disabled

One of the most significant things rehabilitation professionals can do to stop the spread of HIV is to educate their patients as to the modes of transmission and means of preventing transmission. High-risk behaviors must be strongly discouraged, and education in safer sex practices should be included as part of all discussions on sexuality.

The most effective protective measure is the use of a barrier device whenever contact with infectious fluids is anticipated.

This includes the use of condoms, the dental dam for oral sex, and the use of gloves or a finger cot for digital anal penetration. Safe touching should be substituted for scratching, biting, and abrading activities that might lead to inadvertent fluid exposures. Water-soluble lubricants should be used, particularly in insensate areas to reduce the likelihood of inadvertent abrasion. Mutual masturbation may be suggested as an activity that is virtually risk-free. Patients should be reminded to clean and disinfect all enrichment aids (sex toys) using a solution such as 10% chlorine bleach.

When patients experience direct exposure to infectious fluids, prophylaxis should be offered as it is to health-care workers. Because about one-fourth of children delivered vaginally to untreated infected mothers will also be infected, prophylaxis should also be used to reduce vertical transmission. A prospective trial showed that pregnant women who took AZT could decrease the risk of perinatal transmission by 67% (35,36), and several subsequent trials have shown that the risk of mother-to-child transmission can be reduced substantially by perinatal treatment of both mother and neonate (37,38). Prevention of transmission in the adolescent patient demands particular attention (39). The avoidance of HIV transmission among patients who lack the capacity to modify their behavior, such as brain-injured individuals with impaired impulse control, remains a difficult area without clear-cut solutions (40,41).

CLINICAL EVALUATION OF HIV

Serologic Testing

The mainstay of HIV-1 testing involves screening for anti-HIV-1 antibodies with ELISA, with the Western blot test used for confirmation. Serologic testing can only detect infection after seroconversion has occurred, which may take up to 3 to 6 months after acute infection. When ELISA screening and confirmatory Western blot testing are used, the false-positive rate is negligible. Pre- and posttest counseling are advisable to educate patients about the need for repeat testing, as well as modification of high-risk behaviors and, in the event of a positive test, the need to seek specialized medical care. Home test kits, in which samples of saliva, blood, or urine can be collected by the patient at home or in a doctor's office and sent directly to testing laboratories, are available.

Evaluation of the Seropositive Patient

It is particularly important to identify seropositive individuals, both because medical therapy for HIV is highly beneficial and in order to identify the individuals at risk for spreading the infection to others. In patients with unexplained sweats, fevers, or weight loss; skin lesions characteristic of opportunistic infections or malignancy; dyspnea unrelated to intrinsic cardiac or pulmonary disease; or altered neurologic function not attributable to a specific lesion, injury, or toxin, HIV infection must be considered in the differential diagnosis. The presence of other sexually transmitted diseases also should be considered an indication for HIV testing. Even the presence of diseases seen at higher rates in HIV patients, such as tuberculosis (TB), should be considered an indication for testing.

The physical exam should focus on findings often seen in association with HIV. The skin and oral cavity should be carefully examined for mucocutaneous lesions, particularly those associated with Kaposi's sarcoma. The presence of lymphadenopathy or hepatosplenomegaly are also important indicators. Because of the propensity of HIV to involve the nervous sys-

tem, a detailed neurologic examination is essential. Peripheral neuropathies, cognitive disorders, myelopathy, and focal CNS dysfunction may all be seen in association with HIV. Although cognitive dysfunction is not common before the development of AIDS, a neuropsychologic evaluation is helpful to establish a baseline.

The laboratory evaluation should include routine chemistries and a complete blood count. A mild increase in transaminases may be seen, along with an elevated erythrocyte sedimentation rate, anemia, and general cytopenias. Serum protein electrophoresis may demonstrate an increase in immunoglobulins. Lymphocyte evaluation may demonstrate a decrease in CD4-positive lymphocytes or a reversal in the CD4/CD8 ratio. Viral load tests, such as the polymerase chain reaction (PCR) or branched deoxyribonucleic acid (DNA), are important for establishing prognosis and for evaluating the effectiveness of antiretroviral treatments.

TREATMENT STRATEGIES IN AIDS

Because clinically latent stages of HIV-1 infection involve rapid viral replication, strategies now aim to decrease steady-state viral RNA levels. The benefits of decreasing HIV viral load must be weighed against side effects and the risk of developing resistant strains (42,43). Published guidelines are meant to be interpreted by specialized providers (www.hivatis.org) (44). Medications commonly used in HIV along with some of their indications and side effects are summarized in Table 82-2. Numerous important side effects and drug interactions may occur that may limit effectiveness or tolerability of therapy, or result in dangerous iatrogenic complications and disability (45,46).

Antiretroviral Agents

Combination therapy with three or more antiretroviral agents has become the standard of care. Usually combinations consist of either three nucleoside analogue reverse transcriptase (RT) inhibitors or two nucleoside analogue reverse transcriptase inhibitors plus a protease inhibitor or nonnucleoside analogue reverse transcriptase inhibitor. Other combinations can also be effective; however, numerous clinical trials have demonstrated the emergence of resistant strains with monotherapy and dual therapy (47–49).

REVERSE TRANSCRIPTASE INHIBITORS

In 1987, AZT, a nucleoside analog reverse transcriptase inhibitor, was approved by the FDA. Subsequently approved were other nucleoside analogs, including didanosine (ddI), zalcitabine (ddC), stavudine (d4T), lamivudine (3TC), abacavir, and the nucleotide analogue reverse transcriptase inhibitor tenofovir (50–54). These agents act by inhibiting the process of reverse transcription, preventing viral RNA from being transcribed into cellular DNA. Currently there are three nonnucleoside analogue reverse transcriptase inhibitors approved in the United States. These are efavirenz, nevirapine, and delavirdine. As with the nucleoside analogues, they can be highly effective in suppressing the HIV viral load when used in combination with other agents (55–58).

PROTEASE INHIBITORS

As of this writing, six protease inhibitors have been approved by the FDA for HIV infection: saquinavir, indinavir, ritonavir, nelfinavir, amprenavir, and lopinavir, and atazanavir is expected to be approved shortly (53,59–61). These result in the

TABLE 82-2.   Common Drugs Used in HIV

Drug	Common Usage	Side Effects	Drug Interactions
Antiretrovirals (nucleoside analog reverse transcriptase inhibitors)			
Zidovudine (AZT)	Used in combination	Nausea, headache, fatigue, anemia, neutropenia, myopathy	Increased hepatotoxicity of amphotericin B, ganciclovir
Didanosine (ddI)	Used in combination	Painful neuropathy, pancreatitis, mitochondrial toxicity, lactic acidosis	May decrease absorption of other drugs
Zalcitabine (ddC)	Used in combination	Painful neuropathy, pancreatitis, oral ulcers, granulocytopenia, rash, fever, hepatitis	Increased toxicity with foscarnet and valproic acid; alcohol may increase risk of pancreatitis
Lamivudine (3TC)	Used in combination	GI intolerance	
Abacavir	Used in combination	GI intolerance; hypersensitivity reaction may be fatal	
Stavudine (d4T)	Used in combination	Painful neuropathy, hepatic dysfunction, mitochondrial toxicity, lactic acidosis	
Antiretrovirals (nucleotide analogue reverse transcriptase inhibitors)			
Tenofovir	Used in combination	GI	
Antiretrovirals (nonnucleoside analog reverse transcriptase inhibitors)			
Efavirenz	Used in combination	Rash, neurologic and sleep disturbances, lipid abnormalities	Many drug interactions, may decrease protease inhibitor levels
Nevirapine	Used in combination	Rash, hepatitis	May decrease protease inhibitor levels
Delavirdine	Used in combination	Rash	May decrease ddI levels
Antiretrovirals (protease inhibitors)			
Saquinavir	Used in combination	GI distress, elevated LFTs	Decreased bioavailability of calcium channel blockers
Indinavir	Used in combination	Hepatotoxicity, nephrolithiasis, glucose intolerance	As above, plus increased desipramine, rifabutin, ergotamine, and amiodarone levels; prolonged sedation with midazolam and triazolam; decreased OCP effectiveness; fatal arrhythmias with astemizole
Ritonavir	Used in combination or to boost other protease inhibitor levels	GI upset, perioral paresthesias, alteration of taste, headache, elevated LFTs, lipid abnormalities	Similar to indinavir, but may be more pronounced, failure of oral contraception
Nelfinavir	Used in combination	Diarrhea, lipid abnormalities	Decreases some drug levels
Amprenavir	Used in combination	GI disturbance	
Lopinavir/ritonavir	Used in combination	GI disturbance, glucose intolerance, lipid abnormalities	See ritonavir
Prophylactic agents			
Trimethoprim/ sulfamethoxazole	PCP prophylaxis and treatment, toxoplasmosis prophylaxis	Rash, fever, neutropenia, thrombocytopenia, hepatitis, headache, meningitis, hyperkalemia	Potentiation of Coumadin, oral hypoglycemics, and phenytoin; decreased effectiveness of cyclosporine
Dapsone	PCP prophylaxis	Rash, fever, hemolysis in G6PD deficiency	ddI decreases absorption; decreased effectiveness of oral contraceptives
Pentamidine	PCP prophylaxis and treatment	Aerosol: bronchospasm; IV: nephritis, pancreatitis, hypo- or hyperglycemia, rash, neutropenia	Renal failure with amphotericin B; hypocalcemia with foscarnet
Rifabutin	MAC prophylaxis	GI, auditory, iritis	Decreases levels of guanidine, oral contraceptives, phenytoin, methadone, digoxin, cyclosporine, azoles, corticosteroids, beta blockers
Azithromycin	MAC prophylaxis	GI upset	
Common treatments			
Acyclovir	Herpes simplex, zoster	Diarrhea, phlebitis (IV)	
Ganciclovir	CMV	Neutropenia, GI	Increased nephrotoxicity with cyclosporine
Foscarnet	CMV	Nephrotoxicity, seizure, nausea, hypomagnesemia, calcemia and natremia, nephrotoxicity, headache	Hypocalcemia with pentamidine
Cidofovir	CMV	Nephrotoxicity	
Fluconazole	Antifungal: candida and Cryptococcus	Hepatotoxicity, nausea, rash	Decreased absorption with cimetidine; decreased levels with carbamazepine and rifampin; increases phenytoin levels
Ketoconazole	Antifungal: candida	GI upset, pruritus, headache, rash	Fatal arrhythmias with terfenadine and astemizole; decreases rifampin; potentiates Coumadin
Itraconazole	Antifungal: histoplasmosis, aspergilla	Hepatitis, GI upset, rash headache	Fatal arrhythmias with terfenadine and astemizole; decreased levels with carbamazepine; increased sedation with midazolam
Amphotericin B, liposomal ampho B	Antifungal: serious fungal infections	Nephrotoxicity, fever, chills, hypomagnesemia, hypocalcemia	Dosage must be adjusted in renal failure

CMV, cytomegalovirus; GI, gastrointestinal; HIV, human immunodeficiency virus; IV, intravenous; LFT, liver function test; MAC, *Mycobacterium avium* complex; OCP, oral contraceptive preparation; PCP, *Pneumocystis carinii* pneumonia.

production of immature, noninfectious HIV-1 particles by blocking the cleavage of HIV-1 polyproteins into component proteins. Combinations of protease inhibitors and reverse transcriptase inhibitors have been shown to reduce plasma HIV-1 RNA below detectable levels and to reduce morbidity and mortality. The protease inhibitors are often "boosted" to higher plasma levels by the addition of low-dose ritonavir, which is a potent inhibitor of the cytochrome p450 system.

Immune Stimulants

The use of cytokines to stimulate production of CD4 cells has been used in clinical trials (62). Interleukin-2 can stimulate CD4 cell production, but it also increases virus production. The use of stimulating cytokines in conjunction with potent antiretroviral combinations is effective but is not often necessary.

COMMON CAUSES OF DEBILITY

Although HIV itself is felt to be responsible for many forms of functional compromise, particularly in the CNS, a large number of disabling syndromes are associated with opportunistic infections and malignancies. The following sections are organized by the types of impairment syndromes that result and, to the extent practical, in order of the timing of their appearance in HIV infection. A summary of these is listed in Table 82-3.

Respiratory Compromise and Disseminated Infection

PATHOGENIC FUNGI

Endemic pathogenic fungi such as *Histoplasma capsulatum, Blastomyces dermatidis,* and *Coccidioides immitis* can cause disease in normal hosts and particularly in HIV infection and AIDS. Patients often present with slowly progressive wasting, fevers, weight loss, or ulcerations of skin. Bone marrow dysfunction may occur and, occasionally, disseminated intravascular coagulation and death. The chest x-ray may be normal or show a progressive infiltrate. The serum test for *Histoplasma* polysaccharide is specific and sensitive. Treatment consists of induction with amphotericin B and maintenance with itraconazol (63,64).

MYCOBACTERIUM TUBERCULOSIS

TB caused by mycobacterium TB is common and severe, and seen early in the course of AIDS, often at CD4 counts greater than 200 cells/mL (65,66). Symptoms may be subtle. TB may disseminate to a wide variety of organs, including the brain and spine. Guidelines for the diagnosis, treatment, and prophylaxis of infectious TB have been detailed by the CDC and elsewhere (67–69). Of concern, however, are outbreaks of multidrug-resistant TB (70,71).

PNEUMOCYSTIS CARINII PNEUMONIA

Pneumocystis carinii is a funguslike pathogen that causes *Pneumocystis carinii* pneumonia (PCP), the most common AIDS-defining illness in the United States, accounting for about 18% of cases (26,72). Seen throughout the course of the disease, symptoms may develop gradually and include dyspnea on exertion, shortness of breath, cough, weight loss, fevers, and night sweats. Chest x-ray may show a diffuse alveolar infiltrate, and serum lactate dehydrogenase may be elevated. Diagnosis is most often made by identification of *Pneumocystis* organisms in expectorated sputum or from bronchoscopic specimens.

A room air blood gas with $PaO_2 \leq 70$ mm Hg indicates severe disease, which is treated with steroids in addition to intravenous trimethoprim/sulfa, primaquine with either clindamycin or dapsone, or intravenous pentamidine. Trimetrexate plus dapsone may also be used. Prophylaxis with trimethoprim/sulfa or dapsone is a mainstay of AIDS treatment when CD4 counts are less than 200.

MYCOBACTERIUM AVIUM COMPLEX

Mycobacterium avium complex, an atypical mycobacterial infection, is one of the most common opportunistic infections in AIDS patients in the United States, with an incidence of 18% to 43% in untreated patients (73–75). It may be present as a nonpathogenic colonizer or may cause disease in the bone marrow, lungs, liver, colon, and, rarely, the CNS, and occurs late in the course of the disease. The course may be indolent with fevers, night sweats, weight loss and wasting, cough, diarrhea, abdominal pains, lymphadenopathy, and lymph node pain.

Effective drug combinations for treatment of *Mycobacterium avium* complex include clarithromycin, with ethambutol as an alternative. Rifabutin, clofazimine, ethambutol, ciprofloxacin, azithromycin, and aminoglycosides (amikacin) have also been used (76). Clarithromycin has been shown to be effective in preventing disseminated *Mycobacterium avium* complex (77). Primary prophylaxis against *Mycobacterium avium* complex with azithromycin is recommended for those with CD4 counts less than 50 to 75 cells/μL (78).

Gastrointestinal and Swallowing Disorders

Gastrointestinal disease in AIDS is common and presents with diarrhea, weight loss, biliary disorders, abdominal pain, dysphagia, and oral disease (79–82). A wide range of causes are seen, including infections with cytomegalovirus (CMV), herpes simplex virus, *Mycobacterium avium* complex, intestinal parasites, and malignancies such as Kaposi's sarcoma and non-Hodgkin's lymphoma. Drug reactions are also a frequent cause. Dysphagia is due to a treatable cause in 90% of cases and is most often caused by *Candida albicans,* herpes simplex virus, or CMV esophagitis. Other causes include hairy leukoplakia, Kaposi's sarcoma, human papillomavirus infection, and neurogenic causes. The Sicca syndrome, seen often in association with lymphadenopathy, may be treated symptomatically with increased fluids, artificial tears, and careful attention to oral hygiene. Colitis often presents with abdominal pain and bloody or mucous diarrhea and is most often caused by CMV, which responds to treatment with ganciclovir (83). *Clostridium difficile, Campylobacter jejuni, Entamoeba histolytica,* and *Shigella flexneri* are also seen in colitis in AIDS patients.

HIV-RELATED LIVER DISEASE

Over the past several years, liver disease has risen to prominence in HIV patients. Many antiretroviral therapies are hepatotoxic, and a high percentage of HIV patients are infected with hepatitis B or C. It has recently been recognized that a higher percentage of HIV patients develop chronic infections than non–HIV-infected individuals and that these may progress more rapidly to cirrhosis. Treatment for hepatitis C with interferon and ribavirin is commonly used in HIV patients, and

TABLE 82-3. Common Functional Impairment Syndromes in HIV

Cause of Impairment	When Seen	Features	Prognosis	Management
Respiratory compromise and disseminated infection				
Pathogenic fungi	Pre-AIDS and AIDS	Wasting, fevers, etc.	Benign or fulminate	Antifungal agents
mTB	Early AIDS	Nonspecific fever, cough, etc.	Fair, good with HAART	Antituberculin therapy
PCP	Throughout AIDS	Nonspecific fever, cough, etc.	Good except in late AIDS	TMPX, dapsone, pentamidine; prophylaxis in all AIDS
MAC	Late AIDS	Fever, night sweats, weight loss, etc.	Poor but better with HAART	Clarithromycin, ethambutol, etc; combination therapy. prophylaxis when CD4 count is <50–75
GI and swallowing disorders				
Neurogenic swallowing disorders	Throughout AIDS, especially late	Related to underlying neurologic disorder	Related to underlying disorder	Video fluoroscopy, modified swallow, parenteral nutrition
Sicca syndrome		Impaired lacrimation and salivation	Benign course	Symptomatic treatment (artificial tears, oral lubricants, etc.)
Candidiasis	Pre-AIDS and AIDS	Oral plaques, dysphagia	Good with treatment	Topical antifungal agents; systemic agents in severe cases
Kaposi's sarcoma	Throughout AIDS	Characteristic lesions	Slow progression	Appropriate chemotherapy
Intestinal parasites	Late AIDS	Diarrhea	Good if diagnosed	Antiparasitic agents
Weakness and fatigue				
Chronic fatigue	Pre-AIDS and AIDS	Many causes	Fair	Energy conservation and pacing
Fibromyalgia	Any stage of HIV	Pain and fatigue	Good	Standard measures (NSAIDs, etc.)
Myopathy (polymyositis)	Any stage of HIV	Proximal weakness	Good	Steroids, exercise as tolerated
AIDS wasting syndrome	Late AIDS	Proximal weakness	Poor	Supportive care, anabolic steroids, human growth hormone
Pain syndromes and neuropathies				
Arthritis and arthralgias		Psoriasis associated, Reiter's syndrome, reactive and HIV	Similar to idiopathic varieties	Similar to idiopathic varieties (NSAIDs, injections, joint preservation, etc.)
Distal symmetric neuropathy	Increased with decreased CD4 count	Distal numbness, pain, and decreased strength	Responds to symptomatic therapy	Tricyclics, neuroleptics, heat/cold, gait aids, orthotics
Segmental neuropathies	Early or late	Zoster, mononeuritis simplex/multiplex, vasculitis, etc.	Variable	Similar to that in non-HIV patients
Drug-induced neuropathies, vitamin deficiencies	Related to drugs	Didanosine, zalcitabine, stavudine, vincristine, dapsone, rifampin, isoniazide, ethambutol	Good	Cessation or alterations of medications, vitamin supplementation, symptomatic management
Plantar Kaposi's sarcoma	Throughout AIDS	Characteristic lesions	Good	Radiation, custom insoles, etc.
Cognitive dysfunction				
HIV dementia	Late AIDS, but occasionally seen at presentation	Decreased memory, dysphagia, associated myelopathy	Poor	Antiretrovirals, memory book, adaptive strategies, decreased stimulation, etc.
Cryptococcal meningitis	Throughout AIDS	Fever, headache, meningismus, etc.	About 50% respond to treatment	Amphotericin B, followed by lifetime fluconazole
Neurosyphilis	Throughout AIDS	Nonspecific CNS	Fair, frequent relapse	High-dose PCN
Encephalitis (herpesviruses)	Throughout AIDS	Headache, seizure, altered consciousness, focal signs	May be self-limited, fair to good with antiviral treatment	Acyclovir for HSV, ganciclovir or foscarnet for CMV
Focal lesions (see below)	Throughout AIDS	Focal signs	Lesion specific	See below
Metabolic/iatrogenic dementia	Throughout HIV	Nonspecific CNS	Good	Proper diagnosis and correction of underlying problem

(Continued on next page)

hepatitis B can be treated with the reverse transcriptase inhibitors lamivudine and tenofovir (84,85).

CANDIDIASIS
Oral candidiasis (thrush) occurs in 43% to 93% of AIDS patients (86). It most often appears as creamy white, yellow, or erythematous patches on the palate, tongue, and buccal mucosa and causes angular cheilitis and fissures at the corners of the mouth. With more severe immunodeficiency, candida may extend into the pharynx and esophagus. It presents more often in patients with CD4 counts less than 200 cells/mL, but can occur at higher counts as well. Candidiasis may be treated with oral nystatin suspension, clotrimazole troche, or fluconazole or other azoles.

TABLE 82-3.   Common Functional Impairment Syndromes in HIV (Continued)

Cause of Impairment	When Seen	Features	Prognosis	Management
Focal brain disorders				
Cerebral toxoplasmosis	Throughout AIDS	Focal signs, altered consciousness, ring-enhancing lesions	Good with treatment	Pyrimethamine and folinic acid, plus sulfadiazine or clindamycin; prophylaxis when CD4 count is <100
PML	Advanced AIDS	Focal signs, altered consciousness	Very poor except in rare cases	Antiretrovirals
Primary CNS lymphoma	Advanced AIDS	Similar to above, occasional paraneoplastic signs	Extremely poor	Palliative radiation extends both quality and quantity of life
Other metastatic disease	Throughout AIDS	Similar to above	Lesion-specific	Appropriate to lesion
CNS abscesses	Throughout AIDS	Similar to above	Lesion-specific	Drainage of abscess, antimicrobials, antituberculin agents
CMV retinitis	Advanced AIDS	Visual field loss	Progressive	Ganciclovir and foscarnet
Radiculopathies and myelopathies				
Inflammatory demyelinating polyneuropathies	Early in HIV	Guillain-Barré, CIDP; may be associated with nucleoside analogues	Very good	Same as in idiopathic forms
CMV polyradiculopathy	Late AIDS	Flaccid paralysis	Arrested if treatment started quickly	Ganciclovir, foscarnet, rehabilitative interventions as in SCI
Vacuolar myelopathy	Late AIDS	Progressive paraparesis	Poor for recovery	As in other forms of SCI
Other myelitis	Throughout AIDS	Tropical spastic paraparesis (HTLV-1), herpesviruses, meningitis, Pott's disease	Poor	As in other forms of SCI
Pediatric HIV				
LIP	Common throughout AIDS	Nonspecific with variable course	Usually benign	Corticosteroids, symptomatic management for exacerbations
HIV encephalopathy	Common and progressive with AIDS	Static, progressive, or progressive/plateau	Variable	Rehabilitative Interventions similar to spastic diplegic CP

AIDS, acquired immunodeficiency syndrome; CIDP, chronic inflammatory demyelinating polyneuropathy; CMV, cytomegalovirus; CNS, central nervous system; CP, cerebral palsy; GI, gastrointestinal; HAART, highly active antiretroviral therapy; HIV, human immunodeficiency virus; HSV, herpes simplex virus; HTLV, human T-cell lymphotrophic virus; LIP, lymphoid interstitial pneumonitis; MAC, *Mycobacterium avium* complex; mTB, *Mycobacterium tuberculosis*; NSAIDs, nonsteroidal antiinflammatory drugs; PCN, penicillin; PCP, *Pneumocystis carinii* pneumonia; PML, primary multifocal leukoencephalopathy; SCI, spinal cord injury; TMPX, trimethoprim/sulfamethoxazole.

KAPOSI'S SARCOMA

Kaposi's sarcoma is a highly vascular malignant lesion containing endothelial cells and spindle-shaped mesenchymal cells. It can involve skin, oral mucosa, and visceral organs and often appears as dark blue or purple papules or nodules. Cosmetically, lesions can be treated by laser bleaching and spot radiation. Often, Kaposi's sarcoma will regress with immune reconstitution on antiretroviral therapy (87). More severe disease has been treated with antiretrovirals and drugs such as foscarnet (88), localized radiation, immunotherapy with interferon-alpha, cytotoxic chemotherapy, and liposomal doxorubicin (89, 90). Intralesional human chorionic gonadotropin has also been effective (91). Associated edema may be controlled with the use of compressive garments, and painful lesions in the feet may be managed with the use of soft insoles and by unweighting the affected extremity.

INTESTINAL PARASITES

Cryptosporidium parvum is an intracellular protozoan usually seen with CD4 counts less than 200. It is responsible for approximately 1% of AIDS deaths (92). Oral paromomycin or azithromycin may be effective in decreasing diarrhea and stabilizing body weight (93). Microsporidiosis causes similar symptoms and may be treated with albendazole (94). Other in-testinal parasites include *Isospora belli*, *Entamoeba histolytica*, and *Giardia lamblia* (95,96).

Weakness and Fatigue in HIV

Persons with HIV are often fatigued for a variety of reasons, including fibromyalgia, pulmonary dysfunction, anemia, encephalopathy, endocrine dysfunction, myopathies, cardiomyopathy, psychiatric disorders, and depression. Fibromyalgia is commonly seen, and the response to traditional measures is generally good. Fatigue may also result from the effects of antiretroviral therapy. The importance of preventative measures cannot be overemphasized with this population, including the use of light exercise to tolerance, early mobilization after an acute illness, and other measures to prevent common complications of immobility. Psychostimulants and anabolic steroids may also play a role (2,97–109).

HIV-RELATED CARDIAC DISEASE

Although the mechanisms involved are not clear, HIV-related cardiomyopathy is common (110). Other causes of cardiac dysfunction include pericardial disease, infectious and noninfectious endocarditis, metastatic Kaposi's sarcoma, and lymphoma. When symptomatic, management is similar to that of congestive heart failure of other causes, with the use of vasodilators, diuretics, and digitalis preparations. Exercise is instituted as tolerated in a similar fashion.

HIV NEPHROPATHY

An HIV-related nephropathy has been described (111). It is characterized by fluid and electrolyte abnormalities, acid-base imbalance, and proteinuria. Acute renal failure is usually the result of hypovolemia and ischemia or iatrogenic factors from the toxic effects of diagnostic agents and medications.

MYOPATHIES

HIV myopathy may present at any stage of infection, usually as proximal muscle weakness most prominently in the thighs, particularly after exertion (112,113). Myalgia occurs in 25% to 50% of cases (114). Weight loss is common. Creatinine kinase is usually elevated, and electromyography demonstrates abundant spontaneous activity with short-duration, low-amplitude polyphasic motor unit action potentials (115). Confirmation can usually be obtained from muscle biopsy, which demonstrates focal necrosis with regeneration. Prednisone has been reported to improve strength (116). The role of exercise is thought to be similar to that in non–HIV-associated myopathies.

Mitochondrial disease and associated myopathies are common in association with antiretroviral therapy and may even persist in newborns whose mothers have undergone therapy for HIV (117–119). Nemaline myopathy has also been described and is clinically and electrophysiologically indistinguishable from HIV myopathy. Other myopathies may be toxic, autoimmune, or related to Coxasacki virus or human T-cell lymphotrophic virus type I (HTLV-I) coinfection (120). These must be distinguished from the AIDS wasting syndrome, which presents insidiously, late in the course of disease, with symmetrical proximal muscle weakness. Beneficial effects from anabolic steroids, growth hormone, and, particularly, exercise have been described (102,121–124).

Pain Syndromes and Neuropathies

ARTHRITIC DISORDERS

Arthralgias arising from a variety of ill-defined causes are common in association with HIV and with antiretroviral treatment (117,125). Arthritis is also relatively frequent, with psoriasis-associated arthritis, Reiter's syndrome, and reactive arthritis all being described (126–128). Septic arthritis, however, is a fairly rare complication of AIDS (129). The prognosis and management is comparable to that of idiopathic arthritides.

AVASCULAR NECROSIS

Numerous reports have surfaced in recent years of avascular necrosis of the hips in patients with HIV (130–134). Early speculation that this is associated with the use of protease inhibitors has proven to be false (135). Some reports have demonstrated a positive correlation with steroid use (136,137). Of more concern is that radiologic evidence of avascular necrosis has been demonstrated in individuals with HIV who are asymptomatic for hip pain or dysfunction (138). It is not known how many of these if any will develop pain and impairment in mobility as a result of avascular necrosis; however, the potential for collapse of the femoral head must be considered. Presumably, those who are symptomatic can be managed similarly to those with avascular necrosis from other causes.

OTHER RHEUMATOLOGIC DISORDERS

Vasculitis is an unusual finding in HIV, with a reported incidence of 0.4% to 1% (139). Unfortunately, the prognosis is generally poor. Polyarteritis nodosa and an adult Kawasaki-like syndrome have also been described (140,141).

DISTAL SYMMETRIC NEUROPATHY

Peripheral neuropathies are frequently seen in HIV, with a distal symmetrical polyneuropathy being demonstrable on EMG in 35% of AIDS cases (142–147). Symptomatic in about 18% of patients with AIDS, its incidence increases with increasing viral load, and pathologic evidence can be found in nearly all cases on sural nerve biopsy or at autopsy. More common in adults, it has also been reported in children (148,149). It remains essential, however, to rule out treatable causes of neuropathy.

On biopsy, a "dying back" of distal fibers is seen, with loss of both myelinated and nonmyelinated fibers. In some cases, perivascular mononuclear inflammatory infiltrates are seen. Electromyographically, sensory nerve action potentials are reduced in amplitude initially, and F waves are abnormal. In time, denervation potentials become evident in distal muscle groups, and long-duration polyphasic motor unit action potentials, decreased recruitment, and increased amplitude may be seen (115,150).

The treatment of symptomatic peripheral neuropathies has included everything from traditional medications used in treating painful neuropathies to applied vibration and acupuncture (151–156).

OTHER SENSORIMOTOR NEUROPATHIES

Drug-induced neuropathies commonly result from the antiretroviral drugs didanosine, zalcitabine, and stavudine. Other drugs commonly used in AIDS patients that can cause neuropathies include vincristine, dapsone, rifampin, isoniazide, and ethambutol (157–159). Mononeuropathy simplex and multiplex may occur early in HIV as a limited peripheral neuropathy that must be distinguished from segmental herpes zoster, also a common cause of painful neuropathy (160). A multifocal neuropathy associated with severe weakness and disability, and often with fever and cachexia, also may be seen in advanced AIDS. EMG is consistent with both axonal loss and demyelination (115). Motor neuron disease has rarely been reported in patients with HIV, and there is little direct evidence of an association between the two (161).

AUTONOMIC NEUROPATHY

Autonomicneuropathy is commonly found in association with HIV infection, particularly in advanced AIDS (162–166). Patients may experience orthostatic hypotension, syncope, impotence, decreased sweating, impaired gastric motility, and diarrhea. As always, it is important to rule out iatrogenic causes from the use of common medications.

Cognitive Dysfunction in HIV

HIV-ASSOCIATED DEMENTIA

The most common cause of cognitive dysfunction is HIV-associated dementia, also known as the AIDS dementia complex, subacute encephalitis, and HIV encephalopathy (167–170). Although it is usually not seen until advanced disease, it may be present in 3% to 7% of cases at the time of diagnosis and will eventually be found in 15% to 20% of those with advanced disease, making it the leading cause of dementia in young adults (171). Ironically, the incidence in individuals undergoing HAART with CD4 counts greater than 200 cells/mL may actually be increasing (172). Although poorly understood, monocytes and dopaminergic pathways have been implicated (173–178). Alcohol and cocaine may play a role in hastening the progression of dementia (179). Although electrophysiologic abnormalities can be demonstrated on evoked potential testing in a majority of individuals with HIV and abnormalities are evident in functional imaging studies (180), cognitive dysfunction does not usually become evident before the development of AIDS, and the existence of subtle cognitive changes in early disease remains controversial (181,182).

CRYPTOCOCCAL MENINGITIS

Cryptococcus is an important fungal pathogen in patients with CD4 counts less than 200 cells/mL (183). The incidence has declined since the advent of HAART (184). Infection most often presents with meningitis, and symptoms include fever, headache, neck stiffness, and memory loss. Patients may show signs of lethargy, confusion, meningismus, or cranial nerve palsies. Signs and symptoms in AIDS patients, however, are often mild (185). Cryptococcal antigen may be detected in the cerebrospinal fluid (CSF) or serum for diagnosis. Initial treatment is with amphotericin B or fluconazole followed by fluconazole maintenance (186–189). Prophylaxis with low-dose fluconazole may be of use in high-risk patients (190).

OTHER CAUSES OF COGNITIVE DYSFUNCTION

Treponema pallidum may cause chronic meningitis, neuropathy, or dementia when infecting the CNS of AIDS patients (neurosyphilis) (191,192). CSF pleocytosis is often seen, and a CSF Venereal Disease Research Laboratory test (VDRL) may be positive, but sensitivity is low. Treatment is usually with intravenous penicillin G, but relapses are common.

Varicella zoster, a common cause of pneumonia and skin eruptions in AIDS patients, also results in a variety of neurologic syndromes, including painful nerve palsies, transverse myelitis, ascending myelitis, encephalitis, and leukoencephalopathy (193–195). In contrast to herpes simplex virus encephalitis, herpes zoster encephalitis rarely causes focal neurologic signs, deep alterations in consciousness, or seizures. The usual duration of neurologic symptoms is approximately 16 days, and the outcome is generally better than that with the other CNS infections. PCR assay for herpes zoster virus may aid in diagnosis and management. Acute mononucleosis caused by Epstein-Barr virus is also common, often leading to encephalitis, acute cerebellar syndrome, transverse or ascending myelitis, or acute psychosis (196).

Other causes of cognitive dysfunction include cytomegalovirus encephalitis, aseptic meningitis, and cerebral vasculitis (139,160,197–199). Cognitive dysfunction also may result from disorders that cause focal CNS syndromes. As always, with any dementia workup, it is essential to rule out iatrogenic and other potentially treatable causes.

Focal Brain Lesions Found in HIV

The focal deficits seen in association with AIDS are related directly to the areas of the brain affected and may include blindness, hemiparesis, ataxia, aphasia, dysarthria, and cranial nerve deficits (160,200–203). Movement disorders, including hemichorea-ballismus, segmental myoclonus, postural tremor, parkinsonism, and dystonia, also may be found.

TOXOPLASMOSIS

Cerebral toxoplasmosis is the most common CNS mass lesion in AIDS, occurring in 3% to 40% of cases (160,204–206). Without prophylaxis, 30% of previously toxoplasma-seropositive AIDS patients may relapse when the CD4 count drops below 50 cells/mL. Most patients present with focal or nonfocal neurologic signs produced by space-occupying lesions. Headaches, confusion, lethargy, and seizures are common. Contrast-enhanced head computed tomography or magnetic resonance imaging reveals single or multiple ring-enhancing lesions that may be distinguished from lymphoma by biopsy or radiolabeled thallium uptake (203,207–209).

A common diagnostic strategy is to initiate antitoxoplasma therapy and observe for clinical response, which is often dramatic. Treatment regimens include pyrimethamine and folinic acid plus either sulfadiazine or clindamycin. Patients with a positive antitoxoplasma immunoglobulin G antibody should take prophylaxis when their CD4 count is less than 100 cells/mL (210). Trimethoprim/sulfa, often used for *Pneumocystis carinii* pneumonia prophylaxis, is effective, as is clindamycin plus pyrimethamine.

PROGRESSIVE MULTIFOCAL LEUKOENCEPHALOPATHY

Progressive multifocal leukoencephalopathy is a white matter disease associated with infection by the JC virus (200). It occurs in approximately 4% of AIDS patients. Single or multifocal lesions confined to the white matter without the presence of a mass effect or contrast enhancement may be seen on magnetic resonance imaging. Diagnosis can be made based on radiographic appearance or more definitively by biopsy (211). The median survival is on the order of 2 to 4 months, although in approximately 10% of cases, a more benign course is seen, and spontaneous remissions may even occur after HAART is added (212–214).

CNS LYMPHOMA

CNS lymphoma is associated with late-stage AIDS and CD4 counts of less than 100 cells/mL. It may present as a mass lesion with confusion, headache, memory loss, or focal neurologic signs. Untreated, it usually progresses to death in 1 month or less. Palliative radiation can temporarily improve symptoms and extend survival, with an increased quality of life in 75% of cases (215). Associated paraneoplastic syndromes are common. Rarely, other malignancies and metastatic lesions may be seen in the brain, particularly from Kaposi's sarcoma (216).

CMV RETINOPATHY

CMV is one of the most common pathogens in AIDS patients, with more than 90% of patients showing evidence of past exposure and as many as 40% of those with advanced disease developing active CMV disease (217). About 85% of CMV disease in AIDS patients presents as retinitis, which usually affects those with CD4 counts less than 50 cells/mL. Productive infection of the retina can cause full thickness necrosis, although patients may be asymptomatic and gradual visual loss may be unnoticed until vision is significantly impaired. Ophthalmologic examination shows characteristic perivascular yellow-white lesions that are frequently associated with retinal hemorrhage (218). These must be distinguished from cotton wool spots, which are white, fluffy, superficial infarcts of the nerve fiber layer that usually spontaneously regress and do not lead to blindness.

The mainstay of treatment has typically involved a combination of ganciclovir, a nucleoside analogue, and foscarnet, a pyrophosphate analogue (218–220). Cidofovir is a newer agent with a long half-life and can suppress CMV up to 3 weeks after a single administration with probenacid (221,222). Intravitreal injection of ganciclovir and cidofovir, as well as intraocular implants of timed-release devices with ganciclovir or foscarnet, have also been used with success (223–225). Complications are common with all of these drugs (see Table 82-2). Although the incidence is decreasing as a result of HAART, those infected continue to have a poor prognosis, and drug resistance is common (219,220,226,227). Eventual progression to blindness can occur, making early institution of visual retraining and blind rehabilitation particularly important.

OTHER CAUSES OF FOCAL CNS SYNDROMES

Herpes simplex virus I may infect the brain in AIDS patients, causing an encephalitis characterized by the acute onset of headache, behavioral changes with focal neurologic signs, seizures, and coma. Although an increased incidence of thromboembolic cerebrovascular events has been reported, it is not clear that the incidence is greater than that of the general population (228–231). This is in contrast to cerebral vasculitis, which does have an association with AIDS. Primary CNS angiitis is a rare and usually fatal disorder that has a predilection for small cortical vessels (199,232,233). Bacterial and fungal abscesses may also cause focal neurologic deficits (234). TB is of particular concern and may require biopsy for diagnosis. Antituberculin therapy is often initiated in those with a positive purified protein derivative and a new focal lesion when the diagnosis is uncertain (235).

Radiculopathies and Myelopathies

INFLAMMATORY DEMYELINATING NEUROPATHIES

HIV is a major cause of inflammatory demyelinating polyneuropathies and must always be considered in the differential (157,236–238). Guillain-Barré syndrome, or acute inflammatory demyelinating neuropathy, occurs early, often around the time of seroconversion, and is clinically and histopathologically indistinguishable from the idiopathic form. It is managed similarly. In some cases, chronic inflammatory demyelinating polyneuropathy or relapsing polyneuropathy may be seen.

Nerve conduction studies are significant for prolonged sensory and motor latencies with patchy slowing to less than 60% to 70% of normal (115). Marked reduction in motor action potential amplitude or even motor conduction block may be indicative of focal demyelination. F wave and H reflexes are often markedly delayed or absent. The EMG needle exam usually fails to show abnormal spontaneous activity, although denervation potentials with diminished recruitment may sometimes be seen in weak distal muscles.

CMV POLYRADICULOPATHY

CMV causes a common and debilitating peripheral neuropathy in which CMV infects the nerve roots and ganglia (237,239). Patients present with back and lower-extremity sensory changes and weakness that may rapidly progress to flaccid paralysis (236,240). It can be rapidly fatal unless treatment is started within the first 24 to 48 hours (197,237,239). Treatment is effective in halting progression, although patients are often left with severe deficits that may require rehabilitation.

Findings include loss of lower-extremity deep-tendon reflexes, saddle anesthesia, and urinary retention, whereas upper-extremity strength is preserved. Diffuse spontaneous activity is seen on EMG, with decreased recruitment but near-normal conduction velocities (115). The CSF often has a pleocy-tosis with neutrophils and may show elevated protein and inclusion cells, which may stain positive for CMV antigens (197,236). Improvement on treatment with ganciclovir has been described (147,236,241,242). Foscarnet also can be effective.

VACUOLAR MYELOPATHY

Vacuolar myelopathy is the most common cause of spinal cord dysfunction in HIV, being found in 11% to 22% of AIDS cases and demonstrable in as many as 40% of cases at autopsy (160,243,244). It is strongly associated with HIV dementia and shares a virtually identical histopathology. Patients present with progressive paraparesis, ataxia, posterior column sensory loss, spasticity, and neurogenic bowel and bladder.

Spinal cord dysfunction may also result from viral myelitis secondary to varicella zoster virus, herpes simplex virus, CMV, and HTLV-I. Spinal cord disorders may also be seen with tuberculin involvement (Pott's disease), multiple sclerosis, and aseptic, cryptococcal, and lymphomatous meningitis (244,245).

PEDIATRIC HIV

Pediatric cases of HIV differ significantly from their adult counterparts (246,247). More than 80% of cases of HIV infection in children are the result of perinatal transmission, with transmission from blood products being less frequent. The most effective strategy to minimize vertical transmission is prophylactic treatment of the mother as well as the newborn (37,248). Because of transplacental transmission of antibodies, however, most infants of HIV-positive mothers will initially be seropositive at birth, with signs of infection developing in approximately 80% of those with disease at a median age of 5 months. Significant advances in medical management over the past 5 years, however, have resulted in a substantial decrease in the progression to AIDS and an improvement in survival (249).

Opportunistic Infections

In contrast to adults, opportunistic infections of the nervous system are extremely uncommon (250). AIDS-defining criteria in children include recurrent bacterial infections, opportunistic infections, lymphoid interstitial pneumonitis, malignancies, cardiomyopathies, hepatitis, nephropathy, and encephalopathy. Infants with AIDS often present with hepatosplenomegaly, lymphadenopathy, diarrhea, oral candidiasis, parotid enlargement, delayed developmental milestones, and failure to thrive.

More than 80% of HIV-infected children eventually develop either acute or chronic lung diseases. Although most are acute infectious processes, chronic diseases, such as lymphoid interstitial pneumonitis, may occur in 30% to 50% (251–253). The etiology and natural history of lymphoid interstitial pneumonitis are incompletely understood. Although some patients are asymptomatic with infiltrates on chest x-ray, others experience a slowly progressive course with exacerbations caused by lung infections, and some may progress to chronic respiratory decompensation and hypoxemia. HIV-infected children with lymphoid interstitial pneumonitis are believed to have a better long-term prognosis than those with other pulmonary infections. Corticosteroids are used to suppress the lymphocytic infiltrate.

HIV Encephalopathy

The most common neurologic disorder seen in children is HIV encephalopathy (254–257). This may be static, progressive, or progressive with a plateau. Static encephalopathy is characterized by delayed acquisition of developmental skills and is seen in 25% of those with CNS deficits. With progressive encephalopathy, on the other hand, the pace of development becomes progressively slower and may halt altogether or show signs of regression. The clinical picture is not unlike that of spastic diplegic cerebral palsy, but with progressive deficits.

Other children may demonstrate more subtle neurodevelopmental deficits, including easy fatigability, mild depression, expressive language deficits, and mild regression in school performance. The response to antiretroviral therapies has been reported to be good. Uncommon neurologic disorders that may be encountered in children include CNS lymphoma, corticospinal tract degeneration, and, rarely, myelopathy, myopathy, and peripheral neuropathy (148).

PSYCHOSOCIAL AND VOCATIONAL ISSUES

HIV remains one of the most stigmatized diseases of our time. As in oncologic rehabilitation, patients may be faced with issues of death and dying but with appropriate therapy, hope, and long-term survival. Discrimination remains a particular problem because of the infectious nature of the disease and to public misperceptions and prejudice. The health of the caregiver, if there is one, is of particular concern when developing rehabilitation strategies. As always, rehabilitation professionals must deal with the patient in the context of their surroundings and their external support network.

Before the onset of symptoms, 70% to 90% of people with HIV are still employed (258). Even in the first year after the onset of symptoms, fewer than one-third leave the workforce. People with HIV commonly experience workplace discrimination and, with advancing symptoms, may experience a diminished work capacity. Significant controversy exists regarding persons with HIV in the health-care field. Those who are forced to leave the workforce face a potential loss of health insurance. In all other respects, vocational rehabilitation of the HIV patient is similar to that of the patient with cancer or multiple sclerosis, but always keeping in mind the potential for full recovery and long-term health.

THE FUTURE OF HIV REHABILITATION

The management of HIV is one of the most rapidly changing fields of medicine, with entirely new treatment strategies often becoming available in a period of months rather than years. By the time this is published, it is likely that new medications not discussed here will be in common usage. The complexion of HIV rehabilitation continues to evolve rapidly, and the future of HIV rehabilitation is thus largely unknown. As a cure still does not seem to be imminent, however, it is reasonable to expect a need for rehabilitation interventions for the foreseeable future.

Most HIV strategists currently view HIV as being managed as a chronic disease similar to diabetes mellitus. Although not curable, its progression will be held in check by medical therapies. This comparison to diabetes may be particularly apt in the case of rehabilitation. Although the most serious morbidity and mortality of diabetes is avoidable, even with stringent control of blood glucose, amputation, blindness, and peripheral neuropathy remain common sequelae that often respond to rehabilitation interventions. Although new HIV treatments are indeed remarkable in their ability to arrest development of functional impairments and disability, they introduce toxicities of their own that may lead to yet a new set of impairments.

It has now become apparent that long-term viral suppression with antiretrovirals is achievable for most HIV patients, but that it requires an incredible 95% adherence to treatment regimens (259). Missed doses may allow viral replication to produce drug-resistant strains. Much of the effort in care for patients is expended in encouraging and enabling this high-level adherence. Adherence is an integral part of HIV treatment programs.

In the last edition of this book, we speculated that rehabilitation professionals might face a future practice consisting of otherwise healthy individuals with HIV and a variety of disabling conditions such as Guillain-Barré syndrome, polymyositis, distal symmetric polyneuropathy, HIV dementia, and vacuolar myelopathy. Although the numbers remain limited, many have in fact noted an increase in potentially disabling conditions in otherwise healthy individuals with HIV, leading some to call for more emphasis on rehabilitation (3,260–263). Remarkably, exercise has been shown to play a significant role in improving not only the aerobic capacity but also immune system function in individuals with HIV (264–269). The role of rehabilitation may thus be critical not only in keeping these people functional in their communities, but in maintaining their health as well.

REFERENCES

1. O'Connell PG, Levinson SF. Experience with rehabilitation in the acquired immunodeficiency syndrome. *Am J Phys Med Rehabil* 1991;70:195–200.
2. O'Dell MW, Hubert HB, Lubeck DP, et al. Physical disability in a cohort of persons with AIDS: data from the AIDS Time-Oriented Health Outcome Study. *AIDS* 1996;10:667–673.
3. O'Dell MW, Hubert HB, Lubeck DP, et al. Pre-AIDS physical disability: data from the AIDS Time-Oriented Health Outcome Study [see comments]. *Arch Phys Med Rehabil* 1998;79:1200–1205.
4. Crystal S, Sambamoorthi U. Functional impairment trajectories among persons with HIV disease: a hierarchical linear models approach. *Health Serv Res* 1996;31:469–488.
5. Fleishman JA, Crystal S. Functional status transitions and survival in HIV disease: evidence from the AIDS Costs and Service Utilization Survey. *Med Care* 1998;36:533–543.
6. Missmer SA, Spiegelman D, Gorbach SL, et al. Predictors of change in the functional status of children with human immunodeficiency virus infection. *Pediatrics* 2000;106:E24.
7. Wilson IB, Cleary PD. Clinical predictors of functioning in persons with acquired immunodeficiency syndrome. *Med Care* 1996;34:610–623.
8. Wilson IB, Cleary PD. Clinical predictors of declines in physical functioning in persons with AIDS: results of a longitudinal study. *J Acquir Immune Defic Syndr* 1997;16:343–349.
9. Cunningham WE, Shapiro MF, Hays RD, et al. Constitutional symptoms and health-related quality of life in patients with symptomatic HIV disease. *Am J Med* 1998;104:129–136.
10. Grimes DE, Cole FL. Self-help and life quality in persons with HIV disease. *AIDS Care* 1996;8:691–699.
11. Peterman AH, Cella D, Mo F, et al. Psychometric validation of the revised Functional Assessment of Human Immunodeficiency Virus Infection (FAHI) quality of life instrument. *Qual Life Res* 1997;6:572–584.
12. Fauci AS, Pantaleo G, Stanley S, et al. Immunopathogenic mechanisms of HIV infection. *Ann Intern Med* 1996;124:654–663.
13. Pantaleo G, Graziosi C, Demarest JF, et al. HIV infection is active and progressive in lymphoid tissue during the clinically latent stage of disease. *Nature* 1993;362:355–358.
14. Pantaleo G, Graziosi C, Fauci AS. New concepts in the immunopathogenesis of human immunodeficiency virus infection. *N Engl J Med* 1993;328:327–335.
15. Havlir DV, Richman DD. Viral dynamics of HIV: implications for drug development and therapeutic strategies. *Ann Intern Med* 1996;124:984–994.
16. Koup RA, Safrit JT, Cao Y, et al. Temporal association of cellular immune responses with the initial control of viremia in primary human immunodeficiency virus type 1 syndrome. *J Virol* 1994;68:4650–4655.
17. Embretson J, Zupancic M, Ribas JL, et al. Massive covert infection of helper T lymphocytes and macrophages by HIV during the incubation period of AIDS. *Nature* 1993;362:359–362.
18. Mellors JW, Kingsley LA, Rinaldo CRJ, et al. Quantitation of HIV-1 RNA in plasma predict outcome after seroconversion. *Ann Intern Med* 1995;122:573–579.
19. Henrard DR, Phillips JF, Muenz LR, et al. Natural history of HIV-1 cell-free viremia. *JAMA* 1995;274:554–558.
20. O'Brien TR, Blattner WA, Waters D, et al. Serum HIV-1 RNA levels and time to development of AIDS in the multicenter hemophilia cohort study. *JAMA* 1996;276:105–110.

21. Wei X, Ghosh SK, Taylor ME, et al. Viral dynamics in human immunodeficiency virus type 1 infection. *Nature* 1995;373:117–122.

22. Perelson AS, Neumann AU, Markowitz M, et al. HIV-1 dynamics in vivo: virion clearance rate, infected cell lifetime, and viral generation time. *Science* 1996;271:1582–1586.

23. Najera I, Richman DD, Olivares I, et al. Natural occurrence of drug resistance mutations in the reverse transcriptase of human immunodeficiency virus type 1 isolates. *AIDS Res Hum Retroviruses* 1994;10:1479–1488.

24. Centers for Disease Control and Prevention. 1993 revised classification system for HIV infection and expanded surveillance case definition for AIDS among adolescents and adults. *MMWR* 1992;41:RR–17.

25. UNAIDS/WHO. AIDS epidemic update. In: *AIDS epidemic update*. Geneva World Health Organization, 2001:1–36.

26. Centers for Disease Control and Prevention. *HIV/AIDS Surveillance Report* 2001;13:1.

27. Tokars JI, Chamberland ME, Schable CA, et al. A survey of occupational blood contact and HIV infection among orthopedic surgeons. The American Academy of Orthopaedic Surgeons Serosurvey Study Committee. *JAMA* 1992;268:489–494.

28. Tokars JI, Marcus R, Culver DH, et al. Surveillance of HIV infection and zidovudine use among health care workers after occupational exposure to HIV-infected blood. The CDC Cooperative Needlestick Surveillance Group [see comments]. *Ann Intern Med* 1993;118:913–919.

29. Gerberding JL. Management of occupational exposures to blood-borne viruses. *N Engl J Med* 1995;332:444–451.

30. Centers for Disease Control and Prevention. Case-control study of HIV seroconversion in health-care workers after percutaneous exposure to HIV-infected blood—France, United Kingdom, and United States, January 1988–August 1994. *MMWR* 1995;44:929–933.

31. Centers for Disease Control and Prevention. Serious adverse events attributed to nevirapine regimens for postexposure prophylaxis after HIV exposures—worldwide, 1997–2000. *MMWR* 2001;49:1153–1156.

32. U. S. Public Health Service. Updated U.S. Public Health Service guidelines for the management of occupational exposures to HBV, HCV, and HIV and recommendations for postexposure prophylaxis. *MMWR Recomm Rep* 2001; 50:1–52.

33. New York State Department of Health AIDS Institute. *HIV prophylaxis following occupational exposure*. Albany, NY: New York State Department of Health, 2002.

34. Public Health Service Task Force. *Recommendations for use of antiretroviral drugs in pregnant HIV-1-infected women for maternal health and interventions to reduce perinatal HIV-1 transmission in the United States*. Bethesda, MD: National Library of Medicine, 2002.

35. Connor EM, Sperling RS, Gelber R, et al. Reduction of maternal-infant transmission of human immunodeficiency virus type 1 with zidovudine treatment. Pediatric AIDS Clinical Trials Group Protocol 076 Study Group. *N Engl J Med* 1994;3331:1173–1180.

36. Mauskopf JA, Paul JE, Wichman DS, et al. Economic impact of treatment of HIV-positive pregnant women and their newborns with zidovudine. *JAMA* 1996;276:132–138.

37. Guay LA, Musoke P, Fleming T, et al. Intrapartum and neonatal single-dose nevirapine compared with zidovudine for prevention of mother-to-child transmission of HIV-1 in Kampala, Uganda: HIVNET 012 randomised trial. *Lancet* 1999;354:795–802.

38. Mofenson LM, Munderi P. Safety of antiretroviral prophylaxis of perinatal transmission for HIV-infected pregnant women and their infants. *J Acquir Immune Defic Syndr* 2002;30:200–215.

39. Rotheram-Borus MJ, Mahler KA, Rosario M. AIDS prevention with adolescents [Review]. *AIDS Educ Prev* 1995;7:320–336.

40. Auerbach V, Jann B. Neurorehabilitation and HIV Infection: clinical dilemmas. *J Head Trauma Rehabil* 1989;4:23–31.

41. Boccellari A, Zeifert P. Management of neurobehavioral impairment in HIV-1 infection. *Psychiatr Clin North Am* 1994;17:183–203.

42. Carr A, Cooper DA. Adverse effects of antiretroviral therapy. *Lancet* 2000; 356:1423–1430.

43. Smith KY. Selected metabolic and morphologic complications associated with highly active antiretroviral therapy. *J Infect Dis* 2002;185:S123–127.

44. Public Health Service Task Force. Guidelines for the use of antiretroviral agents in HIV-infected adults and adolescents. Bethesda, MD: National Library of Medicine, 2002.

45. Bartlett JA, Benoit SL, Johnson VA, et al. Lamivudine plus zidovudine compared with zalcitabine plus zidovudine in patients with HIV infection. *Ann Intern Med* 1996;125:161–172.

46. Schapiro JM, Winters MA, Stewart F, et al. The effect of high-dose saquinavir on viral load and CD4+ T-cell counts in HIV-infected patients. *Ann Intern Med* 1996;124:1039–1050.

47. Concorde Coordinating Committee. Concorde: MRC/ANS randomised double-blind controlled trial of immediate and deferred zidovudine in symptom-free HIV infection. *Lancet* 1994;343:871–881.

48. Volberding PA, Lagakos SW, Grimes JM, et al. The duration of zidovudine benefit in persons with asymptomatic HIV infection. Prolonged evaluation of protocol 019 of the AIDS clinical Trials Group. *JAMA* 1994;272:437–442.

49. Hammer S, Katzenstein D, Hughes M, et al. Nucleoside monotherapy vs combination therapy in HIV-infected adults: a randomized, double-blind, placebo-controlled trial in persons with CD4 cell. A trial comparing nucleoside monotherapy with combination therapy in HIV-infected adults with CD4 cell counts from 200 to 500 per cubic millimeter. *N Engl J Med* 1996; 335:1081–1090.

50. Katlama C, Ingrand D, Loveday C, et al. Safety and efficacy of lamivudine-zidovudine combination therapy in antiretroviral-naive patients: a randomized controlled comparison with zidovudine monotherapy. *JAMA* 1996;276: 118–125.

51. Cihlar T, Birkus G, Greenwalt DE, et al. Tenofovir exhibits low cytotoxicity in various human cell types: comparison with other nucleoside reverse transcriptase inhibitors. *Antiviral Res* 2002;54:37–45.

52. Opravil M, Hirschel B, Lazzarin A, et al. A randomized trial of simplified maintenance therapy with abacavir, lamivudine, and zidovudine in human immunodeficiency virus infection. *J Infect Dis* 2002;185:1251–1260.

53. Falloon J, Ait-Khaled M, Thomas DA, et al. HIV-1 genotype and phenotype correlate with virological response to abacavir, amprenavir and efavirenz in treatment-experienced patients. *AIDS* 2002;16:387–396.

54. Hetherington S, Hughes AR, Mosteller M, et al. Genetic variations in HLA-B region and hypersensitivity reactions to abacavir. *Lancet* 2002;359:1121–1122.

55. Arribas J. Comparison of NNRTIs in antiretroviral-naive patients. *Int J STD AIDS* 2001;12:3–9.

56. Maggiolo F. Comparison of NNRTIs in antiretroviral-experienced patients. *Int J STD AIDS* 2001;12:10–17.

57. Nelson M. The role of NNRTIs in antiretroviral combination therapy: an introduction. *Int J STD AIDS* 2001;12:1–2.

58. Moyle G. The emerging roles of non-nucleoside reverse transcriptase inhibitors in antiretroviral therapy. *Drugs* 2001;61:19–26.

59. Eron JJ Jr. HIV-1 protease inhibitors. *Clin Infect Dis* 2000;30:S160–170.

60. Moyle GJ, Back D. Principles and practice of HIV-protease inhibitor pharmacoenhancement. *HIV Med* 2001;2:105–113.

61. Yu K, Daar ES. Dual protease inhibitor therapy in the management of the HIV-1. *Exp Opin Pharmacother* 2000;1:1331–1342.

62. Paredes R, Lopez Benaldo de Quiros JC, Fernandez-Cruz E, et al. The potential role of interleukin-2 in patients with HIV infection. *AIDS Rev* 2002;4:36–40.

63. Wheat LJ, Hafner R, Wulfsohn M, et al. Prevention of relapse of histoplasmosis with itraconazole in patients with the acquired immunodeficiency syndrome. *Ann Intern Med* 1993;118:610–616.

64. Wheat LJ, Hafner RE, Korzun AH, et al. Itraconazole treatment of disseminated histoplasmosis in patients with the acquired immunodeficiency syndrome. *Am J Med* 1995;98:336–342.

65. Chaisson RE, Schecter GF, Theuer CP, et al. Tuberculosis-acquired immunodeficiency syndrome: clinical feature, response to therapy, and survival. *Am Rev Respir Dis* 1987;136:570–574.

66. Selwyn PA, Hartel D, Lewis VA, et al. A prospective study of the risk of tuberculosis among intravenous drug users with human immunodeficiency virus infection. *N Engl J Med* 1989;320:545–550.

67. Centers for Disease Control and Prevention. Guidelines for preventing the transmission of Mycobacterium tuberculosis in health-care facilities. *MMWR* 1994;43(RR-13):1–132.

68. Barnes PF, Lakey DL, Burman WJ. Tuberculosis in patients with HIV infection. *Infect Dis Clin North Am* 2002;16:107–126.

69. Decker CF, Lazarus A. Tuberculosis and HIV infection: how to safely treat both disorders concurrently. *Postgrad Med* 2000;108:57–60, 65–68.

70. Kent JH. The epidemiology of multidrug-resistant tuberculosis in the United States. *Med Clin North Am* 1993;77:1391–1409.

71. Centers for Disease Control and Prevention. Multidrug-resistant tuberculosis outbreak on an HIV ward—Madrid, Spain, 1991–1995. *MMWR* 1996;45: 330–333.

72. Centers for Disease Control and Prevention. USPHS/IDSA guidelines for the prevention of opportunistic infections in persons infected with HIV: a summary. *MMWR* 1995;44(RR-8):1–39.

73. Horsburgh CR Jr. The pathophysiology of disseminated Mycobacterium avium complex disease in AIDS. *J Infect Dis* 1999;179:S461–465.

74. Shafran SD. Prevention and treatment of disseminated Mycobacterium avium complex infection in human immunodeficiency virus-infected individuals. *Int J Infect Dis* 1998;3:39–47.

75. Wright J. Current strategies for the prevention and treatment of disseminated Mycobacterium avium complex infection in patients with AIDS. *Pharmacotherapy* 1998;18:738–747.

76. Shafran SD, Singer J, Zarowny DP, et al. A comparison of two regimens for the treatment of mycobacterium avium complex bacteremia in AIDS: rifabutin, ethambutol, and clarithromycin versus rifampin, ethambutol, clofazimine and ciprofloxacin. *N Engl J Med* 1996;335:377–383.

77. Pierce M, Crampton S, Henry D, et al. A randomized trial of clarithromycin as prophylaxis against disseminated mycobacterium avium complex infection in patients with advanced acquired immunodeficiency syndrome. *N Engl J Med* 1996;335:384–391.

78. Havlir DV, Dube MP, Sattler FR, et al. Prophylaxis against disseminated mycobacterium avium complex with weekly azithromycin, daily rifabutin or both. *N Engl J Med* 1996;335:392–398.

79. Cohen J, West AB, Bini EJ. Infectious diarrhea in human immunodeficiency virus. *Gastroenterol Clin North Am* 2001;30:637–664.

80. Duse AG. Nosocomial infections in HIV-infected/AIDS patients. *J Hosp Infect* 1999;43:S191–201.

81. Monkemuller KE, Wilcox CM. Investigation of diarrhea in AIDS. *Can J Gastroenterol* 2000;14:933–940.

82. Pensa E, Borum ML. Opportunistic infections: gastric infections in HIV/AIDS. *AIDS Reader* 2000;10:347–349, 54, 56–58.

83. Dieterich DT, Kotler DP, Busch OF, et al. Ganciclovir treatment of cytomegalovirus colitis in AIDS: a randomized, double-blind, placebo-controlled multicenter study. *J Infect Dis* 1993;167:278–282.

84. Garcia-Samaniego J, Soriano V, Miro JM, et al. Management of chronic viral hepatitis in HIV-infected patients: Spanish Consensus Conference. October 2000. *HIV Clin Trials* 2002;3:99–114.
85. Puoti M, Airoldi M, Bruno R, et al. Hepatitis B virus co-infection in human immunodeficiency virus-infected subjects. *AIDS Rev* 2002;4:27–35.
86. Sangeorzan JA, Bradley SF, He X, et al. Epidemiology of oral candidiasis in HIV-infected patients: colonization, infection, treatment and emergence of fluconazole resistance. *Am J Med* 1994;97:339–346.
87. Monticelli A, Lewi D, Salomon H, et al. Regression of AIDS-related Kaposi's sarcoma following combined antiretroviral treatment. *Rev Argent Microbiol* 2000;32:206–208.
88. Morfeldt L, Torssander J. Long-term remission of Kaposi's sarcoma following foscarnet treatment in HIV-infected patients. *Scand J Infect Dis* 1994;26:749–752.
89. Dezube BJ. New therapies for the treatment of AIDS-related Kaposi sarcoma [Review]. *Curr Opin Oncol* 2000;12:445–449.
90. Nunez M, Saballs P, Valencia ME, et al. Response to liposomal doxorubicin and clinical outcome of HIV-1-infected patients with Kaposi's sarcoma receiving highly active antiretroviral therapy. *HIV Clin Trials* 2001;2:429–437.
91. Gill PS, Lundadi-Iskandar Y, Louie S, et al. The effects of preparations of human chorionic gonadotropin on AIDS-related Kaposi's sarcoma. *N Engl J Med* 1996;335:1261–1269.
92. Centers for Disease Control and Prevention. Assessing the public health threat associated with waterborne cryptosporidiosis: report of a workshop. *MMWR Recomm Rep* 1995;44:RR-6.
93. White AC, Chappell CL, Hayat CS, et al. Paromomycin for cryptosporidiosis in AIDS—a prospective double-blind trial. *J Infect Dis* 1994;70:419–424.
94. Weber R, Bryan RT. Microsporidial infections in immunodeficient and immunocompetent patients. *Clin Infect Dis* 1994;19:517–521.
95. Benator DA, French AL, Beaudet LM, et al. Isospora belli infection associated with acalculous cholecystitis in a patient with AIDS. *Ann Intern Med* 1994;121:663–664.
96. Miao YM, Gazzard BG. Management of protozoal diarrhoea in HIV disease. *HIV Med* 2000;1:194–199.
97. Adinolfi A. Assessment and treatment of HIV-related fatigue. *J Assoc Nurses AIDS Care* 2001;12:29–34; quiz 35–38.
98. Barroso J. A review of fatigue in people with HIV infection. *J Assoc Nurses AIDS Care* 1999;10:42–49.
99. Breitbart W, McDonald MV, Rosenfeld B, et al. Fatigue in ambulatory AIDS patients. *J Pain Symptom Manage* 1998;15:159–167.
100. Breitbart W, Rosenfeld B, Kaim M, et al. A randomized, double-blind, placebo-controlled trial of psychostimulants for the treatment of fatigue in ambulatory patients with human immunodeficiency virus disease. *Arch Intern Med* 2001;161:411–420.
101. Corless IB, Bunch EH, Kemppainen JK, et al. Self-care for fatigue in patients with HIV. *Oncol Nurs Forum* 2002;29:E60–69.
102. Darko DF, Mitler MM, Miller JC. Growth hormone, fatigue, poor sleep, and disability in HIV infection. *Neuroendocrinology* 1998;67:317–324.
103. Ferrando S, Evans S, Goggin K, et al. Fatigue in HIV illness: relationship to depression, physical limitations, and disability. *Psychosom Med* 1998;60:759–764.
104. Groopman JE. Fatigue in cancer and HIV/AIDS. *Oncology (Huntingt)* 1998;12:335–344; discussion 45–46, 51.
105. Newshan G, Leon W. The use of anabolic agents in HIV disease. *Int J STD AIDS* 2001;12:141–144.
106. O'Dell MW, Meighen M, Riggs RV. Correlates of fatigue in HIV infection prior to AIDS: a pilot study. *Disabil Rehabil* 1996;18:249–254.
107. Rose L, Pugh LC, Lears K, et al. The fatigue experience: persons with HIV infection. *J Adv Nurs* 1998;28:295–304.
108. Smith BA, Neidig JL, Nickel JT, et al. Aerobic exercise: effects on parameters related to fatigue, dyspnea, weight and body composition in HIV-infected adults. *AIDS* 2001;15:693–701.
109. Wagner GJ, Rabkin R. Effects of dextroamphetamine on depression and fatigue in men with HIV: a double-blind, placebo-controlled trial. *J Clin Psychiatry* 2000;61:436–440.
110. Barbaro G, Fisher SD, Lipshultz SE. Pathogenesis of HIV-associated cardiovascular complications. *Lancet Infect Dis* 2001;1:115–124.
111. Strauss J, Zilleruelo G, Abitbol C, et al. Human immunodeficiency virus nephropathy. *Pediatric Nephrol* 1993;7:220–225.
112. Al-Tawfiq JA, Sarosi GA, Cushing HE. Pyomyositis in the acquired immunodeficiency syndrome. *South Med J* 2000;93:330–334.
113. Masanes F, Pedrol E, Grau JM, et al. Symptomatic myopathies in HIV-1 infected patients untreated with antiretroviral agents—a clinico-pathological study of 30 consecutive patients. *Clin Neuropathol* 1996;15:221–225.
114. Simpson DM, Citak KA, Godfrey E, et al. Myopathies associated with human immunodeficiency virus and zidovudine: can their effects be distinguished? *Neurology* 1993;43:971–976.
115. Ma DM. Electrodiagnosis of neuromuscular disease in HIV infection. In: O'Dell MW, ed. *HIV-related disability: assessment and management.* Philadelphia: Hanley and Belfus, Inc., 1993:s73–82.
116. Hassett J, Tagliati M, Godbold J, et al. A placebo-controlled study of prednisone in HIV-associated myopathy *Neurology* 1994;44[Suppl 2]:A250.
117. Florence E, Schrooten W, Verdonck K, et al. Rheumatological complications associated with the use of indinavir and other protease inhibitors. *Ann Rheum Dis* 2002;61:82–84.
118. White AJ. Mitochondrial toxicity and HIV therapy [Review]. *Sex Transm Infect* 2001;77:158–173.
119. Blanche S, Tardieu M, Rustin P, et al. Persistent mitochondrial dysfunction and perinatal exposure to antiretroviral nucleoside analogues. *Lancet* 1999;354:1084–1089.
120. Cupler EJ, Leon-Monzon M, Miller J, et al. Inclusion body myositis in HIV-1 and HTLV-1 infected patients. *Brain* 1996;119:1887–1893.
121. Roubenoff R. Acquired immunodeficiency syndrome wasting, functional performance, and quality of life. *Am J Managed Care* 2000;6:1003–1016.
122. Roubenoff R, Wilson IB. Effect of resistance training on self-reported physical functioning in HIV infection. *Med Sci Sports Exerc* 2001;33:1811–1817.
123. Wagner G, Rabkin J, Rabkin R. Exercise as a mediator of psychological and nutritional effects of testosterone therapy in HIV+ men. *Med Sci Sports Exerc* 1998;30:811–817.
124. Yarasheski KE, Roubenoff R. Exercise treatment for HIV-associated metabolic and anthropomorphic complications. *Exerc Sport Sci Rev* 2001;29:170–174.
125. Cuellar ML. HIV infection-associated inflammatory musculoskeletal disorders. *Rheum Dis Clin North Am* 1998;24:403–421.
126. Reveille JD. The changing spectrum of rheumatic disease in human immunodeficiency virus infection. *Semin Arthritis Rheum* 2000;30:147–166.
127. Cuellar ML, Espinoza LR. Rheumatic manifestations of HIV-AIDS. *Best Pract Res Clin Rheum* 2000;14:579–593.
128. Weitzul S, Duvic M. HIV-related psoriasis and Reiter's syndrome. *Semin Cutan Med Surg* 1997;16:213–218.
129. Malin JK, Patel NJ. Arthropathy and HIV infection: a muddle of mimicry. *Postgrad Med* 1993;93:143–146, 49–50.
130. Rademaker J, Dobro JS, Solomon G. Osteonecrosis and human immunodeficiency virus infection. *J Rheumatol* 1997;24:601–604.
131. Monier P, McKown K, Bronze MS. Osteonecrosis complicating highly active antiretroviral therapy in patients infected with human immunodeficiency virus. *Clin Infect Dis* 2000;31:1488–1492.
132. Bonfanti P, Grabbuti A, Carradori S, et al. Osteonecrosis in protease inhibitor-treated patients. *Orthopedics* 2001;24:271–272.
133. Brown P, Crane L. Avascular necrosis of bone in patients with human immunodeficiency virus infection: report of 6 cases and review of the literature. *Clin Infect Dis* 2001;32:1221–1226.
134. Ries MD, Barcohana B, Davidson A, et al. Association between human immunodeficiency virus and osteonecrosis of the femoral head. *J Arthroplasty* 2002;17:135–139.
135. Scribner AN, Troia-Cancio PV, Cox BA, et al. Osteonecrosis in HIV: a case-control study. *J Acquir Immune Defic Syndr* 2000;25:19–25.
136. Glesby MJ, Hoover DR, Vaamonde CM. Osteonecrosis in patients infected with human immunodeficiency virus: a case-control study. *J Infect Dis* 2001;184:519–523.
137. Blacksin MF, Kloser PC, Simon J. Avascular necrosis of bone in human immunodeficiency virus infected patients. *Clin Imaging* 1999;23:314–318.
138. Miller KD, Masur H, Jones EC, et al. High prevalence of osteonecrosis of the femoral head in HIV-infected adults. *Ann Intern Med* 2002;137:17–25.
139. Chetty R. Vasculitides associated with HIV infection. *J Clin Pathol* 2001;54:275–278.
140. Font C, Miro O, Pedrol E, et al. Polyarteritis nodosa in human immunodeficiency virus infection: report of four cases and review of the literature. *British J Rheum* 1996;35:796–799.
141. Johnson RM, Little JR, Storch GA. Kawasaki-like syndromes associated with human immunodeficiency virus infection. *Clin Infect Dis* 2001;32:1628–1634.
142. Bouhassira D, Attal N, Willer JC, et al. Painful and painless peripheral sensory neuropathies due to HIV infection: a comparison using quantitative sensory evaluation. *Pain* 1999;80:265–272.
143. Pardo CA, McArthur JC, Griffin JW. HIV neuropathy: insights in the pathology of HIV peripheral nerve disease. *J Peripher Nerv Syst* 2001;6:21–27.
144. Simpson DM, Haidich AB, Schifitto G, et al. Severity of HIV-associated neuropathy is associated with plasma HIV-1 RNA levels. *AIDS* 2002;16:407–412.
145. Verma A. Epidemiology and clinical features of HIV-1 associated neuropathies. *J Peripher Nerv Syst* 2001;6:8–13.
146. Williams D, Geraci A, Simpson DD. AIDS and AIDS-treatment neuropathies. *Curr Pain Headache Rep* 2002;6:125–130.
147. Wulff EA, Wang AK, Simpson DM. HIV-associated peripheral neuropathy: epidemiology, pathophysiology and treatment. *Drugs* 2000;59:1251–1260.
148. Araujo AP, Nascimento OJ, Garcia OS. Distal sensory polyneuropathy in a cohort of HIV-infected children over five years of age. *Pediatrics* 2000;106:E35.
149. Floeter MK, Civitello LA, Everett CR, et al. Peripheral neuropathy in children with HIV infection. *Neurology* 1997;49:207–212.
150. Bradley WG, Shapshak P, Delgado S, et al. Morphometric analysis of the peripheral neuropathy of AIDS. *Muscle Nerve.* 1998;21:1188–1195.
151. Kemper CA, Kent G, Burton S, et al. Mexiletine for HIV-infected patients with painful peripheral neuropathy: a double-blind, placebo-controlled, crossover treatment trial. *J Acquir Immune Defic Syndr* 1998;19:367– 372.
152. Kieburtz K, Simpson D, Yiannoutsos C, et al. A randomized trial of amitriptyline and mexiletine for painful neuropathy in HIV infection. AIDS Clinical Trial Group 242 Protocol Team. *Neurology* 1998;51:1682–1688.
153. Paice JA, Ferrans CE, Lashley FR, et al. Topical capsaicin in the management of HIV-associated peripheral neuropathy. *J Pain Symptom Manage* 2000;19:45–52.
154. Paice JA, Shott S, Oldenburg FP, et al. Efficacy of a vibratory stimulus for the relief of HIV-associated neuropathic pain. *Pain* 2000;84:291–296.

155. Schifitto G, Yiannoutsos C, Simpson DM, et al. Long-term treatment with recombinant nerve growth factor for HIV-associated sensory neuropathy. *Neurology* 2001;57:1313–1316.

156. Shlay JC, Chaloner K, Max MB, et al. Acupuncture and amitriptyline for pain due to HIV-related peripheral neuropathy: a randomized controlled trial. Terry Beirn Community Programs for Clinical Research on AIDS. *JAMA* 1998;280:1590–1595.

157. Simpson DM, Tagliati M. Neurologic manifestations of HIV infection [published erratum appears in *Ann Intern Med* 1995 ;122(4):317]. *Ann Intern Med* 1994;121:769–785.

158. Dalakas MC. Peripheral neuropathy and antiretroviral drugs. *J Peripher Nerv Syst* 2001;6:14–20.

159. Reliquet V, Mussini JM, Chennebault JM, et al. Peripheral neuropathy during stavudine-didanosine antiretroviral therapy. *HIV Med* 2001;2:92–96.

160. Simpson DM, Berger JR. Neurologic manifestations of HIV infection. *Med Clin North Am* 1996;80:1363–1394.

161. Simpson DM. Neuromuscular complications of human immunodeficiency virus infection. *Semin Neurol* 1992;12:34–42.

162. Becker K, Gorlach I, Frieling T, et al. Characterization and natural course of cardiac autonomic nervous dysfunction in HIV-infected patients. *AIDS* 1997;11:751–757.

163. Gluck T, Degenhardt E, Scholmerich J, et al. Autonomic neuropathy in patients with HIV: course, impact of disease stage, and medication. *Clin Auton Res* 2000;10:17–22.

164. Konturek JW, Fischer H, van der Voort IR, et al. Disturbed gastric motor activity in patients with human immunodeficiency virus infection. *Scand J Gastroenterol* 1997;32:221–225.

165. Neild PJ, Nijran KS, Yazaki E, et al. Delayed gastric emptying in human immunodeficiency virus infection: correlation with symptoms, autonomic function, and intestinal motility. *Dig Dis Sci* 2000;45:1491–1499.

166. Rogstad KE, Shah R, Tesfaladet G, et al. Cardiovascular autonomic neuropathy in HIV infected patients. *Sex Transm Infect* 1999;75:264–267.

167. Navia BA. Clinical and biologic features of the AIDS dementia complex [Review]. *Neuroimaging Clin N Am* 1997;7:581–592.

168. Brew BJ. AIDS dementia complex. *Neurol Clin* 1999;17:861–881.

169. Ferrando SJ. Diagnosis and treatment of HIV-associated neurocognitive disorders. *New Directions for Mental Health Services* 2000;87:25–35.

170. Tardieu M. HIV-1-related central nervous system diseases. *Curr Opin Neurol* 1999;377–381.

171. McArthur JC, Sacktor N, Selnes O. Human immunodeficiency virus-associated dementia. *Semin Neurol* 1999;19:129–150.

172. Sacktor N, Lyles RH, Skolasky R, et al. HIV-associated neurologic disease incidence changes: Multicenter AIDS Cohort Study, 1990–1998. *Neurology* 2001;56:257–260.

173. Berger JR, Arendt G. HIV dementia: the role of the basal ganglia and dopaminergic systems. *J Psychopharmacol* 2000;14:214–221.

174. Gartner S, Liu Y. Insights into the role of immune activation in HIV neuropathogenesis. *J Neurovirol* 2002;8:69–75.

175. Gray F, Adle-Biassette H, Chretien F, et al Neuropathology and neurodegeneration in human immunodeficiency virus infection: pathogenesis of HIV-induced lesions of the brain, correlations with HIV-associated disorders and modifications according to treatments. *Clin Neuropathol* 2001;20:146–155.

176. Lipton SA. Neuropathogenesis of acquired immunodeficiency syndrome dementia. *Curr Opin Neurol* 1997;10:247–253.

177. Lopez OL, Smith G, Meltzer CC, et al. Dopamine systems in human immunodeficiency virus-associated dementia. *Neuropsychiatry Neuropsychol Behav Neurol* 1999;12:184–192.

178. Nath A. Pathobiology of human immunodeficiency virus dementia. *Semin Neurol* 1999;19:113–127.

179. Tyor WR, Middaugh LD. Do alcohol and cocaine abuse alter the course of HIV-associated dementia complex?. *J Leukoc Biol* 1999;65:475–481.

180. Navia BA, Gonzalez RG. Functional imaging of the AIDS dementia complex and the metabolic pathology of the HIV-1-infected brain. *Neuroimaging Clin N Am* 1997;7:431–445.

181. Goodkin K, Wilkie FL, Concha M, et al. Subtle neuropsychological impairment and minor cognitive-motor disorder in HIV-1 infection: neuroradiological, neurophysiological, neuroimmunological, and virological correlates. *Neuroimaging Clin N Am* 1997;7:561–579.

182. White DA, Heaton RK, Monsch AU. Neuropsychological studies of asymptomatic human immunodeficiency virus-type-1 infected individuals. The HNRC Group. HIV Neurobehavioral Research Center. *J Int Neuropsychol Soc* 1995;1:304–15.

183. Oursler KA, Moore RD, Chaisson RE. Risk factors for cryptococcal meningitis in HIV-infected patients. *AIDS Res Hum Retroviruses* 1999;15:625–631.

184. Manfredi R, Pieri F, Pileri SA, et al. The changing face of AIDS-related opportunism: cryptococcosis in the highly active antiretroviral therapy (HAART) era. Case reports and literature review. *Mycopathologia* 1999;148: 73–78.

185. Powderly WG. Cryptococcal meningitis and AIDS. *Clin Infect Dis* 1993;17: 837–842.

186. Robinson PA, Bauer M, Leal MA, et al. Early mycological treatment failure in AIDS-associated cryptococcal meningitis. *Clin Infect Dis* 1999;28:82–92.

187. van der Horst CM, Saag MS, Cloud GA, et al. Treatment of cryptococcal meningitis associated with the acquired immunodeficiency syndrome. National Institute of Allergy and Infectious Diseases Mycoses Study Group and AIDS Clinical Trials Group. *N Engl J Med* 1997;337:15–21.

188. Zeind CS, Cleveland KO, Menon M, et al. Cryptococcal meningitis in patients with the acquired immunodeficiency syndrome. *Pharmacotherapy* 1996;16:547–561.

189. Powderly WG. Recent advances in the management of cryptococcal meningitis in patients with AIDS. *Clin Infect Dis* 1996;22:S119–123.

190. Singh N, Barnish MJ, Berman S, et al. Low-dose fluconazole as primary prophylaxis for cryptococcal infection in AIDS patients with CD4 cell counts of 100/mm3: demonstration of efficacy in a positive, multicenter trial. *Clin Infect Dis* 1996;23:1282–1286.

191. van Voorst Vader PC. Syphilis management and treatment. *Dermatol Clin* 1998;16:699–711, xi.

192. Flood JM, Weinstock HS, Guroy ME, et al. Neurosyphilis during the AIDS epidemic, San Francisco, 1985–1992 [see comments]. *J Infect Dis* 1998;177: 931–940.

193. de Silva SM, Mark AS, Gilden DH, et al. Zoster myelitis: improvement with antiviral therapy in two cases. *Neurology* 1996;47:929–931.

194. Brown M, Scarborough M, Brink N, et al. Varicella zoster virus-associated neurological disease in HIV-infected patients. *Int J STD AIDS* 2001;12:79–83.

195. Iten A, Chatelard P, Vuadens P, et al. Impact of cerebrospinal fluid PCR on the management of HIV-infected patients with varicella-zoster virus infection of the central nervous system. *J Neurovirol* 1999;5:172–180.

196. Okano M, Gross TG. A review of Epstein-Barr virus infection in patients with immunodeficiency disorders. *Am J Med Sci* 2000;319:392–396.

197. Cinque P, Cleator GM, Weber T, et al. Diagnosis and clinical management of neurological disorders caused by cytomegalovirus in AIDS patients. European Union Concerted Action on Virus Meningitis and Encephalitis. *J Neurovirol* 1998;4:120–132.

198. McCutchan JA. Cytomegalovirus infections of the nervous system in patients with AIDS [Review]. *Clin Infect Dis* 1995;20:747–754.

199. Brannagan TH III. Retroviral-associated vasculitis of the nervous system. *Neurol Clin* 1997;15:927–944.

200. Skiest DJ. Focal neurological disease in patients with acquired immunodeficiency syndrome. *Clin Infect Dis* 2002;34:103–115.

201. Cohen BA. Neurologic complications of HIV infection. *Primary Care: Clinics in Office Practice* 1997;24:575–595.

202. Weisberg LA. Neurologic abnormalities in human immunodeficiency virus infection. *South Med J* 2001;94:266–275.

203. Smirniotopoulos JG, Koeller KK, Nelson AM, et al. Neuroimaging—autopsy correlations in AIDS. *Neuroimaging Clin N Am* 1997;7:615–637.

204. Wright D, Schneider A, Berger JR. Central nervous system opportunistic infections. *Neuroimaging Clin N Am* 1997;7:513–525.

205. Roullet E. Opportunistic infections of the central nervous system during HIV-1 infection (emphasis on cytomegalovirus disease). *J Neurol* 1999;246: 237–243.

206. Cohen BA. Neurologic manifestations of toxoplasmosis in AIDS. *Semin Neurol* 1999;19:201–211.

207. Provenzale JM, Jinkins JR. Brain and spine imaging findings in AIDS patients. *Radiol Clin North Am* 1997;35:1127–1166.

208. Walot I, Miller BL, Chang L, et al. Neuroimaging findings in patients with AIDS. *Clin Infect Dis* 1996;22:906–919.

209. Borggreve F, Dierckx RA, Crols R, et al. Repeat thallium-201 SPECT in cerebral lymphoma. *Funct Neurol* 1993;8:95–101.

210. Carmichael C. Prevention and treatment of common HIV-associated opportunistic complications. *Primary Care: Clinics in Office Practice* 1997;24:561–574.

211. von Einsiedel RW, Fife TD, Aksamit AJ, et al. Progressive multifocal leukoencephalopathy in AIDS: a clinicopathological study and review of the literature. *J Neurol* 1993;240:391–406.

212. Dworkin MS, Wan PC, Hanson DL, et al. Progressive multifocal leukoencephalopathy: improved survival of human immunodeficiency virus-infected patients in the protease inhibitor era. *J Infect Dis* 1999;180: 621–625.

213. Albrecht H, Hoffmann C, Degen O, et al. Highly active antiretroviral therapy significantly improves the prognosis of patients with HIV-associated progressive multifocal leukoencephalopathy. *AIDS* 1998;12:1149–1154.

214. Teofilo E, Gouveia J, Brotas V, et al. Progressive multifocal leukoencephalopathy regression with highly active antiretroviral therapy. *AIDS* 1998;12:449.

215. Sparano JA. Clinical aspects and management of AIDS-related lymphoma [Review]. *Eur J Cancer* 2001;37:1296–1305.

216. Buttner A, Weis S. Non-lymphomatous brain tumors in HIV-1 infection: a review. *J Neurooncol* 1999;41:81–88.

217. Bowen EF, Griffiths PD, Davey CC, et al. Lessons from the natural history of cytomegalovirus. *AIDS* 1996;10:S37–41.

218. Friedberg DN. Cytomegalovirus retinitis: diagnosis and status of systemic therapy. *J Acquir Immune Defic Syndr* 1997;14:S1–6.

219. Kuppermann BD. Therapeutic options for resistant cytomegalovirus retinitis. *J Acquir Immune Defic Syndr* 1997;14:S13–21.

220. Spector SA. Current therapeutic challenges in the treatment of cytomegalovirus retinitis. *J Acquir Immune Defic Syndr* 1997;14:S32–35.

221. Lalezari JP. Cidofovir: a new therapy for cytomegalovirus retinitis [Review]. *J Acquir Immune Defic Syndr* 1997;14:S22–26.

222. Lalezari JP, Kuppermann BD. Clinical experience with cidofovir in the treatment of cytomegalovirus retinitis. *J Acquir Immune Defic Syndr* 1997;14: S27–31.

223. Martin DF, Parks DJ, Mellow SD, et al. Treatment of cytomegalovirus retinitis with an intraocular sustained-release ganciclovir implant: a randomized controlled clinical trial. *Arch Ophthalmol* 1994;112:1531–1539.

224. Rahhal FM, Arevalo JF, Chavez de la Paz E, et al. Treatment of cytomegalovirus retinitis with intravitreous cidofovir in patients with AIDS: a preliminary report. *Ann Intern Med* 1996;125:98–103.

225. Smith CL. Local therapy for cytomegalovirus retinitis. *Ann Pharmacother* 1998;32:248–255.

226. Jouan M, Katlama C. Management of CMV retinitis in the era of highly active antiretroviral therapy. *Int J Antimicrob Agents* 1999;13:1–7.

227. Rauz S, Murray PI. Changing patterns of HIV related ocular disease. *Sexu Transm Infect* 1999;75:18–20.

228. Connor MD, Lammie GA, Bell JE, et al. Cerebral infarction in adult AIDS patients: observations from the Edinburgh HIV Autopsy Cohort. *Stroke* 2000; 31:2117–2126.

229. Qureshi AI, Janssen RS, Karon JM, et al. Human immunodeficiency virus infection and stroke in young patients. *Arch Neurol* 1997;54:1150–1153.

230. Gillams AR, Allen E, Hrieb K, et al. Cerebral infarction in patients with AIDS. *Am J Neuroradiology* 1997;18:1581–1585.

231. Pinto AN. AIDS and cerebrovascular disease. *Stroke* 1996;27:538–543.

232. Calabrese LH. Vasculitis and infection with the human immunodeficiency virus. *Rheum Dis Clin North Am* 1991;17:131–147.

233. Calabrese LH, Furlan AJ, Gragg LA, et al. Primary angiitis of the central nervous system: diagnostic criteria and clinical approach. *Cleve Clin J Med* 1992;59:293–306.

234. Marra CM. Bacterial and fungal brain infections in AIDS. *Semin Neurol* 1999; 19:177–184.

235. Sanchez-Portocarrero J, Perez-Cecilia E, Romero-Vivas J. Infection of the central nervous system by Mycobacterium tuberculosis in patients infected with human immunodeficiency virus (the new neurotuberculosis). *Infection* 1999;27:313–317.

236. So YT, Olney RK. Acute lumbosacral polyradiculopathy in acquired immunodeficiency syndrome: experience in 23 patients. *Ann Neurol* 1994;35:53–58.

237. Corral I, Quereda C, Casado JL, et al. Acute polyradiculopathies in HIV-infected patients. *J Neurol* 1997;244:499–504.

238. Qureshi AI, Cook AA, Mishu HP, et al. Guillain-Barré syndrome in immunocompromised patients: a report of three patients and review of the literature. *Muscle Nerve* 1997;20:1002–1007.

239. Anders HJ, Goebel FD. Cytomegalovirus polyradiculopathy in patients with AIDS. *Clin Infect Dis* 1998;27:345–352.

240. Cohen BA, McArthur JC, Grohman S, et al. Neurologic prognosis of cytomegalovirus polyradiculopathy in AIDS. *Neurology* 1993;43:493–499.

241. Miller RG, Storey JR, Greco CM. Ganciclovir in the treatment of progressive AIDS-related polyradiculopathy. *Neurology* 1990;40:569–574.

242. Fuller GN, Gill SK, Guiloff RJ, et al. Ganciclovir for lumbosacral polyradiculopathy in AIDS. *Lancet* 1990;335:48–49.

243. Di Rocco A, Simpson DM. AIDS-associated vacuolar myelopathy. *AIDS Patient Care and STDs* 1998;12:457–461.

244. Budka H. Neuropathology of myelitis, myelopathy, and spinal infections in AIDS. *Neuroimaging Clin N Am* 1997;7:639–650.

245. Di Rocco A. Diseases of the spinal cord in human immunodeficiency virus infection. *Semin Neurol* 1999;19:151–155.

246. Luzuriaga K, Sullivan JL. Pediatric HIV-1 infection: advances and remaining challenges. *AIDS Rev* 2002;4:21–26.

247. Wiznia AA, Lambert G, Pavlakis S. Pediatric HIV infection. *Med Clin North Am* 1996;80:1309–1336.

248. Minkoff H, Mofenson LM. The role of obstetric interventions in the prevention of pediatric human immunodeficiency virus infection. *Am J Obstet Gynecol* 1994;171:1167–1175.

249. Laufer M, Scott GB. Medical management of HIV disease in children. *Pediatr Clin North Am* 2000;47:127–153.

250. Pavlakis SG, Frank Y, Nocyze M, et al. Acquired immunodeficiency syndrome and the developing nervous system. *Adv Pediatr* 1994;41:427–451.

251. Connor EM, Andiman WA. Lymphoid interstitial pneumonitis. In: Pizzo PA, Wilfert CM, eds. *Pediatric AIDS*. Baltimore: Williams and Wilkins, 1994:467–481.

252. Fishback N, Koss M. Update on lymphoid interstitial pneumonitis. *Curr Opin Pulm Med* 1996;2:429–433.

253. Gonzalez CE, Samakoses R, Boler AM, et al. Lymphoid interstitial pneumonitis in pediatric AIDS: natural history of the disease. *Ann NY Acad Sci* 2000;918:358–361.

254. Binder H, Castagnino M. Rehabilitation considerations in pediatric HIV infection. In: O'Dell MW, ed. *HIV-related disability: assessment and management*. Philadelphia: Hanley and Belfus, Inc., 1993:s175–187.

255. Mintz M. Neurological and developmental problems in pediatric HIV infection. *J Nutr* 1996;126:2663S–2673S.

256. Gelbard HA, Epstein LG. HIV-1 encephalopathy in children. *Curr Opin Pediatr* 1995;7:655–662.

257. Belman AL. Pediatric neuro-AIDS: update. *Neuroimaging Clin N Am* 1997;7:593–613.

258. Vachon RA. Employment assistance and vocational rehabilitation for people with HIV or AIDS: policy, practice and prospects. In: O'Dell MW, ed. *HIV-related disability: assessment and management*. Philadelphia: Hanley and Belfus, Inc., 1993:s189–201.

259. Turner BJ. Adherence to antiretroviral therapy by human immunodeficiency virus-infected patients. *J Infect Dis* 2002;185:S143–151.

260. Gisslen M, Hagberg L. Antiretroviral treatment of central nervous system HIV-1 infection: a review. *HIV Med* 2001;2:97–104.

261. Booss J. Chronic-treated HIV: a neurologic disease. *J Urban Health* 2000;77:204–212.

262. O'Dell MW. HIV-related neurological disability and prospects for rehabilitation. *Disabil Rehabil* 1996;18:285–292.

263. O'Dell MW, Levinson SF, Riggs RV. Focused review: physiatric management of HIV-related disability. *Arch Phys Med Rehabil* 1996;77:S66–73.

264. Jones SP, Doran DA, Leatt PB, et al. Short-term exercise training improves body composition and hyperlipidaemia in HIV-positive individuals with lipodystrophy. *AIDS* 2001;15:2049–2051.

265. LaPerriere A, Klimas N, Fletcher MA, et al. Change in CD4+ cell enumeration following aerobic exercise training in HIV-1 disease: possible mechanisms and practical applications. *Intl J Sports Med* 1997;18:S56–61.

266. Perna FM, LaPerriere A, Klimas N, et al. Cardiopulmonary and CD4 cell changes in response to exercise training in early symptomatic HIV infection. *Med Sci Sports Exerc* 1999;31:973–979.

267. Stringer WW, Berezovskaya M, O'Brien WA, et al. The effect of exercise training on aerobic fitness, immune indices, and quality of life in HIV+ patients. *Med Sci Sports Exerc* 1998;30:11–16.

268. Stringer WW. HIV and aerobic exercise: current recommendations. *Sports Med* 1999;28:389–395.

269. Yarasheski KE, Tebas P, Stanerson B, et al. Resistance exercise training reduces hypertriglyceridemia in HIV-infected men treated with antiviral therapy. *J Appl Physiol* 2001;90:133–138.

CHAPTER 83

Cardiac Rehabilitation

Subhash K. Shah

Cardiac rehabilitation (CR) is an individualized, comprehensive program developed by using various principles of rehabilitation medicine with the aim to maintain, restore, and increase the optimal physical, medical, psychological, social, emotional, vocational, and economic status of patients with cardiovascular diseases (CVDs). It requires a patient's active participation and involves medical evaluation, exercise prescription, cardiac risk reduction and modification, education, and counseling. The goals of CR are to change the natural history of the disease, to reduce mortality and morbidity, to increase the patient's functional capacity, and ultimately to limit or reverse the pathological process leading to CVD. Secondary prevention of CVD and exercise training remain the cornerstones of CR. In combination with other strategies, such as smoking cessation and a prudent low-fat diet, CR has been shown to reduce symptoms, increase cardiopulmonary fitness, improve lipid profile, ameliorate high blood pressure, counter obesity, control adult-onset diabetes, enhance fibrinolysis, improve endothelial dysfunction, alleviate depression, improve quality of life, reduce the incidence of sudden death and recurrent fatal myocardial infarction (MI), and lead to regression of pathological process of arteriosclerosis (1–6).

CR is offered to patients recovering from MI; those with stable chronic heart failure (HF); and those who have undergone coronary artery bypass graft surgery (CABG), heart transplantation, angioplasty, pacemaker and left ventricular assistive device insertion, valve surgery, and ventricular aneurysmectomy; and even to patients who are awaiting cardiac transplantation. A number of recent studies have shown that a CR program, which includes all the above features (i.e., cardiac risk reduction, lifestyle alteration, and exercise training), can lower morbidity and mortality, and even regress the pathological process of arteriosclerosis (1,2,3,7).

Figure 83-1 shows core components of CR. CR was first introduced as an exercise program, but various levels of prevention—i.e., primary, secondary, and tertiary—have since been added. Despite major recent advances in other areas of cardiology, relatively little has changed in the methods and approaches of CR.

The exact historical origin of CR is not known, but the eighteenth-century English physician, William Heberden, documented the case of a patient suffering from angina, "who sets himself to take a task sawing wood every day and was nearly cured" (8). In 1854, the Irish doctor William Stokes stated, "The symptoms of disability of the heart are often removable by regulated course of gymnastic or by walking exercises" (9). A London surgeon, John Hilton, is credited with the value of strict bed rest (10). Unfortunately, Hilton's precept was carried to the extreme, and prolonged bed rest or immobilization became the cornerstone of medical care for the patient with CVD.

In the 1950s, Drs. Levine and Lown questioned the wisdom of bed rest. They introduced "arm chair treatment" for the "heart attack" patient (11). This involved sitting up in the chair by the bed a few days after the admission, and the era of early mobilization and CR started. Chapman and Fraser of the University of Minnesota catheterized the patient recovering from MI during treadmill exercise and demonstrated that the cardiovascular response was normal. That paved the way for the introduction of an exercise training program (12). In 1973, seven coronary patients from Toronto, who had received supervised exercise training, entered the Boston Marathon. Their completion of the run without a mishap was a medical milestone (13). Figure 83-2 illustrates various major treatment shifts for CVD. Multiple individuals have since contributed to the development of CR, including Drs. H. K. Hellerstein, Phillip Ades, Leonore Zohman, Nanette Wegner, Michael Pollock, Barry A. Franklin, Gary Balady, Gerald Fletcher, Carl J. Lavie, and many more. Most of the information presented in this chapter has been adapted from their intensive work.

Despite a steady decline in CVD over the last quarter century, it remains the number-one cause of mortality in the United States. Sixty-three million people have one or more types of CVD. Thirty million are men, and 32 million are women. Twenty-five million are older than 65 years of age. High blood pressure accounts for 50 million, coronary atherosclerotic heart disease accounts for 12.6 million, MI for 7.5 million, angina for 6.5 million, and congestive heart failure (CHF) for 4.8 million. In 1999, about 1 million deaths were attributed to coronary artery disease (CAD). CAD accounts for 40% of all deaths, or 1 in every 2.5 deaths. It is estimated that 2,600 deaths per day, or one death every 33 seconds, is due to CVD. Thirty-three percent of all deaths occur before the age of 75. According to various analyses, if all forms of major CVD events were eliminated, life expectancy would increase by 7 years. The total cost of CVD was estimated to be $330 billion in 2002 (14). Of the countries where death records are kept, the Russian Federation has the highest rate of death from CVD; Japan has the lowest rate for men; and France has the lowest rate for women.

Evidence-based medicine promotes that a patient's treatment be guided by the results of high-quality research. Clinical guidelines for CR have been developed by the Agency for Healthcare Research and Quality (15). For various reasons,

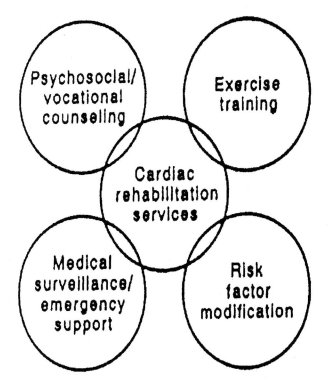

Figure 83-1. Core components of a contemporary cardiac rehabilitation program. (Redrawn with permission from Franklin BA. *ACSM's guidelines for exercise testing and prescription*, 6th ed. Baltimore: American College of Sports Medicine, 2000;81).

studies assessing the efficacy of CR have been disappointing and somewhat contradictory. Some of the reasons relate to methodological issues (such as preselection bias, heterogeneity of the selected population, nonrandomization studies, and the fact that most of the available data is limited to MI patients). Earlier CR programs were exclusively exercise based and paid limited attention to known CVD risk factors. This one-dimensional approach is likely one of the reasons the mortality data from earlier studies did not show any significant improvements with CR. In contrast, in the 1980s, CR programs began to incorporate interventions designed to modify CVD risk factors

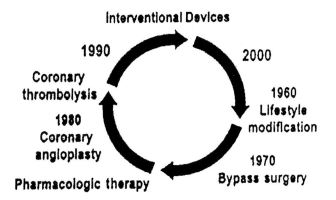

Figure 83-2. In the 1960s, treatment of heart disease largely involved early ambulation and exercise training. Since then, bypass surgery, intensive pharmacotherapy, angioplasty, thrombolytics, and interventional devices (e.g., coronary stents) have emerged. However, recent studies have shown that aggressive risk factor reduction, including exercise training, can stabilize and even reverse the atherosclerotic process. (Redrawn with permission from Franklin BA. *ACSM's guidelines for exercise testing and prescription*, 6th ed. Baltimore: American College of Sports Medicine, 2000;194).

(nutritional counseling, advice regarding lifestyle changes, and drug therapy). The primary goals were preventing and decreasing disability resulting from CVD, and preventing subsequent coronary event, hospitalization, and death. Currently, well-established CR centers employ an interdisciplinary team approach that has been shown to be efficient and effective. In spite of this, only 10% to 12% of appropriate patients are referred to formal CR programs. The following sections discuss the underlying scientific foundation for cardiovascular exercise.

EXERCISE PHYSIOLOGY

Ergometry is determined by the physical factors of force, work, power, and the metabolic equivalent (MET). Loosely defined, the MET can be thought of as a way of quantifying exercise with respect to "how much and how hard." A proper exercise prescription requires the ability to measure and estimate energy expended. Basic definitions for exercise prescription include (16):

1. Mass [m] $\times$ acceleration [a] = force [f] kilo pound [kp]; newton [N]; 1 kp = 9.81 N
2. Force [f] $\times$ distance [d] = work; kp.m.; N.m; joules [J]
3. Work divided by time [t] = power [P]; kpm/min; or J/min; watts [W]
4. *MET* is total energy spent [E]; the unit of E is Kcals [calories]
5. *Calorie* (kilocalories) is the amount of energy required to raise the temperature of 1 kilogram of water by 1° centigrade.
    Kilocalories/min = [METs $\times$ body weight in kilogram $\times$ 3.5/200]. 5 kilocalories = 1 liter of oxygen consumed
6. MET (metabolic equivalent of power) 1 MET = 3.5 cc of O_2/kg/min in a seated person at rest, or 1 MET = 1.2 Kcals/min
7. VO_2 refers to the volume of O_2 consumed per minute. It is a metabolic equivalent of power.
8. $\dot{V}O_2$ refers to the rate of oxygen uptake; $\dot{V}O_{2max}$ is the greatest amount of oxygen a person can take in from inspired air while performing dynamic exercise involving a large part of total muscle mass.
9. *Ventilatory threshold* is the measure of related work effort, and it represents the point at which the ventilation abruptly increases despite linear increases in oxygen uptake and work rate.
10. *Strength* refers to the maximum force that can be generated.
11. *Endurance* refers to the ability to continue specified task.
12. *Absolute power* refers to non–weight bearing activities, i.e., cycle ergometry measured in watts or kpm/min.
13. *Relative power* refers to the weight-bearing activities, i.e., jogging, measured as either MET or VO_2.
14. *Physical activity* is the skeletal muscle contraction resulting in bodily movement that requires energy utilization.
15. *Physical fitness* is a set of attributes that enables an individual to perform physical activity.
16. *Physical exercise* is defined as planned physical activity with the goal of achieving or preserving physical fitness.
17. *Afterload* refers to the resistance against which the heart contracts and is dependent on the ventricle end diastolic volume, aortic impedance, and peripheral vascular resistance.
18. *Preload* is the ventricular filling pressure, which can be changed by blood volume, venous return, myocardial contractility, and ventricular compliance.

19. *Ejection fraction* (EF) is the ratio of left ventricular stroke volume (SV) to end-diastolic volume. EF is usually about 60% to 70% (measured by angiography).

20. *Cardiac index* is the ratio of cardiac output (CO) = heart rate (HR) × SV to square meter of body surface area. Normal value is 2.6 to 4.2 liters per minute per square meter of basal body surface area.

In a healthy subject, the cardiovascular response to maximum dynamic exercise is illustrated by the following:

1. There is a fourfold increase in CO from 5 liters to 20 liters per minute. CO is increased by an augmentation in SV mediated via the Frank-Starling mechanism (increased preload increases fiber length to a certain extent leading to increased force generated with each contraction) and HR. The increase in CO in latter phases of exercise is primarily due to an increase in HR, which can increase up to 300%.

2. Peripherally, there is a threefold increase in oxygen extraction.

3. Total calculated peripheral resistance decreases and systolic blood pressure, mean arterial pressure, and pulse pressure usually increases. Diastolic blood pressure may remain unchanged or may minimally decrease.

4. The steady state conditions are usually reached within minutes after the onset of exercise, and after this occurs, HR, CO, blood pressure, and pulmonary ventilation are maintained at a relatively constant level.

5. Sympathetic discharge is maximal and parasympathetic stimulation is minimal, resulting in vasoconstriction of most of the circulatory system except for that in exercising muscles and in cerebral and coronary circulation.

6. The pulmonary bed can accommodate a sixfold increase in CO without a significant increase in pulmonary artery pressure. Thus, pulmonary pressure is not the limiting determinant of peak exercise capacity.

7. In the postexercise phase, hemodynamics return to the baseline within minutes of exercise termination. Vagal reactivation is an important postexercise cardiac deceleration mechanism. Vagal reactivation is accelerated in well-trained athletes, but blunted in deconditioned patients.

Maximum Oxygen Uptake

The ability to measure or estimate the energy expenditure during exercise is one of the cornerstones behind exercise testing and prescription. Exercise is a metabolic event and generates heat. The rate of heat production during exercise is directly proportional to the energy expended. Because direct calorimetry is difficult to perform on humans, a process of indirect calorimetry of $\dot{V}O_2$ uptake is instead used. $\dot{V}O_2$ is defined as the rate of O_2 utilization as expressed in volume/time. VO_2 is calculated by measuring oxygen from the expired air at the mouth. For any given constant submaximal workload, the VO_2 increases over the first 2 to 4 minutes, approaching a steady-state level. With increasing workload, it reaches a point at which increasing the work further does not produce any increase in VO_2. This point is $\dot{V}O_{2max}$. Exercise intensity is usually expressed as a percentage of $\dot{V}O_{2max}$, the rate at which there is maximum O_2 intake. If the various steady states of VO_2 levels are plotted against the workload, the result is a positive slope with a short horizontal plateau at the top, representing the $\dot{V}O_{2max}$ as seen in Figure 83-3. The effect of post training on VO_2 is illustrated in Figure 83-4. The slope of the line represents the mechanical efficiency of the exercise being performed (16). $\dot{V}O_{2max}$ is the rate of O_2 uptake during the maximum exercise,

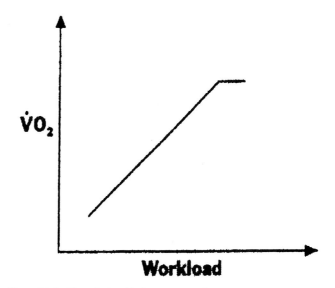

Figure 83-3. The relationship between steady-state oxygen consumption ($\dot{V}O_2$) and workload. (Redrawn with permission from Gonzalez EG. *Downey and Darling's physiological basis of rehabilitation medicine*, 3rd ed. Boston: Butterworth-Heinemann, 2001;172.

and it represents the O_2 consumption by whole body during the work of skeletal muscles. It represents the amount of oxygen transported and used in cellular metabolism.

During staged exercise testing, VO_2 usually remains relatively stable after the second minute of each level of intensity of exercise. VO_2 usually underestimates the energy expenditure from anaerobic metabolism but more accurately reflects the energy used during aerobic metabolism.

The major determinant of $\dot{V}O_{2max}$ is the product of maximum CO and the maximum difference between the arterial and venous oxygen. The oxygen transport system is $\dot{V}O_2$. $\dot{V}O_2$ equals SV × HR × (A − vo$_2$), where SV stands for stroke volume, HR for heart rate, and A − vo$_2$ is arteriovenous oxygen difference. With aerobic training $\dot{V}O_{2max}$ is increased, but at rest and during any given submaximal load, it remains unchanged.

This basic training effect appears to be true for both sexes and different ethnic groups. In a moderately active young man,

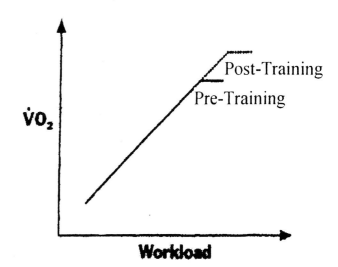

Figure 83-4. The effect of training on the relationship between oxygen consumption ($\dot{V}O_2$) and workload. (Redrawn with permission from Gonzalez EG. *Downey and Darling's physiological basis of rehabilitation medicine*, 3rd ed. Boston: Butterworth-Heinemann, 2001;176.)

$\dot{V}O_{2max}$ is about 12 METs, whereas a distance runner can have a $\dot{V}O_{2max}$ of 18 to 24 METs. $\dot{V}O_2$ is dependent on age. At age 20, it is maximum and age 60, it is two-thirds of that at age 20. Men have a higher value than women. The lower $\dot{V}O_{2max}$ in women is attributed to their smaller muscle mass, lower hemoglobin, blood volume, and smaller SV compared with men.

$\dot{V}O_{2max}$ is determined by genetic makeup. It can increase 10% to 12% with vigorous activity started early in childhood (17). After 3 weeks of bed rest, there is a 20% to 25% decrease in $\dot{V}O_{2max}$ during physical activity. $\dot{V}O_{2max}$ is affected by degree of impairment caused by CVD.

In clinical practice, the relative rate of oxygen used and the intensity of exercise is usually expressed as percentage of $\dot{V}O_{2max}$. $\dot{V}O_2$ is expressed in milliliter/kilogram of body mass per unit time. The absolute O_2 uptake is in liter units. One liter of O_2 yields the liberation of 5 kilocalories or 20.9 calories of energy. The $\dot{V}O_{2max}$ offers the best measure for cardiovascular fitness and exercise capacity.

Stroke Volume

SV is the quantity of blood pumped with each heartbeat. Response of SV to exercise is more variable than the CO or HR responses. In a supine position, SV may increase, decrease, or stay the same with increases in workload. If there is a change from the resting level, the SV levels out at 30% to 40% of $\dot{V}O_{2max}$ (18). Resting SV in the upright position is approximately 60% of that of supine but never reaches the supine value. Thus, in supine position, SV is close to the maximum.

The major determinant of the SV is the diastolic filling volume. The relationship between SV and O_2 consumption ($\dot{V}O_2$) can be seen in Figure 83-5. An increase in SV is mostly related to a combination of increased blood volume and prolonged diastolic filling time. In the early phase of exercise, the CO increases as a result of an increase in SV by the Frank-Starling homeostatic mechanism. With aerobic training, the SV is usually greater at rest after submaximal or maximal exercise, as shown Figure 83-6. The increase in SV is reciprocal to the decrease in HR, which allows longer diastolic filling time. SV is also augmented by increased venous return secondary to exercise-induced increase in blood volume.

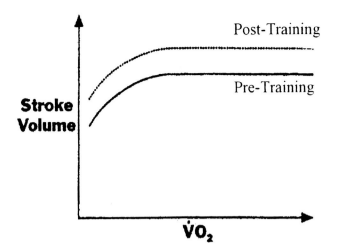

Figure 83-6. The effect of training on the relationship between stroke volume and oxygen consumption ($\dot{V}O_2$). (Redrawn with permission from Gonzalez EG. *Downey and Darling's physiological basis of rehabilitation medicine*, 3rd ed. Boston: Butterworth-Heinemann, 2001;177.)

Heart Rate Response

HR reflects the number of times myocardial contraction occurs per unit time. The relationship between HR and $\dot{V}O_2$ is also linear (Fig. 83-7). Maximum HR (HR_{max}) is a function of age, whereas the level of the physical conditioning determines the slope of the line. The immediate response to exercise is an increased HR that is due to a decrease in vagal tone. With continued exercise, further increase in HR is due to increases in sympathetic outflow to the heart and systemic blood vessels (19). During dynamic exercise, the HR increases linearly with workload and $\dot{V}O_2$, and it reaches a steady state within minutes at a constant workload.

There are many factors that influence HR response to exercise: position, type of exercises (dynamic exercise increases HR more than isometric or resistive exercises), state of health, blood volume, sinus node function, medications, environment, and age (19,20). Certain physical conditions such as deconditioning or prolonged bed rest cause an accelerated HR response to exercise. The decline in HR that is due to age is prob-

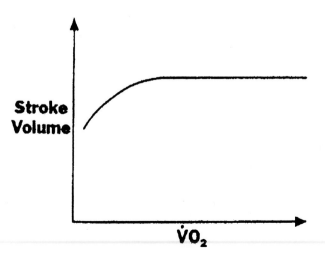

Figure 83-5. The relationship between stroke volume and oxygen consumption ($\dot{V}O_2$). (Redrawn with permission from Gonzalez EG. *Downey and Darling's physiological basis of rehabilitation medicine*, 3rd ed. Boston: Butterworth-Heinemann, 2001;173.)

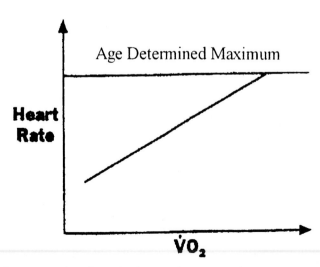

Figure 83-7. The relationship between heart rate and oxygen consumption ($\dot{V}O_2$). (Redrawn with permission from Gonzalez EG. *Downey and Darling's physiological basis of rehabilitation medicine*, 3rd ed. Boston: Butterworth-Heinemann, 2001;172.)

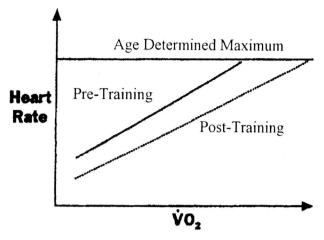

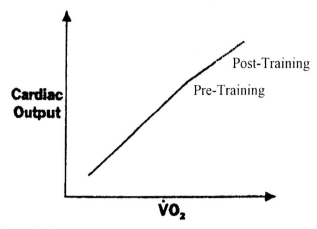

Figure 83-8. The effect of training on the relationship between heart rate and oxygen consumption ($\dot{V}O_2$). (Redrawn with permission from Gonzalez EG. *Downey and Darling's physiological basis of rehabilitation medicine*, 3rd ed. Boston: Butterworth-Heinemann, 2001;176.)

Figure 83-10. The effect of training on the relationship between cardiac output and oxygen consumption ($\dot{V}O_2$). (Redrawn with permission from Gonzalez EG. *Downey and Darling's physiological basis of rehabilitation medicine*, 3rd ed. Boston: Butterworth-Heinemann, 2001;176.)

ably related to neural influences; exercise training causes the HR to be lower at rest and at submaximal workload, but the maximal HR does not change (Fig. 83-8). Resting bradycardia of exercise training is the most noticeable and clinically important change that occurs with aerobic training.

The HR_{max} can be estimated by subtracting the age of the person from 220. This value can then be used in the Karvonen formula to calculate the target heart rate (THR): THR equals the maximum minus the HR at rest (HR_{rest}) multiplied by 50% to 80% plus HR_{rest}

$$THR = (HR_{max} - HR_{rest}) \times (50\% \text{ to } 80\%) + HR_{rest}.$$

Cardiac Output

CO is the product of SV and HR. It is expressed as liters of blood pumped per minute by the heart. The relationship between CO and $\dot{V}O_2$ is linear (Fig. 83-9) (16). With an increase in age, the line shifts downward, but there is no significant change in the slope. The maximum CO increases with training, but there is no change in CO at rest or with submaximal work-

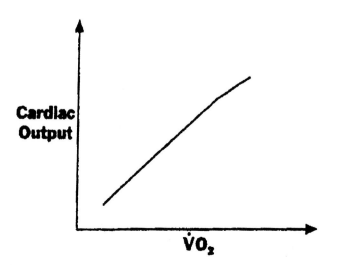

Figure 83-9. The relationship between cardiac output and oxygen consumption ($\dot{V}O_2$). (Redrawn with permission from Gonzalez EG. *Downey and Darling's physiological basis of rehabilitation medicine*, 3rd ed. Boston: Butterworth-Heinemann, 2001;172.)

loads (Fig. 83-10). However, there is a difference in how the submaximal CO is generated and distributed.

Distribution of peripheral blood flow is different in a trained subject, compared with an untrained subject. For example, in a trained subject, less blood is shunted to working muscles than in an untrained subject because the trained individual is able to extract oxygen more efficiently. This change in the distribution produces less of an increase in the total peripheral resistance and thus less afterload for the heart and a lower systolic blood pressure response to exercise.

Myocardial Oxygen Uptake

The myocardial oxygen uptake ($M\dot{V}O_2$) has a significant influence on clinical decision making. The major determinants of $M\dot{V}O_2$ consumption are myocardial mass and myocardial tension (T), which refer to the force developed by myocardial contraction. $M\dot{V}O_2$ is directly proportional to pressure (P) and radius (r) of the ventricle and is inversely proportional to thickness of the ventricle wall (H).

LaPlace's Law states that the myocardial tension (T) is proportional to the product of $P \times r/H$. Contractility refers to the velocity of myocardial fiber shortening or the rise in the rate of ventricular pressure ($\delta P/\delta T$). The oxygen supply of the myocardium is dependent on the oxygen content of the blood. The oxygen content of the blood is determined by arterial and venous oxygen difference, which is related to hemoglobin concentration and blood oxygen saturation. O_2 content equals 1.34 times the hemoglobin in gram percent, multiplied by percent of O_2 saturation divided by 100.

The $M\dot{V}O_2$ rises in a linear fashion when plotted against $\dot{V}O_2$ or other measures of workload (Fig. 83-11). It is limited by $\dot{V}O_{2max}$ or by anginal threshold when O_2 demand exceeds supply and the patient is symptomatic. With aerobic training, there is a decrease in $M\dot{V}O_2$ at rest and at any submaximal workload, but there is no change in the maximum $\dot{V}O_2$ as illustrated in Figure 83-12. Pharmacologic interventions also have an effect on resting and submaximal $\dot{V}O_2$, but not on $\dot{V}O_{2max}$. Angioplasty or bypass surgery can raise or eliminate the anginal threshold.

Patients with CVD can develop angina pectoris, arrhythmia, MI, or sudden death when the myocardial VO_2 required by an activity exceeds the maximum oxygen delivered by the coronary circulation. Blood pressure, HR, ventricle wall tension,

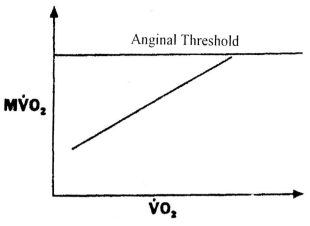

Figure 83-11. The relationship between myocardial oxygen consumption ($M\dot{V}O_2$) and total body oxygen consumption ($\dot{V}O_2$). (Redrawn with permission from Gonzalez EG. *Downey and Darling's physiological basis of rehabilitation medicine*, 3rd ed. Boston: Butterworth-Heinemann, 2001; 173.)

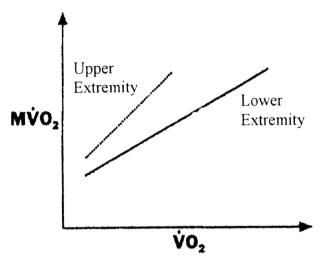

Figure 83-13. A comparison of the relationship between myocardial oxygen demand ($M\dot{V}O_2$) and total body oxygen consumption ($\dot{V}O_2$) for upper- and lower-extremity work. (Redrawn with permission from Gonzalez EG. *Downey and Darling's physiological basis of rehabilitation medicine*, 3rd ed. Boston: Butterworth-Heinemann, 2001;175.)

rate of fiber shortening, venous return, and the systemic arterial pressure (afterload) all influence myocardial $\dot{V}O_2$. It has been shown empirically that only HR and systolic blood pressure need to be measured to obtain a reasonable assessment of $M\dot{V}O_2$.

The rate pressure product (RPP) is calculated by multiplying the HR by the systolic blood pressure and then dividing by 100. The RPP correlates well with the myocardial $\dot{V}O_2$ when directly measured by cardiac catheterization under a variety of clinical situations. The RPP increases in a linear fashion with $\dot{V}O_2$ until anginal threshold is reached (see Fig. 83-11). The anginal threshold is the point at which there is evidence of imbalance between myocardial $\dot{V}O_2$ and available oxygen supply as manifested by anginal pain or ischemic electrocardiogram (ECG) changes.

The level of $M\dot{V}O_2$ is higher when work is performed with the upper extremities compared with the lower extremities (Fig. 83-13). The effect of posture varies with exercise intensity. With lower intensity exercise, the $M\dot{V}O_2$ is higher for supine than upright exercise at same $\dot{V}O_2$, but at higher intensities, the situation is reversed, as illustrated in Figure 83-14. This is im-

portant in rehabilitation when prescribing supine mat exercises for the patients who have coexisting CAD. Supine exercise may create a higher $M\dot{V}O_{2max}$ demand than ambulation or other upright activities, especially if the exercise involves an isometric component, such as bridging. One can use low-intensity exercise in supine posture to increase the range of observable cardiac response during exercise testing of hemiparetic or other patients with limited exercise capacity.

Coronary flow is dependent on coronary arterial pressure, resistance, diastolic time, and aortic pressure. Coronary vascular reserve has a capacity to increase flow five to six times the resting value. More prolonged exercise programs may enhance coronary perfusion because of a combination of reductions in HR and improvements in coronary blood flow capacity. This increase in coronary blood flow is multifactorial and includes contributions from metabolic, endothelial, myogenic, and neu-

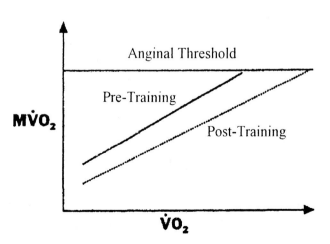

Figure 83-12. The effect of training on the relationship between myocardial oxygen demand ($M\dot{V}O_2$) and total body oxygen consumption ($\dot{V}O_2$). (Redrawn with permission from Gonzalez EG. *Downey and Darling's physiological basis of rehabilitation medicine*, 3rd ed. Boston: Butterworth-Heinemann, 2001;177.)

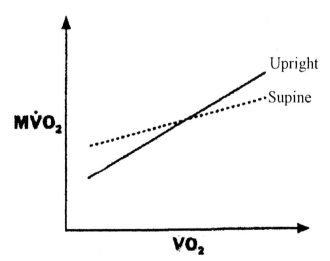

Figure 83-14. A comparison of the relationship between myocardial oxygen demand ($M\dot{V}O_2$) and total body oxygen consumption ($\dot{V}O_2$) for upright and supine work. (Redrawn with permission from Gonzalez EG. *Downey and Darling's physiological basis of rehabilitation medicine*, 3rd ed. Boston: Butterworth-Heinemann, 2001;175.)

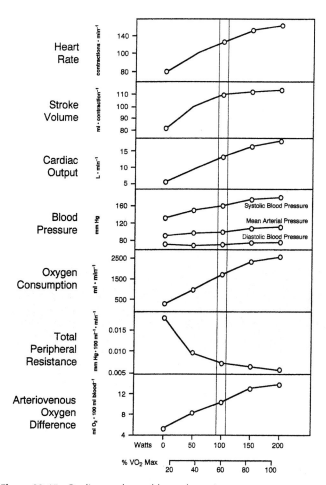

Figure 83-15. Cardiovascular and hemodynamic responses to acute exercise in the untrained subject. The *boxed area* represents the lactate threshold. Work rate is plotted along the X axis. V O $_2$max indicates maximum oxygen consumption. (Redrawn with permission from Durstine LJ, Pate RR, Branch JD. Cardio respiratory responses to acute exercise. In: Durstine JL, King AC, Painter PL, et al., eds. *ACSM resource manual for guidelines for exercise testing and prescription,* 2nd ed. Philadelphia: Lea & Febiger, 1993:66–74).

rohumoral systems. The up-regulation of nitrous oxide synthetase production seen with regular exercise contributes to an improved vasodilatory response (21).

The relationship of various cardiac parameters with $\dot{V}O_{2max}$ is summarized in Figure 83-15.

Arterial Blood Pressure Response

Systolic blood pressure rises with increase in dynamic work as a result of increased CO, whereas diastolic pressure usually remains about the same or moderately lower. After maximum exercise, there is usually a decline in systolic pressure, which normally reaches the resting level within 6 minutes and remains lower than the preexercise level for several hours (22). Figure 83-16 shows the physiologic response to various exercise levels in healthy men.

Skeletal Muscle Response

The skeletal muscle response to exercise requires use of both aerobic and anaerobic metabolic pathways. Major sources of

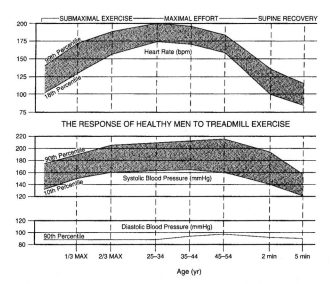

Figure 83-16. The hemodynamic responses of more than 700 healthy men to maximal treadmill exercise. Bands represent 80% of the population, with 10% having values exceeding the upper limit and 10% having lower values. (Redrawn with permission from Wolthius RA, Froelicher VF, Fischer J, et al. The response of healthy men to treadmill exercise. *Circulation* 1977;55:153–157.)

energy are glycogen, glucose, and fatty acids. At rest and at low levels of exercise, the energy is divided equally between fat and carbohydrate, but at maximum work, the sole source of energy is from carbohydrates and glycogen. Exercise training cannot change contractility or glycolytic capacity.

In CVD patients, the beneficial effects of aerobic exercises are seen both peripherally (skeletal muscle and vascular) and centrally (cardiac). Aerobic is defined as living, active, or occurring in the presence of oxygen. Aerobic exercises are the exercises during which energy needed is supplied by inspired oxygen. The skeletal muscle physiologic adaptation includes an increase in fiber area and oxidative enzyme activity (23). The vascular adaptation includes an increase in density of skeletal muscle capillaries and improvement in endothelial dependent vasodilatation in both epicardial and resistive coronary arteries (21). Cardiac adaptation includes and increase in cardiac dimension, SV, CO, and afterload corrected indexes of left ventricular function (23,24).

In a healthy individual, it has been shown that the cardiac chamber dimension increases by 20% and cardiac mass may increase as much as 70%. Increase in coronary flow and collateralization have not been directly demonstrated in humans. Echocardiographic studies have shown an increase in proximal coronary artery size, which is proportional to the increase in cardiac mass. Angiographic studies have shown increased dilating capacity in the left coronary artery. Thus, cardiac function appears to be mainly enhanced by training, left ventricle contractility, and SV increase.

The beneficial effect of training is somewhat dependent on the muscle groups undergoing the training. For example, in lower-extremity training, the HR and blood pressure will increase with leg work, but not as much with arm work. This is important when vocational or avocational training is considered. Thus, an exercise program involving the lower extremities (e.g., treadmill) will not be as beneficial as upper-extremity training would be to the individual who performs vocational activities involving the upper extremities. Both HR and systolic blood pressure are higher for any given submaximal $\dot{V}O_2$ if work is performed with the upper extremities. Thus, $\dot{V}O_{2max}$

determined by arm ergometry is usually less than $\dot{V}O_{2max}$ determined by leg ergometry.

FORMS OF EXERCISE

The physiologic effect of exercise depends on the type of exercise, intensity, duration, and frequency. Exercises can be categorized into isometric (static), isotonic (dynamic or locomotory), and resistive (a combination of isometric and isotonic) (25). Most daily activities involve a combination of all three types of exercises.

Isometric muscle contraction (static) is characterized by muscle contraction without any significant change in fiber length. No external work is accomplished, but substantial energy is used, and total peripheral resistance is increased. Both systolic pressure and diastolic pressure rise substantially. CO is not increased as much as with isotonic exercises because increased resistance in the active muscle group limits blood flow. Isometric exercises increase muscle strength and bulk, which is generally desirable for competitive athletes and for patients with atrophy from musculoskeletal injuries. Isometric work imposes greater pressure load than volume load on the left ventricle. An example of an isometric exercise is the handgrip.

Isotonic exercise (dynamic or locomotory) involves shortening of the muscle fiber with relatively little increase in muscle tension. Isotonic work imposes volume load on the left ventricle. Isotonic exercise produces a major "training effect" via a peripheral effect as discussed earlier. The magnitude of the training effect depends on the intensity, duration, and frequency of the exercise. Aerobic training requires rhythmic repetitive use of large muscle groups for prolonged periods. With isotonic exercise, there is a significant increase in both CO and oxygen consumption and a decrease in peripheral resistance. There is no significant change in diastolic pressure with it, but diastolic volume increases.

Resistive exercises such as free weight lifting are a combination of isometric and isotonic exercises that produce muscle contraction with movement. Resistance exercise training that involves activities that use low or moderate repetitive movement against resistance has been accepted as a component of CR. Before initiating a resistance-training program, the patient should be carefully screened for cardiovascular limitations and for prevention of exacerbation of preexisting neuromusculoskeletal problems. Patients should also be educated regarding specific components of resistance training programs, including proper technique, number and type of exercises, and safety precautions. The program should include a single set of 8 to 10 different exercises—for example, the chest press, shoulder press, triceps extension, biceps curls, pull down, low-back extension, abdominal crunch–curl up, quadriceps extension or leg press, leg curls, and calf raises—that train the major muscle groups.

To achieve a balanced increase in both muscular strength and endurance, 8 to 12 repetitions are recommended for healthy participants younger than 60 years of age, and 10 to 15 repetitions at a lower relative resistance are recommended for cardiac patients and healthy persons older than 60 years of age (26). Injury prevention is the reason for increasing the rate of repetitions at lower relative effort for the older or frail subject. Previous injury is the single greatest cause of musculoskeletal injury with resistance training. Higher-intensity effort (especially poor effort with fewer repetitions using heavier weights) can adversely affect knee and shoulder–rotator cuff area (27). Most daily activities involve a combination of all three types of exercises.

PREVENTATIVE VALUE OF REGULAR EXERCISE

There are more than 100 published reports with nearly 75 percent of them supporting an inverse relationship between physical activity and/or fitness, and the risk of initial fatal or nonfatal MI (28). The sedentary person has twice the incidence of death from CAD as compared with their more active counterpart. There is a fivefold increased risk of death from CVD in a nonfit person compared with fit individuals. It has been suggested that a minimum of 30 minutes of moderate-intensity physical activity (either continuous or in 10-minute increments, preferably 7 days a week) is recommended to reduce the risk of a CVD event (29). This is equivalent to 1.5 miles per day of brisk walking at an energy cost of about 150 calories per day for an average size person. The beneficial effects of exercise and cardiorespiratory fitness "against CVD" can be explained on multiple biological mechanisms (30). Some of them can be classified as:

1. *Anti-atherogenic effect:* Physical activity is associated with less severe CVD, larger coronary lumen diameter and reduced progression of arteriosclerosis (31). These beneficial effects are due to reduction in body fat, particularly in those with excess upper body and abdominal fat, reduction in elevated blood pressure, decreased elevation of plasma triglycerides and associated small dense LDL particles, increase in HDL cholesterol levels, and improvement in insulin sensitivity and glucose use (32).
2. *Antithrombotic effect* (33,34): With exercise, there is reduction in plasma fibrinogen levels, an increase in mean tissue plasminogen activator, an increase in active tissue plasminogen activator, and a reduction of plasminogen activator inhibitors. Available data also suggest that short-term exercise can lead to increased platelet activity, especially in sedentary individuals, but regular long-term exercise may abolish or reduce this response.
3. *Endothelial effect:* Endothelial-dependent dilatation is impaired in patients with coronary arteriosclerosis and patients with coronary risk factors. The emerging evidence suggests that aerobic exercise improves endothelial function (35).
4. *Autonomic system effect:* Improved measures of variability with exercise training have been shown in patients with chronic HF and patients after MI (21,36). Those who were physically trained and physically fit also had a higher sympathetic activity.
5. *Antiischemic effect:* Exercise training may improve the relative balance between myocardial oxygen supply and demand, and thereby result in antiischemic effect. Increased metabolic capacity and improved mechanical performance of the myocardium are well established and well sustained with endurance exercise training (30). The slowing of heart rate with training allows more time during diastole for coronary blood flow to perfuse the myocardium.
6. *Antiarrhythmic effect:* There is an increased risk of ventricular fibrillation with strenuous exercises in patients with CVD. Physically active men with CVD have lower rates of sudden death (31). Exercise improves the supply-to-demand ratio of $M\dot{V}O_2$; decreased adrenergic output decreases chanced arrhythmias.
7. *Blood pressure effect:* Studies (37) have shown an average reduction of 10 mm Hg in systolic and 7.5 mm Hg in diastolic blood pressures with regular exercise. Exercise reduces the incidence of hypertension and helps to normalize blood pressure in mildly hypertensive individuals.

8. *Glucose effect:* Exercise has the beneficial effect of decreasing glucose production by the liver and improving glucose utilization of exercising muscles, increasing sensitivity to insulin (38). Exercise training is an important contributor to weight loss, although the effect of exercise is quite variable. Most controlled exercise training studies have shown only modest weight loss, about 2 to 3 kg in an exercise group, but when diet is added to the exercise program, the average weight loss is 8.5 kg, most of which was is body fat, whereas diet alone results in lesser weight loss of about 5.1 kg (39).

9. *Lipid effects:* There is much variability in the results of exercise with respect to lipid lowering. An analysis of 95 studies, most of which were nonrandomized controlled trials, concluded that exercise leads to reduction in 6.3% in total cholesterol, 10.1% in low-density lipoprotein (LDL) cholesterol, and a 5% increase in HDL (40).

EXERCISE TOLERANCE TESTING

Exercise tolerance testing (ETT) for CR can be classified into functional ETT and diagnostic ETT (41). Functional ETT is especially important for CR, as it evaluates physical work capacity and cardiovascular function. The results of functional ETT are used for exercise prescriptions, setting vocational activity limits, and evaluation of effects of medications or other cardiac interventions. In contrast, the diagnostic ETT is terminated once the diagnostic information is available. Also, in contrast to the functional ETT, which is performed with the patients on their cardiac medications, the medications may mask or confirm the results of the diagnostic ETT. In both tests, the patient is encouraged to provide a maximal effort as most of the diagnostic information is obtained during the latter parts of the test. The usual recommendation is to achieve, if possible, at least 85% of the maximum THR.

Subject Preparation

The following are practical guidelines for an ETT:

1. Obtain informed consent.
2. The patient should be instructed not to eat or smoke for at least 3 hours before the test.
3. The patient should be appropriately dressed, including appropriate footwear.
4. No unaccustomed physical effort should be performed for at least 12 hours before the testing.
5. Because diagnostic ETT results may differ with certain medication, particularly β-blockers, decisions regarding discontinuation should be individualized and based on the clinical information needed from the test.
6. A brief history and physical examination should be performed to rule out any contraindications (Table 83-1). Special attention should be paid to detection of cardiac murmur, gallops, unstable angina, decompensated CHF, valvular disease, congenital heart disease (CHD), and any neuromuscular or orthopedic limitations that could interfere with the testing protocol. It is also especially important to rule out aortic stenosis and listen for pulmonary rales.
7. A 12-lead electrocardiogram should be obtained before the testing, and blood pressure should be recorded in the seated position for cycle ergometry and in a standing position for

TABLE 83-1. Absolute and Relative Contraindications to Exercise Testing	
Absolute Contraindications	**Relative Contraindications**[a]
Acute myocardial infarction or recent change on resting ECG	Less serious noncardiac disorder
Active unstable angina	Significant arterial or pulmonary hypertension
Serious cardiac arrhythmias	Tachyarrhythmias, bradyarrhythmias
Acute pericarditis	Moderate valvular or myocardial heart disease
Endocarditis	Drug effect or electrolyte abnormalities
Severe aortic stenosis	Left main coronary obstructive or its equivalent
Severe left ventricular dysfunction	Hypertrophic cardiomyopathy
Acute pulmonary embolus or pulmonary infarction	Psychiatric disease
Acute or serious noncardiac disorder	
Severe physical handicap or disability	

[a]Under certain circumstances and with appropriate precautions, relative contraindications can be superceded.
Reprinted with permission from Fletcher GF, Froelicher VF, Hartley, et al. *Exercise standards: a statement for health professionals.* Dallas: American Heart Association, 1991:2289.

treadmill exercise, so as to rule out any vasoregulatory abnormality.

Equipment and Protocols

Various equipment and protocols are used for exercise testing as outlined in the American Heart Association (AHA)'s "Guidelines for Clinical Exercise Testing in the Laboratory" (41). The various testing protocols and their relation to METs are summarized in Figure 83-17. Of note, in the United States, treadmill testing is more popular, whereas bicycle ergometry is used more often in Europe.

Bicycle ergometry is usually less expensive, occupies less space, and is especially useful for patients with gait and balance problems, claudication, obesity (weight limit on treadmill being less than 350 pounds), who fear treadmill ambulation, or who plan to train on a bicycle. Although it is non–weight bearing, it has good correlation with treadmill testing and can even be performed in a supine position using a recumbent bicycle. The major limitation of cycle ergometry testing is quadriceps discomfort and fatigue. The energy output is measured in watts. One watt is equivalent to 6-kilopound meter per minute (kpm/min). Another limitation is that there is an artificial elevation of RPP and systolic blood pressure at a given level of submaximal $\dot{V}O_2$.

Upper-extremity ergometry is particularly useful in patients with spinal cord injury, various types of paralyses, arthropathies, and other vascular and neurologic disabilities. It is also particularly useful for manual laborers or those who plan on performing exercises (e.g., swimming) that primarily involve the upper extremities. A disadvantage of upper-extremity er-

FUNCTIONAL CLASS	CLINICAL STATUS	O₂ COST ml/kg/min	METS	BICYCLE ERGOMETER	BRUCE MODIFIED 3 min MPH / %GR	BRUCE 3 min MPH / %GR	NAUGHTON	METS
NORMAL AND I	HEALTHY, DEPENDENT ON AGE, ACTIVITY			1 WATT = 6.1 Kpm/min FOR 70 KG BODY WEIGHT Kpm/min: 6.0 22 / 5.5 20 / 5.0 18				
		56.0	16					16
		52.5	15					15
		49.0	14	1500				14
		45.5	13	1350	4.2 16	4.2 16		13
		42.0	12	1200				12
	SEDENTARY HEALTHY	38.5	11	1050	3.4 14	3.4 14	2 min Stages MPH %GR	11
		35.0	10					10
		31.5	9	900			2 17.5	9
		28.0	8	750	2.5 12	2.5 12	2 14.0	8
		24.5	7					7
II	LIMITED	21.0	6	600			2 10.5	6
		17.5	5	450	1.7 10	1.7 10	2 7.0	5
III	SYMPTOMATIC	14.0	4	300	1.7 5		2 3.5	4
		10.5	3	150			2 0	3
		7.0	2		1.7 0		1 0	2
IV		3.5	1					

Figure 83-17. Relation of metabolic equivalents (METs) to stages in the various testing protocols. Functional class refers to New York Heart Association class; kpm, kilopond-meter; MPH, miles per hour; %GR, percent grade. (Redrawn with permission from Fletcher GF, Froelicher VF, Hartley, et al. *Exercise standards: a statement for health professionals.* Dallas: American Heart Association, 1991:2289.)

gometry is that it causes a greater RPP increase than treadmill testing.

Arm and leg ergometry is used for spanning the workload over greater muscle mass, which could be especially useful in patients with angina or CHF, as they may not become symptomatic during more limited workloads.

A major advantage of treadmill ETT is that there are various well-standardized and readily available protocols, including the Bruce, Cornell, Weber, Balke-Ware, and Naughton. A ramp

TABLE 83-2. Borg Scales for Rating Perceived Exertion

15-Grade Scale		10-Grade Scale	
6	No exertion at all	0	Nothing
7	Extremely light		
8		0.5	Very, very light (just noticeable)
9	Very light		
10		1	Very light
11	Light		
12		2	Light (weak)
13	Somewhat hard		
14		3	Moderate
15	Hard (heavy)	4	
16		5	Heavy (strong)
17	Very hard	6	
18		7	Very heavy
19	Extremely hard	8	
20	Maximal exertion	9	
		10	Very, very heavy (maximal)

Patient Instructions: This is a scale for rating perceived exertion. Perceived exertion is the overall effort or distress of your body during exercise. The number 0 (6 if using the 15-grade scale) represents no perceived exertion or leg discomfort and 10 (20 if using the 15-grade scale) represents the greatest amount of exertion that you have ever experienced. At various times during the exercise test you will be asked to select a number that indicates your rating perceived exertion at the time. Do you have any questions?

Borg RPE. *CR 10 scale.* © Gunnar Borg, 1970, 1985, 1994, 1998 (90).

TABLE 83-3. Frequently Used Angina and Dyspnea Rating Scales

5-Grade Angina Scale		10-Grade Angina/Dyspnea Scale	
0	No Angina	11	Nothing
1	Light, barely noticeable	11.5	Very, very slight
2	Moderate, bothersome	12	Very slight
3	Severe, very uncomfortable	13	Slight
4	Most pain ever experienced	14	Moderate
		15	Somewhat severe
5-Grade Dyspnea Scale		17	Severe
0	No dyspnea		
1	Mild, noticeable	18	Very severe
2	Mild, some difficulty	19	
3	Moderate difficulty, but can continue	20	
4	Severe difficulty, cannot continue	21	Very, very severe Maximal

Adapted from American College of Sports Medicine. *Guidelines for graded exercise testing and prescription,* 5th ed. Baltimore: Williams & Wilkins, 1995 and American Association of Cardiovascular and Pulmonary Rehabilitation. *Guidelines for cardiac rehabilitation program,* 2nd ed. Champaign, IL: Human Kinetics, 1994;64.

protocol can also be used for subjects at relatively low treadmill speeds. Disadvantages are the weight limitations for the treadmill and the difficulty that some patients have in using the treadmill. This is especially true in some patients with lower-extremity musculoskeletal disorders.

The 6-minute walk test is a functional test that can be used to evaluate exercise capacity in a patient with marked left ventricular dysfunction or peripheral vascular disease. Patients are instructed to walk down a 100-foot corridor at their own pace and attempt to cover as much distance as possible in 6 minutes. At the end of the 6-minute interval, the total distance walked is determined, and the symptoms experienced by the patient are recorded. This type of protocol uses submaximal level of stress and correlates modestly with $\dot{V}O_{2max}$.

The Borg scale of perceived exertion is a good tool for rating the patient's exertion perception (Table 83-2) (90). The subjective rating of the intensity of exertion perceived by the person exercising is a good indicator of fatigue, and it seems to be consistent from test to test for that person. In general, a Borg rating of more than 18 indicates the patient has performed maximal exercise, and values of more than 15 to 16 suggest that the aerobic threshold has been exceeded. This scale is useful for patients who cannot be tested on other devices. A limitation is that the patient must be cognitively intact.

Levels of anginal discomfort or dyspnea, in those known or suspected of having CAD, are also excellent subjective end points. Table 83-3 shows the details of the angina and dyspnea rating scales.

EXERCISE TESTING WITH IMAGING MODALITIES

The advantage of an imaging modality is that it can be used on even the most deconditioned or physically impaired patients without presenting any additional risk beyond the exercise performed during the test. It is also useful for patients who are anxious and demonstrate poor effort on standard protocols. Patients with resting ECG baseline abnormalities (e.g., left bundle branch block or ST depression of more than 1 mm) can also be tested with imaging modalities. Asymptomatic patients with abnormal standard exercise tolerance tests are also candidates for exercise testing with imaging modalities.

Exercise Echocardiography

The overall sensitivity of exercise echocardiography for detecting CAD ranges from 71% to 97% with greater sensitivity in multivessel disease. Specificity ranges from 64% to 100%. The images are taken at rest and compared with those obtained during and at the termination of the exercise test. According to the guidelines published by the American College of Cardiology (ACC) and AHA, exercise echocardiography is a good tool for clinical use (42).

Exercise Nuclear Imaging

Exercise testing with nuclear imaging uses a myocardial perfusion imaging agent, such as thallium-201, technetium 99m (Tc 99m)-sestamibi, or tetrofosmin. Sestamibi has a half-life of 6 hours, compared with 73 hours of thallium, and also has higher photon energy. The perfusion defects that are present during exercise but not seen at rest indicate myocardial ischemia. Sestamibi can be also used on a stress test protocol or rest protocol (43).

Pharmacologic Stress Testing

Patients who are unable to undergo exercise testing because of anxiety, severe deconditioning, peripheral vascular disease, orthopedic disability, neurologic diseases, or comorbid illnesses often benefit from pharmacologic stress imaging procedures. Adrenergic agents, such as dobutamine, increase myocardial contractility, and blood pressure. A problem of nausea, headache, tremor, anxiety, angina and atypical chest pain, arterial and ventricular arrhythmia, and hypertension or hypotension can occur during adrenergic testing (44). Vasodilators, such as adenosine or dipyridamole, can be used to assess coronary perfusion during nuclear imaging or echocardiography. They should not be used in patients with second- and third-degree atrioventricular block or in patients with bronchospastic disease, such as asthma or severe chronic obstructive lung disease. The imaging test is also useful for a patient who has a positive treadmill test but is asymptomatic.

If the above tests cannot be performed, one can use what is called a "nonstandard test." This involves ECG or Holter monitoring during the rehabilitation process for patients with hemiplegia, paraplegia, amputation, etc. The testing can be submaximal or maximal. The submaximal test is usually done with a low level of activity. It detects any problems of arrhythmia or any symptomatic changes and determines the level of activity for exercise prescription.

EXERCISE PRESCRIPTION

Exercise for the cardiac patient must be prescribed with as much care as a drug prescription. Fundamentals for developing an exercise program are shown in Table 83-4.

The prescription should specify exercise doses (which are determined by intensity, frequency, and duration of exercise), the type of exercise, and the rate of progression of exercise intensity. A sample prescription is shown in Figure 83-18. Coronary patients should not exercise at levels higher than documented to produce an appropriate cardiovascular response during testing. The hallmark of rehabilitative exercise training is individualized, medically supervised physical activity.

TABLE 83-4. Fundamentals in Developing an Exercise Prescription

Obtain the maximum exercise heart rate—preferably with exercise testing.
Designate a target heart at a level 60–80% of the maximum heart rate.
Begin at a low level (60–70%) and progress over 4–6 wk to the <80% level.
Exercise activity should be done for 30–60 min. 4–6 times weekly, preferably on most days.
Exercise sessions should incorporate aerobic activity, such as walking, jogging, cycling, or water aerobics, with appropriate warm-up and cool-down.
Resistance activities such as light weights should be used on a less frequent basis—2–3 times weekly.

Reprinted with permission from Fletcher GF, Oken KR, Safford RE. Comprehensive Rehabilitation of Patients with Coronary Artery Disease. In: Braunwald E, Zipes DP, Libby P, eds. Heart Disease, 6th ed. Philadelphia: W.B. Saunders, 2001:1409.

In general, patients with CVD have a different exercise response than healthy subjects. They demonstrate decreased resting CO and a smaller increase in CO related to increasing oxygen uptakes. The SV response to exercise may be variable and may not maintain relationships between the increased intensity of workload and HR responses. The degree of the abnormality cannot be predicted by exercise response, even though there is some relation of anatomic obstruction of CAD to exercise. Therefore, it may be inappropriate to use age-predicted THR for CVD patients. Their HR response to exercise will be influenced by various clinical factors, such as cardiovascular mor-

MD ____________

Name ________ Age ________ Starting Date ________

Clinical Status: Normal
Arrhythmia Angina CABG CAD HTN MI PTCA VR

Note: This prescription is valid only if you remain on the same medications (type and dose), and you are in the same clinical status as on the day your exercise test was conducted.

Contraindications: Angina at rest, fever, illness
Temperature and weather extremes (below 30°F or more than 80° with high humidity)

Activities to avoid: Sudden strenuous lifting or carrying
Exertion that leads to holding your breath

Exercise Type: Aerobic types of exercise that are continuous, dynamic and repetitive in nature

Frequency: ______ times/day ______ days/week

Duration: Total duration of exercise session: ______ min

To be divided as follows:

Warm-up: (light flexibility/stretching routine) ______ min

Aerobic training activity: ______ to ______ min

Cool-down: (slow walking and stretching): ______ min

Intensity:

Target heart rate ______ to ______ beats/min

______ to ______ beats/10 sec

Perceived exertion should not exceed "somewhat hard"

Re-évaluation

Your next graded exercise test is due: ____________
Call our office to schedule an appointment. Phone: ____________

Exercise Physiologist ____________

Figure 83-18. Exercise prescription form. (Redrawn with permission from Franklin BA, McCullough PA, Timmis GC. Exercise. In: Hennekens CH, ed. *Clinical trials in cardiovascular disease*. Philadelphia: WB Saunders, 1999:278–295.)

bidities, medications, various therapies, and prior levels of training or fitness.

Intensity Of Exercise

Intensity and duration of exercise determine the total caloric expenditure during a training session and are inversely related. This inverse relationship allows the same amount of energy expenditure with high-intensity exercises for shorter duration or low-intensity exercises for longer durations.

The Centers for Disease Control and Prevention (CDC), AHA, and the American College of Sports Medicine recommend that total exercise expenditure of 700 to 2,000 calories per week is desirable (45). Technically, all clinical ETT results should be reported in METs and not in minutes of exercise. In this way, the results from different protocols and exercise modalities can be compared directly.

The intensity of the exercise is usually expressed as a percent of functional aerobic capacity. It should be the minimum level required to produce a "training effect," yet below the metabolic load that evokes significant symptomatic cardiac events (ECG changes, blood pressure abnormalities, etc.). For most MI patients, the threshold of intensity of exercise training probably lies between 40% and 60% of $\dot{V}O_{2max}$ and is directly proportional to pretraining $\dot{V}O_{2max}$ or to the level of habitual physical activity. The optimal intensity of aerobic exercise training probably occurs between 57% and 78% of $\dot{V}O_{2max}$, which corresponds to 70% to 85% HR_{max}. It should be below the ventilatory threshold. The oxygen uptake and HR correlate linearly with dynamic exercises involving large muscle groups. A predetermined THR has become an index of exercise intensity.

Various methods may be used to determine the range of exercise intensity to be prescribed. Some of them are as follows:

1. *HR method:* This is one of the oldest methods of setting the THR. HR_{max} can be first estimated by subtracting the patient's age from 220 with ±1 standard deviation, i.e., 10–12 beats/min. THR can then be calculated by:

   - Plotting HR against either $\dot{V}O_2$ or exercise intensity. This is called the direct method. This is useful for patients with low fitness levels, those with CVD or pulmonary problems, and those taking medications (β-blockers). It also allows prescribing the THR below the point of adverse signs or symptoms noted during ETT. Low-level activity can be compensated either by increasing the frequency or duration of the training.

   - Percentage of HR_{max} is another simple way of computing THR. It is prescribed as a percentage of HR_{max} obtained preferably with ETT. It usually designates THR at the level of 60% to 80% of the HR_{max}. For example, if a person's HR_{max} is 200 beats/min, the THR range will be 120–160 beats/min (60%–80% of HR_{max}). This method underestimates oxygen consumption equivalent value by about 15%. Considerable new data also suggest that exercise intensity at 50% to 70% of THR range will produce comparable improvements in functional capacity and endurance. This lowering of the THR has allowed for unsupervised exercise and greater safety because of the lower risk of cardiovascular complications. These lower rates are less likely to produce discomfort and may improve long-term exercise compliance.

   - HR reserve method (HRR) or Karvonen method involves subtracting resting heart rate (HR_{rest}) from HR_{max} to obtain the value for HRR. Then 60% and 80% values of HRR

are computed, and each of these values is added to HR_{rest} to obtain the THR range.

$$THR\ range = [(HR_{max} - HR_{rest}) \times 0.60 + HR_{rest}]\ to\ [(HR_{max} - HR_{rest}) \times 0.80 + HR_{rest}]$$

For example: If an individual's HR_{max} was 200 beats/min and HR_{rest} was 70 beats/min, then

$$THR\ range = [(200 - 70) \times 0.60 + 70]\ to\ [(200 - 70) \times 0.80 + 70]$$

$$= [(130 \times 0.6 = 78) + 70 = 148]\ to\ [(130 \times 0.8 = 104) + 70 = 174]$$

$$THR\ range = 148\ to\ 174\ beats/min$$

If for any reason HR cannot be determined, one can modify the Karvonen formula to use blood pressure as follows:

$$TSBP = (SBP_{max} - SBP_{rest}) \times 0.50 + SBP_{rest}\ to\ (SBP_{max} - SBP_{rest}) \times 0.80 + SBP_{rest}$$

Where TSBP = training systolic blood pressure, SBP = systolic blood pressure, SBP_{max} = maximum SBP during ET, SPB_{rest} = SPB at rest.

2. *METs method:* Straight percentage of $\dot{V}O_{2max}$, for example, if a person had a measured $\dot{V}O_{2max}$ of 10 METs, the prescribed intensity could be set at 6–8 METs, corresponding to 60% to 80% of $\dot{V}O_{2max}$ respectively.

3. Rating of perceived exertion (RPE): RPE is an adjunct to monitoring HR. Borg RPE uses a 10–15 grade scale (see Table 83-2). A rating of 11–15 on both scales usually corresponds to appropriate exercise training. It is useful for patients with difficulty with HR palpation and in patients in whom HR response to exercise may have been altered because of medication (46).

4. *Oxygen consumption method:* Oxygen consumption method involves measuring expired gases during ETT. Sixty percent

---

TABLE 83-5. Duke Activity Status Index

Can You:	Weight
1. Take care of yourself, that is, eat, dress, bathe or use the toilet?	2.75
2. Walk indoors, such as around your house?	1.75
3. Walk a block or two on level ground?	2.75
4. Climb a flight of stairs or walk up a hill?	5.50
5. Run a short distance?	8.00
6. Do light work around the house like dusting or washing dishes?	2.70
7. Do moderate work around the house like vacuuming, sweeping floors, or carrying groceries?	3.50
8. Do heavy work around the house like scrubbing floors or lifting or moving heavy furniture?	8.00
9. Do yard work like raking leaves, weeding, or pushing a power mower?	4.50
10. Have sexual relations?	5.25
11. Participate in moderate recreational activities like golf, bowling, dancing, doubles tennis, or throwing a baseball or football?	6.00
12. Participate in strenuous sports like swimming, singles tennis, football, basketball, or skiing?	5.3

DASI = the sum of weight for "yes" replies. VO_{2peak} ($mL \cdot kg^{-1} \cdot min^{-1}$) = 0.43 × DASI + 9.6

Reprinted with permission from Franklin BA. American College of Sports Medicine, *Guidelines for exercise testing and prescription*, 6th ed. Baltimore: American College of Sports Medicine, 2000;141.

TABLE 83-6. Exercise Prescription According to the Characteristics of the Patient

Characteristic	Training Regimen	Intensity	Type of Exercise	Frequency of Sessions no./wk.	Duration of Each Session min.
Age <65 yr, not overweight	High-intensity aerobic	75–85% of maximal heart rate	Walking, jogging, cycling, rowing	3 or 4	30–45 (continuous or interval)
Age >65 yr	Low-intensity aerobic and resistance	65–75% of maximal heart rate	Walking, cycling, rowing	3 or 4	30 (may be intermittent)
Overweight	Aerobic—high caloric expenditure	65–80% of maximal heart rate	Walking	5 or 6	45–60
Age >65 yr and disabled, engaged in physical work, or overweight	Resistance	50–75% of single repetition maximal lift	Weight machine and dumbbells, with the focus on the upper legs, shoulders, and arms	2 or 3	10–20 (10 repetitions of each 5 to 7 exercises)

Reprinted with permission from Adespa. Medical Progress. *N Engl J Med* 2001;345(12):895.

to 70% of maximum oxygen consumption corresponds to maximum HR obtained during ETT.

5. *Work method:* Training sessions should be at two-thirds of the maximal MET level attained during the ETT, or 25 watts (150 kpm) lower than the maximum level attained on cycle ergometer testing, or the highest speed reached at a 10% grade on the treadmill.

6. *Exercise intensity prescription without ETT:*
   - Post MI THR should be less than 120 beats/min or HR_{rest} plus 20 beats/min (arbitrary limit). In the postsurgery patient, it should be the HR_{rest} plus 30 beats/min (arbitrary limit) and to the tolerance of the patient if the patient is asymptomatic.
   - Patient questionnaires, such as the Duke Activity Status Index (47) as outlined in Table 83-5 and Veterans Specific Activity Questionnaire (48), can be used to estimate an individual's activity status and functional capacity.
   - One can use characteristics of the patients as outlined in Table 83-6 or by classification of physical activity intensity as shown in Table 83-7.

Case Study: A 30-year-old man weighing 180 pounds has a history of an uncomplicated MI 6 months ago and now wishes to begin an exercise program. He wants to start walking, using the treadmill or using a bicycle ergometer. He feels comfortable walking at 3.5 mph. His HR_{rest} is 60 beats/min. His HR_{max} would be 190 beats/min and $\dot{V}O_{2max}$ was 48 cc/kg/min. A decision was made to start him on exercise intensity of 70% $\dot{V}O_{2max}$ (49).

What is his target $\dot{V}O_{2max}$?

$$\text{Target } \dot{V}O_{2max} = (\text{intensity of exercise}) \times (\dot{V}O_{2max})$$
$$= 0.70 \times 48 = 33.6 \text{ cc/kg/min}$$

What is appropriate THR according to HRR method?

$$THR = (HR_{max} - HR_{rest}) \times (\text{exercise intensity}) + HR_{rest}$$
$$= (190 - 60) \times (0.70) + 60 = 151 \text{ beats/min}$$

What should be the grade (steepness) of treadmill if he walks at 3.5 mph?

Convert mph to meters/min = 3.5 × 26.8 = 93.8 m/min

TABLE 83-7. Classification of Physical Activity Intensity

	Endurance-Type Activity							Strength-Type Exercise/Relative Intensity*
	Relative Intensity			Absolute Intensity in Healthy Adults (Age), METs				
Intensity	$\dot{V}O_{2\,max,}$%	Maximum Heart Rate, %	RPE†	Young (20–39)	Middle-Aged (40–64)	Old (65–79)	Very Old (80+)	RPE†	Maximum Voluntary Contraction, %
---	---	---	---	---	---	---	---	---	---
Very light	<20	<35	<10	<2.4	<2.0	<1.6	<1.0	<10	<30
Light	20–39	35–54	10–11	2.4–4.7	2.0–3.9	1.6–3.1	1.1–1.9	10–11	30–49
Moderate	40–59	55–69	12–13	4.8–7.1	4.0–5.9	3.2–4.7	2.0–2.9	12–13	50–69
Hard	60–84	70–89	14–16	7.2–10.1	6.0–8.4	4.8–6.7	3.0–4.25	14–16	70–84
Very hard	≥85	≥90	17–19	≥10.2	≥8.5	≥6.8	≥4.25	17–19	≥85
Maximum‡	100	100	20	12.0	10.0	8.0	5.0	20	100

*Based on 8 to 12 repetitions for persons <50–60 years old and 10 to 15 repetitions for persons aged ≥50–60 years.
†Borg rating of Relative Perceived Exertion (RPE), 6–20 scale.
‡Maximum values are mean values achieved during maximum exercise by healthy adults. Absolute intensity values are approximate mean values for men. Mean values for women are ~1 to 2 METs lower than those for men.
Adapted from American College of Sports Medicine position stand: the recommended quantity and quality of exercise for developing and maintaining cardiorespiratory and muscular fitness, and flexibility in healthy adults. *Med Sci Sports Exerc* 1998;30:975–991.

For walking: $\dot{V}O_2 = (0.1 \times speed) + (1.8 \times speed \times fraction\ grade) + 3.5$

$33.6 = 0.1 \times 93.8 + (1.8 \times 93.8 \times fraction\ grade) + 3.5$
$30.1 = 9.38 + 168.8 \times (fraction\ grade)$
$20.7 = 168.8 \times (fraction\ grade)$
$0.123 = fraction\ grade = 12.3\%\ grade$

What is his target work rate on bicycle ergometer?

Body mass in kg = lbs/2.2 = 180/2.2 = 81.8 kg

For bike: $\dot{V}O_2 = 7 + 1.8$ (work rate/body mass)

$33.6 = 7 + 1.8$ (work rate)/81.8
$26.6 = 1.8$ (work rate)/81.8
$2,176 = 1.8$ (work rate)
$1,209$ kg/m/min = work rate

What resistance setting should be used if he is comfortable at 60 rpm pedaling speed?

Work rate = (resistance setting) × (D) × (pedal speed)

Where D is the distance in meter (m) the flywheel of bike travels per one pedal revolution (in a Monarch bike, it is 6 m).

$$1,209 = (resistance\ setting) \times 6 \times 60 = 360 \times (resistance\ setting)$$
$$3.36\ kg = resistance\ setting$$

What will be his caloric expenditure during 30 minutes of exercise?

Net $\dot{V}O_2$ = Target $\dot{V}O_2 - 3.5 = 33.6 - 3.5 = 30.1$ cc/kg/min

VO_2 in L/min = (Net VO_2 cc/kg/min) × body mass in kg/1,000
$$= 30.1 \times 81.8/1000 = 2.46\ L/min$$

1 L of O_2 consumption = 5 kilocalories; kcal/min
$$= 2.46 \times 5 = 12.3$$

Total exercise time = 30 min

Total calories spent = 30 × 12.3 = 369 Kcal

Duration of Exercise

Duration of exercise improvement can be achieved while exercising by varying lengths of time per session. The duration depends on the level of fitness of the individual and the intensity of the exercise. The usual duration when exercise is at 70% of maximum HR is about 20 to 30 minutes at a conditioned level. In poorly conditioned individuals, daily exercises of 3 to 5 minutes duration can bring improvement (50). Although training for 10 to 15 minutes improves cardiorespiratory fitness, a duration of 30 minutes is more effective. After 30 minutes, further training increases the chances of musculoskeletal overuse syndromes.

Frequency of Exercise

All studies agree on the importance of training frequency to bring about cardiovascular improvement. Some studies have shown that improvement was not different whether the training frequency was 2 or 5 days per week, but the most consistent benefit appears to occur with a frequency of 3 times per week for 12 weeks or more. There is no contraindication to exercise every day, but as the number of sessions increases, the likelihood of musculoskeletal injury also increases (49).

Types of Exercises

Cardiovascular conditioning should include isotonic, rhythmic, and aerobic exercises; use large muscle groups; and not involve a significant isometric component. In recent years, strength training (isometric resistive training exercises) and circuit weight training have been added to the ongoing aerobic training exercises and have been found to be a very low risk for patients with good ventricular function (51,52). In addition to improved muscle strength, a combined circuit weight training–aerobic training program also improves the patient's ability to perform activities of daily living (ADLs) and enhances self-image (53,54).

Each type of exercise brings about specific metabolic and physiologic adaptations, resulting in a specific training effect. Aerobic training leads to improvement in endurance, provided it involves large muscle groups (55). Power training is isometric. Results include increases in strength but not increases in endurance. All types of training are felt to be important in rehabilitation to improve ADLs and job-related performance. Because of the relative consistency of oxygen consumption, walking, jogging, and bicycling are the most popular forms of exercises. The older individual often prefers walking or bicycling over jogging. Swimming is a good exercise but is not preferred for the patient with CAD as it increases the HR too high in comparison with estimated HR on exercise testing. It also masks symptoms of HR_{max} and related cardiac symptoms. In bicycling exercise, gripping of the handles should be avoided. Rope skipping is better than running for aerobic exercise because it requires at least 9.5 to 12.5 METs. The key to calisthenics exercise is to alternate rapidly between exercises of one extremity to exercises involving all four extremities. Cross-country skiing is more effective than running, but weather can be a limiting factor and it may be too strenuous for the cardiac patient. Aerobic dancing requires the equivalent of more than 9 METs and it is not popular with MI patients.

Format of an Exercise Session

The training sessions of an exercise program should follow a specific format. There should be an initial warm-up phase, a training phase (i.e., a stimulus phase during which the exercise is performed at the prescribed intensity and duration that induces training effect), and a cool-down phase after the period of training. A warm-up phase usually lasts for about 10 minutes. The stimulus phase is usually about 15 to 30 minutes, and cool-down phase is 10 to 15 minutes. The format of a typical aerobic exercise session is illustrated in Figure 83-19.

The purpose of the warm-up phase is to provide a smooth transition from rest to aerobic endurance training, to increase the joint readiness, to theoretically open the existing collateral circulation, and to prevent any sudden changes in peripheral resistance before the maximum contraction of the skeletal muscle required by the exercise occurs. The CO and oxygen uptake do not begin to approach the steady state until 2 minutes after the onset of work, and the blood pressure response is delayed. This provides time for autoregulation of the cardiovascular system to get ready for conditioning. The warm-up period is usually at a lower-intensity level compared with the exercise to be performed and gradually increases to the prescribed intensity, or it may be in the form of limbering-up exercise. It should include both musculoskeletal and cardiorespiratory activities.

In the cool-down phase, there is a gradual reduction in exercise intensity to allow the redistribution of the blood from the extremities to the other tissue, and to prevent sudden reduction

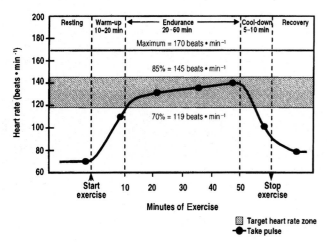

Figure 83-19. Format of a typical aerobic exercise session illustrating the warm-up, endurance, and cool-down phases along with a representative heart rate response. At the conclusion of warm-up, heart rate approached the lower limit of the target zone for training, corresponding to 10% to 85% of the peak heart rate achieved during maximum exercise testing. (Redrawn with permission from Franklin BA. *ACSM's guidelines for exercise testing and prescription*, 6th ed. Baltimore: American College of Sports Medicine, 2000;176).

in venous return, thereby diminishing the possibility of postexercise hypotension or even syncope. It also reduces the development of joint stiffness and muscle soreness. It allows the autoregulating system to go back to the resting level, gives time for dissipation of the heat generated with the exercise and removal of lactic acid, and decreases a certain rise of postexercise catecholamine level.

Common sense should be used for an exercise environment. Exercise should not be done in extreme temperatures. It should be done along with someone else in case help is needed. The individual should not go beyond the established limit of the exercise prescription. Strenuous sustained isometric exercise in particular should be avoided.

RISK OF EXERCISE

Exercise carries both potential risks and benefits. Three of the major exercise risk factors are age, presence of heart disease, and intensity of exercise. Screening procedures can be used to identify individuals at risk for an exercise-related cardiac event. It is generally believed that the benefits of exercise greatly exceed the risks and thus the individual should be encouraged to exercise.

Most of the studies of exercise-related mortality were not randomized controlled trials, and the contribution of all potential variables to sudden death or sudden cardiac arrest cannot be determined. Sudden death is rare in a healthy individual. In an individual younger than 35 years, sudden cardiac death is usually attributed to hypertrophic cardiomyopathy or CHD, whereas coronary atherosclerotic heart disease is more likely the cause for those older than the age of 40. The incidence of major cardiovascular complications during an outpatient cardiac exercise program has been estimated to be 1 in 60,000 participant hours (56). The risk of death, acute MI, or other events requiring hospitalization during or immediately after an exercise test is less than or equal to 0.01%, 0.04%, and 0.2%, respectively. The incidence is lowest during activities that are largely controlled, such as walking, cycling, or treadmill walking (57).

Those who have continuous ECG monitoring have the lowest rates of sudden cardiac arrest compared with those who are unmonitored or only intermittently monitored. In subjects with heart disease, jogging seems to be associated with a greater incidence of sudden cardiac arrest compared with other activities (58). This is probably related to exercise intensity. Jogging at even the lowest pace may generate $\dot{V}O_2$ demand that exceeds 80% of maximum for many untrained individuals.

Exercise can be an important trigger for MI. Approximately 4% to 20% of MIs occur during or soon after exertion (59,60). The chance of an MI occurring during exercise is seven times more than sudden cardiac death. There is an inverse relationship between regular physical activity and MI. The incidence of MI in a sedentary person is much higher than in the individual who regularly exercises five times per week.

Studies indicate that the intensity and nature of impact of physical activity are the two most important factors in determining the frequency of musculoskeletal injuries. These are common and include direct injuries, such as bruises, sprains, and strains, and indirect problems, such as an exacerbation of arthritis and low back pain. Low-impact exercises, such as walking, cycling, and swimming, cause less stress on the bones and joints, whereas the high-impact exercises of running, jogging, and aerobic dancing cause repeated impact on the joints, particularly of both lower extremities.

The rate of occurrence of adverse events has not increased appreciably in spite of the inclusion of elderly patients, patients with increased risks of chronic HF, or those with heart transplants. Patients should be educated about the development of "athletic heart," cardiac ischemia, arrhythmia, sudden death, heat cramps, heat exhaustion, heat stroke, overuse syndromes, muscular imbalance, lack of flexibility, and improper use of equipment.

COMPONENTS OF CARDIAC REHABILITATION AND SECONDARY PREVENTION PROGRAMS

The core components of CR and secondary prevention programs include evaluation, intervention, and determination of expected outcome from the patient assessment. Patient assessment must include a medical history, physical examination, and ETT. The program should incorporate nutritional counseling, lipid management, hypertension management, smoking cessation, weight management, diabetes management, psychosocial management, physical activity counseling, and exercise training (61). Risk reduction in clinical practice is multifactorial because of the frequent coexistence of risk factors. Figure 83-20 shows a decision tree for CR services (35).

Evaluation of long-term benefit of primary prevention is difficult because of selection bias. The AHA in their most recent position paper advocated that institution of an exercise program of moderate intensity around 40% to 60% of maximum $\dot{V}O_2$ performed for 20 to 30 minutes three to four times per week was sufficient for primary prevention (61).

The major risk factors for CVD include cigarette smoking, hypertension (blood pressure of more than 140/90 mm Hg or simply being on hypertensive medication), HDL cholesterol less than 40 mg per deciliter, family history of premature CHD (in first-degree male relative less than 55 years of age and in first-degree female relative less than 65 years of age), and the life habits of obesity, physical inactivity, and atherogenic diet. The emerging risk factors are lipoprotein, homocystinemia, prothrombotic and proinflammatory factors, impaired fasting glucose, evidence of subclinical atherosclerotic disease, C-reac-

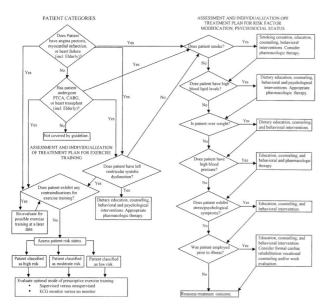

Figure 83-20. Decision tree for cardiac rehabilitation services: ◇, decision points; ▢, interventions. Adapted from material provided by Health Economics Research, Inc. ,Waltham, MA.

tive protein, small dense LDL, hypertriglyceridemia, and apoprotein B.

LDL cholesterol is a major risk category in CVD patients with an equivalent of 100 and increases to 130 in the presence of two risk factors. The management and classification of various categories of LDL cholesterol are summarized in Table 83-8 (62).

One program reported a 22% smoking-cessation rate at 1 year that cost approximately $400 per patient (clinic visits plus drug cost). It was estimated that the cost of a net year of life gained (YLG) by the program was $6,128, which compares favorably with the cost of pneumococcal vaccine in the elderly which was $1,500 YLG. In contrast, treatment of mild to moderate hypertension was $11,300–$24,000 YLG, heart transplantation was $16,200 YLG, and breast cancer screening $26,800 YLG (63).

Comprehensive evaluation of standard risk factors, in addition to the patient's age, allows for clinical assessment for risk of future CAD development. Tables 83-9 and 83-10 summarize data from the Framingham Heart Study's 10-year risk assessment for CAD development, CAD death, nonfatal MI, or unstable angina (64). The Framingham Heart Study, the Multiple Risk Factor Intervention Trials (MRFIT), and the nurse's health study have yielded important information about risk factors for future CAD development (65). These studies estimate that

approximately 30% of all CAD deaths in the United States each year are attributable to cigarette smoking as an independent risk factor. CAD risk definitely declines with smoking cessation, even after many years of heavy smoking. Furthermore, the risk of reinfarction also declines with smoking cessation (66).

The Framingham Heart Study also clarified several misconceptions about blood pressure (37,67). The study found the following:

- Elderly subjects do not tolerate hypertension better than younger subjects.
- Systolic hypertension is not benign, even in elderly. Elevated systolic blood pressure is a greater predictor of CAD risk than diastolic blood pressure.
- The pulse pressure (the difference between the systolic blood pressure and diastolic blood pressure) as a noninvasive measure of arterial stiffness is a powerful predictor of CAD morbidity and mortality.

Both the Framingham Heart Study and MRFIT showed a powerful continued dose relationship between total cholesterol and risk of CAD morbidity and mortality with no critical cutoff where normal ends and abnormal begins. There was a strongly positive association between LDL cholesterol and CAD development. An even more powerful inverse protective relationship of HDL cholesterol and CAD was found. The risk of CAD development within any cholesterol level is markedly influenced by prior existing risk factors (67).

Type II diabetes is a powerful risk factor for CAD development. Risk of death due to an MI, however, in a diabetic patient as compared with a nondiabetic patient is similar. The patients with type II diabetes without previous MI have as high a risk of MI over 7 years as the nondiabetic patient with a previous MI. This is particularly important in a metabolic syndrome characterized by atherogenic dyslipidemia (elevated triglycerides, increased LDL, and decreased HDL), hypertension, insulin resistance, and obesity. This metabolic syndrome can be identified by a waist circumference of at least 40 inches in men and 35 inches in women, increased triglycerides of more than 150 mg, HDL cholesterol of less than 40 mg in men and less than 50 mg in women, a blood pressure of more than 130/85 mm Hg, and fasting blood glucose of 110 mg (68,69).

The previously mentioned factors are influenced by diet and lifestyle (70). Recent data suggests a healthy lifestyle leads to low CAD development. In the nurse's health study, women were grouped according to smoking habits, dietary intake, alcohol consumption, and body mass index and exercise habit (71,72). Women in the low-risk category had a relatively lower risk of coronary events (0.17) as compared with all other women. Eighty-two percent of the coronary events in this group were attributable to lack of adherence to a healthy lifestyle.

TABLE 83-8. LDL Cholesterol Goals (mg/dL) for Patients in Major Risk Categories			
Category	**LDL Goal**	**Initiate TLC***	**Consider Drug**
CHD or risk equivalent	<100	≥100	≥130 (100–129 optional)
2+ risk factors	<130	≥130	≥130
0–1 risk factor	<160	≥160	≥190 (160–189 optional)

*TLC, Therapeutic Lifestyle Changes

TABLE 83-9. Scoring Risk Factors for Men and Women*

Age (yr)	Men	Women	TC (mg/dL)	Men	Women	Glucose (mg/dL)	Men	Women
≤34	−1	−9	<160	−3	−2	<110	0	0
35–39	0	−4	160–199	0	0	110–126	1	2
40–44	1	0	200–239	1	1	>126	2	4
45–49	2	3	240–279	2	2			
50–54	3	6	≥280	3	3			
55–59	4	7						
60–64	5	8						
65–69	6	9						
70–74	7	10						

Smoker	Men	Women	HDL-C (mg/dL)	Men	Women	SBP (mm Hg)	Men	Women
No	0	0	<35	2	5	<120	0	−3
Yes	2	2	35–44	1	2	120–129	0	0
			45–49	0	1	130–139	1	1
			50–59	−1	0	140–159	2	2
			≥60	−2	−3	≥160	3	3

*A symposium held in conjunction with the Primary Medicine Today–PM–Med Midwest 2002 Meeting, Sponsored by The Johns Hopkins University School of Medicine, Baltimore, Maryland.
HDL-C, high density-lipoprotein cholesterol; SBP, systolic blood pressure; TC, total cholesterol.
Courtesy of Dr. Steven P. Schulman.

REHABILITATION FOLLOWING MYOCARDIAL INFARCTION IN PATIENTS WITH CORONARY ATHEROSCLEROTIC DISEASE

Physical inactivity is associated with the development and progression of CAD. Physiologic changes that occur with exercise training lessen myocardial ischemia at rest and during submaximal exercise. However, certain precautionary guidelines are necessary to avoid a cardiac event during exercise. Exercise supervision can be performed by a physician who has the basic knowledge to interpret the 12-lead exercise electrocardiogram, perform and interpret standard exercise testing, understand nuclear imaging technique, and interpret the formal workup of cardiac testing. The physician should also have knowledge of ECG monitoring online or via electronic telemetry and a basic understanding of certain cardiac medications (particularly β-blockers, digitalis, calcium channel blockers, angiotensin-converting enzymes inhibitors, coronary vasodilators, antiarrhythmics, anticoagulants, and lipid lowering medications). The physician should also be familiar with the technique and interpretation of the data from cardiac catheterization, angiographic testing, echocardiography, and Holter monitoring. The physician should understand the concepts of thrombolysis, coronary angioplasty, stenting, arthrectomy, and endarterectomy. He or she should be expert in cardiac exercise prescription and pro-

gression. For long-term follow-up, the doctor should be knowledgeable regarding the basic cardiac prudent dietary concepts and the role of the dietitian; be knowledgeable about vocational assessment, impairment, and disability evaluation; be familiar with team approach; and have a working knowledge of advanced life support.

A hospital stay for acute coronary syndrome is now shortened to 3 to 5 days, and even less for uncomplicated cases. The shorter stay has added the problems of diminished time for counseling in general, and specifically for risk-factor reduction and exercise training. In the past, the program was divided into various phases, which included phase I (acute in-hospital phase beginning with intensive cardiac care unit), phase II (convalescent phase, continuation of the program at home), phase III (training phase using aerobic conditioning to increase the patient's physical work capacity), and phase IV (maintenance phase). In contrast, the recent recommendation from the task force for cardiac rehab has divided the program in two phases: inpatient or hospital phase and outpatient phase (73,74).

Inpatient or Hospital Phase

Table 83-11 summarizes a sample CR clinical pathway used for the inpatient hospital stay. The program is initiated by per-

TABLE 83-10. Absolute Risk of Hard CAD Events/10 Years (CAD Death, MI, Unstable Angina)*

Risk Points	1	2	3	4	5	6	7	8	9	10	11	12	13	14	15	16	17
Men	2	3	4	5	6	7	9	13	16	20	25	30	35	45			
Women	1	2	2	2	2	2	3	3	3	4	7	8	11	13	15	18	20

*A symposium held in conjunction with the Primary Medicine Today–PM–Med Midwest 2002 Meeting, Sponsored by The Johns Hopkins University School of Medicine, Baltimore, Maryland.
Courtesy of Dr. Steven P. Schulman.

**TABLE 83-11.   Sample Rehabilitation Services in Clinical Pathway;
Uncomplicated Myocardia Infarction Average Length of Stay = Five Days***

	Day 1	Day 2	Day 3	Day 4
Consults		Cardiac rehabilitation to assess		
Activity	Bedrest until stable; then OOB in chair; bedside commode	routine CCU activities; sitting warm-ups; walk in room	Up in room; standing warm-ups; walk 5–10 minutes in hall 2–3 times/day (supervision as needed)	Up in room; standing warm-ups; walk 5–10 minutes in hall 3–4 times/day; walk down flight of stairs with supervision
Education	Orient to ER, CCU; explain tests, answer questions	Basic explanation of event and treatment plan	Assess readiness to learn; when ready, teach survival lesson #1 = signs/symptoms recognition, NTG use, emergency plan	Assess readiness to learn; when ready, teach survival lesson = safety factors, do's & don'ts for home
Discharge Planning				

*Documentation of activity and education must be provided for each day.
Reprinted with permission from Williams MA. *Guidelines for cardiac rehabilitation and secondary prevention programs*, 3rd ed. Champaign, IL: American Association of Cardiovascular and Pulmonary Rehabilitation, 1999;28.

forming low-level activities (i.e., 1–2 METs) and gradually increasing the workload as tolerated. It should be supervised for appropriateness and safety. The program primarily involves self-feeding, bathing, use of a bedside commode, sitting at the bedside, and exercises to maintain muscle tone and joint mobility. During this time, monitoring is performed on the ECG, and the patient is questioned regarding symptoms such as chest pain, dyspnea, and palpitations. Gradually, the MET levels are increased to 2 or 3, increased sitting time in the chair is required, and rhythmic repetitive movements of the arms and legs are performed. Walking time and distance are also increased. At discharge, plans are made for the patient to be followed in an outpatient exercise program.

Outpatient or Ambulatory Phase

The elements of CR for the outpatient phase are illustrated in Table 83-12. About 70% of survivors of MI are younger than 70 years of age. The patient with a low-risk coronary event usually progresses rapidly with increase in intensity and duration of exercises. The patient can continue CR without supervision. Coronary patients who are elderly and those with significant morbidity, myocardial ischemia, HF, complication of MI or CABG surgery, or severe angina may require exercise supervision of variable duration.

The basic principles of exercise prescription include emphasis on an appropriate level of frequency, intensity, duration, mode, and progression. Exercise should be done on a regular basis and supervised to ensure safety. This may include ECG monitoring when appropriate. The stimulus phase of exercise usually involves large muscle group activities performed at least three times a week. Each session lasts about 15 to 30 minutes, preceded by a warm-up and followed by a cool-down period. The intensity of exercise is designated by exercise prescription, with moderate intensive activity equaling approximately 40% to 60% of $\dot{V}O_{2max}$. This is effective for increasing both submaximal and maximal endurance. The goal of the exercise intensity is to go up to 80% to 95% of $\dot{V}O_{2max}$. It is associated with low incidence of sudden cardiac arrest. For the warm-up period, flexibility exercises, such as properly selected stretching, may be useful. Flexibility activities should focus on improvement of joint range of motion. Particular attention should be focused on the lower back and posterior thigh region in an attempt to reduce the development of low back pain (26). Walking or running, bicycling, stair stepping, or cross-country skiing and swimming are good examples of dynamic aerobic exercises. A useful approach to the activity prescription is to identify the desired rating of perceived exertion as discussed earlier (Borg scale). The influence of risk-factor reduction for resistive exercises is less than that of traditional aerobic exercises. The increase in strength and potential for increase in

TABLE 83-12.   Elements of Cardiac Rehabilitation

Inpatient	Outpatient			
Identification of Patient	Evaluation	Prescribed Exercise	Modification of Risk Factors	Specification of Long-Term Goals
Smoking cessation and prevention of relapse	Medical history	Aerobic training (high caloric or interval)	Education	Physical
Initial assessment of physical activity	Assessment of risk factors	Resistance training	Nutritional counseling	Vocational
Outpatient referral	Exercise stress test	On-site or at-home exercise program	Exercise	Psychological
	Vocational counseling		Medication	Clinical

Reprinted with permission from Ades PA. Medical progress. *N Engl J Med* 2001;345(12):898.

muscle mass with resistive exercises may improve an individual's physical ability. Particularly in older individuals, resistance exercises may improve the ability to perform ADLs.

The duration of the ambulatory phase varies according to the patient's needs but it is usually about 4 to 6 weeks. After graduating from a supervised program, the patient usually enrolls in a maintenance program and attends usually two to three times per week. The goal is primarily a supervised group session to enhance the educational process, to ensure participant tolerance to the program, to confirm that progress is occurring, and to make appropriate changes in the exercise prescription.

A 1995 report on CR from the medical association of cardiovascular and pulmonary rehabilitation and National Institutes of Health (75) points out that the safety and effectiveness of unsupervised CR exercise must be determined for various populations of CVD patients. The economic constraints and logistics often limit the availability of supervised training. Suggestions were made that patients should have a monitored program if they:

- Have severely depressed left ventricular function, less than 25% of EF
- Have severe or complicated MI
- Have ischemia or ECG changes during exercise program
- Have angina and angina equivalent
- Have arrhythmia during cardiac exercise recovery
- Are less than 6 months post-MI, angioplasty, or heart surgery, especially if they had a complicated hospital course; are deconditioned and will exercise at a high intensity
- Require monitoring of more than HR or are unable to count their own HR
- Have other significant conditions, i.e., diabetes, stroke, amputee, etc.
- Need the services of other CR disciplines

Patients who have completed the monitored program would probably be best off remaining in a supervised setting if they continue to be symptomatic on exertion or if the exercise ECG shows significant arrhythmia. Those without such complications can be enrolled in an exercise program near their work or at home, or at YMCA, etc.

SPECIAL SITUATIONS

Heart Transplantation

There is no evidence of any adverse effect of supervised exercise training in the heart transplant patient. CR has been found to be beneficial with respect to an effective increase in aerobic capacity, a peripheral training effect, and muscular strengthening (76).

There are two types of cardiac transplantations. One is an orthotopic transplantation. The patient receives a new heart and thus is functioning with a denervated heart. The other is a heterotropic transplantation, whereby the diseased heart is not removed and the new heart is implanted in the chest parallel to the original one.

The impaired chronotropic response of the denervated allograft is manifested by high-resting HR, decreased HR reserve, a slower increase in HR at the start of exercise, a diminished maximum HR or peak HR, and a prolonged gradual return of HR to preexercise level after cessation of exercises (76). The allograft is dependent on elevated levels of circulating catecholamines to increase stroke volume and HR during exercise. Biochemical and physiologic evidence of reinervation following human cardiac transplantation is mounting, but such reinervation usually is clinically insignificant. In addition to chronotropic incompetence of diastolic dysfunction, a peripheral abnormality in oxygen utilization and transportation has been reported (77). The left ventricular EF, CO, oxygen uptake, and aerobic thresholds are also lower. Patients who have waited for a heart transplant have shown decreased oxidative enzymatic activity and type I fiber and capillary density in their muscles (78).

The initiation of supervised CR will vary according to the preoperative clinical status and postoperative course of the patient. Because of the abnormal exercise physiology of the cardiac transplant patient, modification of the standard exercise prescription needs to be done.

The HR and blood pressure responses in these patients are often blunted during the initial phase of exercise. An exercise test protocol should be selected that provides a slow increase in workload intensity to allow time for the denervated heart to respond to circulating catecholamines. The THR is problematic because of the denervation and diminished HRR of the denervated heart. Many authorities have therefore recommended use of the Borg rating of perceived exertion. When the rating of perceived exertion is used, an initial target of 11 to 13 is appropriate for those disabled by chronic HF or postoperative recovery. Ideally, the rating of perceived exertion that matches a maximum 60% to 70% of peak oxygen consumption can be used as the end point. However, individuals may vary considerably in the percentage of maximum HR or peak oxygen consumption, and some have suggested that exercise training be predicated on a fixed-distance, fixed-speed prescription that is fine-tuned by the perceived exertion rating. The exercise prescription should advance as the patient's peak oxygen consumption improves with training. In the immediate postoperative phase, one can start with active and passive range-of-motion exercises. Usually the training can start 2 to 6 weeks after surgery and should continue for at least 6 to 8 weeks.

The technique of cardiac transplantation has improved over the last decade, and the number of patients receiving a transplant has increased. The 5- and 10-year survival rates are now 82% and 74% respectively. The transplant itself usually resolves the cardiac disability, but the patient may also have significant musculoskeletal and neurologic symptoms, including weakness, fatigue, low back pain, side effects from antirejection drugs, and psychological needs (i.e., anxiety, depression), that may complicate the recovery process. CR can be really useful in helping to alleviate these problems and help the patient adjust to the disability.

Heart Failure

It is estimated that 4.7 million Americans have HF, with roughly 550,000 new cases diagnosed every year. The total hospital admissions and discharges due to HF have increased from 377,000 in 1979 to 978,000 in 1998. In 1997, 3.7 billion dollars ($5,501 per discharge) were paid on behalf of the Medicare beneficiary for congestive heart failure (CHF) (79). HF is simply the inability of the heart to pump sufficient blood to meet the demand of the body. It is a complex syndrome of interaction among neuroendocrine, genetic, biodynamic, and molecular systems. CHF can be thought of as a state of neurohormonal imbalance in which the activity of potentially harmful pathways outweighs that of favorable ones. It involves myocardial injury resulting from ischemia, toxin, volume and/or pressure load, or a genetic imperfection. Remodeling involves myocyte hypertrophy, interstitial fibrosis, myocyte dropout, and changes in genetic expression of cardiac-related proteins (80). CHF is essentially a cardiocirculatory syndrome in which the tone of peripheral blood vessels modulates the cardiac function. For example, immediately after MI, the noninfarcted myocardium undergoes progressive eccentric hypertrophy for months and years while the infarcted area thins and bulges. Although the hypertrophy has a beneficial compensatory effect, the heart outgrows its energy supply. The genetic changes within the hypertrophic myocyte results in calcium overload, leading to systolic and diastolic dysfunction. The majority of the cardiac cells are nonmyocytes, i.e., fibroblasts. They release growth factors and other agents that influence the myocytes' growth and function. The extracellular matrix increases dynamically along with the interstitial fibrosis, causing the contractile abnormality and diastolic stiffness said to be the major component in remodeling. This involves neurohormonal modulation, and it is believed that it may become more important in the future for understanding the pathophysiology of CHF. For example, angiotensin II causes vasoconstriction, promotes salt and water retention, stimulates argenine vasopressin leading to further water retention and increased vasoconstriction. It also has an effect on sympathetic nerve that promotes release of norepinephrine and other neurotransmitters which stimulate and/or remodel through direct effect the blood vessel walls causing endothelial dysfunction, formation of foam cells and plaques, accumulation of extracellular matrix, release of plasminogen activator inhibitor I, thus leading to a thrombus within vessel walls.

The atrial natriuretic peptides (ANP) and the brain natriuretic peptides (BNP) are the circulatory peptides produced principally by atria and ventricles, respectively. Both peptides increase sodium and water extraction, suppress renin and aldosterone secretion, and lead to venous and arterial dilatation. It may also favorably influence autonomic function and have a direct and indirect antimitotic effect in the heart and blood vessels. Diffuse ANP and BNP have a beneficial hemodynamic, neurohormonal, and renal action in patients with HF. ANP and BNP are metabolized by neural endopeptidase.

Endothelin-I is a major endothelial isopeptide produced in human cardiovascular system and kidney. It is 10 times more potent a vasoconstrictor than angiotensin II in human arteries and has a myocardial, renal, and growth effect similar to angiotensin II. Arginine vasopressin is a powerful vasoconstrictor and a potent antidiuretic agent. Arginine vasopressin acts via V1 receptor, found on the blood vessels and myocardium, and V2 receptor, responsible for the action of peptide on water reabsorption in the renal tubules. There are various new medications being developed to change the deleterious effect of the neurohormonal mechanism and augment the effect of favorable ones. Compelling evidence has been provided that the pharmacologic modulation of hormonal systems has led to improved morbidity and mortality in HF (81).

There is a growing clinical consensus that exercise training may beneficially alter the clinical course of HF. Even though the specific mechanisms responsible for exercise-induced benefit are not clear, there are suggestions that regular endurance exercise reduces the central sympathetic tone, increases parasympathetic activity, decreases plasma rennin activity, improves baroreflex sensitivity, and may indirectly modulate the neurohormonal mechanism described earlier (82).

Surprisingly, the functional capacity of some HF patients may have no relationship to the resting left ventricle ejection. Some HF patients may achieve physical work capacity similar to subjects with normal resting EFs. This helps to confirm the notion that a decreased reduction in EF is not a contraindication to CR. The major effect of exercise in HF is a peripheral "training effect," but there is some controversy regarding a central effect. The peripheral exercise effect produces a positive improvement in the tone and condition of the peripheral vasculature in CHF patients. Exercise activity is now recommended as a component of a comprehensive approach to the patient with HF (83).

The preferred protocol for cardiovascular exercise testing for CHF patients is a modified ramp protocol of progressive exercise load of 0.2 to 0.4 METs per 30-second stage. Patients with poor exercise tolerance should be tested with a continuous protocol that does not exceed 1 to 2 METs per 3-minute stage. Those patients who are unable to do this exercise protocol may need to be tested by other modalities, as mentioned previously. Exercise assessment, such as the 6-minute walk test, is useful in assessing exercise tolerance and monitoring progress during the therapy.

In HF patients, there is an inconsistency of monitoring the exercise parameters, including HR, blood pressure, and perceived exertion. Unstable angina, decompensated CHF, and complicated arrhythmias are contraindications for CR. During exercise, if there is an increase in symptoms associated with CHF, including dyspnea, weakness, and abnormal blood pressure responses, particularly hypotension with signs and symptoms of exertional intolerance, the exercise should be terminated.

In HF, dynamic exercises are preferable to an isometric one because of the high probability of complications, including sudden death. The patient with HF should have a supervised and monitored exercise program until the patient is able to self-monitor after having had no major complications noted during the supervised period. One should also monitor medication compliance, blood pressure, and HR response to exercise.

A number of studies have shown that patients with CHF who have undergone CR have increased oxygen transport, peak oxygen consumption, increased ventilatory aerobic threshold, peak CO, improved physical work capacity, submaximal exercise tolerance, skeletal muscle aerobic enzyme activity, muscle strength and endurance, parasympathetic nervous system activity, and respiratory muscle function (84). In aggregate, this can make a difference between dependence and independence. This is an important topic to the physiatrist who is involved in CR, as the number of CHF patients, particularly those with comorbidity, is increasing in rehabilitation units (85–89).

Cardiac Rehabilitation Following Coronary Artery Bypass Graft

The principles of CR for patients who have undergone heart surgery such as CABG and valve replacement are essentially the same as for MI. The major goals in this situation are to control coronary risk factors and improve total well-being of the patient.

Patients who have undergone CAGB have the advantage of increased ischemic threshold, improved left ventricle function, and improved coronary flow, all leading to improved cardiac and functional capacity. Because of this, CABG patients usually start the CR program earlier than MI patients. The extent of healing of the surgical incision from CABG can be the most limiting factor for exercise. A sternotomy usually requires 4 to 6 weeks for healing, but low-level activities are usually acceptable 24 to 48 hours after surgery. Upper-body exercises that cause sternal tension should be avoided for as long as 3 months after the surgery (27). The CABG patient can also exercise and ambulate at a slightly higher level of intensity and duration than the MI patient. CABG patients can perform upper-extremity range-of-motion exercises unless one hears a clicking sound (occurs in 5% of the patients), as this suggests possible sternal instability. In such a situation, one should avoid upper-extremity exercise. In the postoperative period, CABG patients tend to have tachycardia and increased fatigue secondary to hypovolemia and decreased hemoglobin after surgery.

The length of stay for the CABG patient has decreased to less than a week, and mobilization starts on postoperative day one. This includes sitting, active range-of-motion exercises, and transferring. This prevents further deconditioning, limits the possibility of deep vein thrombosis, and decreases potential pulmonary complications. The patient is encouraged to gradually increase ambulation from 200 to 300 feet as tolerated. Monitoring with ECG telemetry is usually done during the early part of the mobilization. The patient is then taught self-monitoring during a home exercise program and gradually returns to his or her previous level of activity.

A symptom-limited ETT can be performed 3 to 4 weeks after the surgery to determine the level of exercise capacity. Depending on the exercise tolerance, one can establish a low-, moderate-, or high-intensity program. A low-intensity program usually involves 2 to 4 METs of activity and a THR that is usually of 65% to 75% of the HR_{max}. A moderate-intensity program is 3 to 6.5 METs with a THR of 70% to 80% of HR_{max}, and a high-intensity program is about 5 to 8.5 METs with a THR of about 75% to 85% of HR_{max}.

For patients on various medications (including β–blockers) or those who are unable to participate in an ETT, a THR of 20 beats above the resting HR can be set. In short, the program has to be individualized depending on the clinical status of the patient.

Cardiac Rehabilitation in Women

CVD remains the leading cause of death in women older than the age of 50 (50% for CVD versus 4% for breast cancer). CAD onset is 10 years later than in men. Women are more likely to present with angina rather than MI and are more likely to have HF and cardiac rupture than men. Angina is also less likely to improve after bypass and angioplasty. The operative mortality for women is 2.7 times higher than for men. After MI, women have a higher rate of morbidity, rehospitalization, and mortality from CHF even though they have a better average EF than men. Diabetes mellitus increases morbidity in women with CAD more than in men. The levels of HDL and triglyceride are better predictors of CAD risk in women. Hormone replacement therapy (HRT) is an ongoing controversy, as shown by results from the Post Menopausal/Progestin Intervention (PEPI) study (91), the Heart and Estrogen/Progestin Replacement (HERS) study (92), the ongoing Women's Health Initiative (WHI) study (93), and the Raloxifene Use for the Heart (RUTH) study (94). The ACC/AHA guidelines recommend that postmenopausal women taking HRT may continue with the hormonal treatment even during an acute coronary syndrome, but HRT should *not* be initiated for secondary prevention of coronary events. Although exercise training benefits men and women equally, women are referred less frequently to CR. In women, return to work is delayed, and depression, disability, and anxiety are reported more often. Women show better adherence to exercise programs and healthy lifestyle changes. ETTs are frequently false positive in women, so instead pharmacologic stress testing (i.e., dobutamine, dipyridamole, and stress echocardiography) are more reliable and used more often. Thallium scans have limited value because of overlying breast tissue.

TABLE 83-13. Indices of Body Weight and Composition

Body Mass Index* (kg/m²)	Men	Women
Ideal	21–25	21–25
Obese	≥27.8–30	≥27.3–30
Markedly Obese	>30–40	>30–40
Morbidly Obese	>40	>40
Waist-to-Hip Ratio**		
Ideal	<0.90	<0.80
At risk	>0.95	>0.85
% Body Fat***		
Ideal	12–18	18–25

*Body weight in kg divided by (height in meters)³
**Widest circumference measured at waist (level of umbilicus) divided by widest circumference measured at hips (mid-buttock level)
***Can be determined from skin caliper method, hydrostatic weighing, DEXA, or bio-impedance analysis
Reprinted with permission from Williams MA. *Guidelines for cardiac rehabilitation and secondary prevention programs*, 3rd ed. Champaign, IL: American Association of Cardiovascular and Pulmonary Rehabilitation, 1999;126.

Cardiac Rehabiliation in an Obese Patient

Reduction of weight is one of the key components of CR. Exercise training is an important contributor to weight loss, although the effect is variable (95). If the goal is to lose weight, the patient may need a higher level of exercise than what is usually prescribed. The patient needs a basic evaluation for various indices of body weight (Table 83-13) (96).

Most controlled exercise training studies have shown only moderate weight loss of approximately 2 to 3 kg in an exercise group, but with calorie restriction added to the exercise program, the average weight loss was about 8.5 kg, most of which was body fat. Diet alone results in less weight loss, about 5.1 kg (97). These data strongly support the role of both exercise and diet in a weight-loss program. Exercise principles for obese patients include low-impact exercises, such as brisk walking, that are performed at less intensity but increased frequency and duration.

Cardiac Rehabilitation in Percutaneous Coronary Intervention

There are no specific studies that have evaluated the safety of exercise training within days after percutaneous coronary intervention. It is recommended that the subject begin or resume exercise no sooner than 5 to 7 days after the procedure. This gives time for the catheterization sites to heal and remain stable. Exercise testing may be of considerable value in assessing new or different symptoms in the patient with incomplete revascularization.

Cardiac Rehabilitation in Patients with Peripheral Arterial Disease

Peripheral arterial disease (PAD) shares the traditional risk factors for arteriosclerosis and often coexists with CAD. It may also be symptomatic or clinically silent (98). The intermittent claudication rating scale can be used for evaluation and follow-up of the patient, as shown in Table 83-14. PAD and CAD often coexist, and CAD is usually the more limiting of the illnesses. It has been shown that aggressive risk-factor modification is

TABLE 83-14. Intermittent Claudication Rating Scale	
0	No claudication pain
1	Initial, minimal pain
2	Moderate, bothersome pain
3	Intense pain
4	Maximal pain, cannot continue

Adapted from American College of Sports Medicine. *Guidelines for graded exercise testing and prescription,* 5th ed. Baltimore: Williams & Wilkins, 1995 and American Association of Cardiovascular and Pulmonary Rehabilitation, *Guidelines for cardiac rehabilitation program,* 2nd ed. Champaign, IL: Human Kinetics, 1994;64.

needed not only to slow the pace of PAD, but also to reduce cardiovascular events.

Patients with PAD may not complete the standard ETT because of claudication and limited endurance. In these patients, screening by pharmacologic stress testing or angiography is advisable to rule out any silent CAD.

The initial therapeutic intervention for most patients with claudication is a walking program. Thirty to 45 minutes of walking performed 4 or more days weekly has been reported to increase walking distance by 200% or more (99). The mode of exercise may need to be altered to limit the likelihood that the claudication might prevent a peripheral training effect.

The results of most of the studies done on patients with PAD are small and often are nonrandomized and difficult to interpret. A recent metaanalysis of such studies included only 112 patients and concluded that an increase in pain-free walking distance at the end of the exercise program was 140 meters with an increase in total walking distance of 180 meters (100). Thus, although exercise programs are safe and improve physical conditioning, secondary prevention measures are more important, and the magnitude of the treatment effect cannot be defined.

Cardiac Rehabilitation in Diabetes Mellitus

Diabetes mellitus is a major risk factor for the development of CHD and bodes ill for patients with CVD. The mechanisms by which diabetes mellitus adversely affects the prognosis for CHD are diverse. They may include factors such as more rapid progression of CHD, a decreased vasodilatory reserve of coronary arteries, endothelial dysfunction, hypercoagulable state, possible abnormal metabolism, myocardial substrate, and increased multivessel coronary disease. In diabetes mellitus, low exercise capacity independently predicts mortality and acute medical admission for cardiac complications, especially HF, angina, acute MI, or cardiac arrhythmia. Aerobic exercise training has been shown to increase insulin sensitivity in both obese hyperinsulinemic and nonobese patients. The exact mechanism is not known, but it is suggested that it increases the number of insulin receptors and also increases insulin receptor binding (101).

The major benefit of CR is weight loss and a decrease in the atherogenic tendencies of insulin resistance. There are several factors to be considered in CR for diabetic patients.

- *Glucose control:* Adrenergic response to exercise can exacerbate hyperglycemia, and conversely, the patient treated with insulin or oral hypoglycemic medications can experience hypoglycemia during or after exercise. Monitoring of the blood sugar before and after the exercise training is important.

Simple means to address the changes in hyperglycemia or hypoglycemia should be available to the physician and should include 4 to 5 grams of oral glucose tablets, a glucagon injection kit, and blood glucose testing instrumentation. A patient should not proceed or continue to exercise if there is poor glycemic control (i.e., blood sugar exceeding 300 mg/dL and/or ketonuria) (101,102).

- *Autonomic neuropathy:* Exercise training in patients with autonomic neuropathy should be conducted to minimize the adverse consequences of orthostatic hypotension, silent ischemia, and arrhythmia. Patients should be adequately hydrated before exercise and should avoid exercise after a meal or during the morning when the orthostatic hypotension is more likely. They should also adjust their antihypertensive medication and the environmental temperature. They should use compressive stockings, and the exercise should be done in a supervised environment. The target for exercise should be predicted on perceived exertion rather than HR in the patient with autonomic neuropathy because of decreased HR_{max} capacity and resting tachycardia. A moderate level of perceived exertion should be sought over 2 to 4 weeks of gradual training (103).
- *Somatic neuropathy:* This puts the patient at a higher risk for injury because of decreased sensation. The patient should be taught about proper foot care and proper fitting of shoes. Non–weight-bearing exercise, such as swimming, bicycling, rowing, or armchair calisthenics, may be appropriate for patients with a concomitant lower-extremity disorder, such as a Charcot joint or severe neuropathy.
- *Proliferative-nonproliferative retinopathy:* The exact details regarding exercise are not available, but many authors have suggested limiting the diabetic patient with severe nonproliferative neuropathy in a similar fashion to those with proliferative disease (101).

Cardiac Rehabilitation in Patients with End-Stage Renal Disease

The effects of exercise in patients with end-stage renal disease (ESRD) have been studied for patients both with and without concomitant CAD. A small study of dialysis patients free of obvious CAD suggested that an interdialysis exercise program improved quality of life, blood pressure, and some measures of metabolic function (104). CAD is the leading cause of morbidity and mortality in the patient with ESRD. The safety of CR in patients with ESRD and with a recent acute coronary event has not been established. Limited data suggest that there is a potential for hemodynamic compromise with exercise in a patient with ESRD. In a 1-month multicenter study of chronic hemodialysis patients, 76% manifested ventricular arrhythmia, 69% demonstrated supraventricular arrhythmia on 48-hour ambulatory monitoring, and 39% manifested multiple episodes of complex ventricular ectopy (105). The frequency of ventricular arrhythmia increased significantly during the second hour of dialysis and lasted up to 5 hours after dialysis. There is both a higher incidence of ischemia during exercise training and a higher incidence of silent ischemia in a patient with ESRD. This makes a supervised and monitored exercise program prudent for these patients. The benefit of exercise training in ESRD after a major coronary event is similar to that found for the cardiac population at large. Many patients with ESRD have reduced exercise capacity as a result of age, malnutrition, comorbidity, deconditioning, immobility, and advanced CVD. The exercise target rate of 50% to 70% of that achieved on a screening maximum exercise test showed improvement in exercise capacity and symptoms. Again, because of the relatively high likelihood of a cardiac event, it is prudent to schedule exercise training in a supervised and monitored environment.

Cardiac Rehabilitation in Pulmonary Disease

The general principles of CR are applicable to the patient with severe chronic obstructive pulmonary disease (COPD). These patients need to have exercise testing performed with oxygen and need a monitored supervised program because they are in a high-risk group. These patients will often show less improvement in their peak VO_2 with CR compared with non-COPD cardiac patients (106).

Cardiac Rehabilitation in Elderly Patients

Older adults (more than 85 years of age) are the fastest growing group of elderly, and approximately half of this entire group has some CVD. The population of people aged 65 years and older in the United States is increasing at a growth rate twice that of the total population (107,108).

In the elderly, maximal end diastolic volume increases, whereas HR_{max}, left ventricle EF, CO, and aerobic capacity are all lower than in the younger individual. There is an 8% to 10% decline in maximum oxygen consumption per year in the non-trained elderly population. They also show a reduced HR_{max} of 1 beat per minute per year of age, a moderate rapid increase in systolic blood pressure with exercise, and an attenuated elevation of left ventricle EF with exercise. Ischemia often cannot be reliably detected in the elderly because of the frequent absence of chest pain. In addition, dyspnea may be related to an underlying pulmonary disorder rather than an anginal equivalent. There is an increased potential for exercise related myocardial ischemia and arrhythmia in this age group and an overall increased risk for adverse events. There is a gradual decline in physiologic function, with accelerated decline in cardiovascular function and muscle strength that is due to deconditioning from a decrease in physical activity (104). By maintaining a physically active lifestyle, the decline can be blunted by about 25%. Sedentary older persons can increase their aerobic work capacity and muscle strength with exercise training, but older persons show a lesser degree of improvement when they begin their physical conditioning at an older age as compared with the young.

An elderly person's ability to function independently is a critical factor. Overall, exercise training should be done to enhance health-related fitness while simultaneously striving for reduced risk for various chronic diseases and improve overall quality of life. Considerable evidence shows that both endurance- and resistance-type exercise can significantly improve functional capacity and provide assistance for functional independence and overall well being (27).

Psychosocial limitations for participation in CR are important issues in the elderly. ETT should be done to evaluate functional capacity in this age group before prescription of exercises. An exercise test may not be required in an older, apparently healthy person desiring to participate in a low- to moderate-intensity activity such as walking.

Exercise prescription guidelines in the elderly need to be modified with respect to intensity, frequency, duration, and mode of exercise compared with younger individuals. Exercise capacity of the elderly, both before and after exercise training, is usually lower than in the younger person. In addition, the elderly generally have musculoskeletal limitations, particularly as a result of arthritis and deconditioning of specific muscle groups. It is important to recommend activities that require low levels of energy expenditure (around 40% to 50% of VO_{2max}),

particularly during the first weeks of a program. It is often best to prescribe mild increases at the time of program progression. In general, the elderly are encouraged to increase the frequency of exercise but maintain a short duration. There is an increased potential for musculoskeletal injury with high-intensity exercises.

Many of the elderly may not be able to perform the continuous protocol treadmill test and may therefore be forced to use a discontinuous protocol. Alternatively, they can be tested on a cycle ergometer. ECG telemetric monitoring of a patient while walking at his or her own pace for 6 to 12 minutes, or to the level of tolerance, may be sufficient as a preexercise stress test for deconditioned elderly. A 600-foot walk (three times back and forth in a 100-foot hospital corridor) raises a person's HR to the target heart zone for exercise training as determined from a treadmill stress test on the same patient. The principles for exercise prescription in the elderly are the same as for other cardiac patients. Particularly important for the elderly are the limbering exercises that increase joint flexibility and improve agility. They may need to rely on the upper extremities to maintain independence for locomotion by use of an ambulatory aid. A combination of endurance and low-level resistance exercise is suitable for the elderly. Because of reduced cardiac reserve and decreased ability to sweat efficiently, there is a need for a rest period during physical activity. Exercise and other moderate work should be avoided during hot, humid weather. Education of the elderly regarding compliance with exercises and medication should be emphasized.

Some elderly patients also have a pacemaker and/or cardioverter defibrillator. In these patients, exercise principles are the same as for other CR patients. The exercise target rate ranges for the patient with an implanted cardioverter defibrillator should be set at 20 to 30 beats per minute below the threshold rate of the device.

Cardiac Rehabilitation for the Physically Disabled

Many patients seen in both inpatient and outpatient physiatric settings have CVD comorbidity. Because many of the patients also have concomitant musculoskeletal problems, this can be quite challenging.

It may not always be feasible to conduct a peak or symptom-limited exercise test in this group of patients. Alternatively, a symptom-related rating scale could be used. These include the perceived exertion scale of Borg and a scale for angina, dyspnea, or claudication. A dipyridamole thallium stress test could be helpful in determining the integrity of coronary circulation before the beginning of a rehabilitation program (109). One can also use the RPP (HR × systolic pressure) or simply check the HR_{rest} and not allow it to go beyond 20 beats from the baseline with exercise. Oxymetry may be used to supplement this evaluation.

The two most common physical disabilities associated with CVD are stroke and lower-extremity dysvascular amputation. Patients with these conditions are often quite anxious at the start of a program. This tends to adversely affect their cardiac capacity. Furthermore, some patients who appear medically stable may decompensate when they perform a high level of physical activity. Monitoring the patient's initial performance by ECG telemetry may be very useful in guiding therapy. If ECG telemetry is not available, simple ECG monitoring is usually acceptable.

Stroke patients often have CVD and PAD. Functional impairments in this disabled group include those that are due to paresis, paralysis, spasticity, and sensory perceptual dysfunction (110). Aerobic exercise training in the disabled stroke patient is safe (111,112) and reduces the energy expenditure and cardiac demands of a designated activity (113). These patients may perform a variety of aerobic activities, and stationary arm-leg cycle ergometry may be used. Activities should be modified to satisfy the needs of the individual. Limited data suggests that left ventricular EF improves after upper-extremity training. A reduction of risk for stroke later in life has been documented to be due to exercise patterns in early years (114,115). A trained hemiplegic patient who ambulates with or without a lower-extremity orthosis walks at a speed that is 40% to 45% slower than the normal individual, yet the energy cost of ambulation is 50% to 65% higher. Monitoring of the patient during training to negotiate stairs, use ambulatory aids, establish wheelchair activities, and perform upper-extremity strengthening exercises is useful. Monitoring may convince the patient that physical rehabilitation training is feasible and will improve the patient's psychological comfort.

The reduced exercise capacity of patients with spinal cord injury is multifactorial. These factors include loss of muscle pump action causing decreased venous return, muscle weakness or atrophy, altered respiratory system function, small cardiac chamber size, greater use of type II overType I muscle fibers, sedentary lifestyle, impaired autonomic nervous system, impaired neurosystem control, and altered hormonal effects. There is also potential secondary comorbidity in the form of infection, skin breakdown, etc. Wheelchair propulsion, arm ergometry, wheelchair cycling using arm cranks, and hybrid exercises involving arm ergometry combined with lower-extremity functional electrical stimulation can be used as modes of aerobic exercise for spinal cord injury patients.

In cardiac amputee patients, before starting preprosthetic ambulation training, the cardiac capacity to walk on only one extremity can be assessed by upper-extremity ergometry. By knowing the weight of the individual, one can test the patient at a specific work stage. For example, for a 50- to 70-kg person, one can test the patient to more than 150 kpm, 3.5 METs; the 70- to 81-kg person to 225 kpm, 4 to 5 METs; the 80- to 120-kg person to 300 kpm, 5 METs. Prosthetic ambulation even in a trained individual is a high-energy-cost physical activity. The energy cost of amputee ambulation is tabulated in Table 83-15.

Compared with the average energy cost of normal ambulation at 3 METs, prosthetic ambulation requires a 9% to 28% increase for the unilateral below-knee amputee, a 40% to 65% increase for the unilateral above-knee amputee, a 125% increase for the hemipelvectomy patient, and a whopping 280% increase for the bilateral above-knee amputee. Knowing the New York Heart Association functional computation classification,

one can estimate the cardiac functional capacity and the patient's ability to ambulate with a prosthesis by referring to Table 83-16.

Except for some unilateral below-knee amputees, class III patients usually function at a wheelchair level. Class II patients, except bilateral above-knee amputees, may have the capacity to walk with a prosthesis. Monitoring can be a way to convince the patient with lower-extremity amputation that it is safe to proceed with prosthesis training or that prosthetic training is contraindicated and that functioning at the wheelchair level is consistent with a person's cardiac capacity.

PSYCHOLOGICAL ASPECTS OF CARDIAC REHABILITATION

Many patients with successful physical recovery following MI or cardiac surgery have residual psychological impairments. Emotional stress increases blood pressure and serum lipids, decreases endothelial dependent vasodilatation, and causes paradoxical coronary artery constriction (116). The concept of the type A personality and the relationship to CVD remains controversial, although the hostility component of type A behavior is regarded as the most adverse feature for CVD. High levels of anger and hostility are associated with increased cardiac morbidity and mortality (117). Major psychological problems with CVD patients are denial, anxiety, depression, dependence, and unrecognized cognitive dysfunction. Denial of presenting symptoms may limit or delay access to care and affect outcomes adversely. Anxiety, which is often the initial psychological manifestation during hospitalization, is related to the fear of dying and fears for the future. During this time, the patient may contemplate their potential inability to resume former family, occupational, and community roles. This may lead to depression.

Anxiety and depression are the most common psychological complications of MI and contribute to the failure to make satisfactory life adjustments, return to work, resume sexual function, and engage in social activities after discharge. Depression is associated with increased mortality and morbidity after a cardiac event and is present in 30% to 50% of MI patients. Patients with depression are five times more likely to die during the initial 6 months following MI than nondepressed patients (118). A major problem with depression is the frequent occurrence of social isolation, which may serve as an independent risk factor. Six-month mortality of patients living alone is double that of patients who live with others. Follow-up studies of patients with angiographically documented coronary disease showed a 50% mortality rate among those more socially isolated compared with 17% among those living with others.

Education, counseling, and initiation of physical activity appear to help limit this psychological problem (119). However, many patients remain psychologically disabled because they inappropriately perceive an excess severity of their disability and vulnerability to death. A resumption of physical activity provides reassurance and restores self-confidence. It has been shown that even with a low level of exercise in older and sicker coronary patients, there is physical and psychological benefit. Peer support in a group program should be encouraged.

CR programs improve anxiety and depression in the short term, but proof of the long-term benefit is lacking, except for a few isolated studies (120). A practical approach includes vigorous measures to encourage patients to return to work because this provides reassurance, helps to focus attention away from health problems, and may address the concerns of low-income patients who have higher mortality after MI (121,122).

TABLE 83-15. Energy Cost of Amputee Ambulation[a]

	Increase (%)	MET
No prosthesis, with crutches	50	4.5
Unilateral BK with prosthesis	9–28	3.3–3.8
Unilateral AK with prosthesis	40–65	4.2–5.8
Bilateral BK with prosthesis	41–100	4.2–6.0
BK plus AK with prosthesis	75	5.3
Bilateral AK with prosthesis	280	11.4
Unilateral hip disarticulation with prosthesis	82	5.5
Hemipelvectomy with prosthesis	125	6.75
No prosthesis, with crutches	75	5.3

AK, above the knee; BK, below the knee amputation
[a]Based on percentage increase above cost of normal (3 METs)

TABLE 83-16. Correlation of the Energy Cost of Ambulation According to the Level of Amputation with the Estimated Work Capacity According to Cardiac Functional Class

Cardiac Class	MET	Amputee Ambulation	MET
Class IV	<2	—	—
Class III	<2 to <5	Wheelchair	2.0–3.0
		Unilateral BK with prosthesis	3.3–3.8
Class II	>5 to <7	No prosthesis with crutches	4.5
		Unilateral AK with prosthesis	4.2–5.0
		Bilateral AK with prosthesis	4.2–6.0
		BK plus AK with prostheses	5.3
		Hip disarticulation with prosthesis	5.5
		Hemipelvectomy with prosthesis	6.75
Class I	>7	Bilateral AK with prostheses	11.4

AK, above the knee; BK, below the knee amputation

Ideally, a CR program should also include psychological evaluation of the spouse or significant other. They should be screened for psychological stress, and those in distress should be offered intervention that focuses on assisting them to deal with specific stress related to their experience with their spouse's heart disease. Many instruments are available to evaluate psychological status, including the brief summary inventory, global severity index, heart disease hassle scale, coping strategy inventory, Miller intimacy scale, and McMaster Family Assessment Device.

CARDIAC REHABILITATION AND SEXUAL ACTIVITY

Resumption of sexual activity is one of the major concerns of the patient with MI or heart surgery. Of primary concern is whether they can resume sexual activity at least at the same level before the cardiac event. For men, anxiety about being able to perform as well as before the cardiac event may lead them to request sildenafil (Viagra). After MI, approximately one-fourth of patients report cessation of sexual activity, one-fourth of patients report no change in sexual activity, and half report a decreased amount of sexual activity.

The energy requirement for sexual intercourse between normal middle-aged couples is about 3 to 4 METs and at the point of orgasm is 4 to 5 METs. Patients can resume sexual activity if they can achieve a physical activity capacity of 5 METs or more. One way to test this level is to do standard ETT. Another way is to estimate patients physical capacity to perform various physical activities as shown in Figure 83-21. One of the most com-

monly used principles is exercise capacity to ascend and descend two flights of stairs (two-flight test) (123). It has been recommended that stair climbing be preceded by several minutes of rapid walking. Sexual activity between long-married couples normally does not incur HR above 117 beats per minute and may cause less ST depression or ischemia than other ADLs, such as watching an exciting sport on television, driving, or working at the office. Extramarital, clandestine sex preceded by heavy eating or drinking may place excessive demands on a damaged myocardium. This may lead to a declaration that a cardiac patient may return to lovemaking with his wife in 6 weeks and "with his mistress in 6 months."

In men, CVD can manifest as erectile dysfunction, which is defined as the persistent inability to attain and maintain penile erection sufficient to permit satisfactory sexual intercourse. It can have both psychogenic and organic causes (i.e., neurogenic, endocrinologic, and vasculogenic), or a mix of both. It is estimated that 10 to 12 million men in the United States have severe erectile dysfunction and another 10 million have partial erectile dysfunction. Most of them are older than 65 years of age. With normal aging, there are fewer spontaneous erections, more stimulation is needed, the firmness of erection decreases, and less forceful ejaculation occurs. There is also a longer refractory time. One potential advantage is that erections usually last longer.

Sexual dysfunction among women with CVD has been largely neglected in medicine. A study by Yaacov Drory suggested that the impact of the first acute MI on the frequency and satisfaction with sexual activity did not significantly differ between men and women (124). Both women and men reported a statistically significant decrease in frequency and satisfaction with sexual activity after MI. There are changes in sexuality in aging women. It takes longer to lubricate, and there is less lubrication. The vaginal tissue tends to be more sensitive because of atrophic changes. Physiological changes are less intense. Specifically, there is a decreased intensity of muscle spasm associated with orgasm; however, the orgasm may be psychologically as intense as when the woman was younger.

Patients usually can return to sexual activity by 12 weeks, but more than 50% return to these activities within 3 weeks of an acute MI (125). Drory (126) found that recovered cardiac patients who did not have ischemia on exercise stress testing had no ischemia during intercourse. Patients with a positive stress test might have high chances of ischemia or an increase in HR during sexual activity. The latter group deserves counseling and may require additional medications and cardiac monitor-

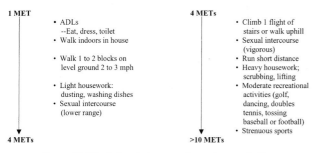

1 MET

- ADLs
  - -Eat, dress, toilet
- Walk indoors in house

- Walk 1 to 2 blocks on level ground 2 to 3 mph

- Light housework: dusting, washing dishes
- Sexual intercourse (lower range)

4 METs

4 METs

- Climb 1 flight of stairs or walk uphill
- Sexual intercourse (vigorous)
- Run short distance
- Heavy housework; scrubbing, lifting
- Moderate recreational activities (golf, dancing, doubles tennis, tossing baseball or football)
- Strenuous sports

>10 METs

Figure 83-21. Estimated energy for various activities.

TABLE 83-17.   Risk of Myocardial Infarction Triggered by Sexual Activity

- Analysis of 1,774 MI survivors
    858 were sexually active; 27 had sex within 2 hours of MI
- Risk of acute MI triggered by sexual activity increased by
    2.5x for all patients
    2.1x for patients with prior angina
    2.9x for patients with prior MI
- Baseline risk for MI is approximately 1 per million per hour (Framingham)

Muller JE, et al. *JAMA* 1996;275:1405–1409.

ing. In one study, the percentage (10 of 88 patients) of ectopic activity during intercourse was the same as in daily activities (127).

The components of cardiac and sexual rehabilitation include exercise, dietary counseling, smoking cessation, weight management, and psychological support. Resumption of sexual activity is often recommended to occur about 3 to 6 weeks after stabilization. Monitoring medications for side effects is done, and counseling for distressed couples is offered. A graded exercise tolerance test may be added to help boost self-confidence, reduce the patient's and the partner's fears, encourage communication and sensuality, and caution particularly if symptoms reoccur, i.e., coital angina, intense prolonged fatigue or prolong palpitation, or dizziness after sexual activity.

In a sense, the patient has not only suffered an MI, but also an "ego infarction." This is particularly true in men and needs to be addressed at length. Dr. Muller and associates (128) studied whether sexual activity can actually trigger a coronary event. Their conclusion came from a survey of more than 1,774 MI survivors, 850 of whom were sexually active, and 27 of whom had sex within 2 hours of suffering an MI. The risk of acute MI triggered by sexual activity is increased by 2.5 times for all patients, 2.1 times for patients with prior angina, and 2.9 times for patients with a prior MI. The baseline risk for MI is approximately 1 per 1,000,000 hours of sexual activity. Table 83-17 lists the risks of an acute MI triggered by sexual activity. It is suggested that regular exercise reduces or eliminates the risk of MI during or immediately after sexual activity.

No convincing data are available for any particular sexual position that appears to be more or less safe than any other. Few data are available about sex with unfamiliar partners or with nonspouse partners.

Sexual rehabilitation starts with the clinician treating the cardiac condition. The patient may have concerns that there is a disconnection with the partner that may not be reestablished. The patient should be educated, and fear should be minimized. The key principle for the patient is to relax and go slow in reestablishing a sexual relationship, with an emphasis on reestablishing a romantic relationship as well as physically intimate relationship. Foreplay is felt to be helpful. The patient should also be well rested before sexual activity, and food and drink should be avoided 1 to 3 hours before the sexual activity.

The clinician should pay close attention to medications, particularly antipsychotic, antidepressant, and antihypertensive medications that may act on neurotransmitter pathways and lead to sexual dysfunction. The AHA and ACC suggest caution when prescribing sildenafil for patients with active ischemia or HF, or with borderline low blood pressure or blood volume (129). Similar caution is recommended for patients receiving complicated multidrug regimens or antihypertensive medications, patients with liver or kidney disease, and patients receiving drugs metabolized by cytochrome-P450 3A4 isoenzyme

(e.g., erythromycin or cimetidine should also be monitored). To address this concern, caution is advised in prescribing sildenafil to CVD patients even though controlled data are not available. Particular caution is advised for patients who have MI, stroke, arrhythmia within 6 months of MI, resting hypotension (blood pressure less than 90/50 mm Hg) or hypertension (more than 170 to 110 mm Hg), or cardiac failure and CAD causing unstable angina. Clinicians should also pay attention to the vasodilatory effect of sildenafil, especially when considered with respect to the effects of sexual activity.

CARDIAC REHABILITATION AND VOCATIONAL REHABILITATION

CVD is the leading disorder in the United States for which individuals receive disability benefits under the Social Security System. In fact, one-fourth of men and women receiving social security disability allowances have a permanent disability that is due to CVD. The indirect health-care cost of disability, including decreased productivity, loss of income, welfare payment, and unemployment insurance costs, must be considered when the cost benefit of CR is determined. There is a variable correlation between return to work and resumption of premorbid lifestyle with cardiac functional improvement. Psychological status appears to be the major determinant. A number of studies have shown that a patient's preillness perception about ability to return to work appears to be very important (130).

Many nonmedical factors negatively influence the resumption of employment, including old age, adequate nonwork income, anxiety or depression, activity-induced symptoms, lower social class, less education, job involving high level of physical activity, and preoccupation of coronary illness as job related. Medical reasons for failure to return to work include unwarranted medical restrictions and lack of professional assurance of safety. Patients who fail to resume employment within 6 months after a coronary event are unlikely to ever do so. In the case of an uncomplicated cardiac event in a patient who is younger than 65 years of age and employed at the time of MI, there is an 80% chance of return to work within 2 to 3 months. Continued employment is a problem, however, as there is a 20% decline in continued employment between 6 months to 1 year. Comparative data are not available for complicated MIs, but estimated return to work is about 25% to 33% (131).

An evaluation to determine the capacity to return to gainful employment should involve an assessment of the clinical status of the patient as well as the type of work required on the job. A major goal of CR is the resumption of gainful employment and a change in occupation if needed.

The level of performance attained on an ETT is also predictive of whether a job is too strenuous for the patient. An ETT performed for risk stratification can also be used for work evaluation. This helps to decrease apprehension on the part of the patient, family, physician, and employer. Extrapolation of the exercise data to the job requirements should include an analysis of the job to be performed in different environments and its associated intellectual demands, travel requirements, and emotional stress. If results of an ETT are not available, the New York Heart Association cardiovascular functional classification can be used in an attempt to correlate this with the metabolic cost of work (131).

In the United States, most occupational activities require less than 5 METs. In the 15% of individuals in the workforce whose work involves heavy manual labor (132), exercise data should not be used as the sole criterion for recommendation regarding return to work. Heavy labor can increase myocardial work and thus may increase myocardial ischemia, arrhythmia, and sudden cardiac arrest. It may also pose a problem for employers who are liable for workers compensation if complications that are due to heart disease occur on the job. The person who can perform 7 METs or higher activity without limitation or abnormal response should be able to return to most jobs except heavy industrial work. Those who can exercise at 5 METs or greater, but less than 7 METs, can perform most jobs and most household chores. Those who exercise at or less than 3 METs may not be suitable for return to employment. A CR program can increase capacity by as much as 50% after 2 to 3 months of reconditioning. Recommendation for full-time work should be for a work level at approximately 30% of the major physical work capacity. Guidelines are available for assessing and establishing employment for the patient with CVD (133).

COMPLIANCE WITH CARDIAC REHABILITATION

In patients with CVD, exercise adherence is low, despite the fact that exercise has been shown to improve short-term clinical outcomes. In a prospective study of 255 consecutive patients enrolled in a community-based CR, the adherence rate was 51% for men and 63% for women (15). In a training level comparison trial, exercise attendance during the first year averaged 64% in a low-intensity exercise group, and 55.5% in a high-intensity group. Moore et al. (133a) found that of 40 women with a cardiac event who completed CR program, only 50% continued to exercise 3 months after completion of the program. Behavioral science probably holds the key to improving adherence to prescribed rehabilitation programs. Behavioral change seems to involve an intrinsic process that dramatically alters the way the patient views necessary changes expected of them. Cognition (i.e., education) is only one component in the dynamic process of behavior modification (134).

According to cognitive behavioral theory, maladaptive behavior is the product of faulty or irrational thinking. The cognitive component is designed to modify how an individual thinks about or perceives a situation. Behavioral therapy is based on the idea that new and constructive behavior can be learned through teaching and reinforcement.

In social cognitive theory, behavior is a concept of self-efficacy. Self-efficacy is an individual's confidence in his or her ability to perform a given task and is the product of both efficacy expectation (an individual's perception of his or her ability to achieve a specific level of performance) and outcome expectation (an individual's evaluation of the probable consequences of specific behavior). Efficacy expectations are derived from four different sources, including performance mastery, vicarious experiences, verbal persuasion, and physiological state. The health professional involved in CR can support all four of these factors so as to improve compliance.

In a health behavior model, the individual will adopt a given healthy behavior if the individual believes that the behavior will help ward off a perceived health threat. It heavily relies on subjective perception of health status rather than objective or clinical measures. Major factors are motivation to act, perceived cost, benefits of action, and cues to action.

The exercise belief model suggests that exercise behavior is influenced by perceived control over exercise behavior, attitude toward exercise and self-concept, and value related to exercise. The transtheoretical model (stages of change in a completed model) suggests that the health behavior varies in individuals based on cognitive and performance factors. Individuals can be staged along a continuum consisting of five different levels: (a) precontemplation—no intent to begin exer-

cising; (b) contemplation—not exercising but considering beginning the exercises in the future; (c) preparation—beginning exercises on a limited or inconsistent basis; (d) action—exercise on a regular basis (three or more 20-minute exercise sessions per week for less than 6 months); (e) maintenance—exercise on a regular basis, as in the action level, but for 6 or more months. Several processes can facilitate action, including contingency management relationship assistance, counter conditioning, and stimulus control (135).

Past experiences of success or failure at a given task influence the individual's perception of what he or she can achieve. Successful performance of specific tasks increases efficacy expectation, whereas failed performance reduces expectations. Clearly building a base of success early in the therapeutic exercise training program is essential to improving exercise maintenance over a long period (136,137).

CARDIAC REHABILITATION AND COMPLIMENTARY MEDICINE

Evidence continues to mount that demonstrates the positive value of spiritual and religious factors in the maintenance of health (138). A survey demonstrated that religious involvement is important to many Americans. Ninety-five percent said that they believe in God, and approximately 40% said that they attend weekly church services; in fact, almost 75% percent of Americans maintain that their religion plays a central role in how they live. In addition, as many as 40% of persons older than 60 years report that they use religion as the primary coping strategy when hospitalized with medical illness. One survey showed that 40% of the patients felt that their caregiver, particularly doctor, should discuss pertinent religious issues with them.

There is confusion, however, between religious commitment and spirituality. It is easy to define religious commitment, which usually refers to shared behavioral practices within an organized community of people of the same faith. Spirituality usually refers to the sense of connection with life and other people that implies a meaning of connection to something greater than individual self. It is hypothesized that spirituality acts as a unifying force that integrates the individual's physical, cognitive, emotional, and social experiences. Second, spirituality helps to create a sense of meaning and purpose that serves as a motivator. Third, spiritual experience is used to create a common bond among individuals. Fourth, spirituality reflects faith in a higher power that may not be seen or easily described, but can be felt nonetheless.

Matthews et al. (139) suggest that the following questions be added to the physician's initial patient interview. Specifically, they recommend to first ask the question, "Is your religion or faith helpful to you in handling your illnesses?" If the answer is yes, a follow-up questions might be, "What can I do to support your faith and religious commitment?" This facilitates the patient to talk more about how their faith supports their health. Studies suggest that people benefit from religious and spiritual activities when they feel ill. The effectiveness of prayer in the setting of CVD was assessed by a Duke University study (140). One hundred and fifty angioplasty patients at a local Veteran Affairs hospital were randomly assigned to five 30-member groups. All five groups received the usual and customary care, whereas three also received nontraditional therapies, such as stress-management training, guided imagery training, and therapeutic touch. The fourth group of patients had their names sent to people around the world who were willing to pray for them. The people who did the praying were in

Jerusalem, Nepal, France, and Baltimore, were of different faiths, and prayed for each of the 30 people in the group by name. In this double-blind study, the patient's progress was monitored through electrocardiogram, blood pressure, HR, and clinical outcome. Those patients who received prayer in addition to their usual medical care did 50% to 100% better during their hospitalization than those in the control group. The group receiving other alternative treatment—i.e., imagery training, therapeutic touch, or stress management—saw improvement that ranged between 30% and 50% over the control group (141).

In 1988, Byrd studied 393 patients randomized into a prospective double-blind protocol at San Francisco Hospital (142). Each subject in the treatment group was prayed for daily by two or three Christian intercessors who were informed only of the first name, diagnosis, and general condition of each patient. In addition, those praying received an update on general progress of each patient. All the praying was done outside the hospital. Neither the researcher collecting the data nor the patient knew who was prayed for. People in the group who were prayed for did substantially better on a number of outcome variables than those who were not prayed for. At the end of the 10 months, the subjects in the prayer group required less ventilator assistance, antibiotics, and diuretics than those in the control group. In addition, patients in the prayer group spent less time in the coronary care unit, and their overall course of treatment was rated better.

In a 25-year longitudinal study of Seventh Day Adventists, Adventist men live more than 6 years longer and Adventist women live almost 4 years longer than the national norm. In particular, the mortality rate of heart disease was 66% lower for the Seventh Day Adventist than the national norm. Active Mormons also had lower rates for mortality than national norms, particularly with respect to smoking-related cancer and CVDs.

Recently, the use of principle oriental medicine has come into vogue. Preliminary studies have shown some beneficial effect. Nei Ching, the Yellow Emperor's classic on internal medicine written about 300 B.C., attempts to answer many questions, including some theories such as the transmission of essence of light, the seasons of pattern of the viscera, and the five elements, i.e., fire, earth, wind, water, and metal. There is a reference to acupuncture for prevention and treatment of cardiac diseases (143). Preliminary data using acupuncture in angina and CHF are exciting and promising (144,145). Although double-blind scientific results are not available, one should keep an open mind to a system based on more than 2,500 years of experience.

CARDIAC REHABILITATION AND COST-EFFECTIVENESS

In this era of managed care, outcome-based intervention and cost are important considerations. A comprehensive economic analysis of CR and secondary prevention includes not only the direct cost of CR intervention, but also indirect cost and cost savings attributed to the treatment benefits (146). Unfortunately, no single study is comprehensive, randomized, and well controlled, and study results from different parts of the country are varied. The effect of CR on subsequent rehabilitation rehospitalization costs in 580 patients over a mean follow-up of 21 months was shown to be $739 lower than for control patients (147). A randomized study of 8 weeks of CR interventions that focused on anxious and depressed patients after MI noted a cost-effectiveness of $9,200 per quality adjusted life year (148). It is similar to the cost-effectiveness of well-estab-lished medical interventions, such as CABG for left CAD and beta blockade after MI, but CR is more cost-effective than other accepted practices, such as angiotensin-converting enzymes inhibitors for hypertension and statins for hypercholesteremia (149).

In conclusion, evidence regarding the health benefits of CR are overwhelming; however, there are many questions unanswered. Research needs to be continued and supported. For example, no single prospective randomized controlled trial has compared the benefits of high- versus low-dose intensity of exercises on the fitness level or modifiable cardiovascular risk factors. The CR mechanisms responsible for reduction in total mortality and cardiovascular events are probably multiple, and the specific contribution of each element of CR is not known.

REFERENCES

1. Niebauer J, Harmbrecht R, Velich T, et al. Attenuated progression of coronary artery disease after 6 years of multifactorial risk intervention: role of physical exercise. *Circulation* 1997;96:2534–2541.
2. Gould KL, Ornish D, Kirkeeide R, et al. Improved stenosis geometry by quantitative coronary arteriography after vigorous risk factor modification. *Am J Cardiol* 1992;69:845–853.
3. Ornish D, Scherwitz LW, Billings JH, et al. Intensive lifestyle changes for reversal of coronary heart disease. *JAMA* 1999;281:1380.
4. National Institutes of Health. Leon AS, ed. *Physical activity and cardiovascular health: a national consensus.* Champaign, IL: Human Kinetics, 1997.
5. Kavanagh T. *Take heart.* Toronto: Key Porter Books, Ltd, 1998.
6. Pashkow FJ. Issues in contemporary cardiac rehabilitation: a historical perspective. *J Am Coll Cardiol* 1993;21:822–834.
7. Ornish D, Brown SE, Scherwitz LW, et al. Can lifestyle changes reverse coronary heart disease? The lifestyle heart trial. *Lancet* 1990;336:129–133.
8. Heberden W. *Commentaries on the history and cure of diseases.* London: T Payne, 1802.
9. Stokes W. *The diseases of the heart and the aorta.* Dublin: Hodges and Smith, 1854.
10. Hilton J. *Rest and pain.* London: G Bell & Sons Ltd., 1863.
11. Levine SA, Lown B. "Armchair" treatment of acute coronary thrombosis. *JAMA* 1952;148:1365–1369.
12. Chapman C, Fraser R. Studies on the effect of exercise on cardiovascular function: cardiovascular responses to exercise inpatients with healed myocardial infarction. *Circulation* 1954;9:34–51.
13. Kavanagh T, Shepahard RJ, Pandit V. Marathon running after myocardial infarction. *JAMA* 1974;229:1602–1605.
14. The American Heart Association. *2001 Heart and stroke statistical update.* Dallas: American Heart Association, 2000.
15. Wenger NK, Froelicker ES, Smith LK, et al. Cardiac rehabilitation clinical practice. Washington, D.C.: U.S. Department of Health and Human Services, 1995:9–26, 27–47, 100–102, 121–128.
16. Moldover JR, Stein J, Krug PG. Cardiopulmonary physiology. In: Gonzalez EG, Myers SJ, eds. *Physiological basis of rehabilitation medicine,* 3rd ed. Boston: Butterworth-Heinemann, 2001:169–177; 0–7506–7179–3.
17. Bouchard C, Daw EW, Rice T, et al. Familial resemblance for VO_{2max} the sedentary state: The HERITAGE family study. *Med Sci Sports Exerc* 1998;30: 252–258.
18. McLaren PF, Nurhayati Y, Boutcher SH. Stroke volume response to cycle ergometry in trained and untrained older men. *Eur J Appl Occup Physiol* 1997; 75(6):537–542.
19. Tulppo MP, Makikallio TH, Seppanen T, et al. Vagal modulation of heart rate during exercise: effects of age and physical fitness. *Am J Physiol* 1998;274(2 pt. 2):H424–H429.
20. Fitzgerald MD, Tanaka H, Tran ZV, et al. Age-related declines in maximal aerobic capacity in regularly exercising vs. sedentary women: a meta-analysis. *J Appl Physiol* 1997;83:160–165.
21. Hambrecht R, Wolf A, Gielen S, et al. Effect of exercise on coronary endothelial function in patients with coronary artery disease. *N Engl J Med* 2000; 342:454–460.
22. Schuit AJ, van-Amelsvoort LG, Verheij TC, et al. Exercise training and heart rate variability in older people. *Med Sci Sports Exerc* 1999;31:816–821.
23. Ades PA, Waldmann ML, Meyer WL, et al. Skeletal muscle and cardiovascular adaptations to exercise conditioning in older coronary patients. *Circulation* 1996; 94:323–330.
24. Hagberg JM. Physiologic adaptations to prolonged high-intensity exercise training in inpatients with coronary artery disease. *Med Sci Sports Exerc* 1991;23:661–667.
25. MacDougall J. Blood pressure responses to resistive static and dynamic exercise. In: Fletcher G, ed. *Cardiovascular response to exercise.* Mount Kisco, NY: Futura, 1994:155–173.
26. American College of Sports Medicine Position Stand: the recommended quantity and quality of exercise for developing and maintaining cardiores-

piratory and muscular fitness, and flexibility in healthy adults. *Med Sci Sports Exerc* 1998;30:975–991.

27. Pollock ML, Franklin BA, Balady GJ, et al. Resistance exercise in individuals with and without cardiovascular disease: benefits, rationale, safety, and prescription: an advisory from the Committee on Exercise, Rehabilitation, and Prevention, Council on Clinical Cardiology, American Heart Association. *Circulation* 2000;101:828–833.

28. Fletcher GF, Balady GJ, Amsterdam EA. Exercise standards for testing and training: a statement for healthcare professionals from the American Heart Association. *Circulation* 2001;104:1694–1740.

29. NIH Consensus Development Panel on Physical Activity and Cardiovascular Health. Physical Activity and Cardiovascular Health. *JAMA* 1996;276:241–246.

30. Leon AS, Richardson M. Exercise, health, and disease. In: Roberts SO, Roversg RA, Hanson P, eds. *Clinical exercise testing and prescription: theory and application.* Boca Raton, FL: CRC Press, 1997:281–302.

31. Squires RW. Mechanisms by which exercise training may improve the clinical status of cardiac patients. In: Pollock ML, Schmidt DH, eds. *Heart disease and rehabilitation,* 3rd ed. Champaign, IL: Human Kinetics, 1995:147–160.

32. Bouchard C, Despres JP. Physical activity and health: atherosclerotic, metabolic, and hypertensive diseases. *Res Q Exerc Sport* 1995;66:268–275.

33. Rao GHR. Effect of exercise on platelet of physiology and pharmacology. In: Somani SM, ed. *Pharmacology and toxicology.* Boca Raton, FL: CRC Press, 1996:211–223.

34. Stratton JR, Chandler WL, Schwartz RS, et al. Effects of physical conditioning on fibrinolytic variables and fibrinogen in young and old healthy adults. *Circulation* 1991;83:1692–1697.

35. Charo S, Gokce N, Vita JA. Endothelial dysfunction and coronary risk reduction. *J Cardiopulm Rehabil* 1998;18:60–67.

36. Goldsmith RL, Bigger JR Jr, Steinman RC, et al. Comparison of 24-hour parasympathetic activity in endurance-trained and untrained young men. *J Am Coll Cardiol* 1992;20:552–558.

37. Kokkinos PF, Papademetriou V. Exercise and hypertension. *Coron Artery Dis* 2000;11:99–102.

38. Wasserman DH, Zinman B. Fuel homeostasis. In: Ruderman N, Devlin JT, eds. *The health professional's guide to diabetes and exercise.* Alexandria, VA: American Diabetes Association, 1995:29–47.

39. Schoeller DA, Shay K, Kushner RF. How much physical activity is needed to minimize weight gain in previously obese women? *Am J Clin Nutr* 1997;66:551–556.

40. King AC, Haskell WL, Young DR, et al. Long-term effects of varying intensities and formats of physical activity on participation rates, fitness, and lipoproteins in men and women aged 50 to 65 years. *Circulation* 1995;91:2596–2604.

41. Pina IL, Balady GJ, Hanson P, et al. Guidelines for clinical exercise testing laboratories: a statement for healthcare professionals from the Committee on Exercise and Cardiac Rehabilitation, American Heart Association. *Circulation* 1995;91:912–921.

42. Cheitlin MD, Alpert JS, Armstrong WF, et al. ACC/AHA guidelines for the clinical application of echocardiography: a report of the American College of Cardiology/American Heart Association Task Force on Practice Guidelines (Committee of Clinical Application of Echocardiography), developed in collaboration with the American Society of Echocardiography. *Circulation* 1997;95:1686–1744.

43. Ritchie JL, Bateman TM, Bonow RO, et al. Guidelines for clinical use of cardiac radionuclide imaging: report of the American College of Cardiology/American Heart Association Task Force on Assessment of Diagnostic and Therapeutic Cardiovascular Procedures (Committee on Radionuclide Imaging), developed in collaboration with the American Society of Nuclear Cardiology. *J Am Coll Cardiol* 1995;25:521–547.

44. Secknus MA, Marwick TH. Evolution of dobutamine echocardiography protocols and indications: safety and side effects in 3,011 studies over 5 years. *J Am Coll Cardiol* 1997;29:1234–1240.

45. Pate RR, Pratt M, Blair SN, et al. Physical activity and public health: a recommendation from the Centers for Disease Control and Prevention and the American College of Sports Medicine. *JAMA* 1995;273:402–407.

46. Whaley MH, Brubaker PH, Kaminsky LA, et al. Validity of rating of perceived exertion during graded exercise testing in apparently healthy adults and cardiac patients. *J Cardiopulm Rehabil* 1997;17:261–267.

47. Hlatky MA, Boineau RE, Hiffinbotham MB, et al. A brief self-administered questionnaire to determine functional capacity (the Duke Activity Status Index). *Am J Cardiol* 1989;64:651–654.

48. Meyer JN, Do D, Herbert W, et al. A monogram to predict exercise capacity from a specific activity questionnaire and clinical data. *Am J Cardiol* 1994;73:591–596.

49. Franklin B. American College of Sports Medicine. *Guidelines for exercise testing prescription,* 6th ed. Indianapolis: ACSM, 2000.

50. Haskell WL. Health consequences of physical activity: understanding and challenges regarding dose-response. *Med Sci Sports Exerc* 1994;26:649–660.

51. Wenger NK. Rehabilitation of the patient with coronary heart disease. In: Sclant RG, Alexander RW, eds. *The heart, arteries and veins,* 6th ed. New York: McGraw-Hill, 1994:1223–1237.

52. Stewart KJ. Weight training in coronary artery disease and hypertension. *Prog Cardiovasc Dis* 1992;35:159–168.

53. Faigenbaum AD, Skrinar GS, Cesare WF, et al. Physiologic and symptomatic responses of cardiac patients to resistance exercise. *Arch Phys Med Rehabil* 1990;71:395–398.

54. Haennel RG, Quinney HA, Kappagoda CT. Effects of hydraulic circuit training following coronary artery bypass surgery. *Med Sci Sports Exerc* 1991;23:158–165.

55. Lillegard WA, Terrio JD. Appropriate strength training. *Med Clin North Am* 1994;78:457–477.

56. Franklin BA, Bonzheim K, Gordon S, et al. Safety and medically supervised outpatient cardiac rehabilitation exercise therapy: a 16-year follow-up. *Chest* 1998;114:902–906.

57. Hakim AA, Petrovitch H, Burchfiel CM, et al. Effects of walking on mortality among nonsmoking retired men. *N Engl J Med* 1998;338:94–99.

58. Burke AP, Farb A, Malcom GT, et al. Plaque rupture and sudden death related to exertion in men with coronary artery disease. *JAMA* 1999;281:921–926.

59. Mittleman MA, Maclure M, Tofler GH, et al. Triggering of acute myocardial infarction by heavy physical exertion: protection against triggering by regular exertion: Determinants of Myocardial Infarction Onset Study Investigators. *N Engl J Med* 1993;329:1677–1683.

60. Willich SN, Lewis M, Lowel H, et al. Physical exertion as a trigger of acute myocardial infarction: triggers and mechanisms of Myocardial Infarction Study Group. *N Engl J Med* 1993;329:1684–1690.

61. Balady GG, Ades PA, Comoss P, et al. Core components of cardiac rehabilitation—secondary prevention program; a statement for health care professionals from the American Heart Association and the American Association of Cardiovascular and Pulmonary Rehabilitation Writing Group 2000;102:1069–1073.

62. Third Report of the National Cholesterol Education Program (NCEP) Expert Panel on Detection, Evaluation and Treatment of High Blood Cholesterol in Adults (Adult Treatment Panel). Executive Summary. US Department of Health and Human Services; Public Health Service; National Institutes of Health; National Heart, Lung and Blood Institutes. NIH Publication NO. 01–3670. May, 2001.

63. Croghan IT, Offord KP, Evans RW, et al. Cost effectiveness of treating nicotine dependence: the Mayo Clinic experience. *Mayo Clin Proc* 1997;72:917–924.

64. D'Agostino RB Sr, Grundy S, Sullivan LM, et al. Validation of the Framingham coronary heart disease prediction scores: results of a multiple ethnic groups investigation. *JAMA* 2001;286:180–187.

65. MacMahon S, Peto R, Culter J, et al. Blood pressure, stroke, and coronary heart disease, Part 1. Prolonged differences in blood pressure: prospective observational studies corrected for the regression dilution bias. *Lancet* 1990;335:765–774.

66. Ockene IS, Miller NH. Cigarette smoking, cardiovascular disease, and stroke: a statement for health care professionals from the American Heart Association, American Heart Association Task Force on Risk Reduction. *Circulation* 1997;96:3243–3247.

67. Expert Panel on Detection, Evaluation, and Treatment of High Blood Cholesterol in Adults. Executive summary of the Third Report of the National Cholesterol Education Programs (NCEP) Expert Panel of Detection, Evaluation, and Treatment of High Blood Cholesterol in Adults (Adult Treatment Panel III). *JAMA* 2001;285:2486–2497.

68. UK Prospective Diabetes Study Group. Tight blood pressure control and risk of macrovascular and microvascular complications in type 2 diabetes (UKPDS 38). *BMJ* 1998;317:703–713.

69. Haffner SM, Lehto S, Ronnemaa T, et al. Mortality from coronary heart disease in subjects with type 2 diabetes and in nondiabetic subjects with and without prior myocardial infarction. *N Engl J Med* 1998;339:229–234.

70. Stampfer MJ, Hu FB, Manson JE, et al. Primary prevention of coronary heart disease in women through diet and lifestyle. *N Engl J Med* 2000;343:16–22.

71. Wilson K, Gibson N, Willan A, et al. Effect of smoking cessation on mortality after myocardial infarction: meta-analysis of cohort studies. *Arch Intern Med* 2000;160:939–944.

72. Fiore MC, Bailey WC, Cohen SJ, et al. *Treating tobacco use and dependence.* Clinical Practice Guideline. Rockville, MD: U.S. Department of Health and Human Services Public Service, June 2000.

73. Hertanu JS, Moldover JR. Cardiovascular, pulmonary, and cancer rehabilitation. 1. Cardiac rehabilitation. *Arch Phys Med Rehabil* 1996;77[Suppl3]:S38–S44.

74. Stone JA, Cyr C, Friesen M, et al. Canadian guidelines for cardiac rehabilitation and atherosclerotic heart disease prevention: a summary. *Can J Cardiol* 2001;17[Suppl B]:3B–30B.

75. Wenger NK, Froelecher ES, Smith LK. *Cardiac rehabilitation.* Clinical Practice Guideline No. 17. Rockville, MD: Public Health Service, 1995.

76. Kobashigawa JA, Leaf DA, Lee N, et al. A controlled trial of exercise rehabilitation after heart transplantation. *N Engl J Med* 1999;340:272–277.

77. Von Scheidt W, Neudert J, Erdmann E, et al. Contractility of the transplanted, denervated human heart. *Am Heart J* 1991;121:1480–1488.

78. Bussieres LM, Pflugfelder PW, Taylor AW, et al. Changes in skeletal muscle morphology and biochemistry after cardiac transplantation. *Am J Cardiol* 1997;79:630–634.

79. American Heart Association. *2001 Heart and Stroke Statistical Update.* Dallas: AHA, 2000.

80. Dubach P, Myers J, Dziekan G, et al. Effect of exercise training on myocardial remodeling in patients with reduced left ventricular function after myocardial infarction: application of magnetic resonance imaging. *Circulation* 1997;95:2060–2067.

81. McMurray J, Pfeffer MA. New therapeutic options in congestive heart failure: Part I. *Circulation* 2002;105:2099–2106.

82. Shemesh J, Grossman E, Peleg E, et al. Norepinephrine and atrial natriuretic peptide responses to exercise testing in rehabilitated and nonrehabilitated men with ischemic cardiomyopathy after healing of anterior wall acute myocardial infarction. *Am J Cardiol* 1995;75:1072–1074.

83. Belardinelli R, Georgiou D, Cianci G, et al. Randomized, controlled trial of long-term moderate exercise training in chronic heart failure: effects on functional capacity, quality of life and clinical outcome. *Circulation* 1999;99: 1173–1182.

84. Maiorana A, O'Driscoll G, Cheetham C, et al. Combined aerobic and resistance exercise training improves functional capacity and strength in CHF. *J Appl Physiol* 2000;88:1565–1570.

85. Humphrey R, Bartels MN. Exercise, cardiovascular disease and chronic heart failure. *Arch Phys Med Rehabil* 2001;82[Suppl 1]S76–S81.

86. Sturm B, Quittan M, Wiesinger GF, et al. Moderate-intensity training with elements of step aerobics in patients with severe chronic heart failure. *Arch Phys Med Rehabil* 1999;80:746–750.

87. Kokkinos PF, Choucair W, Graves P, et al. Chronic heart failure and exercise. *Am Heart J* 2000;140:21–28.

88. Grady KL, Dracup K, Kennedy G, et al. Team management of patients with heart failure: a statement for healthcare professionals from the Cardiovascular Nursing Council of the American Heart Association. *Circulation* 2000;102: 2443–2456.

89. Whellan D, Shaw L, et al. Cardiac rehabilitation and survival in patients with left ventricular systolic dysfunction. *Am Heart J* 2001;142:160–166.

90. Pollock ML, Wilmore JH. Exercise in health and disease: Evaluation and prescription for prevention and rehabilitation, 2nd ed. Philadelphia: WB Saunders, 1990.

91. The Writing Group for the PEPI Trial. Effects of estrogen or estrogen/progestin regimens on heart disease risk factors in postmenopausal women: the Postmenopausal Estrogen/Progestin Interventions (PEPI) Trial (published erratum). *JAMA* 1995;274:199–208.

92. Hulley S, Grady D, Bush T, et al. Randomized trial of estrogen plus progestin for secondary prevention of coronary heart disease in postmenopausal women. Heart and Estrogen/Progestin Replacement Study (HERS) Research group. JAMA 1998; 280:605–613.

93. National Institutes of Health, National Heart, Lung, and Blood Institute. Women's Health Initiative. Available at www.nhlbi.nih.gov/health/public/heart/other/whi/wmn/hlt.htm. Accessed 17 May 2002.

94. Mosca L, Barrett CE, Wenger NK, et al. Design and methods of the Raloxifene Use for the Heart (RUTH) study. *Am J Cardiol* 2001;88:392–395.

95. Savage PD, Brochu M, Scott P, et al. Low caloric expenditure in cardiac rehabilitation. *Am Heart J* 2000;140:527–533.

96. Brochu M, Poehlman ET, Ades PA. Obesity, body fat distribution, and coronary artery disease. *J Cardiopulm Rehabil* 2000;20:96–108.

97. Harvey-Berino J. Weight loss in the clinical setting: applications for cardiac rehabilitation. *Coron Artery Dis* 1998;9:795–798.

98. Burek KA, Sutton-Tyrrell K, Brooks MM, et al. Prognostic importance of lower extremity arterial disease in patients undergoing coronary revasularization in the Bypass Angioplasty Revascularization Investigation (BARI). *J Am Coll Cardiol* 1999;34:716–721.

99. Patterson RB, Pinto B, Marcus B, et al. Value of a supervised exercise program for the therapy of arterial claudication. *J Vasc Surg* 1997;25:312–319.

100. Girolami B, Bernardi E, Prins MH, et al. Treatment of intermittent claudication with physical training, smoking cessation, pentoxifylline or nafronyl: a meta-analysis. *Arch Intern Med* 1999;159:337–345.

101. American Diabetes Association. Position statement: diabetes mellitus and exercise. *Diabetes Care* 1998;21[Suppl 1]:S40–S44.

102. Smith DA, Crandall J. Exercising training in special populations. In: Wenger NK, Smith LK, Froelicher ED, eds. *Cardiac rehabilitation: a guide to practice in the 21ˢᵗ century*. New York: Marcel Dekker, 1999:141–149, 0–8247–6092–1.

103. Dylewicz P, Bienkowska A, Szczensniak L, et al. Beneficial effect of short-term endurance training on glucose metabolism during rehabilitation after coronary bypass surgery. *Chest* 2000;117:47–51.

104. Lo CY, Li L, Lo WK, et al. Benefits of exercise training in patients on continuous ambulatory peritoneal dialysis. *Am J Kidney Dis* 1998;32:1011–1018.

105. Gruppo Emodialisi e Patologie Cardiovascular. Multicentre, cross-sectional study of ventricular arrhythmias in chronically haemodialysed patients. *Lancet* 1988;2:305–309.

106. Wijkstra PJ. Pulmonary rehabilitation at home (editorial). *Thorax* 1996;51: 117–118.

107. Ades PA. Cardiac rehabilitation in older coronary patients. *J Am Geriatric Soc* 1999;47:98–105.

108. Wannamethee SG, Shaper AG, Walker M. Physical activity and mortality in older men with diagnosed coronary heart disease. *Circulation* 2000;102: 1358–1363.

109. Fletcher BJ, Dunbar SB, Felner JM, et al. Exercise testing and training in physically disabled men with clinical evidence of coronary artery disease. *Am J Cardiol* 1994;73:170–174.

110. Potempa K, Braun LT, Tinknell T, et al. Benefits of aerobic exercise after stroke. *Sports Med* 1996;21:337–346.

111. Monga TN, Deforge DA, Williams J, et al. Cardiovascular responses to acute exercise in patients with cerebrovascular accidents. *Arch Phys Med Rehabil* 1988;69:937–940.

112. Fletcher BJ, Dunbar S, Coleman J, et al. Cardiac precautions for non-acute inpatient settings. *Am J Phys Med Rehabil* 1993;72:140–143.

113. Macko RF, DeSouza CA, Tretter LD, et al. Treadmill aerobic exercise training reduces the energy expenditure and cardiovascular demands of hemiparetic gait in chronic stroke patients: a preliminary report. *Stroke* 1997;28:326–330.

114. Abbott RD, Rodriquez BL, Burchfiel CM, et al. Physical activity in older middle-aged men and reduced risk of stroke: the Honolulu Heart Program. *Am J Epidemiol* 1994;139:881–893.

115. Shinton R, Sagar G. Lifelong exercise and stroke. *BMJ* 1993;307:231–234.

116. Frasure-Smith N, Lesperance F, Gravel G, et al. Social support, depression, and mortality during the first year after myocardial infarction. *Circulation* 2000;101:1919–1924.

117. Helmers KF, Krantz DS, Howell RH, et al. Hostility and myocardial ischemia in coronary artery disease patients: evaluation by gender and ischemic index. *Psychosom Med* 1993;55:29–36.

118. Frasure-Smith N, Lesperance F, Talajic M. Depression following myocardial infarction: impact on 6-month survival. *JAMA* 1993;270:1819–1825.

119. Linden W, Stossel C, Maurice J. Psychosocial interventions for patients with coronary artery disease: a meta-analysis. *Arch Intern Med* 1996;745–752.

120. Oldridge N, Guyatt G, Jones N, et al. Effects on quality of life with comprehensive rehabilitation after acute myocardial infarction. *Am J Cardiol* 1991; 67:1084–1089.

121. Williams RB, Barefoot JC, Califf RM, et al. Prognostic importance of social and economic resources among medically treated patients with angiograpically documented coronary artery disease. *JAMA* 1992;267:520–524.

122. Salomaa V, Niemela M, Miettinen H, et al. Relationship of socioeconomic status to the incidence and prehospital, 28-day, and 1-year mortality rates of acute coronary events in the FINMONICA myocardial infarction register study. *Circulation* 2000;101:1913–1918.

123. Taylor HA. Sexual activity and the cardiovascular patient: guidelines. *Am J Cardiol* 1999;84:6N–10N.

124. Drory Y, Kravetz S, Weingarten M. Comparison of sexual activity of women and men after a first acute myocardial infarction. *Am J Cardiol* 2000;85:1283–1287.

125. Froelicher ES, Kee LL, Newton KM, et al. Return to work, sexual activity and other activities after acute myocardial infarction. *Heart Lung* 1994;23: 423–435.

126. Drory Y, Shapira I, Fishman EZ, et al. Myocardial ischemia during sexual activity in patients with coronary artery disease. *Am J Cardiol* 1995;75:835–837.

127. Drory Y, Fishman EZ, Shapira I, et al. Ventricular arrhythmia during sexual activity in patients with coronary artery disease. *Chest* 1996;109:922–924.

128. Muller JE, Mittleman A, Maclure M, et al. Triggering myocardial infarction by sexual activity: low absolute risk and prevention by regular physical exertion. Determinants of Myocardial Infarction Onset Study Investigators. *JAMA* 1996;275:1405–1409.

129. ACC/AHA Expert consensus document. Use of sildenafil (Viagra) in patients with cardiovascular disease. *J Am Coll Cardiol* 1999;33:273–282.

130. Rost K, Smith GR. Return to work after an initial myocardial infarction and subsequent emotional distress. *Arch Intern Med* 1992;152:381–385.

131. Hellerstein HK. Vocational aspects of rehabilitation: work evaluation. In: Wenger NK, Hellerstein HK, eds. *Rehabilitation of the coronary patients*, 3rd ed. New York: Churchill-Livingston, 1992:523, 0–443–08765–2.

132. American Association of Cardiovascular Pulmonary Rehabilitation. *Guidelines for cardiac rehabilitation and secondary prevention programs: promoting health and preventing disease*, 3rd ed. Champaign, IL: Human Kinetics, 1999.

133. 20th Bethesda Conference: Insurability and employability of the patient with ischemic heart disease, October 3–4, 1989. *J Am Coll Cardiol* 1989;14: 1003–1044.

133a. Moore SM, Roland CM, Pashkow FJ, et al. Women's patterns of exercise following cardiac rehabilitation. *Nurs Res* 1998;47:318–324.

134. Burke LE, Dunbar-Jacob JM, Hill MN. Compliance with cardiovascular disease prevention strategies: a review of the research. *Ann Behav Med* 1997; 19:239–263.

135. Carlson JJ, Johnson JA, Franklin BA, et al. Program participation, exercise adherence, cardiovascular outcomes, and program cost of traditional versus modified cardiac rehabilitation. *Am J Cardiol* 2000;86:17–23.

136. McAuley E, Courneya KS, Rudolph DL, et al. Enhancing exercise adherence in middle-aged males and females. *Prev Med* 1994;23:498–506.

137. King AC, Sallis JF, Dunn AL, et al. Overview of the Activity Counseling Trial (ACT) intervention for promoting physical activity in primary health care settings: Activity Counseling Trial Research Group. *Med Sci Sports Exerc* 1998;30:1086–1096.

138. Luskin F. Review of the effect of spiritual and religious factors on mortality and morbidity with a focus on cardiovascular and pulmonary disease. *J Cardiopulm Rehabil* 2000; 20:8–15.

139. Matthews DA, McCullough ME, Larson DB, et al. Religious commitment and health status: a review of the research and implications for family medicine. *Arch Fam Med* 1998;7:118–124.

140. Krucoff M, Crater S. Effect of intercessory prayer on disease outcome. Presented at the Seventy-First Annual Conference of the American Heart Association, Dallas, Texas, November 1998.

141. Craigie FC, Larson DB, Liu IY. References to religion in the Journal of Family Practice: dimensions and valence of spirituality. *J Fam Pract* 1990;30: 477–478, 480.

142. Byrd T. Positive therapeutic effects of intercessory prayer in a coronary care unit population. *South Med J* 1988;81:826–829.

143. Chiu YJ, Chi A, Reid IA. Cardiovascular and endocrine effects of acupuncture in hypertensive patients. *Clin Exp Hypertens* 1997;19:1047–1063.

144. Ballegaard S, Johannessen A, Karpatschof B, et al. Addition of acupuncture and self-care education in the treatment of patients with severe angina pec-

toris may be cost beneficial: an open prospective study. *J Altern Complement Med* 1999;5:405–413.

145. Ho FM, Huang PJ, Lo HM, et al. Effect of acupuncture at nei-kuan on left ventricular function in patients with coronary artery disease. *Am J Chin Med* 1999;27:149–156.

146. Ades PA, Pashkow FJ, Nestor JR. Cost-effectiveness of cardiac rehabilitation after myocardial infarction. *J Cardiopulm Rehabil* 1997;17:222–231.

147. Ades PA, Huang D, Weaver SO. Cardiac rehabilitation participation predicts lower rehospitalization costs. *Am Heart J* 1992;123:916–921.

148. Oldridge N, Furlong W, Feeny D, et al. Economic evaluation of cardiac rehabilitation soon after acute myocardial infarction. *Am J Cardiol* 1993;72:154–161.

149. Kupersmith J, Homes-Rovner M, Hogan A, et al. Cost-effectiveness analysis in heart disease, Part III. Ischemia, congestive heart failure, and arrhythmias. *Prog Cardiovasc Dis* 1995;37:307–346.

CHAPTER 84

Rehabilitation of the Patient with Respiratory Dysfunction

John R. Bach

Pulmonary rehabilitation has been defined as "a multidimensional continuum of services directed to persons with pulmonary disease and their families, usually by an interdisciplinary team of specialists, with the goal of achieving and maintaining the individual's maximum level of independence and functioning in the community" (1). Interventions can include exercise, education, emotional support, oxygen, noninvasive mechanical ventilation, optimization of airway secretion clearance, promoting compliance with medical care to reduce numbers of exacerbations and hospitalizations, and returning to work and/or a more active and emotionally satisfying life. These goals are appropriate for any patients with diminished respiratory reserve whether due to obstructive or intrinsic pulmonary diseases (oxygenation impairment) or neuromuscular weakness (ventilatory impairment). The former are normally eucapnic or hypocapnic, often despite severe hypoxia, and significant hypercapnia occurs only during episodes of acute respiratory failure or with end-stage disease. For the latter, hypercapnia usually precedes significant hypoxia or oxyhemoglobin desaturation (dSpO$_2$), and *ventilatory dysfunction* causes the abnormality in blood oxygenation. Many useful techniques for managing the latter have historically been described, developed, or initially adapted by physiatrists in the United States (2–7) and elsewhere (8) and deserve wider application by our field.

REHABILITATION OF PATIENTS WITH OBSTRUCTIVE LUNG DISEASE

Chronic obstructive pulmonary disease (COPD) affects 10% to 40% of all Americans and is the fifth leading cause of death in the United States. Its incidence is increasing rapidly with the aging of the general population. It is the fourth largest cause of major activity limitation (9).

Pathophysiology

Patients with primarily oxygenation impairment have an increased A-a gradient with or without hypercapnia. The A-a gradient increases whenever there is decreased diffusion or increased blood flow. The increased blood flow that occurs with increased physical activity can exacerbate the A-a oxygen gradient and cause or exacerbate dyspnea. Arterial PO$_2$ decreases before there is an observed rise in PaCO$_2$ because of the greater rate of carbon dioxide diffusion. Thus, hypoxia in the presence of eucapnia or hypocapnia is characteristic of intrinsic lung diseases like emphysema, pulmonary fibrosis, and pneumonia and is characteristic of either respiratory insufficiency or failure. Unlike for patients with ventilation impairment that is due to respiratory muscle dysfunction, the hypoxia of patients with an increased A-a gradient can not be reversed by assisted ventilation or airway secretion elimination by noninvasive means. Respiratory failure develops during periods of acute decompensation in pulmonary function that is due to intrinsic lung or airways disease with deterioration in arterial blood gases and a decrease in blood pH to less than 7.25.

Emphysema, chronic bronchitis, asthmatic bronchitis, cystic fibrosis (CF), and bronchopulmonary dysplasia are the most common causes of COPD and oxygenation impairment. These conditions usually have significant elements of both airway obstruction and parenchymal lung disease. COPD often results from a combination of genetic predisposition and environmental factors in which allergic diatheses (e.g., asthma), respiratory infections (e.g., bronchopneumonitis), chemical inflammation (cigarette smoke, asbestosis), and possibly metabolic abnormalities (e.g. alpha$_1$ antitrypsin deficiency) play a role.

Cigarette smoking is the most frequent cause of chronic bronchitis-emphysema. In the 1990 report of the Surgeon General, smoking was estimated to have caused 57,000 deaths from COPD, 143,000 deaths from cardiovascular disease, and 138,000 deaths from lung and other cancers, at a financial burden of $50 billion or 10% of annualized health-care costs in the United States (10). Smokers are 3.5 to 25 times more likely (depending on the amounts smoked) to die of COPD than nonsmokers (11). One in 15 succumb to lung cancer. On the average, 30- to 35-year-olds who smoke 10 to 20 cigarettes per day die 5 years sooner than nonsmokers. One- to two-pack-a-day smokers of the same age die 6.5 years sooner (12). Smoking cessation has been associated with improvement in symptoms (13), decreased ratio of loss of pulmonary function (14), decreased risk of respiratory tract infection (15), and a long-term decreased reduction in rate of loss of forced expiratory volumes (16). Despite this, fewer than 15% of smokers who saw physicians in 1996 were offered assistance to quit smoking, and only 3% had a follow-up appointment to address tobacco use (17). This is true despite the fact that bupropion SR, nicotine patches, gum, inhalers, and nasal sprays have all been shown to be effective in facilitating smoking cessation (18).

Emphysema is characterized by distention of air spaces distal to terminal nonrespiratory bronchioles with destruction of alveolar walls. This occurs because of the unimpeded action of neutrophil-derived elastase. This enzyme is present in polymorphonuclear leukocytes, which occur in large numbers at the bases of normal human lungs. The neutrophil-derived elastase is extremely proteolytic and punches holes in biologic membranes, allowing neutrophil entry. Alpha 1-antiprotease, which primarily inactivates neutrophil-derived elastase, normally protects the lungs but is destroyed by cigarette smoke and other toxins that also cause chronic inflammation and impair mucociliary clearance (19). Ultimately, there is loss of lung recoil, excessive airway collapse on exhalation, and chronic airflow obstruction.

Chronic bronchitis and CF are characterized by enlargement of tracheobronchial mucous glands and chronic mucous hypersecretion and chest infections. Chronic bronchitis is distinguished from asthmatic bronchitis by its irreversibility, lack of bronchial hyperreactivity, lack of responsiveness to bronchodilators, and distinctive abnormalities in ventilation-perfusion (20). Mucous hypersecretion occurs, blocks airways, and sets the stage for recurrent infection, airway and alveolar damage, and irreversible airflow obstruction. Asthmatics develop hypertrophy of bronchial muscle, mucosal edema, infiltration with mononuclear cells and eosinophils, and changes in basement membrane. Chronic bronchitis can develop from asthma.

The gas exchange surface of the lung, which under normal circumstances has the area of a tennis court and maintains normal blood gases throughout a 20-fold range of metabolic demand, is greatly reduced in patients with intrinsic lung disease. Gas exchange is dependent on ventilation, perfusion, and diffusion, all of which are commonly affected. Oxygen and carbon dioxide diffusion across the respiratory exchange membrane of the lung is a function of the gas partial pressures and the respiratory exchange membrane area, and is inversely related to membrane thickness (21). Exchange normally takes place in one-third of the pulmonary capillary blood transit time. With decreased diffusion or increased blood flow, arterial pO_2 is significantly lower than alveolar pO_2. Arterial pO_2 falls before there is an observed rise in pCO_2 because of the greater rate of diffusion of CO_2. Thus, hypoxia in the presence of normal or hyperventilation (pCO_2 less than 45 mm Hg) is characteristic of intrinsic lung disease. Such patients may develop overt respiratory failure with or without hypercapnia. Pulmonary vascular resistance increases in the presence of generalized or local pulmonary tissue hypoxia, especially in the presence of acidosis. Widespread alveolar hypoventilation leads to severe pulmonary artery hypertension and right ventricular failure.

Peripheral chemoreceptors in the aortic and carotid bodies sense pO_2, pCO_2, and pH. Central receptors on the surface of the medulla respond to hydrogen ion levels in the cerebrospinal fluid (21). Response to pCO_2 is reduced by drugs, heavy mechanical loads, and elevated bicarbonate levels. Hypercapnia is caused by the resort to shallow breathing to avoid respiratory muscle fatigue (22). Hypercapnic COPD patients also have weaker respiratory muscles than eucapnic patients (23,24).

Patient Evaluation

In addition to the elements of the patient evaluation noted in Table 84-1, any medical, physical, financial, or psychological factors that might interfere with a rehabilitation program need to be noted. Various dyspnea assessment surveys can be used

TABLE 84-1. Patient Evaluation

Family history of pulmonary diseases
Symptom progression and impact on function
Exacerbation and hospitalization history
Nutritional status and weight changes
Medications, substance abuse
Physical examination for hyperresonant chest, poor breath and cardiac sounds
Radiographic low, flattened diaphragm, long, narrow heart shadow, increased retrosternal translucency, and narrowing of peripheral pulmonary vessels
Gas diffusion capacities decreased in emphysema, normal in bronchitis
Air trapping
Low maximum midexpiratory flow rates and increased midexpiratory times
Normal or increased lung compliance and increased flow work
Generally increased residual volume and total lung capacity
Clinical exercise testing
A 3-, 6-, or 12-minute walk
Assessment of the ventilatory anaerobic threshold and maximum exercise tolerance for a precise exercise regimen

to objectify the extent of dyspnea and the effects of rehabilitation (25–28). In addition, the presence of any coughing, wheezing, chest pains, neurologic or psychological disturbances, allergies, previous communicable diseases, and injuries is explored. Dyspnea and acute exacerbations of respiratory insufficiency occur because of trapping of airway secretions and, ultimately, respiratory tract infections. Hospitalization rates, morbidity, and mortality correlate with the extent of hypercapnia (29) and can decrease with treatment and rehabilitation. Recognition of weight changes is a good means for detecting nutritional imbalance or changes in hydration status or edema. Arterial blood gases may be normal at rest but abnormal during exercise. Early on, resting hypoxemia is absent but ventilation is high with low or normal pCO_2 in emphysema.

Undernutrition reduces hepatic protein synthesis. Poor nutrition can be characterized by low protein values. Serum albumin and iron transport protein (transferrin) levels reflect protein availability to the liver for protein synthesis. Both protein and transferrin have half-lives just less than 2 weeks. Therefore, their serum levels reflect long-term changes in protein status (30). Serum albumin level correlates better with hypoxia than do spirometric values and is a good predictor of rehabilitation potential (31).

Measures of the urinary nitrogen level, a measurement of nitrogen metabolism, are accomplished by a 24-hour urine collection. Other tests that assess nutritional status include total iron binding capacity, cholesterol, and serum vitamin levels, especially of vitamins A, C, and E. This is especially important because COPD and neuromuscular disease (NMD) patients have a high incidence of vitamin deficiencies. Delayed cutaneous hypersensitivity is a function of cell-mediated immunity and is the immune response most sensitive to nutritional deprivation. Hypophosphatemia, hypomagnesemia, hypocalcemia, and hypokalemia may also cause respiratory muscle weakness, which is reversible following replacement (32). Social, educational, and vocational histories and any relevant environmental factors are explored.

The chronic bronchitic often has a plethoric complexion with a wet cough, wheeze, basal rales, and sputum production with infective exacerbations. Characteristically, there is greater than 100 mL of sputum production per day for over 3 months for at least 2 consecutive years. There is often an increase in

PaO_2 and $PaCO_2$ with exercise, the former because of improvement in ventilation-perfusion ratios. There is a tendency to develop polycythemia, edema, and cor pulmonale. The great majority of COPD patients have elements of both bronchitis and emphysema, and about 10% of COPD patients have a component of reversible bronchospasm.

The pulmonary function studies of COPD patients demonstrate air trapping, low-maximum midexpiratory flow rates and increased midexpiratory times, normal or increased lung compliance, and increased flow work. Residual volume and total lung capacity are generally increased. Exertional dyspnea tends to occur when the forced expiratory volume in 1 second (FEV_1) is less than 1500 mL. FEV_1 decreases by 45 to 75 mL per year for COPD patients (33), a rate up to three times normal. Arterial oxygen tensions may be posturally related, significantly decreased with the patient supine (34), and desaturation may be episodically severe during sleep (35). The patient is assessed for sleep blood gas alterations when daytime hypercapnia is present or there are symptoms suggestive of nocturnal hypercapnia.

Thirty percent of COPD patients with FEV_1 less than 750 mL die within 1 year and 50% within 3 years (33). However, pulmonary function impairment does not predict the overall extent of the patient's functional impairment. Clinical exercise testing, on the other hand, measures the functional reserve of all mechanisms taking part in oxygen and carbon dioxide transport and yields information regarding the capacity to perform exercise, the factors that limit exercise, the reasons for exercise-related symptoms, and the diagnosis (36). It permits the clinician to determine whether the primary disability is pulmonary, cardiac, or related to exercise-induced bronchospasm (37). The latter two diagnoses and even the presence of purely restrictive pulmonary syndromes are commonly mistaken for COPD and, therefore, may be mismanaged. Clinical exercise testing can also be useful for documenting patient progress when performed both before and after the rehabilitation program.

Clinical exercise testing, whether by using a treadmill, stationary bicycle, or upper-extremity ergometer, includes monitoring of the following: vital signs, electrocardiography, oxygen consumption, carbon dioxide production, the respiratory quotient, the ventilatory equivalent, minute ventilation, and metabolic rate. The respiratory quotient is the ratio of the carbon dioxide produced divided by the oxygen consumed. The ventilatory equivalent is equal to the volume of air breathed for 1 liter of oxygen consumed. A metabolic equivalent (MET) is the resting metabolic rate per kilogram of body weight (i.e., 1 MET = 3.5 mL 0_2/kg/min). Other useful measures for noninvasively assessing cardiac function include the oxygen pulse, a measure of the mL of oxygen consumed per heart beat (37). A clinical exercise test should advance until oxygen consumption fails to increase, maximum allowable heart rate for age is reached (usually $220 -$ age in years), or electrocardiographic changes, chest pain, severe dyspnea, or intolerable fatigue occurs. A minute ventilation 37.5 times the patient's FEV_1 can be the goal (38). Arterial blood gas analyses and oximetry are performed to determine need for supplemental oxygen therapy to maintain SpO_2 greater than 90% during reconditioning exercise or greater than 60 mm Hg long term (39).

When energy cost studies are not available, maximum exercise tolerance may be estimated from pulmonary function data (40). A 3-, 6-, or 12-minute walk test can also provide useful information. The patient is instructed to gradually increase walking speed and duration on subsequent walking tests. The test is simple and may be performed daily in the hospital or at home (41).

Any motivated COPD patient who has respiratory symptoms that limit activities of daily living (ADLs) and who has adequate medical, neuromusculoskeletal, financial, and psychosocial status to permit active participation is a candidate for rehabilitation. Active patients who are still able to walk several blocks but who have noted yearly decreases in exercise tolerance or who have recently begun to require ongoing medical attention for pulmonary symptoms or complications are ideal candidates.

Organization of a Comprehensive Rehabilitation Program

The pulmonary rehabilitation multidisciplinary team can consist of a physiatrist and pulmonologist; respiratory, physical, and occupational therapists; an exercise physiologist; a psychiatrist or psychologist; a social worker; a vocational counselor; and a dietitian. However, in the present fiscal environment, an effective small program may have only one specifically trained therapist or nurse under physician supervision (38,42). Consultants can be contacted on an individual basis for patients with difficult-to-address nutritional, psychological, or equipment issues. Because, other than perhaps for smoking cessation (43), there is no evidence that inpatient programs are more effective than outpatient programs (42–45), the former should be reserved for severely debilitated patients (46), for ventilator weaning (47), or for optimizing the ventilatory aid regimen while initiating other aspects of comprehensive rehabilitation. Table 84-2 is a sample therapeutic prescription for an ambulatory, moderately affected COPD patient.

Therapeutic Interventions

MEDICATIONS

The patient's medical regimen is optimized prior to the re-conditioning exercise program. Bronchodilators include β (preferably β-2) agonists, anticholinergics, and theophyllines (48). Most bronchodilators can be delivered orally or as aerosolized solutions. Orally administered β agonists are used when aerosolized medications are ineffective or when metered-dose inhalers can not be efficiently used. Bronchodilators are used to decrease airflow limitation, including reversible bronchospasm, so as to facilitate airway secretion elimination and improve dyspnea and exercise tolerance. One-half and two-thirds of 33 double-blind, randomized, placebo-controlled studies showed significant positive effects of anticholinergics and short-acting β-2 mimetics (especially salbutamol), respectively, on exercise capacity. On the other hand, although theophylline can act as a bronchodilator and has been reported to alleviate diaphragm fatigue (49), increase cardiac output, inhibit mast-cell degranulation, and enhance mucociliary clearance for COPD patients, the majority of studies examining theophylline use on exercise outcomes were negative (50). Greater than 20% improvement in FEV_1 is significant with bronchodilator use, but many physicians use bronchodilators with no apparent effect on FEV_1. Mast-cell membrane stabilizing medications can prevent release of bronchoconstrictor substances for some patients.

Medications that can impair respiratory function are considered, e.g. nonselective β-blocker antihypertensive agents. Systemic glucocorticoid use should generally be discontinued in favor of the use of synthetic steroid inhalers. However, although the latter can be very beneficial for a considerable minority of patients, the overall outcomes of therapy do not justify the widespread use of this treatment in light of increasing

TABLE 84-2.   A Sample Therapeutic Prescription for a Patient with Chronic Obstructive Pulmonary Disease

Diagnosis:
Chronic obstructive pulmonary disease
Prognosis:
Favorable, patient on stable self-medication program
Goals:
- Improve endurance and efficiency
- Optimize oxygen needs and control of secretions
- Increase independence in ambulation and self-care activities
- Reduce anxiety and improve self-esteem through enhanced body awareness
Precautions:
- Supplemental oxygen needed during exercise
- Discontinue and notify physician if patients becomes severely dyspneic or develops chest pain with exercise
Respiratory therapy:
- Conduct ear oximetry at rest and during exercise to determine portable oxygen flow rate needed to maintain oxygen saturation higher than 90%
- Instruct patient in diaphragmatic and pursed-lip breathing
- Instruct patient and family in postural drainage techniques
- Instruct patient and family in portable oxygen use
- Instruct in use of metered-dose inhaler before exercise
- Instruct in use of nocturnal bilevel positive airway pressure
Physical therapy:
- Assess baseline endurance, using 12-minute walk test
- Begin incremental exercise program to improve endurance through ambulation and stair climbing. Begin with 5-minute sessions, followed by rest periods between sessions. When patient tolerates 20 minutes of total exercise per day, begin consolidating the sessions. Initial treatments on daily basis during weeks 1 and 2, taper to three times per week over weeks 3 and 4, and then taper to home program with self-monitoring in weeks 5 and 6.
- Review proper body mechanics and coordinate with breathing patterns, using diaphragmatic and pursed-lip breathing when appropriate
Occupational therapy:
- Assess upper-extremity mobility, strength, and endurance
- Evaluate basic and advanced self-care activities, and provide adaptive aids to improve independence with dressing, hygiene, bathing, cooking, and other chores
- Train the patient in energy conservation and work simplification techniques
- Evaluate home environment and make recommendations for workspace modifications and equipment to improve safety, efficiency, and independence
- Provide relaxation exercise training with visual imagery techniques

recognition of potential adverse systemic effects of high-dose inhaled corticosteroids (51). Other medications, such as expectorants, mucolytics, and antibiotics, are used along with humidification, ample fluid intake, and facilitated airway secretion elimination as warranted. Low-flow nasal supplemental oxygen can be provided to decrease dyspnea, enhance performance, and exert a cardioprotective effect on patients with coronary artery disease. Early medical attention is important during intercurrent respiratory tract infections (52).

COUNSELING AND GENERAL MEDICAL CARE

Dyspnea often causes fear and panic. This may worsen tachypnea while increasing dead space ventilation, the work of breathing, hyperinflation, and air trapping. Relaxation exercises, such as Jacobson exercises and biofeedback, may be used to decrease tension and anxiety (53,54). Diaphragmatic and pursed-lip breathing (described later) also aid in relaxation.

COPD patients perceive impairment in quality of life. Depression has been reported in 50% of patients, and there is often severe reduction in social interaction (55). Integrating psychosocial support with multimodal pulmonary rehabilitation optimizes intervention (56). Loss of employment and physical independence may also need to be addressed.

COPD patients tend to overuse medications during periods of respiratory distress and underuse them otherwise. They are counseled on adhering to their medication regimens (57) and on avoiding atmospheric or vocational pollutants and other aggravating factors, such as pollen, aerosols, excessive humidity, stress, and respiratory tract pathogens. Yearly flu vaccinations are recommended; and pneumococcal vaccines are used one time or every 6 years for high-risk cases. High-altitude travel

may require an additional 0.5 L/min of supplemental oxygen administration for those already requiring supplemental oxygen; otherwise, oxygen therapy generally need not be used only for short flights (58). Good hydration should be maintained with ample fluid intake.

NUTRITION

Significant weight loss occurs in 19% to 71% of COPD patients (32). In one study, 30 of 50 consecutive COPD patients presenting with acute respiratory failure had evidence of significant undernutrition using a multiparameter nutritional index, and impaired nutritional status was more prevalent in those patients requiring mechanical ventilation (74% vs. 43%) (59).

Several studies indicate that not reduced caloric intake but the hypermetabolism that results from the high work of breathing is the primary cause of malnutrition in patients with COPD (60). However, despite the hypercatabolic state, patients with COPD may also decrease food intake because of dyspnea, gastrointestinal side effects of medications, anorexia, and difficulty with meal preparation that is due to related energy expenditure. Folate and B_{12} deficiencies, as well as other forms of avitaminoses, are common in these patients. Lowered antioxidant levels can also potentiate emphysematous changes in lung parenchyma.

Decreased nutrient intake can also be related to eating difficulties resulting from cognitive impairments or from the loss of appetite associated with depression, medications, bloating, and shortness of breath or tachypnea. Indwelling tracheostomy tubes also impair swallowing.

Undernutrition complicating COPD has been associated with increased morbidity and mortality. It has been associated with an increased susceptibility to infection that is due in part to impaired cell-mediated immunity, reduced secretory immunoglobulin A, depressed pulmonary alveolar macrophage function, and increased colonization and adherence of bacteria in the upper and lower airways. Patients with significant nutritional impairment are more frequently colonized by *Pseudomonas* species (61,62). In addition, malnutrition can also adversely affect lung repair, surfactant synthesis, control of ventilation and response to hypoxia, respiratory muscle function and lung mechanics (63), and water homeostasis. It can lead to respiratory muscle atrophy and decreased exercise capacity, cor pulmonale, increased rate of hospitalization for pulmonary-related problems, hypercapnic respiratory failure, and difficulty in weaning from mechanical ventilation (59,64,65). Likewise, inappropriate nutrition, such as increasing carbohydrate intake, can exacerbate hypercapnia.

Short-term refeeding of malnourished patients can improve respiratory muscle endurance and increase respiratory muscle strength in the absence of demonstrable changes in skeletal muscle function (66). However, bloating and abdominal distention that is due to a low diaphragm can result in dyspnea during normal meals (67). For this reason, patients are advised to take small mouthfuls of food, eat slowly, and take smaller and more frequent meals. SpO_2 can be evaluated while eating. If desaturation occurs, supplemental oxygen is used or increased. For those with marginal ventilatory reserve, a dietary regimen high in calories derived from fat can decrease hypercapnia. Although short-term refeeding can be beneficial, refeeding programs lasting more than 2 weeks have not consistently resulted in increases in body weight. Growth hormone has not been shown to be useful. Possible beneficial effects of anabolic steroids as adjuncts to nutritional support and exercise have been suggested but not confirmed (68).

INHALERS

More than 60% of COPD patients use their metered-dose inhalers incorrectly (69). Training in the proper use of inhalers, "spacers," nebulizers, and ventilatory equipment is critical; otherwise, medications are often largely deposited uselessly on the tongue.

BREATHING RETRAINING

Shallow, rapid breathing is commonly seen in anxious and often dyspneic patients. This increases dead-space ventilation and airflow through narrowed airways, thus increasing the flow work of breathing. Patients with chronic airflow obstruction also have an altered pattern of ventilatory muscle recruitment in which the most effective ventilatory pressure is generated by the rib-cage inspiratory muscles rather than by the diaphragm, with significant contribution by expiratory muscles (70). Diaphragmatic breathing and pursed-lip exhalation can help to reverse these tendencies. These techniques are usually initiated in the supine or 15% to 25% head-down position. Deep, essentially diaphragmatic breathing is guided by having the patient place one hand over the abdomen and the other on the thorax just below the clavicle. He should breathe deeply through the nose while distending the abdomen forward as appreciated by movement of the hand on the abdomen. Movement of the rib cage and, thus, the hand on the thorax should be kept to a minimum. Small weights can be placed on the abdomen to provide some resistance training and enhance the patient's focus. During exhalation, the abdominal muscles and the hand on the abdomen should compress the abdominal contents, and exhalation should be via pursed lips (71). Classically, a lighted candle is put several feet in front of the patient, and

the patient flickers the flame while exhaling. This equalizes pleural and bronchial pressures, thus preventing collapse of smaller bronchi and decreasing air trapping. The combination of diaphragmatic and pursed-lip breathing decreases the respiratory rate, coordinates the breathing pattern, and can improve blood gases (72). It should be used often, particularly during routine ADLs or exercise. When used correctly, it can help maintain the cadence of breathing. It can also improve exercise performance by relaxing accessory muscles and improving breathing efficiency.

Air-shifting techniques may be useful to decrease microatelectasis. Air shifting involves taking a deep inspiration that is held with the glottis closed for 5 seconds, during which time the air shifts to lesser-ventilated areas of the lung. The subsequent expiration is via pursed lips. This technique may be most beneficial when performed several times per hour.

AIRWAY SECRETION ELIMINATION

Airway secretion clearance is crucial because exacerbations of COPD are caused by trapping of airway secretions in the peripheral airways. The patient's cough may be weak or ineffective as a result of airway collapse in more central airways than is normal, and frequent bouts of coughing are fatiguing. The high expulsive pressures generated during coughing attempts can exacerbate both air trapping and secretion retention. "Huffing," or frequent short expulsive bursts following a deep breath, is often an effective and more comfortable alternative to coughing. Chest percussion and postural drainage can be useful for patients with chronic bronchitis or others with greater than 30 mL of sputum production per day (73), although caution must be taken to increase oxygen delivery as necessary during treatment.

Autogenic drainage involves breathing with low tidal volumes between the functional residual capacity and residual volume to mobilize secretions in small airways. This is followed by taking increasingly larger tidal volumes and forced expirations to transport mucus to the mouth (74).

Application of positive expiratory pressure (PEP) breathing is based on the theory that mucus in small airways is more effectively mobilized by coughing or forced expirations if alveolar pressure and volume behind mucous plugs are increased. PEP is applied by breathing through a face mask or mouthpiece with an inspiratory tube containing a one-way valve and an expiratory tube containing a variable expiratory resistance. Expiratory pressures of 10 to 20 cm H_2O are maintained throughout expiration. PEP increases functional residual capacity, reducing resistance to airflow in collateral and small airways (75,76). The results of studies on the clinical benefits of PEP breathing have been inconclusive (77) for both CF (78–82), and COPD (82,83).

Flutter breathing is a combination of PEP and oscillation applied at the mouth. The patient expires through a small pipe. A small stainless steel ball rests on the expiratory end of the pipe; it is pushed upward during expiration, producing PEP, and falls downward again, interrupting flow. The mucus-mobilizing effect is thought to be due to widening of the airways because of the increased expiratory pressure and the airflow oscillations that are due to the oscillating ball (84). For this too, however, the results of clinical trials have been conflicting (85). Pryor and colleagues (86), in fact, found that use of the active cycle of breathing technique resulted in a significantly greater amount of expectorated mucus than flutter breathing in a study of CF patients. On the other hand, Bellone et al. reported that use of Flutter combined with expiration with an open glottis in the lateral posture resulted in greater sputum clearance than chest percussion and postural drainage (87). In a recent study of 23 patients with severe COPD, the bronchodilator response to combined ipratropium and salbutamol delivered by metered-dose inhaler was significantly increased, the increases prolonged, and 6-minute walk was better improved by preinhaler use of a Flutter device (88). Flutter alone but not sham also resulted in significant improvements in forced expiratory volume in 1 second (FEV_1) and forced vital capacity (FVC). Despite this, use of the Flutter device is demanding, and it cannot always be easily used by patients with severe disease. Controlled studies need to be done before widely recommending this technique.

With currently available technology, mechanical vibration or oscillation can be mechanically applied to the thorax or directly to the airway to facilitate airway secretion elimination. Vibration is possible at frequencies up to 170 Hz applied under a soft plastic shell to the thorax and abdomen (the Hayek Oscillator™, Breasy Medical Equipment Inc., Stamford, CT). Another device delivers rapid burst airflows at up to 25 Hz under a vest covering the chest and upper abdomen (THAIRapy System, American Biosystems, Inc., St. Paul, MN). The effects of mechanical chest percussion and vibration appear to be frequency dependent (89–91). In most animal studies, frequencies between 10 to 15 Hz appear to best facilitate mucous transport (89,91,92), especially the transport of a thicker mucous layer (93). Warwick and Hansen (94) found long-term increases in FVC and forced expiratory flows for CF patients treated with high-frequency chest-wall compression as compared with receiving manual chest percussion alone. Others have reported improvement in pulmonary function (95) and in gas exchange during high-frequency oscillation (95–98), and Sibuya et al. (98) found that chest-wall vibration decreased dyspnea. Most studies on COPD and CF patients, however, have failed to demonstrate objective clinical benefits from percussion or vibration on mucous transport (99–102). Side effects of percussion and vibration can include increasing obstruction to airflow for some patients with COPD (103,104). In an animal model, the application of vibration and percussion was also associated with the development of atelectasis (105). Despite conflicting studies, the THAIRapy Vest has become popular for CF and familial dysautonomia patients, and attempts are being made to show a decreased hospitalization rate with its daily use. Patients with airways disease and daily airways secretion encumbrance usually feel that its use is beneficial.

The Percussionator (Percussionaire Corp., Sandpoint, ID) can deliver aerosolized medications while providing high-flow percussive minibursts of air directly to the airways at rates of 2.5 to 5 Hz. This intrapulmonary percussive ventilation, too, has been reported to be more effective than chest percussion and postural drainage in the treatment of postoperative atelectasis and secretion mobilization in COPD patients (106,107). The majority of patients using this technique also have felt that it was helpful (108).

Patterson and coworkers (109) found in a 10-year study of CF patients that good patient compliance with methods to assist in mobilizing airway secretions was associated with a slower rate of loss of pulmonary function. Patient compliance with mucus-mobilizing interventions is generally poor, however (110–112). There is greater patient compliance for the use of simpler methods that can be used independently. Some expensive mechanical oscillators are difficult to use independently, and little has been documented concerning long-term safety and efficacy. Thus, they should only be used when there is convincing evidence of clinical benefit. Because there is no evidence that the expensive methods are more effective than simple handheld vibrators costing only about $400 [Jeannie Rub Percussor, Morfan Inc., Mishawaka, IN (Fig, 84-1) or Neo-Cussor General Physical Therapy, St. Louis, MO], the latter should be favored for routine clinical use.

INSPIRATORY RESISTIVE EXERCISES

Inspiratory resistive exercises, including maximum sustained ventilation, inspiratory resistive loading, and inspiratory threshold loading, can improve the endurance of respiratory muscles (113–115). Typically, patients breathe through these devices for a total of 30 minutes daily for 8 to 10 weeks. The settings of the devices are adjusted to increase difficulty as patients improve and the program advances.

Levine and associates conducted an evaluation of the isocapnic hyperpnea method and determined that no more benefits could be derived from it than could be achieved using periodic intermittent positive pressure breathing treatments, a regimen that was considered equivalent to placebo (116). However, Ries et al. randomly assigned 18 patients to either a home isocapnic hyperventilation training program or a walking program and found that the former led to improvements in ventilatory muscle endurance and exercise performance and significant improvements in VO_{2max}, whereas walking exercise improved exercise endurance but did not improve ventilatory muscle endurance (117).

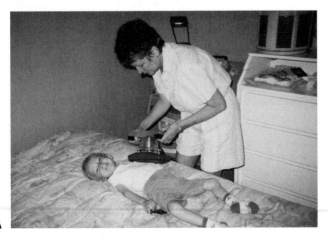
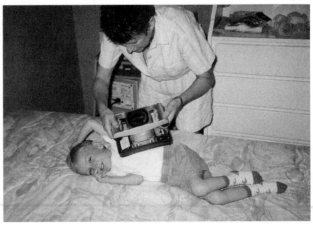

A   B

Figure 84-1. A,B: Jeanie Rub Vibrator M69–315A used on a 6-year-old boy with spinal muscular atrophy type 2 (Morfam Inc., Mishawaka, IN).

Twenty-one controlled studies of inspiratory resistive loading involving 259 COPD patients documented significant improvements in inspiratory muscle strength and endurance (118). The mean increase in strength (increase in maximum inspiratory pressure) was 19%. However, it recently became apparent that many of the subjects of inspiratory resistive training consciously or unconsciously reduced their inspiratory flow rates and lengthened their inspiratory time to reduce the severity of the imposed loads. Consequently, "targeted" or threshold inspiratory muscle training has been recommended over the simpler flow-resistive training to assure adequate intensity of inspiratory muscle activity during training.

With targeted training, the subject is provided feedback regarding the inspiratory flow rates through the resistor or the inspiratory pressure generated by flow through the resistor; with threshold training, the subject is unable to generate flow through the device until a predetermined pressure is achieved. Six of the nine controlled studies of the use of targeted or threshold resistor devices in COPD reported significantly greater improvements in inspiratory muscle function in the subjects than in the controls (118). In three of the six studies in which it was assessed, exercise tolerance was greater for trained subjects than for controls. In one controlled study comparing exercise reconditioning plus threshold inspiratory muscle training with exercise reconditioning alone, the former resulted in significantly greater increases in inspiratory muscle strength and endurance and in exercise tolerance (119). Exercise tolerance seemed to be improved particularly for those with electromyographic changes indicating inspiratory muscle fatigue with exercise (120). One controlled, well-designed, but small study of threshold inspiratory exercise for CF patients demonstrated significant improvements in inspiratory muscle strength, FVC, total lung capacity, and exercise tolerance in the experimental group (121). In another controlled study of patients taking corticosteroids, inspiratory muscle training appeared to prevent the weakness that would have otherwise resulted from the steroid use (122). In another uncontrolled study, besides improvement in respiratory muscle strength, dyspnea was also reportedly decreased (115). Indeed, in a recent study, the combination of inspiratory muscle training along with bronchodilator therapy and reconditioning exercise was demonstrated to very significantly reduce dyspnea by comparison to the use of bronchodilators and general exercise without inspiratory muscle training (123). In general, improvements in inspiratory muscle function and in exercise tolerance were greater for the targeted and threshold studies than for the flow-resistor studies.

When COPD patients failed to demonstrate significantly greater improvements from inspiratory muscle training than did untrained or sham-trained subjects, it may have been because of lack of cooperation with such a tedious and uncomfortable exercise, the presence of chronic inspiratory muscle fatigue, inadequate nutritional status, or concomitant drug therapy (corticosteroids or β-adrenergic blocking agents or agonists), which could prevent or diminish a positive response to a training regimen (118). A recent 6-month controlled study of inspiratory muscle training for asthmatics indicated not only improved inspiratory muscle strength and endurance but also improvement in asthma symptoms, hospitalization, and emergency department contact rates, school or work attendance, and medication consumption (124).

Despite the generally positive results of inspiratory training programs on inspiratory muscle strength and endurance, the positive effects have not been shown to translate into fewer COPD exacerbations or in decreased risk of pulmonary complications or mortality. It is also not clear which regimen of inspiratory resistance training offers the best results, nor whether the benefits are long term. Thus, although controlled trials of inspiratory muscle training have thus far failed to demonstrate a major benefit in a broad range of patients, highly motivated and adequately nourished patients do appear to benefit from training. Improvements are consistently observed and readily demonstrable, and training is inexpensive and lends itself well to home-based exercise programs and the logging of daily results.

RESPIRATORY MUSCLE REST

Relatively minor changes in the pattern of breathing or respiratory muscle loading can place many patients in the critical zone for developing acute respiratory muscle fatigue and failure. Interspersing periods of exercise and muscle rest is a basic principle of rehabilitation. Hypercapnia is an indication of limited reserve before the appearance of overt fatigue and may indicate the need for periods of respiratory muscle assistance or rest before using strengthening exercise (125). Diaphragm rest can be achieved by assisted ventilation using either body ventilators or mouth or nasal ventilation.

Despite high ventilation rates in COPD, ventilatory response to both hypercapnia and hypoxia may be reduced. This is often exacerbated during sleep. The increase in pulmonary vascular resistance that occurs in the presence of pulmonary tissue hypoxia is exacerbated by acidosis. When this situation becomes severe, it may lead to right ventricular failure. The use of oxygen therapy alone may exacerbate CO_2 retention and acidosis.

Two groups of patients may be suited to ventilatory assistance at home. The first and smaller group includes those who require aid around the clock, usually by tracheostomy, but who are medically and psychologically stable. However, these patients tend to require frequent hospital readmission and to have a poorer prognosis than ventilator assisted individuals with NMD. The second group may benefit from nocturnal assistance alone.

There have been numerous reports of the success of various regimens of daytime or nocturnal negative pressure body ventilator (NPBV) use in normalizing arterial blood gases, increasing maximum inspiratory and expiratory pressures, maximal transdiaphragmatic pressure, quality of life, 12-minute walking distance, respiratory muscle endurance, and decreasing dyspnea (126). However, these methods cause obstructive apneas during sleep in the majority of users (127,128). More recently, it has been shown that noninvasive positive pressure ventilation, whether provided by portable volume-cycled ventilator or pressure-limited bilevel positive airway pressure (BiPAP) machine, can rest inspiratory muscles, assist ventilation, and splint open the airway to prevent sleep apneas and airway collapse (129).

Belman and associates reported greater diaphragm relaxation by nasal ventilation than by use of NPBVs (130). Marino demonstrated reversal of nocturnal ventilatory insufficiency for COPD patients using nasal ventilation (131), and others have used assisted ventilation via oral-nasal interfaces as an alternative to intubation and tracheostomy for COPD patients in acute exacerbation (132). Nasal BiPAP has the additional benefit of the expiratory positive airway pressure countering auto–positive end-expiratory pressure (PEEP) in these patients who have a tendency to trap air. This decreases their work of breathing. A number of studies have reported long-term improvements in daytime blood gases with the use of nocturnal nasal ventilation for hypercapnic COPD patients (126,133,134), and it has been suggested that nocturnal ventilator use can also decrease dyspnea, improve quality of life (135), and improve survival (133). Without acutely altering nocturnal PaO_2 or $PaCO_2$ levels, nocturnal nasal BiPAP was also reported to improve sleep efficiency and total sleep time in hypercapnic COPD patients (136). In another study of 49 hypercapnic patients with COPD, while hospitalization rates were decreased by both long-term oxygen therapy (LTOT) as well as by LTOT with nocturnal nasal ventilation by BiPAP, only the latter group had a significant decrease in intensive-care admissions and a significant improvement in 6-minute walk distance (137). Although it is widely considered appropriate to offer nocturnal BiPAP for hypercapnic COPD patients, little or no benefit has been reported with nocturnal use for nonhypercapnic patients, and the role of nocturnal noninvasive ventilation for COPD patients in general remains controversial (138).

SUPPLEMENTAL OXYGEN THERAPY

Supplemental oxygen therapy is indicated for patients with pO_2 continuously less than 55 to 60 mm Hg (39). Home oxygen therapy can decrease pulmonary hypertension, polycythemia, and perception of effort during exercise, and it can prolong life (139,140). Patients with COPD have also been shown to have increased sympathetic modulation and reduced baroreflex sensitivity. Supplemental oxygen has been shown to significantly and favorably alter autonomic modulation and decrease blood pressure and pulse (141). In addition, cognitive function can be improved and hospital needs reduced.

An international consensus on the current status and indications for long-term oxygen therapy recently suggested that the prescription be based on (142):

1. An appropriately documented diagnosis
2. Concurrent optimal use of other rehabilitative approaches, such as pharmacotherapy, smoking abstinence, and exercise training
3. Properly documented chronic hypoxemia

Oxygen therapy should be given with caution to hypercapnic patients whether or not they are using noninvasive ventilation (143).

There is also a possible need for supplemental oxygen during exercise. Many patients exhibit exercise hypoxemia. Often the decrease in SpO_2 occurs within the first minute, after which SpO_2 stabilizes; but occasionally there is a progressive decline in SpO_2 with exercise. In a study of 38 subjects in whom the mean resting SpO_2 was 93±3%, a decrease in SpO_2 of 4.7±3.6% (range 1%–18%) was observed during submaximal exercise (144). Decreases in SpO_2 are noted at physical activity levels comparable to those necessary to perform ADLs.

In a crossover study of 12 subjects with severe COPD (145), four patients more than doubled their duration of exercise while receiving 40% oxygen, but in only two of these was desaturation observed in the absence of oxygen. Bradley et al. (146) reported that in subjects with mild hypoxemia and exercise desaturation, supplemental oxygen by nasal prongs did not influence maximum work rate but did influence endurance. Davidson and associates noted that oxygen increased mean walking endurance time by 59% and 6-minute walking distance by 17%. Moreover, submaximal cycle time at a constant workload was increased by 51% at a flow rate of 2 L/m and by 88% at 4 L/m, suggesting a dose response curve (147). The exercise response to oxygen could not be predicted from the degree of desaturation, resting pulmonary function tests, echocardiographic measurements of right ventricular systolic pressure, or other clinical parameters (145). In fact, in nonhypoxemic COPD patients performing moderate exercise, oxygen supplementation decreases ventilatory requirement by its direct effect on chemoreceptor inhibition (148). Thus, exercise tolerance can be increased by oxygen therapy without improving oxygen consumption or utilization. Marcus et al. also reported significantly greater exercise tolerance in CF patients receiving oxygen (149).

The most widely accepted guideline for prescribing oxygen use during exercise is that of exercise-induced SpO_2 below 90%. However, it seems reasonable to recommend that measurements of dyspnea and exercise tolerance be undertaken with and without supplemental oxygen to determine which individuals are less short of breath or walk further (have greater exercise tolerance) when given supplemental oxygen. Because of the inconsistencies in patient response to oxygen therapy, patients should be individually evaluated (150). Certainly, exercise-induced decreases in SpO_2 below 90% when combined with increased exercise tolerance with oxygen therapy warrants the prescription of oxygen therapy during exercise.

Inspiratory phase or pulsed oxygen therapy, especially when delivered transtracheally, avoids waste and decreases discomfort and drying of mucous membranes. Oxygen flow delivery is 0.25–0.4 l/min compared to 2–4 l/min when delivered via nasal cannulas or face masks (151,152). Oxygen therapy should be used in combination with mechanical ventilation for patients with concomitant carbon dioxide retention.

RECONDITIONING EXERCISE

Because of decreased efficiency of gas exchange, there is an abnormally high ventilatory requirement and a rapid increase in breathing frequency by comparison to tidal volume during exercise. The COPD patient's maximal exercise ventilation (VE_{max}) is close to or exceeds maximum voluntary ventilation. Cardiac output rises normally with exercise, but exercise can cease at relatively low heart rates because of the ventilatory limitation associated with dyspnea. Hypoxia (153)—and in severely limited patients, hypercapnia—may occur with exercise. Thus, not all patients can attain the 60% to 70% of predicted maximum heart rate and the minute oxygen consumption needed for cardiac or aerobic exercise training. Even when the ventilatory anaerobic threshold (VAT) can not be achieved, however, maximum symptom-limited oxygen consumption does correlate with ability to perform ADLs, and it can be significantly increased with exercise training (154).

Independent of LTOT, it has been suggested that rehabilitation with exercise reconditioning may prolong survival for COPD patients (155). For 149 patients, 89% of whom had COPD and mean age of 69 years, age, sex, body mass index, and primary diagnosis were not related to survival after completion of a pulmonary rehabilitation program. However, a higher postrehabilitation functional activities score, a longer postrehabilitation 6-min walk distance, and being married were strongly associated with increased survival (156). Gerardi et al. also demonstrated that postrehabilitation 12-min walk was a strong predictor of survival and much better than PaO_2, $PaCO_2$, FEV_1, and nutritional status (157). Thus, exercise tolerance is extremely important for predicting survival.

In normal male subjects, as well as in COPD patients, the intensity of training is the most important factor in improving maximum oxygen consumption (VO_2 max). Greater exercise tolerance results from high- rather than low-intensity programs. Punzal et al. demonstrated that moderately to severely affected COPD patients could exercise at 95% of the baseline maximum treadmill workload. At training weeks 1, 4, and 8, they can train at 85%, 84%, and 86%, respectively, of initial baseline maximum. Maximum treadmill workload, VO_{2max}, and endurance exercise time can be increased and symptoms decreased in this manner (158). The minority of patients who did not reach the anaerobic threshold were able to train at a higher percentage of maximum exercise tolerance than patients who reached anaerobic threshold, but the increase in exercise performance was similar for both groups. Indeed, moderate to severely affected COPD patients can perform exercise training successfully at intensity levels that represent higher percentages of maximum than typically recommended in normal individuals or other patients (158). Although both men and women benefit from short-term (3-month) exercise therapy with improvements in dyspnea, fatigue, and emotional function, men but not women continued to benefit from long-term exercise therapy (159).

The VAT is defined as the highest VO_2 during exercise above which sustained lactic acidosis occurs. The VAT can be consistently achievable for patients with less than very advanced disease, including for patients with 0.5 L of FEV_1. The parameters of a 45-minute, maximally intense, bilevel training prescription can be derived from bilevel exercise in cycles of 4 minutes of exercise at the VAT (lower level) and 1 minute at the VO_2 max (upper level) (160). For the minority of cases for whom the VAT can not be achieved, bilevel exercise can be provided by using the maximum VO_2 attained for the upper (1-minute) level and 40% of this figure for the lower (4-minute) level. These intensities can be maintained for 45 minutes in a maximally intense endurance exercise program using a Square Wave Endurance Exercise Trainer, essentially a cycle ergometer.

Imprecisely prescribed exercise regimens—for example, when too intense to be tolerated for 45-minute sessions—will result in patients failing to complete the prescribed sessions and deriving suboptimal benefits on endurance. Others, for whom the prescription is submaximalm will be able to complete the 45-minute sessions but at exercise intensities inadequate for optimally effective reconditioning. Submaximal exercise programs have not been demonstrated to increase VO_{2max} or reduce lactate production. Increases in VO_{2max} can result in both lower ventilation requirement at given exercise levels and increased exercise tolerance.

Some advocate guiding initial exercise intensity by parameters of clinical exercise testing, e.g., heart rate at ventilation levels of 37.5 times the FEV_1 (38). Such patients benefiting from high-intensity exercise training can increase exercise ventilation and sustain it at a high percentage of their maximum voluntary ventilation. With training, they can exceed the levels attained during initial exercise testing (117). For example, 34 patients in one study could walk at a work level of 86% of their baseline maximum for a mean duration of 22 minutes (117). Carter et al. also trained patients at near their ventilatory limits and reported mean peak exercise ventilation of 94% to 100% of measured maximum voluntary ventilation (161). Training above the anaerobic threshold leads to a reduced ventilatory requirement during exercise and, therefore, improved maximum exercise tolerance (162).

Walking, stair climbing, calisthenics, bicycling, and pool activities may be used for reconditioning. The patient is made responsible for a progressive program. As a minimum, we recommend the purchase of a stationary bicycle for the patient's home and its daily use. A daily 12-minute walk is recommended, as well as daily 15-minute sessions of inspiratory muscle training. A daily log of time and distance walked and bicycled and of the inspiratory resistance tolerated during 15-minute inspiratory training sessions provides feedback to both the patient and physician. In general, the pulse should return to baseline 5 to 10 minutes after exercise. Increased endurance for exercise can occur independently of changes in ventilatory

muscle endurance. A typical program consists of weekly reevaluations for 10 to 12 weeks, during which the patient logs are reviewed and exercise parameters modified. Educational and peer groups sessions reinforce the activities. Such a program is inexpensive, minimally intrusive, and optimizes the chances for continued independent adherence to the protocol following the 10- to 12-week supervision period.

UPPER-EXTREMITY EXERCISE

Upper-extremity reconditioning is part of any comprehensive program. Many arm and shoulder muscles are also accessory muscles of respiration and, as such, are very active for patients with COPD. The overlap in function explains why COPD patients are particularly short of breath when performing upper-extremity ADLs.

It is widely felt that only muscles that are trained respond to the training (163) and that little or no carryover of benefit to upper-extremity function is possible from lower-extremity exercise. Belman and Kendregan, for example, demonstrated a significant increase in arm cycle endurance for an arm-trained group and leg cycle endurance for a leg-trained group, without crossover effect (164). Since then, several other studies have demonstrated benefits in gas exchange, strength, endurance, and performance in ADLs when arm cranking is added to leg exercise as part of comprehensive programs of rehabilitation (165–168). Training of the upper extremities in COPD reduces the increased metabolic demand and ventilation associated with arm elevation and reduces dyspnea (167). Although upper-extremity training increases endurance for arm exercise, no apparent effects have been demonstrated on ADLs (155). However, further studies on upper-extremity exercise training are required before firm conclusions can be drawn concerning performance of ADLs.

The possibility of crossover effects of exercise is controversial. Because it has been shown that highly trained swimmers have a relatively high VO_{2max} when running, it seems possible that long-term endurance training may generate adaptations that are in part transferable to other modes of endurance exercise. In fact, although crossover benefits of training are not widely recognized (164) (quite possibly because of the submaximal nature of most exercise prescriptions), a program of maximally tolerable daily 45-minute exercise sessions has resulted in significantly decreased dyspnea at rest (p<0.01), decreased blood lactate at submaximal (40-watt) exercise levels (p<0.001); increased VO_{2max} and total physical work (p<0.01), increased maximum inspiratory and expiratory pressures (p<0.01), and increased grip and forearm strength and endurance (p<0.01); and it increased maximum voluntary ventilation while decreasing the ventilatory equivalent at the VO_{2max} and during the exercise (p<0.001) (160).

Unsupported upper-extremity activities range from typing, lifting, reaching, and carrying to athletic activities and personal daily care (eating, grooming, cleaning). Unsupported arm exercise shifts work to the diaphragm, leading to earlier fatigue (165). In a randomized controlled trial comparing supported arm exercise with unsupported arm exercise within a general rehabilitation program for COPD patients, the group performing the unsupported upper-extremity exercise demonstrated significantly greater improvements and reduced oxygen consumption during upper-extremity exercise than the supported upper-extremity exercise group (166). Five other studies have recently substantiated the greater benefits to be derived from unsupported rather than supported upper-extremity exercise (165).

The Results of Pulmonary Rehabilitation

In a review of 48 pulmonary rehabilitation studies that included exercise reconditioning, exercise tolerance improved significantly in all 48 studies, including 14 controlled studies (42). It improved equally significantly (proportionally) in patients with mild or advanced (hypercapnic) (169) disease. Consistent improvements included decreases in the ventilatory equivalent or the ventilation/oxygen consumption ratio, increases in work efficiency (external work per unit of oxygen consumed) and thus in exercise tolerance, ambulation capacity, general well-being, and dyspnea tolerance. The patients developed better performance strategies and greater confidence in performing the tests. In many programs, decreases in blood lactate levels were also observed in combination with higher maximum oxygen consumption (VO_{2max}), implying a physiologic training effect as well as improved motivation and effort. Maximum tolerated intensity exercise regimens yielded better results than low-intensity exercise for proportionally longer periods (160,170,171).

In general, peak performance appeared to be reached in 26 to 51 weeks and lasted for as long as 5 years (170–173). Quality-of-life measures (45,174–176), hospitalization rates, postoperative pulmonary complications (177), and physical functioning were likewise reported to be significantly improved in the majority of both the controlled and the repetitive measure studies (42). Outcomes were equivalent for inpatient and outpatient programs, although many of the outpatient programs were predominantly home based. Pulmonary function parameters, such as FEV_1, did not significantly improve in 31 of 35 studies (42).

Thus, virtually all studies indicate that pulmonary rehabilitation including exercise training results in significant increases in ambulation capacity and exercise endurance for COPD patients, as well as for many patients with other intrinsic lung pathology (178). The often-reported decreased resting oxygen consumption and carbon dioxide production may, at least in part, account for the significant decrease in perception of dyspnea, the general increase in functional performance, and in the often-found improved sense of well-being.

One study of 120 advanced hypercapnic COPD patients, 117 of whom with FEV_1 less than 1 L, demonstrated significant increases in PaO_2, vital capacity (VC), FEV_1, maximum inspiratory pressures, and ambulation tolerance with pulmonary rehabilitation, including exercise reconditioning. Maximum expiratory pressures did not change significantly. The higher the initial $PaCO_2$, the more $PaCO_2$ fell and PaO_2 rose during the rehabilitation program. The patients' improvement in performance of ADLs correlated with increased walking distance. Thus, hypercapnia is not a contraindication to intensive rehabilitation, and the use of rigorous reconditioning exercise does not precipitate respiratory muscle fatigue in this population (169). Indeed, because improvements in both physiologic and psychologic parameters are not directly related to lung function, the benefits of rehabilitation can extend to all patients with COPD, regardless of the severity of preexisting pulmonary disease (154).

In one study of 61 of 80 bedridden ventilator-dependent COPD patients in a respiratory care unit, 60 underwent a stepwise rehabilitation program consisting of skeletal and respiratory muscle training and early ambulation. Twenty percent of both the rehabilitation and nonrehabilitation patients died while in the unit. However, all but nine of the rehabilitation patients were weaned from invasive mechanical ventilation after a mean stay of 38±14 days (47). Six-minute walk distances and mean inspiratory pressure increased significantly more in the rehabilitation group.

Following the acute rehabilitation period, continued surveillance and attention to abstinence from smoking, bronchial hygiene, breathing retraining, physical reconditioning, oxygen therapy, and airway secretion mobilization have been shown to reduce hospital admissions, the length of hospital stays, and cost (179). As noted, the benefits of pulmonary rehabilitation on exercise performance and quality of life persist for up to 5 years (170–173,180–183). Pulmonary function parameters, dyspnea, exercise tolerance, and quality of life are not further improved long-term by yearly repeated 2-month outpatient pulmonary rehabilitation interventions, but rates of hospitalizations and acute exacerbations are further decreased by repeated interventions (184). The principles of rehabilitation for COPD are being increasingly applied to patients with asthma with similar outcomes (185).

REHABILITATION OF PATIENTS WITH RESTRICTIVE PULMONARY IMPAIRMENT AND SLEEP-DISORDERED BREATHING

Pathophysiology

Despite total respiratory muscle paralysis, patients with primarily lung ventilation impairment on the basis of respiratory muscle weakness or central hypoventilation can avoid episodes of respiratory failure with the use of physical medicine inspiratory and expiratory muscle aids. Ventilatory insufficiency is defined by hypercapnia in the presence of a normal arterial-alveolar A-a gradient. It is hypercapnia not caused by intrinsic lung disease or irreversible upper- or lower-airway obstruction as in COPD. These patients can have airway obstruction from bronchial mucous plugging that causes an elevated A-a gradient. However, the mucous plugging is reversible by using expiratory (cough) aids. Symptomatic hypercapnic patients benefit from the use of noninvasive ventilation for at least part of the day, most often overnight. With progressive ventilatory muscle weakness, withdrawal of periods of daily or nightly aid for these patients eventually results in ventilatory failure.

Ventilatory muscle failure is the inability of the inspiratory and expiratory muscles to sustain one's respiration without resort to ventilator use. Ventilatory insufficiency leading to failure can be nocturnal only and result from diaphragm failure with the patient unable to breathe when supine, can result from a lack of central ventilatory drive, or can result from severe generalized respiratory muscle dysfunction. Many patients with ventilatory insufficiency survive for years without ventilator use at the cost of increasing hypercapnia, its associated symptoms and dangers, and a compensatory metabolic alkalosis that depresses central ventilatory drive. The alkalosis allows the brain to accommodate to hypercapnia without overt symptoms of acute ventilatory failure. When such patients are treated with noninvasive intermittent positive pressure ventilation (IPPV)—"ventilatory assistance,"—blood gases normalize and the alkalosis resolves as the kidneys excrete excess bicarbonate ions. Then, because of the need to take bigger breaths to maintain normal $PaCO_2$ and blood pH levels, the ventilator user becomes intolerably short of breath when discontinuing ventilator use and, at least temporarily, loses any significant breathing tolerance. Without ventilator use, the patient develops increasingly severe hypercapnia that eventually results in coma that is due to carbon dioxide narcosis or ventilatory arrest. Thus, patients with ventilatory muscle dysfunction can require daily periods of, and at times, continuous, ventilatory support. Some patients with ventilatory muscle failure and no measurable VC with their breathing muscles use only nocturnal aid and rely on glossopharyngeal breathing (GPB) to ventilate their lungs during daytime hours.

For patients with primarily ventilatory impairment, respiratory morbidity and mortality are a direct result of respiratory muscle dysfunction and can be avoided by assisting respiratory muscles so long as bulbar muscle dysfunction is not so severe that the SpO_2 remains below 95% because of continuous aspiration of saliva. Such patients develop essentially irreversible upper-airway obstruction and require tracheostomy tubes to protect the airway. In general, this scenario occurs for bulbar amyotrophic lateral sclerosis (ALS) patients who have lost the ability to speak and for few other patients with NMDs.

Epidemiology

There are 500,000 people in the United States, or 0.15% of the population, with pediatric NMDs (186) and many more with thoracic wall restrictive lung disease. One out of 3,500 boys is born with Duchenne muscular dystrophy (DMD), one in 5,000 children have spinal muscular atrophy (SMA), and 1 in 1,800 people develop ALS. It has been estimated that of the patients who had acute poliomyelitis, 1.63 million with a median age of 57 were still alive in 1987. Many of these patients have ventilatory insufficiency and require ventilator use today. Respiratory muscle dysfunction amenable to treatment by respiratory muscle aids also occurs in people with the diagnoses listed in Table 84-3.

Surveys of the United States, Western Europe, and Japan indicate that the use of home mechanical ventilation is increasing rapidly (186). Most people who appear to require more than nocturnal ventilator use, however, and those who have difficulty weaning when intubated during chest infections generally undergo tracheotomy. This often occurs because of failure

to introduce physical medicine aids. Likewise, 90% of episodes of acute respiratory failure for young patients with NMD occur as a result of inability to generate effective PCFs during otherwise benign upper-respiratory infections (187). These episodes are usually avoidable.

What Are Physical Medicine Respiratory Muscle Aids?

Inspiratory and expiratory muscle aids are devices and techniques that involve the manual or mechanical application of forces to the body or intermittent pressure changes to the airway to assist inspiratory or expiratory muscle function. The devices that act on the body include NPBVs that create pressure changes around the thorax and abdomen. Negative pressure applied to the airway during expiration or coughing assists coughing just as positive pressure applied to the airway during inhalation (noninvasive ventilation) assists the inspiratory muscles. Continuous positive airway pressure (CPAP) does not assist ventilation and is rarely useful for patients with primarily ventilatory impairment.

Patient Evaluation

Patients with diminished ventilatory reserve who are able to walk chiefly report exertional dyspnea. Eventually, morning headaches, fatigue, sleep disturbances, and hypersomnolence develop (188). For wheelchair users, symptoms may be minimal, except during intercurrent respiratory infections when anxiety, inability to fall asleep, and dyspnea become problems.

The patient is observed for increased rate, decreased depth, or irregularity of breathing. Purely diaphragmatic breathing or

---

TABLE 84-3. Conditions with Functional Bulbar Musculature that Can Result in Chronic Alveolar Hypoventilation

Myopathies
Muscular dystrophies
Dystrophinopathies: Duchenne and Becker dystrophies
Other muscular dystrophies: limb-girdle, Emery-Dreifuss, facioscapulohumeral, congenital, childhood autosomal recessive, and myotonic dystrophy non-Duchenne myopathies
Congenital, metabolic, inflammatory, and mitochondrial myopathies Myopathies of systemic disease, such as carcinomatous myopathy, cachexia/anorexia nervosa, medication-associated diseases of the myoneural junction
Mixed connective tissue disease
Neurological disorders
Spinal muscular atrophies
Motor neuron diseases
Poliomyelitis
Neuropathies
Hereditary sensory motor neuropathies
Familial hypertrophic interstitial polyneuropathy
Phrenic neuropathies
Guillain-Barré syndrome
Multiple sclerosis
Disorders of supraspinal tone, such as Friedreich's ataxia
Myelopathies of rheumatoid, infectious, spondylitic, vascular, traumatic, or idiopathic etiology
Tetraplegia associated with pancuronium bromide, botulism
Static encephalopathies, syringomyelia, myelomeningocele
Sleep-disordered breathing, including obesity hypoventilation, central hypoventilation syndromes, hypoventilation associated with diabetic microangiopathy, familial dysautonomia, Prader-Willi syndrome
Kyphoscoliosis, idiopathic or from osteogenesis imperfecta, rigid spine syndrome, spondyloepiphyseal dysplasia congenita, tuberculosis, central nervous system disease
Restrictive lung disease associated with lung resection, tuberculosis, Milroy's disease, congenital diaphragmatic hernia, vocal cord paralysis, postlaryngotracheal reconstruction
Endocrine abnormalities as with hypothyroidism, acromegaly
Mixed ventilatory-respiratory impairment like chronic obstructive pulmonary disease, cystic fibrosis

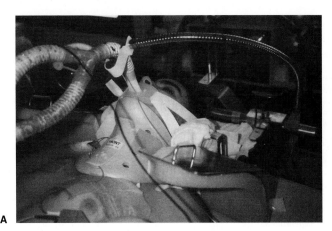
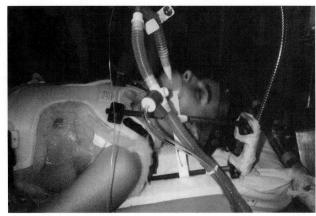

A   B

Figure 84-2. 15-year-old patient with acute high-level spinal cord injury, continuously ventilator dependent from 12 hours postinjury. Never intubated, he uses lipseal intermittent positive pressure ventilation (IPPV) while sleeping (seen here) and a simple mouth piece for IPPV while awake, without ventilator-free breathing ability, for 10 days before weaning from ventilator use. Because there is no neck movement, the lipseal is used with a single Velcro strap to the posterior poster rather than the customary two straps.

asymmetric movement of the abdomen or thorax are often present. Hypophonia, nasal alae flaring, use of auxiliary respiratory musculature, peribuccale or generalized cyanosis, flushing or pallor, hypertension, difficulty controlling airway secretions, dysphagia, regurgitation of fluids through the nose, nasality of speech, cor pulmonale, confusion, and fluid retention may all be signs of ventilatory insufficiency.

Maximum inspiratory and expiratory pressures generated at the mouth correlate best with inspiratory and expiratory muscle strength. Maximum voluntary ventilation gauges respiratory muscle endurance. The VC gives an indication of both of these parameters and is simple, easy to measure, objective, and very reproducible. Because hypoventilation is often worst during sleep, the supine rather than sitting position VC is the most important indicator of ventilatory dysfunction. Spirometry is also useful for monitoring progress with GPB and air stacking. A patient's maximum insufflation capacity (MIC) is determined by giving the patient the largest volume of air that can be held with a closed glottis, usually from a volume-cycled ventilator or Cough Assist™, or by teaching the patient to stack volumes of air consecutively delivered from a manual resuscitator or volume-cycled ventilator. The patient holds the stacked volumes with a closed glottis until the lungs are expanded as much as possible and then expels the air into the spirometer. Patients who learn GPB can often air stack consecutive GPB gulps to or beyond the MIC independently of mechanical assistance (189). A nasal interface or lipseal can be used for air stacking when the lips are too weak for effective air stacking via the mouth (Fig. 84-2).

PCFs are measured using a peak flow meter (Access Peak Flow Meter, Healthscan Products Inc., Cedar Grove, NJ). PCFs of 160 L/m are the minimum needed to eliminate airway secretions (190), and this is the best indicator for tracheostomy tube removal irrespective of remaining pulmonary function (Fig. 84-3) (191). Indeed, almost 50% of patients with ALS can survive despite continuous ventilator dependence using strictly noninvasive aids (192). Patients with VCs less than 1,500 mL have assisted PCF measured from a maximally stacked volume of air and with an abdominal thrust delivered simultaneously with glottic opening.

For the stable patient without intrinsic pulmonary disease, arterial blood gas sampling is unnecessary. Besides the discomfort, 25% of patients hyperventilate as a result of anxiety or pain during the procedure (110). Noninvasive continuous blood gas monitoring, including capnography and oximetry, yield more useful information, particularly during sleep.

Nocturnal noninvasive blood gas monitoring is performed for patients with diminished supine VC, especially for those with rapidly evolving conditions and symptoms suggestive of hypoventilation. The oximeter and the capnograph, which measures end-tidal pCO_2, must be capable of summarizing and printing out the data (188). These studies are most conveniently performed in the home. Any symptomatic patient with decreased VC, multiple nocturnal $dSpO_2$s below 95%, and elevated nocturnal $PaCO_2$ requires treatment for nocturnal hypoventilation.

For symptomatic patients with normal VC, an unclear pattern of oxyhemoglobin desaturation, and no apparent carbon dioxide retention, sleep disordered breathing is suspected. This is particularly true when loud high-pitched snoring, interrupted breathing, and hypersomnolence dominate the picture (193). These patients undergo polysomnography and are con-

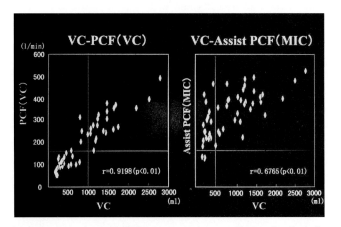

Figure 84-3. Peak cough flows increase from ineffective levels (below 160 L/m) to effective levels by maximally insufflating the patient and then providing an abdominal thrust. (With permission and appreciation to Dr. Yuka Ishikawa). Dept. of Pediatrics Yakumo Byoin National Sanatorium, Yakumo-cho Hikkardo.

sidered for CPAP therapy. Obesity-hypoventilation patients are treated with nocturnal ventilatory support, as are NMD patients. When concurrent obstructive or interstitial lung disease is documented by pulmonary function studies, capnography is correlated to $PaCO_2$.

The Intervention Objectives

The intervention goals are to maintain lung and chest-wall compliance and to promote normal lung and chest-wall growth for children by mobilization, to maintain normal alveolar ventilation around the clock, and to maximize cough flows. The long-term goals are to avert episodes of acute respiratory failure during intercurrent chest infections, avoid hospitalizations, and prolong survival without resorting to tracheotomy. All goals can be attained by evaluating, training, and equipping patients in the outpatient setting and at home.

GOAL ONE: MAINTAIN PULMONARY COMPLIANCE, LUNG GROWTH, AND CHEST-WALL MOBILITY

Pulmonary compliance is lost because the ability to expand the lungs to the predicted inspiratory capacity is lost as the VC decreases. As the VC decreases, the largest breath that one can take can only expand a small portion of the lungs. Like limb articulations and other soft tissues, regular range-of-motion (ROM) is required to prevent chest-wall contractures and lung restriction. This can only be achieved by providing deep insufflations, air stacking, or nocturnal noninvasive ventilation (194). The extent to which the MIC is greater than the VC predicts the capacity of the patient to be maintained by noninvasive rather than tracheostomy ventilatory support (190). This is because the MIC vs. VC difference, like assisted PCF, is a function of bulbar muscle integrity.

The primary objectives in using air stacking or maximum insufflations for lung and chest-wall ROM are to increase the MIC, to maximize PCF (see Fig. 84-3), to maintain or improve pulmonary compliance, to prevent or eliminate atelectasis, and to master noninvasive IPPV. In 278 spirometry evaluations of NMD patients able to air stack, we found mean sitting VC to be 1190.5 mL, a mean supine of 974.9 mL, and a mean MIC of 1820.7 mL. The higher volumes increase both unassisted and manually assisted PCF, and they permit the patient to raise voice volume as desired.

Because any patient who can air stack is also able to use noninvasive IPPV, if such a patient is intubated for respiratory failure, he or she can be extubated directly to continuous noninvasive IPPV regardless of whether the patient regained any breathing tolerance. Extubation of a patient with little or no breathing tolerance who has not been trained in noninvasive IPPV can result in panic, ventilator dyssynchrony, asphyxia, and possible reintubation.

Before patients' VCs decrease to 70% of predicted normal, they are instructed to air stack 10 to 15 times at least two or three times daily. Thus, the first respiratory equipment that is prescribed for patients with ventilatory impairment is often a manual resuscitator. In general, because of the importance of air stacking, patients without air trapping who have less than normal VC use volume-cycled ventilators rather than pressure-limited ventilators unless the pressure-limited ventilator can attain the 50 to 80 cm H_2O pressures required for insufflation to the MIC.

Infants can not air stack or cooperate to receive maximal insufflations. All SMA type 1 babies, SMA type 2 infants and others with infantile NMD who have paradoxical chest-wall movement require nocturnal high-span bi-level positive airway pressure to prevent pectus excavatum and promote lung growth (195). Although widely thought to be fatal before age 2, management of SMA1 according to a recently described noninvasive respiratory aid protocol allows many of these patients to survive early childhood. They have fewer medical difficulties and hospitalizations as they get older (195). In addition to nocturnal aid, deep insufflations can be provided via oral-nasal interface for children older than 1 year of age along with concomitant abdominal compression to prevent abdominal expansion while directing the air into the upper thorax. These insufflations need to be timed to the child's inspirations. Children can become cooperative with deep insufflation therapy by 14 to 30 months of age.

GOAL TWO: CONTINUOUSLY MAINTAIN NORMAL ALVEOLAR VENTILATION BY ASSISTING INSPIRATORY MUSCLES AS NEEDED

I. The Nocturnal Inspiratory Muscle Aids
   A. Negative Pressure Body Ventilators

The NPBVs available today include the iron lung, the Porta-Lung™, chest-shell ventilator, and various wrap-style ventilators. They are only practical for use during sleep. Although NPBVs have been used by patients with little or no VC for decades, they become ineffective with aging and decreasing pulmonary compliance (127). Such patients are switched to noninvasive IPPV (196,197). Although NPBVs continue to be used in a few centers (including ours) as a "bridge" to noninvasive IPPV while extubating unweanable patients (198,199), it is debatable whether their long-term use is ever warranted today.

   B. Noninvasive Intermittent Positive Pressure Ventilation

IPPV can be noninvasively delivered via mouthpieces and nasal and oral-nasal interfaces for nocturnal ventilatory support. Although for acutely ill patients, introduction of noninvasive ventilation needs to be done in the hospital setting, the great majority of noninvasive IPPV users are introduced to it in the clinic and home setting.

   1. Mouthpiece Intermittent Positive Pressure Ventilation

Many patients with little or no measurable VC, and no upper-extremity function, who have used ventilators without alarms have kept simple 15- or 22-mm angled mouthpieces (Respironics Inc., Murrysville, PA) between their teeth and received mouthpiece IPPV for continuous ventilatory support for years without losing the mouthpiece and dying from asphyxia. However, these patients invariably have disturbed sleep architecture and many nocturnal $dSpO_2$s. When using mouthpiece IPPV during sleep, a lipseal retention system with two cloth straps with Velcro closures is strongly recommended (Mallincrodt, Pleasanton, CA) (see Fig. 84-2). The retention straps of an Adam circuit (Mallincrodt Inc., Pleasanton, CA) can be substituted for the cloth straps.

The lipseal can provide an essentially closed system of noninvasive ventilatory support. Mouthpiece IPPV with lipseal retention is delivered during sleep with little insufflation leakage out of the mouth and with virtually no risk of the mouthpiece falling out of the mouth. A new strapless lipseal system called the Oracle (Fisher-Paykel Inc., New Zealand) is on the market. Yet another newly described lipseal is made of transparent silicon. It has no intraoral mouth piece but a similar retention strap system (Masque Buccal, Metamed, France) (200). Orthodontic bite plates and custom fabricated acrylic lipseals can also increase comfort and efficacy, and eliminate the orthodontic deformity that can otherwise occur in some long-term continuous mouthpiece IPPV users.

Generally, symptoms from nasal insufflation leakage during lipseal IPPV remain subclinical because the typically used high ventilator insufflation volumes of 1,000 to 2,000 mL compensate, at least in part, for nasal leakage. Whether using nocturnal nasal or lipseal IPPV in a regimen of 24-hour noninvasive IPPV, and despite the maintenance of normal daytime alveolar ventilation, 3% to 10% of patients with no breathing tolerance (5 of 161) (201) have episodes of excessive insufflation leakage and transient dSpO$_2$s during sleep. These can result in arousals with shortness of breath. The patient may also report recurrence of morning headaches, fatigue, and perhaps nightmares and anxiety. The nasal ventilation user can be switched to lipseal IPPV. Lipseal IPPV users can have their systems "closed" by having their nostrils plugged with cotton and covered by a Band-Aid during sleep. Another practical solution is to set the ventilator's low pressure alarm at a level that by its sounding stimulates the patient sufficiently to shorten periods of excessive insufflation leakage during sleep. Commonly, a low-pressure alarm setting of 10 to 15 cm H$_2$O pressure is used for this purpose, and the patient develops conditioned reflexes to prevent prolonged excessive leak associated dSpO$_2$s and hypoventilation.

2. Nasal Intermittent Positive Pressure Ventilation

Nasal is preferred over lipseal IPPV by more than two out of three patients who use IPPV only for sleep (188). Nasal IPPV with PEEP can be provided by portable pressure or volume-cycled ventilators. There are now numerous commercially available nasal interfaces (CPAP masks). Each interface design applies pressure differently to the paranasal area. One can not predict which model will be most effective and preferred by any particular patient. Nasal bridge pressure and insufflation leakage into the eyes are common symptoms with several of these generic models. Such difficulties resulted in the fabrication of interfaces that mold themselves to facial tissues and custom-molded interface designs (6,188,202–205). No patient should be offered and expected to use only one nasal interface

anymore than one should be offered only lipseal or oral-nasal interfaces. Alternating IPPV interfaces nightly alternates skin pressure sites, minimizes discomfort, and is to be encouraged.

Excessive insufflation leakage via the mouth is prevented by keeping ventilatory drive intact by maintaining normal daytime CO$_2$ and avoiding supplemental O$_2$ and sedatives. However, in the presence of daytime hypercapnia and excessive nocturnal dSpO$_2$s and bothersome arousals, for patients not wishing to switch to lipseal IPPV, a chin strap or plugged lipseal without mouthpiece can be used to decrease oral leakage. In the presence of nasal congestion, patients either use decongestants to permit nasal IPPV or they switch to mouthpiece and lipseal IPPV; on rare occasions, they use a body ventilator. Most often, the patient continues nasal IPPV using decongestants.

Oral-nasal interfaces can have strap retention systems like those for mouthpiece or nasal IPPV or can be custom fabricated and strapless and retained by bite plates (206). Because effective ventilatory support can usually be provided by either nasal or mouthpiece/lipseal IPPV, oral-nasal interfaces are infrequently used for long-term assisted ventilation.

Although mouthpiece and nasal IPPV are usually used as open systems and the user relies on central nervous system reflexes to prevent excessive insuffla-

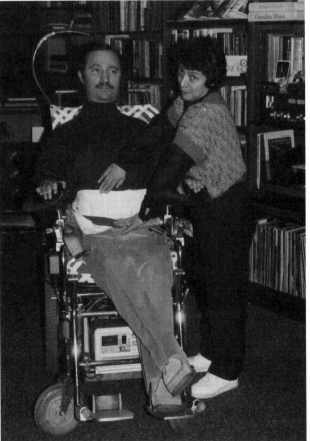

Figure 84-4. A postpolio survivor with no measurable vital capacity since 1952 using an intermittent abdominal pressure ventilator (Exsufflation Belt™, Respironics International Inc., Murrysville, PA) during daytime hours and lipseal IPPV nightly since 1956. The air bladder inside the girdle is connected to the ventilator circuit (seen here), then the girdle is placed under the clothes and over the patient's abdomen.

tion leakage during sleep (188,207), essentially closed noninvasive IPPV systems include lipseal with nasal pledgets, strap-retained oral-nasal interfaces, and strapless oro-nasal interfaces.

II. The Daytime Inspiratory Muscle Aids

A. Body Ventilators

The intermittent abdominal pressure ventilator (IAPV) involves the intermittent inflation of an elastic air sac that is contained in a corset or belt worn beneath the patient's outer clothing (Fig. 84-4) (Exsufflation Belt™, Respironics Inc., Murrysville, PA). The sac is cyclically inflated by a positive pressure ventilator. Bladder inflation moves the diaphragm upward. During bladder deflation, gravity causes the abdominal contents and diaphragm to return to the resting position, and inspiration occurs passively. A trunk angle of 30 degrees or more from the horizontal is necessary for it to be effective. If the patient has any inspiratory capacity or is capable of GPB, he or she can add volumes of air autonomously taken in to that taken in mechanically. The IAPV generally augments tidal volumes by about 300 mL, but volumes as high as 1,200 mL have been reported (208). Patients with less than 1 hour of breathing tolerance usually prefer to use the IAPV rather than use noninvasive IPPV during daytime hours.

B. Mouthpiece Intermittent Positive Pressure Ventilation

Mouthpiece IPPV is the most important method of daytime ventilatory support. Some patients keep the mouthpiece between their teeth all day. Most patients prefer to have the mouthpiece held near the mouth. A metal clamp attached to a wheelchair can be used for this purpose, or the mouthpiece can be fixed onto motorized wheelchair controls—most often, sip and puff, chin, or tongue controls (Fig, 84-5). The ventilator is set for large tidal volumes, often 1,000 to 2,000 mL. The patient grabs the mouthpiece with his mouth and supplements or sub-

stitutes for inadequate autonomous breath volumes. The patient varies the volume of air taken from ventilator cycle to ventilator cycle and breath to breath to vary speech volume and cough flows as well as to air stack to fully expand the lungs.

To use mouthpiece IPPV effectively and conveniently, adequate neck rotation and oral motor function are necessary to grab the mouthpiece and receive IPPV without insufflation leakage. To prevent the latter, the soft palate must move posteriocaudally to seal off the nasopharynx. In addition, the patient must open the glottis and vocal cords, dilate the hypopharynx, and maintain airway patency to receive the air. These normally reflex movements may require a few minutes to relearn for patients who have been receiving IPPV via a tracheostomy tube.

C. Nasal Intermittent Positive Pressure Ventilation

Because patients prefer to use mouthpiece IPPV or the IAPV for daytime use (188,208), nasal IPPV is most practical only for nocturnal use. Daytime nasal IPPV is indicated for infants and for those who can not grab or retain a mouthpiece because of oral muscle weakness, inadequate jaw opening, or insufficient neck movement. Nevertheless, 24-hour nasal IPPV can be a viable and desirable alternative to tracheostomy, even for some patients with severe lip and oropharyngeal muscle weakness (188). Nasal IPPV users learn to close their mouths or seal off the oropharynx with their soft palates and tongues to prevent oral insufflation leakage.

Complications of Noninvasive Intermittent Positive Pressure Ventilation and Barotrauma

Besides orthodontic deformities and skin pressure from the interface, other potential difficulties include allergy to the plastic lipseal or silicone interfaces (13% vs. 5% for nonsilicone interfaces), dry mouth (65%), eye irritation from air leakage (about 24%), nasal congestion (25%) and dripping (35%), sinusitis (8%), nose bleeding (4% to 19%), gum discomfort (20%) and receding from nasal interface or lipseal pressure, maxillary flattening in children, aerophagia (209), and, as for invasive ventilation, barotrauma. In addition, occasional patients express claustrophobia. Proper interface selection eliminates or minimizes discomfort.

Pressure drop-off through the narrow air passages of the nose is normally between 2 and 3 cm H_2O. Suboptimal humidification dries out and irritates nasal mucous membranes, causes sore throat, and results in vasodilatation and nasal congestion. Increased airflow resistance to 8 cm H_2O can be caused by the loss of humidity that is due to unidirectional airflow with expiration via the mouth during nasal CPAP or IPPV (210). This problem can not be ameliorated by using a cold pass-over humidifier, but the increase in airway resistance can be reduced by 50% by warming the inspired air to body temperature and humidifying it with the use of a hot-water bath humidifier (210). Decongestants can also relieve sinus irritation and nasal congestion. Switching to lipseal IPPV can relieve most if not all difficulties associated with nasal IPPV. There are no absolute contraindications to the long-term use of noninvasive inspiratory muscle aids (211). Relative contraindications are listed in Table 84-4.

Abdominal distention tends to occur sporadically in noninvasive IPPV users. The air usually passes as flatus once the patient gets up or is placed into a wheelchair in the morning. When severe, it can present as intestinal pseudoobstruction with diminished bowel sounds and increased ventilator dependence. A rectal tube can usually decompress the colon; a gas-

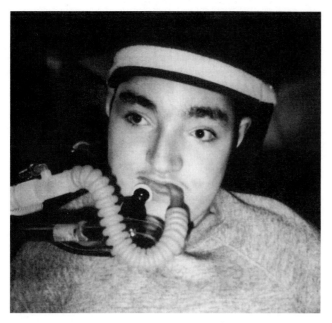

Figure 84-5. Thirty-five-year-old man with Duchenne muscular dystrophy who has used 24-hour mouthpiece IPPV for 21 years, now with less than 1 minute of breathing tolerance. The mouthpiece is fixed adjacent to the chin/tongue controls of his motorized wheelchair.

TABLE 84-4. Relative Contraindications for Long-Term Noninvasive Intermittent Positive Pressure Ventilation (IPPV)

1. Lack of cooperation or use of heavy sedation or narcotics
2. Need for high levels of supplemental oxygen therapy
3. SpO_2 can not be maintained above 94% despite noninvasive IPPV and optimal use of assisted coughing techniques when needed
4. Ssubstance abuse or uncontrollable seizures
5. Unassisted or assisted peak cough flows can not exceed 2.7 L/s (for adults)
6. Conditions that interfere with the use of IPPV interfaces, i.e., facial fractures, inadequate bite for mouthpiece entry, presence of beards that hamper airtight interface seal,
7. Inadequate caregiver support.

trostomy tube, when present, can be burped; or a nasogastric tube can be passed to relieve the problem.

Barotrauma results from rupture of the boundary between the alveoli and the bronchovascular sheath. Although its incidence has been cited as 4% to 15% for intensive care unit invasive ventilation users with primarily respiratory impairment (212), in 139 patients it has been reported to occur in 60% of those with acute respiratory distress syndrome but was absent for those with congestive heart failure or neurologic disease (213). We have had one case in 800 ventilator users.

Inspissated secretions can be life-threatening (214,215). Secretion encumbrance for patients with primarily ventilatory impairment results from failure to teach assisted coughing. Chronic aspiration of saliva to the extent of lowering baseline SpO_2 can overwhelm normally sterile airways and lead to pneumonia (216), tracheitis, bronchitis (217), and chronic lung disease (216). The indication for tracheostomy is assisted PCF less than 160 L/m and SpO_2 baseline less than 95% as a result of chronic airway secretion aspiration. This is rare other than for averbal bulbar-ALS patients.

GOAL THREE: PROVIDE FUNCTIONAL COUGHS BY ASSISTING EXPIRATORY MUSCLES

I. Why Are Expiratory Muscle Aids Needed?

Bulbar, inspiratory, and expiratory muscles are needed for effective coughing. The latter are predominantly the abdominal and intercostal muscles. Clearing airway secretions and airway mucus can be a continual problem for patients who can not swallow saliva or food without aspiration. For patients with respiratory muscle dysfunction and functional bulbar musculature, it becomes a problem during chest infections, following general anesthesia, and during any other periods of bronchial hypersecretion.

II. Manually Assisted Coughing

Assisted PCF can be greatly increased in patients receiving maximal insufflations before manual thrusts for assisted coughing (218). In 364 evaluations of our NMD patients able to air stack, the mean VC in the sitting position was 996.9 mL, the mean MIC was 1647.6 mL, and although PCFs were 2.3 L/s (less than 2.7 L/s or the minimum needed to eliminate airway secretions) mean assisted PCF were 3.9 L/s.

Techniques of manually assisted coughing involve different hand and arm placements for expiratory cycle thrusts (Fig. 84-6). An epigastric thrust with one hand while applying counterpressure across the chest to avoid paradoxical chest expansion with the other arm and hand further increases assisted PCF for 20% of patients (219). Manually assisted coughing is usually ineffective in the presence of severe scoliosis because of a combination of restricted lung capacity and the inability to effect diaphragm movement by abdominal thrusting because of severe rib-cage and diaphragm deformity. Abdominal compressions should not be used for 1 to 1.5 hours following a meal. When inadequate, and especially when inadequacy is due to difficulty air stacking, the most effective alternative for generating optimal PCF and clearing airway secretions is the use of mechanical insufflation-exsufflation (MI-E).

The inability to generate more than 2.7 L/s or 160 L/m of assisted PCF despite having a VC or MIC greater than 1 L usually indicates fixed upper-airway obstruction or severe bulbar muscle weakness and hypopharyngeal collapse during coughing attempts. Vocal cord adhesions or paralysis may have resulted from a previous translaryngeal intubation or tracheostomy (220). Because some lesions, especially the presence of obstructing granulation tissue, can be corrected surgically, laryngoscopic examination is warranted.

III. Mechanical Insufflation-Exsufflation

A. Introduction of Mechanical Insufflation-Exsufflation

MI-Es (Cough Assist™, J. H. Emerson Co., Cambridge, MA) deliver deep insufflations followed immediately by deep exsufflations. The insufflation and exsufflation pressures and delivery times are indepen-

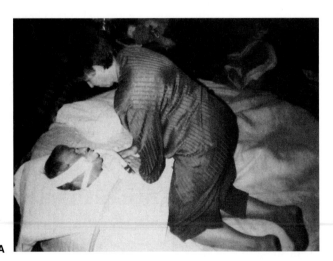
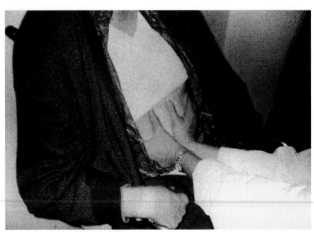

A   B

Figure 84-6. Hand placement for manually assisted coughing.

dently adjustable. Insufflation to exsufflation pressures of +40 to −40 cm H_2O are usually the most effective and preferred by most patients. Onset of insufflation generates an insufflation flow peak and a lung insufflation of more than 2 L. Mechanical exsufflation generates two exsufflation flow notches. One occurs when the insufflation pressure stops and is due to the elastic recoil of the lung. The second one, a bit greater, is caused by the exsufflation pressure itself. Except after a meal, an abdominal thrust is applied in conjunction with the exsufflation (MAC, or mechanically assisted coughing). MI-E can be provided via an oral-nasal mask, a simple mouthpiece, or via a translaryngeal or tracheostomy tube. When delivered via the latter, the cuff, when present, should be inflated. The Cough Assist™ can be manually or automatically cycled. Manual cycling facilitates caregiver-patient coordination of inspiration and expiration with insufflation and exsufflation, but it requires hands to deliver an abdominal thrust, to hold the mask on the patient, and to cycle the machine.

One treatment consists of about five cycles of MI-E or MAC followed by a short period of normal breathing or ventilator use to avoid hyperventilation. Insufflation and exsufflation pressures are almost always from +35 to +60 cm H_2O to −35 to −60 cm H_2O. Most patients use 35 to 45 cm H_2O pressures for insufflations and exsufflations. In experimental models, +40 to −40 cm H_2O pressures have been shown to provide maximum forced deflation VCs and flows (221). Insufflation and exsufflation times are adjusted to provide maximum chest expansion and rapid lung emptying. In general, 2 to 4 seconds are required. Multiple treatments are given in one sitting until no further secretions are expulsed and any secretion or mucus-induced $dSpO_2$s are reversed. Use can be required as frequently as every few minutes around the clock during chest infections.

The use of MI-E via the upper airway can be effective for children as young as 11 months of age. Patients this young can become accustomed to MI-E and permit its effective use by not crying or closing their glottises. Between 2.5 and 5 years of age, most children become able to cooperate and cough on queue with MI-E. Exsufflation-timed abdominal thrusts are also used for infants.

Whether via the upper airway or via indwelling airway tubes, routine airway suctioning misses the left main stem bronchus about 90% of the time (222). MI-E, on the other hand, provides the same exsufflation flows in both left and right airways without the discomfort or airway trauma of tracheal suctioning. Patients prefer MI-E to suctioning for comfort and effectiveness, and they find it less tiring (223). Deep suctioning, whether via airway tube or via the upper airway, can be discontinued for most patients.

B. Efficacy of MI-E

The efficacy of MI-E was demonstrated both clinically and on animal models (224). Flow generation is adequate in both proximal and distal airways to eliminate respiratory tract debris (225,226). VC, pulmonary flow rates, and SpO_2 when abnormal improve immediately with clearing of airway secretions and mucus by MI-E (227,228). An increase in VC of 15% to 42% was noted immediately following treatment in 67 patients with "obstructive dyspnea," and a 55% increase in VC was noted following MI-E in patients with neuromuscular conditions (229). We have observed 15% to 400% (200 to 800 mL) improvements in VC and normalization

of SpO_2 as MI-E eliminates airway mucus for ventilator-assisted NMD patients with chest infections (219).

C. Indications for MI-E

Of the three muscle groups required for effective coughing, MI-E can only take the place of the inspiratory and expiratory muscles. Thus, it can not be used to avert tracheotomy very long if bulbar function is inadequate to prevent airway collapse, as is often the case in advanced bulbar ALS. On the other hand, patients with completely intact bulbar muscle function, such as most ventilator users with traumatic tetraplegia, can usually air stack to volumes of 3 L or more, and, unless very scoliotic or obese, a properly delivered abdominal thrust can often result in assisted PCF of 6 to 9 L/s. These flows should be more than adequate to clear the airways and prevent pneumonia and respiratory failure without need for MI-E. Thus, the patients who need MI-E the most are those whose bulbar muscle function can maintain adequate airway patency but is insufficient to permit optimal air stacking for assisted PCF more than 250 to 300 L/m. This is typical of most non-bulbar ALS/NMD patients. The most typical example of patients who can consistently avoid hospitalization and respiratory failure by using MI-E during intercurrent chest infections is DMD patients (228). Patients with respiratory muscle weakness complicated by scoliosis and inability to capture the asymmetric diaphragm by abdominal thrusting also greatly benefit from MI-E.

Glossopharyngeal Breathing

Both inspiratory and, indirectly, expiratory muscle function can be assisted by GPB (189). GPB can provide an individual with weak inspiratory muscles and no VC or breathing tolerance with normal alveolar ventilation and perfect safety when not using a ventilator or in the event of sudden ventilator failure day or night (189,230). The technique involves the use of the glottis to add to an inspiratory effort by projecting (gulping) boluses of air into the lungs. The glottis closes with each "gulp." One breath usually consists of 6 to 9 gulps of 40 to 200 mL each (Fig. 84-7). During the training period, the efficiency of GPB can be monitored by spirometrically measuring the milliliters of air per gulp, gulps per breath, and breaths per minute. A training manual (231) and numerous videos are available (232), the best of which was produced in 1999 (233).

Although severe oropharyngeal muscle weakness can limit the usefulness of GPB, we have managed 13 DMD ventilator users who had no breathing tolerance other than by GPB. Approximately 60% of ventilator users with no autonomous ability to breathe and good bulbar muscle function (230,234) can use GPB and discontinue ventilator use for minutes to up to all day. Although potentially extremely useful, GPB is rarely taught because there are few health-care professionals familiar with the technique. GPB is also rarely useful in the presence of an indwelling tracheostomy tube. It can not be used when the tube is uncapped as it is during tracheostomy IPPV, and even when capped, the gulped air tends to leak around the outer walls of the tube and out the stoma as airway volumes and pressures increase during the GPB air-stacking process. The safety and versatility afforded by GPB are key reasons to eliminate tracheostomy in favor of noninvasive aids.

Because of their generally intact bulbar musculature, spinal cord injury (SCI) patients are ideal candidates to master GPB. High-level SCI patients typically use it for ventilator-free breathing. In some centers, these patients are decannulated to

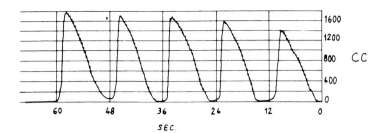

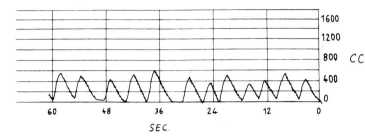

CC

Figure 84-7. Normal minute ventilation (60 to 90 mL per gulp, 6 to 8 gulps per breath, 12 breaths per minute) throughout daytime hours by glossopharyngeal breathing (GPB) for an individual with no measurable vital capacity otherwise. Maximum glossopharyngeal single breath capacities can exceed 3000 mL for such individuals.

free them from the fear of ventilator failure or accidental ventilator disconnection (230,234). Some patients with no measurable VC have awoken at night, breathing glossopharyngeally, to find that their ventilators had failed, a scenario not possible for tracheostomy IPPV users. Mouthpiece IPPV is not indicated for patients who can not rotate the neck to grab a mouthpiece. Although electrophrenic pacing can occasionally be used for continuous ventilatory support for such patients, it is best for daytime aid to free the patient from need for a mouthpiece, nasal interface, IAPV, or tracheostomy tube. When combined with nocturnal noninvasive IPPV, SCI patients can be decannulated, permitting mastery of GPB (Table 84-5) and the security and benefits that accompany decannulation.

Maintenance of Respiratory Muscle Strength and Endurance

In the few studies of respiratory muscle exercise performed on NMD patients, short daily sessions of inspiratory resistive exercise alone were reported to have no effect on spirometry or maximum inspiratory or expiratory pressures (235,236) but did improve respiratory muscle endurance (235,236,238). However, the degree of improvement in endurance correlated significantly with the level of VC and maximum inspiratory pressure at the outset of training, and no patient with less than 30% of predicted VC improved (238). This is the level of VC at which point patients often require nocturnal ventilatory aid and have considerable difficulty during respiratory tract infections (239). There is also no evidence that beginning an exercise program earlier would preserve more muscle function for the time when the patient requires aid, nor that the improvement in endurance for relatively strong patients (mean VC 54% to 59% in the patients studied) delays the occurrence of pulmonary complications as suggested (235). Indeed, there is some evidence to the contrary. Mildly affected ALS patients were reported to respond to a respiratory muscle-resistive exercise program with a decrease in VC and inspiratory pressures (238). There may also be a greater subsequent rate of loss of muscle strength in any temporarily strengthened muscles. The training itself may be hazardous for advanced patients. Thus, for those most likely to have respiratory complications, the use of resistance exercise is likely to be of little or no value.

Oximetry Monitoring and Feedback Protocol

For a patient with chronic alveolar hypoventilation who has not been using ventilatory support, or the patient being weaned from tracheostomy IPPV, introduction to and use of mouthpiece or nasal IPPV is facilitated by oximetry feedback. An SpO_2 alarm may be set from 93% to 94%. The patient sees that by taking slightly deeper breaths, SpO_2 will exceed 95% within seconds. He or she is instructed to maintain SpO_2 above 94% all day (228). This can be achieved by unassisted breathing for a period of time, and once tiring, by mouthpiece or nasal IPPV. With time, the patient requires increasing periods of IPPV to maintain adequate ventilation (SpO_2 greater than 94%). In this manner, an oximeter may also help to reset central ventilatory drive.

Oximetry feedback is especially important during the management of respiratory tract infections. The cough of infants and small children who can never sit is inadequate to prevent chest cold–triggered pneumonia and respiratory failure. Children who can sit are usually protected from this until after 2

TABLE 84-5. Management of Patients with Spinal Cord Injury				
Level*	VC ml	Bulbar muscles**	Daytime	Nocturnal
Above C1	0	inadequate/inadequate	TIPPV	TIPPV
C2–C3	< 200	adequate/inadequate	EPR	N/MIPPV
Below C2	> 200	adequate/adequate	MIPPV/IAPV	N/MIPPV

*Motor levels
**Adequate neck function involves sufficient oral and neck muscular control to rotate, flex, and extend the neck to grab and use a mouthpiece for IPPV; adequate bulbar function is indicated by the ability to generate assisted PCF >160 L/m and to prevent aspiration of saliva to the degree that the SpO_2 baseline decreases below 95%.
EPR, electrophrenic pacing; IAPV, intermittent abdominal pressure ventilator; MIPPV, mouthpiece intermittent positive pressure ventilation; NIPPV, nasal intermittent positive pressure ventilation; TIPPV, tracheostomy intermittent positive pressure ventilation.

years of age. Older children and adults whose assisted PCF decreases below 300 L/m are also at high risk for chest cold–triggered acute respiratory failure. Such patients require continuous SpO_2 monitoring and are taught that any dip in SpO_2 below 95% is due either to underventilation, or bronchial mucous plugging, and if these two causes are not quickly addressed, to atelectasis or pneumonia. They are instructed to use noninvasive IPPV to maintain normal ventilation and manually or mechanically assisted coughing to reverse mucous plug associated oxyhemoglobin desaturations. In this way, most episodes that would otherwise cause acute respiratory failure are successfully managed at home.

Although noninvasive ventilation is initiated for any patient with symptomatic inspiratory muscle weakness or alveolar hypoventilation, some patients require an oximeter, portable ventilator, and expiratory (cough) aids. For young patients with weak coughs and frequent chest colds that can trigger pneumonia and respiratory failure, oximeters and Cough-Assist™ devices need to be in the home at all times. For adults with infrequent chest colds, rapid access to this equipment may be all that is necessary. Likewise, with intact bulbar muscle function, manually assisted coughing may be sufficient to generate effective cough flows, whereas with complete bulbar muscle paralysis, even MAC may not spare patients from respiratory failure. Because clinical involvement ranges between these extremes, clinical guidelines are useful for institution of training and equipping patients (Table 84-6).

Treatment of Sleep-Disordered Breathing

Significant weight reduction can improve the central and obstructive apneas and hypopneas of sleep disordered breathing (240) in the morbidly obese. CPAP can be effective for patients with primarily obstructive events, but it is not adequate for those who have restricted pulmonary volumes and hypercapnia. Mask discomfort and air leakage into the eyes can make the use of CPAP via CPAP masks intolerable for about 35% of patients (241).

Independently varying inspiratory positive airway pressures (IPAP) and expiratory positive airway pressures (EPAP) with bilevel positive airway pressure machines can be effective for hypercapnic patients. The greater the pulse pressure difference—that is, the difference between the IPAP and EPAP—the greater the inspiratory muscle assistance. Often 20 to 30 cm H_2O IPAP and minimum EPAP are most effective. Custom-molded nasal interfaces are used for patients who require better fit than can be accorded by commercially available CPAP masks (206). Portable volume ventilators are used instead of BiPAP to deliver nasal IPPV for hypercapnic morbidly obese patients who require greater inspiratory muscle assist at higher peak ventilator pressures than can be provided by BiPAP.

Another convenient long-term solution, effective for many obstructive sleep apnea syndrome patients, is the use of an orthodontic splint that brings the mandible and tongue forward, thus, helping to splint open the hypopharynx (242). Uvulopalatopharyngoplasty and mandibular advancement procedures have also been used but are usually ineffective (243–245).

Invasive Ventilatory Support

The use of noninvasive aids can be contraindicated by the presence of any of the following: depressed cognitive function, orthopedic conditions interfering with the application of noninvasive IPPV interfaces and exsufflation techniques, pulmonary disease necessitating high fiO_2, or uncontrolled seizures or substance abuse (241,246). Also, the presence of a nasogastric tube can hamper the fitting of a nasal interface and the use of mouthpiece or nasal IPPV by interfering with both soft palate closure of the pharynx and seal at the nose. Although tracheostomy IPPV can extend survival for patients with neuromuscular ventilatory failure (247), morbidity and mortality outcomes are not as favorable as by noninvasive approaches (187). Tracheotomy is indicated for severe bulbar ALS patients (190), rarely if ever for DMD patients (228), and rarely for SMA patients. It has been found that even SMA type 1 children have less long-term morbidity when managed without tracheostomy tubes (195). Patients with DMD, even those who are continuously ventilator dependent on noninvasive IPPV, can avoid hospitalizations and pulmonary morbidity and mortality for decades and tracheotomy indefinitely when properly managed by using respiratory muscle aids (248).

When tracheostomy IPPV is continued despite the fact that oropharyngeal muscles are sufficient for swallowing and speaking, either cuffless tubes or tracheostomy cuff deflation are used up to 24 hours a day (112). Delivered air volumes are increased to compensate leak and support speech and one-way valves used to further facilitate verbal communication (109). Tracheostomy buttons are useful to optimize air passage through the upper airway for autonomous breathing as well as during transition from tracheostomy to noninvasive IPPV (234).

Quality of Life

Misconceptions about the undesirability of "'going on a respirator' have far-reaching negative effects for persons now happily being supported on a respirator, and mitigate the positive effects it could have for some types of chronically impaired persons whose quality of life also could be enhanced by the use of a ventilator" (249). Although it would seem that intelligent, self-directed individuals should be fully informed about therapeutic options, in the frenzy of seeking a less expensive healthcare delivery system, some physicians have suggested elimi-

---

TABLE 84-6. Milestones for Use of Noninvasive Aids

Infants and Children	Indication	Intervention
	paradoxical breathing	nocturnal high span BiPAP, oximetry
Children	never able to walk	Cough-Assist™
	symptomatic and can air stack	volume-cycled noninvasive IPPV
	symptomatic and can not air stack	volume-cycled noninvasive IPPV
Adults	assisted PCF <160 L/m asymptomatic	oximetry
	& symptomatic assisted PCF <130 L/m	high span BiPAP oximetry
	asympatomatic	rapid access to Cough-Assist™
	& symptomatic	volume-cycled noninvasive IPPV

PCF, peak cough flows symptomatic or asymptomatic for alveolar hypoventilation.

nating the patient from the decision-making process. As recently as 1989, it has been recommended that a physician's assessment of patients' quality of life be done "independent of the patient's feelings" to guide the clinician in whether to institute mechanical ventilation (250).

Poor quality of life is usually given as the reason for withholding ventilator use (251). However, no quality-of-life criteria can be appropriately applied to all individuals. Life satisfaction depends, rather, on personal preferences (252) and on subjective satisfaction in physical, mental, and social situations, even though these may be deficient in some manner. Thus, not quality of life but potential satisfaction with life should be considered. It is particularly appropriate that the life satisfaction of individuals who are living the consequences of having chosen to use ventilators be considered when deciding about such ethically and financially complex matters as ventilator use for others. Interestingly, data indicate that severely disabled, long-term postpoliomyelitis, DMD, and SCI ventilator users (251) generally have very positive views of their lives and life satisfaction. These individuals find quality of life in interpersonal activities, and they are very significantly more satisfied with life than health-care professional estimates suggest (252). Crucial for this is often the availability of personal attendant–care services. Thus, in the face of calls to limit entitlement spending, it should be noted that a society willing to provide free room, board, health care, legal and educational services, vocational training, and cable television for murderers, rapists, drug dealers, and other felons at exorbitant cost has the ethical responsibility to provide attendant-care services to those in need, some of whom are crime victims themselves.

Our specialty needs to do more than instruct the patient and his/her family; it must advocate for them to assure that they have access to appropriate community resources. We especially need to advocate for our patients against those who would detract from their personal freedom, even when that freedom incurs reasonable risk. "The Bush administration estimates that America spends more than $200 billion annually to keep people dependent (institutionalized) . . . that amounts to about $50,000 a person each year. But personal attendant services can serve as many as five people for the same amount while providing the individual with the opportunity to live an independent, productive, and meaningful life" (253).

REFERENCES

1. Fishman AP. The chest physician and physiatrist: perspectives on the scientific basis of pulmonary rehabilitation and related research. In: Bach JR, ed. *Pulmonary rehabilitation: the obstructive and paralytic conditions.* Philadelphia: Hanley & Belfus, 1996:1–12.
2. Alberion G, Alba A, Lee M, Solomon M. Pulmonary care of Duchenne type of dystrophy. *N Y State J Med* 1973;73:1206–1207.
3. Alexander MA, Johnson EW, Petty J, Stauch D. Mechanical ventilation of patients with late stage Duchenne muscular dystrophy: management in the home. *Arch Phys Med Rehabil* 1979;60:289–292.
4. Curran FJ, Colbert AP. Night ventilation by body respirators for patients in chronic respiratory failure due to late stage Duchenne muscular dystrophy. *Arch Phys Med Rehabil* 1981;62:270–274.
5. Dail C, Rodgers M, Guess V, Adkins HV. *Glossopharyngeal breathing manual.* Downey, CA: Professional Staff Association of Rancho Los Amigos Hospital, 1979.
6. McDermott I, Bach JR, Parker C, Sortor S. Custom-fabricated interfaces for intermittent positive pressure ventilation. *Int J Prosthodont* 1989;2:224–233.
7. Splaingard ML, Frates RC, Jefferson LS, et al. Home negative pressure ventilation: report of 20 years of experience in patients with neuromuscular disease. *Arch Phys Med Rehabil* 1985;66:239–242.
8. Delaubier A. Traitement de l'insuffisaire respiratoire chronique dans les dystrophies musculaires. In: *Memoires de certificat d'etudes superieures de reeducation et readaptation fonctionnelles.* Paris: Universite R Descarte, 1984:1–124.
9. Higgins ITT. Epidemiology of bronchitis and emphysema. In: Fishman AP, ed. *Pulmonary diseases and disorders,* 2nd ed. New York: McGraw-Hill, 1988: 70–90.
10. U.S. Department of Health and Human Services. *The health benefits of smoking cessation: a report of the Surgeon General.* DHHS Publication No. (CDC) 90–8416.Atlanta, GA: U.S. Department of Health and Human Services, Public Health Service, Centers for Disease Control, Center for Chronic Disease Prevention and Health Promotion, Office of Smoking and Health, 1990.
11. Fishman AP. The spectrum of chronic obstructive disease of the airways. In: Fishman AP, ed. *Pulmonary diseases and disorders.* New York: McGraw-Hill, 1988;2:1159–1171.
12. Department of Health Education and Welfare. *Smoking and health: a report of the Surgeon General.* DHEW Publication No. (PHS) 79–50066. Washington, DC: 1979.
13. Leeder SR, Colley JRT, Corkhill R, et al. Change in respiratory symptom prevalence in adults who alter their smoking habits. *Am J Epidemiol* 1977; 105:522–529.
14. Buist AS, Nagy JM, Sexton GJ. The effect of smoking cessation on pulmonary function: a 30-month follow-up of two smoking cessation clinics. *Am Rev Respir Dis* 1979;120:953–957.
15. Kark JD, Leguish M, Rannon L. Cigarette smoking as a risk factor for epidemic A (HI,NI) influenza in young men. *N Engl J Med* 1982;307:1042–1046.
16. Bosse R, Sparrow D, Rose CL, et al. Longitudinal effect of age and smoking cessation on pulmonary function. *Am Rev Respir Dis* 1981;123:378–381.
17. Goldstein MG, Niaura R, Willey-Lessne C, et al. Physicians counseling smokers: a population-based survey of patients' perceptions of health care provider-delivered smoking cessation interventions. *Arch Intern Med* 1997;157:1313–1319.
18. Anderson JE, Jorenby DE, Scott WJ, Fiore MC. Treating tobacco use and dependence: an evidence-based clinical practice guideline for tobacco cessation. *Chest* 2002;121:932–941.
19. Hillberg RE. Chronic obstructive pulmonary disease: causes and clinicopathologic considerations. In: Bach JR, ed. *Pulmonary rehabilitation: the obstructive and paralytic conditions.* Philadelphia: Hanley & Belfus, 1996:27–38.
20. Tager IB. Chronic bronchitis. In: Fishman AP, ed. *Pulmonary diseases and disorders.* New York: McGraw-Hill, 1988:1543–1551.
21. Slonim NB, Hamilton LH, eds. *Respiratory physiology,* 5th ed. St. Louis: C. V. Mosby, 1987.
22. Begin P, Grassino A. Inspiratory muscle dysfunction and chronic hypercapnia in chronic obstructive pulmonary disease. *Am Rev Respir Dis* 1991;143: 905–912.
23. Rochester DF, Braun NMT. Determinants of maximal inspiratory pressure in chronic obstructive pulmonary disease. *Am Rev Respir Dis* 1985;132:42–47.
24. Stubbing DG, Pengelly LD, Morse JLC, Jones NL. Pulmonary mechanics during exercise in subjects with chronic airflow obstruction. *J Appl Physiol* 1980;49:511–515.
25. Holden DA, Stelmach KD, Curtis PS, et al. The impact of a rehabilitation program on functional status of patients with chronic lung disease. *Respir Care* 1990;35:332–341.
26. Mahler DA, Weinberg DH, Wells CK, Feinstein AR. The measurement of dyspnea: contents, interobserver agreement, and physiologic correlates of two new clinical indexes. *Chest* 1984;85:751–758.
27. Moser K, Bokinsky G, Savage R, et al. Results of a comprehensive rehabilitation program: physiologic and functional effects on patients with chronic obstructive pulmonary disease. *Arch Intern Med* 1980;140:1596–1601.
28. Stoller JK, Ferranti R, Feinstein AR. Further specification and evaluation of a new clinical index for dyspnea. *Am Rev Respir Dis* 1986;134:1129–1134.
29. Boushy SF, Thompson HK Jr, North LB, et al. Prognosis in chronic obstructive pulmonary disease. *Am Rev Respir Dis* 1973;108:1373–1383.
30. Axen KV. Nutrition in chronic obstructive pulmonary disease. In: Haas F, Axen K, eds. *Pulmonary therapy and rehabilitation principles and practice,* 2nd ed. Baltimore: Williams & Wilkins, 1991:95–105.
31. Ferranti RD, Roberto M, Brown C Jr, Cohelo C. Oral intake, oxygen, dyspnea, dysphagia and other considerations for the COPD patient. In: Ferranti RD, ed. *Current topics in rehabilitation.* Verona, Italy: Bi & Gi Publishers, 1992:181–190.
32. Lewis MI. Nutrition and chronic obstructive pulmonary disease: a clinical overview. In: Bach JR, ed. *Pulmonary rehabilitation: the obstructive and paralytic conditions.* Philadelphia: Hanley & Belfus, 1996:156–172.
33. Burrows B. An overview of obstructive lung diseases. *Med Clin N Am* 1981;65:455–471.
34. Stokes DC, Wohl MEB, Khaw KT, Strieder DJ. Postural hypoxemia in cystic fibrosis. *Chest* 1985;87:785–791.
35. Flick MR, Block AJ. Continuous in-vivo monitoring of arterial oxygenation in chronic obstructive lung disease. *Ann Intern Med* 1977;86:725–730.
36. Jones NL. Current concepts: new tests to assess lung function. *N Engl J Med* 1975;293:541–544.
37. Jones NL, Campbell EJM. *Clinical exercise testing,* 2nd ed. Philadelphia: W. B. Saunders, 1982:158.
38. Reina-Rosenbaum R, Bach JR, Penek J. The cost/benefits of outpatient based pulmonary rehabilitation. *Arch Phys Med Rehabil* 1997;78:240–244.
39. Goldstein RS. Supplemental oxygen in chronic respiratory disease. In: Bach JR, ed. *Pulmonary rehabilitation: the obstructive and paralytic conditions.* Philadelphia: Hanley & Belfus, 1996:55–84.
40. Carlson DJ, Ries AL, Kaplan RM. Prediction of maximum exercise tolerance in patients with COPD. *Chest* 1991;100:307–311.
41. Guyatt GH, Thompson PJ, Berman LB, et al. How should we measure function in patients with chronic heart and lung disease? *J Chron Dis* 1985;38: 517–524.

42. Bach JR. *The effectiveness of pulmonary rehabilitation.* Report to the Office of Civilian Health and Medical Programs for the Uniform Services, Washington, D.C., 1995.

43. Guilmette TJ, Motta SI, Shadel WG, et al. Promoting smoking cessation in the rehabilitation setting. *Am J Phys Med Rehabil* 2001; 80:560–562.

44. Hernandez MTE, Rubio TM, Ruiz FO, et al. Results of a home-based training program for patients with COPD. *Chest* 2000;118:106–114.

45. Finnerty JP, Keeping I, Bullough I, Jones J. The effectiveness of outpatient pulmonary rehabilitation in chronic lung disease: a randomized controlled trial. *Chest* 2001;119:1705–1710.

46. Votto J, Bowen J, Scalise P, et al. Short-stay comprehensive inpatient pulmonary rehabilitation for advanced chronic obstructive pulmonary disease. *Arch Phys Med Rehabil* 1996;77:1115–1118.

47. Nava S. Rehabilitation of patients admitted to a respirator intensive care unit. *Arch Phys Med Rehabil* 1998;79:849–854.

48. Murciano D, Aubier M, Lecocguic Y, Pariente R. Effects of theophylline on diaphragmatic strength and fatigue in patients with chronic obstructive pulmonary disease. *N Engl J Med* 1984;311:349–353.

49. Vitres N, Aubier M, Musciano D, et al. Effects of aminophylline on diaphragmatic fatigue during acute respiratory failure. *Am Rev Respir Dis* 1984; 129:396–402.

50. Liesker JJW, Wijkstra PJ, Ten Hacken NHT, et al. A systematic review of the effects of bronchodilators on exercise capacity in patients with COPD. *Chest* 2002;121:597–608.

51. Nishimura K, Koyama H, Ikeda A, et al. The effect of high-dose inhaled beclomethasone dipropionate in patients with stable COPD. *Chest* 1999;115:31–37.

52. Nicotra MB, Rivera M, Awe RJ. Antibiotic therapy of acute exacerbations of chronic bronchitis: a controlled study using tetracycline. *Ann Intern Med* 1982;97:18–21.

53. Haas A, Pineda H, Haas F, Axen K. *Pulmonary therapy and rehabilitation: principles and practice.* Baltimore: Williams & Wilkens, 1979;124–125.

54. Kahn AU. Effectiveness of biofeedback and counter conditioning in the treatment of bronchial asthma. *J Psychosom Res* 1977;21:97–104.

55. Light RW, Marrill EJ, Despars JA, et al. Prevalence of depression and anxiety in patients with COPD: relationships to functional capacity. *Chest* 1985;87:35–38.

56. Dudley DL, Glaser EM, Jorgenson BN, et al. Psychosocial concomitants in chronic obstructive pulmonary disease II: psychosocial treatment. *Chest* 1980;77:544–551.

57. Dolce JJ, Crisp C, Manzella B, et al. Medication adherence patterns in chronic obstructive pulmonary disease. *Chest* 1991;99:837–841.

58. Stoller JK. Travel for the technology-dependent individual. *Respir Care* 1994;39:347–362.

59. Laaban J-P, Kouchakji B, Dore M-F, et al. Nutritional status of patients with chronic obstructive pulmonary disease and acute respiratory failure. *Chest* 1993;103:1362–1368.

60. Fitting JW. Energy expenditure in chronic lung disease. In: Ferranti RD, Rampulla C, Fracchia C, Ambrosino N, eds. *Nutrition and ventilatory function.* New York: Springer-Verlag, 1992:45–52.

61. Mohsenin V, Ferranti R, Loke JS. Nutrition for the respiratory insufficient patient. *Eur Respir J* 1989;2:663s–665s.

62. Niederman MS, Merrill WW, Ferranti RD, et al. Nutritional status and bacterial binding in the lower respiratory tract in patients with chronic tracheostomy. *Ann Intern Med* 1984;100:795–800.

63. Frankfort JD, Fischer CE, Stansbury DW, et al. Effects of high- and low-carbohydrate meals on maximum exercise performance in chronic airflow obstruction. *Chest* 1991;100:792–795.

64. Memsic L, Silberman AW, Silberman H. Malnutrition and respiratory distress: who's at risk. *J Respir Dis* 1990;11:529–535.

65. Juan G, Calverley P, Talamo C. Effect of carbon dioxide on diaphragmatic function in human beings. *N Engl J Med* 1984;310:874–877.

66. Whittaker JS, Ryan CR, Buckley PA, Road JD. The effects of refeeding on peripheral and respiratory muscle function in malnourished chronic obstructive pulmonary disease patients. *Am Rev Respir Dis* 1990;142:283–288.

67. Wilson DO, Rogers RM, Openbrier D. Nutritional aspects of chronic obstructive pulmonary disease. *Clin Chest Med* 1986;7:643–656.

68. Ferreira IM, Brooks D, Lacasse Y, Goldstein RS. Nutritional intervention in COPD: a systematic overview. *Chest* 2001;119:353–363.

69. De Blaquiere P, Christensen DB, Carter WB, Martin TR. Use and misuse of metered-dose inhalers by patients with chronic lung disease. *Am Rev Respir Dis* 1989;140:910–916.

70. Fartinez FJ, Couser JI, Celli BR. Factors influencing ventilatory muscle recruitment in patients with chronic airflow obstruction. *Am Rev Respir Dis* 1990;142:276–282.

71. Haas A, Pineda H, Haas F, Axen K. *Pulmonary therapy and rehabilitation: principles and practice.* Baltimore: Williams & Wilkens 1979:128–131.

72. Mueller RE, Petty TL, Filley GF. Ventilation and arterial blood gas changes induced by pursed-lip breathing. *J Appl Physiol* 1970;28:784–789.

73. Kirilloff LH, Owens GR, Rogers RM, Mazzocco MC. Does chest physical therapy work? *Chest* 1985;88:436–444.

74. Schoi MH. Autogenic drainage: a modern approach to physiotherapy in cystic fibrosis. *J R Soc Med* 1989;82[Suppl 16]:32–37.

75. Menkes HA, Traystman RJ. State of the art: collateral ventilation. *Am Rev Respir Dis* 1977;116:287–309.

76. Peters RM. Pulmonary physiologic studies of the perioperative period. *Chest* 1979;76:576–584.

77. Falk M, Kelstrup M, Andersen JB, et al. Improving the ketchup bottle method with positive expiratory pressure, PEP: a controlled study in patients with cystic fibrosis. *Eur J Respir Dis* 1984;65:57–66.

78. Hofmeyer JL, Webber BA, Hodson ME. Evaluation of positive expiratory pressure as an adjunct to chest physiotherapy in the treatment of cystic fibrosis. *Thorax* 1986;41:951–954.

79. Mortensen J, Falk M, Groth S, Jensen C. The effects of postural drainage and positive expiratory pressure physiotherapy on tracheobronchial clearance in cystic fibrosis. *Chest* 1991;100:1350–1357.

80. Tyrrell JC, Hiller EJ, Martin J. Face mask physiotherapy in cystic fibrosis. *Arch Dis Child* 1986;61:598–611.

81. van Asperen PP, Jackson L, Hennessy P, Brown J. Comparison of positive expiratory pressure (PEP) mask with postural drainage in patients with cystic fibrosis. *Aust Paediatr J* 1987;23:283–284.

82. van der Schans CP, van der Mark ThW, de Vries G, et al. Effect of positive expiratory pressure breathing in patients with cystic fibrosis. *Thorax* 1991;46:252–256.

83. Olsni L, Midgren B, Honblad Y, Wollmer P. Chest physiotherapy in chronic obstructive pulmonary disease: forced expiratory technique combined with either postural drainage or positive expiratory pressure breathing. *Respir Med* 1994;88:435–440.

84. Schibler A, Casaulta C, Kraemer R. Rational of oscillatory breathing in patients with cystic fibrosis. *Paediatr Pulmonol* 1992;8:301S.

85. Konstan MW, Stern RC, Doershuk CF. Efficacy of the Flutter device for airway mucus clearance in patients with cystic fibrosis. *J Pediatr* 1994;124:689–693.

86. Pryor JA, Webber BA, Hodson ME, Warner JO. The Flutter VRP1 as an adjunct to chest physiotherapy in cystic fibrosis. *Respir Med* 1994;88:677–681.

87. Bellone A, Lascioli R, Raschi S, et al. Chest physical therapy in patients with acute exacerbation of chronic bronchitis: effectiveness of three methods. *Arch Phys Med Rehabil* 2000;81:558–560.

88. Wolkove N, Kamel H, Rotaple M, Baltzan MA Jr. Use of a mucus clearance device enhances the bronchodilator response in patients with stable COPD. *Chest* 2002;121:702–707.

89. King M, Phillips DM, Gross D, et al. Enhanced tracheal mucus clearance with high frequency chest wall compression. *Am Rev Respir Dis* 1983;128:511–515.

90. Radford R, Barutt J, Billingsley JG, et al. A rational basis for percussion augmented mucociliary clearance. *Respir Care* 1982;27:556–563.

91. Rubin EM, Scantlen GE, Chapman GA, et al. Effect of chest wall oscillation on mucus clearance: comparison of two vibrators. *Pediatr Pulmonol* 1989;6:123–127.

92. Flower KA, Eden RI, Lomax L, et al. New mechanical aid to physiotherapy in cystic fibrosis. *BMJ* 1979;2:630–631.

93. Chang HK, Weber ME, King M. Mucus transport by high frequency nonsymmetrical airflow. *J Appl Physiol* 1988;65:1203–1209.

94. Warwick WJ, Hansen LG. The long-term effect of high-frequency chest compression therapy on pulmonary complications of cystic fibrosis. *Pediatr Pulmonol* 1991;11:265–271.

95. Christensen EF, Nedergaard, Dahl R. Long-term treatment of chronic bronchitis with positive expiratory pressure mask and chest physiotherapy. *Chest* 1990;97:645–650.

96. Holody B, Goldberg HS. The effect of mechanical vibration physiotherapy on arterial oxygenation in acutely ill patients with atelectasis or pneumonia. *Am Rev Respir Dis* 1981;124:372–375.

97. Piquet J, Brochard L, Isabey D, et al. High frequency chest wall oscillation in patients with chronic air-flow obstruction. *Am Rev Respir Dis* 1987;136:1355–1359.

98. Sibuya M, Yamada M, Kanamaru A, et al. Effect of chest wall vibration on dyspnea in patients with chronic respiratory disease. *Am J Respir Crit Care Med* 1994;149:1235–1240.

99. Pryor JA, Parker RA, Webber BA. A comparison of mechanical and manual percussion as adjuncts to postural drainage in the treatment of cystic fibrosis in adolescents and adults. *Physiother* 1981;6:140–141.

100. Sutton PP, Parker RA, Webber BA, et al. Assessment of the forced expiration technique, postural drainage and directed coughing in chest physiotherapy. *Eur J Respir Dis* 1983;64:62–68.

101. van Hengstum M, Festen J, Beurskens C, et al. No effect of oral high frequency oscillation combined with forced expiration maneuvers on tracheobronchial clearance in chronic bronchitis. *Eur Respir J* 1990;3:14–18.

102. van der Schans CP, Piers DA, Postma DS. Effect of manual percussion on tracheobronchial clearance in patients with chronic airflow obstruction and excessive tracheobronchial secretions. *Thorax* 1986;41:448–452.

103. Campbell AH, O'Connell JM, Wilson F. The effect of chest physiotherapy upon the FEV_1 in chronic bronchitis. *Med J Aust* 1975;1:33–35.

104. Zapletal A, Stefanova J, Horak J, et al. Chest physiotherapy and airway obstruction in patients with cystic fibrosis—a negative report. *Eur J Respir Dis* 1983;64:426–433.

105. Zidulka A, Chrome JF, Wight DW, et al. Clapping or percussion causes atelectasis in dogs and influences gas exchange. *J Appl Physiol* 1989;66:2833–2838.

106. Toussaint M, De Win H, Steens M, Soudon P. A new technique in secretion clearance by the percussionaire for patients with neuromuscular disease. In: *Programme des journées internationales de ventilation à domicile.* Lyon, France: Hopital de la Croix Rousse, 1993:27(abst).

107. Thangathuria D, Holm AP, Mikhail M, et al. HFV in management of a patient with severe bronchorrhea. *Respiratory Management* 1988;1:31–33.

108. McInturff SL, Shaw LI, Hodgkin JE, et al. Intrapulmonary percussive ventilation in the treatment of COPD. *Respir Care* 1985;30:885.

109. Patterson JM, Budd J, Goetz D, et al. Family correlates of a 10-year pulmonary health trend in cystic fibrosis. *Pediatrics* 1993;91:383–389.

110. Currie DC, Munro C, Gaskell D, et al. Practice, problems and compliance with postural drainage: a survey of chronic sputum producers. *Br J Dis Chest* 1986;80:249–253.

111. Passero MA, Remor B, Salomon J. Patient-reported compliance with cystic fibrosis therapy. *Clin Pediatr Phila* 1981;20:264–268.

112. Fong SL, Dales RE, Tierney MG. Compliance among adults with cystic fibrosis. *DICP* 1990;24:689–692.

113. Pardy RL, Reid WD, Belman MJ. Respiratory muscle training. *Clin Chest Med* 1989;9:287–295.

114. Belman MJ. Exercise in chronic obstructive pulmonary disease. *Clin Chest Med* 1986;7:585–597.

115. Nield MA. Inspiratory muscle training protocol using a pressure threshold device: effect on dyspnea in chronic obstructive pulmonary disease. *Arch Phys Med Rehabil* 1999;80:100–102.

116. Levine S, Weiser P, Gillen J. Evaluation of a ventilatory muscle endurance training program in the rehabilitation of patients with chronic obstructive pulmonary disease. *Am Rev Respir Dis* 1986;133:400–406.

117. Ries AL, Moser KM. Comparison of isocapnic hyperventilation and walking exercise training at home in pulmonary rehabilitation. *Chest* 1986;90:285–289.

118. Aldrich TK. Inspiratory muscle training in COPD. In: Bach JR, ed. *Pulmonary rehabilitation: the obstructive and paralytic conditions.* Philadelphia: Hanley & Belfus, 1996:285–301.

119. Weiner P, Azgad Y, Ganam R. Inspiratory muscle training combined with general exercise reconditioning in patients with COPD. *Chest* 1992;102:1351–1356.

120. Pardy RL, Rivington RM, Despas PJ, Macklem PT. Effects of inspiratory muscle training on exercise performance in chronic airflow limitation. *Am Rev Respir Dis* 1981;123:426–433.

121. Sawyer EH, Clanton TL. Improved pulmonary function and exercise tolerance with inspiratory muscle conditioning in children with cystic fibrosis. *Chest* 1993;104:490–497.

122. Weiner P, Azgad Y, Weiner M. Inspiratory muscle training during treatment with corticosteroids in humans. *Chest* 1995;107:1041–1044.

123. Weiner P, Magadle R, Berar-Yanay N, et al. The cumulative effect of long-acting bronchodilators, exercise, and inspiratory muscle training on the perception of dyspnea in patients with advanced COPD. *Chest* 2000;118:672–678.

124. Weiner P, Azgad Y, Ganam R, Weiner M. Inspiratory muscle training in patients with bronchial asthma. *Chest* 1992;102:1357–1361.

125. Braun NMT, Faulkner J, Hughes RL, et al. When should respiratory muscles be exercised? *Chest* 1983;84:76–84.

126. Hill NS. Home noninvasive ventilation in patients with lung disease. In: Bach JR, ed. *Noninvasive mechanical ventilation.* Philadelphia: Hanley & Belfus 2002:241–258.

127. Bach JR, Penek J. Obstructive sleep apnea complicating negative pressure ventilatory support in patients with chronic paralytic/restrictive ventilatory dysfunction. *Chest* 1991;99:1386–1393.

128. Levy RD, Bradley TD, Newman SL, et al. Negative pressure ventilation: effects on ventilation during sleep in normal subjects. *Chest* 1989;65:95–99.

129. Elliott MW. Noninvasive ventilation: mechanisms of action. In: Bach JR, ed. *Noninvasive mechanical ventilation.* Philadelphia: Hanley & Belfus 2002:73–82.

130. Belman MJ, Soo Hoo GW, Kuei JH, Shadmehr R. Efficacy of positive vs negative pressure ventilation in unloading the respiratory muscles. *Chest* 1990;98:850–856.

131. Marino W. Intermittent volume cycled mechanical ventilation via nasal mask in patients with respiratory failure due to COPD. *Chest* 1991;99:681–684.

132. Meduri GU, Abou-Shala N, Fox RC, et al. Noninvasive face mask mechanical ventilation in patients with acute hypercapnic respiratory failure. *Chest* 1991;100:445–454.

133. Sivasothy P, Smith IE, Shneerson JM. Mask intermittent positive pressure ventilation in chronic hypercapnic respiratory failure due to chronic obstructive pulmonary disease. *Eur Respir J* 1998;11:34–40.

134. Anton A, Guell R. Home mechanical ventilation: do we know when and how to use it? *Chest* 2000;118:1525–1526.

135. Janssens JP, de Muralt B, Titelion V. Management of dyspnea in severe chronic obstructive pulmonary disease. *J Pain Symptom Manage* 2000;19:378–392.

136. Krachman SL, Quaranta AJ, Berger TJ, Criner GJ. Effects of noninvasive positive pressure ventilation on gas exchange and sleep in COPD patients. *Chest* 1997;112:623–628.

137. Sturani EC, Porta R, Scarduelli C, et al. Outcome of COPD patients performing nocturnal non-invasive mechanical ventilation. *Respir Med* 1998;92:1215–1222.

138. Casanova C, Celli BR, Tost L, et al. Long-term controlled trial of nocturnal nasal positive pressure ventilation in patients with severe COPD. *Chest* 2000;118:1582–1590.

139. Anthonisen NR. Home oxygen therapy in chronic obstructive pulmonary disease. *Clin Chest Med* 1986;7:673–677.

140. Nixon PA, Orenstein DM, Curtis SE, Ross EA. Oxygen supplementation during exercise in cystic fibrosis. *Am Rev Respir Dis* 1990;142:807–811.

141. Bartels MN, Gonzalez JM, Kim W, DeMeersman RE. Oxygen supplementation and cardiac-autonomic modulation in COPD. *Chest* 2000;118:691–696.

142. Pierson DJ. Current status of home oxygen in the U.S.A. In: Kira S, Petty TL, eds. *Progress in domiciliary respiratory care—current status and perspective.* New York: Elsevier Science BV, 1994:93–98.

143. Sassoon CSH, Hassell KT, Mahutte CK. Hyperoxic-induced hypercapnia in stable chronic obstructive pulmonary disease. *Am Rev Respir Dis* 1987;135:907–911.

144. D'Urzo AD, Mateika J, Bradley TD, et al. Correlates of arterial oxygenation during exercise in severe chronic obstructive pulmonary disease. *Chest* 1989;95:13–17.

145. Dean NC, Brown JK, Himelman RB, et al. Oxygen may improve dyspnea and endurance in patients with chronic obstructive pulmonary disease and only mild hypoxemia. *Am Rev Respir Dis* 1992;146:941–945.

146. Bradley BL, Garner AE, Billiu D, et al. Oxygen assisted exercise in chronic obstructive lung disease: the effect on exercise capacity and arterial blood gas tensions. *Am Rev Respir Dis* 1978;118:239–243.

147. Davidson AC, Leach R, George RJD, Geddes DM. Supplemental oxygen and exercise ability in chronic obstructive airways disease. *Thorax* 1988;43:965–971.

148. Somfay A, Porszdsz J, Sang-Moo L, Casaburi R. Effect of hyperoxia on gas exchange and lactate kinetics following exercise onset in nonhypoxemic COPD patients. *Chest* 2002;121:393–400.

149. Marcus CL, Bader D, Stabile MW, et al. Supplemental oxygen and exercise performance in patients with cystic fibrosis with severe pulmonary disease. *Chest* 1992;101:52–57.

150. Jolly EC, DiBoscio V, Aguirre L, et al. Effects of supplemental oxygen during activity in patients with advanced COPD without severe resting hypoxemia. *Chest* 2001;120:437–443.

151. O'Donohue WJ. The future of home oxygen therapy. *Respir Care* 1988;33:1125–1130.

152. Tiep BL, Christopher KL, Spofford BT, et al. Pulsed nasal and transtracheal oxygen delivery. *Chest* 1990;97:364–368.

153. Dantzker DR, D'Alonzo GE. The effect of exercise on pulmonary gas exchange in patients with severe chronic obstructive pulmonary disease. *Am Rev Respir Dis* 1986;134:1135–1139.

154. Niederman MS, Clemente PH, Fein AM, et al. Benefits of a multidisciplinary pulmonary rehabilitation program: improvements are independent of lung function. *Chest* 1991;99:798–804.

155. Make BJ, Glenn K. Outcomes of pulmonary rehabilitation. In: Bach JR, ed. *Pulmonary rehabilitation: the obstructive and paralytic/restrictive pulmonary syndromes.* Philadelphia: Hanley & Belfus 1996:173–191.

156. Brown JB, Votto JJ, Thrall RS, et al. Functional status and survival following pulmonary rehabilitation. *Chest* 2000;118:697–703.

157. Gerardi DA, Lovett L, Benoit-Connors ML, et al. Variables related to increased mortality following out-patient pulmonary rehabilitation. *Eur Respir J* 1996;9:431–435.

158. Punzal PA, Ries AL, Kaplan RM, Prewitt LM. Maximum intensity exercise training in patients with chronic obstructive pulmonary disease. *Chest* 1991;100:618–623.

159. Foy CG, Rejeski WJ, Berry MJ, et al. Gender moderates the effects of exercise therapy on health-related quality of life among COPD patients. *Chest* 2001;119:70–76.

160. Gimenez M, Servera E, Vergara P, et al. Endurance training in patients with chronic obstructive pulmonary disease: a comparison of high versus moderate intensity. *Arch Phys Med Rehabil* 2000;81:102–109.

161. Carter R, Nicotra B, Clark L, et al. Exercise conditioning in the rehabilitation of patients with chronic obstructive pulmonary disease. *Arch Phys Med Rehabil* 1988;69:118–122.

162. Casaburi R, Wasserman K, Patessio A, et al. A new perspective in pulmonary rehabilitation: anaerobic threshold as a discriminant in training. *Eur Respir J* 1989;2:618s–623s.

163. Lacasse Y, Guyatt GH, Goldstein RS. The components of a respiratory rehabilitation program: a systematic overview. *Chest* 1997;111:1077–1088.

164. Belman M, Kendregan BA. Exercise training fails to increase skeletal muscle enzymes in patients with chronic obstructive pulmonary disease. *Am Rev Respir Dis* 1981;36:256–261.

165. Celli B, Gotlief S. Biofeedback and upper extremity exercise in COPD. In: Bach JR, ed. *Pulmonary rehabilitation: the obstructive and paralytic/restrictive pulmonary syndromes.* Philadelphia: Hanley & Belfus, 1996:285–301.

166. Martinez FJ, Vogel PD, Dupont DN, et al. Supported arm exercise vs. unsupported arm exercise in the rehabilitation of patients with severe chronic airflow obstruction. *Chest* 1993;103:1397–1402.

167. Couser J, Martinez F, Celli, BR. Pulmonary rehabilitation that includes arm exercise reduces metabolic and ventilatory requirements for simple arm elevation. *Chest* 1993;103:37–41.

168. Lake FR, Herndersen K, Briffa T. Upper limb and lower limb exercise training in patients with chronic airflow obstruction. *Chest* 1990;97:1077–1082.

169. Foster S, Lopez D, Thomas HM. Pulmonary rehabilitation in COPD patients with elevated pCO2. *Am Rev Respir Dis* 1988;138:1519–1523.

170. Ries AL, Kaplan RM, Limberg TM, Prewitt LM. Effects of pulmonary rehabilitation on physiologic and psychosocial outcomes in patients with chronic obstructive pulmonary disease. *Ann Intern Med* 1995;122:823–832.

171. Casaburi R, Patessio A, Ioli F, et al. Reductions in exercise lactic acidosis and ventilation as a result of exercise training in patients with obstructive lung disease. *Am Rev Respir Dis* 1991;143:9–18.

172. Wijkstra PJ, TenVergert EM, van Altena R, et al. Long term benefits of rehabilitation at home on quality of life and exercise tolerance in patients with chronic obstructive pulmonary disease. *Thorax* 1995; 0:824–828.

173. Tydeman DE, Chandler AR, Graveling BM, et al. An investigation into the effects of exercise tolerance training of patients with chronic airways obstruction. *Physiotherapy* 1984;70:261–264.

174. Tu SP, McDonell MB, Spertus JA, et al. A new self-administered questionnaire to monitor health-related quality of life in patients with COPD. *Chest* 1997;112:614–622.

175. Fuchs-Climent D, LeGallais D, Varray A, et al. Factor analysis of quality of life, dyspnea, and physiologic variables in patients with chronic obstructive pulmonary disease before and after rehabilitation. *Am J Phys Med Rehabil* 2001;80:113–120.

176. Boueri FMV, Bucher-Bartelson BL, Glenn KA, Make BJ. Quality of life measured with a generic instrument improves following pulmonary rehabilitation in patients with COPD. *Chest* 2001;119:77–84.

177. Chumillas S, Ponce JL, Delgado F, et al. Prevention of postoperative pulmonary complications through respiratory rehabilitation: a controlled clinical study. *Arch Phys Med Rehabil* 1998;79:5–9.

178. de Jong W, Grevink RG, Roorda RJ, et al. Effect of a home exercise training program in patients with cystic fibrosis. *Chest* 1994;105:463–468.

179. Roselle S, D'Amico FJ. The effect of home respiratory therapy on hospital readmission rates of patients with chronic obstructive pulmonary disease. *Respir Care* 1990;35:1208–1213.

180. Holle RHO, Williams DV, Vandree JC, et al. Increased muscle efficiency and sustained benefits in an outpatient community hospital-based pulmonary rehabilitation program. *Chest* 1988;94:1161–1168.

181. Ilowite J, Niederman M, Fein A, et al. Can benefits seen in pulmonary rehabilitation be sustained long term? *Chest* 1991;100:182.

182. Mall RW, Medieros M. Objective evaluation of results of a pulmonary rehabilitation program in a community hospital. *Chest* 1988;94:1156–1160.

183. Vale F, Reardon J, ZuWallack R. Is improvement sustained following pulmonary rehabilitation? *Chest* 1991;100:56s.

184. Foglio K, Bianchi L, Ambrosino N. Is it really useful to repeat outpatient pulmonary rehabilitation programs in patients with chronic airway obstruction?: A 2-year controlled study. *Chest* 2001;119:1696–1704.

185. Cambach W, Wagenaar RC, Koelman TW, et al. The long-term effects of pulmonary rehabilitation in patients with asthma and chronic obstructive pulmonary disease: a research synthesis. *Arch Phys Med Rehabil* 1999;80:103–111.

186. Bach JR, Niranjan V. Noninvasive ventilation in pediatrics. In: Bach JR, ed. *Noninvasive mechanical ventilation.* Philadelphia: Hanley & Belfus 2002:203–222.

187. Bach JR, Rajaraman R, Ballanger F, et al. Neuromuscular ventilatory insufficiency: the effect of home mechanical ventilator use vs. oxygen therapy on pneumonia and hospitalization rates. *Am J Phys Med Rehabil* 1998; 77:8–19.

188. Bach JR, Alba AS. Management of chronic alveolar hypoventilation by nasal ventilation. *Chest* 1990;97:52–57.

189. Bach JR, Alba AS, Bodofsky E, et al. Glossopharyngeal breathing and noninvasive aids in the management of post-polio respiratory insufficiency. *Birth Defects* 1987;23:99–113.

190. Bach JR. Amyotrophic lateral sclerosis: predictors for prolongation of life by noninvasive respiratory aids. *Arch Phys Med Rehabil* 1995;76:828–832.

191. Bach JR, Saporito LR. Indications and criteria for decannulation and transition from invasive to noninvasive long-term ventilatory support. *Respir Care* 1994;39:515–531.

192. Bach JR. Amyotrophic lateral sclerosis: prolongation of life by noninvasive respiratory aids. *Chest* 2002;122:92–98.

193. Williams AJ, Yu G, Santiago S, Stein M. Screening for sleep apnea using pulse oximetry and a clinical score. *Chest* 1991;100:631–635.

194. Bach JR, Kang SW. Disorders of ventilation: weakness, stiffness, and mobilization. *Chest* 2000;117:301–303.

195. Bach JR, Baird JS, Plosky D, et al. Spinal muscular atrophy type 1: management and outcomes. *Pediatr Pulmonol* 2002;34:16–22.

196. Bach JR. Inappropriate weaning and late onset ventilatory failure of individuals with traumatic quadriplegia. *Paraplegia* 1993;31:430–438.

197. Bach JR, Alba AS, Bohatiuk G, et al. Mouth intermittent positive pressure ventilation in the management of post-polio respiratory insufficiency. *Chest* 1987;91:859–864.

198. Frederick C. Noninvasive mechanical ventilation with the iron lung. *Crit Care Nurs Clin North Am* 1994;6:831–840.

199. Corrado A, Gorini M, De Paola E, et al. Iron lung treatment of acute on chronic respiratory failure: 16 years of experience. *Monaldi Arch Chest Dis* 1994;49:552–555.

200. Lherm T. Ventilation postopératoire non invasive par masque buccal. *Ann Fr Anesth Reanim* 1998;17:344–347.

201. Bach JR, Alba AS, Saporito LR. Intermittent positive pressure ventilation via the mouth as an alternative to tracheostomy for 257 ventilator users. *Chest* 1993;103:174–182.

202. Bach JF, Alba A, Mosher R, Delaubier A. Intermittent positive pressure ventilation via nasal access in the management of respiratory insufficiency. *Chest* 1987;92:168–170.

203. Leger P, Jennequin J, Gerard M, Robert D. Home positive pressure ventilation via nasal mask for patients with neuromuscular weakness or restrictive lung or chest-wall disease. *Respir Care* 1989;34:73–79.

204. Leger SS, Leger P. The art of interface: tools for administering noninvasive ventilation. *Med Klin* 1999;94:35–39.

205. Sekino H, Ohi M, Chin K, et al. Long-term artificial ventilation by nasal intermittent positive pressure ventilation: 6 cases of domiciliary assisted ventilation. *Nihon Kyobu Shikkan Gakkai Zasshi* 1993;31:1377–1384.

206. Bach JR, McDermott I. Strapless oral-nasal interfaces for positive pressure ventilation. *Arch Phys Med Rehabil* 1990;71:908–911.

207. Bach JR, Robert D, Leger P, Langevin B. Sleep fragmentation in kyphoscoliotic individuals with alveolar hypoventilation treated by nasal IPPV. *Chest* 1995;107:1552–1558.

208. Bach JR, Alba AS. Total ventilatory support by the intermittent abdominal pressure ventilator. *Chest* 1991;99:630–636.

209. Pepin JL, Leger P, Veale D, et al. Side effects of nasal continuous positive airway pressure in sleep apnea syndrome: study of 193 patients in two French sleep centers. *Chest* 1995;107:375–381.

210. Richards GN, Cistulli PA, Gunnar Ungar R, et al. Mouth leak with nasal continuous positive airway pressure increases nasal airway resistance. *Am J Respir Crit Care Med* 1996;154:182–186.

211. Bach JR. Update and perspectives on noninvasive respiratory muscle aids, part 1—. The inspiratory muscle aids. *Chest* 1994;105:1230–1240.

212. Marcy TW. Barotrauma: detection, recognition, and management. *Chest* 1993;104:578–584.

213. Gammon RB, Shin MS, Buchalter SE. Pulmonary barotrauma in mechanical ventilation. *Chest* 1992;102:568–572.

214. Wood KE, Flaten AL, Backes WJ. Inspissated secretions: a life-threatening complication of prolonged noninvasive ventilation. *Respir Care* 2000;45:491–493.

215. Hill NS. Complications of noninvasive ventilation. *Respir Care* 2000;45: 480–481.

216. Arvedson J, Rogers B, Buck G, et al. Silent aspiration prominent in children with dysphagia. *Int J Pediatr Otorhinolaryngol* 1994;28:173–181.

217. Loughlin GM. Respiratory consequences of dysfunctional swallowing and aspiration. *Dysphagia* 1989;3:126–130.

218. Kirby NA, Barnerias MJ, Siebens AA. An evaluation of assisted cough in quadriparetic patients. *Arch Phys Med Rehabil* 1966;47:705–710.

219. Bach JR. Mechanical insufflation-exsufflation: comparison of peak expiratory flows with manually assisted and unassisted coughing techniques. *Chest* 1993;104:1553–1562.

220. Richard I, Giraud M, Perrouin-Verbe B, et al. Laryngo-tracheal stenosis after intubation or tracheostomy in neurological patients. *Arch Phys Med Rehabil* 1996;77:493–497.

221. Newth CJL, Asmler B, Anderson GP, Morley J. The effects of varying inflation and deflation pressures on the maximal expiratory deflation flow-volume relationship in anesthetized Rhesus monkeys. *Am Rev Respir Dis* 1991;144:807–813.

222. Fishburn MJ, Marino RJ, Ditunno JF Jr. Atelectasis and pneumonia in acute spinal cord injury. *Arch Phys Med Rehabil* 1990;71:197–200.

223. Garstang SV, Kirshblum SC, Wood KE. Patient preference for in-exsufflation for secretion management with spinal cord injury. *J Spinal Cord Med* 2000;23:80–85.

224. Bickerman HA. Exsufflation with negative pressure: elimination of radiopaque material and foreign bodies from bronchi of anesthetized dogs. *Arch Intern Med* 1954;93:698–704.

225. Leiner GC, Abramowitz S, Small MJ, et al. Expiratory peak flow rate: standard values for normal subjects. *Am Rev Respir Dis* 1963;88:644.

226. Siebens AA, Kirby NA, Poulos DA. Cough following transection of spinal cord at C-6. *Arch Phys Med Rehabil* 1964;45:1–8.

227. Bach JR, Smith WH, Michaels J, et al. Airway secretion clearance by mechanical exsufflation for post-poliomyelitis ventilator assisted individuals. *Arch Phys Med Rehabil* 1993;74:170–177.

228. Bach JR, Ishikawa Y, Kim H. Prevention of pulmonary morbidity for patients with Duchenne muscular dystrophy. *Chest* 1997;112:1024–1028.

229. Barach AL, Beck GJ. Exsufflation with negative pressure: physiologic and clinical studies in poliomyelitis, bronchial asthma, pulmonary emphysema and bronchiectasis. *Arch Intern Med* 1954;93:825–841.

230. Bach JR. New approaches in the rehabilitation of the traumatic high level quadriplegic. *Am J Phys Med Rehabil* 1991;70:13–20.

231. Dail C, Rodgers M, Guess V, Adkins HV. *Glossopharyngeal breathing.* Downey, CA: Rancho Los Amigos Department of Physical Therapy, 1979.

232. Dail CW, Affeldt JE. *Glossopharyngeal breathing* [video]. Los Angeles: Department of Visual Education, College of Medical Evangelists, 1954.

233. Webber B, Higgens J. Glossopharyngeal breathing: what, when and how? [video] Aslan Studios Ltd., Holbrook, Horsham, West Sussex, England, 1999.

234. Bach JR, Alba AS. Noninvasive options for ventilatory support of the traumatic high level quadriplegic. *Chest* 1990;98:613–619.

235. DiMarco AF, Kelling JS, DiMarco MS, et al. The effects of inspiratory resistive training on respiratory muscle function in patients with muscular dystrophy. *Muscle Nerve* 1985;8:284–290.

236. Martin AJ, Stern L, Yeates J, et al. Respiratory muscle training in Duchenne muscular dystrophy. *Devp Med Child Neurol* 1986;28:314–318.

237. Rodillo E, Noble-Jamieson CM, Aber V, et al. Respiratory muscle training in Duchenne muscular dystrophy. *Arch Dis Child* 1989;64:736–738.

238. Smith PEM, Coakley JH, Edwards RHT. Respiratory muscle training in Duchenne muscular dystrophy [Letter]. *Muscle Nerve* 1988;11:784–85.

239. Schiffman PL, Belsh JM. Effect of inspiratory resistance and theophylline on respiratory muscle strength in patients with amyotrophic lateral sclerosis. *Am Rev Respir Dis* 1989;139:1418–1423.

240. Lombard R Jr, Zwillich CW. Medical therapy of obstructive sleep apnea. *Med Clin North Am* 1985;69:1317–1335.
241. Waldhorn RE, Herrick TW, Nguyen MC, et al. Long-term compliance with nasal continuous positive airway pressure therapy of obstructive sleep apnea. *Chest* 1990;97:33–38.
242. Clark GT, Nakano M. Dental appliances for the treatment of obstructive sleep apnea. *J Am Dent Assoc* 1989;118:611–619.
243. Katsantonis GP, Walsh JK, Schweitzer PK, Friedman WH. Further evaluation of uvulopalatopharyngoplasty in the treatment of obstructive sleep apnea syndrome. Otolaryngol Head Neck Surg 1985;93:244–250.
244. Riley RW, Powell NB, Guilleminault C, Mino-Murcia G. Maxillary, mandibular, and hyoid advancement: an alternative to tracheostomy in obstructive sleep apnea syndrome. *Otolaryngol Head Neck Surg* 1986; 94:584–588.
245. Thawley SE. Surgical treatment of obstructive sleep apnea. *Med Clin North Am* 1985;69:1337–1358.
246. Bach JR, Saporito LR. Criteria for extubation and tracheostomy tube removal for patients with ventilatory failure: a different approach to weaning. *Chest* 1996;110:1566–1571.
247. Bach JR. Conventional approaches to managing neuromuscular ventilatory failure. In: Bach JR, ed. *Pulmonary rehabilitation: the obstructive and paralytic conditions.* Philadelphia: Hanley & Belfus 1996:285–301.
248. Gomez-Merino E, Bach JR. Duchenne muscular dystrophy: prolongation of life by noninvasive respiratory muscle aids. *Am J Phys Med Rehabil* 2002;81:411–415.
249. Purtilo RB. Ethical issues in the treatment of chronic ventilator-dependent patients. *Arch Phys Med Rehabil* 1986;67:718–721.
250. Dracup K, Raffin T. Withholding and withdrawing mechanical ventilation: assessing quality of life. *Am Rev Respir Dis* 1989;140:S44–S46.
251. Bach JR, Barnett V. Psychosocial, vocational, quality of life and ethical issues In: Bach JR, ed. *Pulmonary rehabilitation: the obstructive and paralytic conditions.* Philadelphia: Hanley & Belfus 1996:395–411.
252. Jonsen R, Siegler M, Winslade WJ. *Clinical ethics: a practical approach to ethical decisions in clinical medicine.* New York: Macmillan, 1982.
253. Starkloff M. Disabled and despondent. *Rehabilitation Gazette* 1993;33:7–8.

CHAPTER 85

Burn Rehabilitation

Phala A. Helm, Karen Kowalske, and Marjorie Head

The incidence and severity of burn injury have decreased dramatically over the last 20 years but continue to be a major cause of traumatic injury and death. Approximately 1.25 million burn injuries occur each year, resulting in 5,500 fatalities and 51,000 hospital admissions. The overall number of hospital admissions continues to decline, with a shift to day surgery and comprehensive outpatient treatment. National fire prevention programs, including the increased use of smoke detectors, coincide with a reduction in burn injuries and deaths. Declines in deaths due to burn are also a result of improvement in patient care and the delivery of care in national burn centers (1). In the mid-1960s, burn injuries of 50% of the total body surface area (TBSA) had a 50% mortality rate. The mortality rate for the same injury is now about 10%, and survival of a 70% TBSA burn is now about 50% at major burn centers (2). The head and neck and upper extremities are the most frequently involved body areas burned. Injuries to these areas result in functional and cosmetic deficits that result in severe impairment and disability (3).

Rehabilitation of the burn injured must begin soon after burn to try to prevent deformities and poor functional outcomes. Total time in rehabilitation may be up to 2 years, depending on severity of injury, compliance issues due to pain and discomfort, and other psychological factors that interfere with treatment. Interdisciplinary rehabilitation treatment with specialized personnel is currently the standard in 80% to 90% of major burn centers (4). In recent years other skin disorders have been routinely referred for treatment at burn centers. Toxic epidermal necrolysis is a devastating medication-induced desquamation disorder that has frequently been referred for treatment. The clinical course of this disorder is similar to partial-thickness burns, and management is similar. Toxic epidermal necrolysis is a reaction triggered by exposure to certain drugs causing extensive damage to the skin and mucous membranes (5). The most common etiologic agents are antibiotics, anticonvulsants, and nonsteroidal antiinflammatory drugs. Necrotizing fasciitis, a rapidly progressing bacterial infection affecting full-thickness skin down to the fascia, is also treated in burn centers. This progressive problem can result in massive tissue loss requiring extensive grafting. Rehabilitation management of both toxic epidermal necrolysis and necrotizing fasciitis is similar to partial- and full-thickness burns.

Classification of the burn injury is important for planning the patient's treatment regimen. Burns may be classified by causative agent, depth, and percentage of TBSA burned (Table 85-1). Other factors considered are body part burned, age of patient, preexisting illnesses, and associated injuries such as smoke inhalation and fractures (6).

PATHOPHYSIOLOGY

Normal Skin

The epidermis and dermis constitute the two layers of skin. Epidermal cells begin in the basal layer and gradually move to the surface. As the cells approach the surface, they undergo keratinization and flatten, leaving a thin layer of keratin fiber on the surface that provides a protective barrier to bacterial invasion and fluid loss. The epidermal cells line not only the basal layer of the epidermis but also the hair follicles and sweat glands, which are deep in the dermis. The dermis consists of vascular connective tissue that supports and provides nutrition to the epidermis and skin appendages and the sweat glands, hair follicles, and sebaceous glands (Fig. 85-1). The dermis gives the skin strength and elasticity by an interlacing of collagen and elastic fibers. The skin thickness varies with age and body location, with thicker skin over the back and posterior neck and thinner skin over the medial aspect of the arms and legs.

Local Effects of Heat Injury

Thermal destruction of the skin causes a chain of events that may be classified as local and systemic. The amount of tissue destroyed depends on local and systemic reactions to heat damage, the duration and intensity of thermal exposure, and the characteristics of the area burned. In children the rete pegs are not well developed in most body areas, and in the elderly they have become thin and atrophic, thus increasing the damage with burn injury because of fewer protective layers of epithelium (7).

It is very difficult, even for the most experienced, to determine with certainty the depth of burn for 3 to 5 days after injury. Shortly after the burn injury, histamine is released into the local area, causing intense vasoconstriction, and within a few hours there is vasodilatation and increased capillary permeability, which permits plasma to escape into the wound. Damaged cells swell. Platelets and leukocytes aggregate, causing thrombotic ischemia and further damage.

Partial- and full-thickness burns impair the body's defenses against infection and cause loss of massive amounts of body

TABLE 85-1. Burn Classification

A. Causative agent
  1. Thermal
    a. Heat
    b. Cold
  2. Electrical
  3. Chemical
  4. Radiation
B. Depth of burn
  1. Older terminology
    a. First degree; epidermis injured
    b. Second degree; dermis partially damaged
    c. Third degree; all dermis destroyed
    d. Fourth degree; muscle, nerve, and bond damaged
  2. Newer terminology
    a. Superficial partial thickness; epidermis and upper part of dermis injured
    b. Deep partial thickness; epidermis and large upper portion of dermis injured
    c. Full thickness; all skin destroyed
C. Size of burn: rule of nines
  1. Head = 9% BSA
  2. Each upper extremity = 9% BSA
  3. Each lower extremity = 18% BSA
  4. Anterior trunk = 18% BSA
  5. Posterior trunk = 18% BSA
  6. Perineum = 1% BSA
D. American Burn Board classification
  1. Minor
    a. <15% BSA partial thickness (10% in child)
    b. <2% BSA full thickness (not involving eyes, ears, face, or perineum)
  2. Moderate[a]
    a. 15% to 20% BSA (10% to 20% in child)
    b. 2% to 10% BSA full thickness (not involving eyes, ears, face, or perineum)
  3. Major[a]
    a. >25% BSA partial thickness (20% in child); ≥10% BSA full thickness
    b. All burns to eyes, ears, face, and perineum
    c. All electrical
    d. All inhalation
    e. All burns with fracture or major tissue trauma
    f. All with poor risk secondary to age or illness

[a]Most moderate and all major burns should be hospitalized; BSA, body surface area

ANATOMY OF THE SKIN

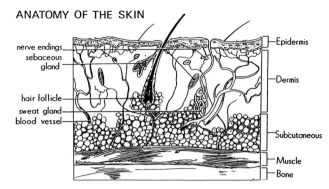

Figure 85-1. Anatomy of the skin.

tence is depressed for many reasons, including depression of immunoglobulin (7).

Skin Regeneration and Scarring

Spontaneous reepithelialization is impossible with a full-thickness burn injury because of destruction of the dermal appendages. Full-thickness burns result in hair loss, sensory impairment, loss of normal skin lubrication, and heat intolerance because of destruction of sweat glands.

Healing and regeneration of skin in partial-thickness burns arise from the epithelial linings of the hair follicles and sweat glands. Depending on the depth, healing is completed within 14 to 21 days. The new skin again becomes active as a temperature regulator and a barrier against bacteria. After epithelialization there is continued healing with regeneration of the peripheral nerves, sometimes associated with symptoms of pain and itching. Although epithelium covers the wound, dermal scarring occurs in the burn wound on a continuous basis for several months after injury. The healing process is ongoing from 6 months to 2 years until the skin is mature. By that point the vascularity of the wound has returned to near normal, and there is no further collagen deposition in the wound.

PATIENT MANAGEMENT

Acute Phase

RESUSCITATION

An immediate estimate of the total percentage of surface area burned is a priority in management to determine if intravenous fluid therapy is needed to prevent or treat burn shock. A shift of body fluids to involved areas can cause intravascular hypovolemia and massive edema of both injured and uninjured tissues. If treatment is inadequate, acute renal failure and death can occur. Several formulas are available for calibrating fluid requirements (e.g., Brooke, Evans, and Parkland formulas); however, the formulas serve only as guidelines, and individual adjustments must be made based on the patient's response. It is important that the fluids contain sodium and that fluid replacement be completed within 48 hours.

ESCHAROTOMY

An escharotomy is an incision through the burned tissue to relieve increased tissue pressure (Fig. 85-2). Massive edema of the extremities can cause neurovascular compromise, which could result in amputation. To prevent compartment syn-

fluids through open wounds. The evaporation results in heat loss and a large caloric drain on the patient. Bacterial contamination of the burn wound may occur immediately with resulting burn wound sepsis.

Systemic Effects of Heat Injury

Some of the major systemic effects of burns include acute hypovolemia, with loss of fluid into the extravascular compartment and subsequent burn shock; pulmonary changes with hyperventilation; and markedly increased oxygen consumption. The high incidence of upper-airway obstruction is related to direct damage by inhalation of noxious gases, and because of this patients are subject to pneumonia. Blood viscosity increases, and platelets increase their adhesiveness, which decreases bleeding in the wounds but increases the risk of deep vein thrombosis. Acute gastric dilation and gastrointestinal ileus commonly occur in the first 3 days following a burn. Immunologic compe-

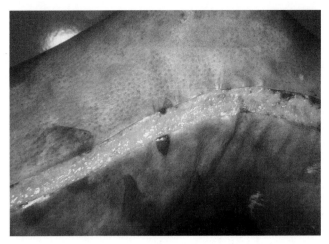

Figure 85-2. Escharotomy of the lower extremity.

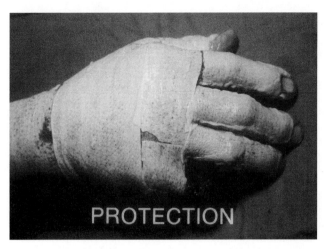

Figure 85-3. Skin substitute—pigskin.

dromes, fasciotomies are recommended. Early assessment of blood flow is essential. This can be evaluated by physical examination, Doppler studies, and measurement of tissue pressures with a wick catheter. If tissue pressure is used as a guide, escharotomy is indicated when tissue pressure exceeds 40 mm Hg. Escharotomies are done on other parts of the body, such as the chest when chest expansion is limited and interferes with breathing.

WOUND COVERAGE

Topical Antibacterial Agents

After resuscitation, the burn wound is cleaned, devitalized tissue is removed, and a topical antibacterial agent is applied. A number of effective topical agents are used for the prevention of burn wound sepsis. Among the various agents available are mafenide, silver nitrate, gentamicin, neomycin, povidone-iodine, and silver sulfadiazine, which is in widest use because of its comfort and fewer side effects. No single agent is universally effective, and no one agent is superior to another in terms of patient survival.

SKIN SUBSTITUTES

Burn survival has significantly improved over the past four decades. Burns with greater TBSA involvement have fewer donor sites; consequently, temporary skin coverage is necessary for survival.

Biological Dressings

A biological dressing is a skin substitute used for temporary coverage of the burn wound. These skin substitutes are skin grafts from cadavers, human fetal membranes (i.e., homografts or allografts), and skin grafts from pigs (i.e., heterografts or xenografts) (Fig. 85-3). The recommended uses for these dressings are for immediate coverage of a superficial partial-thickness burn, as a test dressing (i.e., if it adheres, the wound bed is ready for autografting), and for wound coverage after excision of burn eschar. In addition, closing a wound with a biological dressing prevents fluid loss, decreases pain, inhibits bacterial growth on clean wounds, and encourages growth of granulation tissue. The biological dressing should be changed every several days until the wound is healed or ready for autografting. If left in place too long it becomes incorporated into the burn wound, making removal extremely difficult. It also can become dry and adhere to the wound, restricting range of mo-

tion. The disadvantage of xenografts is that they do not establish vessel-to-vessel connection and will undergo avascular necrosis and sloughs.

Synthetic Dressings

Synthetic skin substitutes were developed to cover open wounds until the wound healed or until it could be autografted. They are used in place of xenografts or homografts. For the synthetic skin to be an effective replacement for certain biological dressings it had to meet certain criteria. A product was needed that was readily available, nonallergenic, relatively inexpensive, and easily removable and that had a permeable membrane. One additional criterion was that it come in large sheets that would conform to various tissue planes. A product that met these criteria, and that is widely used, is Biobrane (Dow B. Hickam, Sugarland, TX). It consists of an epidermal analogue composed of a thin sheet of silastic and a dermal analogue composed of type 1 porcine gel. Biobrane has been found to function as well as porcine xenograft. The disadvantage of Biobrane is that it has to be stapled in place (8). Another bilaminate skin substitute is Integra. The epidermal analogue is a silastic film and the dermal analog is a net of collagen fibrils covered in chondroitin-6-sulfate. The dermal layer can become vascularized after it is applied to an excised burn wound. When vascularization is adequate, a thin cutaneous autograft can be applied. The disadvantage to Integra is its susceptibility to infection and the potential for greater scar formation.

Cultured Epidermal Autographs

Over the past decade, techniques have been developed to cover an excised wound immediately after injury with artificial skin. A material that has been developed is cultured epidermal autografts (CEA) consisting of sheets of cultured keratinocytes. Clinical evaluation of cultured epidermal autografts has shown that adherence is generally good in burns of 50% TBSA or less. However, as the burn size increases, rejection increases proportionally (9). The result is a permanent skin replacement with functioning dermis and epidermis. This procedure is primarily employed in cases of very large, full-thickness or deep partial-thickness injuries with minimal donor sites for grafting are available. A drawback to this procedure is the requirement for immobility of the body part involved for 3 weeks, which increases risk of contractures. In addition, scarring has been observed to be worse (10).

SURGICAL MANAGEMENT

Debridement

Debridement is the removal of devitalized tissue (i.e., eschar down to a viable tissue level) to prepare the wound bed for definitive coverage. Debridement of blisters in partial-thickness burns is always debatable because some feel wound healing is faster with debridement and others feel blisters should be left intact. A Study by Ono et al. on cytokines in burn blister fluid reported that retention fluid from blisters of partial-thickness burns contains large amounts of growth factors and cytokines that stimulate the wound-healing process. It was suggested that the blister wall be maintained intact and that, even if the blister ruptures, the physiologic environment be re-created by using hydrocolloid to retain the exudate (11). Removal of eschar aids in healing by preventing bacterial proliferation. Types of debridement include mechanical with scissors and forceps and wet to dry dressings; enzymatic; and surgical tangential, fascial, and full-thickness excisions.

MECHANICAL DEBRIDEMENT

Removal of dressings when they are dry is effective in debridement of dead tissue because it adheres to the dressing however may be quite painful. Mechanical debridement is best accomplished either during hydrotherapy or immediately following. All areas should be cleaned gently to remove topical agents so that the wound is completely visible before sharp debridement begins. Hydrotherapy without wound care is poor patient management.

Wet-to-dry dressings also can be very effective in removal of eschar or exudate. Coarse mesh gauze, soaked in warmed antibacterial solution or normal saline, is applied to the wound and left to dry. With this technique the eschar softens, sticks to the dressing, and then is debrided as the dressing is removed.

ENZYMATIC DEBRIDEMENT

An enzymatic debriding agent such as Accuzyme will selectively digest necrotic tissue without harming viable tissue. Because there is increased fluid drainage through the wound with enzymatic debridement, no more than 20% of the body surface area should be treated at one time. Other side effects include bleeding, body temperature elevation, and pain. The enzymatics should not be used in conjunction with hexachlorophene or iodine preparations because enzyme activity will be impaired (12).

SURGICAL DEBRIDEMENT

The two primary surgical techniques used for wound debridement are fascial and tangential (i.e., sequential excision) (Fig. 85-4). Fascial excision removes nonviable burn tissue and a variable amount of viable tissue and is reserved for patients with very deep burns. It is believed that skin grafts adhere much better to fascia than to fat. The problem with fascial excision is that fat does not regenerate; this can cause severe cosmetic deformities (Fig. 85-5).

The most widely used technique in surgical debridement is eschar removal by tangential excision, usually performed at 1 to 10 days following a burn. The principle of tangential excision is to shave thin layers of burn eschar sequentially until viable tissue is apparent. There can be a significant amount of blood loss, and different methods are used to control this. Tourniquets are used for the extremities by the more experienced surgeon, but there is the danger of sacrificing normal tissue by excising too deeply. Some surgeons control bleeding with microcrystalline collagen, thrombin, epinephrine, and

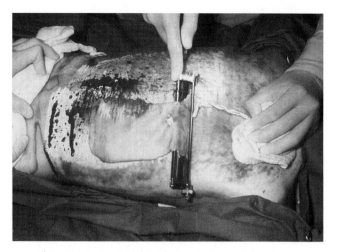

Figure 85-4. Surgical debridement by tangential excision.

electrocautery. Heimbach reports that early excision and grafting, compared with the standard nonoperative treatment, has led to decreased hospital stay, slight decline in overall patient mortality, decreased systemic sepsis, and fewer deaths from burn wound sepsis (13).

Skin Grafting

With the exception of small wounds, all full-thickness wounds require skin grafting. Deep partial-thickness wounds that are slow to heal also may require skin grafting. Grafting of deep partial-thickness wounds may prevent the development of thick scar tissue. Autografting is the removal of skin from one part of the body and its transfer to another part. Split-thickness skin grafts are used primarily, whereas full-thickness grafts are used more for reconstructive procedures. It should be noted that split-thickness autografts have no dermal appendages.

There are a variety of split-thickness skin grafts, each with different indications for use. The Tanner mesh graft is expandable skin that can be used to cover large wounds (Fig. 85-6). Expansion of the skin can be varied, with better cosmetic results with 1.5:1 expansion than, for example, with 6:1. Postage-stamp grafting is the application of squares or rectangles of various dimensions spread evenly over the wound. This type of grafting often leaves a poor cosmetic result because of hypertrophic scarring of the uncovered areas. Sheet grafting is an-

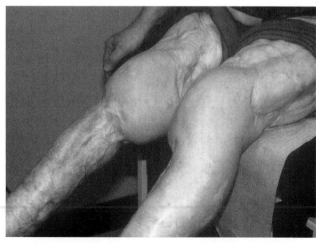

Figure 85-5. Cosmetic deformity following fascial excision.

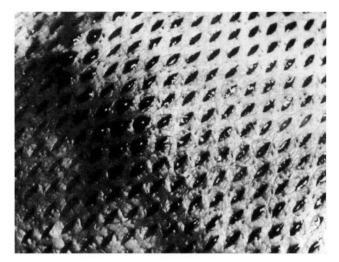

Figure 85-6. Tanner mesh split-thickness skin graft.

other method used and involves using a piece of split-thickness skin without meshing or cutting it into small squares. This method is used on smaller burn wounds and on the face, neck, and hands for better cosmetic results. The part grafted should be immobilized for at least 3 days.

Rehabilitation

WOUND CARE

Wound care, debridement, and subsequent skin care are extremely important considerations for functional and cosmetic outcome, and therefore have a direct bearing on rehabilitation. Aggressive wound care is important to delineate wounds before early surgical intervention, to protect and promote good granulation tissue until grafting, or to promote rapid healing in mid to deep partial-thickness wounds, which tend to have prolonged healing times and subsequently increased scarring (14). The goals of wound care are to prevent or control infection; to preserve as much tissue as possible; and to prepare the wound for earliest possible closure by primary healing or grafting.

Cleaning techniques include local care, spray or nonsubmersion hydrotherapy, and submersion with or without agitation of the water. The choice depends on the depth of injury, extent and location of the wound, and overall condition of the patient. All areas should be scrubbed gently but thoroughly. When manual debridement is indicated, it should be done after the cleaning process. Daily wound care, which must be aggressive and vigorous, should always be done with as little trauma as possible to the wound and granulation tissue.

POSITIONING

In the acute-care period, contracture prevention by proper positioning is fundamental to the overall program. The burn patient obviously is extremely uncomfortable and seeks relief by moving the extremities and trunk into a relaxed position to remove the stretch from the burned tissue. To do so he or she primarily flexes and adducts the extremities into a position of comfort. Because contractures develop rapidly in these patients, antideformity positioning should begin immediately. It is only logical to stress abduction and extension (Fig. 85-7). The alternating of positions so that opposing deformities or pain problems are not created by trying to prevent these flexion–adduction contractures is often forgotten. To aid in positioning,

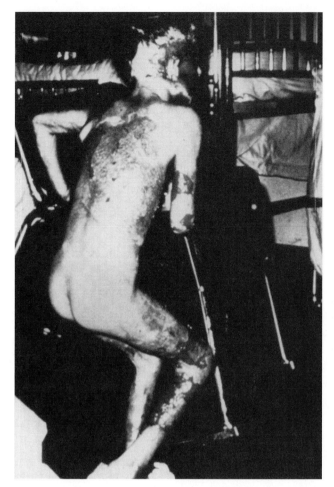

Figure 85-7. Therapeutic positioning. (From Helm PA, Kevorkian GC, Lushbaugh MS, et al. Burn injury: rehabilitation management in 1982. *Arch Phys Med Rehabil* 1982;63:6–16.)

the addition of orthopedic frames and shoulder boards to the bed allows for innovative techniques.

Another salient issue in positioning is the type of bed used. Often, air-fluidized beds are used on burn units for relief of pressure in decubitus prevention and for more even distribution of pressure over wounds and grafts. Although the pressure is better distributed, contractures can be encouraged because the patient sinks into the bed or often assumes a fetal position. The Roho mattress can be as effective as an air-fluidized bed for pressure distribution and is superior in preventing contractures.

SPLINTING AND CASTING

If voluntary positioning becomes a problem, as with the elderly, the noncompliant, and children, splinting becomes an important adjunct to care. If normal range of motion is maintained, there is no need to apply splints, with two major exceptions. Exposed tendons (Fig. 85-8) should be splinted in a slack position in an attempt to prevent rupture, whereas exposed joints should be splinted for protection. Opposite deformities can be created by prolonged immobilization with splinting; therefore frequent assessments of joint range of motion are necessary. The major splints used in the acute phase are as follows:

Resting hand splints to decrease edema and prevent claw hand deformity

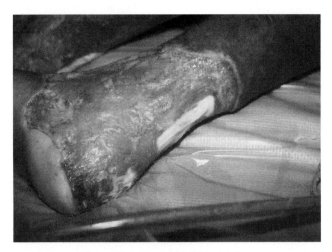

Figure 85-8. Exposed Achilles tendon.

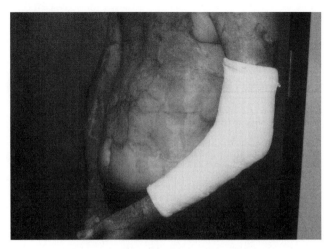

Figure 85-10. Serial casting of the elbow.

Dorsiflexion splints to the ankles for tight heel cords and peroneal nerve palsies (Fig. 85-9)

Velcro band around thighs to prevent "frog leg" position, particularly in children

Elbow extension splints for limited elbow extension with the precaution that the patient have close to full elbow flexion

Serial plaster of Paris casting is an alternative to splinting, especially for children and the noncompliant adult (Figs. 85-10 and 85–11).

The following are reasons for casting (15):

- Provides long-duration stretch to tissues using minimal force.
- Provides protection for exposed tendons.
- Applies static stretch and pressure to remodel scar.
- Cannot be removed easily by the patient.
- Is inexpensive.
- Can be applied easily.
- Can be applied over open wounds.

In a study of 35 refractory contractures in which casting was used for a mean total of 13 days, with casts changed every 3.3 days, range of motion increased from a mean of 56% of normal to a mean of 86% of normal. Full range of motion was attained in nine of 15 elbows and seven of 10 knees. Ankle and wrist range of motion did not improve as much (16). The transparent

face mask frequently is applied early in the acute phase. The plastic mask is made from a plaster model of the face and is applied over new grafts and over newly healed skin (Figs. 85-12 to 85-14). Its advantages include conforming well to the contours of the face, transparency to allow viewing of the skin to verify appropriate pressure distribution, and, when worn properly, prevention of severe cosmetic deformities. Many centers are using silicone face masks immediately after grafting and before application of the transparent face mask.

EXERCISE AND AMBULATION

Throughout convalescence, gentle, sustained stretch of burned tissue is more effective than multiple repetitive movements. Before the therapist begins an exercise program, the area to receive treatment must be viewed directly; otherwise, an inadvertent tissue injury can occur. Exercise programs may be indicated three to four times daily to more involved areas. Without exception the patient should exercise independently between therapy sessions. Active exercises to the lower extremities, whether burned or not, assist in the prevention of thrombophlebitis. Range-of-motion exercises while the patient is anesthetized in the surgical suite permit evaluation of the true range of motion because of lack of patient's resistance (17). Escharotomies, heterografts, synthetic dressings, and tangential

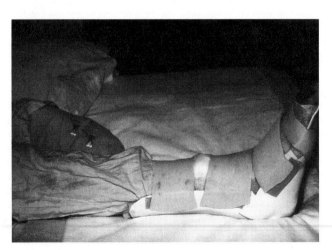

Figure 85-9. Dorsiflexion splint.

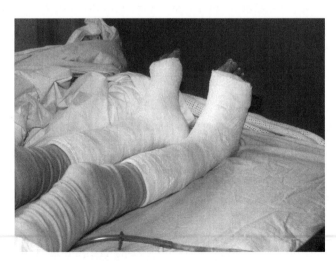

Figure 85-11. Serial casting of the ankles.

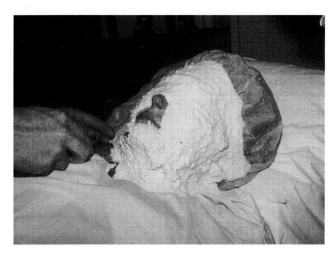

Figure 85-12. Plaster applied to patient to make mold of face.

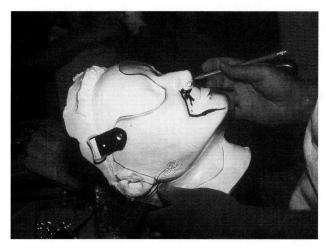

Figure 85-14. Transparent mask fitted to the mold.

excisions are not contraindications for exercise. However, exercises should be discontinued for 3 days to joints proximal and distal to autografted and, sometimes, homografted areas.

In the acute period, trunk mobilization is needed to prevent the robot-type posture that frequently occurs. Burns to the anterior trunk can cause rounding and elevation of the shoulders with a sunken chest and limited trunk rotary movements. To counteract these problems, vigorous trunk flexion–extension and rotation exercises and bilateral shoulder horizontal abduction exercises are necessary (Figs. 85-15 and 85-16). Every part of the body that has received a burn should be exercised in some manner.

Assistive devices, if needed to get or keep the patient ambulatory, should be used. A wheeled walker with an adjustable overhead attached bar can be used for patients with upper-extremity burns to help stretch and increase range of motion of shoulders and elbows as well as reduce edema in the arms. Ambulatory patients have fewer problems with lower-extremity contractures and endurance. Patients with burns to the feet requiring deep excision or partial foot amputations should be fitted early with total-contact sandals (Fig. 85-17), extra-depth shoes, molded insoles, or inserts. Early application of proper footwear prevents later secondary complications of knee, hip, and back pain.

The historical consensus has been that 1 to 2 weeks of bed rest is necessary after lower-extremity grafting. This protocol was expensive and contributed to deconditioning and weakness (18). In a study, 100 consecutive lower-extremity burn admissions were excised and grafted. A dome paste boot (Unna boot) was applied within 24 hours, and ambulation was initiated 4 hours later with full weight bearing. Excellent to satisfactory graft take occurred in 96% of cases, and independent ambulation was achieved in 11 days. Similar results were obtained by Burnsworth et al. (19). Thus, early ambulation (within 1 day with Unna boot) after lower-extremity grafting facilitates functional outcome without risk to graft take. It has also been shown by Kowalske that full weight-bearing ambulation 3 days after grafting without Unna boot does not change graft loss and allows earlier hospital discharge (20). Another method that provides early ambulation with either partial-thickness or full-thickness thermal injury is plaster of Paris casting. This is of particular benefit in individuals with insensate extremities, as seen in diabetics. Diabetics with burns to the plantar aspect of their feet may ambulate in total-contact casts while their wounds are healing (Figs. 85-18 and 85-19). This casting technique is also useful for maintaining range of motion in children following release of toe contractures. Casts are generally changed on a weekly basis.

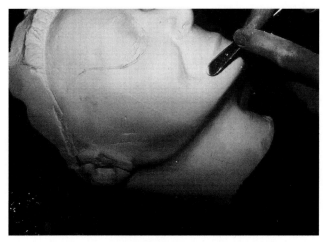

Figure 85-13. Positive mold of face.

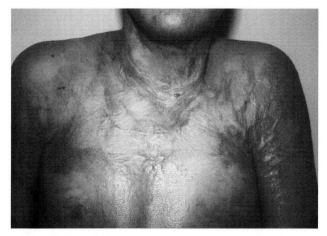

Figure 85-15. Burn scars in a relaxed position across chest and axillas.

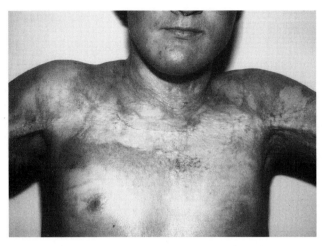

Figure 85-16. Burn scars on a stretch in horizontally abducted position.

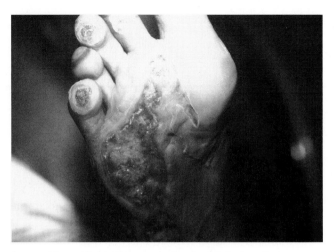

Figure 85-18. Burns to the foot in a diabetic patient.

HAND BURNS

Burn injuries to the hands have a profound effect on the patient's return to normal function; therefore hand therapy is stressed during both acute and postacute phases. A comprehensive medical/surgical hand treatment protocol including splinting, casting, postgraft immobilization, web spacers, compression gloves, and exercise in warm water or silicone gel produces good functional recovery and reduces need for reconstructure surgery (21). A similar protocol was described by Sheridan et al. with good functional results if tendon, joint capsule, or bone involvement was absent (22). It has also been observed that early grafting of the hands has resulted in good hand function, whereas a delay in grafting may not show good results.

Edema

Edema is a major cause of the typical clawed burned hand with hyperextension of the metacarpophalangeal (MCP) joints, flexion of the proximal and distal interphalangeal (IP) joints, and the thumb in adduction and external rotation. The protein-rich edema fluid appears to form a gel after about 12 hours, leading to obstruction of local lymphatic vessels and impairing edema

clearance. Antideformity positioning is best achieved with a resting hand splint, positioning the wrist in slight extension (Fig. 85–46A,B), the MCP joints in 60- to 90-degree flexion, the proximal and distal IP joints in full extension, and the thumb in palmar abduction. It may be necessary to wear the splints continuously until edema resolves and the patient is actively using his or her hands. Edema also is treated through elevation and active exercise. Immediately following injury, the arms may be elevated with Robert Jones skeletal traction, with bedside troughs, or with nighttime stands.

A complication of the pneumatic tourniquet with prolonged application, as reported by Bruner, has adverse effects on tissues of the hand, called the postischemic hand syndrome (23). Bruner's findings of puffiness of the hand and fingers, stiffness of the hand and finger joints, color changes in the hand (e.g., congested in the dependent position), subjective sensations of numbness, and objective evidence of weakness without real paralysis are frequently encountered in the postoperative burn patient (23).

Exposed Tendons, Joints, and Bone

Exposed tendons in the hand can be a serious problem because they have a tendency to dehydrate rapidly, denature, and sub-

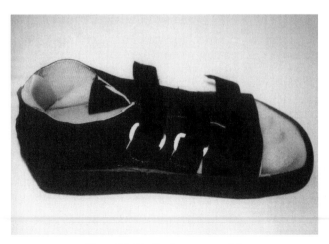

Figure 85-17. Total contact sandal.

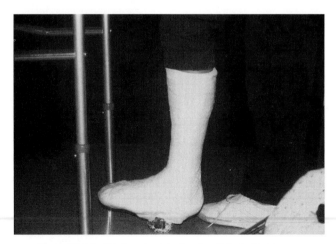

Figure 85-19. Total contact casting for diabetic foot burns.

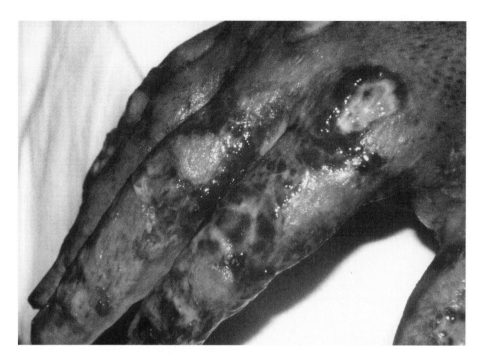

Figure 85-20. Exposed tendons in the hand.

sequently rupture (Fig. 85-20). Exposed tendons should therefore be covered with a moist dressing to prevent drying. Continuous splinting or casting should be used to maintain the tendon in a slack position until permanent wound closure is obtained. Tendons that appear denatured or charred may ultimately revascularize and should not be debrided prematurely. If the dorsal hood mechanism is exposed, the IP joints should be splinted in extension until wound closure. Exercise should be "tendon glide" only. If the dorsal hood ruptures, the typical boutonniere deformity develops (Fig. 85-21). Immediately after rupture, immobilization of the finger for 6 weeks in extension may allow scar tissue to form across the extensor surface and provide a substitute for the destroyed extensor mechanism at 6 weeks. Active motion can then be started (24). If the extensor digitorum longus tendon ruptures at the distal interphalangeal (DIP) joint, a mallet finger deformity occurs (Fig. 85-22). The DIP joint should be splinted or casted in extension for 3 to 4 weeks so the tendon can reattach. Swan neck deformities due to volar

plate rupture or intrinsic muscle tightness can also occur and severely limit hand function (Fig. 85-23). If joint capsules are exposed but not open, they may be gently exercised actively and protectively splinted. If the joint is open or draining, it will probably undergo spontaneous ankylosis; therefore functional positioning should be encouraged. Bone that is exposed must be covered with moist dressings to prevent desiccation of the periosteum. Some surgeons drill burr holes in exposed bone to stimulate granulation tissue formation for eventual bone coverage (Fig. 85-24).

Exercise

Primary considerations in exercising the burned hand include intrinsic muscle stretching by mobilizing the metacarpals and stretching the intrinsic muscles by hyperextension of the MCP joint in combination with flexion of the proximal IP joint (Fig.

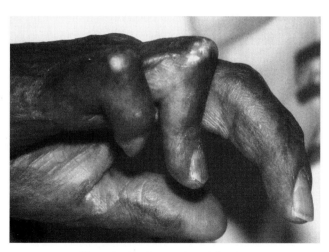

Figure 85-21. Boutonniere deformity.

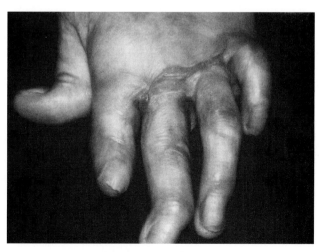

Figure 85-22. Mallet finger.

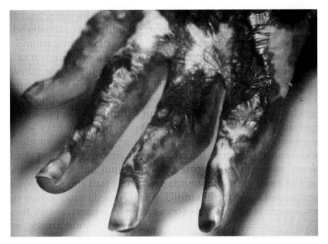

Figure 85-23. Swan neck deformity.

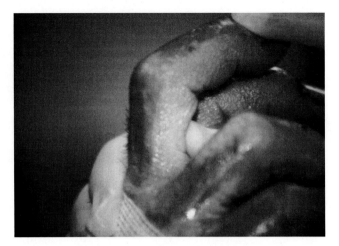

Figure 85-25. Intrinsic muscle stretching.

85-25). Traction applied to the joints with passive movement allows for additional ligamentous stretch.

Splinting

It is not unusual for the burned hand to require customized splinting. Dynamic, as well as static, splinting is used. Custom-conforming splints are used primarily on the flexor surfaces of the hand in patients who have developed contractures or banding over the palmar aspect. The pressure of the splint produces softening, flattening, and lengthening of the scar band. Splints may be used for serial splinting, with the splint being applied at maximum tension and constant pressure; as the contracture improves, the splint is remodeled. Dynamic splinting can be effective in correcting contractures. Nail hooks, leather loops over the phalanges, flexion wrap, or a flexion glove may be used for dynamic stretch in extension contractures (see Fig. 85–46F,G later in this chapter). A custom-made elastomer foam insert placed at the first web space is helpful in maintaining the space and in decreasing an adduction contracture of the thumb. Successful splinting of the hand requires therapist innovation as well as significant patient cooperation.

Rehabilitation of a child's hand is different from that of the adult's and bears special mention. The child's hand is small,

making it difficult to fabricate properly fitting hand orthoses, and children have a tendency to flex the hand, causing splint movement and thus producing pressure ulcers. Unfortunately, the young child cannot express pain complaints appropriately. For dorsal hand burns it may be necessary to position the MCP as well as the IP joints in extension. In the uncooperative child, serial casting is very beneficial, and passive range-of-motion exercises are critical. Play activities become a much more important feature of the exercise program (25).

ELECTRICAL INJURIES

Mechanism of Injury

Electrical injuries constitute 2% to 3% of most burn unit admissions; however, they are the most devastating types of thermal injury. These injuries are arbitrarily divided into low-voltage, those no greater than 500 to 1,000 volts, and high-voltage, those greater than 1,000 volts. Home injuries usually involve 110 to 220 volts with 60-cycle current and cause little cutaneous damage. Deep muscle damage is very rare. These low-voltage accidents, however, can be associated with cardiac standstill or rhythm irregularities. The most common low-voltage burn injury is in the child who bites an electrical cord and sustains a

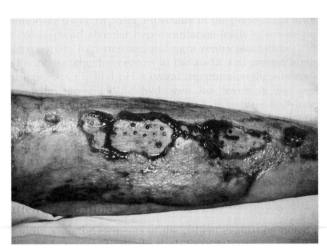

Figure 85-24. Burr holes in bone.

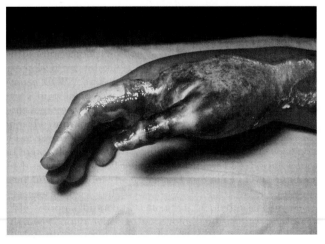

Figure 85-26. Electrical injury.

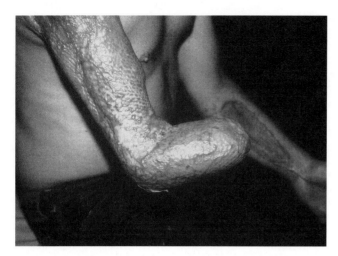

Figure 85-27. Transradial amputation from an electrical injury.

burn of the commissure of the lips. Generally, the greater the voltage, the greater the amperage and, consequently, the more severe the injury. As current flows through the body, electrical energy is converted to heat. Damage is related primarily to tissue resistance and sensitivity to heat. The most resistant or nonconductive tissue is bone, followed by cartilage, tendon, skin, muscle, blood, and nerve. Blood vessels and nerves offer little resistance, which produces higher current flow. These structures also seem to be particularly sensitive to heat damage and sustain injury because of their low resistance (26–28).

Soft-Tissue and Bone Damage

Tissue destruction is always greatest in areas of the body with small volume, such as fingers, toes, wrists, or ankles (Fig. 85-26). The physician must therefore be knowledgeable about this iceberg-type injury, in which the cutaneous injury may give no indication of the possible underlying muscle, bone, and nerve damage.

The acute surgical treatment is early diagnosis and debridement of necrotic tissue. In all burn patients, the greatest number of amputations occur from electrical injuries (Figs. 85-27 and 85-28) (29). Burn amputations can present with many pre-

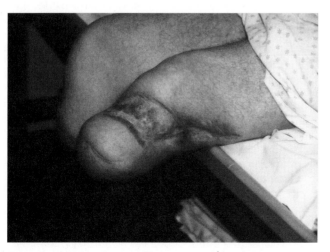

Figure 85-28. Bilateral transtibial amputation from an electrical injury.

and postprosthetic problems, including skin fragility and breakdown, painful scars, bone spurs, joint contractures, and muscle weakness. These situations can delay prosthetic fitting, but eventually most patients achieve successful prosthetic use. Also, wounds on other parts of the body can adversely affect successful prosthetic use. These problems must be addressed concurrently with prosthetic fitting and training (30).

Localized Nerve and Central Nervous System Injury

Localized neuropathies may occur both in tissues that are directly burned and in tissue through which electrical energy passes. Radiculopathies, as a result of neck hyperextension as the current flows through the body, may appear immediately following injury or later in the convalescent period. Patients who have had current pass through their legs often complain of weakness manifested by inability to stand for long periods of time and general lack of stamina. Electrodiagnostic tests are worthwhile to diagnose subtle peripheral neuropathies that are common following electrical injury.

Central nervous system damage may result in memory loss, personality changes, and spinal cord pathology. Symptoms of central nervous system injury may not be evident for up to 2 years following injury; therefore long-term patient follow-up is needed.

Cataracts

Electrical contact on the head or shoulders or visual exposure to the flash may predispose a patient to cataracts. Cataracts may form within 1 month or as late as 3 years following injury. Therefore serial eye examinations should be performed for at least 3 years after injury.

NEUROLOGIC INJURIES

Localized Neuropathies

Peripheral neurologic complications in the burn patient are not uncommon; however, they frequently are undiagnosed because neurologic assessments are difficult in patients with multiple concurrent problems. To a great extent, most nerve injuries are preventable; therefore a clear understanding of their etiology is essential. Certain patients are predisposed to peripheral nerve compromise because their nerves are diseased, as seen in diabetics and alcoholics. Elderly patients develop neuropathies because their peripheral nerves do not tolerate pressure well and because they are less mobile; therefore they maintain prolonged positions that place their nerves at risk (31–33).

BRACHIAL PLEXUS

The burn patient may assume several bed positions and intraoperative positions that put the brachial plexus at risk. In conjunction with these at-risk positions, loss of muscle tone in the anesthetized patient and immobility of the patient in bed add to the problem of positioning risks. Several authors have reported possible mechanisms of injury to the plexus during anesthesia. Jackson and Keats reported that plexus stretch injury could occur in patients positioned supine with shoulders abducted 90 degrees or more and externally rotated (34). In addition, if the upper arm is posteriorly displaced (i.e., hung below table level), added tension is placed on the plexus.

The mechanism creating the injury is compression of the plexus between the clavicle and first rib, which causes tension

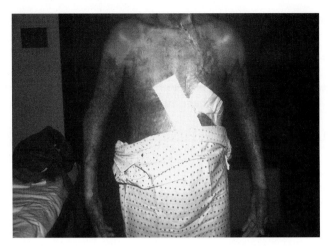

Figure 85-29. Bilateral brachial plexus injury secondary to prone positioning.

and stretch with these particular shoulder and arm movements (34). Ewing wrote that when the humerus is abducted in external rotation, its head forms a prominence in the axilla where the nerve trunks pass; the nerves may become angulated with resultant stretching (35). The nerve trunks to the upper extremity are anchored at the vertebral column and by fascial attachments in the axilla; they pass under a tendinous arch formed by the insertion of the pectoralis minor. Even though nerves are extensible, there is a limit to their stretch (35). Dhuner reported that a brachial plexus injury occurred in as little as 40 minutes in the operating room (36). Other at-risk positions are prone and side-lying (Fig. 85-29). In the prone position, the patient lies with arms abducted 90 degrees or more and externally rotated (36). Patients positioned on one side with the opposite arm abducted, elbow extended, and then suspended from an intravenous pole or overhead frame can develop a traction injury to the brachial plexus. This position may be used in the surgical suite for grafting of the axilla or lateral chest wall; for bed positioning, to decrease edema of the extremity; or for prevention of axillary contractures.

To prevent compression or stretch injury to the brachial plexus, some have recommended positioning the supine patient in 15 inches of arm horizontal adduction, lifting the clavicle off the first rib. One or two pillows under the chest of the prone-lying patient will adduct the extremities and lift the clavicle off the first rib.

Another possible problem is a stretch injury of the plexus after an axillary contracture release, particularly if the contracture has been long-standing. All structures can become tight with prolonged limited mobility; therefore the surgeon often chooses to do staged releases to try to prevent a stretch injury from occurring. In a stretch injury, the upper trunk (i.e., C5 and C6 of the brachial plexus) is involved primarily. Generally, the patient recovers completely, but it may take several months.

SUPRASCAPULAR NERVE

Injury to the suprascapular nerve often is overlooked because function is not markedly impaired and the burn usually involves the posterior shoulder girdle on the side of injury. The suprascapular nerve passes through a fibroosseous tunnel of the suprascapular notch to innervate the supraspinatus and infraspinatus. As reported by Rask, hyperprotraction of the shoulder overstretches the nerve, with resultant swelling and unrelenting pain in the shoulder region. A hyperprotracted position can occur when the patient tries to stretch the skin in the

posterior shoulder girdle by forward flexion and horizontal adduction of the arm. Injury can be prevented by stabilizing the scapula (37).

ULNAR NERVE

The primary area of involvement of the ulnar nerve in the burn patient is at the elbow in the cubital tunnel. The roof of the tunnel is the arcuate ligament, which extends from a fixed point on the medial epicondyle to a movable attachment on the olecranon. The floor of the tunnel is formed by the medial ligament of the elbow. Wadsworth reports that the capacity of the tunnel is maximal with elbow extension when the arcuate ligament is slack (38). When the elbow is flexed to 90 degrees the arcuate ligament becomes taut and the medial ligament bulges, decreasing the capacity of the tunnel and putting the nerve at risk. He also noted that pronation of the forearm could cause surface contact with the cubital tunnel, whereas supination of the forearm lifts the tunnel containing the ulnar nerve away from the surface. Unfortunately, many burn patients assume the position of elbow flexion and forearm pronation, causing elbow flexion pronation contractures; this probably accounts for the majority of ulnar neuropathies. In the operating suite, the patient frequently is positioned in the same manner. An injury at this level usually spares the flexor carpi ulnaris and ulnar half of the flexor digitorum profundus because the fibers to these muscles are located deep in the central part of the nerve. Another circumstance predisposing a patient to an ulnar neuropathy is subluxation of the ulnar nerve onto the medial epicondyle, thereby essentially leaving it unprotected from pressure. In cases of heterotopic bone at the elbow, entrapment of the ulnar nerve in an osseous tunnel has been reported (39).

RADIAL NERVE

The radial nerve is involved most frequently in the burn patient by compression in the spiral groove, where the nerve winds around the humerus and virtually lies on bone. Compression injuries at this level may be secondary to the arm resting on the side rails of the bed, hanging over the edge of the operating table, or slipping off the edge of an arm board. In these cases, the triceps muscle usually is spared because it is innervated at a higher level. Restraints at the distal forearm–wrist level can injure the superficial cutaneous branch of the radial nerve, causing paresthesia of the dorsum of the hand and thumb.

MEDIAN NERVE

Most injuries to the median nerve occur at the wrist level and may be caused by edema acutely or by the extremes of positioning used to gain range of motion. Prolonged or repeated hyperextension of the wrist compresses the nerve at the carpal tunnel, which can cause paresthesia in the thumb index, middle, and ring fingers and weakness of the thenar muscles. Sustained stretch to the wrist in a hyperextended position, either with splints or in exercise programs, should be performed with caution.

FEMORAL NERVE

Femoral nerve dysfunction in the burn patient is uncommon; however, the femoral nerve has been known to be injured in the femoral triangle after hematoma formation, secondary to obtaining femoral blood samples. Femoral blood withdrawal often is necessary in the extensively burned patient. The nerve also is susceptible to injury in patients on anticoagulant therapy who have had a retroperitoneal hemorrhage. Mant et al. studied 76 patients receiving heparin anticoagulation for venous thromboembolism and found a 7% incidence of retroperitoneal hemorrhage (40). Reinstein et al. studied femoral nerve dysfunction after retroperitoneal hemorrhage with computed tomography and were able to localize the hematoma (41). They found that localization of the hematoma within the tight iliacus muscle compartment could produce femoral nerve injury by compressing the nerve against the taut psoas tendon. It is reported that 75% of the patients experience complete recovery of nerve function with conservative management (41).

PERONEAL NERVE

The peroneal nerve has several peculiarities that make it vulnerable to injury. Berry and Richardson showed that the nerve is applied to the periosteum of the fibula for a total of 10 cm; is exposed over the bony prominence for about 4 cm, covered only by skin and fascia; and has limited longitudinal mobility of about 0.5 cm (42). Although compression injuries of the peroneal nerve are notoriously associated with the lateral decubitus position, metal stirrups, and leg straps, less attention is given to positions of the leg that cause stretch injuries. When a patient maintains a position of externally rotated hips, flexion of the knees, and inverted feet (i.e., frog leg), either because the bed is too short, because a urinal is placed between the thighs for men, or because there are tender medial thigh or perineum burns, the peroneal nerve is placed on a stretch and can be injured in a matter of hours because of its limited longitudinal mobility. This type of injury usually involves the common peroneal nerve, and moderate-to-good recovery is reported at 3 months (42). Another source of injury that cannot be ignored is pressure at the fibular head from heavy, bulky dressings. Windowing of the dressings over the fibular head helps relieve pressure.

TOURNIQUET PARALYSIS

Most articles on tourniquet paralysis usually state that since the pneumatic tourniquet has been employed, it has virtually eliminated the danger of nerve palsy. However, the pneumatic tourniquet used to establish a bloodless field has not prevented this complication to the extent reported. Aho et al. report that faulty gauges on pneumatic tourniquets can sometimes be the cause of the problem (43). Tourniquet inflation to 500 mm Hg instead of the intended 250 mm Hg can cause direct pressure injury of the nerve at the cuff edge. The radial nerve is most vulnerable, but ulnar and median nerves also can be damaged (Fig. 85-30). Sunderland reports that the nerve lesions heal in 3 to 6 months and are only exceptionally permanently damaged

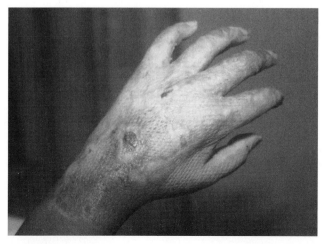

Figure 85-30. Ulnar nerve injury caused by a tourniquet.

(44). In cases of paralysis, the tourniquet time has varied from 28 minutes to 2 hours and 40 minutes (23,43).

Peripheral Neuropathy

Generalized peripheral neuropathy is the most common peripheral neurologic disorder seen in the burn patient. It usually occurs in patients with burns of more than 20% of the TBSA, with the exception of electrical injuries, in which the total body surface burn may be less. The incidence ranges from 15%, as determined by Henderson, Koepke, and Feller, to 29%, as reported by Helm et al. (31,45,46). The etiology of peripheral neuropathies is uncertain; however, metabolic complications and neurotoxic drugs have been implicated. The patient may have symptoms of paresthesia and signs of mild to moderate weakness in the muscles of the distal extremities. On manual muscle testing, most patients eventually appear to recover their strength, although they complain of lack of endurance and easy fatigability for years after the burn (31,45,46).

Multiple mononeuropathy was found in nine of 121 persons with more than 40% TBSA burn injury (47). Multiple mononeuropathy is defined as an asymmetric neuropathy that involves two or more nerves that result from multiple crush syndrome. Multiple crush syndrome represents the summation of the effects of neurotoxins, metabolic factors, and/or compression. At 1 year, lower-extremity multiple mononeuropathies achieved good functional recovery; upper-extremity results were less satisfactory. The intervention utilized with these patients included sensory education, range of motion exercise, and splinting.

BONE AND JOINT CHANGES

Bone Growth

Growth disturbances in burns may result from premature fusion of the entire epiphyseal plate or only a portion of the plate and subsequent growth arrest. Premature fusion of the epiphyseal plate can cause bone shortening and should be a consideration in children who have scar tissue crossing joints, or especially who have persistent joint contractures. Partial epiphyseal plate fusion may cause bone deviation and deformity (48). Pressure treatment of scar tissue as reported by Leung et al. can cause regressed skeletal growth in the chin and thoracic cage from wearing a face mask and body suit. The face was noted to be "birdlike" because of the slow-growing mandible and the thoracic cage, developing a roundish appearance (49). Shortened legs, hands, and feet have occurred (Fig. 85-31).

Growth stimulation also has been found by some investigators and is described as growth spurts in children and increased shoe size in adults. It is postulated that skeletal growth is stimulated through stasis or passive hyperemia or a chronic inflammatory process.

Osteophytes

Evans and Smith report that osteophytes are the most frequently observed skeletal alteration in adult burn patients. They are most often seen at the elbow and occur along the articular margins of the olecranon or coronoid process (50,51).

New Bone Formation

HETEROTOPIC OSSIFICATION

New bone formation begins as heterotopic calcification and is seen on plain film as a fluffy shadow. In at least 50% of patients

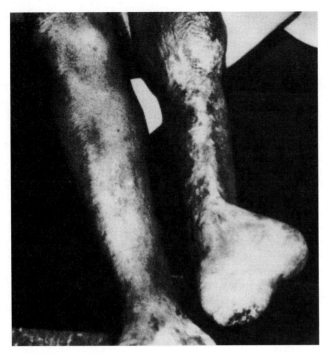

Figure 85-31. Growth disturbance in a 56-year-old patient who was burned at 6 years of age.

this calcification will be absorbed; in the remainder it can ossify. Calcification and ossification have been reported to occur as early as 5 to 6 weeks following a burn but usually develop in 3 to 4 months. Teperman et al. reported that bone scans assist in making early diagnosis (52). Positive bone scans preceded positive radiologic findings by 3 weeks. Rarely are there any detectable chemical changes by laboratory tests. One of the earliest signs of heterotopic ossification is loss of joint range of motion; this change can precede radiologic findings by 5 days (52). The most common site involved is the elbow, followed by the hip in children and the shoulder in adults.

Patients who are predisposed to the development of heterotopic ossification are those with full-thickness burns to the upper extremities and burns of more than 20% of the TBSA. Other commonalities for development are immobility, repeated minor trauma, and pressure, particularly over the medial epicondyle. The incidence of true heterotopic ossification probably ranges between 0.1% and 3.1% (52).

Once the diagnosis of heterotopic ossification has been made, forceful passive movements of the extremity are contraindicated because this type of exercise can make the condition worse. Only gentle movement within the patient's active range should be performed. Operative treatment is indicated if there is no spontaneous resolution of the heterotopic calcification. Most surgeons will not operate until the bone is mature, which can take 12 to 18 months. A retrospective review of 1,478 burn admissions indicated that 18 developed heterotopic ossification; 10 of these recovered full range of motion with the preceding treatment protocol within 6 months of diagnosis. The remaining eight received surgery followed by rehabilitation, and all developed functional range of motion with no recurrence after 3 years (53).

REDUCTION IN BONE MASS

Significant growth delays occur in children for up to 3 years after survival from a burn injury. A more recent study has shown that children who sustain a severe thermal injury have an acute loss of bone mass that is maintained (54). The mecha-

nism for loss of bone mass is not completely understood but is thought to be related to immobilization, increased production of endogenous corticosteroids, and aluminum loading. In those children with severe burns (40% to 100%) of the TBSA the incidence of fractures appeared to be higher than in unburned children (55).

BONY CHANGES IN ELECTRICAL BURNS

New bone formation at amputation sites in the electrical burn has been reported to involve long bones, or more specifically, above-elbow, below-elbow, above-knee, and below-knee residual limbs. Helm et al. reported that 23 of 28 (82%) patients with long-bone amputations developed new bone at the amputation site. Of the 61 amputations studied, 78% of upper-extremity and 90% of lower-extremity long-bone amputations had new bone formation. The average time from amputation to diagnosis of new bone was 38 weeks. Five patients (11.6%) required surgical revision of the stump, and an additional three patients (7%) required replacement of their prosthesis secondary to new bone formation. The cause of this high rate of new bone formation in the electrical amputee has not been determined. However, the effect of high voltage on bone may be similar to long-term low-voltage/amperage stimulation for promoting callus formation at fracture sites (56).

Vrabec and Kolar studied bone changes in the electrical burn and described bony changes that are directly related to the action of the passage of electric current as bone splitting, bone pearls from the melting of bone minerals, bony necrosis, and periosteal new bone caused by inflammatory reaction as a result of avulsion of the periosteum. Other authors have reported lucent holes in the bone and bone swelling (57).

SCOLIOSIS AND KYPHOSIS

Asymmetric burns of the trunk, hips, and shoulder girdle can cause the patient to favor the side of the body burned and shift weight to the same side. A functional scoliosis can develop because of the pain in maintaining correct posture, and the functional scoliosis can change to a structural scoliosis with vertebral wedging if a child has a growth spurt before this is corrected (Fig. 85-32) (58). Burns on the anterior neck, shoulders, and chest wall may produce a rounding of the shoulders and sunken chest. This is caused by burn scar shortening and by the patient assuming a protective posture. The result can be a kyphotic thoracic spine if not corrected with proper exercise and positioning programs. Surgical excision usually is not successful for correcting this abnormality.

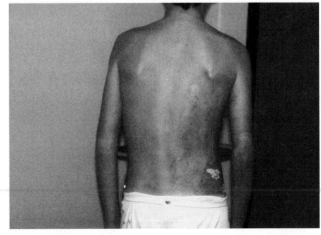

Figure 85-32. Scoliosis caused by asymmetric burns of the trunk.

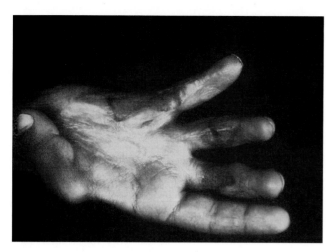

Figure 85-33. Subluxation of the thumb.

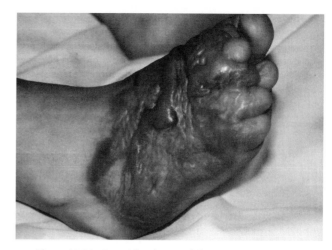

Figure 85-34. Dorsal foot burn with hyperextension of toes.

SEPTIC ARTHRITIS

Septic arthritis can be overlooked easily in the severely burned patient because of lack of usual clinical signs and symptoms. Some septic joints are pain-free, and some are covered with burn wounds that mask the usual fusiform swelling and local tenderness.

The two primary causes of a septic joint in burns are penetrating burns into joints and bacteremia. Septic arthritis may cause gross dislocation because of capsular laxity or cartilage and bone destruction (52), or it may result in severe restriction of movement or ankylosis. It occurs most frequently in the joints of the hands, hips, knees, and wrists.

SUBLUXATIONS AND DISLOCATIONS

Joint subluxation in the hands and feet is seen commonly in burn patients (Fig. 85-33). Generally, the burn is over the dorsal aspect, and as the burn wound contracts, it pulls the joint into hyperextension. If this is allowed to persist, the joint will sublux. This is more commonly seen in the MCP and metatarsophalangeal (MTP) joints. An ulnar neuropathy can accentuate the problem in the fourth and fifth digits. A hyperextended thumb at the MCP joint also can easily sublux. Prevention of this injury in the hand begins in the acute phase of treatment by splinting the MCP joints in flexion to approximately 60 to 90 degrees, thereby keeping the collateral ligament on a stretch. This is done in conjunction with an exercise program stressing joint flexion. The MTP joints of the toes become more of a problem after healing, as the burn scar contracts, especially in children (Fig. 85-34). Simple application of surgical high-top shoes with a metatarsal bar worn 24 hours a day keeps the toes in an antideformity position.

Hip dislocation can be a problem in children if the hip is allowed to remain in an adducted and flexed position. Shoulder dislocations are reported to occur in extreme positions of abduction and extension.

LONG-TERM REHABILITATION

The postacute rehabilitative phase of treatment can be five to 10 times longer than the acute phase. It is during this period that the patient undergoes a multitude of physical and emotional changes. It is also usually during this time that the patient and family realize how devastating this insult has been to the body. They frequently react in adverse ways that can affect outcome if proper support is not available. The physicians and therapists assume a new role when rehabilitation, rather than survival, is the primary issue.

Skin and Wound Care

Rarely does the patient leave the hospital with completely healed wounds and donor sites. Therefore continuation of the wound care program with hydrotherapy, debridement, and dressing changes is necessary. Once the wounds are healed or only spotty areas are open, hydrotherapy should be discontinued because of the drying effect on the skin, which will cause the skin to crack and make it more susceptible to bacterial invasion.

Additional problems can occur after healing, such as skin breakdown, blistering, ulceration, and allergic reactions. Newly formed skin is especially fragile, and even the slightest trauma, such as a result of stretching exercises, pressure from splints and garments, or minor bumps, can cause abrasions and blisters (Fig. 85-35). Blisters may form in reepithelialized areas of burns or in grafted areas and typically start within 2 to 6 weeks of wound closure. As the skin matures, blistering usually diminishes. Blisters can be drained with a sterile needle and flattened with a dressing (Figs. 85-36 and 85-37). If denuded areas are created by large blisters, Betadine and saline mixture 50:50 is a good drying agent. These areas usually will dry, crust, and heal. All open wounds, however, should be gently cleaned with a mild soap. Ulcerations or chronic open wounds usually develop in tight bands of scar tissue in the axilla and cubital and popliteal fossae. These wounds generally are deep, and repeated splitting of the wounds with exercise prolongs heal-

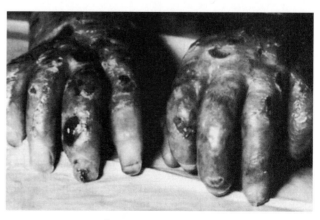

Figure 85-35. Fragile skin.

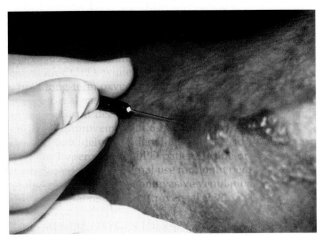

Figure 85-36. Drain blisters with sterile needle.

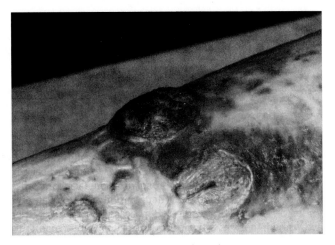

Figure 85-38. Marjolin's ulcer.

ing and causes increased scarring. If the wound is clean, application of a biological dressing and placing the part at rest will speed the healing process. Malignant changes can occur in chronic open wounds caused by burns and are referred to as Marjolin's ulcer (Fig. 85-38). The mechanism for the change is seen in wounds that repeatedly open and close, in scars that are traumatized repeatedly, and in wounds that never fully close. Most cases are squamous cell carcinoma. This type of cancer has a propensity for the extremities, particularly in flexion creases where blood supply is decreased and trauma increased (59).

Allergic reactions after healing that produce moist, weeping wounds can be frustrating because finding the irritating agent is sometimes difficult. Domoboro solution applied daily as a soak for 10 to 15 minutes will aid in drying the weeping lesions. Also, Calmoseptine Ointment (Calmoseptine Inc., Hunting Beach, CA) applied sparingly over the affected areas promotes drying and healing. The most common agents that cause these reactions have been skin lubricants, particularly those products with mineral oil; pressure garments; and various soaps used to cleanse the skin. All these agents should be discontinued for 2 to 4 days before beginning substitution with different products, one at a time.

Healed partial-thickness burns are said to lack natural lubrication for 6 to 8 weeks. Skin lubrication comes from two sources: sebaceous gland secretion and lipids from epidermal cells. Sebaceous secretion returns in partial-thickness burns, since skin appendages survive; however, in full-thickness burns that have been grafted skin appendages do not reform. Therefore topical agents are used to moisturize the skin. Emollients that contain both water to hydrate the skin and a lipid to retard its evaporation are recommended (60). Dryness and decreased elasticity contribute to skin problems, such as cracking, pruritus, and skin breakdown.

Patients who are treated in settings where there is no hands-on technique suffer from hypersensitive skin and scars. Skin lubrication helps alleviate some of these problems and should be considered an essential part of the overall treatment program performed by the therapists. Massage of healed burn wounds can accomplish skin lubrication, decrease skin hypersensitivity, and increase skin suppleness. A variety of lotions have been found to be nonirritating, such as aloe vera moisturizers, vitamin E ointment, and cocoa butter. Application of lotion after refrigeration is helpful.

Itching

Pruritis can be a very serious problem for many patients. A study by Tyack et al. on functional outcome in children found that itching was one of the primary impairments that contributed to reduced functional outcome after a burn injury. In another study, severity of itching was not related to the age of the patient, or if the patient was grafted, but was related to TBSA involved and the time it took for the wounds to close. It

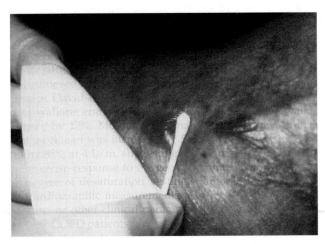

Figure 85-37. Flatten blisters after drainage.

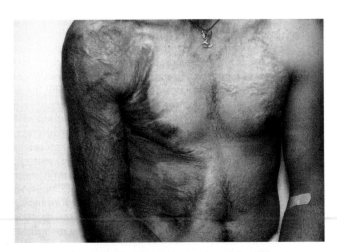

Figure 85-39. Hyperpigmentation of the skin.

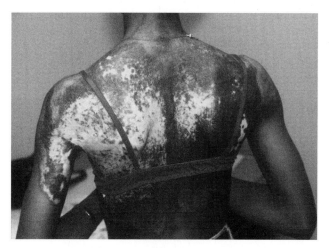

Figure 85-40. Hypopigmentation of the skin.

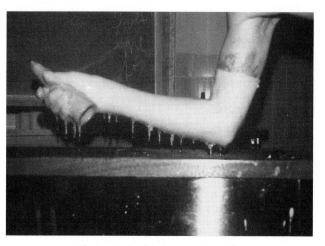

Figure 85-42. Application of paraffin.

was also noted that patients with burns of more than 40% TBSA would likely have a problem with itching and that legs were at greatest risk for itching, followed by the arms. The face did not itch (61). Pruritic symptoms frequently require oral antihistamine medication as well as pressure garments to make the patient more comfortable (14). New creams developed over the last few years appear promising as a topical aid in controlling itching. Zeta Provace (Swiss-American Products, Inc. Dallas, TX) and Prudoxin (DPT Laboratories, San Antonio, TX) are two that have been used with good results.

Skin Color Changes

A study by de Chalain et al. on burn skin color changes after superficial burns showed variable changes the first 3 years after injury. Subsequently, there was cumulative hyperpigmentation at the burn site as long as the melanocyte-bearing deep dermis had not been destroyed (Fig. 85-39). Deeper burn injuries may cause hypopigmentation or depigmentation (Fig. 85-40). Pigmentary changes may improve with time, but they may be permanent (62). Avoidance of sunlight exposure for 6 months or longer is recommended after wound healing to avoid sunburn and hyperpigmentation. Sunscreen products with a sun protection factor of at least 15 are recommended. Waterproof products may be effective for only 80 minutes (60). Hydroquinone cream has been used to help fade hypopigmented areas.

Exercise

TECHNIQUES

Maintaining range of motion of a joint after healing or grafting is more difficult than in the acute phase. Burn scars contract, form bands, and thicken, and joint range of motion is affected. Remolding of the burn scar is possible while the scar is actively undergoing internal changes, such as collagen degradation and deposition and myofibroblastic activity. Once the burn scar matures, stretching a skin contracture is of less benefit.

By far the most effective stretching technique for skin contractures is slow, sustained stretch (Fig. 85-41). The part being stretched should be visible and should be palpated along the line of pull to ensure that the skin does not tear. Stretching can be done manually with weights, traction, splinting, and serial casting. The technique of applying paraffin to the part being mobilized and allowing 30 minutes of sustained stretch has been very rewarding in gaining range of motion. At the same time it decreases joint discomfort and lubricates the skin (Fig. 85-42). The paraffin temperature must be lowered to 116° to 118°F to prevent burning of the skin (63).

Another important principle in the exercise program is to put the entire length of a burn scar on a total stretch (Fig. 85-43). In other words, if a scar crosses multiple joints, all involved joints are stretched simultaneously. A joint does not have full range of motion unless full range is obtained in combined movements.

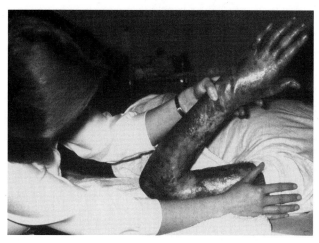

Figure 85-41. Slow sustained stretch on burn scars.

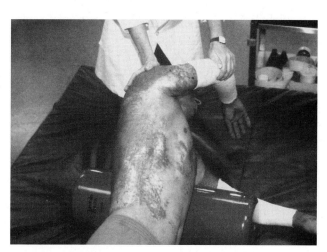

Figure 85-43. Burn scar on a stretch.

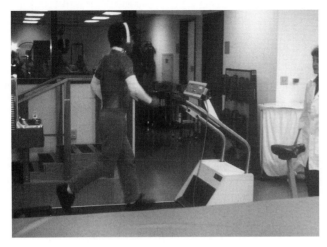

Figure 85-44.

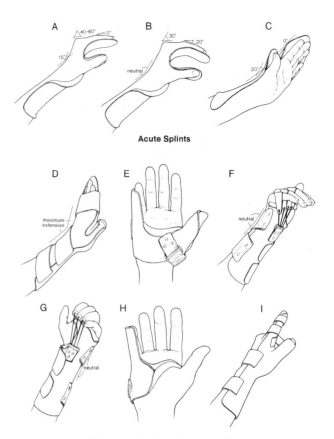

Acute Splints

Figure 85-46. Convalescent splints.

Finally, all patients should be on a generalized strengthening program for reconditioning after prolonged inactivity. Resistive exercises of opposing muscle groups also are beneficial in contracture prevention and treatment. Exercises for endurance and coordination frequently are overlooked in burn rehabilitation but are an essential aspect of the total program (Figs. 85-44 and 85-45).

A recent study has shown that patients with severe burns of more than 30% TBSA had weaker muscles years after the burn, suggesting either inability to fully recover or insufficient rehabilitation. The strength deficits were more marked at the faster velocities, suggesting a preferential atrophy of fast-twitch fibers. It was also shown that a cardiovascular fitness protocol with isokinetic strengthening was more effective than isometric and isotonic strengthening (64).

SPECIALIZED SPLINTING
Without the benefit of custom-made splints and casting, exercise programs would be in vain. A joint contracture may be stretched to full range, but maintaining that range depends in part on static and dynamic positioning accomplished with splinting and casting (Fig. 85-46). Hence, the mistake often is made to splint joints in full extension for prolonged periods because the patient looks anatomically correct; however, function

is sacrificed. This unfortunately is true especially for elbows, which often are placed in extension.

Experienced therapists are able to make splints that control more than one joint and, at the same time, apply pressure over thick bands of scar tissue. Major areas of concern in the convalescent period are hands. Difficult areas requiring specialized splints include the following:

Palmar contractures (Fig. 85-46C,D)
Cupping of the palm (Fig. 85-46E)
Fifth-digit flexion contracture (Fig. 85-46H)
Tight thumb-index web space (Fig. 85-46I)
Ruptured extensor hood mechanism
Neck flexion contracture
Hip flexion abduction–external rotation in children
Ankle-dorsiflexion contractures

MODALITIES
Certain modalities commonly used in rehabilitation medicine clinics have been found useful in treating specific burn complications. Electrical stimulation, using an alternating current, is helpful in treating tendon adherence to underlying scar tissue. The transcutaneous electrical stimulator is useful for treatment of various pain problems, particularly those involving the shoulder from prolonged or faulty positioning.

Ultrasound has been used to treat painful joints and facilitate better tolerance of range-of-motion exercise. It has also been applied along with ice massage to decrease hypertrophic scar pain. In a prospective randomized double-blind study, the effectiveness of ultrasound with passive stretching versus placebo ultrasound with passive stretching was investigated. The results indicated no difference in range of motion or per-

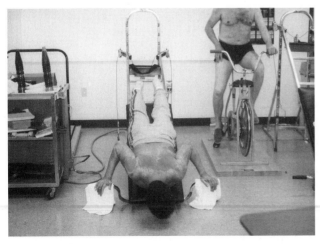

Figure 85-45. Exercises for endurance and strengthening.

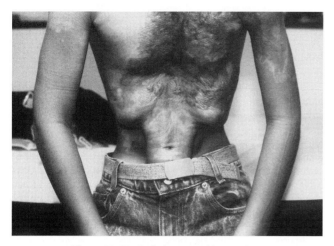

Figure 85-47. Early hypertrophic scarring.

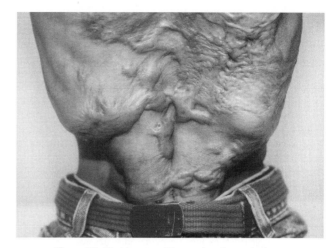

Figure 85-48. Hypertrophic scarring 2 months later.

ceived pain between these two groups. This suggests that although widely used, ultrasound may not have an effect on functional improvement of contractures (65).

Intermittent compression units or similar devices are valuable in reducing edema in extremities, primarily the edematous hand. Posthealing hand edema secondary to circumferential burns of the forearm, hands with reflex sympathetic dystrophy, and hands with postischemic hand syndrome usually respond well to elevation and compression. Persistent edema can be devastating, because it can result in a "frozen hand."

Continuous passive motion (CPM) machines can never take the place of the hands-on exercises by the therapists. Occasionally, CPM is indicated with a patient who resists the exercise program from fear of pain, in children who seem to relax better with CPM, in those who need additional range-of-motion treatments for exceptionally tight areas, and in patients following excision of heterotopic ossification.

Burn Sequelae

HYPERTROPHIC SCARRING
It is well known that hypertrophic scar and scar contracture can result from deep partial- and full-thickness burns (Figs. 85-

47 and 85-48). Many factors contribute to the severity of hypertrophic scarring: depth of burn, healing time, grafting, age of patient, and skin character. An excellent review on hypertrophic scarring and the effects of pressure was done by Jensen and Parshley (66). They reported on areas of the skin affected by the scar, noting that the epidermis was not thickened and did not contribute to the depth of the hypertrophic scar. They also reported, "the regenerated epidermis lacks rete pegs and interconnections that attach it to the dermis; hence it is cosmetically abnormal with respect to color, texture, and friability and is prone to abrasion with minor trauma" (66). They noted that changes in the dermis involving fibroblasts, myofibroblasts, mast cells, collagen, mucopolysaccharides, and vasculature cause a metabolically active abnormal mass of thick tissue. In hypertrophic scars, collagen forms large nodules rather than loose, wavy bundles as seen in normal dermis. In granulation tissue and hypertrophic scars, capillaries proliferate and are thought to have a mediating effect on hypertrophic scar formation. The mechanism for contraction of hypertrophic scar is thought to be the myofibroblast (56).

Patients with extensive scarring or with contractures may require reconstructive surgeries. Thin scar bands can be released by the Z-plasty technique. Thick bands require release and grafting. Scarring on the face, neck, and trunk can be treated with tissue expansion and reconstruction (Fig. 85-49).

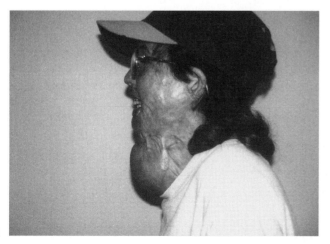

A

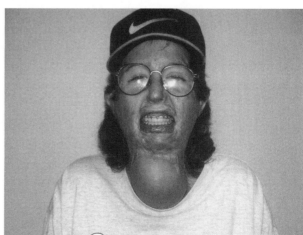

B

Figure 85-49. Tissue expanders

It has been known for years that external pressure in the form of special garments that provide at least 25 mm Hg or more of pressure (i.e., above capillary pressure) can flatten scar tissue if worn continuously until the scars lose redness and soften. Burn scars that lose their redness within 8 to 10 weeks may not become hypertrophic. It is postulated that pressure inhibits blood flow with occlusion of vessels in the scar, affecting fibroblastic activity and reducing tissue water content. Prolonged pressure also may have detrimental effects, and the clinician should therefore be certain there are indications for its use. Obstructive sleep apnea has been described in two patients secondary to pressure garments used to treat severe facial and upper-body burn. Complex sleep polysonography confirmed obstructive sleep apnea with desaturations sufficient to result in physiologic dysfunction that significantly improved with removal of the garments. It was also noted that nocturnal desaturations were associated with noisy breathing, gasping, restlessness, and early-morning headaches (67).

Potential Problems in Pediatric Patients
Caused by Pressure and Scarring
The following are some potential problems in pediatric patients that result from pressure and scarring (68):

- Scar contractures of the mandible may affect dental occlusion.
- Mandibular contractures may cause difficulty with lip closure and subsequent drooling.
- Pressure garments may cause mandibular hypoplasia.
- Mouth burns have been associated with dental changes, including cross bite, crowding, and retrusion of bite.
- Pressure garments may affect facial growth.
- Severe neck contractures can elongate the mandible.

In a study of 100 patients with burn injury to determine factors associated with risk of hypertrophic scar development, 38 developed hypertrophic scars in 63 of 245 anatomic areas. Incidence was greater in African-Americans, especially if healing required more than 10 days. Healing time also predicted scar formation; that is, 33% scarred if healing required 14 to 21 days, whereas 78% scarred if healing required more than 21 days.

Burn scars that lose their redness within 8 to 10 weeks may not become hypertrophic (69).

Approximately 15% of burn unit admissions are elderly patients (65 years and older). Burn depth in the elderly has a tendency to be deeper because of thinner skin. The rate of wound healing is decreased, and the elderly do not scar as much as younger patients. Often they choose not to wear pressure garments because (a) they are uncomfortable, (b) they are not concerned about scars, and (c) they have difficulty putting them on (70). Children heal more quickly than adults but also have a greater propensity for hypertrophic scarring. Pressure therapy is critical but does have many challenges. It is difficult to fit gloves on very small hands. Vests have a tendency to ride up and need to be anchored through the groin. It is impossible to get buttock pressure for children still in diapers. Pressure garments may impair facial growth (68).

Silicone gel sheeting has been reported to assist in scar treatment without pressure assistance. To investigate the effectiveness of silicone gel, a sample of ten adults with 14 scarred areas was studied. Each was its own control, as one scarred area on each person was treated with silicone gel and another scarred area was treated without silicone, both for a period of 8 weeks. Based on elastometry, skin biopsy, texture, color, thickness, durability, and itching, the silicone-treated areas were more improved at 4 weeks, 8 weeks, and 4 weeks after treatment was stopped than the control scars (71). This suggests that silicone gel may be an effective intervention for hypertrophic scars.

A study was conducted on the use of frictional massage 10 minutes a day over a 3-month period in a group of 30 pediatric patients with hypertrophic scarring. The study failed to demonstrate any appreciable effects on the vascularity, pliability, and height of the hypertrophic scarring, although the patients did report decrease in pruritus (72).

OTHER RESIDUAL DEFECTS
After the surgeon has completed all the reconstructive procedures and the patient is, from a medical standpoint, totally rehabilitated, certain residual defects affect the remainder of the burn patient's life (Table 85-2).

TABLE 85-2.   Burn Sequelae

Defect	Cause
Hypopigmentation, Hyperpigmentation	Melanin abnormality and donor site choice
Sensory impairment	Sensory nerve fibers fail to penetrate thick scar tissue Damaged in full-thickness burns
Abnormal skin lubrication	Loss of sebaceous glands because of depth of burns
Abnormal hair growth	Hair follicle damage
Abnormal sweating, heat intolerance	Unable to penetrate heavy scar tissue
Cold intolerance	Loss of sweat glands as a result of depth of burn
Pruritis	Dry skin from lack of lubrication
Fragile skin	Loss of normal elasticity; thin
Ingrown hairs, pustules	Hair cannot penetrate thick scar and becomes infected
Permanent tanning	If exposed to direct sunlight before 12 to 18 months after a burn
Marjolin ulcer	Chronic recurring ulcers Poorly nourished scar tissue Permanent scarring
Cosmesis	Flattened facies Body part amputated
Joint pain	Repeated minor trauma to hands and knees Joint pinning
Psychological, social Fatigability Lack of endurance	All of the above

PSYCHOSOCIAL ISSUES IN BURN REHABILITATION

Burn injury is one of the most psychologically devastating injuries know to man. Burns are traumatic, functionally impairing, excruciatingly painful, and disfiguring. This combination produces a significant stress on even the healthiest psyches. Psychological distress following burn injury is relatively common, with 30% to 50% continuing to have some psychological complications in the first year following injury (73). The impact of these problems varies, but most are mild and do not interfere with daily functioning (74). Unfortunately, the rate of premorbid psychopathology is higher in burn patients than in the general population, including depression, character disorders, and substance abuse. This group tends to stay in the hospital longer and is at much greater risk of postburn psychological difficulties (75).

Early following the injury, it is critical that pain be adequately managed. Failure to manage pain can result in escalating anxiety with associated increased difficulty in managing the wound care experience. If anxiety becomes problematic, this can be managed with anxiolytic medication, biofeedback, relaxation techniques, hypnosis, or distraction therapy. The clinician must remember that anxiolytics are an adjuvant to narcotics and should never be used in isolation. Sleep disturbance is common following burn injury. Pain and itching interfere with sleep. Psychological stressors also interrupt the normal sleep–wake cycle. Nightmares are common, particularly in those patients who are injured by electricity. Posttraumatic stress disorder following burn injury occurs in 30% to 60% of patients during acute hospitalization. Persistent posttraumatic stress disorder is rare but can be seen particularly in those patients who were injured by electricity (75).

As the patient approaches discharge, the blur of the acute care hospitalization fades and confrontation with the outside world begins. This is a time of significant emotional challenge for patients. Once an individual is outside of the protective hospital environment, confrontation with functional impairments and cosmetic changes begins. Family relationships are altered as a previously independent family member takes on a dependent role. This is a challenge both for the burn survivor and for the caregiver. This is a time when patients need to be monitored closely for emerging depression. Additional challenges are related to loss of one's societal role, including work challenges, cosmetic factors, sexual functioning, and resumption of recreational activities. Although this improves with time, there is a trend for decreased socialization for those with visible scars (75).

Most burn patients perceive themselves as having a good quality of life following injury, with most reporting no psychological or physical problems except for those with large burns in which decreases in level of activity are seen (76). Surprisingly, children with burn injuries seem to adjust well psychologically and socially. Unfortunately, their parents report an increase in stress in their own lives, which they attribute to their children (77).

Difficulty with community integration primarily occurs in the first 6 months following a burn (78) and correlates with preburn factors as well as burn injury characteristics. Mean return to work ranges from 14.3 to 17 weeks, with 66% back to work at 6 months and 90% back to work at 24 months (79,80). Interestingly, only 37% had returned to the same job with the same employer (80). The probability of returning to work is reduced by a psychiatric history and extremity burns and is inversely proportional to the TBSA burned (80). This reinforces the fact that although burn patients do well in general with social reintegration and return to work, a considerable life disruption is associated with major burns (Table 85-3).

TABLE 85-3. Common Causes of Burns

Burn Cause	Burn Prevention
Scald burns from bathing	Set hot water temperature at 124° or lower.
Radiator burns	Do not remove cap on hot radiator.
Automobile failure to start	Do not *prime* carburetor.
Grease fire in kitchen	Do not carry burning grease outside–smother burning grease with soda or flour.
Scald burns from hot liquid on range	Turn all pot handles inward so child cannot reach.
Burning candles	Do not reach over. Do not wear loose clothing close to burning candles. Place in protective container.
Burning trash	Do not throw combustible liquids on trash to start the fire. Keep garden hose in area where trash is burned.
BBQ pit fires	Do not start fire with combustible liquids.
Lawn mower fires	Wait until mower is cool before adding gas.
Hot irons	Keep children out of areas with hot irons.
House fires	Do not smoke in bed. Check smoke detector battery frequently. Do not use combustible cleaning solutions in area around hot water heater.
Vaporizers	Do not use hot water vaporizers close to child's bed.
Electric blankets	Can catch fire.
Methamphetamine lab explosions	You know the answer.
Insensate extremities	Do not soak in hot water. Do not walk on hot cement. Do not warm feet with heating pad or next to a radiator.

CONCLUSION

The basic components of an interdisciplinary burn rehabilitation program are wound care, range of motion, pressure garments, splinting and casting, conditioning and strengthening, psychological assessment and intervention, and long-term medical rehabilitation follow-up. The effectiveness of this approach to burn injury has been indirectly demonstrated by the significant reduction in reconstruction surgery admissions (81). The following is a synopsis of burn rehabilitation planning during both acute and postdischarge phases of treatment.

Inpatient rehabilitation begins on the day of admission or within the first 24 hours. The rehabilitation burn team normally consists of a physician, physical therapist, occupational therapist, social worker, and psychologist and/or psychiatrist. The patient is generally seen once or twice daily, 6 days per week, by both the physical and occupational therapist. The typical inpatient treatment should involve

1. Positioning with special devices in bed and chair.
2. Passive, active, and active assistive exercises.
3. Casting and splinting of body parts to prevent contractures.
4. Range of motion under anesthesia as indicated.
5. Transfer activities.
6. Ambulation/assistive devices.
7. Early application of pressure.

Patients are then discharged to a rehabilitation facility, usually those with larger debilitating burns, or to an outpatient clinic for follow-up therapy. Problems that require outpatient treatment include open wounds, contractures, fragile hypersensitive skin, early hypertrophic scarring, itching, pain, weakness, deconditioning, and psychological/emotional reactions. A typical rehabilitation program for a 25% burn injury to the upper and lower extremities would be treatment for 5 days per week for 5 to 6 hours per day and would include

1. Wound care and dressing changes.
2. Paraffin and sustained stretch to all healed areas over joints with tightness.
3. Active and active assistive exercises to all joints involved.
4. Serial casting or splinting of major contractures.
5. Massage to healed skin to desensitize and loosen scar tissue.
6. Evaluative activities of daily living and modification with assistive devices as needed.
7. Conditioning program consisting of treadmill, upper-body ergometer, and bike.
8. Individualized strengthening programs for mononeuropathies.
9. Fitting with compression garments to control scarring (two sets). (Order new garments every 3 to 4 months, as they tend to wear out or become loose and ineffective.)
10. Silicon gel sheeting for hypertrophic scars.
11. Prescription for prosthetic or orthotic devices where needed.

This program could last anywhere from 4 to 6 months. It would decrease in number of days treated per week as the patient improves. It could last for a year or more if the burn injury is more severe. Rechecks by the physician prescribing treatment should occur every 2 weeks initially and every 1 to 2 months for the first 1 to 2 years.

The psychological/emotional needs of individuals with burn injury also require attention. Problems identified during acute hospitalization should be properly addressed. These problems may take on greater significance after discharge, when the individual is faced with beginning the process of community reentry. Because burn injury results in documented psychological sequelae that can be disruptive to functional independence and compliance with treatment, it is recommended that individuals with burn injury be evaluated after discharge and at regular intervals to identify any problems. If they do exist, short-term psychotherapy (5–15 sessions) is suggested. Relaxation training and biofeedback can be used adjunctively for sleep, pain, or other stress-related problems.

Follow-up rehabilitation is required after reconstructive procedures such as contracture release. Wound care and range-of-motion exercises are usually restarted to assist with wound closure and prevent contracture recurrence. Specialized splinting or casting may be necessary to maintain proper positioning at night. In most cases this postreconstructive surgery rehabilitation period is much shorter (e.g., 5 to 6 weeks).

REFERENCES

1. Brigham PA, McLoughlin, E. Burn incidence and medical care use in the United States: estimates, trends, and data sources. *J Burn Care Rehabil* 1996; 17:95–106.
2. Feller IJ. Introduction—statement of the problem. In: Fisher SV, Helm PA, eds. *Comprehensive rehabilitation of burns*. Baltimore: Williams & Wilkins, 1984:4.
3. Demling RH. Preface. In: LaLonde C. ed. *Burn trauma*. New York: Thieme, 1989:x.
4. Cromes GF, Helm PA. The status of burn rehabilitation services in the United States: results of a national survey. *J Burn Care Rehabil* 1992;13:656–662.
5. Schulz JT, Sheridan RL, Ryan CM, et al. A 10-year experience with toxic epidermal necrolysis. *J Burn Care Rehabil* 2000;21:199–204.
6. Solem ID. Classification. In: Fisher SV, Helm PA, eds. *Comprehensive rehabilitation of burns*. Baltimore: Williams & Wilkins, 1984:9–15.
7. Dimick AR. Pathophysiology. In: Fisher SV, Helm PA, eds. *Comprehensive rehabilitation of burns*. Baltimore: Williams & Wilkins, 1984:16–27.
8. Robson M. Synthetic burn dressings: round table discussion. *J Burn Care Rehalibil* 1985;66:66–73.
9. Pruitt BA. The evolutionary development of biologic dressings and skin substitutes. *J Burn Care Rehabil* 1997;182:S2–S5.
10. Tompkins RG, Burke JF. Progress in burn treatment and the use of artificial skin. *World J Surg* 1990;14:819–824.
11. Ono I, Gunji H, Zhang JZ, et al. A study of cytokines in burn blister fluid related to wound healing. *Burns* 1995;21:352–355.
12. Dimick AR. Debridement: surgical, mechanical, and biochemical. In: Dimick AR, ed. *Practical approaches to burn management*. Deerfield, IL: Flint Laboratories, Division of Travenol Laboratories, 1977:21–26.
13. Heimbach DM, Engrav LH. *Surgical management of the burn wound*. New York: Raven Press, 1984.
14. Head MD. Wound and skin care. In: Fisher SV, Helm PA, eds. *Comprehensive rehabilitation of burns*. Baltimore: Williams & Wilkins, 1984:148–176.
15. Staley M, Serghiour M. Casting guidelines, tips, and techniques: proceedings for the 1997 American Burn Association PT/OT Casting Workshop. *J Burn Care Rehabil* 1998;19:254–260.
16. Bennett GB, Helm PA, Purdue GF, et al. Serial casting: a method for treating burn contractures. *J Burn Care Rehabil* 1989;6:543–545.
17. Blassingame WM, Bennett GB, Helm PA, et al. Range of motion of the shoulder performed while patient is anesthetized. *J Burn Care Rehabil* 1989;10: 539–542.
18. Grube BJ, Engrav LH, Heimbach DM. Early ambulation and discharge in 100 patients with burns of the foot treated by grafts. *J Trauma* 1992;13:662–664.
19. Burnsworth B, Krob MJ, Langer-Schnepp M. Immediate ambulation of patients with lower-extremity grafts. *J Burn Care Rehabil* 1992;1:89–92.
20. Kowalske KJ, Purdue G, Hunt J, et al. Early ambulation following skin grafting of lower extremity burns: a randomized control trial. *Proc Am Burn Assoc* 1993;25:102.
21. Pegg SP, Cavaye D, Fowler D, et al. Results of early excision and grafting in hand burns. *Burns* 1984;11:99–103.
22. Sheridan RL, Hurley J, Smith MA, et al. The acutely burned hand: management and outcome based on a ten-year experience with 1047 acute hand burns. *J Trauma* 1995;38:406–411.
23. Bruner JM. Safety factors in the use of the pneumatic tourniquet for hemostasis in surgery of the hand. *J Bone Joint Surg* 1951;33A:221–224.
24. Helm PA, Kevorkian GC, Lushbaugh MS, et al. Burn injury rehabilitation management in 1982. *Arch Phys Med Rehabil* 1982;63:6–16.
25. Pullium GF. Splinting and positioning. In: Fisher SV, Helm PA, eds. *Comprehensive rehabilitation of burns*. Baltimore: Williams & Wilkins, 1984:64–95.
26. Artz CP. Electrical injury. In: Artz CP, Moncrief J, Pruitt BA Jr, eds. *Burns: a team approach*. Philadelphia: WB Saunders, 1979:351–362.
27. Hunt JL. Electrical injuries. In: Fisher SV, Helm PA, eds. *Comprehensive rehabilitation of burns*. Baltimore: Williams & Wilkins, 1984:249–266.
28. Hunt JL, Mason AD, Masterson TS, et al. The pathophysiology of acute electrical injuries. *J Trauma* 1976;16:335–340.
29. Meier RH III. Amputation and prosthetic fitting. In: Fisher SV, Helm PA, eds. *Comprehensive rehabilitation of burns*. Baltimore: Williams & Wilkins, 1984: 267–310.
30. Ward RS, Hayes-Lundy C, Schnebly WA, et al. Prosthetic use in patients with burns and associated limb amputations. *J Burn Care Rehabil* 1990;11:361–364.
31. Helm PA, Johnson ER, Carlton AM. Peripheral neurological problems in the acute burn patient. *Burns* 1977;3:123–125.
32. Helm PA, Pandian G, Heck E. Neuromuscular problems in the burn patient: cause and prevention. *Arch Phys Med Rehabil* 1985;66:451–453.
33. Kowalske K, Holahavanahalli R, Helm P. Neuropathy following burn injury. *J Burn Care Rehabil* 2001;44:354–357.
34. Jackson L, Keats AS. Mechanism of brachial plexus palsy following anesthesia. *Anesthesiology* 1965;26:190–194.
35. Ewing MR. Postoperative paralysis in the upper extremity: report of five cases. *Lancet* 1950;1:99–103.
36. Dhuner KG. Nerve injuries following operations: a survey of cases occurring during a six year period. *Anesthesiology* 1950;11:289–293.
37. Rask MR. Suprascapular nerve entrapment: a report of two cases treated with suprascapular notch resection. *Clin Orthop* 1977;123:73–75.
38. Wadsworth TG. The external compression syndrome of the ulnar nerve at the cubital tunnel. *Clin Orthop* 1977;124:189–204.
39. Edlich RF, Horowitz JH, Rheuban KS, et al. Heterotopic calcification and ossification in burn patients. *Curr Concepts Trauma Care* 1985;8:4–9.
40. Mant MJ, O'Brien BD, Thong KL, et al. Haemorrhagic complications of heparin therapy. *Lancet* 1977;1:1133–1135.
41. Reinstein L, Alevizatos AC, Twardzik FG, et al. Femoral nerve dysfunction after retroperitoneal hemorrhage: pathophysiology revealed by computed tomography. *Arch Phys Med Rehabil* 1984;65:37–40.
42. Berry H, Richardson PM. Common peroneal nerve palsy: a clinical and electrophysiological review. *J Neurol Neurosurg Psychiatry* 1976;39:1162–1171.
43. Aho K, Sainio K, Kianta M, et al. Pneumatic tourniquet paralysis: case report. *J Bone Joint Surg* 1983;65B:441–443.
44. Sunderland S. *Nerves and nerve injuries*. Edinburgh: F & S Livingstone, 1968.
45. Helm PA. Neuromuscular considerations. In: Fisher SV, Helm PA, eds. *Comprehensive rehabilitation of burns*. Baltimore: Williams & Wilkins, 1984:235–241.
46. Henderson B, Koepke GH, Feller I. Peripheral polyneuropathy among patients with burn. *Arch Phys Med Rehabil* 1971;52:149–151.

47. Dagum AB, Eng BS, Peters WJ, et al. Severe multiple mononeuropathy in patients with major thermal burns. *J Burn Care Rehabil* 1993;14:440–445.

48. Jackson DM. Destructive burns: some orthopaedic complications. *Burns* 1980;7:105–122.

49. Leung KS, Cheng JCY, Ma GFY, et al. Complications of pressure therapy for post-burn hypertrophic scars: biochemical analysis based on 5 patients. *Burns* 1984;10:434–438.

50. Evans EB. Bone and joint changes secondary to burns. In: Lewis SR, ed. *Symposium on the treatment of burns*. St Louis: CV Mosby, 1973:76–78.

51. Evans EB, Smith JR. Bone and joint changes following burns: a roentgenographic study preliminary report. *J Bone Joint Surg* 1959;41A:785–799.

52. Teperman PS, Hilbert L, Peters WJ, et al. Heterotopic ossifications in burns. *J Burn Care Rehabil* 1984;5:283–287.

53. Crawford CM, Varghese G, Mani MM, et al. Heterotopic ossification: are range of motion exercises contraindicated? *J Burn Care Rehabil* 1986;7:323–327.

54. Rutan RL, Herndon DN. Growth delay in postburn pediatric patients. *Arch Surg* 1990;125:392–395.

55. Klein GL, Herndon DN, Langman CB, et al. Long-term reduction in bone mass after severe burn injury in children. *J Pediatr* 1999;126:252–256.

56. Helm PA, Walker SC. New bone formation at amputation sites in electrically burn-injured patients. *Arch Phys Med Rehabil* 1987;68:284–286.

57. Vrabec R, Kolar J. Bone changes caused by electric current. In: *Transactions of the Fourth International Congress of Plastic and Reconstructive Surgery, Rome, 1967*. Amsterdam: Excerpta Medica, 1969:215–217.

58. Evans EB. Scoliosis and kyphosis. In: Feller I, Crabb WC, eds. *Reconstruction and rehabilitation of the burned patient*. Ann Arbor, MI: National Institute for Burn Medicine, 1979:264.

59. Ozek C, Celik N, Bilkay U, et al. Marjolin's ulcer of the scalp: report of 5 cases and review of literature. *J Burn Care Rehabil* 2001;22:65–69.

60. Poh-Fitzpatrick M. Skin care of the healed burned patient. *Clin Plast Surg* 1992;19:745–751.

61. Vitale M, Fields-Blache C, Luterman A. Severe itching in the patient with burns. *J Burn Care Rehabil* 1991;12:330–333.

62. De Chalain TMB, Tang C, Thomson HG. Burn area color changes after superficial burns in childhood: can they be predicted? *J Burn Care Rehabil* 1998;19:39–47.

63. Head M, Helm P. Paraffin and sustained stretching in the treatment of burn contracture. *Burns* 1977;4:136–139.

64. St-Pierre DMM, Choinière M, Forget R, et al. Muscle strength in individuals with healed burns. *Arch Phys Med Rehabil* 1998;79:155–161.

65. Ward RS, Hayes-Lundy C, Reddy R, et al. Evaluation of topical therapeutic ultrasound to improve response to physical therapy and lessen scar contracture after burn injury. *J Burn Care Rehabil* 1994;15:74–79.

66. Jensen LL, Parshley PF. Postburn scar contractures: histology and effects of pressure treatment. *J Burn Care Rehabil* 1984;5:119–123.

67. Hubbard M, Masters IB, Williams GR, et al. Severe obstructive sleep apnoea secondary to pressure garments used in the treatment of hypertrophic burn scars. *Eur Respir J* 2000;16:1205–1207.

68. Staley M, Richard R, Billmire D, et al. Head/face/neck burns: therapist considerations for the pediatric patient. *J Burn Care Rehabil* 1997;18:164–171.

69. Deitch EA, Wheelahan TM, Rose MP, et al. Hypertrophic burn scars: analysis of variables. *J Trauma* 1983;10:895–898.

70. Staley M, Richard R. The elderly patient with burns: treatment conditions. *J Burn Care Rehabil* 1993;14:559–565.

71. Ahn ST, Monafo WW, Mustoe TA. Topical silicone gel: a new treatment for hypertrophic scars. *Surgery* 1989;4:781–787.

72. Patino O, Novick C, Merko A, et al. Message in hypertrophic scars. *J Burn Care Rehabil* 1999;20:268–271.

73. Adler A. Neuropsychiatric complication in victims of Boston's Cocoanut Grove disaster. *JAMA* 1943;123:1098.

74. Andreasen NJC, Norris AS, Hartford CE. Incidence of long-term psychiatric complication in severely burned adults. *Ann Surg* 1970;174:785–793.

75. Patterson DR, Everett JJ, Bombardier CH, et al. Psychological effects of severe burn injuries. *Psychol Bull* 1993;113:362–378.

76. Cobb N, Maxwell G, Silverstein P. Patient perception of quality of life after burn injury. Results of an eleven-year survey. *J Burn Care Rehabil* 1990;11:330–333.

77. Blakeney P, Meyer W, Moore P, et al. Psychosocial sequelae of pediatric burns involving 80% or greater total body surface area. *J Burn Care Rehabil* 1993;14:685–689.

78. Esselman PC, Ptacek JT, Kowalske KJ, et al. Community integration after burn injuries. *J Burn Care Rehabil* 2001;22:221–227.

79. Saffle JR, Tuohig GM, Sullivan JJ, et al. Return to work as a measure of outcome in adults hospitalized for acute burn treatment. *J Burn Care Rehabil* 1996;17:353–361.

80. Brych SB, Engrav LH, Rivara FP, et al. Time off work and return to work rates after burns: systematic review of the literature and a large two-center series. *J Burn Care Rehabil* 2001;22:401–405.

81. Prasad JK, Bowden ML, Thompson PD. A review of reconstructive surgery needs of 3167 survivors of burn injury. *Burns* 1991;17:302–305.

CHAPTER 86

Rehabilitation of the Patient with Visual Impairment

Stanley F. Wainapel and Marla Bernbaum

Visual impairment and blindness have been notably overlooked in the rehabilitation medicine literature (1,2), and only once prior to the third edition of the present textbook has a chapter in a rehabilitation medicine textbook dealt with this topic (3). The relative neglect of vision rehabilitation by physiatrists is both surprising and unjustified in the context of historical associations and epidemiologic trends, both of which suggest the need for a greater degree of involvement.

THE HISTORICAL CONTEXT

World War II was a turning point in human history as well as a turning point in the development of both vision and medical rehabilitation. The extensive and severe casualties from battle occurred at a time when antibiotics and other medical and surgical techniques saved the lives of many soldiers who would otherwise have succumbed to their injuries. Society was then faced with a tremendous challenge as veterans with limb amputations, traumatic brain injuries, and traumatic spinal cord injuries attempted to take up their social roles as workers and family members. The response by the health-care system was the creation of a multidisciplinary and functionally oriented approach that emphasized psychosocial and vocational goals compatible with the needs of these young and predominantly male veterans. Adding life to years rather than years to life (4) became the motto of the physicians who pioneered this approach, and by 1947 the American Board of Physical Medicine and Rehabilitation had been established.

At the same time and under the same circumstances, a large number of veterans blinded by combat injuries entered society with equally urgent needs for retraining and social reintegration. The response of the vision care system was the development of a multidisciplinary and functionally oriented approach that emphasized psychosocial and vocational goals. By 1948 the first civilian vision rehabilitation program had been established at the Veterans Administration Hospital in Hines, Illinois. That program was located within the Department of Rehabilitation Medicine (5).

The parallels between vision rehabilitation and medical rehabilitation are obvious from their shared roots, but the similarities go deeper. The professionals who comprise the rehabilitation team (physical therapist, occupational therapist, etc.) have their counterparts within the vision rehabilitation team, and physiatric areas of expertise such as orthotics and prosthetics have clear homologs for visually impaired patients (Table 86-1). There are notable differences between the two systems, however, and they explain why the systems have tended to diverge from their conjoint origins into parallel but distinct paths over the last 50 years. When vision loss is an isolated sensory deficit affecting a single organ and unassociated with other medical problems, the major focus tends to be on social and vocational issues rather than on comprehensive medical management. When vision loss is part of multiple traumatic events or part of a medical problem (e.g., diabetes mellitus), the approach needs to be comprehensive. Because vision loss is often the only problem, vision rehabilitation services have tended to be funded under social service and vocational sources, and the agencies providing vision rehabilitation have remained separate from the medical mainstream. To some extent this was not a problem when the patient was an otherwise healthy young person such as the blind veteran around whose needs the programs were developed. But this paradigm is increasingly inadequate for the new generation of individuals with visual impairments (older and with associated comorbidities), whose care will make it essential that medical and vision rehabilitation systems join forces after a half-century of relative insularity. The new challenge does not come from the ravages of war but from the ravages of age.

THE EPIDEMIOLOGIC CONTEXT

In 1900 only 4% of the American population was 65 years of age or older; by 1994 that percentage had more than tripled, to 12.6%, which represents 33 million individuals(6), and it will continue to increase as the "baby boom" generation ages during the early twenty-first century. The physiologic changes of aging are protean and affect all body systems or organs (7), and the visual system is no exception. Thus the new "epidemic" of visual impairment will occur among the geriatric population.

Epidemiologic surveys confirm this conclusion. Nelson and Dimitrova (8) have analyzed data from the 1990 Health Interview Survey; 4.3 million Americans had difficulty reading ordinary newspaper print (the equivalent of less than 20/70 corrected visual acuity) even when using reading glasses, and

TABLE 86-1. Comparisons Between Medical and Vision Rehabilitation

Rehabilitation Medicine	Vision Rehabilitation
Physical therapy	Orientation and mobility
Occupational therapy	Rehabilitation teaching
Social work	Social work
Rehabilitation counseling	Rehabilitation counseling
Orthotics	Vision enhancement
Prosthetics	Vision substitution

TABLE 86-2. Prevalence of Severe Visual Impairment in the United States, 1990

Age	Number with Visual Impairment	Prevalence
0–17	95,410	1.5/1,000
18–44	349,350	3.2/1,000
45–54	340,510	13.5/1,000
55–64	600,600	28.4/1,000
65–74	1,068,290	59.0/1,000
75–85	1,190,520	118.4/1,000
85+	648,680	210.6/1,000
Total	4,293,360	17.3/1,000

Adapted from Nelson KA, Dimitrova E. Severe visual impairment in the United States and in each state, 1990. *J Vis Impairment Blind* 1993;87:80–86; reprinted by permission of the American Foundation of the Blind.

about two-thirds of these were 65 or older (Table 86-2). It is worth noting that this prevalence of visual impairment is greater than that for stroke and lower-limb amputation combined. Because both of the latter conditions are frequent diagnoses among the elderly, it is not surprising to find them associated with vision problems, producing the blind amputee (9,10) or the blind stroke patient (11).

The prevalence of visual impairment among rehabilitation medicine inpatients has been reported to be about 7% in a retrospective survey of 191 consecutive admissions to an inpatient unit (12). These patients were older than the average but had a length of stay (LOS) that was actually shorter than that for the entire unit's mean LOS (Table 86-3). Vision loss was a comorbidity that did not adversely affect outcome, probably because these patients had lost vision a number of years before the current admission and had adjusted to their impairment.

THE FUNCTIONAL CONTEXT

It is not sufficient for visual impairment to be prevalent for it to warrant closer attention from the physiatrist. It must also result in significant limitation in the level of activity and participation. A number of studies have documented that vision loss has adverse effects on mobility, self-care, and social function (13–20).

Vision is one of the three essential components for normal upright stance; vestibular function and proprioception are the other two (13). Loss of this stabilizing influence has been impli-

cated in falls by several authors (14–16), and Felson (17) has graphically demonstrated a greater than twofold increased risk of hip fractures among members of the Framingham Eye Study cohort, a longitudinal study of an unselected general community population.

Deficits in basic and/or instrumental activities of daily living (ADL) have been documented in those with isolated visual impairment in a number of settings in the United States as well as Europe. Carabellese and co-workers (18) studied a large urban Italian community sample of those 70 years of age or older, measuring their self-care status and dividing the sample into groups based on the presence or absence of self-reported visual or hearing impairments. Visual impairment alone produced statistically significant losses in ADL and IADL function. Branch and co-workers (19) found IADL deficits in a more heterogeneous sample of older residents of Massachusetts but failed to find statistically significant basic ADL losses. Others (20) have documented that visually impaired people have lower perceived health status and suffer from a sense of social isolation.

The rationale for physiatrists' increased awareness of and attention to vision-related issues is clear. Visual impairment is

TABLE 86-3. Length of Stay in Rehabilitation Facility for Patients with Visual Impairment

Sex	Age	Rehabilitation Diagnosis	Vision Diagnosis	Length of Stay (days)	Discharge Status
F	78	CVA, R hemi	Cataracts	56	Home
F	82	Pelvic fracture	Macular degeneration	17	Home
F	81	Back pain	Macular degeneration	50	Home
F	81	Back pain	Macular degeneration	28	Home
F	82	Gait disorder	Cataracts, macular degeneration	15	Surgery
F	82	S/P VP shunt	Cataracts, macular degeneration	17	Medicine
M	79	Bilateral BKA	Cataracts, glaucoma	24	Home
M	89	CVA, R hemi	Glaucoma	25	Home
M	84	CVA, R hemi	Glaucoma	30	Home
F	69	L BKA	Diabetic retinopathy	30	Home
F	70	CVA, L hemi	Diabetic retinopathy	72	Skilled nursing facility

BKA, below-knee amputation; CVA, cerebrovascular accident; L hemi, left hemiparesis; R hemi, right hemiparesis; VP, ventriculo-peritoneal.
From Wainapel S, Kwon YS, Fazzari PJ. Severe visual impairment on a rehabilitation unit: incidence and implications. *Arch Phys Med Rehabil* 1989; 70:439–441; reprinted by permission of WB Saunders, Co.

| TABLE 86-4. Changes in the Eye Associated with Aging ||
Functional Change	Physiological Change
Visual acuity	Morphologic change in choroid, pigment epithelium, or retina
	Decreased function of rods, cones, or other neural elements
Extraocular motion	Difficulty in gazing upward and maintaining convergence
Intraocular pressure	Increased pressure
Refractive power	Increased hyperopia and myopia
	Presbyopia
	Increased lens size
	Nuclear sclerosis (lens)
	Ciliary muscle atrophy
Tear secretion	Decreased tearing
	Decreased lacrimal gland function
	Decreased goblet cell secretion
Corneal function	Loss of endothelial integrity
	Posterior surface pigmentation

From Kane RL, Ouslander JG, Abrass IB. Sensory impairment. In: *Essentials of clinical geriatrics, 2nd ed.*; reprinted by permission of McGraw-Hill, Inc.

a frequent concomitant of the aging process, producing significant disability in its own right. It occurs with some frequency among patients seen by the physiatrist. It affects balance, gait, and self-care activities. It can also occur as part of the syndromes produced by three common rehabilitation medicine diagnoses: stroke, traumatic brain injury, and multiple sclerosis.

VISION PROBLEMS ASSOCIATED WITH AGING

As the eye ages, it undergoes many physiologic and morphologic changes, which are summarized in Table 86-4. Familiar changes include the arcus senilis, the loss of accommodation after age 40, which produces the need for reading glasses, and the development of clouding of the crystalline lens, which can lead to full-blown cataract formation. Other changes are often quite significant. The pupil becomes smaller with age and limits the amount of light reaching the retina. By age 60, the retina receives less than one-third the light it did at age 20 (7). Ptosis of the upper eyelid can produce a reduction of the upper visual field. Nuclear sclerosis produces heightened glare sensitivity, and yellowing of the lens leads to color distortions.

The great majority of visual impairments in the elderly are caused by one of four diagnoses: cataract, age-related macular degeneration (AMD), glaucoma, and diabetic retinopathy (21). A detailed discussion of their etiology, pathophysiology, and medical/surgical management is beyond the scope of this chapter, but a brief summary of their characteristics is included, since the physiatrist will be likely to see many patients with these disorders. An excellent concise guide to the aging eye and its management has been published by the New York Lighthouse and is highly recommended as a reference (22). Figures 86-1 through 86-4 present visual simulations of the identical objects as they would appear to a person with these disorders.

Cataract is an opacification of the normally clear crystalline lens. It is extremely common with advancing age but may not require specific treatment unless it produces symptoms that impact on the patient's life style and normal activities. Three

major types of cataract are distinguished: (a) central (nuclear) cataract, the most common variety; (b) peripheral (cortical) cataract, which is associated with increased age; and (c) posterior (subcapsular) cataract, which occurs most commonly in diabetics or patients receiving corticosteroids (23). Common symptoms include blurred vision, glare sensitivity, and yellow vision. Treatment is surgical and usually takes the form of extracapsular lens extraction or phacoemulsification of the lens, each of which leaves the capsule intact and permits the implantation of an intraocular lens (23).

The intraocular lens produces much less magnification or distortion than the older techniques of cataract glasses or contact lenses. The surgery is performed on an ambulatory basis and has an extremely high success rate that approaches 90% in patients without comorbid conditions. Follow-up studies have documented that elderly patients experience improved self-care status and even improvement of mental status following intraocular lens implant surgery (24,25).

The most frequent cause of blindness among the elderly is AMD, especially among those 75 years of age or older. In this condition the macula suffers damage with a resulting loss of central visual field but preservation of peripheral vision (see Fig. 86-2). Detail vision for facial recognition, reading, and close-up observation is severely affected, but mobility is relatively preserved because peripheral vision remains intact. Two types of AMD have been delineated: (a) nonexudative ("dry") AMD, which may be relatively benign and nonprogressive; and (b) exudative ("wet") AMD, which frequently progresses to total loss of macular function. Although laser photocoagulation surgery has been of some benefit in selected cases of exudative AMD, most patients have no surgical or medical option at the present time. Fortunately, the disease is self-limited, and the patient can be reassured that he or she will not become totally blind, nor will his or her mobility be impaired.

The visual deficit of glaucoma results from damage to the optic nerve from increased intraocular pressure related to abnormal mechanisms of fluid flow between the anterior and posterior chambers of the eye. It presents in one of two ways: (a) a rapidly progressive vision loss with pain from acute angle closure, a true ophthalmologic emergency; or (b) an insidious and silently progressive disease that gradually constricts the peripheral visual fields with resulting "tunnel vision" (see Fig. 86-3) and, if unrecognized, ultimate total vision loss. Early detection is essential for the second type, which is called open-angle glaucoma; intraocular pressure should be regularly measured in every elderly patient to facilitate early detection and treatment. The management of glaucoma can be purely medical, using various eye drops with anticholinergic or β-adrenergic effects but sometimes requires a surgical procedure, usually a laser iridotomy, that reestablishes normal drainage of the aqueous humor.

Diabetic retinopathy is an important cause of blindness in young and middle-aged patients as well as the elderly. Its clinical manifestations can be more variable than the preceding three disorders, but they usually produce central deficits that affect visual acuity (see Fig. 86-4). It is discussed in more detail in the following section.

VISION PROBLEMS IN THE YOUNG AND MIDDLE-AGED

As shown in Table 86–2, visual impairment is relatively uncommon below the age of 55, but when it does occur, its effects can be particularly devastating, interfering with a person's ability

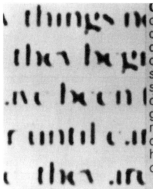
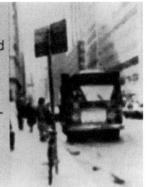

Cataract - An opacity of the lens results in diminished acuity, but does not affect the field of vision. There is no scotoma, but the person's vision is hazy overall, particularly in glaring light. With cataracts and corneal disease, print appears hazy or lacking in contrast.

Figure 86-1. Simulation of visual consequences of cataract. (From Faye EE, Stuen CS. *The aging eye and low vision.* New York: The Lighthouse, 1992. Reprinted by permission of The Lighthouse, Inc.)

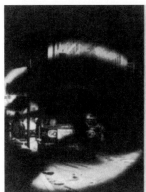
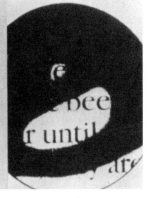

Macular Degeneration The deterioration of the macula, the central area of the retina, is prevalent among older patients. This illustration shows the area of decreased central vision, called a central scotoma. With macular degeneration, print appears distorted and segments of words may be missing.

Figure 86-2. Simulation of visual consequences of macular degeneration. (From Faye EE, Stuen CS. *The aging eye and low vision.* New York: The Lighthouse, 1992. Reprinted by permission of The Lighthouse, Inc.)

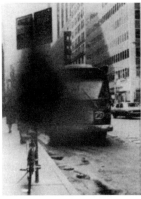

Glaucoma - Chronic elevated eye pressure in susceptible individuals may cause optic nerve atrophy and loss of peripheral vision. Early detection and close medical monitoring can help reduce complications. In advanced glaucoma, print may appear faded and words may be difficult to read.

Figure 86-3. Simulation of visual consequences of glaucoma. (From Faye EE, Stuen CS. *The aging eye and low vision.* New York: The Lighthouse, 1992. Reprinted by permission of The Lighthouse, Inc.)

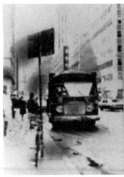
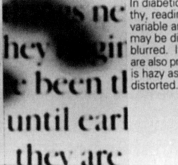

Diabetic Retinopathy - The leaking of retinal blood vessels may occur in advanced or long-term diabetes and affect the macula or the entire retina and vitreous. Not all diabetics develop retinal changes, but the likelihood of retinopathy and cataracts increases with the length of time a person has diabetes.

In diabetic retinopathy, reading vision is variable and print may be distorted or blurred. If cataracts are also present, print is hazy as well as distorted.

Figure 86-4. Simulation of visual consequences of diabetic retinopathy. (From Faye EE, Stuen CS. *The aging eye and low vision.* New York: The Lighthouse, 1992. Reprinted by permission of The Lighthouse, Inc.)

to complete educational studies, obtain employment, or continue in the usual social role. Causes of vision loss are more variable than among the elderly, with diabetic retinopathy being by far the most prevalent. Retinopathy of prematurity, which was formerly called retrolental fibroplasia, is occurring more frequently in recent years because of the improved care of premature infants who would have previously died. Other causes of blindness or visual impairment in infants and children include congenital cataracts, rubella syndrome, and anoxic brain damage with cerebral palsy. Tapetoretinal degenerative disorders, of which retinitis pigmentosa (RP) is the most prevalent, characteristically manifest themselves in childhood or early adulthood with symptoms of night blindness and "tunnel vision" from loss of peripheral visual fields with preservation of central vision, similar to the effects of open-angle glaucoma (see Fig. 86-3). This type of vision loss produces significant difficulty in mobility while leaving reading and detail vision unimpaired. The course of RP is dependent on the particular variant of the disease, but in general there is progressive narrowing of visual field that may progress to total blindness by middle age. Cataract formation may also contribute to the loss of residual central vision in RP.

A relatively new cause of vision loss in the young adult is that associated with cytomegalovirus (CMV) retinitis in patients with acquired immunodeficiency syndrome (AIDS). This infection has been a relatively late manifestation of the disease and has carried a grave prognosis for prolonged survival, but recent advances in treatment using intraocular ganciclovir have extended survival in these patients. Other opportunistic infections of the central nervous system such as cryptococcal meningitis and toxoplasmosis may also produce visual sequelae.

Diabetes mellitus is the leading cause of visual impairment in American adults between the ages of 20 and 74 years and, overall, accounts for 12% of new cases of blindness (26). Development of diabetic retinopathy correlates with disease duration as well as with the degree of blood glucose control (27). After 15 years, background retinopathy is present in 97% of individuals with insulin-dependent diabetes mellitus (IDDM), 80% of individuals with non–insulin-dependent diabetes mellitus (NIDDM) who are insulin treated, and 55% of individuals with NIDDM who are not insulin requiring (26). Small hemorrhages, microaneurysms, and lipid exudates are visible within the retina, although vision is usually unaffected. However, in 8% of individuals, the macula is involved, resulting in moderate to severe visual impairment (28). Early laser photocoagulation can reduce vision loss by 60% (29–31).

Within 15 years of diagnosis, proliferative retinopathy occurs in 30% of individuals with IDDM, 10% to 15% of those with insulin-requiring NIDDM, and 5% of non–insulin-requiring individuals (26). Proliferative retinopathy involves blockages of the microvascular circulation nourishing the retina, leading to the formation of new and abnormal (neovascular) vessels (28). These fragile vessels rupture and hemorrhage easily. They may also grow out of the retina into the vitreous humor, with subsequent traction tears, detachments, and scarring of the retina. Optimal control of the blood glucose can prevent or delay the progression of retinopathy (27). Early intervention with laser photocoagulation can reduce the incidence of serious vision loss (29–31). Individuals who already have severe visual impairment with extensive hemorrhages, fibrosis, or retinal detachments are treated with surgical vitrectomy to remove vitreous hemorrhage and opacities and to release mechanical traction on the retina. Vitrectomy can be very effective in restoring visual acuity, but there is a 25% complication rate, which may lead to further compromise of vision (31,32).

The patient with diabetic retinopathy is a classic example in which the medical and vision rehabilitation systems must interface for optimal outcome. The many medical complications associated with diabetes mellitus—peripheral neuropathy, autonomic neuropathy, peripheral vascular disease, and nephropathy, among others—demand close medical attention, whereas the physical disabilities that can accompany these conditions—lower-limb amputations, weakness, and/or sensory disturbances—warrant the participation of the physiatrist. When one adds the presence of severe visual impairment to the preceding scenario, it becomes quite evident that vision rehabilitation personnel need to become more familiar with medical rehabilitation issues, whereas physiatrists need to understand the basic principles of vision rehabilitation in order to adequately serve such a patient.

AN OVERVIEW OF VISION REHABILITATION PRINCIPLES AND PRACTICE

As has already been illustrated (see Table 86-1), vision rehabilitation has many similarities to the medical rehabilitation model. In the case of the individual with visual impairment or blindness, the process can be divided into the following components:

1. Assessment and classification of the degree and type of visual impairment.
2. Referral to vision rehabilitation system and providers.
3. Devices and techniques to enhance residual vision.
4. Devices and techniques that substitute for lost vision.

Assessment and Classification

Vision assessment should be as routine a part of the physiatrist's evaluation as the peripheral sensory examination. The thoroughness of this assessment cannot be expected to equal that of the ophthalmologist or optometrist (33), but it is essential to rule out this important sensory disability in all rehabilitation medicine patients. A high index of suspicion should be present when examining patients with stroke, multiple sclerosis, traumatic brain injury, or underlying diabetes mellitus. The high prevalence of visual impairment among the elderly, which reaches 27% in those aged 85 or older (34), should be recalled. History taking should include functionally oriented questions about vision: difficulty in reading, night vision problems, glare sensitivity in sunlight, mobility problems related to narrow visual fields, or difficulty in ADL related to vision loss (e.g., diabetics unable to draw up or self-administer insulin). The physical examination should include evaluation of extraocular movements, which can be affected in brainstem stroke or multiple sclerosis. Visual acuity can be measured using a portable Snellen eye chart, and even without one it is possible to use a newspaper as a rough screening tool. Inability to read the latter corresponds to a visual acuity of less than 20/70. Visual field testing with confrontation at the bedside is a useful method to determine the presence of hemianopia, but more accurate formal perimetry testing is often indicated when subtler deficits are present or suspected. A full ophthalmologic consultation should be requested when any of the preceding screening tests reveal vision deficits.

Classification of visual impairment is of more than academic significance; it determines the patient's eligibility for state-funded vision rehabilitation services. Two main levels of impairment are usually recognized for classification, based on corrected visual acuity and extent of visual fields. *Legal blindness* is defined as corrected acuity of less than 20/200 or visual field of less than 20 degrees in the better eye. *Low vision* is defined as corrected acuity between 20/70 and 20/200 or visual field deficit with residual field of greater than 20 degrees in the better eye. These definitions clearly have major limitations because they exclude patients with significant vision problems who would not meet their criteria. For example, a diabetic who is totally blind in one eye and has 20/60 corrected acuity in the remaining eye would not be considered legally blind. Nevertheless, such a patient would require extensive vision rehabilitation.

Visual impairments can also be classified into acuity or visual field deficits. The former can be subdivided into discrete deficits such as scotomas or diffuse deficits such as those produced by cataract. The latter can be subdivided into central deficits such as those resulting from AMD or concentric deficits such as those produced by glaucoma or RP.

Referral for Vision Rehabilitation

The vision rehabilitation system varies from state to state, but in general it is administered by the Department of Social Services or a similar agency. Funding for treatment comes from this source rather than from third-party insurance carriers, as is the case with most medical care. This distinction is extremely important in light of the previously discussed overlaps between visual and medical disabilities. Certification of legal blindness by an ophthalmologist or optometrist is sent to the appropriate state agency, which then institutes an evaluation by a social worker or rehabilitation counselor, who then determines which rehabilitation services should be provided. This case-management model provides the following major treatment options (see Table 86-1):

1. *Orientation and mobility (O&M) instructor:* The equivalent of a physical therapist for the visually impaired or blind patient, the O&M instructor (formerly referred to as a peripatologist) teaches ambulation and navigation techniques that allow the patient to safely negotiate indoor and outdoor environments using a variety of assistive devices such as the long white cane or guide dog.
2. *Rehabilitation teacher:* The equivalent of an occupational therapist, this professional teaches special ADL and IADL techniques that enable the visually impaired person to function independently. In addition to prescribing self-help devices, the rehabilitation teacher may also instruct the patient in reading and writing Braille.
3. *Low-vision specialist:* An optometrist is usually consulted for formal low-vision evaluation and prescription of devices that enhance or substitute for vision.
4. *Communication/computer specialist:* This individual concentrates on skills that will improve reading and writing, such as Braille and computer adaptations.
5. *Social worker:* As with their medical rehabilitation counterparts, social workers assist the patient and family with psychosocial issues.
6. *Rehabilitation counselor:* As with their counterparts in medical rehabilitation, rehabilitation counselors assist the patient in the areas of education and employment.

This multidisciplinary team provides input as well as specific services for the patient. Treatments are usually given at a specialized nonresidential facility, although in some cases they may be performed in the patient's own home.

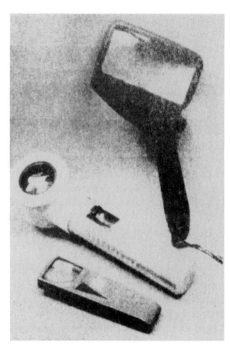

Figure 86-5. Hand-held magnifiers. (Photograph by permission of Resources for Rehabilitation, Lexington, MA.)

Enhancement of Residual Vision

Vision enhancement, often referred to as low-vision rehabilitation, is a complex subject that is exhaustively discussed in books by Faye (35) and by Cole and Rosenthal (36). In general, there are basic components: (a) optical devices or techniques that provide magnification of the image; (b) devices or techniques to alter the visual field; (c) nonoptical aids that modify environmental factors such as glare, lighting, and contrast.

Ordinary spectacles and contact lenses are the most ubiquitous magnification devices, although their range of enlargement is relatively modest. Magnifiers come in many shapes and sizes, but they share the advantage of being portable and relatively inexpensive. Hand-held devices (Fig. 86-5) require functional use of the upper extremities (a potential problem for arthritics, hemiplegics, or parkinsonian patients) and must have their focal length adjusted for maximal effect. Stand magnifiers eliminate these difficulties (Fig. 86-6). Adding built-in halogen illumination to a stand magnifier provides even greater visibility (Fig. 86-7). Monocular or binocular spectacle-mounted telescopic lenses are prescribed for patients to facilitate reading (Fig. 86-8) or even for driving. Hand-held monocular telescopes can assist with distance vision, as in the case of patients having difficulty reading street signs. Visual fatigue and a limited field of vision are shared disadvantages of magnifiers and telescopes. The closed-circuit television videomagnifier (CCTV) offers a wide range of magnification from 3 to 60 times normal while minimizing reading fatigue and maximizing the field of view (Fig. 86-9). The reversal of image that gives a black background with white foreground increases contrast and further heightens visibility. The main problem with the CCTV is its relatively high cost and its size, although portable models are now available. Enlarged-print books, magazines, and computer output are another magnification option for patients with low vision.

Expansion or shifting of the visual field is the second treatment option for enhancing vision. Reversing a pair of binoculars or opera glasses is a simple expedient to increase the nar-

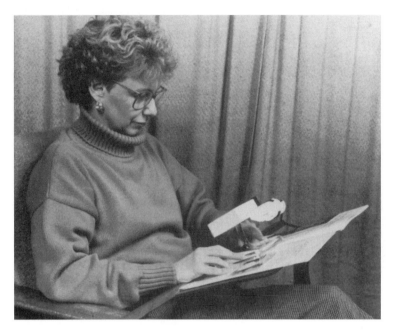

Figure 86-6. Stand magnifier.

row visual fields produced by RP or glaucoma. Prisms or minification lenses are also used for this purpose. Fresnell prisms can divert vision from impaired areas to intact ones, as in the case of stroke or head injury with homonymous hemianopia. A mirror mounted on a pair of glasses (Fig. 86-10) is an alternative option that can be made more cosmetic by mounting it behind the lenses. Central visual field defects produced by AMD may be compensated for by learning the technique of eccentric viewing, in which a new fixation point is trained to substitute for the macula (36).

Modification of external factors within the environment can markedly improve visual function, and conversely, a lack of attention to them can cause great difficulty despite adequate magnification. The nonoptical aids that are used to reduce glare, heighten contrast, and optimize illumination are often simple and quite inexpensive. Glare can be reduced by sunglasses, especially those whose tinting blocks the passage of the blue part of the visible spectrum (orange and yellow tints are particularly effective); a hat or cap with a brim or a simple visor can also decrease glare from light coming from above the

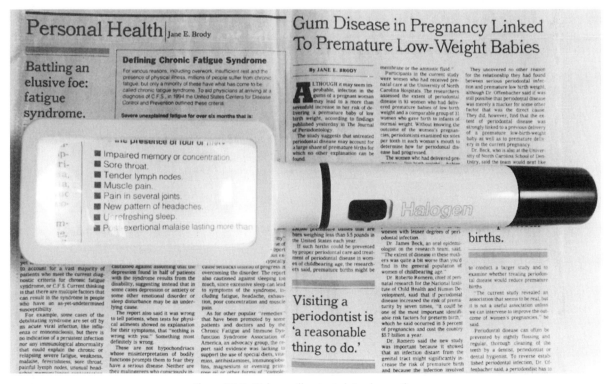

Figure 86-7. Halogen-illuminated stand magnifier.

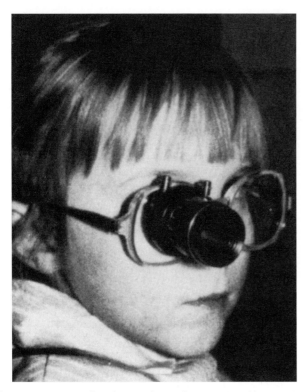

Figure 86-8. Monocular telescope for reading. (Reprinted by permission of Resources for Rehabilitation, Lexington, MA.)

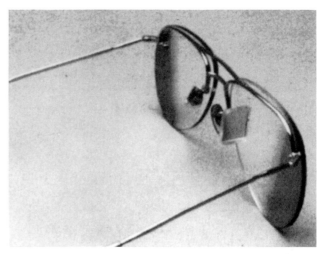

Figure 86-10. Spectacle-mounted mirror for homonymous hemianopia. (From Cole RG, Rosenthal BP. *Remediation and management of low vision.* St Louis: CV Mosby, 1996. Reprinted by permission of Mosby-Year Book Publishers.)

viewer. Indirect lighting is also indicated. The amount of illumination that suffices for each patient will vary with age and underlying condition, but it is essential to have an adjustable lighting source for any near-vision activities, such as reading, writing, or sewing. Impaired night vision can be enhanced by the use of illumination devices originally developed for underwater or wartime activities. Contrast-enhancing devices include sharply contrasting colors on adjacent surfaces, paper with thick and dark lines, felt-tipped or boldly writing pens, and tinted glasses. Typoscopes are made from dark-colored material into which a series of apertures are cut that guide the

user to the right position for signing his or her name, writing a check, or addressing an envelope. They can also be extremely helpful for visual tracking while reading (Fig. 86-11).

Substitution for Lost Vision

Vision enhancement is useful only when there is sufficient residual vision to be enhanced. Often, however, so little remains that it only provides cues about light, shapes, and movement. Although only 12% of the visually impaired population have no light perception (8), a larger proportion have nonfunctional vision, and for these individuals it is necessary to resort to substitutes for vision. New techniques need to be learned for mobility, self-care, and reading/writing. The O&M instructor and the rehabilitation teacher now assume a major role in the rehabilitation process. Mobility techniques, tactile substitution, vocal substitution, and specialized ADL techniques are used by these professionals to foster an independent life style.

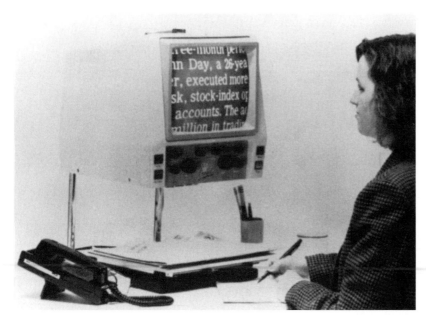

Figure 86-9. Closed-circuit television video magnifier (CCTV). (Reprinted by permission of VTek, Santa Monica, CA.)

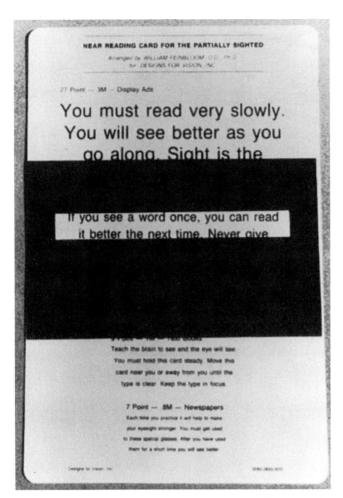

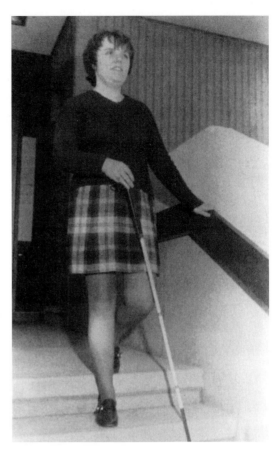

Figure 86-12. Stair climbing with long white cane. (From Cole RG, Rosenthal BP. *Remediation and management of low vision.* St Louis: CV Mosby, 1996. Reprinted by permission of Mosby-Year Book Publishers.)

Figure 86-11. Typoscope for enhanced contrast for reading. (From Cole RG, Rosenthal BP. *Remediation and management of low vision.* St Louis: CV Mosby, 1996. Reprinted by permission of Mosby-Year Book Publishers.)

Many options are available for improving the mobility of a blind person (37,38). The most frequently used techniques are a sighted guide, the long white cane, the guide dog, and various electronic or sonic navigation aids. Sighted guide technique is the correct way for a sighted person to assist one who is blind: the blind person places his or her hand just above the guide's elbow and then walks a step behind, allowing the guide's body movements to be communicated before turning, ascending/descending stairs, or negotiating curbs. The long white cane serves as an extension of the sense of touch, warning the blind traveler of upcoming obstacles or terrain changes as it is tapped about two paces in front of the user (the cane is usually 4 to 5 feet long). When used correctly, it allows movement in potentially hazardous circumstances such as descending stairs (Fig. 86-12). The laser cane, though more expensive and difficult to master, provides increased feedback about distant drop-offs and obstacles at head level by sending out three separate light beams, which trigger vibratory signals on the cane when such obstacles are detected (Fig. 86-13). The guide dog allows a greater degree of freedom of movement than the cane as well as a sense of companionship and security, but it requires intensive training of both dog and user, entails extra responsibility for the animal's care, and may be too strenuous for older or frailer individuals. Ultrasonic navigation aids can be worn over the chest by wheelchair users, mounted on walkerettes or wheelchairs, held in the hand, or mounted on a pair of glasses

(38). The most recent advance in electronic navigation is global positioning systems, which involve satellite tracking and computer localization with synthetic speech output. Surgical implantation of computer chips into the retina for vision substitution remains in its experimental stage at this time.

Tactile substitution is used in a wide variety of ways by blind persons. The best known is Braille, a tactile language system developed in France and based on permutations of a series of six small raised dots, which have the form seen on an ordinary domino. With practice it is possible to detect the more than 250 variations that are the basis of grade 2 Braille, which makes fluent reading possible. However, most blind people, particularly those whose vision loss was acquired in later life, will find it difficult to master, although a simpler form (grade 1) can be used for writing labels or brief notes. Written Braille and Braille output from computers are important communication tools, especially in persons with early-onset vision loss. Other tactile techniques include raised-line diagrams (for reading maps or illustrations); raised-dot marking of kitchen utensils to facilitate such activities as weighing, measuring, and using oven or toaster; watches with covers that can be swung away to permit the hands to be felt for keeping time; and raised letters or numbers for use by those unable to learn Braille.

Vocal substitution covers a wide range of techniques and resources in which any type of sound provides feedback or information for the blind individual. Recorded books and magazines are an invaluable source of pleasure and information for thousands of visually impaired people who do not have access to Braille. The Talking Book Program of the Library of Congress has recorded versions of most fiction and many nonfic-

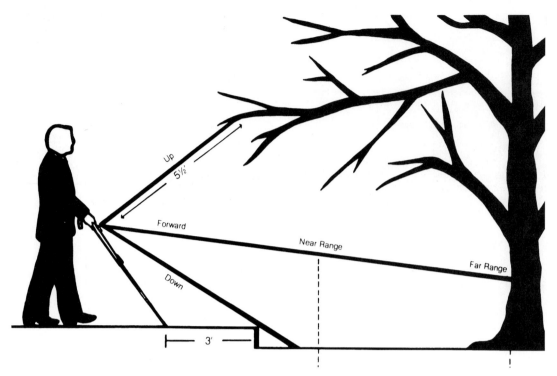

Figure 86-13. Laser cane. (Reprinted with permission of Nurion Industries, Inc., Paoli, PA.)

tion books in a convenient four-track cassette format recorded at half speed, which allows 6 hours of material on each cassette. Cassettes are sent to participants in plastic containers, and these are returned to the local library distributor free of charge via the mail. A modified cassette recorder is required to play these tapes; a large one is provided to users of the program, and smaller, more portable ones can be purchased for $150 to $250. Within the next few years the recording system will be updated to reflect digital technology, with the resultant modification of the playback devices. A physician, optometrist, or vision rehabilitation professional can certify that a patient has difficulty reading print; legal blindness is not a requirement, and the program is also available to those with dyslexia or neuromuscular problems that interfere with normal reading. Recordings for the Blind and Dyslexic of Princeton, New Jersey, supplements the Talking Books program with more than 75,000 recorded books, many of which are textbooks that can be used by students with print disabilities.

Synthetic speech technology is another form of vocal substitution that has greatly facilitated the lives of visually impaired people, spawning a host of devices that announce their data in clearly audible form: watches, calculators, weight scales, thermometers, glucometers, and even sphygmomanometers. The synthetic speech, screen-reading, and optical character recognition (OCR) software that have been developed in recent years are revolutionizing the field of computer technology for blind individuals, and it is now possible for such a person to read documents using a scanner and to perform other computer activities such as word processing and use of the Internet (Fig. 86-14).

Other ADL techniques for the blind combine tactile and vocal substitution strategies. For example, a liquid level indicator emits a tone when a cup of tea or coffee is filled to near the top; coins are identified by touch; dollar bill denominations are made identifiable by folding specific denominations in different patterns; clothing is color-coded using Braille labeling; and food preparation is simplified by using a measuring cup, weight scale, and timer that are marked with raised dots to indicate divisions of volume, weight, and time.

TREATING COMBINED VISUAL AND NEUROMUSCULAR DISABILITIES

The need for closer coordination between vision and medical rehabilitation systems is exemplified in a number of instances in which a neuromuscular impairment coexists with or includes a visual impairment. In some cases the two developed separately, as in the blind person who subsequently suffers an amputation of the lower extremity or a cerebrovascular accident (CVA). Altner, Rusin, and DeBoer (9) have demonstrated that blind amputees generally become prosthetic users and noted a 66% success rate among 12 such patients. Fisher (10) has added two more cases, both of which had positive outcomes. Wainapel (11) reviewed 220 consecutive stroke admissions to a general rehabilitation medicine unit, seven of whom had preexisting blindness. Although these patients were older and had a more lengthy hospital course, most of them became ambulatory, and four were discharged to their homes. These articles emphasize that blindness plus a second disability is no contraindication to rehabilitation; in fact, it is possible that the prior experience of a disability and its successful rehabilitation might be beneficial in terms of adaptation to a second disability.

Stroke is also associated with its own types of visual impairment, including perceptual—motor problems caused by right-sided brain damage and homonymous hemianopia from damage to the optic radiation on either side. The latter condition may severely interfere with mobility, self-care, and safety. The patient needs to be aware of the presence of this field deficit and to compensate for it by turning the head toward the af-

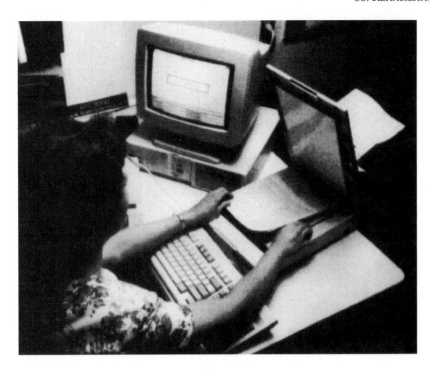

Figure 86-14. Computer and scanner for the visually impaired individual. (From Cole RG, Rosenthal BP. *Remediation and management of low vision.* St Louis: CV Mosby, 1996. Reprinted by permission of Mosby-Year Book Publishers.)

fected side. Prisms or a spectacle-mounted mirror (see Fig. 86-10) can deflect vision from the impaired to the normal portions of the visual field. More recently, it has been suggested that monocular eye patching combined with computer-generated stimulation of the affected visual field may produce beneficial results (39).

Traumatic brain injury (TBI) is also associated with visual disturbances, some of which are similar to those seen with CVA. However, the greater degree of cognitive impairment with TBI makes diagnosis of these problems more difficult. Gianutsos, Ramsey, and Perlin (40) performed visual screening on 55 severely brain-injured patients in a long-term-care facility and found that more than half of them had visual impairments (e.g., visual field loss, visual neglect, deficits in depth perception.). Of the 26 sent to a rehabilitative optometrist, all but two were benefited by this intervention, and many patients showed increased participation in their rehabilitation program following treatment. The optometric examination in such patients is quite difficult and often time-consuming. The participation of a cognitive therapist can be of great help during this exam. This kind of cooperation between the vision and medical rehabilitation systems is precisely what is needed for these complex clinical challenges.

The visual consequences of multiple sclerosis include diplopia, blurred vision, nystagmus, and even monocular or binocular blindness as a result of optic neuritis. Vision enhancement and substitution techniques for such patients may be difficult or impossible because of associated weakness, spasticity, and ataxia of the upper extremities. Standing magnifiers are preferable to hand-held ones, and recorded material is definitely more accessible than Braille. Computers may have to be voice-activated because of loss of finger dexterity and coordination. Similar obstacles face the diabetic patient whose retinopathy is combined with peripheral neuropathy. Additionally, diabetics develop autonomic dysfunction that can impact negatively on exercise programs and therapy in the rehabilitation setting. In one study of 29 visually impaired diabetics, 28 had parasympathetic neuropathy manifested by abnormal heart rate changes with respiration, 23 had sympathetic neuropathy

manifested by abnormal cardiovascular responses to tilting, and nine developed frank orthostatic hypotension (41). In some of these patients it is advisable to perform physical therapy and occupational therapy as well as general exercise programs in the seated or recumbent position.

ADAPTATIONS FOR THERAPEUTIC AND RECREATIONAL EXERCISE

It is imperative that visually impaired individuals have the same opportunity for physical activity as their sighted counterparts. Although a physical fitness program is recognized as an important component of the education curriculum for visually impaired children, many progress to adolescence and adulthood without the opportunity to develop healthy exercise habits (42). Adults with acquired visual deficits often withdraw from previous activities and are apprehensive to undertake new forms of exercise. Because of social isolation, lack of access, or discomfort with unfamiliar settings, they do not join exercise classes or utilize community exercise facilities. A complete rehabilitation program for visually impaired individuals should encourage lifelong exercise habits and should offer instruction in adaptive exercise training for its benefits on aerobic capacity, balance, and obesity prevention. A comprehensive exercise program design must address (a) modifications of the exercise environment and equipment, (b) safety precautions for unstable eye disease, and (c) accommodations for special problems imposed by concurrent disease and disability.

Environmental Modifications

Visually impaired individuals are more apt to have a positive experience on initiation of an exercise program if they are comfortable with the program personnel and the physical setting. The exercise instructor and support staff should receive sensitivity training and should learn sighted guide techniques. Visually impaired participants should receive hands-on orientation to the exercise facility and equipment. Location of exercise stations, locker rooms, and rest rooms must be included in the orientation.

During warm-up and cool-down exercises, those with severe visual impairments need to be stationed near a wall, chair, or other solid object that can be used as a center for spatial orientation and support. Exercise routines should be described verbally, and movements should be demonstrated individually until the routines are mastered. Participants can select from multiple aerobic options such as walking, running, stationary bicycling, and swimming. Visually impaired people can participate in dance aerobics when time is allowed for proper demonstration of movements (42). Existing indoor and outdoor tracks for walking and running can be modified by installing a guide rope along the perimeter of the track. A single-lane track can be improvised by stringing a guide rope along the length of the exercise room or designating an area adjacent to a long, straight segment of wall. By maintaining hand contact with the rope or wall, even a totally blind individual will feel more confident and safe and will be able to focus efforts more effectively on the exercise activity. At home, one may establish a guide rope to walk repetitive laps along a driveway or yard or designate an indoor walking lane along an uncluttered hallway or other wall space. Those who have honed cane-travel skills can select safe low-traffic walking routes.

Those who prefer other forms of indoor exercise, at home or at a public facility, can choose from a variety of aerobic exercise equipment, including treadmills, step trainers, stationary bicycles, cross-country ski synthesizers, rowing machines, and exercise gliders. Before using equipment, the visually impaired person should have an opportunity to manually explore all moving parts and controls. Dial settings and touch panels can be marked with Braille or raised dots. Swimming is another excellent aerobic option. Blind swimmers may have difficulty maintaining orientation and staying within the boundaries of designated lap lanes. To overcome this problem, they can align themselves with conventional floating lane markers and periodically brush a hand against the lane marker to maintain a straight course (43–47).

Precautions for Unstable Eye Conditions

Individuals who have had recent eye surgery or those with unstable eye conditions may be advised to curtail physical activities. However, in diseases such as proliferative diabetic retinopathy, the condition may be chronic. Prolonged inactivity will lead to severe cardiovascular and musculoskeletal deconditioning (44,48). If appropriate precautions are taken, an exercise training program can be designed to promote cardiovascular and general fitness without aggravating the pathologic eye condition (43,44). The role of exercise in inducing retinal hemorrhage is uncertain. However, abnormalities in systemic blood pressure and local blood flow to the eye have been observed in patients with proliferative diabetic retinopathy (49). Hence, it seems wise to limit blood pressure excursions during exercise. In one exercise program involving 29 participants with proliferative diabetic retinopathy, no visual deterioration was noted when systolic blood pressures were maintained below 200 mm Hg and were not allowed to exceed the baseline by an increment greater than 50 mm Hg (44,48).

There are no definitive studies, but cautious recommendations for those with active diabetic retinopathy and other unstable eye conditions are (a) to keep the head elevated (avoid forward bending from the waist), (b) to avoid the supine or prone position, (c) to avoid contact sports, (d) to avoid vigorous bouncing exercises (e.g., jumping, jogging), and (e) to avoid isometric exercises and heavy weight lifting with the associated Valsalva maneuver.

To adhere to these recommendations, an exercise program can be developed in which warm-up and cool-down exercises are performed from an erect sitting or standing position. Preferred aerobic selections would include low-impact activities such as walking, stationary bicycling, and rowing (43,44).

Special Considerations for Diabetes Mellitus

Diabetes is the leading cause of blindness for middle-aged and older adults in the United States. Rehabilitation specialists involved in designing exercise programs and mobility training for persons with diabetes and visual impairment will need to consider other concurrent complications of the disease. Even when precautions are taken to minimize deterioration of the eye disease, there will be concerns about blood glucose excursions during exercise as well as cardiac, renal, and neurologic dysfunction.

Exercise can induce low blood sugar in those receiving insulin or oral antiglycemic medications. Previously inactive individuals may experience low blood sugar even with low to moderate levels of activity (41). Because insulin and other medications are planned to match food ingestion, exercise and mobility training sessions should be planned to avoid delays or omissions of meals. The instructor or the participant should carry a source of carbohydrate such as fruit juice, hard candy, or glucose tablets. These items should be ingested if the individual develops symptoms of low blood sugar (weakness, shaking, sweating, palpitations, headaches, confusion), and the training session should be discontinued until these symptoms completely resolve. Some people with very high blood sugar will experience fatigue or have difficulty concentrating, necessitating postponement of the training session. Others will have no obvious symptoms and will have no difficulty in continuing with the planned session.

Manifestations of diabetic neuropathy may include diminished sensations in the hands and feet as well as loss of muscle strength and balance. Autonomic nervous system dysfunction may result in orthostatic hypotension and poor exercise tolerance, related to abnormal cardiac and circulatory responses. Those with these problems may need to perform all exercises stationed near a wall or solid piece of furniture or may need to carry out exercise routines from a seated position. Those with orthostatic hypotension, who are unable to remain standing for sustained periods, may select aerobic activities such as rowing or bicycling from a semirecumbent position. The latter can be achieved by seating the individual in an armchair placed behind the seat of a conventional stationary bicycle, or through the use of a semirecumbent bicycle (41,44).

Sensory loss to the feet combined with circulatory problems places the individual at high risk for foot injury, which may lead to infection or amputation. Those with severe neuropathy or existing foot injuries should avoid weight-bearing exercise, although light cycling, rowing, and upper-body activities may be appropriate. In all cases, it is essential that footwear be comfortable, properly fitted, and adequately protective. The feet should be inspected before and after each exercise session for signs of pressure and friction injury. Abrasions and blisters should receive appropriate medical attention and should be observed until completely healed (50,51).

Participation in exercise and mobility training may be limited by heart and kidney disease, which frequently accompany failing vision. Individuals should be evaluated by a physician before initiating an exercise program. Aerobic activity should be selected according to the individual's abilities and needs.

The heart rate and blood pressure should be monitored throughout the exercise session. Individuals should be taught how to measure their own pulse rates, and they should be given guidelines to curtail exercise if the heart rate or blood pressure exceeds preset limits. Aerobic programs should begin at low levels, and the length and level of the exercise should be gradually incremented as the individual develops improved strength and cardiovascular conditioning. Once individuals have learned the principles of safe exercise and appropriate goals have been determined, they may continue to exercise independently using home equipment or walking in safe environments.

A model 12-week program including three exercise sessions per week was designed specifically to meet the needs of visually impaired individuals with diabetes mellitus (43,44). All the precautions and principles discussed were incorporated into the exercise program. There were moderate improvements in diabetes control with decreased insulin requirements. There were moderate improvements in exercise performance, opening the potential for other work and leisure activities. Patients with the poorest baseline conditioning derived the most cardiovascular benefit (48). Improvements in psychosocial function were also observed, which may have been related to enhanced self-confidence, better balance and coordination, and facilitation of social interactions (43,44,47,52). Other exercise programs have been described for patients with diabetes and visual impairment, although outcome data have not been reported (45,46).

Those with other neuromuscular problems and systemic disease in conjunction with visual impairment may benefit from similar adaptations to exercise. Specific needs should be analyzed so that individualized exercise programs can be developed. The final objective of every exercise training program should be to teach the participants safe and practical exercise routines that can be maintained in the home environment and that will enhance general health and the ability to undertake occupational and leisure activities.

CONCLUSIONS: BRIDGING TWO WORLDS

The worlds of rehabilitation medicine and vision rehabilitation, which commingled their expertise in the postwar years, have since then gone their separate ways. Both have produced their own specialists and unique therapeutic approaches to the disabilities and handicaps of their target populations. Both continue to have distinct scholarly journals (*Journal of Vision Impairment and Blindness, Journal of Vision Rehabilitation*). And both have established distinct roles as advocates for their patients. But the commonalities are stronger than the distinctions, and contemporary trends favor a return to the earlier intimacy between these worlds. The aging population guarantees an ever-increasing supply of patients with combinations of visual and superimposed medical disabilities; in such cases, a more eclectic treatment approach is necessary to address the multiple functional losses that ensue. Neither system can adequately address this challenge on its own. Similarly, the visual impairments produced by such common rehabilitation diagnoses as CVA, TBI, MS, and IDDM demand greater knowledge of vision rehabilitation options by physiatrists. Finally, the increasing role of managed care in medical decision making and service reimbursement encourages the concept of the physiatrist as primary care physician for people with physical disabilities. Such a conceptual model would be unthinkable if the practitioner were to remain ignorant of the rehabilitation methods appropriate for a group of more than 4 million people.

A provocative recent article by Massof and co-workers (53) demonstrates that the rehabilitation paradigm can be applied to the vision care system and can be used to justify reimbursement of vision rehabilitation services by third-party payers such as Medicare or Medicaid. Physiatrists are ideally suited for the role of medical coordinator of these patients by virtue of their training, their patient-centered and functionally oriented approach, and their traditional role as advocates for those with disabilities. This is a wonderful opportunity to expand physiatric involvement into an area with which it has long historical associations. A half-century after the global conflict that spurred their simultaneous evolution into modern specialties, the two worlds need to commingle their respective identities once again, and both of them ought to be the stronger and more effective from their association.

RESOURCES

American Council of the Blind (ACB)
1155 15th Street NW, Suite 720
Washington, DC 20005
800–424–8666 (3 P.M. to 5:30 P.M.)
202–467–5081

American Foundation for the Blind (AFB)
11 Penn Plaza, Suite 300
New York, NY 10001
800–232–5463
212–502–7600

American Printing House for the Blind (APH)
1839 Frankfort Avenue
Louisville, KY 40206
800–223–1839
502–895–2405

Blinded Veterans Association
477 H Street NW
Washington, DC 20001–2694
800 669–7079
202–371–8880

Council of Citizens with Low Vision International (CCLVI)
6511 26th Street West
Bradenton, FL 34207
800–733–2258
Library of Congress

National Library Service for the Blind and Physically
  Handicapped
1291 Taylor Street NW
Washington, DC 20542
800–424–8567
202–707–5100

The Lighthouse, Inc.
111 East 59th Street
New York, NY 10022
800–334–5497
212–821–9200

National Association for Visually Handicapped
22 West 21st Street
New York, NY 10010
212–889–3141

National Federation of the Blind (NFB)
1800 Johnson Street
Baltimore, MD 21230
410–659–9314

Recordings for the Blind and Dyslexic
The Anne T. MacDonald Center
20 Roszel Road
Princeton, NJ 08540
800–221–4792
609–452–0606

REFERENCES

1. Wainapel SF. Vision rehabilitation: an overlooked subject in physiatric training and practice. *Am J Phys Med Rehabil* 1995;74:313–314.
2. Lupinacci M. Physiatric management of the visually impaired disabled patient. *Curr Concepts Rehabil Med* 1990;5:6–13.
3. Goodpasture RC. Rehabilitation of the blind. In: Krusen FH, Kottke FJ, Ellwood PM, eds. *Handbook of physical medicine and rehabilitation*, 2nd ed. Philadelphia: WB Saunders, 1971.
4. Rusk HA. *A world to care for.* New York: Random House, 1977.
5. Koestler FA. *The unseen minority: a history of the blind in America.* New York: American Foundation for the Blind, 1976.
6. National Center for Health Statistics, Centers for Disease Control and Prevention. Health United States, 1993. Hyattsville, MD: US Public Health Service, 1994. DHHS Publication No. 94–1232.
7. Faye EE, Stuen CS, eds. *The aging eye and low vision: a study guide for physicians.* New York: The Lighthouse, Inc., 1992.
8. Nelson KA, Dimitrova E. Severe visual impairment in the United States and in each state, 1990. *J Vis Impairment Blind* 1993;87:80–86.
9. Altner PE, Rusin JJ, DeBoer A. Rehabilitation of blind patients with lower extremity amputations. *Arch Phys Med Rehabil* 1980;61:82–85.
10. Fisher R. Rehabilitation of the blind amputee: a rewarding experience. *Arch Phys Med Rehabil* 1987;68:382–383.
11. Wainapel SF. Rehabilitation of the blind stroke patient. *Arch Phys Med Rehabil* 1984;65:487–489.
12. Wainapel SF, Kwon YS, Fazzari PJ. Severe visual impairment on a rehabilitation unit: incidence and implications. *Arch Phys Med Rehabil* 1989;70:439–441.
13. Tobis JS, Block M, Steinhaus-Donham C, et al. Falling among the sensorially impaired elderly. *Arch Phys Med Rehabil* 1990;71:144–147.
14. Tinetti M, Inouye S, Gill T, et al. Shared risk factors for falls, incontinence, and functional dependence. *JAMA* 1995;273:1348–1353.
15. Stones MV, Kozma A. Balance and age in the sighted and blind. *Arch Phys Med Rehabil* 1987;68:85–89.
16. Cohn TE, Lasley DJ. Visual depth illusion and falls in the elderly. *Clin Geriatr Med* 1985;1:601–620.
17. Felson D, Anderson JJ, Hannan MT, et al. Impaired vision and hip fracture: the Framingham Study. *J Am Geriatr Soc* 1989;37:495–500.
18. Carabellese C, Appollonio I, Rozzini R, et al. Sensory impairment and quality of life in community elderly population. *J Am Geriatr Soc* 1993;41:401–407.
19. Branch LG, Horowitz A, Carr C. The implications for everyday life of incident self-reported visual decline among people over age 65 living in the community. *Gerontologist* 1989;29:359–365.
20. Gillman AE, Simmel A, Simon EP. Visual handicap in the aged: self-reported visual disability and the quality of life of residents of public housing for the elderly. *J Vis Impairment Blind* 1986;80:588–590.
21. Kahn HA, Liebowitz HM, Ganley JP. The Framingham Eye Study: outline and major prevalence findings. *Am J Epidemiol* 1977;106:17–32.
22. Faye EE, Stuen CS. *The aging eye and low vision.* New York: The Lighthouse, 1992.
23. Obstbaum SA. Clinical crossroads: an 82 year old woman with cataracts. *JAMA* 1996;275:1675–1680.
24. Steinberg EP, Tielsch JM, Schein OD. National study of cataract surgery outcomes: variations in four month postoperative outcomes as reflected in multiple outcome measures. *Ophthalmology* 1994;101:1142–1152.
25. Applegate WB, Miller ST, Elam JT, et al. Impact of cataract surgery with lens implantation on vision and physical function in elderly patients. *JAMA* 1987;257:1064–1066.
26. Klein R, Klein BEK. Vision disorders in diabetes. In: National Diabetes Data Group, eds. *Diabetes in America*, 2nd ed. Bethesda: National Institutes of Health, 1995:293–337.
27. Diabetes Control and Complications Trial Research Group. The effect of intensive treatment of diabetes on the development and progression of long-term complications in insulin-dependent diabetes mellitus. *N Engl J Med* 1993;329:977–986.
28. Ferris FL 3rd. Diabetic retinopathy. *Diabetes Care* 1993;16:322–325.
29. Diabetic Retinopathy Study Research Group. Preliminary report on effects of photocoagulation therapy. *Am J Ophthalmol* 1976;81:383–396.
30. Early Treatment Diabetic Retinopathy Study Research Group. Photocoagulation for diabetic macular edema. Early Treatment Diabetic Retinopathy Study report number 1. *Arch Ophthalmol* 1985;103:1796–1806.
31. Raskin P, Arauz-Pacheco C. The treatment of diabetic retinopathy: a view for the internist. *Ann Intern Med* 1992;117:226–233.
32. Kohner EM. Diabetic retinopathy. *Br Med J* 1993;307:1195–1199.
33. Rosenthal BP, Cole RG. *Functional assessment of low vision.* St Louis: CV Mosby, 1996.
34. Havlik RJ. *Aging in the eighties. Impaired senses for sound and light in persons aged 65 years and over.* Preliminary data from the Supplement on Aging to the National Health Interview Survey;United States, Jan–June, 1984. Advanced Data from Vital and Health Statistics. DHHS Publication (PHS) 86–1250. Hyattsville, MD: U.S. Department of Health and Human Services, 1986.
35. Faye EE. *Clinical low vision.* Boston: Little, Brown, 1984.
36. Cole RG, Rosenthal BP. *Remediation and management of low vision.* St Louis: CV Mosby, 1996.
37. Walsh R, Blasch BB. *Foundations of orientation and mobility.* New York: American Foundation for the Blind, 1983.
38. Coleman CL, Weinstock RF. Physically handicapped blind people: adaptive mobility techniques. *J Vis Impairment Blind* 1984;78:113–117.
39. Butter C, Kirsch N. Combined and separate effects of eye patching and visual stimulation on unilateral neglect following stroke. *Arch Phys Med Rehabil* 1992;73:1133–1139.
40. Gianutsos R, Ramsey G, Perlin R. Rehabilitative optometric services for survivors of acquired brain injury. *Arch Phys Med Rehabil* 1988;69:573–578.
41. Bernbaum M, Albert SG, Cohen JD. Exercise training in individuals with diabetic retinopathy and blindness. *Arch Phys Med Rehabil* 1989;70:605–611.
42. Ponchillia SV, Powell LL, Felski KA, et al. The effectiveness of aerobic exercise instruction for totally blind women. *J Vis Impairment Blind* 1992;86:174–177.
43. Bernbaum M, Albert SG, Brusca SR, et al. A team approach. Promoting diabetes self-management and independence in the visually impaired: a model clinical program. *Diabetes Educ* 1988;14:51–54.
44. Bernbaum M, Albert SG, Brusca SR, et al. A model clinical program for patients with diabetes and vision impairment. *Diabetes Educ* 1989;15:325–330.
45. Dods J. Two exercise programs for people with diabetes and visual impairment. *J Vis Impairment Blind* 1993;87:365–367.
46. Weitzman DM. Promoting healthful exercise for visually impaired persons with diabetes. *J Vis Impairment Blind* 1993;87:361–364.
47. Albert SG, Bernbaum M. Exercise for patients with diabetic retinopathy. *Diabetes Care* 1995;18:130–132.
48. Bernbaum M, Albert SG, Cohen JD, et al. Cardiovascular conditioning in individuals with diabetic retinopathy. *Diabetes Care* 1989;12:740–742.
49. Albert SG, Gomez CR, Russell S, et al. Cerebral and ophthalmic artery hemodynamic responses in diabetes mellitus. *Diabetes Care* 1993;16:476–482.
50. Caputo GM, Cavanagh PR, Ulbrecht JS, et al. Assessment and management of foot disease in patients with diabetes. *N Engl J Med* 1994;331:854–860.
51. Plummer ES, Albert SG. Foot care assessment in patients with diabetes mellitus: a screening algorithm for patient education and referral. *Diabetes Educ* 1995;21:47–51.
52. Bernbaum M, Albert SG, Duckro PN. Psychosocial profiles in patients with visual impairment due to diabetic retinopathy. *Diabetes Care* 1988;11:551–557.
53. Massof RW, Dagnelie G, Deremeik JT, et al. Low vision rehabilitation in the US health care system. *J Vis Rehabil* 1995;9:3–31.

CHAPTER 87

Auditory Rehabilitation with Cochlear Implants

Teresa A. Zwolan and Paul R. Kileny

A cochlear implant (CI) is an electric auditory prosthesis used to rehabilitate hearing loss when a conventional hearing aid is not effective. The following sections present specific, well-defined criteria for cochlear implant candidates. However, there is some overlap between the candidacy criteria for traditional hearing aids and cochlear implants. Structural differences between cochlear implants and hearing aids are presented in Fig. 87-1. A hearing aid can be used to compensate for hearing loss resulting from a partial loss of cochlear hair cells utilizing the underlying principle that this compensation will be achieved by increasing the intensity of sounds delivered to the ear. While this amplification effort results in increased audibility, it does not always result in improved speech understanding or environmental sound identification. This is particularly true in patients who have lost the majority of hair cells in a certain cochlear region, as in severe high-frequency hearing loss.

Some patients who receive no benefit from conventional acoustic amplification because of loss of hair cells have adequate afferent auditory neural elements to allow the individual to receive an auditory response in the brain with electrical stimulation of the nerves. Theoretically, this is because the CI delivers patterned electrical stimulation to neural elements beyond the cochlear hair cells. It appears that even in the presence of substantial or complete hair cell loss the auditory nerve remains relatively intact, enabling patients to perceive well-distributed electrical information. However, hair cell loss is often accompanied by cochlear nerve degeneration, and this may result in a reduction in the number of auditory nerve fibers available for electrical stimulation by a cochlear implant.

Sensorineural hearing loss tends to have a greater effect on the patient's ability to detect high-frequency sounds than it does on their ability to perceive low-frequency sounds. With conventional amplification, relatively little compensation can be offered in the high-frequency range to patients with a significant high-frequency loss. This lack of effective high-frequency amplification results in poor speech discrimination with a hearing aid because of the relatively high frequency spectral content of consonant sounds. The same is not the case with electrical stimulation because these hair cells are not necessary for successful cochlear implant performance and because one does not have to deal with limitations imposed by basilar membrane mechanics. Thus it is actually easier to provide high-frequency information through electrical stimulation than to do so through amplification of the auditory signal.

Before the advent of cochlear implants, rehabilitation options for patients with severe to profound hearing loss and poor speech understanding were limited. The CI is designed and developed to fill this need in hearing rehabilitation. The success of cochlear implants has led to improvements in technology, including improvements in safety and efficacy, allowing for the expansion of candidacy criteria to include younger patients and patients with greater amounts of residual hearing.

HOW COCHLEAR IMPLANTS WORK

Three CI systems are currently available for use in the United States. All three have received FDA approval for use in adults and in children as young as 12 months of age. These systems include the Clarion device, manufactured by Advanced Bionics of Sylmar, California (www.advancedbionics.com), the Nucleus device, manufactured by Cochlear Pty. Ltd. of Australia (www.cochlear.com), and the Combi 40+ device, manufactured by MedEl, Inc. of Innsbruck, Austria (www.medel.com). All three systems consist of surgically implanted internal components and externally worn speech processor and headset components.

Internal Device Components

The internal device consists of a receiving coil, an internal processor, and an electrode array. The receiving coil is surgically placed in the mastoid bone and is composed of a magnet (for attachment of the external headset) and an antenna. The receiving coil and internal processor are housed in either a silastic or ceramic case. An example of the Nucleus Contour internal receiver and electrode array is provided in Fig. 87-2.

All three of the currently available devices have more than one intracochlear electrode and are referred to as multichannel. These devices take advantage of the tonotopic organization of the cochlea and provide differently processed information to various locations within the cochlea. The total number of electrodes in use depends on several factors, including the number of electrodes available on the array, the speech-processing strategy in use, and the psychophysical responses of the patient. The number of stimulating electrodes used in currently available systems varies from eight to 22.

Hearing Aid vs. Cochlear Implant

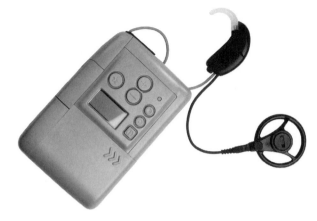

Figure 87-1. Schematic representation comparing a conventional hearing aid to a cochlear implant.

External Components

The external components of cochlear implant systems collect, analyze, process, and transmit auditory information to the internal components. External components include a microphone, speech processor, and transmitter coil. The microphone, which is usually housed on the headset, picks up sound from the environment and sends it to the speech processor. The speech processor converts the sound to an electrical signal coded for transmission to the internal device. The signal is then

Figure 87-3. Nucleus 24 multichannel cochlear implant, SPRINT speech processor and headset. (Courtesy of Cochlear Ltd.)

sent to the transmitter. This transmitter is located on the outside of the CI user's head and is held in place and aligned with the internal receiving coil by external and internal magnets. The integrated circuit within the cochlear implant receives the information from the transmitter, decodes the signal, and delivers electrical stimulation to the intracochlear electrodes.

Speech Processor Features

Both body-worn and ear-level style speech processors are currently available for cochlear implant users (Figs. 87-3 and 87-4). Although they vary in size and weight, the available speech processors have several features in common, including the ability to store more than one program; the availability of an external input port that enables the user to connect to assistive listening devices; separate dials to control volume, microphone sensitivity, and power; and the availability of private or public alarms to alert users or their parents when the battery is low or the device has been disconnected. Speech processors are powered by either alkaline or rechargeable batteries.

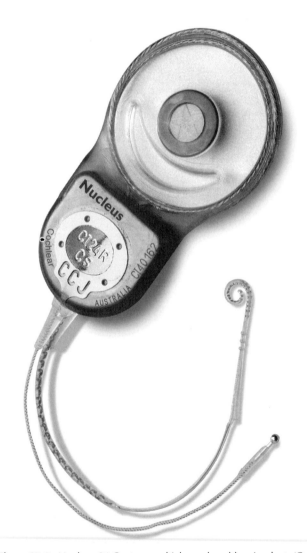

Figure 87-2. Nucleus 24 Contour multichannel cochlear implant. (Courtesy of Cochlear Ltd.)

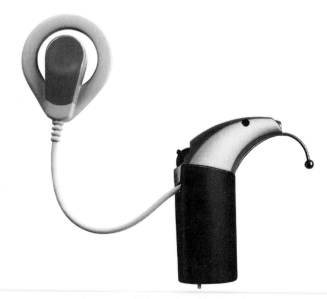

Figure 87-4. Nucleus 24 multichannel cochlear implant ESPRIT 3G ear level speech processor. (Courtesy of Cochlear Ltd.)

Speech-Processing Strategies

The specific type of information delivered to the CI user depends on several factors, including the integrated circuit within the implant, the characteristics of the electrode array, and the speech-processing strategy. The speech-processing strategy determines the features of the speech signal that will be delivered to the patient and the manner in which this information will be relayed to the electrode array.

EVALUATION AND DETERMINATION OF CANDIDACY

Candidacy requirements for a cochlear implant have changed greatly over the past several years. Such requirements will continue to evolve as advances are made in device technology, surgical technique, and speech-processing strategies. Referral guidelines for CI evaluation of children or adults are provided in Table 87-1. Determination of candidacy for a cochlear implant is most often made by a team of qualified professionals, including: an otologic surgeon, an audiologist, a speech-language pathologist, and a psychologist. The opinions of other professionals, such as deaf educators and classroom teachers, are also often taken into account when determining CI candidacy.

The evaluation process involves several appointments. First, the patient is seen by the audiologist for audiologic testing to determine the type and severity of the hearing loss. Next, a hearing aid evaluation, which includes evaluation of speech perception skills, is performed to evaluate the patient's hearing skills when using appropriate amplification. The patient may be seen for electrophysiologic testing, such as the Auditory Brainstem Response (ABR), to verify the results obtained audiologically. ABR is particularly useful with very young children.

TABLE 87-1. Guidelines for When to Refer an Adult or a Child for Cochlear Implant Evaluation

Patients should be referred for cochlear implant evaluation when they demonstrate the following.

Adults
A moderate to profound hearing loss in the low frequencies and severe hearing loss in the mid to high speech frequencies.
Difficulty understanding speech when unable to see the speaker's face, such as when using the telephone.
A monosyllabic word score, obtained with appropriate amplification, of less than 40% correct; or a sentence recognition score, obtained with appropriate amplification, of less than 60% correct.
A profound sensorineural hearing loss. Patients should *not* be ruled out for a cochlear implant based on the finding of no residual hearing.
Adults should *not* be ruled out for candidacy based on their age. Many adults in their 80s demonstrate great success with cochlear implants.

Children
Bilateral severe to profound sensorineural hearing loss. If identified at birth, a child should be referred to a cochlear implant center by 3 months of age. This will facilitate long-term monitoring and regular testing by the implant center to definitively determine candidacy by the time the child is 12 months of age.
Little or no benefit from amplification, as demonstrated by a lack of progress on simple auditory tasks.
For older children who can perform such testing, a monosyllabic word score less than 40% correct.

Next, the patient undergoes a medical evaluation by an implant surgeon, which will include computed tomography (CT) or magnetic resonance imaging (MRI) of the brain and skull to visualize the mastoid development, the inner ear structures, and the vestibulo-cochlear nerves. Additional preoperative appointments may also include speech-language and neuropsychologic evaluations.

Current adult candidacy criteria indicate that cochlear implants are useful in patients who have bilateral pre-, peri-, or postlinguistic sensorineural hearing impairment and who obtain limited benefit from appropriate binaural hearing aids. These individuals typically have moderate to profound hearing loss in the low frequencies and profound ($\geq$90 dB HL) hearing loss in the mid to high speech frequencies. Limited benefit from amplification is defined by test scores of 50% or less correct in the ear to be implanted, and 60% or less in the best-aided condition, on tape-recorded tests of open-set sentence recognition (1).

Current pediatric candidacy criteria indicate that devices are useful for children 12 to 24 months of age who have a bilateral profound sensorineural deafness and demonstrate limited benefit from appropriate binaural hearing aids. Children 2 years of age and older may be candidates if they demonstrate severe to profound hearing loss bilaterally. In younger children, limited benefit is defined as lack of progress in the development of simple auditory skills in conjunction with appropriate amplification and participation in intensive aural habilitation over a 3- to 6-month period (1). Because very young children may not be able to participate in speech perception testing, lack of benefit from amplification is additionally based on parental response to clinician-administered questionnaires such as the Meaningful Auditory Integration Scale (MAIS) (2) or the Infant Toddler (IT)-MAIS (3). Children who can participate in speech perception testing should obtain a score less than or equal to 30% correct on the open-set Lexical Neighborhood Test (LNT) or the Multisyllabic Lexical Neighborhood Test (MLNT) (4). Some implant manufacturers also recommend a 3- to 6-month hearing aid trial for children with no previous hearing aid experience.

SURGICAL PROCEDURE

Most centers perform cochlear implant surgery as an outpatient procedure. The surgery lasts 2 to 5 hours, depending on the surgeon's experience, the device selected, and the complexity of the patient's anatomy. Children and adults often return to their normal routines within 1 week of surgery. Risks include a remote possibility of infection, temporary or permanent facial paralysis on the operated side, mild temporary taste disturbances, tinnitus, vertigo, and loss of residual hearing in the implanted ear.

Specifically, a postauricular incision is made and the receiver-stimulator portion of the internal device is placed in a well that has been cut into the skull behind the mastoid bone. The bone between the tympanic membrane and the facial nerve is removed until the round window and the cochlear promontory are visualized. A cochleostomy is made into the basal turn of the scala tympani just anterior to the round window and the electrode array is inserted into the cochlea. The receiver-stimulator of the internal device is then secured into the well behind the mastoid. The incision is closed and a pressure dressing is placed over the ear for 24 hours.

Cochlear implant recipients must avoid various medical and surgical procedures that could damage the implanted device or the functioning auditory nerve fibers that transmit the electrical signal to the brain. These include the use of monopolar electrosurgical instruments in the region of the head or neck, diathermy, neurostimulation, ionizing radiation therapy involving the area of the implant, electroconvulsive therapy, and magnetic resonance imaging (MRI).

POSTOPERATIVE FOLLOW-UP

The patient returns to the clinic approximately 4 weeks after surgery for initial programming of the device. This waiting period allows for healing and reduction of swelling around the incision. Programming of the device is performed while the patient's speech processor is connected to a computer that is run by the implant audiologist. Sounds are delivered to the patient through the cochlear implant via the computer. Testing begins with determination of the softest level of sound (threshold) that can be heard when each electrode is stimulated. The upper level of stimulation is then determined for each electrode. Depending on the type of device used, this level of stimulation may be "most comfortable" ("M" level) or "loud but comfortable" ("C" level). This psychophysical information is then used in the program for the speech-processing strategy.

The number of return patient visits for continued programming depends on several factors, such as the age of the child, programming needs, and proximity to the clinic. In most cases, children return twice a month for the first 3 months, monthly for the next 3 months, and then every 3 months to program their speech processor. Adults are usually seen twice the first month and at the 3-, 6-, and 12-month intervals. Once the patient has used the device for 1 year, most centers recommend that children return every 6 months and that adults return annually for speech perception testing and programming of the speech processor.

POSTOPERATIVE RESULTS IN ADULTS

Performance of adults with cochlear implants is greatly affected by several factors, including age at onset of deafness, length of deafness, and primary communication method. Patients who lost their hearing before the development of speech and language skills are referred to as prelingually deafened adults. Typically, these patients demonstrate poorer speech perception skills with an implant than postlingually deafened adults (5–7). They demonstrate little change in postoperative speech recognition scores over time when traditional open- and closed-set speech perception tests are used, and also progress slowly in speech perception and speech production skills when provided with intensive rehabilitation (8). Because of these factors, prelingually deafened adults demonstrate a higher device nonuse rate than postlingually deafened adults. However, many prelingually deafened adults use their device regularly, are satisfied with their device, and report that the cochlear implant improves both their expressive and receptive communication skills (7).

In contrast, most postlingually deafened adults demonstrate greatly improved communication skills when using their CI. Although the open-set speech recognition scores obtained by postlingually deafened adults vary greatly from individual to individual, most patients obtain scores in the 70% to 80% correct range on open-set sentence tests and scores in the 30% to 40% correct range on monosyllabic word tests [personal communication, Mary Joe Osberger, Advanced Bionics (9)].

Many postlingually deafened adults understand speech so well that they can converse interactively over a standard telephone.

POSTOPERATIVE RESULTS IN CHILDREN

Several factors are known to impact a child's performance with a cochlear implant, such as age at onset of profound deafness, age at implant, etiology of deafness, additional handicaps, and educational placement. Several investigators have demonstrated that the age at onset of profound deafness and age at implantation have a strong impact on performance with a cochlear implant. In general, patients who receive their implant at younger ages tend to perform better on speech perception tests than children implanted at older ages (10,11). Additionally, some recent studies indicate that children with greater amounts of residual hearing at the time of implant tend to demonstrate greater overall gains in speech perception with an implant than children with little or no preoperative residual hearing (12).

The status of the cochlea has also been found to affect performance. Patients who present with congenital malformations or cochlear ossification are still considered to be candidates for a cochlear implant (13,14). However, patients who present with such anomalies frequently demonstrate poorer speech recognition skills after implant than do patients with normal cochleae (15,16).

Some children may demonstrate disabilities in addition to their deafness that may or may not affect their performance with a cochlear implant. Noncognitive disabilities, such as blindness and cerebral palsy, are not likely to impact the child's eventual performance with a cochlear implant. Cognitive disabilities, on the other hand, are likely to affect performance with a CI and should be considered in the decision regarding candidacy.

There is great controversy in the literature regarding the effect that educational placement has on a child's performance with a cochlear implant. Several investigators have reported that children enrolled in oral communication programs tend to demonstrate greater gains in speech perception skills with a cochlear implant than children educated in a total communication setting (17,18). One issue that is strongly agreed on, however, is that children will perform optimally with a cochlear implant if their school supports the child in her use of the device, if they offer aggressive auditory management and treatment, and if they provide an optimal auditory environment that promotes and encourages auditory development.

CLINICAL INVESTIGATIONS AND FUTURE DEVELOPMENTS

The introduction of cochlear implants into clinical practice has revolutionized the rehabilitation opportunities for patients with a severe to profound hearing loss. Previously, the opportunity for auditory rehabilitation was limited or nonexistent for such patients. Over the years, there has been a series of advances in terms of both device efficacy and clinical criteria for implantation. Today we are implanting patients with more residual hearing than at the outset, and the age limit is much lower. These changes are due to improved device performance and demonstrated safety, which have enhanced the benefit-to-risk ratio.

Cochlear implants have changed over the years in a number of areas, including speech-processing strategy, electrode and electrode carrier design, and speech processor utility and design. Currently, there are continuing efforts to improve performance, especially for patients where performance is relatively poor, and to include patient categories where prosthetic rehabilitation of hearing may have been previously unavailable. For example, patients diagnosed with neurofibromatosis II and acoustic neuromas eventually undergo bilateral resection of their acoustic neuromas (usually consecutively, but sometimes years apart). In most cases, these patients are not candidates for a CI. The reasons for this are (a) these patients incur a mixed sensory and neural hearing loss brought about by increased compression and attenuation of the cochlear nerve by the growing tumor as well as by cochlear ischemia due to compression of the labyrinthine artery and (b) the surgical resection of these tumors, especially if they are relatively large, entails resection of the cochlear nerve. Thus hearing rehabilitation through intracochlear stimulation of the auditory nerve is not plausible. The only alternative for these patients is to bypass the cochlea and the cochlear nerve and to deliver the electrical stimulation to the cochlear nucleus in the brainstem. This is the principle of the auditory brainstem implant (ABI).

The Nucleus 24 ABI is the only auditory brainstem implant currently available in the United States. This device received FDA approval for use in adults and children 12 years of age and older in 2001. The electrode array of the ABI is distributed on a small silastic pad that is placed over the lateral surface of the dorsal cochlear nucleus. Unfortunately, the speech recognition skills of patients with ABIs are poorer than those obtained by patients with cochlear implants. This is due to the difficulty of precise electrode placement and the inability to stabilize the device over the cochlear nucleus. During the surgical procedure, placement is determined by electrophysiologic measures indicating the presence of an auditory evoked response with activation of the ABI. Although the device is stabilized before closure, the implant can migrate from this optimal placement. Work is currently under way to create an electrode pad that partially penetrates the cochlear nucleus.

Another area of clinical research in prosthetic auditory rehabilitation involves bilateral cochlear implantation. Clinical trials are currently under way in children and adults to evaluate the effects of binaural implantation. Early results obtained in these trials indicate improved sound localization in space, and improvements in speech perception in noisy backgrounds when compared with a unilateral implant. Concerns have been raised regarding the feasibility, efficacy, and cost-effectiveness of this approach to rehabilitation.

Investigation also includes the development of totally implantable cochlear implants. All components of such a CI would be internal, including the microphone and the power source. Technology for an implanted microphone currently exists, with a device implanted underneath the skin of the external ear canal. This has the added advantage of utilizing the acoustics of the ear canal in the same way as with normal hearing. Such a device will also have cosmetic advantages. It is anticipated that such an implant will become available by 2008.

CI PROGRAMS: RESOURCES AND FINANCIAL ASPECTS

Hearing rehabilitation with a cochlear implant is a complex undertaking requiring specialized equipment and expertise. The cumulative nature of a cochlear implant program should be taken into account when considering space needs. Unlike other types of surgical rehabilitation of hearing loss, where only one or two follow-up visits may be needed, a CI patient remains dependent on the implant program for the rest of his life. Patients are often accompanied by more than one family member or friend, and the public area should accommodate this number of visitors. In addition, it is important to provide facilities that would allow the observation of treatment without interference. Ideally, a cochlear implant facility should be equipped with closed-circuit video systems to allow several people to observe a given treatment room. Such facilities are also valuable for training clinicians and to allow visiting teachers to observe the treatment.

Hearing rehabilitation with a cochlear implant requires several pieces of equipment, including standard audiologic test equipment and a soundproof booth for pre- and postoperative testing. If the program includes pediatric patients, it is necessary to have equipment available for electrophysiologic (ABR) testing and appropriate behavioral conditioning equipment, such as visual reinforcement audiometry tools and objects for conditioned play audiometry. The programming equipment for cochlear implants is specific for each device but primarily consists of an interface box that connects to a standard computer. Electrophysiologic equipment may be used in conjunction with programming equipment to help evaluate device integrity, define programming parameters, and trouble-shoot problems that arise.

CONCLUSION

The introduction of cochlear implants has greatly expanded the treatment options available for patients with a severe to profound hearing loss. Great improvements in CI technology have occurred over the past several years and will continue to occur in the near future. Therefore it is important for professionals to remain informed of changes in device candidacy as well as device options for their patients.

REFERENCES

1. Cochlear Corporation Nucleus 24 Package Insert, 2001; Australia.
2. Robbins AM, Renshaw JJ, Berry SW. Evaluating meaningful auditory integration in profoundly hearing-impaired children. Am J Otol 1991;12[Suppl]:144–150.
3. Zimmerman-Phillips S, Murad C. Programming features of the Clarion Multi-Strategy Cochlear Implant. Ann Otol Rhinol Laryngol 1999;108:17–21.
4. Kirk KI, Pisoni DB, Osberger MJ. Lexical effects on spoken word recognition by pediatric cochlear implant users. Ear Hearing 1995;16:470–481.
5. Waltzman SB, Cohen NL, Shapiro WH. Use of a multichannel cochlear implant in the congenitally deaf and prelingually deaf population. Laryngoscope 1992;102:395–399.
6. Skinner MW, Binzer SM, Fears BT, et al. Study of the performance of four prelinguistically or perilinguistically deaf patients with a multi-electrode intracochlear implant. Laryngoscope 1992;102:797–806.
7. Zwolan TA, Kileny PR, Telian SA. Self report of cochlear implant use and satisfaction by prelingually deafened adults. Ear Hearing 1996;17:198–210.
8. Zwolan TA. Factors affecting auditory performance with a cochlear implant by prelingually deafened adults. Presentation at the 100th NIH Consensus Development Conference: Cochlear Implants in Adults and Children, 1995. National Institutes of Health, Washington, DC.
9. Arndt PA, Staller SJ, Holden LK. Application of advanced speech encoding strategies in cochlear implant recipients, 1999. 11th Annual Meeting of the American Academy of Audiology, Miami.
10. Kileny PR, Zwolan TA, Ashbaugh CJ. The influence of age at implantation on performance with a cochlear implant in children. Otol Neurotol 2001;22:42–46.
11. Cheng AK, Grant GD, Niparko JK. Meta-analysis of pediatric cochlear implant literature. Ann Otolaryngol Rhinolaryngol 1999;108[Suppl]:124–128.
12. Zwolan TA, Ashbaugh CJ, Zimmerman-Phillips S, et al. Cochlear implantation of children with minimal open-set speech recognition skills. Ear Hearing 1997;18:240–251.

13. Tucci DD, Telian SA, Zimmerman-Phillips S, et al. Cochlear implantation in patients with cochlear malformations. *Arch Otolaryngol Head Neck Surg* 1995;121:833–838.

14. Balkany T, Gantz BJ, Steenerson RL, et al. Systematic approach to electrode insertion in the ossified cochlea. *Otolaryngol Head Neck Surg* 1996;114:4–11.

15. El-Kashlan H, Ashbaugh C, Zwolan TA, et al. Cochlear implantation in prelingually deaf children with ossified cochleae. *Otol Neurotol* 2003;24:596–600.

16. Eisenman D, Ashbaugh CA, Zwolan TA, et al. Implantation of the malformed cochlea: a matched pairs analysis. *Otol Neurotol* 2001;22:834–841.

17. Ash SD, Hodges AV, Butts SL, et al. Speech perception abilities in pediatric cochlear implant recipients receiving total communication, oral, and auditory verbal training. 1997; Vth International Cochlear Implant Conference, New York.

18. Miyamoto RT, Kirk KI, Svirsky MA, et al. Communication skills in pediatric cochlear implant recipients. *Acta Otolaryngol* 1999;119:219–224.

CHAPTER 88

Transplantation Medicine: A Rehabilitation Perspective

Ross D. Zafonte, Barbara Pippin, Michael Munin, and Noc Thai

INTRODUCTION

History

The modern field of transplantation traces its origins to a successful renal auto-transplant in a dog performed in 1902. The development of vascular anastomosis, which underlies organ transplantation, was developed by Alexis Carrel (1,2), who is known as the father of transplantation, although this was not his eventual career. For this development he was awarded the Nobel Prize. Medawar discovered that allograft rejection is an immunologic process. This classic series of studies foreshadowed the future by including descriptions of tolerance, a goal of transplantation (3–5). Progress in the field was fostered by the development of an understanding of the histocompatibility complex (MHC), which in humans is referred to as the HLA allele, and the recognition that the HLA is the immunologic target of rejection (6). Developments in the understanding of cellular immunity and pharmacologic manipulation have allowed for the growth of the clinical field of transplantation medicine. Transplantation medicine is essentially only 30 years old, with the first successful trial in kidney transplantation in the 1970s and liver transplantation in 1980 by Thomas Starzl (7,8). These developments where supported by the development of immunosuppression agents such as cyclosporine and FK-506 (7,9). In fact, small bowel transplantation has only been recently approved by the Food and Drug Administration (FDA) as an acceptable treatment for short-gut syndrome. Nonetheless, the field has advanced to such an extent that transplant surgery is almost considered routine.

The Transplantation Process

The reception of a transplant allograft in many ways represents a complete medical renaissance of an individual. The transplant patient is likely an extremely deconditioned, malnourished, cachectic individual with one, if not more, end-stage organ disease, whether it is cirrhosis, lung disease, or cardiac disease. Having withstood the often long and unavoidably bloody operation with its attendant risks (i.e., prolonged anesthesia, prolonged paralysis, single positioning), these patients are further deconditioned and commit themselves to a lifetime of immunosuppression, with its associated side effects (infection, rejection, steroids). Such patients often have associated

musculoskeletal and neuromotor impairments, making rehabilitation an important part of their care.

Despite these seemingly insurmountable obstacles, the transplant patient is often able to return to be a highly functional, productive member of society. Transplant patients are running marathons, having babies, and returning to work as a state governor.

ISSUES RELATED TO TRANSPLANTATION

Of importance to the rehabilitation specialist is a series of medical issues that influence the outcome of those with a transplant.

Immunosuppression

Immunosuppression is a double-edged sword. While rescuing the transplant patient from the wave of rejection, immunosuppressive drugs, in addition to exposing these patients to infection, have significant direct toxicities (Table 88-1). Most transplant centers rely on the three-drug cocktail: cyclosporine, azathioprine, and prednisone. At our center the Transplantation Institute has replaced cyclosporine with tacrolimus and has dropped the use of prednisone in most patients (1,2). Of interest, many patients at our institution require only monotherapy with tacrolimus, and theories regarding the taper of immunosuppressive medications are being espoused (10). Other medications, including rapamycin (11) and mycophenolate mofetil, may also be used in transplant patients undergoing rehabilitation. Whatever the "primary cocktail" combination, the crucial component to immunosuppression resides in the calcineurin inhibitors, cyclosporine or tacrolimus. Cyclosporine and tacrolimus work by inhibiting calcineurin, a phosphatase that acts on nuclear regulatory factor, the end effect of which is the inhibition of interleukin-2 (IL-2), a cytokine critical in T-cell activation and thus rejection (11).

Cyclosporine

Cyclosporine in combination with prednisone and azathioprine in the early 1980s allowed for the high rate of graft acceptance seen today, and thus is the mainstay of immunosuppression in many transplant centers. Cyclosporine is a unique agent

TABLE 88-1. Major Immunosuppressive Agents

Immunosuppressive	Mechanism	Role	Side Effects
Cyclosporine	Inhibits IL-2	Primary	Neurotoxicity Nephrotoxicity Electrolyte imbalance
Tacrolimus	Inhibits IL-2	Primary	Neurotoxicity Nephrotoxicity Electrolyte imbalance
Sirolimus	Inhibits IL-2	Primary/adjunct	Neutropenia Hyperlipidemia Concerns regarding bronchial anastomosis
Steroids	Cytokine inhibitor	Adjunct	Muscle wasting Poor wound healing Osteoporosis
Azathioprine	Purine synthesis inhibitor	Adjunct	Pancytopenia GI distress
Mycophenolic acid	Purine synthesis inhibitor	Adjunct	Pancytopenia GI distress

that on introduction nearly doubled the 1-year graft survival among those receiving kidney transplantation (12). Working via the inhibition of calcineurin, cyclosporine acts to freeze antigen-activated lymphocytes at an early phase and potentially allows for a deescalation of the cycle of response (11,12). Both the drug and its metabolites are eliminated via the liver as a primary step and the kidney as a secondary clearance step (13).

CONCERNS

Several medications interact with cyclosporine, especially those that act at the cytochrome P450 system. Anticonvulsant therapy leads to decreased levels, and several antibiotics and ketoconazole markedly increase levels of cyclosporine. Of importance is the fact that St. John's wort interacts with cyclosporine to cause a decrease in cyclosporine blood levels. In several cases, this has led to transplant rejection.

The main concern with cyclosporine is nephrotoxicity, occurring in 18% of patients (14,15). Cyclosporine appears to inhibit renal function via multiple mechanisms, including vasoconstriction via endothelins and thromboxane stimulation, direct toxicity of vascular endothelium, causing acute microvascular disease and inducing a chronic interstitial fibrosis (15,16). The two former mechanisms may be reversible with reduction or cessation of cyclosporine, whereas the latter may progress to renal failure or, fortunately in many cases, may stabilize. Loss of renal function remains significant, with 9.5% requiring dialysis at 13 years after a liver transplant (15,16). There is great variation in patient susceptibility to cyclosporine-induced nephrotoxicity, although those with underlying renal impairment appear predisposed to renal failure from cyclosporine. Urine output and creatinine remain the first line of nephrotoxicity detection. Elevation of creatinine should prompt a nephrology or transplantation consultation with possible plans to lower cyclosporine if rejection is not a problem.

Neurotoxicity remains the other major side effect of cyclosporine, ranging from peripheral neuropathy, tremors, and dysesthesias, which are very common, to seizures and severe encephalopathy (17–20). The fine motor tremor associated with cyclosporine therapy can often be accommodated via adjustment of medication and accommodation of the patient. Headaches secondary to cyclosporine therapy have been reported, and a demyelinating neuropathy can be produced by the medication (21).

Hypertension is associated with the use of cyclosporine therapy. It appears to be driven by sodium and water retention and as well as by increased intracellular calcium (22,23). Other complications include electrolyte abnormalities with mild hyperkalemia, which sometimes requires treatment (24,25). Lipid profile dysfunction is also noted with cyclosporine therapy. Hypomagnesemia is common and may need oral replacement, as it predisposes the transplant patient to seizures. Hypertrichosis and gingival hyperplasia are not severe but can be cosmetically troublesome (26).

Tacrolimus

Tacrolimus (FK 506) was introduced in the 1990s and is considered more potent than cyclosporine. This agent has been reported to be as much as 100 times more potent than cyclosporine (27). Tacrolimus is a metabolite of the fungus Streptomyces tsukubaensis. It is a macrolide, highly plasma bound and processed in a variable fashion via the liver in the cytochrome P450 system (28,29). Tacrolimus immunosuppressive action is similar to that of cyclosporine, working via the calcineurin system. Tacrolimus has allowed for steroid-free therapy and has permitted small bowel transplantation to be more acceptable (30). Several large trials have examined the efficacy of tacrolimus in preventing rejection after liver transplantation (31). The incidence of acute rejection and chronic rejection appeared to be lowered by the use of tacrolimus. There also appeared to be more retransplantations required in the nontacrolimus-treated group (32,33). A study by Jain and colleagues of more than 1,000 liver transplant patients concluded that chronic rejection occurred rarely among patients maintained long term on tacrolimus-based immunosuppressive therapy (33). The Multicenter Tacrolimus Rescue Trial has shown that among transplant patients receiving cyclosporine who are experiencing chronic rejection, many can be salvaged by transfer to tacrolimus (34). An additional potential benefit of tacrolimus is that it has been shown to demonstrate a reduction in serum cholesterol when compared with cyclosporine (35,36).

CONCERNS

Tacrolimus, being also a calcineurin inhibitor, has a toxic profile remarkably similar to that of cyclosporine, although neurotoxicity is more prevalent (37,38). Susceptibility to neurotoxicity may have a genetic relationship. In a study by Yamauchi the genotype of six patients who had experienced neurotoxicity after liver transplantation was examined (39). The authors found a relationship between neurotoxicity associated with polymorphism in the ABCB1 gene (39). The neurologic seque-lae are of concern, although debate exists as to how much this profile of side effects occurs among those taking tacrolimus when compared with the population utilizing cyclosporine for immunosuppression (37). Shimono utilized diffusion-weighted MRI imaging to evaluate those that developed neurotoxicity following organ transplantation (40). He noted that 35.7% had white matter abnormalities, 7.1% had putamenal hemorrhage, and 57.1% had normal findings on MRI (40). Bartynski evalu-ated 22 patients with neurotoxic reaction. He also noted the significance of white matter lesions in this population (41). Pa-tients often have tremors initially, although personal observa-tion suggests that there may be an acclimation to the drug. For persistent tremor that affects activities of daily living, low-dose clonazepam may be helpful.

Sirolimus

Sirolimus (Rapamune) is a newer immunosuppressive that in-hibits the cell cycle and the activation of IL-2 (42,43). This agent is produced by *Streptomyces hygroscopicus*. Sirolimus is still finding its place in immunosuppression as either a primary drug or an adjunct with tacrolimus or cyclosporine. Its mecha-nism of action is different from that of either cyclosporine or tacrolimus in that it does not inhibit calcineurin (44). Sirolimus appears to prevent the translation of mRNA influencing cell cycle regulation (45–47). Sirolimus, being nonnephrotoxic, is a viable alternative in patients who develop renal insufficiency caused by calcineurin inhibitors (42,48–50). In a retrospective review, patients who were more than 3 years post transplanta-tion were selected to evaluate the role of sirolimus. Patients who had proteinuria, those administered any other nephro-toxic agents, and those with a creatinine clearance of less than 20 mL/min were excluded. Renal insufficiency was defined as mild, moderate, or severe. In the 16 patients these authors stud-ied there was significant improvement in serum blood urea nitrogen and serum creatinine levels 6 months after switching to sirolimus therapy. No patient developed cellular rejection or other graft-related complications (51). Among liver trans-plant recipients with chronic renal insufficiency, conversion to sirolimus-based immunosuppression may allow complete with-drawal of other agents, leading to some improvement in renal function. Another recent study evaluated the safety and effi-cacy of sirolimus plus steroids as a maintenance regimen with or without small-dose cyclosporine adjunctive therapy in renal transplantation (52). A total of 133 recipients of kidney allograft transplantations recruited in the United Kingdom and Ireland were enrolled into the study. Patient and graft survival were 97.7% and 95.5%, respectively, whereas the biopsy-proven acute rejection rate in the first 6 months was 19.5%. Incidents of acute rejection rates comprised 22 episodes (16.5%) during the first 3 months of the study and four episodes (3%) after ran-domization. These data demonstrate that withdrawal of cy-closporine from a small-dose sirolimus maintenance regimen is safe and is associated with an improvement in renal function (52). The study also suggests that the addition of small-dose-cyclosporine to a sirolimus maintenance regimen does not in-crease immunosuppressive efficacy.

CONCERNS
Sirolimus causes neutropenia and hyperlipidemia and may predispose patients to more infection. Its antiproliferative

properties can also delay healing (53). It is also noted to cause thrombocytopenia and has been suggested to have a pro-thrombotic activity. Sirolimus increases the levels of cyclo-sporine when used in combination. Even though sirolimus is not primarily nephrotoxic, dual treatment groups have noted an increased incidence of nephrotoxicity (54). Combination sirolimus–tacrolimus may cause nephrotoxicity in some pa-tients by mechanisms that are presently unexplained. Siroli-mus appears to prolong delayed graft function (DGF). It may not be the optimal immunosuppressive choice in the DGF set-ting (55). A recent report of delayed wound healing in a person treated with sirolimus who received a liver transplant has been noted, and late wound dehiscence can occur (56).

Corticosteroids

Corticosteroids have been used in transplantation medicine since the early days of solid-organ transplantation. These agents affect the functional capacity and the concentration of active leukocytes (57). This tends to occur via the regulation of cytokine gene transcription. These agents have value as adju-vant therapy, at times of stress, and in the treatment of mild to moderate acute rejection. Several attempts have been made at discontinuing steroid therapy. The most successful of these programs have been in tacrolimus-based paradigms (58,59).

Corticosteroids have long been a cornerstone of orthotopic liver transplant immunosuppression. Newer, more potent agents have successfully allowed for more rapid tapering and discontinuation of corticosteroids in liver transplant recipients. Washburn hypothesized that corticosteroids can be safely avoided after the first postoperative day using these newer agents (59). Thirty adult orthotopic liver transplant recipients were prospectively enrolled in a randomized open-label proto-col. The incidence of biopsy-proven acute rejection requiring steroid therapy was 6.7% in both the steroid and the "no steroid" groups. Serum cholesterol level was significantly lower in the "no steroid" group at 6 months after transplanta-tion. Serum triglycerides were also lower, but the difference was not significant. Boots et al. evaluated the role of steroids in renal transplantation; they compared tapering in 3 to 6 months, with stopping steroids 1 week after transplantation (60). The results of this trial were noted to be comparable in patient and graft survival with a similar incidence of acute rejections. The incidence of new-onset diabetes may be reduced among those receiving early taper from steroids sooner (60). The immuno-suppressive benefit of adding enteral prednisone to tacrolimus seems to be limited.

CONCERNS
The side effects of long-term steroid use are well described and are significant in transplant patients. These include poor wound healing, glucose intolerance, osteoporosis, anasarca, muscle wasting and myopathy, and emotional liability. Lipid abnormalities have also been described. Genotypic testing noted that the presence of an apolipoprotein E4 allele wors-ened HDL, triglycerides, and cholesterol (61). Thus apolipo-protein E4 has a larger impact than apolipoprotein E2 on fast-ing-lipid profile in transplant candidates. There have been occasional reports of acute respiratory and skeletal muscle weakness in intensive care unit patients treated with massive doses of corticosteroids for rejection prophylaxis or treatment. Compared with the pretreatment condition, approximately 45% of patients showed acute generalized muscle weakness that recovered after approximately 2 months (62). If given a "risk-free" choice, the majority of recipients prefer withdrawal of steroids (63).

Alternative Agents

Azathioprine and mycophenolic acid are adjunctive immuno-suppressive agents that inhibit purine synthesis, thereby generally inhibiting immune cells, particularly lymphocytes. These agents have been noted to block *de novo* purine synthesis by blocking key enzymes. This process is required by T- and B-lymphocytes for proliferation (64). The role of mycophenolic acid as adjunct therapy in preventing rejection has been established among those with renal and heart transplantation (65). Mycophenolate combined with cyclosporine and prednisone significantly lowers acute rejection frequency in the early post–renal transplantation phase (66). A comparative retrospective analysis of the 5-year results with mycophenolate was performed by Offerman (67). Both the total population and subgroups showed a nonsignificant trend toward better graft survival with mycophenolate, evident at 2 years and persisting for 5 years. Extrapolation indicates that on combination therapy with mycophenolate, approximately 10% more patients will be alive at 10 years with a functional graft. These agents are also employed in the treatment of acute rejection (67). Side effects include gastrointestinal distress, neutropenia, and pancytopenia. Thymoglobulin was noted to be effective as induction therapy in high-risk pancreas transplant recipients and resulted in initial reversal of rejection in 74% of patients. Dose adjustments were required in more than half the cases and were usually due to leukopenia. Infections occurring subsequent to thymoglobulin were not uncommon and reflected the immunosuppressive burden of the patient population (68).

Monoclonal Antibody Agents

A major thrust of transplantation research is to find more effective and less broadly toxic immunosuppressive agents. One potential way is the use of monoclonal antibodies directed to the IL-2 receptor. Several monoclonal antibodies have been introduced; these agents target the IL-2 receptor. Daclizumab and basiliximab focus on the α_2 chains of the IL-2 receptor (69,70). Pediatric patients appear to be among those that benefit the most from anti-IL-2 receptor therapy (71). Immunoprophylaxis with daclizumab has been shown to be effective in the prevention of acute rejection in kidney transplant patients. Niemeyer initiated a pilot study in 28 liver transplant patients in which daclizumab was administered intravenously. At 4 years following the transplant no lymphoproliferative disease was observed (72). Immunoprophylaxis with a two-dose daclizumab regimen appears safe, effective, and well tolerated, and does not lead to increased opportunistic infections. Such agents are utilized in combination with the agents previously described (72–75). A two-dose regimen appears to be as effective as the five-dose regimen in preventing acute rejection and is associated with the lowest acute rejection rates and the highest rate of event-free survival (no rejection or graft loss). However, the benefits of daclizumab compared with no antibody induction await larger sample size accrual (76).

Gene Therapy

One major complication facing organ transplant recipients is the requirement for life-long systemic immunosuppression to prevent rejection, which is associated with an increased incidence of malignancy and susceptibility to opportunistic infections. Presently, exciting investigations into the role of gene therapy for immunosuppression are under way. Gene therapy has the potential to eliminate problems associated with immunosuppression by allowing the production of immunomod-ulatory proteins in the donor grafts, resulting in local rather than systemic immunosuppression (77,78). Gene therapy may also make xenografts more practical. Alternatively, gene therapy approaches could eliminate the requirement for general immunosuppression by allowing the induction of donor-specific tolerance. Gene therapy interventions may also be able to prevent graft damage owing to nonimmune-mediated graft loss or injury and may prevent chronic rejection (77–79).

INFECTION

Immunosuppression places these patients at extreme risk for opportunistic infections, which has probably remained the significant cause of morbidity and mortality in the transplant recipient. Since the immunosuppressive regimen includes medications that suppress both T- and B-cell action, these patients are vulnerable to many types of infections: bacterial, viral, fungal, tuberculosis, and pneumocystis. Such infections are often not seen in immunocompetent individuals. Despite the fact that aggressive pretransplantation infectious evaluation is part of every protocol, infections are common. Moreover, immuno-suppressives, especially prednisone, may mask infectious etiologies, making the diagnosis of infection difficult in transplant patients (80). Fever and leukocytosis are still the most common signs of infection, although their absence does not rule it out. Systemic infections may present with a low-grade fever or no fever at all. It is not uncommon for a transplant patient to have two simultaneous opportunistic infections. Again because of the immunosuppression, once a patient begins to show signs of infection, the course to fulminant sepsis and possibly death can be brief and dramatic (81–83). Vigilance and a high index of suspicion are the rule in detecting infections in transplant patients. During the past decade ever-increasing numbers of patients have undergone renal, pancreatic, small bowel, hepatic, cardiac, or lung transplantation as therapy for various types of renal disease requiring dialytic therapy. Significant improvements in patient and allograft survival have been observed in all categories. Unfortunately, despite such improved results, the risks of infection related to immunosuppression continue to be substantial. Dunn performed a review of transplant-related nonsocial infections (84). These authors noted that suppression of host defenses by exogenous immunosuppressive agents renders patients susceptible to invasion by either resident or environmental bacterial, fungal, viral, and protozoal microbes or parasites (84). In such patients, invasion of organisms that produce mild infection in nonimmuno-suppressed individuals can produce severe, lethal disease. Thus in an ideal world, immunosuppression could be decreased or eliminated in such patients.

Posttransplantation infections can be divided into three main etiologic categories based on time after surgery: During the first 3 or 4 weeks after transplant, infections are related to technical and mechanical problems (i.e., line infections, abscess, cholangitis from biliary stenosis, bowel obstruction, wound infections). In a second phase, the first to sixth months following transplant, cytomegalovirus (CMV) accounts for two-thirds of infections. Beyond 6 months, infections are similar to that seen in the general population (85,86). The typical transplant patient receiving acute inpatient rehabilitation is in the first category, although now, with long-term transplant survivors, physiatrists are also treating posttransplant patients with other medical problems, such as hip replacement in a patient with an allograft.

Along with factors related to immunosuppression, those receiving transplant may have prolonged hospitalization and thus secondary infection. Common pathogens include *Aspergillus, Staphylococcus, Clostridium difficile, Pseudomonas aeruginosa*, and *Legionella*. Viral infections are also quite possible and include CMV, Epstein-Barr virus, herpes simplex, varicella zoster, and hepatitis B and C (87).

Pulmonary infections are the most common cause of morbidity in the lung transplant population. Prompt recognition and treatment are necessary to prevent poor outcomes. An understanding of the temporal relationship between immunosuppression and the risk for developing infection can assist the clinician with appropriate treatment. Bacterial pneumonia is common within the first 4 months of transplantation, whereas CMV infection or disease becomes prevalent after the discontinuation of prophylaxis in at-risk patients (88,89). Fungal infections, especially aspergillosis, can be fatal if not treated early, and the risk for infection is present throughout the transplant period. Community-acquired viral infections present with upper-respiratory symptoms and wheezing that may lead to a chronic decline in lung function. Suspicion of a pulmonary infection in these immunosuppressed individuals should lead to an urgent diagnostic bronchoscopy and empiric antimicrobial therapy (87).

Cytomegalovirus is the most common infection in transplant patients and deserves significant attention. CMV is usually found latent in either recipient or donor and becomes active in the milieu of immune inhibition found in transplant patients (88,89). The most virulent CMV infection is seen when a CMV naïve recipient succumbs to CMV carried from the donor in the allograft. CMV can be widely disseminated, and infection can occur anywhere in the body. Fever, leukopenia, and generalized malaise are the most common symptoms, although pneumonitis, hepatitis, cholecystitis, and colitis with occasional gastrointestinal bleeding are not uncommon (89). Posttransplant CMV infection has been associated with posttransplant arteriopathy and can signify invasive infection (90). In many transplant centers, a fever work-up includes CMV culture and antigen detection. In our center all transplant patients receive prophylaxis with acyclovir (200 mg PO BID), and active treatment is initially with intravenous (IV) ganciclovir (5 mg/kg for 3 to 4 weeks, followed by maintenance dose orally for a specified period of time, usually months) (91). Treatment is continued until the patient has three consecutive CMV antigen-negative tests. CMV antigen detection is done weekly at our institution for all patients within the first month of their operation.

Fungal infections are also more common in the immunosuppressed (usually steroids are integral part of the regimen) transplant patients than the general population. The clinician has to be vigilant because fungal infections can be so devastating. Feltis has noted mycotic aneurysms after transplantation (92). Unfortunately, the diagnosis is usually made late—symptoms may be mild and nonspecific, even with dissemination. Mortality associated with disseminated fungal infections is high, whereas that associated with limited fungal infections is low (93). Although the risk factors for invasive fungal infections in liver transplant patients are well identified, early diagnosis is challenging, and commonly used diagnostic methods lack sensitivity and specificity (93). The incidence of fungal infections following liver transplantation appears to be falling. Mortality and morbidity associated with fungal infections suggest that future developments should focus on enhancing earlier diagnosis, implementing more effective and less toxic antifungal therapy recipients (94,95). Early fungal infections are related to surgical complications, whereas the period of 1 to 6 months reflects opportunistic, relapsed, or residual infections. Fungal infections of greater than 6 months and thereafter are usually associated with treatments for chronic rejection or bronchial airway mechanical abnormalities (96). Most fungal infections in lung transplant recipients involve *Aspergillus* species, followed by species of *Candida, Pneumocystis*, and *Cryptococcus*; geographically restricted agents; and newly emerging fungal pathogens. Virulent infections such as caused by *Aspergillus* or mucor mycosis are usually fatal. *Aspergillus* can be widely disseminated and may not grow in culture despite systemic infection (97).

Of note, those persons receiving lung transplant for cystic fibrosis appear to be at particular risk of infections caused by *Aspergillus* (97). The isolation of *Aspergillus fumigatus* from respiratory tract specimens in heart transplant recipients appears to be highly predictive of invasive aspergillosis (98). The presence of *Aspergillus* "fungus balls" lesions in the brain usually means death, and lung involvement requires resection for any chance of survival. Mucormycosis spreads by the nasal sinuses into the brain, where infection portends death. If the infection is caught early enough, cure requires aggressive debridement and resection of facial tissues.

REJECTION

Rejection involves a continuum of responses that are important to understand. Transplant rejection has been classified as hyperacute, acute, subacute, and chronic. Hyperacute rejection occurs when the recipient has antibodies to antigens present on the transplanted organs. This elicits an aggressive immune response, resulting in organ failure. This response type has generally been limited by extensive routine cross matching. Acute rejection is a relatively intense inflammatory response to the new organ. The inflammation that occurs has been described as similar to that seen in hypersensitivity types of reactions (99). The result of this reaction is the deposition of a large number of inflammatory cells within the graft. The clinical syndrome manifests itself as rubor edema fever and pain. Transplanted organ functional laboratories may also become acutely impaired. Despite potent immunosuppression, more chronic forms of rejection are still common, usually within the first 3 months of transplantation. Symptoms such as fever and leukocytosis are sometimes present, although rejection often occurs in the absence of these symptoms. Usually, subacute and chronic rejection are heralded by a rise in allograft laboratory value, such as increased creatinine in those with renal transplantation, increase in bilirubin or liver function enzymes in those with liver transplantation, and elevation in amylase and lipase among those with pancreas transplants. Tissue biopsy, usually obtained percutaneously, with histologic examination remains the gold standard for the diagnosis of rejection. The incidence of chronic rejection varies by type of solid-organ transplantation. The incidence of chronic rejection has been reported to be as high as 50% in the lung transplantation population and as low as 5% among those receiving liver transplantation (100,101).

Chronic allograft nephropathy is the most common cause of renal transplant loss. It is characterized by loss of function and replacement of tissue by fibrotic material (100). The pathogenesis is not clear but seems to be multifactorial and involves events both early and late after transplantation.

Once the diagnosis of acute rejection is confirmed, treatment is initially with high-dose steroids and a steroid taper will resolve 80% to 85% of allograft rejection. Steroid-resistant rejection can be treated with antibodies, OKT3, thymoglobulin; this will resolve 95% of all rejections. Resolution is characterized by the normalizing of laboratory value, so that follow-up biopsy is

TABLE 88-2.   Rejection Symptoms

Type	Symptom	Treatment
Hyperacute	• Occurs in OR during initial transplantation surgery. • Secondary to preformed antibodies. • Graft is lost.	• Graft replacement/retransplantation
Acute Chronic	• T-cell-mediated antigraft inflammatory infiltrate • May see increase. • ↑LFT in liver. • ↑Glucose in pancreas. • ↑BUN with creatinine in kidney. • ↑Heart/lung biopsy may reveal ↑ inflammation. • There may be ↑ need for oxygen. • ↑Shortness of breath. • ↑Edema.	• Solumedrol; if steroid resistant thymoglobulin or OKT3 • Organ replacement is treatment of choice. • Possibly ↑ FK506 or give steroid bolus.

usually not necessary. Solumedrol administration and a steroid taper can be given in the rehabilitation unit without affecting the patient's level of activity. Antibody treatment will require closer monitoring and is best done upon transfer to a specialized transplant service.

A new and exciting concept is that of tolerogenic immunosuppression. Under this concept individuals develop a partial tolerance to the transplanted organ and thus require less immunosuppression without associated rejection. This concept focuses on the principle of recipient pretreatment and minimum use of posttransplant immunosuppression. Starzl and colleagues evaluated 82 patients awaiting various solid-organ transplants (102). Posttransplant patients were maintained on sirolimus and subsequently tapered dose after 4 months of therapy. Immunosuppression-related morbidity was virtually eliminated and transplant graft survival at 1 year was 89% (Table 88-2).

MALIGNANCY

Immunosuppressive therapy for organ transplant recipients is complicated by high rates of malignant diseases, one of these being Kaposi's sarcoma (KS) (103). A review of 1,075 patients who underwent kidney transplantation between 1985 and 2002 noted that a total of 52 malignant diseases was observed in 50 patients (4.7%) during the posttransplantation period (104). Kaposi's sarcoma was identified in 16 of these 50 individuals. One recipient had concomitant lymphoma and KS. The lesions of seven patients were limited to the skin, five patients had lesions that involved the skin and gastrointestinal tract, and four patients had disseminated disease (104). The combination of immunosuppressive drug withdrawal and chemotherapy appears to be very effective in patients with limited disease, but the results in cases of generalized disease have been poor (105).

Posttransplant lymphoproliferative disease (PTLD) is a lymphoid neoplasm that has been associated with immunosuppressive therapy (106). The exact mechanism of this malignancy in the posttransplant population is not well understood. However, as predicted and subsequently verified in 1968, an increased incidence of certain de novo malignancies has been observed, particularly about lymphoid neoplasms (107). Jain et al. performed a retrospective review of 4,000 consecutive patients who underwent liver transplantation (108). The 1-year patient survival for liver transplant patients with PTLD was 85%. The actuarial 20-year survival was estimated at 45%. The overall median time to PTLD presentation was 10 months, and children had an incidence of PTLD that was threefold higher

than that of adults (108). Patient survival was better in children, in patients transplanted in the era of tacrolimus immunosuppression, in patients with polymorphic PTLD, and in those with limited disease.

The overall incidence of PTLD in pediatric liver transplant recipients has been reported to be 4% to 11%. The long-term risk of PTLD associated with primary tacrolimus therapy was determined by Cacciarelli (109). These authors evaluated 131 pediatric recipients who underwent liver transplantation and received primary tacrolimus therapy. Pretransplant Epstein-Barr virus (EBV) serologies were negative in 82% and positive in 12% of the patients (109). The cumulative long-term risk of PTLD was found to increase over time. Mortality from PTLD was 12%. A suggestion of a causal relationship exists between PTLD and EBV status. EBV surveillance should occur early after transplantation (109).

Recurrent and de novo malignancies are the second leading causes of late death in liver transplant recipients, following age-related cardiovascular complications (106). The greatest incidence of de novo malignancies is seen in cancers associated with chronic viral infections, such as possible Epstein-Barr virus–associated posttransplant lymphoproliferative disease, and skin cancers, including squamous cell carcinoma and Kaposi's sarcoma (106).

SOLID-ORGAN TRANSPLANTATION

Liver Transplantation

The achievement of liver transplantation by Thomas E. Starzl is one of the remarkable technical surgical accomplishments and remains one of the most major operations in surgery. As such, it is metabolically demanding on the patient. When operating on patients with portal hypertension and all of its stigmata, including friable varices, hypocoagulability can be challenging. Because of the multiple vascular anastomoses (inferior vena cava (IVC), portal vein, hepatic artery), and the extensive dissection in the right upper quadrant, bleeding postoperatively can also be significant. Usually two to four Jackson-Pratt drains are placed to drain the suprahepatic space, where bleeding from the IVC anastomosis can occur; to drain the subhepatic space, where the infrahepatic IVC, portal, and hepatic artery anastomosis may bleed; and near the hilum, to detect bile leaks from the biliary anastomosis (110). These drains are usually removed by 1 week, although some may stay longer if they are draining copious amounts of ascites postoperatively. T-tube stenting across the biliary anastomosis is also commonly done, and these are removed months after liver transplantation but can be capped if the bilirubin has normalized to allow internal drainage of bile. Most patients in rehabilitation units will have T tubes but not drains.

Vital signs and laboratory values for CBC, LFTs, and immunosuppressive levels taken two or three times per week are sufficient for routine screening. Fever, leukocytosis, and sudden leukopenia should prompt a fever work-up, including CMV titer and culture (111). An elevated total bilirubin is the most sensitive indicator of rejection, although its increase in face of rising AST, ALT, and gGTP may signify rejection or infection (hepatitis), or vascular or biliary complications. Hepatic artery aneurysm and thrombosis are important complications after transplantation (112,113). Persistence of ascites or the sudden development of ascites in a recent liver transplant patient should prompt an examination of the vasculature of the liver allografts to rule out outflow obstruction or portal vein thrombosis (113). An abdominal ultrasound Doppler to assess the hepatic vessels is the first step toward diagnosis. A T-tube cholangiogram should be obtained, and if these studies are unrevealing, a biopsy to rule out rejection should be performed (114,115). These studies are usually completed, with the results returned to the transplant team's primary care. It is obvious that a close coordination between the physiatrist and transplant surgeon is critical to the optimal care of the patient.

Renal Transplant

The kidney allograft is placed in the iliac fossa in the retroperitoneal position. The renal artery and vein are anastomosed to the iliac artery and vein, respectively, and the ureter is implanted onto the bladder medially. Lasting only 2 to 4 hours, renal transplantation is not associated with much blood loss. Drains are not usually placed, and in rare situations in which the renal bed is drained, they are removed within 3 to 5 days. Foley catheters are kept in for 5 to 7 days to decompress the bladder and protect the ureteral anastomosis.

Graft function is assessed by urine output and creatinine levels. Urine output of less than 50 mL/hour should prompt an investigation into the cause, keeping in mind that the usual cause is hypovolemia. A fluid challenge should be the first step. The goal for urine output in a renal transplant is approximately 2 L/day. A rise in creatinine signifies renal derangement that could be hydronephrosis, urinary tract infection, rejection, or immunosuppressive toxicity. Doppler ultrasound is the first test to obtain to rule out anatomic abnormality such as hydronephrosis from stricture of the ureterovesicular anastomosis. It can also rule out a perinephric collection that is compressing the allograft and preventing perfusion (116,117). Finally, the ultrasound can examine the vessels to assess patency and flow and to rule out thrombosis or stenosis (118,119). A simple urinalysis and culture will answer the question of a urinary tract infection. A history of trough levels of immunosuppression may suggest drug toxicity, although tacrolimus or cyclosporin nephropathy can occur with normal levels. A renal biopsy will rule out rejection or drug toxicity (116). First-line therapy for rejection is steroids and antibodies (OKT3, thymoglobulin) if the creatinine does not fall to baseline.

Finally, most renal transplant patients are diabetics and/or have hypertension and are vulnerable to cardiac disease (120). Almost all renal patients undergo a cardiac work-up, including a dobutamine echo, but this work-up is not foolproof. Incidences of myocardial ischemia occur with intraoperative graft reperfusion when blood pressure drops, and at postoperative days 3 to 4 when the patient is mobilizing fluid from the interstitial back to the intravascular space (121). These problems are managed by standard medical guidelines.

Pancreas Transplant

Pancreas transplantation is usually offered to type I diabetics with severe diabetic organ damage. End-stage renal failure, severe gastroparesis, neuropathy, retinopathy, and especially hypoglycemic unawareness are indications for pancreas transplantation. Patients are offered simultaneous kidney pancreas transplant, pancreas transplant after having a kidney allograft, or pancreas transplant alone (122). The pancreas allograft is typically placed in the iliac fossa, more commonly on the right because of anatomic advantage, and the exocrine drainage can be to the small bowel or to the bladder. There is a general trend to use enteric drainage due to the complications of bladder drainage, such as pain, urinary tract infection, and bicarbonate loss (123).

There are very strict criteria for the selection of donor pancreas organ and recipient simply because the pancreas is a fragile organ prone to many potential morbidities. For instance, donor or recipient with an age above 45 is associated with increased morbidity and mortality (123). Isolated pancreas graft survival, which has the worst outcome of the three options, is only 75% at 1 year and 66% at 5 years, although there has been steady improvement in the last 10 years. Overall morbidity (fistulas, leaks, bleeds, pancreatitis, infection, necrosis, abscess) can be up to 80% (122,124,125). Unlike the situation with kidney or liver transplantation, only a small number of transplant programs in the United States perform more than 30 pancreas transplants per year.

The postoperative management of a pancreas transplant patient can be very challenging for the surgeon and physiatrist alike. The usual course for the pancreas recipient can be "stormy" in the first month, during which time daily or every-other-day labs, including electrolytes, CBC, amylase, and lipase, should be drawn. Fasting blood glucoses should be obtained four times per day, and c-peptide levels should be measured weekly to access pancreas function. These patients can take a regular diet, and fasting glucoses should be less than 150, and preferably less than 100. Recent surgery as well as the heterotopic placement of a pancreas allograft makes these patients prone to ileus, or diarrhea, making nutrition potentially problematic in the early postoperative course.

Venous thrombosis, which occurs in 10% to 15% of all pancreas transplants, usually occurs during the first 2 weeks after the operation but can occur anytime (124). A sudden and persistent rise in the blood glucose (>200) should prompt an immediate pancreas ultrasound and nuclear flow scan to rule out thrombosis, and immediate notification of the transplant service, as this situation can be dangerous.

Enteric leak at the anastomosis can also occur in 10% of all pancreatic transplants and can be fatal. Leaks usually occur within the first month after transplant. Fever, abdominal pain, signs of sepsis, and leukocytosis are the usual manifestations of this problem. A CT scan without IV contrast is usually obtained to rule out leakage, and if positive the transplant service should be notified immediately, because this is a surgical emergency. The presence of steroids and immunosuppression, which can mask peritonitis, makes this diagnosis difficult.

Pancreatitis and its complications, such as fistulas, pseudocyst, and necrosis, can and do often occur, and at anytime after transplantation (125). All these conditions can increase the amylase and lipase levels, which are also indicators of rejection. Again ultrasound is the first test obtained to rule collections and to examine vascular flow in the pancreas. Once a collection is ruled out, a pancreas biopsy should be performed, if technically possible, to delineate pancreatitis from graft rejection. Mild pancreatitis can be observed or treated with Sandostatin. More severe pancreatitis, in which there is tenderness over the graft, is best treated by making the patient NPO (nothing by mouth), and administering total parenteral nutrition (TPN) and Sandostatin.

Percutaneous biopsy is the only way to diagnose conclusively pancreas rejection, but this can be technically difficult to perform (126–128). Those patients with simultaneous pancreas and kidney from the same donor have the advantage of the kidney as a sentinel organ for rejection. Kidneys are less technically demanding to biopsy, and the creatinine level serves as another marker of rejection. An increase in amylase and lipase is the best marker of allograft rejection, although the differential diagnosis is not small. Moreover, in a small number of cases, there is pancreas rejection without an increase in lipase (129). The pancreas is not as resilient as other types of allograft, so rejection should be treated aggressively. Mild rejection is usually treated with steroid therapy. Antibody treatment is used for steroid-resistant rejection or for moderate to severe pancreas rejection, depending on the judgment of the surgeon.

Small Bowel Transplant

Small bowel transplantation is reserved for patients with irreversible intestinal failure who no longer can be maintained on TPN. Small bowel transplant can be offered alone, in combination with liver allograft, or as part of a multivisceral transplant, which includes liver, pancreas, stomach, and small bowel. Short gut syndrome (midgut volvulus, necrotizing enterocolitis), intestinal dysmotility, or enterocyte failure (radiation enteritis, autoimmune enteropathy) are some indications for small bowel transplants (130). Chronic TPN can cause liver disease for cholestasis, adding the need for a liver transplant with the small bowel. Finally, extensive thrombosis of visceral vessels may necessitate a multivisceral transplantation.

The small bowel transplant patient is usually malnourished, cachectic, and deconditioned. The rehabilitation team can expect intestinal transplant patients to have an ostomy stoma, gastrostomy tube, and jejunostomy tube. The gastrostomy tube is usually clamped unless the patient experiences vomiting or bloating, at which time the gastrostomy tube can be unclamped for decompression. During the postoperative period enteral nutrition is required and oral intake is often ad lib. Occasionally, intestinal absorption remains suboptimal and TPN is still required. Patients require frequent biopsies via colonoscopy as well as careful clinical and tissue observation for rejection (131). Persistent diarrhea because of dumping syndrome is extremely common and can be controlled with Immodium and tincture of opium. Nutrition consultation is usually necessary and helpful. The psychiatric manifestation, narcotic dependency from chronic abdominal pain and TPN can hamper optimal rehabilitation (132). For this reason intestinal transplant patients especially require neuropsychological evaluation and counseling. An appropriate goal during the rehabilitation phase is transition from intravenous pain medication to orally dosed medication as long as absorption is adequate.

Lung Transplantation

Hardy completed the first human lung transplant in 1963. During the next decade several attempts at human lung transplantation were completed; however, survival was short (133–135).

In the early 1980s several reports of long-term successful lung transplantation surfaced. The first was a series of combined heart–lung transplants. These had the advantage of ensuring adequate bronchial perfusion. Evolution of technique has allowed for single and double lung transplantation while avoiding bronchial airway ischemia. The waiting list for lung transplantation in the United States now exceeds 3,000.

Those with pulmonary fibrosis, chronic obstructive pulmonary disease, pulmonary hypertension, and chronic bronchitis often present as candidates for transplantation while in there 60s and 70s. Many have comorbidities and should be carefully screened for malignancies. Among younger patients, those with cystic fibrosis may require transplantation (136). Such patients may have comorbidities associated with brittle diabetes or hepatobiliary dysfunction. Although not absolute, general contraindications to lung transplantation are considered to be hepatic disease, severe renal dysfunction, and coronary or left ventricular heart disease not treatable with surgery or concomitant heart–lung transplant. Also of concern are those individuals with a history of malignancy. Those patients with tumors that have a propensity for late recurrence should have a longer disease-free period before lung transplantation is considered. Several premorbid conditions have been noted to impact outcome among those receiving lung transplantation (135). Of interest to the rehabilitation community is the notion that premorbid functional status has been shown to be a strong predictor of survival among those receiving lung transplantation. Among those who require pretransplant invasive ventilation, 1-year posttransplant survival is less than 50% (137). Both morbid obesity and poor nutrition may result in increased morbidity and mortality. Patients with severe osteopenia and osteoporosis may experience impaired quality of life. Almost one-half the patients with cystic fibrosis and obstructive lung disease presenting for transplantation have metabolic bone dysfunction (136). The role of living donor transplantation has continued to grow. When selecting donor sites among living donors the lower lobe is often chosen because of anatomic considerations and functional capacity.

In the immediate postoperative period attempts are made to limit peak ventilatory pressures to 35 mm hg or less. Attempts are made to wean the patient quickly from high FiO_2 in order to reduce oxygen toxicity. Complications with the bronchial anastomosis can occur, and tracheal dehiscence or airway necrosis will result in extensive pulmonary compromise (138,139). Recent reports regarding the role of sirolimus in bronchial anastomotic complications have raised further concerns. Progressive strictures or bronchomalacia can be common and are often recognized by direct visualization of a greater than 50% obstruction of the airway. Posttransplant bronchoscopy will focus on the evaluation of anastomotic areas and is often helpful in evaluating for secondary infection (138–141). Ischemia and/or reperfusion injury complicates some 15% of lung transplantations and is usually manifested early on (142,143). This syndrome appears to manifest itself in a way similar to that of adult respiratory distress syndrome.

During the typical rehabilitation phase pulmonary artery thrombosis and deep venous thrombosis have occurred in as many as 12% of lung transplant recipients (144). Chest CT imaging may also provide a useful diagnostic adjunct (145). The possibility of neoplasm should be considered in the differential of slowly growing infiltrates in this population. Chronic rejection can be manifested by obliterative bronchiolitis (146, 147). Those with obliterative bronchiolitis demonstrate significant decrements in Fev_1, and management is focused on progressive immunosuppressive therapies (147). Postoperative delirium has commonly occurred in lung transplant recipients and appears to be associated with prolonged cardiopulmonary bypass, the administration of cyclosporine, and other nonspecific factors.

Primary bilateral lung transplantation or combined lung and heart transplantation interrupts the vagus nerve and thus the normal stretch receptor input. Despite this interruption, breathing at rest should retain the classical pattern similar to that of normal subjects. Perhaps more important is the fact that cough response to airway irritants is relatively impaired. Those receiving heart–lung or bilateral lung transplants achieve relatively normal total lung capacity, but this may be impaired secondary to sternotomy for the transplantation itself. Among those with single lung transplantation, final pulmonary function becomes rate limited by the function of the remaining diseased lung.

Fink has noticed that exercise capacity can increase up to 10 years after lung transplantation (148). Peripheral mechanisms have been suggested as a source of improvement in exercise capacity (149). Stable lung transplant patients often remain with exercise capacity deficits, and much of this is secondary to expiratory and lower limb muscle weakness. Wang has noticed that such persons have a lower proportion of type I fibers and that they have higher lactate and inosine monophosphate ratios indicating a greater dependence on anaerobic metabolism (150). Schwaiblmair evaluated 103 consecutive recipients of single-lung, bilateral-lung, and heart–lung transplants. Cardiopulmonary exercise testing noted severe exercise intolerance and markedly impaired output parameters (151). Work capacity, oxygen pulse, tidal volume, and peak minute ventilation did not differ in patients following single-, double-lung, or heart–lung transplantation (151). These authors noted that despite the persistent limitations in aerobic capacity and work rate seen in many of the recipients, cardiopulmonary performance is reasonably well restored shortly after lung and heart–lung transplantation, further suggesting a peripheral component to the exercise dysfunction (151).

Studies of lung transplant recipients have found low maximum oxygen consumptions because of an as yet unexplained mechanism (152). Six lung transplant recipients and six age- and sex-matched, healthy control subjects were studied to assess the possibility of a mitochondrial myopathy in lung transplant recipients (152). The transplant group had significantly lower percent-predicted maximum oxygen consumption than the control group. The authors felt that lung transplant recipients have an impaired maximal exercise capacity because of a disorder of peripheral oxygen utilization (152). A proposed etiology is that this peripheral weakness may be caused by a cyclosporine-induced mitochondrial myopathy (152). Cardiopulmonary exercise studies of lung transplant recipients have found low maximum oxygen consumptions because of an as yet unexplained mechanism. A study of lung transplant recipients noted a significantly lower percent predicted maximum oxygen consumption than the control group and earlier onset of the anaerobic threshold (153). Lung transplant recipients also appear to have an impaired maximal exercise capacity because of a disorder of peripheral oxygen utilization, perhaps related to a myopathic component (153). Hall has suggested that exercise capacity is limited due to disorders of potassium regulation that explain the peripheral muscle weakness (154). Ross has noted persistent ventilation perfusion (V/Q) mismatches among those with lung transplantation during active exercise (155). Evans has also noted a persistent decrease in VO_{2max} after lung transplantation that may be related to abnormalities of skeletal muscle oxidative capacity (156). Such deficits may be longstanding, and data have suggested that after 6 and 12 months, indices of skeletal and respiratory mus-

cle function and VO_{2max} improve further, but still remain lower than normal values (157). These authors concluded that in patients with heart–lung transplantation, skeletal and respiratory muscle function as well as exercise performance are reduced after surgery and that muscle function may improve with time but still appears impaired at 18 months.

Rehabilitation offers techniques for enhanced coughing and mucociliary clearance, and provides treatment of the musculoskeletal system via exercise that appears to enhance peripheral muscle capacity. Kesten even suggests a value in a preoperative rehabilitation program for those awaiting transplantation (158). Those providing exercise and inpatient rehabilitation to such person should be aware of the need for close oxygen monitoring and for frequent rest periods until capacity is increased. The rehabilitation environment should also have capacity to deal with pulmonary secretions, as this is a cause of secondary complications. Stiebellehner performed a study of a training program (AET) in comparison with normal daily activities to evaluate exercise capacity in lung transplant recipients (159). Nine lung transplant recipients were examined, and all underwent incremental bicycle ergometry. Identical exercise tests were performed after 11 weeks of normal daily activities and then after a 6-week AET. Normal daily activities had no effect on exercise performance (159). The AET induced a significant decrease in resting minute ventilation, and at an identical, submaximal level of exercise a significant decrease in minute ventilation was also noted. Thus in a carefully monitored setting an AET improves submaximal and peak exercise performance significantly.

Heart Transplantation

Cardiac transplantation is a therapy of choice for end-stage heart disease. Despite major advances with organ preservation and immunosuppression, the physiology of the cardiac allograft is not normal, and this decreases exercise tolerance and functional performance. The physiatrist should have a basic understanding of the major physiologic changes after heart transplantation, the beneficial effects of exercise, and indications for both immediate acute inpatient rehabilitation and long-term rehabilitation follow-up.

The most common indications for heart transplantation surgery are cardiomyopathy, end-stage coronary artery disease, and inability to be weaned from temporary cardiac-assist devices after myocardial infarction or nontransplant cardiac surgery (160). Recipient selection criteria are stringent, and approximately one-quarter of patients found suitable for transplants die of cardiac disease before a suitable donor organ becomes available. Left ventricular-assist devices and artificial hearts can be used as interim support. The heart is transplanted in an orthotopic position with aortic, pulmonary artery, and pulmonary vein. Venous return is provided by a single anastomosis joining the retained posterior wall of the recipient's right atrium to that of the donor organ. More recently, the bicaval anastomosis technique has been used in performing heart transplantation (161). This technique differs from the standard mid-atrial anastomosis by keeping both atria intact and performing anastomoses in both the cava and pulmonary veins. This technique apparently avoids desynchronized atrial contractions and may improve cardiac performance by contributing more blood flow to the ventricles.

Cardiac transplantation involves removing the diseased heart and leaving an atrial cuff, which results in the complete denervation of the donor heart with loss of both afferent and efferent nerve connections. Impairments in chronotropic responsiveness and ventricular function caused by surgical interruption of postganglionic sympathetic fibers at the time of transplantation have been regarded as the major reasons for diminished exercise performance (162). The donor heart rate will not respond to vagolytic muscle relaxants, anticholinergics, anticholinesterases, digoxin, nifedipine, or nitroprusside (161). Because of these mechanisms the resting heart rate of the denervated heart varies between 90 and 110 beats per minute because of the loss of vagal tone (161). Since the resting heart rate is usually elevated, the resting stroke volume is small. The denervated heart requires mechanisms other than neural to maintain normal function in activities of daily living.

The Frank-Starling mechanism remains a major factor to maintain exercise performance in the transplanted heart (161). With this mechanism, increase in venous return allows for an increased preload that subsequently increases left ventricular end diastolic volume to result in an increase in the stroke volume. Thus the assurance of adequate preload is especially important after heart transplantation.

While the effects of denervation after heart transplantation are well described, it has become increasingly clear that denervation is not a persistent phenomenon. In a recent study by Bengel and colleagues using positron emission tomography and a catecholamine analog technique, partial restoration of myocardial sympathetic innervation was measured and then correlated with improvements in the capacity for exercise (162). In 29 heart transplant recipients, increased sympathetic activity was significantly correlated with the change in global ejection fraction in response to stress. The improvements in chronotropic response to exercise resulted in significantly better exercise performance in those patients who had innervation compared with those who had persistent denervation without recovery of sympathetic tone (163). Of those who obtain this physiologic adaptation, patients who had undergone heart transplantation earlier seem to have had more sympathetic recovery. Others have noted similar findings, although the exact mechanism of recovery is not fully understood (163,164) (Table 88-3).

In the transplanted heart the initial response to exercise is an increased stroke volume secondary to the increased venous return, which is due to a combination of muscle and thoracic pumping and decreased peripheral vascular resistance (161). Through this mechanism stroke volume can be increased up to 20%, thus increasing cardiac output via a Frank-Starling mechanism. With vigorous exercise, further increases of cardiac output are mediated by chronotropic and inotropic responses to circulating catecholamines (161). This contrasts to the normal heart in which increased stroke volume and heart rate occur simultaneously rather than sequentially.

When prescribing an exercise program, it is important to understand that resting heart rate is increased yet there is a delay in heart rate elevation when beginning vigorous activity. There is also delayed return of resting heart rate after cessation of exercise, decreased resting left ventricular ejection fraction, reduced exercise cardiac output, reduced maximal power output, and reduced anaerobic threshold (161). From a practical perspective, heart transplant patients may require 6 to 10 minutes of steady work to increase heart rate compared with 2 to 3 minutes in subjects without a denervated heart. Isometric exercise in cardiac transplant patients does not increase cardiac output because of denervation (165). However, there is the expected increase in blood pressure due to an increase in α-adrenergic tone mediated by the central nervous system and not from increased circulating catecholamines.

Exercise training after heart transplantation increases the capacity of physical work without increasing the peak heart rate. This should theoretically permit individuals to do more work than before training at the same level of exertion. Yet patients undergoing heart transplantation have preoperative inactivity and postoperative deconditioning that affects exercise tolerance (166). One study estimates that the transplant patient has a 10% to 50% reduction in body mass due to prolonged preoperative physical inactivity combined with high corticosteroid administration (167). Consequently, maximal work output is reduced and maximal oxygen uptake is only two-thirds of the normal age-matched population.

Although physical exercise has become an important part of the standard therapy for patients who have had an acute myocardial infarction and cardiac surgery, the role after heart transplantation has only recently been defined. In a randomized controlled trial, patients were enrolled approximately 2 weeks after transplantation surgery to an intensive rehabilitation protocol or to a control group that only received written guidelines for exercise (166). The exercise program was multifaceted and included supervision by a physical therapist according to each patient's specific needs. Strengthening exercises consisted primarily of closed-chain resistive exercises such as bridging with lifting of the hips while keeping the knees in a flexed, supine position. Other activities included half-squats, toe raises, ab-

TABLE 88-3. Summary of Precautions and Exercise Function During Early and Later Exercise Training[a]

Routine Precautions During Initial Rehabilitation	Early Cardiovascular Changes	Later Cardiovascular Changes
Sternal incision protection	Elevated resting heart rate	Improvement of exercise parameters with training
Cardiovascular monitoring using pulse rate, BP, pulse oxymetry and Borg Rating of Perceived Exertion	Stroke volume increases before heart rate increases during exercise	Improvement in sympathetic tone to transplanted organ in some individuals
Ensure adequate preload	Delayed heart rate cool down after cessation of exercise	Improved left ventricular ejection fraction with training
Monitor for depression and other psychiatric symptoms, peripheral neuropathy, osteoporotic fractures	Decreased peak heart rate	Possible development of hypertension
Minimize exercise training during episodes of acute graft rejection	Decreased left ventricular ejection fraction	Possible development of coronary artery disease in transplanted heart

[a]See text for full details.

dominal flexion, and pelvic tilts. Flexibility exercises, which emphasize chest expansion and thoracic mobility, included thigh stretches, trunk twists, scapular squeezes, and shoulder rolls. Aerobic exercise consisted of walking on a motorized treadmill or paddling on a bicycle ergometer. The goal of this exercise training was at least 30 minutes of continuous exercise at moderate intensity. Patients visited a cardiac rehabilitation clinic one to three times per week, but the authors did note that some were unable to attend more than once a week because of transportation difficulty and graft rejection. Routine transvenous endomyocardial biopsy is used to diagnose rejection, because other signs and symptoms are often absent and rejection can be detected before graft function deteriorates. Patients who did have rejection were instructed not to exercise until follow-up endomyocardial biopsy showed resolution of rejection that usually required 2 weeks. Before discharge from the rehabilitation protocol, patients of both groups received written guidelines primarily focusing on active-assist range-of-motion exercises, flexibility, and lower-extremity strengthening. Patients who participated in the exercise-training program increased their capacity for physical work as compared with controlled patients who did not undergo exercise training. Niset and Kavanagh have also shown improvements in physiologic parameters with a prescribed exercise program (168,169). Proximal weakness measured by sitting to standing rates improved in both the experimental and control groups between the baseline evaluation and the 6-month follow-up; the improvement among the exercising patients was almost three times as large. Exercise training is well tolerated, and studies have not demonstrated higher incidents of rejection (165,170). The take-home message is that exercise training should be considered standard postoperative care for heart transplant recipients.

One study by Joshi and Kevorkian documented how inpatient rehabilitation can benefit cardiac transplant recipients (171). This study did include a selection bias to those with more severe complications. Hence it may not reflect the typical patient who receives a cardiac transplant. In this cohort, a number of secondary medical problems were noted during the inpatient rehabilitation protocol. Specifically, six out of 12 patients had hypertension, five of 12 had dysphagia, four of 12 had decubitus ulcers, three of 12 had peripheral neuropathy, three of 12 had elevated blood sugars, two of 12 had hemiparesis, and two of 12 had psychiatric disorders requiring antidepressant therapy. There was also one patient who sustained an osteoporotic vertebral compression fracture. Even with these deficits, significant gains in the Modified Barthel Index were documented (171).

The inpatient rehabilitation protocol should avoid strenuous upper-limb exercises and teach proper positioning of the upper limbs during transfers or bed maneuvers. Specifically, patients should be instructed to keep their hands forward on the anterior thigh rather than reaching in an abducted posture to stabilize the upper torso during sit-to-stand maneuvers. In addition, patients should routinely have blood pressure, pulse rate, and pulse oximetry monitored during therapy. The Borg rating of perceived exertion is also used to keep the self-report below a rating of 13 (somewhat hard) during exercise. Of the 12 patients in the Joshi and Kervorkian series, 10 were discharged to community, with the remaining two discharged back to acute care because of medical or surgical complications (171). Patients in this study were also discharged from acute inpatient rehabilitation to phase II and phase III cardiac rehabilitation programs that share similarities to outpatient cardiac rehabilitation programs prescribed for patients recovering from myocardial infarction and coronary artery bypass grafting.

Lastly, patients may be seen in acute rehabilitation who are longstanding cardiac transplant recipients admitted to the hospital for other diagnoses and then requiring rehabilitative services. It is important to remember that the development of coronary artery disease in the transplanted heart can be observed in 50% of recipients, and the presence of ischemic cardiac disease should be considered when prescribing a rehabilitation protocol (161). Heart transplantation is a life-saving technique for those with end-stage cardiac disease. Rehabilitation is extremely important and now is considered to be the standard of care postoperatively. It is important for the rehabilitation physician to understand the concept of the denervated heart but to realize that this state can improve over time via mechanisms that are not fully understood. Isometric and resistive exercise training is an important part of the rehabilitation protocol and has been shown to be safe in heart transplant recipients. Inpatient rehabilitation is useful for a subset of patients who are severely deconditioned or have other medical comorbid illnesses. Precautions should include routine measurement of cardiac parameters and avoidance of pressure at the sternal incision. Cardiac rehabilitation programs appear to be worthwhile not only in the acute phase but also in the more subacute phases of recovery to improve overall workload and quality of life in these individuals.

REHABILITATION ISSUES

Deconditioning

Patients on a transplant waiting list are severely deconditioned from their underlying disease and associated adverse physiologic effects of these diseases. For example, a typical patient with liver failure is a gaunt, cachectic, jaundiced, edematous, ascitic individual. Failure of this vital organ interferes with synthetic function (albumin, acute-phase reactants, clotting factors) as well as metabolism of amino acids, glucose, and fat, making this patient malnourished, coagulopathic, edematous, and immunosuppressed. The combination of protein wasting (usually from muscle) and increased weight from edema and ascites is damaging to patient conditioning. Compounding this state is the mechanical impingement to respiration from the massive ascites among those with hepatic dysfunction. Many of these patients also have pulmonary and renal manifestation of liver diseases (hepatorenal syndrome, hepatopulmonary syndrome) and often require prolonged intensive-care stay while waiting for donor organs, further exacerbating an already suboptimal condition.

Similar states of severe deconditioning are also seen in patients with other end organ failure. It is easy to imagine the result of short-gut syndrome (malnutrition), obliterative lung disease, and heart failure. Even among those with renal dysfunction, dialysis hinders full activity and is wrought with complications. These patients are anemic, have poor healing, and are hypertensive. In diabetics awaiting pancreas transplants, the insulin supplement does not replace all factors, however undefined, produced by this organ. Thus these patients are also malnourished and usually have associated morbidities, such as atherosclerotic disease and poor healing, both of which hinder postoperative recovery.

The very act of surgery itself places a physiologic demand on these patients. Transplantation surgeries are usually complex, time-consuming, and bloody. The long duration under anesthesia and the paralysis of the patient in a single position no doubt has physical implications with regard to postoperative deconditioning and rehabilitation (172). Similarly, cardiopulmonary bypass in lung and heart transplant creates additional stresses on a patient and can produce cognitive dysfunction. The inexorable catabolic state seen in all postoperative surgical patients further weakens an already malnourished and protein-depleted patient.

Neurocognitive Concerns

Transplant recipients have been noted to experience variety of neurocognitive dysfunctions. Ghaus et al. performed a study to evaluate such concerns among those with liver transplantation (173). They reviewed 41 consecutive patients who had 45 procedures for liver transplantation. Encephalopathy occurred after 28 procedures (62%) with immediate onset and no significant recovery before death or retransplantation in 11 (24%), slow recovery in eight (18%), and delayed onset (1 to 50 days, average 11) in six (13%) (173). Intermittent confusion and agitation with full recovery followed three, and focal and generalized seizures followed five (11%) procedures, with multifocal myoclonus in two and status epilepticus in one. Isolated focal seizures were noted and all patients with seizures had encephalopathy. Brain imaging showed atrophy in three instances, intracerebral hemorrhage in two, multiple infarctions in one, and intracerebral and subarachnoid hemorrhage with infarction in one. Neurologic complications after transplantation were associated with increased mortality (173). Postoperative hypomagnesemia was associated with the development of nervous system complications. In another study of 40 patients who received liver transplantation, Buis noted transient confusion among 48% of those receiving transplantation for alcoholic liver disease but transient confusion occurred among only 6% of those who required transplantation secondary to hepatitis C (174). Studies of diffusion-weighted imaging and recovery imaging (FLAIR) have noted hyperintense lesions on FLAIR imaging. Psychological consequences of transplantation are also an important consideration for the rehabilitation team. Patients often benefit from psychological evaluation while in rehabilitation. Rothenhausler performed a study of 75 subjects to explore the prevalence of psychiatric disorders among orthotopic liver transplantation recipients and to investigate how psychiatric morbidity was linked to health-related quality of life (HRQOL) (175). Psychiatric morbidity was assessed using the Structural Clinical Interview for the *DSM-III-R*. A probable psychiatric diagnosis according to the *Diagnostic and Statistical Manual,* version III, revised (*DSM-III-R*) was noted in 22.7% of the sample: 2.7% had full posttraumatic stress disorder (PTSD); 2.7%, major depressive disorder (MDD); and 16%, partial PTSD. Patients with PTSD symptoms demonstrated lower cognitive performance, higher severity of depressive symptoms, and more unfavorable perception of social support (175). Liver transplant–related PTSD symptomatology was associated with maximal decrements in HRQOL. The duration of intensive care treatment, the number of medical complications, and the occurrence of acute rejection were positively correlated with the risk of PTSD symptoms subsequent to liver transplantation (175). Neuropsychological performance is also an important consideration after transplantation. Temple and others examined the relationship between cardiac function and cognitive test performance among candidates for heart transplant. Increasing hemodynamic pressure variables, such as pulmonary artery systolic pressure, were associated with decreased cognitive performance on a measure of psychomotor speed and attention (176). In contrast, cardiac output and cardiac index appeared not to be significantly related to cognitive performance (176). Of note, these authors found that poor performance on cognitive tests among heart transplant candidates appears to be attentionally mediated (176). Activities of daily living are often affected by cognition disorders after transplantation. Putzke evaluated the ability of heart transplant patients to perform day-to-day tasks (medication management, dietary regulation) (177). They studied a series of 75 heart transplant candidates and 38 controls to examine the predictive validity of demographic, neuropsychologic, and cardiac function variables to a performance-based measure of instrumental activities of daily living capacity. The instrumental activities of daily living capacity were most consistently predicted by long-standing verbal ability and psychomotor speed and mental flexibility. In contrast, cardiac function measures (cardiac output, mean atrial pressure) were largely unrelated to the patient's activities of daily living performance (177).

Neuropathy and Myopathy

Severe acute polyneuropathy complicating transplantation is not uncommon. Rezaiguia-Delclaux reported three cases of severe acute motor deficit after orthotopic liver transplantation (178). In a context of graft dysfunction these patients developed acute quadriplegia concomitant with early allograft failure. In these three patients, electrophysiologic signs of sensorimotor axonal polyneuropathy were found.

El-Sabrout noted that peripheral neurologic complications occur frequently in solid-organ transplant recipients (179). Recent evidence supports the role of the immune system in initiating and perpetuating the ongoing neural damage in this entity. Infectious agents may initiate the immune attack, and these authors reported on a series of transplant patients with a Gullain-Barré–like syndrome associated with CMV (179). Cyclosporine has now also been associated with a generalized sensorimotor neuropathy (180). An important consideration has been the improvement in function that may occur after transplantation. Lee et al. studied nerve conduction velocity changes among patients with severe liver syndrome (181). Twenty-five patients admitted for a liver transplantation were involved in this study. All patients underwent nerve conduction study before liver transplantation and 6 months after liver transplantation. The sensory amplitudes and motor conduction velocities substantially improved after transplantation (181).

Immunosuppressive medications have also been associated with acute myopathy and exercise impairment (182). Critical illness myopathy has been associated with those receiving liver transplant, and acute myopathy following transplantation has been reported to produce a teraplegia-like picture (183). Campellone reviewed the problems associated with acute myopathy among transplant recipients (184). One hundred consecutive adult patients were prospectively assessed for muscle weakness after otrhotopic liver transplant, and electrodiagnostic studies and muscle biopsies were performed. Seven patients developed acute persistent weakness after orthotopic liver transplant. Electrodiagnostic studies were consistent with a necrotizing myopathy. Histopathologic evaluation in five revealed a necrotizing myopathy with loss of myosin-thick filaments (184). A higher initial index of illness severity, dialysis requirement, and higher doses of glucocorticoids were associated with development of myopathy. Patients with myopathy subsequently remained in the intensive care unit longer than unaffected patients. Stephenson and colleagues performed a study to determine the exercise impairment that occurs in liver transplant recipients. They noted that liver transplant recipients exhibit impaired peak exercise performance similar to that observed after other solid-organ transplants, probably as a re-

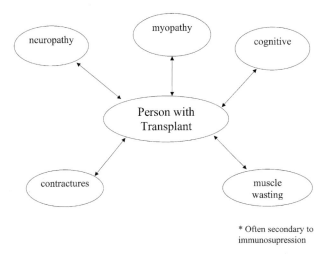

* Often secondary to
immunosupression

Figure 88-1. Rehabilitation issues of transplant recipients.

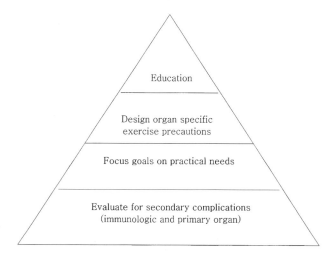

Figure 88-2. The pyramid of rehabilitation care for the person with transplant.

sult of chronic deconditioning or myopathy related to immunosuppressive medications (185) (Fig. 88-1).

QUALITY-OF-LIFE ISSUES

The initial focus in organ transplantation clinical research was demonstrating acceptable technical and survival outcomes. However, quality of life after transplantation has now become an important parameter. Bucuvalas performed a study of 77 pediatric liver transplant recipients 5 to 18 years of age, all of whom had had liver transplant at least 6 months previously (186). These authors evaluated quality-of-life issues. Health-related quality of life (HRQOL) in pediatric liver transplant recipients was lower than that reported for healthy children but similar to that for children with other chronic illness. Age at transplantation and maternal education predicted psychosocial function. HRQOL was decreased in a population of pediatric liver transplant recipients compared with the general population and similar to that for children with chronic illness. Forsberg et al. performed a study of the coping strategies of adult liver transplant recipients (187). The group showed a homogeneous pattern of change in coping strategies. This prospective study indicated that coping style changed primarily at an individual level during the first year after liver transplantation, whereas changes in coping strategies were not common for the group. The usual coping strategy during the first posttransplant year was confrontational coping. A German study evaluated the quality of life among those who had participated as liver donors 1 year after surgery (188). Donors viewed living related liver transplant positively. Quality of life after donation did not change. However, donors had a prolonged period of physical rehabilitation, and 41% experienced financial disadvantages (Fig. 88-2).

NOVEL CONCEPTS

Recent advances have allowed for the transplantation of neural and cartilaginous tissues with early success. Bentley has recently described a randomized study demonstrating the potential efficacy of chondrocyte implantation in the knee (189). Meniscal allograft transplantation appears efficacious among younger patients with focal knee dysfunction (190). These tissues are unique in that they appear to be privileged, and thus

do not require extensive immunosuppression. Kondziolka and Meltzer have described neuronal transplantation in humans for chronic motor dysfunction following stroke (191–193). These preliminary studies have noted clinical improvements in motor function and integration of the neuronal transplant when assessed via imaging techniques. Several authors have postulated on the role of neuronal transplantation in the treatment of spinal cord injury (194–196). The role of these implants may be via direct growth or perhaps via neurotrophic growth factors. The rehabilitation of those with neurologic and musculoskeletal disorders may be changed by these novel transplantation concepts in the near future.

CONCLUSION

Transplant medicine has made tremendous strides during the last 30 years. Those surviving transplantation are often left with neuromusculoskeletal disorders that require rehabilitation intervention. Many of the associated complications of transplantation are mediated via immunosuppressive therapy. Novel concepts such as tolerogenic therapy may help to moderate such effects. The rehabilitation specialist will continue to play a key role in helping to ameliorate the mobility and cognitive issues associated with solid-organ transplant.

REFERENCES

1. Carrel A. The transplantation of organs: a preliminary communication 1905. *Yale J Biol Med* 2001;74:239–241.
2. Carrel A, Guthrie CC. Anastomosis of blood vessels by the patching method and transplantation of the kidney 1906 [classical article]. *Yale J Biol Med* 2001;74:243–247.
3. Medawar P. The future of transplantation biology and medicine. *Transplant Proc* 1969;1:666–669.
4. Medawar PB. Tolerance reconsidered—a critical survey. *Transplant Proc* 1973;5:7–9.
5. Medawar P. Transplantation biology: an appraisal. *Mt Sinai J Med* 1974; 41:760–764.
6. Dausset J. The biological implications of the main histocompatibility system: the HL-A system. *C R Seances Soc Biol Fil* 1974;168:160–172.
7. Starzl TE, Weil R 3rd, Iwatsuki S, et al. The use of cyclosporine A and prednisone in cadaver kidney transplantation. *Surg Gynecol Obstet* 1980;151: 17–26.
8. Starzl TE, Iwatsuki S, Klintmalm G, et al. Liver transplantation, 1980, with particular reference to cyclosporine-A. *Transplant Proc* 1981;13(1 Pt 1):281–285.

9. Todo S, Fung JJ, Starzl TE, et al. Liver, kidney, and thoracic organ transplantation under FK 506. *Ann Surg* 1990;212:295–305.

10. Chakrabarti P, Wong HY, Toyofuku A, et al. Outcome after steroid withdrawal in adult renal transplant patients receiving tacrolimus-based immunosuppression. *Transplant Proc* 2001;33:1235–1236.

11. Shapiro R, Scantlebury VP, Jordan ML, et al. A pilot trial of tacrolimus, sirolimus, and steroids in renal transplant recipients. *Transplant Proc* 2002; 34:1651–1652.

12. Ho S, Clipstone N, Timmermann L, et al. The mechanism of action of cyclosporine A and FK 506. *Clin Immunol Immunopathol* 1996;80:S40–S45.

13. Gonwa TA, Mai ML, Melton LB, et al. End-stage renal disease (ESRD) after orthotopic liver transplantation using calcineurin-based immunotherapy: risk of development and treatment. *Transplantation* 2001;72:1934–1939.

14. Platz KP, Mueller AR, Blumhardt G, et al. Nephrotoxicity after orthotopic liver transplantation in cyclosporine A and FK 506-treated patients. *Transpl Int* 1994;7[Suppl 1]:S52–S57.

15. Prevot A, Semama DS, Tendron A, et al. Endothelin, angiotensin II and adenosine in acute cyclosporine A nephrotoxicity. *Pediatr Nephrol* 2000;14: 927–934.

16. Forpomes O, Combe C, Cambar J, et al. Cyclosporin-A- and angiotensin-II-induced vasoreactivity in isolated glomeruli and cultured mesangial cells, 4 and 24 h after renal mass reduction: role of vasodilatory prostaglandins. *Nephron* 1997;76:337–344.

17. Mueller AR, Platz KP, Schattenfroh N, et al. Neurotoxicity after orthotopic liver transplantation in cyclosporin A- and FK 506-treated patients. *Transpl Int* 1994;7:281–289.

18. Wijdicks EF, Plevak DJ, Wiesner RH, et al. Causes and outcome of seizures in liver transplant recipients. *Neurology* 1996;47:1523–1525.

19. Wijdicks EF, Wiesner RH, Krom RA. Neurotoxicity in liver transplant recipients with cyclosporine immunosuppression. *Neurology* 1995;45:1962–1964.

20. Mueller AR, Platz KP, Bechstein WO, et al. Neurotoxicity after orthotopic liver transplantation. A comparison between cyclosporine and FK506. *Transplantation* 1994;58:155–170.

21. Bronster DJ, Emre S, Mor E, et al. Neurologic complications of orthotopic liver transplantation. *Mt Sinai J Med* 1994;61:63–69.

22. El-Agroudy AE, Bakr MA, Hassan NA, et al. Characteristics of long-term live-donor renal allograft survivors. *Am J Nephrol* 2003;23:165–171.

23. Shaltout H, Abdel-Rahman A. cyclosporine induces progressive attenuation of baroreceptor heart rate response and cumulative pressor response in conscious unrestrained rats. *J Pharmacol Exp Ther* 2003;305:966–973.

24. Caliskan Y, Kalayoglu-Besisik S, Sargin D, et al. Cyclosporine-associated hyperkalemia: report of four allogeneic blood stem-cell transplant cases. *Transplantation* 2003;75:1069–1072.

25. Aker S, Heering P, Kinne-Saffran E, et al. Different effects of cyclosporine A and FK506 on potassium transport systems in MDCK cells. *Exp Nephrol* 2001;9:332–340.

26. Kwun WH, Suh BY, Kwun KB. Effect of azithromycin in the treatment of cyclosporine-induced gingival hyperplasia in renal transplant recipients. *Transplant Proc* 2003;35:311–312.

27. Fletchner S. Minimizing calcineurin inhibitor drugs in renal transplantation. *Transplant Proc* 2003;35[Suppl]:S11–21.

28. Armstrong VW, Oellerich M. New developments in the immunosuppressive drug monitoring of cyclosporine, tacrolimus, and azathioprine. *Clin Biochem* 2001;34:9–16.

29. Lecointre K, Furlan V, Taburet AM. In vitro effects of tacrolimus on human cytochrome P450. *Fundam Clin Pharmacol* 2002;16:455–460.

30. Todo S, Tzakis A, Reyes J, et al. Clinical small bowel or small bowel plus liver transplantation under FK 506. *Transplant Proc* 1991;23:3093–3095.

31. Oellerich M, Armstrong VW, Schutz E, et al. Therapeutic drug monitoring of cyclosporine and tacrolimus. Update on Lake Louise Consensus Conference on cyclosporine and tacrolimus. *Clin Biochem* 1998;31:309–316.

32. Jain A, Venkataramanan R, Lever J, et al. FK 506 in small bowel transplant recipients: pharmacokinetics and dosing. *Transplant Proc* 1994;26:1609–1610.

33. Jain A, Mazariegos G, Pokharna R, et al. The absence of chronic rejection in pediatric primary liver transplant patients who are maintained on tacrolimus-based immunosuppression: a long-term analysis. *Transplantation* 2003;75:1020–1025.

34. Klein A. Tacrolimus rescue in liver transplant patients with refractory rejection or intolerance or malabsorption of cyclosporine. The US Multicenter FK506 Liver Study Group. *Liver Transpl Surg* 1999;5:502–508.

35. Ben-Ari Z, Mor E, Bar-Nathan N, et al. Comparison of tacrolimus with cyclosporin as primary immunosuppression in patients with hepatitis C virus infection after liver transplantation. *Transplant Proc* 2003;35:612–613.

36. Artz MA, Boots JM, Ligtenberg G, et al. Randomized conversion from cyclosporine to tacrolimus in renal transplant patients: improved lipid profile and unchanged plasma homocysteine levels. *Transplant Proc* 2002;34:1793–1794.

37. Plosker GL, Foster RH. Tacrolimus: a further update of its pharmacology and therapeutic use in the management of organ transplantation. *Drugs* 2000;59:323–389.

38. Veroux P, Veroux M, Puliatti C, et al. Tacrolimus-induced neurotoxicity in kidney transplant recipients. *Transplant Proc* 2002;34:3188–3190.

39. Yamauchi A, Ieiri I, Kataoka Y, et al. Neurotoxicity induced by tacrolimus after liver transplantation: relation to genetic polymorphisms of the ABCB1 (MDR1) gene. *Transplantation* 2002;74:571–572.

40. Shimono T, Miki Y, Toyoda H, et al. MR imaging with quantitative diffusion mapping of tacrolimus-induced neurotoxicity in organ transplant patients. *Eur Radiol* 2003;13:986–993.

41. Bartynski WS, Zeigler Z, Spearman MP, et al. Etiology of cortical and white matter lesions in cyclosporin-A and FK-506 neurotoxicity. *Am J Neuroradiol* 2001;22:1901–1914.

42. Kahan BD, Chang J, Sehgel S. Preclinical eval of a potent new immunosuppressive agent: Rapamycin. *Transplantation* 1991;52:155–191.

43. Morris RE. Rapamycin: FK 506's fraternal twin or distant cousin. *Immunol Today* 1991;12:137–140.

44. Kniepeiss D, Iberer F, Grasser B, et al. Sirolimus in patients after liver transplantation. *Transplant Proc* 2003;35:815–816.

45. Neff GW, Montalbano M, Tzakis AG. Ten years of sirolimus therapy in orthotopic liver transplant recipients. *Transplant Proc* 2003;35[3 Suppl]:S209–S216.

46. Trotter JF. Sirolimus in liver transplantation. *Transplant Proc* 2003;35[Suppl]: S193–S200.

47. Stegall MD, Larson TS, Prieto M, et al. Kidney transplantation without calcineurin inhibitors using sirolimus. *Transplant Proc* 2003;35[Suppl]:S125.

48. Sehgal SN. Sirolimus: its discovery, biological properties, and mechanism of action. *Transplant Proc* 2003;35[3 Suppl]:S7–S14.

49. Camardo J. The Rapamune era of immunosuppression 2003: the journey from the laboratory to clinical transplantation. *Transplant Proc* 2003;35[3 Suppl]:S18–S24.

50. Neff GW, Montalbano M, Slapak-Green G, et al. A retrospective review of sirolimus (Rapamune) therapy in orthotopic liver transplant recipients diagnosed with chronic rejection. *Liver Transpl* 2003;9:477–483.

51. Nair S, Eason J, Loss G., Sirolimus monotherapy in nephrotoxicity due to calcineurin inhibitors in liver transplant recipients. *Liver Transpl* 2003;9: 126–129.

52. Baboolal K. A phase III prospective, randomized study to evaluate concentration-controlled sirolimus (rapamune) with cyclosporine dose minimization or elimination at six months in *de novo* renal allograft recipients. *Transplantation* 2003;75:1404–1408.

53. Guilbeau JM. Delayed wound healing with sirolimus after liver transplant. *Ann Pharmacother* 2002;36:139.

54. Alsina J, Grinyo JM. New immunosuppressive agent: expectations and controversies. *Transplantation* 2003;75:741–742.

55. McTaggart RA, Gottlieb D, Brooks J, et al. Sirolimus prolongs recovery from delayed graft function after cadaveric renal transplantation. *Am J Transplant* 2003;3:416–423.

56. Mathis AS. Comment: delayed wound healing with sirolimus after liver transplant. *Ann Pharmacother* 2003;37:453.

57. Pascual M, Theruvath T, Kawai T, et al. Strategies to improve long-term outcomes after renal transplantation. *N Engl J Med* 2002;346:580–590.

58. Pascual J, Ortuno J. Simple tacrolimus-based immunosuppressive regimens following renal transplantation: a large multicenter comparison between double and triple therapy. *Transplant Proc* 2002;34:89–91.

59. Washburn K, Speeg KV, Esterl R, et al. Steroid elimination 24 hours after liver transplantation using daclizumab, tacrolimus, and mycophenolate mofetil. *Transplantation* 2001;72:1675–1679.

60. Boots JM, Christiaans MH, van Duijnhoven EM, et al. Early steroid withdrawal in renal transplantation with tacrolimus dual therapy: a pilot study. *Transplant Proc* 2002; 34:1698–1699.

61. Balakrishnan S, Colling C, Burkman T, et al. Apolipoprotein E gene polymorphism alters lipids before pancreas transplantation. *Transplantation* 2002;74:974–977.

62. Nava S, Fracchia C, Callegari G, et al. Weakness of respiratory and skeletal muscles after a short course of steroids in patients with acute lung rejection. *Eur Respir J* 2002;20:497–499.

63. Prasad GV, Nash MM, McFarlane PA, et al. Renal transplant recipient attitudes toward steroid use and steroid withdrawal. *Clin Transplant* 2003;17: 135–139.

64. Aw MM, Brown NW, Itsuka T, et al. Mycophenolic acid pharmacokinetics in pediatric liver transplant recipients. *Liver Transpl* 2003;9:38.

65. Tsai MK, Hu RH, Lee CJ, et al. Efficacy of low-dose mycophenolate mofetil therapy for Taiwanese renal transplantation patients receiving primary cyclosporine immunosuppression. *J Formos Med Assoc* 2002;101:616–621.

66. Offermann G. Five-year results of renal transplantation on immunosuppressive triple therapy with mycophenolate mofetil. *Clin Transplant* 2003;17: 43–46.

67. Vasquez EM, Sifontis NM, Pollak R, et al. Impact of mycophenolate mofetil on recurrent rejection in kidney transplant patients. *Clin Transplant* 2001;15:253–257.

68. Trofe J, Stratta RJ, Egidi MF, et al. Thymoglobulin for induction or rejection therapy in pancreas allograft recipients: a single centre experience. *Clin Transplant* 2002;16[Suppl 7]:34–44.

69. Church AC. Clinical advances in therapies targeting the interleukin-2 receptor. *QJM* 2003;96:91–102.

70. Adu D, Cockwell P, Ives NJ, et al. Interleukin-2 receptor monoclonal antibodies in renal transplantation: meta-analysis of randomized trials. *BMJ* 2003;326:789.

71. Ciancio G, Burke GW, Suzart K, et al. Effect of daclizumab, tacrolimus, and mycophenolate mofetil in pediatric first renal transplant recipients. *Transplant Proc* 2002;34:1944–1945.

72. Niemeyer G, Koch M, Light S, et al. Long-term safety, tolerability and efficacy of daclizumab (Zenapax) in a two-dose regimen in liver transplant recipients. *Am J Transplant* 2002;2:454–460.

73. Koch M, Niemeyer G, Patel I, et al. Pharmacokinetics, pharmacodynamics, and immunodynamics of daclizumab in a two-dose regimen in liver transplantation. *Transplantation* 2002;73:1640–1646.

74. Fanlike J, Wolff S, Mantle R, et al. Staggered immunosuppression with the interleukin-2 receptor antagonist daclizumab combined with tacrolimus, prednisolone, and mycophenolate mofetil after orthotopic liver transplantation: a pilot efficacy and safety study. *Transplant Proc* 2002;34:1242–1244.

75. Baczkowska T, Kukula K, Nowacka-Cieciura E, et al. Use of daclizumab in the immunosuppression of high-risk kidney and kidney/pancreas recipients: Warsaw Transplantation Center experience. *Transplant Proc* 2002;34: 551–552.

76. Stratta RJ, Alloway RR, Hodge E, et al. A multicenter, open-label, comparative trial of two daclizumab dosing strategies versus no antibody induction in simultaneous kidney–pancreas transplantation: 6-month interim analysis. *Transplant Proc* 2002;34:1903–1905.

77. Bagley J, Iacomini J. Gene therapy progress and prospects: gene therapy in organ transplantation. *Gene Ther* 2003;10:605–611.

78. Cotterell AA, Kenyon NS. Alternatives to immunosuppressive drugs in human islet transplantation. *Curr Diab Rep* 2002;2:377–382.

79. Sehon AH, Lang GM. Avoiding untoward immune responses to novel gene products. *J Liposome Res* 2002;12A:199–204.

80. Manfredi R, Chiodo F. Management of relapsing cytomegalovirus disease in transplant recipients: diagnostic and therapeutic dilemmas. *Transpl Infect Dis* 2001;3:51–53.

81. Angelis M, Cooper JT, Freeman RB. Impact of donor infections on outcome of orthotopic liver transplantation. *Liver Transpl* 2003;9:451–462.

82. Kulkarni S, Naureckas E, Cronin DC. Solid-organ transplant recipients treated with drotrecogin alfa (activated) for severe sepsis. *Transplantation* 2003;75:899–901.

83. Pietrantoni C, Minai OA, Yu NC, et al. Respiratory failure and sepsis are the major causes of ICU admissions and mortality in survivors of lung transplants. *Chest* 2003;123:504–509.

84. Dunn DL. Hazardous crossing: immunosuppression and nosocomial infections in solid organ transplant recipients. *Surg Infect (Larchmt)* 2001;2:103–110.

85. Paya CV. Prevention of fungal infection in transplantation. *Transpl Infect Dis* 2002;4[Suppl 3]:46–51.

86. Bhorade SM, Lurain NS, Jordan A, et al. Emergence of ganciclovir-resistant cytomegalovirus in lung transplant recipients. *J Heart Lung Transplant* 2002;21:1274–1282.

87. Chan KM, Allen SA. Infectious pulmonary complications in lung transplant recipients. *Semin Respir Infect* 2002;17:291–302.

88. Rubin RH. Cytomegalovirus in solid organ transplantation. *Transpl Infect Dis* 2001;3[Suppl 2]:1–5.

89. Rubin RH. Importance of CMV in the transplant population. *Transpl Infect Dis* 1999;1[Suppl 1]:3–7.

90. Vamvakopoulos J, Hayry P. Cytomegalovirus and transplant arteriopathy: evidence for a link is mounting, but the jury is still out there. *Transplantation* 2003;75:742–743.

91. Fishman JA, Doran MT, Volpicelli SA, et al. Dosing of intravenous ganciclovir for the prophylaxis and treatment of cytomegalovirus infection in solid organ transplant recipients. *Transplantation* 2000;15:389–394.

92. Feltis BA, Lee DA, Beilman GJ. Mycotic aneurysm of the descending thoracic aorta caused by *Pseudomonas aeruginosa* in a solid organ transplant recipient: case report and review. *Surg Infect (Larchmt)* 2002;3:29–33.

93. Fung JJ. Fungal infection in liver transplantation. *Transpl Infect Dis* 2002; 4[Suppl 3]:18–23.

94. Wu G, Vilchez RA, Eidelman B, et al. Cryptococcal meningitis: an analysis among 5,521 consecutive organ transplant recipients. *Transpl Infect Dis* 2002;4:183–188.

95. Vilchez RA, Fung J, Kusne S. Cryptococcosis in organ transplant recipients: an overview. *Am J Transplant* 2002;2:575–580.

96. Kubak BM. Fungal infection in lung transplantation. *Transpl Infect Dis* 2002;4[Suppl 3]:24–31.

97. Helmi M, Love RB, Welter D, et al. *Aspergillus* infection in lung transplant recipients with cystic fibrosis: risk factors and outcomes comparison to other types of transplant recipients. *Chest* 2003;123:800–808.

98. Munoz P, Alcala L, Sanchez Conde M, et al. The isolation of *Aspergillus fumigatus* from respiratory tract specimens in heart transplant recipients is highly predictive of invasive aspergillosis. *Transplantation* 2003;75:326–329.

99. Book WM, Kelley L, Gravanis MB. Fulminant mixed humoral and cellular rejection in a cardiac transplant recipient: a review of the histological findings and literature. *J Heart Lung Transplant* 2003;22:604–607.

100. Scherer A, Krause A, Walker JR, et al. Early prognosis of the development of renal chronic allograft rejection by gene expression profiling of human protocol biopsies. *Transplantation* 2003;75:1323–1330.

101. Paraskevas S, Kandaswamy R, Humar A, et al. Predicting long-term kidney graft survival: can new trials be performed? *Transplantation* 2003;75:1256–1259.

102. Starzl TE, Murase N, Abu-Elmagd K, et al. Tolerogenic immunosuppression for organ transplantation. *Lancet* 2003;361:1502–1510.

103. Euvrard S, Kanitakis J, Claudy A. Skin cancers after organ transplantation. *N Engl J Med* 2003;348:1681–1691.

104. Haberal M, Moray G, Colak T, et al. Immunosuppressive therapy and Kaposi's sarcoma after kidney transplantation. *Tissue Antigens* 2002;60:558–564.

105. Munoz P, Alvarez P, de Ory F, et al. Incidence and clinical characteristics of Kaposi sarcoma after solid organ transplantation in Spain: importance of seroconversion against HHV-8. *Medicine (Baltimore)* 2002;81:293–304.

106. Fung JJ, Jain A, Kwak EJ, et al. De novo malignancies after liver transplantation: a major cause of late death. *Liver Transpl* 2001;7[11 Suppl 1]:S109–S118.

107. Guthery SL, Heubi JE, Bucuvalas JC, et al. Posttransplant lymphoproliferative disorder in pediatric liver transplant recipients using objective case ascertainment. *Transplantation* 2003;75:987–993.

108. Jain A, Nalesnik M, Reyes J, et al. Posttransplant lymphoproliferative disorders in liver transplantation: a 20-year experience. *Ann Surg* 2002;236:429–436.

109. Cacciarelli TV, Green M, Jaffe R, et al. Management of posttransplant lymphoproliferative disease in pediatric liver transplant recipients receiving primary tacrolimus (FK506) therapy. *Transplantation* 1998;66:1047–1052.

110. Kurdow R, Marks HG, Kraemer-Hansen H, et al. Recurrence of primary biliary cirrhosis after orthotopic liver transplantation. *Hepatogastroenterology* 2003;50:322–325.

111. Angelis M, Cooper JT, Freeman RB. Impact of donor infections on outcome of orthotopic liver transplantation. *Liver Transpl* 2003;9:451–462.

112. Leelaudomlipi S, Bramhall SR, Gunson BK, et al. Hepatic-artery aneurysm in adult liver transplantation. *Transpl Int* 2003;16:257–261.

113. Bernardos A, Serrano J, Gomez MA, et al. Portal vein thrombosis: an emergency solution for blood flow in liver transplantation. *Transpl Int* 2003;16: 500–501.

114. Farmer DG, Anselmo DM, Ghobrial RM, et al. Liver transplantation for fulminant hepatic failure: experience with more than 200 patients over a 17-year period. *Ann Surg* 2003;237:666–676

115. Neuberger J. Liver transplantation for cholestatic liver disease. *Curr Treat Options Gastroenterol* 2003;6:113–121.

116. Moons P, Vanrenterghem Y, Van Hooff JP, et al. Health-related quality of life and symptom experience in tacrolimus-based regimens after renal transplantation: a multicentre study. *Transpl Int* 2003;16:653–664.

117. Mosallaci M, Ghahramani N, Malek-Hosseini SA, et al. Renal transplantation in diabetic nephropathy. *Transplant Proc* 2003;35:149–151.

118. Salgado OJ, Henriquez C, Rosales B, et al. Renal Doppler sonographic and histologic findings in post-transplant primary cytomegalovirus disease. *J Clin Ultrasound* 2000;28:430–434.

119. Nakatani T, Uchida J, Han YS, et al. Renal allograft arteriovenous fistula and large pseudoaneurysm. *Clin Transplant* 2003;17:9–12.

120. Hypolite IO, Bucci J, Hshieh P, et al. Acute coronary syndromes after renal transplantation in patients with end-stage renal disease resulting from diabetes. *Am J Transplant* 2002;2:274–281.

121. Marcen R, Morales JM, Fernandez-Juarez G, et al. Risk factors of ischemic heart disease after renal transplantation. *Transplant Proc* 2002;34:394–395.

122. Ben-Haim M, Spector D, Merhav H, et al. Pancreas transplantation 120. Late intra-abdominal surgical complications after pancreas transplantation with Roux-en-Y enteric drainage. *J Gastrointest Surg* 2003;7:295.

123. Reddy KS, Ranjan D, Johnston TD. Pancreas transplantation: current status and experience at the University of Kentucky. *J Ky Med Assoc* 2002; 100:278–281.

124. MacMillan N, Fernandez-Cruz L, Ricart MJ, et al. Venous graft thrombosis in clinical pancreas transplantation: options for a rescue treatment. *Transplant Proc* 1998;30:425–426.

125. Ciancio G, Lo Monte A, Julian JF, et al. Vascular complications following bladder drained, simultaneous pancreas–kidney transplantation: the University of Miami experience. *Transpl Int* 2000;13[Suppl 1]:S187–S190.

126. Kayler LK, Merion RM, Rudich SM, et al. Evaluation of pancreatic allograft dysfunction by laparoscopic biopsy. *Transplantation* 2002;74:1287–1289.

127. Klassen DK, Weir MR, Cangro CB, et al. Pancreas allograft biopsy: safety of percutaneous biopsy—results of a large experience. *Transplantation* 2002;73: 553–555.

128. Lee BC, McGahan JP, Perez RV, et al. The role of percutaneous biopsy in detection of pancreatic transplant rejection. *Clin Transplant* 2000;14:493–498.

129. Drachenberg CB, Papadimitriou JC, Klassen DK, et al. Chronic pancreas allograft rejection: morphologic evidence of progression in needle biopsies and proposal of a grading scheme. *Transplant Proc* 1999;31:614.

130. Abu-Elmagd K, Bond G. The current status and future outlook of intestinal transplantation. *Minerva Chir* 2002;57:543–560.

131. Wu T, Abu-Elmagd K, Bond G, et al. A schema for histologic grading of small intestine allograft acute rejection. *Transplantation* 2003;75:1241–1248.

132. Hasegawa T, Sasaki T, Kimura T, et al. Effects of isolated small bowel transplantation on liver dysfunction caused by intestinal failure and long-term total parenteral nutrition. *Pediatr Transplant* 2002;6:235–239.

133. Hardy JD. The first lung transplant in man (1963) and the first heart transplant in man (1964). *Transplant Proc* 1999;31:25–29.

134. Mendeloff EN. The history of pediatric heart and lung transplantation. *Pediatr Transplant* 2002;6:270–279.

135. Beilby S, Moss-Morris R, Painter L. Quality of life before and after heart, lung and liver transplantation. *N Z Med J* 2003;116(1171):U381.

136. Liou TG, Cahill BC, Adler FR, et al. Selection of patients with cystic fibrosis for lung transplantation. *Curr Opin Pulm Med* 2002;8:535–541.

137. Meyers BF, Lynch JP, Battafarano RJ, et al. Lung transplantation is warranted for stable, ventilator-dependent recipients. *Ann Thorac Surg* 2000;70: 1675–1678.

138. Chhajed PN, Malouf MA, Tamm M, et al. Interventional bronchoscopy for the management of airway complications following lung transplantation. *Chest* 2001;120:1894–1899.

139. Griffith BP, Magee MJ, Gonzalez IF, et al. Anastomotic pitfalls in lung transplantation. *J Thorac Cardiovasc Surg* 1994;107:743–753.

140. Alvarez A, Algar J, Santos F, et al. Airway complications after lung transplantation: a review of 151 anastomosis. *Eur J Cardiothorac Surg* 2001;19: 381–387.

141. Herrera JM, McNeil KD, Higgins RS, et al. Airway complications after lung transplantation: treatment and long-term outcome. *Ann Thorac Surg* 2001;71: 989–993.

142. De Perrot M, Liu M, Waddell TK, et al. Ischemia–reperfusion-induced lung injury. *Am J Respir Crit Care Med* 2003;167:490–511.

143. Della Rocca G, Pierconti F, Costa MG, et al. Severe reperfusion lung injury after double lung transplantation. *Crit Care* 2002;6:240–244.

144. Schulman LL, Anandarangam T, Leibowitz DW, et al. Four-year prospective study of pulmonary venous thrombosis after lung transplantation. *J Am Soc Echocardiogr* 2001;14:806–812.

145. Goudarzi BM, Bonvino S. Critical care issues in lung and heart transplantation. *Crit Care Clin* 2003;19:209–231.

146. Nathan SD, Barnett SD, Wohlrab J, et al. Bronchiolitis obliterans syndrome: utility of the new guidelines in single lung transplant recipients. *J Heart Lung Transplant* 2003;22:427–432.

147. Frost AE. Bronchiolitis obliterans: the Achilles heel of lung transplantation. *Verh K Acad Geneeskd Belg* 2002;64:303–319.

148. Fink G, Lebzelter J, Blau C, et al. The sky is the limit: exercise capacity 10 years post-heart–lung transplantation. *Transplant Proc* 2000;32:733–734.

149. Van Der Woude BT, Kropmans TJ, Douma KW, et al. Peripheral muscle force and exercise capacity in lung transplant candidates. *Int J Rehabil Res* 2002;25: 351–355.

150. Wang XN, Williams TJ, McKenna MJ, et al. Skeletal muscle oxidative capacity, fiber type, and metabolites after lung transplantation. *Am J Respir Crit Care Med* 1999;160:57–63.

151. Schwaiblmair M, Reichenspurner H, Muller C, et al. Cardiopulmonary exercise testing before and after lung and heart–lung transplantation. *Am J Respir Crit Care Med* 1999;159(4 Pt 1):1277–1283.

152. Tirdel GB, Girgis R, Fishman RS, et al. Metabolic myopathy as a cause of the exercise limitation in lung transplant recipients. *J Heart Lung Transplant* 1998;17:1231–1237.

153. Lands LC, Smountas AA, Mesiano G, et al. Maximal exercise capacity and peripheral skeletal muscle function following lung transplantation. *J Heart Lung Transplant* 1999;18:113–120.

154. Hall MJ, Snell GI, Side EA, et al. Exercise, potassium, and muscle deconditioning post-thoracic organ transplantation. *J Appl Physiol* 1994;77:2784–2790.

155. Ross DJ, Kass RM, Mohsenifar Z. Assessment of regional VA/Q relationships by SPECT after single lung transplantation. *Transplant Proc* 1998;30: 180–186.

156. Evans AB, Al-Himyary AJ, Hrovat MI, et al. Abnormal skeletal muscle oxidative capacity after lung transplantation by 31P-MRS. *Am J Respir Crit Care Med* 1997;155:615–621.

157. Evans RW, Manninen DL, Dong FB, et al. Determinants of heart–lung transplantation outcomes: results of a consensus survey. *Ann Thorac Surg* 1993; 56:343–345.

158. Kesten S. Advances in lung transplantation. *Dis Mon* 1999;45:101–114.

159. Stiebellehner L, Quittan M, End A, et al. Aerobic endurance training program improves exercise performance in lung transplant recipients. *Chest* 1998;113:906–912.

160. Beens MH, Berkow R., eds. *Merck manual of diagnosis and therapy*, 17th ed. Merck, Inc., New Jersey, USA, 1999.

161. Kobashigawa J. Physiology of the transplanted heart. In: Norman D, Turk L, ed. *Primer on transplantation*. Mt. Laurel, NJ: American Society of Transplantation, 2001:358–363

162. Bengel FM, Ueperfuhr P, Schiepel N, et al. Effect of sympathetic reinnervation on cardiac performance after heart transplantation. *N Engl J Med* 2001; 345:731–738.

163. Marconi C, Marzorati M, Fiocchi R, et al. Age related heart response to exercise in heart transplant recipients. Functional significance. *Pflugers Arch* 2002;443:698–706.

164. Ferretti G, Marconi C, Achilli G, et al. The heart rate response to exercise and circulating catecholamines in heart transplant recipients *Pflugers Arch* 2002;443:370–376.

165. Oliver D, Pflugfelder PW, McCart NN, et al. Acute cardiovascular responses to leg press resistance exercise in heart transplant recipients. *Int J Cardiol* 2001;81:61–74.

166. Kobashigawa JA, Leaf DA, Lee N, et al. A controlled trial of exercise rehabilitation after heart transplantation *N Engl J Med* 1999;340:272–277.

167. Braith RW, Welsch MA, Mills RM, et al. Resistance exercise prevents glucocorticoid-induced myopathy in a heart transplant recipients. *Med Sci Sports Exerc* 1998;30:483–489.

168. Niset G, Hermans L, Depelchin P. Exercise and heart transplantation: a review. *Sports Med* 1991;12:359–379.

169. Kavanagh T, Yacoub MH, Mertens DJ. Cardiorespiratory responses to exercise training after orthotopic cardiac transplantation. *Circulation* 1988;77: 162–171.

170. Schmidt A, Pleiner J, Payerle-Eder M. Regular physical exercise improves endothelial function in heart transplant recipients. *Clin Transpl* 2002;16:137–143.

171. Joshi A, Kevorkian CG. Rehabilitation after cardiac transplantation, case series and literature review. *Am J Phys Med Rehabil* 1997;76:249–254.

172. Buckels JA, Buist L, Aertz R, et al. Liver transplantation: the first 200 grafts in Birmingham. *Clin Transpl* 1988;39–43.

173. Ghaus N, Bohlega S, Rezeig M. Neurological complications in liver transplantation. *J Neurol* 2001;248:1042–1048.

174. Buis CI, Wiesner RH, Krom RA, et al. Acute confusional state following liver transplantation for alcoholic liver disease. *Neurology* 2002;59:601–605.

175. Rothenhausler HB, Ehrentraut S, Kapfhammer HP, et al. Psychiatric and psychosocial outcome of orthotopic liver transplantation. *Psychother Psychosom* 2002;71:285–297.

176. Temple RO, Putzke JD, Boll TJ. Neuropsychological performance as a function of cardiac status among heart transplant candidates: a replication. *Percept Mot Skills* 2000;91(3 Pt 1):821–825.

177. Putzke JD, Williams MA, Daniel FJ, et al. Activities of daily living among heart transplant candidates: neuropsychological and cardiac function predictors. *J Heart Lung Transplant* 2000;19:995–1006.

178. Rezaiguia-Delclaux S, Lefaucheur JP, Zakkouri M, et al. Severe acute polyneuropathy complicating orthotopic liver allograft failure. *Transplantation* 2002;74:880–882.

179. El-Sabrout RA, Radovancevic B, Ankoma-Sey V, et al. Guillain-Barre syndrome after solid organ transplantation. *Transplantation* 2001;71:1311–1316.

180. Chan CY, DasGupta K, Baker AL. Cyclosporin A: drug discontinuation for the management of long-term toxicity after liver transplantation. *Hepatology* 1996;24:1085–1089.

181. Lee JH, Jung WJ, Choi KH, et al. Nerve conduction study on patients with severe liver syndrome and its change after transplantation. *Clin Transpl* 2002;16:430–432.

182. Lacomis D. Critical illness myopathy. *Curr Rheumatol Rep* 2002;4:403–408.

183. Miro O, Salmeron JM, Masanes F, et al. Acute quadriplegic myopathy with myosin-deficient muscle fibres after liver transplantation: defining the clinical picture and delimiting the risk factors. *Transplantation* 1999;67:1144–1151.

184. Campellone JV, Lacomis D, Kramer DJ, et al. Acute myopathy after liver transplantation. *Neurology* 1998;50:46–53.

185. Stephenson AL, Yoshida EM, Abboud RT, et al. Impaired exercise performance after successful liver transplantation. *Transplantation* 2001;72:1161–1164.

186. Bucuvalas JC, Britto M, Krug S, et al. Health-related quality of life in pediatric liver transplant recipients: a single-center study. *Liver Transpl* 2003;9: 62–71.

187. Forsberg A, Backman L, Svensson E. Liver transplant recipients' ability to cope during the first 12 months after transplantation—a prospective study. *Scand J Caring Sci* 2002;16:345–352.

188. Karliova M, Malago M, Valentin-Gamazo C, et al. Living-related liver transplantation from the view of the donor: a 1-year follow-up survey. *Transplantation* 2002;73:1799–1804.

189. Bentley G, Biant LC, Carrington RW, et al. A prospective, randomized comparison of autologous chondrocyte implantation versus mosaicplasty for osteochondral defects in the knee. *J Bone Joint Surg Br* 2003;85:223–230.

190. Yoldas EA, Sekiya JK, Irrgang JJ, et al. Arthroscopically assisted meniscal allograft transplantation with and without combined anterior cruciate ligament reconstruction. *Knee Surg Sports Traumatol Arthrosc* 2003;11:173–182.

191. Kondziolka D, Wechsler L, Gebel J, et al. Neuronal transplantation for motor stroke: from the laboratory to the clinic. *Phys Med Rehabil Clin N Am* 2003;14 [1 Suppl]:S153–S160.

192. Meltzer CC, Kondziolka D, Villemagne VL, et al. Serial [18F] fluorodeoxyglucose positron emission tomography after human neuronal implantation for stroke. *Neurosurgery* 2001;49:586–591.

193. Kondziolka D, Steinberg G, Wechsler L, et al. Neurotransplantation for basal ganglia stroke: results from a phase 2 trial. American Society for Stereotactic and Functional Neurosurgery, New York, May 18–21, 2003.

194. Ramon-Cueto A, Santos-Benito FF. Cell therapy to repair injured spinal cords: olfactory ensheathing glia transplantation. *Restor Neurol Neurosci* 2001;19:149–156.

195. Schwab ME. Repairing the injured spinal cord. *Science* 2002;295:1029–1031.

196. Bregman BS, Coumans JV, Dai HN, et al. Transplants and neurotrophic factors increase regeneration and recovery of function after spinal cord injury. *Prog Brain Res* 2002;137:257–273.

Index